OTHER TITLES OF INTEREST

CODING AND REIMBURSEMENT

Collections Made Easy!
CPT Coders Choice®, Thumb Indexed
CPT TimeSaver®, Ring Binder, Tab Indexed
CPT & HCPCS Coding Made Easy!
HCPCS Coders Choice®
Health Insurance Carrier Directory
ICD-9-CM, Coders Choice®, Thumb Indexed
ICD-9-CM, TimeSaver® Ring Binder, Tab Indexed
ICD-9-CM Coding Made Easy!
Physicians Fees
Medicare Rules and Regulations
Reimbursement Manual for the Medical Office

PRACTICE MANAGEMENT

365 Ways to Manage the Business Called Private Practice
Computerizing Your Medical Office
Designing and Building Your Professional Office
Effective Laboratory Supervision
Encyclopedia of Practice and Financial Management
Health Information Management
Hospital and Health Facilities Directory
Managing Medical Office Personnel
Marketing Healthcare
Marketing Strategies for Physicians
Medical Practice Handbook
Medical Risk Management
Medical Staff Privileges
On-Line Systems: How to Access and Use Databases
Patient Satisfaction
Performance Standards for the Laboratory
Physician's Office Laboratory
Professional and Practice Development
Promoting Your Medical Practice
Remodeling Your Professional Office
Software, Systems and Services Directory
Starting in Medical Practice

AVAILABLE FROM YOUR LOCAL MEDICAL BOOK STORE OR CALL 1-800-MED-SHOP

OTHER TITLES OF INTEREST

FINANCIAL MANAGEMENT

A Physician's Guide to Financial Independence
Business Ventures for Physicians
Financial Planning Workbook for Physicians
Financial Valuation of Your Practice
Personal Money Management for Physicians
Personal Pension Plan Strategies for Physicians
Securing Your Assets
Selling or Buying a Medical Practice

RISK MANAGEMENT

Belli: For Your Malpractice Defense
Law, Liability and Ethics
Malpractice Depositions
Malpractice: Managing Your Defense
Preventing Emergency Malpractice
Testifying in Court

DICTIONARIES AND OTHER REFERENCE

Drug Interactions Index
Isler's Pocket Dictionary
Medical Acronyms and Abbreviations
Medical Phrase Index
Medico-Legal Glossary
Spanish/English Handbook

MEDICAL REFERENCE AND CLINICAL

Gastroenterology: Problems in Primary Care
Medical Procedures for Referral
Neurology: Problems in Primary Care
Orthopaedics: Problems in Primary Care
Patient Care Emergency Handbook
Patient Care Flowchart Manual
Patient Care Procedures for Your Practice
Sexually Transmitted Diseases

AVAILABLE FROM YOUR LOCAL MEDICAL BOOK STORE OR CALL 1-800-MED-SHOP

ICD•9•CM

International Classification of Diseases
9th Revision
Clinical Modification
Fourth Edition

Color Coded

1996

PMIC

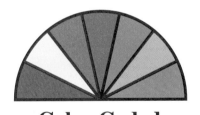

Volumes 1 & 2

ISBN 1-57066-035-2 (Soft cover)
ISBN 1-57066-037-9 (Hard cover)

Volumes 1, 2, & 3

ISBN 1-57066-036-0 (Soft cover)
ISBN 1-57066-034-4 (Timesaver Binder)

Practice Management Information Corporation [PMIC]
4727 Wilshire Boulevard, Suite 300
Los Angeles, California 90010
1-800-MED-SHOP

Printed in the United States of America

Preface

Health care professionals have long used coding systems to describe procedures, services, and supplies. However, most described the reason for the procedure, service or supply with a diagnostic statement. Of those health care professionals who do code the diagnosis, either due to a requirement for a computer billing system and/or electronic claims filing, many do not code completely or accurately. With the passage of the Medicare Catastrophic Coverage Act of 1988, diagnostic coding using ICD-9-CM became mandatory for Medicare claims. In the area of health care reimbursement rules and regulations, the typical progression is that changes required for Medicare are followed shortly by similar changes for Medicaid and private insurance carriers.

To some professionals, the requirement to use diagnostic coding may seem a burden or simply another excuse for Medicare intermediaries to delay or deny payment. However, it is important to understand that the proper use of coding systems for both procedures and diagnoses gives the professional absolute control over his or her billing and reimbursement. Accurate diagnosis coding is not easy. It requires a good working knowledge of medical terminology and a fundamental understanding of ICD-9-CM. In addition, the coder must know the rules and regulations required to comply with Medicare requirements for coding.

This edition of the *International Classification of Diseases, 9th Revision, Clinical Modification (ICD-9-CM)* is published by Practice Management Information Corporation in recognition of its responsibility to promulgate this classification throughout the United States for morbidity coding and billing purposes. The *International Classification of Diseases, 9th Revision*, originally published by the World Health Organization (WHO) is the foundation of the *ICD-9-CM* and continues to be the classification employed in cause-of-death coding in the United States.

The *ICD-9-CM* is recommended for use in all clinical settings, but is required for reporting diagnoses and diseases to all U.S. Public Health Service and Health Care Financing Administration programs. This version faithfully follows and contains the same information found in the U.S. Public Health Service and Health Care Financing Administration version of the *ICD-9-CM.*

All official authorized addenda effective October 1, 1995 have been included in this edition. A new revision will be available approximately September 15th of each year. Revised editions may be purchased from:

Practice Management Information Corp.
4727 Wilshire Blvd., Suite 300
Los Angeles, CA 90010
1-800-MED-SHOP

Disclaimer

This publication is identical in content to U.S. Department of Health and Human Services Publication No. (PHS) 91-1260 with the exception that this publication includes special symbols to indicate additions and revisions from the previous edition and special symbols to facilitate identification of diagnostic codes that require 4th or 5th digit specificity, the use of color coding to alert the user to special coding considerations, and thumb indexing to make locating codes easier. This publication is revised annually so that we may present the most current information possible. Though all of the information is carefully researched and checked for accuracy and completeness, the publisher accepts no responsibility with regard to errors, omissions, misuse or misinterpretation.

Table of Contents

Table of Contents

Table of Contents

Table of Contents

(1) These listings appear only in the three volume edition

Introduction to ICD-9-CM

ICD-9-CM is an acronym for *International Classification of Diseases, 9th Revision, Clinical Modification*, published under different names since 1900. ICD-9-CM is a statistical classification system that arranges diseases and injuries into groups according to established criteria. Most ICD-9-CM codes are numeric and consist of three, four or five numbers and a description. The codes are revised approximately every 10 years by the World Health Organization and annual updates are published by HCFA.

HISTORICAL PERSPECTIVE

The *International Classification of Diseases, 9th Revision, Clinical Modification* (ICD-9-CM) is based on the official version of the World Health Organization's (WHO) 9th Revision, International Classification of Diseases (ICD-9). ICD-9 is designed for the classification of morbidity and mortality information for statistical purposes, and for the indexing of medical records by disease and operations, and for data storage and retrieval. ICD-9-CM replaced the Eighth Revision International Classification of Diseases, Adapted for Use in the United States commonly referred to as ICDA.

The concept of extending the International Classification of Diseases for use in hospital indexing was originally developed in response to a need for a more efficient basis for storage and retrieval of diagnostic data. In 1950, the U.S. Public Health Service and the Veterans Administration began independent tests of the International Classification of Diseases for hospital indexing purposes. In the following year, the Columbia Presbyterian Medical Center in New York City adopted the International Classification of Diseases, 6th Revision for use in its medical record department. A few years later, the Commission on Professional and Hospital Activities adopted the International Classification of Diseases for use in hospitals participating in the Professional Activity Study (PAS).

In view of the growing interest in the use of the International Classification of Diseases for hospital indexing, a study was undertaken in 1956 by the American Medical Association and the American Medical Record Association of the relative efficiencies of coding systems for diagnostic indexing. Following this study, the major uses of the International Classification of Diseases for hospital indexing purposes consolidated their experiences and an adaptation was published in December 1959. A revision containing the first "Classification of Operations and Treatments" was published in 1962.

In 1968, following a study by the American Hospital Association, the United States Public Health Service published the Eighth Revision International Classification of Diseases, Adapted for Use in the United States. This publication became commonly known as ICDA, and served as the basis for coding diagnostic data for official morbidity and mortality statistics in the United States.

ICD-9-CM Background

In February 1977, a committee was convened by the National Center for Health Statistics to provide advice and counsel for the development of clinical modification of the ICD-9. The organizations represented on the committee included:

American Association of Health Data Systems
American Hospital Association
American Medical Record Association
Association for Health Records
Council on Clinical Classifications, sponsored by:

American Academy of Pediatrics
American College of Obstetricians and Gynecologists
American College of Physicians
American College of Surgeons
American Psychiatric Association

Commission on Professional and Hospital Activities
Health Care Financing Administration
WHO Center for Classification of Diseases

The resulting ICD-9-CM is a clinical modification of the World Health Organization's International Classification of Diseases, 9th Revision (ICD-9). The term "clinical" is used to emphasize the modifications intent; namely, to serve as a useful tool in the area of classification of morbidity data for indexing of medical records, medical care review, ambulatory and other medical care programs, as well as for basic health statistics.

In use since January 1979, ICD-9-CM provides a diagnostic coding system that is more precise than those needed only for statistical groupings and trend analysis. Official addenda (updates) to ICD-9-CM were issued in October 1986, 1987 and 1988 by the Health Care Financing Administration. A special addendum was published by the U.S.
Public Health Service in January 1988 containing codes for AIDS and AIDS related illnesses.

Use of ICD-9-CM Codes for Professional Billing

Until passage of the Medicare Catastrophic Coverage Act of 1988, health care professionals were not required to report ICD-9-CM codes when billing government or private insurance carriers for reimbursement. The exception to this requirement was for those health care professionals who filed insurance claims electronically and those who used "code driven" computer billing services or computer systems.

Most health care professionals simply included the text or description of the injury, illness, sign or symptom that was the reason for the encounter. Insurance carriers who used ICD-9-CM coding had to code the diagnostic statements prior to input into their computer systems for reimbursement processing.

A specific requirement of the Medicare Catastrophic Coverage Act of 1988 required health care professionals to include ICD-9-CM codes on their Medicare claim forms effective April 1, 1989. A two-month grace period, to June 1, 1989, was allowed at the request of the American Medical Association, to allow health care professionals additional time to develop the knowledge and systems necessary to implement the requirement.

TERMINOLOGY

There are terms used throughout this publication that are important for a proper understanding of ICD-9-CM. The following terms are defined specifically as they are used for ICD-9-CM with the knowledge that some terms may have other definitions and meanings.

acute refers to the condition that is the primary reason for the current encounter.

addenda official updates to ICD-9-CM published continuously since 1986, that become effective on October 1st of each year.

adverse any response to a drug that is noxious and unintended and occurs with proper dosage.

aftercare an encounter for something planned in advance, for example, cast removal.

AHFS American Hospital Formulary Service.

alphabetic the portion of ICD-9-CM that lists definitions and codes in alphabetic order. Also called Volume 2.

category refers to diagnoses codes listed within a specific three-digit category, for example category 250, Diabetes Mellitus.

cause that which brings about any condition or produces any effect.

chronic continuing over a long period of time or recurring frequently.

coding the process of transferring written or verbal descriptions of diseases, injuries and procedures into numerical designations.

combination a code that combines a diagnosis with an associated secondary process or complication.

complication the occurrence of two or more diseases in the same patient at the same time.

concurrent when a patient is being treated by more than one provider for different care conditions at the same time.

conventions refers to the use of certain abbreviations, punctuation, symbols, type faces, and other instructions that must be clearly understood in order to use ICD-9-CM.

CPT Current Procedural Terminology. Listing of codes and descriptions for procedures, services and supplies published by the American Medical Association. Used to bill insurance carriers.

diagnosis a written description of the reason(s) for the procedure, service, supply or encounter.

down coding the process where insurance carriers reduce the value of a procedure, and the resulting reimbursement, due to either 1) a mismatch of CPT code and description or 2) ICD-9-CM code does not justify the procedure or level of service.

E codes specific ICD-9-CM codes used to identify the cause of injury, poisoning and other adverse effects.

eponyms medical procedures or conditions named after a person or a place.

etiology the cause(s) or origin of a disease.

HCFA Health Care Financing Administration. The government agency that administers the Medicare and Medicaid programs.

HCFA1500 Uniform Health Insurance Claim Form used for billing services to Medicare and other insurance carriers.

hierarchy a system that ranks items one above another.

ICD-9-CM International Classification of Diseases, 9th Revision, Clinical Modification.

ICD-10 International Classification of Diseases, 10th Revision

late effect a residual effect (condition produced) after the acute phase of an illness or injury has ended.

main term refers to listings in the Alphabetic Index appearing BOLDFACE type.

manifestation characteristic signs or symptoms of an illness.

multiple refers to the need to use more than one ICD-9-CM code to fully identify coding a condition.

primary code the ICD-9-CM code that defines the main reason for the current encounter.

residual the long-term condition(s) resulting from a previous acute illness or injury.

rule out refers to a method used to indicate that a condition is probable, suspected, or questionable but unconfirmed. ICD-9-CM has no provisions for the use of this term.

secondary code(s) listed after the primary code that further indicate the cause(s) codefor the current encounter or define the need for higher levels of care.

sections refers to portions of the Tabular List that are organized in groups of three-digit code numbers. For example, Malignant Neoplasm of Lip, Oral Cavity and Pharynx (140-149).

sequencing the process of listing ICD-9-CM codes in the proper order.

specificity refers to the requirement to code to the highest number of digits possible, 3, 4 or 5, when choosing an ICD-9-CM code.

sub term refers to listings appearing in the Alphabetic Index under MAIN TERMS and always indented two spaces to the right.

subcategories refers to groupings of four-digit codes listed under three-digit categories.

tabular list the portion of ICD-9-CM that lists codes and definitions in numeric order. Also referred to as Volume 1.

V codes specific ICD-9-CM codes used to identify encounters for reasons other than illness or injury, for example, immunization.

Volume 1 see TABULAR LIST

Volume 2 see ALPHABETIC INDEX

Volume 3 procedure codes used only for hospital coding. Volume 3 contains both a numeric listing and alphabetic index.

FORMAT OF ICD-9-CM

The *International Classification of Diseases, 9th Revision, Clinical Modification* was originally published as a three volume set (2nd edition). Newer versions of ICD-9-CM, Fourth Edition, are available as two separate books (Volume 1 and Volume 2) and as a single book containing Volume 1 and Volume 2, or Volumes 1, 2 and 3 depending on the publisher.

The Third Edition of ICD-9-CM includes all official addenda from October 1986 through October 1988. The Fourth Edition of ICD-9-CM includes all official addenda from October 1986 through October 1994. Most publishers who print the ICD-9-CM now offer an annual version, usually published in December of each year, that includes all of the addenda through October of the same year.

The Tabular List (Volume 1)

The Tabular List (Volume 1) is a numeric listing of diagnosis codes and descriptions consisting of 17 chapters that classify diseases and injuries, two sections containing supplementary codes (V codes and E codes) and six appendices.

Classification of Diseases and Injuries

The Classification of Diseases and Injuries includes the following 17 chapters:

Chapter 1	Infectious and Parasitic Diseases (001-139)
Chapter 2	Neoplasms (140-239)
Chapter 3	Endocrine, Nutritional and Metabolic Diseases, and Immunity Disorders (240-279)
Chapter 4	Diseases of the Blood and Blood-Forming Organs (280-289)
Chapter 5	Mental Disorders (290-319)
Chapter 6	Diseases of the Nervous System and Sense Organs
Chapter 7	Diseases of the Circulatory System (390-459)
Chapter 8	Diseases of the Respiratory System (460-519)
Chapter 9	Diseases of the Digestive System (520-579)
Chapter 10	Diseases of the Genitourinary System (580-629)
Chapter 11	Complications of Pregnancy, Childbirth, and the Puerperium (630-676)
Chapter 12	Diseases of the Skin and Subcutaneous Tissue (680-709)
Chapter 13	Diseases of the Musculoskeletal System and Connective Tissue (710-739)
Chapter 14	Congenital Anomalies (740-759)
Chapter 15	Certain Conditions Originating in the Perinatal Period (760-779)
Chapter 16	Symptoms, Signs and Ill-defined Conditions (780-799)
Chapter 17	Injury and Poisoning (800-999)

Each chapter of the Tabular List (Volume 1) is structured into four components; namely:

Sections: groups of three-digit code numbers

Categories: three-digit code numbers

Subcategories: four-digit code numbers

Fifth-Digit Subclassifications: five-digit code numbers

Supplementary Classifications

There are two supplementary classifications included in the Tabular List (Volume 1). These are:

V Codes	Supplementary Classification of Factors Influencing Health Status and Contact with Health Services (V01-V82)
E Codes	Supplementary Classification of External Causes of Injury and Poisoning (E800-E999)

Appendices

The Tabular List (Volume 1) includes six appendices. These are:

Appendix 1	Morphology of Neoplasms
Appendix 2	Glossary of Mental Disorders
Appendix 3	Classification of Drugs by American Hospital Formulary Service List Number and their ICD-9-CM Equivalents
Appendix 4	Classification of Industrial Accidents According to Agency
Appendix 5	List of Three-Digit Categories
Appendix 6	Supplementary Classification of External Causes of Injury and Poisoning

Specifications for the Tabular List

1. Three-digit rubrics and their contents are unchanged from *ICD-9*.
2. The sequence of three-digit rubrics is unchanged from *ICD-9*.
3. Three-digit rubrics are not added to the main body of the classification.

4. Unsubdivided three-digit rubrics are subdivided where necessary to:

   a) Add clinical detail

   b) Isolate terms for clinical accuracy

5. The modification in *ICD-9-CM* is accomplished by the addition of a fifth digit to existing *ICD-9* rubrics, except as noted under #7 below.

6. Four-digit rubrics are added to subdivided three-digit codes only when there is no other means of achieving desired detail. These codes, unique to *ICD-9-CM* (28 three-digit categories) are marked with the symbol in the Tabular List.

7. The optional dual classification in *ICD-9* is modified.

   a) Duplicate rubrics are deleted:

      1) Four-digit manifestation categories duplicating etiology entries.

      2) Manifestation inclusion terms duplicating etiology entries.

   b) Manifestations of diseases are identified, to the extent possible, by creating five digit codes in the etiology rubrics.

   c) When the manifestation of a disease cannot be included in the etiology rubrics, provision for its identification is made by retaining the *ICD-9* rubrics used for classifying manifestations of disease.

8. The format of *ICD-9-CM* is revised from that used in *ICD-9*.

   a) American spelling of medical terms is used.

   b) Inclusion terms are indented beneath the titles of codes.

   c) Codes not to be used for primary tabulation of disease are printed in italics with the notation, "code also underlying disease."

The Alphabetical Index (Volume 2)

The Alphabetic Index (Volume 2) of ICD-9-CM consists of an alphabetic list of terms and codes, two supplementary Sections following the alphabetic listing, plus three special tables found within the alphabetic listing. The Alphabetic Index (Volume 2) is structured as follows:

MAIN TERMS:	appear in **BOLDFACE** type
SUBTERMS:	are always indented two spaces to the right under main terms
CARRY-OVER LINES:	are always indented more than two spaces from the level of the preceding line

Supplementary Sections

The supplementary sections following the Alphabetic Index are:

TABLE OF DRUGS AND CHEMICALS

This table contains a classification of drugs and other chemical substances to identify poisoning states and external causes of adverse effects.

INDEX TO EXTERNAL CAUSES OF INJURIES & POISONINGS (E-CODES)

This section contains the index to the codes that classify environmental events, circumstances, and other conditions as the cause of injury and other adverse effects.

Special Tables

The two special tables, located within the Alphabetic Index, and found under the main terms as underlined below, are:

Hypertension Table

Neoplasm Table

Specifications for the Alphabetic Index

1. Format of the Alphabetic Index follows the format of the *ICD-9*.
2. Main terms in the Alphabetic Index are printed in bold face type.
3. When two codes are required to indicate etiology and manifestation, the optional manifestation code appears in brackets, e.g., diabetic cataract 250.5 [366.41].

Procedures: Tabular List and Alphabetic Index (Volume 3)

The Procedures: Tabular List and Alphabetic Index (Volume 3) consists of two sections of codes that define procedures instead of diagnoses. Frequently used incorrectly by health care professionals, codes from Volume 3 are intended only for use by hospitals. The fourth edition of ICD-9-CM printed by the U.S. Government Printing Office does not include Volume 3.

The *ICD-9-CM* Procedure Classification is a modification of WHO's Fascicle V, Surgical Procedures," and is published as Volume 3 of *ICD-9-CM*. It contains both a Tabular List and an Alphabetic Index. Greater detail has been added to the *ICD-9-CM* Procedure Classification necessitating expansion of the codes from three to four digits. Approximately 90% of the rubrics refer to surgical procedures with the remaining 10% accounting for other investigative and therapeutic procedures.

Tabular List of Procedures

Includes 16 chapters containing codes and descriptions for surgical procedures and miscellaneous diagnostic and therapeutic procedures.

Alphabetic Index to Procedures

Provides an alphabetic index to the Tabular List of Volume 3

Specifications for the Procedure Classification

1. The *ICD-9-CM* Procedure Classification is published in its own volume containing both a Tabular List and an Alphabetic Index.

2. The classification is a modification of Fascicle V "Surgical Procedures" of the *ICD-9* Classification of Procedures in Medicine, working from the draft dated Geneva, 30 September-6 October 1975, and labeled WHO/ICD-9/Rev. Conf. 75.4.

3. All three-digit rubrics in the range 01-86 are maintained as they appear in Fascicle V, whenever feasible.

4. Nonsurgical procedures are segregated from the surgical procedures and confined to the rubrics 87-99, whenever feasible.

5. Selected detail contained in the remaining fascicles of the *ICD-9 Classification of Procedures in Medicine* is accommodated where possible.

6. The structure of the classification is based on anatomy rather than surgical specialty.

7. The *ICD-9-CM* Procedure Classification is numeric only, i.e., no alphabetic characters are used.

8. The classification is based on a two-digit structure with two decimal digits where necessary.

9. Compatibility with the *ICD-9 Classification of Procedures in Medicine* was not maintained when a different axis was deemed more clinically appropriate.

CONVENTIONS USED IN THE TABULAR LIST

The ICD-9-CM Tabular List (Volume 1) makes use of certain abbreviations, punctuation, symbols, and other conventions that must be clearly understood. The purpose of these conventions is to first, provide special coding instructions, and second, to conserve space.

Abbreviations

NOS	Not Otherwise Specified. Equivalent to Unspecified. This abbreviation refers to a lack of sufficient detail in the statement of diagnosis to be able to assign it to a more specific sub division within the classification.
NEC	Not Elsewhere Classified. Used with ill-defined terms to alert the coder that a specified form of the condition is classified differently. The category number for the term including NEC is to be used only when the coder lacks the information necessary to code the term to a more specific category.

Punctuation

( ) PARENTHESIS are used to enclose supplementary words that may be present or absent in a statement of disease without effecting the code assignment.

[ ] SQUARE BRACKETS are used to enclose synonyms, alternate wordings or explanatory phrases.

: COLONS are used after an incomplete phrase or term that requires one or more of the modifiers indented under it to make it assignable to a given category. EXCEPTION to this rule pertains to the abbreviation NOS.

{ } BRACES are used to connect a series of terms to a common stem. Each term on the left of the brace is incomplete and must be completed by a term to the right of the brace.

Symbols

□ The LOZENGE symbol appearing in the left margin preceding a four-digit code indicates that the code and description are not the same in ICD-9-CM as in ICD-9. May be ignored for coding purposes.

● A filled BLACK CIRCLE preceding a code indicates that the code is new to this revision of ICD-9-CM. A symbol key appears on all left-hand pages of the Tabular List, Volume 1.

▲ A filled BLACK TRIANGLE preceding a code indicates that there is a revision to the text or notes of an existing code. A symbol key appears on all left-hand pages of the Tabular List, Volume 1.

④ ⑤ A circle containing the number 4 or the number 5 preceding a code indicates that a fourth or fifth digit is required for coding to the highest level of specificity. Valid digits are in [brackets] under each code. Definitions of valid fifth digits are found under the major category.

Other conventions

Type Face:

BOLD: Bold type face is used for all codes and titles in the Tabular List.

Italics: Italicized type face is used for all exclusion notes and to identify those rubrics that are not to be used for primary tabulations of disease.

Format: ICD-9-CM uses an indented format for ease in reference.

Instructional Notations

Instructional terms define what is, or what is not, included in a given subdivision. This is accomplished by using both inclusion and exclusion terms.

INCLUDES: Indicates separate terms, as, modifying adjectives, sites and conditions, entered under a subdivision, such as a category, to further define or give examples of, the content of the category.

Excludes: Exclusion terms are enclosed in a box and are printed in italics to draw attention to their presence. The importance of this instructional term is its use as a guideline to direct the coder to the proper code assignment. In other words, all terms following the word EXCLUDES: are to be coded elsewhere as indicated in each instance.

NOTES These are used to define terms and give coding instructions. Often used to list the fifth-digit subclassifications for certain categories.

SEE Acts as a cross reference and, is an explicit direction to look elsewhere. This instructional term must always be followed. (Cross references provide the user with other possible modifiers for a term, or, its synonyms.)

SEE CATEGORY A variation of the instructional term SEE. This refers the coder to a specific category. You must *always* follow this instructional term.

SEE ALSO A direction given to look elsewhere if the main term or subterm(s) are not sufficient to code the information you have.

CODE FIRST This instructional note is used for those codes not intended to be used as a principal diagnosis, or not to be sequenced before the underlying disease. The note requires that the underlying disease (etiology) be coded first with the code the note is applied to being coded second. This note appears only in the tabular list (Vol. 1).

USE ADDITIONAL CODE This instruction is placed in the Tabular List in those categories where the coder may wish to add further information, by using an additional code, to give a more complete picture of the diagnosis or procedure.

Related terms

AND Whenever this term appears in a title, it should be interpreted as "and/or."

WITH When this term is used in a title it indicates a requirement that both parts of the title must be present in the diagnostic statement.

COLOR CODING

All PMIC versions of ICD-9-CM include color-coding to alert the user to special coding situations or conditions that require additional attention. The use of color-coding is found in the Tabular List of Volume 1 and the Tabular List of Volume 3. The color is applied as solid rectangular bars over the codes only so that the descriptions remain clear and legible. The color codes and definitions are printed at the bottom of all right-sided pages of Volume 1 and Volume 3.

Volume 1

Three digit codes. Coding to fourth or fifth digit specificity is required.

Unspecified code. Descriptions include the term "unspecified". Use only if a more specific diagnosis is not known or available.

Nonspecific code. Descriptions include the term "nonspecific, unspecified, other specified or other". A report *may* be required by insurance carriers.

Manifestation codes. Used only to code the manifestation of an underlying disease. Code the underlying disease first.

Medicare secondary payer (MSP) alert. Diagnoses that may trigger a post-payment review by Medicare. Medicare is usually the secondary payer for these diagnoses.

Volume 3*

Noncovered operating room procedure. An operating room procedure that is not covered by Medicare.

Non-operating room procedure. A procedure that is not performed in the operating room that affects DRG assignment.

Bilateral procedure.

Valid operating room procedure. Prompts a change in DRG assignment.

Nonspecific operating room procedure. Choose a more precise code if possible.

*These colors appear only in the three-volume edition

ICD-9-CM CODING FUNDAMENTALS

Learning and following the basic steps of ICD-9-CM coding will increase your chances of better and faster reimbursement from third party payers, as well as establish meaningful profiles for future reimbursement rates. To become a proficient coder, two basic principles must be considered.

- It is imperative that you use both the Alphabetic Index (Volume 2) and the Tabular List (Volume 1) when locating and assigning codes. Coding only from the Alphabetic Index will cause you to miss any additional information provided only in the Tabular List: such as, exclusions, instructions to use additional codes or the need for a fifth-digit.

- The level of specificity is important in all coding situations. So, a three-digit code that has subdivisions indicates you must use the appropriate subdivision code. Also, any time a fifth-digit subclassification is provided, you must use the fifth-digit code.

Nine Steps for Accurate ICD-9-CM Coding

1. Locate the main term within the diagnostic statement.

2. Locate that main term in the Alphabetic Index (Volume 2). Keep in mind that the primary arrangement for main terms is by condition in the Alphabetic Index (Volume 2); main terms can be referred to in outmoded, ill-defined and lay terms as well as proper medical terms; main terms can be expressed in broad or specific terms, as nouns, adjectives or eponyms and can be with or without modifiers. Certain conditions may be listed under more than one main term.

3. Remember to refer to all notes under the main term. Be guided by the instructions in any notes appearing in a box immediately after the main term.

4. Examine any modifiers appearing in parentheses next to the main term. See if any of these modifiers apply to any of the qualifying terms used in the diagnostic statement.

5. Take note of the subterms indented beneath the main term. Subterms differ from main terms in that they provide greater specificity becoming more specific the further they are indented to the right of the main term in 2-space increments and, they provide the anatomical sites affected by the disease or injury.

6. Be sure to follow any cross reference instructions. These instructional terms ("see" or "see also") must be followed to locate the correct code.

7. Confirm the code selection in the Tabular List (Volume 1). make certain you have selected the appropriate classification in accordance with the diagnosis.

8. Follow instructional terms in the Tabular List (Volume 1). Watch for exclusion terms, notes and fifth-digit instructions that apply to the code number you are verifying. It is necessary to search not only the selected code number for

instructions but also, the category, section and chapter in which the code number is collapsible. Many times the instructional information is located one or more pages preceding the actual page you find the code number on.

9. Finally, assign the code number you have determined to be correct. Repeat the above steps until all codes have been assigned.

MEDICARE REQUIREMENTS FOR ICD-9-CM CODING

The Medicare Catastrophic Coverage Act of 1988 (PL 100-330) requires that health care professionals submit an appropriate diagnosis code, using the International Classification of Diseases, 9th Revision, Clinical Modification (ICD-9-CM) for each procedure, service, or supply billed under Medicare Part B.

To comply with the regulations, health care professionals must convert the reason(s) for the procedures, services or supplies, performed or issued, from written diagnostic statements that may include specific diagnoses, signs, symptoms and/or complaints, into ICD-9-CM diagnosis codes. The Health Care Financing Administration originally set the implementation date for this requirement as April 1, 1989, however, it was subsequently delayed until June 1, 1989, at the request of the American Medical Association, to give health care providers additional time to prepare for the change.

HCFA Guidelines for Using ICD-9-CM Codes

The Health Care Financing Administration (HCFA) has prepared guidelines for using ICD-9-CM codes and instructions on how to report them on claim forms. In addition, HCFA has directed your medicare intermediary to provide you with a written copy of these instructions. The basic HCFA guidelines are summarized below, however, it is very important that you obtain a copy of the guidelines from your Medicare intermediary as implementation of HCFA requirements varies from one intermediary to another.

1. Indicate on the claim form or itemized statement the appropriate code(s) from the ICD-9-CM code range 001.0 through V82.9 to identify diagnoses, symptoms, conditions, problems, complaints or other reason(s) for the procedure, service or supply provided.

   A. In choosing codes to describe the reason for the encounter, the health care professional will frequently be using codes within the range from 001.0 through 999.9, the section of ICD-9-CM for the classification of diseases and injuries (e.g. infectious and parasitic diseases; neoplasms; signs, symptoms and ill-defined conditions). Codes that describe symptoms as opposed to diagnoses are acceptable if this is the highest level of certainty documented by the physician.

   B. ICD-9-CM also provides codes to deal with visits for circumstances other than a disease or injury, such as an encounter for a laboratory test only. These codes are found in the V-code section and range from V01.0 through V82.9.

2. The ICD-9-CM code for the diagnosis, condition, problem, or other reason for the encounter documented in the medical record as the main reason for the procedure, service or supply provided should be listed first. Additional ICD-9-CM codes that describe any current coexisting conditions are then listed. Do not include codes for conditions that were previously treated and no longer exist.

3. ICD-9-CM codes should be used at their highest level of specificity.

   A. Assign three digit codes only if there are no four digit codes within the coding category.

   B. Assign four digit codes only if there is no fifth digit subclassification for that category.

   C. Assign the fifth digit subclassification code for those categories where it exists.

   Claims submitted with three or four digit codes where four and five digit codes are available may be returned to you by the Medicare intermediary for proper coding. It is recognized that a very specific diagnosis may not be known at the time of the initial encounter. However, that is not an acceptable reason to submit a three digit code when four or five digits are available.

   For example, if the patient has chronic bronchitis, ICD-9-CM code 491, and the physician has not yet documented whether the bronchitis is simple, mucopurulent, or obstructive, the code for unspecified chronic bronchitis, ICD-9-CM code 491.9, should be listed.

4. Diagnoses documented as "probable," "suspected," "questionable," or "rule out" should not be coded as if the diagnosis is confirmed. The condition(s) should be coded to the highest degree of certainty for the encounter, such as describing symptoms, signs, abnormal test results, or other reasons for the encounter.

5. Chronic disease(s) treated on an ongoing basis may be coded and reported as many times as the patient receives treatment and care for the condition(s).

6. When patients receive ancillary diagnostic services only during an encounter, the appropriate "V code" for the service should be listed first, and the diagnosis or problem for which the diagnostic procedures are being performed should be listed second.

   A. V codes will be used frequently by radiologists who perform radiological examinations on referrals. For example, ICD-9-CM code V72.5, Radiological examination, not elsewhere classified, describes the reason for the encounter and should be listed first on the claim form or statement. If the reason for the referral is known, a second ICD-9-CM code that describes the signs or symptoms for which the examination was ordered should be listed.

   B. Failure to list a second ICD-9-CM code in addition to the V code may result in claim delays or denials. The ICD-9-CM code V72.5, Radio-logical examination, not elsewhere classified, includes referrals for routine chest x-rays that are not covered by the Medicare program. Medicare intermediaries may establish screening programs to verify that the referrals were not for routine chest x-rays.

By supplying a second ICD-9-CM code to describe the reason for the referral, these claims can be clearly identified by the Medicare intermediary as referrals to evaluate symptoms, signs or diagnoses. The mission of a second ICD-9-CM code may lead to requests for additional information from Medicare intermediaries prior to processing the claim.

7. For patients receiving only ancillary therapeutic services during an encounter, list the appropriate V code first, followed by the ICD-9-CM code for the diagnosis or problem for which the services are being performed. For example, a patient with multiple sclerosis presenting for rehabilitation services would be coded using code V57.1, Other physical therapy, or code V57.89, Other care involving use of rehabilitation procedures, followed by code 340, multiple sclerosis.

8. For surgical procedures, use the ICD-9-CM code for the diagnosis for which the surgery was performed. If the postoperative diagnosis is known to be different at the time the claim is filed, use the ICD-9-CM code for the post-operative diagnosis.

9. Code all documented conditions that coexist at the time of the visit that require or affect patient care, treatment or management. Do not code conditions that were previously treated and no longer exist.

Completing the HCFA1500 Claim Form

Health care professionals using the Uniform Health Insurance Claim Form, HCFA1500, to file claims for services provided to Medicare beneficiaries must list a minimum of one ICD-9-CM code and may list up to four total ICD-9-CM codes on the claim form.

The ICD-9-CM code for the diagnosis, condition, problem or other reason for the encounter is listed first, followed by up to three additional codes that describe any coexisting conditions. At times, there may be several conditions that equally resulted in the encounter. In these cases, the health care professional is free to select the one that will be listed first.

The ICD-9-CM codes are listed in Box 23 of the "old" HCFA1500 (10/84) claim form and Box 21 of the "new" HCFA1500 (12/90) claim form (see example). In addition, in Box 24 D of both versions of the form, you must indicate by a number from 1 to 4, or combination of numbers, which diagnoses from Box 23 support the procedure, service or supply listed in Box 24 C.

Due to space limitations on the claim form you may use only up to four ICD-9-CM codes for diagnoses, conditions, or signs and symptoms. Frequently the patient may have more than four conditions present at the time of the encounter, however, you must choose only four codes to be listed on the claim form.

If you strongly believe that additional diagnostic information is needed by the Medicare intermediary for proper claim processing you may attach additional supporting documentation to your manual claim. Keep in mind that in most cases the additional documentation will be ignored by the claims examiners, and, in other cases will result in reimbursement delay while someone reviews your documentation.

Medicare Penalties for Non-compliance

The Medicare Catastrophic Coverage Act of 1988 mandates submission of an appropriate ICD-9-CM diagnosis code or codes for each procedure, service, or supply furnished by the health care professional to Medicare Part B beneficiaries. The Act further specifies that compliance is mandatory and that penalties may be assessed for noncompliance.

The penalties for noncompliance differ depending upon whether or not the health care professional has agreed to accept assignment or not.

1. For health care professionals who accept assignment on a Medicare claim and who fail to include ICD-9-CM codes as required will have their claim(s) returned for proper coding and may be subject to post-payment review by the Medicare intermediary, as well as payment denials.

2. For health care professionals who do not accept assignment, the penalties are more severe.

   A. If the original claim form does not include ICD-9-CM codes as required, and the health care professional refuses to provide the codes promptly on request to the Medicare intermediary, the professional may be subject to a civil monetary penalty in an amount not to exceed $2,000, per claim.

   B. If the health care professional continuously fails to provide ICD-9-CM codes as requested, the professional may be subject to the sanction process described in section 1842 (j) (2) (A), that mandates that the professional may be barred from participation in the Medicare program for a period not to exceed five years.

CODING AND BILLING ISSUES

Diagnosis Codes Must Support Procedure Codes

Each service or procedure performed for a patient should be represented by a diagnosis that would substantiate those particular services or procedures as necessary in the investigation or treatment of their condition based on currently accepted standards of practice by the medical profession.

Place (Location) of Service

The actual setting that the services are rendered in for particular diagnoses plays an important part in reimbursement. Many people became accustomed to using Emergency Rooms for any type of illness or injury. By utilizing highly specialized places of service for conditions that were not true emergencies, third party payer were being billed with CPT codes indicating emergency services were rendered. Since the cost of services rendered on an emergency basis is considerably more expensive than those services in an non-emergency situation, third party payers began watching for those claims with diagnoses that did not indicate that a true emergency existed. Payment then was based on what the cost would have been had the patient been treated in the proper setting.

Level of Service Provided

The patient's condition and the treatment of that condition must be billed according to the criteria, as published by the AMA, for each level of service (i.e., minimal, brief, limited, intermediate, extended, comprehensive). Many practices bill the office visit level that they know will pay better rather than to consider the criteria that must be met to use a particular level of service. Again, the patient's diagnosis enters into this concept as well as it is often the diagnosis that indicates the complexity of the level of service to be used.

Frequency of Services

Many times claims are submitted for a patient with the same diagnosis and the same procedure(s) time after time. When the diagnosis indicates a chronic condition and the claims do not indicate any change in the patient's treatment or, give any indication that the patient's condition has been altered (i.e., exacerbated, other symptomology) the third party payer may deny payment based on the frequency of services for the reported condition.

Down Coding

Down coding is the process of reducing a code from one of a higher value to one of a lower value that results in lowered reimbursement. In the area of procedure coding, this process results in the loss of millions of dollars annually by health care professionals and their patients.

With procedure coding, down coding claims is easily resolved by either providing a procedure description that matches that of Current Procedural Terminology (CPT) exactly, or, even better, by eliminating all procedure descriptions from your claim forms, that forces the insurance carrier to allow full value for your procedure, service, or supply. With diagnosis coding, the issue is not mismatch of description to code, as the description is not required, but that the ICD-9-CM code(s) provide justification for the procedure, service or supply or the level of service provided.

A key point to remember is that if there are any current coexisting conditions that may complicate the treatment for the primary condition, it is very important to include the ICD-9-CM codes for the coexisting conditions that will help to justify the level of service provided.

Concurrent Care

Reimbursement problems often arise when a patient is being treated by different professionals, within the same billing entity (medical group or clinic), for different problems at the same time. This is known as concurrent care. For example, a patient may be hospitalized by a clinic's general surgeon for an operation and may also be seen while hospitalized by the group's cardiologist for an unrelated cardiac condition.

If you submit claims for daily hospital visits by both of the above professionals without explanation, most insurance carriers would reject one daily visit as an apparent "duplication" of service. Prior to publication of the 1992 edition of CPT, the key to obtaining proper reimbursement for concurrent care was first, to use the procedure modifier - 75, Concurrent Care, Services Rendered by More than One Physician, and second, to submit a different ICD-9-CM code for the services provided by each physician, that support and justify the need for those services.

Note that modifier -75 was deleted in the 1992 edition of CPT, therefore, when using the new CPT Evaluation and Management codes to bill Medicare, the ICD-9-CM code becomes the key factor for proper reimbursement of concurrent care.

ICD-10

Since 1948, the World Health Organization has revised the *International Classification of Diseases* approximately every 10 years, with a modified version appearing in the United States about one to three years following the WHO publication. Based on the regular schedule, *ICD-10* should have been released in 1987. However, due to difficulties in coordinating the international committees, the first volume of *ICD-10*, the Tabular List, was not published until June of 1992.

Implementation of ICD-10 in the United States

Prior to being implemented in the United States, *ICD-10* must be converted to "American" English and pass through a variety of private and government committees, agencies, associations and organizations. As of this printing, the official position of the Health Care Financing Administration (HCFA) is that *ICD-10* will not be mandated for Medicare claims until "at least the year 2,000."

Summary of Changes in ICD-10

1. All codes in the *ICD-10* are alphanumeric, just like the V-codes and E-codes are in the *ICD-9-CM*.

2. Explanatory notes and instructions are greatly expanded.

3. Main categories are increased from about 1,200 to over 2,000.

4. Separate chapters have been added for diseases of the eye and ear.

5. There are new categories for coding post-procedural disorders.

6. There is greater coding precision for drug-induced conditions.

WHERE TO GET ANSWERS TO QUESTIONS ABOUT ICD-9-CM

Questions regarding the use and interpretation of the *International Classification of Diseases, 9th Revision, Clinical Modification* should be directed in writing to any of the organizations listed below.

Coding Advice/Central Office on ICD-9-CM
American Hospital Association
840 N. Lake Shore Drive, #10E
Chicago, Illinois 60611

World Health Organization Collaborating Center
for Classification of Diseases in North America
National Center for Health Statistics
Department of Health and Human Services
6525 Belcrest Road
Hyattsville, Maryland 20782

Morbidity Classification Branch
National Center for Health Statistics
Department of Health and Human Services
6525 Belcrest Road
Hyattsville, Maryland 20782

Health Care Financing Administration (HCFA)
Division of Prospective Payment
C5-06-27
7500 Security Blvd.
Baltimore, MD 21244-1850

Comments, questions or suggestions regarding the PMIC version of *ICD-9-CM* should be directed in writing to:

Managing Editor
Practice Management Information Corporation
4727 Wilshire Boulevard, Suite 300
Los Angeles, California 90010

DISEASES: TABULAR LIST
VOLUME 1

1. INFECTIOUS AND PARASITIC DISEASES (001-139)

Note: Categories for "late effects" of infectious and parasitic diseases are to be found at 137-139.
Includes: diseases generally recognized as communicable or transmissible as well as a few diseases of unknown but possibly infectious origin

Excludes: *acute respiratory infections (460-466)*
carrier or suspected carrier of infectious organism (V02.0-V02.9)
certain localized infections
influenza (487.0-487.8)

INTESTINAL INFECTIOUS DISEASES (001-009)

Excludes: *helminthiases (120.0-129)*

001 Cholera

001.0 Due to Vibrio cholerae

001.1 Due to Vibrio cholerae el tor

001.9 Cholera, unspecified

002 Typhoid and paratyphoid fevers

002.0 Typhoid fever
Typhoid (fever) (infection) [any site]

002.1 Paratyphoid fever A

002.2 Paratyphoid fever B

002.3 Paratyphoid fever C

002.9 Paratyphoid fever, unspecified

003 Other salmonella infections
Includes: infection or food poisoning by Salmonella [any serotype]

003.0 Salmonella gastroenteritis
Salmonellosis

003.1 Salmonella septicemia

003.2 Localized salmonella infections

003.20 Localized salmonella infection, unspecified

003.21 Salmonella meningitis

003.22 Salmonella pneumonia

003.23 Salmonella arthritis

003.24 Salmonella osteomyelitis

003.29 Other

003.8 Other specified salmonella infections

003.9 Salmonella infection, unspecified

004 Shigellosis
Includes: bacillary dysentery

004.0 Shigella dysenteriae
Infection by group A Shigella (Schmitz) (Shiga)

004.1 Shigella flexneri
Infection by group B Shigella

004.2 Shigella boydii
Infection by group C Shigella

004.3 Shigella sonnei
Infection by group D Shigella

004.8 Other specified shigella infections

004.9 Shigellosis, unspecified

005 Other food poisoning (bacterial)

Excludes: *salmonella infections (003.0-003.9)*
toxic effect of:
food contaminants (989.7)
noxious foodstuffs (988.0-988.9)

005.0 Staphylococcal food poisoning
Staphylococcal toxemia specified as due to food

005.1 Botulism
Food poisoning due to Clostridium botulinum

005.2 Food poisoning due to Clostridium perfringens [C. welchii]
Enteritis necroticans

005.3 Food poisoning due to other Clostridia

005.4 Food poisoning due to Vibrio parahaemolyticus

005.8 Other bacterial food poisoning
Food poisoning due to Bacillus cereus

Excludes: *salmonella food poisoning (003.0-003.9)*

● **005.81 Food poisoning due to Vibrio vulnificus**

● **005.89 Other bacterial food poisoning**

005.9 Food poisoning, unspecified

006 Amebiasis
Includes: infection due to Entamoeba histolytica

Excludes: *amebiasis due to organisms other than Entamoeba histolytica (007.8)*

006.0 Acute amebic dysentery without mention of abscess
Acute amebiasis

006.1 Chronic intestinal amebiasis without mention of abscess
Chronic:
amebiasis
amebic dysentery

006.2 Amebic nondysenteric colitis

006.3 Amebic liver abscess
Hepatic amebiasis

006.4 Amebic lung abscess
Amebic abscess of lung (and liver)

006.5 Amebic brain abscess
Amebic abscess of brain (and liver) (and lung)

006.6 Amebic skin ulceration
Cutaneous amebiasis

006.8 Amebic infection of other sites
Amebic:
appendicitis
balanitis
Ameboma

Excludes: *specific infections by free-living amebae (136.2)*

006.9 Amebiasis, unspecified
Amebiasis NOS

007 Other protozoal intestinal diseases
Includes: protozoal:
colitis
diarrhea
dysentery

007.0 Balantidiasis
Infection by Balantidium coli

007.1 Giardiasis
Infection by Giardia lamblia
Lambliasis

007.2 Coccidiosis
Infection by Isospora belli and Isospora hominis
Isosporiasis

007.3 Intestinal trichomoniasis

007.8 Other specified protozoal intestinal diseases
Amebiasis due to organisms other than Entamoeba histolytica

007.9 Unspecified protozoal intestinal disease
Flagellate diarrhea
Protozoal dysentery NOS

008 Intestinal infections due to other organisms
Includes: any condition classifiable to 009.0-009.3 with mention of the responsible organisms

Excludes: *food poisoning by these organisms (005.0-005.9)*

● Code new to this edition ▲ Revision of existing code ④ ⑤ Fourth or fifth digit required

008.0 Escherichia coli [E. coli]

008.00 E. coli, unspecified
E. coli enteritis NOS

008.01 Enteropathogenic E. coli

008.02 Enterotoxigenic E. coli

008.03 Enteroinvasive E. coli

008.04 Enterohemorrhagic E. coli

008.09 Other intestinal E. coli infections

008.1 Arizona group of paracolon bacilli

008.2 Aerobacter aerogenes
Enterobacter aerogenes

008.3 Proteus (mirabilis) (morganii)

008.4 Other specified bacteria

008.41 Staphylococcus
Staphylococcal enterocolitis

008.42 Pseudomonas

008.43 Campylobacter

008.44 Yersinia enterocolitica

008.45 Clostridium difficile
Pseudomembranous colitis

008.46 Other anaerobes
Anaerobic enteritis NOS
Gram-negative anaerobes
Bacteroides (fragilis)

008.47 Other Gram-negative bacteria
Gram-negative enteritis NOS

Excludes: *Gram-negative anaerobes (008.46)*

008.49 Other

008.5 Bacterial enteritis, unspecified

008.6 Enteritis due to specified virus

008.61 Rotavirus

008.62 Adenovirus

008.63 Norwalk virus
Norwalk-like agent

008.64 Other small round viruses [SRV's]
Small round virus NOS

008.65 Calcivirus

008.66 Astrovirus

008.67 Enterovirus NEC
Coxsackie virus
Echovirus

Excludes: *poliovirus (045.0-045.9)*

008.69 Other viral enteritis
Torovirus

008.8 Other organism, not elsewhere classified
Viral:
enteritis NOS
gastroenteritis

Excludes: *influenza with involvement of gastrointestinal tract (487.8)*

009 Ill-defined intestinal infections

Excludes: *diarrheal disease or intestinal infection due to specified organism (001.0-008.8)*
diarrhea following gastrointestinal surgery (564.4)
intestinal malabsorption (579.0-579.9)
ischemic enteritis (557.0-557.9)
other noninfectious gastroenteritis and colitis (558.1-558.9)
regional enteritis (555.0-555.9)
ulcerative colitis (556)

009.0 Infectious colitis, enteritis, and gastroenteritis

Colitis, Enteritis, Gastroenteritis } septic

Dysentery:
- NOS
- catarrhal
- hemorrhagic

009.1 Colitis, enteritis, and gastroenteritis of presumed infectious origin

Excludes: *colitis NOS (558.9)*
enteritis NOS (558.9)
gastroenteritis NOS (558.9)

009.2 Infectious diarrhea

Diarrhea:
- dysenteric
- epidemic

Infectious diarrheal disease NOS

009.3 Diarrhea of presumed infectious origin

Excludes: *diarrhea NOS (787.91)*

TUBERCULOSIS (010-018)

Includes: infection by Mycobacterium tuberculosis (human) (bovine)

Excludes: *congenital tuberculosis (771.2)*
late effects of tuberculosis (137.0-137.4)

The following fifth-digit subclassification is for use with categories 010-018:

- **0 unspecified**
- **1 bacteriological or histological examination not done**
- **2 bacteriological or histological examination unknown (at present)**
- **3 tubercle bacilli found (in sputum) by microscopy**
- **4 tubercle bacilli not found (in sputum) by microscopy, but found by bacterial culture**
- **5 tubercle bacilli not found by bacteriological examination, but tuberculosis confirmed histologically**
- **6 tubercle bacilli not found by bacteriological or histological examination but tuberculosis confirmed by other methods [inoculation of animals]**

⑤ **010 Primary tuberculous infection**

Excludes: *nonspecific reaction to tuberculin skin test without active tuberculosis (795.5)*
positive PPD (795.5)
positive tuberculin skin test without active tuberculosis (795.5)

010.0 Primary tuberculous complex

010.1 Tuberculous pleurisy in primary progressive tuberculosis

010.8 Other primary progressive tuberculosis

Excludes: *tuberculous erythema nodosum (017.1)*

010.9 Primary tuberculous infection, unspecified

⑤ **011 Pulmonary tuberculosis**

Use additional code, if desired, to identify any associated silicosis (502)

011.0 Tuberculosis of lung, infiltrative

011.1 Tuberculosis of lung, nodular

011.2 Tuberculosis of lung with cavitation

011.3 Tuberculosis of bronchus

Excludes: *isolated bronchial tuberculosis (012.2)*

011.4 Tuberculous fibrosis of lung

011.5 Tuberculous bronchiectasis

011.6 Tuberculous pneumonia [any form]

011.7 Tuberculous pneumothorax

011.8 Other specified pulmonary tuberculosis

011.9 Pulmonary tuberculosis, unspecified

Respiratory tuberculosis NOS
Tuberculosis of lung NOS

⑤ **012 Other respiratory tuberculosis**

Excludes: *respiratory tuberculosis, unspecified (011.9)*

012.0 Tuberculous pleurisy
Tuberculosis of pleura
Tuberculous empyema
Tuberculous hydrothorax

Excludes: *pleurisy with effusion without mention of cause (511.9)*
tuberculous pleurisy in primary progressive tuberculosis (010.1)

012.1 Tuberculosis of intrathoracic lymph nodes
Tuberculosis of lymph nodes:
hilar
mediastinal
tracheobronchial
Tuberculous tracheobronchial adenopathy

Excludes: *that specified as primary (010.0-010.9)*

012.2 Isolated tracheal or bronchial tuberculosis

012.3 Tuberculous laryngitis
Tuberculosis of glottis

012.8 Other specified respiratory tuberculosis
Tuberculosis of:
mediastinum
nasopharynx
Tuberculosis of:
nose (septum)
sinus [any nasal]

⑤ **013 Tuberculosis of meninges and central nervous system**

013.0 Tuberculous meningitis
Tuberculosis of meninges (cerebral) (spinal)
Tuberculous:
leptomeningitis
meningoencephalitis

Excludes: *tuberculoma of meninges (013.1)*

013.1 Tuberculoma of meninges

□ **013.2 Tuberculoma of brain**
Tuberculosis of brain (current disease)

□ **013.3 Tuberculous abscess of brain**

□ **013.4 Tuberculoma of spinal cord**

□ **013.5 Tuberculous abscess of spinal cord**

□ **013.6 Tuberculous encephalitis or myelitis**

□ **013.8 Other specified tuberculosis of central nervous system**

013.9 Unspecified tuberculosis of central nervous system
Tuberculosis of central nervous system NOS

⑤ **014 Tuberculosis of intestines, peritoneum, and mesenteric glands**

014.0 Tuberculous peritonitis
Tuberculous ascites

014.8 Other
Tuberculosis (of):
anus
intestine (large) (small)
mesenteric glands
rectum
retroperitoneal (lymph nodes)
Tuberculous enteritis

⑤ **015 Tuberculosis of bones and joints**
Use additional code, if desired, to identify manifestation, as:
tuberculous:
arthropathy (711.4)
necrosis of bone (730.8)
osteitis (730.8)
osteomyelitis (730.8)
synovitis (727.01)
tenosynovitis (727.01)

015.0 Vertebral column
Pott's disease

Use additional code, if desired, to identify manifestation, as:
curvature of spine [Pott's] (737.4)
kyphosis (737.4)
spondylitis (720.81)

015.1 Hip

015.2 Knee

□ **015.5 Limb bones**
Tuberculous dactylitis

□ **015.6 Mastoid**
Tuberculous mastoiditis

□ **015.7 Other specified bone**

015.8 Other specified joint

015.9 Tuberculosis of unspecified bones and joints

⑤ **016 Tuberculosis of genitourinary system**

016.0 Kidney
Renal tuberculosis

Use additional code, if desired, to identify manifestation, as:
tuberculous:
nephropathy (583.81)
pyelitis (590.81)
pyelonephritis (590.81)

□ **016.1 Bladder**

□ **016.2 Ureter**

□ **016.3 Other urinary organs**

□ **016.4 Epididymis**

□ **016.5 Other male genital organs**

Use additional code, if desired, to identify manifestation, as:
tuberculosis of:
prostate (601.4)
seminal vesicle (608.81)
testis (608.81)

□ **016.6 Tuberculous oophoritis and salpingitis**

□ **016.7 Other female genital organs**
Tuberculous:
cervicitis
endometritis

016.9 Genitourinary tuberculosis, unspecified

⑤ **017 Tuberculosis of other organs**

017.0 Skin and subcutaneous cellular tissue
Lupus:
exedens
vulgaris
Scrofuloderma
Tuberculosis:
colliquativa
cutis
lichenoides
papulonecrotica
verrucosa cutis

Excludes: *lupus erythematosus (695.4)*
disseminated (710.0)
lupus NOS (710.0)
nonspecific reaction to tuberculin skin test without active tuberculosis (795.5)
positive PPD (795.5)
positive tuberculin skin test without active tuberculosis (795.5)

017.1 Erythema nodosum with hypersensitivity reaction in tuberculosis
Bazin's disease
Erythema:
induratum
nodosum, tuberculous
Tuberculosis indurativa

Excludes: *erythema nodosum NOS (695.2)*

017.2 Peripheral lymph nodes
Scrofula
Scrofulous abscess
Tuberculous adenitis

Excludes: *tuberculosis of lymph nodes:*
bronchial and mediastinal (012.1)
mesenteric and retroperitoneal (014.8)
tuberculous tracheobronchial adenopathy (012.1)

017.3 Eye
Use additional code, if desired, to identify manifestation, as:
tuberculous:
chorioretinitis, disseminated (363.13)
episcleritis (379.09)
interstitial keratitis (370.59)
iridocyclitis, chronic (364.11)
keratoconjunctivitis (phlyctenular) (370.31)

017.4 Ear
Tuberculosis of ear
Tuberculous otitis media

Excludes: *tuberculous mastoiditis (015.6)*

017.5 Thyroid gland

017.6 Adrenal glands
Addison's disease, tuberculous

017.7 Spleen

□ **017.8 Esophagus**

□ **017.9 Other specified organs**
Use additional code, if desired, to identify manifestation, as:
tuberculosis of:
endocardium [any valve] (424.91)
myocardium (422.0)
pericardium (420.0)

⑤ **018 Miliary tuberculosis**
Includes: tuberculosis:
disseminated
generalized
miliary, whether of a single specified site, multiple sites, or unspecified site
polyserositis

018.0 Acute miliary tuberculosis

018.8 Other specified miliary tuberculosis

018.9 Miliary tuberculosis, unspecified

ZOONOTIC BACTERIAL DISEASES (020-027)

020 Plague
Includes: infection by Yersinia [Pasteurella] pestis

020.0 Bubonic

020.1 Cellulocutaneous

020.2 Septicemic

020.3 Primary pneumonic

020.4 Secondary pneumonic

020.5 Pneumonic, unspecified

020.8 Other specified types of plague
Abortive plague
Ambulatory plague
Pestis minor

020.9 Plague, unspecified

021 Tularemia
Includes: deerfly fever
infection by Francisella [Pasteurella] tularensis
rabbit fever

021.0 Ulceroglandular tularemia

021.1 Enteric tularemia
Tularemia:
cryptogenic
intestinal
typhoidal

021.2 Pulmonary tularemia
Bronchopneumonic tularemia

021.3 Oculoglandular tularemia

021.8 Other specified tularemia
Tularemia:
generalized or disseminated
glandular

021.9 Unspecified tularemia

022 Anthrax

022.0 Cutaneous anthrax
Malignant pustule

022.1 Pulmonary anthrax
Respiratory anthrax
Wool-sorters' disease

022.2 Gastrointestinal anthrax

022.3 Anthrax septicemia

022.8 Other specified manifestations of anthrax

022.9 Anthrax, unspecified

023 Brucellosis
Includes: fever:
Malta
Mediterranean
undulant

023.0 Brucella melitensis

023.1 Brucella abortus

023.2 Brucella suis

023.3 Brucella canis

023.8 Other brucellosis
Infection by more than one organism

023.9 Brucellosis, unspecified

024 Glanders
Infection by:
Actinobacillus mallei
Malleomyces mallei
Pseudomonas mallei
Farcy
Malleus

025 Melioidosis
Infection by:
Malleomyces pseudomallei
Pseudomonas pseudomallei
Whitmore's bacillus
Pseudoglanders

026 Rat-bite fever

026.0 Spirillary fever
Rat-bite fever due to Spirillum minor [S. minus]
Sodoku

026.1 Streptobacillary fever
Epidemic arthritic erythema
Haverhill fever
Rat-bite fever due to Streptobacillus moniliformis

026.9 Unspecified rat-bite fever

027 Other zoonotic bacterial diseases

027.0 Listeriosis
Infection } by Listeria monocytogenes
Septicemia }

Use additional code, if desired, to identify manifestation, as meningitis (320.7)

Excludes: congenital listeriosis (771.2)

● Code new to this edition
▲ Revision of existing code
④ ⑤ Fourth or fifth digit required

027.1 Erysipelothrix infection
Erysipeloid (of Rosenbach)
Infection } by Erysipelothrix insidiosa [E. rhusiopathiae]
Septicemia } by Erysipelothrix insidiosa [E. rhusiopathiae]

027.2 Pasteurellosis
Pasteurella pseudotuberculosis infection
Mesenteric adenitis } by Pasteurella multocida [P. septica]
Septic infection (cat bite) (dog bite) } by Pasteurella multocida [P. septica]

Excludes: *infection by:*
Francisella [Pasteurella] tularensis (021.0-021.9)
Yersinia [Pasteurella] pestis (020.0-020.9)

027.8 Other specified zoonotic bacterial diseases

027.9 Unspecified zoonotic bacterial disease

OTHER BACTERIAL DISEASES (030-041)

Excludes: *bacterial venereal diseases (098.0-099.9)*
bartonellosis (088.0)

030 Leprosy
Includes: Hansen's disease
infection by Mycobacterium leprae

030.0 Lepromatous [type L]
Lepromatous leprosy (macular) (diffuse) (infiltrated) (nodular) (neuritic)

030.1 Tuberculoid [type T]
Tuberculoid leprosy (macular) (maculoanesthetic) (major) (minor) (neuritic)

030.2 Indeterminate [group I]
Indeterminate [uncharacteristic] leprosy (macular) (neuritic)

030.3 Borderline [group B]
Borderline or dimorphous leprosy (infiltrated) (neuritic)

030.8 Other specified leprosy

030.9 Leprosy, unspecified

031 Diseases due to other mycobacteria

031.0 Pulmonary
Infection by Mycobacterium:
avium
intracellulare [Battey bacillus]
kansasii
Battey disease

031.1 Cutaneous
Buruli ulcer
Infection by Mycobacterium:
marinum [M. balnei]
ulcerans

031.8 Other specified mycobacterial diseases

031.9 Unspecified diseases due to mycobacteria
Atypical mycobacterium infection NOS

032 Diphtheria
Includes: infection by Corynebacterium diphtheriae

032.0 Faucial diphtheria
Membranous angina, diphtheritic

032.1 Nasopharyngeal diphtheria

032.2 Anterior nasal diphtheria

032.3 Laryngeal diphtheria
Laryngotracheitis, diphtheritic

032.8 Other specified diphtheria

032.81 Conjunctival diphtheria
Pseudomembranous diphtheritic conjunctivitis

032.82 Diphtheritic myocarditis

032.83 Diphtheritic peritonitis

032.84 Diphtheritic cystitis

032.85 Cutaneous diphtheria

Add 4th or 5th digit | Nonspecific code | Unspecified code | Manifestation code

032.89 Other

032.9 Diphtheria, unspecified

033 Whooping cough
Includes: pertussis

Use additional code, if desired, to identify any associated pneumonia (484.3)

033.0 Bordetella pertussis [B. pertussis]

033.1 Bordetella parapertussis [B. parapertussis]

033.8 Whooping cough due to other specified organism
Bordetella bronchiseptica [B. bronchiseptica]

033.9 Whooping cough, unspecified organism

034 Streptococcal sore throat and scarlet fever

034.0 Streptococcal sore throat
Septic:
angina
sore throat
Streptococcal:
angina
laryngitis
pharyngitis
tonsillitis

034.1 Scarlet fever
Scarlatina

Excludes: *parascarlatina (057.8)*

035 Erysipelas

Excludes: *postpartum or puerperal erysipelas (670)*

036 Meningococcal infection

036.0 Meningococcal meningitis
Cerebrospinal fever (meningococcal)
Meningitis:
cerebrospinal
epidemic

036.1 Meningococcal encephalitis

036.2 Meningococcemia
Meningococcal septicemia

036.3 Waterhouse-Friderichsen syndrome, meningococcal
Meningococcal hemorrhagic adrenalitis
Meningococcic adrenal syndrome
Waterhouse-Friderichsen syndrome NOS

036.4 Meningococcal carditis

036.40 Meningococcal carditis, unspecified

036.41 Meningococcal pericarditis

036.42 Meningococcal endocarditis

036.43 Meningococcal myocarditis

036.8 Other specified meningococcal infections

036.81 Meningococcal optic neuritis

036.82 Meningococcal arthropathy

036.89 Other

036.9 Meningococcal infection, unspecified
Meningococcal infection NOS

037 Tetanus

Excludes: *tetanus:*
complicating:
abortion (634-638 with .0, 639.0)
ectopic or molar pregnancy (639.0)
neonatorum (771.3)
puerperal (670)

038 Septicemia

Excludes: *bacteremia (790.7)*
during labor (659.3)
following ectopic or molar pregnancy (639.0)
following infusion, injection, transfusion, or vaccination (999.3)
postpartum, puerperal (670)
that complicating abortion (634-638 with .0, 639.0)

038.0 Streptococcal septicemia

038.1 Staphylococcal septicemia

038.2 Pneumococcal septicemia

038.3 Septicemia due to anaerobes
Septicemia due to bacteroides

Excludes: *gas gangrene (040.0)*
that due to anaerobic streptococci (038.0)

038.4 Septicemia due to other gram-negative organisms

038.40 Gram-negative organism, unspecified
Gram-negative septicemia NOS

038.41 Hemophilus influenzae [H. influenzae]

038.42 Escherichia coli [E. coli]

038.43 Pseudomonas

038.44 Serratia

038.49 Other

038.8 Other specified septicemias

Excludes: *septicemia (due to):*
anthrax (022.3)
gonococcal (098.89)
herpetic (054.5)
meningococcal (036.2)
septicemic plague (020.2)

038.9 Unspecified septicemia
Septicemia NOS

Excludes: *bacteremia NOS (790.7)*

039 Actinomycotic infections

Includes: actinomycotic mycetoma
infection by Actinomycetales, such as species of Actinomyces, Actinomadura, Nocardia, Streptomyces
maduromycosis (actinomycotic)
schizomycetoma (actinomycotic)

039.0 Cutaneous
Erythrasma
Trichomycosis axillaris

039.1 Pulmonary
Thoracic actinomycosis

039.2 Abdominal

039.3 Cervicofacial

039.4 Madura foot

Excludes: *madura foot due to mycotic infection (117.4)*

039.8 Of other specified sites

039.9 Of unspecified site
Actinomycosis NOS
Maduromycosis NOS
Nocardiosis NOS

040 Other bacterial diseases

Excludes: *bacteremia NOS (790.7)*
bacterial infection NOS (041.9)

040.0 Gas gangrene
Gas bacillus infection or gangrene
Infection by Clostridium:
histolyticum
oedematiens
perfringens [welchii]
septicum
sordellii
Malignant edema
Myonecrosis, clostridial
Myositis, clostridial

040.1 Rhinoscleroma

040.2 Whipple's disease
Intestinal lipodystrophy

040.3 Necrobacillosis

040.8 Other specified bacterial diseases

040.81 Tropical pyomyositis

040.89 Other

041 Bacterial infection in conditions classified elsewhere and of unspecified site

Note: This category is provided to be used as an additional code where it is desired to identify the bacterial agent in diseases classified elsewhere. This category will also be used to classify bacterial infections of unspecified nature or site.

Excludes: *bacteremia NOS (790.7)*
septicemia (038.0-038.9)

041.0 Streptococcus

041.00 Streptococcus, unspecified

041.01 Group A

041.02 Group B

041.03 Group C

041.04 Group D

041.05 Group G

041.09 Other Streptococcus

041.1 Staphylococcus

041.10 Staphylococcus, unspecified

041.11 Staphylococcus aureus

041.19 Other Staphylococcus

041.2 Pneumococcus

041.3 Friedländer's bacillus
Infection by Klebsiella pneumoniae

041.4 Escherichia coli [E. coli]

041.5 Hemophilus influenzae [H. influenzae]

041.6 Proteus (mirabilis) (morganii)

041.7 Pseudomonas

041.8 Other specified bacterial infections

041.81 Mycoplasma
Eaton's agent
Pleuropneumonia-like organisms [PPLO]

041.82 Bacillus fragilis

041.83 Clostridium perfringens

041.84 Other anaerobes
Gram-negative anaerobes
Bacteroides (fragilis)

Excludes *Helicobacter pylori (041.86)*

041.85 Other Gram-negative organisms
Aerobacter aerogenes
Gram-negative bacteria NOS
Mima polymorpha
Serratia

Excludes: *Gram-negative anaerobes (041.84)*

● **041.86 Helicobacter pylori (H. pylori)**

041.89 Other specified bacteria

041.9 Bacterial infection, unspecified

HUMAN IMMUNODEFICIENCY VIRUS (HIV) INFECTION (042)

042 Human immunodeficiency virus [HIV] disease

Acquired immune deficiency syndrome
Acquired immunodeficiency syndrome
AIDS
AIDS-like syndrome
AIDS-related complex
ARC
HIV infection, symptomatic

Use additional code(s) to identify all manifestations of HIV

Use additional code, if desired, to identify HIV-2 infection (079.53)

Excludes: *asymptomatic HIV infection status (V08)*
exposre to HIV virus (V01.7)
nonspecific serologic evidence of HIV (795.71)

POLIOMYELITIS AND OTHER NON-ARTHROPOD-BORNE VIRAL DISEASES OF CENTRAL NERVOUS SYSTEM (045-049)

⑤ **045 Acute poliomyelitis**

Excludes: *late effects of acute poliomyelitis (138)*

The following fifth-digit subclassification is for use with category 045:

0 poliovirus, unspecified type

1 poliovirus type I

2 poliovirus type II

3 poliovirus type III

045.0 Acute paralytic poliomyelitis specified as bulbar

Infantile paralysis (acute) } specified as bulbar
Poliomyelitis (acute) (anterior) } specified as bulbar
Polioencephalitis (acute) (bulbar)
Polioencephalomyelitis (acute) (anterior) (bulbar)

045.1 Acute poliomyelitis with other paralysis

Paralysis:
acute atrophic, spinal infantile, paralytic
Poliomyelitis (acute) } with paralysis except bulbar
anterior } with paralysis except bulbar
epidemic

045.2 Acute nonparalytic poliomyelitis

Poliomyelitis (acute) } specified as nonparalytic
anterior } specified as nonparalytic
epidemic } specified as nonparalytic

045.9 Acute poliomyelitis, unspecified

Infantile paralysis } unspecified whether paralytic or nonparalytic
Poliomyelitis (acute) } unspecified whether paralytic or nonparalytic
anterior } unspecified whether paralytic or nonparalytic
epidemic } unspecified whether paralytic or nonparalytic

046 Slow virus infection of central nervous system

046.0 Kuru

046.1 Jakob-Creutzfeldt disease

Subacute spongiform encephalopathy

046.2 Subacute sclerosing panencephalitis

Dawson's inclusion body encephalitis
Van Bogaert's sclerosing leukoencephalitis

046.3 Progressive multifocal leukoencephalopathy

Multifocal leukoencephalopathy NOS

046.8 Other specified slow virus infection of central nervous system

046.9 Unspecified slow virus infection of central nervous system

047 Meningitis due to enterovirus

Includes: meningitis:
abacterial
aseptic
viral

Excludes: *meningitis due to:*
adenovirus (049.1)
arthropod-borne virus (060.0-066.9)
leptospira (100.81)
virus of:
herpes simplex (054.72)
herpes zoster (053.0)
lymphocytic choriomeningitis (049.0)
mumps (072.1)
poliomyelitis (045.0-045.9)
any other infection specifically classified elsewhere

047.0 Coxsackie virus

047.1 ECHO virus
Meningo-eruptive syndrome

047.8 Other specified viral meningitis

047.9 Unspecified viral meningitis
Viral meningitis NOS

048 Other enterovirus diseases of central nervous system
Boston exanthem

049 Other non-arthropod-borne viral diseases of central nervous system

Excludes: *late effects of viral encephalitis (139.0)*

049.0 Lymphocytic choriomeningitis
Lymphocytic:
meningitis (serous) (benign)
meningoencephalitis (serous) (benign)

049.1 Meningitis due to adenovirus

049.8 Other specified non-arthropod-borne viral diseases of central nervous system
Encephalitis:
acute:
inclusion body
necrotizing
epidemic
Encephalitis:
lethargica
Rio Bravo
von Economo's disease

049.9 Unspecified non-arthropod-borne viral diseases of central nervous system
Viral encephalitis NOS

VIRAL DISEASES ACCOMPANIED BY EXANTHEM (050-057)

Excludes: *arthropod-borne viral diseases (060.0-066.9)*
Boston exanthem (048)

050 Smallpox

050.0 Variola major
Hemorrhagic (pustular) smallpox
Malignant smallpox
Purpura variolosa

050.1 Alastrim
Variola minor

050.2 Modified smallpox
Varioloid

050.9 Smallpox, unspecified

051 Cowpox and paravaccinia

051.0 Cowpox
Vaccinia not from vaccination

Excludes: *vaccinia (generalized) (from vaccination) (999.0)*

051.1 Pseudocowpox
Milkers' node

051.2 Contagious pustular dermatitis
Ecthyma contagiosum
Orf

051.9 Paravaccinia, unspecified

052 Chickenpox

052.0 Postvaricella encephalitis
Postchickenpox encephalitis

052.1 Varicella (hemorrhagic) pneumonitis

052.7 With other specified complications

052.8 With unspecified complication

052.9 Varicella without mention of complication
Chickenpox NOS
Varicella NOS

053 Herpes zoster
Includes: shingles
zona

053.0 With meningitis

053.1 With other nervous system complications

053.10 With unspecified nervous system complication

053.11 Geniculate herpes zoster
Herpetic geniculate ganglionitis

053.12 Postherpetic trigeminal neuralgia

053.13 Postherpetic polyneuropathy

053.19 Other

053.2 With ophthalmic complications

053.20 Herpes zoster dermatitis of eyelid
Herpes zoster ophthalmicus

053.21 Herpes zoster keratoconjunctivitis

053.22 Herpes zoster iridocyclitis

053.29 Other

053.7 With other specified complications

053.71 Otitis externa due to herpes zoster

053.79 Other

053.8 With unspecified complication

053.9 Herpes zoster without mention of complication
Herpes zoster NOS

054 Herpes simplex
Excludes: congenital herpes simplex (771.2)

054.0 Eczema herpeticum
Kaposi's varicelliform eruption

054.1 Genital herpes

054.10 Genital herpes, unspecified
Herpes progenitalis

054.11 Herpetic vulvovaginitis

054.12 Herpetic ulceration of vulva

054.13 Herpetic infection of penis

054.19 Other

054.2 Herpetic gingivostomatitis

054.3 Herpetic meningoencephalitis
Herpes encephalitis
Simian B disease

054.4 With ophthalmic complications

054.40 With unspecified ophthalmic complication

054.41 Herpes simplex dermatitis of eyelid

054.42 Dendritic keratitis

054.43 Herpes simplex disciform keratitis

054.44 Herpes simplex iridocyclitis

Add 4th or 5th digit | Nonspecific code | Unspecified code | Manifestation code

054.49 **Other**

054.5 **Herpetic septicemia**

054.6 **Herpetic whitlow**
Herpetic felon

054.7 **With other specified complications**

054.71 **Visceral herpes simplex**

054.72 **Herpes simplex meningitis**

054.73 **Herpes simplex otitis externa**

054.79 **Other**

054.8 **With unspecified complication**

054.9 **Herpes simplex without mention of complication**

055 Measles
Includes: morbilli
rubeola

055.0 **Postmeasles encephalitis**

055.1 **Postmeasles pneumonia**

055.2 **Postmeasles otitis media**

055.7 **With other specified complications**

055.71 **Measles keratoconjunctivitis**
Measles keratitis

055.79 **Other**

055.8 **With unspecified complication**

055.9 **Measles without mention of complication**

056 Rubella
Includes: German measles

Excludes: *congenital rubella (771.0)*

056.0 **With neurological complications**

056.00 **With unspecified neurological complication**

056.01 **Encephalomyelitis due to rubella**
Encephalitis } due to rubella
Meningoencephalitis } due to rubella

056.09 **Other**

056.7 **With other specified complications**

056.71 **Arthritis due to rubella**

056.79 **Other**

056.8 **With unspecified complications**

056.9 **Rubella without mention of complication**

057 Other viral exanthemata

057.0 **Erythema infectiosum [fifth disease]**

057.8 **Other specified viral exanthemata**
Dukes (-Filatow) disease
Exanthema subitum [sixth disease]
Fourth disease
Parascarlatina
Pseudoscarlatina
Roseola infantum

057.9 **Viral exanthem, unspecified**

ARTHROPOD-BORNE VIRAL DISEASES (060-066)

Use additional code, if desired, to identify any associated meningitis (321.2)

Excludes: *late effects of viral encephalitis (139.0)*

060 Yellow fever

060.0 **Sylvatic**
Yellow fever:
jungle
sylvan

060.1 **Urban**

060.9 **Yellow fever, unspecified**

● Code new to this edition ▲ Revision of existing code ④ ⑤ Fourth or fifth digit required

061 Dengue
Breakbone fever

Excludes: *hemorrhagic fever caused by dengue virus (065.4)*

062 Mosquito-borne viral encephalitis

062.0 Japanese encephalitis
Japanese B encephalitis

062.1 Western equine encephalitis

062.2 Eastern equine encephalitis

Excludes: *Venezuelan equine encephalitis (066.2)*

062.3 St. Louis encephalitis

062.4 Australian encephalitis
Australian arboencephalitis
Australian X disease
Murray Valley encephalitis

062.5 California virus encephalitis
Encephalitis:
California
La Crosse
Tahyna fever

062.8 Other specified mosquito-borne viral encephalitis
Encephalitis by Ilheus virus

062.9 Mosquito-borne viral encephalitis, unspecified

063 Tick-borne viral encephalitis
Includes: diphasic meningoencephalitis

063.0 Russian spring-summer [taiga] encephalitis

063.1 Louping ill

063.2 Central European encephalitis

063.8 Other specified tick-borne viral encephalitis
Langat encephalitis
Powassan encephalitis

063.9 Tick-borne viral encephalitis, unspecified

064 Viral encephalitis transmitted by other and unspecified arthropods
Arthropod-borne viral encephalitis, vector unknown
Negishi virus encephalitis

Excludes: *viral encephalitis NOS (049.9)*

065 Arthropod-borne hemorrhagic fever

065.0 Crimean hemorrhagic fever [CHF Congo virus]
Central Asian hemorrhagic fever

065.1 Omsk hemorrhagic fever

065.2 Kyasanur Forest disease

065.3 Other tick-borne hemorrhagic fever

065.4 Mosquito-borne hemorrhagic fever
Chikungunya hemorrhagic fever
Dengue hemorrhagic fever

Excludes: *Chikungunya fever (066.3)*
dengue (061)
yellow fever (060.0-060.9)

065.8 Other specified arthropod-borne hemorrhagic fever
Mite-borne hemorrhagic fever

065.9 Arthropod-borne hemorrhagic fever, unspecified
Arbovirus hemorrhagic fever NOS

066 Other arthropod-borne viral diseases

066.0 Phlebotomus fever
Changuinola fever
Sandfly fever

066.1 Tick-borne fever
Nairobi sheep disease
Tick fever:
American mountain
Colorado
Tick fever:
Kemerovo
Quaranfil

Add 4th or 5th digit | Nonspecific code | Unspecified code | Manifestation code

066.2 Venezuelan equine fever
Venezuelan equine encephalitis

066.3 Other mosquito-borne fever
Fever (viral):
Bunyamwera
Bwamba
Chikungunya
GuamaR Mayaro
Mucambo
O'nyong-nyong
Fever (viral):
Oropouche
Pixuna
Rift valley
Ross river
Wesselsbron
West Nile
Zika

Excludes: *dengue (061)*
yellow fever (060.0-060.9)

066.8 Other specified arthropod-borne viral diseases
Chandipura fever
Piry fever

066.9 Arthropod-borne viral disease, unspecified
Arbovirus infection NOS

OTHER DISEASES DUE TO VIRUSES AND CHLAMYDIAE (070-079)

070 Viral hepatitis
Includes: viral hepatitis (acute) (chronic)
Excludes: *cytomegalic inclusion virus hepatitis (078.5)*

The following fifth-digit subclassification is for use with categories 070.2 and 070.3:
0 acute or unspecified, without mention of hepatitis delta
1 acute or unspecified, with hepatitis delta
2 chronic, without mention of hepatitis delta
3 chronic, with hepatitis delta

070.0 Viral hepatitis A with hepatic coma

070.1 Viral hepatitis A without mention of hepatic coma
Infectious hepatitis

⑤ **070.2 Viral hepatitis B with hepatic coma**

⑤ **070.3 Viral hepatitis B without mention of hepatic coma**
Serum hepatitis

070.4 Other specified viral hepatitis with hepatic coma

▲ **070.41 Acute or unspecified hepatitis C with hepatic coma**

070.42 Hepatitis delta without mention of active hepatitis B disease with hepatic coma
Hepatitis delta with hepatitis B carrier state

070.43 Hepatitis E with hepatic coma

070.44 Chronic hepatitis C with hepatic coma

070.49 Other specified viral hepatitis with hepatic coma

070.5 Other specified viral hepatitis without mention of hepatic coma

070.51 Acute or unspecified hepatitis C without mention of hepatic coma

070.52 Hepatitis delta without mention of active hepatitis B disease or hepatic coma

070.53 Hepatitis E without mention of hepatic coma

070.54 Chronic hepatitis C without mention of hepatic coma

070.59 Other specified viral hepatitis without mention of hepatic coma

070.6 Unspecified viral hepatitis with hepatic coma

070.9 Unspecified viral hepatitis without mention of hepatic coma
Viral hepatitis NOS

071 Rabies
Hydrophobia
Lyssa

072 Mumps

072.0 Mumps orchitis

072.1 Mumps meningitis

072.2 Mumps encephalitis
Mumps meningoencephalitis

072.3 Mumps pancreatitis

072.7 Mumps with other specified complications

072.71 Mumps hepatitis

072.72 Mumps polyneuropathy

072.79 Other

072.8 Mumps with unspecified complication

072.9 Mumps without mention of complication

Epidemic parotitis
Infectious parotitis

073 Ornithosis

Includes: parrot fever
psittacosis

073.0 With pneumonia

Lobular pneumonitis due to ornithosis

073.7 With other specified complications

073.8 With unspecified complication

073.9 Ornithosis, unspecified

074 Specific diseases due to Coxsackie virus

Excludes: *Coxsackie virus:*
infection NOS (079.2)
meningitis (047.0)

074.0 Herpangina

Vesicular pharyngitis

074.1 Epidemic pleurodynia

Bornholm disease
Devil's grip
Epidemic:
myalgia
myositis

074.2 Coxsackie carditis

074.20 Coxsackie carditis, unspecified

074.21 Coxsackie pericarditis

074.22 Coxsackie endocarditis

074.23 Coxsackie myocarditis

Aseptic myocarditis of newborn

074.3 Hand, foot, and mouth disease

Vesicular stomatitis and exanthem

074.8 Other specified diseases due to Coxsackie virus

Acute lymphonodular pharyngitis

075 Infectious mononucleosis

Glandular fever
Monocytic angina
Pfeiffer's disease

076 Trachoma

Excludes: *late effect of trachoma (139.1)*

076.0 Initial stage

Trachoma dubium

076.1 Active stage

Granular conjunctivitis (trachomatous)
Trachomatous:
follicular conjunctivitis
pannus

076.9 Trachoma, unspecified

Trachoma NOS

077 Other diseases of conjunctiva due to viruses and Chlamydiae

Excludes: *ophthalmic complications of viral diseases classified elsewhere*

077.0 Inclusion conjunctivitis

Paratrachoma
Swimming pool conjunctivitis

Excludes: *inclusion blennorrhea (neonatal) (771.6)*

077.1 Epidemic keratoconjunctivitis

Shipyard eye

077.2 Pharyngoconjunctival fever

Add 4th or 5th digit | Nonspecific code | Unspecified code | Manifestation code

Viral pharyngoconjunctivitis

077.3 Other adenoviral conjunctivitis
Acute adenoviral follicular conjunctivitis

077.4 Epidemic hemorrhagic conjunctivitis
Apollo:
conjunctivitis
disease
Conjunctivitis due to enterovirus type 70
Hemorrhagic conjunctivitis (acute) (epidemic)

077.8 Other viral conjunctivitis
Newcastle conjunctivitis

077.9 Unspecified diseases of conjunctiva due to Viruses and Chlamydiae

077.98 Due to Chlamydiae

077.99 Due to viruses
Viral conjunctivitis NOS

078 Other diseases due to viruses and Chlamydiae

Excludes: *viral infection NOS (079.0-079.9)*
viremia NOS (790.8)

078.0 Molluscum contagiosum

078.1 Viral warts

078.10 Viral warts, unspecified
Condyloma NOS
Verruca:
NOS
vulgaris
Warts (infectious)

078.11 Condyloma acuminatum

078.19 Other specified viral warts
Genital warts NOS
Verruca:
plana
plantaris

078.2 Sweating fever
Miliary fever
Sweating disease

078.3 Cat-scratch disease
Benign lymphoreticulosis (of inoculation)
Cat-scratch fever

078.4 Foot and mouth disease
Aphthous fever
Epizootic:
aphthae
stomatitis

078.5 Cytomegaloviral disease
Cytomegalic inclusion disease
Salivary gland virus disease

Use additional code, if desired, to identify manifestation, as:
cytomegalic inclusion virus:
hepatitis (573.1)
pneumonia (484.1)

Excludes: *congenital cytomegalovirus infection (771.1)*

078.6 Hemorrhagic nephrosonephritis
Hemorrhagic fever:
epidemic
Korean
Hemorrhagic fever:
Russian
with renal syndrome

078.7 Arenaviral hemorrhagic fever
Hemorrhagic fever:
Argentine
Bolivian
Hemorrhagic fever:
Junin virus
Machupo virus

078.8 Other specified diseases due to viruses and Chlamydiae

Excludes: *epidemic diarrhea (009.2)*
lymphogranuloma venereum (099.1)

078.81 Epidemic vertigo

078.82 Epidemic vomiting syndrome
Winter vomiting disease

078.88 Other specified diseases due to Chlamydiae

078.89 Other specified diseases due to viruses
Epidemic cervical myalgia
Marburg disease
Tanapox

079 Viral and chlamydial infection in conditions classified elsewhere and of unspecified site

Note: This category is provided to be used as an additional code where it is desired to identify the viral agent in diseases classifiable elsewhere. This category will also be used to classify virus infection of unspecified nature or site.

079.0 Adenovirus

079.1 ECHO virus

079.2 Coxsackievirus

079.3 Rhinovirus

079.4 Human papilloma virus

079.5 Retrovirus

Excludes: *human immunodeficiency virus, type 1 [HIV-1] (042)*
human T-cell lymphotrophic virus, type III [HTLV-III] (042)
lymphadenopathy-associated virus [LAV] (042)

079.50 Retrovirus, unspecified

079.51 Human T-cell lymphotrophic virus, type I [HTLV-I]

079.52 Human T-cell lymphotrophic virus, type II [HTLV-II]

079.53 Human immunodeficiency virus, type 2 [HIV-2]

079.59 Other specified retrovirus

079.8 Other specified viral and chlamydial infections

● **079.81 Hantavirus**

079.88 Other specified chlamydial infection

079.89 Other specified viral infection

079.9 Unspecified viral and chlamydial infections

Excludes: *viremia NOS (790.8)*

079.98 Unspecified chlamydial infection
Chlamydial infection NOS

079.99 Unspecified viral infection
Viral infection NOS

RICKETTSIOSES AND OTHER ARTHROPOD-BORNE DISEASES (080-088)

Excludes: *arthropod-borne viral diseases (060.0-066.9)*

080 Louse-borne [epidemic] typhus
Typhus (fever):
classical
epidemic
Typhus (fever):
exanthematic NOS
louse-borne

081 Other typhus

081.0 Murine [endemic] typhus
Typhus (fever):
endemic
flea-borne

081.1 Brill's disease
Brill-Zinsser disease
Recrudescent typhus (fever)

081.2 Scrub typhus
Japanese river fever
Kedani fever
Mite-borne typhus
Tsutsugamushi

081.9 Typhus, unspecified
Typhus (fever) NOS

082 Tick-borne rickettsioses

Add 4th or 5th digit | Nonspecific code | Unspecified code | Manifestation code

082.0 Spotted fevers
Rocky mountain spotted fever
São Paulo fever

082.1 Boutonneuse fever
African tick typhus
India tick typhus
Kenya tick typhus
Marseilles fever
Mediterranean tick fever

082.2 North Asian tick fever
Siberian tick typhus

082.3 Queensland tick typhus

082.8 Other specified tick-borne rickettsioses
Lone star fever

082.9 Tick-borne rickettsiosis, unspecified
Tick-borne typhus NOS

083 Other rickettsioses

083.0 Q fever

083.1 Trench fever
Quintan fever
Wolhynian fever

083.2 Rickettsialpox
Vesicular rickettsiosis

083.8 Other specified rickettsioses

083.9 Rickettsiosis, unspecified

084 Malaria

Note: Subcategories 084.0-084.6 exclude the listed conditions with mention of pernicious complications (084.8-084.9).

Excludes: *congenital malaria (771.2)*

084.0 Falciparum malaria [malignant tertian]
Malaria (fever):
by Plasmodium falciparum
subtertian

084.1 Vivax malaria [benign tertian]
Malaria (fever) by Plasmodium vivax

084.2 Quartan malaria
Malaria (fever) by Plasmodium malariae
Malariae malaria

084.3 Ovale malaria
Malaria (fever) by Plasmodium ovale

084.4 Other malaria
Monkey malaria

084.5 Mixed malaria
Malaria (fever) by more than one parasite

084.6 Malaria, unspecified
Malaria (fever) NOS

084.7 Induced malaria
Therapeutically induced malaria

Excludes: *accidental infection from syringe, blood transfusion, etc. (084.0-084.6, above, according to parasite species)*
transmission from mother to child during delivery (771.2)

084.8 Blackwater fever
Hemoglobinuric:
fever (bilious)
malaria
Malarial hemoglobinuria

084.9 Other pernicious complications of malaria
Algid malaria
Cerebral malaria

Use additional code, if desired, to identify complication, as:
malarial:
hepatitis (573.2)
nephrosis (581.81)

085 Leishmaniasis

085.0 Visceral [kala-azar]

Dumdum fever
Infection by Leishmania:
  donovani
  infantum
Leishmaniasis:
  dermal, post-kala-azar
  Mediterranean
  visceral (Indian)

085.1 Cutaneous, urban

Aleppo boil
Baghdad boil
Delhi boil
Infection by Leishmania tropica (minor)
Leishmaniasis, cutaneous:
  dry form
  late
  recurrent
  ulcerating
Oriental sore

085.2 Cutaneous, Asian desert

Infection by Leishmania tropica major
Leishmaniasis, cutaneous:
  acute necrotizing
  rural
  wet form
  zoonotic form

085.3 Cutaneous, Ethiopian

Infection by Leishmania ethiopica
Leishmaniasis, cutaneous:
  diffuse
  lepromatous

085.4 Cutaneous, American

Chiclero ulcer
Infection by Leishmania mexicana
Leishmaniasis tegumentaria diffusa

085.5 Mucocutaneous (American)

Espundia
Infection by Leishmania braziliensis
Uta

085.9 Leishmaniasis, unspecified

086 Trypanosomiasis

Use additional code, if desired, to identify manifestations, as:
  trypanosomiasis:
    encephalitis (323.2)
    meningitis (321.3)

086.0 Chagas' disease with heart involvement

American trypanosomiasis } with heart involvement
Infection by Trypanosoma cruzi } with heart involvement
Any condition classifiable to 086.2

086.1 Chagas' disease with other organ involvement

American trypanosomiasis } with involvement of organ other than heart
Infection by Trypanosoma cruzi } with involvement of organ other than heart
Any condition classifiable to 086.2

086.2 Chagas' disease without mention of organ involvement

American trypanosomiasis
Infection by Trypanosoma cruzi

086.3 Gambian trypanosomiasis

Gambian sleeping sickness
Infection by Trypanosoma gambiense

086.4 Rhodesian trypanosomiasis

Infection by Trypanosoma rhodesiense
Rhodesian sleeping sickness

086.5 African trypanosomiasis, unspecified

Sleeping sickness NOS

086.9 Trypanosomiasis, unspecified

087 Relapsing fever

Includes: recurrent fever

087.0 Louse-borne

087.1 Tick-borne

087.9 Relapsing fever, unspecified

088 Other arthropod-borne diseases

088.0 Bartonellosis
Carrión's disease
Oroya fever
Verruga peruana

088.8 Other specified arthropod-borne diseases

088.81 Lyme Disease
Erythema chronicum migrans

088.82 Babesiosis
Babesiasis

088.89 Other

088.9 Arthropod-borne disease, unspecified

SYPHILIS AND OTHER VENEREAL DISEASES (090-099)

Excludes: *nonvenereal endemic syphilis (104.0)*
urogenital trichomoniasis (131.0)

090 Congenital syphilis

090.0 Early congenital syphilis, symptomatic
Congenital syphilitic:
choroiditis
coryza (chronic)
hepatomegaly
mucous patches
periostitis
splenomegaly
Syphilitic (congenital):
epiphysitis
osteochondritis
pemphigus
Any congenital syphilitic condition specified as early or manifest less than two years after birth

090.1 Early congenital syphilis, latent
Congenital syphilis without clinical manifestations, with positive serological reaction and negative spinal fluid test, less than two years after birth

090.2 Early congenital syphilis, unspecified
Congenital syphilis NOS, less than two years after birth

090.3 Syphilitic interstitial keratitis
Syphilitic keratitis:
parenchymatous
punctata profunda

Excludes: *interstitial keratitis NOS (370.50)*

090.4 Juvenile neurosyphilis
Use additional code, if desired, to identify any associated mental disorder

090.40 Juvenile neurosyphilis, unspecified
Congenital neurosyphilis
Dementia paralytica juvenilis
Juvenile:
general paresis
tabes
taboparesis

090.41 Congenital syphilitic encephalitis

090.42 Congenital syphilitic meningitis

090.49 Other

090.5 Other late congenital syphilis, symptomatic
Gumma due to congenital syphilis
Hutchinson's teeth
Syphilitic saddle nose
Any congenital syphilitic condition specified as late or manifest two years or more after birth

090.6 Late congenital syphilis, latent
Congenital syphilis without clinical manifestations, with positive serological reaction and negative spinal fluid test, two years or more after birth

090.7 Late congenital syphilis, unspecified
Congenital syphilis NOS, two years or more after birth

090.9 Congenital syphilis, unspecified

091 Early syphilis, symptomatic

Excludes: *early cardiovascular syphilis (093.0-093.9)*
early neurosyphilis (094.0-094.9)

091.0 Genital syphilis (primary)
Genital chancre

091.1 Primary anal syphilis

091.2 Other primary syphilis
Primary syphilis of:
breast
fingers
Primary syphilis of:
lip
tonsils

091.3 Secondary syphilis of skin or mucous membranes
Condyloma latum
Secondary syphilis of:
anus
mouth
pharynx
Secondary syphilis of:
skin
tonsils
vulva

091.4 Adenopathy due to secondary syphilis
Syphilitic adenopathy (secondary)
Syphilitic lymphadenitis (secondary)

091.5 Uveitis due to secondary syphilis

091.50 Syphilitic uveitis, unspecified

091.51 Syphilitic chorioretinitis (secondary)

091.52 Syphilitic iridocyclitis (secondary)

091.6 Secondary syphilis of viscera and bone

091.61 Secondary syphilitic periostitis

091.62 Secondary syphilitic hepatitis
Secondary syphilis of liver

091.69 Other viscera

091.7 Secondary syphilis, relapse
Secondary syphilis, relapse (treated) (untreated)

091.8 Other forms of secondary syphilis

091.81 Acute syphilitic meningitis (secondary)

091.82 Syphilitic alopecia

091.89 Other

091.9 Unspecified secondary syphilis

092 Early syphilis, latent
Includes: syphilis (acquired) without clinical manifestations, with positive serological reaction and negative spinal fluid test, less than two years after infection

092.0 Early syphilis, latent, serological relapse after treatment

092.9 Early syphilis, latent, unspecified

093 Cardiovascular syphilis

093.0 Aneurysm of aorta, specified as syphilitic
Dilatation of aorta, specified as syphilitic

093.1 Syphilitic aortitis

093.2 Syphilitic endocarditis

093.20 Valve, unspecified
Syphilitic ostial coronary disease

093.21 Mitral valve

093.22 Aortic valve
Syphilitic aortic incompetence or stenosis

093.23 Tricuspid valve

093.24 Pulmonary valve

093.8 Other specified cardiovascular syphilis

093.81 Syphilitic pericarditis

093.82 Syphilitic myocarditis

093.89 Other

093.9 Cardiovascular syphilis, unspecified

094 Neurosyphilis
Use additional code, if desired, to identify any associated mental disorder

094.0 Tabes dorsalis
Locomotor ataxia (progressive)
Posterior spinal sclerosis (syphilitic)
Tabetic neurosyphilis

Use additional code, if desired, to identify manifestation, as:
neurogenic arthropathy [Charcot's joint disease] (713.5)

094.1 General paresis
Dementia paralytica
General paralysis (of the insane) (progressive)
Paretic neurosyphilis
Taboparesis

094.2 Syphilitic meningitis
Meningovascular syphilis

Excludes: *acute syphilitic meningitis (secondary) (091.81)*

094.3 Asymptomatic neurosyphilis

094.8 Other specified neurosyphilis

094.81 Syphilitic encephalitis

094.82 Syphilitic Parkinsonism

094.83 Syphilitic disseminated retinochoroiditis

094.84 Syphilitic optic atrophy

094.85 Syphilitic retrobulbar neuritis

094.86 Syphilitic acoustic neuritis

094.87 Syphilitic ruptured cerebral aneurysm

094.89 Other

094.9 Neurosyphilis, unspecified
Gumma (syphilitic) } of central nervous system NOS
Syphilis (early) (late) } of central nervous system NOS
Syphiloma

095 Other forms of late syphilis, with symptoms
Includes: gumma (syphilitic)
syphilis, late, tertiary, or unspecified stage

095.0 Syphilitic episcleritis

095.1 Syphilis of lung

095.2 Syphilitic peritonitis

095.3 Syphilis of liver

095.4 Syphilis of kidney

095.5 Syphilis of bone

095.6 Syphilis of muscle
Syphilitic myositis

095.7 Syphilis of synovium, tendon, and bursa
Syphilitic:
bursitis
synovitis

095.8 Other specified forms of late symptomatic syphilis

Excludes: *cardiovascular syphilis (093.0-093.9)*
neurosyphilis (094.0-094.9)

095.9 Late symptomatic syphilis, unspecified

096 Late syphilis, latent
Syphilis (acquired) without clinical manifestations, with positive serological reaction and negative spinal fluid test, two years or more after infection

097 Other and unspecified syphilis

097.0 Late syphilis, unspecified

097.1 Latent syphilis, unspecified
Positive serological reaction for syphilis

097.9 Syphilis, unspecified
Syphilis (acquired) NOS

Excludes: *syphilis NOS causing death under two years of age (090.9)*

098 Gonococcal infections

098.0 Acute, of lower genitourinary tract

Gonococcal:
- Bartholinitis (acute)
- urethritis (acute)
- vulvovaginitis (acute)

Gonorrhea (acute):
- NOS
- genitourinary (tract) NOS

098.1 Acute, of upper genitourinary tract

098.10 Gonococcal infection (acute) of upper genitourinary tract, site unspecified

098.11 Gonococcal cystitis (acute)
Gonorrhea (acute) of bladder

098.12 Gonococcal prostatitis (acute)

098.13 Gonococcal epididymo-orchitis (acute)
Gonococcal orchitis (acute)

098.14 Gonococcal seminal vesiculitis (acute)
Gonorrhea (acute) of seminal vesicle

098.15 Gonococcal cervicitis (acute)
Gonorrhea (acute) of cervix

098.16 Gonococcal endometritis (acute)
Gonorrhea (acute) of uterus

098.17 Gonococcal salpingitis, specified as acute

098.19 Other

098.2 Chronic, of lower genitourinary tract

Gonococcal:
- Bartholinitis
- urethritis
- vulvovaginitis

Gonorrhea:
- NOS
- genitourinary (tract)

Any condition classifiable to 098.0

} specified as chronic or with duration of two months or more

098.3 Chronic, of upper genitourinary tract

Includes: any condition classifiable to 098.1 stated as chronic or with a duration of two months or more

098.30 Chronic gonococcal infection of upper genitourinary tract, site unspecified

098.31 Gonococcal cystitis, chronic
Any condition classifiable to 098.11, specified as chronic
Gonorrhea of bladder, chronic

098.32 Gonococcal prostatitis, chronic
Any condition classifiable to 098.12, specified as chronic

098.33 Gonococcal epididymo-orchitis, chronic
Any condition classifiable to 098.13, specified as chronic
Chronic gonococcal orchitis

098.34 Gonococcal seminal vesiculitis, chronic
Any condition classifiable to 098.14, specified as chronic
Gonorrhea of seminal vesicle, chronic

098.35 Gonococcal cervicitis, chronic
Any condition classifiable to 098.15, specified as chronic
Gonorrhea of cervix, chronic

098.36 Gonococcal endometritis, chronic
Any condition classifiable to 098.16, specified as chronic

098.37 Gonococcal salpingitis (chronic)

098.39 Other

098.4 Gonococcal infection of eye

098.40 Gonococcal conjunctivitis (neonatorum)
Gonococcal ophthalmia (neonatorum)

098.41 Gonococcal iridocyclitis

098.42 Gonococcal endophthalmia

098.43 Gonococcal keratitis

098.49 Other

098.5 Gonococcal infection of joint

098.50 Gonococcal arthritis
Gonococcal infection of joint NOS

098.51 Gonococcal synovitis and tenosynovitis

098.52 Gonococcal bursitis

098.53 Gonococcal spondylitis

098.59 Other
Gonococcal rheumatism

098.6 Gonococcal infection of pharynx

098.7 Gonococcal infection of anus and rectum
Gonococcal proctitis

098.8 Gonococcal infection of other specified sites

098.81 Gonococcal keratosis (blennorrhagica)

098.82 Gonococcal meningitis

098.83 Gonococcal pericarditis

098.84 Gonococcal endocarditis

098.85 Other gonococcal heart disease

098.86 Gonococcal peritonitis

098.89 Other
Gonococcemia

099 Other venereal diseases

099.0 Chancroid
Bubo (inguinal):
chancroidal
due to Hemophilus ducreyi
Chancre:
Ducrey's
simple
soft
Ulcus molle (cutis) (skin)

099.1 Lymphogranuloma venereum
Climatic or tropical bubo
(Durand-) Nicolas- Favre disease
Esthiomene
Lymphogranuloma inguinale

099.2 Granuloma inguinale
Donovanosis
Granuloma pudendi (ulcerating)
Granuloma venereum
Pudendal ulcer

099.3 Reiter's disease
Reiter's syndrome

099.4 Other nongonococcal urethritis [NGU]

099.40 Unspecified
Nonspecific urethritis

099.41 Chlamydia trachomatis

099.49 Other specified organism

099.5 Other venereal diseases due to Chlamydia trachomatis

Excludes: *Chlamydia trachomatis infection of conjunctiva (076.0-076.9, 077.0, 077.9)*
Lymphogranuloma venereum (099.1)

099.50 Unspecified site

099.51 Pharynx

099.52 Anus and rectum

099.53 Lower genitourinary sites

Excludes: *urethra (099.41)*

Use additional code, if desired, to specify site of infection, such as:
bladder (595.4)
cervix (616.0)
vagina and vulva (616.11)

099.54 Other genitourinary sites
Use additional code, if desired, to specify site of infection, such as:
pelvic inflammatory disease NOS (614.9)
testis and epididymis (604.91)

099.55 Unspecified genitourinary site

● Code new to this edition ▲ Revision of existing code ④ ⑤ Fourth or fifth digit required

099.56 Peritoneum
Perihepatitis

099.59 Other specified site

099.8 Other specified venereal diseases

099.9 Venereal disease, unspecified

OTHER SPIROCHETAL DISEASES (100-104)

100 Leptospirosis

100.0 Leptospirosis icterohemorrhagica
Leptospiral or spirochetal jaundice (hemorrhagic)
Weil's disease

100.8 Other specified leptospiral infections

100.81 Leptospiral meningitis (aseptic)

100.89 Other
Fever:
- Fort Bragg
- pretibial
- swamp

Infection by Leptospira:
- australis
- bataviae
- pyrogenes

100.9 Leptospirosis, unspecified

101 Vincent's angina
Acute necrotizing ulcerative:
- gingivitis
- stomatitis

Fusospirochetal pharyngitis
Spirochetal stomatitis
Trench mouth
Vincent's:
- gingivitis
- infection [any site]

102 Yaws
Includes: frambesia
pian

102.0 Initial lesions
Chancre of yaws
Frambesia, initial or primary
Initial frambesial ulcer
Mother yaw

102.1 Multiple papillomata and wet crab yaws
Butter yaws
Frambesioma
Pianoma
Planter or palmer papilloma of yaws

102.2 Other early skin lesions
Early yaws (cutaneous) (macular) (papular) (maculopapular) (micropapular)
Frambeside of early yaws
Cutaneous yaws, less than five years after infection

102.3 Hyperkeratosis
Ghoul hand
Hyperkeratosis, palmer or plantar (early) (late) due to yaws
Worm-eaten soles

102.4 Gummata and ulcers
Nodular late yaws (ulcerated)
Gummatous frambeside

102.5 Gangosa
Rhinopharyngitis mutilans

102.6 Bone and joint lesions
Goundou
Gumma, bone
Gummatous osteitis or periostitis
} of yaws (late)

Hydrarthrosis
Osteitis
Periostitis (hypertrophic)
} of yaws (early) (late)

102.7 Other manifestations
Juxta-articular nodules of yaws
Mucosal yaws

102.8 Latent yaws
Yaws without clinical manifestations, with positive serology

102.9 Yaws, unspecified

Add 4th or 5th digit | Nonspecific code | Unspecified code | Manifestation code

103 Pinta

103.0 Primary lesions

Chancre (primary) / Papule (primary) / Pintid } of pinta [carate]

103.1 Intermediate lesions

Erythematous plaques / Hyperchromic lesions / Hyperkeratosis } of pinta [carate]

103.2 Late lesions

Cardiovascular lesions / Skin lesions: achromic, cicatricial, dyschromic / Vitiligo } of pinta [carate]

103.3 Mixed lesions

Achromic and hyperchromic skin lesions of pinta [carate]

103.9 Pinta, unspecified

104 Other spirochetal infection

104.0 Nonvenereal endemic syphilis

Bejel
Njovera

104.8 Other specified spirochetal infections

Excludes: *relapsing fever (087.0-087.9)*
syphilis (090.0-097.9)

104.9 Spirochetal infection, unspecified

MYCOSES (110-118)

Use additional code, if desired, to identify manifestation, as:
arthropathy (711.6)
meningitis (321.0-321.1)
otitis externa (380.15)

Excludes: *infection by Actinomycetales, such as species of Actinomyces, Actinomadura, Nocardia, Streptomyces (039.0-039.9)*

110 Dermatophytosis

Includes: infection by species of Epidermophyton, Microsporum, and Trichophyton tinea, any type except those in 111

110.0 Of scalp and beard

Kerion
Sycosis, mycotic
Trichophytic tinea [black dot tinea], scalp

110.1 Of nail

Dermatophytic onychia
Onychomycosis
Tinea unguium

110.2 Of hand

Tinea manuum

110.3 Of groin and perianal area

Dhobie itch
Eczema marginatum
Tinea cruris

110.4 Of foot

Athlete's foot
Tinea pedis

110.5 Of the body

Herpes circinatus
Tinea imbricata [Tokelau]

110.6 Deep seated dermatophytosis

Granuloma trichophyticum
Majocchi's granuloma

110.8 Of other specified sites

110.9 Of unspecified site

Favus NOS
Microsporic tinea NOS
Ringworm NOS

111 Dermatomycosis, other and unspecified

111.0 Pityriasis versicolor
Infection by Malassezia [Pityrosporum] furfur
Tinea flava
Tinea versicolor

111.1 Tinea nigra
Infection by Cladosporium species
Keratomycosis nigricans
Microsporosis nigra
Pityriasis nigra
Tinea palmaris nigra

111.2 Tinea blanca
Infection by Trichosporon (beigelii) cutaneum
White piedra

111.3 Black piedra
Infection by Piedraia hortai

111.8 Other specified dermatomycoses

111.9 Dermatomycosis, unspecified

112 Candidiasis
Includes: infection by Candida species
moniliasi

Excludes: *neonatal monilial infection (771.7)*

112.0 Of mouth
Thrush (oral)

112.1 Of vulva and vagina
Candidal vulvovaginitis
Monilial vulvovaginitis

112.2 Of other urogenital sites
Candidal balanitis

112.3 Of skin and nails
Candidal intertrigo
Candidal onychia
Candidal perionyxis [paronychia]

112.4 Of lung
Candidal pneumonia

112.5 Disseminated
Systemic candidiasis

112.8 Of other specified sites

112.81 Candidal endocarditis

112.82 Candidal otitis externa
Otomycosis in moniliasis

112.83 Candidal meningitis

112.84 Candidal esophagitis

112.85 Candidal enteritis

112.89 Other

112.9 Of unspecified site

114 Coccidioidomycosis
Includes: infection by Coccidioides (immitis)
Posada-Wernicke disease

114.0 Primary coccidioidomycosis (pulmonary)
Acute pulmonary coccidioidomycosis
Coccidioidomycotic pneumonitis
Desert rheumatism
Pulmonary coccidioidomycosis
San Joaquin Valley fever

114.1 Primary extrapulmonary coccidioidomycosis
Chancriform syndrome
Primary cutaneous coccidioidomycosis

114.2 Coccidioidal meningitis

114.3 Other forms of progressive coccidioidomycosis
Coccidioidal granuloma
Disseminated coccidioidomycosis

114.4 Chronic pulmonary coccidioidomycosis

114.5 Pulmonary coccidioidomycosis, unspecified

114.9 Coccidioidomycosis, unspecified

⑤ **115 Histoplasmosis**

The following fifth-digit subclassification is for use with category 115:

- **0 without mention of manifestation**
- **1 meningitis**
- **2 retinitis**
- **3 pericarditis**
- **4 endocarditis**
- **5 pneumonia**
- **9 other**

115.0 Infection by Histoplasma capsulatum
American histoplasmosis
Darling's disease
Reticuloendothelial cytomycosis
Small form histoplasmosis

115.1 Infection by Histoplasma duboisii
African histoplasmosis
Large form histoplasmosis

115.9 Histoplasmosis, unspecified
Histoplasmosis NOS

116 Blastomycotic infection

116.0 Blastomycosis
Blastomycotic dermatitis
Chicago disease
Cutaneous blastomycosis
Disseminated blastomycosis
Gilchrist's disease
Infection by Blastomyces [Ajellomyces] dermatitidis
North American blastomycosis
Primary pulmonary blastomycosis

116.1 Paracoccidioidomycosis
Brazilian blastomycosis
Infection by Paracoccidioides [Blastomyces] brasiliensis
Lutz-Splendore-Almeida disease
Mucocutaneous-lymphangitic paracoccidioidomycosis
Pulmonary paracoccidioidomycosis
South American blastomycosis
Visceral paracoccidioidomycosis

116.2 Lobomycosis
Infections by Loboa [Blastomyces] loboi
Keloidal blastomycosis
Lobo's disease

117 Other mycoses

117.0 Rhinosporidiosis
Infection by Rhinosporidium seeberi

117.1 Sporotrichosis
Cutaneous sporotrichosis
Disseminated sporotrichosis
Infection by Sporothrix [Sporotrichum] schenckii
Lymphocutaneous sporotrichosis
Pulmonary sporotrichosis
Sporotrichosis of the bones

117.2 Chromoblastomycosis
Chromomycosis
Infection by Cladosporidium carrionii, Fonsecaea compactum, Fonsecaea pedrosoi, Phialophora verrucosa

117.3 Aspergillosis
Infection by Aspergillus species, mainly A. fumigatus, A. flavus group, A. terreus group

● Code new to this edition ▲ Revision of existing code ④ ⑤ Fourth or fifth digit required

117.4 Mycotic mycetomas
Infection by various genera and species of Ascomycetes and Deuteromycetes, such as Acremonium [Cephalosporium] falciforme, Neotestudina rosatii, Madurella grisea, Madurella mycetomii, Pyrenochaeta romeroi, Zopfia [Leptosphaeria] senegalensis
Madura foot, mycotic
Maduromycosis, mycotic

Excludes: *actinomycotic mycetomas (039.0-039.9)*

117.5 Cryptococcosis
Busse-Buschke's disease
European cryptococcosis
Infection by Cryptococcus neoformans
Pulmonary cryptococcosis
Systemic cryptococcosis
Torula

117.6 Allescheriosis [Petriellidosis]
Infections by Allescheria [Petriellidium] boydii [Monosporium apiospermum]

Excludes: *mycotic mycetoma (117.4)*

117.7 Zygomycosis [Phycomycosis or Mucormycosis]
Infection by species of Absidia, Basidiobolus, Conidiobolus, Cunninghamella, Entomophthora, Mucor, Rhizopus, Saksenaea

117.8 Infection by dematiacious fungi, [Phaehyphomycosis]
Infection by dematiacious fungi, such as Cladosporium trichoides [bantianum], Dreschlera hawaiiensis, Phialophora gougerotii, Phialophora jeanselmi

117.9 Other and unspecified mycoses

118 Opportunistic mycoses
Infection of skin, subcutaneous tissues, and/or organs by a wide variety of fungi generally considered to be pathogenic to compromised hosts only (e.g., infection by species of Alternaria, Dreschlera, Fusarium)

HELMINTHIASES (120-129)

120 Schistosomiasis [bilharziasis]

120.0 Schistosoma haematobium
Vesical schistosomiasis NOS

120.1 Schistosoma mansoni
Intestinal schistosomiasis NOS

120.2 Schistosoma japonicum
Asiatic schistosomiasis NOS
Katayama disease or fever

120.3 Cutaneous
Cercarial dermatitis
Infection by cercariae of Schistosoma
Schistosome dermatitis
Swimmers' itch

120.8 Other specified schistosomiasis
Infection by Schistosoma:
- bovis
- intercalatum
- mattheii

Infection by Schistosoma spindale
Schistosomiasis chestermani

120.9 Schistosomiasis, unspecified
Blood flukes NOS
Hemic distomiasis

121 Other trematode infections

121.0 Opisthorchiasis
Infection by:
- cat liver fluke
- Opisthorchis (felineus) (tenuicollis) (viverrini)

121.1 Clonorchiasis
Biliary cirrhosis due to clonorchiasis
Chinese liver fluke disease
Hepatic distomiasis due to Clonorchis sinensis
Oriental liver fluke disease

121.2 Paragonimiasis
Infection by Paragonimus
Lung fluke disease (oriental)
Pulmonary distomiasis

121.3 Fascioliasis
Infection by Fasciola:
- gigantica
- hepatica

Liver flukes NOS
Sheep liver fluke infection

121.4 Fasciolopsiasis
Infection by Fasciolopsis [buski]
Intestinal distomiasis

121.5 Metagonimiasis
Infection by Metagonimus yokogawai

121.6 Heterophyiasis
Infection by:
Heterophyes heterophyes
Stellantchasmus falcatus

121.8 Other specified trematode infections
Infection by:
Dicrocoelium dendriticum
Echinostoma ilocanum
Gastrodiscoides hominis

121.9 Trematode infection, unspecified
Distomiasis NOS
Fluke disease NOS

122 Echinococcosis
Includes: echinococciasis
hydatid disease
hydatidosis

122.0 Echinococcus granulosus infection of liver

122.1 Echinococcus granulosus infection of lung

122.2 Echinococcus granulosus infection of thyroid

122.3 Echinococcus granulosus infection, other

122.4 Echinococcus granulosus infection, unspecified

122.5 Echinococcus multilocularis infection of liver

122.6 Echinococcus multilocularis infection, other

122.7 Echinococcus multilocularis infection, unspecified

122.8 Echinococcosis, unspecified, of liver

122.9 Echinococcosis, other and unspecified

123 Other cestode infection

123.0 Taenia solium infection, intestinal form
Pork tapeworm (adult) (infection)

123.1 Cysticercosis
Cysticerciasis
Infection by Cysticercus cellulosae [larval form of Taenia solium]

123.2 Taenia saginata infection
Beef tapeworm (infection)
Infection by Taeniarhynchus saginatus

123.3 Taeniasis, unspecified

123.4 Diphyllobothriasis, intestinal
Diphyllobothrium (adult) (latum) (pacificum) infection
Fish tapeworm (infection)

123.5 Sparganosis [larval diphyllobothriasis]
Infection by:
Diphyllobothrium larvae
Sparganum (mansoni) (proliferum)
Spirometra larvae

123.6 Hymenolepiasis
Dwarf tapeworm (infection)
Hymenolepis (diminuta) (nana) infection
Rat tapeworm (infection)

123.8 Other specified cestode infection
Diplogonoporus (grandis) } infection
Dipylidium (caninum) } infection
Dog tapeworm (infection)

123.9 Cestode infection, unspecified
Tapeworm (infection) NOS

124 Trichinosis
Trichinella spiralis infection
Trichinellosis
Trichiniasis

125 Filarial infection and dracontiasis

125.0 Bancroftian filariasis

Chyluria, Elephantiasis, Infection, Lymphadenitis, Lymphangitis } due to Wuchereria bancrofti

Wuchereriasis

125.1 Malayan filariasis

Brugia filariasis, Chyluria, Elephantiasis, Infection, Lymphadenitis, Lymphangitis } due to Brugia [Wuchereria] malayi

125.2 Loiasis

Eyeworm disease of Africa
Loa loa infection

125.3 Onchocerciasis

Onchocerca volvulus infection
Onchocercosis

125.4 Dipetalonemiasis

Infection by:
- Acanthocheilonema perstans
- Dipetalonema perstans

125.5 Mansonella ozzardi infection

Filariasis ozzardi

125.6 Other specified filariasis

Dirofilaria infection
Infection by:
- Acanthocheilonema streptocerca
- Dipetalonema streptocerca

125.7 Dracontiasis

Guinea-worm infection
Infection by Dracunculus medinensis

125.9 Unspecified filariasis

126 Ancylostomiasis and necatoriasis

Includes: cutaneous larva migrans due to Ancylostoma
hookworm (disease) (infection)
uncinariasis

126.0 Ancylostoma duodenale

126.1 Necator americanus

126.2 Ancylostoma braziliense

126.3 Ancylostoma ceylanicum

126.8 Other specified Ancylostoma

126.9 Ancylostomiasis and necatoriasis, unspecified

Creeping eruption NOS
Cutaneous larva migrans NOS

127 Other intestinal helminthiases

127.0 Ascariasis

Ascaridiasis
Infection by Ascaris lumbricoides
Roundworm infection

127.1 Anisakiasis

Infection by Anisakis larva

127.2 Strongyloidiasis

Infection by Strongyloides stercoralis

Excludes: trichostrongyliasis (127.6)

127.3 Trichuriasis

Infection by Trichuris trichiuria
Trichocephaliasis
Whipworm (disease) (infection)

127.4 Enterobiasis
Infection by Enterobius vermicularis
Oxyuriasis
Oxyuris vermicularis infection
Pinworn (disease) (infection)
Threadworm infection

127.5 Capillariasis
Infection by Capillaria philippinensis

Excludes: *infection by Capillaria hepatica (128.8)*

127.6 Trichostrongyliasis
Infection by Trichostrongylus species

127.7 Other specified intestinal helminthiasis
Infection by:
Oesophagostomum apiostomum and related species
Ternidens diminutus
other specified intestinal helminth
Physalopteriasis

127.8 Mixed intestinal helminthiasis
Infection by intestinal helminths classified to more than one of the categories 120.0-127.7
Mixed helminthiasis NOS

127.9 Intestinal helminthiasis, unspecified

128 Other and unspecified helminthiases

128.0 Toxocariasis
Larva migrans visceralis
Toxocara (canis) (cati) infection
Visceral larva migrans syndrome

128.1 Gnathostomiasis
Infection by Gnathostoma spinigerum and related species

128.8 Other specified helminthiasis
Infection by:
Angiostrongylus cantonensis
Capillaria hepatica
other specified helminth

128.9 Helminth infection, unspecified
Helminthiasis NOS
Worms NOS

129 Intestinal parasitism, unspecified

OTHER INFECTIOUS AND PARASITIC DISEASES (130-136)

130 Toxoplasmosis
Includes: infection by toxoplasma gondii
toxoplasmosis (acquired)

Excludes: *congenital toxoplasmosis (771.2)*

130.0 Meningoencephalitis due to toxoplasmosis
Encephalitis due to acquired toxoplasmosis

130.1 Conjunctivitis due to toxoplasmosis

130.2 Chorioretinitis due to toxoplasmosis
Focal retinochoroiditis due to acquired toxoplasmosis

130.3 Myocarditis due to toxoplasmosis

130.4 Pneumonitis due to toxoplasmosis

130.5 Hepatitis due to toxoplasmosis

130.7 Toxoplasmosis of other specified sites

130.8 Multisystemic disseminated toxoplasmosis
Toxoplasmosis of multiple sites

130.9 Toxoplasmosis, unspecified

131 Trichomoniasis
Includes: infection due to Trichomonas (vaginalis)

131.0 Urogenital trichomoniasis

131.00 Urogenital trichomoniasis, unspecified
Fluor (vaginalis) } trichomonal or due to Trichomonas (vaginalis)
Leukorrhea (vaginalis) } trichomonal or due to Trichomonas (vaginalis)

131.01 Trichomonal vulvovaginitis
Vaginitis, trichomonal or due to Trichomonas (vaginalis)

131.02 Trichomonal urethritis

131.03 Trichomonal prostatitis

131.09 Other

131.8 Other specified sites

Excludes: *intestinal (007.3)*

131.9 Trichomoniasis, unspecified

132 Pediculosis and phthirus infestation

132.0 Pediculus capitis [head louse]

132.1 Pediculus corporis [body louse]

132.2 Phthirus pubis [pubic louse]
Pediculus pubis

132.3 Mixed infestation
Infestation classifiable to more than one of the categories 132.0-132.2

132.9 Pediculosis, unspecified

133 Acariasis

133.0 Scabies
Infestation by Sarcoptes scabiei
Norwegian scabies
Sarcoptic itch

133.8 Other acariasis
Chiggers
Infestation by:
Demodex folliculorum
Trombicula

133.9 Acariasis, unspecified
Infestation by mites NOS

134 Other infestation

134.0 Myiasis
Infestation by:
Dermatobia (hominis)
fly larvae
Gasterophilus (intestinalis)
Infestation by:
maggots
Oestrus ovis

134.1 Other arthropod infestation
Infestation by:
chigoe
sand flea
Tunga penetrans
Jigger disease
Scarabiasis
Tungiasis

134.2 Hirudiniasis
Hirudiniasis (external) (internal)
Leeches (aquatic) (land)

134.8 Other specified infestations

134.9 Infestation, unspecified
Infestation (skin) NOS
Skin parasites NOS

135 Sarcoidosis
Besnier-Boeck- Schaumann disease
Lupoid (miliary) of Boeck
Lupus pernio (Besnier)
Lymphogranulomatosis, benign (Schaumann's)
Sarcoid (any site):
NOS
Boeck
Darier-Roussy
Uveoparotid fever

136 Other and unspecified infectious and parasitic diseases

136.0 Ainhum
Dactylolysis spontanea

136.1 Behçet's syndrome

136.2 Specific infections by free-living amebae
Meningoencephalitis due to Naegleria

136.3 Pneumocystosis
Pneumonia due to Pneumocystis carinii

136.4 Psorospermiasis

136.5 Sarcosporidiosis
Infection by Sarcocystis lindemanni

136.8 Other specified infectious and parasitic diseases
Candiru infestation

136.9 Unspecified infectious and parasitic diseases
Infectious disease NOS
Parasitic disease NOS

LATE EFFECTS OF INFECTIOUS AND PARASITIC DISEASES (137-139)

137 Late effects of tuberculosis

Note: This category is to be used to indicate conditions classifiable to 010-018 as the cause of late effects, which are themselves classified elsewhere. The "late effects" include those specified as such, as sequelae, or as due to old or inactive tuberculosis, without evidence of active disease.

137.0 Late effects of respiratory or unspecified tuberculosis

137.1 Late effects of central nervous system tuberculosis

137.2 Late effects of genitourinary tuberculosis

137.3 Late effects of tuberculosis of bones and joints

137.4 Late effects of tuberculosis of other specified organs

138 Late effects of acute poliomyelitis

Note: This category is to be used to indicate conditions classifiable to 045 as the cause of late effects, which are themselves classified elsewhere. The "late effects" include conditions specified as such, or as sequelae, or as due to old or inactive poliomyelitis, without evidence of active disease.

139 Late effects of other infectious and parasitic diseases

Note: This category is to be used to indicate conditions classifiable to categories 001-009, 020-041, 046-136 as the cause of late effects, which are themselves classified elsewhere. The "late effects" include conditions specified as such; they also include sequela of diseases classifiable to the above categories if there is evidence that the disease itself is no longer present.

139.0 Late effects of viral encephalitis
Late effects of conditions classifiable to 049.8-049.9, 062-064

139.1 Late effects of trachoma
Late effects of conditions classifiable to 076

139.8 Late effects of other and unspecified infectious and parasitic diseases

● Code new to this edition ▲ Revision of existing code ④ ⑤ Fourth or fifth digit required

2. NEOPLASMS (140-239)

Notes:

1. Content
This chapter contains the following broad groups:

140-195	**Malignant neoplasms, stated or presumed to be primary, of specified sites, except of lymphatic and hematopoietic tissue**
196-198	**Malignant neoplasms, stated or presumed to be secondary, of specified sites**
199	**Malignant neoplasms, without specification of site**
200-208	**Malignant neoplasms, stated or presumed to be primary, of lymphatic and hematopoietic tissue**
210-229	**Benign neoplasms**
230-234	**Carcinoma in situ**
235-238	**Neoplasms of uncertain behavior [see Note, page 92]**
239	**Neoplasms of unspecified nature**

2. Functional activity
All neoplasms are classified in this chapter, whether or not functionally active. An additional code from Chapter 3 may be used, if desired, to identify such functional activity associated with any neoplasm, e.g.:
catecholamine-producing malignant pheochromocytoma of adrenal:
code 194.0, additional code 255.6
basophil adenoma of pituitary with Cushing's syndrome:
code 227.3, additional code 255.0

3. Morphology [Histology]
For those wishing to identify the histological type of neoplasms, a comprehensive coded nomenclature, which comprises the morphology rubrics of the ICD-Oncology, is given on pages 529-542.

4. Malignant neoplasms overlapping site boundaries
Categories 140-195 are for the classification of primary malignant neoplasms according to their point of origin. A malignant neoplasm that overlaps two or more subcategories within a three-digit rubric and whose point of origin cannot be determined should be classified to the subcategory .8 "Other." For example, "carcinoma involving tip and ventral surface of tongue" should be assigned to 141.8. On the other hand, "carcinoma of tip of tongue, extending to involve the ventral surface" should be coded to 141.2, as the point of origin, the tip, is known. Three subcategories (149.8, 159.8, 165.8) have been provided for malignant neoplasms that overlap the boundaries of three-digit rubrics within certain systems. Overlapping malignant neoplasms that cannot be classified as indicated above should be assigned to the appropriate subdivision of category 195 (Malignant neoplasm of other and ill-defined sites).

MALIGNANT NEOPLASM OF LIP, ORAL CAVITY, AND PHARYNX (140-149)

Excludes: *carcinoma in situ (230.0)*

140 Malignant neoplasm of lip

Excludes: *skin of lip (173.0)*

140.0 Upper lip, vermilion border
Upper lip:
NOS
external
lipstick area

140.1 Lower lip, vermilion border
Lower lip:
NOS
external
lipstick area

140.3 Upper lip, inner aspect
Upper lip:
buccal aspect
frenulum
Upper lip:
mucosa
oral aspect

140.4 Lower lip, inner aspect
Lower lip:
buccal aspect
frenulum
Lower lip:
mucosa
oral aspect

140.5 Lip, unspecified, inner aspect
Lip, not specified whether upper or lower:
buccal aspect
frenulum
mucosa
oral aspect

140.6 Commissure of lip
Labial commissure

140.8 Other sites of lip
Malignant neoplasm of contiguous or overlapping sites of lip whose point of origin cannot be determined

140.9 Lip, unspecified, vermilion border
Lip, not specified as upper or lower:
NOS
external
lipstick area

141 Malignant neoplasm of tongue

141.0 Base of tongue
Dorsal surface of base of tongue
Fixed part of tongue NOS

141.1 Dorsal surface of tongue
Anterior two-thirds of tongue, dorsal surface
Dorsal tongue NOS
Midline of tongue

Excludes: *dorsal surface of base of tongue (141.0)*

141.2 Tip and lateral border of tongue

141.3 Ventral surface of tongue
Anterior two-thirds of tongue, ventral surface
Frenulum linguae

141.4 Anterior two-thirds of tongue, part unspecified
Mobile part of tongue NOS

141.5 Junctional zone
Border of tongue at junction of fixed and mobile parts at insertion of anterior tonsillar pillar

141.6 Lingual tonsil

141.8 Other sites of tongue
Malignant neoplasm of contiguous or overlapping sites of tongue whose point of origin cannot be determined

141.9 Tongue, unspecified
Tongue NOS

142 Malignant neoplasm of major salivary glands
Includes: salivary ducts

Excludes: *malignant neoplasm of minor salivary glands:*
NOS (145.9)
buccal mucosa (145.0)
soft palate (145.3)
tongue (141.0-141.9)
tonsil, palatine (146.0)

142.0 Parotid gland

142.1 Submandibular gland
Submaxillary gland

142.2 Sublingual gland

142.8 Other major salivary glands
Malignant neoplasm of contiguous or overlapping sites of salivary glands and ducts whose point of origin cannot be determined

142.9 Salivary gland, unspecified
Salivary gland (major) NOS

143 Malignant neoplasm of gum
Includes: alveolar (ridge) mucosa
gingiva (alveolar) (marginal)
interdental papillae

Excludes: malignant odontogenic neoplasms (170.0-170.1)

143.0 Upper gum

143.1 Lower gum

143.8 Other sites of gum
Malignant neoplasm of contiguous or overlapping sites of gum whose point of origin cannot be determined

143.9 Gum, unspecified

144 Malignant neoplasm of floor of mouth

144.0 Anterior portion
Anterior to the premolar-canine junction

144.1 Lateral portion

144.8 Other sites of floor of mouth
Malignant neoplasm of contiguous or overlapping sites of floor of mouth whose point of origin cannot be determined

144.9 Floor of mouth, part unspecified

145 Malignant neoplasm of other and unspecified parts of mouth

Excludes: mucosa of lips (140.0-140.9)

145.0 Cheek mucosa
Buccal mucosa
Cheek, inner aspect

145.1 Vestibule of mouth
Buccal sulcus (upper) (lower)
Labial sulcus (upper) (lower)

145.2 Hard palate

145.3 Soft palate

Excludes: nasopharyngeal [posterior] [superior] surface of soft palate (147.3)

145.4 Uvula

145.5 Palate, unspecified
Junction of hard and soft palate
Roof of mouth

145.6 Retromolar area

145.8 Other specified parts of mouth
Malignant neoplasm of contiguous or overlapping sites of mouth whose point of origin cannot be determined

145.9 Mouth, unspecified
Buccal cavity NOS
Minor salivary gland, unspecified site
Oral cavity NOS

146 Malignant neoplasm of oropharynx

146.0 Tonsil
Tonsil:
NOS
faucial
palatine

Excludes: lingual tonsil (141.6)
pharyngeal tonsil (147.1)

146.1 Tonsillar fossa

146.2 Tonsillar pillars (anterior) (posterior)
Faucial pillar
Glossopalatine fold
Palatoglossal arch
Palatopharyngeal arch

146.3 Vallecula
Anterior and medial surface of the pharyngoepiglottic fold

146.4 Anterior aspect of epiglottis
Epiglottis, free border [margin] Glossoepiglottic fold(s)

Excludes: *epiglottis:*
NOS (161.1)
suprahyoid portion (161.1)

146.5 Junctional region
Junction of the free margin of the epiglottis, the aryepiglottic fold, and the pharyngoepiglottic fold

146.6 Lateral wall of oropharynx

146.7 Posterior wall of oropharynx

146.8 Other specified sites of oropharynx
Branchial cleft
Malignant neoplasm of contiguous or overlapping sites of oropharynx whose point of origin cannot be determined

146.9 Oropharynx, unspecified

147 Malignant neoplasm of nasopharynx

147.0 Superior wall
Roof of nasopharynx

147.1 Posterior wall
Adenoid
Pharyngeal tonsil

147.2 Lateral wall
Fossa of Rosenmüller
Opening of auditory tube
Pharyngeal recess

147.3 Anterior wall
Floor of nasopharynx
Nasopharyngeal [posterior] [superior] surface of soft palate
Posterior margin of nasal septum and choanae

147.8 Other specified sites of nasopharynx
Malignant neoplasm of contiguous or overlapping sites of nasopharynx whose point of origin cannot be determined

147.9 Nasopharynx, unspecified
Nasopharyngeal wall NOS

148 Malignant neoplasm of hypopharynx

148.0 Postcricoid region

148.1 Pyriform sinus
Pyriform fossa

148.2 Aryepiglottic fold, hypopharyngeal aspect
Aryepiglottic fold or interarytenoid fold:
NOS
marginal zone

Excludes: *aryepiglottic fold or interarytenoid fold, laryngeal aspect (161.1)*

148.3 Posterior hypopharyngeal wall

148.8 Other specified sites of hypopharynx
Malignant neoplasm of contiguous or overlapping sites of hypopharynx whose point of origin cannot be determined

148.9 Hypopharynx, unspecified
Hypopharyngeal wall NOS
Hypopharynx NOS

149 Malignant neoplasm of other and ill-defined sites within the lip, oral cavity, and pharynx

149.0 Pharynx, unspecified

149.1 Waldeyer's ring

149.8 Other
Malignant neoplasms of lip, oral cavity, and pharynx whose point of origin cannot be assigned to any one of the categories 140-148

Excludes: *"book leaf" neoplasm [ventral surface of tongue and floor of mouth] (145.8)*

149.9 Ill-defined

MALIGNANT NEOPLASM OF DIGESTIVE ORGANS AND PERITONEUM (150-159)

Excludes: *carcinoma in situ (230.1-230.9)*

150 Malignant neoplasm of esophagus

150.0 Cervical esophagus

150.1 Thoracic esophagus

150.2 Abdominal esophagus

Excludes: *adenocarcinoma (151.0)*
cardio-esophageal junction (151.0)

150.3 Upper third of esophagus
Proximal third of esophagus

150.4 Middle third of esophagus

150.5 Lower third of esophagus
Distal third of esophagus

Excludes: *adenocarcinoma (151.0)*
cardio-esophageal junction (151.0)

150.8 Other specified part
Malignant neoplasm of contiguous or overlapping sites of esophagus whose point of origin cannot be determined

150.9 Esophagus, unspecified

151 Malignant neoplasm of stomach

151.0 Cardia
Cardiac orifice
Cardio-esophageal junction

Excludes: *squamous cell carcinoma (150.2, 150.5)*

151.1 Pylorus
Prepylorus
Pyloric canal

151.2 Pyloric antrum
Antrum of stomach NOS

151.3 Fundus of stomach

151.4 Body of stomach

151.5 Lesser curvature, unspecified
Lesser curvature, not classifiable to 151.1-151.4

151.6 Greater curvature, unspecified
Greater curvature, not classifiable to 151.0-151.4

151.8 Other specified sites of stomach
Anterior wall, not classifiable to 151.0-151.4
Posterior wall, not classifiable to 151.0-151.4
Malignant neoplasm of contiguous or overlapping sites of stomach whose point of origin cannot be determined

151.9 Stomach, unspecified
Carcinoma ventriculi
Gastric cancer

152 Malignant neoplasm of small intestine, including duodenum

152.0 Duodenum

152.1 Jejunum

152.2 Ileum

Excludes: *ileocecal valve (153.4)*

152.3 Meckel's diverticulum

152.8 Other specified sites of small intestine
Duodenojejunal junction
Malignant neoplasm of contiguous or overlapping sites of small intestine whose point of origin cannot be determined

152.9 Small intestine, unspecified

153 Malignant neoplasm of colon

153.0 Hepatic flexure

153.1 Transverse colon

153.2 Descending colon
Left colon

153.3 Sigmoid colon
Sigmoid (flexure)

Excludes: rectosigmoid junction (154.0)

153.4 Cecum
Ileocecal valve

153.5 Appendix

153.6 Ascending colon
Right colon

153.7 Splenic flexure

153.8 Other specified sites of large intestine
Malignant neoplasm of contiguous or overlapping sites of colon whose point of origin cannot be determined

Excludes: ileocecal valve (153.4)
rectosigmoid junction (154.0)

153.9 Colon, unspecified
Large intestine NOS

154 Malignant neoplasm of rectum, rectosigmoid junction, and anus

154.0 Rectosigmoid junction
Colon with rectum
Rectosigmoid (colon)

154.1 Rectum
Rectal ampulla

154.2 Anal canal
Anal sphincter

Excludes: skin of anus (172.5, 173.5)

154.3 Anus, unspecified

Excludes: anus:
margin (172.5, 173.5)
skin (172.5, 173.5)
perianal skin (172.5, 173.5)

154.8 Other
Anorectum
Cloacogenic zone
Malignant neoplasm of contiguous or overlapping sites of rectum, rectosigmoid junction, and anus whose point of origin cannot be determined

155 Malignant neoplasm of liver and intrahepatic bile ducts

155.0 Liver, primary
Carcinoma:
liver, specified as primary
hepatocellular
liver cell
Hepatoblastoma

155.1 Intrahepatic bile ducts
Canaliculi biliferi
Interlobular:
bile ducts
biliary canals
Intrahepatic:
biliary passages
canaliculi
gall duct

Excludes: hepatic duct (156.1)

155.2 Liver, not specified as primary or secondary

156 Malignant neoplasm of gallbladder and extrahepatic bile ducts

156.0 Gallbladder

156.1 Extrahepatic bile ducts
Biliary duct or passage NOS
Common bile duct
Cystic duct
Hepatic duct
Sphincter of Oddi

156.2 Ampulla of Vater

● Code new to this edition
▲ Revision of existing code
④ ⑤ Fourth or fifth digit required

156.8 Other specified sites of gallbladder and extrahepatic bile ducts
Malignant neoplasm of contiguous or overlapping sites of gallbladder and extrahepatic bile ducts whose point of origin cannot be determined

156.9 Biliary tract, part unspecified
Malignant neoplasm involving both intrahepatic and extrahepatic bile ducts

157 Malignant neoplasm of pancreas

157.0 Head of pancreas

157.1 Body of pancreas

157.2 Tail of pancreas

157.3 Pancreatic duct
Duct of:
Santorini
Wirsung

157.4 Islets of Langerhans
Islets of Langerhans, any part of pancreas

Use additional code, if desired, to identify any functional activity

157.8 Other specified sites of pancreas
Ectopic pancreatic tissue
Malignant neoplasm of contiguous or overlapping sites of pancreas whose point of origin cannot be determined

157.9 Pancreas, part unspecified

158 Malignant neoplasm of retroperitoneum and peritoneum

158.0 Retroperitoneum
Periadrenal tissue
Perinephric tissue
Perirenal tissue
Retrocecal tissue

158.8 Specified parts of peritoneum
Cul-de-sac (of Douglas)
Mesentery
Mesocolon
Omentum
Malignant neoplasm of contiguous or overlapping sites of retroperitoneum and peritoneum whose point of origin cannot be determined
Peritoneum:
parietal
pelvic
Rectouterine pouch

158.9 Peritoneum, unspecified

159 Malignant neoplasm of other and ill-defined sites within the digestive organs and peritoneum

159.0 Intestinal tract, part unspecified
Intestine NOS

159.1 Spleen, not elsewhere classified
Angiosarcoma } of spleen
Fibrosarcoma } of spleen

Excludes: *Hodgkin's disease (201.0-201.9)*
lymphosarcoma (200.1)
reticulosarcoma (200.0)

159.8 Other sites of digestive system and intra-abdominal organs
Malignant neoplasm of digestive organs and peritoneum whose point of origin cannot be assigned to any one of the categories 150-158

Excludes: *anus and rectum (154.8)*
cardio-esophageal junction (151.0)
colon and rectum ORANGE (154.0)

159.9 Ill-defined
Alimentary canal or tract NOS
Gastrointestinal tract NOS

Excludes: *abdominal NOS (195.2)*
intra-abdominal NOS (195.2)

MALIGNANT NEOPLASM OF RESPIRATORY AND INTRATHORACIC ORGANS (160-165)

Excludes: *carcinoma in situ (231.0-231.9)*

160 Malignant neoplasm of nasal cavities, middle ear, and accessory sinuses

160.0 Nasal cavities

Cartilage of nose
Conchae, nasal
Internal nose
Septum of nose
Vestibule of nose

Excludes: *nasal bone (170.0)*
nose NOS (195.0)
olfactory bulb (192.0)
posterior margin of septum and choanae (147.3)
skin of nose (172.3, 173.3)
turbinates (170.0)

160.1 Auditory tube, middle ear, and mastoid air cells

Antrum tympanicum
Eustachian tube
Tympanic cavity

Excludes: *auditory canal (external) (172.2, 173.2)*
bone of ear (meatus) (170.0)
cartilage of ear (171.0)
ear (external) (skin) (172.2, 173.2)

160.2 Maxillary sinus

Antrum (Highmore) (maxillary)

160.3 Ethmoidal sinus

160.4 Frontal sinus

160.5 Sphenoidal sinus

160.8 Other

Malignant neoplasm of contiguous or overlapping sites of nasal cavities, middle ear, and accessory sinuses whose point of origin cannot be determined

160.9 Accessory sinus, unspecified

161 Malignant neoplasm of larynx

161.0 Glottis

Intrinsic larynx
Laryngeal commissure (anterior) (posterior)
True vocal cord
Vocal cord NOS

161.1 Supraglottis

Aryepiglottic fold or interarytenoid fold, laryngeal aspect
Epiglottis (suprahyoid portion) NOS
Extrinsic larynx
False vocal cords
Posterior (laryngeal) surface of epiglottis
Ventricular bands

Excludes: *anterior aspect of epiglottis (146.4)*
aryepiglottic fold or interarytenoid fold:
NOS (148.2)
hypopharyngeal aspect (148.2)
marginal zone (148.2)

161.2 Subglottis

161.3 Laryngeal cartilages

Cartilage:
arytenoid
cricoid

Cartilage:
cuneiform
thyroid

161.8 Other specified sites of larynx

Malignant neoplasm of contiguous or overlapping sites of larynx whose point of origin cannot be determined

161.9 Larynx, unspecified

162 Malignant neoplasm of trachea, bronchus, and lung

162.0 Trachea

Cartilage } of trachea
Mucosa } of trachea

● Code new to this edition ▲ Revision of existing code ④ ⑤ Fourth or fifth digit required

162.2 Main bronchus
Carina
Hilus of lung

162.3 Upper lobe, bronchus or lung

162.4 Middle lobe, bronchus or lung

162.5 Lower lobe, bronchus or lung

162.8 Other parts of bronchus or lung
Malignant neoplasm of contiguous or overlapping sites of bronchus or lung whose point of origin cannot be determined

162.9 Bronchus and lung, unspecified

163 Malignant neoplasm of pleura

163.0 Parietal pleura

163.1 Visceral pleura

163.8 Other specified sites of pleura
Malignant neoplasm of contiguous or overlapping sites of pleura whose point of origin cannot be determined

163.9 Pleura, unspecified

164 Malignant neoplasm of thymus, heart, and mediastinum

164.0 Thymus

164.1 Heart
Endocardium
Epicardium
Myocardium
Pericardium

Excludes: *great vessels (171.4)*

164.2 Anterior mediastinum

164.3 Posterior mediastinum

164.8 Other
Malignant neoplasm of contiguous or overlapping sites of thymus, heart, and mediastinum whose point of origin cannot be determined

164.9 Mediastinum, part unspecified

165 Malignant neoplasm of other and ill-defined sites within the respiratory system and intrathoracic organs

165.0 Upper respiratory trace, part unspecified

165.8 Other
Malignant neoplasm of respiratory and intrathoracic organs whose point of origin cannot be assigned to any one of the categories 160-164

165.9 Ill-defined sites within the respiratory system
Respiratory tract NOS

Excludes: *intrathoracic NOS (195.1)*
thoracic NOS (195.1)

MALIGNANT NEOPLASM OF BONE, CONNECTIVE TISSUE, SKIN, AND BREAST (170-176)

Excludes: *carcinoma in situ:*
breast (233.0)
skin (232.0-232.9)

170 Malignant neoplasm of bone and articular cartilage
Includes: cartilage (articular) (joint)
periosteum

Excludes: *bone marrow NOS (202.9)*
cartilage:
ear (171.0)
eyelid (171.0)
larynx (161.3)
nose (160.0)
synovia (171.0-171.9)

170.0 Bones of skull and face, except mandible

Bone:
- ethmoid
- frontal
- malar
- nasal
- occipital
- orbital
- parietal
- sphenoid
- temporal
- zygomatic

Maxilla (superior)
Turbinate
Upper jaw bone
Vomer

Excludes: *carcinoma, any type except intraosseous or odontogenic:*
maxilla, maxillary (sinus) (160.2)
upper jaw bone (143.0)
jaw bone (lower) (170.1)

170.1 Mandible

Inferior maxilla
Jaw bone NOS
Lower jaw bone

Excludes: *carcinoma, any type except intraosseous or odontogenic:*
jaw bone NOS (143.9)
lower (143.1)
upper jaw bone (170.0)

170.2 Vertebral column, excluding sacrum and coccyx

Spinal column
Spine
Vertebra

Excludes: *sacrum and coccyx (170.6)*

170.3 Ribs, sternum, and clavicle

Costal cartilage
Costovertebral joint
Xiphoid process

170.4 Scapula and long bones of upper limb

Acromion
Bones NOS of upper limb
Humerus
Radius
Ulna

170.5 Short bones of upper limb

Carpal
Cuneiform, wrist
Metacarpal
Navicular, of hand
Phalanges of hand
Pisiform
Scaphoid (of hand)
Semilunar or lunate
Trapezium
Trapezoid
Unciform

170.6 Pelvic bones, sacrum, and coccyx

Coccygeal vertebra
Ilium
Ischium
Pubic bone
Sacral vertebra

170.7 Long bones of lower limb

Bones NOS of lower limb
Femur
Fibula
Tibia

170.8 Short bones of lower limb

Astragalus [talus]
Calcaneus
Cuboid
Cuneiform, ankle
Metatarsal
Navicular (of ankle)
Patella
Phalanges of foot
Tarsal

170.9 Bone and articular cartilage, site unspecified

171 Malignant neoplasm of connective and other soft tissue

Includes: blood vessel
bursa
fascia
fat
ligament, except uterine
muscle
peripheral, sympathetic, and parasympathetic nerves and ganglia
synovia
tendon (sheath)

Excludes: *cartilage (of):*
articular (170.0-170.9)
larynx (161.3)
nose (160.0)
connective tissue:
breast (174.0-175.9)
internal organs—code to malignant neoplasm of the site [e.g., leiomyosarcoma of stomach, 151.9]
heart (164.1)
uterine ligament (183.4)

171.0 Head, face, and neck
Cartilage of:
ear
eyelid

171.2 Upper limb, including shoulder
Arm
Finger
Forearm
Hand

171.3 Lower limb, including hip
Foot
Leg
Popliteal space
Thigh
Toe

171.4 Thorax
Axilla
Diaphragm
Great vessels

Excludes: *heart (164.1)*
mediastinum (164.2-164.9)
thymus (164.0)

171.5 Abdomen
Abdominal wall
Hypochondrium

Excludes: *peritoneum (158.8)*
retroperitoneum (158.0)

171.6 Pelvis
Buttock
Groin
Inguinal region
Perineum

Excludes: *pelvic peritoneum (158.8)*
retroperitoneum (158.0)
uterine ligament, any (183.3-183.5)

171.7 Trunk, unspecified
Back NOS
Flank NOS

171.8 Other specified sites of connective and other soft tissue
Malignant neoplasm of contiguous or overlapping sites of connective tissue whose point of origin cannot be determined

171.9 Connective and other soft tissue, site unspecified

172 Malignant melanoma of skin

Includes: melanocarcinoma
melanoma (skin) NOS

Excludes: *skin of genital organs (184.0-184.9, 187.1-187.9)*
sites other than skin—code to malignant neoplasm of the site

172.0 Lip

Excludes: *vermilion border of lip (140.0-140.1, 140.9)*

172.1 Eyelid, including canthus

Add 4th or 5th digit | Nonspecific code | Unspecified code | Manifestation code

172.2 Ear and external auditory canal
Auricle (ear)
Auricular canal, external
External [acoustic] meatus
Pinna

172.3 Other and unspecified parts of face
Cheek (external)
Chin
Eyebrow
Forehead
Nose, external
Temple

172.4 Scalp and neck

172.5 Trunk, except scrotum
Axilla
Breast
Buttock
Groin
Perianal skin
Perineum
Umbilicus

Excludes: *anal canal (154.2)*
anus NOS (154.3)
scrotum (187.7)

172.6 Upper limb, including shoulder
Arm
Finger
Forearm
Hand

172.7 Lower limb, including hip
Ankle
Foot
Heel
Knee
Leg
Popliteal area
Thigh
Toe

172.8 Other specified sites of skin
Malignant melanoma of contiguous or overlapping sites of skin whose point of origin cannot be determined

172.9 Melanoma of skin, site unspecified

173 Other malignant neoplasm of skin
Includes: malignant neoplasm of:
sebaceous glands
sudoriferous, sudoriparous glands
sweat glands

Excludes: *Kaposi's sarcoma (176.0-176.9)*
malignant melanoma of skin (172.0-172.9)
skin of genital organs (184.0-184.9, 187.1-187.9)

173.0 Skin of lip

Excludes: *vermilion border of lip (140.0-140.1, 140.9)*

173.1 Eyelid, including canthus

Excludes: *cartilage of eyelid (171.0)*

173.2 Skin of ear and external auditory canal
Auricle (ear)
Auricular canal, external
External meatus
Pinna

Excludes: *cartilage of ear (171.0)*

173.3 Skin of other and unspecified parts of face
Cheek, external
Chin
Eyebrow
Forehead
Nose, external
Temple

173.4 Scalp and skin of neck

173.5 Skin of trunk, except scrotum

Axillary fold
Perianal skin
Skin of:
  abdominal wall
  anus
  back
  breast
Skin of:
  buttock
  chest wall
  groin
  perineum
Umbilicus

Excludes: *anal canal (154.2)*
anus NOS (154.3)
skin of scrotum (187.7)

173.6 Skin of upper limb, including shoulder

Arm
Finger
Forearm
Hand

173.7 Skin of lower limb, including hip

Ankle
Foot
Heel
Knee
Leg
Popliteal area
Thigh
Toe

173.8 Other specified sites of skin

Malignant neoplasm of contiguous or overlapping sites of skin whose point of origin cannot be determined

173.9 Skin, site unspecified

174 Malignant neoplasm of female breast

Includes:
breast (female)
connective tissue
soft parts
Paget's disease of:
  breast
  nipple

Excludes: *skin of breast (172.5, 173.5)*

174.0 Nipple and areola

174.1 Central portion

174.2 Upper-inner quadrant

174.3 Lower-inner quadrant

174.4 Upper-outer quadrant

174.5 Lower-outer quadrant

174.6 Axillary tail

174.8 Other specified sites of female breast

Ectopic sites
Inner breast
Lower breast
Malignant neoplasm of contiguous or overlapping sites of breast whose point of origin cannot be determined
Midline of breast
Outer breast
Upper breast

174.9 Breast (female), unspecified

175 Malignant neoplasm of male breast

Excludes: *skin of breast (172.5, 173.5)*

175.0 Nipple and areola

175.9 Other and unspecified sites of male breast

Ectopic breast tissue, male

176 Kaposi's sarcoma

176.0 Skin

176.1 Soft Tissue

Includes:
blood vessel
connective tissue
fascia
ligament
lymphatic(s) NEC
muscle

Excludes: *lymph glands and nodes (176.5)*

176.2 Palate

176.3 Gastrointestinal sites

Add 4th or 5th digit | Nonspecific code | Unspecified code | Manifestation code

176.4 Lung

176.5 Lymph nodes

176.8 Other specified sites
Includes: oral cavity NEC

176.9 Unspecified
Viscera NOS

MALIGNANT NEOPLASM OF GENITOURINARY ORGANS (179-189)

Excludes: carcinoma in situ (233.1-233.9)

179 Malignant neoplasm of uterus, part unspecified

180 Malignant neoplasm of cervix uteri
Includes: invasive malignancy [carcinoma]

Excludes: carcinoma in situ (233.1)

180.0 Endocervix
Cervical canal NOS
Endocervical canal
Endocervical gland

180.1 Exocervix

180.8 Other specified sites of cervix
Cervical stump
Squamocolumnar junction of cervix
Malignant neoplasm of contiguous or overlapping sites of cervix uteri whose point of origin cannot be determined

180.9 Cervix uteri, unspecified

181 Malignant neoplasm of placenta
Choriocarcinoma NOS
Chorioepithelioma NOS

Excludes: chorioadenoma (destruens) (236.1)
hydatidiform mole (630)
malignant (236.1)
invasive mole (236.1)
male choriocarcinoma NOS (186.0-186.9)

182 Malignant neoplasm of body of uterus

Excludes: carcinoma in situ (233.2)

182.0 Corpus uteri, except isthmus
Cornu
Endometrium
Fundus
Myometrium

182.1 Isthmus
Lower uterine segment

182.8 Other specified sites of body of uterus
Malignant neoplasm of contiguous or overlapping sites of body of uterus whose point of origin cannot be determined

Excludes: uterus NOS (179)

183 Malignant neoplasm of ovary and other uterine adnexa

Excludes: Douglas' cul-de-sac (158.8)

183.0 Ovary
Use additional code, if desired, to identify any functional activity

183.2 Fallopian tube
Oviduct
Uterine tube

183.3 Broad ligament
Mesovarium
Parovarian region

183.4 Parametrium
Uterine ligament NOS
Uterosacral ligament

183.5 Round ligament

183.8 Other specified sites of uterine adnexa
Tubo-ovarian
Utero-ovarian
Malignant neoplasm of contiguous or overlapping sites of ovary and other uterine adnexa whose point of origin cannot be determined

183.9 Uterine adnexa, unspecified

● Code new to this edition
▲ Revision of existing code
④ ⑤ Fourth or fifth digit required

184 Malignant neoplasm of other and unspecified female genital organs

Excludes: *carcinoma in situ (233.3)*

184.0 Vagina
Gartner's duct
Vaginal vault

184.1 Labia majora
Greater vestibular [Bartholin's] gland

184.2 Labia minora

184.3 Clitoris

184.4 Vulva, unspecified
External female genitalia NOS
Pudendum

184.8 Other specified sites of female genital organs
Malignant neoplasm of contiguous or overlapping sites of female genital organs whose point of origin cannot be determined

184.9 Female genital organ, site unspecified
Female genitourinary tract NOS

185 Malignant neoplasm of prostate

Excludes: *seminal vesicles (187.8)*

186 Malignant neoplasm of testis

Use additional code, if desired, to identify any functional activity

186.0 Undescended testis
Ectopic testis
Retained testis

186.9 Other and unspecified testis
Testis:
NOS
descended
scrotal

187 Malignant neoplasm of penis and other male genital organs

187.1 Prepuce
Foreskin

187.2 Glans penis

187.3 Body of penis
Corpus cavernosum

187.4 Penis, part unspecified
Skin of penis NOS

187.5 Epididymis

187.6 Spermatic cord
Vas deferens

187.7 Scrotum
Skin of scrotum

187.8 Other specified sites of male genital organs
Seminal vesicle
Tunica vaginalis
Malignant neoplasm of contiguous or overlapping sites of penis and other male genital organs whose point of origin cannot be determined

187.9 Male genital organ, site unspecified
Male genital organ or tract NOS

188 Malignant neoplasm of bladder

Excludes: *carcinoma in situ (233.7)*

188.0 Trigone of urinary bladder

188.1 Dome of urinary bladder

188.2 Lateral wall of urinary bladder

188.3 Anterior wall of urinary bladder

188.4 Posterior wall of urinary bladder

188.5 Bladder neck
Internal urethral orifice

188.6 Ureteric orifice

188.7 Urachus

188.8 Other specified sites of bladder
Malignant neoplasm of contiguous or overlapping sites of bladder whose point of origin cannot be determined

188.9 Bladder, part unspecified
Bladder wall NOS

189 Malignant neoplasm of kidney and other and unspecified urinary organs

189.0 Kidney, except pelvis
Kidney NOS
Kidney parenchyma

189.1 Renal pelvis
Renal calyces
Ureteropelvic junction

189.2 Ureter

Excludes: *ureteric orifice of bladder (188.6)*

189.3 Urethra

Excludes: *urethral orifice of bladder (188.5)*

189.4 Paraurethral glands

189.8 Other specified sites of urinary organs
Malignant neoplasm of contiguous or overlapping sites of kidney and other urinary organs whose point of origin cannot be determined

189.9 Urinary organ, site unspecified
Urinary system NOS

MALIGNANT NEOPLASM OF OTHER AND UNSPECIFIED SITES (190-199)

Excludes: *carcinoma in situ (234.0-234.9)*

190 Malignant neoplasm of eye

Excludes: *carcinoma in situ (234.0)*
eyelid (skin) (172.1, 173.1)
cartilage (171.0)
optic nerve (192.0)
orbital bone (170.0)

190.0 Eyeball, except conjunctiva, cornea, retina, and choroid
Ciliary body
Crystalline lens
Iris
Sclera
Uveal tract

190.1 Orbit
Connective tissue of orbit
Extraocular muscle
Retrobulbar

Excludes: *bone of orbit (170.0)*

190.2 Lacrimal gland

190.3 Conjunctiva

190.4 Cornea

190.5 Retina

190.6 Choroid

190.7 Lacrimal duct
Lacrimal sac
Nasolacrimal duct

190.8 Other specified sites of eye
Malignant neoplasm of contiguous or overlapping sites of eye whose point of origin cannot be determined

190.9 Eye, part unspecified

191 Malignant neoplasm of brain

Excludes: *cranial nerves (192.0)*
retrobulbar area (190.1)

191.0 Cerebrum, except lobes and ventricles
Basal ganglia
Cerebral cortex
Corpus striatum
Globus pallidus
Hypothalamus
Thalamus

191.1 Frontal lobe

191.2 Temporal lobe
Hippocampus — Uncus

191.3 Parietal lobe

191.4 Occipital lobe

191.5 Ventricles
Choroid plexus — Floor of ventricle

191.6 Cerebellum NOS
Cerebellopontine angle

191.7 Brain stem
Cerebral peduncle — Midbrain
Medulla oblongata — Pons

191.8 Other parts of brain
Corpus callosum
Tapetum
Malignant neoplasm of contiguous or overlapping sites of brain whose point of origin cannot be determined

191.9 Brain, unspecified
Cranial fossa NOS

192 Malignant neoplasm of other and unspecified parts of nervous system

Excludes: peripheral, sympathetic, and parasympathetic nerves and ganglia (171.0-171.9)

192.0 Cranial nerves
Olfactory bulb

192.1 Cerebral meninges
Dura (mater) — Meninges NOS
Falx (cerebelli) (cerebri) — Tentorium

192.2 Spinal cord
Cauda equina

192.3 Spinal meninges

192.8 Other specified sites of nervous system
Malignant neoplasm of contiguous or overlapping sites of other parts of nervous system whose point of origin cannot be determined

192.9 Nervous system, part unspecified
Nervous system (central) NOS

Excludes: meninges NOS (192.1)

193 Malignant neoplasm of thyroid gland
Sipple's syndrome — Thyroglossal duct
Use additional code, if desired, to identify any functional activity

194 Malignant neoplasm of other endocrine glands and related structures
Use additional code, if desired, to identify any functional activity

Excludes: islets of Langerhans (157.4)
ovary (183.0)
testis (186.0-186.9)
thymus (164.0)

194.0 Adrenal gland
Adrenal cortex — Suprarenal gland
Adrenal medulla

194.1 Parathyroid gland

194.3 Pituitary gland and craniopharyngeal duct
Craniobuccal pouch — Rathke's pouch
Hypophysis — Sella turcica

194.4 Pineal gland

194.5 Carotid body

194.6 Aortic body and other paraganglia
Coccygeal body — Para-aortic body
Glomus jugulare

194.8 Other
Pluriglandular involvement NOS
Note: If the sites of multiple involvements are known, they should be coded separately.

194.9 Endocrine gland, site unspecified

Add 4th or 5th digit — Nonspecific code — Unspecified code — Manifestation code

195 Malignant neoplasm of other and ill-defined sites

Includes: malignant neoplasms of contiguous sites, not elsewhere classified, whose point of origin cannot be determined

Excludes: *malignant neoplasm:*
lymphatic and hematopoietic tissue (200.0-208.9)
secondary sites (196.0-198.8)
unspecified site (199.0-199.1)

195.0 Head, face, and neck
Cheek NOS
Jaw NOS
Nose NOS
Supraclavicular region NOS

195.1 Thorax
Axilla
Chest (wall) NOS
Intrathoracic NOS

195.2 Abdomen
Intra-abdominal NOS

195.3 Pelvis
Groin
Inguinal region NOS
Presacral region
Sacrococcygeal region
Sites overlapping systems within pelvis, as:
rectovaginal (septum)
rectovesical (septum)

195.4 Upper limb

195.5 Lower limb

195.8 Other specified sites
Back NOS
Flank NOS
Trunk NOS

196 Secondary and unspecified malignant neoplasm of lymph nodes

Excludes: *any malignant neoplasm of lymph nodes, specified as primary (200.0-202.9)*
Hodgkin's disease (201.0-201.9)
lymphosarcoma (200.1)
reticulosarcoma (200.0)
other forms of lymphoma (202.0-202.9)

196.0 Lymph nodes of head, face, and neck
Cervical
Cervicofacial
Scalene
Supraclavicular

196.1 Intrathoracic lymph nodes
Bronchopulmonary
Intercostal
Mediastinal
Tracheobronchial

196.2 Intra-abdominal lymph nodes
Intestinal
Mesenteric
Retroperitoneal

196.3 Lymph nodes of axilla and upper limb
Brachial
Epitrochlear
Infraclavicular
Pectoral

196.5 Lymph nodes of inguinal region and lower limb
Femoral
Groin
Popliteal
Tibial

196.6 Intrapelvic lymph nodes
Hypogastric
Iliac
Obturator
Parametrial

196.8 Lymph nodes of multiple sites

196.9 Site unspecified
Lymph nodes NOS

197 Secondary malignant neoplasm of respiratory and digestive systems

Excludes: *lymph node metastasis (196.0-196.9)*

197.0 Lung
Bronchus

197.1 Mediastinum

197.2 Pleura

197.3 Other respiratory organs
Trachea

197.4 Small intestine, including duodenum

197.5 Large intestine and rectum

197.6 Retroperitoneum and peritoneum

197.7 Liver, specified as secondary

197.8 Other digestive organs and spleen

198 Secondary malignant neoplasm of other specified sites

Excludes: *lymph node metastasis (196.0-196.9)*

198.0 Kidney

198.1 Other urinary organs

198.2 Skin
Skin of breast

198.3 Brain and spinal cord

198.4 Other parts of nervous system
Meninges (cerebral) (spinal)

198.5 Bone and bone marrow

198.6 Ovary

198.7 Adrenal gland
Suprarenal gland

198.8 Other specified sites

198.81 Breast

Excludes: *skin of breast (198.2)*

198.82 Genital organs

198.89 Other

Excludes: *retroperitoneal lymph nodes (196.2)*

199 Malignant neoplasm without specification of site

199.0 Disseminated

Carcinomatosis
Generalized:
cancer
malignancy
Multiple cancer

} unspecified site (primary) (secondary)

199.1 Other

Cancer
Carcinoma
Malignancy

} unspecified site (primary) (secondary)

MALIGNANT NEOPLASM OF LYMPHATIC AND HEMATOPOIETIC TISSUE (200-208)

Excludes: *secondary neoplasm of:*
bone marrow (198.5)
spleen (197.8)
secondary and unspecified neoplasm of lymph nodes (196.0-196.9)

The following fifth-digit subclassification is for use with categories 200-202:

0 unspecified site, extranodal and solid organ sites

1 lymph nodes of head, face, and neck

2 intrathoracic lymph nodes

3 intra-abdominal lymph nodes

4 lymph nodes of axilla and upper limb

5 lymph nodes of inguinal region and lower limb

6 intrapelvic lymph nodes

7 spleen

8 lymph nodes of multiple sites

⑤ 200 Lymphosarcoma and reticulosarcoma

200.0 Reticulosarcoma

Lymphoma (malignant):
  histiocytic (diffuse):
    nodular
    pleomorphic cell type
  reticulum cell type
Reticulum cell sarcoma:
  NOS
  pleomorphic cell type

200.1 Lymphosarcoma

Lymphoblastoma (diffuse)
Lymphoma (malignant):
  lymphoblastic (diffuse)
  lymphocytic (cell type) (diffuse)
  lymphosarcoma type
Lymphosarcoma:
  NOS
  diffuse NOS
  lymphoblastic (diffuse)
  lymphocytic (diffuse)
  prolymphocytic

Excludes: *lymphosarcoma:*
  follicular or nodular (202.0)
  mixed cell type (200.8)
lymphosarcoma cell leukemia (207.8)

200.2 Burkitt's tumor or lymphoma

Malignant lymphoma, Burkitt's type

200.8 Other named variants

Lymphoma (malignant):
  lymphoplasmacytoid type
  mixed lymphocytic-histiocytic (diffuse)
Lymphosarcoma, mixed cell type (diffuse)
Reticulolymphosarcoma (diffuse)

⑤ 201 Hodgkin's disease

201.0 Hodgkin's paragranuloma

201.1 Hodgkin's granuloma

201.2 Hodgkin's sarcoma

201.4 Lymphocytic-histiocytic predominance

201.5 Nodular sclerosis

Hodgkin's disease, nodular sclerosis:
  NOS
  cellular phase

201.6 Mixed cellularity

201.7 Lymphocytic depletion

Hodgkin's disease, lymphocytic depletion:
  NOS
  diffuse fibrosis
  reticular type

201.9 Hodgkin's disease, unspecified

Hodgkin's:
  disease NOS
  lymphoma NOS
Malignant:
  lymphogranuloma
  lymphogranulomatosis

⑤ 202 Other malignant neoplasms of lymphoid and histiocytic tissue

202.0 Nodular lymphoma

Brill-Symmers disease
Lymphoma:
  follicular (giant)
  lymphocytic, nodular
Lymphosarcoma:
  follicular (giant)
  nodular
Reticulosarcoma, follicular or nodular

202.1 Mycosis fungoides

202.2 Sézary's disease

202.3 Malignant histiocytosis

Histiocytic medullary reticulosis
Malignant:
  reticuloendotheliosis
  reticulosis

202.4 Leukemic reticuloendotheliosis

Hairy-cell leukemia

● Code new to this edition ▲ Revision of existing code ④ ⑤ Fourth or fifth digit required

202.5 Letterer-Siwe disease
Acute:
differentiated progressive histiocytosis
histiocytosis X (progressive)
infantile reticuloendotheliosis
reticulosis of infancy

Excludes: *Hand-Schüller-Christian disease (277.8)*
histiocytosis (acute) (chronic) (277.8)
histiocytosis X (chronic) (277.8)

202.6 Malignant mast cell tumors
Malignant:
mastocytoma
mastocytosis
Mast cell sarcoma
Systemic tissue mast cell disease

Excludes: *mast cell leukemia (207.8)*

202.8 Other lymphomas
Lymphoma (malignant):
NOS
diffuse

Excludes: *benign lymphoma (229.0)*

202.9 Other and unspecified malignant neoplasms of lymphoid and histiocytic tissue
Malignant neoplasm of bone marrow NOS

⑤ **203 Multiple myeloma and immunoproliferative neoplasms**
The following fifth-digit subclassification is for use with category 203
0 without mention of remission
1 in remission

203.0 Multiple myeloma
Kahler's disease
Myelomatosis

Excludes: *solitary myeloma (238.6)*

203.1 Plasma cell leukemia
Plasmacytic leukemia

203.8 Other immunoproliferative neoplasms

⑤ **204 Lymphoid leukemia**
Includes:
leukemia:
lymphatic
lymphoblastic
leukemia:
lymphocytic
lymphogenous

The following fifth-digit subclassification is for use with category 204
0 without mention of remission
1 in remission

204.0 Acute

Excludes: *acute exacerbation of chronic lymphoid leukemia (204.1)*

204.1 Chronic

204.2 Subacute

204.8 Other lymphoid leukemia
Aleukemic leukemia:
lymphatic
lymphocytic
lymphoid

204.9 Unspecified lymphoid leukemia

⑤ **205 Myeloid leukemia**
Includes:
leukemia:
granulocytic
myeloblastic
myelocytic
Tmyelogenous
leukemia:
myelomonocytic
myelosclerotic
myelosis

The following fifth-digit subclassification is for use with category 205
0 without mention of remission
1 in remission

Add 4th or 5th digit | Nonspecific code | Unspecified code | Manifestation code

205.0 Acute
Acute promyelocytic leukemia

Excludes: *acute exacerbation of chronic myeloid leukemia (205.1)*

205.1 Chronic
Eosinophilic leukemia
Neutrophilic leukemia

205.2 Subacute

205.3 Myeloid sarcoma
Chloroma
Granulocytic sarcoma

205.8 Other myeloid leukemia
Aleukemic leukemia:
granulocytic
myelogenous
myeloid
Aleukemic myelosis

205.9 Unspecified myeloid leukemia

⑤ **206 Monocytic leukemia**
Includes: leukemia:
histiocytic
monoblastic
monocytoid

The following fifth-digit subclassification is for use with category 206

0 without mention of remission

1 in remission

206.0 Acute

Excludes: *acute exacerbation of chronic monocytic leukemia (206.1)*

206.1 Chronic

206.2 Subacute

206.8 Other monocytic leukemia
Aleukemic:
monocytic leukemia
monocytoid leukemia

206.9 Unspecified monocytic leukemia

⑤ **207 Other specified leukemia**

Excludes: *leukemic reticuloendotheliosis (202.4)*
plasma cell leukemia (203.1)

The following fifth-digit subclassification is for use with category 207

0 without mention of remission

1 in remission

207.0 Acute erythremia and erythroleukemia
Acute erythremic myelosis
Di Guglielmo's disease
Erythremic myelosis

207.1 Chronic erythremia
Heilmeyer-Schöner disease

207.2 Megakaryocytic leukemia
Megakaryocytic myelosis
Thrombocytic leukemia

207.8 Other specified leukemia
Lymphosarcoma cell leukemia

⑤ **208 Leukemia of unspecified cell type**

The following fifth-digit subclassification is for use with category 208

0 without mention of remission

1 in remission

208.0 Acute
Acute leukemia NOS
Blast cell leukemia
Stem cell leukemia

Excludes: *acute exacerbation of chronic unspecified leukemia (208.1)*

208.1 Chronic
Chronic leukemia NOS

● Code new to this edition
▲ Revision of existing code
④ ⑤ Fourth or fifth digit required

208.2 Subacute
Subacute leukemia NOS

208.8 Other leukemia of unspecified cell type

208.9 Unspecified leukemia
Leukemia NOS

BENIGN NEOPLASMS (210-229)

210 Benign neoplasm of lip, oral cavity, and pharynx

Excludes: *cyst (of):*
jaw (526.0-526.2, 526.89)
oral soft tissue (528.4)
radicular (522.8)

210.0 Lip
Frenulum labii
Lip (inner aspect) (mucosa) (vermilion border)

Excludes: *labial commissure (210.4)*
skin of lip (216.0)

210.1 Tongue
Lingual tonsil

210.2 Major salivary glands
Gland:
parotid
sublingual
submandibular

Excludes: *benign neoplasms of minor salivary glands:*
NOS (210.4)
buccal mucosa (210.4)
lips (210.0)
palate (hard) (soft) (210.4)
tongue (210.1)
tonsil, palatine (210.5)

210.3 Floor of mouth

210.4 Other and unspecified parts of mouth
Gingiva
Gum (upper) (lower)
Labial commissure
Oral cavity NOS
Oral mucosa
Palate (hard) (soft)
Uvula

Excludes: *benign odontogenic neoplasms of bone (213.0-213.1)*
developmental odontogenic cysts (526.0)
mucosa of lips (210.0)
nasopharyngeal [posterior] [superior] surface of soft palate (210.7)

210.5 Tonsil
Tonsil (faucial) (palatine)

Excludes: *lingual tonsil (210.1)*
pharyngeal tonsil (210.7)
tonsillar:
fossa (210.6)
pillars (210.6)

210.6 Other parts of oropharynx
Branchial cleft or vestiges
Epiglottis, anterior aspect
Fauces NOS
Mesopharynx NOS
Tonsillar:
fossa
pillars
Vallecula

Excludes: *epiglottis:*
NOS (212.1)
suprahyoid portion (212.1)

210.7 Nasopharynx
Adenoid tissue
Lymphadenoid tissue
Pharyngeal tonsil
Posterior nasal septum

Add 4th or 5th digit | Nonspecific code | Unspecified code | Manifestation code

210.8 Hypopharynx

Arytenoid fold
Laryngopharynx
Postcricoid region
Pyriform fossa

210.9 Pharynx, unspecified

Throat NOS

211 Benign neoplasm of other parts of digestive system

211.0 Esophagus

211.1 Stomach

Body, Cardia, Fundus } stomach
Cardiac orifice
Pylorus

211.2 Duodenum, jejunum, and ileum

Small intestine NOS

Excludes: *ampulla of Vater (211.5)*
ileocecal valve (211.3)

211.3 Colon

Appendix
Cecum
Ileocecal valve
Large intestine NOS

Excludes: *rectosigmoid junction (211.4)*

211.4 Rectum and anal canal

Anal canal or sphincter
Anus NOS
Rectosigmoid junction

Excludes: *anus:*
margin (216.5)
skin (216.5)
perianal skin (216.5)

211.5 Liver and biliary passages

Ampulla of Vater
Common bile duct
Cystic duct
Gallbladder
Hepatic duct
Sphincter of Oddi

211.6 Pancreas, except islets of Langerhans

211.7 Islets of Langerhans

Islet cell tumor

Use additional code, if desired, to identify any functional activity

211.8 Retroperitoneum and peritoneum

Mesentery
Mesocolon
Omentum
Retroperitoneal tissue

211.9 Other and unspecified site

Alimentary tract NOS
Digestive system NOS
Gastrointestinal tract NOS
Intestinal tract NOS
Intestine NOS
Spleen, not elsewhere classified

212 Benign neoplasm of respiratory and intrathoracic organs

212.0 Nasal cavities, middle ear, and accessory sinuses

Cartilage of nose
Eustachian tube
Nares
Septum of nose
Sinus:
ethmoidal
frontal
maxillary
sphenoidal

Excludes: *auditory canal (external) (216.2)*
bone of:
ear (213.0)
nose [turbinates] (213.0)
cartilage of ear (215.0)
ear (external) (skin) (216.2)
nose NOS (229.8)
skin (216.3)
olfactory bulb (225.1)
polyp of:
accessory sinus (471.8)
ear (385.30-385.35)
nasal cavity (471.0)
posterior margin of septum and choanae (210.7)

● Code new to this edition ▲ Revision of existing code ④ ⑤ Fourth or fifth digit required

212.1 Larynx
Cartilage:
arytenoid
cricoid
cuneiform
thyroid
Epiglottis (suprahyoid portion) NOS
Glottis
Vocal cords (false) (true)

Excludes: *epiglottis, anterior aspect (210.6)*
polyp of vocal cord or larynx (478.4)

212.2 Trachea

212.3 Bronchus and lung
Carina
Hilus of lung

212.4 Pleura

212.5 Mediastinum

212.6 Thymus

212.7 Heart

Excludes: *great vessels (215.4)*

212.8 Other specified sites

212.9 Site unspecified
Respiratory organ NOS
Upper respiratory tract NOS

Excludes: *intrathoracic NOS (229.8)*
thoracic NOS (229.8)

213 Benign neoplasm of bone and articular cartilage
Includes: cartilage (articular) (joint)
periosteum

Excludes: *cartilage of:*
ear (215.0)
eyelid (215.0)
larynx (212.1)
nose (212.0)
exostosis NOS (726.91)
synovia (215.0-215.9)

213.0 Bones of skull and face

Excludes: *lower jaw bone (213.1)*

213.1 Lower jaw bone

213.2 Vertebral column, excluding sacrum and coccyx

213.3 Ribs, sternum, and clavicle

213.4 Scapula and long bones of upper limb

213.5 Short bones of upper limb

213.6 Pelvic bones, sacrum, and coccyx

213.7 Long bones of lower limb

213.8 Short bones of lower limb

213.9 Bone and articular cartilage, site unspecified

214 Lipoma
Includes: angiolipoma
fibrolipoma
hibernoma
lipoma (fetal) (infiltrating) (intramuscular)
myelolipoma
myxolipoma

214.0 Skin and subcutaneous tissue of face

214.1 Other skin and subcutaneous tissue

214.2 Intrathoracic organs

214.3 Intra-abdominal organs

214.4 Spermatic cord

214.8 Other specified sites

214.9 Lipoma, unspecified site

215 Other benign neoplasm of connective and other soft tissue

Includes:

blood vessel
bursa
fascia
ligament
muscle
peripheral, sympathetic, and parasympathetic nerves and ganglia
synovia
tendon (sheath)

Excludes: *cartilage:*
articular (213.0-213.9)
larynx (212.1)
nose (212.0)
connective tissue of:
breast (217)
internal organ, except lipoma and hemangioma — code to benign neoplasm of the site
lipoma (214.0-214.9)

215.0 Head, face, and neck

215.2 Upper limb, including shoulder

215.3 Lower limb, including hip

215.4 Thorax

Excludes: *heart (212.7)*
mediastinum (212.5)
thymus (212.6)

215.5 Abdomen

Abdominal wall
Hypochondrium

215.6 Pelvis

Buttock
Groin
Inguinal region
Perineum

Excludes: *uterine:*
leiomyoma (218.0-218.9)
ligament, any (221.0)

215.7 Trunk, unspecified

Back NOS
Flank NOS

215.8 Other specified sites

215.9 Site unspecified

216 Benign neoplasm of skin

Includes:

blue nevus
dermatofibroma
hydrocystoma
pigmented nevus
syringoadenoma
syringoma

Excludes: *skin of genital organs (221.0-222.9)*

216.0 Skin of lip

Excludes: *vermilion border of lip (210.0)*

216.1 Eyelid, including canthus

Excludes: *cartilage of eyelid (215.0)*

216.2 Ear and external auditory canal

Auricle (ear)
Auricular canal, external
External meatus
Pinna

Excludes: *cartilage of ear (215.0)*

216.3 Skin of other and unspecified parts of face

Cheek, external
Eyebrow
Nose, external
Temple

216.4 Scalp and skin of neck

216.5 Skin of trunk, except scrotum

Axillary fold
Perianal skin
Skin of:
abdominal wall
anus
back
breast
Skin of:
buttock
chest wall
groin
perineum
Umbilicus

Excludes: *anal canal (211.4)*
anus NOS (211.4)
skin of scrotum (222.4)

216.6 Skin of upper limb, including shoulder

216.7 Skin of lower limb, including hip

216.8 Other specified sites of skin

216.9 Skin, site unspecified

217 Benign neoplasm of breast

Breast (male) (female)
connective tissue
glandular tissue
soft parts

Excludes: *adenofibrosis (610.2)*
benign cyst of breast (610.0)
fibrocystic disease (610.1)
skin of breast (216.5)

218 Uterine leiomyoma

Includes: fibroid (bleeding) (uterine)
uterine:
fibromyoma
myoma

218.0 Submucous leiomyoma of uterus

218.1 Intramural leiomyoma of uterus

Interstitial leiomyoma of uterus

218.2 Subserous leiomyoma of uterus

Subperitoneal leiomyoma of uterus

218.9 Leiomyoma of uterus, unspecified

219 Other benign neoplasm of uterus

219.0 Cervix uteri

219.1 Corpus uteri

Endometrium
Fundus
Myometrium

219.8 Other specified parts of uterus

219.9 Uterus, part unspecified

220 Benign neoplasm of ovary

Use additional code, if desired, to identify any functional activity (256.0-256.1)

Excludes: *cyst:*
corpus albicans (620.2)
corpus luteum (620.1)
endometrial (617.1)
follicular (atretic) (620.0)
graafian follicle (620.0)
ovarian NOS (620.2)
retention (620.2)

221 Benign neoplasm of other female genital organs

Includes: adenomatous polyp
benign teratoma

Excludes: *cyst:*
epoophoron (752.11)
fimbrial (752.11)
Gartner's duct (752.11)
parovarian (752.11)

221.0 Fallopian tube and uterine ligaments
Oviduct
Parametrium
Uterine ligament (broad) (round) (uterosacral)
Uterine tube

221.1 Vagina

221.2 Vulva
Clitoris
External female genitalia NOS
Greater vestibular [Bartholin's] gland
Labia (majora) (minora)
Pudendum

Excludes: *Bartholin's (duct) (gland) cyst (616.2)*

221.8 Other specified sites of female genital organs

221.9 Female genital organ, site unspecified
Female genitourinary tract NOS

222 Benign neoplasm of male genital organs

222.0 Testis
Use additional code, if desired, to identify any functional activity

222.1 Penis
Corpus cavernosum
Glans penis
Prepuce

222.2 Prostate

Excludes: *adenomatous hyperplasia of prostate (600)*
prostatic:
adenoma (600)
enlargement (600)
hypertrophy (600)

222.3 Epididymis

222.4 Scrotum
Skin of scrotum

222.8 Other specified sites of male genital organs
Seminal vesicle
Spermatic cord

222.9 Male genital organ, site unspecified
Male genitourinary tract NOS

223 Benign neoplasm of kidney and other urinary organs

223.0 Kidney, except pelvis
Kidney NOS

Excludes: *renal:*
calyces (223.1)
pelvis (223.1)

223.1 Renal pelvis

223.2 Ureter

Excludes: *ureteric orifice of bladder (223.3)*

223.3 Bladder

223.8 Other specified sites of urinary organs

223.81 Urethra

Excludes: *urethral orifice of bladder (223.3)*

223.89 Other
Paraurethral glands

223.9 Urinary organ, site unspecified
Urinary system NOS

224 Benign neoplasm of eye

Excludes: *cartilage of eyelid (215.0)*
eyelid (skin) (216.1)
optic nerve (225.1)
orbital bone (213.0)

224.0 Eyeball, except conjunctiva, cornea, retina, and choroid
Ciliary body
Iris
Sclera
Uveal tract

224.1 Orbit

Excludes: *bone of orbit (213.0)*

224.2 Lacrimal gland

224.3 Conjunctiva

224.4 Cornea

224.5 Retina

Excludes: *hemangioma of retina (228.03)*

224.6 Choroid

224.7 Lacrimal duct
Lacrimal sac
Nasolacrimal duct

224.8 Other specified parts of eye

224.9 Eye, part unspecified

225 Benign neoplasm of brain and other parts of nervous system

Excludes: *hemangioma (228.02)*
neurofibromatosis (237.7)
peripheral, sympathetic, and parasympathetic nerves and ganglia (215.0-215.9)
retrobulbar (224.1)

225.0 Brain

225.1 Cranial nerves

225.2 Cerebral meninges
Meninges NOS
Meningioma (cerebral)

225.3 Spinal cord
Cauda equina

225.4 Spinal meninges
Spinal meningioma

225.8 Other specified sites of nervous system

225.9 Nervous system, part unspecified
Nervous system (central) NOS

Excludes: *meninges NOS (225.2)*

226 Benign neoplasm of thyroid glands
Use additional code, if desired, to identify any functional activity

227 Benign neoplasm of other endocrine glands and related structures
Use additional code, if desired, to identify any functional activity

Excludes: *ovary (220)*
pancreas (211.6)
testis (222.0)

227.0 Adrenal gland
Suprarenal gland

227.1 Parathyroid gland

227.3 Pituitary gland and craniopharyngeal duct (pouch)
Craniobuccal pouch
Hypophysis
Rathke's pouch
Sella turcica

227.4 Pineal gland
Pineal body

227.5 Carotid body

227.6 Aortic body and other paraganglia
Coccygeal body
Glomus jugulare
Para-aortic body

227.8 Other

227.9 Endocrine gland, site unspecified

Add 4th or 5th digit | Nonspecific code | Unspecified code | Manifestation code

228 Hemangioma and lymphangioma, any site

Includes: angioma (benign) (cavernous) (congenital) NOS
cavernous nevus
glomus tumor
hemangioma (benign) (congenital)

Excludes: *benign neoplasm of spleen, except hemangioma and lymphangioma (211.9)*
glomus jugulare (227.6)
nevus:
NOS (216.0-216.9)
blue or pigmented (216.0-216.9)
vascular (757.32)

228.0 Hemangioma, any site

228.00 Of unspecified site

228.01 Of skin and subcutaneous tissue

228.02 Of intracranial structures

228.03 Of retina

228.04 Of intra-abdominal structures
Peritoneum
Retroperitoneal tissue

228.09 Of other sites
Systemic angiomatosis

228.1 Lymphangioma, any site
Congenital lymphangioma
Lymphatic nevus

229 Benign neoplasm of other and unspecified sites

229.0 Lymph nodes

Excludes: *lymphangioma (228.1)*

229.8 Other specified sites
Intrathoracic NOS
Thoracic NOS

229.9 Site unspecified

CARCINOMA IN SITU (230-234)

Includes: Bowen's disease
erythroplasia
Queyrat's erythroplasia

Excludes: *leukoplakia—see Alphabetic Index*

230 Carcinoma in situ of digestive organs

230.0 Lip, oral cavity, and pharynx
Gingiva
Hypopharynx
Mouth [any part]
Nasopharynx
Oropharynx
Salivary gland or duct
Tongue

Excludes: *aryepiglottic fold or interarytenoid fold, laryngeal aspect (231.0)*
epiglottis:
NOS (231.0)
suprahyoid portion (231.0)
skin of lip (232.0)

230.1 Esophagus

230.2 Stomach
Body, Cardia, Fundus } of stomach
Cardiac orifice
Pylorus

230.3 Colon
Appendix
Cecum
Ileocecal valve
Large intestine NOS

Excludes: *rectosigmoid junction (230.4)*

230.4 Rectum
Rectosigmoid junction

230.5 Anal canal
Anal sphincter

230.6 Anus, unspecified

Excludes: *anus:*
margin (232.5)
skin (232.5)
perianal skin (232.5)

230.7 Other and unspecified parts of intestine
Duodenum
Ileum
Jejunum
Small intestine NOS

Excludes: *ampulla of Vater (230.8)*

230.8 Liver and biliary system
Ampulla of Vater
Common bile duct
Cystic duct
Gallbladder
Hepatic duct
Sphincter of Oddi

230.9 Other and unspecified digestive organs
Digestive organ NOS
Gastrointestinal tract NOS
Pancreas
Spleen

231 Carcinoma in situ of respiratory system

231.0 Larynx
Cartilage:
arytenoid
cricoid
cuneiform
thyroid
Epiglottis:
NOS
posterior surface
suprahyoid portion
Vocal cords (false) (true)

Excludes: *aryepiglottic fold or interarytenoid fold:*
NOS (230.0)
hypopharyngeal aspect (230.0)
marginal zone (230.0)

231.1 Trachea

231.2 Bronchus and lung
Carina
Hilus of lung

231.8 Other specified parts of respiratory system
Accessory sinuses
Middle ear
Nasal cavities
Pleura

Excludes: *ear (external) (skin) (232.2)*
nose NOS (234.8)
skin (232.3)

231.9 Respiratory system, part unspecified
Respiratory organ NOS

232 Carcinoma in situ of skin
Includes: pigment cells

232.0 Skin of lip

Excludes: *vermilion border of lip (230.0)*

232.1 Eyelid, including canthus

232.2 Ear and external auditory canal

232.3 Skin of other and unspecified parts of face

232.4 Scalp and skin of neck

232.5 Skin of trunk, except scrotum
Anus, margin
Axillary fold
Perianal skin
Skin of:
abdominal wall
anus
back
breast
buttock
chest wall
groin
perineum
Umbilicus

Excludes: *anal canal (230.5)*
anus NOS (230.6)
skin of genital organs (233.3, 233.5-233.6)

232.6 Skin of upper limb, including shoulder

232.7 Skin of lower limb, including hip

232.8 Other specified sites of skin

232.9 Skin, site unspecified

233 Carcinoma in situ of breast and genitourinary system

233.0 Breast

Excludes: *Paget's disease (174.0-174.9)*
skin of breast (232.5)

233.1 Cervix uteri

233.2 Other and unspecified parts of uterus

233.3 Other and unspecified female genital organs

233.4 Prostate

233.5 Penis

233.6 Other and unspecified male genital organs

233.7 Bladder

233.9 Other and unspecified urinary organs

234 Carcinoma in situ of other and unspecified sites

234.0 Eye

Excludes: *cartilage of eyelid (234.8)*
eyelid (skin) (232.1)
optic nerve (234.8)
orbital bone (234.8)

234.8 Other specified sites
Endocrine gland [any]

234.9 Site unspecified
Carcinoma in situ NOS

NEOPLASMS OF UNCERTAIN BEHAVIOR (235-238)

Note: Categories 235-238 classify by site certain histo-morphologically well-defined neoplasms, the subsequent behavior of which cannot be predicted from the present appearance.

235 Neoplasm of uncertain behavior of digestive and respiratory systems

235.0 Major salivary glands
Gland:
parotid
sublingual
submandibular

Excludes: *minor salivary glands (235.1)*

235.1 Lip, oral cavity, and pharynx
Gingiva
Hypopharynx
Minor salivary glands
Mouth
Nasopharynx
Oropharynx
Tongue

Excludes: *aryepiglottic fold or interarytenoid fold, laryngeal aspect (235.6)*
epiglottis:
NOS (235.6)
suprahyoid portion (235.6)
skin of lip (238.2)

235.2 Stomach, intestines, and rectum

235.3 Liver and biliary passages
Ampulla of Vater
Bile ducts [any]
Gallbladder
Liver

235.4 Retroperitoneum and peritoneum

235.5 Other and unspecified digestive organs
Anal:
canal
sphincter
Anus NOS
Esophagus
Pancreas
Spleen

Excludes: *anus:*
margin (238.2)
skin (238.2)
perianal skin (238.2)

235.6 Larynx

Excludes: *aryepiglottic fold or interarytenoid fold:*
NOS (235.1)
hypopharyngeal aspect (235.1)
marginal zone (235.1)

235.7 Trachea, bronchus, and lung

235.8 Pleura, thymus, and mediastinum

235.9 Other and unspecified respiratory organs
Accessory sinuses
Middle ear
Nasal cavities
Respiratory organ NOS

Excludes: *ear (external) (skin) (238.2)*
nose (238.8)
skin (238.2)

236 Neoplasm of uncertain behavior of genitourinary organs

236.0 Uterus

236.1 Placenta
Chorioadenoma (destruens)
Invasive mole
Malignant hydatid(iform) mole

236.2 Ovary
Use additional code, if desired, to identify any functional activity

236.3 Other and unspecified female genital organs

236.4 Testis
Use additional code, if desired, to identify any functional activity

236.5 Prostate

236.6 Other and unspecified male genital organs

236.7 Bladder

236.9 Other and unspecified urinary organs

236.90 Urinary organ, unspecified

236.91 Kidney and ureter

236.99 Other

237 Neoplasm of uncertain behavior of endocrine glands and nervous system

237.0 Pituitary gland and craniopharyngeal duct
Use additional code, if desired, to identify any functional activity

237.1 Pineal gland

237.2 Adrenal gland
Suprarenal gland
Use additional code, if desired, to identify any functional activity

237.3 Paraganglia
Aortic body
Carotid body
Coccygeal body
Glomus jugulare

237.4 Other and unspecified endocrine glands
Parathyroid gland
Thyroid gland

237.5 Brain and spinal cord

237.6 Meninges
Meninges:
NOS
cerebral
spinal

237.7 Neurofibromatosis
von Recklinghausen's disease

237.70 Neurofibromatosis, unspecified

237.71 Neurofibromatosis, Type I [von Recklinghausen's disease]

237.72 Neurofibromatosis, Type II [acoustic neurofibromatosis]

237.9 Other and unspecified parts of nervous system
Cranial nerves

Excludes: *peripheral, sympathetic, and parasympathetic nerves and ganglia (238.1)*

Add 4th or 5th digit | Nonspecific code | Unspecified code | Manifestation code

238 Neoplasm of uncertain behavior of other and unspecified sites and tissues

238.0 Bone and articular cartilage

Excludes: *cartilage:*
ear (238.1)
eyelid (238.1)
larynx (235.6)
nose (235.9)
synovia (238.1)

238.1 Connective and other soft tissue
Peripheral, sympathetic, and parasympathetic nerves and ganglia

Excludes: *cartilage (of):*
articular (238.0)
larynx (235.6)
nose (235.9)
connective tissue of breast (238.3)

238.2 Skin

Excludes: *anus NOS (235.5)*
skin of genital organs (236.3, 236.6)
vermilion border of lip (235.1)

238.3 Breast

Excludes: *skin of breast (238.2)*

238.4 Polycythemia vera

238.5 Histiocytic and mast cells
Mast cell tumor NOS
Mastocytoma NOS

238.6 Plasma cells
Plasmacytoma NOS
Solitary myeloma

238.7 Other lymphatic and hematopoietic tissues
Disease:
lymphoproliferative (chronic) NOS
myeloproliferative (chronic) NOS
Idiopathic thrombocythemia
Megakaryocytic myelosclerosis
Myelodysplastic syndrome
Myelosclerosis with myeloid metaplasia
Panmyelosis (acute)

Excludes: *myelofibrosis (289.8)*
myelosclerosis NOS (289.8)
myelosis:
NOS (205.9)
megakaryocytic (207.2)

238.8 Other specified sites
Eye
Heart

Excludes: *eyelid (skin) (238.2)*
cartilage (238.1)

238.9 Site unspecified

NEOPLASMS OF UNSPECIFIED NATURE (239)

239 Neoplasms of unspecified nature

Note: Category 239 classifies by site neoplasms of unspecified morphology and behavior. The term "mass," unless otherwise stated, is not to be regarded as a neoplastic growth.

Includes: "growth" NOS
neoplasm NOS
new growth NOS
tumor NOS

239.0 Digestive system

Excludes: *anus:*
margin (239.2)
skin (239.2)
perianal skin (239.2)

239.1 Respiratory system

● Code new to this edition
▲ Revision of existing code
④ ⑤ Fourth or fifth digit required

239.2 Bone, soft tissue, and skin

Excludes: *anal canal (239.0)*
anus NOS (239.0)
bone marrow (202.9)
cartilage:
larynx (239.1)
nose (239.1)
connective tissue of breast (239.3)
skin of genital organs (239.5)
vermilion border of lip (239.0)

239.3 Breast

Excludes: *skin of breast (239.2)*

239.4 Bladder

239.5 Other genitourinary organs

239.6 Brain

Excludes: *cerebral meninges (239.7)*
cranial nerves (239.7)

239.7 Endocrine glands and other parts of nervous system

Excludes: *peripheral, sympathetic, and parasympathetic nerves and ganglia (239.2)*

239.8 Other specified sites

Excludes: *eyelids (skin) (239.2)*
cartilage (239.2)
great vessels (239.2)
optic nerve (239.7)

239.9 Site unspecified

3. ENDOCRINE, NUTRITIONAL AND METABOLIC DISEASES, AND IMMUNITY DISORDERS (240-279)

Excludes: *endocrine and metabolic disturbances specific to the fetus and newborn (775.0-775.9)*

Note: All neoplasms, whether functionally active or not, are classified in Chapter 2. Codes in Chapter 3 (i.e., 242.8, 246.0, 251-253, 255-259) may be used, if desired, to identify such functional activity associated with any neoplasm, or by ectopic endocrine tissue.

DISORDERS OF THYROID GLAND (240-246)

240 Simple and unspecified goiter

240.0 Goiter, specified as simple
Any condition classifiable to 240.9, specified as simple

240.9 Goiter, unspecified
Enlargement of thyroid
Goiter or struma:
NOS
diffuse colloid
endemic
Goiter or struma:
hyperplastic
nontoxic (diffuse)
parenchymatous
sporadic

Excludes: *congenital (dyshormonogenic) goiter (246.1)*

241 Nontoxic nodular goiter

Excludes: *adenoma of thyroid (226)*
cystadenoma of thyroid (226)

241.0 Nontoxic uninodular goiter
Thyroid nodule
Uninodular goiter (nontoxic)

241.1 Nontoxic multinodular goiter
Multinodular goiter (nontoxic)

241.9 Unspecified nontoxic nodular goiter
Adenomatous goiter
Nodular goiter (nontoxic) NOS
Struma nodosa (simplex)

⑤ **242 Thyrotoxicosis with or without goiter**

Excludes: *neonatal thyrotoxicosis (775.3)*

The following fifth-digit subclassification is for use with category 242:

0 without mention of thyrotoxic crisis or storm

1 with mention of thyrotoxic crisis or storm

242.0 Toxic diffuse goiter
Basedow's disease
Exophthalmic or toxic goiter NOS
Graves' disease
Primary thyroid hyperplasia

242.1 Toxic uninodular goiter
Thyroid nodule } toxic or with hyperthyroidism
Uninodular goiter }

242.2 Toxic multinodular goiter
Secondary thyroid hyperplasia

242.3 Toxic nodular goiter, unspecified
Adenomatous goiter } toxic or with hyperthyroidism
Nodular goiter }
Struma nodosa }
Any condition classifiable to 241.9 specified as toxic or with hyperthyroidism

242.4 Thyrotoxicosis from ectopic thyroid nodule

242.8 Thyrotoxicosis of other specified origin
Overproduction of thyroid-stimulating hormone [TSH]
Thyrotoxicosis:
factitia
from ingestion of excessive thyroid material

Use additional E code, if desired, to identify cause, if drug-induced

242.9 Thyrotoxicosis without mention of goiter or other cause
Hyperthyroidism NOS
Thyrotoxicosis NOS

Add 4th or 5th digit | Nonspecific code | Unspecified code | Manifestation code

243 Congenital hypothyroidism
Congenital thyroid insufficiency
Cretinism (athyrotic) (endemic)

Use additional code, if desired, to identify associated mental retardation

Excludes: *congenital (dyshormonogenic) goiter (246.1)*

244 Acquired hypothyroidism
Includes: athyroidism (acquired)
hypothyroidism (acquired)
myxedema (adult) (juvenile)
thyroid (gland) insufficiency (acquired)

244.0 Postsurgical hypothyroidism

244.1 Other postablative hypothyroidism
Hypothyroidism following therapy, such as irradiation

244.2 Iodine hypothyroidism
Hypothyroidism resulting from administration or ingestion of iodide

Use additional E code, if desired, to identify drug

244.3 Other iatrogenic hypothyroidism
Hypothyroidism resulting from:
P-aminosalicylic acid [PAS]
Phenylbutazone
Resorcinol
Iatrogenic hypothyroidism NOS

Use additional E code, if desired, to identify drug

244.8 Other specified acquired hypothyroidism
Secondary hypothyroidism NEC

244.9 Unspecified hypothyroidism
Hypothyroidism } primary or NOS
Myxedema }

245 Thyroiditis

245.0 Acute thyroiditis
Abscess of thyroid
Thyroiditis:
nonsuppurative, acute
pyogenic
suppurative

Use additional code, if desired, to identify organism

245.1 Subacute thyroiditis
Thyroiditis:
de Quervain's
giant cell
Thyroiditis:
granulomatous
viral

245.2 Chronic lymphocytic thyroiditis
Hashimoto's disease
Struma lymphomatosa
Thyroiditis:
autoimmune
lymphocytic (chronic)

245.3 Chronic fibrous thyroiditis
Struma fibrosa
Thyroiditis:
invasive (fibrous)
ligneous
Riedel's

245.4 Iatrogenic thyroiditis

Use additional code, if desired, to identify cause

245.8 Other and unspecified chronic thyroiditis
Chronic thyroiditis:
NOS
nonspecific

245.9 Thyroiditis, unspecified
Thyroiditis NOS

246 Other disorders of thyroid

246.0 Disorders of thyrocalcitonin secretion
Hypersecretion of calcitonin or thyrocalcitonin

246.1 Dyshormonogenic goiter
Congenital (dyshormonogenic) goiter
Goiter due to enzyme defect in synthesis of thyroid hormone
Goitrous cretinism (sporadic)

246.2 Cyst of thyroid

Excludes: *cystadenoma of thyroid (226)*

246.3 Hemorrhage and infarction of thyroid

246.8 Other specified disorders of thyroid
Abnormality of thyroid-binding globulin
Atrophy of thyroid
Hyper-TBG-nemia
Hypo-TBG-nemia

246.9 Unspecified disorder of thyroid

DISEASES OF OTHER ENDOCRINE GLANDS (250-259)

⑤ **250 Diabetes mellitus**

Excludes: *gestational diabetes (648.8)*
hyperglycemia NOS (790.6)
neonatal diabetes mellitus (775.1)
nonclinical diabetes (790.2)
that complicating pregnancy, childbirth, or the puerperium (648.0)

The following fifth-digit subclassification is for use with category 250:

0 type II [non-insulin dependent type] [NIDDM type] [adult-onset type] or unspecified type, not stated as uncontrolled

1 type I [insulin dependent type] [IDDM] [juvenile type], not stated as uncontrolled

2 type II [non-insulin dependent type] [NIDDM] [adult-onset type] or unspecified type, uncontrolled

3 type I [insulin dependent type] [IDDM] [juvenile type], uncontrolled

250.0 Diabetes mellitus without mention of complication
Diabetes mellitus without mention of complication or manifestation classifiable to 250.1-250.9
Diabetes (mellitus) NOS

250.1 Diabetes with ketoacidosis
Diabetic:
acidosis } without mention of coma
ketosis } without mention of coma

□ **250.2 Diabetes with hyperosmolarity**
Hyperosmolar (nonketotic) coma

□ **250.3 Diabetes with other coma**
Diabetic coma (with ketoacidosis)
Diabetic hypoglycemic coma
Insulin coma NOS

Excludes: *diabetes with hyperosmolar coma (250.2)*

□ **250.4 Diabetes with renal manifestations**
Use additional code, if desired, to identify manifestation, as:
diabetic:
nephropathy NOS (583.81)
nephrosis (581.81)
intercapillary glomerulosclerosis (581.81)
Kimmelstiel-Wilson syndrome (581.81)

□ **250.5 Diabetes with ophthalmic manifestations**
Use additional code, if desired, to identify manifestation, as:
diabetic:
blindness (369.00-369.9)
cataract (366.41)
glaucoma (365.44)
retinal edema (362.83)
retinopathy (362.01-362.02)

Add 4th or 5th digit | Nonspecific code | Unspecified code | Manifestation code

□ **250.6 Diabetes with neurological manifestations**

Use additional code, if desired, to identify manifestation, as:
diabetic:
amyotrophy (358.1)
mononeuropathy (354.0-355.9)
neurogenic arthropathy (713.5)
peripheral autonomic neuropathy (337.1)
polyneuropathy (357.2)

□ **250.7 Diabetes with peripheral circulatory disorders**

Use additional code, if desired, to identify manifestation, as:
diabetic:
gangrene (785.4)
peripheral angiopathy (443.81)

□ **250.8 Diabetes with other specified manifestations**

Diabetic hypoglycemia
Hypoglycemic shock

Use additional code, if desired, to identify manifestation, as:
diabetic bone changes (731.8)

Use additional E code, if desired, to identify cause, if drug-induced.

Excludes: *intercurrent infections in diabetic patients*

250.9 Diabetes with unspecified complication

251 Other disorders of pancreatic internal secretion

251.0 Hypoglycemic coma

Iatrogenic hyperinsulinism
Non-diabetic insulin coma

Use additional E code, if desired, to identify cause, if drug-induced

Excludes: *hypoglycemic coma in diabetes mellitus (250.3)*

251.1 Other specified hypoglycemia

Use additional E code, if desired, to identify cause, if drug-induced

Hyperinsulinism:
NOS
ectopic
functional
Hyperplasia of pancreatic islet beta cells NOS

Excludes: *hypoglycemia in diabetes mellitus (250.8)*
hypoglycemia in infant of diabetic mother (775.0)
hypoglycemic coma (251.0)
neonatal hypoglycemia (775.6)

251.2 Hypoglycemia, unspecified

Hypoglycemia:
NOS
reactive
spontaneous

Excludes: *hypoglycemia:*
with coma (251.0)
in diabetes mellitus (250.8)
leucine-induced (270.3)

251.3 Postsurgical hypoinsulinemia

Hypoinsulinemia following complete or partial pancreatectomy
Postpancreatectomy hyperglycemia

251.4 Abnormality of secretion of glucagon

Hyperplasia of pancreatic islet alpha cells with glucagon excess

251.5 Abnormality of secretion of gastrin

Hyperplasia of pancreatic alpha cells with gastrin excess
Zollinger-Ellison syndrome

251.8 Other specified disorders of pancreatic internal secretion

251.9 Unspecified disorder of pancreatic internal secretion

Islet cell hyperplasia NOS

252 Disorders of parathyroid gland

252.0 Hyperparathyroidism
Hyperplasia of parathyroid
Osteitis fibrosa cystica generalisata
von Recklinghausen's disease of bone

Excludes: *ectopic hyperparathyroidism (259.3)*
secondary hyperparathyroidism (of renal origin) (588.8)

252.1 Hypoparathyroidism
Parathyroiditis (autoimmune)
Tetany:
parathyroid
parathyroprival

Excludes: *pseudohypoparathyroidism (275.4)*
pseudo-pseudohypoparathyroidism (275.4)
tetany NOS (781.7)
transitory neonatal hypoparathyroidism (775.4)

252.8 Other specified disorders of parathyroid gland
Cyst } of parathyroid gland
Hemorrhage }

252.9 Unspecified disorder of parathyroid gland

253 Disorders of the pituitary gland and its hypothalamic control
Includes: the listed conditions whether the disorder is in the pituitary or the hypothalamus

Excludes: *Cushing's syndrome (255.0)*

253.0 Acromegaly and gigantism
Overproduction of growth hormone

253.1 Other and unspecified anterior pituitary hyperfunction
Forbes-Albright syndrome

Excludes: *overproduction of:*
ACTH (255.3)
thyroid-stimulating hormone [TSH] (242.8)

253.2 Panhypopituitarism
Cachexia, pituitary
Necrosis of pituitary (postpartum)
Pituitary insufficiency NOS
Sheehan's syndrome
Simmonds' disease

Excludes: *iatrogenic hypopituitarism (253.7)*

253.3 Pituitary dwarfism
Isolated deficiency of (human) growth hormone [HGH]
Lorain-Levi dwarfism

253.4 Other anterior pituitary disorders
Isolated or partial deficiency of an anterior pituitary hormone, other than growth hormone
Prolactin deficiency

253.5 Diabetes insipidus
Vasopressin deficiency

Excludes: *nephrogenic diabetes insipidus (588.1)*

253.6 Other disorders of neurohypophysis
Syndrome of inappropriate secretion of antidiuretic hormone [ADH]

Excludes: *ectopic antidiuretic hormone secretion (259.3)*

253.7 Iatrogenic pituitary disorders
Hypopituitarism:
hormone-induced
hypophysectomy-induced
postablative
radiotherapy-induced

Use additional E code, if desired, to identify cause

253.8 Other disorders of the pituitary and other syndromes of diencephalohypophyseal origin
Abscess of pituitary
Adiposogenital dystrophy
Cyst of Rathke's pouch
Fröhlich's syndrome

Excludes: *craniopharyngioma (237.0)*

Add 4th or 5th digit | Nonspecific code | Unspecified code | Manifestation code

253.9 Unspecified
Dyspituitarism

254 Diseases of thymus gland

Excludes: *aplasia or dysplasia with immunodeficiency (279.2)*
hypoplasia with immunodeficiency (279.2)
myasthenia gravis (358.0)

254.0 Persistent hyperplasia of thymus
Hypertrophy of thymus

254.1 Abscess of thymus

254.8 Other specified diseases of thymus gland
Atrophy } of thymus
Cyst } of thymus

Excludes *thymoma (212.6)*

254.9 Unspecified disease of thymus gland

255 Disorders of adrenal glands
Includes: the listed conditions whether the basic disorder is in the adrenals or is pituitary-induced

255.0 Cushing's syndrome
Adrenal hyperplasia due to excess ACTH
Cushing's syndrome:
NOS
iatrogenic
idiopathic
pituitary-dependent
Ectopic ACTH syndrome
Iatrogenic syndrome of excess cortisol
Overproduction of cortisol

Use additional E code, if desired, to identify cause, if drug-induced

Excludes: *congenital adrenal hyperplasia (255.2)*

255.1 Hyperaldosteronism
Aldosteronism (primary) (secondary)
Bartter's syndrome
Conn's syndrome

255.2 Adrenogenital disorders
Adrenogenital syndromes, virilizing or feminizing, whether acquired or associated with congenital adrenal hyperplasia consequent on inborn enzyme defects in hormone synthesis
Achard-Thiers syndrome
Congenital adrenal hyperplasia
Female adrenal pseudohermaphroditism
Male:
macrogenitosomia praecox
sexual precocity with adrenal hyperplasia
Virilization (female) (suprarenal)

Excludes: *adrenal hyperplasia due to excess ACTH (255.0)*
isosexual virilization (256.4)

255.3 Other corticoadrenal overactivity
Acquired benign adrenal androgenic overactivity
Overproduction of ACTH

255.4 Corticoadrenal insufficiency
Addisonian crisis
Addison's disease NOS
Adrenal:
atrophy (autoimmune)
calcification
Adrenal:
crisis
hemorrhage
infarction
insufficiency NOS

Excludes: *tuberculous Addison's disease (017.6)*

255.5 Other adrenal hypofunction
Adrenal medullary insufficiency

Excludes: *Waterhouse-Friderichsen syndrome (meningococcal) (036.3)*

255.6 Medulloadrenal hyperfunction
Catecholamine secretion by pheochromocytoma

255.8 Other specified disorders of adrenal glands
Abnormality of cortisol-binding globulin

255.9 Unspecified disorder of adrenal glands

● Code new to this edition ▲ Revision of existing code ④ ⑤ Fourth or fifth digit required

256 Ovarian dysfunction

256.0 Hyperestrogenism

256.1 Other ovarian hyperfunction
Hypersecretion of ovarian androgens

256.2 Postablative ovarian failure
Ovarian failure:
iatrogenic
postirradiation
postsurgical

256.3 Other ovarian failure
Premature menopause NOS
Primary ovarian failure

256.4 Polycystic ovaries
Isosexual virilization
Stein-Leventhal syndrome

256.8 Other ovarian dysfunction

256.9 Unspecified ovarian dysfunction

257 Testicular dysfunction

257.0 Testicular hyperfunction
Hypersecretion of testicular hormones

257.1 Postablative testicular hypofunction
Testicular hypofunction:
iatrogenic
postirradiation
postsurgical

257.2 Other testicular hypofunction
Defective biosynthesis of testicular androgen
Eunuchoidism:
NOS
hypogonadotropic
Failure:
Leydig's cell, adult
seminiferous tubule, adult
Testicular hypogonadism

Excludes: *azoospermia (606.0)*

257.8 Other testicular dysfunction
Goldberg-Maxwell syndrome
Male pseudohermaphroditism with testicular feminization
Testicular feminization

257.9 Unspecified testicular dysfunction

258 Polyglandular dysfunction and related disorders

258.0 Polyglandular activity in multiple endocrine adenomatosis
Wermer's syndrome

258.1 Other combinations of endocrine dysfunction
Lloyd's syndrome
Schmidt's syndrome

258.8 Other specified polyglandular dysfunction

258.9 Polyglandular dysfunction, unspecified

259 Other endocrine disorders

259.0 Delay in sexual development and puberty, not elsewhere classified
Delayed puberty

259.1 Precocious sexual development and puberty, not elsewhere classified
Sexual precocity:
NOS
constitutional
cryptogenic
idiopathic

259.2 Carcinoid syndrome
Hormone secretion by carcinoid tumors

259.3 Ectopic hormone secretion, not elsewhere classified
Ectopic:
antidiuretic hormone secretion [ADH]
hyperparathyroidism

Excludes: *ectopic ACTH syndrome (255.0)*

259.4 Dwarfism, not elsewhere classified
Dwarfism:
NOS
constitutional

Excludes: *dwarfism:*
achondroplastic (756.4)
intrauterine (759.7)
nutritional (263.2)
pituitary (253.3)
renal (588.0)
progeria (259.8)

259.8 Other specified endocrine disorders
Pineal gland dysfunction
Progeria
Werner's syndrome

259.9 Unspecified endocrine disorder
Disturbance:
endocrine NOS
hormone NOS
Infantilism NOS

NUTRITIONAL DEFICIENCIES (260-269)

Excludes: *deficiency anemias (280.0-281.9)*

260 Kwashiorkor
Nutritional edema with dyspigmentation of skin and hair

261 Nutritional marasmus
Nutritional atrophy
Severe calorie deficiency
Severe malnutrition NOS

262 Other severe protein-calorie malnutrition
Nutritional edema without mention of dyspigmentation of skin and hair

263 Other and unspecified protein-calorie malnutrition

263.0 Malnutrition of moderate degree

263.1 Malnutrition of mild degree

263.2 Arrested development following protein-calorie malnutrition
Nutritional dwarfism
Physical retardation due to malnutrition

263.8 Other protein-calorie malnutrition

263.9 Unspecified protein-calorie malnutrition
Dystrophy due to malnutrition
Malnutrition (calorie) NOS

Excludes: *nutritional deficiency NOS (269.9)*

264 Vitamin A deficiency

264.0 With conjunctival xerosis

264.1 With conjunctival xerosis and Bitot's spot
Bitot's spot in the young child

264.2 With corneal xerosis

264.3 With corneal ulceration and xerosis

264.4 With keratomalacia

264.5 With night blindness

264.6 With xerophthalmic scars of cornea

264.7 Other ocular manifestations of vitamin A deficiency
Xerophthalmia due to vitamin A deficiency

264.8 Other manifestations of vitamin A deficiency
Follicular keratosis } due to vitamin A deficiency
Xeroderma } due to vitamin A deficiency

264.9 Unspecified vitamin A deficiency
Hypovitaminosis A NOS

265 Thiamine and niacin deficiency states

265.0 Beriberi

265.1 Other and unspecified manifestations of thiamine deficiency
Other vitamin B_1 deficiency states

● Code new to this edition
▲ Revision of existing code
④ ⑤ Fourth or fifth digit required

265.2 Pellagra
Deficiency:
niacin (-tryptophan)
nicotinamide
nicotinic acid
vitamin PP
Pellagra (alcoholic)

266 Deficiency of B-complex components

266.0 Ariboflavinosis
Riboflavin [vitamin B_2] deficiency

266.1 Vitamin B_6 deficiency
Deficiency:
pyridoxal
pyridoxamine
pyridoxine
Vitamin B_6 deficiency syndrome

Excludes: *vitamin B_6-responsive sideroblastic anemia (285.0)*

266.2 Other B-complex deficiencies
Deficiency:
cyanocobalamin
folic acid
vitamin B_{12}

Excludes: *combined system disease with anemia (281.0-281.1)*
deficiency anemias (281.0-281.9)
subacute degeneration of spinal cord with anemia (281.0-281.1)

266.9 Unspecified vitamin B deficiency

267 Ascorbic acid deficiency
Deficiency of vitamin C
Scurvy

Excludes: *scorbutic anemia (281.8)*

268 Vitamin D deficiency

Excludes: *vitamin D-resistant:*
osteomalacia (275.3)
rickets (275.3)

268.0 Rickets, active

Excludes: *celiac rickets (579.0)*
renal rickets (588.0)

268.1 Rickets, late effect
Any condition specified as due to rickets and stated to be a late effect or sequela of rickets

Use additional code, if desired, to identify the nature of late effect

268.2 Osteomalacia, unspecified

268.9 Unspecified vitamin D deficiency
Avitaminosis D

269 Other nutritional deficiencies

269.0 Deficiency of vitamin K

Excludes: *deficiency of coagulation factor due to vitamin K deficiency (286.7)*
vitamin K deficiency of newborn (776.0)

269.1 Deficiency of other vitamins
Deficiency:
vitamin E
vitamin P

269.2 Unspecified vitamin deficiency
Multiple vitamin deficiency NOS

269.3 Mineral deficiency, not elsewhere classified
Deficiency:
calcium, dietary
iodine

Excludes: *deficiency:*
calcium NOS (275.4)
potassium (276.8)
sodium (276.1)

269.8 Other nutritional deficiency

Excludes: *failure to thrive (783.4)*
feeding problems (783.3)
newborn (779.3)

269.9 Unspecified nutritional deficiency

OTHER METABOLIC AND IMMUNITY DISORDERS (270-279)

Use additional code, if desired, to identify any associated mental retardation

270 Disorders of amino-acid transport and metabolism

Excludes: *abnormal findings without manifest disease (790.0-796.9)*
disorders of purine and pyrimidine metabolism (277.1-277.2)
gout (274.0-274.9)

270.0 Disturbances of amino-acid transport
Cystinosis
Cystinuria
Fanconi (-de Toni) (-Debré) syndrome
Glycinuria (renal)
Hartnup disease

270.1 Phenylketonuria [PKU]
Hyperphenylalaninemia

270.2 Other disturbances of aromatic amino-acid metabolism
Albinism
Alkaptonuria
Alkaptonuric ochronosis
Disturbances of metabolism of tyrosine and tryptophan
Homogentisic acid defects
Hydroxykynureninuria
Hypertyrosinemia
Indicanuria
Kynureninase defects
Oasthouse urine disease
Ochronosis
Tyrosinosis
Tyrosinuria
Waardenburg syndrome

Excludes: *vitamin B_6-deficiency syndrome (266.1)*

270.3 Disturbances of branched-chain amino-acid metabolism
Disturbances of metabolism of leucine, isoleucine, and valine
Hypervalinemia
Intermittent branched-chain ketonuria
Leucine-induced hypoglycemia
Leucinosis
Maple syrup urine disease

270.4 Disturbances of sulphur-bearing amino-acid metabolism
Cystathioninemia
Cystathioninuria
Disturbances of metabolism of methionine, homocystine, and cystathionine
Homocystinuria
Hypermethioninemia
Methioninemia

270.5 Disturbances of histidine metabolism
Carnosinemia
Histidinemia
Hyperhistidinemia
Imidazole aminoaciduria

270.6 Disorders of urea cycle metabolism
Argininosuccinic aciduria
Citrullinemia
Disorders of metabolism of ornithine, citrulline, argininosuccinic acid, arginine, and ammonia
Hyperammonemia
Hyperornithinemia

270.7 Other disturbances of straight-chain amino-acid metabolism

Glucoglycinuria
Glycinemia (with methyl-malonic acidemia)
Hyperglycinemia
Hyperlysinemia
Pipecolic acidemia
Saccharopinuria
Other disturbances of metabolism of glycine, threonine, serine, glutamine, and lysine

270.8 Other specified disorders of amino-acid metabolism

Alaninemia
Ethanolaminuria
Glycoprolinuria
Hydroxyprolinemia
Hyperprolinemia
Iminoacidopathy
Prolinemia
Prolinuria
Sarcosinemia

270.9 Unspecified disorder of amino-acid metabolism

271 Disorders of carbohydrate transport and metabolism

Excludes: *abnormality of secretion of glucagon (251.4)*
diabetes mellitus (250.0-250.9)
hypoglycemia NOS (251.2)
mucopolysaccharidosis (277.5)

271.0 Glycogenosis

Amylopectinosis
Glucose-6-phosphatase deficiency
Glycogen storage disease
McArdle's disease
Pompe's disease
von Gierke's disease

271.1 Galactosemia

Galactose-1-phosphate uridyl transferase deficiency
Galactosuria

271.2 Hereditary fructose intolerance

Essential benign fructosuria
Fructosemia

271.3 Intestinal disaccharidase deficiencies and disaccharide malabsorption

Intolerance or malabsorption (congenital) (of):
glucose-galactose
lactose
sucrose-isomaltose

271.4 Renal glycosuria

Renal diabetes

271.8 Other specified disorders of carbohydrate transport and metabolism

Essential benign pentosuria
Fucosidosis
Glycolic aciduria
Hyperoxaluria (primary)
Mannosidosis
Oxalosis
Xylosuria
Xylulosuria

271.9 Unspecified disorder of carbohydrate transport and metabolism

272 Disorders of lipoid metabolism

Excludes: *localized cerebral lipidoses (330.1)*

272.0 Pure hypercholesterolemia

Familial hypercholesterolemia
Fredrickson Type IIa hyperlipoproteinemia
Hyperbetalipoproteinemia
Hyperlipidemia, Group A
Low-density-lipoid-type [LDL] hyperlipoproteinemia

272.1 Pure hyperglyceridemia

Endogenous hyperglyceridemia
Fredrickson Type IV hyperlipoproteinemia
Hyperlipidemia, Group B
Hyperprebetalipoproteinemia
Hypertriglyceridemia, essential
Very-low-density-lipoid-type [VLDL] hyperlipoproteinemia

272.2 Mixed hyperlipidemia

Broad- or floating-betalipoproteinemia
Fredrickson Type IIb or III hyperlipoproteinemia
Hypercholesterolemia with endogenous hyperglyceridemia
Hyperbetalipoproteinemia with prebetalipoproteinemia
Tubo-eruptive xanthoma
Xanthoma tuberosum

272.3 Hyperchylomicronemia
Bürger-Grütz syndrome
Fredrickson type I or V hyperlipoproteinemia
Hyperlipidemia, Group D
Mixed hyperglyceridemia

272.4 Other and unspecified hyperlipidemia
Alpha-lipoproteinemia
Combined hyperlipidemia
Hyperlipidemia NOS
Hyperlipoproteinemia NOS

272.5 Lipoprotein deficiencies
Abetalipoproteinemia
Bassen-Kornzweig syndrome
High-density lipoid deficiency
Hypoalphalipoproteinemia
Hypobetalipoproteinemia (familial)

272.6 Lipodystrophy
Barraquer-Simons disease
Progressive lipodystrophy

Use additional E code, if desired, to identify cause, if iatrogenic

Excludes: *intestinal lipodystrophy (040.2)*

272.7 Lipidoses
Chemically-induced lipidosis
Disease:
  Anderson's
  Fabry's
  Gaucher's
  I cell [mucolipidosis I]
  lipoid storage NOS
  Neimann-Pick
  pseudo-Hurler's or mucolipidosis III
Disease:
  triglyceride storage, Type I or II
  Wolman's or triglyceride storage, Type III
Mucolipidosis II
Primary familial xanthomatosis

Excludes: *cerebral lipidoses (330.1)*
Tay-Sachs disease (330.1)

272.8 Other disorders of lipoid metabolism
Hoffa's disease or liposynovitis prepatellaris
Launois-Bensaude's lipomatosis
Lipoid dermatoarthritis

272.9 Unspecified disorder of lipoid metabolism

273 Disorders of plasma protein metabolism

Excludes: *agammaglobulinemia and hypogammaglobulinemia (279.0 -279.2)*
coagulation defects (286.0-286.9)
hereditary hemolytic anemias (282.0-282.9)

273.0 Polyclonal hypergammaglobulinemia
Hypergammaglobulinemic purpura:
  benign primary
  Waldenström's

273.1 Monoclonal paraproteinemia
Benign monoclonal hypergammaglobulinemia [BMH]
Monoclonal gammopathy:
  NOS
  associated with lymphoplasmacytic dyscrasias
  benign
Paraproteinemia:
  benign (familial)
  secondary to malignant or inflammatory disease

273.2 Other paraproteinemias
Cryoglobulinemic:
  purpura
  vasculitis
Mixed cryoglobulinemia

273.3 Macroglobulinemia
Macroglobulinemia (idiopathic) (primary)
Waldenström's macroglobulinemia

273.8 Other disorders of plasma protein metabolism
Abnormality of transport protein
Bisalbuminemia

273.9 Unspecified disorder of plasma protein metabolism

274 Gout

Excludes: *lead gout (984.0-984.9)*

274.0 Gouty arthropathy

274.1 Gouty nephropathy

274.10 Gouty nephropathy, unspecified

274.11 Uric acid nephrolithiasis

274.19 Other

274.8 Gout with other specified manifestations

274.81 Gouty tophi of ear

274.82 Gouty tophi of other sites
Gouty tophi of heart

274.89 Other
Use additional code, if desired, to identify manifestations, as:
gouty:
iritis (364.11)
neuritis (357.4)

274.9 Gout, unspecified

275 Disorders of mineral metabolism

Excludes: *abnormal findings without manifest disease (790.0-796.9)*

275.0 Disorders of iron metabolism
Bronzed diabetes
Hemochromatosis
Pigmentary cirrhosis (of liver)

Excludes: *anemia:*
iron deficiency (280.0-280.9)
sideroblastic (285.0)

275.1 Disorders of copper metabolism
Hepatolenticular degeneration
Wilson's disease

275.2 Disorders of magnesium metabolism
Hypermagnesemia
Hypomagnesemia

275.3 Disorders of phosphorus metabolism
Familial hypophosphatemia
Hypophosphatasia
Vitamin D-resistant:
osteomalacia
rickets

275.4 Disorders of calcium metabolism
Calcinosis
Hypercalcemia
Hypercalcinuria
Nephrocalcinosis
Pseudohypoparathyroidism
Pseudo-pseudohypoparathyroidism

Excludes: *parathyroid disorders (252.0-252.9)*
vitamin D deficiency (268.0-268.9)

275.8 Other specified disorders of mineral metabolism

275.9 Unspecified disorder of mineral metabolism

276 Disorders of fluid, electrolyte, and acid-base balance

Excludes: *diabetes insipidus (253.5)*
familial periodic paralysis (359.3)

276.0 Hyperosmolality and/or hypernatremia
Sodium [Na] excess
Sodium [Na] overload

276.1 Hyposmolality and/or hyponatremia
Sodium [Na] deficiency

276.2 Acidosis
Acidosis:
NOS
lactic
metabolic
respiratory

Excludes: *diabetic acidosis (250.1)*

Add 4th or 5th digit | Nonspecific code | Unspecified code | Manifestation code

276.3 Alkalosis
Alkalosis:
NOS
metabolic
respiratory

276.4 Mixed acid-base balance disorder
Hypercapnia with mixed acid-base disorder

276.5 Volume depletion
Dehydration
Depletion of volume of plasma or extracellular fluid
Hypovolemia

Excludes: *hypovolemic shock:*
postoperative (998.0)
traumatic (958.4)

276.6 Fluid overload
Fluid retention

Excludes: *ascites (789.5)*
localized edema (782.3)

276.7 Hyperpotassemia
Hyperkalemia
Potassium [K]:
excess
intoxication
overload

276.8 Hypopotassemia
Hypokalemia
Potassium [K] deficiency

276.9 Electrolyte and fluid disorders not elsewhere classified
Electrolyte imbalance
Hyperchloremia
Hypochloremia

Excludes: *electrolyte imbalance:*
associated with hyperemesis gravidarum (643.1)
complicating labor and delivery (669.0)
following abortion and ectopic or molar pregnancy (634-638 with .4, 639.4)

277 Other and unspecified disorders of metabolism

277.0 Cystic fibrosis
Fibrocystic disease of the pancreas
Mucoviscidosis

277.00 Without mention of meconium ileus

277.01 With meconium ileus
Meconium:
ileus (of newborn)
obstruction of intestine in mucoviscidosis

277.1 Disorders of porphyrin metabolism
Hematoporphyria
Hematoporphyrinuria
Hereditary coproporphyria
Porphyria
Porphyrinuria
Protocoproporphyria
Protoporphyria
Pyrroloporphyria

277.2 Other disorders of purine and pyrimidine metabolism
Hypoxanthine-guanine-phosphoribosyltransferase deficiency [HG-PRT deficiency]
Lesch-Nyhan syndrome
Xanthinuria

Excludes: *gout (274.0-274.9)*
orotic aciduric anemia (281.4)

277.3 Amyloidosis
Amyloidosis:
NOS
inherited systemic
nephropathic
neuropathic (Portuguese) (Swiss)
secondary
Benign paroxysmal peritonitis
Familial Mediterranean fever
Hereditary cardiac amyloidosis

277.4 Disorders of bilirubin excretion

Hyperbilirubinemia:
- congenital
- constitutional

Syndrome:
- Crigler-Najjar
- Dubin-Johnson
- Gilbert's
- Rotor's

Excludes: *hyperbilirubinemias specific to the perinatal period (774.0-774.7)*

277.5 Mucopolysaccharidosis

Gargoylism
Hunter's syndrome
Hurler's syndrome
Lipochondrodystrophy
Maroteaux-Lamy syndrome
Morquio-Brailsford disease
Osteochondrodystrophy
Sanfilippo's syndrome
Scheie's syndrome

277.6 Other deficiencies of circulating enzymes

Alpha 1-antitrypsin deficiency
Hereditary angioedema

277.8 Other specified disorders of metabolism

Hand-Schüller-Christian disease
Histiocytosis (acute) (chronic)
Histiocytosis X (chronic)

Excludes: *histiocytosis:*
- *acute differentiated progressive (202.5)*
- *X, acute (progressive) (202.5)*

277.9 Unspecified disorder of metabolism

Enzymopathy NOS

278 Obesity and other hyperalimentation

Excludes: *hyperalimentation NOS (783.6)*
poisoning by vitamins NOS (963.5)
polyphagia (783.6)

278.0 Obesity

Excludes: *adiposogenital dystrophy (253.8)*
obesity of endocrine origin NOS (259.9)

● **278.00 Obesity, unspecified**

Obesity NOS

● **278.01 Morbid obesity**

278.1 Localized adiposity

Fat pad

278.2 Hypervitaminosis A

278.3 Hypercarotinemia

278.4 Hypervitaminosis D

278.8 Other hyperalimentation

279 Disorders involving the immune mechanism

279.0 Deficiency of humoral immunity

279.00 Hypogammaglobulinemia, unspecified

Agammaglobulinemia NOS

279.01 Selective IgA immunodeficiency

279.02 Selective IgM immunodeficiency

279.03 Other selective immunoglobulin deficiencies

Selective deficiency of IgG

279.04 Congenital hypogammaglobulinemia

Agammaglobulinemia:
- Bruton's type
- X-linked

279.05 Immunodeficiency with increased IgM

Immunodeficiency with hyper-IgM:
- autosomal recessive
- X-linked

279.06 Common variable immunodeficiency
Dysgammaglobulinemia (acquired) (congenital) (primary)
Hypogammaglobulinemia:
acquired primary
congenital non-sex-linked
sporadic

279.09 Other
Transient hypogammaglobulinemia of infancy

279.1 Deficiency of cell-mediated immunity

279.10 Immunodeficiency with predominant T-cell defect, unspecified

279.11 DiGeorge's syndrome
Pharyngeal pouch syndrome
Thymic hypoplasia

279.12 Wiskott-Aldrich syndrome

279.13 Nezelof's syndrome
Cellular immunodeficiency with abnormal immunoglobulin deficiency

279.19 Other

Excludes: *ataxia-telangiectasia (334.8)*

279.2 Combined immunity deficiency
Agammaglobulinemia:
autosomal recessive
Swiss-type
x-linked recessive
Severe combined immunodeficiency [SCID]
Thymic:
alymphoplasia
aplasia or dysplasia with immunodeficiency

Excludes: *thymic hypoplasia (279.11)*

279.3 Unspecified immunity deficiency

279.4 Autoimmune disease, not elsewhere classified
Autoimmune disease NOS

Excludes: *transplant failure or rejection (996.80-996.89)*

279.8 Other specified disorders involving the immune mechanism
Single complement [C_1-C_9] deficiency or dysfunction

279.9 Unspecified disorder of immune mechanism

4. DISEASES OF THE BLOOD AND BLOOD-FORMING ORGANS (280-289)

Excludes: *anemia complicating pregnancy or the puerperium (648.2)*

280 Iron deficiency anemias

Includes: anemia:
- asiderotic
- hypochromic-microcytic
- sideropenic

Excludes: *familial microcytic anemia (282.4)*

280.0 Secondary to blood loss (chronic)
Normocytic anemia due to blood loss

Excludes: *acute posthemorrhagic anemia (285.1)*

280.1 Secondary to inadequate dietary iron intake

280.8 Other specified iron deficiency anemias
Paterson-Kelly syndrome
Plummer-Vinson syndrome
Sideropenic dysphagia

280.9 Iron deficiency anemia, unspecified
Anemia:
- achlorhydric
- chlorotic
- idiopathic hypochromic
- iron [Fe] deficiency NOS

281 Other deficiency anemias

281.0 Pernicious anemia
Anemia:
- Addison's
- Biermer's
- congenital pernicious

Congenital intrinsic factor [Castle's] deficiency

Excludes: *combined system disease without mention of anemia (266.2)*
subacute degeneration of spinal cord without mention of anemia (266.2)

281.1 Other vitamin B_{12} deficiency anemia
Anemia:
- vegan's
- vitamin B_{12} deficiency (dietary)
- due to selective vitamin B_{12} malabsorption with proteinuria

Syndrome:
- Imerslund's
- Imerslund-Gräsbeck

Excludes: *combined system disease without mention of anemia (266.2)*
subacute degeneration of spinal cord without mention of anemia (266.2)

281.2 Folate-deficiency anemia
Congenital folate malabsorption
Folate or folic acid deficiency anemia:
- NOS
- dietary
- drug-induced

Goat's milk anemia
Nutritional megaloblastic anemia (of infancy)

Use additional E code, if desired, to identify drug

281.3 Other specified megaloblastic anemias not elsewhere classified
Combined B_{12} and folate-deficiency anemia
Refractory megaloblastic anemia

281.4 Protein-deficiency anemia
Amino-acid-deficiency anemia

281.8 Anemia associated with other specified nutritional deficiency
Scorbutic anemia

281.9 Unspecified deficiency anemia
Anemia:
- dimorphic
- macrocytic
- megaloblastic NOS

Anemia:
- nutritional NOS
- simple chronic

282 Hereditary hemolytic anemias

282.0 Hereditary spherocytosis
Acholuric (familial) jaundice
Congenital hemolytic anemia (spherocytic)
Congenital spherocytosis
Minkowski-Chauffard syndrome
Spherocytosis (familial)

Excludes: *hemolytic anemia of newborn (773.0-773.5)*

282.1 Hereditary elliptocytosis
Elliptocytosis (congenital)
Ovalocytosis (congenital) (hereditary)

282.2 Anemias due to disorders of glutathione metabolism
Anemia:
- 6-phosphogluconic dehydrogenase deficiency
- enzyme deficiency, drug-induced
- erythrocytic glutathione deficiency
- glucose-6-phosphate dehydrogenase [G-6-PD] deficiency
- glutathione-reductase deficiency
- hemolytic nonspherocytic (hereditary), type I

Disorder of pentose phosphate pathway
Favism

282.3 Other hemolytic anemias due to enzyme deficiency
Anemia:
- hemolytic nonspherocytic (hereditary), type II
- hexokinase deficiency
- pyruvate kinase [PK] deficiency
- triosephosphate isomerase deficiency

282.4 Thalassemias
Cooley's anemia
Hereditary leptocytosis
Mediterranean anemia (with other hemoglobinopathy)
Microdrepanocytosis
Sickle-cell thalassemia
Thalassemia (alpha) (beta) (intermedia) (major) (minima) (minor) (mixed) (trait) (with other hemoglobinopathy)
Thalassemia-Hb-S disease

Excludes: *sickle-cell:*
- *anemia (282.60-282.69)*
- *trait (282.5)*

282.5 Sickle-cell trait
Hb-AS genotype
Hemoglobin S [Hb-S] trait
Heterozygous:
- hemoglobin S
- Hb-S

Excludes: *that with other hemoglobinopathy (282.60-282.69)*
that with thalassemia (282.4)

282.6 Sickle-cell anemia

Excludes: *sickle-cell thalassemia (282.4)*
sickle-cell trait (282.5)

282.60 Sickle-cell anemia, unspecified

282.61 Hb-S disease without mention of crisis

282.62 Hb-S disease with mention of crisis
Sickle-cell crisis NOS

282.63 Sickle-cell/Hb-C disease
Hb-S/Hb-C disease

282.69 Other
Disease:
- Hb-S/Hb-D
- Hb-S/Hb-E

Disease:
- sickle-cell/Hb-D
- sickle-cell/Hb-E

● Code new to this edition ▲ Revision of existing code ④ ⑤ Fourth or fifth digit required

282.7 Other hemoglobinopathies
Abnormal hemoglobin NOS
Congenital Heinz-body anemia
Disease:
  Hb-Bart's
  hemoglobin C [Hb-C]
  hemoglobin D [Hb-D]
  hemoglobin E [Hb-E]
  hemoglobin Zurich [Hb-Zurich]
Hemoglobinopathy NOS
Hereditary persistence of fetal hemoglobin [HPFH]
Unstable hemoglobin hemolytic disease

Excludes: *familial polycythemia (289.6)*
hemoglobin M [Hb-M] disease (289.7)
high-oxygen-affinity hemoglobin (289.0)

282.8 Other specified hereditary hemolytic anemias
Stomatocytosis

282.9 Hereditary hemolytic anemia, unspecified
Hereditary hemolytic anemia NOS

283 Acquired hemolytic anemias

283.0 Autoimmune hemolytic anemias
Autoimmune hemolytic anemias (cold type) (warm type)
Chronic cold hemagglutinin disease
Cold agglutinin disease or hemoglobinuria
Hemolytic anemia:
  cold type (secondary) (symptomatic)
  drug-induced
  warm type (secondary) (symptomatic)

Use additional E code, if desired, to identify cause, if drug-induced

Excludes: *Evans' syndrome (287.3)*
hemolytic disease of newborn (773.0-773.5)

283.1 Non-autoimmune hemolytic anemias

283.10 Non-autoimmune hemolytic anemia, unspecified

283.11 Hemolytic-uremic syndrome

283.19 Other non-autoimmune hemolytic anemias
Hemolytic anemia:
  mechanical
  microangiopathic
  toxic

Use additional E code, if desired, to identify cause

283.2 Hemoglobinuria due to hemolysis from external causes
Acute intravascular hemolysis
Hemoglobinuria:
  from exertion
  march
  paroxysmal (cold) (nocturnal)
  due to other hemolysis
Marchiafava-Micheli syndrome

Use additional E code, if desired, to identify cause

283.9 Acquired hemolytic anemia, unspecified
Acquired hemolytic anemia NOS
Chronic idiopathic hemolytic anemia

284 Aplastic anemia

284.0 Constitutional aplastic anemia
Aplasia, (pure) red cell:
  congenital
  of infants
  primary
Blackfan-Diamond syndrome
Familial hypoplastic anemia
Fanconi's anemia
Pancytopenia with malformations

284.8 Other specified aplastic anemias

Aplastic anemia (due to):
- chronic systemic disease
- drugs
- infection
- radiation
- toxic (paralytic)

Pancytopenia (acquired)

Red cell aplasia (acquired) (adult) (pure) (with thymoma)

Use additional E code, if desired, to identify cause

284.9 Aplastic anemia, unspecified

Anemia:
- aplastic (idiopathic) NOS
- aregenerative
- hypoplastic NOS

Anemia:
- nonregenerative
- refractory

Medullary hypoplasia

285 Other and unspecified anemias

285.0 Sideroblastic anemia

Anemia:
- hypochromic with iron loading
- sideroachrestic
- sideroblastic
  - acquired
  - congenital
  - hereditary
  - primary
  - refractory
  - secondary (drug-induced) (due to disease)
  - sex-linked hypochromic
  - vitamin B_6-responsive

Pyridoxine-responsive (hypochromic) anemia

Use additional E code, if desired, to identify cause, if drug induced

285.1 Acute posthemorrhagic anemia

Anemia due to acute blood loss

Excludes: *anemia due to chronic blood loss (280.0)*
blood loss anemia NOS (280.0)

285.8 Other specified anemias

Anemia:
- dyserythropoietic (congenital)
- dyshematopoietic (congenital)
- leukoerythroblastic
- von Jaksch's

Infantile pseudoleukemia

285.9 Anemia, unspecified

Anemia:
- NOS
- essential
- normocytic, not due to blood loss

Anemia:
- profound
- progressive
- secondary

Oligocythemia

Excludes: *anemia (due to):*
blood loss:
acute (285.1)
chronic or unspecified (280.0)
iron deficiency (280.0-280.9)

286 Coagulation defects

286.0 Congenital factor VIII disorder

Antihemophilic globulin [AHG] deficiency

Factor VIII (functional) deficiency

Hemophilia:
- NOS
- A
- classical
- familial
- hereditary

Subhemophilia

Excludes: *factor VIII deficiency with vascular defect (286.4)*

● Code new to this edition ▲ Revision of existing code ④ ⑤ Fourth or fifth digit required

286.1 Congenital factor IX disorder
Christmas disease
Deficiency:
  factor IX (functional)
  plasma thromboplastin component [PTC]
Hemophilia B

286.2 Congenital factor XI deficiency
Hemophilia C
Plasma thromboplastin antecedent [PTA] deficiency
Rosenthal's disease

286.3 Congenital deficiency of other clotting factors
Congenital afibrinogenemia
Deficiency:
  AC globulin factor:
    I [fibrinogen]
    II [prothrombin]
    V [labile]
    VII [stable]
    X [Stuart-Prower]
    XII [Hageman]
    XIII [fibrin stabilizing]
Deficiency:
  Laki-Lorand factor
  proaccelerin
Disease:
  Owren's
  Stuart-Prower
Dysfibrinogenemia (congenital)
Dysprothrombinemia (constitutional)
Hypoproconvertinemia
Hypoprothrombinemia (hereditary)
Parahemophilia

286.4 von Willebrand's disease
Angiohemophilia (A) (B)
Constitutional thrombopathy
Factor VIII deficiency with vascular defect
Pseudohemophilia type B
Vascular hemophilia
von Willebrand's (-Jürgens') disease

Excludes: *factor VIII deficiency:*
  NOS (286.0)
  with functional defect (286.0)
hereditary capillary fragility (287.8)

286.5 Hemorrhagic disorder due to circulating anticoagulants
Antithrombinemia
Antithromboplastinemia
Antithromboplastinogenemia
Hyperheparinemia
Increase in:
  anti-VIIIa
  anti-IXa
  anti-Xa
  anti-XIa
  antithrombin
Systemic lupus erythematosus [SLE] inhibitor

Use additional E code, if desired, to identify cause, if drug induced

286.6 Defibrination syndrome
Afibrinogenemia, acquired
Consumption coagulopathy
Diffuse or disseminated intravascular coagulation [DIC syndrome]
Fibrinolytic hemorrhage, acquired
Hemorrhagic fibrinogenolysis
Pathologic fibrinolysis
Purpura:
  fibrinolytic
  fulminans

Excludes: *that complicating:*
  abortion (634-638 with .1, 639.1)
  pregnancy or the puerperium (641.3, 666.3)
disseminated intravascular coagulation in newborn (776.2)

286.7 Acquired coagulation factor deficiency
Deficiency of coagulation factor due to:
  liver disease
  vitamin K deficiency
Hypoprothrombinemia, acquired

Excludes: *vitamin K deficiency of newborn (776.0)*

Use additional E-code, if desired, to identify cause, if drug induced

Add 4th or 5th digit | Nonspecific code | Unspecified code | Manifestation code

286.9 Other and unspecified coagulation defects
Defective coagulation NOS
Deficiency, coagulation factor NOS
Delay, coagulation
Disorder:
  coagulation
  hemostasis

Excludes: *abnormal coagulation profile (790.92)*
hemorrhagic disease of newborn (776.0)
that complicating:
  abortion (634-638 with .1, 639.1)
  pregnancy or the puerperium (641.3, 666.3)

287 Purpura and other hemorrhagic conditions

Excludes: *hemorrhagic thrombocythemia (238.7)*
purpura fulminans (286.6)

287.0 Allergic purpura
Peliosis rheumatica
Purpura:
  anaphylactoid
  autoimmune
  Henoch's
Purpura:
  nonthrombocytopenic:
    hemorrhagic
    idiopathic
  rheumatica
  Schönlein-Henoch
  vascular
Vasculitis, allergic

Excludes: *hemorrhagic purpura (287.3)*
purpura annularis telangiectodes (709.1)

287.1 Qualitative platelet defects
Thrombasthenia (hemorrhagic) (hereditary)
Thrombocytasthenia
Thrombocytopathy (dystrophic)
Thrombopathy (Bernard-Soulier)

Excludes: *von Willebrand's disease (286.4)*

287.2 Other nonthrombocytopenic purpuras
Purpura:
  NOS
  senile
  simplex

287.3 Primary thrombocytopenia
Evans' syndrome
Megakaryocytic hypoplasia
Purpura, thrombocytopenic
  congenital
  hereditary
  idiopathic
Thrombocytopenia:
  congenital
  hereditary
  primary
Tidal platelet dysgenesis

Excludes: *thrombotic thrombocytopenic purpura (446.6)*
transient thrombocytopenia of newborn (776.1)

287.4 Secondary thrombocytopenia
Posttransfusion purpura
Thrombocytopenia (due to):
  dilutional
  drugs
  extracorporeal circulation of blood
  massive blood transfusion
  platelet alloimmunization

Use additional E code, if desired, to identify cause

Excludes: *transient thrombocytopenia of newborn (776.1)*

287.5 Thrombocytopenia, unspecified

287.8 Other specified hemorrhagic conditions
Capillary fragility (hereditary)
Vascular pseudohemophilia

287.9 Unspecified hemorrhagic conditions
Hemorrhagic diathesis (familial)

288 Diseases of white blood cells

Excludes: *leukemia (204.0-208.9)*

288.0 Agranulocytosis

Infantile genetic agranulocytosis
Kostmann's syndrome
Neutropenia:
- NOS
- cyclic
- drug-induced
- immune
- periodic
- toxic

Neutropenic splenomegaly

Use additional E code, if desired, to identify drug or other cause

Excludes: *transitory neonatal neutropenia (776.7)*

288.1 Functional disorders of polymorphonuclear neutrophils

Chronic (childhood) granulomatous disease
Congenital dysphagocytosis
Job's syndrome
Lipochrome histiocytosis (familial)
Progressive septic granulomatosis

288.2 Genetic anomalies of leukocytes

Anomaly (granulation) (granulocyte) or syndrome:
- Alder's (-Reilly)
- Chédiak-Steinbrinck (-Higashi)
- Jordan's
- May-Hegglin
- Pelger-Huet

Hereditary:
- hypersegmentation
- hyposegmentation
- leukomelanopathy

288.3 Eosinophilia

Eosinophilia
- allergic
- hereditary
- idiopathic
- secondary

Eosinophilic leukocytosis

Excludes: *Löffler's syndrome (518.3)*
pulmonary eosinophilia (518.3)

288.8 Other specified disease of white blood cells

Leukemoid reaction
- lymphocytic
- monocytic
- myelocytic

Leukocytosis
Lymphocytopenia
Lymphocytosis (symptomatic)
Lymphopenia
Monocytosis (symptomatic)
Plasmacytosis

Excludes: *immunity disorders (279.0-279.9)*

288.9 Unspecified disease of white blood cells

289 Other diseases of blood and blood-forming organs

289.0 Polycythemia, secondary

High-oxygen-affinity hemoglobin
Polycythemia:
- acquired
- benign
- due to:
  - fall in plasma volume
  - high altitude
- emotional
- erythropoietin
- hypoxemic
- nephrogenous
- relative
- spurious
- stress

Excludes: *polycythemia:*
- *neonatal (776.4)*
- *primary (238.4)*
- *vera (238.4)*

Add 4th or 5th digit | Nonspecific code | Unspecified code | Manifestation code

289.1 Chronic lymphadenitis
Chronic:
adenitis } any lymph node, except mesenteric
lymphadenitis } any lymph node, except mesenteric

Excludes: *acute lymphadenitis (683)*
mesenteric (289.2)
enlarged glands NOS (785.6)

289.2 Nonspecific mesenteric lymphadenitis
Mesenteric lymphadenitis (acute) (chronic)

289.3 Lymphadenitis, unspecified, except mesenteric

289.4 Hypersplenism
"Big spleen" syndrome
Dyssplenism
Hypersplenia

Excludes: *primary splenic neutropenia (288.0)*

289.5 Other diseases of spleen

289.50 Disease of spleen, unspecified

289.51 Chronic congestive splenomegaly

289.59 Other
Lien migrans
Perisplenitis
Splenic:
abscess
atrophy
cyst
Splenic:
fibrosis
infarction
rupture, nontraumatic
Splenitis
Wandering spleen

Excludes: *bilharzial splenic fibrosis (120.0-120.9)*
hepatolienal fibrosis (571.5)
splenomegaly NOS (789.2)

289.6 Familial polycythemia
Familial:
benign polycythemia
erythrocytosis

289.7 Methemoglobinemia
Congenital NADH [DPNH]-methemoglobin-reductase deficiency
Hemoglobin M [Hb-M] disease
Methemoglobinemia:
NOS
acquired (with sulfhemoglobinemia)
hereditary
toxic
Stokvis' disease
Sulfhemoglobinemia

Use additional E code, if desired, to identify cause

289.8 Other specified diseases of blood and blood-forming organs
Hypergammaglobulinemia
Myelofibrosis
Pseudocholinesterase deficiency

289.9 Unspecified diseases of blood and blood-forming organs
Blood dyscrasia NOS
Erythroid hyperplasia

5. MENTAL DISORDERS (290-319)

In the International Classification of Diseases, 9th Revision (*ICD-9*), the corresponding Chapter V, "Mental Disorders," includes a glossary which defines the contents of each category. The introduction to Chapter V in *ICD-9* indicates that the glossary is intended so that psychiatrists can make the diagnosis based on the descriptions provided rather than from the category titles. Lay coders are instructed to code whatever diagnosis the physician records.

Chapter 5, "Mental Disorders," in *ICD-9-CM* uses the standard classification format with inclusion and exclusion terms, omitting the glossary as part of the main text.

The mental disorders section of *ICD-9-CM* has been expanded to incorporate additional psychiatric disorders not listed in *ICD-9*. The glossary from *ICD-9* does not contain all these terms. It now appears in Appendix B, pages 543-564 which also contains descriptions and definitions for the terms added in *ICD-9-CM*. Some of these were provided by the American Psychiatric Association's Task Force on Nomenclature and Statistics who are preparing the *Diagnostic and Statistical Manual*, Third Edition (DSM-III), and others from *A Psychiatric Glossary*.

The American Psychiatric Association provided invaluable assistance in modifying Chapter 5 of *ICD-9-CM* to incorporate detail useful to American clinicians and gave permission to use material from the aforementioned sources.

1. **Manual of the *International Statistical Classification of Diseases, Injuries, and Causes of Death*, 9th Revision, World Health Organization, Geneva, Switzerland, 1975.**
2. **American Psychiatric Association, Task Force on Nomenclature and Statistics, Robert L. Spitzer, M.D., Chairman.**
3. ***A Psychiatric Glossary*, Fourth Edition, American Psychiatric Association, Washington, D.C., 1975.**

PSYCHOSES (290-299)

Excludes: *mental retardation (317-319)*

ORGANIC PSYCHOTIC CONDITIONS (290-294)

Includes: psychotic organic brain syndrome

Excludes: *nonpsychotic syndromes of organic etiology (310.0-310.9)*
psychoses classifiable to 295-298 and without impairment of orientation, comprehension, calculation, learning capacity, and judgement, but associated with physical disease, injury, or condition affecting the brain [e.g., following childbirth] (295.0-298.8)

290 Senile and presenile organic psychotic conditions

Use additional code to identify the associated neurological conditions, as:
Alzheimer's disease (331.0)
Jakob-Creutzfeldt disease (046.1)
Pick's disease of the brain (331.1)

Excludes: *dementia not classified as senile, presenile, or arteriosclerotic (294.1)*
psychoses classifiable to 295-298 occurring in the senium without dementia or delirium (295.0-298.8)
senility with mental changes of nonpsychotic severity (310.1)
transient organic psychotic conditions (293.0-293.9)

290.0 Senile dementia, uncomplicated

Senile dementia:
NOS
simple type

Excludes: *mild memory disturbances, not amounting to dementia, associated with senile brain disease (310.1)*
senile dementia with:
delirium or confusion (290.3)
delusional [paranoid] features (290.20)
depressive features (290.21)

290.1 Presenile dementia

Brain syndrome with presenile brain disease
Dementia in:
Alzheimer's disease
Jakob-Creutzfeldt disease
Pick's disease of the brain

Excludes: *arteriosclerotic dementia (290.40-290.43)*
dementia associated with other cerebral conditions (294.1)

290.10 Presenile dementia, uncomplicated
Presenile dementia:
NOS
simple type

290.11 Presenile dementia with delirium
Presenile dementia with acute confusional state

290.12 Presenile dementia with delusional features
Presenile dementia, paranoid type

290.13 Presenile dementia with depressive features
Presenile dementia, depressed type

290.2 Senile dementia with delusional or depressive features

Excludes: *senile dementia:*
NOS (290.0)
with delirium and/or confusion (290.3)

290.20 Senile dementia with delusional features
Senile dementia, paranoid type
Senile psychosis NOS

290.21 Senile dementia with depressive features

290.3 Senile dementia with delirium
Senile dementia with acute confusional state

Excludes: *senile:*
dementia NOS (290.0)
psychosis NOS (290.20)

290.4 Arteriosclerotic dementia
Multi-infarct dementia or psychosis

Use additional code to identify cerebral atherosclerosis (437.0)

Excludes: *suspected cases with no clear evidence of arteriosclerosis (290.9)*

290.40 Arteriosclerotic dementia, uncomplicated
Arteriosclerotic dementia:
NOS
simple type

290.41 Arteriosclerotic dementia with delirium
Arteriosclerotic dementia with acute confusional state

290.42 Arteriosclerotic dementia with delusional features
Arteriosclerotic dementia, paranoid type

290.43 Arteriosclerotic dementia with depressive features
Arteriosclerotic dementia, depressed type

290.8 Other specified senile psychotic conditions
Presbyophrenic psychosis

290.9 Unspecified senile psychotic condition

291 Alcoholic psychoses

Excludes: *alcoholism without psychosis (303.0-303.9)*

291.0 Alcohol withdrawal delirium
Alcoholic delirium
Delirium tremens

291.1 Alcohol amnestic syndrome
Alcoholic polyneuritic psychosis
Korsakoff's psychosis, alcoholic
Wernicke-Korsakoff syndrome (alcoholic)

291.2 Other alcoholic dementia
Alcoholic dementia NOS
Alcoholism associated with dementia NOS
Chronic alcoholic brain syndrome

291.3 Alcohol withdrawal hallucinosis
Alcoholic:
hallucinosis (acute)
psychosis with hallucinosis

Excludes: *alcohol withdrawal with delirium (291.0)*
schizophrenia (295.0-295.9) and paranoid states (297.0-297.9) taking the form of chronic hallucinosis with clear consciousness in an alcoholic

● Code new to this edition
▲ Revision of existing code
④ ⑤ Fourth or fifth digit required

291.4 Idiosyncratic alcohol intoxication
Pathologic:
alcohol intoxication
drunkenness

Excludes: *acute alcohol intoxication (305.0)*
in alcoholism (303.0)
simple drunkenness (305.0)

291.5 Alcoholic jealousy
Alcoholic:
paranoia
psychosis, paranoid type

Excludes: *nonalcoholic paranoid states (297.0-297.9)*
schizophrenia, paranoid type (295.3)

291.8 Other specified alcoholic psychosis
Alcohol:
abstinence syndrome or symptoms
withdrawal syndrome or symptoms

Excludes: *alcohol withdrawal:*
delirium (291.0)
hallucinosis (291.3)
delirium tremens (291.0)

291.9 Unspecified alcoholic psychosis
Alcoholic:
mania NOS
psychosis NOS
Alcoholism (chronic) with psychosis

292 Drug psychoses
Includes: drug-induced mental disorders
organic brain syndrome associated with consumption of drugs

Use additional code for any associated drug dependence (304.0-304.9)

Use additional E code, if desired, to identify drug

292.0 Drug withdrawal syndrome
Drug:
abstinence syndrome or symptoms
withdrawal syndrome or symptoms

292.1 Paranoid and/or hallucinatory states induced by drugs

292.11 Drug-induced organic delusional syndrome
Paranoid state induced by drugs

292.12 Drug-induced hallucinosis
Hallucinatory state induced by drugs

Excludes: *states following LSD or other hallucinogens, lasting only a few days or less ["bad trips"] (305.3)*

292.2 Pathological drug intoxication
Drug reaction:
NOS
idiosyncratic
pathologic
} resulting in brief psychotic states

Excludes: *expected brief psychotic reactions to hallucinogens ["bad trips"] (305.3)*
physiological side-effects of drugs (e.g., dystonias)

292.8 Other specified drug-induced mental disorders

292.81 Drug-induced delirium

292.82 Drug-induced dementia

292.83 Drug-induced amnestic syndrome

292.84 Drug-induced organic affective syndrome
Depressive state induced by drugs

292.89 Other
Drug-induced organic personality syndrome

292.9 Unspecified drug-induced mental disorder
Organic psychosis NOS due to or associated with drugs

293 Transient organic psychotic conditions

Includes: transient organic mental disorders not associated with alcohol or drugs

Use additional code to identify the associated physical or neurological condition

Excludes: *confusional state or delirium superimposed on senile dementia (290.3)*
dementia due to:
alcohol (291.0-291.9)
arteriosclerosis (290.40-290.43)
drugs (292.82)
senility (290.0)

293.0 Acute delirium

Acute:
confusional state
infective psychosis
organic reaction
posttraumatic organic psychosis
psycho-organic syndrome

Acute psychosis associated with endocrine, metabolic, or cerebrovascular disorder

Epileptic:
confusional state
twilight state

293.1 Subacute delirium

Subacute:
confusional state
infective psychosis
organic reaction
posttraumatic organic psychosis

Subacute:
psycho-organic syndrome
psychosis associated with endocrine or metabolic disorder

293.8 Other specified transient organic mental disorders

293.81 Organic delusional syndrome

Transient organic psychotic condition, paranoid type

293.82 Organic hallucinosis syndrome

Transient organic psychotic condition, hallucinatory type

293.83 Organic affective syndrome

Transient organic psychotic condition, depressive type

293.89 Other

293.9 Unspecified transient organic mental disorder

Organic psychosis:
infective NOS
posttraumatic NOS
transient NOS

Psycho-organic syndrome

294 Other organic psychotic conditions (chronic)

Includes: organic psychotic brain syndromes (chronic), not elsewhere classified

294.0 Amnestic syndrome

Korsakoff's psychosis or syndrome (nonalcoholic)

Excludes: *alcoholic:*
amnestic syndrome (291.1)
Korsakoff's psychosis (291.1)

294.1 Dementia in conditions classified elsewhere

Code first any underlying physical condition, as:
cerebral lipidoses (330.1)
epilepsy (345.0-345.9)
general paresis [syphilis] (094.1)
hepatolenticular degeneration (275.1)
Huntington's chorea (333.4)
multiple sclerosis (340)
polyarteritis nodosa (446.0)
syphilis (094.1)

Excludes: *dementia:*
arteriosclerotic (290.40-290.43)
presenile (290.10-290.13)
senile (290.0)
epileptic psychosis NOS (294.8)

● Code new to this edition ▲ Revision of existing code ④ ⑤ Fourth or fifth digit required

294.8 Other specified organic brain syndromes (chronic)
Epileptic psychosis NOS
Mixed paranoid and affective organic psychotic states

Use additional code for associated epilepsy (345.0-345.9)

Excludes: *mild memory disturbances, not amounting to dementia (310.1)*

294.9 Unspecified organic brain syndrome (chronic)
Organic psychosis (chronic)

OTHER PSYCHOSES (295-299)

Use additional code to identify any associated physical disease, injury, or condition affecting the brain with psychoses classifiable to 295-298

⑤ 295 Schizophrenic disorders

Includes: schizophrenia of the types described in 295.0-295.9 occurring in children

Excludes: *childhood type schizophrenia (299.9)*
infantile autism (299.0)

The following fifth-digit subclassification is for use with category 295:

0 unspecified
1 subchronic
2 chronic
3 subchronic with acute exacerbation
4 chronic with acute exacerbation
5 in remission

295.0 Simple type
Schizophrenia simplex

Excludes: *latent schizophrenia (295.5)*

295.1 Disorganized type
Hebephrenia
Hebephrenic type schizophrenia

295.2 Catatonic type
Catatonic (schizophrenia):
agitation
excitation
excited type
stupor
withdrawn type

Schizophrenic:
catalepsy
catatonia
flexibilitas cerea

295.3 Paranoid type
Paraphrenic schizophrenia

Excludes: *involutional paranoid state (297.2)*
paranoia (297.1)
paraphrenia (297.2)

295.4 Acute schizophrenic episode
Oneirophrenia
Schizophreniform:
attack
disorder
psychosis, confusional type

Excludes: *acute forms of schizophrenia of:*
catatonic type (295.2)
hebephrenic type (295.1)
paranoid type (295.3)
simple type (295.0)
undifferentiated type (295.8)

295.5 Latent schizophrenia
Latent schizophrenic reaction
Schizophrenia:
borderline
incipient

Schizophrenia:
prepsychotic
prodromal
pseudoneurotic
pseudopsychopathic

Excludes: *schizoid personality (301.20-301.22)*

Add 4th or 5th digit | Nonspecific code | Unspecified code | Manifestation code

295.6 Residual schizophrenia
Chronic undifferentiated schizophrenia
Restzustand (schizophrenic)
Schizophrenic residual state

295.7 Schizo-affective type
Cyclic schizophrenia
Mixed schizophrenic and affective psychosis
Schizo-affective psychosis
Schizophreniform psychosis, affective type

295.8 Other specified types of schizophrenia
Acute (undifferentiated) schizophrenia
Atypical schizophrenia
Cenesthopathic schizophrenia

Excludes: *infantile autism (299.0)*

295.9 Unspecified schizophrenia
Schizophrenia:
NOS
mixed NOS
undifferentiated NOS
Schizophrenic reaction NOS
Schizophreniform psychosis NOS

296 Affective psychoses
Includes: episodic affective disorders

Excludes: *neurotic depression (300.4)*
reactive depressive psychosis (298.0)
reactive excitation (298.1)

The following fifth-digit subclassification is for use with categories 296.0-296.6:

0 unspecified

1 mild

2 moderate

3 severe, without mention of psychotic behavior

4 severe, specified as with psychotic behavior

5 in partial or unspecified remission

6 in full remission

□ ⑤ **296.0 Manic disorder, single episode**
Hypomania (mild) NOS
Hypomanic psychosis
Mania (monopolar) NOS
Manic-depressive psychosis or reaction:
hypomanic
manic
} single episode or unspecified

Excludes: *circular type, if there was a previous attack of depression (296.4)*

□ ⑤ **296.1 Manic disorder, recurrent episode**
Any condition classifiable to 296.0, stated to be recurrent

Excludes: *circular type, if there was a previous attack of depression (296.4)*

□ ⑤ **296.2 Major depressive disorder, single episode**
Depressive psychosis
Endogenous depression
Involutional melancholia
Manic-depressive psychosis or reaction, depressed type
Monopolar depression
Psychotic depression
} single episode or unspecified

Excludes: *circular type, if previous attack was of manic type (296.5)*
depression NOS (311)
reactive depression (neurotic) (300.4)
psychotic (298.0)

□ ⑤ **296.3 Major depressive disorder, recurrent episode**
Any condition classifiable to 296.2, stated to be recurrent

Excludes: *circular type, if previous attack was of manic type (296.5)*
depression NOS (311)
reactive depression (neurotic) (300.4)
psychotic (298.0)

□ ⑤ **296.4 Bipolar affective disorder, manic**
Bipolar disorder, now manic
Manic-depressive psychosis, circular type but currently manic

Excludes: *brief compensatory or rebound mood swings (296.99)*

□ ⑤ **296.5 Bipolar affective disorder, depressed**
Bipolar disorder, now depressed
Manic-depressive psychosis, circular type but currently depressed

Excludes: *brief compensatory or rebound mood swings (296.99)*

□ ⑤ **296.6 Bipolar affective disorder, mixed**
Manic-depressive psychosis, circular type, mixed

□ **296.7 Bipolar affective disorder, unspecified**
Atypical bipolar affective disorder NOS
Manic-depressive psychosis, circular type, current condition not specified as either manic or depressive

□ **296.8 Manic-depressive psychosis, other and unspecified**

296.80 Manic-depressive psychosis, unspecified
Manic-depressive:
reaction NOS
syndrome NOS

296.81 Atypical manic disorder

296.82 Atypical depressive disorder

296.89 Other
Manic-depressive psychosis, mixed type

□ **296.9 Other and unspecified affective psychoses**

Excludes: *psychogenic affective psychoses (298.0-298.8)*

296.90 Unspecified affective psychosis
Affective psychosis NOS
Melancholia NOS

296.99 Other specified affective psychoses
Mood swings:
brief compensatory
rebound

297 Paranoid states
Includes: paranoid disorders

Excludes: *acute paranoid reaction (298.3)*
alcoholic jealousy or paranoid state (291.5)
paranoid schizophrenia (295.3)

297.0 Paranoid state, simple

297.1 Paranoia
Chronic paranoid psychosis
Sander's disease
Systematized delusions

Excludes: *paranoid personality disorder (301.0)*

297.2 Paraphrenia
Involutional paranoid state
Late paraphrenia
Paraphrenia (involutional)

297.3 Shared paranoid disorder
Folie à deux
Induced psychosis or paranoid disorder

297.8 Other specified paranoid states
Paranoia querulans
Sensitiver Beziehungswahn

Excludes: *acute paranoid reaction or state (298.3)*
senile paranoid state (290.20)

297.9 Unspecified paranoid state
Paranoid:
disorder NOS
psychosis
Paranoid:
reaction NOS
state NOS

298 Other nonorganic psychoses
Includes: psychotic conditions due to or provoked by:
emotional stress
environmental factors as major part of etiology

298.0 Depressive type psychosis
Psychogenic depressive psychosis
Psychotic reactive depression
Reactive depressive psychosis

Excludes: *manic-depressive psychosis, depressed type (296.2-296.3)*
neurotic depression (300.4)
reactive depression NOS (300.4)

298.1 Excitative type psychosis
Acute hysterical psychosis
Psychogenic excitation
Reactive excitation

Excludes: *manic-depressive psychosis, manic type (296.0-296.1)*

298.2 Reactive confusion
Psychogenic confusion
Psychogenic twilight state

Excludes: *acute confusional state (293.0)*

298.3 Acute paranoid reaction
Acute psychogenic paranoid psychosis
Bouffée délirante

Excludes: *paranoid states (297.0-297.9)*

298.4 Psychogenic paranoid psychosis
Protracted reactive paranoid psychosis

298.8 Other and unspecified reactive psychosis
Brief reactive psychosis NOS
Hysterical psychosis
Psychogenic psychosis NOS
Psychogenic stupor

Excludes: *acute hysterical psychosis (298.1)*

298.9 Unspecified psychosis
Atypical psychosis
Psychosis NOS

⑤ **299 Psychoses with origin specific to childhood**
Includes: pervasive developmental disorders

Excludes: *adult type psychoses occurring in childhood, as:*
affective disorders (296.0-296.9)
manic-depressive disorders (296.0-296.9)
schizophrenia (295.0-295.9)

The following fifth-digit subclassification is for use with category 299:

0 current or active state

1 residual state

299.0 Infantile autism
Childhood autism
Infantile psychosis
Kanner's syndrome

Excludes: *disintegrative psychosis (299.1)*
Heller's syndrome (299.1)
schizophrenic syndrome of childhood (299.9)

299.1 Disintegrative psychosis
Heller's syndrome

Use additional code to identify any associated neurological disorder

Excludes: *infantile autism (299.0)*
schizophrenic syndrome of childhood (299.9)

299.8 Other specified early childhood psychoses
Atypical childhood psychosis
Borderline psychosis of childhood

Excludes: *simple stereotypies without psychotic disturbance (307.3)*

299.9 Unspecified
Child psychosis NOS
Schizophrenia, childhood type NOS
Schizophrenic syndrome of childhood NOS

Excludes: *schizophrenia of adult type occurring in childhood (295.0-295.9)*

NEUROTIC DISORDERS, PERSONALITY DISORDERS, AND OTHER NONPSYCHOTIC MENTAL DISORDERS (300-316)

300 Neurotic disorders

300.0 Anxiety states

Excludes: *anxiety in:*
acute stress reaction (308.0)
transient adjustment reaction (309.24)
neurasthenia (300.5)
psychophysiological disorders (306.0-306.9)
separation anxiety (309.21)

300.00 Anxiety state, unspecified
Anxiety:
neurosis
reaction
state (neurotic)
Atypical anxiety disorder

300.01 Panic disorder
Panic:
attack
state

300.02 Generalized anxiety disorder

300.09 Other

300.1 Hysteria

Excludes: *adjustment reaction (309.0-309.9)*
anorexia nervosa (307.1)
gross stress reaction (308.0-308.9)
hysterical personality (301.50-301.59)
psychophysiologic disorders (306.0-306.9)

300.10 Hysteria, unspecified

300.11 Conversion disorder
Astasia-abasia, hysterical
Conversion hysteria or reaction
Hysterical:
blindness
deafness
paralysis

300.12 Psychogenic amnesia
Hysterical amnesia

300.13 Psychogenic fugue
Hysterical fugue

300.14 Multiple personality
Dissociative identity disorder

300.15 Dissociative disorder or reaction, unspecified

300.16 Factitious illness with psychological symptoms
Compensation neurosis
Ganser's syndrome, hysterical

Add 4th or 5th digit | Nonspecific code | Unspecified code | Manifestation code

300.19 Other and unspecified factitious illness
Factitious illness (with physical symptoms) NOS

Excludes: *multiple operations or hospital addiction syndrome (301.51)*

300.2 Phobic disorders

Excludes: *anxiety state not associated with a specific situation or object (300.0-300.09)*
obsessional phobias (300.3)

300.20 Phobia, unspecified
Anxiety-hysteria NOS
Phobia NOS

300.21 Agoraphobia with panic attacks
Fear of:
open spaces, streets, travel } with panic attacks

300.22 Agoraphobia without mention of panic attacks
Any condition classifiable to 300.21 without mention of panic attacks

300.23 Social phobia
Fear of:
eating in public
public speaking
washing in public

300.29 Other isolated or simple phobias
Acrophobia
Animal phobias
Claustrophobia
Fear of crowds

300.3 Obsessive-compulsive disorders
Anancastic neurosis
Compulsive neurosis
Obsessional phobia [any]

Excludes: *obsessive-compulsive symptoms occurring in:*
endogenous depression (296.2-296.3)
organic states (e.g., encephalitis)
schizophrenia (295.0-295.9)

300.4 Neurotic depression
Anxiety depression
Depression with anxiety
Depressive reaction
Dysthymic disorder
Neurotic depressive state
Reactive depression

Excludes: *adjustment reaction with depressive symptoms (309.0-309.1)*
depression NOS (311)
manic-depressive psychosis, depressed type (296.2-296.3)
reactive depressive psychosis (298.0)

300.5 Neurasthenia
Fatigue neurosis
Nervous debility
Psychogenic:
asthenia
general fatigue

Use additional code to identify any associated physical disorder

Excludes: *anxiety state (300.00-300.09)*
neurotic depression (300.4)
psychophysiological disorders (306.0-306.9)
specific nonpsychotic mental disorders following organic brain damage (310.0-310.9)

300.6 Depersonalization syndrome
Depersonalization disorder
Derealization (neurotic)
Neurotic state with depersonalization episode

Excludes: *depersonalization associated with:*
anxiety (300.00-300.09)
depression (300.4)
manic-depressive disorder or psychosis (296.0-296.9)
schizophrenia (295.0-295.9)

300.7 Hypochondriasis
Atypical somatoform disorder
Body dysmorphic disorder

Excludes: *hypochondriasis in:*
hysteria (300.10-300.19)
manic-depressive psychosis, depressed type (296.2-296.3)
neurasthenia (300.5)
obsessional disorder (300.3)
schizophrenia (295.0-295.9)

300.8 Other neurotic disorders

300.81 Somatization disorder
Briquet's disorder

300.89 Other
Occupational neurosis, including writers' cramp
Psychasthenia
Psychasthenic neurosis

300.9 Unspecified neurotic disorder
Neurosis NOS
Psychoneurosis NOS

301 Personality disorders
Includes: character neurosis
Use additional code to identify any associated neurosis or psychosis, or physical condition

Excludes: *nonpsychotic personality disorder associated with organic brain syndromes (310.0-310.9)*

301.0 Paranoid personality disorder
Fanatic personality
Paranoid personality (disorder)
Paranoid traits

Excludes: *acute paranoid reaction (298.3)*
alcoholic paranoia (291.5)
paranoid schizophrenia (295.3)
paranoid states (297.0-297.9)

301.1 Affective personality disorder

Excludes: *affective psychotic disorders (296.0-296.9)*
neurasthenia (300.5)
neurotic depression (300.4)

301.10 Affective personality disorder, unspecified

301.11 Chronic hypomanic personality disorder
Chronic hypomanic disorder
Hypomanic personality

301.12 Chronic depressive personality disorder
Chronic depressive disorder
Depressive character or personality

301.13 Cyclothymic disorder
Cycloid personality
Cyclothymia
Cyclothymic personality

301.2 Schizoid personality disorder

Excludes: *schizophrenia (295.0-295.9)*

301.20 Schizoid personality disorder, unspecified

301.21 Introverted personality

301.22 Schizotypal personality

301.3 Explosive personality disorder
Aggressive:
  personality
  reaction
Aggressiveness
Emotional instability (excessive)
Pathological emotionality
Quarrelsomeness

Excludes: *dyssocial personality (301.7)*
hysterical neurosis (300.10-300.19)

301.4 Compulsive personality disorder
Anancastic personality
Obsessional personality

Excludes: *obsessive-compulsive disorder (300.3)*
phobic state (300.20-300.29)

301.5 Histrionic personality disorder

Excludes: *hysterical neurosis (300.10-300.19)*

301.50 Histrionic personality disorder, unspecified
Hysterical personality NOS

301.51 Chronic factitious illness with physical symptoms
Hospital addiction syndrome
Multiple operations syndrome
Munchausen syndrome

301.59 Other histrionic personality disorder
Personality:
emotionally unstable
labile
psychoinfantile

301.6 Dependent personality disorder
Asthenic personality
Inadequate personality
Passive personality

Excludes: *neurasthenia (300.5)*
passive-aggressive personality (301.84)

301.7 Antisocial personality disorder
Amoral personality
Asocial personality
Dyssocial personality
Personality disorder with predominantly sociopathic or asocial manifestation

Excludes: *disturbance of conduct without specifiable personality disorder (312.0-312.9)*
explosive personality (301.3)

301.8 Other personality disorders

301.81 Narcissistic personality

301.82 Avoidant personality

301.83 Borderline personality

301.84 Passive-aggressive personality

301.89 Other
Personality:
eccentric
"haltlose" type
immature
Personality:
masochistic
psychoneurotic

Excludes: *psychoinfantile personality (301.59)*

301.9 Unspecified personality disorder
Pathological personality NOS
Personality disorder NOS
Psychopathic:
constitutional state
personality (disorder)

302 Sexual deviations and disorders

Excludes: *sexual disorder manifest in:*
organic brain syndrome (290.0-294.9, 310.0-310.9)
psychosis (295.0-298.9)

302.0 Ego-dystonic homosexuality
Ego-dystonic lesbianism
Homosexual conflict disorder

Excludes: *homosexual pedophilia (302.2)*

302.1 Zoophilia
Bestiality

302.2 Pedophilia

302.3 Transvestism

Excludes: *trans-sexualism (302.5)*

302.4 Exhibitionism

● Code new to this edition
▲ Revision of existing code
④ ⑤ Fourth or fifth digit required

302.5 Trans-sexualism

Excludes: *transvestism (302.3)*

302.50 With unspecified sexual history

302.51 With asexual history

302.52 With homosexual history

302.53 With heterosexual history

302.6 Disorders of psychosexual identity

Feminism in boys
Gender identity disorder of childhood

Excludes: *gender identity disorder in adult (302.85)*
homosexuality (302.0)
trans-sexualism (302.50-302.53)
transvestism (302.3)

302.7 Psychosexual dysfunction

Excludes: *impotence of organic origin (607.84)*
normal transient symptoms from ruptured hymen
transient or occasional failures of erection due to fatigue, anxiety, alcohol, or drugs

302.70 Psychosexual dysfunction, unspecified

302.71 With inhibited sexual desire

302.72 With inhibited sexual excitement

Frigidity   Impotence

302.73 With inhibited female orgasm

302.74 With inhibited male orgasm

302.75 With premature ejaculation

302.76 With functional dyspareunia

Dyspareunia, psychogenic

302.79 With other specified psychosexual dysfunctions

302.8 Other specified psychosexual disorders

302.81 Fetishism

302.82 Voyeurism

302.83 Sexual masochism

302.84 Sexual sadism

302.85 Gender identity disorder of adolescent or adult life

302.89 Other

Nymphomania   Satyriasis

302.9 Unspecified psychosexual disorder

Pathologic sexuality NOS   Sexual deviation NOS

⑤ **303 Alcohol dependence syndrome**

Use additional code to identify any associated condition, as:
alcoholic psychoses (291.0-291.9)
drug dependence (304.0-304.9)
physical complications of alcohol, such as:
cerebral degeneration (331.7)
cirrhosis of liver (571.2)
epilepsy (345.0-345.9)
gastritis (535.3)
hepatitis (571.1)
liver damage NOS (571.3)

Excludes: *drunkenness NOS (305.0)*

The following fifth-digit subclassification is for use with category 303:

0 unspecified

1 continuous

2 episodic

3 in remission

303.0 Acute alcoholic intoxication
Acute drunkenness in alcoholism

303.9 Other and unspecified alcohol dependence
Chronic alcoholism
Dipsomania

⑤ **304 Drug dependence**

Excludes: *nondependent abuse of drugs (305.1-305.9)*

The following fifth-digit subclassification is for use with category 304:

0 unspecified
1 continuous
2 episodic
3 in remission

304.0 Opioid type dependence
Heroin
Meperidine
Methadone
Morphine
Opium
Opium alkaloids and their derivatives
Synthetics with morphine-like effects

304.1 Barbiturate and similarly acting sedative or hypnotic dependence
Barbiturates
Nonbarbiturate sedatives and tranquilizers with a similar effect:
chlordiazepoxide
diazepam
glutethimide
meprobamate
methaqualone

304.2 Cocaine dependence
Coca leaves and derivatives

304.3 Cannabis dependence
Hashish
Hemp
Marihuana

304.4 Amphetamine and other psychostimulant dependence
Methylphenidate
Phenmetrazine

304.5 Hallucinogen dependence
Dimethyltryptamine [DMT]
Lysergic acid diethylamide [LSD] and derivatives
Mescaline
Psilocybin

304.6 Other specified drug dependence
Absinthe addiction
Glue sniffing

Excludes: *tobacco dependence (305.1)*

304.7 Combinations of opioid type drug with any other

304.8 Combinations of drug dependence excluding opioid type drug

304.9 Unspecified drug dependence
Drug addiction NOS
Drug dependence NOS

⑤ **305 Nondependent abuse of drugs**

Note: Includes cases where a person, for whom no other diagnosis is possible, has come under medical care because of the maladaptive effect of a drug on which he is not dependent and that he has taken on his own initiative to the detriment of his health or social functioning.

Excludes: *alcohol dependence syndrome (303.0-303.9)*
drug dependence (304.0-304.9)
drug withdrawal syndrome (292.0)
poisoning by drugs or medicinal substances (960.0-979.9)

The following fifth-digit subclassification is for use with codes 305.0, 305.2-305.9:

0 unspecified
1 continuous
2 episodic
3 in remission

305.0 Alcohol abuse
Drunkenness NOS
Excessive drinking of alcohol NOS
"Hangover" (alcohol)
Inebriety NOS

Excludes: *acute alcohol intoxication in alcoholism (303.0)*
alcoholic psychoses (291.0-291.9)
physical complications of alcohol, such as:
cirrhosis of liver (571.2)
epilepsy (345.00-345.91)
gastritis (535.3)

305.1 Tobacco use disorder
Tobacco dependence

Excludes: *history of tobacco use (V15.82)*

305.2 Cannabis abuse

305.3 Hallucinogen abuse
Acute intoxication from hallucinogens ["bad trips"]
LSD reaction

305.4 Barbiturate and similarly acting sedative or hypnotic abuse

305.5 Opioid abuse

305.6 Cocaine abuse

305.7 Amphetamine or related acting sympathomimetic abuse

305.8 Antidepressant type abuse

305.9 Other, mixed, or unspecified drug abuse
"Laxative habit"
Misuse of drugs NOS
Nonprescribed use of drugs or patent medicinals

306 Physiological malfunction arising from mental factors
Includes: psychogenic:
physical symptoms } not involving tissue damage
physiological manifestations } not involving tissue damage

Excludes: *hysteria (300.11-300.19)*
physical symptoms secondary to a psychiatric disorder classified elsewhere
psychic factors associated with physical conditions involving tissue damage classified elsewhere (316)
specific nonpsychotic mental disorders following organic brain damage (310.0-310.9)

306.0 Musculoskeletal
Psychogenic paralysis
Psychogenic torticollis

Excludes: *Gilles de la Tourette's syndrome (307.23)*
paralysis as hysterical or conversion reaction (300.11)
tics (307.20-307.22)

306.1 Respiratory
Psychogenic:
air hunger
cough
hiccough
Psychogenic:
hyperventilation
yawning

Excludes: *psychogenic asthma (316 and 493.9)*

306.2 Cardiovascular
Cardiac neurosis
Cardiovascular neurosis
Neurocirculatory asthenia
Psychogenic cardiovascular disorder

Excludes: *psychogenic paroxysmal tachycardia (316 and 427.2)*

306.3 Skin
Psychogenic pruritus

Excludes: *psychogenic:*
alopecia (316 and 704.00)
dermatitis (316 and 692.9)
eczema (316 and 691.8 or 692.9)
urticaria (316 and 708.0-708.9)

306.4 Gastrointestinal

Aerophagy
Cyclical vomiting, psychogenic
Diarrhea, psychogenic
Nervous gastritis
Psychogenic dyspepsia

Excludes: *cyclical vomiting NOS (536.2)*
globus hystericus (300.11)
mucous colitis (316 and 564.1)
psychogenic:
cardiospasm (316 and 530.0)
duodenal ulcer (316 and 532.0-532.9)
gastric ulcer (316 and 531.0-531.9)
peptic ulcer NOS (316 and 533.0-533.9)
vomiting NOS (307.54)

306.5 Genitourinary

Excludes: *enuresis, psychogenic (307.6)*
frigidity (302.72)
impotence (302.72)
psychogenic dyspareunia (302.76)

306.50 Psychogenic genitourinary malfunction, unspecified

306.51 Psychogenic vaginismus
Functional vaginismus

306.52 Psychogenic dysmenorrhea

306.53 Psychogenic dysuria

306.59 Other

306.6 Endocrine

306.7 Organs of special sense

Excludes: *hysterical blindness or deafness (300.11)*
psychophysical visual disturbances (368.16)

306.8 Other specified psychophysiological malfunction
Bruxism
Teeth grinding

306.9 Unspecified psychophysiological malfunction
Psychophysiologic disorder NOS
Psychosomatic disorder NOS

307 Special symptoms or syndromes, not elsewhere classified

Note: This category is intended for use if the psychopathology is manifested by a single specific symptom or group of symptoms which is not part of an organic illness or other mental disorder classifiable elsewhere.

Excludes: *those due to mental disorders classified elsewhere*
those of organic origin

307.0 Stammering and stuttering

Excludes: *dysphasia (784.5)*
lisping or lalling (307.9)
retarded development of speech (315.31-315.39)

307.1 Anorexia nervosa

Excludes: *eating disturbance NOS (307.50)*
feeding problem (783.3)
of nonorganic origin (307.59)
loss of appetite (783.0)
of nonorganic origin (307.59)

307.2 Tics

Excludes: *nail-biting or thumb-sucking (307.9)*
stereotypies occurring in isolation (307.3)
tics of organic origin (333.3)

307.20 Tic disorder, unspecified

307.21 Transient tic disorder of childhood

307.22 Chronic motor tic disorder

307.23 Gilles de la Tourette's disorder
Motor-verbal tic disorder

307.3 Stereotyped repetitive movements

Body-rocking
Head banging
Spasmus nutans
Stereotypies NOS

Excludes: *tics (307.20-307.23)*
of organic origin (333.3)

307.4 Specific disorders of sleep of nonorganic origin

Excludes: *narcolepsy (347)*
those of unspecified cause (780.50-780.59)

307.40 Nonorganic sleep disorder, unspecified

307.41 Transient disorder of initiating or maintaining sleep

Hyposomnia, Insomnia, Sleeplessness } associated with acute or intermittent emotional reactions or conflicts

307.42 Persistent disorder of initiating or maintaining sleep

Hyposomnia, insomnia, or sleeplessness associated with:
- anxiety
- conditioned arousal
- depression (major) (minor)
- psychosis

307.43 Transient disorder of initiating or maintaining wakefulness

Hypersomnia associated with acute or intermittent emotional reactions or conflicts

307.44 Persistent disorder of initiating or maintaining wakefulness

Hypersomnia associated with depression (major) (minor)

307.45 Phase-shift disruption of 24-hour sleep-wake cycle

Irregular sleep-wake rhythm, nonorganic origin
Jet lag syndrome
Rapid time-zone change
Shifting sleep-work schedule

307.46 Somnambulism or night terrors

307.47 Other dysfunctions of sleep stages or arousal from sleep

Nightmares:
- NOS
- REM-sleep type

Sleep drunkenness

307.48 Repetitive intrusions of sleep

Repetitive intrusion of sleep with:
- atypical polysomnographic features
- environmental disturbances
- repeated REM-sleep interruptions

307.49 Other

"Short-sleeper"
Subjective insomnia complaint

307.5 Other and unspecified disorders of eating

Excludes: *anorexia:*
nervosa (307.1)
of unspecified cause (783.0)
overeating, of unspecified cause (783.6)
vomiting:
NOS (787.0)
cyclical (536.2)
psychogenic (306.4)

307.50 Eating disorder, unspecified

307.51 Bulimia

Overeating of nonorganic origin

307.52 Pica

Perverted appetite of nonorganic origin

307.53 Psychogenic rumination

Regurgitation, of nonorganic origin, of food with reswallowing

Excludes: *obsessional rumination (300.3)*

307.54 Psychogenic vomiting

307.59 Other
Infantile feeding disturbances } of nonorganic origin
Loss of appetite } of nonorganic origin

307.6 Enuresis
Enuresis (primary) (secondary) of nonorganic origin

Excludes: *enuresis of unspecified cause (788.3)*

307.7 Encopresis
Encopresis (continuous) (discontinuous) of nonorganic origin

Excludes: *encopresis of unspecified cause (787.6)*

307.8 Psychalgia

307.80 Psychogenic pain, site unspecified

307.81 Tension headache

Excludes: *headache:*
NOS (784.0)
migraine (346.0-346.9)

307.89 Other
Psychogenic backache

Excludes: *pains not specifically attributable to a psychological cause (in):*
back (724.5)
joint (719.4)
limb (729.5)
lumbago (724.2)
rheumatic (729.0)

307.9 Other and unspecified special symptoms or syndromes, not elsewhere classified
Hair plucking
Lalling
Lisping
Masturbation
Nail-biting
Thumb-sucking

308 Acute reaction to stress
Includes: catastrophic stress
combat fatigue
gross stress reaction (acute)
transient disorders in response to exceptional physical or mental stress which usually subside within hours or days

Excludes: *adjustment reaction or disorder (309.0-309.9)*
chronic stress reaction (309.1-309.9)

308.0 Predominant disturbance of emotions
Anxiety } as acute reaction to exceptional [gross] stress
Emotional crisis } as acute reaction to exceptional [gross] stress
Panic state } as acute reaction to exceptional [gross] stress

308.1 Predominant disturbance of consciousness
Fugues as acute reaction to exceptional [gross] stress

308.2 Predominant psychomotor disturbance
Agitation states } as acute reaction to exceptional [gross] stress
Stupor } as acute reaction to exceptional [gross] stress

308.3 Other acute reactions to stress
Acute situational disturbance
Brief or acute posttraumatic stress disorder

Excludes: *prolonged posttraumatic emotional disturbance (309.81)*

308.4 Mixed disorders as reaction to stress

308.9 Unspecified acute reaction to stress

309 Adjustment reaction
Includes: adjustment disorders
reaction (adjustment) to chronic stress

Excludes: *acute reaction to major stress (308.0-308.9)*
neurotic disorders (300.0-300.9)

● Code new to this edition
▲ Revision of existing code
④ ⑤ Fourth or fifth digit required

309.0 Brief depressive reaction
Adjustment disorder with depressed mood
Grief reaction

Excludes: *affective psychoses (296.0-296.9)*
neurotic depression (300.4)
prolonged depressive reaction (309.1)
psychogenic depressive psychosis (298.0)

309.1 Prolonged depressive reaction

Excludes: *affective psychoses (296.0-296.9)*
brief depressive reaction (309.0)
neurotic depression (300.4)
psychogenic depressive psychosis (298.0)

309.2 With predominant disturbance of other emotions

309.21 Separation anxiety disorder

309.22 Emancipation disorder of adolescence and early adult life

309.23 Specific academic or work inhibition

309.24 Adjustment reaction with anxious mood

309.28 Adjustment reaction with mixed emotional features
Adjustment reaction with anxiety and depression

309.29 Other
Culture shock

309.3 With predominant disturbance of conduct
Conduct disturbance } as adjustment reaction
Destructiveness } as adjustment reaction

Excludes: *destructiveness in child (312.9)*
disturbance of conduct NOS (312.9)
dyssocial behavior without manifest psychiatric disorder (V71.01-V71.02)
personality disorder with predominantly sociopathic or asocial manifestations (301.7)

309.4 With mixed disturbance of emotions and conduct

309.8 Other specified adjustment reactions

309.81 Prolonged posttraumatic stress disorder
Chronic posttraumatic stress disorder
Concentration camp syndrome

Excludes: *posttraumatic brain syndrome:*
nonpsychotic (310.2)
psychotic (293.0-293.9)

309.82 Adjustment reaction with physical symptoms

309.83 Adjustment reaction with withdrawal
Elective mutism as adjustment reaction
Hospitalism (in children) NOS

309.89 Other

309.9 Unspecified adjustment reaction
Adaptation reaction NOS
Adjustment reaction NOS

310 Specific nonpsychotic mental disorders due to organic brain damage

Excludes: *neuroses, personality disorders, or other nonpsychotic conditions occurring in a form similar to that seen with functional disorders but in association with a physical condition (300.0-300.9, 301.0-301.9)*

310.0 Frontal lobe syndrome
Lobotomy syndrome
Postleucotomy syndrome [state]

Excludes: *postcontusion syndrome (310.2)*

310.1 Organic personality syndrome
Cognitive or personality change of other type, of nonpsychotic severity
Mild memory disturbance
Organic psychosyndrome of nonpsychotic severity
Presbyophrenia NOS
Senility with mental changes of nonpsychotic severity

Add 4th or 5th digit | Nonspecific code | Unspecified code | Manifestation code

310.2 Postconcussion syndrome
Postcontusion syndrome or encephalopathy
Posttraumatic brain syndrome, nonpsychotic
Status postcommotio cerebri

Excludes: *frontal lobe syndrome (310.0)*
postencephalitic syndrome (310.8)
any organic psychotic conditions following head injury (293.0—294.0)

310.8 Other specified nonpsychotic mental disorders following organic brain damage
Postencephalitic syndrome
Other focal (partial) organic psychosyndromes

310.9 Unspecified nonpsychotic mental disorder following organic brain damage

311 Depressive disorder, not elsewhere classified
Depressive disorder NOS
Depressive state NOS
Depression NOS

Excludes: *acute reaction to major stress with depressive symptoms (308.0)*
affective personality disorder (301.10-301.13)
affective psychoses (296.0-296.9)
brief depressive reaction (309.0)
depressive states associated with stressful events (309.0-309.1)
disturbance of emotions specific to childhood and adolescence, with misery and unhappiness (313.1)
mixed adjustment reaction with depressive symptoms (309.4)
neurotic depression (300.4)
prolonged depressive adjustment reaction (309.1)
psychogenic depressive psychosis (298.0)

312 Disturbance of conduct, not elsewhere classified

Excludes: *adjustment reaction with disturbance of conduct (309.3)*
drug dependence (304.0-304.9)
dyssocial behavior without manifest psychiatric disorder (V71.01-V71.02)
personality disorder with predominantly sociopathic or asocial manifestations (301.7)
sexual deviations (302.0-302.9)

The following fifth-digit subclassification is for use with categories 312.0-312.2:

0 unspecified

1 mild

2 moderate

3 severe

□ ⑤ **312.0 Undersocialized conduct disorder, aggressive type**
Aggressive outburst
Anger reaction
Unsocialized aggressive disorder

□ ⑤ **312.1 Undersocialized conduct disorder, unaggressive type**
Childhood truancy, unsocialized
Solitary stealing
Tantrums

□ ⑤ **312.2 Socialized conduct disorder**
Childhood truancy, socialized
Group delinquency

Excludes: *gang activity without manifest psychiatric disorder (V71.01)*

□ **312.3 Disorders of impulse control, not elsewhere classified**

312.30 Impulse control disorder, unspecified

312.31 Pathological gambling

312.32 Kleptomania

312.33 Pyromania

312.34 Intermittent explosive disorder

312.35 Isolated explosive disorder

312.39 Other

□ **312.4 Mixed disturbance of conduct and emotions**
Neurotic delinquency

Excludes: *compulsive conduct disorder (312.3)*

312.8 Other specified disturbances of conduct, not elsewhere classified

312.81 Conduct disorder, childhood onset type

312.82 Conduct disorder, adolescent onset type

312.89 Other conduct disorder

312.9 Unspecified disturbance of conduct
Delinquency (juvenile)

313 Disturbance of emotions specific to childhood and adolescence

Excludes: *adjustment reaction (309.0-309.9)*
emotional disorder of neurotic type (300.0-300.9)
masturbation, nail-biting, thumb-sucking, and other isolated symptoms (307.0-307.9)

313.0 Overanxious disorder
Anxiety and fearfulness } of childhood and adolescence
Overanxious disorder } of childhood and adolescence

Excludes: *abnormal separation anxiety (309.21)*
anxiety states (300.00-300.09)
hospitalism in children (309.83)
phobic state (300.20-300.29)

313.1 Misery and unhappiness disorder

Excludes: *depressive neurosis (300.4)*

313.2 Sensitivity, shyness, and social withdrawal disorder

Excludes: *infantile autism (299.0)*
schizoid personality (301.20-301.22)
schizophrenia (295.0-295.9)

313.21 Shyness disorder of childhood
Sensitivity reaction of childhood or adolescence

313.22 Introverted disorder of childhood
Social withdrawal } of childhood or adolescence
Withdrawal reaction } of childhood or adolescence

313.23 Elective mutism

Excludes: *elective mutism as adjustment reaction (309.83)*

313.3 Relationship problems
Sibling jealousy

Excludes: *relationship problems associated with aggression, destruction, or other forms of conduct disturbance (312.0-312.9)*

313.8 Other or mixed emotional disturbances of childhood or adolescence

313.81 Oppositional disorder

313.82 Identity disorder

313.83 Academic underachievement disorder

313.89 Other

313.9 Unspecified emotional disturbance of childhood or adolescence

314 Hyperkinetic syndrome of childhood

Excludes: *hyperkinesis as symptom of underlying disorder—code the underlying disorder*

314.0 Attention deficit disorder

314.00 Without mention of hyperactivity
Predominantly inattentive type

314.01 With hyperactivity
Combined type
Overactivity NOS
Predominantly hyperactive/impulsive type
Simple disturbance of attention with overactivity

314.1 Hyperkinesis with developmental delay
Developmental disorder of hyperkinesis

Use additional code to identify any associated neurological disorder

314.2 Hyperkinetic conduct disorder
Hyperkinetic conduct disorder without developmental delay

Excludes: *hyperkinesis with significant delays in specific skills (314.1)*

314.8 Other specified manifestations of hyperkinetic syndrome

314.9 Unspecified hyperkinetic syndrome
Hyperkinetic reaction of childhood or adolescence NOS
Hyperkinetic syndrome NOS

315 Specific delays in development

Excludes: *that due to a neurological disorder (320.0-389.9)*

315.0 Specific reading disorder

315.00 Reading disorder, unspecified

315.01 Alexia

315.02 Developmental dyslexia

315.09 Other
Specific spelling difficulty

315.1 Specific arithmetical disorder
Dyscalculia

315.2 Other specific learning difficulties

Excludes: *specific arithmetical disorder (315.1)*
specific reading disorder (315.00-315.09)

315.3 Developmental speech or language disorder

315.31 Developmental language disorder
Developmental aphasia
Word deafness

Excludes: *acquired aphasia (784.3)*
elective mutism (309.83, 313.0, 313.23)

315.39 Other
Developmental articulation disorder
Dyslalia

Excludes: *lisping and lalling (307.9)*
stammering and stuttering (307.0)

315.4 Coordination disorder
Clumsiness syndrome
Dyspraxia syndrome
Specific motor development disorder

315.5 Mixed development disorder

315.8 Other specified delays in development

315.9 Unspecified delay in development
Developmental disorder NOS

316 Psychic factors associated with diseases classified elsewhere
Psychologic factors in physical conditions classified elsewhere

Use additional code to identify the associated physical condition, as:
psychogenic:
- asthma (493.9)
- dermatitis (692.9)
- duodenal ulcer (532.0-532.9)
- eczema (691.8, 692.9)
- gastric ulcer (531.0-531.9)
- mucous colitis (564.1)
- paroxysmal tachycardia (427.2)
- ulcerative colitis (556)
- urticaria (708.0-708.9)

psychosocial dwarfism (259.4)

Excludes: *physical symptoms and physiological malfunctions, not involving tissue damage, of mental origin (306.0-306.9)*

MENTAL RETARDATION (317-319)

Use additional code(s) to identify any associated psychiatric or physical condition(s)

317 Mild mental retardation
High-grade defect
IQ 50-70
Mild mental subnormality

318 Other specified mental retardation

318.0 Moderate mental retardation
IQ 35-49
Moderate mental subnormality

318.1 Severe mental retardation
IQ 20-34
Severe mental subnormality

318.2 Profound mental retardation
IQ under 20
Profound mental subnormality

319 Unspecified mental retardation
Mental deficiency NOS
Mental subnormality NOS

6. DISEASES OF THE NERVOUS SYSTEM AND SENSE ORGANS (320-389)

INFLAMMATORY DISEASES OF THE CENTRAL NERVOUS SYSTEM (320-326)

320 Bacterial meningitis

Includes:

arachnoiditis, leptomeningitis, meningitis, meningoencephalitis, meningomyelitis, pachymeningitis } bacterial

320.0 Hemophilus meningitis

Meningitis due to Hemophilus influenzae [H. influenzae]

320.1 Pneumococcal meningitis

320.2 Streptococcal meningitis

320.3 Staphylococcal meningitis

320.7 Meningitis in other bacterial diseases classified elsewhere

Code first underlying disease, as:

actinomycosis (039.8)
listeriosis (027.0)
typhoid fever (002.0)
whooping cough (033.0-033.9)

Excludes: meningitis (in):

epidemic (036.0)
gonococcal (098.82)
meningococcal (036.0)
salmonellosis (003.21)
syphilis:
NOS (094.2)
congenital (090.42)
meningovascular (094.2)
secondary (091.81)
tuberculous (013.0)

320.8 Meningitis due to other specified bacteria

320.81 Anaerobic meningitis

Bacteroides (fragilis)
Gram-negative anaerobes

320.82 Meningitis due to Gram-negative bacteria, not elsewhere classified

Aerobacter aerogenes
Escherichia coli [E. coli]
Friedlander bacillus
Klebsiella pneumoniae
Proteus morganii
Pseudomonas

Excludes: Gram-negative anaerobes (320.81)

320.89 Meningitis due to other specified bacteria

Bacillus pyocyaneus

320.9 Meningitis due to unspecified bacterium

Meningitis:
bacterial NOS
purulent NOS

Meningitis:
pyogenic NOS
suppurative NOS

321 Meningitis due to other organisms

Includes:

arachnoiditis, leptomeningitis, meningitis, pachymeningitis } due to organisms other than bacteria

321.0 Cryptococcal meningitis

Code first underlying disease (117.5)

321.1 Meningitis in other fungal diseases

Code first underlying disease (110.0-118)

Excludes: meningitis in:

Add 4th or 5th digit | Nonspecific code | Unspecified code | Manifestation code

candidiasis (112.83)
coccidioidomycosis (114.2)
histoplasmosis (115.01, 115.11, 115.91)

321.2 Meningitis due to viruses not elsewhere classified
Code first underlying disease, as:
meningitis due to arbovirus (060.0-066.9)

Excludes: *meningitis (due to):*
abacterial (047.0-047.9)
adenovirus (049.1)
aseptic NOS (047.9)
Coxsackie (virus) (047.0)
ECHO virus (047.1)
enterovirus (047.0-047.9)
herpes simplex virus (054.72)
herpes zoster virus (053.0)
lymphocytic choriomeningitis virus (049.0)
mumps (072.1)
viral NOS (047.9)
meningo-eruptive syndrome (047.1)

321.3 Meningitis due to trypanosomiasis
Code first underlying disease (086.0-086.9)

321.4 Meningitis in sarcoidosis
Code first underlying disease (135)

321.8 Meningitis due to other nonbacterial organisms classified elsewhere
Code first underlying disease

Excludes: *leptospiral meningitis (100.81)*

322 Meningitis of unspecified cause
Includes:
arachnoiditis, leptomeningitis, meningitis, pachymeningitis } with no organism specified as cause

322.0 Nonpyogenic meningitis
Meningitis with clear cerebrospinal fluid

322.1 Eosinophilic meningitis

322.2 Chronic meningitis

322.9 Meningitis, unspecified

323 Encephalitis, myelitis, and encephalomyelitis
Includes: acute disseminated encephalomyelitis
meningoencephalitis, except bacterial
meningomyelitis, except bacterial
myelitis (acute):
ascending
transverse

Excludes: *bacterial:*
meningoencephalitis (320.0-320.9)
meningomyelitis (320.0-320.9)

323.0 Encephalitis in viral diseases classified elsewhere
Code first underlying disease, as:
cat-scratch disease (078.3)
infectious mononucleosis (075)
ornithosis (073.7)

Excludes: *encephalitis (in):*
arthropod-borne viral (062.0-064)
herpes simplex (054.3)
mumps (072.2)
poliomyelitis (045.0-045.9)
rubella (056.01)
slow virus infections of central nervous system (046.0-046.9)
other viral diseases of central nervous system (049.8-049.9)
viral NOS (049.9)

323.1 Encephalitis in rickettsial diseases classified elsewhere
Code first underlying disease (080-083.9)

● Code new to this edition ▲ Revision of existing code ④ ⑤ Fourth or fifth digit required

323.2 ***Encephalitis in protozoal diseases classified elsewhere***
Code first underlying disease, as:
malaria (084.0-084.9)
trypanosomiasis (086.0-086.9)

323.4 ***Other encephalitis due to infection classified elsewhere***
Code first underlying disease

Excludes: *encephalitis (in):*
meningococcal (036.1)
syphilis:
NOS (094.81)
congenital (090.41)
toxoplasmosis (130.0)
tuberculosis (013.6)
meningoencephalitis due to free-living ameba [Naegleria] (136.2)

323.5 Encephalitis following immunization procedures
Encephalitis } postimmunization or postvaccinal
Encephalomyelitis } postimmunization or postvaccinal

Use additional E code, if desired, to identify vaccine

323.6 ***Postinfectious encephalitis***
Code first underlying disease

Excludes: *encephalitis:*
postchickenpox (052.0)
postmeasles (055.0)

323.7 ***Toxic encephalitis***
Code first underlying cause, as:
carbon tetrachloride (982.1)
hydroxyquinoline derivatives (961.3)
lead (984.0-984.9)
mercury (985.0)
thallium (985.8)

323.8 Other causes of encephalitis

323.9 Unspecified cause of encephalitis

324 Intracranial and intraspinal abscess

324.0 Intracranial abscess
Abscess (embolic):
cerebellar
cerebral

Abscess (embolic) of brain [any part]:
epidural
extradural
otogenic
subdural

Excludes: *tuberculous (013.3)*

324.1 Intraspinal abscess
Abscess (embolic) of spinal cord [any part]:
epidural
extradural
subdural

Excludes: *tuberculous (013.5)*

324.9 Of unspecified site
Extradural or subdural abscess NOS

325 Phlebitis and thrombophlebitis of intracranial venous sinuses
Embolism
Endophlebitis
Phlebitis, septic or suppurative } of cavernous, lateral, or other intracranial or unspecified intracranial venous sinus
Thrombophlebitis } of cavernous, lateral, or other intracranial or unspecified intracranial venous sinus
Thrombosis } of cavernous, lateral, or other intracranial or unspecified intracranial venous sinus

Excludes: *that specified as:*
complicating pregnancy, childbirth, or the puerperium (671.5)
of nonpyogenic origin (437.6)

Add 4th or 5th digit | Nonspecific code | Unspecified code | Manifestation code

326 Late effects of intracranial abscess or pyogenic infection

Note: This category is to be used to indicate conditions whose primary classification is to 320-325 [excluding 320.7, 321.0-321.8, 323.0-323.4, 323.6-323.7] as the cause of late effects, themselves classifiable elsewhere. The "late effects" include conditions specified as such, or as sequelae, which may occur at any time after the resolution of the causal condition.

Use additional code, if desired, to identify condition, as:
hydrocephalus (331.4)
paralysis (342.0-342.9, 344.0-344.9)

HEREDITARY AND DEGENERATIVE DISEASES OF THE CENTRAL NERVOUS SYSTEM (330-337)

Excludes: *hepatolenticular degeneration (275.1)*
multiple sclerosis (340)
other demyelinating diseases of central nervous system (341.0-341.9)

330 Cerebral degenerations usually manifest in childhood

Use additional code, if desired, to identify associated mental retardation

330.0 Leukodystrophy
Krabbe's disease
Leukodystrophy:
NOS
globoid cell
Leukodystrophy:
metachromatic
sudanophilic
Pelizaeus-Merzbacher disease
Sulfatide lipidosis

330.1 Cerebral lipidoses
Amaurotic (familial) idiocy
Disease:
Batten
Jansky-Bielschowsky
Disease:
Kufs'
Spielmeyer-Vogt
Tay-Sachs
Gangliosidosis

330.2 Cerebral degeneration in generalized lipidoses
Code first underlying disease, as:
Fabry's disease (272.7)
Gaucher's disease (272.7)
Neimann-Pick disease (272.7)
sphingolipidosis (272.7)

330.3 Cerebral degeneration of childhood in other diseases classified elsewhere
Code first underlying disease, as:
Hunter's disease (277.5)
mucopolysaccharidosis (277.5)

330.8 Other specified cerebral degenerations in childhood
Alpers' disease or gray-matter degeneration
Infantile necrotizing encephalomyelopathy
Leigh's disease
Subacute necrotizing encephalopathy or encephalomyelopathy

330.9 Unspecified cerebral degeneration in childhood

331 Other cerebral degenerations

331.0 Alzheimer's disease

331.1 Pick's disease

331.2 Senile degeneration of brain

Excludes: *senility NOS (797)*

331.3 Communicating hydrocephalus

Excludes: *congenital hydrocephalus (741.0, 742.3)*

331.4 Obstructive hydrocephalus
Acquired hydrocephalus NOS

Excludes: *congenital hydrocephalus (741.0, 742.3)*

331.7 ***Cerebral degeneration in diseases classified elsewhere***
Code first underlying disease, as:
alcoholism (303.0-303.9)
beriberi (265.0)
cerebrovascular disease (430-438)
congenital hydrocephalus (741.0, 742.3)
neoplastic disease (140.0-239.9)
myxedema (244.0-244.9)
vitamin B_{12} deficiency (266.2)

Excludes: *cerebral degeneration in:*
Jakob-Creutzfeldt disease (046.1)
progressive multifocal leukoencephalopathy (046.3)
subacute spongiform encephalopathy (046.1)

331.8 Other cerebral degeneration

331.81 Reye's syndrome

331.89 Other
Cerebral ataxia

331.9 Cerebral degeneration, unspecified

332 Parkinson's disease

332.0 Paralysis agitans
Parkinsonism or Parkinson's disease:
NOS
idiopathic
primary

332.1 Secondary Parkinsonism
Parkinsonism due to drugs

Use additional E code, if desired, to identify drug, if drug-induced

Excludes: *Parkinsonism (in):*
Huntington's disease (333.4)
progressive supranuclear palsy (333.0)
Shy-Drager syndrome (333.0)
syphilitic (094.82)

333 Other extrapyramidal disease and abnormal movement disorders
Includes: other forms of extrapyramidal, basal ganglia, or striatopallidal disease

Excludes: *abnormal movements of head NOS (781.0)*

333.0 Other degenerative diseases of the basal ganglia
Atrophy or degeneration:
olivopontocerebellar [Déjérine-Thomas syndrome]
pigmentary pallidal [Hallervorden-Spatz disease]
striatonigral
Parkinsonian syndrome associated with:
idiopathic orthostatic hypotension
symptomatic orthostatic hypotension
Progressive supranuclear ophthalmoplegia or palsy
Shy-Drager syndrome

333.1 Essential and other specified forms of tremor
Benign essential tremor
Familial tremor

Use additional E code, if desired, to identify drug, if drug-induced

Excludes: *tremor NOS (781.0)*

333.2 Myoclonus
Familial essential myoclonus
Progressive myoclonic epilepsy
Unverricht-Lundborg disease

Use additional E code, if desired, to identify drug, if drug-induced

333.3 Tics of organic origin

Excludes: *Gilles de la Tourette's syndrome (307.23)*
habit spasm (307.22)
tic NOS (307.20)

Use additional E code, if desired, to identify drug, if drug-induced

333.4 Huntington's chorea

Add 4th or 5th digit | Nonspecific code | Unspecified code | Manifestation code

333.5 Other choreas
Hemiballism(us)
Paroxysmal choreo-athetosis

Excludes: *Sydenham's or rheumatic chorea (392.0-392.9)*

Use additional E code, if desired, to identify drug, if drug-induced

333.6 Idiopathic torsion dystonia
Dystonia:
deformans progressiva
musculorum deformans
(Schwalbe-) Ziehen-Oppenheim disease

333.7 Symptomatic torsion dystonia
Athetoid cerebral palsy [Vogt's disease]
Double athetosis (syndrome)

Use additional E code, if desired, to identify drug, if drug-induced

333.8 Fragments of torsion dystonia

Use additional E code, if desired, to identify drug, if drug-induced

333.81 Blepharospasm

333.82 Orofacial dyskinesia

333.83 Spasmodic torticollis

Excludes: *torticollis:*
NOS (723.5)
hysterical (300.11)
psychogenic (306.0)

333.84 Organic writers' cramp

Excludes: *psychogenic (300.89)*

333.89 Other

333.9 Other and unspecified extrapyramidal diseases and abnormal movement disorders

333.90 Unspecified extrapyramidal disease and abnormal movement disorder

333.91 Stiff-man syndrome

333.92 Neuroleptic malignant syndrome
Use additional E code to identify drug

333.93 Benign shuddering attacks

333.99 Other
Restless legs

334 Spinocerebellar disease

Excludes: *olivopontocerebellar degeneration (333.0)*
peroneal muscular atrophy (356.1)

334.0 Friedreich's ataxia

334.1 Hereditary spastic paraplegia

334.2 Primary cerebellar degeneration
Cerebellar ataxia:
Marie's
Sanger-Brown
Dyssynergia cerebellaris myoclonica
Primary cerebellar degeneration:
NOS
hereditary
sporadic

334.3 Other cerebellar ataxia
Cerebellar ataxia NOS

Use additional E code, if desired, to identify drug, if drug-induced

334.4 Cerebellar ataxia in diseases classified elsewhere
Code first underlying disease, as:
alcoholism (303.0-303.9)
myxedema (244.0-244.9)
neoplastic disease (140.0-239.9)

334.8 Other spinocerebellar diseases
Ataxia-telangiectasia [Louis-Bar syndrome]
Corticostriatal-spinal degeneration

334.9 Spinocerebellar disease, unspecified

335 Anterior horn cell disease

335.0 Werdnig-Hoffmann disease
Infantile spinal muscular atrophy
Progressive muscular atrophy of infancy

335.1 Spinal muscular atrophy

335.10 Spinal muscular atrophy, unspecified

335.11 Kugelberg-Welander disease
Spinal muscular atrophy:
familial
juvenile

335.19 Other
Adult spinal muscular atrophy

335.2 Motor neuron disease

335.20 Amyotrophic lateral sclerosis
Motor neuron disease (bulbar) (mixed type)

335.21 Progressive muscular atrophy
Duchenne-Aran muscular atrophy
Progressive muscular atrophy (pure)

335.22 Progressive bulbar palsy

335.23 Pseudobulbar palsy

335.24 Primary lateral sclerosis

335.29 Other

335.8 Other anterior horn cell diseases

335.9 Anterior horn cell disease, unspecified

336 Other diseases of spinal cord

336.0 Syringomyelia and syringobulbia

336.1 Vascular myelopathies
Acute infarction of spinal cord (embolic) (nonembolic)
Arterial thrombosis of spinal cord
Edema of spinal cord
Hematomyelia
Subacute necrotic myelopathy

336.2 Subacute combined degeneration of spinal cord in diseases classified elsewhere
Code first underlying disease, as:
pernicious anemia (281.0)
other vitamin B_{12} deficiency anemia (281.1)
vitamin B_{12} deficiency (266.2)

336.3 Myelopathy in other diseases classified elsewhere
Code first underlying disease, as:
myelopathy in neoplastic disease (140.0-239.9)

Excludes: *myelopathy in:*
intervertebral disc disorder (722.70-722.73)
spondylosis (721.1, 721.41-721.42, 721.91)

336.8 Other myelopathy
Myelopathy:
drug-induced
radiation-induced

Use additional E code, if desired, to identify cause

336.9 Unspecified disease of spinal cord
Cord compression NOS
Myelopathy NOS

Excludes: *myelitis (323.0-323.9)*
spinal (canal) stenosis (723.0, 724.00-724.09)

337 Disorders of the autonomic nervous system
Includes: disorders of peripheral autonomic, sympathetic, parasympathetic, or vegetative system

Excludes: *familial dysautonomia [Riley-Day syndrome] (742.8)*

337.0 Idiopathic peripheral autonomic neuropathy
Carotid sinus syncope or syndrome
Cervical sympathetic dystrophy or paralysis

Add 4th or 5th digit | Nonspecific code | Unspecified code | Manifestation code

337.1 *Peripheral autonomic neuropathy in disorders classified elsewhere*
Code first underlying disease, as:
amyloidosis (277.3)
diabetes (250.6)

337.2 Reflex sympathetic dystrophy

337.20 Reflex sympathetic dystrophy, unspecified

337.21 Reflex sympathetic dystrophy of the upper limb

337.22 Reflex sympathetic dystrophy of the lower limb

337.29 Reflex sympathetic dystrophy of other specified site

337.9 Unspecified disorder of autonomic nervous system

OTHER DISORDERS OF THE CENTRAL NERVOUS SYSTEM (340-349)

340 Multiple sclerosis
Disseminated or multiple sclerosis:
NOS
brain stem
cord
generalized

341 Other demyelinating diseases of central nervous system

341.0 Neuromyelitis optica

341.1 Schilder's disease
Baló's concentric sclerosis
Encephalitis periaxialis:
concentrica [Baló's]
diffusa [Schilder's]

341.8 Other demyelinating diseases of central nervous system
Central demyelination of corpus callosum
Central pontine myelinosis
Marchiafava (-Bignami) disease

341.9 Demyelinating disease of central nervous system, unspecified

⑤ **342 Hemiplegia and hemiparesis**

Note: This category is to be used when hemiplegia (complete) (incomplete) is reported without further specification, or is stated to be old or long-standing but of unspecified cause. The category is also for use in multiple coding to identify these types of hemiplegia resulting from any cause.

The following fifth-digits are for use with codes 342.0-342.9

0 affecting unspecified site

1 affecting dominant site

2 affecting nondominant site

Excludes: *congenital (343.1)*
infantile NOS (343.4)

342.0 Flaccid hemiplegia

342.1 Spastic hemiplegia

342.8 Other specified hemiplegia

342.9 Hemiplegia, unspecified

343 Infantile cerebral palsy
Includes: cerebral:
palsy NOS
spastic infantile paralysis
congenital spastic paralysis (cerebral)
Little's disease
paralysis (spastic) due to birth injury:
intracranial
spinal

Excludes: *hereditary cerebral paralysis, such as:*
hereditary spastic paraplegia (334.1)
Vogt's disease (333.7)
spastic paralysis specified as noncongenital or noninfantile (344.0-344.9)

343.0 Diplegic
Congenital diplegia
Congenital paraplegia

● Code new to this edition
▲ Revision of existing code
④ ⑤ Fourth or fifth digit required

343.1 Hemiplegic
Congenital hemiplegia

Excludes: *infantile hemiplegia NOS (343.4)*

343.2 Quadriplegic
Tetraplegic

343.3 Monoplegic

343.4 Infantile hemiplegia
Infantile hemiplegia (postnatal) NOS

343.8 Other specified infantile cerebral palsy

343.9 Infantile cerebral palsy, unspecified
Cerebral palsy NOS

344 Other paralytic syndromes

Note: This category is to be used when the listed conditions are reported without further specification or are stated to be old or long-standing but of unspecified cause. The category is also for use in multiple coding to identify these conditions resulting from any cause.

Includes: paralysis (complete) (incomplete), except as classifiable to 342 and 343

Excludes: *congenital or infantile cerebral palsy (343.0-343.9)*
hemiplegia (342.0-342.9)
congenital or infantile (343.1, 343.4)

344.0 Quadriplegia and quadriparesis

344.00 Quadriplegia, unspecified

344.01 C1-C4, complete

344.02 C1-C4, incomplete

344.03 C5-C7, complete

344.04 C5-C7, incomplete

344.09 Other

344.1 Paraplegia
Paralysis of both lower limbs
Paraplegia (lower)

344.2 Diplegia of upper limbs
Diplegia (upper)
Paralysis of both upper limbs

344.3 Monoplegia of lower limb
Paralysis of lower limb

344.30 affecting unspecified side

344.31 affecting dominant side

344.32 affecting nondominant side

344.4 Monoplegia of upper limb
Paralysis of upper limb

344.40 affecting unspecified side

344.41 affecting dominant side

344.42 affecting nondominant side

344.5 Unspecified monoplegia

344.6 Cauda equina syndrome

344.60 Without mention of neurogenic bladder

344.61 With neurogenic bladder
Acontractile bladder
Autonomic hyperreflexia of bladder
Cord bladder
Detrusor hyperreflexia

344.8 Other specified paralytic syndromes

344.81 Locked-in state

344.89 Other specified paralytic syndrome

344.9 Paralysis, unspecified

345 Epilepsy

The following fifth-digit subclassification is for use with categories 345.0, 345.1, 345.4-345.9:

0 without mention of intractable epilepsy

1 with intractable epilepsy

Excludes: *progressive myoclonic epilepsy (333.2)*

⑤ **345.0 Generalized nonconvulsive epilepsy**

Absences:
  atonic
  typical
Minor epilepsy
Petit mal
Pykno-epilepsy
Seizures:
  akinetic
  atonic

⑤ **345.1 Generalized convulsive epilepsy**

Epileptic seizures:
  clonic
  myoclonic
  tonic
  tonic-clonic
Grand mal
Major epilepsy

Excludes: *convulsions:*
  NOS (780.3)
  infantile (780.3)
  newborn (779.0)
infantile spasms (345.6)

345.2 Petit mal status

Epileptic absence status

345.3 Grand mal status

Status epilepticus NOS

Excludes: *epilepsia partialis continua (345.7)*
status:
  psychomotor (345.7)
  temporal lobe (345.7)

⑤ **345.4 Partial epilepsy, with impairment of consciousness**

Epilepsy:
  limbic system
  partial:
    secondarily generalized
    with memory and ideational disturbances
  psychomotor
  psychosensory
  temporal lobe
Epileptic automatism

⑤ **345.5 Partial epilepsy, without mention of impairment of consciousness**

Epilepsy:
  Bravais-Jacksonian NOS
  focal (motor) NOS
  Jacksonian NOS
  motor partial
  partial NOS
Epilepsy:
  sensory-induced
  somatomotor
  somatosensory
  visceral
  visual

⑤ **345.6 Infantile spasms**

Hypsarrhythmia
Lightning spasms
Salaam attacks

Excludes: *salaam tic (781.0)*

⑤ **345.7 Epilepsia partialis continua**

Kojevnikov's epilepsy

⑤ **345.8 Other forms of epilepsy**

Epilepsy:
  cursive [running]
  gelastic

⑤ **345.9 Epilepsy, unspecified**

Epileptic convulsions, fits, or seizures NOS

Excludes: *convulsive seizure or fit NOS (780.3)*

⑤ **346 Migraine**

The following fifth-digit subclassification is for use with category 346:

0 without mention of intractable migraine

1 with intractable migraine, so stated

346.0 Classical migraine
Migraine preceded or accompanied by transient focal neurological phenomena
Migraine with aura

346.1 Common migraine
Atypical migraine
Sick headache

346.2 Variants of migraine
Cluster headache
Histamine cephalgia
Horton's neuralgia
Migraine:
abdominal
basilar
Migraine:
lower half
retinal
Neuralgia:
ciliary
migrainous

346.8 Other forms of migraine
Migraine:
hemiplegic
ophthalmoplegic

346.9 Migraine, unspecified

347 Cataplexy and narcolepsy

348 Other conditions of brain

348.0 Cerebral cysts
Arachnoid cyst
Porencephalic cyst
Porencephaly, acquired
Pseudoporencephaly

Excludes: *porencephaly (congenital) (742.4)*

348.1 Anoxic brain damage

Excludes: *that occurring in:*
abortion (634-638 with .7, 639.8)
ectopic or molar pregnancy (639.8)
labor or delivery (668.2, 669.4)
that of newborn (767.0, 768.0-768.9, 772.1-772.2)

Use additional E code, if desired, to identify cause

348.2 Benign intracranial hypertension
Pseudotumor cerebri

Excludes: *hypertensive encephalopathy (437.2)*

348.3 Encephalopathy, unspecified

348.4 Compression of brain
Compression } brain (stem)
Herniation } brain (stem)
Posterior fossa compression syndrome

348.5 Cerebral edema

348.8 Other conditions of brain
Cerebral:
calcification
fungus

348.9 Unspecified condition of brain

349 Other and unspecified disorders of the nervous system

349.0 Reaction to spinal or lumbar puncture
Headache following lumbar puncture

349.1 Nervous system complications from surgically implanted device

Excludes: *immediate postoperative complications (997.0)*
mechanical complications of nervous system device (996.2)

349.2 Disorders of meninges, not elsewhere classified
Adhesions, meningeal (cerebral) (spinal)
Cyst, spinal meninges
Meningocele, acquired
Pseudomeningocele, acquired

Add 4th or 5th digit | Nonspecific code | Unspecified code | Manifestation code

349.8 Other specified disorders of nervous system

349.81 Cerebrospinal fluid rhinorrhea

Excludes: *cerebrospinal fluid otorrhea (388.61)*

349.82 Toxic encephalopathy
Use additional E code, if desired, to identify cause

349.89 Other

349.9 Unspecified disorders of nervous system
Disorder of nervous system (central) NOS

DISORDERS OF THE PERIPHERAL NERVOUS SYSTEM (350-359)

Excludes: *diseases of:*
acoustic [8th] nerve (388.5)
oculomotor [3rd, 4th, 6th] nerves (378.0-378.9)
optic [2nd] nerve (377.0-377.9)
peripheral autonomic nerves (337.0-337.9)
neuralgia / *neuritis* / *radiculitis* } NOS or "rheumatic" (729.2)
peripheral neuritis in pregnancy (646.4)

350 Trigeminal nerve disorders
Includes: disorders of 5th cranial nerve

350.1 Trigeminal neuralgia
Tic douloureux
Trifacial neuralgia
Trigeminal neuralgia NOS

Excludes: *postherpetic (053.12)*

350.2 Atypical face pain

350.8 Other specified trigeminal nerve disorders

350.9 Trigeminal nerve disorder, unspecified

351 Facial nerve disorders
Includes: disorders of 7th cranial nerve

Excludes: *that in newborn (767.5)*

351.0 Bell's palsy
Facial palsy

351.1 Geniculate ganglionitis
Geniculate ganglionitis NOS

Excludes: *herpetic (053.11)*

351.8 Other facial nerve disorders
Facial myokymia
Melkersson's syndrome

351.9 Facial nerve disorder, unspecified

352 Disorders of other cranial nerves

352.0 Disorders of olfactory [1st] nerve

352.1 Glossopharyngeal neuralgia

352.2 Other disorders of glossopharyngeal [9th] nerve

352.3 Disorders of pneumogastric [10th] nerve
Disorders of vagal nerve

Excludes: *paralysis of vocal cords or larynx (478.30-478.34)*

352.4 Disorders of accessory [11th] nerve

352.5 Disorders of hypoglossal [12th] nerve

352.6 Multiple cranial nerve palsies
Collet-Sicard syndrome
Polyneuritis cranialis

352.9 Unspecified disorder of cranial nerves

353 Nerve root and plexus disorders

Excludes: *conditions due to:*
intervertebral disc disorders (722.0-722.9)
spondylosis (720.0-721.9)
vertebrogenic disorders (723.0-724.9)

353.0 Brachial plexus lesions
Cervical rib syndrome
Costoclavicular syndrome
Scalenus anticus syndrome
Thoracic outlet syndrome

Excludes: *brachial neuritis or radiculitis NOS (723.4)*
that in newborn (767.6)

353.1 Lumbosacral plexus lesions

353.2 Cervical root lesions, not elsewhere classified

353.3 Thoracic root lesions, not elsewhere classified

353.4 Lumbosacral root lesions, not elsewhere classified

353.5 Neuralgic amyotrophy
Parsonage-Aldren-Turner syndrome

353.6 Phantom limb (syndrome)

353.8 Other nerve root and plexus disorders

353.9 Unspecified nerve root and plexus disorder

354 Mononeuritis of upper limb and mononeuritis multiplex

354.0 Carpal tunnel syndrome
Median nerve entrapment
Partial thenar atrophy

354.1 Other lesion of median nerve
Median nerve neuritis

354.2 Lesion of ulnar nerve
Cubital tunnel syndrome
Tardy ulnar nerve palsy

354.3 Lesion of radial nerve
Acute radial nerve palsy

354.4 Causalgia of upper limb

Excludes: *causalgia:*
NOS (355.9)
lower limb (355.71)

354.5 Mononeuritis multiplex
Combinations of single conditions classifiable to 354 or 355

354.8 Other mononeuritis of upper limb

354.9 Mononeuritis of upper limb, unspecified

355 Mononeuritis of lower limb and unspecified site

355.0 Lesion of sciatic nerve

Excludes: *sciatica NOS (724.3)*

355.1 Meralgia paresthetica
Lateral cutaneous femoral nerve of thigh compression or syndrome

355.2 Other lesion of femoral nerve

355.3 Lesion of lateral popliteal nerve
Lesion of common peroneal nerve

355.4 Lesion of medial popliteal nerve

355.5 Tarsal tunnel syndrome

355.6 Lesion of plantar nerve
Morton's metatarsalgia, neuralgia, or neuroma

355.7 Other mononeuritis of lower limb

355.71 Causalgia of lower limb

Excludes: *causalgia:*
NOS (355.9)
upper limb (354.4)

355.79 Other mononeuritis of lower limb

355.8 Mononeuritis of lower limb, unspecified

355.9 Mononeuritis of unspecified site
Causalgia NOS

Excludes: *causalgia:*
lower limb (355.71)
upper limb (354.4)

356 Hereditary and idiopathic peripheral neuropathy

356.0 Hereditary peripheral neuropathy
Déjérine-Sottas disease

356.1 Peroneal muscular atrophy
Charcot-Marie-Tooth disease
Neuropathic muscular atrophy

356.2 Hereditary sensory neuropathy

356.3 Refsum's disease
Heredopathia atactica polyneuritiformis

356.4 Idiopathic progressive polyneuropathy

356.8 Other specified idiopathic peripheral neuropathy
Supranuclear paralysis

356.9 Unspecified

357 Inflammatory and toxic neuropathy

357.0 Acute infective polyneuritis
Guillain-Barré syndrome
Postinfectious polyneuritis

357.1 Polyneuropathy in collagen vascular disease
Code first underlying disease, as:
disseminated lupus erythematosus (710.0)
polyarteritis nodosa (446.0)
rheumatoid arthritis (714.0)

357.2 Polyneuropathy in diabetes
Code first underlying disease (250.6)

357.3 Polyneuropathy in malignant disease
Code first underlying disease (140.0-208.9)

357.4 Polyneuropathy in other diseases classified elsewhere
Code first underlying disease, as:
amyloidosis (277.3)
beriberi (265.0)
deficiency of B vitamins (266.0-266.9)
diphtheria (032.0-032.9)
hypoglycemia (251.2)
pellagra (265.2)
porphyria (277.1)
sarcoidosis (135)
uremia (585)

Excludes: *polyneuropathy in:*
herpes zoster (053.13)
mumps (072.72)

357.5 Alcoholic polyneuropathy

357.6 Polyneuropathy due to drugs
Use additional E code, if desired, to identify drug

357.7 Polyneuropathy due to other toxic agents
Use additional E code, if desired, to identify toxic agent

357.8 Other

357.9 Unspecified

358 Myoneural disorders

358.0 Myasthenia gravis

358.1 Myasthenic syndromes in diseases classified elsewhere
Amyotrophy } from stated cause classified elsewhere
Eaton-Lambert syndrome } from stated cause classified elsewhere
Code first underlying disease, as:
botulism (005.1)
diabetes mellitus (250.6)
hypothyroidism (244.0-244.9)
malignant neoplasm (140.0-208.9)
pernicious anemia (281.0)
thyrotoxicosis (242.0-242.9)

358.2 Toxic myoneural disorders
Use additional E code, if desired, to identify toxic agent

358.8 Other specified myoneural disorders

358.9 Myoneural disorders, unspecified

359 Muscular dystrophies and other myopathies

Excludes: *idiopathic polymyositis (710.4)*

359.0 Congenital hereditary muscular dystrophy
Benign congenital myopathy
Central core disease
Centronuclear myopathy
Myotubular myopathy
Nemaline body disease

Excludes: *arthrogryposis multiplex congenita (754.89)*

359.1 Hereditary progressive muscular dystrophy
Muscular dystrophy:
NOS
distal
Duchenne
Erb's
fascioscapulohumeral
Muscular dystrophy:
Gower's
Landouzy-Déjérine
limb-girdle
ocular
oculopharyngeal

359.2 Myotonic disorders
Dystrophia myotonica
Eulenburg's disease
Myotonia congenita
Paramyotonia congenita
Steinert's disease
Thomsen's disease

359.3 Familial periodic paralysis
Hypokalemic familial periodic paralysis

359.4 Toxic myopathy
Use additional E code, if desired, to identify toxic agent

359.5 Myopathy in endocrine diseases classified elsewhere
Code first underlying disease, as:
Addison's disease (255.4)
Cushing's syndrome (255.0)
hypopituitarism (253.2)
myxedema (244.0-244.9)
thyrotoxicosis (242.0-242.9)

359.6 Symptomatic inflammatory myopathy in diseases classified elsewhere
Code first underlying disease, as:
amyloidosis (277.3)
disseminated lupus erythematosus (710.0)
malignant neoplasm (140.0-208.9)
polyarteritis nodosa (446.0)
rheumatoid arthritis (714.0)
sarcoidosis (135)
scleroderma (710.1)
Sjögren's disease (710.2)

359.8 Other myopathies

359.9 Myopathy, unspecified

DISORDERS OF THE EYE AND ADNEXA (360-379)

360 Disorders of the globe
Includes: disorders affecting multiple structures of eye

360.0 Purulent endophthalmitis

360.00 Purulent endophthalmitis, unspecified

360.01 Acute endophthalmitis

360.02 Panophthalmitis

360.03 Chronic endophthalmitis

360.04 Vitreous abscess

360.1 Other endophthalmitis

360.11 Sympathetic uveitis

360.12 Panuveitis

360.13 Parasitic endophthalmitis NOS

360.14 Ophthalmia nodosa

360.19 Other
Phacoanaphylactic endophthalmitis

360.2 Degenerative disorders of globe

360.20 Degenerative disorder of globe, unspecified

360.21 Progressive high (degenerative) myopia
Malignant myopia

360.23 Siderosis

360.24 Other metallosis
Chalcosis

360.29 Other

Excludes: *xerophthalmia (264.7)*

360.3 Hypotony of eye

360.30 Hypotony, unspecified

360.31 Primary hypotony

360.32 Ocular fistula causing hypotony

360.33 Hypotony associated with other ocular disorders

360.34 Flat anterior chamber

360.4 Degenerated conditions of globe

360.40 Degenerated globe or eye, unspecified

360.41 Blind hypotensive eye
Atrophy of globe   Phthisis bulbi

360.42 Blind hypertensive eye
Absolute glaucoma

360.43 Hemophthalmos, except current injury

Excludes: *traumatic (871.0-871.9, 921.0-921.9)*

360.44 Leucocoria

360.5 Retained (old) intraocular foreign body, magnetic

Excludes: *current penetrating injury with magnetic foreign body (871.5)*
retained (old) foreign body of orbit (376.6)

360.50 Foreign body, magnetic, intraocular, unspecified

360.51 Foreign body, magnetic, in anterior chamber

360.52 Foreign body, magnetic, in iris or ciliary body

360.53 Foreign body, magnetic, in lens

360.54 Foreign body, magnetic, in vitreous

360.55 Foreign body, magnetic, in posterior wall

360.59 Foreign body, magnetic, in other or multiple sites

360.6 Retained (old) intraocular foreign body, nonmagnetic
Retained (old) foreign body:
NOS
nonmagnetic

Excludes: *current penetrating injury with (nonmagnetic) foreign body (871.6)*
retained (old) foreign body in orbit (376.6)

360.60 Foreign body, intraocular, unspecified

360.61 Foreign body in anterior chamber

360.62 Foreign body in iris or ciliary body

360.63 Foreign body in lens

360.64 Foreign body in vitreous

360.65 Foreign body in posterior wall

360.69 Foreign body in other or multiple sites

360.8 Other disorders of globe

360.81 Luxation of globe

360.89 Other

360.9 Unspecified disorder of globe

361 Retinal detachments and defects

361.0 Retinal detachment with retinal defect
Rhegmatogenous retinal detachment

Excludes: *detachment of retinal pigment epithelium (362.42-362.43)*
retinal detachment (serous) (without defect) (361.2)

361.00 Retinal detachment with retinal defect, unspecified

361.01 Recent detachment, partial, with single defect

361.02 Recent detachment, partial, with multiple defects

361.03 Recent detachment, partial, with giant tear

361.04 Recent detachment, partial, with retinal dialysis
Dialysis (juvenile) of retina (with detachment)

361.05 Recent detachment, total or subtotal

361.06 Old detachment, partial
Delimited old retinal detachment

361.07 Old detachment, total or subtotal

361.1 Retinoschisis and retinal cysts

Excludes: *juvenile retinoschisis (362.73)*
microcystoid degeneration of retina (362.62)
parasitic cyst of retina (360.13)

361.10 Retinoschisis, unspecified

361.11 Flat retinoschisis

361.12 Bullous retinoschisis

361.13 Primary retinal cysts

361.14 Secondary retinal cysts

361.19 Other
Pseudocyst of retina

361.2 Serous retinal detachment
Retinal detachment without retinal defect

Excludes: *central serous retinopathy (362.41)*
retinal pigment epithelium detachment (362.42-362.43)

361.3 Retinal defects without detachment

Excludes: *chorioretinal scars after surgery for detachment (363.30-363.35)*
peripheral retinal degeneration without defect (362.60-362.66)

361.30 Retinal defect, unspecified
Retinal break(s) NOS

361.31 Round hole of retina without detachment

361.32 Horseshoe tear of retina without detachment
Operculum of retina without mention of detachment

361.33 Multiple defects of retina without detachment

361.8 Other forms of retinal detachment

361.81 Traction detachment of retina
Traction detachment with vitreoretinal organization

361.89 Other

361.9 Unspecified retinal detachment

362 Other retinal disorders

Excludes: *chorioretinal scars (363.30-363.35)*
chorioretinitis (363.0-363.2)

362.0 Diabetic retinopathy
Code first diabetes (250.5)

362.01 Background diabetic retinopathy
Diabetic retinal microaneurysms
Diabetic retinopathy NOS

362.02 Proliferative diabetic retinopathy

362.1 Other background retinopathy and retinal vascular changes

362.10 Background retinopathy, unspecified

Add 4th or 5th digit | Nonspecific code | Unspecified code | Manifestation code

362.11 Hypertensive retinopathy

362.12 Exudative retinopathy
Coats' syndrome

362.13 Changes in vascular appearance
Vascular sheathing of retina
Use additional code for any associated atherosclerosis (440.8)

362.14 Retinal microaneurysms NOS

362.15 Retinal telangiectasia

362.16 Retinal neovascularization NOS
Neovascularization:
choroidal
subretinal

362.17 Other intraretinal microvascular abnormalities
Retinal varices

362.18 Retinal vasculitis
Eales' disease
Retinal:
arteritis
endarteritis
Retinal:
perivasculitis
phlebitis

362.2 Other proliferative retinopathy

362.21 Retrolental fibroplasia

362.29 Other nondiabetic proliferative retinopathy

362.3 Retinal vascular occlusion

362.30 Retinal vascular occlusion, unspecified

362.31 Central retinal artery occlusion

362.32 Arterial branch occlusion

362.33 Partial arterial occlusion
Hollenhorst plaque
Retinal microembolism

362.34 Transient arterial occlusion
Amaurosis fugax

362.35 Central retinal vein occlusion

362.36 Venous tributary (branch) occlusion

362.37 Venous engorgement
Occlusion:
incipient } of retinal vein
partial }

362.4 Separation of retinal layers

Excludes: *retinal detachment (serous) (361.2)*
rhegmatogenous (361.00-361.07)

362.40 Retinal layer separation, unspecified

362.41 Central serous retinopathy

362.42 Serous detachment of retinal pigment epithelium
Exudative detachment of retinal pigment epithelium

362.43 Hemorrhagic detachment of retinal pigment epithelium

362.5 Degeneration of macula and posterior pole

Excludes: *degeneration of optic disc (377.21-377.24)*
hereditary retinal degeneration [dystrophy] (362.70-362.77)

362.50 Macular degeneration (senile), unspecified

362.51 Nonexudative senile macular degeneration
Senile macular degeneration:
atrophic
dry

362.52 Exudative senile macular degeneration
Kuhnt-Junius degeneration
Senile macular degeneration:
disciform
wet

362.53 Cystoid macular degeneration
Cystoid macular edema

● Code new to this edition
▲ Revision of existing code
④ ⑤ Fourth or fifth digit required

362.54 Macular cyst, hole, or pseudohole

362.55 Toxic maculopathy
Use additional E code, if desired, to identify drug, if drug induced

362.56 Macular puckering
Preretinal fibrosis

362.57 Drusen (degenerative)

362.6 Peripheral retinal degenerations

Excludes: *hereditary retinal degeneration [dystrophy] (362.70-362.77)*
retinal degeneration with retinal defect (361.00-361.07)

362.60 Peripheral retinal degeneration, unspecified

362.61 Paving stone degeneration

362.62 Microcystoid degeneration
Blessig's cysts
Iwanoff's cysts

362.63 Lattice degeneration
Palisade degeneration of retina

362.64 Senile reticular degeneration

362.65 Secondary pigmentary degeneration
Pseudoretinitis pigmentosa

362.66 Secondary vitreoretinal degenerations

362.7 Hereditary retinal dystrophies

362.70 Hereditary retinal dystrophy, unspecified

362.71 Retinal dystrophy in systemic or cerebroretinal lipidoses
Code first underlying disease, as:
cerebroretinal lipidoses (330.1)
systemic lipidoses (272.7)

362.72 Retinal dystrophy in other systemic disorders and syndromes
Code first underlying disease, as:
Bassen-Kornzweig syndrome (272.5)
Refsum's disease (356.3)

362.73 Vitreoretinal dystrophies
Juvenile retinoschisis

362.74 Pigmentary retinal dystrophy
Retinal dystrophy, albipunctate
Retinitis pigmentosa

362.75 Other dystrophies primarily involving the sensory retina
Progressive cone (-rod) dystrophy
Stargardt's disease

362.76 Dystrophies primarily involving the retinal pigment epithelium
Fundus flavimaculatus
Vitelliform dystrophy

362.77 Dystrophies primarily involving Bruch's membrane
Dystrophy:
hyaline
pseudoinflammatory foveal
Hereditary drusen

362.8 Other retinal disorders

Excludes: *chorioretinal inflammations (363.0-363.2)*
chorioretinal scars (363.30-363.35)

362.81 Retinal hemorrhage
Hemorrhage:
preretinal
retinal (deep) (superficial)
subretinal

362.82 Retinal exudates and deposits

362.83 Retinal edema
Retinal:
cotton wool spots
edema (localized) (macular) (peripheral)

362.84 Retinal ischemia

362.85 Retinal nerve fiber bundle defects

362.89 Other retinal disorders

362.9 Unspecified retinal disorder

363 Chorioretinal inflammations, scars, and other disorders of choroid

363.0 Focal chorioretinitis and focal retinochoroiditis

Excludes: *focal chorioretinitis or retinochoroiditis in:*
histoplasmosis (115.02, 115.12, 115.92)
toxoplasmosis (130.2)
congenital infection (771.2)

363.00 Focal chorioretinitis, unspecified
Focal:
choroiditis or chorioretinitis NOS
retinitis or retinochoroiditis NOS

363.01 Focal choroiditis and chorioretinitis, juxtapapillary

363.03 Focal choroiditis and chorioretinitis of other posterior pole

363.04 Focal choroiditis and chorioretinitis, peripheral

363.05 Focal retinitis and retinochoroiditis, juxtapapillary
Neuroretinitis

363.06 Focal retinitis and retinochoroiditis, macular or paramacular

363.07 Focal retinitis and retinochoroiditis of other posterior pole

363.08 Focal retinitis and retinochoroiditis, peripheral

363.1 Disseminated chorioretinitis and disseminated retinochoroiditis

Excludes: *disseminated choroiditis or chorioretinitis in secondary syphilis (091.51)*
neurosyphilitic disseminated retinitis or retinochoroiditis (094.83)
retinal (peri)vasculitis (362.18)

363.10 Disseminated chorioretinitis, unspecified
Disseminated:
choroiditis or chorioretinitis NOS
retinitis or retinochoroiditis NOS

363.11 Disseminated choroiditis and chorioretinitis, posterior pole

363.12 Disseminated choroiditis and chorioretinitis, peripheral

363.13 Disseminated choroiditis and chorioretinitis, generalized
Code first any underlying disease, as:
tuberculosis (017.3)

363.14 Disseminated retinitis and retinochoroiditis, metastatic

363.15 Disseminated retinitis and retinochoroiditis, pigment epitheliopathy
Acute posterior multifocal placoid pigment epitheliopathy

363.2 Other and unspecified forms of chorioretinitis and retinochoroiditis

Excludes: *panophthalmitis (360.02)*
sympathetic uveitis (360.11)
uveitis NOS (364.3)

363.20 Chorioretinitis, unspecified
Choroiditis NOS
Retinitis NOS
Uveitis, posterior NOS

363.21 Pars planitis
Posterior cyclitis

363.22 Harada's disease

363.3 Chorioretinal scars
Scar (postinflammatory) (postsurgical) (posttraumatic):
choroid
retina

363.30 Chorioretinal scar, unspecified

363.31 Solar retinopathy

363.32 Other macular scars

363.33 Other scars of posterior pole

363.34 Peripheral scars

363.35 Disseminated scars

363.4 Choroidal degenerations

363.40 Choroidal degeneration, unspecified
Choroidal sclerosis NOS

363.41 Senile atrophy of choroid

363.42 Diffuse secondary atrophy of choroid

363.43 Angioid streaks of choroid

363.5 Hereditary choroidal dystrophies
Hereditary choroidal atrophy:
partial [choriocapillaris]
total [all vessels]

363.50 Hereditary choroidal dystrophy or atrophy, unspecified

363.51 Circumpapillary dystrophy of choroid, partial

363.52 Circumpapillary dystrophy of choroid, total
Helicoid dystrophy of choroid

363.53 Central dystrophy of choroid, partial
Dystrophy, choroidal:
central areolar
circinate

363.54 Central choroidal atrophy, total
Dystrophy, choroidal:
central gyrate
serpiginous

363.55 Choroideremia

363.56 Other diffuse or generalized dystrophy, partial
Diffuse choroidal sclerosis

363.57 Other diffuse or generalized dystrophy, total
Generalized gyrate atrophy, choroid

363.6 Choroidal hemorrhage and rupture

363.61 Choroidal hemorrhage, unspecified

363.62 Expulsive choroidal hemorrhage

363.63 Choroidal rupture

363.7 Choroidal detachment

363.70 Choroidal detachment, unspecified

363.71 Serous choroidal detachment

363.72 Hemorrhagic choroidal detachment

363.8 Other disorders of choroid

363.9 Unspecified disorder of choroid

364 Disorders of iris and ciliary body

364.0 Acute and subacute iridocyclitis

Anterior uveitis Cyclitis Iridocyclitis Iritis	acute subacute

Excludes: *gonococcal (098.41)*
herpes simplex (054.44)
herpes zoster (053.22)

364.00 Acute and subacute iridocyclitis, unspecified

364.01 Primary iridocyclitis

364.02 Recurrent iridocyclitis

364.03 Secondary iridocyclitis, infectious

364.04 Secondary iridocyclitis, noninfectious
Aqueous:
cells
fibrin
flare

364.05 Hypopyon

364.1 Chronic iridocyclitis

Excludes: *posterior cyclitis (363.21)*

364.10 Chronic iridocyclitis, unspecified

364.11 ***Chronic iridocyclitis in diseases classified elsewhere***
Code first underlying disease, as:
sarcoidosis (135)
tuberculosis (017.3)

Excludes: *syphilitic iridocyclitis (091.52)*

364.2 Certain types of iridocyclitis

Excludes: *posterior cyclitis (363.21)*
sympathetic uveitis (360.11)

364.21 Fuchs' heterochromic cyclitis

364.22 Glaucomatocyclitic crises

364.23 Lens-induced iridocyclitis

364.24 Vogt-Koyanagi syndrome

364.3 Unspecified iridocyclitis
Uveitis NOS

364.4 Vascular disorders of iris and ciliary body

364.41 Hyphema
Hemorrhage of iris or ciliary body

364.42 Rubeosis iridis
Neovascularization of iris or ciliary body

364.5 Degenerations of iris and ciliary body

364.51 Essential or progressive iris atrophy

364.52 Iridoschisis

364.53 Pigmentary iris degeneration
Acquired heterochromia } of iris
Pigment dispersion syndrome } of iris
Translucency } of iris

364.54 Degeneration of pupillary margin
Atrophy of sphincter } of iris
Ectropion of pigment epithelium } of iris

364.55 Miotic cysts of pupillary margin

364.56 Degenerative changes of chamber angle

364.57 Degenerative changes of ciliary body

364.59 Other iris atrophy
Iris atrophy (generalized) (sector shaped)

364.6 Cysts of iris, ciliary body, and anterior chamber

Excludes: *miotic pupillary cyst (364.55)*
parasitic cyst (360.13)

364.60 Idiopathic cysts

364.61 Implantation cysts
Epithelial down-growth, anterior chamber
Implantation cysts (surgical) (traumatic)

364.62 Exudative cysts of iris or anterior chamber

364.63 Primary cyst of pars plana

364.64 Exudative cyst of pars plana

364.7 Adhesions and disruptions of iris and ciliary body

Excludes: *flat anterior chamber (360.34)*

364.70 Adhesions of iris, unspecified
Synechiae (iris) NOS

364.71 Posterior synechiae

364.72 Anterior synechiae

364.73 Goniosynechiae
Peripheral anterior synechiae

364.74 Pupillary membranes
Iris bombé
Pupillary:
occlusion
seclusion

364.75 Pupillary abnormalities
Deformed pupil
Ectopic pupil
Rupture of sphincter, pupil

364.76 Iridodialysis

364.77 Recession of chamber angle

364.8 Other disorders of iris and ciliary body
Prolapse of iris NOS

Excludes: *prolapse of iris in recent wound (871.1)*

364.9 Unspecified disorder of iris and ciliary body

365 Glaucoma

Excludes: *blind hypertensive eye [absolute glaucoma] (360.42)*
congenital glaucoma (743.20-743.22)

365.0 Borderline glaucoma [glaucoma suspect]

365.00 Preglaucoma, unspecified

365.01 Open angle with borderline findings
Open angle with:
borderline intraocular pressure
cupping of optic discs

365.02 Anatomical narrow angle

365.03 Steroid responders

365.04 Ocular hypertension

365.1 Open-angle glaucoma

365.10 Open-angle glaucoma, unspecified
Wide-angle glaucoma NOS

365.11 Primary open angle glaucoma
Chronic simple glaucoma

365.12 Low tension glaucoma

365.13 Pigmentary glaucoma

365.14 Glaucoma of childhood
Infantile or juvenile glaucoma

365.15 Residual stage of open angle glaucoma

365.2 Primary angle-closure glaucoma

365.20 Primary angle-closure glaucoma, unspecified

365.21 Intermittent angle-closure glaucoma
Angle-closure glaucoma:
interval
subacute

365.22 Acute angle-closure glaucoma

365.23 Chronic angle-closure glaucoma

365.24 Residual stage of angle-closure glaucoma

365.3 Corticosteroid-induced glaucoma

365.31 Glaucomatous stage

365.32 Residual stage

365.4 Glaucoma associated with congenital anomalies, dystrophies, and systemic syndromes

365.41 Glaucoma associated with chamber angle anomalies
Code first associated disorder, as:
Axenfeld's anomaly (743.44)
Rieger's anomaly or syndrome (743.44)

365.42 Glaucoma associated with anomalies of iris
Code first associated disorder, as:
aniridia (743.45)
essential iris atrophy (364.51)

365.43 Glaucoma associated with other anterior segment anomalies
Code first associated disorder, as:
microcornea (743.41)

Add 4th or 5th digit | Nonspecific code | Unspecified code | Manifestation code

365.44 ***Glaucoma associated with systemic syndromes***
Code first associated disease, as:
neurofibromatosis (237.7)
Sturge-Weber (-Dimitri) syndrome (759.6)

365.5 Glaucoma associated with disorders of the lens

365.51 Phacolytic glaucoma
Use additional code for associated hypermature cataract (366.18)

365.52 Pseudoexfoliation glaucoma
Use additional code for associated pseudoexfoliation of capsule (366.11)

365.59 Glaucoma associated with other lens disorders
Use additional code for associated disorder, as:
dislocation of lens (379.33-379.34)
spherophakia (743.36)

365.6 Glaucoma associated with other ocular disorders

365.60 Glaucoma associated with unspecified ocular disorder

365.61 Glaucoma associated with pupillary block
Use additional code for associated disorder, as:
seclusion of pupil [iris bombé] (364.74)

365.62 Glaucoma associated with ocular inflammations
Use additional code for associated disorder, as:
glaucomatocyclitic crises (364.22)
iridocyclitis (364.0-364.3)

365.63 Glaucoma associated with vascular disorders
Use additional code for associated disorder, as:
central retinal vein occlusion (362.35)
hyphema (364.41)

365.64 Glaucoma associated with tumors or cysts
Use additional code for associated disorder, as:
benign neoplasm (224.0-224.9)
epithelial down-growth (364.61)
malignant neoplasm (190.0-190.9)

365.65 Glaucoma associated with ocular trauma
Use additional code for associated condition, as:
contusion of globe (921.3)
recession of chamber angle (364.77)

365.8 Other specified forms of glaucoma

365.81 Hypersecretion glaucoma

365.82 Glaucoma with increased episcleral venous pressure

365.89 Other specified glaucoma

365.9 Unspecified glaucoma

366 Cataract

Excludes: *congenital cataract (743.30-743.34)*

366.0 Infantile, juvenile, and presenile cataract

366.00 Nonsenile cataract, unspecified

366.01 Anterior subcapsular polar cataract

366.02 Posterior subcapsular polar cataract

366.03 Cortical, lamellar, or zonular cataract

366.04 Nuclear cataract

366.09 Other and combined forms of nonsenile cataract

366.1 Senile cataract

366.10 Senile cataract, unspecified

366.11 Pseudoexfoliation of lens capsule

366.12 Incipient cataract
Cataract:
coronary
immature NOS
punctate
Water clefts

366.13 Anterior subcapsular polar senile cataract

366.14 Posterior subcapsular polar senile cataract

366.15 Cortical senile cataract

366.16 Nuclear sclerosis
Cataracta brunescens
Nuclear cataract

366.17 Total or mature cataract

366.18 Hypermature cataract
Morgagni cataract

366.19 Other and combined forms of senile cataract

366.2 Traumatic cataract

366.20 Traumatic cataract, unspecified

366.21 Localized traumatic opacities
Vossius' ring

366.22 Total traumatic cataract

366.23 Partially resolved traumatic cataract

366.3 Cataract secondary to ocular disorders

366.30 Cataracts complicata, unspecified

366.31 Glaucomatous flecks (subcapsular)
Code first underlying glaucoma (365.0-365.9)

366.32 Cataract in inflammatory disorders
Code first underlying condition, as:
chronic choroiditis (363.0-363.2)

366.33 Cataract with neovascularization
Code first underlying condition, as:
chronic iridocyclitis (364.10)

366.34 Cataract in degenerative disorders
Sunflower cataract
Code first underlying condition, as:
chalcosis (360.24)
degenerative myopia (360.21)
pigmentary retinal dystrophy (362.74)

366.4 Cataract associated with other disorders

366.41 Diabetic cataract
Code first diabetes (250.5)

366.42 Tetanic cataract
Code first underlying disease, as:
calcinosis (275.4)
hypoparathyroidism (252.1)

366.43 Myotonic cataract
Code first underlying disorder (359.2)

366.44 Cataract associated with other syndromes
Code first underlying condition, as:
craniofacial dysostosis (756.0)
galactosemia (271.1)

366.45 Toxic cataract
Drug-induced cataract
Use additional E code, if desired, to identify drug or other toxic substance

366.46 Cataract associated with radiation and other physical influences
Use additional E code, if desired, to identify cause

366.5 After-cataract

366.50 After-cataract, unspecified
Secondary cataract NOS

366.51 Soemmering's ring

366.52 Other after-cataract, not obscuring vision

366.53 After-cataract, obscuring vision

366.8 Other cataract
Calcification of lens

366.9 Unspecified cataract

367 Disorders of refraction and accommodation

367.0 Hypermetropia
Far-sightedness
Hyperopia

367.1 Myopia
Near-sightedness

367.2 Astigmatism

367.20 Astigmatism, unspecified

367.21 Regular astigmatism

367.22 Irregular astigmatism

367.3 Anisometropia and aniseikonia

367.31 Anisometropia

367.32 Aniseikonia

367.4 Presbyopia

367.5 Disorders of accommodation

367.51 Paresis of accommodation
Cycloplegia

367.52 Total or complete internal ophthalmoplegia

367.53 Spasm of accommodation

367.8 Other disorders of refraction and accommodation

367.81 Transient refractive change

367.89 Other
Drug-induced } disorders of refraction and accommodation
Toxic } disorders of refraction and accommodation

367.9 Unspecified disorder of refraction and accommodation

368 Visual disturbances

Excludes: *electrophysiological disturbances (794.11-794.14)*

368.0 Amblyopia ex anopsia

368.00 Amblyopia, unspecified

368.01 Strabismic amblyopia
Suppression amblyopia

368.02 Deprivation amblyopia

368.03 Refractive amblyopia

368.1 Subjective visual disturbances

368.10 Subjective visual disturbance, unspecified

368.11 Sudden visual loss

368.12 Transient visual loss
Concentric fading
Scintillating scotoma

368.13 Visual discomfort
Asthenopia
Eye strain
Photophobia

368.14 Visual distortions of shape and size
Macropsia
Metamorphopsia
Micropsia

368.15 Other visual distortions and entoptic phenomena
Photopsia
Refractive:
diplopia
polyopia
Visual halos

368.16 Psychophysical visual disturbances
Visual:
agnosia
disorientation syndrome
hallucinations

368.2 Diplopia
Double vision

368.3 Other disorders of binocular vision

368.30 Binocular vision disorder, unspecified

368.31 Suppression of binocular vision

368.32 Simultaneous visual perception without fusion

368.33 Fusion with defective stereopsis

368.34 Abnormal retinal correspondence

368.4 Visual field defects

368.40 Visual field defect, unspecified

368.41 Scotoma involving central area

Scotoma:
- central
- centrocecal
- paracentral

368.42 Scotoma of blind spot area

Enlarged:
- angioscotoma
- blind spot

Paracecal scotoma

368.43 Sector or arcuate defects

Scotoma:
- arcuate
- Bjerrum
- Seidel

368.44 Other localized visual field defect

Scotoma:
- NOS
- ring

Visual field defect:
- nasal step
- peripheral

368.45 Generalized contraction or constriction

368.46 Homonymous bilateral field defects

Hemianopsia (altitudinal) (homonymous)
Quadrant anopia

368.47 Heteronymous bilateral field defects

Hemianopsia:
- binasal
- bitemporal

368.5 Color vision deficiencies

Color blindness

368.51 Protan defect

Protanomaly
Protanopia

368.52 Deutan defect

Deuteranomaly
Deuteranopia

368.53 Tritan defect

Tritanomaly
Tritanopia

368.54 Achromatopsia

Monochromatism (cone) (rod)

368.55 Acquired color vision deficiencies

368.59 Other color vision deficiencies

368.6 Night blindness

Hemeralopia
Nyctalopia

368.60 Night blindness, unspecified

368.61 Congenital night blindness

Hereditary night blindness
Oguchi's disease

368.62 Acquired night blindness

Excludes: *that due to vitamin A deficiency (264.5)*

368.63 Abnormal dark adaptation curve

Abnormal threshold } of cones or rods
Delayed adaptation } of cones or rods

368.69 Other night blindness

368.8 Other specified visual disturbances

Blurred vision NOS

368.9 Unspecified visual disturbance

369 Blindness and low vision

Note: Visual impairment refers to a functional limitation of the eye (e.g., limited visual acuity or visual field). It should be distinguished from visual disability, indicating a limitation of the abilities of the individual (e.g., limited reading skills, vocational skills), and from visual handicap, indicating a limitation of personal and socioeconomic independence (e.g., limited mobility, limited employability.)

The levels of impairment defined in the table on page 174 are based on the recommendations of the WHO Study Group on Prevention of Blindness (Geneva, November 6-10, 1972; WHO Technical Report Series 518), and of the International Council of Ophthalmology (1976).

Note that definitions of blindness vary in different settings.

For international reporting WHO defines blindness as profound impairment. This definition can be applied to blindness of one eye (369.1, 369.6) and to blindness of the individual (369.0).

For determination of benefits in the U.S.A., the definition of legal blindness as severe impairment is often used. This definition applies to blindness of the individual only.

Excludes: *correctable impaired vision due to refractive errors (367.0-367.9)*

369.0 Profound impairment, both eyes

369.00 Impairment level not further specified
Blindness:
NOS according to WHO definition
both eyes

369.01 Better eye: total impairment; lesser eye: total impairment

369.02 Better eye: near-total impairment; lesser eye: not further specified

369.03 Better eye: near-total impairment; lesser eye: total impairment

369.04 Better eye: near-total impairment; lesser eye: near-total impairment

369.05 Better eye: profound impairment; lesser eye: not further specified

369.06 Better eye: profound impairment; lesser eye: total impairment

369.07 Better eye: profound impairment; lesser eye: near-total impairment

369.08 Better eye: profound impairment; lesser eye: profound impairment

369.1 Moderate or severe impairment, better eye, profound impairment lesser eye

369.10 Impairment level not further specified
Blindness, one eye, low vision other eye

369.11 Better eye: severe impairment; lesser eye: blind, not further specified

369.12 Better eye: severe impairment; lesser eye: total impairment

369.13 Better eye: severe impairment; lesser eye: near-total impairment

369.14 Better eye: severe impairment; lesser eye: profound impairment

369.15 Better eye: moderate impairment; lesser eye: blind, not further specified

369.16 Better eye: moderate impairment; lesser eye: total impairment

369.17 Better eye: moderate impairment; lesser eye: near-total impairment

369.18 Better eye: moderate impairment; lesser eye: profound impairment

369.2 Moderate or severe impairment, both eyes

369.20 Impairment level not further specified
Low vision, both eyes NOS

369.21 Better eye: severe impairment; lesser eye: not further specified

369.22 Better eye: severe impairment; lesser eye: severe impairment

369.23 Better eye: moderate impairment; lesser eye: not further specified

369.24 Better eye: moderate impairment; lesser eye: severe impairment

369.25 Better eye: moderate impairment; lesser eye: moderate impairment

369.3 Unqualified visual loss, both eyes

Excludes: *blindness NOS:*
legal [U.S.A. definition] (369.4)
WHO definition (369.00)

□ **369.4 Legal blindness, as defined in U.S.A.**
Blindness NOS according to U.S.A. definition

Excludes: *legal blindness with specification of impairment level (369.01-369.08, 369.11-369.14, 369.21-369.22)*

369.6 Profound impairment, one eye

369.60 Impairment level not further specified
Blindness, one eye

369.61 One eye: total impairment; other eye: not specified

369.62 One eye: total impairment; other eye: near-normal vision

369.63 One eye: total impairment; other eye: normal vision

369.64 One eye: near-total impairment; other eye: not specified

369.65 One eye: near-total impairment; other eye: near-normal vision

369.66 One eye: near-total impairment; other eye: normal vision

369.67 One eye: profound impairment; other eye: not specified

369.68 One eye: profound impairment; other eye: near-normal vision

369.69 One eye: profound impairment; other eye: normal vision

369.7 Moderate or severe impairment, one eye

369.70 Impairment level not further specified
Low vision, one eye

369.71 One eye: severe impairment; other eye: not specified

369.72 One eye: severe impairment; other eye: near-normal vision

369.73 One eye: severe impairment; other eye: normal vision

369.74 One eye: moderate impairment; other eye: not specified

369.75 One eye: moderate impairment; other eye: near-normal vision

369.76 One eye: moderate impairment; other eye: normal vision

369.8 Unqualified visual loss, one eye

369.9 Unspecified visual loss

370 Keratitis

370.0 Corneal ulcer

Excludes: *that due to vitamin A deficiency (264.3)*

370.00 Corneal ulcer, unspecified

370.01 Marginal corneal ulcer

370.02 Ring corneal ulcer

370.03 Central corneal ulcer

370.04 Hypopyon ulcer
Serpiginous ulcer

Add 4th or 5th digit | Nonspecific code | Unspecified code | Manifestation code

Classification		LEVELS OF VISUAL IMPAIRMENT					Additional Descriptors which may be encountered
"legal"	WHO	Visual Acuity and/or Visual Field Limitation (*whichever is worse*)					
	(NEAR-) NORMAL VISION	**RANGE OF NORMAL VISION**					
		20/10	20/13	20/16	20/20	20/25	
		2.0	1.6	1.25	1.0	0.8	
		NEAR-NORMAL VISION					
			20/30	20/40	20/50	20/60	
		0.7	0.6	0.5	0.4	0.3	
	LOW VISION	**MODERATE VISUAL IMPAIRMENT**					Moderate low vision
		20/70	20/80	20/100	20/125	20/160	
			0.25	0.20	0.16	0.12	
LEGAL BLINDNESS		**SEVERE VISUAL IMPAIRMENT**					Severe low vision, "legal" blindness
			20/200	20/250	20/320	20/400	
			0.10	0.08	0.06	0.05	
		Visual Field:	20 degrees or less				
	BLINDNESS	**PROFOUND VISUAL IMPAIRMENT**					Profound low vision, moderate blindness
			20/500	20/630	20/800	20/1000	
			0.04	0.03	0.025	0.02	
		Count Fingers at:	less than 3m (10 ft)				
		Visual Field:	10 degrees or less				
		NEAR-TOTAL VISUAL IMPAIRMENT					Severe blindness
		Visual Acuity:	less than 0.02 (20/1000)				
		Count Fingers at:	1m (3 ft) or less				
(USA) both eyes	(WHO) one or both eyes	Hand Movements:	5m (15 ft) or less				Near-total blindness
		Light projection, light perception					
		Visual Field:	5 degrees or less				
		TOTAL VISUAL IMPAIRMENT					Total blindness
		No light perception (NLP)					

Visual acuity refers to best achievable acuity with correction
Non-listed Snellen fractions may be classified by converting to the nearest decimal equivalent, e.g., 10/200=0.05, 6/30=0.20
CF (count fingers) without designation of distance, may be classified to profound impairment.
HM (hand motion) without designation of distance, may be classified to near-total impairment.
Visual field measurements refer to the largest field diameter for a 1/100 white test object.

370.05 Mycotic corneal ulcer

370.06 Perforated corneal ulcer

370.07 Mooren's ulcer

370.2 Superficial keratitis without conjunctivitis

Excludes: *dendritic [herpes simplex] keratitis (054.42)*

370.20 Superficial keratitis, unspecified

370.21 Punctate keratitis
Thygeson's superficial punctate keratitis

370.22 Macular keratitis
Keratitis:
- areolar
- nummular

Keratitis:
- stellate
- striate

370.23 Filamentary keratitis

370.24 Photokeratitis
Snow blindness
Welders' keratitis

370.3 Certain types of keratoconjunctivitis

370.31 Phlyctenular keratoconjunctivitis
Phlyctenulosis
Use additional code for any associated tuberculosis (017.3)

● Code new to this edition ▲ Revision of existing code ④ ⑤ Fourth or fifth digit required

370.32 Limbar and corneal involvement in vernal conjunctivitis
Use additional code for vernal conjunctivitis (372.13)

370.33 Keratoconjunctivitis sicca, not specified as Sjögren's

Excludes: *Sjögren's syndrome (710.2)*

370.34 Exposure keratoconjunctivitis

370.35 Neurotrophic keratoconjunctivitis

370.4 Other and unspecified keratoconjunctivitis

370.40 Keratoconjunctivitis, unspecified
Superficial keratitis with conjunctivitis NOS

370.44 Keratitis or keratoconjunctivitis in exanthema
Code first underlying condition (050.0-052.9)

Excludes: *herpes simplex (054.43)*
herpes zoster (053.21)
measles (055.71)

370.49 Other

Excludes: *epidemic keratoconjunctivitis (077.1)*

370.5 Interstitial and deep keratitis

370.50 Interstitial keratitis, unspecified

370.52 Diffuse interstitial keratitis
Cogan's syndrome

370.54 Sclerosing keratitis

370.55 Corneal abscess

370.59 Other

Excludes: *disciform herpes simplex keratitis (054.43)*
syphilitic keratitis (090.3)

370.6 Corneal neovascularization

370.60 Corneal neovascularization, unspecified

370.61 Localized vascularization of cornea

370.62 Pannus (corneal)

370.63 Deep vascularization of cornea

370.64 Ghost vessels (corneal)

370.8 Other forms of keratitis

370.9 Unspecified keratitis

371 Corneal opacity and other disorders of cornea

371.0 Corneal scars and opacities

Excludes: *that due to vitamin A deficiency (264.6)*

371.00 Corneal opacity, unspecified
Corneal scar NOS

371.01 Minor opacity of cornea
Corneal nebula

371.02 Peripheral opacity of cornea
Corneal macula not interfering with central vision

371.03 Central opacity of cornea
Corneal:
leucoma } interfering with central vision
macula

371.04 Adherent leucoma

371.05 Phthisical cornea
Code first underlying tuberculosis (017.3)

371.1 Corneal pigmentations and deposits

371.10 Corneal deposit, unspecified

371.11 Anterior pigmentations
Stähli's lines

371.12 Stromal pigmentations
Hematocornea

371.13 Posterior pigmentations
Krukenberg spindle

371.14 Kayser-Fleischer ring

371.15 Other deposits associated with metabolic disorders

371.16 Argentous deposits

371.2 Corneal edema

371.20 Corneal edema, unspecified

371.21 Idiopathic corneal edema

371.22 Secondary corneal edema

371.23 Bullous keratopathy

371.24 Corneal edema due to wearing of contact lenses

371.3 Changes of corneal membranes

371.30 Corneal membrane change, unspecified

371.31 Folds and rupture of Bowman's membrane

371.32 Folds in Descemet's membrane

371.33 Rupture in Descemet's membrane

371.4 Corneal degenerations

371.40 Corneal degeneration, unspecified

371.41 Senile corneal changes
Arcus senilis
Hassall-Henle bodies

371.42 Recurrent erosion of cornea

Excludes: *Mooren's ulcer (370.07)*

371.43 Band-shaped keratopathy

371.44 Other calcerous degenerations of cornea

371.45 Keratomalacia NOS

Excludes: *that due to vitamin A deficiency (264.4)*

371.46 Nodular degeneration of cornea
Salzmann's nodular dystrophy

371.48 Peripheral degenerations of cornea
Marginal degeneration of cornea [Terrien's]

371.49 Other
Discrete colliquative keratopathy

371.5 Hereditary corneal dystrophies

371.50 Corneal dystrophy, unspecified

371.51 Juvenile epithelial corneal dystrophy

371.52 Other anterior corneal dystrophies
Corneal dystrophy:
- microscopic cystic
- ring-like

371.53 Granular corneal dystrophy

371.54 Lattice corneal dystrophy

371.55 Macular corneal dystrophy

371.56 Other stromal corneal dystrophies
Crystalline corneal dystrophy

371.57 Endothelial corneal dystrophy
Combined corneal dystrophy
Cornea guttata
Fuchs' endothelial dystrophy

371.58 Other posterior corneal dystrophies
Polymorphous corneal dystrophy

371.6 Keratoconus

371.60 Keratoconus, unspecified

371.61 Keratoconus, stable condition

371.62 Keratoconus, acute hydrops

● Code new to this edition ▲ Revision of existing code ④ ⑤ Fourth or fifth digit required

371.7 Other corneal deformities

371.70 Corneal deformity, unspecified

371.71 Corneal ectasia

371.72 Descemetocele

371.73 Corneal staphyloma

371.8 Other corneal disorders

371.81 Corneal anesthesia and hypoesthesia

371.82 Corneal disorder due to contact lens

Excludes: *corneal edema due to contact lens (371.24)*

371.89 Other

371.9 Unspecified corneal disorder

372 Disorders of conjunctiva

Excludes: *keratoconjunctivitis (370.3-370.4)*

372.0 Acute conjunctivitis

372.00 Acute conjunctivitis, unspecified

372.01 Serous conjunctivitis, except viral

Excludes: *viral conjunctivitis NOS (077.9)*

372.02 Acute follicular conjunctivitis
Conjunctival folliculosis NOS

Excludes: *conjunctivitis:*
adenoviral (acute follicular) (077.3)
epidemic hemorrhagic (077.4)
inclusion (077.0)
Newcastle (077.8)
epidemic keratoconjunctivitis (077.1)
pharyngoconjunctival fever (077.2)

372.03 Other mucopurulent conjunctivitis
Catarrhal conjunctivitis

Excludes: *blennorrhea neonatorum (gonococcal) (098.40)*
neonatal conjunctivitis (771.6)
ophthalmia neonatorum NOS (771.6)

372.04 Pseudomembranous conjunctivitis
Membranous conjunctivitis

Excludes: *diphtheritic conjunctivitis (032.81)*

372.05 Acute atopic conjunctivitis

372.1 Chronic conjunctivitis

372.10 Chronic conjunctivitis, unspecified

372.11 Simple chronic conjunctivitis

372.12 Chronic follicular conjunctivitis

372.13 Vernal conjunctivitis

372.14 Other chronic allergic conjunctivitis

372.15 Parasitic conjunctivitis
Code first underlying disease, as:
filariasis (125.0-125.9)
mucocutaneous leishmaniasis (085.5)

372.2 Blepharoconjunctivitis

372.20 Blepharoconjunctivitis, unspecified

372.21 Angular blepharoconjunctivitis

372.22 Contact blepharoconjunctivitis

372.3 Other and unspecified conjunctivitis

372.30 Conjunctivitis, unspecified

372.31 Rosacea conjunctivitis
Code first underlying rosacea dermatitis (695.3)

372.33 *Conjunctivitis in mucocutaneous disease*
Code first underlying disease, as:
erythema multiforme (695.1)
Reiter's disease (099.3)

Excludes: *ocular pemphigoid (694.61)*

372.39 Other

372.4 Pterygium

Excludes: *pseudopterygium (372.52)*

372.40 Pterygium, unspecified

372.41 Peripheral pterygium, stationary

372.42 Peripheral pterygium, progressive

372.43 Central pterygium

372.44 Double pterygium

372.45 Recurrent pterygium

372.5 Conjunctival degenerations and deposits

372.50 Conjunctival degeneration, unspecified

372.51 Pinguecula

372.52 Pseudopterygium

372.53 Conjunctival xerosis

Excludes: *conjunctival xerosis due to vitamin A deficiency (264.0, 264.1, 264.7)*

372.54 Conjunctival concretions

372.55 Conjunctival pigmentations
Conjunctival argyrosis

372.56 Conjunctival deposits

372.6 Conjunctival scars

372.61 Granuloma of conjunctiva

372.62 Localized adhesions and strands of conjunctiva

372.63 Symblepharon
Extensive adhesions of conjunctiva

372.64 Scarring of conjunctiva
Contraction of eye socket (after enucleation)

372.7 Conjunctival vascular disorders and cysts

372.71 Hyperemia of conjunctiva

372.72 Conjunctival hemorrhage
Hyposphagma
Subconjunctival hemorrhage

372.73 Conjunctival edema
Chemosis of conjunctiva
Subconjunctival edema

372.74 Vascular abnormalities of conjunctiva
Aneurysm(ata) of conjunctiva

372.75 Conjunctival cysts

372.8 Other disorders of conjunctiva

372.9 Unspecified disorder of conjunctiva

373 Inflammation of eyelids

373.0 Blepharitis

Excludes: *blepharoconjunctivitis (372.20-372.22)*

373.00 Blepharitis, unspecified

373.01 Ulcerative blepharitis

373.02 Squamous blepharitis

373.1 Hordeolum and other deep inflammation of eyelid

373.11 Hordeolum externum
Hordeolum NOS
Stye

● Code new to this edition ▲ Revision of existing code ④ ⑤ Fourth or fifth digit required

373.12 Hordeolum internum
Infection of meibomian gland

373.13 Abscess of eyelid
Furuncle of eyelid

373.2 Chalazion
Meibomian (gland) cyst

Excludes: *infected meibomian gland (373.12)*

373.3 Noninfectious dermatoses of eyelid

373.31 Eczematous dermatitis of eyelid

373.32 Contact and allergic dermatitis of eyelid

373.33 Xeroderma of eyelid

373.34 Discoid lupus erythematosus of eyelid

373.4 Infective dermatitis of eyelid of types resulting in deformity
Code first underlying disease, as:
leprosy (030.0-030.9)
lupus vulgaris (tuberculous) (017.0)
yaws (102.0-102.9)

373.5 Other infective dermatitis of eyelid
Code first underlying disease, as:
actinomycosis (039.3)
impetigo (684)
mycotic dermatitis (110.0-111.9)
vaccinia (051.0)
postvaccination (999.0)

Excludes: *herpes:*
simplex (054.41)
zoster (053.20)

373.6 Parasitic infestation of eyelid
Code first underlying disease, as:
leishmaniasis (085.0-085.9)
loiasis (125.2)
onchocerciasis (125.3)
pediculosis (132.0)

373.8 Other inflammations of eyelids

373.9 Unspecified inflammation of eyelid

374 Other disorders of eyelids

374.0 Entropion and trichiasis of eyelid

374.00 Entropion, unspecified

374.01 Senile entropion

374.02 Mechanical entropion

374.03 Spastic entropion

374.04 Cicatricial entropion

374.05 Trichiasis without entropion

374.1 Ectropion

374.10 Ectropion, unspecified

374.11 Senile ectropion

374.12 Mechanical ectropion

374.13 Spastic ectropion

374.14 Cicatricial ectropion

374.2 Lagophthalmos

374.20 Lagophthalmos, unspecified

374.21 Paralytic lagophthalmos

374.22 Mechanical lagophthalmos

374.23 Cicatricial lagophthalmos

374.3 Ptosis of eyelid

374.30 Ptosis of eyelid, unspecified

374.31 Paralytic ptosis

374.32 Myogenic ptosis

374.33 Mechanical ptosis

374.34 Blepharochalasis
Pseudoptosis

374.4 Other disorders affecting eyelid function

Excludes: *blepharoclonus (333.81)*
blepharospasm (333.81)
facial nerve palsy (351.0)
third nerve palsy or paralysis (378.51-378.52)
tic (psychogenic) (307.20-307.23)
organic (333.3)

374.41 Lid retraction or lag

374.43 Abnormal innervation syndrome
Jaw-blinking
Paradoxical facial movements

374.44 Sensory disorders

374.45 Other sensorimotor disorders
Deficient blink reflex

374.46 Blepharophimosis
Ankyloblepharon

374.5 Degenerative disorders of eyelid and periocular area

374.50 Degenerative disorder of eyelid, unspecified

374.51 Xanthelasma
Xanthoma (planum) (tuberosum) of eyelid
Code first underlying condition (272.0-272.9)

374.52 Hyperpigmentation of eyelid
Chloasma
Dyspigmentation

374.53 Hypopigmentation of eyelid
Vitiligo of eyelid

374.54 Hypertrichosis of eyelid

374.55 Hypotrichosis of eyelid
Madarosis of eyelid

374.56 Other degenerative disorders of skin affecting eyelid

374.8 Other disorders of eyelid

374.81 Hemorrhage of eyelid

Excludes: *black eye (921.0)*

374.82 Edema of eyelid
Hyperemia of eyelid

374.83 Elephantiasis of eyelid

374.84 Cysts of eyelids
Sebaceous cyst of eyelid

374.85 Vascular anomalies of eyelid

374.86 Retained foreign body of eyelid

374.87 Dermatochalasis

374.89 Other disorders of eyelid

374.9 Unspecified disorder of eyelid

375 Disorders of lacrimal system

375.0 Dacryoadenitis

375.00 Dacryoadenitis, unspecified

375.01 Acute dacryoadenitis

375.02 Chronic dacryoadenitis

375.03 Chronic enlargement of lacrimal gland

● Code new to this edition ▲ Revision of existing code ④ ⑤ Fourth or fifth digit required

375.1 Other disorders of lacrimal gland

375.11 Dacryops

375.12 Other lacrimal cysts and cystic degeneration

375.13 Primary lacrimal atrophy

375.14 Secondary lacrimal atrophy

375.15 Tear film insufficiency, unspecified
Dry eye syndrome

375.16 Dislocation of lacrimal gland

375.2 Epiphora

375.20 Epiphora, unspecified as to cause

375.21 Epiphora due to excess lacrimation

375.22 Epiphora due to insufficient drainage

375.3 Acute and unspecified inflammation of lacrimal passages

Excludes: neonatal dacryocystitis (771.6)

375.30 Dacryocystitis, unspecified

375.31 Acute canaliculitis, lacrimal

375.32 Acute dacryocystitis
Acute peridacryocystitis

375.33 Phlegmonous dacryocystitis

375.4 Chronic inflammation of lacrimal passages

375.41 Chronic canaliculitis

375.42 Chronic dacryocystitis

375.43 Lacrimal mucocele

375.5 Stenosis and insufficiency of lacrimal passages

375.51 Eversion of lacrimal punctum

375.52 Stenosis of lacrimal punctum

375.53 Stenosis of lacrimal canaliculi

375.54 Stenosis of lacrimal sac

375.55 Obstruction of nasolacrimal duct, neonatal

Excludes: congenital anomaly of nasolacrimal duct (743.65)

375.56 Stenosis of nasolacrimal duct, acquired

375.57 Dacryolith

375.6 Other changes of lacrimal passages

375.61 Lacrimal fistula

375.69 Other

375.8 Other disorders of lacrimal system

375.81 Granuloma of lacrimal passages

375.89 Other

375.9 Unspecified disorder of lacrimal system

376 Disorders of the orbit

376.0 Acute inflammation of orbit

376.00 Acute inflammation of orbit, unspecified

376.01 Orbital cellulitis
Abscess of orbit

376.02 Orbital periostitis

376.03 Orbital osteomyelitis

376.04 Tenonitis

376.1 Chronic inflammatory disorders of orbit

376.10 Chronic inflammation of orbit, unspecified

376.11 Orbital granuloma
Pseudotumor (inflammatory) of orbit

376.12 Orbital myositis

376.13 Parasitic infestation of orbit
Code first underlying disease, as:
hydatid infestation of orbit (122.3, 122.6, 122.9)
myiasis of orbit (134.0)

376.2 Endocrine exophthalmos
Code first underlying thyroid disorder (242.0-242.9)

376.21 Thyrotoxic exophthalmos

376.22 Exophthalmic ophthalmoplegia

376.3 Other exophthalmic conditions

376.30 Exophthalmos, unspecified

376.31 Constant exophthalmos

376.32 Orbital hemorrhage

376.33 Orbital edema or congestion

376.34 Intermittent exophthalmos

376.35 Pulsating exophthalmos

376.36 Lateral displacement of globe

376.4 Deformity of orbit

376.40 Deformity of orbit, unspecified

376.41 Hypertelorism of orbit

376.42 Exostosis of orbit

376.43 Local deformities due to bone disease

376.44 Orbital deformities associated with craniofacial deformities

376.45 Atrophy of orbit

376.46 Enlargement of orbit

376.47 Deformity due to trauma or surgery

376.5 Enophthalmos

376.50 Enophthalmos, unspecified as to cause

376.51 Enophthalmos due to atrophy of orbital tissue

376.52 Enophthalmos due to trauma or surgery

376.6 Retained (old) foreign body following penetrating wound of orbit
Retrobulbar foreign body

376.8 Other orbital disorders

376.81 Orbital cysts
Encephalocele of orbit

376.82 Myopathy of extraocular muscles

376.89 Other

376.9 Unspecified disorder of orbit

377 Disorders of optic nerve and visual pathways

377.0 Papilledema

377.00 Papilledema, unspecified

377.01 Papilledema associated with increased intracranial pressure

377.02 Papilledema associated with decreased ocular pressure

377.03 Papilledema associated with retinal disorder

377.04 Foster-Kennedy syndrome

377.1 Optic atrophy

377.10 Optic atrophy, unspecified

377.11 Primary optic atrophy

Excludes: *neurosyphilitic optic atrophy (094.84)*

377.12 Postinflammatory optic atrophy

377.13 Optic atrophy associated with retinal dystrophies

377.14 Glaucomatous atrophy [cupping] of optic disc

377.15 Partial optic atrophy
Temporal pallor of optic disc

● Code new to this edition
▲ Revision of existing code
④ ⑤ Fourth or fifth digit required

377.16 Hereditary optic atrophy
Optic atrophy:
dominant hereditary
Leber's

377.2 Other disorders of optic disc

377.21 Drusen of optic disc

377.22 Crater-like holes of optic disc

377.23 Coloboma of optic disc

377.24 Pseudopapilledema

377.3 Optic neuritis

Excludes: *meningococcal optic neuritis (036.81)*

377.30 Optic neuritis, unspecified

377.31 Optic papillitis

377.32 Retrobulbar neuritis (acute)

Excludes: *syphilitic retrobulbar neuritis (094.85)*

377.33 Nutritional optic neuropathy

377.34 Toxic optic neuropathy
Toxic amblyopia

377.39 Other

Excludes: *ischemic optic neuropathy (377.41)*

377.4 Other disorders of optic nerve

377.41 Ischemic optic neuropathy

377.42 Hemorrhage in optic nerve sheaths

377.49 Other
Compression of optic nerve

377.5 Disorders of optic chiasm

377.51 Associated with pituitary neoplasms and disorders

377.52 Associated with other neoplasms

377.53 Associated with vascular disorders

377.54 Associated with inflammatory disorders

377.6 Disorders of other visual pathways

377.61 Associated with neoplasms

377.62 Associated with vascular disorders

377.63 Associated with inflammatory disorders

377.7 Disorders of visual cortex

Excludes: *visual:*
agnosia (368.16)
hallucinations (368.16)
halos (368.15)

377.71 Associated with neoplasms

377.72 Associated with vascular disorders

377.73 Associated with inflammatory disorders

377.75 Cortical blindness

377.9 Unspecified disorder of optic nerve and visual pathways

378 Strabismus and other disorders of binocular eye movements

Excludes: *nystagmus and other irregular eye movements (379.50-379.59)*

378.0 Esotropia
Convergent concomitant strabismus

Excludes: *intermittent esotropia (378.20-378.22)*

378.00 Esotropia, unspecified

378.01 Monocular esotropia

378.02 Monocular esotropia with A pattern

378.03 Monocular esotropia with V pattern

378.04 Monocular esotropia with other noncomitancies
Monocular esotropia with X or Y pattern

378.05 Alternating esotropia

378.06 Alternating esotropia with A pattern

378.07 Alternating esotropia with V pattern

378.08 Alternating esotropia with other noncomitancies
Alternating esotropia with X or Y pattern

378.1 Exotropia
Divergent concomitant strabismus

Excludes: *intermittent exotropia (378.20, 378.23-378.24)*

378.10 Exotropia, unspecified

378.11 Monocular exotropia

378.12 Monocular exotropia with A pattern

378.13 Monocular exotropia with V pattern

378.14 Monocular exotropia with other noncomitancies
Monocular exotropia with X or Y pattern

378.15 Alternating exotropia

378.16 Alternating exotropia with A pattern

378.17 Alternating exotropia with V pattern

378.18 Alternating exotropia with other noncomitancies
Alternating exotropia with X or Y pattern

378.2 Intermittent heterotropia

Excludes: *vertical heterotropia (intermittent) (378.31)*

378.20 Intermittent heterotropia, unspecified
Intermittent:
esotropia NOS
exotropia NOS

378.21 Intermittent esotropia, monocular

378.22 Intermittent esotropia, alternating

378.23 Intermittent exotropia, monocular

378.24 Intermittent exotropia, alternating

378.3 Other and unspecified heterotropia

378.30 Heterotropia, unspecified

378.31 Hypertropia
Vertical heterotropia (constant) (intermittent)

378.32 Hypotropia

378.33 Cyclotropia

378.34 Monofixation syndrome
Microtropia

378.35 Accommodative component in esotropia

378.4 Heterophoria

378.40 Heterophoria, unspecified

378.41 Esophoria

378.42 Exophoria

378.43 Vertical heterophoria

378.44 Cyclophoria

378.45 Alternating hyperphoria

378.5 Paralytic strabismus

378.50 Paralytic strabismus, unspecified

378.51 Third or oculomotor nerve palsy, partial

378.52 Third or oculomotor nerve palsy, total

378.53 Fourth or trochlear nerve palsy

378.54 Sixth or abducens nerve palsy

378.55 External ophthalmoplegia

378.56 Total ophthalmoplegia

378.6 Mechanical strabismus

378.60 Mechanical strabismus, unspecified

378.61 Brown's (tendon) sheath syndrome

378.62 Mechanical strabismus from other musculofascial disorders

378.63 Limited duction associated with other conditions

378.7 Other specified strabismus

378.71 Duane's syndrome

378.72 Progressive external ophthalmoplegia

378.73 Strabismus in other neuromuscular disorders

378.8 Other disorders of binocular eye movements

Excludes: *nystagmus (379.50-379.56)*

378.81 Palsy of conjugate gaze

378.82 Spasm of conjugate gaze

378.83 Convergence insufficiency or palsy

378.84 Convergence excess or spasm

378.85 Anomalies of divergence

378.86 Internuclear ophthalmoplegia

378.87 Other dissociated deviation of eye movements
Skew deviation

378.9 Unspecified disorder of eye movements
Ophthalmoplegia NOS   Strabismus NOS

379 Other disorders of eye

379.0 Scleritis and episcleritis

Excludes: *syphilitic episcleritis (095.0)*

379.00 Scleritis, unspecified
Episcleritis NOS

379.01 Episcleritis periodica fugax

379.02 Nodular episcleritis

379.03 Anterior scleritis

379.04 Scleromalacia perforans

379.05 Scleritis with corneal involvement
Scleroperikeratitis

379.06 Brawny scleritis

379.07 Posterior scleritis
Sclerotenonitis

379.09 Other
Scleral abscess

379.1 Other disorders of sclera

Excludes: *blue sclera (743.47)*

379.11 Scleral ectasia
Scleral staphyloma NOS

379.12 Staphyloma posticum

379.13 Equatorial staphyloma

379.14 Anterior staphyloma, localized

379.15 Ring staphyloma

379.16 Other degenerative disorders of sclera

379.19 Other

379.2 Disorders of vitreous body

379.21 Vitreous degeneration
Vitreous:
- cavitation
- detachment
- liquefaction

379.22 Crystalline deposits in vitreous
Asteroid hyalitis Synchysis scintillans

379.23 Vitreous hemorrhage

379.24 Other vitreous opacities
Vitreous floaters

379.25 Vitreous membranes and strands

379.26 Vitreous prolapse

379.29 Other disorders of vitreous

Excludes: *vitreous abscess (360.04)*

379.3 Aphakia and other disorders of lens

Excludes: *after-cataract (366.50-366.53)*

379.31 Aphakia

379.32 Subluxation of lens

379.33 Anterior dislocation of lens

379.34 Posterior dislocation of lens

379.39 Other disorders of lens

379.4 Anomalies of pupillary function

379.40 Abnormal pupillary function, unspecified

379.41 Anisocoria

379.42 Miosis (persistent), not due to miotics

379.43 Mydriasis (persistent) not due to mydriatics

379.45 Argyll Robertson pupil, atypical
Argyll Robertson phenomenon or pupil, nonsyphilitic

Excludes: *Argyll Robertson pupil (syphilitic) (094.89)*

379.46 Tonic pupillary reaction
Adie's pupil or syndrome

379.49 Other
Hippus
Pupillary paralysis

379.5 Nystagmus and other irregular eye movements

379.50 Nystagmus, unspecified

379.51 Congenital nystagmus

379.52 Latent nystagmus

379.53 Visual deprivation nystagmus

379.54 Nystagmus associated with disorders of the vestibular system

379.55 Dissociated nystagmus

379.56 Other forms of nystagmus

379.57 Deficiencies of saccadic eye movements
Abnormal optokinetic response

379.58 Deficiencies of smooth pursuit movements

379.59 Other irregularities of eye movements
Opsoclonus

379.8 Other specified disorders of eye and adnexa

379.9 Unspecified disorder of eye and adnexa

379.90 Disorder of eye, unspecified

379.91 Pain in or around eye

379.92 Swelling or mass of eye

379.93 Redness or discharge of eye

379.99 Other ill-defined disorders of eye

Excludes: *blurred vision NOS (368.8)*

● Code new to this edition ▲ Revision of existing code ④ ⑤ Fourth or fifth digit required

DISEASES OF THE EAR AND MASTOID PROCESS (380-389)

380 Disorders of external ear

380.0 Perichondritis of pinna
Perichondritis of auricle

380.00 Perichondritis of pinna, unspecified

380.01 Acute perichondritis of pinna

380.02 Chronic perichondritis of pinna

380.1 Infective otitis externa

380.10 Infective otitis externa, unspecified
Otitis externa (acute):
NOS
circumscribed
diffuse
hemorrhagica
infective NOS

380.11 Acute infection of pinna

Excludes: *furuncular otitis externa (680.0)*

380.12 Acute swimmers' ear
Beach ear
Tank ear

380.13 Other acute infections of external ear
Code first underlying disease, as:
erysipelas (035)
impetigo (684)
seborrheic dermatitis (690)

Excludes: *herpes simplex (054.73)*
herpes zoster (053.71)

380.14 Malignant otitis externa

380.15 Chronic mycotic otitis externa
Code first underlying disease, as:
aspergillosis (117.3)
otomycosis NOS (111.9)

Excludes: *candidal otitis externa (112.82)*

380.16 Other chronic infective otitis externa
Chronic infective otitis externa NOS

380.2 Other otitis externa

380.21 Cholesteatoma of external ear
Keratosis obturans of external ear (canal)

Excludes: *cholesteatoma NOS (385.30-385.35)*
postmastoidectomy (383.32)

380.22 Other acute otitis externa
Acute otitis externa:
actinic
chemical
contact
eczematoid
reactive

380.23 Other chronic otitis externa
Chronic otitis externa NOS

380.3 Noninfectious disorders of pinna

380.30 Disorder of pinna, unspecified

380.31 Hematoma of auricle or pinna

380.32 Acquired deformities of auricle or pinna

Excludes: *cauliflower ear (738.7)*

380.39 Other

Excludes: *gouty tophi of ear (274.81)*

380.4 Impacted cerumen
Wax in ear

380.5 Acquired stenosis of external ear canal
Collapse of external ear canal

380.50 Acquired stenosis of external ear canal, unspecified as to cause

380.51 Secondary to trauma

380.52 Secondary to surgery

380.53 Secondary to inflammation

380.8 Other disorders of external ear

380.81 Exostosis of external ear canal

380.89 Other

380.9 Unspecified disorder of external ear

381 Nonsuppurative otitis media and Eustachian tube disorders

381.0 Acute nonsuppurative otitis media
Acute tubotympanic catarrh
Otitis media, acute or subacute:
catarrhal
exudative
transudative
with effusion

Excludes: *otitic barotrauma (993.0)*

381.00 Acute nonsuppurative otitis media, unspecified

381.01 Acute serous otitis media
Acute or subacute secretory otitis media

381.02 Acute mucoid otitis media
Acute or subacute seromucinous otitis media
Blue drum syndrome

381.03 Acute sanguinous otitis media

381.04 Acute allergic serous otitis media

381.05 Acute allergic mucoid otitis media

381.06 Acute allergic sanguinous otitis media

381.1 Chronic serous otitis media
Chronic tubotympanic catarrh

381.10 Chronic serous otitis media, simple or unspecified

381.19 Other
Serosanguinous chronic otitis media

381.2 Chronic mucoid otitis media
Glue ear

Excludes: *adhesive middle ear disease (385.10-385.19)*

381.20 Chronic mucoid otitis media, simple or unspecified

381.29 Other
Mucosanguinous chronic otitis media

381.3 Other and unspecified chronic nonsuppurative otitis media
Otitis media, chronic:
allergic
exudative
secretory
Otitis media, chronic:
seromucinous
transudative
with effusion

381.4 Nonsuppurative otitis media, not specified as acute or chronic
Otitis media:
allergic
catarrhal
exudative
mucoid
Otitis media:
secretory
seromucinous
serous
transudative
with effusion

381.5 Eustachian salpingitis

381.50 Eustachian salpingitis, unspecified

381.51 Acute Eustachian salpingitis

381.52 Chronic Eustachian salpingitis

381.6 Obstruction of Eustachian tube
Stenosis } of Eustachian tube
Stricture }

381.60 Obstruction of Eustachian tube, unspecified

381.61 Osseous obstruction of Eustachian tube
Obstruction of Eustachian tube from cholesteatoma, polyp, or other osseous lesion

381.62 Intrinsic cartilagenous obstruction of Eustachian tube

381.63 Extrinsic cartilagenous obstruction of Eustachian tube
Compression of Eustachian tube

381.7 Patulous Eustachian tube

381.8 Other disorders of Eustachian tube

381.81 Dysfunction of Eustachian tube

381.89 Other

381.9 Unspecified Eustachian tube disorder

382 Suppurative and unspecified otitis media

382.0 Acute suppurative otitis media
Otitis media, acute:
necrotizing NOS
purulent

382.00 Acute suppurative otitis media without spontaneous rupture of ear drum

382.01 Acute suppurative otitis media with spontaneous rupture of ear drum

382.02 Acute suppurative otitis media in diseases classified elsewhere
Code first underlying disease, as:
influenza (487.8)
scarlet fever (034.1)

Excludes: postmeasles otitis (055.2)

382.1 Chronic tubotympanic suppurative otitis media
Benign chronic suppurative otitis media } (with anterior perforation of ear drum)
Chronic tubotympanic disease }

382.2 Chronic atticoantral suppurative otitis media
Chronic atticoantral disease } (with posterior or superior marginal perforation of ear drum)
Persistent mucosal disease }

382.3 Unspecified chronic suppurative otitis media
Chronic purulent otitis media

Excludes: tuberculous otitis media (017.4)

382.4 Unspecified suppurative otitis media
Purulent otitis media NOS

382.9 Unspecified otitis media
Otitis media:
NOS
acute NOS
chronic NOS

383 Mastoiditis and related conditions

383.0 Acute mastoiditis
Abscess of mastoid
Empyema of mastoid

383.00 Acute mastoiditis without complications

383.01 Subperiosteal abscess of mastoid

383.02 Acute mastoiditis with other complications
Gradenigo's syndrome

383.1 Chronic mastoiditis
Caries of mastoid
Fistula of mastoid

Excludes: tuberculous mastoiditis (015.6)

383.2 Petrositis
Coalescing osteitis }
Inflammation } of petrous bone
Osteomyelitis }

383.20 Petrositis, unspecified

Add 4th or 5th digit | Nonspecific code | Unspecified code | Manifestation code

383.21 Acute petrositis

383.22 Chronic petrositis

383.3 Complications following mastoidectomy

383.30 Postmastoidectomy complication, unspecified

383.31 Mucosal cyst of postmastoidectomy cavity

383.32 Recurrent cholesteatoma of postmastoidectomy cavity

383.33 Granulations of postmastoidectomy cavity
Chronic inflammation of postmastoidectomy cavity

383.8 Other disorders of mastoid

383.81 Postauricular fistula

383.89 Other

383.9 Unspecified mastoiditis

384 Other disorders of tympanic membrane

384.0 Acute myringitis without mention of otitis media

384.00 Acute myringitis, unspecified
Acute tympanitis NOS

384.01 Bullous myringitis
Myringitis bullosa hemorrhagica

384.09 Other

384.1 Chronic myringitis without mention of otitis media
Chronic tympanitis

384.2 Perforation of tympanic membrane
Perforation of ear drum:
NOS
persistent posttraumatic
postinflammatory

Excludes: *traumatic perforation [current injury] (872.61)*

384.20 Perforation of tympanic membrane, unspecified

384.21 Central perforation of tympanic membrane

384.22 Attic perforation of tympanic membrane
Pars flaccida

384.23 Other marginal perforation of tympanic membrane

384.24 Multiple perforations of tympanic membrane

384.25 Total perforation of tympanic membrane

384.8 Other specified disorders of tympanic membrane

384.81 Atrophic flaccid tympanic membrane
Healed perforation of ear drum

384.82 Atrophic nonflaccid tympanic membrane

384.9 Unspecified disorder of tympanic membrane

385 Other disorders of middle ear and mastoid

Excludes: *mastoiditis (383.0-383.9)*

385.0 Tympanosclerosis

385.00 Tympanosclerosis, unspecified as to involvement

385.01 Tympanosclerosis involving tympanic membrane only

385.02 Tympanosclerosis involving tympanic membrane and ear ossicles

385.03 Tympanosclerosis involving tympanic membrane, ear ossicles, and middle ear

385.09 Tympanosclerosis involving other combination of structures

385.1 Adhesive middle ear disease
Adhesive otitis
Otitis media:
chronic adhesive
fibrotic

Excludes: *glue ear (381.20-381.29)*

385.10 Adhesive middle ear disease, unspecified as to involvement

385.11 Adhesions of drum head to incus

385.12 Adhesions of drum head to stapes

385.13 Adhesions of drum head to promontorium

385.19 Other adhesions and combinations

385.2 Other acquired abnormality of ear ossicles

385.21 Impaired mobility of malleus
Ankylosis of malleus

385.22 Impaired mobility of other ear ossicles
Ankylosis of ear ossicles, except malleus

385.23 Discontinuity or dislocation of ear ossicles

385.24 Partial loss or necrosis of ear ossicles

385.3 Cholesteatoma of middle ear and mastoid
Cholesterosis, Epidermosis, Keratosis, Polyp } of (middle) ear

Excludes: *cholesteatoma:*
external ear canal (380.21)
recurrent of postmastoidectomy cavity (383.32)

385.30 Cholesteatoma, unspecified

385.31 Cholesteatoma of attic

385.32 Cholesteatoma of middle ear

385.33 Cholesteatoma of middle ear and mastoid

385.35 Diffuse cholesteatosis

385.8 Other disorders of middle ear and mastoid

385.82 Cholesterin granuloma

385.83 Retained foreign body of middle ear

385.89 Other

385.9 Unspecified disorder of middle ear and mastoid

386 Vertiginous syndromes and other disorders of vestibular system

Excludes: *vertigo NOS (780.4)*

386.0 Ménière's disease
Endolymphatic hydrops
Lermoyez's syndrome
Ménière's syndrome or vertigo

386.00 Ménière's disease, unspecified
Ménière's disease (active)

386.01 Active Ménière's disease, cochleovestibular

386.02 Active Ménière's disease, cochlear

386.03 Active Ménière's disease, vestibular

386.04 Inactive Ménière's disease
Ménière's disease in remission

386.1 Other and unspecified peripheral vertigo

Excludes: *epidemic vertigo (078.81)*

386.10 Peripheral vertigo, unspecified

386.11 Benign paroxysmal positional vertigo
Benign paroxysmal positional nystagmus

386.12 Vestibular neuronitis
Acute (and recurrent) peripheral vestibulopathy

386.19 Other
Aural vertigo
Otogenic vertigo

386.2 Vertigo of central origin
Central positional nystagmus
Malignant positional vertigo

386.3 Labyrinthitis

386.30 Labyrinthitis, unspecified

386.31 Serous labyrinthitis
Diffuse labyrinthitis

386.32 Circumscribed labyrinthitis
Focal labyrinthitis

386.33 Suppurative labyrinthitis
Purulent labyrinthitis

386.34 Toxic labyrinthitis

386.35 Viral labyrinthitis

386.4 Labyrinthine fistula

386.40 Labyrinthine fistula, unspecified

386.41 Round window fistula

386.42 Oval window fistula

386.43 Semicircular canal fistula

386.48 Labyrinthine fistula of combined sites

386.5 Labyrinthine dysfunction

386.50 Labyrinthine dysfunction, unspecified

386.51 Hyperactive labyrinth, unilateral

386.52 Hyperactive labyrinth, bilateral

386.53 Hypoactive labyrinth, unilateral

386.54 Hypoactive labyrinth, bilateral

386.55 Loss of labyrinthine reactivity, unilateral

386.56 Loss of labyrinthine reactivity, bilateral

386.58 Other forms and combinations

386.8 Other disorders of labyrinth

386.9 Unspecified vertiginous syndromes and labyrinthine disorders

387 Otosclerosis
Includes: otospongiosis

387.0 Otosclerosis involving oval window, nonobliterative

387.1 Otosclerosis involving oval window, obliterative

387.2 Cochlear otosclerosis
Otosclerosis involving:
otic capsule
round window

387.8 Other otosclerosis

387.9 Otosclerosis, unspecified

388 Other disorders of ear

388.0 Degenerative and vascular disorders of ear

388.00 Degenerative and vascular disorders, unspecified

388.01 Presbyacusis

388.02 Transient ischemic deafness

388.1 Noise effects on inner ear

388.10 Noise effects on inner ear, unspecified

388.11 Acoustic trauma (explosive) to ear
Otitic blast injury

388.12 Noise-induced hearing loss

388.2 Sudden hearing loss, unspecified

388.3 Tinnitus

388.30 Tinnitus, unspecified

388.31 Subjective tinnitus

388.32 Objective tinnitus

388.4 Other abnormal auditory perception

388.40 Abnormal auditory perception, unspecified

388.41 Diplacusis

388.42 Hyperacusis

388.43 Impairment of auditory discrimination

388.44 Recruitment

● Code new to this edition ▲ Revision of existing code ④ ⑤ Fourth or fifth digit required

388.5 Disorders of acoustic nerve
Acoustic neuritis
Degeneration } of acoustic or eighth nerve
Disorder } of acoustic or eighth nerve

Excludes: *acoustic neuroma (225.1)*
syphilitic acoustic neuritis (094.86)

388.6 Otorrhea

388.60 Otorrhea, unspecified
Discharging ear NOS

388.61 Cerebrospinal fluid otorrhea

Excludes: *cerebrospinal fluid rhinorrhea (349.81)*

388.69 Other
Otorrhagia

388.7 Otalgia

388.70 Otalgia, unspecified
Earache NOS

388.71 Otogenic pain

388.72 Referred pain

388.8 Other disorders of ear

388.9 Unspecified disorder of ear

389 Hearing loss

389.0 Conductive hearing loss
Conductive deafness

389.00 Conductive hearing loss, unspecified

389.01 Conductive hearing loss, external ear

389.02 Conductive hearing loss, tympanic membrane

389.03 Conductive hearing loss, middle ear

389.04 Conductive hearing loss, inner ear

389.08 Conductive hearing loss of combined types

389.1 Sensorineural hearing loss
Perceptive hearing loss or deafness

Excludes: *abnormal auditory perception (388.40-388.44)*
psychogenic deafness (306.7)

389.10 Sensorineural hearing loss, unspecified

389.11 Sensory hearing loss

389.12 Neural hearing loss

389.14 Central hearing loss

389.18 Sensorineural hearing loss of combined types

389.2 Mixed conductive and sensorineural hearing loss
Deafness or hearing loss of type classifiable to 389.0 with type classifiable to 389.1

389.7 Deaf mutism, not elsewhere classifiable
Deaf, nonspeaking

389.8 Other specified forms of hearing loss

389.9 Unspecified hearing loss
Deafness NOS

7. DISEASES OF THE CIRCULATORY SYSTEM (390-459)

ACUTE RHEUMATIC FEVER (390-392)

390 Rheumatic fever without mention of heart involvement
Arthritis, rheumatic, acute or subacute
Rheumatic fever (active) (acute)
Rheumatism, articular, acute or subacute

Excludes: *that with heart involvement (391.0-391.9)*

391 Rheumatic fever with heart involvement

Excludes: *chronic heart diseases of rheumatic origin (393.0-398.9) unless rheumatic fever is also present or there is evidence of recrudescence or activity of the rheumatic process*

391.0 Acute rheumatic pericarditis
Rheumatic:
fever (active) (acute) with pericarditis
pericarditis (acute)
Any condition classifiable to 390 with pericarditis

Excludes: *that not specified as rheumatic (420.0-420.9)*

391.1 Acute rheumatic endocarditis
Rheumatic:
endocarditis, acute
fever (active) (acute) with endocarditis or valvulitis
valvulitis acute
Any condition classifiable to 390 with endocarditis or valvulitis

391.2 Acute rheumatic myocarditis
Rheumatic fever (active) (acute) with myocarditis
Any condition classifiable to 390 with myocarditis

391.8 Other acute rheumatic heart disease
Rheumatic:
fever (active) (acute) with other or multiple types of heart involvement
pancarditis, acute
Any condition classifiable to 390 with other or multiple types of heart involvement

391.9 Acute rheumatic heart disease, unspecified
Rheumatic:
carditis, acute
fever (active) (acute) with unspecified type of heart involvement
heart disease, active or acute
Any condition classifiable to 390 with unspecified type of heart involvement

392 Rheumatic chorea
Includes: Sydenham's chorea

Excludes: *chorea:*
NOS (333.5)
Huntington's (333.4)

392.0 With heart involvement
Rheumatic chorea with heart involvement of any type classifiable to 391

392.9 Without mention of heart involvement

CHRONIC RHEUMATIC HEART DISEASE (393-398)

393 Chronic rheumatic pericarditis
Adherent pericardium, rheumatic
Chronic rheumatic:
mediastinopericarditis
myopericarditis

Excludes: *pericarditis NOS or not specified as rheumatic (423.0-423.9)*

394 Diseases of mitral valve

Excludes: *that with aortic valve involvement (396.0-396.9)*

394.0 Mitral stenosis
Mitral (valve):
obstruction (rheumatic)
stenosis NOS

394.1 Rheumatic mitral insufficiency
Rheumatic mitral:
incompetence
regurgitation

Excludes: *that not specified as rheumatic (424.0)*

394.2 Mitral stenosis with insufficiency
Mitral stenosis with incompetence or regurgitation

394.9 Other and unspecified mitral valve diseases
Mitral (valve):
disease (chronic)
failure

395 Diseases of aortic valve

Excludes: *that not specified as rheumatic (424.1)*
that with mitral valve involvement (396.0-396.9)

395.0 Rheumatic aortic stenosis
Rheumatic aortic (valve) obstruction

395.1 Rheumatic aortic insufficiency
Rheumatic aortic:
incompetence
regurgitation

395.2 Rheumatic aortic stenosis with insufficiency
Rheumatic aortic stenosis with incompetence or regurgitation

395.9 Other and unspecified rheumatic aortic diseases
Rheumatic aortic (valve) disease

396 Diseases of mitral and aortic valves
Includes: involvement of both mitral and aortic valves, whether specified as rheumatic or not

396.0 Mitral valve stenosis and aortic valve stenosis
Atypical aortic (valve) stenosis
Mitral and aortic (valve) obstruction (rheumatic)

396.1 Mitral valve stenosis and aortic valve insufficiency

396.2 Mitral valve insufficiency and aortic valve stenosis

396.3 Mitral valve insufficiency and aortic valve insufficiency
Mitral and aortic (valve):
incompetence
regurgitation

396.8 Multiple involvement of mitral and aortic valves
Stenosis and insufficiency of mitral or aortic valve with stenosis or insufficiency, or both, of the other valve

396.9 Mitral and aortic valve diseases, unspecified

397 Diseases of other endocardial structures

397.0 Diseases of tricuspid valve
Tricuspid (valve) (rheumatic):
disease
insufficiency
obstruction
regurgitation
stenosis

397.1 Rheumatic diseases of pulmonary valve

Excludes: *that not specified as rheumatic (424.3)*

397.9 Rheumatic diseases of endocardium, valve unspecified
Rheumatic:
endocarditis (chronic)
valvulitis (chronic)

Excludes: *that not specified as rheumatic (424.90-424.99)*

398 Other rheumatic heart disease

398.0 Rheumatic myocarditis
Rheumatic degeneration of myocardium

Excludes: *myocarditis not specified as rheumatic (429.0)*

398.9 Other and unspecified rheumatic heart diseases

398.90 Rheumatic heart disease, unspecified
Rheumatic:
carditis
heart disease NOS

Excludes: *carditis not specified as rheumatic (429.89)*
heart disease NOS not specified as rheumatic (429.9)

398.91 Rheumatic heart failure (congestive)
Rheumatic left ventricular failure

398.99 Other

HYPERTENSIVE DISEASE (401-405)

Excludes: *that complicating pregnancy, childbirth, or the puerperium (642.0-642.9)*
that involving coronary vessels (410.00-414.9)

401 Essential hypertension
Includes: high blood pressure
hyperpiesia
hyperpiesis
hypertension (arterial) (essential) (primary) (systemic)
hypertensive vascular:
degeneration
disease

Excludes: *elevated blood pressure without diagnosis of hypertension (796.2)*
pulmonary hypertension (416.0-416.9)
that involving vessels of:
brain (430-438)
eye (362.11)

401.0 Malignant

401.1 Benign

401.9 Unspecified

402 Hypertensive heart disease
Includes: hypertensive:
cardiomegaly
cardiopathy
cardiovascular disease
heart (disease) (failure)
any condition classifiable to 428, 429.0-429.3, 429.8, 429.9 due to hypertension

402.0 Malignant

402.00 Without congestive heart failure

402.01 With congestive heart failure

402.1 Benign

402.10 Without congestive heart failure

402.11 With congestive heart failure

402.9 Unspecified

402.90 Without congestive heart failure

402.91 With congestive heart failure

⑤ **403 Hypertensive renal disease**
The following fifth-digit subclassification is for use with category 403:

0 without mention of renal failure

1 with renal failure
Includes: arteriolar nephritis
arteriosclerosis of:
kidney
renal arterioles
arteriosclerotic nephritis (chronic) (interstitial)
hypertensive:
nephropathy
renal failure
uremia (chronic)
nephrosclerosis
renal sclerosis with hypertension
any condition classifiable to 585, 586, or 587 with any condition classifiable to 401

Excludes: *acute renal failure (584.5-584.9)*

continued

400

Add 4th or 5th digit | Nonspecific code | Unspecified code | Manifestation code

renal disease stated as not due to hypertension
renovascular hypertension (405.0-405.9 with fifth-digit 1)

403.0 Malignant

403.1 Benign

403.9 Unspecified

⑤ **404 Hypertensive heart and renal disease**

The following fifth-digit subclassification is for use with category 404:

- **0 without mention of congestive heart failure or renal failure**
- **1 with congestive heart failure**
- **2 with renal failure**
- **3 with congestive heart failure and renal failure**

Includes: disease:
cardiornal
cardiovascular renal
any condition classifiable to 402 with any condition classifiable to 403

404.0 Malignant

404.1 Benign

404.9 Unspecified

405 Secondary hypertension

405.0 Malignant

405.01 Renovascular

405.09 Other

405.1 Benign

405.11 Renovascular

405.19 Other

405.9 Unspecified

405.91 Renovascular

405.99 Other

ISCHEMIC HEART DISEASE (410-414)

Includes: that with mention of hypertension

Use additional code, if desired, to identify presence of hypertension (401.0-405.9)

⑤ **410 Acute myocardial infarction**

Includes: cardiac infarction
coronary (artery):
embolism
occlusion
rupture
thrombosis
infarction of heart, myocardium, or ventricle
rupture of heart, myocardium, or ventricle
any condition classifiable to 414.1-414.9 specified as acute or with a stated duration of 8 weeks or less

The following fifth-digit subclassification is for use with category 410:

0 episode of care unspecified

Use when the source document does not contain sufficient information for the assignment of fifth digit 1 or 2.

1 initial episode of care

Use fifth digit 1 to designate the first episode of care (regardless of facility site) for a newly diagnosed myocardial infarction. The fifth digit 1 is assigned regardless of the number of times a patient may be transferred during the initial episode of care

2 subsequent episode of care

Use fifth digit 2 to designate an episode of care following the initial episode when the patient is admitted for further observation, evaluation, or treatment for a myocardial infarction that has received initial treatment, but is still less than 8 weeks old.

410.0 Of anterolateral wall

410.1 Of other anterior wall
Infarction:
anterior (wall) NOS
anteroapical
anteroseptal
} (with contiguous portion of intraventricular septum)

410.2 Of inferolateral wall

410.3 Of inferoposterior wall

410.4 Of other inferior wall
Infarction:
diaphragmatic wall
inferior (wall) NOS
} (with contiguous portion of intraventricular septum)

410.5 Of other lateral wall
Infarction:
apical-lateral
basal-lateral
Infarction:
high lateral
posterolateral

410.6 True posterior wall infarction
Infarction:
posterobasal
strictly posterior

410.7 Subendocardial infarction
Nontransmural infarction

410.8 Of other specified sites
Infarction of:
atrium
papillary muscle
septum alone

410.9 Unspecified site
Acute myocardial infarction NOS
Coronary occlusion NOS

411 Other acute and subacute forms of ischemic heart disease

411.0 Postmyocardial infarction syndrome
Dressler's syndrome

411.1 Intermediate coronary syndrome
Impending infarction
Preinfarction angina
Preinfarction syndrome
Unstable angina

Excludes: *angina (pectoris) (413.9)*
decubitus (413.0)

411.8 Other

411.81 Acute coronary occlusion without myocardial infarction
Coronary (artery):
embolism
occlusion
thrombosis
} without or not resulting in myocardial infarction

411.89 Other
Coronary insufficiency (acute)
Subendocardial ischemia

412 Old myocardial infarction
Healed myocardial infarction
Past myocardial infarction diagnosed on ECG [EKG] or other special investigation, but currently presenting no symptoms

413 Angina pectoris

413.0 Angina decubitus
Nocturnal angina

413.1 Prinzmetal angina
Variant angina pectoris

413.9 Other and unspecified angina pectoris
Angina:
NOS
cardiac
of effort
Anginal syndrome
Status anginosus
Stenocardia
Syncope anginosa

Excludes: *preinfarction angina (411.1)*

414 Other forms of chronic ischemic heart disease

Excludes: *arteriosclerotic cardiovascular disease [ASCVD] (429.2)*
cardiovascular:
arteriosclerosis or sclerosis (429.2)
degeneration or disease (429.2)

414.0 Coronary atherosclerosis
Arteriosclerotic heart disease [ASHD]
Atherosclerotic heart disease
Coronary (artery):
arteriosclerosis
arteritis or endarteritis
atheroma
sclerosis
stricture

Excludes: *embolism of graft (996.72)*
occlusion NOS
thrombus

414.00 Of unspecified vessel

414.01 Of native coronary artery

414.02 Of autologous vein bypass graft

414.03 Of nonautologous biological bypass graft

414.1 Aneurysm of heart

414.10 Of heart (wall)
Aneurysm (arteriovenous):
mural
ventricular

414.11 Of coronary vessels
Aneurysm (arteriovenous) of coronary vessels

414.19 Other
Arteriovenous fistula, acquired, of heart

414.8 Other specified forms of chronic ischemic heart disease
Chronic coronary insufficiency
Ischemia, myocardial (chronic)
Any condition classifiable to 410 specified as chronic, or presenting with symptoms after 8 weeks from date of infarction

Excludes: *coronary insufficiency (acute) (411.89)*

414.9 Chronic ischemic heart disease, unspecified
Ischemic heart disease NOS

DISEASES OF PULMONARY CIRCULATION (415-417)

415 Acute pulmonary heart disease

415.0 Acute cor pulmonale

Excludes: *cor pulmonale NOS (416.9)*

415.1 Pulmonary embolism and infarction
Pulmonary (artery) (vein):
apoplexy
embolism
infarction (hemorrhagic)
thrombosis

Excludes: *that complicating:*
abortion (634-638 with .6, 639.6)
ectopic or molar pregnancy (639.6)
pregnancy, childbirth, or the puerperium (673.0-673.8)

● **415.11 Iatrogenic pulmonary embolism and infarction**

● **415.19 Other**

416 Chronic pulmonary heart disease

416.0 Primary pulmonary hypertension
Idiopathic pulmonary arteriosclerosis
Pulmonary hypertension (essential) (idiopathic) (primary)

416.1 Kyphoscoliotic heart disease

● Code new to this edition
▲ Revision of existing code
④ ⑤ Fourth or fifth digit required

416.8 Other chronic pulmonary heart diseases
Pulmonary hypertension, secondary

416.9 Chronic pulmonary heart disease, unspecified
Chronic cardiopulmonary disease
Cor pulmonale (chronic) NOS

417 Other diseases of pulmonary circulation

417.0 Arteriovenous fistula of pulmonary vessels

Excludes: *congenital arteriovenous fistula (747.3)*

417.1 Aneurysm of pulmonary artery

Excludes: *congenital aneurysm (747.3)*

417.8 Other specified diseases of pulmonary circulation
Pulmonary:
  arteritis
  endarteritis
Rupture } of pulmonary vessel
Stricture } of pulmonary vessel

417.9 Unspecified disease of pulmonary circulation

OTHER FORMS OF HEART DISEASE (420-429)

420 Acute pericarditis
Includes: acute:
  mediastinopericarditis
  myopericarditis
  pericardial effusion
  pleuropericarditis
  pneumopericarditis

Excludes: *acute rheumatic pericarditis (391.0)*
postmyocardial infarction syndrome [Dressler's] (411.0)

420.0 Acute pericarditis in diseases classified elsewhere
Code first underlying disease, as:
  actinomycosis (039.8)
  amebiasis (006.8)
  nocardiosis (039.8)
  tuberculosis (017.9)
  uremia (585)

Excludes: *pericarditis (acute) (in):*
  Coxsackie (virus) (074.21)
  gonococcal (098.83)
  histoplasmosis (115.0-115.9 with fifth-digit 3)
  meningococcal infection (036.41)
  syphilitic (093.81)

420.9 Other and unspecified acute pericarditis

420.90 Acute pericarditis, unspecified
Pericarditis (acute):
  NOS
  infective NOS
  sicca

420.91 Acute idiopathic pericarditis
Pericarditis, acute:
  benign
  nonspecific
  viral

420.99 Other
Pericarditis (acute):
  pneumococcal
  purulent
  staphylococcal
Pericarditis (acute):
  streptococcal
  suppurative
Pneumopyopericardium
Pyopericardium

Excludes: *pericarditis in diseases classified elsewhere (420.0)*

Add 4th or 5th digit | Nonspecific code | Unspecified code | Manifestation code

421 Acute and subacute endocarditis

421.0 Acute and subacute bacterial endocarditis

Endocarditis (acute) (chronic) (subacute):
- bacterial
- infective NOS
- lenta
- malignant
- purulent
- septic
- ulcerative
- vegetative

Infective aneurysm
Subacute bacterial endocarditis [SBE]

Use additional code, if desired, to identify infectious organism [e.g., Streptococcus 041.0, Staphylococcus 041.1]

421.1 Acute and subacute infective endocarditis in diseases classified elsewhere

Code first underlying disease, as:
- blastomycosis (116.0)
- Q fever (083.0)
- typhoid (fever) (002.0)

Excludes: *endocarditis (in):*
- *Coxsackie (virus) (074.22)*
- *gonococcal (098.84)*
- *histoplasmosis (115.0-115.9 with fifth-digit 4)*
- *meningococcal infection (036.42)*
- *monilial (112.81)*

421.9 Acute endocarditis, unspecified

Endocarditis, Myoendocarditis, Periendocarditis } acute or subacute

Excludes: *acute rheumatic endocarditis (391.1)*

422 Acute myocarditis

Excludes: *acute rheumatic myocarditis (391.2)*

422.0 Acute myocarditis in diseases classified elsewhere

Code first underlying disease, as:
- myocarditis (acute):
  - influenzal (487.8)
  - tuberculous (017.9)

Excludes: *myocarditis (acute) (due to):*
- *aseptic, of newborn (074.23)*
- *Coxsackie (virus) (074.23)*
- *diphtheritic (032.82)*
- *meningococcal infection (036.43)*
- *syphilitic (093.82)*
- *toxoplasmosis (130.3)*

422.9 Other and unspecified acute myocarditis

422.90 Acute myocarditis, unspecified

Acute or subacute (interstitial) myocarditis

422.91 Idiopathic myocarditis

Myocarditis (acute or subacute):
- Fiedler's
- giant cell
- isolated (diffuse) (granulomatous)
- nonspecific granulomatous

422.92 Septic myocarditis

Myocarditis, acute or subacute:
- pneumococcal
- staphylococcal

Use additional code, if desired, to identify infectious organism [e.g., Staphylococcus 041.1]

Excludes: *myocarditis, acute or subacute:*
- *in bacterial diseases classified elsewhere (422.0)*
- *streptococcal (391.2)*

422.93 Toxic myocarditis

422.99 Other

423 Other diseases of pericardium

Excludes: *that specified as rheumatic (393)*

423.0 Hemopericardium

423.1 Adhesive pericarditis

Adherent pericardium
Fibrosis of pericardium
Milk spots
Pericarditis:
  adhesive
  obliterative
Soldiers' patches

423.2 Constrictive pericarditis

Concato's disease
Pick's disease of heart (and liver)

423.8 Other specified diseases of pericardium

Calcification } of pericardium
Fistula } of pericardium

423.9 Unspecified disease of pericardium

424 Other diseases of endocardium

Excludes: *bacterial endocarditis (421.0-421.9)*
rheumatic endocarditis (391.1, 394.0-397.9)
syphilitic endocarditis (093.20-093.24)

424.0 Mitral valve disorders

Mitral (valve):
  incompetence } NOS of specified cause, except rheumatic
  insufficiency } NOS of specified cause, except rheumatic
  regurgitation } NOS of specified cause, except rheumatic

Excludes: *mitral (valve):*
  disease (394.9)
  failure (394.9)
  stenosis (394.0)
the listed conditions:
  specified as rheumatic (394.1)
  unspecified as to cause but with mention of:
    diseases of aortic valve (396.0-396.9)
    mitral stenosis or obstruction (394.2)

424.1 Aortic valve disorders

Aortic (valve):
  incompetence } NOS of specified cause, except rheumatic
  insufficiency } NOS of specified cause, except rheumatic
  regurgitation } NOS of specified cause, except rheumatic
  stenosis } NOS of specified cause, except rheumatic

Excludes: *hypertrophic subaortic stenosis (425.1)*
that specified as rheumatic (395.0-395.9)
that of unspecified cause but with mention of diseases of mitral valve (396.0-396.9)

424.2 Tricuspid valve disorders, specified as nonrheumatic

Tricuspid valve:
  incompetence } of specified cause, except rheumatic
  insufficiency } of specified cause, except rheumatic
  regurgitation } of specified cause, except rheumatic
  stenosis } of specified cause, except rheumatic

Excludes: *rheumatic or of unspecified cause (397.0)*

424.3 Pulmonary valve disorders

Pulmonic:
  incompetence NOS
  insufficiency NOS
Pulmonic:
  regurgitation NOS
  stenosis NOS

Excludes: *that specified as rheumatic (397.1)*

424.9 Endocarditis, valve unspecified

424.90 Endocarditis, valve unspecified, unspecified cause
Endocarditis (chronic):
NOS
nonbacterial thrombotic
Valvular:
incompetence
insufficiency
regurgitation
stenosis
Valvulitis (chronic)
} of unspecified valve, unspecified cause

424.91 Endocarditis in diseases classified elsewhere
Code first underlying disease, as:
atypical verrucous endocarditis [Libman-Sacks] (710.0)
disseminated lupus erythematosus (710.0)
tuberculosis (017.9)

Excludes: syphilitic (093.20-093.24)

424.99 Other
Any condition classifiable to 424.90 with specified cause, except rheumatic

Excludes: endocardial fibroelastosis (425.3)
that specified as rheumatic (397.9)

425 Cardiomyopathy
Includes: myocardiopathy

425.0 Endomyocardial fibrosis

425.1 Hypertrophic obstructive cardiomyopathy
Hypertrophic subaortic stenosis (idiopathic)

425.2 Obscure cardiomyopathy of Africa
Becker's disease
Idiopathic mural endomyocardial disease

425.3 Endocardial fibroelastosis
Elastomyofibrosis

425.4 Other primary cardiomyopathies
Cardiomyopathy:
NOS
congestive
constrictive
familial
hypertrophic
Cardiomyopathy:
idiopathic
nonobstructive
obstructive
restrictive
Cardiovascular collagenosis

425.5 Alcoholic cardiomyopathy

425.7 Nutritional and metabolic cardiomyopathy
Code first underlying disease, as:
amyloidosis (277.3)
beriberi (265.0)
cardiac glycogenosis (271.0)
mucopolysaccharidosis (277.5)
thyrotoxicosis (242.0-242.9)

Excludes: gouty tophi of heart (274.82)

425.8 Cardiomyopathy in other diseases classified elsewhere
Code first underlying disease, as:
Friedreich's ataxia (334.0)
myotonia atrophica (359.2)
progressive muscular dystrophy (359.1)
sarcoidosis (135)

Excludes: cardiomyopathy in Chagas' disease (086.0)

425.9 Secondary cardiomyopathy, unspecified

426 Conduction disorders

426.0 Atrioventricular block, complete
Third degree atrioventricular block

426.1 Atrioventricular block, other and unspecified

426.10 Atrioventricular block, unspecified
Atrioventricular [AV] block (incomplete) (partial)

426.11 First degree atrioventricular block
Incomplete atrioventricular block, first degree
Prolonged P-R interval NOS

426.12 Mobitz (type) II atrioventricular block
Incomplete atrioventricular block:
Mobitz (type) II
second degree, Mobitz (type) II

426.13 Other second degree atrioventricular block
Incomplete atrioventricular block:
Mobitz (type) I [Wenckebach's]
second degree:
NOS
Mobitz (type) I
with 2:1 atrioventricular response [block]
Wenckebach's phenomenon

426.2 Left bundle branch hemiblock
Block:
left anterior fascicular
left posterior fascicular

426.3 Other left bundle branch block
Left bundle branch block:
NOS
anterior fascicular with posterior fascicular
complete
main stem

426.4 Right bundle branch block

426.5 Bundle branch block, other and unspecified

426.50 Bundle branch block, unspecified

426.51 Right bundle branch block and left posterior fascicular block

426.52 Right bundle branch block and left anterior fascicular block

426.53 Other bilateral bundle branch block
Bifascicular block NOS
Bilateral bundle branch block NOS
Right bundle branch with left bundle branch block (incomplete) (main stem)

426.54 Trifascicular block

426.6 Other heart block
Intraventricular block:
NOS
diffuse
myofibrillar
Sinoatrial block
Sinoauricular block

426.7 Anomalous atrioventricular excitation
Atrioventricular conduction:
accelerated
accessory
pre-excitation
Ventricular pre-excitation
Wolff-Parkinson-White syndrome

426.8 Other specified conduction disorders

426.81 Lown-Ganong-Levine syndrome
Syndrome of short P-R interval, normal QRS complexes, and supraventricular tachycardias

426.89 Other
Dissociation:
atrioventricular [AV]
interference
isorhythmic
Nonparoxysmal AV nodal tachycardia

426.9 Conduction disorder, unspecified
Heart block NOS
Stokes-Adams syndrome

427 Cardiac dysrhythmias

Excludes: *that complicating:*
abortion (634-638 with .7, 639.8)
ectopic or molar pregnancy (639.8)
labor or delivery (668.1, 669.4)

427.0 Paroxysmal supraventricular tachycardia
Paroxysmal tachycardia:
atrial [PAT]
atrioventricular [AV]
junctional
nodal

427.1 Paroxysmal ventricular tachycardia
Ventricular tachycardia (paroxysmal)

427.2 Paroxysmal tachycardia, unspecified
Bouveret-Hoffmann syndrome
Paroxysmal tachycardia:
NOS
essential

427.3 Atrial fibrillation and flutter

427.31 Atrial fibrillation

427.32 Atrial flutter

427.4 Ventricular fibrillation and flutter

427.41 Ventricular fibrillation

427.42 Ventricular flutter

427.5 Cardiac arrest
Cardiorespiratory arrest

427.6 Premature beats

427.60 Premature beats, unspecified
Ectopic beats
Extrasystoles
Extrasystolic arrhythmia
Premature contractions or systoles NOS

427.61 Supraventricular premature beats
Atrial premature beats, contractions, or systoles

427.69 Other
Ventricular premature beats, contractions, or systoles

427.8 Other specified cardiac dysrhythmias

427.81 Sinoatrial node dysfunction
Sinus bradycardia:
persistent
severe
Syndrome:
sick sinus
tachycardia-bradycardia

Excludes: *sinus bradycardia NOS (427.89)*

427.89 Other
Rhythm disorder:
coronary sinus
ectopic
nodal
Wandering (atrial) pacemaker

Excludes: *carotid sinus syncope (337.0)*
reflex bradycardia (337.0)
tachycardia (785.0)

427.9 Cardiac dysrhythmia, unspecified
Arrhythmia (cardiac) NOS

428 Heart failure

Excludes: *following cardiac surgery (429.4)*
rheumatic (398.91)
that complicating:
abortion (634-638 with .7, 639.8)
ectopic or molar pregnancy (639.8)
labor or delivery (668.1, 669.4)
that due to hypertension (402.0-402.9 with fifth-digit 1)

428.0 Congestive heart failure
Congestive heart disease
Right heart failure (secondary to left heart failure)

428.1 Left heart failure
Acute edema of lung } with heart disease NOS or heart failure
Acute pulmonary edema } with heart disease NOS or heart failure
Cardiac asthma
Left ventricular failure

428.9 Heart failure, unspecified
Cardiac failure NOS
Heart failure NOS
Myocardial failure NOS
Weak heart

429 Ill-defined descriptions and complications of heart disease

429.0 Myocarditis, unspecified
Myocarditis: (with mention of arteriosclerosis)
- NOS
- chronic (interstitial)
- fibroid
- senile

Use additional code, if desired, to identify presence of arteriosclerosis

Excludes: *acute or subacute (422.0-422.9)*
rheumatic (398.0)
acute (391.2)
that due to hypertension (402.0-402.9)

429.1 Myocardial degeneration
Degeneration of heart or myocardium: (with mention of arteriosclerosis)
- fatty
- mural
- muscular

Myocardial: (with mention of arteriosclerosis)
- degeneration disease

Use additional code, if desired, to identify presence of arteriosclerosis

Excludes: *that due to hypertension (402.0-402.9)*

429.2 Cardiovascular disease, unspecified
Arteriosclerotic cardiovascular disease [ASCVD]
Cardiovascular arteriosclerosis
Cardiovascular: (with mention of arteriosclerosis)
- degeneration
- disease
- sclerosis

Use additional code, if desired, to identify presence of arteriosclerosis

Excludes: *that due to hypertension (402.0-402.9)*

429.3 Cardiomegaly
Cardiac:
- dilatation
- hypertrophy

Ventricular dilatation

Excludes: *that due to hypertension (402.0-402.9)*

429.4 Functional disturbances following cardiac surgery
Cardiac insufficiency } following cardiac surgery or due to prosthesis
Heart failure } following cardiac surgery or due to prosthesis
Postcardiotomy syndrome
Postvalvulotomy syndrome

Excludes: *cardiac failure in the immediate postoperative period (997.1)*

429.5 Rupture of chordae tendineae

429.6 Rupture of papillary muscle

Add 4th or 5th digit | Nonspecific code | Unspecified code | Manifestation code

429.7 Certain sequelae of myocardial infarction, not elsewhere classified

Use additional code to identify the associated myocardial infarction:
with onset of 8 weeks or less (410.00-410.92)
with onset of more than 8 weeks (414.8)

Excludes: *congenital defects of heart (745, 746)*
coronary aneurysm (414.11)
disorders of papillary muscle (429.6, 429.81)
postmyocardial infarction syndrome (411.0)
rupture of chordae tendineae (429.5)

429.71 Acquired cardiac septal defect

Excludes: *acute septal infarction (410.00-410.92)*

429.79 Other
Mural thrombus (atrial) (ventricular), acquired, following myocardial infarction

429.8 Other ill-defined heart diseases

429.81 Other disorders of papillary muscle
Papillary muscle:
atrophy
degeneration
dysfunction
Papillary muscle:
incompetence
incoordination
scarring

429.82 Hyperkinetic heart disease

429.89 Other
Carditis

Excludes: *that due to hypertension (402.0-402.9)*

429.9 Heart disease, unspecified
Heart disease (organic) NOS
Morbus cordis NOS

Excludes: *that due to hypertension (402.0-402.9)*

CEREBROVASCULAR DISEASE (430-438)

Includes: with mention of hypertension (conditions classifiable to 401-405)

Use additional code, if desired, to identify presence of hypertension

Excludes: *any condition classifiable to 430-434, 436, 437 occurring during pregnancy, childbirth, or the puerperium, or specified as puerperal (674.0)*

430 Subarachnoid hemorrhage
Meningeal hemorrhage
Ruptured:
berry aneurysm
(congenital) cerebral aneurysm NOS

Excludes: *syphilitic ruptured cerebral aneurysm (094.87)*

431 Intracerebral hemorrhage
Hemorrhage (of):
basilar
bulbar
cerebellar
cerebral
cerebromeningeal
cortical
internal capsule
Hemorrhage (of):
intrapontine
pontine
subcortical
ventricular
Rupture of blood vessel in brain

432 Other and unspecified intracranial hemorrhage

432.0 Nontraumatic extradural hemorrhage
Nontraumatic epidural hemorrhage

432.1 Subdural hemorrhage
Subdural hematoma, nontraumatic

432.9 Unspecified intracranial hemorrhage
Intracranial hemorrhage NOS

● Code new to this edition ▲ Revision of existing code ④ ⑤ Fourth or fifth digit required

⑤ **433 Occlusion and stenosis of precerebral arteries**

The following fifth-digit subclassification is for use with category 433:

0 without mention of cerebral infarction

1 with cerebral infarction

Includes:
embolism, narrowing, obstruction, thrombosis } of basilar, carotid, and vertebral arteries

Excludes: *insufficiency NOS of precerebral arteries (435.0-435.9)*

433.0 Basilar artery

433.1 Carotid artery

433.2 Vertebral artery

433.3 Multiple and bilateral

433.8 Other specified precerebral artery

433.9 Unspecified precerebral artery
Precerebral artery NOS

⑤ **434 Occlusion of cerebral arteries**

The following fifth-digit subclassification is for use with category 434:

0 without mention of cerebral infarction

1 with cerebral infarction

434.0 Cerebral thrombosis
Thrombosis of cerebral arteries

434.1 Cerebral embolism

434.9 Cerebral artery occlusion, unspecified

435 Transient cerebral ischemia

Includes: cerebrovascular insufficiency (acute) with transient focal neurological signs and symptoms
insufficiency of basilar, carotid, and vertebral arteries
spasm of cerebral arteries

Excludes: *acute cerebrovascular insufficiency NOS (437.1)*
that due to any condition classifiable to 433 (433.0-433.9)

435.0 Basilar artery syndrome

435.1 Vertebral artery syndrome

435.2 Subclavian steal syndrome

● **435.3 Vertebrobasilar artery syndrome**

435.8 Other specified transient cerebral ischemias

435.9 Unspecified transient cerebral ischemia
Impending cerebrovascular accident
Intermittent cerebral ischemia
Transient ischemic attack [TIA]

436 Acute, but ill-defined, cerebrovascular disease

Apoplexy, apoplectic:
NOS
attack
cerebral
seizure
Cerebral seizure
Cerebrovascular accident [CVA] NOS
Stroke

Excludes: *any condition classifiable to categories 430-435*

437 Other and ill-defined cerebrovascular disease

437.0 Cerebral atherosclerosis
Atheroma of cerebral arteries
Cerebral arteriosclerosis

437.1 Other generalized ischemic cerebrovascular disease
Acute cerebrovascular insufficiency NOS
Cerebral ischemia (chronic)

437.2 Hypertensive encephalopathy

437.3 Cerebral aneurysm, nonruptured

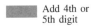

437.4 Cerebral arteritis

437.5 Moyamoya disease

437.6 Nonpyogenic thrombosis of intracranial venous sinus

Excludes: *pyogenic (325)*

437.7 Transient global amnesia

437.8 Other

437.9 Unspecified

Cerebrovascular disease or lesion NOS

438 Late effects of cerebrovascular disease

Note: This category is to be used to indicate conditions in 430-437 as the cause of late effects, themselves classifiable elsewhere. The "late effects" include conditions specified as such, or as sequelae, which may occur at any time after the onset of the causal condition.

Code first sequelae:

aphasia (784.3)
dysphasia (784.5)
hemiplegia (342.0-342.9)
paralysis (344.0-344.9)

DISEASES OF ARTERIES, ARTERIOLES, AND CAPILLARIES (440-448)

440 Atherosclerosis

Includes: arteriolosclerosis
arteriosclerosis (obliterans) (senile)
arteriosclerotic vascular disease
atheroma
degeneration:
arterial
arteriovascular
vascular
endarteritis deformans or obliterans
senile:
arteritis
endarteritis

440.0 Of aorta

440.1 Of renal artery

Excludes: *atherosclerosis of renal arterioles (403.00-403.91)*

440.2 Of native arteries of the extremities

Excludes: *atherosclerosis of bypass graft of the extremities (440.30-440.32)*

440.20 Atherosclerosis of the extremities, unspecified

440.21 Atherosclerosis of the extremities with intermittent claudication

440.22 Atherosclerosis of the extremities with rest pain

Includes: any condition classifiable to 440.21

440.23 Atherosclerosis of the extremities with ulceration

Includes: any condition classifiable to 440.21 and 440.22

440.24 Atherosclerosis of the extremities with gangrene

Includes: any condition classifiable to 440.21, 440.22, and 440.23 with ischemic gangrene 785.4

Excludes: *gas gangrene 040.0*

440.29 Other

440.3 Of bypass graft of the extremities

Excludes: *atherosclerosis of native artery of the extremity (440.21-440.24)*
embolism [occlusion NOS] [thrombus] of graft (996.74)

440.30 Of unspecified graft

440.31 Of autologous vein bypass graft

440.32 Of nonautologous biological bypass graft

440.8 Of other specified arteries

Excludes: *basilar (433.0)*
carotid (433.1)
cerebral (437.0)
coronary (414.0)
mesenteric (557.1)

precerebral (433.0-433.9)
pulmonary (416.0)
vertebral (433.2)

440.9 Generalized and unspecified atherosclerosis
Arteriosclerotic vascular disease NOS

Excludes: *arteriosclerotic cardiovascular disease [ASCVD] (429.2)*

▲ **441 Aortic aneurysm and dissection**

Excludes: *syphilitic aortic aneurysm (093.0)*
traumatic aortic aneurysm (901.0, 902.0)

▲ **441.0 Dissection of aorta**
Dissecting aneurysm of aorta (ruptured)

441.00 Unspecified site

441.01 Thoracic

441.02 Abdominal

441.03 Thoracoabdominal

441.1 Thoracic aneurysm, ruptured

441.2 Thoracic aneurysm without mention of rupture

441.3 Abdominal aneurysm, ruptured

441.4 Abdominal aneurysm without mention of rupture

441.5 Aortic aneurysm of unspecified site, ruptured
Rupture of aorta NOS

441.6 Thoracoabdominal aneurysm, ruptured

441.7 Thoracoabdominal aneurysm, without mention of rupture

□ **441.9 Aortic aneurysm of unspecified site without mention of rupture**
Aneurysm, Dilatation, Hyaline necrosis } of aorta

442 Other aneurysm
Includes: aneurysm (ruptured) (cirsoid) (false) (varicose)
aneurysmal varix

Excludes: *arteriovenous aneurysm or fistula:*
acquired (447.0)
congenital (747.6)
traumatic (900.0-904.9)

442.0 Of artery of upper extremity

442.1 Of renal artery

442.2 Of iliac artery

442.3 Of artery of lower extremity
Aneurysm:
femoral, popliteal } artery

442.8 Of other specified artery

442.81 Artery of neck
Aneurysm of carotid artery (common) (external) (internal)

442.82 Subclavian artery

442.83 Splenic artery

442.84 Other visceral artery
Aneurysm:
celiac, gastroduodenal, gastroepiploic, Hepatic, pancreaticoduodenal, superior mesenteric } artery

442.89 Other
Aneurysm:
mediastinal, spinal } artery

Excludes: *cerebral (nonruptured) (437.3)*
ruptured (430)
coronary (414.11)
heart (414.10)
pulmonary (417.1)

442.9 Of unspecified site

443 Other peripheral vascular disease

443.0 Raynaud's syndrome
Raynaud's:
disease
phenomenon (secondary)

Use additional code, if desired, to identify gangrene (785.4)

443.1 Thromboangiitis obliterans [Buerger's disease]
Presenile gangrene

443.8 Other specified peripheral vascular diseases

443.81 Peripheral angiopathy in diseases classified elsewhere
Code first underlying disease, as:
diabetes mellitus (250.7)

443.89 Other
Acrocyanosis
Acroparesthesia:
simple [Schultze's type]
vasomotor [Nothnagel's type]
Erythrocyanosis
Erythromelalgia

Excludes: *chilblains (991.5)*
frostbite (991.0-991.3)
immersion foot (991.4)

443.9 Peripheral vascular disease, unspecified
Intermittent claudication NOS
Peripheral:
angiopathy NOS
vascular disease NOS
Spasm of artery

Excludes: *spasm of cerebral artery (435.0-435.9)*
Atherosclerosis of the arteries of the extremities (440.20-440.22)

444 Arterial embolism and thrombosis
Includes: infarction:
embolic
thrombotic
occlusion

Excludes: *that complicating:*
abortion (634-638 with .6, 639.6)
ectopic or molar pregnancy (639.6)
pregnancy, childbirth, or the puerperium (673.0-673.8)

444.0 Of abdominal aorta
Aortic bifurcation syndrome
Aortoiliac obstruction
Leriche's syndrome
Saddle embolus

444.1 Of thoracic aorta
Embolism or thrombosis of aorta (thoracic)

444.2 Of arteries of the extremities

444.21 Upper extremity

444.22 Lower extremity
Arterial embolism or thrombosis:
femoral
peripheral NOS
popliteal

Excludes: *iliofemoral (444.81)*

444.8 Of other specified artery

444.81 Iliac artery

● Code new to this edition
▲ Revision of existing code
④ ⑤ Fourth or fifth digit required

444.89 Other

Excludes: *basilar (433.0)*
carotid (433.1)
cerebral (434.0-434.9)
coronary (410.00-410.92)
mesenteric (557.0)
ophthalmic (362.30-362.34)
precerebral (433.0-433.9)
pulmonary (415.1)
renal (593.81)
retinal (362.30-362.34)
vertebral (433.2)

444.9 Of unspecified artery

446 Polyarteritis nodosa and allied conditions

446.0 Polyarteritis nodosa
Disseminated necrotizing periarteritis
Necrotizing angiitis
Panarteritis (nodosa)
Periarteritis (nodosa)

446.1 Acute febrile mucocutaneous lymph node syndrome [MCLS]
Kawasaki disease

446.2 Hypersensitivity angiitis

Excludes: *antiglomerular basement membrane disease without pulmonary hemorrhage (583.89)*

446.20 Hypersensitivity angiitis, unspecified

446.21 Goodpasture's syndrome
Antiglomerular basement membrane antibody-mediated nephritis with pulmonary hemorrhage
Use additional code, if desired, to identify renal disease (583.81)

446.29 Other specified hypersensitivity angiitis

446.3 Lethal midline granuloma
Malignant granuloma of face

446.4 Wegener's granulomatosis
Necrotizing respiratory granulomatosis
Wegener's syndrome

446.5 Giant cell arteritis
Cranial arteritis
Horton's disease
Temporal arteritis

446.6 Thrombotic microangiopathy
Moschcowitz's syndrome
Thrombotic thrombocytopenic purpura

446.7 Takayasu's disease
Aortic arch arteritis
Pulseless disease

447 Other disorders of arteries and arterioles

447.0 Arteriovenous fistula, acquired
Arteriovenous aneurysm, acquired

Excludes: *cerebrovascular (437.3)*
coronary (414.19)
pulmonary (417.0)
surgically created arteriovenous shunt or fistula:
complication (996.1, 996.61-996.62)
status or presence (V45.1)
traumatic (900.0-904.9)

447.1 Stricture of artery

447.2 Rupture of artery
Erosion } of artery
Fistula, except arteriovenous } of artery
Ulcer } of artery

Excludes: *traumatic rupture of artery (900.0-904.9)*

447.3 Hyperplasia of renal artery
Fibromuscular hyperplasia of renal artery

447.4 Celiac artery compression syndrome
Celiac axis syndrome
Marable's syndrome

447.5 Necrosis of artery

447.6 Arteritis, unspecified
Aortitis NOS
Endarteritis NOS

Excludes: *arteritis, endarteritis:*
aortic arch (446.7)
cerebral (437.4)
coronary (414.0)
deformans (440.0-440.9)
obliterans (440.0-440.9)
pulmonary (417.8)
senile (440.0-440.9)
polyarteritis NOS (446.0)
syphilitic aortitis (093.1)

447.8 Other specified disorders of arteries and arterioles
Fibromuscular hyperplasia of arteries, except renal

447.9 Unspecified disorders of arteries and arterioles

448 Disease of capillaries

448.0 Hereditary hemorrhagic telangiectasia
Rendu-Osler-Weber disease

448.1 Nevus, non-neoplastic
Nevus:
araneus
senile
Nevus:
spider
stellar

Excludes: *neoplastic (216.0-216.9)*
port wine (757.32)
strawberry (757.32)

448.9 Other and unspecified capillary diseases
Capillary:
hemorrhage
hyperpermeability
thrombosis

Excludes: *capillary fragility (hereditary) (287.8)*

DISEASES OF VEINS AND LYMPHATICS, AND OTHER DISEASES OF CIRCULATORY SYSTEM (451-459)

451 Phlebitis and thrombophlebitis
Includes: endophlebitis
inflammation, vein
periphlebitis
suppurative phlebitis

Use additional E Code, if desired, to identify drug, if drug-induced

Excludes: *that complicating:*
abortion (634-638 with .7, 639.8)
ectopic or molar pregnancy (639.8)
pregnancy, childbirth, or the puerperium (671.0-671.9)
that due to or following:
implant or catheter device (996.61-996.62)
infusion, perfusion, or transfusion (999.2)

451.0 Of superficial vessels of lower extremities
Saphenous vein (greater) (lesser)

451.1 Of deep vessels of lower extremities

451.11 Femoral vein (deep) (superficial)

451.19 Other
Femoropopliteal vein
Popliteal vein
Tibial vein

451.2 Of lower extremities, unspecified

451.8 Of other sites

Excludes: *intracranial venous sinus (325)*
nonpyogenic (437.6)
portal (vein) (572.1)

451.81 Iliac vein

451.82 Of superficial veins of upper extremities
Antecubital vein
Basilic vein
Cephalic vein

451.83 Of deep veins of upper extremities
Brachial vein
Radial vein
Ulnar vein

451.84 Of upper extremities, unspecified

451.89 Other
Axillary vein
Jugular vein
Subclavian vein
Thrombophlebitis of breast (Mondor's disease)

451.9 Of unspecified site

452 Portal vein thrombosis
Portal (vein) obstruction

Excludes: *hepatic vein thrombosis (453.0)*
phlebitis of portal vein (572.1)

453 Other venous embolism and thrombosis

Excludes: *that complicating:*
abortion (634-638 with .7, 639.8)
ectopic or molar pregnancy (639.8)
pregnancy, childbirth, or the puerperium (671.0-671.9)
that with inflammation, phlebitis, and thrombophlebitis (451.0-451.9)

453.0 Budd-Chiari syndrome
Hepatic vein thrombosis

453.1 Thrombophlebitis migrans

453.2 Of vena cava

453.3 Of renal vein

453.8 Of other specified veins

Excludes: *cerebral (434.0-434.9)*
coronary (410.00-410.92)
intracranial venous sinus (325)
nonpyogenic (437.6)
mesenteric (557.0)
portal (452)
precerebral (433.0-433.9)
pulmonary (415.1)

453.9 Of unspecified site
Embolism of vein
Thrombosis (vein)

454 Varicose veins of lower extremities

Excludes: *that complicating pregnancy, childbirth, or the puerperium (671.0)*

454.0 With ulcer
Varicose ulcer (lower extremity, any part)
Varicose veins with ulcer of lower extremity [any part] or of unspecified site
Any condition classifiable to 454.9 with ulcer or specified as ulcerated

454.1 With inflammation
Stasis dermatitis
Varicose veins with inflammation of lower extremity [any part] or of unspecified site
Any condition classifiable to 454.9 with inflammation or specified as inflamed

454.2 With ulcer and inflammation
Varicose veins with ulcer and inflammation of lower extremity [any part] or of unspecified site
Any condition classifiable to 454.9 with ulcer and inflammation

454.9 Without mention of ulcer or inflammation
Phlebectasia
Varicose veins } of lower extremity [any part] or of unspecified site
Varix }

455 Hemorrhoids
Includes: hemorrhoids (anus) (rectum)
piles
varicose veins, anus or rectum

Excludes: that complicating pregnancy, childbirth or the puerperium (671.8)

455.0 Internal hemorrhoids without mention of complication

455.1 Internal thrombosed hemorrhoids

455.2 Internal hemorrhoids with other complication
Internal hemorrhoids:
bleeding
prolapsed
strangulated
ulcerated

455.3 External hemorrhoids without mention of complication

455.4 External thrombosed hemorrhoids

455.5 External hemorrhoids with other complication
External hemorrhoids:
bleeding
prolapsed
strangulated
ulcerated

455.6 Unspecified hemorrhoids without mention of complication
Hemorrhoids NOS

455.7 Unspecified thrombosed hemorrhoids
Thrombosed hemorrhoids, unspecified whether internal or external

455.8 Unspecified hemorrhoids with other complication
Hemorrhoids, unspecified whether internal or external:
bleeding
prolapsed
strangulated
ulcerated

455.9 Residual hemorrhoidal skin tags
Skin tags, anus or rectum

456 Varicose veins of other sites

456.0 Esophageal varices with bleeding

456.1 Esophageal varices without mention of bleeding

456.2 Esophageal varices in diseases classified elsewhere
Code first underlying cause, as:
cirrhosis of liver (571.0-571.9)
portal hypertension (572.3)

456.20 With bleeding

456.21 Without mention of bleeding

456.3 Sublingual varices

456.4 Scrotal varices
Varicocele

456.5 Pelvic varices
Varices of broad ligament

456.6 Vulval varices
Varices of perineum

Excludes: that complicating pregnancy, childbirth, or the puerperium (671.1)

456.8 Varices of other sites
Varicose veins of nasal septum (with ulcer)

Excludes: placental varices (656.7)
retinal varices (362.17)
varicose ulcer of unspecified site (454.0)
varicose veins of unspecified site (454.9)

457 Noninfectious disorders of lymphatic channels

457.0 Postmastectomy lymphedema syndrome
Elephantiasis } due to mastectomy
Obliteration of lymphatic vessel } due to mastectomy

457.1 Other lymphedema
Elephantiasis (nonfilarial) NOS
Lymphangiectasis
Lymphedema:
acquired (chronic)
praecox
secondary
Obliteration, lymphatic vessel

Excludes: *elephantiasis (nonfilarial):*
congenital (757.0)
eyelid (374.83)
vulva (624.8)

457.2 Lymphangitis
Lymphangitis:
NOS
chronic
subacute

Excludes: *acute lymphangitis (682.0-682.9)*

457.8 Other noninfectious disorders of lymphatic channels
Chylocele (nonfilarial)
Chylous:
ascites
cyst
Lymph node or vessel:
fistula
infarction
rupture

Excludes: *chylocele:*
filarial (125.0-125.9)
tunica vaginalis (nonfilarial) (608.84)

457.9 Unspecified noninfectious disorder of lymphatic channels

458 Hypotension
Includes: hypopiesis

Excludes: *cardiovascular collapse (785.50)*
maternal hypotension syndrome (669.2)
shock (785.50-785.59)
Shy-Drager syndrome (333.0)

458.0 Orthostatic hypotension
Hypotension:
orthostatic (chronic)
postural

458.1 Chronic hypotension
Permanent idiopathic hypotension

● **458.2 Iatrogenic hypotension**
Postoperative hypotension

458.9 Hypotension, unspecified
Hypotension (arterial) NOS

459 Other disorders of circulatory system

459.0 Hemorrhage, unspecified
Rupture of blood vessel NOS
Spontaneous hemorrhage NEC

Excludes: *hemorrhage:*
gastrointestinal NOS (578.9)
in newborn NOS (772.9)
secondary or recurrent following trauma (958.2)
traumatic rupture of blood vessel (900.0-904.9)

459.1 Postphlebitic syndrome

459.2 Compression of vein
Stricture of vein
Vena cava syndrome (inferior) (superior)

459.8 Other specified disorders of circulatory system

459.81 Venous (peripheral) insufficiency, unspecified
Chronic venous insufficiency NOS

459.89 Other

Collateral circulation (venous), any site
Phlebosclerosis
Venofibrosis

459.9 Unspecified circulatory system disorder

8. DISEASES OF THE RESPIRATORY SYSTEM (460-519)

Use additional code, if desired, to identify infectious organism

ACUTE RESPIRATORY INFECTIONS (460-466)

Excludes: *pneumonia and influenza (480.0-487.8)*

460 Acute nasopharyngitis [common cold]

Coryza (acute)
Nasal catarrh, acute
Nasopharyngitis:
  NOS
  acute
  infective NOS
Rhinitis:
  acute
  infective

Excludes: *nasopharyngitis, chronic (472.2)*
pharyngitis:
  acute or unspecified (462)
  chronic (472.1)
rhinitis:
  allergic (477.0-477.9)
  chronic or unspecified (472.0)
sore throat:
  acute or unspecified (462)
  chronic (472.1)

461 Acute sinusitis

Includes: abscess, empyema, infection, inflammation, suppuration } acute, of sinus (accessory) (nasal)

Excludes: *chronic or unspecified sinusitis (473.0-473.9)*

461.0 Maxillary
Acute antritis

461.1 Frontal

461.2 Ethmoidal

461.3 Sphenoidal

461.8 Other acute sinusitis
Acute pansinusitis

461.9 Acute sinusitis, unspecified
Acute sinusitis NOS

462 Acute pharyngitis

Acute sore throat NOS
Pharyngitis (acute):
  NOS
  gangrenous
  infective
  phlegmonous
  pneumococcal
Pharyngitis (acute):
  staphylococcal
  suppurative
  ulcerative
Sore throat (viral) NOS
Viral pharyngitis

Excludes: *abscess:*
  peritonsillar [quinsy] (475)
  pharyngeal NOS (478.29)
  retropharyngeal (478.24)
chronic pharyngitis (472.1)
infectious mononucleosis (075)
that specified as (due to):
  Coxsackie (virus) (074.0)
  gonococcus (098.6)
  herpes simplex (054.79)
  influenza (487.1)
  septic (034.0)
  streptococcal (034.0)

463 Acute tonsillitis

Tonsillitis (acute):
- NOS
- follicular
- gangrenous
- infective
- pneumococcal

Tonsillitis (acute):
- septic
- staphylococcal
- suppurative
- ulcerative
- viral

Excludes: *chronic tonsillitis (474.0)*
hypertrophy of tonsils (474.1)
peritonsillar abscess [quinsy] (475)
sore throat:
acute or NOS (462)
septic (034.0)
streptococcal tonsillitis (034.0)

464 Acute laryngitis and tracheitis

Excludes: *that associated with influenza (487.1)*
that due to Streptococcus (034.0)

464.0 Acute laryngitis

Laryngitis (acute):
- NOS
- edematous
- Hemophilus influenza [H. influenzae]

Laryngitis (acute):
- pneumococcal
- septic
- suppurative
- ulcerative

Excludes: *chronic laryngitis (476.0-476.1)*
influenzal laryngitis (487.1)

464.1 Acute tracheitis

Tracheitis (acute):
- NOS
- catarrhal
- viral

Excludes: *chronic tracheitis (491.8)*

464.10 Without mention of obstruction

464.11 With obstruction

464.2 Acute laryngotracheitis

Laryngotracheitis (acute)
Tracheitis (acute) with laryngitis (acute)

Excludes: *chronic laryngotracheitis (476.1)*

464.20 Without mention of obstruction

464.21 With obstruction

464.3 Acute epiglottitis

Viral epiglottitis

Excludes: *epiglottitis, chronic (476.1)*

464.30 Without mention of obstruction

464.31 With obstruction

464.4 Croup

Croup syndrome

465 Acute upper respiratory infections of multiple or unspecified sites

Excludes: *upper respiratory infection due to:*
influenza (487.1)
Streptococcus (034.0)

465.0 Acute laryngopharyngitis

465.8 Other multiple sites

Multiple URI

465.9 Unspecified site

Acute URI NOS
Upper respiratory infection (acute)

466 Acute bronchitis and bronchiolitis
Includes: that with:
bronchospasm
obstruction

466.0 Acute bronchitis
Bronchitis, acute or subacute:
fibrinous
membranous
pneumococcal
purulent
septic
viral
with tracheitis
Croupous bronchitis
Tracheobronchitis, acute

466.1 Acute bronchiolitis
Bronchiolitis (acute)
Capillary pneumonia

OTHER DISEASES OF THE UPPER RESPIRATORY TRACT (470-478)

470 Deviated nasal septum
Deflected septum (nasal) (acquired)

Excludes: *congenital (754.0)*

471 Nasal polyps

Excludes: *adenomatous polyps (212.0)*

471.0 Polyp of nasal cavity
Polyp:
choanal
nasopharyngeal

471.1 Polypoid sinus degeneration
Woakes' syndrome or ethmoiditis

471.8 Other polyp of sinus
Polyp of sinus:
accessory
ethmoidal
Polyp of sinus:
maxillary
sphenoidal

471.9 Unspecified nasal polyp
Nasal polyp NOS

472 Chronic pharyngitis and nasopharyngitis

472.0 Chronic rhinitis
Ozena
Rhinitis:
NOS
atrophic
granulomatous
Rhinitis:
hypertrophic
obstructive
purulent
ulcerative

Excludes: *allergic rhinitis (477.0-477.9)*

472.1 Chronic pharyngitis
Chronic sore throat
Pharyngitis:
atrophic
granular (chronic)
hypertrophic

472.2 Chronic nasopharyngitis

Excludes: *acute or unspecified nasopharyngitis (460)*

473 Chronic sinusitis
Includes:
abscess, empyema, infection, suppuration } (chronic) of sinus (accessory) (nasal)

Excludes: *acute sinusitis (461.0-461.9)*

473.0 Maxillary
Antritis (chronic)

Add 4th or 5th digit | Nonspecific code | Unspecified code | Manifestation code

473.1 Frontal

473.2 Ethmoidal

Excludes: *Woakes' ethmoiditis (471.1)*

473.3 Sphenoidal

473.8 Other chronic sinusitis
Pansinusitis (chronic)

473.9 Unspecified sinusitis (chronic)
Sinusitis (chronic) NOS

474 Chronic disease of tonsils and adenoids

474.0 Chronic tonsillitis

Excludes: *acute or unspecified tonsillitis (463)*

474.1 Hypertrophy of tonsils and adenoids
Enlargement, Hyperplasia, Hypertrophy } of tonsils or adenoids

474.10 Tonsils with adenoids

474.11 Tonsils alone

474.12 Adenoids alone

474.2 Adenoid vegetations

474.8 Other chronic disease of tonsils and adenoids
Amygdalolith
Calculus, tonsil
Cicatrix of tonsil (and adenoid)
Tonsillar tag
Ulcer, tonsil

474.9 Unspecified chronic disease of tonsils and adenoids
Disease (chronic) of tonsils (and adenoids)

475 Peritonsillar abscess
Abscess of tonsil
Peritonsillar cellulitis
Quinsy

Excludes: *tonsillitis:*
acute or NOS (463)
chronic (474.0)

476 Chronic laryngitis and laryngotracheitis

476.0 Chronic laryngitis
Laryngitis:
catarrhal
hypertrophic
sicca

476.1 Chronic laryngotracheitis
Laryngitis, chronic, with tracheitis (chronic)
Tracheitis, chronic, with laryngitis

Excludes: *chronic tracheitis (491.8)*
laryngitis and tracheitis, acute or unspecified (464.0-464.4)

477 Allergic rhinitis
Includes: allergic rhinitis (nonseasonal) (seasonal)
hay fever
spasmodic rhinorrhea

Excludes: *allergic rhinitis with asthma (bronchial) (493.0)*

477.0 Due to pollen
Pollinosis

477.8 Due to other allergen

477.9 Cause unspecified

478 Other diseases of upper respiratory tract

478.0 Hypertrophy of nasal turbinates

478.1 Other diseases of nasal cavity and sinuses

Abscess, Necrosis, Ulcer } of nose (septum)

Cyst or mucocele of sinus (nasal)

Rhinolith

Excludes: *varicose ulcer of nasal septum (456.8)*

478.2 Other diseases of pharynx, not elsewhere classified

478.20 Unspecified disease of pharynx

478.21 Cellulitis of pharynx or nasopharynx

478.22 Parapharyngeal abscess

478.24 Retropharyngeal abscess

478.25 Edema of pharynx or nasopharynx

478.26 Cyst of pharynx or nasopharynx

478.29 Other

Abscess of pharynx or nasopharynx

Excludes: *ulcerative pharyngitis (462)*

478.3 Paralysis of vocal cords or larynx

478.30 Paralysis, unspecified

Laryngoplegia   Paralysis of glottis

478.31 Unilateral, partial

478.32 Unilateral, complete

478.33 Bilateral, partial

478.34 Bilateral, complete

478.4 Polyp of vocal cord or larynx

Excludes: *adenomatous polyps (212.1)*

478.5 Other diseases of vocal cords

Abscess, Cellulitis, Granuloma, Leukoplakia } of vocal cords

Chorditis (fibrinous) (nodosa) (tuberosa)

Singers' nodes

478.6 Edema of larynx

Edema (of):
- glottis
- subglottic
- supraglottic

478.7 Other diseases of larynx, not elsewhere classified

478.70 Unspecified disease of larynx

478.71 Cellulitis and perichondritis of larynx

478.74 Stenosis of larynx

478.75 Laryngeal spasm

Laryngismus (stridulus)

478.79 Other

Abscess, Necrosis, Obstruction, Pachyderma, Ulcer } of larynx

Excludes: *ulcerative laryngitis (464.0)*

478.8 Upper respiratory tract hypersensitivity reaction, site unspecified

Excludes: *hypersensitivity reaction of lower respiratory tract, as:*
extrinsic allergic alveolitis (495.0-495.9)
pneumoconiosis (500-505)

478.9 Other and unspecified diseases of upper respiratory tract
Abscess } of trachea
Cicatrix } of trachea

PNEUMONIA AND INFLUENZA (480-487)

Excludes: *pneumonia:*
allergic or eosinophilic (518.3)
aspiration:
NOS (507.0)
newborn (770.1)
solids and liquids (507.0-507.8)
congenital (770.0)
lipoid (507.1)
passive (514)
rheumatic (390)

480 Viral pneumonia

480.0 Pneumonia due to adenovirus

480.1 Pneumonia due to respiratory syncytial virus

480.2 Pneumonia due to parainfluenza virus

480.8 Pneumonia due to other virus not elsewhere classified

Excludes: *congenital rubella pneumonitis (771.0)*
influenza with pneumonia, any form (487.0)
pneumonia complicating viral diseases classified elsewhere (484.1-484.8)

480.9 Viral pneumonia, unspecified

481 Pneumococcal pneumonia [Streptococcus pneumoniae pneumonia]
Lobar pneumonia, organism unspecified

482 Other bacterial pneumonia

482.0 Pneumonia due to Klebsiella pneumoniae

482.1 Pneumonia due to Pseudomonas

482.2 Pneumonia due to Hemophilus influenzae [H. influenzae]

482.3 Pneumonia due to Streptococcus

Excludes: *Streptococcus pneumoniae pneumonia (481)*

482.30 Streptococcus, unspecified

482.31 Group A

482.32 Group B

482.39 Other Streptococcus

482.4 Pneumonia due to Staphylococcus

482.8 Pneumonia due to other specified bacteria

Excludes: *pneumonia complicating infectious disease classified elsewhere (484.1-484.8)*

482.81 Anaerobes
Bacteroides (melaninogenicus)
Gram-negative anaerobes

482.82 Escherichia coli [E. coli]

482.83 Other Gram-negative bacteria
Gram-negative pneumonia NOS
Proteus
Serratia marcescens

Excludes: *Gram-negative anaerobes (482.81)*

482.89 Other specified bacteria

482.9 Bacterial pneumonia unspecified

483 Pneumonia due to other specified organism

483.0 Mycoplasma pneumoniae
Eaton's agent
Pleuropneumonia-like organism [PPLO]

483.8 Other specified organism

484 Pneumonia in infectious diseases classified elsewhere

Excludes: *influenza with pneumonia, any form (487.0)*

***484.1* Pneumonia in cytomegalic inclusion disease**
Code first underlying disease (078.5)

***484.3* Pneumonia in whooping cough**
Code first underlying disease (033.0-033.9)

***484.5* Pneumonia in anthrax**
Code first underlying disease (022.1)

***484.6* Pneumonia in aspergillosis**
Code first underlying disease (117.3)

***484.7* Pneumonia in other systemic mycoses**
Code first underlying disease

Excludes: *pneumonia in:*
candidiasis (112.4)
coccidioidomycosis (114.0)
histoplasmosis (115.0-115.9 with fifth-digit 5)

***484.8* Pneumonia in other infectious diseases classified elsewhere**
Code first underlying disease, as:
Q fever (083.0)
typhoid fever (002.0)

Excludes: *pneumonia in:*
actinomycosis (039.1)
measles (055.1)
nocardiosis (039.1)
ornithosis (073.0)
Pneumocystis carinii (136.3)
salmonellosis (003.22)
toxoplasmosis (130.4)
tuberculosis (011.6)
tularemia (021.2)
varicella (052.1)

485 Bronchopneumonia, organism unspecified
Bronchopneumonia:
hemorrhagic
terminal
Pleurobronchopneumonia
Pneumonia:
lobular
segmental

Excludes: *bronchiolitis (acute) (466.1)*
chronic (491.8)
lipoid pneumonia (507.1)

486 Pneumonia, organism unspecified

Excludes: *hypostatic or passive pneumonia (514)*
influenza with pneumonia, any form (487.0)
inhalation or aspiration pneumonia due to foreign materials (507.0-507.8)
pneumonitis due to fumes and vapors (506.0)

487 Influenza

Excludes: *Hemophilus influenzae [H. influenzae]:*
infection NOS (041.5)
laryngitis (464.0)
meningitis (320.0)
pneumonia (482.2)

487.0 With pneumonia
Influenza with pneumonia, any form
Influenzal:
bronchopneumonia
pneumonia

487.1 With other respiratory manifestations
Influenza NOS
Influenzal:
laryngitis
pharyngitis
respiratory infection (upper) (acute)

487.8 With other manifestations
Encephalopathy due to influenza
Influenza with involvement of gastrointestinal tract

Excludes: *"intestinal flu" [viral gastroenteritis] (008.8)*

CHRONIC OBSTRUCTIVE PULMONARY DISEASE AND ALLIED CONDITIONS (490-496)

490 Bronchitis, not specified as acute or chronic
Bronchitis NOS:
catarrhal
with tracheitis NOS
Tracheobronchitis NOS

Excludes: *bronchitis:*
allergic NOS (493.9)
asthmatic NOS (493.9)
due to fumes and vapors (506.0)

491 Chronic bronchitis

Excludes: *chronic obstructive asthma (493.2)*

491.0 Simple chronic bronchitis
Catarrhal bronchitis, chronic
Smokers' cough

491.1 Mucopurulent chronic bronchitis
Bronchitis (chronic) (recurrent):
fetid
mucopurulent
purulent

491.2 Obstructive chronic bronchitis
Bronchitis:
asthmatic, chronic
emphysematous
obstructive (chronic) (diffuse)
Bronchitis with:
chronic airway obstruction
emphysema

Excludes: *asthmatic bronchitis (acute) NOS (493.9)*
chronic obstructive asthma (493.2)

491.20 Without mention of acute exacerbation
Chronic asthmatic bronchitis
Emphysema with chronic bronchitis

491.21 With acute exacerbation
Acute bronchitis with chronic obstructive pulmonary disease [COPD]
Acute and chronic obstructive bronchitis
Chronic asthmatic bronchitis with acute exacerbation
Emphysema with both acute and chronic bronchitis

491.8 Other chronic bronchitis
Chronic:
tracheitis
tracheobronchitis

491.9 Unspecified chronic bronchitis

492 Emphysema

492.0 Emphysematous bleb
Giant bullous emphysema
Ruptured emphysematous bleb
Tension pneumatocele
Vanishing lung

492.8 Other emphysema
Emphysema (lung or pulmonary):
NOS
centriacinar
centrilobular
obstructive
panacinar
Emphysema (lung or pulmonary):
panlobular
unilateral
vesicular
MacLeod's syndrome
Swyer-James syndrome
Unilateral hyperlucent lung

Excludes: *emphysema:*
compensatory (518.2)
due to fumes and vapors (506.4)
interstitial (518.1)
newborn (770.2)
mediastinal (518.1)
surgical (subcutaneous) (998.81)
traumatic (958.7)
with chronic bronchitis (491.20)
with both acute and chronic bronchitis (491.21)

● Code new to this edition ▲ Revision of existing code ④ ⑤ Fourth or fifth digit required

⑤ **493 Asthma**

The following fifth-digit subclassification is for use with category 493:

0 without mention of status asthmaticus

1 with status asthmaticus

493.0 extrinsic asthma

Asthma:
- allergic with stated cause
- atopic
- childhood
- hay
- platinum

Hay fever with asthma

Excludes: *asthma:*
- *allergic NOS (493.9)*
- *detergent (507.8)*
- *miners' (500)*
- *wood (495.8)*

493.1 Intrinsic asthma

Late-onset asthma

493.2 Chronic obstructive asthma

Asthma with chronic obstructive pulmonary disease [COPD]

Excludes: *chronic asthmatic bronchitis (491.2)*
chronic obstructive bronchitis (491.2)

493.9 Asthma, unspecified

Asthma (bronchial) (allergic NOS)

Bronchitis:
- allergic
- asthmatic

494 Bronchiectasis

Bronchiectasis (fusiform) (postinfectious) (recurrent)

Bronchiolectasis

Excludes: *congenital (748.61)*
tuberculous bronchiectasis (current disease) (011.5)

495 Extrinsic allergic alveolitis

Includes: allergic alveolitis and pneumonitis due to inhaled organic dust particles of fungal, thermophilic actinomycete, or other origin

495.0 Farmers' lung

495.1 Bagassosis

495.2 Bird-fanciers' lung

Budgerigar-fanciers' disease or lung

Pigeon-fanciers' disease or lung

495.3 Suberosis

Cork-handlers' disease or lung

495.4 Malt workers' lung

Alveolitis due to Aspergillus clavatus

495.5 Mushroom workers' lung

495.6 Maple bark-strippers' lung

Alveolitis due to Cryptostroma corticale

495.7 "Ventilation" pneumonitis

Allergic alveolitis due to fungal, thermophilic actinomycete, and other organisms growing in ventilation [air conditioning] systems

495.8 Other specified allergic alveolitis and pneumonitis
Cheese-washers' lung
Coffee workers' lung
Fish-meal workers' lung
Furriers' lung
Grain-handlers' disease or lung
Pituitary snuff-takers' disease
Sequoiosis or red-cedar asthma
Wood asthma

495.9 Unspecified allergic alveolitis and pneumonitis
Alveolitis, allergic (extrinsic)
Hypersensitivity pneumonitis

496 Chronic airway obstruction, not elsewhere classified
Note: This code is not to be used with any code from categories 491-493
Chronic:
nonspecific lung disease
obstructive lung disease
obstructive pulmonary disease [COPD] NOS

Excludes: *chronic obstructive lung disease [COPD] specified (as) (with):*
allergic alveolitis (495.0-495.9)
asthma (493.2)
bronchiectasis (494)
bronchitis (491.20-491.21)
with emphysema (491.20-491.21)
emphysema (492.0-492.8)

PNEUMOCONIOSES AND OTHER LUNG DISEASES DUE TO EXTERNAL AGENTS (500-508)

500 Coal workers' pneumoconiosis
Anthracosilicosis
Anthracosis
Black lung disease
Coal workers' lung
Miner's asthma

501 Asbestosis

502 Pneumoconiosis due to other silica or silicates
Pneumoconiosis due to talc
Silicotic fibrosis (massive) of lung
Silicosis (simple) (complicated)

503 Pneumoconiosis due to other inorganic dust
Aluminosis (of lung)
Bauxite fibrosis (of lung)
Berylliosis
Graphite fibrosis (of lung)
Siderosis
Stannosis

504 Pneumonopathy due to inhalation of other dust
Byssinosis
Cannabinosis
Flax-dressers' disease

Excludes: *allergic alveolitis (495.0-495.9)*
asbestosis (501)
bagassosis (495.1)
farmers' lung (495.0)

505 Pneumoconiosis, unspecified

506 Respiratory conditions due to chemical fumes and vapors
Use additional E code, if desired, to identify cause

506.0 Bronchitis and pneumonitis due to fumes and vapors
Chemical bronchitis (acute)

506.1 Acute pulmonary edema due to fumes and vapors
Chemical pulmonary edema (acute)

Excludes: *acute pulmonary edema NOS (518.4)*
chronic or unspecified pulmonary edema (514)

506.2 Upper respiratory inflammation due to fumes and vapors

506.3 Other acute and subacute respiratory conditions due to fumes and vapors

506.4 Chronic respiratory conditions due to fumes and vapors
Emphysema (diffuse) (chronic) } due to inhalation of chemical fumes and vapors
Obliterative bronchiolitis (chronic) (subacute) } due to inhalation of chemical fumes and vapors
Pulmonary fibrosis (chronic) } due to inhalation of chemical fumes and vapors

506.9 Unspecified respiratory conditions due to fumes and vapors
Silo-fillers' disease

507 Pneumonitis due to solids and liquids

Excludes: *fetal aspiration pneumonitis (770.1)*

507.0 Due to inhalation of food or vomitus

Aspiration pneumonia (due to):
- NOS
- food (regurgitated)
- gastric secretions
- milk
- saliva
- vomitus

507.1 Due to inhalation of oils and essences

Lipoid pneumonia (exogenous)

Excludes: *endogenous lipoid pneumonia (516.8)*

507.8 Due to other solids and liquids

Detergent asthma

508 Respiratory conditions due to other and unspecified external agents

Use additional E code, if desired, to identify cause

508.0 Acute pulmonary manifestations due to radiation

Radiation pneumonitis

508.1 Chronic and other pulmonary manifestations due to radiation

Fibrosis of lung following radiation

508.8 Respiratory conditions due to other specified external agents

508.9 Respiratory conditions due to unspecified external agent

OTHER DISEASES OF RESPIRATORY SYSTEM (510-519)

510 Empyema

Use additional code, if desired, to identify infectious organism (041.0-041.9)

Excludes: *abscess of lung (513.0)*

510.0 With fistula

Fistula:
- bronchocutaneous
- bronchopleural
- hepatopleural

Fistula:
- mediastinal
- pleural
- thoracic

Any condition classifiable to 510.9 with fistula

510.9 Without mention of fistula

Abscess:
- pleura
- thorax

Empyema (chest) (lung) (pleura)

Fibrinopurulent pleurisy

Pleurisy:
- purulent
- septic
- seropurulent
- suppurative

Pyopneumothorax

Pyothorax

511 Pleurisy

Excludes: *malignant pleural effusion (197.2)*
pleurisy with mention of tuberculosis, current disease (012.0)

511.0 Without mention of effusion or current tuberculosis

Adhesion, lung or pleura

Calcification of pleura

Pleurisy (acute) (sterile):
- diaphragmatic
- fibrinous
- interlobar

Pleurisy:
- NOS
- pneumococcal
- staphylococcal
- streptococcal

Thickening of pleura

511.1 With effusion, with mention of a bacterial cause other than tuberculosis

Pleurisy with effusion (exudative) (serous):
- pneumococcal
- staphylococcal
- streptococcal
- other specified nontuberculous bacterial cause

511.8 Other specified forms of effusion, except tuberculous
Encysted pleurisy
Hemopneumothorax
Hemothorax
Hydropneumothorax
Hydrothorax

Excludes: *traumatic (860.2-860.5)*

511.9 Unspecified pleural effusion
Pleural effusion NOS
Pleurisy:
  exudative
  serofibrinous
Pleurisy:
  serous
  with effusion NOS

512 Pneumothorax

512.0 Spontaneous tension pneumothorax

512.1 Iatrogenic pneumothorax
Postoperative pneumothorax

512.8 Other spontaneous pneumothorax
Pneumothorax:
  NOS
  acute
  chronic

Excludes: *pneumothorax:*
  congenital (770.2)
  traumatic (860.0-860.1, 860.4-860.5)
  tuberculous, current disease (011.7)

513 Abscess of lung and mediastinum

513.0 Abscess of lung
Abscess (multiple) of lung
Gangrenous or necrotic pneumonia
Pulmonary gangrene or necrosis

513.1 Abscess of mediastinum

514 Pulmonary congestion and hypostasis
Hypostatic:
  bronchopneumonia
  pneumonia
Passive pneumonia
Pulmonary congestion (chronic) (passive)
Pulmonary edema:
  NOS
  chronic

Excludes: *acute pulmonary edema:*
  NOS (518.4)
  with mention of heart disease or failure (428.1)

515 Postinflammatory pulmonary fibrosis
Cirrhosis of lung
Fibrosis of lung (atrophic)
  (confluent) (massive)
  (perialveolar) (peribronchial)
Induration of lung
} chronic or unspecified

516 Other alveolar and parietoalveolar pneumonopathy

516.0 Pulmonary alveolar proteinosis

516.1 Idiopathic pulmonary hemosiderosis
Essential brown induration of lung
Code first underlying disease (275.0)

516.2 Pulmonary alveolar microlithiasis

516.3 Idiopathic fibrosing alveolitis
Alveolar capillary block
Diffuse (idiopathic) (interstitial) pulmonary fibrosis
Hamman-Rich syndrome

516.8 Other specified alveolar and parietoalveolar pneumonopathies
Endogenous lipoid pneumonia
Interstitial pneumonia (desquamative) (lymphoid)

Excludes: *lipoid pneumonia, exogenous or unspecified (507.1)*

516.9 Unspecified alveolar and parietoalveolar pneumonopathy

517 Lung involvement in conditions classified elsewhere

Excludes: *rheumatoid lung (714.81)*

517.1 Rheumatic pneumonia
Code first underlying disease (390)

517.2 Lung involvement in systemic sclerosis
Code first underlying disease (710.1)

517.8 Lung involvement in other diseases classified elsewhere
Code first underlying disease, as:
amyloidosis (277.3)
polymyositis (710.4)
sarcoidosis (135)
Sjögren's disease (710.2)
systemic lupus erythematosus (710.0)

Excludes: *syphilis (095.1)*

518 Other diseases of lung

518.0 Pulmonary collapse
Atelectasis
Collapse of lung
Middle lobe syndrome

Excludes: *atelectasis:*
congenital (partial) (770.5)
primary (770.4)
tuberculous, current disease (011.8)

518.1 Interstitial emphysema
Mediastinal emphysema

Excludes: *surgical (subcutaneous) emphysema (998.81)*
that in fetus or newborn (770.2)
traumatic emphysema (958.7)

518.2 Compensatory emphysema

518.3 Pulmonary eosinophilia
Eosinophilic asthma
Löffler's syndrome
Pneumonia:
allergic
eosinophilic
Tropical eosinophilia

518.4 Acute edema of lung, unspecified
Acute pulmonary edema NOS
Pulmonary edema, postoperative

Excludes: *pulmonary edema:*
acute, with mention of heart disease or failure (428.1)
chronic or unspecified (514)
due to external agents (506.0-508.9)

518.5 Pulmonary insufficiency following trauma and surgery
Adult respiratory distress syndrome
Pulmonary insufficiency following:
shock
surgery
trauma
Shock lung

Excludes: *adult respiratory distress syndrome associated with other conditions (518.82)*
pneumonia:
aspiration (507.0)
hypostatic (514)
respiratory failure in other conditions (518.81)

518.8 Other diseases of lung

518.81 Respiratory failure
Respiratory failure:
NOS
acute
acute and chronic (acute-on-chronic)
chronic

Excludes: *acute respiratory distress (518.82)*
respiratory arrest (799.1)
respiratory failure, newborn (770.8)

518.82 Other pulmonary insufficiency, not elsewhere classified
Acute respiratory distress
Acute respiratory insufficiency
Adult respiratory distress syndrome NEC

Excludes: *adult respiratory distress syndrome associated with trauma and surgery (518.5)*
pulmonary insufficiency following trauma and surgery (518.5)
respiratory distress:
NOS (786.09)
newborn (770.8)
syndrome, newborn (769)
shock lung (518.5)

518.89 Other diseases of lung, not elsewhere classified
Broncholithiasis
Calcification of lung
Lung disease NOS
Pulmolithiasis

519 Other diseases of respiratory system

519.0 Tracheostomy complication
Hemorrhage from } tracheostomy stoma
Sepsis of } tracheostomy stoma

Tracheal stenosis } following tracheostomy
Tracheoesophageal fistula } following tracheostomy

Tracheostomy:
hemorrhage
obstruction
sepsis

519.1 Other diseases of trachea and bronchus, not elsewhere classified
Calcification } of bronchus or trachea
Stenosis } of bronchus or trachea
Ulcer } of bronchus or trachea

519.2 Mediastinitis

519.3 Other diseases of mediastinum, not elsewhere classified
Fibrosis } of mediastinum
Hernia } of mediastinum
Retraction } of mediastinum

519.4 Disorders of diaphragm
Diaphragmitis
Paralysis of diaphragm
Relaxation of diaphragm

Excludes: *congenital defect of diaphragm (756.6)*
diaphragmatic hernia (551-553 with .3)
congenital (756.6)

519.8 Other diseases of respiratory system, not elsewhere classified

519.9 Unspecified disease of respiratory system
Respiratory disease (chronic) NOS

9. DISEASES OF THE DIGESTIVE SYSTEM (520-579)

DISEASES OF ORAL CAVITY, SALIVARY GLANDS, AND JAWS (520-529)

520 Disorders of tooth development and eruption

520.0 Anodontia

Absence of teeth (complete) (congenital) (partial)
Hypodontia
Oligodontia

Excludes: *acquired absence of teeth (525.1)*

520.1 Supernumerary teeth

Distomolar
Fourth molar
Mesiodens
Paramolar
Supplemental teeth

Excludes: *supernumerary roots (520.2)*

520.2 Abnormalities of size and form

Concrescence, Fusion, Gemination } of teeth
Dens evaginatus
Dens in dente
Dens invaginatus
Enamel pearls
Macrodontia
Microdontia
Peg-shaped [conical] teeth
Supernumerary roots
Taurodontism
Tuberculum paramolare

Excludes: *that due to congenital syphilis (090.5)*
tuberculum Carabelli, which is regarded as a normal variation

520.3 Mottled teeth

Dental fluorosis
Mottling of enamel
Nonfluoride enamel opacities

520.4 Disturbances of tooth formation

Aplasia and hypoplasia of cementum
Dilaceration of tooth
Enamel hypoplasia (neonatal) (postnatal) (prenatal)
Horner's teeth
Hypocalcification of teeth
Regional odontodysplasia
Turner's tooth

Excludes: *Hutchinson's teeth and mulberry molars in congenital syphilis (090.5)*
mottled teeth (520.3)

520.5 Hereditary disturbances in tooth structure, not elsewhere classified

Amelogenesis, Dentinogenesis, Odontogenesis } imperfecta
Dentinal dysplasia
Shell teeth

520.6 Disturbances in tooth eruption

Teeth:
- embedded
- impacted
- natal
- neonatal
- primary [deciduous]:
  - persistent
  - shedding, premature

Tooth eruption:
- late
- obstructed
- premature

Excludes: *exfoliation of teeth (attributable to disease of surrounding tissues) (525.0-525.1)*
impacted or embedded teeth with abnormal position of such teeth or adjacent teeth (524.3)

520.7 Teething syndrome

520.8 Other specified disorders of tooth development and eruption

Color changes during tooth formation
Pre-eruptive color changes

Excludes: *posteruptive color changes (521.7)*

520.9 Unspecified disorder of tooth development and eruption

521 Diseases of hard tissues of teeth

521.0 Dental caries
Caries (of):
  arrested
  cementum
  dentin (acute) (chronic)
  enamel (acute) (chronic) (incipient)
Infantile melanodontia
Odontoclasia
White spot lesions of teeth

521.1 Excessive attrition
Approximal wear
Occlusal wear

521.2 Abrasion
Abrasion: dentifrice, habitual, occupational, ritual, traditional } of teeth
Wedge defect NOS } of teeth

521.3 Erosion
Erosion of teeth:
  NOS
  due to:
    medicine
    persistent vomiting
Erosion of teeth:
  idiopathic
  occupational

521.4 Pathological resorption
Internal granuloma of pulp
Resorption of tooth or root (external) (internal)

521.5 Hypercementosis
Cementation hyperplasia

521.6 Ankylosis of teeth

521.7 Posteruptive color changes
Staining [discoloration] of teeth:
  NOS
  due to:
    drugs
    metals
    pulpal bleeding

Excludes: *accretions [deposits] on teeth (523.6)*
pre-eruptive color changes (520.8)

521.8 Other specified diseases of hard tissues of teeth
Irradiated enamel
Sensitive dentin

521.9 Unspecified disease of hard tissues of teeth

522 Diseases of pulp and periapical tissues

522.0 Pulpitis
Pulpal:
  abscess
  polyp
Pulpitis:
  acute
  chronic (hyperplastic) (ulcerative)
  suppurative

522.1 Necrosis of the pulp
Pulp gangrene

522.2 Pulp degeneration
Denticles
Pulp calcifications
Pulp stones

522.3 Abnormal hard tissue formation in pulp
Secondary or irregular dentin

522.4 Acute apical periodontitis of pulpal origin

522.5 Periapical abscess without sinus
Abscess:
  dental
  dentoalveolar

Excludes: *periapical abscess with sinus (522.7)*

522.6 Chronic apical periodontitis
Apical or periapical granuloma
Apical periodontitis NOS

522.7 Periapical abscess with sinus
Fistula:
alveolar process
dental

522.8 Radicular cyst
Cyst:
apical (periodontal)
periapical
radiculodental
residual radicular

Excludes: *lateral developmental or lateral periodontal cyst (526.0)*

522.9 Other and unspecified diseases of pulp and periapical tissues

523 Gingival and periodontal diseases

523.0 Acute gingivitis

Excludes: *acute necrotizing ulcerative gingivitis (101)*
herpetic gingivostomatitis (054.2)

523.1 Chronic gingivitis
Gingivitis (chronic):
NOS
desquamative
hyperplastic
Gingivitis (chronic):
simple marginal
ulcerative
Gingivostomatitis

Excludes: *herpetic gingivostomatitis (054.2)*

523.2 Gingival recession
Gingival recession (generalized) (localized) (postinfective) (postoperative)

523.3 Acute periodontitis
Acute:
pericementitis
pericoronitis
Paradontal abscess
Periodontal abscess

Excludes: *acute apical periodontitis (522.4)*
periapical abscess (522.5, 522.7)

523.4 Chronic periodontitis
Alveolar pyorrhea
Chronic pericoronitis
Pericementitis (chronic)
Periodontitis:
NOS
complex
simplex

Excludes: *chronic apical periodontitis (522.6)*

523.5 Periodontosis

523.6 Accretions on teeth
Dental calculus:
subgingival
supragingival
Deposits on teeth:
betel
materia alba
soft
tartar
tobacco

523.8 Other specified periodontal diseases
Giant cell:
epulis
peripheral granuloma
Gingival:
cysts
enlargement NOS
fibromatosis
Gingival polyp
Periodontal lesions due to traumatic occlusion
Peripheral giant cell granuloma

Excludes: *leukoplakia of gingiva (528.6)*

523.9 Unspecified gingival and periodontal disease

524 Dentofacial anomalies, including malocclusion

524.0 Major anomalies of jaw size

Excludes: *hemifacial atrophy or hypertrophy (754.0)*
unilateral condylar hyperplasia or hypoplasia of mandible (526.89)

524.00 Unspecified anomaly

524.01 Maxillary hyperplasia

524.02 Mandibular hyperplasia

524.03 Maxillary hypoplasia

524.04 Mandibular hypoplasia

524.05 Macrogenia

524.06 Microgenia

524.09 Other specified anomaly

524.1 Anomalies of relationship of jaw to cranial base

524.10 Unspecified anomaly
prognathism
retrognathism

524.11 Maxillary asymmetry

524.12 Other jaw asymmetry

524.19 Other specified anomaly

524.2 Anomalies of dental arch relationship
Crossbite (anterior) (posterior)
Disto-occlusion
Mesio-occlusion
Midline deviation
Open bite (anterior) (posterior)
Overbite (excessive)
deep
horizontal
vertical
Overjet
Posterior lingual occlusion of mandibular teeth
Soft tissue impingement

Excludes: *hemifacial atrophy or hypertrophy (754.0)*
unilateral condylar hyperplasia or hypoplasia of mandible (526.89)

524.3 Anomalies of tooth position
Crowding, Diastema, Displacement, Rotation, Spacing, abnormal } of tooth, teeth
Transposition
Impacted or embedded teeth with abnormal position of such teeth or adjacent teeth

524.4 Malocclusion, unspecified

524.5 Dentofacial functional abnormalities
Abnormal jaw closure
Malocclusion due to:
abnormal swallowing
mouth breathing
tongue, lip, or finger habits

524.6 Temporomandibular joint disorders

Excludes: *current temporomandibular joint:*
dislocation (830.0-830.1)
strain (848.1)

524.60 Temporomandibular joint disorders, unspecified
Temporomandibular joint-pain-dysfunction syndrome [TMJ]

524.61 Adhesions and ankylosis (bony or fibrous)

524.62 Arthralgia of temporomandibular joint

524.63 Articular disc disorder (reducing or non-reducing)

524.69 Other specified temporomandibular joint disorders

524.7 Dental alveolar anomalies

524.70 Unspecified alveolar anomaly

524.71 Alveolar maxillary hyperplasia

524.72 Alveolar mandibular hyperplasia

524.73 Alveolar maxillary hypoplasia

524.74 Alveolar mandibular hypoplasia

524.79 Other specified alveolar anomaly

524.8 Other specified dentofacial anomalies

524.9 Unspecified dentofacial anomalies

525 Other diseases and conditions of the teeth and supporting structures

525.0 Exfoliation of teeth due to systemic causes

525.1 Loss of teeth due to accident, extraction, or local periodontal disease
Acquired absence of teeth

525.2 Atrophy of edentulous alveolar ridge

525.3 Retained dental root

525.8 Other specified disorders of the teeth and supporting structures
Enlargement of alveolar ridge NOS
Irregular alveolar process

525.9 Unspecified disorder of the teeth and supporting structures

526 Diseases of the jaws

526.0 Developmental odontogenic cysts
Cyst:
dentigerous
eruption
follicular
lateral developmental
Cyst:
lateral periodontal
primordial
Keratocyst

Excludes: radicular cyst (522.8)

526.1 Fissural cysts of jaw
Cyst:
globulomaxillary
incisor canal
median anterior maxillary
median palatal
nasopalatine
palatine of papilla

Excludes: cysts of oral soft tissues (528.4)

526.2 Other cysts of jaws
Cyst of jaw:
NOS
aneurysmal
Cyst of jaw:
hemorrhagic
traumatic

526.3 Central giant cell (reparative) granuloma

Excludes: peripheral giant cell granuloma (523.8)

526.4 Inflammatory conditions
Abscess } of jaw (acute) (chronic) (suppurative)
Osteitis } of jaw (acute) (chronic) (suppurative)
Osteomyelitis (neonatal) } of jaw (acute) (chronic) (suppurative)
Periostitis
Sequestrum of jaw bone

Excludes: alveolar osteitis (526.5)

526.5 Alveolitis of jaw
Alveolar osteitis
Dry socket

526.8 Other specified diseases of the jaws

526.81 Exostosis of jaw
Torus mandibularis
Torus palatinus

526.89 Other
Cherubism } of jaw(s)
Fibrous dysplasia } of jaw(s)
Latent bone cyst } of jaw(s)
Osteoradionecrosis of jaw(s)
Unilateral condylar hyperplasia or hypoplasia of mandible

526.9 Unspecified disease of the jaws

527 Diseases of the salivary glands

527.0 Atrophy

527.1 Hypertrophy

527.2 Sialoadenitis

Parotitis:
  NOS
  allergic
  toxic

Sialoangitis
Sialodochitis

Excludes: *epidemic or infectious parotitis (072.0-072.9)*
uveoparotid fever (135)

527.3 Abscess

527.4 Fistula

Excludes: *congenital fistula of salivary glands (750.24)*

527.5 Sialolithiasis

Calculus } of salivary gland or duct
Stone } of salivary gland or duct
Sialodocholithiasis

527.6 Mucocele

Mucous:
  extravasation cyst of salivary gland
  retention cyst of salivary gland
Ranula

527.7 Disturbance of salivary secretion

Hyposecretion
Ptyalism
Sialorrhea
Xerostomia

527.8 Other specified diseases of the salivary glands

Benign lymphoepithelial lesion of salivary gland
Sialectasia
Sialosis
Stenosis } of salivary duct
Stricture } of salivary duct

527.9 Unspecified disease of the salivary glands

528 Diseases of the oral soft tissues, excluding lesions specific for gingiva and tongue

528.0 Stomatitis

Stomatitis:
  NOS
  ulcerative
Vesicular stomatitis

Excludes: *stomatitis:*
  acute necrotizing ulcerative (101)
  aphthous (528.2)
  gangrenous (528.1)
  herpetic (054.2)
  Vincent's (101)

528.1 Cancrum oris

Gangrenous stomatitis
Noma

528.2 Oral aphthae

Aphthous stomatitis
Canker sore
Periadenitis mucosa necrotica recurrens
Recurrent aphthous ulcer
Stomatitis herpetiformis

Excludes: *herpetic stomatitis (054.2)*

528.3 Cellulitis and abscess

Cellulitis of mouth (floor)
Ludwig's angina
Oral fistula

Excludes: *abscess of tongue (529.0)*
cellulitis or abscess of lip (528.5)
fistula (of):
  dental (522.7)
  lip (528.5)
gingivitis (523.0-523.1)

528.4 Cysts

Dermoid cyst, Epidermoid cyst, Epstein's pearl, Lymphoepithelial cyst, Nasoalveolar cyst, Nasolabial cyst — of mouth

Excludes: *cyst:*
- *gingiva (523.8)*
- *tongue (529.8)*

528.5 Diseases of lips

Abscess, Cellulitis, Fistula, Hypertrophy — of lip(s)

Cheilitis:
- NOS
- angular

Cheilodynia
Cheilosis

Excludes: *actinic cheilitis (692.79)*
congenital fistula of lip (750.25)
leukoplakia of lips (528.6)

528.6 Leukoplakia of oral mucosa, including tongue

Leukokeratosis of oral mucosa
Leukoplakia of:
- gingiva
- lips
- tongue

Excludes: *carcinoma in situ (230.0, 232.0)*
leukokeratosis nicotina palati (528.7)

528.7 Other disturbances of oral epithelium, including tongue

Erythroplakia, Focal epithelial hyperplasia, Leukoedema, Leukokeratosis nicotina palati — of mouth or tongue

Excludes: *carcinoma in situ (230.0, 232.0)*
leukokeratosis NOS (702)

528.8 Oral submucosal fibrosis, including of tongue

528.9 Other and unspecified diseases of the oral soft tissues

Cheek and lip biting
Denture sore mouth
Denture stomatitis
Melanoplakia
Papillary hyperplasia of palate
Eosinophilic granuloma, Irritative hyperplasia, Pyogenic granuloma, Ulcer (traumatic) — of oral mucosa

529 Diseases and other conditions of the tongue

529.0 Glossitis

Abscess, Ulceration (traumatic) — of tongue

Excludes: *glossitis:*
- *benign migratory (529.1)*
- *Hunter's (529.4)*
- *median rhomboid (529.2)*
- *Moeller's (529.4)*

529.1 Geographic tongue

Benign migratory glossitis
Glossitis areata exfoliativa

529.2 Median rhomboid glossitis

529.3 Hypertrophy of tongue papillae
Black hairy tongue
Coated tongue
Hypertrophy of foliate papillae
Lingua villosa nigra

529.4 Atrophy of tongue papillae

Bald tongue	Glossodynia exfoliativa
Glazed tongue	Smooth atrophic tongue
Glossitis:	
Hunter's	
Moeller's	

529.5 Plicated tongue
Fissured
Furrowed } tongue
Scrotal

Excludes: *fissure of tongue, congenital (750.13)*

529.6 Glossodynia
Glossopyrosis   Painful tongue

Excludes: *glossodynia exfoliativa (529.4)*

529.8 Other specified conditions of the tongue
Atrophy
Crenated
Enlargement
Hypertrophy } (of) tongue
Glossocele
Glossoptosis

Excludes: *erythroplasia of tongue (528.7)*
leukoplakia of tongue (528.6)
macroglossia (congenital) (750.15)
microglossia (congenital) (750.16)
oral submucosal fibrosis (528.8)

529.9 Unspecified condition of the tongue

DISEASES OF ESOPHAGUS, STOMACH, AND DUODENUM (530-537)

530 Diseases of esophagus

Excludes: *esophageal varices (456.0-456.2)*

530.0 Achalasia and cardiospasm
Achalasia (of cardia)
Aperistalsis of esophagus
Megaesophagus

Excludes: *congenital cardiospasm (750.7)*

530.1 Esophagitis

Abscess of esophagus	Esophagitis:
Esophagitis:	postoperative
NOS	regurgitant
chemical	
peptic	

Use additional E code, if desired, to identify cause, if induced by chemical

Excludes: *tuberculous esophagitis (017.8)*

    530.10 Esophagitis, unspecified

    530.11 Reflux esophagitis

    530.19 Other esophagitis

530.2 Ulcer of esophagus

Ulcer of esophagus	Ulcer of esophagus due to ingestion of:
fungal	aspirin
peptic	chemicals
	medicines

Use additional E code, if desired, to identify cause, if induced by chemical or drug

● Code new	▲ Revision of	④ ⑤ Fourth or fifth
to this edition	existing code	digit required

530.3 Stricture and stenosis of esophagus
Compression of esophagus
Obstruction of esophagus

Excludes: *congenital stricture of esophagus (750.3)*

530.4 Perforation of esophagus
Rupture of esophagus

Excludes: *traumatic perforation of esophagus (862.22, 862.32, 874.4-874.5)*

530.5 Dyskinesia of esophagus
Corkscrew esophagus
Curling esophagus
Esophagospasm
Spasm of esophagus

Excludes: *cardiospasm (530.0)*

530.6 Diverticulum of esophagus, acquired
Diverticulum, acquired:
- epiphrenic
- pharyngoesophageal
- pulsion
- subdiaphragmatic
- traction
- Zenker's (hypopharyngeal)

Esophageal pouch, acquired
Esophagocele, acquired

Excludes: *congenital diverticulum of esophagus (750.4)*

530.7 Gastroesophageal laceration-hemorrhage syndrome
Mallory-Weiss syndrome

530.8 Other specified disorders of esophagus

530.81 Esophageal reflux
Gastroesophageal reflux

Excludes: *reflux esophagitis (530.11)*

530.82 Esophageal hemorrhage

Excludes: *hemorrhage due to esophageal varices (456.0-456.2)*

530.83 Esophageal leukoplakia

530.84 Tracheoesophageal fistula

Excludes: *congenital tracheoesophageal fistula (750.3)*

530.89 Other

Excludes: *Paterson-Kelly syndrome (280.8)*

530.9 Unspecified disorder of esophagus

⑤ **531 Gastric ulcer**
Includes: ulcer (peptic):
- prepyloric
- pylorus
- stomach

Use additional E code, if desired, to identify drug, if drug-induced

Excludes: *peptic ulcer NOS (533.0-533.9)*

The following fifth-digit subclassification is for use with category 531:

0 without mention of obstruction

1 with obstruction

531.0 Acute with hemorrhage

531.1 Acute with perforation

531.2 Acute with hemorrhage and perforation

531.3 Acute without mention of hemorrhage or perforation

531.4 Chronic or unspecified with hemorrhage

531.5 Chronic or unspecified with perforation

531.6 Chronic or unspecified with hemorrhage and perforation

531.7 Chronic without mention of hemorrhage or perforation

531.9 Unspecified as acute or chronic, without mention of hemorrhage or perforation

Add 4th or 5th digit | Nonspecific code | Unspecified code | Manifestation code

⑤ **532 Duodenal ulcer**

Includes: erosion (acute) of duodenum
ulcer (peptic):
duodenum
postpyloric

Use additional E code, if desired, to identify drug, if drug-induced

Excludes: *peptic ulcer NOS (533.0-533.9)*

The following fifth-digit subclassification is for use with category 532:

0 without mention of obstruction

1 with obstruction

532.0 Acute with hemorrhage

532.1 Acute with perforation

532.2 Acute with hemorrhage and perforation

532.3 Acute without mention of hemorrhage or perforation

532.4 Chronic or unspecified with hemorrhage

532.5 Chronic or unspecified with perforation

532.6 Chronic or unspecified with hemorrhage and perforation

532.7 Chronic without mention of hemorrhage or perforation

532.9 Unspecified as acute or chronic, without mention of hemorrhage or perforation

⑤ **533 Peptic ulcer, site unspecified**

Includes: gastroduodenal ulcer NOS
peptic ulcer NOS
stress ulcer NOS

Use additional E code, if desired, to identify drug, if drug-induced

Excludes: *peptic ulcer:*
duodenal (532.0-532.9)
gastric (531.0-531.9)

The following fifth-digit subclassification is for use with category 533:

0 without mention of obstruction

1 with obstruction

533.0 Acute with hemorrhage

533.1 Acute with perforation

533.2 Acute with hemorrhage and perforation

533.3 Acute without mention of hemorrhage and perforation

533.4 Chronic or unspecified with hemorrhage

533.5 Chronic or unspecified with perforation

533.6 Chronic or unspecified with hemorrhage and perforation

533.7 Chronic without mention of hemorrhage or perforation

533.9 Unspecified as acute or chronic, without mention of hemorrhage or perforation

⑤ **534 Gastrojejunal ulcer**

Includes: ulcer (peptic) or erosion:
anastomotic
gastrocolic
gastrointestinal
gastrojejunal
jejunal
marginal
stomal

Excludes: *primary ulcer of small intestine (569.82)*

The following fifth-digit subclassification is for use with category 534:

0 without mention of obstruction

1 with obstruction

534.0 Acute with hemorrhage

534.1 Acute with perforation

534.2 Acute with hemorrhage and perforation

534.3 Acute without mention of hemorrhage or perforation

534.4 Chronic or unspecified with hemorrhage

534.5 Chronic or unspecified with perforation

534.6 Chronic or unspecified with hemorrhage and perforation

534.7 Chronic without mention of hemorrhage or perforation

534.9 Unspecified as acute or chronic, without mention of hemorrhage or perforation

⑤ **535 Gastritis and duodenitis**

The following fifth-digit subclassification is for use with category 535

0 without mention of hemorrhage

1 with hemorrhage

535.0 Acute gastritis

535.1 Atrophic gastritis

Gastritis:
atrophic-hyperplastic
chronic (atrophic)

535.2 Gastric mucosal hypertrophy

Hypertrophic gastritis

535.3 Alcoholic gastritis

535.4 Other specified gastritis

Gastritis:
allergic
bile induced
irritant

Gastritis:
superficial
toxic

535.5 Unspecified gastritis and gastroduodenitis

535.6 Duodenitis

536 Disorders of function of stomach

Excludes: *functional disorders of stomach specified as psychogenic (306.4)*

536.0 Achlorhydria

536.1 Acute dilatation of stomach

Acute distention of stomach

536.2 Persistent vomiting

Habit vomiting
Persistent vomiting [not of pregnancy]
Uncontrollable vomiting

Excludes: *excessive vomiting in pregnancy (643.0-643.9)*
vomiting NOS (787.0)

536.3 Gastroparesis

536.8 Dyspepsia and other specified disorders of function of stomach

Achylia gastrica
Hourglass contraction of stomach
Hyperacidity
Hyperchlorhydria
Hypochlorhydria
Indigestion

Excludes: *achlorhydria (536.0)*
heartburn (787.1)

536.9 Unspecified functional disorder of stomach

Functional gastrointestinal:
disorder
disturbance
irritation

537 Other disorders of stomach and duodenum

537.0 Acquired hypertrophic pyloric stenosis

Constriction, Obstruction, Stricture } of pylorus, acquired or adult

Excludes: *congenital or infantile pyloric stenosis (750.5)*

537.1 Gastric diverticulum

Excludes: *congenital diverticulum of stomach (750.7)*

537.2 Chronic duodenal ileus

Add 4th or 5th digit | Nonspecific code | Unspecified code | Manifestation code

537.3 Other obstruction of duodenum
Cicatrix, Stenosis, Stricture, Volvulus } of duodenum

Excludes: *congenital obstruction of duodenum (751.1)*

537.4 Fistula of stomach or duodenum
Gastrocolic fistula
Gastrojejunocolic fistula

537.5 Gastroptosis

537.6 Hourglass stricture or stenosis of stomach
Cascade stomach

Excludes: *congenital hourglass stomach (750.7)*
hourglass contraction of stomach (536.8)

537.8 Other specified disorders of stomach and duodenum

537.81 Pylorospasm

Excludes: *congenital pylorospasm (750.5)*

537.82 Angiodysplasia of stomach and duodenum without mention of hemorrhage

537.83 Angiodysplasia of stomach and duodenum with hemorrhage

537.89 Other
Gastric or duodenal:
prolapse
rupture
Intestinal metaplasia of gastric mucosa
Passive congestion of stomach

Excludes: *diverticula of duodenum (562.00-562.01)*
gastrointestinal hemorrhage (578.0-578.9)

537.9 Unspecified disorder of stomach and duodenum

APPENDICITIS (540-543)

540 Acute appendicitis

540.0 With generalized peritonitis
Appendicitis (acute): fulminating, gangrenous, obstructive; Cecitis (acute); Rupture of appendix } with: perforation peritonitis (generalized) rupture

Excludes: *acute appendicitis with peritoneal abscess (540.1)*

540.1 With peritoneal abscess
Abscess of appendix
With generalized peritonitis

540.9 Without mention of peritonitis
Acute: appendicitis: fulminating, gangrenous, inflamed, obstructive; cecitis } without mention of perforation, peritonitis, or rupture

541 Appendicitis, unqualified

542 Other appendicitis
Appendicitis:
chronic
recurrent

Appendicitis:
relapsing
subacute

Excludes: *hyperplasia (lymphoid) of appendix (543.0)*

543 Other diseases of appendix

543.0 Hyperplasia of appendix (lymphoid)

543.9 Other and unspecified diseases of appendix
Appendicular or appendiceal:
colic
concretion
fistula
Diverticulum } of appendix
Fecalith } of appendix
Intussusception } of appendix
Mucocele } of appendix
Stercolith } of appendix

HERNIA OF ABDOMINAL CAVITY (550-553)

Includes: hernia:
acquired
congenital, except diaphragmatic or hiatal

⑤ **550 Inguinal hernia**
Includes: bubonocele
inguinal hernia (direct) (double) (indirect) (oblique) (sliding)
scrotal hernia

The following fifth-digit subclassification is for use with category 550:

0 unilateral or unspecified (not specified as recurrent)
Unilateral NOS

1 unilateral or unspecified, recurrent

2 bilateral (not specified as recurrent)
Bilateral NOS

3 bilateral, recurrent

550.0 Inguinal hernia, with gangrene
Inguinal hernia with gangrene (and obstruction)

550.1 Inguinal hernia, with obstruction, without mention of gangrene
Inguinal hernia with mention of incarceration, irreducibility, or strangulation

550.9 Inguinal hernia, without mention of obstruction or gangrene
Inguinal hernia NOS

551 Other hernia of abdominal cavity, with gangrene
Includes: that with gangrene (and obstruction)

551.0 Femoral hernia with gangrene

551.00 Unilateral or unspecified (not specified as recurrent)
Femoral hernia NOS with gangrene

551.01 Unilateral or unspecified, recurrent

551.02 Bilateral (not specified as recurrent)

551.03 Bilateral, recurrent

551.1 Umbilical hernia with gangrene
Parumbilical hernia specified as gangrenous

551.2 Ventral hernia with gangrene

551.20 Ventral, unspecified, with gangrene

551.21 Incisional, with gangrene
Hernia: } specified as gangrenous
postoperative } specified as gangrenous
recurrent, ventral } specified as gangrenous

551.29 Other
Epigastric hernia specified as gangrenous

551.3 Diaphragmatic hernia with gangrene
Hernia: } specified as gangrenous
hiatal (esophageal) (sliding) } specified as gangrenous
paraesophageal } specified as gangrenous
Thoracic stomach } specified as gangrenous

Excludes: *congenital diaphragmatic hernia (756.6)*

551.8 Hernia of other specified sites, with gangrene
Any condition classifiable to 553.8 if specified as gangrenous

551.9 Hernia of unspecified site, with gangrene
Any condition classifiable to 553.9 if specified as gangrenous

552 Other hernia of abdominal cavity, with obstruction, but without mention of gangrene

Excludes: *that with mention of gangrene (551.0-551.9)*

552.0 Femoral hernia with obstruction
Femoral hernia specified as incarcerated, irreducible, strangulated, or causing obstruction

552.00 Unilateral or unspecified (not specified as recurrent)

552.01 Unilateral or unspecified, recurrent

552.02 Bilateral (not specified as recurrent)

552.03 Bilateral, recurrent

552.1 Umbilical hernia with obstruction
Parumbilical hernia specified as incarcerated, irreducible, strangulated, or causing obstruction

552.2 Ventral hernia with obstruction
Ventral hernia specified as incarcerated, irreducible, strangulated, or causing obstruction

552.20 Ventral, unspecified, with obstruction

552.21 Incisional, with obstruction
Hernia:
postoperative } specified as incarcerated, irreducible, strangulated, or causing obstruction
recurrent, ventral }

552.29 Other
Epigastric hernia specified as incarcerated, irreducible, strangulated, or causing obstruction

552.3 Diaphragmatic hernia with obstruction
Hernia:
hiatal (esophageal) (sliding) } specified as incarcerated, irreducible, strangulated, or causing obstruction
paraesophageal }
Thoracic stomach }

Excludes: *congenital diaphragmatic hernia (756.6)*

552.8 Hernia of other specified sites, with obstruction
Any condition classifiable to 553.8 if specified as incarcerated, irreducible, strangulated, or causing obstruction

552.9 Hernia of unspecified site, with obstruction
Any condition classifiable to 553.9 if specified as incarcerated, irreducible, strangulated, or causing obstruction

553 Other hernia of abdominal cavity without mention of obstruction or gangrene

Excludes: *the listed conditions with mention of:*
gangrene (and obstruction) (551.0-551.9)
obstruction (552.0-552.9)

553.0 Femoral hernia

553.00 Unilateral or unspecified (not specified as recurrent)
Femoral hernia NOS

553.01 Unilateral or unspecified, recurrent

553.02 Bilateral (not specified as recurrent)

553.03 Bilateral, recurrent

553.1 Umbilical hernia
Parumbilical hernia

553.2 Ventral hernia

553.20 Ventral, unspecified

553.21 Incisional
Hernia:
postoperative
recurrent, ventral

553.29 Other
Hernia:
epigastric
spigelian

553.3 Diaphragmatic hernia
Hernia:
hiatal (esophageal) (sliding)
paraesophageal
Thoracic stomach

Excludes: *congenital:*
diaphragmatic hernia (756.6)
hiatal hernia (750.6)
esophagocele (530.6)

553.8 Hernia of other specified sites
Hernia:
ischiatic
ischiorectal
lumbar
obturator
pudendal
Hernia:
retroperitoneal
sciatic
Other abdominal hernia of specified site

Excludes: *vaginal enterocele (618.6)*

553.9 Hernia of unspecified site
Enterocele
Epiplocele
Hernia:
NOS
interstitial
Hernia:
intestinal
intra-abdominal
Rupture (nontraumatic)
Sarcoepiplocele

NONINFECTIOUS ENTERITIS AND COLITIS (555-558)

555 Regional enteritis
Includes: Crohn's disease
Granulomatous enteritis

Excludes: *ulcerative colitis (556)*

555.0 Small intestine
Ileitis:
regional
segmental
terminal
Regional enteritis or Crohn's disease of:
duodenum
ileum
jejunum

555.1 Large intestine
Colitis:
granulomatous
regional
transmural
Regional enteritis or Crohn's disease of:
colon
large bowel
rectum

555.2 Small intestine with large intestine
Regional ileocolitis

555.9 Unspecified site
Crohn's disease NOS
Regional enteritis NOS

556 Ulcerative colitis

556.0 Ulcerative (chronic) enterocolitis

556.1 Ulcerative (chronic) ileocolitis

556.2 Ulcerative (chronic) proctitis

556.3 Ulcerative (chronic) proctosigmoiditis

556.4 Pseudopolyposis of colon

556.5 Left-sided ulcerative (chronic) colitis

556.6 Universal ulcerative (chronic) colitis
Pancolitis

556.8 Other ulcerative colitis

556.9 Ulcerative colitis, unspecified
Ulcerative enteritis NOS

557 Vascular insufficiency of intestine

Excludes: *necrotizing enterocolitis of the newborn (777.5)*

557.0 Acute vascular insufficiency of intestine
Acute:
hemorrhagic enterocolitis
ischemic colitis, enteritis, or enterocolitis
massive necrosis of intestine
Bowel infarction
Embolism of mesenteric artery
Fulminant enterocolitis
Hemorrhagic necrosis of intestine
Intestinal gangrene
Intestinal infarction (acute) (agnogenic) (hemorrhagic) (nonocclusive)
Mesenteric infarction (embolic) (thrombotic)
Terminal hemorrhagic enteropathy
Thrombosis of mesenteric artery

557.1 Chronic vascular insufficiency of intestine
Angina, abdominal
Chronic ischemic colitis, enteritis, or enterocolitis
Ischemic stricture of intestine
Mesenteric:
angina
artery syndrome (superior)
vascular insufficiency

557.9 Unspecified vascular insufficiency of intestine
Alimentary pain due to vascular insufficiency
Ischemic colitis, enteritis, or enterocolitis NOS

558 Other noninfectious gastroenteritis and colitis

Excludes: *infectious:*
colitis, enteritis, or gastroenteritis (009.0-009.1)
diarrhea (009.2-009.3)

558.1 Gastroenteritis and colitis due to radiation
Radiation enterocolitis

558.2 Toxic gastroenteritis and colitis
Use additional E code, if desired, to identify cause

558.9 Other and unspecified noninfectious gastroenteritis and colitis
Colitis
Enteritis
Gastroenteritis
Ileitis
Jejunitis
Sigmoiditis
} NOS, allergic, dietetic, or noninfectious

OTHER DISEASES OF INTESTINES AND PERITONEUM (560-569)

560 Intestinal obstruction without mention of hernia

Excludes: *duodenum (537.2-537.3)*
inguinal hernia with obstruction (550.1)
intestinal obstruction complicating hernia (552.0-552.9)
mesenteric:
embolism (557.0)
infarction (557.0)
thrombosis (557.0)
neonatal intestinal obstruction (277.01, 777.1-777.2, 777.4)

560.0 Intussusception
Intussusception (colon) (intestine) (rectum)
Invagination of intestine or colon

Excludes: *intussusception of appendix (543.9)*

560.1 Paralytic ileus
Adynamic ileus
Ileus (of intestine) (of bowel) (of colon)
Paralysis of intestine or colon

Excludes: *gallstone ileus (560.31)*

● Code new to this edition ▲ Revision of existing code ④ ⑤ Fourth or fifth digit required

560.2 Volvulus
Knotting, Strangulation, Torsion, Twist — of intestine, bowel, or colon

560.3 Impaction of intestine

560.30 Impaction of intestine, unspecified
Impaction of colon

560.31 Gallstone ileus
Obstruction of intestine by gallstone

560.39 Other
Concretion of intestine
Enterolith
Fecal impaction

560.8 Other specified intestinal obstruction

▲ **560.81 Intestinal or peritoneal adhesions with obstruction (postoperative) (postinfection)**

Excludes: *adhesions without obstruction (568.0)*

560.89 Other
Mural thickening causing obstruction

Excludes: *ischemic stricture of intestine (557.1)*

560.9 Unspecified intestinal obstruction
Enterostenosis, Obstruction, Occlusion, Stenosis, Stricture — of intestine or colon

Excludes: *congenital stricture or stenosis of intestine (751.1-751.2)*

562 Diverticula of intestine
Use additional code, if desired, to identify any associated:
peritonitis (567.0-567.9)

Excludes: *congenital diverticulum of colon (751.5)*
diverticulum of appendix (543.9)
Meckel's diverticulum (751.0)

562.0 Small intestine

562.00 Diverticulosis of small intestine (without mention of hemorrhage)
Diverticulosis:
duodenum, ileum, jejunum — without mention of diverticulitis

562.01 Diverticulitis of small intestine (without mention of hemorrhage)
Diverticulitis (with diverticulosis):
duodenum
ileum
jejunum
small intestine

562.02 Diverticulosis of small intestine with hemorrhage

562.03 Diverticulitis of small intestine with hemorrhage

562.1 Colon

562.10 Diverticulosis of colon (without mention of hemorrhage)
Diverticulosis:
NOS, intestine (large) — without mention of diverticulitis
Diverticular disease (colon)

562.11 Diverticulitis of colon (without mention of hemorrhage)
Diverticulitis (with diverticulosis):
NOS
colon
intestine (large)

562.12 Diverticulosis of colon with hemorrhage

562.13 Diverticulitis of colon with hemorrhage

564 Functional digestive disorders, not elsewhere classified

Excludes: *functional disorders of stomach (536.0-536.9)*
those specified as psychogenic (306.4)

564.0 Constipation

564.1 Irritable colon

Colitis:
adaptive
membranous
mucous
Enterospasm
Irritable bowel syndrome
Spastic colon

564.2 Postgastric surgery syndromes

Dumping syndrome
Jejunal syndrome
Postgastrectomy syndrome
Postvagotomy syndrome

Excludes: *malnutrition following gastrointestinal surgery (579.3)*
postgastrojejunostomy ulcer (534.0-534.9)

564.3 Vomiting following gastrointestinal surgery

Vomiting (bilious) following gastrointestinal surgery

564.4 Other postoperative functional disorders

Diarrhea following gastrointestinal surgery

Excludes: *colostomy and enterostomy complications (569.60-569.69)*

564.5 Functional diarrhea

Excludes: *diarrhea:*
NOS (787.91)
psychogenic (306.4)

564.6 Anal spasm

Proctalgia fugax

564.7 Megacolon, other than Hirschsprung's

Dilatation of colon

Excludes: *megacolon:*
congenital [Hirschsprung's] (751.3)
toxic (556)

564.8 Other specified functional disorders of intestine

Atony of colon

Excludes: *malabsorption (579.0-579.9)*

564.9 Unspecified functional disorder of intestine

565 Anal fissure and fistula

565.0 Anal fissure

Tear of anus, nontraumatic

Excludes: *traumatic (863.89, 863.99)*

565.1 Anal fistula

Fistula:
anorectal
rectal
rectum to skin

Excludes: *fistula of rectum to internal organs—see Alphabetic Index*
ischiorectal fistula (566)
rectovaginal fistula (619.1)

566 Abscess of anal and rectal regions

Abscess:
ischiorectal
perianal
perirectal
Cellulitis:
anal
perirectal
rectal
Ischiorectal fistula

567 Peritonitis

Excludes: *peritonitis:*
benign paroxysmal (277.3)
pelvic, female (614.5, 614.7)
periodic familial (277.3)
puerperal (670)
with or following:
abortion (634-638 with .0, 639.0)
appendicitis (540.0-540.1)
ectopic or molar pregnancy (639.0)

567.0 ***Peritonitis in infectious diseases classified elsewhere***
Code first underlying disease

Excludes: *peritonitis:*
gonococcal (098.86)
syphilitic (095.2)
tuberculous (014.0)

567.1 Pneumococcal peritonitis

567.2 Other suppurative peritonitis
Abscess (of):
abdominopelvic
mesenteric
omentum
peritoneum
retrocecal
retroperitoneal
subdiaphragmatic
Abscess (of):
subhepatic
subphrenic
Peritonitis (acute):
general
pelvic, male
subphrenic
suppurative

567.8 Other specified peritonitis
Chronic proliferative peritonitis
Fat necrosis of peritoneum
Mesenteric saponification
Peritonitis due to:
bile
urine

567.9 Unspecified peritonitis
Peritonitis:
NOS
of unspecified cause

568 Other disorders of peritoneum

▲ **568.0 Peritoneal adhesions (postoperative) (postinfection)**
Adhesions (of):
abdominal (wall)
diaphragm
intestine
male pelvis
Adhesions (of):
mesenteric
omentum
stomach
Adhesive bands

Excludes: *adhesions:*
pelvic, female (614.6)
with obstruction:
duodenum (537.3)
intestine (560.81)

568.8 Other specified disorders of peritoneum

568.81 Hemoperitoneum (nontraumatic)

568.82 Peritoneal effusion (chronic)

Excludes: *ascites NOS (789.5)*

568.89 Other
Peritoneal:
cyst
granuloma

568.9 Unspecified disorder of peritoneum

569 Other disorders of intestine

569.0 Anal and rectal polyp

Add 4th or 5th digit | Nonspecific code | Unspecified code | Manifestation code

569.1 Rectal prolapse

Procidentia:
- anus (sphincter)
- rectum (sphincter)

Proctoptosis

Prolapse:
- anal canal
- rectal mucosa

Excludes: *prolapsed hemorrhoids (455.2, 455.5)*

569.2 Stenosis of rectum and anus

Stricture of anus (sphincter)

569.3 Hemorrhage of rectum and anus

Excludes: *gastrointestinal bleeding NOS (578.9)*
melena (578.1)

569.4 Other specified disorders of rectum and anus

569.41 Ulcer of anus and rectum

Solitary ulcer, Stercoral ulcer } of anus (sphincter) or rectum (sphincter)

569.42 Anal or rectal pain

569.49 Other

Granuloma, Rupture } of rectum (sphincter)

Hypertrophy of anal papillae
Proctitis NOS

Excludes: *fistula of rectum to:*
- *internal organs—see Alphabetic Index*
- *skin (565.1)*

hemorrhoids (455.0-455.9)
incontinence of sphincter ani (787.6)

569.5 Abscess of intestine

Excludes: *appendiceal abscess (540.1)*

▲ **569.6 Colostomy and enterostomy complications**

● **569.60 Unspecified complication**

● **569.61 Infection of colostomy or enterostomy**

Cellulitis or abscess

Use additional code to identify organism (041.00-041.9)

● **569.69 Other complication**

Malfunction

569.8 Other specified disorders of intestine

569.81 Fistula of intestine, excluding rectum and anus

Fistula:
- abdominal wall
- enterocolic

Fistula:
- enteroenteric
- ileorectal

Excludes: *fistula of intestine to internal organs —see Alphabetic Index*
persistent postoperative fistula (998.6)

569.82 Ulceration of intestine

Primary ulcer of intestine
Ulceration of colon

Excludes: *that with perforation (569.83)*

569.83 Perforation of intestine

569.84 Angiodysplasia of intestine (without mention of hemorrhage)

569.85 Angiodysplasia of intestine with hemorrhage

569.89 Other

Enteroptosis
Granuloma, Prolapse } of intestine
Pericolitis
Perisigmoiditis
Visceroptosis

Excludes: *gangrene of intestine, mesentery, or omentum (557.0)*
hemorrhage of intestine NOS (578.9)
obstruction of intestine (560.0-560.9)

● Code new to this edition ▲ Revision of existing code ④ ⑤ Fourth or fifth digit required

569.9 Unspecified disorder of intestine

OTHER DISEASES OF DIGESTIVE SYSTEM (570-579)

570 Acute and subacute necrosis of liver

Acute hepatic failure
Acute or subacute hepatitis, not specified as infective
Necrosis of liver (acute) (diffuse) (massive) (subacute)
Parenchymatous degeneration of liver
Yellow atrophy (liver) (acute) (subacute)

Excludes: *icterus gravis of newborn (773.0-773.2)*
serum hepatitis (070.2-070.3)
that with:
abortion (634-638 with .7, 639.8)
ectopic or molar pregnancy (639.8)
pregnancy, childbirth, or the puerperium (646.7)
viral hepatitis (070.0-070.9)

571 Chronic liver disease and cirrhosis

571.0 Alcoholic fatty liver

571.1 Acute alcoholic hepatitis
Acute alcoholic liver disease

571.2 Alcoholic cirrhosis of liver
Florid cirrhosis
Laennec's cirrhosis (alcoholic)

571.3 Alcoholic liver damage, unspecified

571.4 Chronic hepatitis

Excludes: *viral hepatitis (acute) (chronic) (070.0-070.9)*

571.40 Chronic hepatitis, unspecified

571.41 Chronic persistent hepatitis

571.49 Other
Chronic hepatitis:
active
aggressive
Recurrent hepatitis

571.5 Cirrhosis of liver without mention of alcohol
Cirrhosis of liver:
NOS
cryptogenic
macronodular
micronodular
Cirrhosis of liver:
posthepatitic
postnecrotic
Healed yellow atrophy (liver)
Portal cirrhosis

571.6 Biliary cirrhosis
Chronic nonsuppurative destructive cholangitis
Cirrhosis:
cholangitic
cholestatic

571.8 Other chronic nonalcoholic liver disease
Chronic yellow atrophy (liver)
Fatty liver, without mention of alcohol

571.9 Unspecified chronic liver disease without mention of alcohol

572 Liver abscess and sequelae of chronic liver disease

572.0 Abscess of liver

Excludes: *amebic liver abscess (006.3)*

572.1 Portal pyemia
Phlebitis of portal vein
Portal thrombophlebitis
Pylephlebitis
Pylethrombophlebitis

572.2 Hepatic coma
Hepatic encephalopathy
Hepatocerebral intoxication
Portal-systemic encephalopathy

572.3 Portal hypertension

572.4 Hepatorenal syndrome

Excludes: *that following delivery (674.8)*

572.8 Other sequelae of chronic liver disease

573 Other disorders of liver

Excludes: *amyloid or lardaceous degeneration of liver (277.3)*
congenital cystic disease of liver (751.62)
glycogen infiltration of liver (271.0)
hepatomegaly NOS (789.1)
portal vein obstruction (452)

573.0 Chronic passive congestion of liver

573.1 Hepatitis in viral diseases classified elsewhere
Code first underlying disease as:
Coxsackie virus disease (074.8)
cytomegalic inclusion virus disease (078.5)
infectious mononucleosis (075)

Excludes: *hepatitis (in):*
mumps (072.71)
viral (070.0-070.9)
yellow fever (060.0-060.9)

573.2 Hepatitis in other infectious diseases classified elsewhere
Code first underlying disease, as:
malaria (084.9)

Excludes: *hepatitis in:*
late syphilis (095.3)
secondary syphilis (091.62)
toxoplasmosis (130.5)

573.3 Hepatitis, unspecified
Toxic (noninfectious) hepatitis

Use additional E code, if desired, to identify cause

573.4 Hepatic infarction

573.8 Other specified disorders of liver
Hepatoptosis

573.9 Unspecified disorder of liver

⑤ **574 Cholelithiasis**

The following fifth-digit subclassification is for use with category 574:

0 without mention of obstruction

1 with obstruction

574.0 Calculus of gallbladder with acute cholecystitis
Biliary calculus, Calculus of cystic duct, Cholelithiasis } with acute cholecystitis
Any condition classifiable to 574.2 with acute cholecystitis

574.1 Calculus of gallbladder with other cholecystitis
Biliary calculus, Calculus of cystic duct, Cholelithiasis } with cholecystitis
Cholecystitis with cholelithiasis NOS
Any condition classifiable to 574.2 with cholecystitis (chronic)

574.2 Calculus of gallbladder without mention of cholecystitis
Biliary:
calculus NOS
colic NOS
Calculus of cystic duct
Cholelithiasis NOS
Colic (recurrent) of gallbladder
Gallstone (impacted)

574.3 Calculus of bile duct with acute cholecystitis
Calculus of bile duct [any], Choledocholithiasis } with acute cholecystitis
Any condition classifiable to 574.5 with acute cholecystitis

574.4 Calculus of bile duct with other cholecystitis
Calculus of bile duct [any], Choledocholithiasis } with cholecystitis (chronic)
Any condition classifiable to 574.5 with cholecystitis (chronic)

● Code new to this edition
▲ Revision of existing code
④ ⑤ Fourth or fifth digit required

574.5 Calculus of bile duct without mention of cholecystitis

Calculus of:
- bile duct [any]
- common duct
- hepatic duct

Choledocholithiasis

Hepatic:
- colic (recurrent)
- lithiasis

575 Other disorders of gallbladder

575.0 Acute cholecystitis

Abscess of gallbladder
Angiocholecystitis
Cholecystitis:
- emphysematous (acute)
- gangrenous
- suppurative

Empyema of gallbladder
Gangrene of gallbladder
} without mention of calculus

Excludes: *that with:*
- *choledocholithiasis (574.3)*
- *cholelithiasis (574.0)*

575.1 Other cholecystitis

Cholecystitis:
- NOS
- chronic

} without mention of calculus

Excludes: *that with:*
- *choledocholithiasis (574.4)*
- *cholelithiasis (574.1)*

575.2 Obstruction of gallbladder

Occlusion
Stenosis
Stricture
} of cystic duct or gallbladder without mention of calculus

Excludes: *that with calculus (574.0-574.2 with fifth-digit 1)*

575.3 Hydrops of gallbladder

Mucocele of gallbladder

575.4 Perforation of gallbladder

Rupture of cystic duct or gallbladder

575.5 Fistula of gallbladder

Fistula:
- cholecystoduodenal
- cholecystoenteric

575.6 Cholesterolosis of gallbladder

Strawberry gallbladder

575.8 Other specified disorders of gallbladder

Adhesions
Atrophy
Cyst
Hypertrophy
Nonfunctioning
Ulcer
Biliary dyskinesia
} (of) { cystic duct, gallbladder }

Excludes: *nonvisualization of gallbladder (793.3)*

575.9 Unspecified disorder of gallbladder

576 Other disorders of biliary tract

Excludes: *that involving the:*
- *cystic duct (575.0-575.9)*
- *gallbladder (575.0-575.9)*

576.0 Postcholecystectomy syndrome

576.1 Cholangitis

Cholangitis:
- NOS
- acute
- ascending
- chronic
- primary

Cholangitis:
- recurrent
- sclerosing
- secondary
- stenosing
- suppurative

576.2 Obstruction of bile duct

Occlusion, Stenosis, Stricture } of bile duct, except cystic duct, without mention of calculus

Excludes: *congenital (751.61)*
that with calculus (574.3-574.5 with fifth-digit 1)

576.3 Perforation of bile duct

Rupture of bile duct, except cystic duct

576.4 Fistula of bile duct

Choledochoduodenal fistula

576.5 Spasm of sphincter of Oddi

576.8 Other specified disorders of biliary tract

Adhesions, Atrophy, Cyst, Hypertrophy, Stasis, Ulcer } of bile duct [any]

Excludes: *congenital choledochal cyst (751.69)*

576.9 Unspecified disorder of biliary tract

577 Diseases of pancreas

577.0 Acute pancreatitis

Abscess of pancreas
Necrosis of pancreas:
  acute
  infective

Pancreatitis:
  NOS
  acute (recurrent)
  apoplectic
  hemorrhagic
  subacute
  suppurative

Excludes: *mumps pancreatitis (072.3)*

577.1 Chronic pancreatitis

Chronic pancreatitis:
  NOS
  infectious
  interstitial

Pancreatitis:
  painless
  recurrent
  relapsing

577.2 Cyst and pseudocyst of pancreas

577.8 Other specified diseases of pancreas

Atrophy, Calculus, Cirrhosis, Fibrosis } of pancreas

Pancreatic:
  infantilism
  necrosis:
    NOS
    aseptic
    fat
Pancreatolithiasis

Excludes: *fibrocystic disease of pancreas (277.00-277.01)*
islet cell tumor of pancreas (211.7)
pancreatic steatorrhea (579.4)

577.9 Unspecified disease of pancreas

578 Gastrointestinal hemorrhage

Excludes: *that with mention of :*
angiodysplasia of stomach and duodenum (537.83)
angiodysplasia of intestine (569.85)
diverticulitis, intestine:
large (562.13)
small (562.03)
diverticulosis, intestine:
large (562.12)
small (562.02)
gastritis and duodenitis (535.0-535.6)
ulcer:
duodenal (532.0-532.9)
gastric (531.0-531.9)
gastrojejunal (534.0-534.9)
peptic (533.0-533.9)

578.0 Hematemesis
Vomiting of blood

578.1 Blood in stool
Melena

Excludes: *occult blood (792.1)*

578.9 Hemorrhage of gastrointestinal tract, unspecified
Gastric hemorrhage
Intestinal hemorrhage

579 Intestinal malabsorption

579.0 Celiac disease
Celiac:
crisis
infantilism
rickets
Gee (-Herter) disease
Gluten enteropathy
Idiopathic steatorrhea
Nontropical sprue

579.1 Tropical sprue
Sprue:
NOS
tropical
Tropical steatorrhea

579.2 Blind loop syndrome
Postoperative blind loop syndrome

579.3 Other and unspecified postsurgical nonabsorption
Hypoglycemia } following gastrointestinal surgery
Malnutrition } following gastrointestinal surgery

579.4 Pancreatic steatorrhea

579.8 Other specified intestinal malabsorption
Enteropathy:
exudative
protein-losing
Steatorrhea (chronic)

579.9 Unspecified intestinal malabsorption
Malabsorption syndrome NOS

10. DISEASES OF THE GENITOURINARY SYSTEM (580-629)

NEPHRITIS, NEPHROTIC SYNDROME, AND NEPHROSIS (580-589)

Excludes: *hypertensive renal disease (403.00-403.91)*

580 Acute glomerulonephritis
Includes: acute nephritis

580.0 With lesion of proliferative glomerulonephritis
Acute (diffuse) proliferative glomerulonephritis
Acute poststreptococcal glomerulonephritis

580.4 With lesion of rapidly progressive glomerulonephritis
Acute nephritis with lesion of necrotizing glomerulitis

580.8 With other specified pathological lesion in kidney

580.81 Acute glomerulonephritis in diseases classified elsewhere
Code first underlying disease, as:
infectious hepatitis (070.0-070.9)
mumps (072.79)
subacute bacterial endocarditis (421.0)
typhoid fever (002.0)

580.89 Other
Glomerulonephritis, acute, with lesion of:
exudative nephritis
interstitial (diffuse) (focal) nephritis

580.9 Acute glomerulonephritis with unspecified pathological lesion in kidney
Glomerulonephritis:
NOS
hemorrhagic
Nephritis
Nephropathy
} specified as acute

581 Nephrotic syndrome

581.0 With lesion of proliferative glomerulonephritis

581.1 With lesion of membranous glomerulonephritis
Epimembranous nephritis
Idiopathic membranous glomerular disease
Nephrotic syndrome with lesion of:
focal glomerulosclerosis
sclerosing membranous glomerulonephritis
segmental hyalinosis

581.2 With lesion of membranoproliferative glomerulonephritis
Nephrotic syndrome with lesion (of):
endothelial
hypocomplementemic persistent
lobular
mesangiocapillary
mixed membranous and proliferative
} glomerulonephritis

581.3 With lesion of minimal change glomerulonephritis
Foot process disease
Lipoid nephrosis
Minimal change:
glomerular disease
glomerulitis
nephrotic syndrome

581.8 With other specified pathological lesion in kidney

581.81 Nephrotic syndrome in diseases classified elsewhere
Code first underlying disease, as:
amyloidosis (277.3)
diabetes mellitus (250.4)
malaria (084.9)
polyarteritis (446.0)
systemic lupus erythematosus (710.0)

Excludes: *nephrosis in epidemic hemorrhagic fever (078.6)*

581.89 Other
Glomerulonephritis with edema and lesion of:
exudative nephritis
interstitial (diffuse) (focal) nephritis

581.9 Nephrotic syndrome with unspecified pathological lesion in kidney
Glomerulonephritis with edema NOS
Nephritis:
nephrotic NOS
with edema NOS
Nephrosis NOS
Renal disease with edema NOS

582 Chronic glomerulonephritis
Includes: chronic nephritis

582.0 With lesion of proliferative glomerulonephritis
Chronic (diffuse) proliferative glomerulonephritis

582.1 With lesion of membranous glomerulonephritis
Chronic glomerulonephritis:
membranous
sclerosing
Focal glomerulosclerosis
Segmental hyalinosis

582.2 With lesion of membranoproliferative glomerulonephritis
Chronic glomerulonephritis:
endothelial
hypocomplementemic persistent
lobular
membranoproliferative
mesangiocapillary
mixed membranous and proliferative

582.4 With lesion of rapidly progressive glomerulonephritis
Chronic nephritis with lesion of necrotizing glomerulitis

582.8 With other specified pathological lesion in kidney

582.81 Chronic glomerulonephritis in diseases classified elsewhere
Code first underlying disease, as:
amyloidosis (277.3)
systemic lupus erythematosus (710.0)

582.89 Other
Chronic glomerulonephritis with lesion of:
exudative nephritis
interstitial (diffuse) (focal) nephritis

582.9 Chronic glomerulonephritis with unspecified pathological lesion in kidney
Glomerulonephritis:
NOS
hemorrhagic
Nephritis
Nephropathy
} specified as chronic

583 Nephritis and nephropathy, not specified as acute or chronic
Includes: "renal disease" so stated, not specified as acute or chronic but with stated pathology or cause

583.0 With lesion of proliferative glomerulonephritis
Proliferative:
glomerulonephritis (diffuse) NOS
nephritis NOS
nephropathy NOS

583.1 With lesion of membranous glomerulonephritis
Membranous:
glomerulonephritis NOS
nephritis NOS
Membranous nephropathy NOS

583.2 With lesion of membranoproliferative glomerulonephritis
Membranoproliferative:
glomerulonephritis NOS
nephritis NOS
nephropathy NOS
Nephritis NOS, with lesion of:
hypocomplementemic persistent
lobular
mesangiocapillary
mixed membranous and proliferative
} glomerulonephritis

● Code new to this edition
▲ Revision of existing code
④ ⑤ Fourth or fifth digit required

583.4 With lesion of rapidly progressive glomerulonephritis
Necrotizing or rapidly progressive:
glomerulitis NOS
glomerulonephritis NOS
nephritis NOS
nephropathy NOS
Nephritis, unspecified, with lesion of necrotizing glomerulitis

583.6 With lesion of renal cortical necrosis
Nephritis NOS } with (renal) cortical necrosis
Nephropathy NOS } with (renal) cortical necrosis
Renal cortical necrosis NOS

583.7 With lesion of renal medullary necrosis
Nephritis NOS } with (renal) medullary [papillary] necrosis
Nephropathy NOS } with (renal) medullary [papillary] necrosis

583.8 With other specified pathological lesion in kidney

583.81 Nephritis and nephropathy, not specified as acute or chronic, in diseases classified elsewhere
Code first underlying disease, as:
amyloidosis (277.3)
diabetes mellitus (250.4)
gonococcal infection (098.19)
Goodpasture's syndrome (446.21)
systemic lupus erythematosus (710.0)
tuberculosis (016.0)

Excludes: *gouty nephropathy (274.10)*
syphilitic nephritis (095.4)

583.89 Other
Glomerulitis, Glomerulonephritis, Nephritis, Nephropathy, Renal disease } with lesion of:
exudative nephritis
interstitial nephritis

583.9 With unspecified pathological lesion in kidney
Glomerulitis, Glomerulonephritis, Nephritis, Nephropathy } NOS

Excludes: *nephropathy complicating pregnancy, labor, or the puerperium (642.0-642.9, 646.2)*
renal disease NOS with no stated cause (593.9)

584 Acute renal failure

Excludes: *following labor and delivery (669.3)*
posttraumatic (958.5)
that complicating:
abortion (634-638 with .3, 639.3)
ectopic or molar pregnancy (639.3)

584.5 With lesion of tubular necrosis
Lower nephron nephrosis
Renal failure with (acute) tubular necrosis
Tubular necrosis:
NOS
acute

584.6 With lesion of renal cortical necrosis

584.7 With lesion of renal medullary [papillary] necrosis
Necrotizing renal papillitis

584.8 With other specified pathological lesion in kidney

584.9 Acute renal failure, unspecified

Add 4th or 5th digit | Nonspecific code | Unspecified code | Manifestation code

585 Chronic renal failure
Chronic uremia

Use additional code, if desired, to identify manifestation as:
uremic:
neuropathy (357.4)
pericarditis (420.0)

Excludes: *that with any condition classifiable to 401 (403.0-403.9 with fifth-digit 1)*

586 Renal failure, unspecified
Uremia NOS

Excludes: *following labor and delivery (669.3)*
posttraumatic renal failure (958.5)
that complicating:
abortion (634-638 with .3, 639.3)
ectopic or molar pregnancy (639.3)
uremia:
extrarenal (788.9)
prerenal (788.9)
with any condition classifiable to 401 (403.0-403.9 with fifth-digit 1)

587 Renal sclerosis, unspecified
Atrophy of kidney
Contracted kidney
Renal:
cirrhosis
fibrosis

Excludes: *nephrosclerosis (arteriolar) (arteriosclerotic) (403.00-403.92)*
with hypertension (403.00-403.92)

588 Disorders resulting from impaired renal function

588.0 Renal osteodystrophy
Azotemic osteodystrophy
Phosphate-losing tubular disorders
Renal:
dwarfism
infantilism
rickets

588.1 Nephrogenic diabetes insipidus

Excludes: *diabetes insipidus NOS (253.5)*

588.8 Other specified disorders resulting from impaired renal function
Hypokalemic nephropathy
Secondary hyperparathyroidism (of renal origin)

Excludes: *secondary hypertension (405.0-405.9)*

588.9 Unspecified disorder resulting from impaired renal function

589 Small kidney of unknown cause

589.0 Unilateral small kidney

589.1 Bilateral small kidneys

589.9 Small kidney, unspecified

OTHER DISEASES OF URINARY SYSTEM (590-599)

590 Infections of kidney

Use additional code, if desired, to identify organism, such as Escherichia coli [E. coli] (041.4)

590.0 Chronic pyelonephritis
Chronic pyelitis
Chronic pyonephrosis
Code first any associated vesicoureteral reflux (593.70-593.73)

590.00 Without lesion of renal medullary necrosis

590.01 With lesion of renal medullary necrosis

590.1 Acute pyelonephritis
Acute pyelitis
Acute pyonephrosis

590.10 Without lesion of renal medullary necrosis

590.11 With lesion of renal medullary necrosis

590.2 Renal and perinephric abscess
Abscess:
kidney
nephritic
perirenal
Carbuncle of kidney

590.3 Pyeloureteritis cystica
Infection of renal pelvis and ureter
Ureteritis cystica

590.8 Other pyelonephritis or pyonephrosis, not specified as acute or chronic

590.80 Pyelonephritis, unspecified
Pyelitis NOS
Pyelonephritis NOS

Excludes: *calculous pyelonephritis (592.9)*

590.81 Pyelitis or pyelonephritis in diseases classified elsewhere
Code first underlying disease, as:
tuberculosis (016.0)

590.9 Infection of kidney, unspecified

Excludes: *urinary tract infection NOS (599.0)*

591 Hydronephrosis
Hydrocalycosis
Hydronephrosis
Hydroureteronephrosis

Excludes: *congenital hydronephrosis (753.2)*
hydroureter (593.5)

592 Calculus of kidney and ureter

Excludes: *nephrocalcinosis (275.4)*

592.0 Calculus of kidney
Nephrolithiasis NOS
Renal calculus or stone
Staghorn calculus
Stone in kidney

Excludes: *uric acid nephrolithiasis (274.11)*

592.1 Calculus of ureter
Ureteric stone
Ureterolithiasis

592.9 Urinary calculus, unspecified
Calculous pyelonephritis

593 Other disorders of kidney and ureter

593.0 Nephroptosis
Floating kidney
Mobile kidney

593.1 Hypertrophy of kidney

593.2 Cyst of kidney, acquired
Cyst (multiple) (solitary) of kidney, not congenital
Peripelvic (lymphatic) cyst

Excludes: *calyceal or pyelogenic cyst of kidney (591)*
congenital cyst of kidney (753.1)
polycystic (disease of) kidney (753.1)

593.3 Stricture or kinking of ureter
Angulation } of ureter (postoperative)
Constriction } of ureter (postoperative)
Stricture of pelviureteric junction

593.4 Other ureteric obstruction
Idiopathic retroperitoneal fibrosis
Occlusion NOS of ureter

Excludes: *that due to calculus (592.1)*

593.5 Hydroureter

Excludes: *congenital hydroureter (753.2)*
hydroureteronephrosis (591)

593.6 Postural proteinuria
Benign postural proteinuria
Orthostatic proteinuria

Excludes: *proteinuria NOS (791.0)*

593.7 Vesicoureteral reflux

Use additional code to identify:
chronic pyelonephritis (590.00-590.01)
renal agenesis (753.0)
renal dysplasia (753.15)

593.70 Unspecified or without reflux nephropathy

593.71 With reflux nephropathy, unilateral

593.72 With reflux nephropathy, bilateral

593.73 With reflux nephropathy NOS

593.8 Other specified disorders of kidney and ureter

593.81 Vascular disorders of kidney

Renal (artery):
embolism
hemorrhage
thrombosis

Renal infarction

593.82 Ureteral fistula

Intestinoureteral fistula

Excludes: *fistula between ureter and female genital tract (619.0)*

593.89 Other

Adhesions, kidney or ureter
Periureteritis
Polyp of ureter
Pyelectasia
Ureterocele

Excludes: *tuberculosis of ureter (016.2)*
ureteritis cystica (590.3)

593.9 Unspecified disorder of kidney and ureter

Renal disease NOS
Salt-losing nephritis or syndrome

Excludes: *cystic kidney disease (753.1)*
nephropathy, so stated (583.0-583.9)
renal disease:
acute (580.0-580.9)
arising in pregnancy or the puerperium (642.1-642.2, 642.4-642.7, 646.2)
chronic (582.0-582.9)
not specified as acute or chronic, but with stated pathology or cause (583.0-583.9)

594 Calculus of lower urinary tract

594.0 Calculus in diverticulum of bladder

594.1 Other calculus in bladder

Urinary bladder stone

Excludes: *staghorn calculus (592.0)*

594.2 Calculus in urethra

594.8 Other lower urinary tract calculus

594.9 Calculus of lower urinary tract, unspecified

Excludes: *calculus of urinary tract NOS (592.9)*

595 Cystitis

Excludes: *prostatocystitis (601.3)*

Use additional code, if desired, to identify organism, such as Escherichia coli [E. coli] (041.4)

595.0 Acute cystitis

Excludes: *trigonitis (595.3)*

595.1 Chronic interstitial cystitis

Hunner's ulcer
Panmural fibrosis of bladder
Submucous cystitis

595.2 Other chronic cystitis

Chronic cystitis NOS
Subacute cystitis

Excludes: *trigonitis (595.3)*

595.3 Trigonitis
Follicular cystitis
Trigonitis (acute) (chronic)
Urethrotrigonitis

595.4 Cystitis in diseases classified elsewhere
Code first underlying disease, as:
actinomycosis (039.8)
amebiasis (006.8)
bilharziasis (120.0-120.9)
Echinococcus infestation (122.3, 122.6)

Excludes: *cystitis:*
diphtheritic (032.84)
gonococcal (098.11, 098.31)
monilial (112.2)
trichomonal (131.09)
tuberculous (016.1)

595.8 Other specified types of cystitis

595.81 Cystitis cystica

595.82 Irradiation cystitis
Use additional E code, if desired, to identify cause

595.89 Other
Abscess of bladder
Cystitis:
bullous
emphysematous
glandularis

595.9 Cystitis, unspecified

596 Other disorders of bladder
Use additional code, if desired, to identify urinary incontinence (625.6, 788.30-788.39)

596.0 Bladder neck obstruction
Contracture (acquired), Obstruction (acquired), Stenosis (acquired) } of bladder neck or vesicourethral orifice

Excludes: *congenital (753.6)*

596.1 Intestinovesical fistula
Fistula:
enterovesical
vesicocolic
Fistula:
vesicoenteric
vesicorectal

596.2 Vesical fistula, not elsewhere classified
Fistula:
bladder NOS
urethrovesical
Fistula:
vesicocutaneous
vesicoperineal

Excludes: *fistula between bladder and female genital tract (619.0)*

596.3 Diverticulum of bladder
Diverticulitis, Diverticulum (acquired) (false) } of bladder

Excludes: *that with calculus in diverticulum of bladder (594.0)*

596.4 Atony of bladder
High compliance bladder, Hypotonicity, Inertia } of bladder

Excludes: *neurogenic bladder (596.54)*

596.5 Other functional disorders of bladder

Excludes: *cauda equina syndrome with neurogenic bladder (344.61)*

596.51 Hypertonicity of bladder
Hyperactivity

596.52 Low bladder compliance

596.53 Paralysis of bladder

Add 4th or 5th digit | Nonspecific code | Unspecified code | Manifestation code

596.54 Neurogenic bladder NOS

596.55 Detrusor sphincter dyssynergia

596.59 Other functional disorder of bladder
Detrusor instability

596.6 Rupture of bladder, nontraumatic

596.7 Hemorrhage into bladder wall
Hyperemia of bladder

Excludes: *acute hemorrhagic cystitis (595.0)*

596.8 Other specified disorders of bladder
Bladder:
calcified
contracted
Bladder:
hemorrhage
hypertrophy

Excludes: *cystocele, female (618.0, 618.2-618.4)*
hernia or prolapse of bladder, female (618.0, 618.2-618.4)

596.9 Unspecified disorder of bladder

597 Urethritis, not sexually transmitted, and urethral syndrome

Excludes: *nonspecific urethritis, so stated (099.4)*

597.0 Urethral abscess
Abscess of:
bulbourethral gland
Cowper's gland
Littré's gland
Abscess:
periurethral
urethral (gland)
Periurethral cellulitis

Excludes: *urethral caruncle (599.3)*

597.8 Other urethritis

597.80 Urethritis, unspecified

597.81 Urethral syndrome NOS

597.89 Other
Adenitis, Skene's glands
Cowperitis
Meatitis, urethral
Ulcer, urethra (meatus)
Verumontanitis

Excludes: *trichomonal (131.02)*

598 Urethral stricture
Includes: pinhole meatus
stricture of urinary meatus

Excludes: *congenital stricture of urethra and urinary meatus (753.6)*

Use additional code, if desired, to identify urinary incontinence (625.6, 788.30-788.39)

598.0 Urethral stricture due to infection

598.00 Due to unspecified infection

598.01 Due to infective diseases classified elsewhere
Code first underlying disease, as:
gonococcal infection (098.2)
schistosomiasis (120.0-120.9)
syphilis (095.8)

598.1 Traumatic urethral stricture
Stricture of urethra:
late effect of injury
postobstetric

Excludes: *postoperative following surgery on genitourinary tract (598.2)*

598.2 Postoperative urethral stricture
Postcatheterization stricture of urethra

598.8 Other specified causes of urethral stricture

598.9 Urethral stricture, unspecified

599 Other disorders of urethra and urinary tract

599.0 Urinary tract infection, site not specified
Pyuria

Use additional code, if desired, to identify organism, such as Escherichia coli [E. coli] (041.4)

● Code new to this edition
▲ Revision of existing code
④ ⑤ Fourth or fifth digit required

599.1 Urethral fistula
Fistula:
urethroperineal
urethrorectal
Urinary fistula NOS

Excludes: *fistula:*
urethroscrotal (608.89)
urethrovaginal (619.0)
urethrovesicovaginal (619.0)

599.2 Urethral diverticulum

599.3 Urethral caruncle
Polyp of urethra

599.4 Urethral false passage

599.5 Prolapsed urethral mucosa
Prolapse of urethra
Urethrocele

Excludes: *urethrocele, female (618.0, 618.2-618.4)*

599.6 Urinary obstruction, unspecified
Obstructive uropathy NOS
Urinary (tract) obstruction NOS

Excludes: *obstructive nephropathy NOS (593.89)*

Use additional code, if desired, to identify urinary incontinence (625.6, 788.30-788.39)

599.7 Hematuria
Hematuria (benign) (essential)

Excludes: *hemoglobinuria (791.2)*

599.8 Other specified disorders of urethra and urinary tract

Excludes: *symptoms and other conditions classifiable to 788.0-788.9, 791.0-791.9*

Use additional code, if desired, to identify urinary incontinence (625.6, 788.30-788.39)

599.81 Urethral hypermobility

599.82 Intrinsic (urethral) sphincter deficiency [ISD]

599.83 Urethral instability

599.84 Other specified disorders of urethra
Rupture of urethra (nontraumatic)
Urethral:
cyst
granuloma

599.89 Other specified disorders of urinary tract

599.9 Unspecified disorder of urethra and urinary tract

DISEASES OF MALE GENITAL ORGANS (600-608)

600 Hyperplasia of prostate
Adenofibromatous hypertrophy of prostate
Adenoma (benign) of prostate
Enlargement (benign) of prostate
Fibroadenoma of prostate
Fibroma of prostate
Hypertrophy (benign) of prostate
Myoma of prostate
Median bar (prostate)
Prostatic obstruction NOS

Excludes: *benign neoplasms of prostate (222.2)*

Use additional code, if desired, to identify urinary incontinence (788.30-788.39)

601 Inflammatory diseases of prostate
Use additional code, if desired, to identify organism, such as Staphylococcus (041.1), or Streptococcus (041.0)

601.0 Acute prostatitis

601.1 Chronic prostatitis

601.2 Abscess of prostate

601.3 Prostatocystitis

600

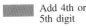

601.4 ***Prostatitis in diseases classified elsewhere***
Code first underlying disease, as:
actinomycosis (039.8)
blastomycosis (116.0)
syphilis (095.8)
tuberculosis (016.5)

Excludes: *prostatitis:*
gonococcal (098.12, 098.32)
monilial (112.2)
trichomonal (131.03)

601.8 **Other specified inflammatory diseases of prostate**
Prostatitis:
cavitary
diverticular
granulomatous

601.9 **Prostatitis, unspecified**
Prostatitis NOS

602 **Other disorders of prostate**

602.0 **Calculus of prostate**
Prostatic stone

602.1 **Congestion or hemorrhage of prostate**

602.2 **Atrophy of prostate**

602.8 **Other specified disorders of prostate**
Fistula, Infarction, Stricture } of prostate
Periprostatic adhesions

602.9 **Unspecified disorder of prostate**

603 **Hydrocele**
Includes: hydrocele of spermatic cord, testis, or tunica vaginalis
Excludes: *congenital (778.6)*

603.0 **Encysted hydrocele**

603.1 **Infected hydrocele**
Use additional code, if desired, to identify organism

603.8 **Other specified types of hydrocele**

603.9 **Hydrocele, unspecified**

604 **Orchitis and epididymitis**
Use additional code, if desired, to identify organism, such as Escherichia coli [E. coli] (041.4), Staphylococcus (041.1), or Streptococcus (041.0)

604.0 **Orchitis, epididymitis, and epididymo-orchitis, with abscess**
Abscess of epididymis or testis

604.9 **Other orchitis, epididymitis, and epididymo-orchitis, without mention of abscess**

604.90 **Orchitis and epididymitis, unspecified**

604.91 ***Orchitis and epididymitis in diseases classified elsewhere***
Code first underlying disease, as:
diphtheria (032.89)
filariasis (125.0-125.9)
syphilis (095.8)

Excludes: *orchitis:*
gonococcal (098.13, 098.33)
mumps (072.0)
tuberculous (016.5)
tuberculous epididymitis (016.4)

604.99 **Other**

605 **Redundant prepuce and phimosis**
Adherent prepuce
Paraphimosis
Phimosis (congenital)
Tight foreskin

● Code new to this edition
▲ Revision of existing code
④ ⑤ Fourth or fifth digit required

606 Infertility, male

606.0 Azoospermia
Absolute infertility
Infertility due to:
germinal (cell) aplasia
spermatogenic arrest (complete)

606.1 Oligospermia
Infertility due to:
germinal cell desquamation
hypospermatogenesis
incomplete spermatogenic arrest

606.8 Infertility due to extratesticular causes
Infertility due to:
drug therapy
infection
obstruction of efferent ducts
radiation
systemic disease

606.9 Male infertility, unspecified

607 Disorders of penis

Excludes: *phimosis (605)*

607.0 Leukoplakia of penis
Kraurosis of penis

Excludes: *carcinoma in situ of penis (233.5)*
erythroplasia of Queyrat (233.5)

607.1 Balanoposthitis
Balanitis

Use additional code, if desired, to identify organism

607.2 Other inflammatory disorders of penis
Abscess, Boil, Carbuncle, Cellulitis } of corpus cavernosum or penis
Cavernitis (penis)

Use additional code, if desired, to identify organism

Excludes: *herpetic infection (054.13)*

607.3 Priapism
Painful erection

607.8 Other specified disorders of penis

607.81 Balanitis xerotica obliterans
Induratio penis plastica

607.82 Vascular disorders of penis
Embolism, Hematoma (nontraumatic), Hemorrhage, Thrombosis } of corpus cavernosum or penis

607.83 Edema of penis

607.84 Impotence of organic origin

Excludes: *nonorganic or unspecified (302.72)*

607.89 Other
Atrophy, Fibrosis, Hypertrophy, Ulcer (chronic) } of corpus cavernosum or penis

607.9 Unspecified disorder of penis

608 Other disorders of male genital organs

608.0 Seminal vesiculitis

Abscess } of seminal vesicle
Cellulitis } of seminal vesicle
Vesiculitis (seminal)

Use additional code, if desired, to identify organism

Excludes: *gonococcal infection (098.14, 098.34)*

608.1 Spermatocele

608.2 Torsion of testis

Torsion of:
- epididymis
- spermatic cord
- testicle

608.3 Atrophy of testis

608.4 Other inflammatory disorders of male genital organs

Abscess, Boil, Carbuncle, Cellulitis } of scrotum, spermatic cord, testis [except abscess], tunica vaginalis, or vas deferens
Vasitis

Use additional code, if desired, to identify organism

Excludes: *abscess of testis (604.0)*

608.8 Other specified disorders of male genital organs

608.81 Disorders of male genital organs in diseases classified elsewhere

Code first underlying disease, as:
- filariasis (125.0-125.9)
- tuberculosis (016.5)

608.83 Vascular disorders

Hematoma (nontraumatic), Hemorrhage } of seminal vesicle, spermatic cord, testis, scrotum, tunica vaginalis, or vas deferens
Thrombosis
Hematocele NOS, male

608.84 Chylocele of tunica vaginalis

608.85 Stricture

Stricture of:
- spermatic cord
- tunica vaginalis
- vas deferens

608.86 Edema

608.89 Other

Atrophy, Fibrosis, Hypertrophy, Ulcer } of seminal vesicle, spermatic cord, testis, scrotum, tunica vaginalis, or vas deferens

Excludes: *atrophy of testis (608.3)*

608.9 Unspecified disorder of male genital organs

DISORDERS OF BREAST (610-611)

610 Benign mammary dysplasias

610.0 Solitary cyst of breast

Cyst (solitary) of breast

610.1 Diffuse cystic mastopathy

Chronic cystic mastitis
Cystic breast
Fibrocystic disease of breast

610.2 Fibroadenosis of breast

Fibroadenosis of breast:
- NOS
- chronic
- cystic

Fibroadenosis of breast:
- diffuse
- periodic
- segmental

610.3 Fibrosclerosis of breast

610.4 Mammary duct ectasia
Comedomastitis
Dust ectasia
Mastitis:
periductal
plasma cell

610.8 Other specified benign mammary dysplasias
Mazoplasia
Sebaceous cyst of breast

610.9 Benign mammary dysplasia, unspecified

611 Other disorders of breast

Excludes: *that associated with lactation or the puerperium (675.0-676.9)*

611.0 Inflammatory disease of breast
Abscess (acute) (chronic) (nonpuerperal) of:
areola
breast
Mammillary fistula
Mastitis (acute) (subacute) (nonpuerperal):
NOS
infective
retromammary
submammary

Excludes: *carbuncle of breast (680.2)*
chronic cystic mastitis (610.1)
neonatal infective mastitis (771.5)
thrombophlebitis of breast [Mondor's disease] (451.89)

611.1 Hypertrophy of breast
Gynecomastia
Hypertrophy of breast:
NOS
massive pubertal

611.2 Fissure of nipple

611.3 Fat necrosis of breast
Fat necrosis (segmental) of breast

611.4 Atrophy of breast

611.5 Galactocele

611.6 Galactorrhea not associated with childbirth

611.7 Signs and symptoms in breast

611.71 Mastodynia
Pain in breast

611.72 Lump or mass in breast

611.79 Other
Induration of breast
Inversion of nipple
Nipple discharge
Retraction of nipple

611.8 Other specified disorders of breast
Hematoma (nontraumatic) } of breast
Infarction } of breast
Occlusion of breast duct
Subinvolution of breast (postlactational) (postpartum)

611.9 Unspecified breast disorder

INFLAMMATORY DISEASE OF FEMALE PELVIC ORGANS (614-616)

Use additional code, if desired, to identify organism, such as Staphylococcus (041.1), or Streptococcus (041.0)

Excludes: *that associated with pregnancy, abortion, childbirth, or the puerperium (630-676.9)*

614 Inflammatory disease of ovary, fallopian tube, pelvic cellular tissue, and peritoneum

Excludes: *endometritis (615.0-615.9)*
major infection following delivery (670)
that complicating:
abortion (634-638 with .0, 639.0)
ectopic or molar pregnancy (639.0)
pregnancy or labor (646.6)

614.0 Acute salpingitis and oophoritis
Any condition classifiable to 614.2, specified as acute or subacute

Add 4th or 5th digit | Nonspecific code | Unspecified code | Manifestation code

614.1 Chronic salpingitis and oophoritis
Hydrosalpinx
Salpingitis:
follicularis
isthmica nodosa
Any condition classifiable to 614.2, specified as chronic

614.2 Salpingitis and oophoritis not specified as acute, subacute, or chronic
Abscess (of):
fallopian tube
ovary
tubo-ovarian
Oophoritis
Perioophoritis
Perisalpingitis
Pyosalpinx
Salpingitis
Salpingo-oophoritisRTubo-ovarian inflammatory disease

Excludes: *gonococcal infection (chronic) (098.37)*
acute (098.17)
tuberculous (016.6)

614.3 Acute parametritis and pelvic cellulitis
Acute inflammatory pelvic disease
Any condition classifiable to 614.4, specified as acute

614.4 Chronic or unspecified parametritis and pelvic cellulitis
Abscess (of):
broad ligament } chronic or NOS
parametrium } chronic or NOS
pelvis, female } chronic or NOS
pouch of Douglas } chronic or NOS
Chronic inflammatory pelvic disease
Pelvic cellulitis, female

Excludes: *tuberculous (016.7)*

614.5 Acute or unspecified pelvic peritonitis, female

▲ **614.6 Pelvic peritoneal adhesions, female (postoperative) (postinfection)**
Adhesions:
peritubal
tubo-ovarian

Use additional code, if desired, to identify any associated infertility (628.2)

614.7 Other chronic pelvic peritonitis, female

Excludes: *tuberculous (016.7)*

614.8 Other specified inflammatory disease of female pelvic organs and tissues

614.9 Unspecified inflammatory disease of female pelvic organs and tissues
Pelvic infection or inflammation, female NOS
Pelvic inflammatory disease [PID]

615 Inflammatory diseases of uterus, except cervix

Excludes: *following delivery (670)*
hyperplastic endometritis (621.3)
that complicating:
abortion (634-638 with .0, 639.0)
ectopic or molar pregnancy (639.0)
pregnancy or labor (646.6)

615.0 Acute
Any condition classifiable to 615.9, specified as acute or subacute

615.1 Chronic
Any condition classifiable to 615.9, specified as chronic

615.9 Unspecified inflammatory disease of uterus
Endometritis
Endomyometritis
Metritis
Myometritis
Perimetritis
Pyometra
Uterine abscess

616 Inflammatory disease of cervix, vagina, and vulva

Excludes: *that complicating:*
abortion (634-638 with .0, 639.0)
ectopic or molar pregnancy (639.0)
pregnancy, childbirth, or the puerperium (646.6)

616.0 Cervicitis and endocervicitis
Cervicitis } with or without mention of erosion or ectropion
Endocervicitis } with or without mention of erosion or ectropion
Nabothian (gland) cyst or follicle

Excludes: *erosion or ectropion without mention of cervicitis (622.0)*

616.1 Vaginitis and vulvovaginitis

616.10 Vaginitis and vulvovaginitis, unspecified
Vaginitis:
NOS
postirradiation
Vulvitis NOS
Vulvovaginitis NOS

Use additional code, if desired, to identify organism, such as Escherichia coli [E. coli] (041.4), Staphylococcus (041.1), or Streptococcus (041.0)

Excludes: *noninfective leukorrhea (623.5)*
postmenopausal or senile vaginitis (627.3)

616.11 Vaginitis and vulvovaginitis in diseases classified elsewhere
Code first underlying disease, as:
pinworm vaginitis (127.4)

Excludes: *herpetic vulvovaginitis (054.11)*
monilial vulvovaginitis (112.1)
trichomonal vaginitis or vulvovaginitis (131.01)

616.2 Cyst of Bartholin's gland
Bartholin's duct cyst

616.3 Abscess of Bartholin's gland
Vulvovaginal gland abscess

616.4 Other abscess of vulva
Abscess } of vulva
Carbuncle } of vulva
Furuncle } of vulva

616.5 Ulceration of vulva

616.50 Ulceration of vulva, unspecified
Ulcer NOS of vulva

616.51 Ulceration of vulva in diseases classified elsewhere
Code first underlying disease, as:
Behçet's syndrome (136.1)
tuberculosis (016.7)

Excludes: *vulvar ulcer (in):*
gonococcal (098.0)
herpes simplex (054.12)
syphilitic (091.0)

616.8 Other specified inflammatory diseases of cervix, vagina, and vulva
Caruncle, vagina or labium
Ulcer, vagina

Excludes: *noninflammatory disorders of:*
cervix (622.0-622.9)
vagina (623.0-623.9)
vulva (624.0-624.9)

616.9 Unspecified inflammatory disease of cervix, vagina, and vulva

OTHER DISORDERS OF FEMALE GENITAL TRACT (617-629)

617 Endometriosis

617.0 Endometriosis of uterus
Adenomyosis
Endometriosis:
cervix
internal
myometrium

Excludes: *stromal endometriosis (236.0)*

617.1 Endometriosis of ovary
Chocolate cyst of ovary
Endometrial cystoma of ovary

617.2 Endometriosis of fallopian tube

617.3 Endometriosis of pelvic peritoneum
Endometriosis:
broad ligament
cul-de-sac (Douglas')
parametrium
round ligament

617.4 Endometriosis of rectovaginal septum and vagina

617.5 Endometriosis of intestine
Endometriosis:
appendix
colon
rectum

617.6 Endometriosis in scar of skin

617.8 Endometriosis of other specified sites
Endometriosis:
bladder
lung
umbilicus
vulva

617.9 Endometriosis, site unspecified

618 Genital prolapse

Use additional code, if desired, to identify urinary incontinence (625.6, 788.31, 788.33-788.39)

Excludes: *that complicating pregnancy, labor, or delivery (654.4)*

618.0 Prolapse of vaginal walls without mention of uterine prolapse
Cystocele
Cystourethrocele
Proctocele, female
Rectocele
Urethrocele, female
Vaginal prolapse
} without mention of uterine prolapse

Excludes: *that with uterine prolapse (618.2-618.4)*
enterocele (618.6)
vaginal vault prolapse following hysterectomy (618.5)

618.1 Uterine prolapse without mention of vaginal wall prolapse
Descensus uteri
Uterine prolapse:
NOS
complete
first degree
second degree
third degree

Excludes: *that with mention of cystocele, urethrocele, or rectocele (618.2-618.4)*

618.2 Uterovaginal prolapse, incomplete

618.3 Uterovaginal prolapse, complete

618.4 Uterovaginal prolapse, unspecified

618.5 Prolapse of vaginal vault after hysterectomy

618.6 Vaginal enterocele, congenital or acquired
Pelvic enterocele, congenital or acquired

618.7 Old laceration of muscles of pelvic floor

618.8 Other specified genital prolapse
Incompetence or weakening of pelvic fundus
Relaxation of vaginal outlet or pelvis

618.9 Unspecified genital prolapse

619 Fistula involving female genital tract

Excludes: *vesicorectal and intestinovesical fistula (596.1)*

619.0 Urinary-genital tract fistula, female
Fistula:
cervicovesical
ureterovaginal
urethrovaginal
urethrovesicovaginal
uteroureteric
uterovesical
vesicocervicovaginal
vesicovaginal

619.1 Digestive-genital tract fistula, female
Fistula:
intestinouterine
intestinovaginal
rectovaginal
rectovulval
sigmoidovaginal
uterorectal

619.2 Genital tract-skin fistula, female
Fistula:
uterus to abdominal wall
vaginoperineal

619.8 Other specified fistulas involving female genital tract
Fistula:
cervix
cul-de-sac (Douglas')
Fistula:
uterus
vagina

619.9 Unspecified fistula involving female genital tract

620 Noninflammatory disorders of ovary, fallopian tube, and broad ligament

Excludes: *hydrosalpinx (614.1)*

620.0 Follicular cyst of ovary
Cyst of graafian follicle

620.1 Corpus luteum cyst or hematoma
Corpus luteum hemorrhage or rupture
Lutein cyst

620.2 Other and unspecified ovarian cyst
Cyst:
NOS
corpus albicans
retention NOS
serous
theca-lutein
} of ovary
Simple cystoma of ovary

Excludes: *cystadenoma (benign) (serous) (220)*
developmental cysts (752.0)
neoplastic cysts (220)
polycystic ovaries (256.4)
Stein-Leventhal syndrome (256.4)

620.3 Acquired atrophy of ovary and fallopian tube
Senile involution of ovary

620.4 Prolapse or hernia of ovary and fallopian tube
Displacement of ovary and fallopian tube
Salpingocele

620.5 Torsion of ovary, ovarian pedicle, or fallopian tube
Torsion:
accessory tube
hydatid of Morgagni

620.6 Broad ligament laceration syndrome
Masters-Allen syndrome

620.7 Hematoma of broad ligament
Hematocele, broad ligament

620.8 Other noninflammatory disorders of ovary, fallopian tube, and broad ligament
Cyst
Polyp
} of broad ligament or fallopian tube
Infarction
Rupture
} of ovary or fallopian tube
Hematosalpinx

Excludes: *hematosalpinx in ectopic pregnancy (639.2)*
peritubal adhesions (614.6)
torsion of ovary, ovarian pedicle, or fallopian tube (620.5)

620.9 Unspecified noninflammatory disorder of ovary, fallopian tube, and broad ligament

621 Disorders of uterus, not elsewhere classified

621.0 Polyp of corpus uteri
Polyp:
endometrium
uterus NOS

Excludes: *cervical polyp NOS (622.7)*

621.1 Chronic subinvolution of uterus

Excludes: *puerperal (674.8)*

Add 4th or 5th digit | Nonspecific code | Unspecified code | Manifestation code

621.2 Hypertrophy of uterus
Bulky or enlarged uterus

Excludes: *puerperal (674.8)*

621.3 Endometrial cystic hyperplasia
Hyperplasia (adenomatous) (cystic) (glandular) of endometrium
Hyperplastic endometritis

621.4 Hematometra
Hemometra

Excludes: *that in congenital anomaly (752.2-752.3)*

621.5 Intrauterine synechiae
Adhesions of uterus
Band(s) of uterus

621.6 Malposition of uterus
Anteversion } of uterus
Retroflexion } of uterus
Retroversion } of uterus

Excludes: *malposition complicating pregnancy, labor, or delivery (654.3-654.4)*
prolapse of uterus (618.1-618.4)

621.7 Chronic inversion of uterus

Excludes: *current obstetrical trauma (665.2)*
prolapse of uterus (618.1-618.4)

621.8 Other specified disorders of uterus, not elsewhere classified
Atrophy, acquired } of uterus
Cyst } of uterus
Fibrosis NOS } of uterus
Old laceration (postpartum) } of uterus
Ulcer } of uterus

Excludes: *bilharzial fibrosis (120.0-120.9)*
endometriosis (617.0)
fistulas (619.0-619.8)
inflammatory diseases (615.0-615.9)

621.9 Unspecified disorder of uterus

622 Noninflammatory disorders of cervix

Excludes: *abnormality of cervix complicating pregnancy, labor, or delivery (654.5-654.6)*
fistula (619.0-619.8)

622.0 Erosion and ectropion of cervix
Eversion } of cervix
Ulcer } of cervix

Excludes: *that in chronic cervicitis (616.0)*

622.1 Dysplasia of cervix (uteri)
Anaplasia of cervix
Cervical atypism

Excludes: *carcinoma in situ of cervix (233.1)*
cervical intraepithelial neoplasia III [CIN III] (233.1)

622.2 Leukoplakia of cervix (uteri)

Excludes: *carcinoma in situ of cervix (233.1)*

622.3 Old laceration of cervix
Adhesions } of cervix
Band(s) } of cervix
Cicatrix (postpartum) } of cervix

Excludes: *current obstetrical trauma (665.3)*

622.4 Stricture and stenosis of cervix
Atresia (acquired) } of cervix
Contracture } of cervix
Occlusion } of cervix
Pinpoint os uteri } of cervix

Excludes: *congenital (752.49)*
that complicating labor (654.6)

622.5 Incompetence of cervix

Excludes: *complicating pregnancy (654.5)*
that affecting fetus or newborn (761.0)

622.6 Hypertrophic elongation of cervix

622.7 Mucous polyp of cervix
Polyp NOS of cervix

Excludes: *adenomatous polyp of cervix (219.0)*

622.8 Other specified noninflammatory disorders of cervix
Atrophy (senile) } of cervix
Cyst } of cervix
Fibrosis } of cervix
Hemorrhage } of cervix

Excludes: *endometriosis (617.0)*
fistula (619.0-619.8)
inflammatory diseases (616.0)

622.9 Unspecified noninflammatory disorder of cervix

623 Noninflammatory disorders of vagina

Excludes: *abnormality of vagina complicating pregnancy, labor, or delivery (654.7)*
congenital absence of vagina (752.49)
congenital diaphragm or bands (752.49)
fistulas involving vagina (619.0-619.8)

623.0 Dysplasia of vagina

Excludes: *carcinoma in situ of vagina (233.3)*

623.1 Leukoplakia of vagina

623.2 Stricture or atresia of vagina
Adhesions (postoperative) (postradiation) of vagina
Occlusion of vagina
Stenosis, vagina

Use additional E code, if desired, to identify any external cause

Excludes: *congenital atresia or stricture (752.49)*

623.3 Tight hymenal ring
Rigid hymen } acquired or congenital
Tight hymenal ring } acquired or congenital
Tight introitus } acquired or congenital

Excludes: *imperforate hymen (752.42)*

623.4 Old vaginal laceration

Excludes: *old laceration involving muscles of pelvic floor (618.7)*

623.5 Leukorrhea, not specified as infective
Leukorrhea NOS of vagina
Vaginal discharge NOS

Excludes: *trichomonal (131.00)*

623.6 Vaginal hematoma

Excludes: *current obstetrical trauma (665.7)*

623.7 Polyp of vagina

623.8 Other specified noninflammatory disorders of vagina
Cyst } of vagina
Hemorrhage } of vagina

623.9 Unspecified noninflammatory disorder of vagina

624 Noninflammatory disorders of vulva and perineum

Excludes: *abnormality of vulva and perineum complicating pregnancy, labor, or delivery (654.8)*
condyloma acuminatum (078.1)
fistulas involving:
perineum—see Alphabetic Index
vulva (619.0-619.8)
vulval varices (456.6)
vulvar involvement in skin conditions (690-709.9)

624.0 Dystrophy of vulva
Kraurosis } of vulva
Leukoplakia } of vulva

Excludes: *carcinoma in situ of vulva (233.3)*

624.1 Atrophy of vulva

624.2 Hypertrophy of clitoris

Excludes: *that in endocrine disorders (255.2, 256.1)*

624.3 Hypertrophy of labia
Hypertrophy of vulva NOS

624.4 Old laceration or scarring of vulva

624.5 Hematoma of vulva

Excludes: *that complicating delivery (664.5)*

624.6 Polyp of labia and vulva

624.8 Other specified noninflammatory disorders of vulva and perineum
Cyst } of vulva
Edema } of vulva
Stricture } of vulva

624.9 Unspecified noninflammatory disorder of vulva and perineum

625 Pain and other symptoms associated with female genital organs

625.0 Dyspareunia

Excludes: *psychogenic dyspareunia (302.76)*

625.1 Vaginismus
Colpospasm
Vulvismus

Excludes: *psychogenic vaginismus (306.51)*

625.2 Mittelschmerz
Intermenstrual pain
Ovulation pain

625.3 Dysmenorrhea
Painful menstruation

Excludes: *psychogenic dysmenorrhea (306.52)*

625.4 Premenstrual tension syndromes
Menstrual:
migraine
molimen
Premenstrual tension NOS

625.5 Pelvic congestion syndrome
Congestion-fibrosis syndrome
Taylor's syndrome

625.6 Stress incontinence, female

Excludes: *mixed incontinence (788.33)*
stress incontinence, male (788.32)

625.8 Other specified symptoms associated with female genital organs

625.9 Unspecified symptom associated with female genital organs

626 Disorders of menstruation and other abnormal bleeding from female genital tract

Excludes: *menopausal and premenopausal bleeding (627.0)*
pain and other symptoms associated with menstrual cycle (625.2-625.4)
postmenopausal bleeding (627.1)

626.0 Absence of menstruation
Amenorrhea (primary) (secondary)

626.1 Scanty or infrequent menstruation
Hypomenorrhea
Oligomenorrhea

626.2 Excessive or frequent menstruation
Heavy periods
Menometrorrhagia
Menorrhagia
Polymenorrhea

Excludes: *premenopausal (627.0)*
that in puberty (626.3)

626.3 Puberty bleeding
Excessive bleeding associated with onset of menstrual periods
Pubertal menorrhagia

626.4 Irregular menstrual cycle
Irregular:
bleeding NOS
menstruation
periods

626.5 Ovulation bleeding
Regular intermenstrual bleeding

626.6 Metrorrhagia
Bleeding unrelated to menstrual cycle
Irregular intermenstrual bleeding

626.7 Postcoital bleeding

626.8 Other
Dysfunctional or functional uterine hemorrhage NOS
Menstruation:
retained
suppression of

626.9 Unspecified

627 Menopausal and postmenopausal disorders

627.0 Premenopausal menorrhagia
Excessive bleeding associated with onset of menopause
Menorrhagia:
climacteric
menopausal
preclimacteric

627.1 Postmenopausal bleeding

627.2 Menopausal or female climacteric states
Symptoms, such as flushing, sleeplessness, headache, lack of concentration, associated with the menopause

627.3 Postmenopausal atrophic vaginitis
Senile (atrophic) vaginitis

627.4 States associated with artificial menopause
Postartificial menopause syndromes
Any condition classifiable to 627.1, 627.2, or 627.3 which follows induced menopause

627.8 Other specified menopausal and postmenopausal disorders
Excludes: premature menopause NOS (256.3)

627.9 Unspecified menopausal and postmenopausal disorder

628 Infertility, female
Includes: primary and secondary sterility

628.0 Associated with anovulation
Anovulatory cycle

Use additional code for any associated Stein-Leventhal syndrome (256.4)

628.1 Of pituitary-hypothalamic origin
Code first underlying cause, as:
adiposogenital dystrophy (253.8)
anterior pituitary disorder (253.0-253.4)

628.2 Of tubal origin
Infertility associated with congenital anomaly of tube
Tubal:
block
occlusion
stenosis

Use additional code for any associated peritubal adhesions (614.6)

628.3 Of uterine origin
Infertility associated with congenital anomaly of uterus
Nonimplantation

Use additional code for any associated tuberculous endometritis (016.7)

628.4 Of cervical or vaginal origin
Infertility associated with:
anomaly of cervical mucus
congenital structural anomaly
dysmucorrhea

628.8 Of other specified origin

628.9 Of unspecified origin

629 Other disorders of female genital organs

629.0 Hematocele, female, not elsewhere classified

Excludes: hematocele or hematoma:
broad ligament (620.7)
fallopian tube (620.8)
that associated with ectopic pregnancy (633.0-633.9)
uterus (621.4)
vagina (623.6)
vulva (624.5)

629.1 Hydrocele, canal of Nuck
Cyst of canal of Nuck (acquired)

Excludes: congenital (752.41)

629.8 Other specified disorders of female genital organs

629.9 Unspecified disorder of female genital organs
Habitual aborter without current pregnancy

11. COMPLICATIONS OF PREGNANCY, CHILDBIRTH, AND THE PUERPERIUM (630-676)

ECTOPIC AND MOLAR PREGNANCY (630-633)

Use additional code from category 639 to identify any complications

630 Hydatidiform mole
Trophoblastic disease NOS
Vesicular mole

Excludes: *choriadenoma (destruens) (236.1)*
chorionepithelioma (181)
malignant hydatidiform mole (236.1)

631 Other abnormal product of conception
Blighted ovum
Mole:
NOS
carneous
Mole:
fleshy
stone

632 Missed abortion
Early fetal death before completion of 22 weeks' gestation with retention of dead fetus
Retained products of conception, not following spontaneous or induced abortion or delivery

Excludes: *failed induced abortion (638.0-638.9)*
fetal death (intrauterine) (late) (656.4)
missed delivery (656.4)
that with abnormal product of conception (630, 631)

633 Ectopic pregnancy
Includes: ruptured ectopic pregnancy

633.0 Abdominal pregnancy
Intraperitoneal pregnancy

633.1 Tubal pregnancy
Fallopian pregnancy
Rupture of (fallopian) tube due to pregnancy
Tubal abortion

633.2 Ovarian pregnancy

633.8 Other ectopic pregnancy
Pregnancy:
cervical
combined
cornual
Pregnancy:
intraligamentous
mesometric
mural

633.9 Unspecified ectopic pregnancy

OTHER PREGNANCY WITH ABORTIVE OUTCOME (634-639)

Note: Use the following fifth-digit subclassification with categories 634-637:

0 Unspecified

1 Incomplete

2 Complete

The following fourth-digit subdivisions are for use with categories 634-638:

.0 Complicated by genital tract and pelvic infection
Endometritis
Salpingo-oophoritis
Sepsis NOS
Septicemia NOS
Any condition classifiable to 639.0, with condition classifiable to 634-638

Excludes: *urinary tract infection (634-638 with .7)*

.1 Complicated by delayed or excessive hemorrhage
Afibrinogenemia
Defibrination syndrome
Intravascular hemolysis
Any condition classifiable to 639.1, with condition classifiable to 634-638

.2 Complicated by damage to pelvic organs and tissues
Laceration, perforation, or tear of:
bladder
uterus
Any condition classifiable to 639.2, with condition classifiable to 634-638

Add 4th or 5th digit | Nonspecific code | Unspecified code | Manifestation code

.3 Complicated by renal failure
Oliguria
Uremia
Any condition classifiable to 639.3, with condition classifiable to 634-638

.4 Complicated by metabolic disorder
Electrolyte imbalance with conditions classifiable to 634-638

.5 Complicated by shock
Circulatory collapse
Shock (postoperative) (septic)
Any condition classifiable to 639.5, with condition classifiable to 634-638

.6 Complicated by embolism
Embolism:
NOS
amniotic fluid
pulmonary
Any condition classifiable to 639.6, with condition classifiable to 634-638

.7 With other specified complications
Cardiac arrest or failure
Urinary tract infection
Any condition classifiable to 639.8, with condition classifiable to 634-638

.8 With unspecified complication

.9 Without mention of complication

⑤ **634 Abortion**
Includes: miscarriage
spontaneous abortion

634.0 Complicated by genital tract and pelvic infection

634.1 Complicated by delayed or excessive hemorrhage

634.2 Complicated by damage to pelvic organs or tissues

634.3 Complicated by renal failure

634.4 Complicated by metabolic disorder

634.5 Complicated by shock

634.6 Complicated by embolism

634.7 With other specified complications

634.8 With unspecified complication

634.9 Without mention of complication

⑤ **635 Legally induced abortion**
Includes: abortion or termination of pregnancy:
elective
legal
therapeutic

Excludes: *menstrual extraction or regulation (V25.3)*

635.0 Complicated by genital tract and pelvic infection

635.1 Complicated by delayed or excessive hemorrhage

635.2 Complicated by damage to pelvic organs or tissues

635.3 Complicated by renal failure

635.4 Complicated by metabolic disorder

635.5 Complicated by shock

635.6 Complicated by embolism

635.7 With other specified complications

635.8 With unspecified complication

635.9 Without mention of complication

⑤ **636 Illegally induced abortion**
Includes: abortion:
criminal
illegal
self-induced

636.0 Complicated by genital tract and pelvic infection

636.1 Complicated by delayed or excessive hemorrhage

636.2 Complicated by damage to pelvic organs or tissues

● Code new to this edition ▲ Revision of existing code ④ ⑤ Fourth or fifth digit required

636.3 Complicated by renal failure

636.4 Complicated by metabolic disorder

636.5 Complicated by shock

636.6 Complicated by embolism

636.7 With other specified complications

636.8 With unspecified complication

636.9 Without mention of complication

⑤ **637 Unspecified abortion**

Includes: abortion NOS
retained products of conception following abortion, not classifiable elsewhere

637.0 Complicated by genital tract and pelvic infection

637.1 Complicated by delayed or excessive hemorrhage

637.2 Complicated by damage to pelvic organs or tissues

637.3 Complicated by renal failure

637.4 Complicated by metabolic disorder

637.5 Complicated by shock

637.6 Complicated by embolism

637.7 With other specified complications

637.8 With unspecified complication

637.9 Without mention of complication

638 Failed attempted abortion

Includes: failure of attempted induction of (legal) abortion

Excludes: *incomplete abortion (634.0-637.9)*

638.0 Complicated by genital tract and pelvic infection

638.1 Complicated by delayed or excessive hemorrhage

638.2 Complicated by damage to pelvic organs or tissues

638.3 Complicated by renal failure

638.4 Complicated by metabolic disorder

638.5 Complicated by shock

638.6 Complicated by embolism

638.7 With other specified complications

638.8 With unspecified complication

638.9 Without mention of complication

639 Complications following abortion and ectopic and molar pregnancies

Note: This category is provided for use when it is required to classify separately the complications classifiable to the fourth-digit level in categories 634-638; for example:

a) when the complication itself was responsible for an episode of medical care, the abortion, ectopic or molar pregnancy itself having been dealt with at a previous episode

b) when these conditions are immediate complications of ectopic or molar pregnancies classifiable to 630-633 where they cannot be identified at fourth-digit level.

639.0 Genital tract and pelvic infection

Endometritis
Parametritis
Pelvic peritonitis
Salpingitis
Salpingo-oophoritis
Sepsis NOS
Septicemia NOS
} following conditions classifiable to 630-638

Excludes: *urinary tract infection (639.8)*

639.1 Delayed or excessive hemorrhage

Afibrinogenemia
Defibrination syndrome
Intravascular hemolysis
} following conditions classifiable to 630-638

Add 4th or 5th digit | Nonspecific code | Unspecified code | Manifestation code

639.2 Damage to pelvic organs and tissues

Laceration, perforation, or tear of: bladder, bowel, broad ligament, cervix, periurethral tissue, uterus, vagina — following conditions classifiable to 630-638

639.3 Renal failure

Oliguria; Renal: failure (acute), shutdown, tubular necrosis; Uremia — following conditions classifiable to 630-638

639.4 Metabolic disorders

Electrolyte imbalance following conditions classifiable to 630-638

639.5 Shock

Circulatory collapse; Shock (postoperative) (septic) — following conditions classifiable to 630-638

639.6 Embolism

Embolism: NOS, air, amniotic fluid, blood-clot, fat, pulmonary, pyemic, septic, soap — following conditions classifiable to 630-638

639.8 Other specified complications following abortion or ectopic and molar pregnancy

Acute yellow atrophy or necrosis of liver; Cardiac arrest or failure; Cerebral anoxia; Urinary tract infection — following conditions classifiable to 630-638

639.9 Unspecified complication following abortion or ectopic and molar pregnancy

Complication(s) not further specified following conditions classifiable to 630-638

COMPLICATIONS MAINLY RELATED TO PREGNANCY (640-648)

Includes: the listed conditions even if they arose or were present during labor, delivery, or the puerperium

The following fifth-digit subclassification is for use with categories 640-648 to denote the current episode of care:

0 unspecified as to episode of care or not applicable

1 delivered, with or without mention of antepartum condition

Antepartum condition with delivery; Delivery NOS; Intrapartum obstetric condition; Pregnancy, delivered — (with mention of antepartum complication during current episode of care)

2 delivered, with mention of postpartum complication

Delivery with mention of puerperal complication during current episode of care

3 antepartum condition or complication

Antepartum obstetric condition, not delivered during the current episode of care

4 postpartum condition or complication

Postpartum or puerperal obstetric condition or complication following delivery that occurred:
- during previous episode of care
- outside hospital, with subsequent admission for observation or care

⑤ **640 Hemorrhage in early pregnancy**

Includes: hemorrhage before completion of 22 weeks' gestation

640.0 Threatened abortion

[0,1,3]

● Code new to this edition ▲ Revision of existing code ④ ⑤ Fourth or fifth digit required

640.8 Other specified hemorrhage in early pregnancy
[0,1,3]

640.9 Unspecified hemorrhage in early pregnancy
[0,1,3]

⑤ 641 Antepartum hemorrhage, abruptio placentae, and placenta previa

641.0 Placenta previa without hemorrhage
[0,1,3]
Low implantation of placenta
Placenta previa noted:
during pregnancy
before labor (and delivered by cesarean delivery)
} without hemorrhage

641.1 Hemorrhage from placenta previa
[0,1,3]
Low-lying placenta
Placenta previa
incomplete
marginal
partial
total
} NOS or with hemorrhage (intrapartum)

Excludes: *hemorrhage from vasa previa (663.5)*

641.2 Premature separation of placenta
[0,1,3]
Ablatio placentae
Abruptio placentae
Accidental antepartum hemorrhage
Couvelaire uterus
Detachment of placenta (premature)
Premature separation of normally implanted placenta

641.3 Antepartum hemorrhage associated with coagulation defects
[0,1,3]
Antepartum or intrapartum hemorrhage associated with:
afibrinogenemia
hyperfibrinolysis
hypofibrinogenemia

641.8 Other antepartum hemorrhage
[0,1,3]
Antepartum or intrapartum hemorrhage associated with:
trauma
uterine leiomyoma

641.9 Unspecified antepartum hemorrhage
[0,1,3]
Hemorrhage:
antepartum NOS
intrapartum NOS
of pregnancy NOS

⑤ 642 Hypertension complicating pregnancy, childbirth, and the puerperium

642.0 Benign essential hypertension complicating pregnancy, childbirth, and the puerperium
[0-4]
Hypertension:
benign essential
chronic NOS
essential
pre-existing NOS
} specified as complicating, or as a reason for obstetric care during pregnancy, childbirth, or the puerperium

642.1 Hypertension secondary to renal disease, complicating pregnancy, childbirth, and the puerperium
[0-4]
Hypertension secondary to renal disease, specified as complicating, or as a reason for obstetric care during pregnancy, childbirth, or the puerperium

642.2 Other pre-existing hypertension complicating pregnancy, childbirth, and the puerperium
[0-4]
Hypertensive:
heart and renal disease
heart disease
renal disease
Malignant hypertension
} specified as complicating, as a reason for obstetric care during pregnancy, childbirth, or the puerperium

642.3 Transient hypertension of pregnancy
[0-4]
Gestational hypertension
Transient hypertension, so described, in pregnancy, childbirth, or the puerperium

Add 4th or 5th digit | Nonspecific code | Unspecified code | Manifestation code

642.4 Mild or unspecified pre-eclampsia
[0-4] Hypertension in pregnancy, childbirth, or the puerperium, not specified as pre-existing, with either albuminuria or edema, or both; mild or unspecified

Pre-eclampsia:	Toxemia (pre-eclamptic):
NOS	NOS
mild	mild

Excludes: *albuminuria in pregnancy, without mention of hypertension (646.2)*
edema in pregnancy, without mention of hypertension (646.1)

642.5 Severe pre-eclampsia
[0-4] Hypertension in pregnancy, childbirth, or the puerperium, not specified as pre-existing, with either albuminuria or edema, or both; specified as severe
Pre-eclampsia, severe
Toxemia (pre-eclamptic), severe

642.6 Eclampsia
[0-4] Toxemia:
eclamptic
with convulsions

642.7 Pre-eclampsia or eclampsia superimposed on pre-existing hypertension
[0-4] Conditions classifiable to 642.4-642.6, with conditions classifiable to 642.0-642.2

642.9 Unspecified hypertension complicating pregnancy, childbirth, or the puerperium
[0-4] Hypertension NOS, without mention of albuminuria or edema, complicating pregnancy, childbirth, or the puerperium

⑤ **643 Excessive vomiting in pregnancy**
Includes:
hyperemesis } arising during pregnancy
vomiting: } arising during pregnancy
persistent } arising during pregnancy
vicious } arising during pregnancy
hyperemesis gravidarum

643.0 Mild hyperemesis gravidarum
[0,1,3] Hyperemesis gravidarum, mild or unspecified, starting before the end of the 22nd week of gestation

643.1 Hyperemesis gravidarum with metabolic disturbance
[0,1,3] Hyperemesis gravidarum, starting before the end of the 22nd week of gestation, with metabolic disturbance, such as:
carbohydrate depletion
dehydration
electrolyte imbalance

643.2 Late vomiting of pregnancy
[0,1,3] Excessive vomiting starting after 22 completed weeks of gestation

643.8 Other vomiting complicating pregnancy
[0,1,3] Vomiting due to organic disease or other cause, specified as complicating pregnancy, or as a reason for obstetric care during pregnancy
Use additional code, if desired, to specify cause

643.9 Unspecified vomiting of pregnancy
[0,1,3] Vomiting as a reason for care during pregnancy, length of gestation unspecified

⑤ **644 Early or threatened labor**

□ **644.0 Threatened premature labor**
[0,3] Premature labor after 22 weeks, but before 37 completed weeks of gestation without delivery

Excludes: *that occurring before 22 completed weeks of gestation (640.0)*

□ **644.1 Other threatened labor**
[0,3] False labor:
NOS } without delivery
after 37 completed weeks of gestation } without delivery
Threatened labor NOS } without delivery

□ **644.2 Early onset of delivery**
[0,1] Onset (spontaneous) of delivery } before 37 completed weeks of gestation
Premature labor with onset of delivery } before 37 completed weeks of gestation

⑤ **645 Prolonged pregnancy**
[0,1,3] Post-term pregnancy
Pregnancy which has advanced beyond 42 weeks of gestation
Use 0 as fourth-digit for this category

● Code new to this edition ▲ Revision of existing code ④ ⑤ Fourth or fifth digit required

⑤ **646 Other complications of pregnancy, not elsewhere classified**

Use additional code(s) to further specify complication

646.0 Papyraceous fetus
[0,1,3]

646.1 Edema or excessive weight gain in pregnancy, without mention of hypertension
[0-4] Gestational edema
Maternal obesity syndrome

Excludes: *that with mention of hypertension (642.0-642.9)*

646.2 Unspecified renal disease in pregnancy, without mention of hypertension
[0-4]
Albuminuria, Nephropathy NOS, Renal disease NOS, Uremia, Gestational proteinuria } in pregnancy or the puerperium, without mention of hypertension

Excludes: *that with mention of hypertension (642.0-642.9)*

646.3 Habitual aborter
[0,1,3]

Excludes: *with current abortion (634.0-634.9)*
without current pregnancy (629.9)

646.4 Peripheral neuritis in pregnancy
[0-4]

646.5 Asymptomatic bacteriuria in pregnancy
[0-4]

646.6 Infections of genitourinary tract in pregnancy
[0-4] Conditions classifiable to 590, 595, 597, 599.0, 616 complicating pregnancy, childbirth, or the puerperium
Conditions classifiable to 614-615 complicating pregnancy or labor

Excludes: *major puerperal infection (670)*

646.7 Liver disorders in pregnancy
[0,1,3]
Acute yellow atrophy of liver (obstetric) (true), Icterus gravis } of pregnancy
Necrosis of liver

Excludes: *hepatorenal syndrome following delivery (674.8)*
viral hepatitis (647.6)

646.8 Other specified complications of pregnancy
[0-4] Fatigue during pregnancy
Herpes gestationis
Insufficient weight gain of pregnancy

646.9 Unspecified complication of pregnancy
[0,1,3]

⑤ **647 Infectious and parasitic conditions in the mother classifiable elsewhere, but complicating pregnancy, childbirth, or the puerperium**

Includes: the listed conditions when complicating the pregnant state, aggravated by the pregnancy, or when a main reason for obstetric care

Excludes: *those conditions in the mother known or suspected to have affected the fetus (655.0-655.9)*

Use additional code(s) to further specify complication

647.0 Syphilis
[0-4] Conditions classifiable to 090-097

647.1 Gonorrhea
[0-4] Conditions classifiable to 098

647.2 Other venereal diseases
[0-4] Conditions classifiable to 099

647.3 Tuberculosis
[0-4] Conditions classifiable to 010-018

647.4 Malaria
[0-4] Conditions classifiable to 084

647.5 Rubella
[0-4] Conditions classifiable to 056

647.6 Other viral diseases
[0-4] Conditions classifiable to 042 and 050-079, except 056

647.8 Other specified infectious and parasitic diseases
[0-4]

647.9 Unspecified infection or infestation
[0-4]

⑤ **648 Other current conditions in the mother classifiable elsewhere, but complicating pregnancy, childbirth, or the puerperium**

Includes: the listed conditions when complicating the pregnant state, aggravated by the pregnancy, or when a main reason for obstetric care

Excludes: *those conditions in the mother known or suspected to have affected the fetus (655.0-655.9)*

Use additional code(s) to identify the condition

648.0 Diabetes mellitus
[0-4] Conditions classifiable to 250

Excludes: *gestational diabetes (648.8)*

648.1 Thyroid dysfunction
[0-4] Conditions classifiable to 240-246

648.2 Anemia
[0-4] Conditions classifiable to 280-285

648.3 Drug dependence
[0-4] Conditions classifiable to 304

648.4 Mental disorders
[0-4] Conditions classifiable to 290-303, 305-316, 317-319

648.5 Congenital cardiovascular disorders
[0-4] Conditions classifiable to 745-747

648.6 Other cardiovascular diseases
[0-4] Conditions classifiable to 390-398, 410-429

Excludes: *cerebrovascular disorders in the puerperium (674.0)*
venous complications (671.0-671.9)

648.7 Bone and joint disorders of back, pelvis, and lower limbs
[0-4] Conditions classifiable to 720-724, and those classifiable to 711-719 or 725-738, specified as affecting the lower limbs

648.8 Abnormal glucose tolerance
[0-4] Conditions classifiable to 790.2
Gestational diabetes

648.9 Other current conditions classifiable elsewhere
[0-4] Nutritional deficiencies [conditions classifiable to 260-269]

NORMAL DELIVERY, AND OTHER INDICATIONS FOR CARE IN PREGNANCY, LABOR, AND DELIVERY (650-659)

The following fifth-digit subclassification is for use with categories 651-659 to denote the current episode of care:

0 unspecified as to episode of care or not applicable
1 delivered, with or without mention of antepartum condition
2 delivered, with mention of postpartum complication
3 antepartum condition or complication
4 postpartum condition or complication

▲ **650 Normal delivery**

Delivery requiring minimal or no assistance, with or without episiotomy, without fetal manipulation [e.g., rotation version] or instrumentation [forceps] of spontaneous, cephalic, vaginal, full-term, single, live born infant. This code is for use as a single diagnosis code and is not to be used with any other code in the range 630-676.

Excludes: *breech delivery (assisted) (spontaneous) NOS (652.2)*
delivery by vacuum extractor, forceps, cesarean section, or breech extraction, without specified complication (669.5-669.7)

Use additional code to indicate outcome of delivery (V27.0)

● Code new to this edition ▲ Revision of existing code ④ ⑤ Fourth or fifth digit required

⑤ **651 Multiple gestation**

651.0 Twin pregnancy
[0,1,3]

651.1 Triplet pregnancy
[0,1,3]

651.2 Quadruplet pregnancy
[0,1,3]

651.3 Twin pregnancy with fetal loss and retention of one fetus
[0,1,3]

651.4 Triplet pregnancy with fetal loss and retention of one or more fetus(es)
[0,1,3]

651.5 Quadruplet pregnancy with fetal loss and retention of one or more fetus(es)
[0,1,3]

651.6 Other multiple pregnancy with fetal loss and retention of one or more fetus(es)
[0,1,3]

651.8 Other specified multiple gestation
[0,1,3]

651.9 Unspecified multiple gestation
[0,1,3]

⑤ **652 Malposition and malpresentation of fetus**
Code first any associated obstructed labor (660.0)

652.0 Unstable lie
[0,1,3]

652.1 Breech or other malpresentation successfully converted to cephalic presentation
[0,1,3] Cephalic version NOS

652.2 Breech presentation without mention of version
[0,1,3] Breech delivery (assisted) (spontaneous) NOS

652.3 Transverse or oblique presentation
[0,1,3] Oblique lie; Transverse lie

Excludes: transverse arrest of fetal head (660.3)

652.4 Face or brow presentation
[0,1,3] Mentum presentation

652.5 High head at term
[0,1,3] Failure of head to enter pelvic brim

652.6 Multiple gestation with malpresentation of one fetus or more
[0,1,3]

652.7 Prolapsed arm
[0,1,3]

652.8 Other specified malposition or malpresentation
[0,1,3] Compound presentation

652.9 Unspecified malposition or malpresentation
[0,1,3]

⑤ **653 Disproportion**
Code first any associated obstructed labor (660.1)

653.0 Major abnormality of bony pelvis, not further specified
[0,1,3] Pelvic deformity NOS

653.1 Generally contracted pelvis
[0,1,3] Contracted pelvis NOS

653.2 Inlet contraction of pelvis
[0,1,3] Inlet contraction (pelvis)

653.3 Outlet contraction of pelvis
[0,1,3] Outlet contraction (pelvis)

653.4 Fetopelvic disproportion
[0,1,3] Cephalopelvic disproportion NOS
Disproportion of mixed maternal and fetal origin, with normally formed fetus

653.5 Unusually large fetus causing disproportion
[0,1,3] Disproportion of fetal origin with normally formed fetus
Fetal disproportion NOS

Excludes: *that when the reason for medical care was concern for the fetus (656.6)*

653.6 Hydrocephalic fetus causing disproportion
[0,1,3]

Excludes: *that when the reason for medical care was concern for the fetus (655.0)*

653.7 Other fetal abnormality causing disproportion
[0,1,3] Conjoined twins
Fetal:
ascites
hydrops
Fetal:
myelomeningocele
sacral teratoma
tumor

653.8 Disproportion of other origin
[0,1,3]

Excludes: *shoulder (girdle) dystocia (660.4)*

653.9 Unspecified disproportion
[0,1,3]

⑤ **654 Abnormality of organs and soft tissues of pelvis**
Includes: the listed conditions during pregnancy, childbirth, or the puerperium
Code first any associated obstructed labor (660.2)

654.0 Congenital abnormalities of uterus
[0-4] Double uterus
Uterus bicornis

654.1 Tumors of body of uterus
[0-4] Uterine fibroids

654.2 Previous cesarean delivery NOS
[0,1,3] Uterine scar from previous cesarean delivery

654.3 Retroverted and incarcerated gravid uterus
[0-4]

654.4 Other abnormalities in shape or position of gravid uterus and of neighboring structures
[0-4] Cystocele
Pelvic floor repair
Pendulous abdomen
Prolapse of gravid uterus
Rectocele
Rigid pelvic floor

654.5 Cervical incompetence
[0-4] Presence of Shirodkar suture with or without mention of cervical incompetence

654.6 Other congenital or acquired abnormality of cervix
[0-4] Cicatricial cervix
Polyp of cervix
Previous surgery to cervix
Rigid cervix (uteri)
Stenosis or stricture of cervix
Tumor of cervix

654.7 Congenital or acquired abnormality of vagina
[0-4] Previous surgery to vagina
Septate vagina
Stenosis of vagina (acquired)
(congenital)
Stricture of vagina
Tumor of vagina

654.8 Congenital or acquired abnormality of vulva
[0-4] Fibrosis of perineum
Persistent hymen
Previous surgery to perineum or vulva
Rigid perineum
Tumor of vulva

Excludes: *varicose veins of vulva (671.1)*

654.9 Other and unspecified
[0-4] Uterine scar NEC

⑤ **655 Known or suspected fetal abnormality affecting management of mother**

Includes: the listed conditions in the fetus as a reason for observation or obstetrical care of the mother, or for termination of pregnancy

655.0 Central nervous system malformation in fetus
[0,1,3] Fetal or suspected fetal:
anencephaly
hydrocephalus
spina bifida (with myelomeningocele)

655.1 Chromosomal abnormality in fetus
[0,1,3]

655.2 Hereditary disease in family possibly affecting fetus
[0,1,3]

655.3 Suspected damage to fetus from viral disease in the mother
[0,1,3] Suspected damage to fetus from maternal rubella

655.4 Suspected damage to fetus from other disease in the mother
[0,1,3] Suspected damage to fetus from maternal:
alcohol addiction
listeriosis
toxoplasmosis

655.5 Suspected damage to fetus from drugs
[0,1,3]

Excludes: fetal distress in labor and delivery due to drug administration (656.3)

655.6 Suspected damage to fetus from radiation
[0,1,3]

655.8 Other known or suspected fetal abnormality, not elsewhere classified
[0,1,3] Suspected damage to fetus from:
environmental toxins
intrauterine contraceptive device

655.9 Unspecified
[0,1,3]

⑤ **656 Other fetal and placental problems affecting management of mother**

656.0 Fetal-maternal hemorrhage
[0,1,3] Leakage (microscopic) of fetal blood into maternal circulation

656.1 Rhesus isoimmunization
[0,1,3] Anti-D [Rh] antibodies
Rh incompatibility

656.2 Isoimmunization from other and unspecified blood-group incompatibility
[0,1,3] ABO isoimmunization

656.3 Fetal distress
[0,1,3] Abnormal fetal:
acid-base balance
heart rate or rhythm
Fetal:
acidemia
bradycardia
tachycardia
Meconium in liquor

656.4 Intrauterine death
[0,1,3] Fetal death:
NOS
after completion of 22 weeks' gestation
late
Missed delivery

Excludes: missed abortion (632)

656.5 Poor fetal growth
[0,1,3] "Light-for-dates"
"Placental insufficiency"
"Small-for-dates"

656.6 Excessive fetal growth
[0,1,3] "Large-for-dates"

656.7 Other placental conditions
[0,1,3] Abnormal placenta
Placental infarct

Excludes: *placental polyp (674.4)*
placentitis (658.4)

656.8 Other specified fetal and placental problems
[0,1,3] Lithopedian

656.9 Unspecified fetal and placental problem
[0,1,3]

⑤ **657 Polyhydramnios**
[0,1,3] Hydramnios
Use 0 as fourth-digit for this category

⑤ **658 Other problems associated with amniotic cavity and membranes**

Excludes: *amniotic fluid embolism (673.1)*

658.0 Oligohydramnios
[0,1,3] Oligohydramnios without mention of rupture of membranes

658.1 Premature rupture of membranes
[0,1,3] Rupture of amniotic sac less than 24 hours prior to the onset of labor

658.2 Delayed delivery after spontaneous or unspecified rupture of membranes
[0,1,3] Prolonged rupture of membranes NOS
Rupture of amniotic sac 24 hours or more prior to the onset of labor

658.3 Delayed delivery after artificial rupture of membranes
[0,1,3]

658.4 Infection of amniotic cavity
[0,1,3] Amnionitis
Chorioamnionitis
Membranitis
Placentitis

658.8 Other
[0,1,3] Amnion nodosum
Amniotic cyst

658.9 Unspecified
[0,1,3]

⑤ **659 Other indications for care or intervention related to labor and delivery, not elsewhere classified**

659.0 Failed mechanical induction
[0,1,3] Failure of induction of labor by surgical or other instrumental methods

659.1 Failed medical or unspecified induction
[0,1,3] Failed induction NOS
Failure of induction of labor by medical methods, such as oxytocic drugs

659.2 Maternal pyrexia during labor, unspecified
[0,1,3]

659.3 Generalized infection during labor
[0,1,3] Septicemia during labor

659.4 Grand multiparity
[0,1,3]

Excludes: *supervision only, in pregnancy (V23.3)*
without current pregnancy (V61.5)

659.5 Elderly primigravida
[0,1,3]

Excludes: *supervision only, in pregnancy (V23.8)*

659.6 Other advanced maternal age
[0,1,3]

Excludes: *elderly primigravida 659.5*

659.8 Other specified indications for care or intervention related to labor and delivery
[0,1,3]

659.9 Unspecified indication for care or intervention related to labor and delivery
[0,1,3]

● Code new to this edition
▲ Revision of existing code
④ ⑤ Fourth or fifth digit required

COMPLICATIONS OCCURRING MAINLY IN THE COURSE OF LABOR AND DELIVERY (660-669)

The following fifth-digit subclassification is for use with categories 660-669 to denote the current episode of care:

0 unspecified as to episode of care or not applicable

1 delivered, with or without mention of antepartum condition

2 delivered, with mention of postpartum complication

3 antepartum condition or complication

4 postpartum condition or complication

⑤ **660 Obstructed labor**

660.0 Obstruction caused by malposition of fetus at onset of labor
[0,1,3] Any condition classifiable to 652, causing obstruction during labor

Use additional code from 652.0-652.9, if desired, to identify condition

660.1 Obstruction by bony pelvis
[0,1,3] Any condition classifiable to 653, causing obstruction during labor

Use additional code from 653.0-653.9, if desired, to identify condition

660.2 Obstruction by abnormal pelvic soft tissues
[0,1,3] Prolapse of anterior lip of cervix
Any condition classifiable to 654, causing obstruction during labor

Use additional code from 654.0-654.9, if desired, to identify condition

660.3 Deep transverse arrest and persistent occipitoposterior position
[0,1,3]

660.4 Shoulder (girdle) dystocia
[0,1,3] Impacted shoulders

660.5 Locked twins
[0,1,3]

660.6 Failed trial of labor, unspecified
[0,1,3] Failed trial of labor, without mention of condition or suspected condition

660.7 Failed forceps or vacuum extractor, unspecified
[0,1,3] Application of ventouse or forceps, without mention of condition

660.8 Other causes of obstructed labor
[0,1,3]

660.9 Unspecified obstructed labor
[0,1,3] Dystocia:
NOS
fetal NOS
maternal NOS

⑤ **661 Abnormality of forces of labor**

661.0 Primary uterine inertia
[0,1,3] Failure of cervical dilation
Hypotonic uterine dysfunction, primary
Prolonged latent phase of labor

661.1 Secondary uterine inertia
[0,1,3] Arrested active phase of labor
Hypotonic uterine dysfunction, secondary

661.2 Other and unspecified uterine inertia
[0,1,3] Atony of uterus
Desultory labor
Irregular labor
Poor contractions
Slow slope active phase of labor

661.3 Precipitate labor
[0,1,3]

661.4 Hypertonic, incoordinate, or prolonged uterine contractions
[0,1,3] Cervical spasm
Contraction ring (dystocia)
Dyscoordinate labor
Hourglass contraction of uterus
Hypertonic uterine dysfunction
Incoordinate uterine action
Retraction ring (Bandl's) (pathological)
Tetanic contractions
Uterine dystocia NOS
Uterine spasm

661.9 Unspecified abnormality of labor
[0,1,3]

⑤ **662 Long labor**

662.0 Prolonged first stage
[0,1,3]

662.1 Prolonged labor, unspecified
[0,1,3]

662.2 Prolonged second stage
[0,1,3]

662.3 Delayed delivery of second twin, triplet, etc.
[0,1,3]

⑤ **663 Umbilical cord complications**

663.0 Prolapse of cord
[0,1,3] Presentation of cord

663.1 Cord around neck, with compression
[0,1,3] Cord tightly around neck

663.2 Other and unspecified cord entanglement, with compression
[0,1,3] Entanglement of cords of twins in mono-amniotic sac
Knot in cord (with compression)

663.3 Other and unspecified cord entanglement, without mention of compression
[0,1,3]

663.4 Short cord
[0,1,3]

663.5 Vasa previa
[0,1,3] Velamentous insertion of umbilical cord

663.6 Vascular lesions of cord
[0,1,3] Bruising of cord
Hematoma of cord
Thrombosis of vessels of cord

663.8 Other umbilical cord complications
[0,1,3]

663.9 Unspecified umbilical cord complication
[0,1,3]

⑤ **664 Trauma to perineum and vulva during delivery**
Includes: damage from instruments
that from extension of episiotomy

664.0 First-degree perineal laceration
[0,1,4] Perineal laceration, rupture, or tear involving:
fourchette
hymen
labia
skin
vagina
vulva

664.1 Second-degree perineal laceration
[0,1,4] Perineal laceration, rupture, or tear (following episiotomy) involving:
pelvic floor
perineal muscles
vaginal muscles

Excludes: *that involving anal sphincter (664.2)*

664.2 Third-degree perineal laceration
[0,1,4] Perineal laceration, rupture, or tear (following episiotomy) involving:
anal sphincter
rectovaginal septum
sphincter NOS

Excludes: *that with anal or rectal mucosal laceration (664.3)*

664.3 Fourth-degree perineal laceration
[0,1,4] Perineal laceration, rupture, or tear as classifiable to 664.2 and involving also:
anal mucosa
rectal mucosa

664.4 Unspecified perineal laceration
[0,1,4] Central laceration

664.5 Vulval and perineal hematoma
[0,1,4]

664.8 Other specified trauma to perineum and vulva
[0,1,4]

664.9 Unspecified trauma to perineum and vulva
[0,1,4]

⑤ **665 Other obstetrical trauma**
Includes: damage from instruments

665.0 Rupture of uterus before onset of labor
[0,1,3]

665.1 Rupture of uterus during labor
[0,1] Rupture of uterus NOS

665.2 Inversion of uterus
[0,2,4]

665.3 Laceration of cervix
[0,1,4]

665.4 High vaginal laceration
[0,1,4] Laceration of vaginal wall or sulcus without mention of perineal laceration

665.5 Other injury to pelvic organs
[0,1,4] Injury to:
bladder
urethra

665.6 Damage to pelvic joints and ligaments
[0,1,4] Avulsion of inner symphyseal cartilage
Damage to coccyx
Separation of symphysis (pubis)

665.7 Pelvic hematoma
[0,1,2,4] Hematoma of vagina

665.8 Other specified obstetrical trauma
[0-4]

665.9 Unspecified obstetrical trauma
[0-4]

⑤ **666 Postpartum hemorrhage**

666.0 Third-stage hemorrhage
[0,2,4] Hemorrhage associated with retained, trapped, or adherent placenta
Retained placenta NOS

666.1 Other immediate postpartum hemorrhage
[0,2,4] Hemorrhage within the first 24 hours following delivery of placenta
Postpartum hemorrhage (atonic) NOS

666.2 Delayed and secondary postpartum hemorrhage
[0,2,4] Hemorrhage:
after the first 24 hours following delivery
associated with retained portions of placenta or membranes
Postpartum hemorrhage specified as delayed or secondary
Retained products of conception NOS, following delivery

666.3 Postpartum coagulation defects
[0,2,4] Postpartum:
afibrinogenemia
fibrinolysis

⑤ **667 Retained placenta or membranes, without hemorrhage**

667.0 Retained placenta without hemorrhage
[0,2,4] Placenta accreta } without hemorrhage
Retained placenta: } without hemorrhage
NOS
total

667.1 Retained portions of placenta or membranes, without hemorrhage
[0,2,4] Retained products of conception following delivery, without hemorrhage

⑤ **668 Complications of the administration of anesthetic or other sedation in labor and delivery**
Includes: complications arising from the administration of a general or local anesthetic, analgesic, or other sedation in labor and delivery

Excludes: *reaction to spinal or lumbar puncture (349.0)*
spinal headache (349.0)

Use additional code(s) to further specify complication

Add 4th or 5th digit | Nonspecific code | Unspecified code | Manifestation code

668.0 Pulmonary complications
[0-4]
Inhalation [aspiration] of stomach contents or secretions
Mendelson's syndrome
Pressure collapse of lung
} following anesthesia or other sedation in labor or delivery

668.1 Cardiac complications
[0-4]
Cardiac arrest or failure following anesthesia or other sedation in labor and delivery

668.2 Central nervous system complications
[0-4]
Cerebral anoxia following anesthesia or other sedation in labor and delivery

668.8 Other complications of anesthesia or other sedation in labor and delivery
[0-4]

668.9 Unspecified complication of anesthesia and other sedation
[0-4]

⑤ **669 Other complications of labor and delivery, not elsewhere classified**

669.0 Maternal distress
[0-4]
Metabolic disturbance in labor and delivery

669.1 Shock during or following labor and delivery
[0-4]
Obstetric shock

669.2 Maternal hypotension syndrome
[0-4]

669.3 Acute renal failure following labor and delivery
[0,2,4]

669.4 Other complications of obstetrical surgery and procedures
[0-4]
Cardiac:
arrest
failure
Cerebral anoxia
} following cesarean or other obstetrical surgery or procedure, including delivery NOS

Excludes: *complications of obstetrical surgical wounds (674.1-674.3)*

669.5 Forceps or vacuum extractor delivery without mention of indication
[0,1]
Delivery by ventouse, without mention of indication

669.6 Breech extraction, without mention of indication
[0,1]

Excludes: *breech delivery NOS (652.2)*

669.7 Cesarean delivery, without mention of indication
[0,1]

669.8 Other complications of labor and delivery
[0-4]

669.9 Unspecified complication of labor and delivery
[0-4]

COMPLICATIONS OF THE PUERPERIUM (670-677)

Note:Categories 671 and 673-676 include the listed conditions even if they occur during pregnancy or childbirth.

The following fifth-digit subclassification is for use with categories 670-676 to denote the current episode of care:

0 unspecified as to episode of care or not applicable
1 delivered, with or without mention of antepartum condition
2 delivered, with mention of postpartum complication
3 antepartum condition or complication
4 postpartum condition or complication

⑤ **670 Major puerperal infection**
[0,2,4]
Puerperal:
- endometritis
- fever
- pelvic:
  - cellulitis
  - sepsis

Puerperal:
- peritonitis
- pyemia
- salpingitis
- septicemia

Use 0 as fourth-digit for this category

Excludes: *infection following abortion (639.0)*
minor genital tract infection following delivery (646.6)
urinary tract infection following delivery (646.6)

⑤ **671 Venous complications in pregnancy and the puerperium**

671.0 Varicose veins of legs
[0-4] Varicose veins NOS

671.1 Varicose veins of vulva and perineum
[0-4]

671.2 Superficial thrombophlebitis
[0-4] Thrombophlebitis (superficial)

671.3 Deep phlebothrombosis, antepartum
[0,1,3] Deep-vein thrombosis, antepartum

671.4 Deep phlebothrombosis, postpartum
[0,2,4] Deep-vein thrombosis, postpartum
Pelvic thrombophlebitis, postpartum
Phlegmasia alba dolens (puerperal)

671.5 Other phlebitis and thrombosis
[0-4] Cerebral venous thrombosis
Thrombosis of intracranial venous sinus

671.8 Other venous complications
[0-4] Hemorrhoids

671.9 Unspecified venous complication
[0-4] Phlebitis NOS
Thrombosis NOS

⑤ **672 Pyrexia of unknown origin during the puerperium**
[0,2,4] Puerperal pyrexia NOS
Use 0 as fourth-digit for this category

⑤ **673 Obstetrical pulmonary embolism**
Includes: pulmonary emboli in pregnancy, childbirth, or the puerperium, or specified as puerperal

Excludes: *embolism following abortion (639.6)*

673.0 Obstetrical air embolism
[0-4]

673.1 Amniotic fluid embolism
[0-4]

673.2 Obstetrical blood-clot embolism
[0-4] Puerperal pulmonary embolism NOS

673.3 Obstetrical pyemic and septic embolism
[0-4]

673.8 Other pulmonary embolism
[0-4] Fat embolism

⑤ **674 Other and unspecified complications of the puerperium, not elsewhere classified**

674.0 Cerebrovascular disorders in the puerperium
[0-4] Any condition classifiable to 430-434, 436-437 occurring during pregnancy, childbirth, or the puerperium, or specified as puerperal

Excludes: *intracranial venous sinus thrombosis (671.5)*

674.1 Disruption of cesarean wound
[0,2,4] Dehiscence or disruption of uterine wound

674.2 Disruption of perineal wound
[0,2,4] Breakdown of perineum
Disruption of wound of:
- episiotomy
- perineal laceration

Secondary perineal tear

674.3 Other complications of obstetrical surgical wounds
[0,2,4] Hematoma | Hemorrhage | Infection } of cesarean section or perineal wound

Excludes: *damage from instruments in delivery (664.0-665.9)*

674.4 Placental polyp
[0,2,4]

674.8 Other
[0,2,4] Hepatorenal syndrome, following delivery
Postpartum:
cardiomyopathy
subinvolution of uterus
uterine hypertrophy

674.9 Unspecified
[0,2,4] Sudden death of unknown cause during the puerperium

⑤ **675 Infections of the breast and nipple associated with childbirth**
Includes: the listed conditions during pregnancy, childbirth, or the puerperium

675.0 Infections of nipple
[0-4] Abscess of nipple

675.1 Abscess of breast
[0-4] Abscess:
mammary
subareolar
submammary

Mastitis:
purulent
retromammary
submammary

675.2 Nonpurulent mastitis
[0-4] Lymphangitis of breast

Mastitis:
NOS
interstitial
parenchymatous

675.8 Other specified infections of the breast and nipple
[0-4]

675.9 Unspecified infection of the breast and nipple
[0-4]

⑤ **676 Other disorders of the breast associated with childbirth and disorders of lactation**
Includes: the listed conditions during pregnancy, the puerperium, or lactation

676.0 Retracted nipple
[0-4]

676.1 Cracked nipple
[0-4] Fissure of nipple

676.2 Engorgement of breasts
[0-4]

676.3 Other and unspecified disorder of breast
[0-4]

676.4 Failure of lactation
[0-4] Agalactia

676.5 Suppressed lactation
[0-4]

676.6 Galactorrhea
[0-4]

Excludes: *galactorrhea not associated with childbirth (611.6)*

676.8 Other disorders of lactation
[0-4] Galactocele

676.9 Unspecified disorder of lactation
[0-4]

677 Late effect of complication of pregnancy, childbirth, and the puerperium
Note: This category is to be used to indicate conditions in 632-648.9 and 651-676.9 as the cause of the late effect, themselves classifiable elsewhere. The "late effects" include conditions specified as such, or as sequelae, which may occur at any time after the puerperium.
Code first any sequelae

12. DISEASES OF THE SKIN AND SUBCUTANEOUS TISSUE (680-709)

INFECTIONS OF SKIN AND SUBCUTANEOUS TISSUE (680-686)

Excludes: *certain infections of skin classified under "Infectious and Parasitic Diseases," such as:*
erysipelas (035)
erysipeloid of Rosenbach (027.1)
herpes:
simplex (054.0-054.9)
zoster (053.0-053.9)
molluscum contagiosum (078.0)
viral warts (078.1)

680 Carbuncle and furuncle
Includes: boil
furunculosis

680.0 Face
Ear [any part]
Face [any part, except eye]
Nose (septum)
Temple (region)

Excludes: *eyelid (373.13)*
lacrimal apparatus (375.31)
orbit (376.01)

680.1 Neck

680.2 Trunk
Abdominal wall
Back [any part, except buttocks]
Breast
Chest wall
Flank
Groin
Pectoral region
Perineum
Umbilicus

Excludes: *buttocks (680.5)*
external genital organs:
female (616.4)
male (607.2, 608.4)

680.3 Upper arm and forearm
Arm [any part, except hand]
Axilla
Shoulder

680.4 Hand
Finger [any]
Thumb
Wrist

680.5 Buttock
Anus
Gluteal region

680.6 Leg, except foot
Ankle
Hip
Knee
Thigh

680.7 Foot
Heel
Toe

680.8 Other specified sites
Head [any part, except face]
Scalp

Excludes: *external genital organs:*
female (616.4)
male (607.2, 608.4)

680.9 Unspecified site
Boil NOS
Carbuncle NOS
Furuncle NOS

681 Cellulitis and abscess of finger and toe
Includes: that with lymphangitis
Use additional code, if desired, to identify organism, such as Staphylococcus (041.1)

681.0 Finger

681.00 Cellulitis and abscess, unspecified

Add 4th or 5th digit | Nonspecific code | Unspecified code | Manifestation code

681.01 Felon

Pulp abscess
Whitlow

Excludes: *herpetic whitlow (054.6)*

681.02 Onychia and paronychia of finger

Panaritium } of finger
Perionychia } of finger

681.1 Toe

681.10 Cellulitis and abscess, unspecified

681.11 Onychia and paronychia of toe

Panaritium } of toe
Perionychia } of toe

681.9 Cellulitis and abscess of unspecified digit

Infection of nail NOS

682 Other cellulitis and abscess

Includes:

abscess (acute) } (with lymphangitis) except of finger or toe
cellulitis (diffuse) } (with lymphangitis) except of finger or toe
lymphangitis, acute } (with lymphangitis) except of finger or toe

Use additional code, if desired, to identify organism, such as Staphylococcus (041.1)

Excludes: *lymphangitis (chronic) (subacute) (457.2)*

682.0 Face

Cheek, external
Chin
Forehead
Nose, external
Submandibular
Temple (region)

Excludes: *ear [any part] (380.10-380.16)*
eyelid (373.13)
lacrimal apparatus (375.31)
lip (528.5)
mouth (528.3)
nose (internal) (478.1)
orbit (376.01)

682.1 Neck

682.2 Trunk

Abdominal wall
Back [any part, except buttock]
Chest wall
Flank
Groin
Pectoral region
Perineum
Umbilicus, except newborn

Excludes: *anal and rectal regions (566)*
breast:
NOS (611.0)
puerperal (675.1)
external genital organs:
female (616.3-616.4)
male (604.0, 607.2, 608.4)
umbilicus, newborn (771.4)

682.3 Upper arm and forearm

Arm [any part, except hand]
Axilla
Shoulder

Excludes: *hand (682.4)*

682.4 Hand, except fingers and thumb

Wrist

Excludes: *finger and thumb (681.00-681.02)*

682.5 Buttock

Gluteal region

Excludes: *anal and rectal regions (566)*

682.6 Leg, except foot

Ankle
Hip
Knee
Thigh

682.7 Foot, except toes
Heel

Excludes: *toe (681.10-681.11)*

682.8 Other specified sites
Head [except face]
Scalp

Excludes: *face (682.0)*

682.9 Unspecified site
Abscess NOS
Cellulitis NOS
Lymphangitis, acute NOS

Excludes: *lymphangitis NOS (457.2)*

683 Acute lymphadenitis
Abscess (acute) / Adenitis, acute / Lymphadenitis, acute } lymph gland or node, except mesenteric

Use additional code, if desired, to identify organism, such as Staphylococcus (041.1)

Excludes: *enlarged glands NOS (785.6)*
lymphadenitis:
chronic or subacute, except mesenteric (289.1)
mesenteric (acute) (chronic) (subacute) (289.2)
unspecified (289.3)

684 Impetigo
Impetiginization of other dermatoses
Impetigo (contagiosa) [any site] [any organism]:
bullous
circinate
neonatorum
simplex
Pemphigus neonatorum

Excludes: *impetigo herpetiformis (694.3)*

685 Pilonidal cyst
Includes:
fistula / sinus } coccygeal or pilonidal

685.0 With abscess

685.1 Without mention of abscess

686 Other local infections of skin and subcutaneous tissue
Use additional code, if desired, to identify any infectious organism (041.0-041.8)

686.0 Pyoderma
Dermatitis:
purulent
septic
suppurative

686.1 Pyogenic granuloma
Granuloma:
septic
suppurative
telangiectaticum

Excludes: *pyogenic granuloma of oral mucosa (528.9)*

686.8 Other specified local infections of skin and subcutaneous tissue
Bacterid (pustular)
Dermatitis vegetans
Ecthyma
Perlèche

Excludes: *dermatitis infectiosa eczematoides (690.18)*
panniculitis (729.30-729.39)

686.9 Unspecified local infection of skin and subcutaneous tissue
Fistula of skin NOS
Skin infection NOS

Excludes: *fistula to skin from internal organs—see Alphabetic Index*

OTHER INFLAMMATORY CONDITIONS OF SKIN AND SUBCUTANEOUS TISSUE (690-698)

Excludes: *panniculitis (729.30-729.39)*

690 Erythematosquamous dermatosis

Excludes: *eczematous dermatitis of eyelid (373.31)*
parakeratosis variegata (696.2)
psoriasis (696.0-696.1)
seborrheic keratosis (702)

● **690.1 Seborrheic dermatitis**

● **690.10 Seborrheic dermatitis, unspecified**
Seborrheic dermatitis NOS

● **690.11 Seborrhea capitis**
Cradle cap

● **690.12 Seborrheic infantile dermatitis**

● **690.18 Other seborrheic dermatitis**

● **690.8 Other erythematosquamous dermatosis**

691 Atopic dermatitis and related conditions

691.0 Diaper or napkin rash
Ammonia dermatitis
Diaper or napkin:
dermatitis
erythema
rash
Psoriasiform napkin eruption

691.8 Other atopic dermatitis and related conditions
Atopic dermatitis
Besnier's prurigo
Eczema:
atopic
flexural
infantile (acute) (chronic)
intrinsic (allergic)
Neurodermatitis:
atopic
diffuse (of Brocq)

692 Contact dermatitis and other eczema

Includes:
dermatitis:
NOS
contact
occupational
venenata
eczema (acute) (chronic):
NOS
allergic
erythematous
occupational

Excludes: *allergy NOS (995.3)*
contact dermatitis of eyelids (373.32)
dermatitis due to substances taken internally (693.0-693.9)
eczema of external ear (380.22)
perioral dermatitis (695.3)
urticarial reactions (708.0-708.9, 995.1)

692.0 Due to detergents

692.1 Due to oils and greases

692.2 Due to solvents
Dermatitis due to solvents of:
chlorocompound
cyclohexane
ester
glycol
hydrocarbon
ketone
} group

692.3 Due to drugs and medicines in contact with skin
Dermatitis (allergic) (contact) due to:
arnica
fungicides
iodine
keratolytics
mercurials
neomycin
pediculocides
phenols
scabicides
any drug applied to skin
Dermatitis medicamentosa due to drug applied to skin

● Code new to this edition
▲ Revision of existing code
④ ⑤ Fourth or fifth digit required

Use additional E code, if desired, to identify drug

Excludes: *allergy NOS due to drugs (995.2)*
dermatitis due to ingested drugs (693.0)
dermatitis medicamentosa NOS (693.0)

692.4 Due to other chemical products

Dermatitis due to:
- acids
- adhesive plaster
- alkalis
- caustics
- dichromate
- insecticide
- nylon
- plastic
- rubber

692.5 Due to food in contact with skin

Dermatitis, contact, due to:
- cereals
- fish
- flour
- fruit
- meat
- milk

Excludes: *dermatitis due to:*
dyes (692.89)
ingested foods (693.1)
preservatives (692.89)

692.6 Due to plants [except food]

Dermatitis due to:
- lacquer tree [Rhus verniciflua]
- poison:
  - ivy [Rhus toxicodendron]
  - oak [Rhus diversiloba]
  - sumac [Rhus venenata]
  - vine [Rhus radicans]
- primrose [Primula]
- ragweed [Senecio jacobae]
- other plants in contact with the skin

Excludes: *allergy NOS due to pollen (477.0)*
nettle rash (708.8)

692.7 Due to solar radiation

692.70 Unspecified dermatitis due to sun

692.71 Sunburn

692.72 Acute dermatitis due to solar radiation

Berloque dermatitis
Photoallergic response
Phototoxic response
Polymorphus light eruption
Acute solar skin damage NOS

Excludes: *sunburn (692.71)*

Use additional E code, if desired, to identify drug, if drug induced

692.73 Actinic reticuloid and actinic granuloma

692.74 Other chronic dermatitis due to solar radiation

solar elastosis
chronic solar skin damage NOS

Excludes: *actinic [solar] keratosis (702.0)*

692.79 Other dermatitis due to solar radiation

Hydroa aestivale
Photodermatitis } (due to sun)
Photosensitiveness } (due to sun)
Solar skin damage NOS

692.8 Due to other specified agents

692.81 Dermatitis due to cosmetics

692.82 Dermatitis due to other radiation

infrared rays
light, except from sun
radiation NOS
ultraviolet rays, except from sun
x-rays

continued

Add 4th or 5th digit | Nonspecific code | Unspecified code | Manifestation code

Excludes: *that due to solar radiation (692.70-692.79)*

692.83 Dermatitis due to metals
jewelry

692.89 Other
Dermatitis due to:
cold weather
dyes
furs
hot weather
preservatives

Excludes: *allergy NOS due to animal hair, dander (animal), or dust (477.8)*
sunburn (692.71)

692.9 Unspecified cause
Dermatitis:
NOS
contact NOS
venenata NOS
Eczema NOS

693 Dermatitis due to substances taken internally

Excludes: *adverse effect NOS of drugs and medicines (995.2)*
allergy NOS (995.3)
contact dermatitis (692.0-692.9)
urticarial reactions (708.0-708.9, 995.1)

693.0 Due to drugs and medicines
Dermatitis medicamentosa NOS

Use additional E code, if desired, to identify drug

Excludes: *that due to drugs in contact with skin (692.3)*

693.1 Due to food

693.8 Due to other specified substances taken internally

693.9 Due to unspecified substance taken internally

Excludes: *dermatitis NOS (692.9)*

694 Bullous dermatoses

694.0 Dermatitis herpetiformis
Dermatosis herpetiformis
Duhring's disease
Hydroa herpetiformis

Excludes: *herpes gestationis (646.8)*
dermatitis herpetiformis:
juvenile (694.2)
senile (694.5)

694.1 Subcorneal pustular dermatosis
Sneddon-Wilkinson disease or syndrome

694.2 Juvenile dermatitis herpetiformis
Juvenile pemphigoid

694.3 Impetigo herpetiformis

694.4 Pemphigus
Pemphigus:
NOS
erythematosus
foliaceus
Pemphigus:
malignant
vegetans
vulgaris

Excludes: *pemphigus neonatorum (684)*

694.5 Pemphigoid
Benign pemphigus NOS
Bullous pemphigoid
Herpes circinatus bullosus
Senile dermatitis herpetiformis

694.6 Benign mucous membrane pemphigoid
Cicatricial pemphigoid
Mucosynechial atrophic bullous dermatitis

694.60 Without mention of ocular involvement

● Code new to this edition
▲ Revision of existing code
④ ⑤ Fourth or fifth digit required

694.61 With ocular involvement
Ocular pemphigus

694.8 Other specified bullous dermatoses
Excludes: *herpes gestationis (646.8)*

694.9 Unspecified bullous dermatoses

695 Erythematous conditions

695.0 Toxic erythema
Erythema venenatum

695.1 Erythema multiforme
Erythema iris
Herpes iris
Lyell's syndrome
Scalded skin syndrome
Stevens-Johnson syndrome
Toxic epidermal necrolysis

695.2 Erythema nodosum
Excludes: *tuberculous erythema nodosum (017.1)*

695.3 Rosacea
Acne:
erythematosa
rosacea
Perioral dermatitis
Rhinophyma

695.4 Lupus erythematosus
Lupus:
erythematodes (discoid)
erythematosus (discoid), not disseminated
Excludes: *lupus (vulgaris) NOS (017.0)*
systemic [disseminated] lupus erythematosus (710.0)

695.8 Other specified erythematous conditions

695.81 Ritter's disease
Dermatitis exfoliativa neonatorum

695.89 Other
Erythema intertrigo
Intertrigo
Pityriasis rubra (Hebra)
Excludes: *mycotic intertrigo (111.0-111.9)*

695.9 Unspecified erythematous condition
Erythema NOS
Erythroderma (secondary)

696 Psoriasis and similar disorders

696.0 Psoriatic arthropathy

696.1 Other psoriasis
Acrodermatitis continua
Dermatitis repens
Psoriasis:
NOS
any type, except arthropathic
Excludes: *psoriatic arthropathy (696.0)*

696.2 Parapsoriasis
Parakeratosis variegata
Parapsoriasis lichenoides chronica
Pityriasis lichenoides et varioliformis

696.3 Pityriasis rosea
Pityriasis circinata (et maculata)

696.4 Pityriasis rubra pilaris
Devergie's disease
Lichen ruber acuminatus
Excludes: *pityriasis rubra (Hebra) (695.89)*

696.5 Other and unspecified pityriasis
Pityriasis:
NOS
alba
streptogenes
Excludes: *pityriasis:*

continued

simplex (690.18)
versicolor (111.0)

696.8 Other

697 Lichen

Excludes: *lichen:*
obtusus corneus (698.3)
pilaris (congenital) (757.39)
ruber acuminatus (696.4)
sclerosus et atrophicus (701.0)
scrofulosus (017.0)
simplex chronicus (698.3)
spinulosus (congenital) (757.39)
urticatus (698.2)

697.0 Lichen planus
Lichen:
planopilaris
ruber planus

697.1 Lichen nitidus
Pinkus' disease

697.8 Other lichen, not elsewhere classified
Lichen:
ruber moniliforme
striata

697.9 Lichen, unspecified

698 Pruritus and related conditions

Excludes: *pruritus specified as psychogenic (306.3)*

698.0 Pruritus ani
Perianal itch

698.1 Pruritus of genital organs

698.2 Prurigo
Lichen urticatus
Prurigo:
NOS
Hebra's
mitis
simplex
Urticaria papulosa (Hebra)

Excludes: *prurigo nodularis (698.3)*

698.3 Lichenification and lichen simplex chronicus
Hyde's disease
Neurodermatitis (circumscripta) (local)
Prurigo nodularis

Excludes: *neurodermatitis, diffuse (of Brocq) (691.8)*

698.4 Dermatitis factitia [artefacta]
Dermatitis ficta
Neurotic excoriation

Use additional code, if desired, to identify any associated mental disorder

698.8 Other specified pruritic conditions
Pruritus:
hiemalis
senilis
Winter itch

698.9 Unspecified pruritic disorder
Itch NOS
Pruritus NOS

OTHER DISEASES OF SKIN AND SUBCUTANEOUS TISSUE (700-709)

Excludes: *conditions confined to eyelids (373.0-374.9)*
congenital conditions of skin, hair, and nails (757.0-757.9)

700 Corns and callosities
Callus
Clavus

701 Other hypertrophic and atrophic conditions of skin

Excludes: *dermatomyositis (710.3)*
hereditary edema of legs (757.0)

continued

scleroderma (generalized) (710.1)

701.0 Circumscribed scleroderma
Addison's keloid
Dermatosclerosis, localized
Lichen sclerosus et atrophicus
Morphea
Scleroderma, circumscribed or localized

701.1 Keratoderma, acquired
Acquired:
ichthyosis
keratoderma palmaris et plantaris
Elastosis perforans serpiginosa
Hyperkeratosis:
NOS
follicularis in cutem penetrans
palmoplantaris climacterica
Keratoderma:
climactericum
tylodes, progressive
Keratosis (blennorrhagica)

Excludes: *Darier's disease [keratosis follicularis] (congenital) (757.39)*
keratosis:
arsenical (692.4)
gonococcal (098.81)

701.2 Acquired acanthosis nigricans
Keratosis nigricans

701.3 Striae atrophicae
Atrophic spots of skin
Atrophoderma maculatum
Atrophy blanche (of Milian)
Degenerative colloid atrophy
Senile degenerative atrophy
Striae distensae

701.4 Keloid scar
Cheloid
Hypertrophic scar
Keloid

701.5 Other abnormal granulation tissue
Excessive granulation

701.8 Other specified hypertrophic and atrophic conditions of skin
Acrodermatitis atrophicans chronica
Atrophia cutis senilis
Atrophoderma neuriticum
Confluent and reticulate papillomatosis
Cutis laxa senilis
Elastosis senilis
Folliculitis ulerythematosa reticulata
Gougerot-Carteaud syndrome or disease

701.9 Unspecified hypertrophic and atrophic conditions of skin
Atrophoderma

702 Other dermatoses

Excludes: *carcinoma in situ (232.0-232.9)*

702.0 Actinic keratosis

702.1 Seborrheic keratosis

702.11 Inflamed seborrheic keratosis

702.19 Other seborrheic keratosis
Seborrheic keratosis NOS

702.8 Other specified dermatoses

703 Diseases of nail

Excludes: *congenital anomalies (757.5)*
onychia and paronychia (681.02, 681.11)

Add 4th or 5th digit
Nonspecific code
Unspecified code
Manifestation code

703.0 Ingrowing nail
Ingrowing nail with infection
Unguis incarnatus

Excludes: *infection, nail NOS (681.9)*

703.8 Other specified diseases of nail
Dystrophia unguium
Hypertrophy of nail
Koilonychia
Leukonychia (punctata) (striata)
Onychauxis
Onychogryposis
Onycholysis

703.9 Unspecified disease of nail

704 Diseases of hair and hair follicles

Excludes: *congenital anomalies (757.4)*

704.0 Alopecia

Excludes: *madarosis (374.55)*
syphilitic alopecia (091.82)

704.00 Alopecia, unspecified
Baldness
Loss of hair

704.01 Alopecia areata
Ophiasis

704.02 Telogen effluvim

704.09 Other
Folliculitis decalvans
Hypotrichosis:
NOS
postinfectional NOS
Pseudopelade

704.1 Hirsutism
Hypertrichosis:
NOS
lanuginosa, acquired
Polytrichia

Excludes: *hypertrichosis of eyelid (374.54)*

704.2 Abnormalities of the hair
Atrophic hair
Clastothrix
Fragilitas crinium
Trichiasis:
NOS
cicatrical
Trichorrhexis (nodosa)

Excludes: *trichiasis of eyelid (374.05)*

704.3 Variations in hair color
Canities (premature)
Grayness, hair (premature)
Heterochromia of hair
Poliosis:
NOS
circumscripta, acquired

704.8 Other specified diseases of hair and hair follicles
Folliculitis:
NOS
abscedens et suffodiens
pustular
Perifolliculitis:
NOS
capitis abscedens et suffodiens
scalp
Sycosis:
NOS
barbae [not parasitic]
lupoid
vulgaris

704.9 Unspecified disease of hair and hair follicles

705 Disorders of sweat glands

705.0 Anhidrosis
Hypohidrosis
Oligohidrosis

705.1 Prickly heat
Heat rash
Miliaria rubra (tropicalis)
Sudamina

705.8 Other specified disorders of sweat glands

705.81 Dyshidrosis
Cheiropompholyx
Pompholyx

705.82 Fox-Fordyce disease

705.83 Hidradenitis
Hidradenitis suppurativa

705.89 Other
Bromhidrosis
Chromhidrosis
Granulosis rubra nasi
Urhidrosis

Excludes: *hidrocystoma (216.0-216.9)*
hyperhidrosis (780.8)

705.9 Unspecified disorder of sweat glands
Disorder of sweat glands NOS

706 Diseases of sebaceous glands

706.0 Acne varioliformis
Acne:
frontalis
necrotica

706.1 Other acne
Acne:
NOS
conglobata
cystic
pustular
vulgaris
Blackhead
Comedo

Excludes: *acne rosacea (695.3)*

706.2 Sebaceous cyst
Atheroma, skin
Keratin cyst
Wen

706.3 Seborrhea

Excludes: *seborrhea:*
capitis (704.8)
sicca (690)
seborrheic keratosis (702)

706.8 Other specified diseases of sebaceous glands
Asteatosis (cutis)
Xerosis cutis

706.9 Unspecified disease of sebaceous glands

707 Chronic ulcer of skin

Excludes: *skin infections (680.0-686.9)*
specific infections classified under "Infectious and Parasitic Diseases" (001.0-136.9)
varicose ulcer (454.0, 454.2)

707.0 Decubitus ulcer
Bed sore
Decubitus ulcer [any site]
Plaster ulcer
Pressure ulcer

707.1 Ulcer of lower limbs, except decubitus
Ulcer, chronic:
neurogenic } of lower limb
trophic } of lower limb

Excludes: *that with atherosclerosis of the extremities (440.23)*

707.8 Chronic ulcer of other specified sites
Ulcer, chronic: } of other specified sites
neurogenic } of other specified sites
trophic

707.9 Chronic ulcer of unspecified site
Chronic ulcer NOS
Trophic ulcer NOS
Tropical ulcer NOS
Ulcer of skin NOS

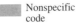

Add 4th or 5th digit | Nonspecific code | Unspecified code | Manifestation code

708 Urticaria

Excludes: *edema:*
angioneurotic (995.1)
Quincke's (995.1)
hereditary angioedema (277.6)
urticaria:
giant (995.1)
papulosa (Hebra) (698.2)
pigmentosa (juvenile) (congenital) (757.33)

708.0 Allergic urticaria

708.1 Idiopathic urticaria

708.2 Urticaria due to cold and heat
Thermal urticaria

708.3 Dermatographic urticaria
Dermatographia
Factitial urticaria

708.4 Vibratory urticaria

708.5 Cholinergic urticaria

708.8 Other specified urticaria
Nettle rash
Urticaria:
chronic
recurrent periodic

708.9 Urticaria, unspecified
Hives NOS

709 Other disorders of skin and subcutaneous tissue

709.0 Dyschromia

709.00 Dyschromia, unspecified

709.01 Vitiligo

709.09 Other

Excludes: *albinism (270.2)*
pigmented nevus (216.0-216.9)
that of eyelid (374.52-374.53)

709.1 Vascular disorders of skin
Angioma serpiginosum
Purpura (primary) annularis telangiectodes

709.2 Scar conditions and fibrosis of skin
Adherent scar (skin)
Cicatrix
Disfigurement (due to scar)
Fibrosis, skin NOS
Scar NOS

Excludes: *keloid scar (701.4)*

709.3 Degenerative skin disorders
Calcinosis:
circumscripta
cutis
Colloid milium
Degeneration, skin
Deposits, skin
Senile dermatosis NOS
Subcutaneous calcification

709.4 Foreign body granuloma of skin and subcutaneous tissue

Excludes: *that of muscle (728.82)*

709.8 Other specified disorders of skin
Epithelial hyperplasia
Menstrual dermatosis
Vesicular eruption

709.9 Unspecified disorder of skin and subcutaneous tissue
Dermatosis NOS

● Code new to this edition
▲ Revision of existing code
④ ⑤ Fourth or fifth digit required

13. DISEASES OF THE MUSCULOSKELETAL SYSTEM AND CONNECTIVE TISSUE (710-739)

The following fifth-digit subclassification is for use with categories 711-712, 715-716, 718-719, and 730:

0 site unspecified

1 shoulder region
Acromioclavicular joint(s)
Glenohumeral joint(s)
Sternoclavicular joint(s)
Clavicle
Scapula

2 upper arm
Elbow joint
Humerus

3 forearm
Radius
Ulna
Wrist joint

4 hand
Carpus
Metacarpus
Phalanges [fingers]

5 pelvic region and thigh
Buttock
Femur
Hip (joint)

6 lower leg
Fibula
Knee joint
Patella
Tibia

7 ankle and foot
Ankle joint
Digits [toes]
Metatarsus
Phalanges, foot
Tarsus
Other joints in foot

8 other specified sites
Head
Neck
Ribs
Skull
Trunk
Vertebral column

9 multiple sites

ARTHROPATHIES AND RELATED DISORDERS (710-719)

Excludes: *disorders of spine (720.0-724.9)*

710 Diffuse diseases of connective tissue

Includes: all collagen diseases whose effects are not mainly confined to a single system

Use additional code, if desired, to identify manifestation, as:
lung involvement (517.8)
myopathy (359.6)

Excludes: *those affecting mainly the cardiovascular system, i.e., polyarteritis nodosa and allied conditions (446.0-446.7)*

710.0 Systemic lupus erythematosus
Disseminated lupus erythematosus
Libman-Sacks disease

Use additional code, if desired, to identify manifestation, as:
endocarditis (424.91)
nephritis (583.81)
chronic (582.81)
nephrotic syndrome (581.81)

Excludes: *lupus erythematosus (discoid) NOS (695.4)*

710.1 Systemic sclerosis
Acrosclerosis
CRST syndrome
Progressive systemic sclerosis
Scleroderma

Excludes: *circumscribed scleroderma (701.0)*

710.2 Sicca syndrome
Keratoconjunctivitis sicca
Sjögren's disease

710.3 Dermatomyositis
Poikilodermatomyositis
Polymyositis with skin involvement

710.4 Polymyositis

710.5 Eosinophilia myalgia syndrome
Toxic oil syndrome

Use additional E code, if desired, to identify drug, if drug induced

710.8 Other specified diffuse diseases of connective tissue
Multifocal fibrosclerosis (idiopathic) NEC
Systemic fibrosclerosing syndrome

710.9 Unspecified diffuse connective tissue disease
Collagen disease NOS

⑤ **711 Arthropathy associated with infections**

Includes:

arthritis arthropathy polyarthritis polyarthropathy	associated with conditions classifiable below

Excludes: *rheumatic fever (390)*

The following fifth-digit subclassification is for use with category 711; valid digits are in [brackets] under each code. For definitions, see the beginning of this chapter:

- **0 site unspecified**
- **1 shoulder region**
- **2 upper arm**
- **3 forearm**
- **4 hand**
- **5 pelvic region and thigh**
- **6 lower leg**
- **7 ankle and foot**
- **8 other specified sites**
- **9 multiple sites**

711.0 Pyogenic arthritis
[0-9]
Arthritis or polyarthritis (due to):
coliform [Escherichia coli]
Hemophilus influenzae [H. influenzae]
pneumococcal
Pseudomonas
staphylococcal
streptococcal
Pyarthrosis

Use additional code, if desired, to identify infectious organism (041.0-041.8)

711.1 Arthropathy associated with Reiter's disease and nonspecific urethritis
[0-9]
Code first underlying disease, as:
nonspecific urethritis (099.4)
Reiter's disease (099.3)

711.2 Arthropathy in Behçet's syndrome
[0-9]
Code first underlying disease (136.1)

711.3 Postdysenteric arthropathy
[0-9]
Code first underlying disease, as:
dysentery (009.0)
enteritis, infectious (008.0-009.3)
paratyphoid fever (002.1-002.9)
typhoid fever (002.0)

Excludes: *salmonella arthritis (003.23)*

● Code new to this edition ▲ Revision of existing code ④ ⑤ Fourth or fifth digit required

711.4 ***Arthropathy associated with other bacterial diseases***
[0-9] *Code first underlying disease, as:*
diseases classifiable to 010-040, 090-099, except as in 711.1, 711.3, and 713.5
leprosy (030.0-030.9)
tuberculosis (015.0-015.9)

Excludes: *gonococcal arthritis (098.50)*
meningococcal arthritis (036.82)

711.5 ***Arthropathy associated with other viral diseases***
[0-9] *Code first underlying disease, as:*
diseases classifiable to 045-049, 050-079, 480, 487
O'nyong nyong (066.3)

Excludes: *that due to rubella (056.71)*

711.6 ***Arthropathy associated with mycoses***
[0-9] *Code first underlying disease (110.0-118)*

711.7 ***Arthropathy associated with helminthiasis***
[0-9] *Code first underlying disease, as:*
filariasis (125.0-125.9)

711.8 ***Arthropathy associated with other infectious and parasitic diseases***
[0-9] *Code first underlying disease, as:*
diseases classifiable to 080-088, 100-104, 130-136

Excludes: *arthropathy associated with sarcoidosis (713.7)*

711.9 **Unspecified infective arthritis**
[0-9] Infective arthritis or polyarthritis (acute) (chronic) (subacute) NOS

⑤ **712** **Crystal arthropathies**
Includes: crystal-induced arthritis and synovitis

Excludes: *gouty arthropathy (274.0)*

The following fifth-digit subclassification is for use with category 712; valid digits are in [brackets] under each code. See beginning of this chapter for definitions:

0 **site unspecified**
1 **shoulder region**
2 **upper arm**
3 **forearm**
4 **hand**
5 **pelvic region and thigh**
6 **lower leg**
7 **ankle and foot**
8 **other specified sites**
9 **multiple sites**

712.1 ***Chondrocalcinosis due to dicalcium phosphate crystals***
[0-9] Chondrocalcinosis due to dicalcium phosphate crystals (with other crystals)
Code first underlying disease (275.4)

712.2 ***Chondrocalcinosis due to pyrophosphate crystals***
[0-9] *Code first underlying disease (275.4)*

712.3 ***Chondrocalcinosis, unspecified***
[0-9] *Code first underlying disease (275.4)*

712.8 **Other specified crystal arthropathies**
[0-9]

712.9 **Unspecified crystal arthropathy**
[0-9]

713 Arthropathy associated with other disorders classified elsewhere

Includes:

arthritis arthropathy polyarthritis polyarthropathy	associated with conditions classifiable below

713.0 Arthropathy associated with other endocrine and metabolic disorders

Code first underlying disease, as:

acromegaly (253.0)
hemochromatosis (275.0)
hyperparathyroidism (252.0)
hypogammaglobulinemia (279.00-279.09)
hypothyroidism (243-244.9)
lipoid metabolism disorder (272.0-272.9)
ochronosis (270.2)

Excludes: *arthropathy associated with:*
amyloidosis (713.7)
crystal deposition disorders, except gout (712.1-712.9)
diabetic neuropathy (713.5)
gouty arthropathy (274.0)

713.1 Arthropathy associated with gastrointestinal conditions other than infections

Code first underlying disease, as:

regional enteritis (555.0-555.9)
ulcerative colitis (556)

713.2 Arthropathy associated with hematological disorders

Code first underlying disease, as:

hemoglobinopathy (282.4-282.7)
hemophilia (286.0-286.2)
leukemia (204.0-208.9)
malignant reticulosis (202.3)
multiple myelomatosis (203.0)

Excludes: *arthropathy associated with Henoch-Schönlein purpura (713.6)*

713.3 Arthropathy associated with dermatological disorders

Code first underlying disease, as:

erythema multiforme (695.1)
erythema nodosum (695.2)

Excludes: *psoriatic arthropathy (696.0)*

713.4 Arthropathy associated with respiratory disorders

Code first underlying disease, as:

diseases classifiable to 490-519

Excludes: *arthropathy associated with respiratory infections (711.0, 711.4-711.8)*

713.5 Arthropathy associated with neurological disorders

Charcot's arthropathy Neuropathic arthritis	associated with diseases classifiable elsewhere

Code first underlying disease, as:

neuropathic joint disease [Charcot's joints]:
NOS (094.0)
diabetic (250.6)
syringomyelic (336.0)
tabetic [syphilitic] (094.0)

713.6 Arthropathy associated with hypersensitivity reaction

Code first underlying disease, as:

Henoch (-Schönlein) purpura (287.0)
serum sickness (999.5)

Excludes: *allergic arthritis NOS (716.2)*

713.7 Other general diseases with articular involvement

Code first underlying disease, as:

amyloidosis (277.3)
familial Mediterranean fever (277.3)
sarcoidosis (135)

● Code new to this edition
▲ Revision of existing code
④ ⑤ Fourth or fifth digit required

713.8 ***Arthropathy associated with other conditions classifiable elsewhere***
Code first underlying disease, as:
conditions classifiable elsewhere except as in 711.1-711.8, 712, and 713.0-713.7

714 Rheumatoid arthritis and other inflammatory polyarthropathies

Excludes: *rheumatic fever (390)*
rheumatoid arthritis of spine NOS (720.0)

714.0 Rheumatoid arthritis
Arthritis or polyarthritis:
atrophic
rheumatic (chronic)

Use additional code, if desired, to identify manifestation, as:
myopathy (359.6)
polyneuropathy (357.1)

Excludes: *juvenile rheumatoid arthritis NOS (714.30)*

714.1 Felty's syndrome
Rheumatoid arthritis with splenoadenomegaly and leukopenia

714.2 Other rheumatoid arthritis with visceral or systemic involvement
Rheumatoid carditis

714.3 Juvenile chronic polyarthritis

714.30 Polyarticular juvenile rheumatoid arthritis, chronic or unspecified
Juvenile rheumatoid arthritis NOS
Still's disease

714.31 Polyarticular juvenile rheumatoid arthritis, acute

714.32 Pauciarticular juvenile rheumatoid arthritis

714.33 Monoarticular juvenile rheumatoid arthritis

714.4 Chronic postrheumatic arthropathy
Chronic rheumatoid nodular fibrositis
Jaccoud's syndrome

714.8 Other specified inflammatory polyarthropathies

714.81 Rheumatoid lung
Caplan's syndrome
Diffuse interstitial rheumatoid disease of lung
Fibrosing alveolitis, rheumatoid

714.89 Other

714.9 Unspecified inflammatory polyarthropathy
Inflammatory polyarthropathy or polyarthritis NOS

Excludes: *polyarthropathy NOS (716.5)*

⑤ 715 Osteoarthrosis and allied disorders

Note: Localized, in the subcategories below, includes bilateral involvement of the same site.
Includes: arthritis or polyarthritis:
degenerative
hypertrophic
degenerative joint disease
osteoarthritis

Excludes: *Marie-Strümpell spondylitis (720.0)*
osteoarthrosis [osteoarthritis] of spine (721.0-721.9)

The following fifth-digit subclassification is for use with category 715; valid digits are in [brackets] under each code. See beginning of this chapter for definitions:

0 site unspecified
1 shoulder region
2 upper arm
3 forearm
4 hand
5 pelvic region and thigh
6 lower leg
7 ankle and foot
8 other specified sites
9 multiple sites

Add 4th or 5th digit | Nonspecific code | Unspecified code | Manifestation code

715.0 Osteoarthrosis, generalized
[0,4,9] Degenerative joint disease, involving multiple joints
Primary generalized hypertrophic osteoarthrosis

715.1 Osteoarthrosis, localized, primary
[0-8] Localized osteoarthropathy, idiopathic

715.2 Osteoarthrosis, localized, secondary
[0-8] Coxae malum senilis

715.3 Osteoarthrosis, localized, not specified whether primary or secondary
[0-8] Otto's pelvis

715.8 Osteoarthrosis involving, or with mention of more than one site, but not specified as generalized
[0,9]

715.9 Osteoarthrosis, unspecified whether generalized or localized
[0-8]

⑤ **716 Other and unspecified arthropathies**

Excludes: *cricoarytenoid arthropathy (478.79)*

The following fifth-digit subclassification is for use with category 716; valid digits are in [brackets] under each code. See beginning of this chapter for definitions:

0 site unspecified

1 shoulder region

2 upper arm

3 forearm

4 hand

5 pelvic region and thigh

6 lower leg

7 ankle and foot

8 other specified sites

9 multiple sites

716.0 Kaschin-Beck disease
[0-9] Endemic polyarthritis

716.1 Traumatic arthropathy
[0-9]

716.2 Allergic arthritis
[0-9]

Excludes: *arthritis associated with Henoch-Schönlein purpura or serum sickness (713.6)*

716.3 Climacteric arthritis
[0-9] Menopausal arthritis

716.4 Transient arthropathy
[0-9]

Excludes: *palindromic rheumatism (719.3)*

716.5 Unspecified polyarthropathy or polyarthritis
[0-9]

716.6 Unspecified monoarthritis
[0-8] Coxitis

716.8 Other specified arthropathy
[0-9]

716.9 Arthropathy, unspecified
[0-9] Arthritis } (acute) (chronic) (subacute)
Arthropathy } (acute) (chronic) (subacute)
Articular rheumatism (chronic)
Inflammation of joint NOS

717 Internal derangement of knee

Includes:

degeneration rupture, old tear, old	of articular cartilage or meniscus of knee

Excludes: *acute derangement of knee (836.0-836.6)*
ankylosis (718.5)
contracture (718.4)
current injury (836.0-836.6)
deformity (736.4-736.6)
recurrent dislocation (718.3)

717.0 Old bucket handle tear of medial meniscus
Old bucket handle tear of unspecified cartilage

717.1 Derangement of anterior horn of medial meniscus

717.2 Derangement of posterior horn of medial meniscus

717.3 Other and unspecified derangement of medial meniscus
Degeneration of internal semilunar cartilage

717.4 Derangement of lateral meniscus

717.40 Derangement of lateral meniscus, unspecified

717.41 Bucket handle tear of lateral meniscus

717.42 Derangement of anterior horn of lateral meniscus

717.43 Derangement of posterior horn of lateral meniscus

717.49 Other

717.5 Derangement of meniscus, not elsewhere classified
Congenital discoid meniscus
Cyst of semilunar cartilage
Derangement of semilunar cartilage NOS

717.6 Loose body in knee
Joint mice, knee
Rice bodies, knee (joint)

717.7 Chondromalacia of patella
Chondromalacia patellae
Degeneration [softening] of articular cartilage of patella

717.8 Other internal derangement of knee

717.81 Old disruption of lateral collateral ligament

717.82 Old disruption of medial collateral ligament

717.83 Old disruption of anterior cruciate ligament

717.84 Old disruption of posterior cruciate ligament

717.85 Old disruption of other ligaments of knee
Capsular ligament of knee

717.89 Other
Old disruption of ligaments of knee NOS

717.9 Unspecified internal derangement of knee
Derangement NOS of knee

⑤ **718 Other derangement of joint**

Excludes: *current injury (830.0-848.9)*
jaw (524.6)

The following fifth-digit subclassification is for use with category 718; valid digits are in [brackets] under each code. See beginning of this chapter for definitions:

0 site unspecified
1 shoulder region
2 upper arm
3 forearm
4 hand
5 pelvic region and thigh
6 lower leg
7 ankle and foot

continued

8 other specified sites

9 multiple sites

718.0 Articular cartilage disorder
[0-5, 7-9] Meniscus:
disorder
rupture, old
tear, old
Old rupture of ligament(s) of joint NOS

Excludes: *articular cartilage disorder:*
in ochronosis (270.2)
knee (717.0-717.9)
chondrocalcinosis (275.4)
metastatic calcification (275.4)

718.1 Loose body in joint
[0-5, 7-9] Joint mice

Excludes: *knee (717.6)*

718.2 Pathological dislocation
[0-9] Dislocation or displacement of joint, not recurrent and not current injury
Spontaneous dislocation (joint)

718.3 Recurrent dislocation of joint
[0-9]

718.4 Contracture of joint
[0-9]

718.5 Ankylosis of joint
[0-9] Ankylosis of joint (fibrous) (osseous)

Excludes: *spine (724.9)*
stiffness of joint without mention of ankylosis (719.5)

718.6 Unspecified intrapelvic protrusion of acetabulum
[0, 5] Protrusio acetabuli, unspecified

718.8 Other joint derangement, not elsewhere classified
[0-9] Flail joint (paralytic) Instability of joint

Excludes: *deformities classifiable to 736 (736.0-736.9)*

718.9 Unspecified derangement of joint
[0-5, 7-9]

Excludes: *knee (717.9)*

⑤ **719 Other and unspecified disorders of joint**

Excludes: *jaw (524.6)*

The following fifth-digit subclassification is for use with category 719; valid digits are in [brackets] under each code. See beginning of this chapter for definitions:

0 site unspecified

1 shoulder region

2 upper arm

3 forearm

4 hand

5 pelvic region and thigh

6 lower leg

7 ankle and foot

8 other specified sites

9 multiple sites

719.0 Effusion of joint
[0-9] Hydrarthrosis
Swelling of joint, with or without pain

Excludes: *intermittent hydrarthrosis (719.3)*

719.1 Hemarthrosis
[0-9]

Excludes: *current injury (840.0-848.9)*

719.2 Villonodular synovitis
[0-9]

719.3 Palindromic rheumatism
[0-9] Hench-Rosenberg syndrome
Intermittent hydrarthrosis

719.4 Pain in joint
[0-9] Arthralgia

719.5 Stiffness of joint, not elsewhere classified
[0-9]

719.6 Other symptoms referable to joint
[0-9] Joint crepitus
Snapping hip

719.7 Difficulty in walking
[0, 5-9]

Excludes: *abnormality of gait (781.2)*

719.8 Other specified disorders of joint
[0-9] Calcification of joint
Fistula of joint

Excludes: *temporomandibular joint-pain-dysfunction syndrome [Costen's syndrome] (524.6)*

719.9 Unspecified disorder of joint
[0-9]

DORSOPATHIES (720-724)

Excludes: *curvature of spine (737.0-737.9)*
osteochondrosis of spine (juvenile) (732.0)
adult (732.8)

720 Ankylosing spondylitis and other inflammatory spondylopathies

720.0 Ankylosing spondylitis
Rheumatoid arthritis of spine NOS
Spondylitis:
Marie-Strümpell
rheumatoid

720.1 Spinal enthesopathy
Disorder of peripheral ligamentous or muscular attachments of spine
Romanus lesion

720.2 Sacroiliitis, not elsewhere classified
Inflammation of sacroiliac joint NOS

720.8 Other inflammatory spondylopathies

720.81 Inflammatory spondylopathies in diseases classified elsewhere
Code first underlying disease, as:
tuberculosis (015.0)

720.89 Other

720.9 Unspecified inflammatory spondylopathy
Spondylitis NOS

721 Spondylosis and allied disorders

721.0 Cervical spondylosis without myelopathy
Cervical or cervicodorsal:
arthritis
osteoarthritis
spondylarthritis

721.1 Cervical spondylosis with myelopathy
Anterior spinal artery compression syndrome
Spondylogenic compression of cervical spinal cord
Vertebral artery compression syndrome

721.2 Thoracic spondylosis without myelopathy
Thoracic:
arthritis
osteoarthritis
spondylarthritis

721.3 Lumbosacral spondylosis without myelopathy
Lumbar or lumbosacral:
arthritis
osteoarthritis
spondylarthritis

721.4 Thoracic or lumbar spondylosis with myelopathy

721.41 Thoracic region
Spondylogenic compression of thoracic spinal cord

721.42 Lumbar region
Spondylogenic compression of lumbar spinal cord

721.5 Kissing spine
Baastrup's syndrome

721.6 Ankylosing vertebral hyperostosis

721.7 Traumatic spondylopathy
Kümmell's disease or spondylitis

721.8 Other allied disorders of spine

721.9 Spondylosis of unspecified site

721.90 Without mention of myelopathy
Spinal:
arthritis (deformans) (degenerative) (hypertrophic)
osteoarthritis NOS
Spondylarthrosis NOS

721.91 With myelopathy
Spondylogenic compression of spinal cord NOS

722 Intervertebral disc disorders

722.0 Displacement of cervical intervertebral disc without myelopathy
Neuritis (brachial) or radiculitis due to displacement or rupture of cervical intervertebral disc
Any condition classifiable to 722.2 of the cervical or cervicothoracic intervertebral disc

722.1 Displacement of thoracic or lumbar intervertebral disc without myelopathy

722.10 Lumbar intervertebral disc without myelopathy
Lumbago or sciatica due to displacement of intervertebral disc
Neuritis or radiculitis due to displacement or rupture of lumbar intervertebral disc
Any condition classifiable to 722.2 of the lumbar or lumbosacral intervertebral disc

722.11 Thoracic intervertebral disc without myelopathy
Any condition classifiable to 722.2 of thoracic intervertebral disc

722.2 Displacement of intervertebral disc, site unspecified, without myelopathy
Discogenic syndrome NOS
Herniation of nucleus pulposus NOS
Intervertebral disc NOS:
extrusion
prolapse
protrusion
rupture
Neuritis or radiculitis due to displacement or rupture of intervertebral disc

722.3 Schmorl's nodes

722.30 Unspecified region

722.31 Thoracic region

722.32 Lumbar region

722.39 Other

722.4 Degeneration of cervical intervertebral disc
Degeneration of cervicothoracic intervertebral disc

722.5 Degeneration of thoracic or lumbar intervertebral disc

722.51 Thoracic or thoracolumbar intervertebral disc

722.52 Lumbar or lumbosacral intervertebral disc

722.6 Degeneration of intervertebral disc, site unspecified
Degenerative disc disease NOS
Narrowing of intervertebral disc or space NOS

722.7 Intervertebral disc disorder with myelopathy

722.70 Unspecified region

722.71 Cervical region

722.72 Thoracic region

722.73 Lumbar region

722.8 Postlaminectomy syndrome

722.80 Unspecified region

722.81 Cervical region

722.82 Thoracic region

722.83 Lumbar region

722.9 Other and unspecified disc disorder
Calcification of intervertebral cartilage or disc
Discitis

722.90 Unspecified region

722.91 Cervical region

722.92 Thoracic region

722.93 Lumbar region

723 Other disorders of cervical region

Excludes: *conditions due to:*
intervertebral disc disorders (722.0-722.9)
spondylosis (721.0-721.9)

723.0 Spinal stenosis in cervical region

723.1 Cervicalgia
Pain in neck

723.2 Cervicocranial syndrome
Barré-Liéou syndrome
Posterior cervical sympathetic syndrome

723.3 Cervicobrachial syndrome (diffuse)

723.4 Brachial neuritis or radiculitis NOS
Cervical radiculitis
Radicular syndrome of upper limbs

723.5 Torticollis, unspecified
Contracture of neck

Excludes: *congenital (754.1)*
due to birth injury (767.8)
hysterical (300.11)
psychogenic (306.0)
spasmodic (333.83)
traumatic, current (847.0)

723.6 Panniculitis specified as affecting neck

723.7 Ossification of posterior longitudinal ligament in cervical region

723.8 Other syndromes affecting cervical region
Cervical syndrome NEC Klippel's disease

723.9 Unspecified musculoskeletal disorders and symptoms referable to neck
Cervical (region) disorder NOS

724 Other and unspecified disorders of back

Excludes: *collapsed vertebra (code to cause, e.g., osteoporosis, 733.00-733.09)*
conditions due to:
intervertebral disc disorders (722.0-722.9)
spondylosis (721.0-721.9)

724.0 Spinal stenosis, other than cervical

724.00 Spinal stenosis, unspecified region

724.01 Thoracic region

724.02 Lumbar region

Add 4th or 5th digit | Nonspecific code | Unspecified code | Manifestation code

724.09 Other

724.1 Pain in thoracic spine

724.2 Lumbago
Low back pain
Low back syndrome
Lumbalgia

724.3 Sciatica
Neuralgia or neuritis of sciatic nerve

Excludes: *specified lesion of sciatic nerve (355.0)*

724.4 Thoracic or lumbosacral neuritis or radiculitis, unspecified
Radicular syndrome of lower limbs

724.5 Backache, unspecified
Vertebrogenic (pain) syndrome NOS

724.6 Disorders of sacrum
Ankylosis } lumbosacral or sacroiliac (joint)
Instability } lumbosacral or sacroiliac (joint)

724.7 Disorders of coccyx

724.70 Unspecified disorder of coccyx

724.71 Hypermobility of coccyx

724.79 Other
Coccygodynia

724.8 Other symptoms referable to back
Ossification of posterior longitudinal ligament NOS
Panniculitis specified as sacral or affecting back

724.9 Other unspecified back disorders
Ankylosis of spine NOS
Compression of spinal nerve root NEC
Spinal disorder NOS

Excludes: *sacroiliitis (720.2)*

RHEUMATISM, EXCLUDING THE BACK (725-729)

Includes: disorders of muscles and tendons and their attachments, and of other soft tissues

725 Polymyalgia rheumatica

726 Peripheral enthesopathies and allied syndromes
Note: Enthesopathies are disorders of peripheral ligamentous or muscular attachments.

Excludes: *spinal enthesopathy (720.1)*

726.0 Adhesive capsulitis of shoulder

726.1 Rotator cuff syndrome of shoulder and allied disorders

726.10 Disorders of bursae and tendons in shoulder region, unspecified
Rotator cuff syndrome NOS
Supraspinatus syndrome NOS

726.11 Calcifying tendinitis of shoulder

726.12 Bicipital tenosynovitis

726.19 Other specified disorders

Excludes: *complete rupture of rotator cuff, nontraumatic (727.61)*

726.2 Other affections of shoulder region, not elsewhere classified
Periarthritis of shoulder
Scapulohumeral fibrositis

726.3 Enthesopathy of elbow region

726.30 Enthesopathy of elbow, unspecified

726.31 Medial epicondylitis

726.32 Lateral epicondylitis
Epicondylitis NOS
Golfers' elbow
Tennis elbow

726.33 Olecranon bursitis
Bursitis of elbow

726.39 Other

726.4 Enthesopathy of wrist and carpus
Bursitis of hand or wrist
Periarthritis of wrist

726.5 Enthesopathy of hip region
Bursitis of hip
Gluteal tendinitis
Iliac crest spur
Psoas tendinitis
Trochanteric tendinitis

726.6 Enthesopathy of knee

726.60 Enthesopathy of knee, unspecified
Bursitis of knee NOS

726.61 Pes anserinus tendinitis or bursitis

726.62 Tibial collateral ligament bursitis
Pellegrini-Stieda syndrome

726.63 Fibular collateral ligament bursitis

726.64 Patellar tendinitis

726.65 Prepatellar bursitis

726.69 Other
Bursitis:
infrapatellar
subpatellar

726.7 Enthesopathy of ankle and tarsus

726.70 Enthesopathy of ankle and tarsus, unspecified
Metatarsalgia NOS

Excludes: Morton's metatarsalgia (355.6)

726.71 Achilles bursitis or tendinitis

726.72 Tibialis tendinitis
Tibialis (anterior) (posterior) tendinitis

726.73 Calcaneal spur

726.79 Other
Peroneal tendinitis

726.8 Other peripheral enthesopathies

726.9 Unspecified enthesopathy

726.90 Enthesopathy of unspecified site
Capsulitis NOS
Periarthritis NOS
Tendinitis NOS

726.91 Exostosis of unspecified site
Bone spur NOS

727 Other disorders of synovium, tendon, and bursa

727.0 Synovitis and tenosynovitis

727.00 Synovitis and tenosynovitis, unspecified
Synovitis NOS
Tenosynovitis NOS

727.01 Synovitis and tenosynovitis in diseases classified elsewhere
Code first underlying disease, as:
tuberculosis (015.0-015.9)

Excludes: crystal-induced (275.4)
gonococcal (098.51)
gouty (274.0)
syphilitic (095.7)

727.02 Giant cell tumor of tendon sheath

727.03 Trigger finger (acquired)

727.04 Radial styloid tenosynovitis
de Quervain's disease

727.05 Other tenosynovitis of hand and wrist

727.06 Tenosynovitis of foot and ankle

727.09 Other

727.1 Bunion

Add 4th or 5th digit | Nonspecific code | Unspecified code | Manifestation code

727.2 Specific bursitides often of occupational origin

Beat:
elbow
hand
knee

Chronic crepitant synovitis of wrist
Miners':
elbow
knee

727.3 Other bursitis

Bursitis NOS

Excludes: *bursitis:*
gonococcal (098.52)
subacromial (726.19)
subcoracoid (726.19)
subdeltoid (726.19)
syphilitic (095.7)
"frozen shoulder" (726.0)

727.4 Ganglion and cyst of synovium, tendon, and bursa

727.40 Synovial cyst, unspecified

Excludes: *that of popliteal space (727.51)*

727.41 Ganglion of joint

727.42 Ganglion of tendon sheath

727.43 Ganglion, unspecified

727.49 Other

Cyst of bursa

727.5 Rupture of synovium

727.50 Rupture of synovium, unspecified

727.51 Synovial cyst of popliteal space

Baker's cyst (knee)

727.59 Other

727.6 Rupture of tendon, nontraumatic

727.60 Nontraumatic rupture of unspecified tendon

727.61 Complete rupture of rotator cuff

727.62 Tendons of biceps (long head)

727.63 Extensor tendons of hand and wrist

727.64 Flexor tendons of hand and wrist

727.65 Quadriceps tendon

727.66 Patellar tendon

727.67 Achilles tendon

727.68 Other tendons of foot and ankle

727.69 Other

727.8 Other disorders of synovium, tendon, and bursa

727.81 Contracture of tendon (sheath)

Short Achilles tendon (acquired)

727.82 Calcium deposits in tendon and bursa

Calcification of tendon NOS
Calcific tendinitis NOS

Excludes: *peripheral ligamentous or muscular attachments (726.0-726.9)*

727.89 Other

Abscess of bursa or tendon

Excludes: *xanthomatosis localized to tendons (272.7)*

727.9 Unspecified disorder of synovium, tendon, and bursa

728 Disorders of muscle, ligament, and fascia

Excludes: *enthesopathies (726.0-726.9)*
muscular dystrophies (359.0-359.1)
myoneural disorders (358.0-358.9)
myopathies (359.2-359.9)
old disruption of ligaments of knee (717.81-717.89)

● Code new to this edition ▲ Revision of existing code ④ ⑤ Fourth or fifth digit required

728.0 Infective myositis
Myositis:
purulent
suppurative

Excludes: *myositis:*
epidemic (074.1)
interstitial (728.81)
syphilitic (095.6)
tropical (040.81)

728.1 Muscular calcification and ossification

728.10 Calcification and ossification, unspecified
Massive calcification (paraplegic)

728.11 Progressive myositis ossificans

728.12 Traumatic myositis ossificans
Myositis ossificans (circumscripta)

728.13 Postoperative heterotopic calcification

728.19 Other
Polymyositis ossificans

728.2 Muscular wasting and disuse atrophy, not elsewhere classified
Amyotrophia NOS
Myofibrosis

Excludes: *neuralgic amyotrophy (353.5)*
progressive muscular atrophy (335.0-335.9)

728.3 Other specific muscle disorders
Arthrogryposis
Immobility syndrome (paraplegic)

Excludes: *arthrogryposis multiplex congenita (754.89)*
stiff-man syndrome (333.91)

728.4 Laxity of ligament

728.5 Hypermobility syndrome

728.6 Contracture of palmar fascia
Dupuytren's contracture

728.7 Other fibromatoses

728.71 Plantar fascial fibromatosis
Contracture of plantar fascia
Plantar fasciitis (traumatic)

728.79 Other
Garrod's or knuckle pads
Nodular fasciitis
Pseudosarcomatous fibromatosis (proliferative) (subcutaneous)

▲ **728.8 Other disorders of muscle, ligament, and fascia**

728.81 Interstitial myositis

728.82 Foreign body granuloma of muscle
Talc granuloma of muscle

728.83 Rupture of muscle, nontraumatic

728.84 Diastasis of muscle
Diastasis recti (abdomen)

Excludes: *diastasis recti complicating pregnancy, labor, and delivery (665.8)*

728.85 Spasm of muscle

● **728.86 Necrotizing fasciitis**
Use additional code to identify:
infectious organism (041.00 - 041.89)
gangrene (785.4), if applicable

728.89 Other
Eosinophilic fasciitis
Use additional E code, if desired, to identify drug, if drug induced

728.9 Unspecified disorder of muscle, ligament, and fascia

729 Other disorders of soft tissues

Excludes: *acroparesthesia (443.89)*
carpal tunnel syndrome (354.0)
disorders of the back (720.0-724.9)
entrapment syndromes (354.0-355.9)
palindromic rheumatism (719.3)
periarthritis (726.0-726.9)
psychogenic rheumatism (306.0)

729.0 Rheumatism, unspecified and fibrositis

729.1 Myalgia and myositis, unspecified
Fibromyositis NOS

729.2 Neuralgia, neuritis, and radiculitis, unspecified

Excludes: *brachial radiculitis (723.4)*
cervical radiculitis (723.4)
lumbosacral radiculitis (724.4)
mononeuritis (354.0-355.9)
radiculitis due to intervertebral disc involvement (722.0-722.2, 722.7)
sciatica (724.3)

729.3 Panniculitis, unspecified

729.30 Panniculitis, unspecified site
Weber-Christian disease

729.31 Hypertrophy of fat pad, knee
Hypertrophy of infrapatellar fat pad

729.39 Other site

Excludes: *panniculitis specified as (affecting):*
back (724.8)
neck (723.6)
sacral (724.8)

729.4 Fasciitis, unspecified

Excludes: *necrotizing fasciitis (728.86)*
nodular fasciitis (728.79)

729.5 Pain in limb

729.6 Residual foreign body in soft tissue

Excludes: *foreign body granuloma:*
muscle (728.82)
skin and subcutaneous tissue (709.4)

729.8 Other musculoskeletal symptoms referable to limbs

729.81 Swelling of limb

729.82 Cramp

729.89 Other

Excludes: *abnormality of gait (781.2)*
tetany (781.7)
transient paralysis of limb (781.4)

729.9 Other and unspecified disorders of soft tissue
Polyalgia

OSTEOPATHIES, CHONDROPATHIES, AND ACQUIRED MUSCULOSKELETAL DEFORMITIES (730-739)

⑤ **730 Osteomyelitis, periostitis, and other infections involving bone**

Excludes: *jaw (526.4-526.5)*
petrous bone (383.2)

Use additional code, if desired, to identify organism, such as Staphylococcus (041.1)

The following fifth-digit subclassification is for use with category 730; valid digits are in [brackets] under each code. See beginning of this chapter for definitions:

0 site unspecified
1 shoulder region
2 upper arm
3 forearm

● Code new to this edition ▲ Revision of existing code ④ ⑤ Fourth or fifth digit required

4 hand

5 pelvic region and thigh

6 lower leg

7 ankle and foot

8 other specified sites

9 multiple sites

730.0 Acute osteomyelitis
[0-9]
Abscess of any bone except accessory sinus, jaw, or mastoid
Acute or subacute osteomyelitis, with or without mention of periostitis

730.1 Chronic osteomyelitis
[0-9]
Brodie's abscess
Chronic or old osteomyelitis, with or without mention of periostitis
Necrosis (acute), Sequestrum } of bone
Sclerosing osteomyelitis of Garré

Excludes: *aseptic necrosis of bone (733.40-733.49)*

730.2 Unspecified osteomyelitis
[0-9]
Osteitis or osteomyelitis NOS, with or without mention of periostitis

730.3 Periostitis without mention of osteomyelitis
[0-9]
Abscess of periosteum, Periostosis } without mention of osteomyelitis

Excludes: *that in secondary syphilis (091.61)*

730.7 Osteopathy resulting from poliomyelitis
[0-9]
Code first underlying disease (045.0-045.9)

730.8 Other infections involving bone in diseases classified elsewhere
[0-9]
Code first underlying disease, as:
tuberculosis (015.0-015.9)
typhoid fever (002.0)

Excludes: *syphilis of bone NOS (095.5)*

730.9 Unspecified infection of bone
[0-9]

731 Osteitis deformans and osteopathies associated with other disorders classified elsewhere

731.0 Osteitis deformans without mention of bone tumor
Paget's disease of bone

731.1 Osteitis deformans in diseases classified elsewhere
Code first underlying disease, as:
malignant neoplasm of bone (170.0-170.9)

731.2 Hypertrophic pulmonary osteoarthropathy
Bamberger-Marie disease

731.8 Other bone involvement in diseases classified elsewhere
Code first underlying disease, as:
diabetes mellitus (250.8)

732 Osteochondropathies

732.0 Juvenile osteochondrosis of spine
Juvenile osteochondrosis (of):
marginal or vertebral epiphysis (of Scheuermann)
spine NOS
Vertebral epiphysitis

Excludes: *adolescent postural kyphosis (737.0)*

732.1 Juvenile osteochondrosis of hip and pelvis
Coxa plana
Ischiopubic synchondrosis (of van Neck)
Osteochondrosis (juvenile) of:
acetabulum
head of femur (of Legg-Calvé-Perthes)
iliac crest (of Buchanan)
symphysis pubis (of Pierson)
Pseudocoxalgia

732.2 Nontraumatic slipped upper femoral epiphysis
Slipped upper femoral epiphysis NOS

732.3 Juvenile osteochondrosis of upper extremity
Osteochondrosis (juvenile) of:
capitulum of humerus (of Panner)
carpal lunate (of Kienbock)
hand NOS
head of humerus (of Haas)
heads of metacarpals (of Mauclaire)
lower ulna (of Burns)
radial head (of Brailsford)
upper extremity NOS

732.4 Juvenile osteochondrosis of lower extremity, excluding foot
Osteochondrosis (juvenile) of:
lower extremity NOS
primary patellar center (of Köhler)
proximal tibia (of Blount)
secondary patellar center (of Sinding-Larsen)
tibial tubercle (of Osgood-Schlatter)
Tibia vara

732.5 Juvenile osteochondrosis of foot
Calcaneal apophysitis
Epiphysitis, os calcis
Osteochondrosis (juvenile) of:
astragalus (of Diaz)
calcaneum (of Sever)
foot NOS
metatarsal
second (of Freiberg)
fifth (of Iselin)
os tibiale externum (Haglund)
tarsal navicular (of Köhler)

732.6 Other juvenile osteochondrosis
Apophysitis, Epiphysitis, Osteochondritis, Osteochondrosis } specified as juvenile, of other site, or site NOS

732.7 Osteochondritis dissecans

732.8 Other specified forms of osteochondropathy
Adult osteochondrosis of spine

732.9 Unspecified osteochondropathy
Apophysitis, Epiphysitis, Osteochondritis, Osteochondrosis } NOS; Not specified as adult or juvenile, of unspecified site

733 Other disorders of bone and cartilage

Excludes: *bone spur (726.91)*
cartilage of, or loose body in, joint (717.0-717.9, 718.0-718.9)
giant cell granuloma of jaw (526.3)
osteitis fibrosa cystica generalisata (252.0)
osteomalacia (268.2)
polyostotic fibrous dysplasia of bone (756.54)
prognathism, retrognathism (524.1)
xanthomatosis localized to bone (272.7)

733.0 Osteoporosis

733.00 Osteoporosis, unspecified
Wedging of vertebra NOS

733.01 Senile osteoporosis
Postmenopausal osteoporosis

733.02 Idiopathic osteoporosis

733.03 Disuse osteoporosis

733.09 Other
Drug-induced osteoporosis
Use additional E code, if desired, to identify drug

● Code new to this edition ▲ Revision of existing code ④ ⑤ Fourth or fifth digit required

733.1 Pathologic fracture
Spontaneous fracture

Excludes: *traumatic fracture (800-829)*

733.10 Pathologic fracture, unspecified site

733.11 Pathologic fracture of humerus

733.12 Pathologic fracture of distal radius and ulna
Wrist NOS

733.13 Pathologic fracture of vertebrae
Collapse of vertebra NOS

733.14 Pathologic fracture of neck of femur
Femur NOS
Hip NOS

733.15 Pathologic fracture of other specified part of femur

733.16 Pathologic fracture of tibia or fibula
Ankle NOS

733.19 Pathologic fracture of other specified site

733.2 Cyst of bone

733.20 Cyst of bone (localized), unspecified

733.21 Solitary bone cyst
Unicameral bone cyst

733.22 Aneurysmal bone cyst

733.29 Other
Fibrous dysplasia (monostotic)

Excludes: *cyst of jaw (526.0-526.2, 526.89)*
osteitis fibrosa cystica (252.0)
polyostotic fibrous dysplasia of bone (756.54)

733.3 Hyperostosis of skull
Hyperostosis interna frontalis
Leontiasis ossium

733.4 Aseptic necrosis of bone

Excludes: *necrosis of bone NOS (730.1)*
osteochondropathies (732.0-732.9)

733.40 Aseptic necrosis of bone, site unspecified

733.41 Head of humerus

733.42 Head and neck of femur
Femur NOS

Excludes: *Legg-Calvé-Perthes disease (732.1)*

733.43 Medial femoral condyle

733.44 Talus

733.49 Other

733.5 Osteitis condensans
Piriform sclerosis of ilium

733.6 Tietze's disease
Costochondral junction syndrome
Costochondritis

733.7 Algoneurodystrophy
Disuse atrophy of bone
Sudeck's atrophy

733.8 Malunion and nonunion of fracture

733.81 Malunion of fracture

733.82 Nonunion of fracture
Pseudoarthrosis (bone)

733.9 Other and unspecified disorders of bone and cartilage

733.90 Disorder of bone and cartilage, unspecified

733.91 Arrest of bone development or growth
Epiphyseal arrest

Add 4th or 5th digit | Nonspecific code | Unspecified code | Manifestation code

733.92 Chondromalacia
Chondromalacia:
NOS
localized, except patella
systemic
tibial plateau

Excludes: *chondromalacia of patella (717.7)*

733.99 Other
Diaphysitis
Hypertrophy of bone
Relapsing polychondritis

734 Flat foot
Pes planus (acquired)
Talipes planus (acquired)

Excludes: *congenital (754.61)*
rigid flat foot (754.61)
spastic (everted) flat foot (754.61)

735 Acquired deformities of toe

Excludes: *congenital (754.60-754.69, 755.65-755.66)*

735.0 Hallux valgus (acquired)

735.1 Hallux varus (acquired)

735.2 Hallux rigidus

735.3 Hallux malleus

735.4 Other hammer toe (acquired)

735.5 Claw toe (acquired)

735.8 Other acquired deformities of toe

735.9 Unspecified acquired deformity of toe

736 Other acquired deformities of limbs

Excludes: *congenital (754.3-755.9)*

736.0 Acquired deformities of forearm, excluding fingers

736.00 Unspecified deformity
Deformity of elbow, forearm, hand, or wrist (acquired) NOS

736.01 Cubitus valgus (acquired)

736.02 Cubitus varus (acquired)

736.03 Valgus deformity of wrist (acquired)

736.04 Varus deformity of wrist (acquired)

736.05 Wrist drop (acquired)

736.06 Claw hand (acquired)

736.07 Club hand, acquired

736.09 Other

736.1 Mallet finger

736.2 Other acquired deformities of finger

736.20 Unspecified deformity
Deformity of finger (acquired) NOS

736.21 Boutonniere deformity

736.22 Swan-neck deformity

736.29 Other

Excludes: *trigger finger (727.03)*

736.3 Acquired deformities of hip

736.30 Unspecified deformity
Deformity of hip (acquired) NOS

736.31 Coxa valga (acquired)

736.32 Coxa vara (acquired)

736.39 Other

736.4 Genu valgum or varum (acquired)

736.41 Genu valgum (acquired)

736.42 Genu varum (acquired)

736.5 Genu recurvatum (acquired)

736.6 Other acquired deformities of knee
Deformity of knee (acquired) NOS

736.7 Other acquired deformities of ankle and foot
Excludes: *deformities of toe (acquired) (735.0-735.9)*
pes planus (acquired) (734)

736.70 Unspecified deformity of ankle and foot, acquired

736.71 Acquired equinovarus deformity
Clubfoot, acquired

Excludes: *clubfoot not specified as acquired (754.5-754.7)*

736.72 Equinus deformity of foot, acquired

736.73 Cavus deformity of foot

Excludes: *that with claw foot (736.74)*

736.74 Claw foot, acquired

736.75 Cavovarus deformity of foot, acquired

736.76 Other calcaneus deformity

736.79 Other
Acquired:
pes } not elsewhere classified
talipes } not elsewhere classified

736.8 Acquired deformities of other parts of limbs

736.81 Unequal leg length (acquired)

736.89 Other
Deformity (acquired):
arm or leg, not elsewhere classified
shoulder

736.9 Acquired deformity of limb, site unspecified

737 Curvature of spine
Excludes: *congenital (754.2)*

737.0 Adolescent postural kyphosis
Excludes: *osteochondrosis of spine (juvenile) (732.0)*
adult (732.8)

737.1 Kyphosis (acquired)

737.10 Kyphosis (acquired) (postural)

737.11 Kyphosis due to radiation

737.12 Kyphosis, postlaminectomy

737.19 Other

Excludes: *that associated with conditions classifiable elsewhere (737.41)*

737.2 Lordosis (acquired)

737.20 Lordosis (acquired) (postural)

737.21 Lordosis, postlaminectomy

737.22 Other postsurgical lordosis

737.29 Other

Excludes: *that associated with conditions classifiable elsewhere (737.42)*

737.3 Kyphoscoliosis and scoliosis

737.30 Scoliosis [and kyphoscoliosis], idiopathic

737.31 Resolving infantile idiopathic scoliosis

737.32 Progressive infantile idiopathic scoliosis

737.33 Scoliosis due to radiation

737.34 Thoracogenic scoliosis

737.39 Other

Excludes: *that associated with conditions classifiable elsewhere (737.43)*
that in kyphoscoliotic heart disease (416.1)

737.4 Curvature of spine associated with other conditions

Code first associated condition, as:
Charcot-Marie-Tooth disease (356.1)
mucopolysaccharidosis (277.5)
neurofibromatosis (237.7)
osteitis deformans (731.0)
osteitis fibrosa cystica (252.0)
osteoporosis (733.00-733.09)
poliomyelitis (138)
tuberculosis [Pott's curvature] (015.0)

737.40 Curvature of spine, unspecified

737.41 Kyphosis

737.42 Lordosis

737.43 Scoliosis

737.8 Other curvatures of spine

737.9 Unspecified curvature of spine

Curvature of spine (acquired) (idiopathic) NOS
Hunchback, acquired

Excludes: *deformity of spine NOS (738.5)*

738 Other acquired deformity

Excludes: *congenital (754.0-756.9, 758.0-759.9)*
dentofacial anomalies (524.0-524.9)

738.0 Acquired deformity of nose

Deformity of nose (acquired)
Overdevelopment of nasal bones

Excludes: *deflected or deviated nasal septum (470)*

738.1 Other acquired deformity of head

738.10 Unspecified deformity

738.11 Zygomatic hyperplasia

738.12 Zygomatic hypoplasia

738.19 Other specified deformity

738.2 Acquired deformity of neck

738.3 Acquired deformity of chest and rib

Deformity:
chest (acquired)
rib (acquired)

Pectus:
carinatum, acquired
excavatum, acquired

738.4 Acquired spondylolisthesis

Degenerative spondylolisthesis
Spondylolysis, acquired

Excludes: *congenital (756.12)*

738.5 Other acquired deformity of back or spine

Deformity of spine NOS

Excludes: *curvature of spine (737.0-737.9)*

738.6 Acquired deformity of pelvis

Pelvic obliquity

Excludes: *intrapelvic protrusion of acetabulum (718.6)*
that in relation to labor and delivery (653.0-653.4, 653.8-653.9)

738.7 Cauliflower ear

738.8 Acquired deformity of other specified site

Deformity of clavicle

738.9 Acquired deformity of unspecified site

739 Nonallopathic lesions, not elsewhere classified
Includes: segmental dysfunction
somatic dysfunction

739.0 Head region
Occipitocervical region

739.1 Cervical region
Cervicothoracic region

739.2 Thoracic region
Thoracolumbar region

739.3 Lumbar region
Lumbosacral region

739.4 Sacral region
Sacrococcygeal region
Sacroiliac region

739.5 Pelvic region
Hip region
Pubic region

739.6 Lower extremities

739.7 Upper extremities
Acromioclavicular region
Sternoclavicular region

739.8 Rib cage
Costochondral region
Costovertebral region
Sternochondral region

739.9 Abdomen and other

14. CONGENITAL ANOMALIES (740-759)

740 Anencephalus and similar anomalies

740.0 Anencephalus
- Acrania
- Amyelencephalus
- Hemianencephaly
- Hemicephaly

740.1 Craniorachischisis

740.2 Iniencephaly

⑤ 741 Spina bifida

Excludes: spina bifida occulta (756.17)

The following fifth-digit subclassification is for use with category 741:

0 unspecified region

1 cervical region

2 dorsal [thoracic] region

3 lumbar region

741.0 With hydrocephalus
- Arnold-Chiari syndrome, type II
- Any condition classifiable to 741.9 with any condition classifiable to 742.3
- Chiari malformation, type II

741.9 Without mention of hydrocephalus
- Hydromeningocele (spinal)
- Hydromyelocele
- Meningocele (spinal)
- Meningomyelocele
- Myelocele
- Myelocystocele
- Rachischisis
- Spina bifida (aperta)
- Syringomyelocele

742 Other congenital anomalies of nervous system

742.0 Encephalocele
- Encephalocystocele
- Encephalomyelocele
- Hydroencephalocele
- Hydromeningocele, cranial
- Meningocele, cerebral
- Meningoencephalocele

742.1 Microcephalus
- Hydromicrocephaly
- Micrencephaly

742.2 Reduction deformities of brain
- Absence, Agenesis, Aplasia, Hypoplasia } of part of brain
- Agyria
- Arhinencephaly
- Holoprosencephaly
- Microgyria

742.3 Congenital hydrocephalus
- Aqueduct of Sylvius:
  - anomaly
  - obstruction, congenital
  - stenosis
- Atresia of foramina of Magendie and Luschka
- Hydrocephalus in newborn

Excludes: hydrocephalus:
- *acquired (331.3-331.4)*
- *due to congenital toxoplasmosis (771.2)*
- *with any condition classifiable to 741.9 (741.0)*

742.4 Other specified anomalies of brain
- Congenital cerebral cyst
- Macroencephaly
- Macrogyria
- Megalencephaly
- Multiple anomalies of brain NOS
- Porencephaly
- Ulegyria

742.5 Other specified anomalies of spinal cord

742.51 Diastematomyelia

742.53 Hydromyelia
- Hydrorhachis

742.59 Other
Amyelia
Atelomyelia
Congenital anomaly of spinal meninges
Defective development of cauda equina
Hypoplasia of spinal cord
Myelatelia
Myelodysplasia

742.8 Other specified anomalies of nervous system
Agenesis of nerve
Displacement of brachial plexus
Familial dysautonomia
Jaw-winking syndrome
Marcus-Gunn syndrome
Riley-Day syndrome

Excludes: *neurofibromatosis (237.7)*

742.9 Unspecified anomaly of brain, spinal cord, and nervous system
Anomaly
Congenital:
disease
lesion
Deformity
} of { brain, nervous system, spinal cord

743 Congenital anomalies of eye

743.0 Anophthalmos

743.00 Clinical anophthalmos, unspecified
Agenesis
Congenital absence
} of eye
Anophthalmos NOS

743.03 Cystic eyeball, congenital

743.06 Cryptophthalmos

743.1 Microphthalmos
Dysplasia
Hypoplasia
} of eye
Rudimentary eye

743.10 Microphthalmos, unspecified

743.11 Simple microphthalmos

743.12 Microphthalmos associated with other anomalies of eye and adnexa

743.2 Buphthalmos
Glaucoma:
congenital
newborn
Hydrophthalmos

Excludes: *glaucoma of childhood (365.14)*
traumatic glaucoma due to birth injury (767.8)

743.20 Buphthalmos, unspecified

743.21 Simple buphthalmos

743.22 Buphthalmos associated with other ocular anomalies
Keratoglobus, congenital
Megalocornea
} associated with buphthalmos

743.3 Congenital cataract and lens anomalies

Excludes: *infantile cataract (366.00-366.09)*

743.30 Congenital cataract, unspecified

743.31 Capsular and subcapsular cataract

743.32 Cortical and zonular cataract

743.33 Nuclear cataract

743.34 Total and subtotal cataract, congenital

743.35 Congenital aphakia
Congenital absence of lens

743.36 Anomalies of lens shape
Microphakia
Spherophakia

743.37 Congenital ectopic lens

743.39 Other

743.4 Coloboma and other anomalies of anterior segment

743.41 Anomalies of corneal size and shape
Microcornea

Excludes: *that associated with buphthalmos (743.22)*

743.42 Corneal opacities, interfering with vision, congenital

743.43 Other corneal opacities, congenital

743.44 Specified anomalies of anterior chamber, chamber angle, and related structures
Anomaly:
  Axenfeld's
  Peters'
  Rieger's

743.45 Aniridia

743.46 Other specified anomalies of iris and ciliary body
Anisocoria, congenital
Atresia of pupil
Coloboma of iris
Corectopia

743.47 Specified anomalies of sclera

743.48 Multiple and combined anomalies of anterior segment

743.49 Other

743.5 Congenital anomalies of posterior segment

743.51 Vitreous anomalies
Congenital vitreous opacity

743.52 Fundus coloboma

743.53 Chorioretinal degeneration, congenital

743.54 Congenital folds and cysts of posterior segment

743.55 Congenital macular changes

743.56 Other retinal changes, congenital

743.57 Specified anomalies of optic disc
Coloboma of optic disc (congenital)

743.58 Vascular anomalies
Congenital retinal aneurysm

743.59 Other

743.6 Congenital anomalies of eyelids, lacrimal system, and orbit

743.61 Congenital ptosis

743.62 Congenital deformities of eyelids
Ablepharon
Absence of eyelid
Accessory eyelid
Congenital:
  ectropion
  entropion

743.63 Other specified congenital anomalies of eyelid
Absence, agenesis, of cilia

743.64 Specified congenital anomalies of lacrimal gland

743.65 Specified congenital anomalies of lacrimal passages
Absence, agenesis of:
  lacrimal apparatus
  punctum lacrimale
Accessory lacrimal canal

743.66 Specified congenital anomalies of orbit

743.69 Other
Accessory eye muscles

743.8 Other specified anomalies of eye

Excludes: *congenital nystagmus (379.51)*
ocular albinism (270.2)
retinitis pigmentosa (362.74)

Add 4th or 5th digit | Nonspecific code | Unspecified code | Manifestation code

743.9 Unspecified anomaly of eye
Congenital:
anomaly NOS } of eye [any part]
deformity NOS } of eye [any part]

744 Congenital anomalies of ear, face, and neck

Excludes: *anomaly of:*
cervical spine (754.2, 756.10-756.19)
larynx (748.2-748.3)
nose (748.0-748.1)
parathyroid gland (759.2)
thyroid gland (759.2)
cleft lip (749.10-749.25)

744.0 Anomalies of ear causing impairment of hearing

Excludes: *congenital deafness without mention of cause (389.0-389.9)*

744.00 Unspecified anomaly of ear with impairment of hearing

744.01 Absence of external ear
Absence of:
auditory canal (external)
auricle (ear) (with stenosis or atresia of auditory canal)

744.02 Other anomalies of external ear with impairment of hearing
Atresia or stricture of auditory canal (external)

744.03 Anomaly of middle ear, except ossicles
Atresia or stricture of osseous meatus (ear)

744.04 Anomalies of ear ossicles
Fusion of ear ossicles

744.05 Anomalies of inner ear
Congenital anomaly of:
membranous labyrinth
organ of Corti

744.09 Other
Absence of ear, congenital

744.1 Accessory auricle
Accessory tragus
Polyotia
Preauricular appendage
Supernumerary:
ear
lobule

744.2 Other specified anomalies of ear

Excludes: *that with impairment of hearing (744.00-744.09)*

744.21 Absence of ear lobe, congenital

744.22 Macrotia

744.23 Microtia

744.24 Specified anomalies of Eustachian tube
Absence of Eustachian tube

744.29 Other
Bat ear
Darwin's tubercle
Pointed ear
Prominence of auricle
Ridge ear

Excludes: *preauricular sinus (744.46)*

744.3 Unspecified anomaly of ear
Congenital:
anomaly NOS } of ear, not elsewhere classified
deformity NOS } of ear, not elsewhere classified

744.4 Branchial cleft cyst or fistula; preauricular sinus

744.41 Branchial cleft sinus or fistula
Branchial:
sinus (external) (internal)
vestige

744.42 Branchial cleft cyst

744.43 Cervical auricle

744.46 Preauricular sinus or fistula

744.47 Preauricular cyst

● Code new to this edition ▲ Revision of existing code ④ ⑤ Fourth or fifth digit required

744.49 Other
Fistula (of):
auricle, congenital
cervicoaural

744.5 Webbing of neck
Pterygium colli

744.8 Other specified anomalies of face and neck

744.81 Macrocheilia
Hypertrophy of lip, congenital

744.82 Microcheilia

744.83 Macrostomia

744.84 Microstomia

744.89 Other

Excludes: *congenital fistula of lip (750.25)*
musculoskeletal anomalies (754.0-754.1, 756.0)

744.9 Unspecified anomalies of face and neck
Congenital:
anomaly NOS } of face [any part] or neck [any part]
deformity NOS }

745 Bulbus cordis anomalies and anomalies of cardiac septal closure

745.0 Common truncus
Absent septum } between aorta and pulmonary artery
Communication (abnormal) } between aorta and pulmonary artery
Aortic septal defect
Common aortopulmonary trunk
Persistent truncus arteriosus

745.1 Transposition of great vessels

745.10 Complete transposition of great vessels
Transposition of great vessels:
NOS
classical

754.11 Double outlet right ventricle
Dextratransposition of aorta
Incomplete transposition of great vessels
Origin of both great vessels from right ventricle
Taussig-Bing syndrome or defect

745.12 Corrected transposition of great vessels

745.19 Other

745.2 Tetralogy of Fallot
Fallot's pentalogy
Ventricular septal defect with pulmonary stenosis or atresia, dextraposition of aorta, and hypertrophy of right ventricle

Excludes: *Fallot's triad (746.09)*

745.3 Common ventricle
Cor triloculare biatriatum
Single ventricle

745.4 Ventricular septal defect
Eisenmenger's defect or complex
Gerbode defect
Interventricular septal defect
Left ventricular-right atrial communication
Roger's disease

Excludes: *common atrioventricular canal type (745.69)*
single ventricle (745.3)

745.5 Ostium secundum type atrial septal defect
Defect:
atrium secundum
fossa ovalis
Lutembacher's syndrome
Patent or persistent:
foramen ovale
ostium secundum

745.6 Endocardial cushion defects

745.60 Endocardial cushion defect, unspecified type

Add 4th or 5th digit | Nonspecific code | Unspecified code | Manifestation code

745.61 Ostium primum defect
Persistent ostium primum

745.69 Other
Absence of atrial septum
Atrioventricular canal type ventricular septal defect
Common atrioventricular canal
Common atrium

745.7 Cor biloculare
Absence of atrial and ventricular septa

745.8 Other

745.9 Unspecified defect of septal closure
Septal defect NOS

746 Other congenital anomalies of heart

Excludes: *endocardial fibroelastosis (425.3)*

746.0 Anomalies of pulmonary valve

Excludes: *infundibular or subvalvular pulmonic stenosis (746.83)*
tetralogy of Fallot (745.2)

746.00 Pulmonary valve anomaly, unspecified

746.01 Atresia, congenital
Congenital absence of pulmonary valve

746.02 Stenosis, congenital

746.09 Other
Congenital insufficiency of pulmonary valve
Fallot's triad or trilogy

746.1 Tricuspid atresia and stenosis, congenital
Absence of tricuspid valve

746.2 Ebstein's anomaly

746.3 Congenital stenosis of aortic valve
Congenital aortic stenosis

Excludes: *congenital:*
subaortic stenosis (746.81)
supravalvular aortic stenosis (747.22)

746.4 Congenital insufficiency of aortic valve
Bicuspid aortic valve
Congenital aortic insufficiency

746.5 Congenital mitral stenosis
Fused commissure } of mitral valve
Parachute deformity } of mitral valve
Supernumerary cusps } of mitral valve

746.6 Congenital mitral insufficiency

746.7 Hypoplastic left heart syndrome
Atresia, or marked hypoplasia, of aortic orifice or valve, with hypoplasia of ascending aorta and defective development of left ventricle (with mitral valve atresia)

746.8 Other specified anomalies of heart

746.81 Subaortic stenosis

746.82 Cor triatriatum

746.83 Infundibular pulmonic stenosis
Subvalvular pulmonic stenosis

746.84 Obstructive anomalies of heart, not elsewhere classified
Uhl's disease

746.85 Coronary artery anomaly
Anomalous origin or communication of coronary artery
Arteriovenous malformation of coronary artery
Coronary artery:
absence
arising from aorta or pulmonary trunk
single

746.86 Congenital heart block
Complete or incomplete atrioventricular [AV] block

746.87 Malposition of heart and cardiac apex
Abdominal heart
Dextrocardia
Ectopia cordis
Levocardia (isolated)
Mesocardia

Excludes: *dextrocardia with complete transposition of viscera (759.3)*

746.89 Other
Atresia } of cardiac vein
Hypoplasia } of cardiac vein
Congenital:
  cardiomegaly
  diverticulum, left ventricle
  pericardial defect

746.9 Unspecified anomaly of heart
Congenital:
  anomaly of heart NOS
  heart disease NOS

747 Other congenital anomalies of circulatory system

747.0 Patent ductus arteriosus
Patent ductus Botalli
Persistent ductus arteriosus

747.1 Coarctation of aorta

747.10 Coarctation of aorta (preductal) (postductal)
Hypoplasia of aortic arch

747.11 Interruption of aortic arch

747.2 Other anomalies of aorta

747.20 Anomaly of aorta, unspecified

747.21 Anomalies of aortic arch
Anomalous origin, right subclavian artery
Dextraposition of aorta
Double aortic arch
Kommerell's diverticulum
Overriding aorta
Persistent:
  convolutions, aortic arch
  right aortic arch
Vascular ring

Excludes: *hypoplasia of aortic arch (747.10)*

747.22 Atresia and stenosis of aorta
Absence } of aorta
Aplasia } of aorta
Hypoplasia } of aorta
Stricture } of aorta
Supra (valvular)-aortic stenosis

Excludes: *congenital aortic (valvular) stenosis or stricture, so stated (746.3)*
hypoplasia of aorta in hypoplastic left heart syndrome (746.7)

747.29 Other
Aneurysm of sinus of Valsalva
Congenital:
  aneurysm } of aorta
  dilation } of aorta

747.3 Anomalies of pulmonary artery
Agenesis } of pulmonary artery
Anomaly } of pulmonary artery
Atresia } of pulmonary artery
Coarctation } of pulmonary artery
Hypoplasia } of pulmonary artery
Stenosis } of pulmonary artery
Pulmonary arteriovenous aneurysm

747.4 Anomalies of great veins

747.40 Anomaly of great veins, unspecified
Anomaly NOS of:
  pulmonary veins
  vena cava

747.41 Total anomalous pulmonary venous connection
Total anomalous pulmonary venous return [TAPVR]:
subdiaphragmatic
supradiaphragmatic

747.42 Partial anomalous pulmonary venous connection
Partial anomalous pulmonary venous return

747.49 Other anomalies of great veins
Absence } of vena cava (inferior) (superior)
Congenital stenosis } of vena cava (inferior) (superior)
Persistent:
left posterior cardinal vein
left superior vena cava
Scimitar syndrome
Transposition of pulmonary veins NOS

747.5 Absence or hypoplasia of umbilical artery
Single umbilical artery

747.6 Other anomalies of peripheral vascular system
Absence } of artery or vein, not elsewhere classified
Anomaly } of artery or vein, not elsewhere classified
Atresia } of artery or vein, not elsewhere classified
Arteriovenous aneurysm (peripheral)
Arteriovenous malformation of the peripheral vascular system
Congenital:
aneurysm (peripheral)
phlebectasia
stricture, artery
varix
Multiple renal arteries

Excludes: *anomalies of:*
cerebral vessels (747.81)
pulmonary artery (747.3)
congenital retinal aneurysm (743.58)
hemangioma (228.00-228.09)
lymphangioma (228.1)

747.60 Anomaly of the peripheral vascular system, unspecified site

747.61 Gastrointestinal vessel anomaly

747.62 Renal vessel anomaly

747.63 Upper limb vessel anomaly

747.64 Lower limb vessel anomaly

747.69 Anomalies of other specified sites of peripheral vascular system

747.8 Other specified anomalies of circulatory system

747.81 Anomalies of cerebrovascular system
Arteriovenous malformation of brain
Cerebral arteriovenous aneurysm, congenital
Congenital anomalies of cerebral vessels

Excludes: *ruptured cerebral (arteriovenous) aneurysm (430)*

747.82 Spinal vessel anomaly
Arteriovenous malformation of spinal vessel

747.89 Other
Aneurysm, congenital, specified site not elsewhere classified

Excludes: *congenital aneurysm:*
coronary (746.85)
peripheral (747.6)
pulmonary (747.3)
retinal (743.58)

747.9 Unspecified anomaly of circulatory system

748 Congenital anomalies of respiratory system

Excludes: *congenital defect of diaphragm (756.6)*

748.0 Choanal atresia
Atresia } of nares (anterior) (posterior)
Congenital stenosis } of nares (anterior) (posterior)

748.1 Other anomalies of nose

Absent nose
Accessory nose
Cleft nose
Deformity of wall of nasal sinus
Congenital:
deformity of nose
notching of tip of nose
perforation of wall of nasal sinus

Excludes: *congenital deviation of nasal septum (754.0)*

748.2 Web of larynx

Web of larynx:
NOS
glottic
subglottic

748.3 Other anomalies of larynx, trachea, and bronchus

Absence or agenesis of:
bronchus
larynx
trachea
Anomaly (of):
cricoid cartilage
epiglottis
thyroid cartilage
tracheal cartilage
Atresia (of):
epiglottis
glottis
larynx
trachea
Cleft thyroid, cartilage, congenital
Congenital:
dilation, trachea
stenosis:
larynx
trachea
tracheocele
Diverticulum:
bronchus
trachea
Fissure of epiglottis
Laryngocele
Posterior cleft of cricoid cartilage (congenital)
Rudimentary tracheal bronchus
Stridor, laryngeal, congenital

748.4 Congenital cystic lung

Disease, lung:
cystic, congenital
polycystic, congenital
Honeycomb lung, congenital

Excludes: *acquired or unspecified cystic lung (518.89)*

748.5 Agenesis, hypoplasia, and dysplasia of lung

Absence of lung (fissures) (lobe)
Aplasia of lung
Hypoplasia of lung (lobe)
Sequestration of lung

748.6 Other anomalies of lung

748.60 Anomaly of lung, unspecified

748.61 Congenital bronchiectasis

748.69 Other

Accessory lung (lobe)
Azygos lobe (fissure), lung

748.8 Other specified anomalies of respiratory system

Abnormal communication between pericardial and pleural sacs
Anomaly, pleural folds
Atresia of nasopharynx
Congenital cyst of mediastinum

748.9 Unspecified anomaly of respiratory system

Anomaly of respiratory system NOS

749 Cleft palate and cleft lip

749.0 Cleft palate

749.00 Cleft palate, unspecified

749.01 Unilateral, complete

749.02 Unilateral, incomplete

Cleft uvula

749.03 Bilateral, complete

749.04 Bilateral, incomplete

749.1 Cleft lip

Cheiloschisis
Congenital fissure of lip
Harelip
Labium leporinum

749.10 Cleft lip, unspecified

749.11 Unilateral, complete

749.12 Unilateral, incomplete

749.13 Bilateral, complete

749.14 Bilateral, incomplete

749.2 Cleft palate with cleft lip
Cheilopalatoschisis

749.20 Cleft palate with cleft lip, unspecified

749.21 Unilateral, complete

749.22 Unilateral, incomplete

749.23 Bilateral, complete

749.24 Bilateral, incomplete

749.25 Other combinations

750 Other congenital anomalies of upper alimentary tract

Excludes: *dentofacial anomalies (524.0-524.9)*

750.0 Tongue tie
Ankyloglossia

750.1 Other anomalies of tongue

750.10 Anomaly of tongue, unspecified

750.11 Aglossia

750.12 Congenital adhesions of tongue

750.13 Fissure of tongue
Bifid tongue
Double tongue

750.15 Macroglossia
Congenital hypertrophy of tongue

750.16 Microglossia
Hypoplasia of tongue

750.19 Other

750.2 Other specified anomalies of mouth and pharynx

750.21 Absence of salivary gland

750.22 Accessory salivary gland

750.23 Atresia, salivary duct
Imperforate salivary duct

750.24 Congenital fistula of salivary gland

750.25 Congenital fistula of lip
Congenital (mucus) lip pits

750.26 Other specified anomalies of mouth
Absence of uvula

750.27 Diverticulum of pharynx
Pharyngeal pouch

750.29 Other specified anomalies of pharynx
Imperforate pharynx

750.3 Tracheoesophageal fistula, esophageal atresia and stenosis
Absent esophagus
Atresia of esophagus
Congenital:
- esophageal ring
- stenosis of esophagus
- stricture of esophagus

Congenital fistula:
- esophagobronchial
- esophagotracheal

Imperforate esophagus
Webbed esophagus

750.4 Other specified anomalies of esophagus

Dilatation, congenital Displacement, congenital Diverticulum Duplication Giant Esophageal pouch	(of) esophagus

Excludes: congenital hiatus hernia (750.6)

750.5 Congenital hypertrophic pyloric stenosis

Congenital or infantile:

constriction hypertrophy spasm stenosis stricture	of pylorus

750.6 Congenital hiatus hernia

Displacement of cardia through esophageal hiatus

Excludes: congenital diaphragmatic hernia (756.6)

750.7 Other specified anomalies of stomach

Congenital:
- cardiospasm
- hourglass stomach

Displacement of stomach

Diverticulum of stomach, congenital

Duplication of stomach

Megalogastria

Microgastria

Transposition of stomach

750.8 Other specified anomalies of upper alimentary tract

750.9 Unspecified anomaly of upper alimentary tract

Congenital:

anomaly NOS deformity NOS	of upper alimentary tract [any part, except tongue]

751 Other congenital anomalies of digestive system

751.0 Meckel's diverticulum

Meckel's diverticulum (displaced) (hypertrophic)

Persistent:
- omphalomesenteric duct
- vitelline duct

751.1 Atresia and stenosis of small intestine

Atresia of:
- duodenum
- ileum
- intestine NOS

Congenital: absence obstruction stenosis stricture Imperforate jejunum	of small intestine or intestine NOS

751.2 Atresia and stenosis of large intestine, rectum, and anal canal

Absence:
- anus (congenital)
- appendix, congenital
- large intestine, congenital
- rectum

Atresia of:
- anus
- colon
- rectum

Congenital or infantile:
- obstruction of large intestine
- occlusion of anus
- stricture of anus

Imperforate:
- anus
- rectum

Stricture of rectum, congenital

751.3 Hirschsprung's disease and other congenital functional disorders of colon

Aganglionosis

Congenital dilation of colon

Congenital megacolon

Macrocolon

751.4 Anomalies of intestinal fixation

Congenital adhesions:
 omental, anomalous
 peritoneal
Jackson's membrane
Malrotation of colon
Rotation of cecum or colon:
 failure of
 incomplete
 insufficient
Universal mesentery

751.5 Other anomalies of intestine

Congenital diverticulum, colon
Dolichocolon
Duplication of:
 anus
 appendix
 cecum
 intestine
Ectopic anus
Megaloappendix
Megaloduodenum
Microcolon
Persistent cloaca
Transposition of:
 appendix
 colon
 intestine

751.6 Anomalies of gallbladder, bile ducts, and liver

751.60 Unspecified anomaly of gallbladder, bile ducts, and liver

751.61 Biliary atresia

Congenital:
 absence, hypoplasia, obstruction, stricture } of bile duct (common) or passage

751.62 Congenital cystic disease of liver

Congenital polycystic disease of liver
Fibrocystic disease of liver

751.69 Other anomalies of gallbladder, bile ducts, and liver

Absence of:
 gallbladder, congenital
 liver (lobe)
Accessory:
 hepatic ducts
 liver
Congenital:
 choledochal cyst
 hepatomegaly
Duplication of:
 biliary duct
 cystic duct
 gallbladder
 liver
Floating:
 gallbladder
 liver
Intrahepatic gallbladder

751.7 Anomalies of pancreas

Absence, Agenesis, Hypoplasia } of pancreas
Accessory pancreas
Annular pancreas
Ectopic pancreatic tissue
Pancreatic heterotopia

Excludes: *diabetes mellitus:*
 congenital (250.0-250.9)
 neonatal (775.1)
fibrocystic disease of pancreas (277.00-277.01)

751.8 Other specified anomalies of digestive system

Absence (complete) (partial) of alimentary tract NOS
Duplication, Malposition, congenital } of digestive organs NOS

Excludes: *congenital diaphragmatic hernia (756.6)*
congenital hiatus hernia (750.6)

751.9 Unspecified anomaly of digestive system

Congenital:
 anomaly NOS, deformity NOS } of digestive system NOS

752 Congenital anomalies of genital organs

Excludes: *syndromes associated with anomalies in the number and form of chromosomes (758.0-758.9)*
testicular feminization syndrome (257.8)

752.0 Anomalies of ovaries

Absence, congenital } (of) ovary
Accessory } (of) ovary
Ectopic } (of) ovary
Streak } (of) ovary

752.1 Anomalies of fallopian tubes and broad ligaments

752.10 Unspecified anomaly of fallopian tubes and broad ligaments

752.11 Embryonic cyst of fallopian tubes and broad ligaments

Cyst:
- epoophoron
- fimbrial

Cyst:
- Gartner's duct
- parovarian

752.19 Other

Absence } (of) fallopian tube or broad ligament
Accessory } (of) fallopian tube or broad ligament
Atresia } (of) fallopian tube or broad ligament

752.2 Doubling of uterus

Didelphic uterus
Doubling of uterus [any degree] (associated with doubling of cervix and vagina)

752.3 Other anomalies of uterus

Absence, congenital } of uterus
Agenesis } of uterus
Aplasia } of uterus
Bicornuate uterus
Uterus unicornis
Uterus with only one functioning horn

752.4 Anomalies of cervix, vagina, and external female genitalia

752.40 Unspecified anomaly of cervix, vagina, and external female genitalia

752.41 Embryonic cyst of cervix, vagina, and external female genitalia

Cyst of:
- canal of Nuck, congenital
- vagina, embryonal
- vulva, congenital

752.42 Imperforate hymen

752.49 Other anomalies of cervix, vagina, and external female genitalia

Absence } of cervix, clitoris, vagina, or vulva
Agenesis } of cervix, clitoris, vagina, or vulva
Congenital stenosis or stricture of:
- cervical canal
- vagina

Excludes: *double vagina associated with total duplication (752.2)*

752.5 Undescended testicle

Cryptorchism
Ectopic testis

752.6 Hypospadias and epispadias

Anaspadias
Congenital chordee

752.7 Indeterminate sex and pseudohermaphroditism

Gynandrism
Hermaphroditism
Ovotestis
Pseudohermaphroditism (male) (female)
Pure gonadal dysgenesis

Excludes: *pseudohermaphroditism:*
- *female, with adrenocortical disorder (255.2)*
- *male, with gonadal disorder (257.8)*
- *with specified chromosomal anomaly (758.0-758.9)*

testicular feminization syndrome (257.8)

752.8 Other specified anomalies of genital organs

Absence of:
- penis
- prostate
- spermatic cord
- vas deferens

Anorchism

Aplasia (congenital) of:
- prostate
- round ligament
- testicle

Atresia of:
- ejaculatory duct
- vas deferens

Curvature of penis (lateral)

Fusion of testes

Hypoplasia of:
- penis
- testis

Monorchism

Paraspadias

Polyorchism

Excludes: *congenital hydrocele (778.6)*
phimosis or paraphimosis (605)

752.9 Unspecified anomaly of genital organs

Congenital:
- anomaly NOS } of genital organ, not elsewhere classified
- deformity NOS } of genital organ, not elsewhere classified

753 Congenital anomalies of urinary system

753.0 Renal agenesis and dysgenesis

Atrophy of kidney:
- congenital
- infantile

Congenital absence of kidney(s)

Hypoplasia of kidney(s)

Code first any associated vesicoureteral reflux (593.70-593.73)

753.1 Cystic kidney disease

Excludes: *acquired cyst of kidney (593.2)*

753.10 Cystic kidney disease, unspecified

753.11 Congenital single renal cyst

753.12 Polycystic kidney, unspecified type

753.13 Polycystic kidney, autosomal dominant

753.14 Polycystic kidney, autosomal recessive

753.15 Renal dysplasia

Code first any associated vesicoureteral reflux (593.70-593.73)

753.16 Medullary cystic kidney

Nephronopthisis

753.17 Medullary sponge kidney

753.19 Other specified cystic kidney disease

Multicystic kidney

753.2 Obstructive defects of renal pelvis and ureter

Atresia of ureter

Congenital:
- dilatation of ureter
- hydronephrosis
- hydroureter
- megaloureter
- occlusion of ureter

Congenital:
- stricture of:
  - ureter
  - ureteropelvic junction
  - ureterovesical orifice
- ureterocele

Impervious ureter

753.3 Other specified anomalies of kidney

Accessory kidney

Congenital:
- calculus of kidney
- displaced kidney

Discoid kidney

Double kidney with double pelvis

Ectopic kidney

Fusion of kidneys

Giant kidney

Horseshoe kidney

Hyperplasia of kidney

Lobulation of kidney

Malrotation of kidney

Trifid kidney (pelvis)

753.4 Other specified anomalies of ureter

Absent ureter

Accessory ureter

Deviation of ureter

Displaced ureteric orifice

Double ureter

Ectopic ureter

Implantation, anomalous of ureter

753.5 Exstrophy of urinary bladder

Ectopia vesicae

Extroversion of bladder

● Code new to this edition ▲ Revision of existing code ④ ⑤ Fourth or fifth digit required

753.6 Atresia and stenosis of urethra and bladder neck

Congenital obstruction:
- bladder neck
- urethra

Congenital stricture of:
- urethra (valvular)
- urinary meatus
- vesicourethral orifice

Imperforate urinary meatus
Impervious urethra
Urethral valve formation

753.7 Anomalies of urachus

Cyst, Fistula, Patent } (of) urachus

Persistent umbilical sinus

753.8 Other specified anomalies of bladder and urethra

Absence, congenital of:
- bladder
- urethra

Accessory:
- bladder
- urethra

Congenital:
- diverticulum of bladder
- hernia of bladder

Congenital urethrorectal fistula
Congenital prolapse of:
- bladder (mucosa)
- urethra

Double:
- urethra
- urinary meatus

753.9 Unspecified anomaly of urinary system

Congenital:
- anomaly NOS, deformity NOS } of urinary system [any part, except urachus]

754 Certain congenital musculoskeletal deformities

Includes: nonteratogenic deformities which are considered to be due to intrauterine malposition and pressure

754.0 Of skull, face, and jaw

Asymmetry of face
Compression facies
Depressions in skull
Deviation of nasal septum, congenital
Dolichocephaly
Plagiocephaly
Potter's facies
Squashed or bent nose, congenital

Excludes: *dentofacial anomalies (524.0-524.9)*
syphilitic saddle nose (090.5)

754.1 Of sternocleidomastoid muscle

Congenital sternomastoid torticollis
Congenital wryneck
Contracture of sternocleidomastoid (muscle)
Sternomastoid tumor

754.2 Of spine

Congenital postural:
- lordosis
- scoliosis

754.3 Congenital dislocation of hip

754.30 Congenital dislocation of hip, unilateral
Congenital dislocation of hip NOS

754.31 Congenital dislocation of hip, bilateral

754.32 Congenital subluxation of hip, unilateral
Congenital flexion deformity, hip or thigh
Predislocation status of hip at birth
Preluxation of hip, congenital

754.33 Congenital subluxation of hip, bilateral

754.35 Congenital dislocation of one hip with subluxation of other hip

754.4 Congenital genu recurvatum and bowing of long bones of leg

754.40 Genu recurvatum

754.41 Congenital dislocation of knee (with genu recurvatum)

754.42 Congenital bowing of femur

754.43 Congenital bowing of tibia and fibula

754.44 Congenital bowing of unspecified long bones of leg

754.5 Varus deformities of feet

Excludes: *acquired (736.71, 736.75, 736.79)*

754.50 Talipes varus
Congenital varus deformity of foot, unspecified
Pes varus

754.51 Talipes equinovarus
Equinovarus (congenital)

754.52 Metatarsus primus varus

754.53 Metatarsus varus

754.59 Other
Talipes calcaneovarus

754.6 Valgus deformities of feet

Excludes: *valgus deformity of foot (acquired) (736.79)*

754.60 Talipes valgus
Congenital valgus deformity of foot, unspecified

754.61 Congenital pes planus
Congenital rocker bottom flat foot
Flat foot, congenital

Excludes: *pes planus (acquired) (734)*

754.62 Talipes calcaneovalgus

754.69 Other
Talipes:
equinovalgus
planovalgus

754.7 Other deformities of feet

Excludes: *acquired (736.70-736.79)*

754.70 Talipes, unspecified
Congenital deformity of foot NOS

754.71 Talipes cavus
Cavus foot (congenital)

754.79 Other
Asymmetric talipes
Talipes:
calcaneus
equinus

754.8 Other specified nonteratogenic anomalies

754.81 Pectus excavatum
Congenital funnel chest

754.82 Pectus carinatum
Congenital pigeon chest [breast]

754.89 Other
Club hand (congenital)
Congenital:
deformity of chest wall
dislocation of elbow
Generalized flexion contractures of lower limb joints, congenital
Spade-like hand (congenital)

755 Other congenital anomalies of limbs

Excludes: *those deformities classifiable to 754.0-754.8*

755.0 Polydactyly

755.00 Polydactyly, unspecified digits
Supernumerary digits

755.01 Of fingers
Accessory fingers

755.02 Of toes
Accessory toes

755.1 Syndactyly
Symphalangy
Webbing of digits

● Code new to this edition ▲ Revision of existing code ④ ⑤ Fourth or fifth digit required

755.10 **Of multiple and unspecified sites**

755.11 **Of fingers without fusion of bone**

755.12 **Of fingers with fusion of bone**

755.13 **Of toes without fusion of bone**

755.14 **Of toes with fusion of bone**

755.2 **Reduction deformities of upper limb**

755.20 **Unspecified reduction deformity of upper limb**
Ectromelia NOS } of upper limb
Hemimelia NOS } of upper limb
Shortening of arm, congenital

755.21 **Transverse deficiency of upper limb**
Amelia of upper limb
Congenital absence of:
fingers, all (complete or partial)
forearm, including hand and fingers
upper limb, complete
Congenital amputation of upper limb
Transverse hemimelia of upper limb

755.22 **Longitudinal deficiency of upper limb, not elsewhere classified**
Phocomelia NOS of upper limb
Rudimentary arm

755.23 **Longitudinal deficiency, combined, involving humerus, radius, and ulna (complete or incomplete)**
Congenital absence of arm and forearm (complete or incomplete) with or without metacarpal deficiency and/or phalangeal deficiency, incomplete
Phocomelia, complete, of upper limb

755.24 **Longitudinal deficiency, humeral, complete or partial (with or without distal deficiencies, incomplete)**
Congenital absence of humerus (with or without absence of some [but not all] distal elements)
Proximal phocomelia of upper limb

755.25 **Longitudinal deficiency, radioulnar, complete or partial (with or without distal deficiencies, incomplete)**
Congenital absence of radius and ulna (with or without absence of some [but not all] distal elements)
Distal phocomelia of upper limb

755.26 **Longitudinal deficiency, radial, complete or partial (with or without distal deficiencies, incomplete)**
Agenesis of radius
Congenital absence of radius (with or without absence of some [but not all] distal elements)

755.27 **Longitudinal deficiency, ulnar, complete or partial (with or without distal deficiencies, incomplete)**
Agenesis of ulna
Congenital absence of ulna (with or without absence of some [but not all] distal elements)

755.28 **Longitudinal deficiency, carpals or metacarpals, complete or partial (with or without incomplete phalangeal deficiency)**

755.29 **Longitudinal deficiency, phalanges, complete or partial**
Absence of finger, congenital
Aphalangia of upper limb, terminal, complete or partial

Excludes: *terminal deficiency of all five digits (755.21)*
transverse deficiency of phalanges (755.21)

755.3 **Reduction deformities of lower limb**

755.30 **Unspecified reduction deformity of lower limb**
Ectromelia NOS } of lower limb
Hemimelia NOS } of lower limb
Shortening of leg, congenital

Add 4th or 5th digit | Nonspecific code | Unspecified code | Manifestation code

755.31 Transverse deficiency of lower limb
Amelia of lower limb
Congenital absence of:
foot
leg, including foot and toes
lower limb, complete
toes, all, complete
Transverse hemimelia of lower limb

755.32 Longitudinal deficiency of lower limb, not elsewhere classified
Phocomelia NOS of lower limb

755.33 Longitudinal deficiency, combined, involving femur, tibia, and fibula (complete or incomplete)
Congenital absence of thigh and (lower) leg (complete or incomplete) with or without metacarpal deficiency and/or phalangeal deficiency, incomplete
Phocomelia, complete, of lower limb

755.34 Longitudinal deficiency, femoral, complete or partial (with or without distal deficiencies, incomplete)
Congenital absence of femur (with or without absence of some [but not all] distal elements)
Proximal phocomelia of lower limb

755.35 Longitudinal deficiency, tibiofibular, complete or partial (with or without distal deficiencies, incomplete)
Congenital absence of tibia and fibula (with or without absence of some [but not all] distal elements)
Distal phocomelia of lower limb

755.36 Longitudinal deficiency, tibia, complete or partial (with or without distal deficiencies, incomplete)
Agenesis of tibia
Congenital absence of tibia (with or without absence of some [but not all] distal elements)

755.37 Longitudinal deficiency, fibular, complete or partial (with or without distal deficiencies, incomplete)
Agenesis of fibula
Congenital absence of fibula (with or without absence of some [but not all] distal elements)

755.38 Longitudinal deficiency, tarsals or metatarsals, complete or partial (with or without incomplete phalangeal deficiency)

755.39 Longitudinal deficiency, phalanges, complete or partial
Absence of toe, congenital
Aphalangia of lower limb, terminal, complete or partial

Excludes: *terminal deficiency of all five digits (755.31)*
transverse deficiency of phalanges (755.31)

755.4 Reduction deformities, unspecified limb
Absence, congenital (complete or partial) of limb NOS
Amelia
Ectromelia
Hemimelia
Phocomelia
} of unspecified limb

755.5 Other anomalies of upper limb, including shoulder girdle

755.50 Unspecified anomaly of upper limb

755.51 Congenital deformity of clavicle

755.52 Congenital elevation of scapula
Sprengel's deformity

755.53 Radioulnar synostosis

755.54 Madelung's deformity

755.55 Acrocephalosyndactyly
Apert's syndrome

755.56 Accessory carpal bones

755.57 Macrodactylia (fingers)

755.58 Cleft hand, congenital
Lobster-claw hand

755.59 Other
Cleidocranial dysostosis
Cubitus:
valgus, congenital
varus, congenital

Excludes: *club hand (congenital) (754.89)*
congenital dislocation of elbow (754.89)

755.6 Other anomalies of lower limb, including pelvic girdle

755.60 Unspecified anomaly of lower limb

755.61 Coxa valga, congenital

755.62 Coxa vara, congenital

755.63 Other congenital deformity of hip (joint)
Congenital anteversion of femur (neck)

Excludes: *congenital dislocation of hip (754.30-754.35)*

755.64 Congenital deformity of knee (joint)
Congenital:
absence of patella
genu valgum [knock-knee]
genu varum [bowleg]
Rudimentary patella

755.65 Macrodactylia of toes

755.66 Other anomalies of toes
Congenital:
hallux valgus
hallux varus
hammer toe

755.67 Anomalies of foot, not elsewhere classified
Astragaloscaphoid synostosis
Calcaneonavicular bar
Coalition of calcaneus
Talonavicular synostosis
Tarsal coalitions

755.69 Other
Congenital:
angulation of tibia
deformity (of):
ankle (joint)
sacroiliac (joint)
fusion of sacroiliac joint

755.8 Other specified anomalies of unspecified limb

755.9 Unspecified anomaly of unspecified limb
Congenital:
anomaly NOS } of unspecified limb
deformity NOS }

Excludes: *reduction deformity of unspecified limb (755.4)*

756 Other congenital musculoskeletal anomalies

Excludes: *those deformities classifiable to 754.0-754.8*

756.0 Anomalies of skull and face bones

Absence of skull bones
Acrocephaly
Congenital deformity of forehead
Craniosynostosis
Crouzon's disease
Hypertelorism
Imperfect fusion of skull
Oxycephaly
Platybasia
Premature closure of cranial sutures
Tower skull
Trigonocephaly

Excludes: *acrocephalosyndactyly [Apert's syndrome] (755.55)*
dentofacial anomalies (524.0-524.9)
skull defects associated with brain anomalies, such as:
anencephalus (740.0)
encephalocele (742.0)
hydrocephalus (742.3)
microcephalus (742.1)

756.1 Anomalies of spine

756.10 Anomaly of spine, unspecified

756.11 Spondylolysis, lumbosacral region
Prespondylolisthesis (lumbosacral)

756.12 Spondylolisthesis

756.13 Absence of vertebra, congenital

756.14 Hemivertebra

756.15 Fusion of spine [vertebra], congenital

756.16 Klippel-Feil syndrome

756.17 Spina bifida occulta

Excludes: *spina bifida (aperta) (741.0-741.9)*

756.19 Other
Platyspondylia
Supernumerary vertebra

756.2 Cervical rib
Supernumerary rib in the cervical region

756.3 Other anomalies of ribs and sternum

Congenital absence of:
rib
sternum
Congenital:
fissure of sternum
fusion of ribs
Sternum bifidum

Excludes: *nonteratogenic deformity of chest wall (754.81-754.89)*

756.4 Chondrodystrophy

Achondroplasia
Chondrodystrophia (fetalis)
Dyschondroplasia
Enchondromatosis
Ollier's disease

Excludes: *lipochondrodystrophy [Hurler's syndrome] (277.5)*
Morquio's disease (277.5)

756.5 Osteodystrophies

756.50 Osteodystrophy, unspecified

756.51 Osteogenesis imperfecta
Fragilitas ossium
Osteopsathyrosis

756.52 Osteopetrosis

756.53 Osteopoikilosis

756.54 Polyostotic fibrous dysplasia of bone

756.55 Chondroectodermal dysplasia
Ellis-van Creveld syndrome

756.56 Multiple epiphyseal dysplasia

756.59 Other
Albright (-McCune)-Sternberg syndrome

756.6 Anomalies of diaphragm
Absence of diaphragm
Congenital hernia:
diaphragmatic
foramen of Morgagni
Eventration of diaphragm

Excludes: *congenital hiatus hernia (750.6)*

756.7 Anomalies of abdominal wall
Omphalocele
Exomphalos
Gastroschisis
Prune belly (syndrome)

Excludes: *umbilical hernia (551-553 with .1)*

756.8 Other specified anomalies of muscle, tendon, fascia, and connective tissue

756.81 Absence of muscle and tendon
Absence of muscle (pectoral)

756.82 Accessory muscle

756.83 Ehlers-Danlos syndrome

756.89 Other
Amyotrophia congenita
Congenital shortening of tendon

756.9 Other and unspecified anomalies of musculoskeletal system
Congenital:
anomaly NOS } of musculoskeletal system, not elsewhere classified
deformity NOS }

757 Congenital anomalies of the integument
Includes: anomalies of skin, subcutaneous tissue, hair, nails, and breast

Excludes: *hemangioma (228.00-228.09)*
pigmented nevus (216.0-216.9)

757.0 Hereditary edema of legs
Congenital lymphedema
Hereditary trophedema
Milroy's disease

757.1 Ichthyosis congenita
Congenital ichthyosis
Harlequin fetus
Ichthyosiform erythroderma

757.2 Dermatoglyphic anomalies
Abnormal palmar creases

757.3 Other specified anomalies of skin

757.31 Congenital ectodermal dysplasia

757.32 Vascular hamartomas
Birthmarks
Port-wine stain
Strawberry nevus

757.33 Congenital pigmentary anomalies of skin
Congenital poikiloderma
Urticaria pigmentosa
Xeroderma pigmentosum

Excludes: *albinism (270.2)*

757.39 Other
Accessory skin tags, congenital
Congenital scar
Epidermolysis bullosa
Keratoderma (congenital)

Excludes: *pilonidal cyst (685.0-685.1)*

757.4 Specified anomalies of hair
Congenital:
alopecia
atrichosis
beaded hair
Congenital:
hypertrichosis
monilethrix
Persistent lanugo

757.5 Specified anomalies of nails

Anonychia
Congenital:
clubnail
koilonychia
Congenital:
leukonychia
onychauxis
pachyonychia

757.6 Specified anomalies of breast

Absent, Accessory, Supernumerary } breast or nipple
Hypoplasia of breast

Excludes: *absence of pectoral muscle (756.81)*

757.8 Other specified anomalies of the integument

757.9 Unspecified anomaly of the integument

Congenital:
anomaly NOS, deformity NOS } of integument

758 Chromosomal anomalies

Includes: syndromes associated with anomalies in the number and form of chromosomes

758.0 Down's syndrome

Mongolism
Translocation Down's syndrome
Trisomy:
21 or 22
G

758.1 Patau's syndrome

Trisomy:
13
D_1

758.2 Edwards' syndrome

Trisomy:
18
E_3

758.3 Autosomal deletion syndromes

Antimongolism syndrome
Cri-du-chat syndrome

758.4 Balanced autosomal translocation in normal individual

758.5 Other conditions due to autosomal anomalies

Accessory autosomes NEC

758.6 Gonadal dysgenesis

Ovarian dysgenesis
Turner's syndrome
XO syndrome

Excludes: *pure gonadal dysgenesis (752.7)*

758.7 Klinefelter's syndrome

XXY syndrome

758.8 Other conditions due to sex chromosome anomalies

Additional sex chromosome
Sex chromosome mosaicism
Syndrome:
triple X
XXX
XYY

758.9 Conditions due to anomaly of unspecified chromosome

759 Other and unspecified congenital anomalies

759.0 Anomalies of spleen

Aberrant, Absent, Accessory } spleen
Congenital splenomegaly
Ectopic spleen
Lobulation of spleen

759.1 Anomalies of adrenal gland

Aberrant, Absent, Accessory } adrenal gland

Excludes: *adrenogenital disorders (255.2)*
congenital disorders of steroid metabolism (255.2)

759.2 Anomalies of other endocrine glands
Absent parathyroid gland
Accessory thyroid gland
Persistent thyroglossal or thyrolingual duct
Thyroglossal (duct) cyst

Excludes: *congenital:*
goiter (246.1)
hypothyroidism (243)

759.3 Situs inversus
Situs inversus or transversus:
abdominalis
thoracis
Transposition of viscera:
abdominal
thoracic

Excludes: *dextrocardia without mention of complete transposition (746.87)*

759.4 Conjoined twins
Craniopagus
Dicephalus
Pygopagus
Thoracopagus
Xiphopagus

759.5 Tuberous sclerosis
Bourneville's disease
Epiloia

759.6 Other hamartoses, not elsewhere classified
Syndrome:
Peutz-Jeghers
Sturge-Weber (-Dimitri)
von Hippel-Lindau

Excludes: *neurofibromatosis (237.7)*

759.7 Multiple congenital anomalies, so described
Congenital:
anomaly, multiple NOS
deformity, multiple NOS

759.8 Other specified anomalies

759.81 Prader-Willi syndrome

759.82 Marfan syndrome

759.83 Fragile X syndrome

759.89 Other
Congenital malformation syndromes affecting multiple systems, not elsewhere classified
Laurence-Moon-Biedl syndrome

759.9 Congenital anomaly, unspecified

15. CERTAIN CONDITIONS ORIGINATING IN THE PERINATAL PERIOD (760-779)

Includes: conditions which have their origin in the perinatal period even though death or morbidity occurs later

Use additional code(s) to further specify condition

MATERNAL CAUSES OF PERINATAL MORBIDITY AND MORTALITY (760-763)

760 Fetus or newborn affected by maternal conditions which may be unrelated to present pregnancy

Includes: the listed maternal conditions only when specified as a cause of mortality or morbidity of the fetus or newborn

Excludes: maternal endocrine and metabolic disorders affecting fetus or newborn (775.0-775.9)

760.0 Maternal hypertensive disorders
Fetus or newborn affected by maternal conditions classifiable to 642

760.1 Maternal renal and urinary tract diseases
Fetus or newborn affected by maternal conditions classifiable to 580-599

760.2 Maternal infections
Fetus or newborn affected by maternal infectious disease classifiable to 001-136 and 487, but fetus or newborn not manifesting that disease

Excludes: congenital infectious diseases (771.0-771.8)
maternal genital tract and other localized infections (760.8)

760.3 Other chronic maternal circulatory and respiratory diseases
Fetus or newborn affected by chronic maternal conditions classifiable to 390-459, 490-519, 745-748

760.4 Maternal nutritional disorders
Fetus or newborn affected by:
maternal disorders classifiable to 260-269
maternal malnutrition NOS

Excludes: fetal malnutrition (764.10-764.29)

760.5 Maternal injury
Fetus or newborn affected by maternal conditions classifiable to 800-995

760.6 Surgical operation on mother

Excludes: cesarean section for present delivery (763.4)
damage to placenta from amniocentesis, cesarean section, or surgical induction (762.1)
previous surgery to uterus or pelvic organs (763.8)

760.7 Noxious influences affecting fetus via placenta or breast milk
Fetus or newborn affected by noxious substance transmitted via placenta or breast milk

Excludes: anesthetic and analgesic drugs administered during labor and delivery (763.5)
drug withdrawal syndrome in newborn (779.5)

760.70 Unspecified noxious substance
Fetus or newborn affected by:
Drug NEC

760.71 Alcohol
Fetal alcohol syndrome

760.72 Narcotics

760.73 Hallucinogenic agents

760.74 Anti-infectives
Antibiotics

760.75 Cocaine

760.76 Diethylstilbestrol (DES)

760.79 Other
Fetus or newborn affected by:
immune sera } transmitted via placenta or breast milk
medicinal agents NEC } transmitted via placenta or breast milk
toxic substance NEC } transmitted via placenta or breast milk

760.8 Other specified maternal conditions affecting fetus or newborn
Maternal genital tract and other localized infection affecting fetus or newborn, but fetus or newborn not manifesting that disease

Excludes: maternal urinary tract infection affecting fetus or newborn (760.1)

760.9 Unspecified maternal condition affecting fetus or newborn

761 Fetus or newborn affected by maternal complications of pregnancy

Includes: the listed maternal conditions only when specified as a cause of mortality or morbidity of the fetus or newborn

761.0 Incompetent cervix

761.1 Premature rupture of membranes

761.2 Oligohydramnios

Excludes: *that due to premature rupture of membranes (761.1)*

761.3 Polyhydramnios

Hydramnios (acute) (chronic)

761.4 Ectopic pregnancy

Pregnancy:
- abdominal
- intraperitoneal
- tubal

761.5 Multiple pregnancy

Triplet (pregnancy)
Twin (pregnancy)

761.6 Maternal death

761.7 Malpresentation before labor

Breech presentation, External version, Oblique lie, Transverse lie, Unstable lie } before labor

761.8 Other specified maternal complications of pregnancy affecting fetus or newborn

Spontaneous abortion, fetus

761.9 Unspecified maternal complication of pregnancy affecting fetus or newborn

762 Fetus or newborn affected by complications of placenta, cord, and membranes

Includes: the listed maternal conditions only when specified as a cause of mortality or morbidity in the fetus or newborn

762.0 Placenta previa

762.1 Other forms of placental separation and hemorrhage

Abruptio placentae
Antepartum hemorrhage
Damage to placenta from amniocentesis, cesarean section, or surgical induction
Maternal blood loss
Premature separation of placenta
Rupture of marginal sinus

762.2 Other and unspecified morphological and functional abnormalities of placenta

Placental:
- dysfunction
- infarction
- insufficiency

762.3 Placental transfusion syndromes

Placental and cord abnormality resulting in twin-to-twin or other transplacental transfusion

Use additional code, if desired, to indicate resultant condition in fetus or newborn:
- fetal blood loss (772.0)
- polycythemia neonatorum (776.4)

762.4 Prolapsed cord

Cord presentation

762.5 Other compression of umbilical cord

Cord around neck
Entanglement of cord
Knot in cord
Torsion of cord

762.6 Other and unspecified conditions of umbilical cord

Short cord
Thrombosis, Varices, Velamentous insertion, Vasa previa } of umbilical cord

Excludes: *infection of umbilical cord (771.4)*
single umbilical artery (747.5)

● Code new to this edition
▲ Revision of existing code
④ ⑤ Fourth or fifth digit required

762.7 Chorioamnionitis
Amnionitis
Membranitis
Placentitis

762.8 Other specified abnormalities of chorion and amnion

762.9 Unspecified abnormality of chorion and amnion

763 Fetus or newborn affected by other complications of labor and delivery
Includes: the listed conditions only when specified as a cause of mortality or morbidity in the fetus or newborn

763.0 Breech delivery and extraction

763.1 Other malpresentation, malposition, and disproportion during labor and delivery
Fetus or newborn affected by:
abnormality of bony pelvis
contracted pelvis
persistent occipitoposterior position
shoulder presentation
transverse lie
conditions classifiable to 652, 653, and 660

763.2 Forceps delivery
Fetus or newborn affected by forceps extraction

763.3 Delivery by vacuum extractor

763.4 Cesarean delivery

Excludes: placental separation or hemorrhage from cesarean section (762.1)

763.5 Maternal anesthesia and analgesia
Reactions and intoxications from maternal opiates and tranquilizers during labor and delivery

Excludes: drug withdrawal syndrome in newborn (779.5)

763.6 Precipitate delivery
Rapid second stage

763.7 Abnormal uterine contractions
Fetus or newborn affected by:
contraction ring
hypertonic labor
hypotonic uterine dysfunction
uterine inertia or dysfunction
conditions classifiable to 661, except 661.3

763.8 Other specified complications of labor and delivery affecting fetus or newborn
Fetus or newborn affected by:
abnormality of maternal soft tissues
destructive operation on live fetus to facilitate delivery
induction of labor (medical)
previous surgery to uterus or pelvic organs
other conditions classifiable to 650-669
other procedures used in labor and delivery

763.9 Unspecified complication of labor and delivery affecting fetus or newborn

OTHER CONDITIONS ORIGINATING IN THE PERINATAL PERIOD (764-779)

The following fifth-digit subclassification is for use with categories 764-765 to denote birthweight:

0 unspecified [weight]
1 less than 500 grams
2 500-749 grams
3 750-999 grams
4 1,000- 1,249 grams
5 1,250-1,499 grams
6 1,500-1,749 grams
7 1,750-1,999 grams
8 2,000-2,499 grams
9 2,500 grams and over

⑤ **764 Slow fetal growth and fetal malnutrition**

Excludes: low birthweight due to short gestation (765.00-765.19)

764.0 "Light-for-dates" without mention of fetal malnutrition
Infants underweight for gestational age
"Small-for-dates"

764.1 "Light-for-dates" with signs of fetal malnutrition
Infants "light-for-dates" classifiable to 764.0, who in addition show signs of fetal malnutrition, such as dry peeling skin and loss of subcutaneous tissue

764.2 Fetal malnutrition without mention of "light-for-dates"
Infants, not underweight for gestational age, showing signs of fetal malnutrition, such as dry peeling skin and loss of subcutaneous tissue
Intrauterine malnutrition

764.9 Fetal growth retardation, unspecified
Intrauterine growth retardation

⑤ **765 Disorders relating to short gestation and unspecified low birthweight**
Includes: the listed conditions, without further specification, as causes of mortality, morbidity, or additional care, in fetus or newborn

Excludes: *low birthweight due to slow fetal growth and fetal malnutrition (764.00-764.99)*

765.0 Extreme immaturity

Note: Usually implies a birthweight of less than 1000 grams and/or a gestation of less than 28 completed weeks.

765.1 Other preterm infants

Note: Usually implies a birthweight of 1000-2499 grams and/or a gestation of 28-37 completed weeks.
Prematurity NOS
Prematurity or small size, not classifiable to 765.0 or as "light-for-dates" in 764

766 Disorders relating to long gestation and high birthweight
Includes: the listed conditions, without further specification, as causes of mortality, morbidity, or additional care, in fetus or newborn

766.0 Exceptionally large baby

Note: Usually implies a birthweight of 4500 grams or more.

766.1 Other "heavy-for-dates" infants
Other fetus or infant "heavy-" or "large-for-dates" regardless of period of gestation

766.2 Post-term infant, not "heavy-for-dates"
Fetus or infant with gestation period of 294 days or more [42 or more completed weeks], not "heavy-" or "large-for-dates"
Postmaturity NOS

767 Birth trauma

767.0 Subdural and cerebral hemorrhage
Subdural and cerebral hemorrhage, whether described as due to birth trauma or to intrapartum anoxia or hypoxia
Subdural hematoma (localized)
Tentorial tear

Use additional code, if desired, to identify cause

Excludes: *intraventricular hemorrhage (772.1)*
subarachnoid hemorrhage (772.2)

767.1 Injuries to scalp
Caput succedaneum
Cephalhematoma
Chignon (from vacuum extraction)
Massive epicranial subaponeurotic hemorrhage

767.2 Fracture of clavicle

767.3 Other injuries to skeleton
Fracture of:
long bones
skull

Excludes: *congenital dislocation of hip (754.30-754.35)*
fracture of spine, congenital (767.4)

● Code new to this edition
▲ Revision of existing code
④ ⑤ Fourth or fifth digit required

767.4 Injury to spine and spinal cord
Dislocation, Fracture, Laceration, Rupture } of spine or spinal cord due to birth trauma

767.5 Facial nerve injury
Facial palsy

767.6 Injury to brachial plexus
Palsy or paralysis:
  brachial
  Erb (-Duchenne)
  Klumpke (-Déjérine)

767.7 Other cranial and peripheral nerve injuries
Phrenic nerve paralysis

767.8 Other specified birth trauma
Eye damage
Hematoma of:
  liver (subcapsular)
  testes
  vulva
Rupture of:
  liver
  spleen
Scalpel wound
Traumatic glaucoma

Excludes: *hemorrhage classifiable to 772.0-772.9*

767.9 Birth trauma, unspecified
Birth injury NOS

768 Intrauterine hypoxia and birth asphyxia
Use only when associated with newborn morbidity classifiable elsewhere

768.0 Fetal death from asphyxia or anoxia before onset of labor or at unspecified time

768.1 Fetal death from asphyxia or anoxia during labor

768.2 Fetal distress before onset of labor, in liveborn infant
Abnormal fetal heart rate or rhythm
Fetal or intrauterine:
  acidosis
  anoxia or hypoxia
Any condition classifiable to 768.4
} first noted before onset of labor, liveborn infant

768.3 Fetal distress first noted during labor, in liveborn infant
Abnormal fetal heart rate or rhythm
Fetal or intrauterine:
  acidosis
  anoxia or hypoxia
Any condition classifiable to 768.4
} first noted during labor or delivery, liveborn infant

768.4 Fetal distress, unspecified, as to time of onset, in liveborn infant
Abnormal fetal heart rate or rhythm
Fetal or intrauterine:
  acidosis
  anoxia
  asphyxia
  distress
  hypercapnia
  hypoxia
} not stated whether first noted before or after onset of labor, liveborn infant

768.5 Severe birth asphyxia
Birth asphyxia with neurologic involvement

768.6 Mild or moderate birth asphyxia
Other specified birth asphyxia (without mention of neurologic involvement)

768.9 Unspecified birth asphyxia in liveborn infant
Anoxia, Asphyxia, Hypoxia } NOS, in liveborn infant

769 Respiratory distress syndrome
Cardiorespiratory distress syndrome of newborn
Hyaline membrane disease (pulmonary)
Idiopathic respiratory distress syndrome [IRDS or RDS] of newborn
Pulmonary hypoperfusion syndrome

Excludes: *transient tachypnea of newborn (770.6)*

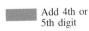

770 Other respiratory conditions of fetus and newborn

770.0 Congenital pneumonia
Infective pneumonia acquired prenatally

Excludes: *pneumonia from infection acquired after birth (480.0-486)*

770.1 Meconium aspiration syndrome
Aspiration of contents of birth canal NOS
Meconium aspiration below vocal cords
Pneumonitis:
fetal aspiration
meconium

770.2 Interstitial emphysema and related conditions
Pneumomediastinum, Pneumopericardium, Pneumothorax } originating in the perinatal period

770.3 Pulmonary hemorrhage
Hemorrhage:
alveolar (lung), intra-alveolar (lung), massive pulmonary } originating in the perinatal period

770.4 Primary atelectasis
Pulmonary immaturity NOS

770.5 Other and unspecified atelectasis
Atelectasis:
NOS, partial, secondary
Pulmonary collapse } originating in the perinatal period

770.6 Transitory tachypnea of newborn
Idiopathic tachypnea of newborn
Wet lung syndrome

Excludes: *respiratory distress syndrome (769)*

770.7 Chronic respiratory disease arising in the perinatal period
Bronchopulmonary dysplasia
Interstitial pulmonary fibrosis of prematurity
Wilson-Mikity syndrome

770.8 Other respiratory problems after birth
Apneic spells NOS, Cyanotic attacks NOS, Respiratory distress NOS, Respiratory failure NOS } originating in the perinatal period

770.9 Unspecified respiratory condition of fetus and newborn

771 Infections specific to the perinatal period
Includes: infections acquired before or during birth or via the umbilicus

Excludes: *congenital pneumonia (770.0)*
congenital syphilis (090.0-090.9)
maternal infectious disease as a cause of mortality or morbidity in fetus or newborn, but fetus or newborn not manifesting the disease (760.2)
ophthalmia neonatorum due to gonococcus (098.40)
other infections not specifically classified to this category

771.0 Congenital rubella
Congenital rubella pneumonitis

771.1 Congenital cytomegalovirus infection
Congenital cytomegalic inclusion disease

771.2 Other congenital infections
Congenital:
herpes simplex
listeriosis
malaria
Congenital:
toxoplasmosis
tuberculosis

771.3 Tetanus neonatorum
Tetanus omphalitis

Excludes: *hypocalcemic tetany (775.4)*

771.4 Omphalitis of the newborn
Infection:
navel cord
umbilical stump

Excludes: *tetanus omphalitis (771.3)*

771.5 Neonatal infective mastitis

Excludes: *noninfective neonatal mastitis (778.7)*

771.6 Neonatal conjunctivitis and dacryocystitis
Ophthalmia neonatorum NOS

Excludes: *ophthalmia neonatorum due to gonococcus (098.40)*

771.7 Neonatal Candida infection
Neonatal moniliasis
Thrush in newborn

771.8 Other infection specific to the perinatal period
Intra-amniotic infection of fetus:
NOS
clostridial
Escherichia coli [E. coli]
Intrauterine sepsis of fetus
Neonatal urinary tract infection
Septicemia [sepsis] of newborn

772 Fetal and neonatal hemorrhage

Excludes: *hematological disorders of fetus and newborn (776.0-776.9)*

772.0 Fetal blood loss
Fetal blood loss from:
cut end of co-twin's cord
placenta
ruptured cord
vasa previa
Fetal exsanguination
Fetal hemorrhage into:
co-twin
mother's circulation

772.1 Intraventricular hemorrhage
Intraventricular hemorrhage from any perinatal cause

772.2 Subarachnoid hemorrhage
Subarachnoid hemorrhage from any perinatal cause

Excludes: *subdural and cerebral hemorrhage (767.0)*

772.3 Umbilical hemorrhage after birth
Slipped umbilical ligature

772.4 Gastrointestinal hemorrhage

Excludes: *swallowed maternal blood (777.3)*

772.5 Adrenal hemorrhage

772.6 Cutaneous hemorrhage
Bruising, Ecchymoses, Petechiae, Superficial hematoma } in fetus or newborn

772.8 Other specified hemorrhage of fetus or newborn

Excludes: *hemorrhagic disease of newborn (776.0)*
pulmonary hemorrhage (770.3)

772.9 Unspecified hemorrhage of newborn

773 Hemolytic disease of fetus or newborn, due to isoimmunization

773.0 Hemolytic disease due to Rh isoimmunization
Anemia, Erythroblastosis (fetalis), Hemolytic disease (fetus) (newborn), Jaundice } due to RH: antibodies, isoimmunization, maternal/fetal incompatibility
Rh hemolytic disease
Rh isoimmunization

773.1 Hemolytic disease due to ABO isoimmunization
ABO hemolytic disease
ABO isoimmunization

Anemia Erythroblastosis (fetalis) Hemolytic disease (fetus) (newborn) Jaundice	due to ABO: antibodies isoimmunization maternal/fetal incompatibility

773.2 Hemolytic disease due to other and unspecified isoimmunization
Erythroblastosis (fetalis) (neonatorum) NOS
Hemolytic disease (fetus) (newborn) NOS
Jaundice or anemia due to other and unspecified blood-group incompatibility

773.3 Hydrops fetalis due to isoimmunization
Use additional code, if desired, to identify type of isoimmunization (773.0-773.2)

773.4 Kernicterus due to isoimmunization
Use additional code, if desired, to identify type of isoimmunization (773.0-773.2)

773.5 Late anemia due to isoimmunization

774 Other perinatal jaundice

774.0 Perinatal jaundice from hereditary hemolytic anemias
Code first underlying disease (282.0-282.9)

774.1 Perinatal jaundice from other excessive hemolysis
Fetal or neonatal jaundice from:
bruising
drugs or toxins transmitted from mother
infection
polycythemia
swallowed maternal blood

Use additional code, if desired, to identify cause

Excludes: *jaundice due to isoimmunization (773.0-773.2)*

774.2 Neonatal jaundice associated with preterm delivery
Hyperbilirubinemia of prematurity
Jaundice due to delayed conjugation associated with preterm delivery

774.3 Neonatal jaundice due to delayed conjugation from other causes

774.30 Neonatal jaundice due to delayed conjugation, cause unspecified

774.31 Neonatal jaundice due to delayed conjugation in diseases classified elsewhere
Code first underlying diseases, as:
congenital hypothyroidism (243)
Crigler-Najjar syndrome (277.4)
Gilbert's syndrome (277.4)

774.39 Other
Jaundice due to delayed conjugation from causes, such as:
breast milk inhibitors
delayed development of conjugating system

774.4 Perinatal jaundice due to hepatocellular damage
Fetal or neonatal hepatitis
Giant cell hepatitis
Inspissated bile syndrome

774.5 Perinatal jaundice from other causes
Code first underlying cause, as:
congenital obstruction of bile duct (751.61)
galactosemia (271.1)
mucoviscidosis (277.00-277.01)

774.6 Unspecified fetal and neonatal jaundice
Icterus neonatorum
Neonatal hyperbilirubinemia (transient)
Physiologic jaundice NOS in newborn

Excludes: *that in preterm infants (774.2)*

774.7 Kernicterus not due to isoimmunization
Bilirubin encephalopathy
Kernicterus of newborn NOS

Excludes: *kernicterus due to isoimmunization (773.4)*

● Code new to this edition ▲ Revision of existing code ④ ⑤ Fourth or fifth digit required

775 Endocrine and metabolic disturbances specific to the fetus and newborn
Includes: transitory endocrine and metabolic disturbances caused by the infant's response to maternal endocrine and metabolic factors, its removal from them, or its adjustment to extrauterine existence

775.0 Syndrome of "infant of a diabetic mother"
Maternal diabetes mellitus affecting fetus or newborn (with hypoglycemia)

775.1 Neonatal diabetes mellitus
Diabetes mellitus syndrome in newborn infant

775.2 Neonatal myasthenia gravis

775.3 Neonatal thyrotoxicosis
Neonatal hyperthyroidism (transient)

775.4 Hypocalcemia and hypomagnesemia of newborn
Cow's milk hypocalcemia
Hypocalcemic tetany, neonatal
Neonatal hypoparathyroidism
Phosphate-loading hypocalcemia

775.5 Other transitory neonatal electrolyte disturbances
Dehydration, neonatal

775.6 Neonatal hypoglycemia

Excludes: infant of mother with diabetes mellitus (775.0)

775.7 Late metabolic acidosis of newborn

775.8 Other transitory neonatal endocrine and metabolic disturbances
Amino-acid metabolic disorders described as transitory

775.9 Unspecified endocrine and metabolic disturbances specific to the fetus and newborn

776 Hematological disorders of fetus and newborn
Includes: disorders specific to the fetus or newborn

776.0 Hemorrhagic disease of newborn
Hemorrhagic diathesis of newborn
Vitamin K deficiency of newborn

Excludes: fetal or neonatal hemorrhage (772.0-772.9)

776.1 Transient neonatal thrombocytopenia
Neonatal thrombocytopenia due to:
- exchange transfusion
- idiopathic maternal thrombocytopenia
- isoimmunization

776.2 Disseminated intravascular coagulation in newborn

776.3 Other transient neonatal disorders of coagulation
Transient coagulation defect, newborn

776.4 Polycythemia neonatorum
Plethora of newborn
Polycythemia due to:
- donor twin transfusion
- maternal-fetal transfusion

776.5 Congenital anemia
Anemia following fetal blood loss

Excludes: anemia due to isoimmunization (773.0-773.2, 773.5)
hereditary hemolytic anemias (282.0-282.9)

776.6 Anemia of prematurity

776.7 Transient neonatal neutropenia
Isoimmune neutropenia
Maternal transfer neutropenia

Excludes: congenital neutropenia (nontransient) (288.0)

776.8 Other specified transient hematological disorders

776.9 Unspecified hematological disorder specific to fetus or newborn

777 Perinatal disorders of digestive system
Includes: disorders specific to the fetus and newborn

Excludes: intestinal obstruction classifiable to 560.0-560.9

Add 4th or 5th digit | Nonspecific code | Unspecified code | Manifestation code

777.1 Meconium obstruction
Congenital fecaliths
Delayed passage of meconium
Meconium ileus NOS
Meconium plug syndrome

Excludes: *meconium ileus in cystic fibrosis (277.01)*

777.2 Intestinal obstruction due to inspissated milk

777.3 Hematemesis and melena due to swallowed maternal blood
Swallowed blood syndrome in newborn

Excludes: *that not due to swallowed maternal blood (772.4)*

777.4 Transitory ileus of newborn

Excludes: *Hirschsprung's disease (751.3)*

777.5 Necrotizing enterocolitis in fetus or newborn
Pseudomembranous enterocolitis in newborn

777.6 Perinatal intestinal perforation
Meconium peritonitis

777.8 Other specified perinatal disorders of digestive system

777.9 Unspecified perinatal disorder of digestive system

778 Conditions involving the integument and temperature regulation of fetus and newborn

778.0 Hydrops fetalis not due to isoimmunization
Idiopathic hydrops

Excludes: *hydrops fetalis due to isoimmunization (773.3)*

778.1 Sclerema neonatorum
Subcutaneous fat necrosis

778.2 Cold injury syndrome of newborn

778.3 Other hypothermia of newborn

778.4 Other disturbances of temperature regulation of newborn
Dehydration fever in newborn
Environmentally-induced pyrexia
Hyperthermia in newborn
Transitory fever of newborn

778.5 Other and unspecified edema of newborn
Edema neonatorum

778.6 Congenital hydrocele
Congenital hydrocele of tunica vaginalis

778.7 Breast engorgement in newborn
Noninfective mastitis of newborn

Excludes: *infective mastitis of newborn (771.5)*

778.8 Other specified conditions involving the integument of fetus and newborn
Urticaria neonatorum

Excludes: *impetigo neonatorum (684)*
pemphigus neonatorum (684)

778.9 Unspecified condition involving the integument and temperature regulation of fetus and newborn

779 Other and ill-defined conditions originating in the perinatal period

779.0 Convulsions in newborn
Fits } in newborn
Seizures }

779.1 Other and unspecified cerebral irritability in newborn

779.2 Cerebral depression, coma, and other abnormal cerebral signs
CNS dysfunction in newborn NOS

779.3 Feeding problems in newborn
Regurgitation of food }
Slow feeding } in newborn
Vomiting }

779.4 Drug reactions and intoxications specific to newborn
Gray syndrome from chloramphenicol administration in newborn

Excludes: *fetal alcohol syndrome (760.71)*
reactions and intoxications from maternal opiates and tranquilizers (763.5)

779.5 Drug withdrawal syndrome in newborn
Drug withdrawal syndrome in infant of dependent mother

Excludes: *fetal alcohol syndrome (760.71)*

779.6 Termination of pregnancy (fetus)
Fetus death due to:
induced abortion
termination of pregnancy

Excludes: *spontaneous abortion (fetus) (761.8)*

779.8 Other specified conditions originating in the perinatal period

779.9 Unspecified condition originating in the perinatal period
Congenital debility NOS
Stillbirth NEC

16. SYMPTOMS, SIGNS, AND ILL-DEFINED CONDITIONS (780-799)

This section includes symptoms, signs, abnormal results of laboratory or other investigative procedures, and ill-defined conditions regarding which no diagnosis classifiable elsewhere is recorded.

Signs and symptoms that point rather definitely to a given diagnosis are assigned to some category in the preceding part of the classification. In general, categories 780-796 include the more ill-defined conditions and symptoms that point with perhaps equal suspicion to two or more diseases or to two or more systems of the body, and without the necessary study of the case to make a final diagnosis. Practically all categories in this group could be designated as "not otherwise specified," or as "unknown etiology," or as "transient." The Alphabetic Index should be consulted to determine which symptoms and signs are to be allocated here and which to more specific sections of the classification; the residual subcategories numbered .9 are provided for other relevant symptoms which cannot be allocated elsewhere in the classification.

The conditions and signs or symptoms included in categories 780-796 consist of: (a) cases for which no more specific diagnosis can be made even after all facts bearing on the case have been investigated; (b) signs or symptoms existing at the time of initial encounter that proved to be transient and whose causes could not be determined; (c) provisional diagnoses in a patient who failed to return for further investigation or care; (d) cases referred elsewhere for investigation or treatment before the diagnosis was made; (e) cases in which a more precise diagnosis was not available for any other reason; (f) certain symptoms which represent important problems in medical care and which it might be desired to classify in addition to a known cause.

SYMPTOMS (780-789)

780 General symptoms

780.0 Alteration of consciousness

Excludes: *coma:*
diabetic (250.2-250.3)
hepatic (572.2)
originating in the perinatal period (779.2)

780.01 Coma

780.02 Transient alteration of awareness

780.03 Persistent vegetative state

780.09 Other

Drowsiness
Semicoma
Unconsciousness
Somnolence
Stupor

780.1 Hallucinations

Hallucinations:
NOS
auditory
gustatory
Hallucinations:
olfactory
tactile

Excludes: *those associated with mental disorders, as functional psychoses (295.0-298.9)*
organic brain syndromes (290.0-294.9, 310.0-310.9)
visual hallucinations (368.16)

780.2 Syncope and collapse

Blackout
Fainting
(Near) (Pre) syncope
Vasovagal attack

Excludes: *carotid sinus syncope (337.0)*
heat syncope (992.1)
neurocirculatory asthenia (306.2)
orthostatic hypotension (458.0)
shock NOS (785.50)

780.3 Convulsions

Convulsions:
NOS
febrile
infantile
Convulsive:
disorder NOS
seizure NOS
Fit NOS

Excludes: *convulsions:*
epileptic (345.10-345.91)
in newborn (779.0)

780.4 Dizziness and giddiness

Light-headedness
Vertigo NOS

Excludes: *Ménière's disease and other specified vertiginous syndromes (386.0-386.9)*

780.5 Sleep disturbances

Excludes: *that of nonorganic origin (307.40-307.49)*

780.50 Sleep disturbance, unspecified

780.51 Insomnia with sleep apnea

780.52 Other insomnia
Insomnia NOS

780.53 Hypersomnia with sleep apnea

780.54 Other hypersomnia
Hypersomnia NOS

780.55 Disruptions of 24-hour sleep-wake cycle
Inversion of sleep rhythm
Irregular sleep-wake rhythm NOS
Non-24-hour sleep-wake rhythm

780.56 Dysfunctions associated with sleep stages or arousal from sleep

780.57 Other and unspecified sleep apnea

780.59 Other

▲ **780.6 Fever**
Chills with fever
Fever NOS
Hyperpyrexia NOS
Pyrexia NOS
Pyrexia of unknown origin

Excludes: *pyrexia of unknown origin (during):*
in newborn (778.4)
labor (659.2)
the puerperium (672)

780.7 Malaise and fatigue
Asthenia NOS
Lethargy
Postviral (asthenic) syndrome
Tiredness

Excludes: *debility, unspecified (799.3)*
fatigue (during):
combat (308.0-308.9)
heat (992.6)
pregnancy (646.8)
neurasthenia (300.5)
senile asthenia (797.5)

780.8 Hyperhidrosis
Diaphoresis
Excessive sweating

780.9 Other general symptoms
Amnesia (retrograde)
Chill(s) NOS
Generalized pain
Hypothermia, not associated with low environmental temperature

Excludes: *hypothermia:*
NOS (accidental) (991.6)
due to anesthesia (995.89)
of newborn (778.2-778.3)
memory disturbance as part of a pattern of mental disorder

781 Symptoms involving nervous and musculoskeletal systems

Excludes: *depression NOS (311)*
disorders specifically relating to:
back (724.0-724.9)
hearing (388.0-389.9)
joint (718.0-719.9)
limb (729.0-729.9)
neck (723.0-723.9)
vision (368.0-369.9)
pain in limb (729.5)

781.0 Abnormal involuntary movements
Abnormal head movements
Fasciculation
Spasms NOS
Tremor NOS

Excludes: *abnormal reflex (796.1)*
chorea NOS (333.5)
infantile spasms (345.60-345.61)
spastic paralysis (342.1, 343.0-344.9)
specified movement disorders classifiable to 333 (333.0-333.9)
that of nonorganic origin (307.2-307.3)

781.1 Disturbances of sensation of smell and taste
Anosmia
Parageusia
Parosmia

781.2 Abnormality of gait
Gait:
ataxic
paralytic
spastic
staggering

Excludes: *ataxia:*
NOS (781.3)
locomotor (progressive) (094.0)
difficulty in walking (719.7)

781.3 Lack of coordination
Ataxia NOS
Muscular incoordination

Excludes: *ataxic gait (781.2)*
cerebellar ataxia (334.0-334.9)
difficulty in walking (719.7)
vertigo NOS (780.4)

781.4 Transient paralysis of limb
Monoplegia, transient NOS

Excludes: *paralysis (342.0-344.9)*

781.5 Clubbing of fingers

781.6 Meningismus
Dupré's syndrome
Meningism

781.7 Tetany
Carpopedal spasm

Excludes: *tetanus neonatorum (771.3)*
tetany:
hysterical (300.11)
newborn (hypocalcemic) (775.4)
parathyroid (252.1)
psychogenic (306.0)

781.8 Neurologic neglect syndrome
Asomatognosia
Hemi-akinesia
Hemi-inattention
Hemispatial neglect
Left-sided neglect
Sensory extinction
Sensory neglect
Visuospatial neglect

781.9 Other symptoms involving nervous and musculoskeletal systems
Abnormal posture

782 Symptoms involving skin and other integumentary tissue

Excludes: *symptoms relating to breast (611.71-611.79)*

782.0 Disturbance of skin sensation
Anesthesia of skin
Burning or prickling sensation
Hyperesthesia
Hypoesthesia
Numbness
Paresthesia
Tingling

782.1 Rash and other nonspecific skin eruption
Exanthem

Excludes: *vesicular eruption (709.8)*

Add 4th or 5th digit | Nonspecific code | Unspecified code | Manifestation code

782.2 Localized superficial swelling, mass, or lump
Subcutaneous nodules

Excludes: *localized adiposity (278.1)*

782.3 Edema
Anasarca
Dropsy
Localized edema NOS

Excludes: *ascites (789.5)*
edema of:
newborn NOS (778.5)
pregnancy (642.0-642.9, 646.1)
fluid retention (276.6)
hydrops fetalis (773.3, 778.0)
hydrothorax (511.8)
nutritional edema (260, 262)

782.4 Jaundice, unspecified, not of newborn
Cholemia NOS
Icterus NOS

Excludes: *jaundice in newborn (774.0-774.7)*
due to isoimmunization (773.0-773.2, 773.4)

782.5 Cyanosis

Excludes: *newborn (770.8)*

782.6 Pallor and flushing

782.61 Pallor

782.62 Flushing
Excessive blushing

782.7 Spontaneous ecchymoses
Petechiae

Excludes: *ecchymosis in fetus or newborn (772.6)*
purpura (287.0-287.9)

782.8 Changes in skin texture
Induration } of skin
Thickening } of skin

782.9 Other symptoms involving skin and integumentary tissues

783 Symptoms concerning nutrition, metabolism, and development

783.0 Anorexia
Loss of appetite

Excludes: *anorexia nervosa (307.1)*
loss of appetite of nonorganic origin (307.59)

783.1 Abnormal weight gain

Excludes: *excessive weight gain in pregnancy (646.1)*
obesity (278.0)

783.2 Abnormal loss of weight

783.3 Feeding difficulties and mismanagement
Feeding problem (elderly) (infant)

Excludes: *feeding disturbance or problems:*
in newborn (779.3)
of nonorganic origin (307.50-307.59)

783.4 Lack of expected normal physiological development
Delayed milestone
Failure to gain weight
Failure to thrive
Lack of growth
Physical retardation
Short stature

Excludes: *delay in sexual development and puberty (259.0)*
specific delays in mental development (315.0-315.9)

783.5 Polydipsia
Excessive thirst

783.6 Polyphagia
Excessive eating
Hyperalimentation NOS

Excludes: *disorders of eating of nonorganic origin (307.50-307.59)*

783.9 Other symptoms concerning nutrition, metabolism, and development
Hypometabolism

Excludes: *abnormal basal metabolic rate (794.7)*
dehydration (276.5)
other disorders of fluid, electrolyte, and acid-base balance (276.0-276.9)

784 Symptoms involving head and neck

Excludes: *encephalopathy NOS (348.3)*
specific symptoms involving neck classifiable to 723 (723.0-723.9)

784.0 Headache
Facial pain
Pain in head NOS

Excludes: *atypical face pain (350.2)*
migraine (346.0-346.9)
tension headache (307.81)

784.1 Throat pain

Excludes: *dysphagia (787.2)*
neck pain (723.1)
sore throat (462)
chronic (472.1)

784.2 Swelling, mass, or lump in head and neck
Space-occupying lesion, intracranial NOS

784.3 Aphasia

Excludes: *developmental aphasia (315.31)*

784.4 Voice disturbance

784.40 Voice disturbance, unspecified

784.41 Aphonia
Loss of voice

784.49 Other
Change in voice
Dysphonia
Hoarseness
Hypernasality
Hyponasality

784.5 Other speech disturbance
Dysarthria
Dysphasia
Slurred speech

Excludes: *stammering and stuttering (307.0)*
that of nonorganic origin (307.0, 307.9)

784.6 Other symbolic dysfunction

Excludes: *developmental learning delays (315.0-315.9)*

784.60 Symbolic dysfunction, unspecified

784.61 Alexia and dyslexia
Alexia (with agraphia)

784.69 Other
Acalculia
Agnosia
Agraphia NOS
Apraxia

784.7 Epistaxis
Hemorrhage from nose
Nosebleed

784.8 Hemorrhage from throat

Excludes: *hemoptysis (786.3)*

784.9 Other symptoms involving head and neck
Choking sensation
Halitosis
Mouth breathing
Sneezing

785 Symptoms involving cardiovascular system

Excludes: *heart failure NOS (428.9)*

785.0 Tachycardia, unspecified
Rapid heart beat

Excludes: *paroxysmal tachycardia (427.0-427.2)*

Add 4th or 5th digit | Nonspecific code | Unspecified code | Manifestation code

785.1 Palpitations
Awareness of heart beat

Excludes: *specified dysrhythmias (427.0-427.9)*

785.2 Undiagnosed cardiac murmurs
Heart murmur NOS

785.3 Other abnormal heart sounds
Cardiac dullness, increased or decreased
Friction fremitus, cardiac
Precordial friction

785.4 Gangrene
Gangrene:
NOS
spreading cutaneous
Phagedena

Use additional code for any associated condition, as:
diabetes (250.7)
Raynaud's syndrome (443.0)

Excludes: *gangrene of certain sites—see Alphabetic Index*
gangrene with atherosclerosis of the extremities (440.24)
gas gangrene (040.0)

785.5 Shock without mention of trauma

785.50 Shock, unspecified
Failure of peripheral circulation

785.51 Cardiogenic shock

785.59 Other
Shock:
endotoxic
gram-negative
Shock:
hypovolemic
septic

Excludes: *shock (due to):*
anesthetic (995.4)
anaphylactic (995.0)
due to serum (999.4)
electric (994.8)
following abortion (639.5)
lightning (994.0)
obstetrical (669.1)
postoperative (998.0)
traumatic (958.4)

785.6 Enlargement of lymph nodes
Lymphadenopathy
"Swollen glands"

Excludes: *lymphadenitis (chronic) (289.1-289.3)*
acute (683)

785.9 Other symptoms involving cardiovascular system
Bruit (arterial)
Weak pulse

786 Symptoms involving respiratory system and other chest symptoms

786.0 Dyspnea and respiratory abnormalities

786.00 Respiratory abnormality, unspecified

786.01 Hyperventilation

Excludes: *hyperventilation, psychogenic (306.1)*

786.02 Orthopnea

786.09 Other
Apnea
Cheyne-Stokes respiration
Respiratory:
distress
insufficiency
Shortness of breath
Tachypnea
Wheezing

Excludes: *respiratory distress:*
following trauma and surgery (518.5)
newborn (770.8)
syndrome (newborn) (769)
adult (518.5)
respiratory failure (518.81)
newborn (770.8)
sleep apnea (780.51, 780.53, 780.57)
transitory tachypnea of newborn (770.6)

786.1 Stridor

Excludes: *congenital laryngeal stridor (748.3)*

786.2 Cough

Excludes: *cough:*
psychogenic (306.1)
smokers' (491.0)
with hemorrhage (786.3)

786.3 Hemoptysis
Cough with hemorrhage
Pulmonary hemorrhage NOS

Excludes: *pulmonary hemorrhage of newborn (770.3)*

786.4 Abnormal sputum
Abnormal: amount, color, odor (of) sputum
Excessive (of) sputum

786.5 Chest pain

786.50 Chest pain, unspecified

786.51 Precordial pain

786.52 Painful respiration
Pain:
anterior chest wall
pleuritic
Pleurodynia

Excludes: *epidemic pleurodynia (074.1)*

786.59 Other
Discomfort in chest
Pressure in chest
Tightness in chest

Excludes: *pain in breast (611.71)*

786.6 Swelling, mass, or lump in chest

Excludes: *lump in breast (611.72)*

786.7 Abnormal chest sounds
Abnormal percussion, chest
Friction sounds, chest
Rales
Tympany, chest

Excludes: *wheezing (786.09)*

786.8 Hiccough

Excludes: *psychogenic hiccough (306.1)*

786.9 Other symptoms involving respiratory system and chest
Breath-holding spell

787 Symptoms involving digestive system

Excludes: *constipation (564.0)*
pylorospasm (537.81)
congenital (750.5)

787.0 Nausea and vomiting
Emesis

Excludes: *hematemesis NOS (578.0)*
vomiting:
bilious, following gastrointestinal surgery (564.3)
cyclical (536.2)
psychogenic (306.4)
excessive, in pregnancy (643.0-643.9)
habit (536.2)
of newborn (779.3)
psychogenic NOS (307.54)

787.01 Nausea with vomiting

787.02 Nausea alone

787.03 Vomiting alone

787.1 Heartburn
Pyrosis
Waterbrash

Excludes: *dyspepsia or indigestion (536.8)*

787.2 Dysphagia
Difficulty in swallowing

787.3 Flatulence, eructation, and gas pain
Abdominal distention (gaseous)
Bloating
Tympanites (abdominal) (intestinal)

Excludes: *aerophagy (306.4)*

787.4 Visible peristalsis
Hyperperistalsis

787.5 Abnormal bowel sounds
Absent bowel sounds
Hyperactive bowel sounds

787.6 Incontinence of feces
Encopresis NOS
Incontinence of sphincter ani

Excludes: *that of nonorganic origin (307.7)*

787.7 Abnormal feces
Bulky stools

Excludes: *abnormal stool content (792.1)*
melena:
NOS (578.1)
newborn (772.4, 777.3)

▲ **787.9 Other symptoms involving digestive system**

Excludes: *gastrointestinal hemorrhage (578.0-578.9)*
intestinal obstruction (560.0-560.9)
specific functional digestive disorders:
esophagus (530.0-530.9)
stomach and duodenum (536.0-536.9)
those not elsewhere classified (564.0-564.9)

● **787.91 Diarrhea**
Diarrhea NOS

● **787.99 Other**
Change in bowel habits
Tenesmus (rectal)

788 Symptoms involving urinary system

Excludes: *hematuria (599.7)*
nonspecific findings on examination of the urine (791.0-791.9)
small kidney of unknown cause (589.0-589.9)
uremia NOS (586)

788.0 Renal colic
Colic (recurrent) of:
kidney
ureter

788.1 Dysuria
Painful urination
Strangury

788.2 Retention of urine

788.20 Retention of urine, unspecified

788.21 Incomplete bladder emptying

788.29 Other specified retention of urine

788.3 Urinary incontinence

Excludes: *that of nonorganic origin (307.6)*

788.30 Urinary incontinence, unspecified
Enuresis NOS

788.31 Urge incontinence

788.32 Stress incontinence, male

Excludes: *stress incontinence (female) (625.6)*

788.33 Mixed incontinence (male) (female)
Urge and stress

788.34 Incontinence without sensory awareness

788.35 Post-void dribbling

788.36 Nocturnal enuresis

788.37 Continuous leakage

788.39 Other urinary incontinence

788.4 Frequency of urination and polyuria

788.41 Urinary frequency
Frequency of micturition

788.42 Polyuria

788.43 Nocturia

788.5 Oliguria and anuria
Deficient secretion of urine
Suppression of urinary secretion

Excludes: *that complicating:*
abortion (634-638 with .3, 639.3)
ectopic or molar pregnancy (639.3)
pregnancy, childbirth, or the puerperium (642.0-642.9, 646.2)

788.6 Other abnormality of urination

788.61 Splitting of urinary stream
Intermittent urinary stream

788.62 Slowing of urinary stream
Weak stream

788.69 Other

788.7 Urethral discharge
Penile discharge
Urethrorrhea

788.8 Extravasation of urine

788.9 Other symptoms involving urinary system
Extrarenal uremia
Vesical:
pain
tenesmus

789 Other symptoms involving abdomen and pelvis

The following fifth-digit subclassification is to be used for codes 789.0, 789.3, 789.4, 789.6

- **0 unspecified site**
- **1 right upper quadrant**
- **2 left upper quadrant**
- **3 right lower quadrant**
- **4 left lower quadrant**
- **5 periumbilic**
- **6 epigastric**
- **7 generalized**
- **9 other specified site**
  multiple sites

Excludes: *symptoms referable to genital organs:*
female (625.0-625.9)
male (607.0-608.9)
psychogenic (302.70-302.79)

789.0 Abdominal pain
Colic:
NOS
infantile
Cramps, abdominal

Excludes: *renal colic (788.0)*

789.1 Hepatomegaly
Enlargement of liver

789.2 Splenomegaly
Enlargement of spleen

789.3 Abdominal or pelvic swelling, mass, or lump
Diffuse or generalized swelling or mass:
abdominal NOS
umbilical

Excludes: *abdominal distention (gaseous) (787.3)*
ascites (789.5)

789.4 Abdominal rigidity

789.5 Ascites
Fluid in peritoneal cavity

789.6 Abdominal tenderness
Rebound tenderness

789.9 Other symptoms involving abdomen and pelvis
Umbilical:
bleeding
discharge

NONSPECIFIC ABNORMAL FINDINGS (790-796)

790 Nonspecific findings on examination of blood

Excludes: *abnormality of:*
platelets (287.0-287.9)
thrombocytes (287.0-287.9)
white blood cells (288.0-288.9)

790.0 Abnormality of red blood cells

Abnormal red cell:
- morphology NOS
- volume NOS

Anisocytosis
Poikilocytosis

Excludes: *anemia:*
- *congenital (776.5)*
- *newborn, due to isoimmunization (773.0-773.2, 773.5)*
- *of premature infant (776.6)*
- *other specified types (280.0-285.9)*

hemoglobin disorders (282.5-282.7)
polycythemia:
- *familial (289.6)*
- *neonatorum (776.4)*
- *secondary (289.0)*
- *vera (238.4)*

790.1 Elevated sedimentation rate

790.2 Abnormal glucose tolerance test

Excludes: *that complicating pregnancy, childbirth, or the puerperium (648.8)*

790.3 Excessive blood level of alcohol

Elevated blood-alcohol

790.4 Nonspecific elevation of levels of transaminase or lactic acid dehydrogenase [LDH]

790.5 Other nonspecific abnormal serum enzyme levels

Abnormal serum level of:
- acid phosphatase
- alkaline phosphatase

Abnormal serum level of:
- amylase
- lipase

Excludes: *deficiency of circulating enzymes (277.6)*

790.6 Other abnormal blood chemistry

Abnormal blood level of:
- cobalt
- copper
- iron
- lithium

Abnormal blood level of:
- magnesium
- mineral
- zinc

Excludes: *abnormality of electrolyte or acid-base balance (276.0-276.9)*
hypoglycemia NOS (251.2)
specific finding indicating abnormality of:
- *amino-acid transport and metabolism (270.0-270.9)*
- *carbohydrate transport and metabolism (271.0-271.9)*
- *lipid metabolism (272.0-272.9)*

uremia NOS (586)

790.7 Bacteremia

Excludes: *septicemia (038)*

Use additional code, if desired, to identify organism (041)

790.8 Viremia, unspecified

790.9 Other nonspecific findings on examination of blood

790.91 Abnormal arterial blood gases

790.92 Abnormal coagulation profile

Abnormal or prolonged:
- bleeding time
- coagulation time
- partial thromboplastin time [PTT]
- prothrombin time [PT]

Excludes: *coagulation (hemorrhagic) disorders (286.0-286.9)*

790.93 Elevated prostate specific antigen (PSA)

790.99 Other

791 Nonspecific findings on examination of urine

Excludes: *hematuria NOS (599.7)*
specific findings indicating abnormality of:
- *amino-acid transport and metabolism (270.0-270.9)*
- *carbohydrate transport and metabolism (271.0-271.9)*

791.0 Proteinuria
Albuminuria
Bence-Jones proteinuria

Excludes: *postural proteinuria (593.6)*
that arising during pregnancy or the puerperium (642.0-642.9, 646.2)

791.1 Chyluria

Excludes: *filarial (125.0-125.9)*

791.2 Hemoglobinuria

791.3 Myoglobinuria

791.4 Biliuria

791.5 Glycosuria

Excludes: *renal glycosuria (271.4)*

791.6 Acetonuria
Ketonuria

791.7 Other cells and casts in urine

791.9 Other nonspecific findings on examination of urine
Crystalluria
Elevated urine levels of:
- 17-ketosteroids
- catecholamines
- indolacetic acid
- vanillylmandelic acid [VMA]

Melanuria

792 Nonspecific abnormal findings in other body substances

Excludes: *that in chromosomal analysis (795.2)*

792.0 Cerebrospinal fluid

792.1 Stool contents
Abnormal stool color
Fat in stool
Mucus in stool
Occult blood
Pus in stool

Excludes: *blood in stool [melena] (578.1)*
newborn (772.4, 777.3)

792.2 Semen
Abnormal spermatozoa

Excludes: *azoospermia (606.0)*
oligospermia (606.1)

792.3 Amniotic fluid

792.4 Saliva

Excludes: *that in chromosomal analysis (795.2)*

792.9 Other nonspecific abnormal findings in body substances
Peritoneal fluid
Pleural fluid
Synovial fluid
Vaginal fluids

793 Nonspecific abnormal findings on radiological and other examination of body structure
Includes: nonspecific abnormal findings of:
thermography
ultrasound examination [echogram]
x-ray examination

Excludes: *abnormal results of function studies and radioisotope scans (794.0-794.9)*

793.0 Skull and head

Excludes: *nonspecific abnormal echoencephalogram (794.01)*

793.1 Lung field
Coin lesion } (of) lung
Shadow } (of) lung

793.2 Other intrathoracic organ
Abnormal:
- echocardiogram
- heart shadow
- ultrasound cardiogram

Mediastinal shift

● Code new to this edition
▲ Revision of existing code
④ ⑤ Fourth or fifth digit required

793.3 Biliary tract
Nonvisualization of gallbladder

793.4 Gastrointestinal tract

793.5 Genitourinary organs
Filling defect:
- bladder
- kidney
- ureter

793.6 Abdominal area, including retroperitoneum

793.7 Musculoskeletal system

793.8 Breast
Abnormal mammogram

793.9 Other
Abnormal:
- placental finding by x-ray or ultrasound method
- radiological findings in skin and subcutaneous tissue

Excludes: abnormal finding by radioisotope localization of placenta (794.9)

794 Nonspecific abnormal results of function studies

Includes: radioisotope:
- scans
- uptake studies

scintiphotography

794.0 Brain and central nervous system

794.00 Abnormal function study, unspecified

794.01 Abnormal echoencephalogram

794.02 Abnormal electroencephalogram [EEG]

794.09 Other
Abnormal brain scan

794.1 Peripheral nervous system and special senses

794.10 Abnormal response to nerve stimulation, unspecified

794.11 Abnormal retinal function studies
Abnormal electroretinogram [ERG]

794.12 Abnormal electro-oculogram [EOG]

794.13 Abnormal visually evoked potential

794.14 Abnormal oculomotor studies

794.15 Abnormal auditory function studies

794.16 Abnormal vestibular function studies

794.17 Abnormal electromyogram [EMG]

Excludes: that of eye (794.14)

794.19 Other

794.2 Pulmonary
Abnormal lung scan
Reduced:
- ventilatory capacity
- vital capacity

794.3 Cardiovascular

794.30 Abnormal function study, unspecified

794.31 Abnormal electrocardiogram [ECG] [EKG]

794.39 Other
Abnormal:
- ballistocardiogram
- phonocardiogram
- vectorcardiogram

794.4 Kidney
Abnormal renal function test

794.5 Thyroid
Abnormal thyroid:
scan
uptake

794.6 Other endocrine function study

794.7 Basal metabolism
Abnormal basal metabolic rate [BMR]

794.8 Liver
Abnormal liver scan

794.9 Other

Bladder	Placenta
Pancreas	Spleen

795 Nonspecific abnormal histological and immunological findings

Excludes: *nonspecific abnormalities of red blood cells (790.0)*

795.0 Nonspecific abnormal Papanicolaou smear of cervix
Dyskaryotic cervical smear

795.1 Nonspecific abnormal Papanicolaou smear of other site

795.2 Nonspecific abnormal findings on chromosomal analysis
Abnormal karyotype

795.3 Nonspecific positive culture findings
Positive culture findings in:
nose
sputum
throat
wound

Excludes: *that of:*
blood (790.7-790.8)
urine (599.0)

795.4 Other nonspecific abnormal histological findings

795.5 Nonspecific reaction to tuberculin skin test without active tuberculosis
Abnormal result of Mantoux test
PPD positive
Tuberculin (skin test):
positive
reactor

795.6 False positive serological test for syphilis
False positive Wassermann reaction

795.7 Other nonspecific immunological findings

Excludes: *isoimmunization, in pregnancy (656.1-656.2)*
affecting fetus or newborn (773.0-773.2)

  795.71 Nonspecific serologic evidence of human immunodeficiency virus [HIV]
Inconclusive human immunodeficiency virus [HIV] test (adult) (infant)

Note: This code is ONLY to be used when a test finding is reported as nonspecific. Asymptomatic positive findings are coded to V08. If any HIV infection symptom or condition is present, see code 042. Negative findings are not coded.

Excludes: *acquired immunodeficiency syndrome [AIDS] (042)*
asymptomatic human immunodeficiency virus, [HIV] infection status (V08)
HIV infection, symptomatic (042)
human immunodeficiency virus [HIV] disease (042)
positive (status) NOS (V08)

  795.79 Other and unspecified nonspecific immunological findings
Raised antibody titer
Raised level of immunoglobulins

796 Other nonspecific abnormal findings

796.0 Nonspecific abnormal toxicological findings
Abnormal levels of heavy metals or drugs in blood, urine, or other tissue

Excludes: *excessive blood level of alcohol (790.3)*

796.1 Abnormal reflex

● Code new to this edition	▲ Revision of existing code	④ ⑤ Fourth or fifth digit required

796.2 Elevated blood pressure reading without diagnosis of hypertension

Note: This category is to be used to record an episode of elevated blood pressure in a patient in whom no formal diagnosis of hypertension has been made, or as an incidental finding.

796.3 Nonspecific low blood pressure reading

796.4 Other abnormal clinical findings

796.9 Other

ILL-DEFINED AND UNKNOWN CAUSES OF MORBIDITY AND MORTALITY (797-799)

797 Senility without mention of psychosis

Old age
Senescence
Senile asthenia
Senile:
  debility
  exhaustion

Excludes: *senile psychoses (290.0-290.9)*

798 Sudden death, cause unknown

798.0 Sudden infant death syndrome

Cot death
Crib death
Sudden death of nonspecific cause in infancy

798.1 Instantaneous death

798.2 Death occurring in less than 24 hours from onset of symptoms, not otherwise explained

Death known not to be violent or instantaneous, for which no cause could be discovered
Died without sign of disease

798.9 Unattended death

Death in circumstances where the body of the deceased was found and no cause could be discovered
Found dead

799 Other ill-defined and unknown causes of morbidity and mortality

799.0 Asphyxia

Excludes: *asphyxia (due to):*
carbon monoxide (986)
inhalation of food or foreign body (932-934.9)
newborn (768.0-768.9)
traumatic (994.7)

799.1 Respiratory arrest

Cardiorespiratory failure

Excludes: *cardiac arrest (427.5)*
failure of peripheral circulation (785.50)
respiratory distress:
  NOS (786.09)
  acute (518.82)
  following trauma and surgery (518.5)
  newborn (770.8)
  syndrome (newborn) (769)
    adult (following trauma and surgery) (518.5)
      other (518.82)
respiratory failure (518.81)
  newborn (770.8)
respiratory insufficiency (786.09)
  acute (518.82)

799.2 Nervousness

"Nerves"

799.3 Debility, unspecified

Excludes: *asthenia (780.7)*
nervous debility (300.5)
neurasthenia (300.5)
senile asthenia (797)

799.4 Cachexia

Wasting disease

Excludes: *nutritional marasmus (261)*

799.8 Other ill-defined conditions

799.9 Other unknown and unspecified cause
Undiagnosed disease, not specified as to site or system involved
Unknown cause of morbidity or mortality

17. INJURY AND POISONING (800-999)

Use additional E code to identify the cause of the injury or poisoning (E800-E999)

Note:

1. The principle of multiple coding of injuries should be followed wherever possible. Combination categories for multiple injuries are provided for use when there is insufficient detail as to the nature of the individual conditions, or for primary tabulation purposes when it is more convenient to record a single code; otherwise, the component injuries should be coded separately.

   Where multiple sites of injury are specified in the titles, the word "with" indicates involvement of both sites, and the word "and" indicates involvement of either or both sites. The word "finger" includes thumb.
2. Categories for "late effect" of injuries are to be found at 905-909.

FRACTURES (800-829)

Excludes: *malunion (733.81)*
nonunion (733.82)
pathologic or spontaneous fracture (733.10-733.19)

The terms "condyle," "coronoid process," "ramus," and "symphysis" indicate the portion of the bone fractured, not the name of the bone involved.

The descriptions "closed" and "open" used in the fourth-digit subdivisions include the following terms:

closed (with or without delayed healing):

comminuted	impacted
depressed	linear
elevated	march
fissured	simple
fracture NOS	slipped epiphysis
greenstick	spiral

open (with or without delayed healing):

compound	puncture
infected	with foreign body
missile	

A fracture not indicated as closed or open should be classified as closed.

FRACTURE OF SKULL (800-804)

The following fifth-digit subclassification is for use with the appropriate codes in categories 800, 801, 803, and 804:

0 unspecified state of consciousness
1 with no loss of consciousness
2 with brief [less than one hour] loss of consciousness
3 with moderate [1-24 hours] loss of consciousness and return to pre-existing conscious level
4 with prolonged [more than 24 hours] loss of consciousness and return to pre-existing conscious level
5 with prolonged [more than 24 hours] loss of consciousness, without return to pre-existing conscious level
6 with loss of consciousness of unspecified duration
9 with concussion, unspecified

⑤ **800 Fracture of vault of skull**
Includes: frontal bone
parietal bone

800.0 Closed without mention of intracranial injury
□ **800.1 Closed with cerebral laceration and contusion**
□ **800.2 Closed with subarachnoid, subdural, and extradural hemorrhage**
□ **800.3 Closed with other and unspecified intracranial hemorrhage**
□ **800.4 Closed with intracranial injury of other and unspecified nature**
□ **800.5 Open without mention of intracranial injury**
□ **800.6 Open with cerebral laceration and contusion**
□ **800.7 Open with subarachnoid, subdural, and extradural hemorrhage**
□ **800.8 Open with other and unspecified intracranial hemorrhage**
□ **800.9 Open with intracranial injury of other and unspecified nature**

⑤ **801 Fracture of base of skull**

Includes:

fossa:
  anterior
  middle
  posterior
occiput bone
orbital roof
sinus:
  ethmoid
  frontal
sphenoid bone
temporal bone

801.0 Closed without mention of intracranial injury

□ **801.1 Closed with cerebral laceration and contusion**

□ **801.2 Closed with subarachnoid, subdural, and extradural hemorrhage**

□ **801.3 Closed with other and unspecified intracranial hemorrhage**

□ **801.4 Closed with intracranial injury of other and unspecified nature**

□ **801.5 Open without mention of intracranial injury**

□ **801.6 Open with cerebral laceration and contusion**

□ **801.7 Open with subarachnoid, subdural, and extradural hemorrhage**

□ **801.8 Open with other and unspecified intracranial hemorrhage**

□ **801.9 Open with intracranial injury of other and unspecified nature**

802 Fracture of face bones

802.0 Nasal bones, closed

802.1 Nasal bones, open

802.2 **Mandible, closed**

Inferior maxilla
Lower jaw (bone)

802.20 Unspecified site

802.21 Condylar process

802.22 Subcondylar

802.23 Coronoid process

802.24 Ramus, unspecified

802.25 Angle of jaw

802.26 Symphysis of body

802.27 Alveolar border of body

802.28 Body, other and unspecified

802.29 Multiple sites

802.3 **Mandible, open**

802.30 Unspecified site

802.31 Condylar process

802.32 Subcondylar

802.33 Coronoid process

802.34 Ramus, unspecified

802.35 Angle of jaw

802.36 Symphysis of body

802.37 Alveolar border of body

802.38 Body, other and unspecified

802.39 Multiple sites

802.4 Malar and maxillary bones, closed

Superior maxilla
Upper jaw (bone)
Zygoma
Zygomatic arch

802.5 Malar and maxillary bones, open

802.6 Orbital floor (blow-out), closed

802.7 Orbital floor (blow-out), open

● Code new to this edition
▲ Revision of existing code
④ ⑤ Fourth or fifth digit required

802.8 Other facial bones, closed
Alveolus
Orbit:
NOS
part other than roof or floor
Palate

Excludes: *orbital:*
floor (802.6)
roof (801.0-801.9)

802.9 Other facial bones, open

⑤ **803 Other and unqualified skull fractures**
Includes: skull NOS
skull multiple NOS

803.0 Closed without mention of intracranial injury
□ **803.1 Closed with cerebral laceration and contusion**
□ **803.2 Closed with subarachnoid, subdural, and extradural hemorrhage**
□ **803.3 Closed with other and unspecified intracranial hemorrhage**
□ **803.4 Closed with intracranial injury of other and unspecified nature**
□ **803.5 Open without mention of intracranial injury**
□ **803.6 Open with cerebral laceration and contusion**
□ **803.7 Open with subarachnoid, subdural, and extradural hemorrhage**
□ **803.8 Open with other and unspecified intracranial hemorrhage**
□ **803.9 Open with intracranial injury of other and unspecified nature**

⑤ **804 Multiple fractures involving skull or face with other bones**

804.0 Closed without mention of intracranial injury
□ **804.1 Closed with cerebral laceration and contusion**
□ **804.2 Closed with subarachnoid, subdural, and extradural hemorrhage**
□ **804.3 Closed with other and unspecified intracranial hemorrhage**
□ **804.4 Closed with intracranial injury of other and unspecified nature**
□ **804.5 Open without mention of intracranial injury**
□ **804.6 Open with cerebral laceration and contusion**
□ **804.7 Open with subarachnoid, subdural, and extradural hemorrhage**
□ **804.8 Open with other and unspecified intracranial hemorrhage**
□ **804.9 Open with intracranial injury of other and unspecified nature**

FRACTURE OF NECK AND TRUNK (805-809)

805 Fracture of vertebral column without mention of spinal cord injury
Includes:
neural arch
spine
spinous process
transverse process
vertebra

The following fifth-digit subclassification is for use with codes 805.0-805.1:

0 cervical vertebra, unspecified level
1 first cervical vertebra
2 second cervical vertebra
3 third cervical vertebra
4 fourth cervical vertebra
5 fifth cervical vertebra
6 sixth cervical vertebra
7 seventh cervical vertebra
8 multiple cervical vertebrae

⑤ **805.0 Cervical, closed**
Atlas
Axis

⑤ **805.1 Cervical, open**

805.2 Dorsal [thoracic], closed

805.3 Dorsal [thoracic], open

805.4 **Lumbar, closed**

805.5 **Lumbar, open**

805.6 **Sacrum and coccyx, closed**

805.7 **Sacrum and coccyx, open**

805.8 **Unspecified, closed**

805.9 **Unspecified, open**

806 **Fracture of vertebral column with spinal cord injury**

Includes: any condition classifiable to 805 with:
complete or incomplete transverse lesion (of cord)
hematomyelia
injury to:
cauda equina
nerve
paralysis
paraplegia
quadriplegia
spinal concussion

806.0 **Cervical, closed**

806.00 **C_1-C_4 level with unspecified spinal cord injury**
Cervical region NOS with spinal cord injury NOS

806.01 **C_1-C_4 level with complete lesion of cord**

806.02 **C_1-C_4 level with anterior cord syndrome**

806.03 **C_1-C_4 level with central cord syndrome**

806.04 **C_1-C_4 level with other specified spinal cord injury**
C_1-C_4 level with:
incomplete spinal cord lesion NOS
posterior cord syndrome

806.05 **C_5-C_7 level with unspecified spinal cord injury**

806.06 **C_5-C_7 level with complete lesion of cord**

806.07 **C_5-C_7 level with anterior cord syndrome**

806.08 **C_5-C_7 level with central cord syndrome**

806.09 **C_5-C_7 level with other specified spinal cord injury**
C_5-C_7 level with:
incomplete spinal cord lesion NOS
posterior cord syndrome

806.1 **Cervical, open**

806.10 **C_1-C_4 level with unspecified spinal cord injury**

806.11 **C_1-C_4 level with complete lesion of cord**

806.12 **C_1-C_4 level with anterior cord syndrome**

806.13 **C_1-C_4 level with central cord syndrome**

806.14 **C_1-C_4 level with other specified spinal cord injury**
C_1-C_4 level with:
incomplete spinal cord lesion NOS
posterior cord syndrome

806.15 **C_5-C_7 level with unspecified spinal cord injury**

806.16 **C_5-C_7 level with complete lesion of cord**

806.17 **C_5-C_7 level with anterior cord syndrome**

806.18 **C_5-C_7 level with central cord syndrome**

806.19 **C_5-C_7 level with other specified spinal cord injury**
C_5-C_7 level with:
incomplete spinal cord lesion NOS
posterior cord syndrome

806.2 **Dorsal [thoracic], closed**

806.20 **T_1-T_6 level with unspecified spinal cord injury**
Thoracic region NOS with spinal cord injury NOS

806.21 **T_1-T_6 level with complete lesion of cord**

806.22 **T_1-T_6 level with anterior cord syndrome**

806.23 **T_1-T_6 level with central cord syndrome**

806.24 **T_1-T_6 level with other specified spinal cord injury**
T_1-T_6 level with:
incomplete spinal cord lesion NOS
posterior cord syndrome

806.25 **T_7-T_{12} level with unspecified spinal cord injury**

806.26 **T_7-T_{12} level with complete lesion of cord**

806.27 **T_7-T_{12} level with anterior cord syndrome**

806.28 **T_7-T_{12} level with central cord syndrome**

806.29 **T_7-T_{12} level with other specified spinal cord injury**
T_7-T_{12} level with:
incomplete spinal cord lesion NOS
posterior cord syndrome

806.3 Dorsal [thoracic], open

806.30 **T_1-T_6 level with unspecified spinal cord injury**

806.31 **T_1-T_6 level with complete lesion of cord**

806.32 **T_1-T_6 level with anterior cord syndrome**

806.33 **T_1-T_6 level with central cord syndrome**

806.34 **T_1-T_6 level with other specified spinal cord injury**
T_1-T_6 level with:
incomplete spinal cord lesion NOS
posterior cord syndrome

806.35 **T_7-T_{12} level with unspecified spinal cord injury**

806.36 **T_7-T_{12} level with complete lesion of cord**

806.37 **T_7-T_{12} level with anterior cord syndrome**

806.38 **T_7-T_{12} level with central cord syndrome**

806.39 **T_7-T_{12} level with other specified spinal cord injury**
T_7-T_{12} level with:
incomplete spinal cord lesion NOS
posterior cord syndrome

806.4 Lumbar, closed

806.5 Lumbar, open

806.6 Sacrum and coccyx, closed

806.60 **With unspecified spinal cord injury**

806.61 **With complete cauda equina lesion**

806.62 **With other cauda equina injury**

806.69 **With other spinal cord injury**

806.7 Sacrum and coccyx, open

806.70 **With unspecified spinal cord injury**

806.71 **With complete cauda equina lesion**

806.72 **With other cauda equina injury**

806.79 **With other spinal cord injury**

806.8 Unspecified, closed

806.9 Unspecified, open

807 Fracture of rib(s), sternum, larynx, and trachea

The following fifth-digit subclassification is for use with codes 807.0-807.1:

0 rib(s), unspecified
1 one rib
2 two ribs
3 three ribs
4 four ribs
5 five ribs
6 six ribs
7 seven ribs
8 eight or more ribs
9 multiple ribs, unspecified

Add 4th or 5th digit | Nonspecific code | Unspecified code | Medicare secondary payer(MSP) alert

⑤ **807.0** **Rib(s), closed**

⑤ **807.1** **Rib(s), open**

807.2 **Sternum, closed**

807.3 **Sternum, open**

807.4 **Flail chest**

807.5 **Larynx and trachea, closed**
Hyoid bone
Thyroid cartilage
Trachea

807.6 **Larynx and trachea, open**

808 **Fracture of pelvis**

808.0 **Acetabulum, closed**

808.1 **Acetabulum, open**

808.2 **Pubis, closed**

808.3 **Pubis, open**

808.4 **Other specified part, closed**

808.41 **Ilium**

808.42 **Ischium**

808.43 **Multiple pelvic fractures with disruption of pelvic circle**

808.49 **Other**
Innominate bone
Pelvic rim

808.5 **Other specified part, open**

808.51 **Ilium**

808.52 **Ischium**

808.53 **Multiple pelvic fractures with disruption of pelvic circle**

808.59 **Other**

808.8 **Unspecified, closed**

808.9 **Unspecified, open**

809 **Ill-defined fractures of bones of trunk**
Includes: bones of trunk with other bones except those of skull and face
multiple bones of trunk

Excludes: *multiple fractures of:*
pelvic bones alone (808.0-808.9)
ribs alone (807.0-807.1, 807.4)
ribs or sternum with limb bones (819.0-819.1, 828.0-828.1)
skull or face with other bones (804.0-804.9)

809.0 **Fracture of bones of trunk, closed**

809.1 **Fracture of bones of trunk, open**

FRACTURE OF UPPER LIMB (810-819)

⑤ **810** **Fracture of clavicle**
Includes: collar bone
interligamentous part of clavicle

The following fifth-digit subclassification is for use with category 810:

0 **unspecified part**
Clavicle NOS

1 **sternal end of clavicle**

2 **shaft of clavicle**

3 **acromial end of clavicle**

810.0 **Closed**

810.1 **Open**

⑤ **811** **Fracture of scapula**
Includes: shoulder blade

The following fifth-digit subclassification is for use with category 811:

0 **unspecified part**

1 **acromial process**
Acromion (process)

continued

● Code new to this edition
▲ Revision of existing code
④ ⑤ Fourth or fifth digit required

2 **coracoid process**

3 **glenoid cavity and neck of scapula**

9 **other**
Scapula body

811.0 Closed

811.1 Open

812 Fracture of humerus

812.0 Upper end, closed

812.00 Upper end, unspecified part
Proximal end
Shoulder

812.01 Surgical neck
Neck of humerus NOS

812.02 Anatomical neck

812.03 Greater tuberosity

812.09 Other
Head
Upper epiphysis

812.1 Upper end, open

812.10 Upper end, unspecified part

812.11 Surgical neck

812.12 Anatomical neck

812.13 Greater tuberosity

812.19 Other

812.2 Shaft or unspecified part, closed

812.20 Unspecified part of humerus
Humerus NOS
Upper arm NOS

812.21 Shaft of humerus

812.3 Shaft or unspecified part, open

812.30 Unspecified part of humerus

812.31 Shaft of humerus

812.4 Lower end, closed
Distal end of humerus
Elbow

812.40 Lower end, unspecified part

812.41 Supracondylar fracture of humerus

812.42 Lateral condyle
External condyle

812.43 Medial condyle
Internal epicondyle

812.44 Condyle(s), unspecified
Articular process NOS
Lower epiphysis NOS

812.49 Other
Multiple fractures of lower end
Trochlea

812.5 Lower end, open

812.50 Lower end, unspecified part

812.51 Supracondylar fracture of humerus

812.52 Lateral condyle

812.53 Medial condyle

812.54 Condyle(s), unspecified

812.59 Other

813 Fracture of radius and ulna

□ **813.0 Upper end, closed**
Proximal end

813.00 Upper end of forearm, unspecified

813.01 Olecranon process of ulna

Add 4th or 5th digit | Nonspecific code | Unspecified code | Medicare secondary payer(MSP) alert

813.02 Coronoid process of ulna

813.03 Monteggia's fracture

813.04 Other and unspecified fractures of proximal end of ulna (alone)
Multiple fractures of ulna, upper end

813.05 Head of radius

813.06 Neck of radius

813.07 Other and unspecified fractures of proximal end of radius (alone)
Multiple fractures of radius, upper end

813.08 Radius with ulna, upper end [any part]

□ **813.1 Upper end, open**

813.10 Upper end of forearm, unspecified

813.11 Olecranon process of ulna

813.12 Coronoid process of ulna

813.13 Monteggia's fracture

813.14 Other and unspecified fractures of proximal end of ulna (alone)

813.15 Head of radius

813.16 Neck of radius

813.17 Other and unspecified fractures of proximal end of radius (alone)

813.18 Radius with ulna, upper end [any part]

813.2 Shaft, closed

813.20 Shaft, unspecified

813.21 Radius (alone)

813.22 Ulna (alone)

813.23 Radius with ulna

813.3 Shaft, open

813.30 Shaft, unspecified

813.31 Radius (alone)

813.32 Ulna (alone)

813.33 Radius with ulna

813.4 Lower end, closed
Distal end

813.40 Lower end of forearm, unspecified

813.41 Colles' fracture
Smith's fracture

813.42 Other fractures of distal end of radius (alone)
Dupuytren's fracture, radius
Radius, lower end

813.43 Distal end of ulna (alone)
Ulna:
head
lower end
Ulna:
lower epiphysis
styloid process

813.44 Radius with ulna, lower end

813.5 Lower end, open

813.50 Lower end of forearm, unspecified

813.51 Colles' fracture

813.52 Other fractures of distal end of radius (alone)

813.53 Distal end of ulna (alone)

813.54 Radius with ulna, lower end

□ **813.8 Unspecified part, closed**

813.80 Forearm, unspecified

813.81 Radius (alone)

813.82 Ulna (alone)

813.83 Radius with ulna

□ **813.9 Unspecified part, open**

813.90 Forearm, unspecified

● Code new to this edition ▲ Revision of existing code ④ ⑤ Fourth or fifth digit required

813.91 Radius (alone)

813.92 Ulna (alone)

813.93 Radius with ulna

⑤ **814 Fracture of carpal bone(s)**

The following fifth-digit subclassification is for use with category 814:

0 carpal bone, unspecified
Wrist NOS

1 navicular [scaphoid] of wrist

2 lunate [semilunar] bone of wrist

3 triquetral [cuneiform] bone of wrist

4 pisiform

5 trapezium bone [larger multangular]

6 trapezoid bone [smaller multangular]

7 capitate bone [os magnum]

8 hamate [unciform] bone

9 other

814.0 Closed

814.1 Open

⑤ **815 Fracture of metacarpal bone(s)**

Includes:hand [except finger]
metacarpus

The following fifth-digit subclassification is for use with category 815:

0 metacarpal bone(s), site unspecified

1 base of thumb [first] metacarpal
Bennett's fracture

2 base of other metacarpal bone(s)

3 shaft of metacarpal bone(s)

4 neck of metacarpal bone(s)

9 multiple sites of metacarpus

815.0 Closed

815.1 Open

⑤ **816 Fracture of one or more phalanges of hand**

Includes: finger(s)
thumb

The following fifth-digit subclassification is for use with category 816:

0 phalanx or phalanges, unspecified

1 middle or proximal phalanx or phalanges

2 distal phalanx or phalanges

3 multiple sites

816.0 Closed

816.1 Open

817 Multiple fractures of hand bones

Includes: metacarpal bone(s) with phalanx or phalanges of same hand

817.0 Closed

817.1 Open

818 Ill-defined fractures of upper limb

Includes: arm NOS
multiple bones of same upper limb

Excludes: multiple fractures of:
metacarpal bone(s) with phalanx or phalanges (817.0-817.1)
phalanges of hand alone (816.0-816.1)
radius with ulna (813.0-813.9)

818.0 Closed

818.1 Open

Add 4th or 5th digit | Nonspecific code | Unspecified code | Medicare secondary payer(MSP) alert

819 Multiple fractures involving both upper limbs, and upper limb with rib(s) and sternum
Includes: arm(s) with rib(s) or sternum
both arms [any bones]

819.0 Closed

819.1 Open

FRACTURE OF LOWER LIMB (820-829)

820 Fracture of neck of femur

820.0 Transcervical fracture, closed

820.00 Intracapsular section, unspecified

820.01 Epiphysis (separation) (upper)
Transepiphyseal

820.02 Midcervical section
Transcervical NOS

820.03 Base of neck
Cervicotrochanteric section

820.09 Other
Head of femur
Subcapital

820.1 Transcervical fracture, open

820.10 Intracapsular section, unspecified

820.11 Epiphysis (separation) (upper)

820.12 Midcervical section

820.13 Base of neck

820.19 Other

820.2 Pertrochanteric fracture, closed

820.20 Trochanteric section, unspecified
Trochanter:
NOS
greater
lesser

820.21 Intertrochanteric section

820.22 Subtrochanteric section

820.3 Pertrochanteric fracture, open

820.30 Trochanteric section, unspecified

820.31 Intertrochanteric section

820.32 Subtrochanteric section

820.8 Unspecified part of neck of femur, closed
Hip NOS
Neck of femur NOS

820.9 Unspecified part of neck of femur, open

821 Fracture of other and unspecified parts of femur

821.0 Shaft or unspecified part, closed

821.00 Unspecified part of femur
Thigh
Upper leg

Excludes: *hip NOS (820.8)*

821.01 Shaft

821.1 Shaft or unspecified part, open

821.10 Unspecified part of femur

821.11 Shaft

821.2 Lower end, closed
Distal end

821.20 Lower end, unspecified part

821.21 Condyle, femoral

821.22 Epiphysis, lower (separation)

821.23 Supracondylar fracture of femur

● Code new to this edition
▲ Revision of existing code
④ ⑤ Fourth or fifth digit required

821.29 Other
Multiple fractures of lower end

821.3 Lower end, open

821.30 Lower end, unspecified part

821.31 Condyle, femoral

821.32 Epiphysis, lower (separation)

821.33 Supracondylar fracture of femur

821.39 Other

822 Fracture of patella

822.0 Closed

822.1 Open

⑤ **823 Fracture of tibia and fibula**

Excludes: *Dupuytren's fracture (824.4-824.5)*
ankle (824.4-824.5)
radius (813.42, 813.52)
Pott's fracture (824.4-824.5)
that involving ankle (824.0-824.9)

The following fifth-digit subclassification is for use with category 823:

0 tibia alone

1 fibula alone

2 fibula with tibia

□ **823.0 Upper end, closed**
Head
Proximal end
Tibia:
condyles
tuberosity

□ **823.1 Upper end, open**

823.2 Shaft, closed

823.3 Shaft, open

□ **823.8 Unspecified part, closed**
Lower leg NOS

□ **823.9 Unspecified part, open**

824 Fracture of ankle

824.0 Medial malleolus, closed
Tibia involving:
ankle
malleolus

824.1 Medial malleolus, open

824.2 Lateral malleolus, closed
Fibula involving:
ankle
malleolus

824.3 Lateral malleolus, open

824.4 Bimalleolar, closed
Dupuytren's fracture, fibula
Pott's fracture

824.5 Bimalleolar, open

824.6 Trimalleolar, closed
Lateral and medial malleolus with anterior or posterior lip of tibia

824.7 Trimalleolar, open

824.8 Unspecified, closed
Ankle NOS

824.9 Unspecified, open

825 Fracture of one or more tarsal and metatarsal bones

825.0 Fracture of calcaneus, closed
Heel bone
Os calcis

825.1 Fracture of calcaneus, open

825.2 Fracture of other tarsal and metatarsal bones, closed

825.20 Unspecified bone(s) of foot [except toes]
Instep

825.21 Astragalus
Talus

825.22 Navicular [scaphoid], foot

825.23 Cuboid

825.24 Cuneiform, foot

825.25 Metatarsal bone(s)

825.29 Other
Tarsal with metatarsal bone(s) only

Excludes: *calcaneus (825.0)*

825.3 Fracture of other tarsal and metatarsal bones, open

825.30 Unspecified bone(s) of foot [except toes]

825.31 Astragalus

825.32 Navicular [scaphoid], foot

825.33 Cuboid

825.34 Cuneiform, foot

825.35 Metatarsal bone(s)

825.39 Other

826 Fracture of one or more phalanges of foot
Includes: toe(s)

826.0 Closed

826.1 Open

827 Other, multiple, and ill-defined fractures of lower limb
Includes: leg NOS
multiple bones of same lower limb

Excludes: *multiple fractures of:*
ankle bones alone (824.4-824.9)
phalanges of foot alone (826.0-826.1)
tarsal with metatarsal bones (825.29, 825.39)
tibia with fibula (823.0-823.9 with fifth-digit 2)

827.0 Closed

827.1 Open

828 Multiple fractures involving both lower limbs, lower with upper limb, and lower limb(s) with rib(s) and sternum
Includes: arm(s) with leg(s) [any bones]
both legs [any bones]
leg(s) with rib(s) or sternum

828.0 Closed

828.1 Open

829 Fracture of unspecified bones

829.0 Unspecified bone, closed

829.1 Unspecified bone, open

DISLOCATION (830-839)

Includes: displacement
subluxation

Excludes: *congenital dislocation (754.0-755.8)*
pathological dislocation (718.2)
recurrent dislocation (718.3)

The descriptions "closed" and "open", used in the fourth-digit subdivisions, include the following terms:

closed:	open:
complete	compound
dislocation NOS	infected
partial	with foreign body
simple	
uncomplicated	

A dislocation not indicated as closed or open should be classified as closed.

830 Dislocation of jaw
Includes: jaw (cartilage) (meniscus)
mandible
maxilla (inferior)
temporomandibular (joint)

830.0 Closed dislocation

830.1 Open dislocation

⑤ **831 Dislocation of shoulder**

Excludes: sternoclavicular joint (839.61, 839.71)
sternum (839.61, 839.71)

The following fifth-digit subclassification is for use with category 831:

0 shoulder, unspecified
Humerus NOS

1 anterior dislocation of humerus

2 posterior dislocation of humerus

3 inferior dislocation of humerus

4 acromioclavicular (joint)
Clavicle

9 other
Scapula

831.0 Closed dislocation

831.1 Open dislocation

⑤ **832 Dislocation of elbow**

The following fifth-digit subclassification is for use with category 832:

0 elbow unspecified

1 anterior dislocation of elbow

2 posterior dislocation of elbow

3 medial dislocation of elbow

4 lateral dislocation of elbow

9 other

832.0 Closed dislocation

832.1 Open dislocation

⑤ **833 Dislocation of wrist**

The following fifth-digit subclassification is for use with category 833:

0 wrist, unspecified part
Carpal (bone) Radius, distal end

1 radioulnar (joint), distal

2 radiocarpal (joint)

3 midcarpal (joint)

4 carpometacarpal (joint)

5 metacarpal (bone), proximal end

9 other
Ulna, distal end

833.0 Closed dislocation

833.1 Open dislocation

⑤ **834 Dislocation of finger**
Includes: finger(s)
phalanx of hand
thumb

The following fifth-digit subclassification is for use with category 834:

0 finger, unspecified part

1 metacarpophalangeal (joint)
Metacarpal (bone), distal end

2 interphalangeal (joint), hand

834.0 Closed dislocation

834.1 Open dislocation

⑤ **835 Dislocation of hip**

The following fifth-digit subclassification is for use with category 835:

0 dislocation of hip, unspecified

1 posterior dislocation

2 obturator dislocation

3 other anterior dislocation

835.0 Closed dislocation

835.1 Open dislocation

836 Dislocation of knee

Excludes: *dislocation of knee:*
old or pathological (718.2)
recurrent (718.3)
internal derangement of knee joint (717.0-717.5, 717.8-717.9)
old tear of cartilage or meniscus of knee (717.0-717.5, 717.8-717.9)

836.0 Tear of medial cartilage or meniscus of knee, current

Bucket handle tear:
NOS } current injury
medial meniscus } current injury

836.1 Tear of lateral cartilage or meniscus of knee, current

836.2 Other tear of cartilage or meniscus of knee, current

Tear of:
cartilage (semilunar) } current injury, not specified as medial or lateral
meniscus } current injury, not specified as medial or lateral

836.3 Dislocation of patella, closed

836.4 Dislocation of patella, open

836.5 Other dislocation of knee, closed

836.50 Dislocation of knee, unspecified

836.51 Anterior dislocation of tibia, proximal end
Posterior dislocation of femur, distal end

836.52 Posterior dislocation of tibia, proximal end
Anterior dislocation of femur, distal end

836.53 Medial dislocation of tibia, proximal end

836.54 Lateral dislocation of tibia, proximal end

836.59 Other

836.6 Other dislocation of knee, open

836.60 Dislocation of knee, unspecified

836.61 Anterior dislocation of tibia, proximal end

836.62 Posterior dislocation of tibia, proximal end

836.63 Medial dislocation of tibia, proximal end

836.64 Lateral dislocation of tibia, proximal end

836.69 Other

837 Dislocation of ankle

Includes:
astragalus
fibula, distal end
navicular, foot
scaphoid, foot
tibia, distal end

837.0 Closed dislocation

837.1 Open dislocation

⑤ **838 Dislocation of foot**

The following fifth-digit subclassification is for use with category 838:

0 foot, unspecified

1 tarsal (bone), joint unspecified

2 midtarsal (joint)

3 tarsometatarsal (joint)

4 metatarsal (bone), joint unspecified

5 metatarsophalangeal (joint)

6 interphalangeal (joint), foot

9 other
Phalanx of foot   Toe(s)

838.0 Closed dislocation

838.1 Open dislocation

839 Other, multiple, and ill-defined dislocations

839.0 Cervical vertebra, closed
Cervical spine   Neck

839.00 Cervical vertebra, unspecified

839.01 First cervical vertebra

839.02 Second cervical vertebra

839.03 Third cervical vertebra

839.04 Fourth cervical vertebra

839.05 Fifth cervical vertebra

839.06 Sixth cervical vertebra

839.07 Seventh cervical vertebra

839.08 Multiple cervical vertebrae

839.1 Cervical vertebra, open

839.10 Cervical vertebra, unspecified

839.11 First cervical vertebra

839.12 Second cervical vertebra

839.13 Third cervical vertebra

839.14 Fourth cervical vertebra

839.15 Fifth cervical vertebra

839.16 Sixth cervical vertebra

839.17 Seventh cervical vertebra

839.18 Multiple cervical vertebrae

839.2 Thoracic and lumbar vertebra, closed

839.20 Lumbar vertebra

839.21 Thoracic vertebra
Dorsal [thoracic] vertebra

839.3 Thoracic and lumbar vertebra, open

839.30 Lumbar vertebra

839.31 Thoracic vertebra

839.4 Other vertebra, closed

839.40 Vertebra, unspecified site
Spine NOS

839.41 Coccyx

839.42 Sacrum
Sacroiliac (joint)

839.49 Other

839.5 Other vertebra, open

839.50 Vertebra, unspecified site

839.51 Coccyx

839.52 Sacrum

839.59 Other

839.6 Other location, closed

839.61 Sternum
Sternoclavicular joint

839.69 Other
Pelvis

839.7 Other location, open

839.71 Sternum

839.79 Other

839.8 Multiple and ill-defined, closed
Arm
Back
Hand
Multiple locations, except fingers or toes alone
Other ill-defined locations
Unspecified location

839.9 Multiple and ill-defined, open

SPRAINS AND STRAINS OF JOINTS AND ADJACENT MUSCLES (804-848)

Includes:

avulsion hemarthrosis laceration rupture sprain strain tear	of:	joint capsule ligament muscle tendon

Excludes: *laceration of tendon in open wounds (880-884 and 890-894 with .2)*

840 Sprains and strains of shoulder and upper arm

840.0 Acromioclavicular (joint) (ligament)

840.1 Coracoclavicular (ligament)

840.2 Coracohumeral (ligament)

840.3 Infraspinatus (muscle) (tendon)

840.4 Rotator cuff (capsule)

840.5 Subscapularis (muscle)

840.6 Supraspinatus (muscle) (tendon)

840.8 Other specified sites of shoulder and upper arm

840.9 Unspecified site of shoulder and upper arm
Arm NOS
Shoulder NOS

841 Sprains and strains of elbow and forearm

841.0 Radial collateral ligament

841.1 Ulnar collateral ligament

841.2 Radiohumeral (joint)

841.3 Ulnohumeral (joint)

841.8 Other specified sites of elbow and forearm

841.9 Unspecified site of elbow and forearm
Elbow NOS

842 Sprains and strains of wrist and hand

842.0 Wrist

842.00 Unspecified site

842.01 Carpal (joint)

842.02 Radiocarpal (joint) (ligament)

842.09 Other
Radioulnar joint, distal

842.1 Hand

842.10 Unspecified site

842.11 Carpometacarpal (joint)

842.12 Metacarpophalangeal (joint)

842.13 Interphalangeal (joint)

842.19 Other
Midcarpal (joint)

843 Sprains and strains of hip and thigh

843.0 Iliofemoral (ligament)

843.1 Ischiocapsular (ligament)

843.8 Other specified sites of hip and thigh

843.9 Unspecified site of hip and thigh
Hip NOS
Thigh NOS

844 Sprains and strains of knee and leg

Excludes: *current tear of cartilage or meniscus of knee (836.0-836.2)*
old tear of cartilage or meniscus of knee (717.0-717.5, 717.8-717.9)

844.0 Lateral collateral ligament of knee

844.1 Medial collateral ligament of knee

844.2 Cruciate ligament of knee

844.3 Tibiofibular (joint) (ligament), superior

844.8 Other specified sites of knee and leg

844.9 Unspecified site of knee and leg
Knee NOS
Leg NOS

845 Sprains and strains of ankle and foot

845.0 Ankle

845.00 Unspecified site

845.01 Deltoid (ligament), ankle
Internal collateral (ligament), ankle

845.02 Calcaneofibular (ligament)

845.03 Tibiofibular (ligament), distal

845.09 Other
Achilles tendon

845.1 Foot

845.10 Unspecified site

845.11 Tarsometatarsal (joint) (ligament)

845.12 Metatarsophalangeal (joint)

845.13 Interphalangeal (joint), toe

845.19 Other

846 Sprains and strains of sacroiliac region

846.0 Lumbosacral (joint) (ligament)

846.1 Sacroiliac ligament

846.2 Sacrospinatus (ligament)

846.3 Sacrotuberous (ligament)

846.8 Other specified sites of sacroiliac region

846.9 Unspecified site of sacroiliac region

847 Sprains and strains of other and unspecified parts of back

Excludes: *lumbosacral (846.0)*

847.0 Neck
Anterior longitudinal (ligament), cervical
Atlanto-axial (joints)
Atlanto-occipital (joints)
Whiplash injury

Excludes: *neck injury NOS (959.0)*
thyroid region (848.2)

847.1 Thoracic

847.2 Lumbar

847.3 Sacrum
Sacrococcygeal (ligament)

847.4 Coccyx

847.9 Unspecified site of back
Back NOS

848 Other and ill-defined sprains and strains

848.0 Septal cartilage of nose

848.1 Jaw
Temporomandibular (joint) (ligament)

848.2 Thyroid region
Cricoarytenoid (joint) (ligament)
Cricothyroid (joint) (ligament)
Thyroid cartilage

848.3 Ribs
Chondrocostal (joint) } without mention of injury to sternum
Costal cartilage }

848.4 Sternum

848.40 Unspecified site

848.41 Sternoclavicular (joint) (ligament)

848.42 Chondrosternal (joint)

848.49 Other
Xiphoid cartilage

848.5 Pelvis
Symphysis pubis

Excludes: *that in childbirth (665.6)*

848.8 Other specified sites of sprains and strains

848.9 Unspecified site of sprain and strain

INTRACRANIAL INJURY, EXCLUDING THOSE WITH SKULL FRACTURE (850-854)

Excludes: *intracranial injury with skull fracture (800-801 and 803-804, except .0 and .5)*
nerve injury (950.0-951.9)
open wound of head without intracranial injury (870.0-873.9)
skull fracture alone (800-801 and 803-804 with .0, .5)

The description "with open intracranial wound", used in the fourth-digit subdivisions, includes those specified as open or with mention of infection or foreign body.

The following fifth-digit subclassification is for use with categories 851-854:

0 unspecified state of consciousness

1 with no loss of consciousness

2 with brief [less than one hour] loss of consciousness

3 with moderate [1-24 hours] loss of consciousness

4 with prolonged [more than 24 hours] loss of consciousness and return to pre-existing conscious level

5 with prolonged [more than 24 hours] loss of consciousness, without return to pre-existing conscious level

6 with loss of consciousness of unspecified duration

9 with concussion, unspecified

850 Concussion
Includes: commotio cerebri

Excludes: *Concussion with:*
cerebral laceration or contusion (851.0-851.9)
cerebral hemorrhage (852-853)
head injury NOS (854)

850.0 With no loss of consciousness
Concussion with mental confusion or disorientation, without loss of consciousness

850.1 With brief loss of consciousness
Loss of consciousness for less than one hour

850.2 With moderate loss of consciousness
Loss of consciousness for 1-24 hours

850.3 With prolonged loss of consciousness and return to pre-existing conscious level
Loss of consciousness for more than 24 hours with complete recovery

850.4 With prolonged loss of consciousness, without return to pre-existing conscious level

850.5 With loss of consciousness of unspecified duration

850.9 Concussion, unspecified

⑤ **851 Cerebral laceration and contusion**

□ **851.0 Cortex (cerebral) contusion without mention of open intracranial wound**

□ **851.1 Cortex (cerebral) contusion with open intracranial wound**

□ **851.2 Cortex (cerebral) laceration without mention of open intracranial wound**

● Code new to this edition ▲ Revision of existing code ④ ⑤ Fourth or fifth digit required

□ **851.3 Cortex (cerebral) laceration with open intracranial wound**

□ **851.4 Cerebellar or brain stem contusion without mention of open intracranial wound**

□ **851.5 Cerebellar or brain stem contusion with open intracranial wound**

□ **851.6 Cerebellar or brain stem laceration without mention of open intracranial wound**

□ **851.7 Cerebellar or brain stem laceration with open intracranial wound**

□ **851.8 Other and unspecified cerebral laceration and contusion, without mention of open intracranial wound**
Brain (membrane) NOS

□ **851.9 Other and unspecified cerebral laceration and contusion, with open intracranial wound**

⑤ **852 Subarachnoid, subdural, and extradural hemorrhage, following injury**

Excludes: *Cerebral contusion or laceration (with hemorrhage) (851.0-851.9)*

□ **852.0 Subarachnoid hemorrhage following injury without mention of open intracranial wound**
Middle meningeal hemorrhage following injury

□ **852.1 Subarachnoid hemorrhage following injury with open intracranial wound**

□ **852.2 Subdural hemorrhage following injury without mention of open intracranial wound**

□ **852.3 Subdural hemorrhage following injury with open intracranial wound**

□ **852.4 Extradural hemorrhage following injury without mention of open intracranial wound**
Epidural hematoma following injury

□ **852.5 Extradural hemorrhage following injury with open intracranial wound**

⑤ **853 Other and unspecified intracranial hemorrhage following injury**

853.0 Without mention of open intracranial wound
Cerebral compression due to injury
Intracranial hematoma following injury
Traumatic cerebral hemorrhage

853.1 With open intracranial wound

⑤ **854 Intracranial injury of other and unspecified nature**

Includes: brain injury NOS
head injury NOS

854.0 Without mention of open intracranial wound

854.1 With open intracranial wound

INTERNAL INJURY OF THORAX, ABDOMEN, AND PELVIS (860-869)

Includes:

blast injuries, blunt trauma, bruise, concussion injuries (except cerebral), crushing, hematoma, laceration, puncture, tear, traumatic rupture } of internal organs

Excludes: *concussion NOS (850.0-850.9)*
flail chest (807.4)
foreign body entering through orifice (930.0-939.9)
injury to blood vessels (901.0-902.9)

The description "with open wound," used in the fourth-digit subdivisions, includes those with mention of infection or foreign body.

860 Traumatic pneumothorax and hemothorax

860.0 Pneumothorax without mention of open wound into thorax

860.1 Pneumothorax with open wound into thorax

860.2 Hemothorax without mention of open wound into thorax

860.3 Hemothorax with open wound into thorax

860.4 Pneumohemothorax without mention of open wound into thorax

860.5 Pneumohemothorax with open wound into thorax

861 Injury to heart and lung

Excludes: *injury to blood vessels of thorax (901.0-901.9)*

861.0 Heart, without mention of open wound into thorax

861.00 Unspecified injury

861.01 Contusion

Cardiac contusion
Myocardial contusion

861.02 Laceration without penetration of heart chambers

861.03 Laceration with penetration of heart chambers

861.1 Heart, with open wound into thorax

861.10 Unspecified injury

861.11 Contusion

861.12 Laceration without penetration of heart chambers

861.13 Laceration with penetration of heart chambers

861.2 Lung, without mention of open wound into thorax

861.20 Unspecified injury

861.21 Contusion

861.22 Laceration

861.3 Lung, with open wound into thorax

861.30 Unspecified injury

861.31 Contusion

861.32 Laceration

862 Injury to other and unspecified intrathoracic organs

Excludes: *injury to blood vessels of thorax (901.0-901.9)*

862.0 Diaphragm, without mention of open wound into cavity

862.1 Diaphragm, with open wound into cavity

862.2 Other specified intrathoracic organs, without mention of open wound into cavity

862.21 Bronchus

862.22 Esophagus

862.29 Other

Pleura
Thymus gland

862.3 Other specified intrathoracic organs, with open wound into cavity

862.31 Bronchus

862.32 Esophagus

862.39 Other

862.8 Multiple and unspecified intrathoracic organs, without mention of open wound into cavity

Crushed chest
Multiple intrathoracic organs

862.9 Multiple and unspecified intrathoracic organs, with open wound into cavity

863 Injury to gastrointestinal tract

Excludes: *anal sphincter laceration during delivery (664.2)*
bile duct (868.0-868.1 with fifth-digit 2)
gallbladder (868.0-868.1 with fifth-digit 2)

863.0 Stomach, without mention of open wound into cavity

863.1 Stomach, with open wound into cavity

863.2 Small intestine, without mention of open wound into cavity

863.20 Small intestine, unspecified site

863.21 Duodenum

863.29 Other

863.3 Small intestine, with open wound into cavity

863.30 Small intestine, unspecified site

863.31 Duodenum

863.39 Other

863.4 Colon or rectum, without mention of open wound into cavity

- **863.40 Colon, unspecified site**
- **863.41 Ascending [right] colon**
- **863.42 Transverse colon**
- **863.43 Descending [left] colon**
- **863.44 Sigmoid colon**
- **863.45 Rectum**
- **863.46 Multiple sites in colon and rectum**
- **863.49 Other**

863.5 Colon or rectum, with open wound into cavity

- **863.50 Colon, unspecified site**
- **863.51 Ascending [right] colon**
- **863.52 Transverse colon**
- **863.53 Descending [left] colon**
- **863.54 Sigmoid colon**
- **863.55 Rectum**
- **863.56 Multiple sites in colon and rectum**
- **863.59 Other**

863.8 Other and unspecified gastrointestinal sites, without mention of open wound into cavity

- **863.80 Gastrointestinal tract, unspecified site**
- **863.81 Pancreas, head**
- **863.82 Pancreas, body**
- **863.83 Pancreas, tail**
- **863.84 Pancreas, multiple and unspecified sites**
- **863.85 Appendix**
- **863.89 Other**
  Intestine NOS

863.9 Other and unspecified gastrointestinal sites, with open wound into cavity

- **863.90 Gastrointestinal tract, unspecified site**
- **863.91 Pancreas, head**
- **863.92 Pancreas, body**
- **863.93 Pancreas, tail**
- **863.94 Pancreas, multiple and unspecified sites**
- **863.95 Appendix**
- **863.99 Other**

⑤ 864 Injury to liver

The following fifth-digit subclassification is for use with category 864:

- **0 unspecified injury**
- **1 hematoma and contusion**
- **2 laceration, minor**
  Laceration involving capsule only, or without significant involvement of hepatic parenchyma [i.e., less than 1 cm deep]
- **3 laceration, moderate**
  Laceration involving parenchyma but without major disruption of parenchyma [i.e., less than 10 cm long and less than 3 cm deep]
- **4 laceration, major**
  Laceration with significant disruption of hepatic parenchyma [i.e., 10 cm long and 3 cm deep]
  Multiple moderate lacerations, with or without hematoma
  Stellate lacerations of liver
- **5 laceration, unspecified**
- **9 other**

864.0 Without mention of open wound into cavity

864.1 With open wound into cavity

⑤ **865 Injury to spleen**

The following fifth-digit subclassification is for use with category 865:

- **0 unspecified injury**
- **1 hematoma without rupture of capsule**
- **2 capsular tears, without major disruption of parenchyma**
- **3 laceration extending into parenchyma**
- **4 massive parenchymal disruption**
- **9 other**

865.0 Without mention of open wound into cavity

865.1 With open wound into cavity

⑤ **866 Injury to kidney**

The following fifth-digit subclassification is for use with category 866:

- **0 unspecified injury**
- **1 hematoma without rupture of capsule**
- **2 laceration**
- **3 complete disruption of kidney parenchyma**

866.0 Without mention of open wound into cavity

866.1 With open wound into cavity

867 Injury to pelvic organs

Excludes: *injury during delivery (664.0-665.9)*

867.0 Bladder and urethra, without mention of open wound into cavity

867.1 Bladder and urethra, with open wound into cavity

867.2 Ureter, without mention of open wound into cavity

867.3 Ureter, with open wound into cavity

867.4 Uterus, without mention of open wound into cavity

867.5 Uterus, with open wound into cavity

867.6 Other specified pelvic organs, without mention of open wound into cavity

Fallopian tube
Ovary
Prostate
Seminal vesicle
Vas deferens

867.7 Other specified pelvic organs, with open wound into cavity

867.8 Unspecified pelvic organs, without mention of open wound into cavity

867.9 Unspecified pelvic organ, with open wound into cavity

⑤ **868 Injury to other intra-abdominal organs**

The following fifth-digit subclassification is for use with category 868:

- **0 unspecified intra-abdominal organ**
- **1 adrenal gland**
- **2 bile duct and gallbladder**
- **3 peritoneum**
- **4 retroperitoneum**
- **9 other and multiple intra-abdominal organs**

868.0 Without mention of open wound into cavity

868.1 With open wound into cavity

869 Internal injury to unspecified or ill-defined organs

Includes: internal injury NOS
multiple internal injury NOS

869.0 Without mention of open wound into cavity

869.1 With open wound into cavity

● Code new to this edition ▲ Revision of existing code ④ ⑤ Fourth or fifth digit required

OPEN WOUND (870-897)

Includes:

animal bite
avulsion
cut
laceration
puncture wound
traumatic amputation

Excludes: *burn (940.0-949.5)*
crushing (925-929.9)
puncture of internal organs (860.0-869.1)
superficial injury (910.0-919.9)
that incidental to:
dislocation (830.0-839.9)
fracture (800.0-829.1)
internal injury (860.0-869.1)
intracranial injury (851.0-854.1)

The description "complicated" used in the fourth-digit subdivisions includes those with mention of delayed healing, delayed treatment, foreign body, or major infection.

OPEN WOUND OF HEAD, NECK, AND TRUNK (870-879)

870 Open wound of ocular adnexa

870.0 Laceration of skin of eyelid and periocular area

870.1 Laceration of eyelid, full-thickness, not involving lacrimal passages

870.2 Laceration of eyelid involving lacrimal passages

870.3 Penetrating wound of orbit, without mention of foreign body

870.4 Penetrating wound of orbit with foreign body

Excludes: *retained (old) foreign body in orbit (376.6)*

870.8 Other specified open wounds of ocular adnexa

870.9 Unspecified open wound of ocular adnexa

871 Open wound of eyeball

Excludes: *2nd cranial nerve [optic] injury (950.0-950.9)*
3rd cranial nerve [oculomotor] injury (951.0)

871.0 Ocular laceration without prolapse of intraocular tissue

871.1 Ocular laceration with prolapse or exposure of intraocular tissue

871.2 Rupture of eye with partial loss of intraocular tissue

871.3 Avulsion of eye
Traumatic enucleation

871.4 Unspecified laceration of eye

871.5 Penetration of eyeball with magnetic foreign body

Excludes: *retained (old) magnetic foreign body in globe (360.50-360.59)*

871.6 Penetration of eyeball with (nonmagnetic) foreign body

Excludes: *retained (old) (nonmagnetic) foreign body in globe (360.60-360.69)*

871.7 Unspecified ocular penetration

871.9 Unspecified open wound of eyeball

872 Open wound of ear

872.0 External ear, without mention of complication

872.00 External ear, unspecified site

872.01 Auricle, ear
Pinna

872.02 Auditory canal

872.1 External ear, complicated

872.10 External ear, unspecified site

872.11 Auricle, ear

872.12 Auditory canal

872.6 Other specified parts of ear, without mention of complication

872.61 Ear drum
Drumhead
Tympanic membrane

872.62 Ossicles

872.63 **Eustachian tube**

872.64 **Cochlea**

872.69 **Other and multiple sites**

872.7 **Other specified parts of ear, complicated**

872.71 **Ear drum**

872.72 **Ossicles**

872.73 **Eustachian tube**

872.74 **Cochlea**

872.79 **Other and multiple sites**

872.8 **Ear, part unspecified, without mention of complication**
Ear NOS

872.9 **Ear, part unspecified, complicated**

873 **Other open wound of head**

Excludes: *that with mention of intracranial injury (851.0-854.1)*

873.0 **Scalp, without mention of complication**

873.1 **Scalp, complicated**

873.2 **Nose, without mention of complication**

873.20 **Nose, unspecified site**

873.21 **Nasal septum**

873.22 **Nasal cavity**

873.23 **Nasal sinus**

873.29 **Multiple sites**

873.3 **Nose, complicated**

873.30 **Nose, unspecified site**

873.31 **Nasal septum**

873.32 **Nasal cavity**

873.33 **Nasal sinus**

873.39 **Multiple sites**

873.4 **Face, without mention of complication**

873.40 **Face, unspecified site**

873.41 **Cheek**

873.42 **Forehead**
Eyebrow

873.43 **Lip**

873.44 **Jaw**

873.49 **Other and multiple sites**

873.5 **Face, complicated**

873.50 **Face, unspecified site**

873.51 **Cheek**

873.52 **Forehead**

873.53 **Lip**

873.54 **Jaw**

873.59 **Other and multiple sites**

873.6 **Internal structures of mouth, without mention of complication**

873.60 **Mouth, unspecified site**

873.61 **Buccal mucosa**

873.62 **Gum (alveolar process)**

873.63 **Tooth (broken)**

873.64 **Tongue and floor of mouth**

873.65 **Palate**

873.69 **Other and multiple sites**

873.7 **Internal structures of mouth, complicated**

873.70 Mouth, unspecified site

873.71 Buccal mucosa

873.72 Gum (alveolar process)

873.73 Tooth (broken)

873.74 Tongue and floor of mouth

873.75 Palate

873.79 Other and multiple sites

873.8 Other and unspecified open wound of head without mention of complication
Head NOS

873.9 Other and unspecified open wound of head, complicated

874 Open wound of neck

874.0 Larynx and trachea, without mention of complication

874.00 Larynx with trachea

874.01 Larynx

874.02 Trachea

874.1 Larynx and trachea, complicated

874.10 Larynx with trachea

874.11 Larynx

874.12 Trachea

874.2 Thyroid gland, without mention of complication

874.3 Thyroid gland, complicated

874.4 Pharynx, without mention of complication
Cervical esophagus

874.5 Pharynx, complicated

874.8 Other and unspecified parts, without mention of complication
Nape of neck
Throat NOS
Supraclavicular region

874.9 Other and unspecified parts, complicated

875 Open wound of chest (wall)

Excludes: *open wound into thoracic cavity (860.0-862.9)*
traumatic pneumothorax and hemothorax (860.1, 860.3, 860.5)

875.0 Without mention of complication

875.1 Complicated

876 Open wound of back
Includes: loin
lumbar region

Excludes: *open wound into thoracic cavity (860.0-862.9)*
traumatic pneumothorax and hemothorax (860.1, 860.3, 860.5)

876.0 Without mention of complication

876.1 Complicated

877 Open wound of buttock
Includes: sacroiliac region

877.0 Without mention of complication

877.1 Complicated

878 Open wound of genital organs (external), including traumatic amputation

Excludes: *injury during delivery (664.0-665.9)*
internal genital organs (867.0-867.9)

878.0 Penis, without mention of complication

878.1 Penis, complicated

878.2 Scrotum and testes, without mention of complication

878.3 Scrotum and testes, complicated

878.4 Vulva, without mention of complication
Labium (majus) (minus)

878.5 Vulva, complicated

878.6 Vagina, without mention of complication

878.7 Vagina, complicated

878.8 Other and unspecified parts, without mention of complication

878.9 Other and unspecified parts, complicated

879 Open wound of other and unspecified sites, except limbs

879.0 Breast, without mention of complication

879.1 Breast, complicated

879.2 Abdominal wall, anterior, without mention of complication

Abdominal wall NOS
Epigastric region
Hypogastric region
Pubic region
Umbilical region

879.3 Abdominal wall, anterior, complicated

879.4 Abdominal wall, lateral, without mention of complication

Flank
Groin
Hypochondrium
Iliac (region)
Inguinal region

879.5 Abdominal wall, lateral, complicated

879.6 Other and unspecified parts of trunk, without mention of complication

Pelvic region
Perineum
Trunk NOS

879.7 Other and unspecified parts of trunk, complicated

879.8 Open wound(s) (multiple) of unspecified site(s) without mention of complication

Multiple open wounds NOS
Open wound NOS

879.9 Open wound(s) (multiple) of unspecified site(s), complicated

OPEN WOUND OF UPPER LIMB (880-887)

⑤ **880 Open wound of shoulder and upper arm**

The following fifth-digit subclassification is for use with category 880:

0 shoulder region
1 scapular region
2 axillary region
3 upper arm
9 multiple sites

880.0 Without mention of complication

880.1 Complicated

880.2 With tendon involvement

⑤ **881 Open wound of elbow, forearm, and wrist**

The following fifth-digit subclassification is for use with category 881:

0 forearm
1 elbow
2 wrist

881.0 Without mention of complication

881.1 Complicated

881.2 With tendon involvement

882 Open wound of hand except finger(s) alone

882.0 Without mention of complication

882.1 Complicated

882.2 With tendon involvement

883 Open wound of finger(s)

Includes: fingernail
thumb (nail)

883.0 Without mention of complication

883.1 Complicated

883.2 With tendon involvement

884 Multiple and unspecified open wound of upper limb

Includes: arm NOS
multiple sites of one upper limb
upper limb NOS

884.0 Without mention of complication

884.1 Complicated

884.2 With tendon involvement

885 Traumatic amputation of thumb (complete) (partial)
Includes: thumb(s) (with finger(s) of either hand)

885.0 Without mention of complication

885.1 Complicated

886 Traumatic amputation of other finger(s) (complete) (partial)
Includes: finger(s) of one or both hands, without mention of thumb(s)

886.0 Without mention of complication

886.1 Complicated

887 Traumatic amputation of arm and hand (complete) (partial)

887.0 Unilateral, below elbow, without mention of complication

887.1 Unilateral, below elbow, complicated

887.2 Unilateral, at or above elbow, without mention of complication

887.3 Unilateral, at or above elbow, complicated

887.4 Unilateral, level not specified, without mention of complication

887.5 Unilateral, level not specified, complicated

887.6 Bilateral [any level], without mention of complication
One hand and other arm

887.7 Bilateral [any level], complicated

OPEN WOUND OF LOWER LIMB (890-897)

890 Open wound of hip and thigh

890.0 Without mention of complication

890.1 Complicated

890.2 With tendon involvement

891 Open wound of knee, leg [except thigh], and ankle
Includes: leg NOS
multiple sites of leg, except thigh

Excludes: *that of thigh (890.0-890.2)*
with multiple sites of lower limb (894.0-894.2)

891.0 Without mention of complication

891.1 Complicated

891.2 With tendon involvement

892 Open wound of foot except toe(s) alone
Includes: heel

892.0 Without mention of complication

892.1 Complicated

892.2 With tendon involvement

893 Open wound of toe(s)
Includes: toenail

893.0 Without mention of complication

893.1 Complicated

893.2 With tendon involvement

894 Multiple and unspecified open wound of lower limb
Includes: lower limb NOS
multiple sites of one lower limb, with thigh

894.0 Without mention of complication

894.1 Complicated

894.2 With tendon involvement

895 Traumatic amputation of toe(s) (complete) (partial)
Includes: toe(s) of one or both feet

895.0 Without mention of complication

895.1 Complicated

896 Traumatic amputation of foot (complete) (partial)

896.0 Unilateral, without mention of complication

896.1 Unilateral, complicated

896.2 Bilateral, without mention of complication

Excludes: *one foot and other leg (897.6-897.7)*

896.3 Bilateral, complicated

897 Traumatic amputation of leg(s) (complete) (partial)

897.0 Unilateral, below knee, without mention of complication

897.1 Unilateral, below knee, complicated

897.2 Unilateral, at or above knee, without mention of complication

897.3 Unilateral, at or above knee, complicated

897.4 Unilateral, level not specified, without mention of complication

897.5 Unilateral, level not specified, complicated

897.6 Bilateral [any level], without mention of complication
One foot and other leg

897.7 Bilateral [any level], complicated

INJURY TO BLOOD VESSELS (900-904)

Includes:
arterial hematoma
avulsion
cut
laceration
rupture
traumatic aneurysm or fistula (arteriovenous)
} of blood vessel, secondary to other injuries e.g., fracture or open wound

Excludes: *accidental puncture or laceration during medical procedure (998.2)*
intracranial hemorrhage following injury (851.0-854.1)

900 Injury to blood vessels of head and neck

900.0 Carotid artery

900.00 Carotid artery, unspecified

900.01 Common carotid artery

900.02 External carotid artery

900.03 Internal carotid artery

900.1 Internal jugular vein

900.8 Other specified blood vessels of head and neck

900.81 External jugular vein
Jugular vein NOS

900.82 Multiple blood vessels of head and neck

900.89 Other

900.9 Unspecified blood vessel of head and neck

901 Injury to blood vessels of thorax

Excludes: *traumatic hemothorax (860.2-860.5)*

901.0 Thoracic aorta

901.1 Innominate and subclavian arteries

901.2 Superior vena cava

901.3 Innominate and subclavian veins

901.4 Pulmonary blood vessels

901.40 Pulmonary vessel(s), unspecified

901.41 Pulmonary artery

901.42 Pulmonary vein

901.8 Other specified blood vessels of thorax

901.81 Intercostal artery or vein

901.82 Internal mammary artery or vein

901.83 Multiple blood vessels of thorax

● Code new to this edition ▲ Revision of existing code ④ ⑤ Fourth or fifth digit required

901.89 Other
Azygos vein Hemiazygos vein

901.9 Unspecified blood vessel of thorax

902 Injury to blood vessels of abdomen and pelvis

902.0 Abdominal aorta

902.1 Inferior vena cava

902.10 Inferior vena cava, unspecified

902.11 Hepatic veins

902.19 Other

902.2 Celiac and mesenteric arteries

902.20 Celiac and mesenteric arteries, unspecified

902.21 Gastric artery

902.22 Hepatic artery

902.23 Splenic artery

902.24 Other specified branches of celiac axis

902.25 Superior mesenteric artery (trunk)

902.26 Primary branches of superior mesenteric artery
Ileo-colic artery

902.27 Inferior mesenteric artery

902.29 Other

902.3 Portal and splenic veins

902.31 Superior mesenteric vein and primary subdivisions
Ileo-colic vein

902.32 Inferior mesenteric vein

902.33 Portal vein

902.34 Splenic vein

902.39 Other
Cystic vein Gastric vein

902.4 Renal blood vessels

902.40 Renal vessel(s), unspecified

902.41 Renal artery

902.42 Renal vein

902.49 Other
Suprarenal arteries

902.5 Iliac blood vessels

902.50 Iliac vessel(s), unspecified

902.51 Hypogastric artery

902.52 Hypogastric vein

902.53 Iliac artery

902.54 Iliac vein

902.55 Uterine artery

902.56 Uterine vein

902.59 Other

902.8 Other specified blood vessels of abdomen and pelvis

902.81 Ovarian artery

902.82 Ovarian vein

902.87 Multiple blood vessels of abdomen and pelvis

902.89 Other

902.9 Unspecified blood vessel of abdomen and pelvis

903 Injury to blood vessels of upper extremity

903.0 Axillary blood vessels

903.00 Axillary vessel(s), unspecified

903.01 Axillary artery

903.02 Axillary vein

903.1 Brachial blood vessels

903.2 Radial blood vessels

903.3 Ulnar blood vessels

903.4 Palmar artery

903.5 Digital blood vessels

903.8 Other specified blood vessels of upper extremity
Multiple blood vessels of upper extremity

903.9 Unspecified blood vessel of upper extremity

904 Injury to blood vessels of lower extremity and unspecified sites

904.0 Common femoral artery
Femoral artery above profunda origin

904.1 Superficial femoral artery

904.2 Femoral veins

904.3 Saphenous veins
Saphenous vein (greater) (lesser)

904.4 Popliteal blood vessels

904.40 Popliteal vessel(s), unspecified

904.41 Popliteal artery

904.42 Popliteal vein

904.5 Tibial blood vessels

904.50 Tibial vessel(s), unspecified

904.51 Anterior tibial artery

904.52 Anterior tibial vein

904.53 Posterior tibial artery

904.54 Posterior tibial vein

904.6 Deep plantar blood vessels

904.7 Other specified blood vessels of lower extremity
Multiple blood vessels of lower extremity

904.8 Unspecified blood vessel of lower extremity

904.9 Unspecified site
Injury to blood vessel NOS

LATE EFFECTS OF INJURIES, POISONINGS, TOXIC EFFECTS, AND OTHER EXTERNAL CAUSES (905-909)

Note: These categories are to be used to indicate conditions classifiable to 800-999 as the cause of late effects, which are themselves classified elsewhere. The “late effects” include those specified as such, or as sequelae, which may occur at any time after the acute injury.

905 Late effects of musculoskeletal and connective tissue injuries

905.0 Late effect of fracture of skull and face bones
Late effect of injury classifiable to 800-804

905.1 Late effect of fracture of spine and trunk without mention of spinal cord lesion
Late effect of injury classifiable to 805, 807-809

905.2 Late effect of fracture of upper extremities
Late effect of injury classifiable to 810-819

905.3 Late effect of fracture of neck of femur
Late effect of injury classifiable to 820

905.4 Late effect of fracture of lower extremities
Late effect of injury classifiable to 821-827

905.5 Late effect of fracture of multiple and unspecified bones
Late effect of injury classifiable to 828-829

905.6 Late effect of dislocation
Late effect of injury classifiable to 830-839

905.7 Late effect of sprain and strain without mention of tendon injury
Late effect of injury classifiable to 840-848, except tendon injury

905.8 Late effect of tendon injury
Late effect of tendon injury due to:
open wound [injury classifiable to 880-884 with .2, 890-894 with .2]
sprain and strain [injury classifiable to 840-848]

905.9 Late effect of traumatic amputation
Late effect of injury classifiable to 885-887, 895-897

Excludes: *late amputation stump complication (997.60-997.69)*

906 Late effects of injuries to skin and subcutaneous tissues

906.0 Late effect of open wound of head, neck, and trunk
Late effect of injury classifiable to 870-879

906.1 Late effect of open wound of extremities without mention of tendon injury
Late effect of injury classifiable to 880-884, 890-894 except .2

906.2 Late effect of superficial injury
Late effect of injury classifiable to 910-919

906.3 Late effect of contusion
Late effect of injury classifiable to 920-924

906.4 Late effect of crushing
Late effect of injury classifiable to 925-929

906.5 Late effect of burn of eye, face, head, and neck
Late effect of injury classifiable to 940-941

906.6 Late effect of burn of wrist and hand
Late effect of injury classifiable to 944

906.7 Late effect of burn of other extremities
Late effect of injury classifiable to 943 or 945

906.8 Late effect of burns of other specified sites
Late effect of injury classifiable to 942, 946-947

906.9 Late effect of burn of unspecified site
Late effect of injury classifiable to 948-949

907 Late effects of injuries to the nervous system

907.0 Late effect of intracranial injury without mention of skull fracture
Late effect of injury classifiable to 850-854

907.1 Late effect of injury to cranial nerve
Late effect of injury classifiable to 950-951

907.2 Late effect of spinal cord injury
Late effect of injury classifiable to 806, 952

907.3 Late effect of injury to nerve root(s), spinal plexus(es), and other nerves of trunk
Late effect of injury classifiable to 953-954

907.4 Late effect of injury to peripheral nerve of shoulder girdle and upper limb
Late effect of injury classifiable to 955

907.5 Late effect of injury to peripheral nerve of pelvic girdle and lower limb
Late effect of injury classifiable to 956

907.9 Late effect of injury to other and unspecified nerve
Late effect of injury classifiable to 957

908 Late effects of other and unspecified injuries

908.0 Late effect of internal injury to chest
Late effect of injury classifiable to 860-862

908.1 Late effect of internal injury to intra-abdominal organs
Late effect of injury classifiable to 863-866, 868

908.2 Late effect of internal injury to other internal organs
Late effect of injury classifiable to 867 or 869

908.3 Late effect of injury to blood vessel of head, neck, and extremities
Late effect of injury classifiable to 900, 903-904

908.4 Late effect of injury to blood vessel of thorax, abdomen, and pelvis
Late effect of injury classifiable to 901-902

908.5 Late effect of foreign body in orifice
Late effect of injury classifiable to 930-939

908.6 Late effect of certain complications of trauma
Late effect of complications classifiable to 958

908.9 Late effect of unspecified injury
Late effect of injury classifiable to 959

909 Late effects of other and unspecified external causes

909.0 Late effect of poisoning due to drug, medicinal or biological substance
Late effect of conditions classifiable to 960-979

Excludes: *late effect of adverse effect of drug, medicinal or biological substance (909.5)*

909.1 Late effect of toxic effects of nonmedical substances
Late effect of conditions classifiable to 980-989

909.2 Late effect of radiation
Late effect of conditions classifiable to 990

909.3 Late effect of complications of surgical and medical care
Late effect of conditions classifiable to 996-999

909.4 Late effect of certain other external causes
Late effect of conditions classifiable to 991-994

909.5 Late effect of adverse effect of drug, medicinal or biological substance

Excludes: *late effect of poisoning due to drug, medicinal or biological substance (909.0)*

909.9 Late effect of other and unspecified external causes
Late effect of conditions classifiable to 995

SUPERFICIAL INJURY (910-919)

Excludes: *burn (blisters) (940.0-949.5)*
contusion (920-924.9)
foreign body:
granuloma (728.82)
inadvertently left in operative wound (998.4)
residual, in soft tissue (729.6)
insect bite, venomous (989.5)
open wound with incidental foreign body (870.0-897.7)

910 Superficial injury of face, neck, and scalp except eye
Includes:

cheek	lip
ear	nose
gum	throat

Excludes: *eye and adnexa (918.0-918.9)*

910.0 Abrasion or friction burn without mention of infection

910.1 Abrasion or friction burn, infected

910.2 Blister without mention of infection

910.3 Blister, infected

910.4 Insect bite, nonvenomous, without mention of infection

910.5 Insect bite, nonvenomous, infected

910.6 Superficial foreign body (splinter) without major open wound and without mention of infection

910.7 Superficial foreign body (splinter) without major open wound, infected

910.8 Other and unspecified superficial injury of face, neck, and scalp without mention of infection

910.9 Other and unspecified superficial injury of face, neck, and scalp, infected

911 Superficial injury of trunk
Includes:

abdominal wall	interscapular region
anus	labium (majus) (minus)
back	penis
breast	perineum
buttock	scrotum
chest wall	testis
flank	vagina
groin	vulva

Excludes: *hip (916.0-916.9)*
scapular region (912.0-912.9)

911.0 Abrasion or friction burn without mention of infection

911.1 Abrasion or friction burn, infected

911.2 Blister without mention of infection

911.3 Blister, infected

911.4 Insect bite, nonvenomous, without mention of infection

911.5 Insect bite, nonvenomous, infected

911.6 Superficial foreign body (splinter) without major open wound and without mention of infection

911.7 Superficial foreign body (splinter) without major open wound, infected

911.8 Other and unspecified superficial injury of trunk without mention of infection

911.9 Other and unspecified superficial injury of trunk, infected

912 Superficial injury of shoulder and upper arm

Includes: axilla; scapular region

912.0 Abrasion or friction burn without mention of infection

912.1 Abrasion or friction burn, infected

912.2 Blister without mention of infection

912.3 Blister, infected

912.4 Insect bite, nonvenomous, without mention of infection

912.5 Insect bite, nonvenomous, infected

912.6 Superficial foreign body (splinter) without major open wound and without mention of infection

912.7 Superficial foreign body (splinter) without major open wound, infected

912.8 Other and unspecified superficial injury of shoulder and upper arm without mention of infection

912.9 Other and unspecified superficial injury of shoulder and upper arm, infected

913 Superficial injury of elbow, forearm, and wrist

913.0 Abrasion or friction burn without mention of infection

913.1 Abrasion or friction burn, infected

913.2 Blister without mention of infection

913.3 Blister, infected

913.4 Insect bite, nonvenomous, without mention of infection

913.5 Insect bite, nonvenomous, infected

913.6 Superficial foreign body (splinter) without major open wound and without mention of infection

913.7 Superficial foreign body (splinter) without major open wound, infected

913.8 Other and unspecified superficial injury of elbow, forearm, and wrist without mention of infection

913.9 Other and unspecified superficial injury of elbow, forearm, and wrist, infected

914 Superficial injury of hand(s) except finger(s) alone

914.0 Abrasion or friction burn without mention of infection

914.1 Abrasion or friction burn, infected

914.2 Blister without mention of infection

914.3 Blister, infected

914.4 Insect bite, nonvenomous, without mention of infection

914.5 Insect bite, nonvenomous, infected

914.6 Superficial foreign body (splinter) without major open wound and without mention of infection

914.7 Superficial foreign body (splinter) without major open wound, infected

914.8 Other and unspecified superficial injury of hand without mention of infection

914.9 Other and unspecified superficial injury of hand, infected

915 Superficial injury of finger(s)

Includes: fingernail; thumb (nail)

915.0 Abrasion or friction burn without mention of infection

915.1 Abrasion or friction burn, infected

915.2 Blister without mention of infection

915.3 Blister, infected

915.4 Insect bite, nonvenomous, without mention of infection

915.5 Insect bite, nonvenomous, infected

915.6 Superficial foreign body (splinter) without major open wound and without mention of infection

915.7 Superficial foreign body (splinter) without major open wound, infected

915.8 Other and unspecified superficial injury of fingers without mention of infection

915.9 Other and unspecified superficial injury of fingers, infected

916 Superficial injury of hip, thigh, leg, and ankle

916.0 Abrasion or friction burn without mention of infection

916.1 Abrasion or friction burn, infected

916.2 Blister without mention of infection

916.3 Blister, infected

916.4 Insect bite, nonvenomous, without mention of infection

916.5 Insect bite, nonvenomous, infected

916.6 Superficial foreign body (splinter) without major open wound and without mention of infection

916.7 Superficial foreign body (splinter) without major open wound, infected

916.8 Other and unspecified superficial injury of hip, thigh, leg, and ankle without mention of infection

916.9 Other and unspecified superficial injury of hip, thigh, leg, and ankle, infected

917 Superficial injury of foot and toe(s)

Includes: heel
toenail

917.0 Abrasion or friction burn without mention of infection

917.1 Abrasion or friction burn, infected

917.2 Blister without mention of infection

917.3 Blister, infected

917.4 Insect bite, nonvenomous, without mention of infection

917.5 Insect bite, nonvenomous, infected

917.6 Superficial foreign body (splinter) without major open wound and without mention of infection

917.7 Superficial foreign body (splinter) without major open wound, infected

917.8 Other and unspecified superficial injury of foot and toes without mention of infection

917.9 Other and unspecified superficial injury of foot and toes, infected

918 Superficial injury of eye and adnexa

Excludes: *burn (940.0-940.9)*
foreign body on external eye (930.0-930.9)

918.0 Eyelids and periocular area

Abrasion
Insect bite
Superficial foreign body (splinter)

918.1 Cornea

Corneal abrasion
Superficial laceration

Excludes: *corneal injury due to contact lens (371.82)*

918.2 Conjunctiva

918.9 Other and unspecified superficial injuries of eye

Eye (ball) NOS

919 Superficial injury of other, multiple, and unspecified sites

Excludes: *multiple sites classifiable to the same three-digit category (910.0-918.9)*

919.0 Abrasion or friction burn without mention of infection

919.1 Abrasion or friction burn, infected

919.2 Blister without mention of infection

919.3 Blister, infected

919.4 Insect bite, nonvenomous, without mention of infection

919.5 Insect bite, nonvenomous, infected

919.6 Superficial foreign body (splinter) without major open wound and without mention of infection

919.7 Superficial foreign body (splinter) without major open wound, infected

919.8 Other and unspecified superficial injury without mention of infection

919.9 Other and unspecified superficial injury, infected

CONTUSION WITH INTACT SKIN SURFACE (920-924)

Includes:
bruise, hematoma } without fracture or open wound

Excludes: *concussion (850.0-850.9)*
hemarthrosis (840.0-848.9)
internal organs (860.0-869.1)
that incidental to:
crushing injury (925-929.9)
dislocation (830.0-839.9)
fracture (800.0-829.1)
internal injury (860.0-869.1)
intracranial injury (850.0-854.1)
nerve injury (950.0-957.9)
open wound (870.0-897.7)

920 Contusion of face, scalp, and neck except eye(s)
Cheek
Ear (auricle)
Gum
Lip
Mandibular joint area
Nose
Throat

921 Contusion of eye and adnexa

921.0 Black eye, not otherwise specified

921.1 Contusion of eyelids and periocular area

921.2 Contusion of orbital tissues

921.3 Contusion of eyeball

921.9 Unspecified contusion of eye
Injury of eye NOS

922 Contusion of trunk

922.0 Breast

922.1 Chest wall

922.2 Abdominal wall
Flank
Groin

922.3 Back
Buttock
Interscapular region

Excludes: *scapular region (923.01)*

922.4 Genital organs
Labium (majus) (minus)
Penis
Perineum
Scrotum
Testis
Vagina
Vulva

922.8 Multiple sites of trunk

922.9 Unspecified part
Trunk NOS

923 Contusion of upper limb

923.0 Shoulder and upper arm

923.00 Shoulder region

923.01 Scapular region

923.02 Axillary region

923.03 Upper arm

923.09 Multiple sites

923.1 Elbow and forearm

923.10 Forearm

923.11 Elbow

923.2 Wrist and hand(s), except finger(s) alone

923.20 Hand(s)

923.21 Wrist

Add 4th or 5th digit | Nonspecific code | Unspecified code | Medicare secondary payer(MSP) alert

923.3 Finger
Fingernail
Thumb (nail)

923.8 Multiple sites of upper limb

923.9 Unspecified part of upper limb
Arm NOS

924 Contusion of lower limb and of other and unspecified sites

924.0 Hip and thigh

924.00 Thigh

924.01 Hip

924.1 Knee and lower leg

924.10 Lower leg

924.11 Knee

924.2 Ankle and foot, excluding toe(s)

924.20 Foot
Heel

924.21 Ankle

924.3 Toe
Toenail

924.4 Multiple sites of lower limb

924.5 Unspecified part of lower limb
Leg NOS

924.8 Multiple sites, not elsewhere classified

924.9 Unspecified site

CRUSHING INJURY (925-929)

Excludes: *concussion (850.0-850.9)*
fractures (800-829)
internal organs (860.0-869.1)
that incidental to:
internal injury (860.0-869.1)
intracranial injury (850.0-854.1)

925 Crushing injury of face, scalp, and neck
Cheek
Ear
Larynx
Pharynx
Throat

925.1 Crushing injury of face and scalp
Cheek
Ear

925.2 Crushing injury of neck
Larynx
Pharynx
Throat

926 Crushing injury of trunk

Excludes: *crush injury of internal organs (860.0-869.1)*

926.0 External genitalia
Labium (majus) (minus)
Penis
Scrotum
Testis
Vulva

926.1 Other specified sites

926.11 Back

926.12 Buttock

926.19 Other
Breast

Excludes: *crushing of chest (860.0-862.9)*

926.8 Multiple sites of trunk

926.9 Unspecified site
Trunk NOS

927 Crushing injury of upper limb

927.0 Shoulder and upper arm

927.00 Shoulder region

927.01 **Scapular region**

927.02 **Axillary region**

927.03 **Upper arm**

927.09 **Multiple sites**

927.1 **Elbow and forearm**

927.10 **Forearm**

927.11 **Elbow**

927.2 **Wrist and hand(s), except finger(s) alone**

927.20 **Hand(s)**

927.21 **Wrist**

927.3 **Finger(s)**

927.8 **Multiple sites of upper limb**

927.9 **Unspecified site**
Arm NOS

928 Crushing injury of lower limb

928.0 **Hip and thigh**

928.00 **Thigh**

928.01 **Hip**

928.1 **Knee and lower leg**

928.10 **Lower leg**

928.11 **Knee**

928.2 **Ankle and foot, excluding toe(s) alone**

928.20 **Foot**
Heel

928.21 **Ankle**

928.3 **Toe(s)**

928.8 **Multiple sites of lower limb**

928.9 **Unspecified site**
Leg NOS

929 Crushing injury of multiple and unspecified sites

Excludes: multiple internal injury NOS (869.0-869.1)

929.0 **Multiple sites, not elsewhere classified**

929.9 **Unspecified site**

EFFECTS OF FOREIGN BODY ENTERING THROUGH ORIFICE (930-939)

Excludes: foreign body:
granuloma (728.82)
inadvertently left in operative wound (998.4, 998.7)
in open wound (800-839, 851-897)
residual, in soft tissues (729.6)
superficial without major open wound (910-919 with .6 or .7)

930 Foreign body on external eye

Excludes: foreign body in penetrating wound of:
eyeball (871.5-871.6)
retained (old) (360.5-360.6)
ocular adnexa (870.4)
retained (old) (376.6)

930.0 **Corneal foreign body**

930.1 **Foreign body in conjunctival sac**

930.2 **Foreign body in lacrimal punctum**

930.8 **Other and combined sites**

930.9 **Unspecified site**
External eye NOS

931 Foreign body in ear
Auditory canal
Auricle

932 Foreign body in nose
Nasal sinus
Nostril

933 Foreign body in pharynx and larynx

933.0 Pharynx
Nasopharynx
Throat NOS

933.1 Larynx
Asphyxia due to foreign body
Choking due to:
food (regurgitated)
phlegm

934 Foreign body in trachea, bronchus, and lung

934.0 Trachea

934.1 Main bronchus

934.8 Other specified parts
Bronchioles
Lung

934.9 Respiratory tree, unspecified
Inhalation of liquid or vomitus, lower respiratory tract NOS

935 Foreign body in mouth, esophagus, and stomach

935.0 Mouth

935.1 Esophagus

935.2 Stomach

936 Foreign body in intestine and colon

937 Foreign body in anus and rectum
Rectosigmoid (junction)

938 Foreign body in digestive system, unspecified
Alimentary tract NOS
Swallowed foreign body

939 Foreign body in genitourinary tract

939.0 Bladder and urethra

939.1 Uterus, any part

Excludes: *intrauterine contraceptive device:*
complications from (996.32, 996.65)
presence of (V45.51)

939.2 Vulva and vagina

939.3 Penis

939.9 Unspecified site

BURNS (940-949)

Includes: burns from:
electrical heating appliance
electricity
flame
hot object
lightning
radiation
chemical burns (external) (internal)
scalds

Excludes: *friction burns (910-919 with .0, .1)*
sunburn (692.71)

940 Burn confined to eye and adnexa

940.0 Chemical burn of eyelids and periocular area

940.1 Other burns of eyelids and periocular area

940.2 Alkaline chemical burn of cornea and conjunctival sac

940.3 Acid chemical burn of cornea and conjunctival sac

940.4 Other burn of cornea and conjunctival sac

940.5 Burn with resulting rupture and destruction of eyeball

940.9 Unspecified burn of eye and adnexa

⑤ **941 Burn of face, head, and neck**

Excludes: *mouth (947.0)*

The following fifth-digit subclassification is for use with category 941:

0 face and head, unspecified site

1 ear [any part]

2 eye (with other parts of face, head, and neck)

3 lip(s)

4 chin

5 nose (septum)

6 scalp [any part]
Temple (region)

7 forehead and cheek

8 neck

9 multiple sites [except with eye] of face, head, and neck

941.0 Unspecified degree

941.1 Erythema [first degree]

941.2 Blisters, epidermal loss [second degree]

941.3 Full-thickness skin loss [third degree NOS]

□ **941.4 Deep necrosis of underlying tissues [deep third degree] without mention of loss of a body part**

□ **941.5 Deep necrosis of underlying tissues [deep third degree] with loss of a body part**

⑤ **942 Burn of trunk**

Excludes: *scapular region (943.0-943.5 with fifth-digit 6)*

The following fifth-digit subclassification is for use with category 942:

0 trunk, unspecified site

1 breast

2 chest wall, excluding breast and nipple

3 abdominal wall
Flank
Groin

4 back [any part]
Buttock
Interscapular region

5 genitalia
Labium (majus) (minus)
Penis
Perineum
Scrotum
Testis
Vulva

9 other and multiple sites of trunk

942.0 Unspecified degree

942.1 Erythema [first degree]

942.2 Blisters, epidermal loss [second degree]

942.3 Full-thickness skin loss [third degree NOS]

□ **942.4 Deep necrosis of underlying tissues [deep third degree] without mention of loss of a body part**

□ **942.5 Deep necrosis of underlying tissues [deep third degree] with loss of a body part**

⑤ **943 Burn of upper limb, except wrist and hand**

The following fifth-digit subclassification is for use with category 943:

0 upper limb, unspecified site

1 forearm

2 elbow

3 upper arm

4 axilla

5 shoulder

6 scapular region

9 multiple sites of upper limb, except wrist and hand

Add 4th or 5th digit | Nonspecific code | Unspecified code | Medicare secondary payer(MSP) alert

943.0 Unspecified degree

943.1 Erythema [first degree]

943.2 Blisters, epidermal loss [second degree]

943.3 Full-thickness skin loss [third degree NOS]

□ 943.4 Deep necrosis of underlying tissues [deep third degree] without mention of loss of a body part

□ 943.5 Deep necrosis of underlying tissues [deep third degree] with loss of a body part

⑤ **944 Burn of wrist(s) and hand(s)**

The following fifth-digit subclassification is for use with category 944:

0 hand, unspecified site
1 single digit [finger (nail)] other than thumb
2 thumb (nail)
3 two or more digits, not including thumb
4 two or more digits including thumb
5 palm
6 back of hand
7 wrist
8 multiple sites of wrist(s) and hand(s)

944.0 Unspecified degree

944.1 Erythema [first degree]

944.2 Blisters, epidermal loss [second degree]

944.3 Full-thickness skin loss [third degree NOS]

□ 944.4 Deep necrosis of underlying tissues [deep third degree] without mention of loss of a body part

□ 944.5 Deep necrosis of underlying tissues [deep third degree] with loss of a body part

⑤ **945 Burn of lower limb(s)**

The following fifth-digit subclassification is for use with category 945:

0 lower limb [leg], unspecified site
1 toe(s) (nail)
2 foot
3 ankle
4 lower leg
5 knee
6 thigh [any part]
9 multiple sites of lower limb(s)

945.0 Unspecified degree

945.1 Erythema [first degree]

945.2 Blisters, epidermal loss [second degree]

945.3 Full-thickness skin loss [third degree NOS]

□ 945.4 Deep necrosis of underlying tissues [deep third degree] without mention of loss of a body part

□ 945.5 Deep necrosis of underlying tissues [deep third degree] with loss of a body part

946 Burns of multiple specified sites

Includes: burns of sites classifiable to more than one three-digit category in 940-945

Excludes: multiple burns NOS (949.0-949.5)

946.0 Unspecified degree

946.1 Erythema [first degree]

946.2 Blisters, epidermal loss [second degree]

946.3 Full-thickness skin loss [third degree NOS]

□ 946.4 Deep necrosis of underlying tissues [deep third degree] without mention of loss of a body part

□ 946.5 Deep necrosis of underlying tissues [deep third degree] with loss of a body part

947 Burn of internal organs

Includes: burns from chemical agents (ingested)

● Code new to this edition ▲ Revision of existing code ④ ⑤ Fourth or fifth digit required

947.0 Mouth and pharynx
Gum
Tongue

947.1 Larynx, trachea, and lung

947.2 Esophagus

947.3 Gastrointestinal tract
Colon
Rectum
Small intestine
Stomach

947.4 Vagina and uterus

947.8 Other specified sites

947.9 Unspecified site

⑤ **948 Burns classified according to extent of body surface involved**

Note: This category is to be used when the site of the burn is unspecified, or with categories 940-947 when the site is specified.

The following fifth-digit subclassification is for use with category 948 to indicate the percent of *body surface* with *third degree* burn; valid digits are in [brackets] under each code:

0 less than 10 percent or unspecified
1 10-19%
2 20-29%
3 30-39%
4 40-49%
5 50-59%
6 60-69%
7 70-79%
8 80-89%
9 90% or more of body surface

948.0 Burn [any degree] involving less than 10 percent of body surface
[0]

948.1 10-19 percent of body surface
[0-1]

948.2 20-29 percent of body surface
[0-2]

948.3 30-39 percent of body surface
[0-3]

948.4 40-49 percent of body surface
[0-4]

948.5 50-59 percent of body surface
[0-5]

948.6 60-69 percent of body surface
[0-6]

948.7 70-79 percent of body surface
[0-7]

948.8 80-89 percent of body surface
[0-8]

948.9 90 percent or more of body surface
[0-9]

949 Burn, unspecified

Includes:
burn NOS
multiple burns NOS

Excludes: *burn of unspecified site but with statement of the extent of body surface involved (948.0-948.9)*

949.0 Unspecified degree

949.1 Erythema [first degree]

949.2 Blisters, epidermal loss [second degree]

949.3 Full-thickness skin loss [third degree NOS]

□ **949.4 Deep necrosis of underlying tissues [deep third degree] without mention of loss of a body part**

□ **949.5 Deep necrosis of underlying tissues [deep third degree] with loss of a body part**

INJURY TO NERVES AND SPINAL CORD (950-957)

Includes:

division of nerve lesion in continuity traumatic neuroma traumatic transient paralysis	(with open wound)

Excludes: *accidental puncture or laceration during medical procedure (998.2)*

950 Injury to optic nerve and pathways

950.0 Optic nerve injury
Second cranial nerve

950.1 Injury to optic chiasm

950.2 Injury to optic pathways

950.3 Injury to visual cortex

950.9 Unspecified
Traumatic blindness NOS

951 Injury to other cranial nerve(s)

951.0 Injury to oculomotor nerve
Third cranial nerve

951.1 Injury to trochlear nerve
Fourth cranial nerve

951.2 Injury to trigeminal nerve
Fifth cranial nerve

951.3 Injury to abducens nerve
Sixth cranial nerve

951.4 Injury to facial nerve
Seventh cranial nerve

951.5 Injury to acoustic nerve
Auditory nerve
Eighth cranial nerve
Traumatic deafness NOS

951.6 Injury to accessory nerve
Eleventh cranial nerve

951.7 Injury to hypoglossal nerve
Twelfth cranial nerve

951.8 Injury to other specified cranial nerves
Glossopharyngeal [9th cranial] nerve
Olfactory [1st cranial] nerve
Pneumogastric [10th cranial] nerve
Traumatic anosmia NOS
Vagus [10th cranial] nerve

951.9 Injury to unspecified cranial nerve

952 Spinal cord injury without evidence of spinal bone injury

952.0 Cervical

952.00 C_1-C_4 level with unspecified spinal cord injury
Spinal cord injury, cervical region NOS

952.01 C_1-C_4 level with complete lesion of spinal cord

952.02 C_1-C_4 level with anterior cord syndrome

952.03 C_1-C_4 level with central cord syndrome

952.04 C_1-C_4 level with other specified spinal cord injury
Incomplete spinal cord lesion at C_1-C_4 level:
NOS
with posterior cord syndrome

952.05 C_5-C_7 level with unspecified spinal cord injury

952.06 C_5-C_7 level with complete lesion of spinal cord

952.07 C_5-C_7 level with anterior cord syndrome

952.08 C_5-C_7 level with central cord syndrome

952.09 **C_5-C_7 level with other specified spinal cord injury**
Incomplete spinal cord lesion at C_5-C_7 level:
NOS
with posterior cord syndrome

952.1 Dorsal [thoracic]

952.10 **T_1-T_6 level with unspecified spinal cord injury**
Spinal cord injury, thoracic region NOS

952.11 **T_1-T_6 level with complete lesion of spinal cord**

952.12 **T_1-T_6 level with anterior cord syndrome**

952.13 **T_1-T_6 level with central cord syndrome**

952.14 **T_1-T_6 level with other specified spinal cord injury**
Incomplete spinal cord lesion at T_1-T_6 level:
NOS
with posterior cord syndrome

952.15 **T_7-T_{12} level with unspecified spinal cord injury**

952.16 **T_7-T_{12} level with complete lesion of spinal cord**

952.17 **T_7-T_{12} level with anterior cord syndrome**

952.18 **T_7-T_{12} level with central cord syndrome**

952.19 **T_7-T_{12} level with other specified spinal cord injury**
Incomplete spinal cord lesion at T_7-T_{12} level:
NOS
with posterior cord syndrome

952.2 Lumbar

952.3 Sacral

952.4 Cauda equina

952.8 Multiple sites of spinal cord

952.9 Unspecified site of spinal cord

953 Injury to nerve roots and spinal plexus

953.0 Cervical root

953.1 Dorsal root

953.2 Lumbar root

953.3 Sacral root

953.4 Brachial plexus

953.5 Lumbosacral plexus

953.8 Multiple sites

953.9 Unspecified site

954 Injury to other nerve(s) of trunk, excluding shoulder and pelvic girdles

954.0 Cervical sympathetic

954.1 Other sympathetic
Celiac ganglion or plexus
Inferior mesenteric plexus
Splanchnic nerve(s)
Stellate ganglion

954.8 Other specified nerve(s) of trunk

954.9 Unspecified nerve of trunk

955 Injury to peripheral nerve(s) of shoulder girdle and upper limb

955.0 Axillary nerve

955.1 Median nerve

955.2 Ulnar nerve

955.3 Radial nerve

955.4 Musculocutaneous nerve

955.5 Cutaneous sensory nerve, upper limb

955.6 Digital nerve

955.7 Other specified nerve(s) of shoulder girdle and upper limb

955.8 Multiple nerves of shoulder girdle and upper limb

955.9 Unspecified nerve of shoulder girdle and upper limb

956 Injury to peripheral nerve(s) of pelvic girdle and lower limb

956.0 Sciatic nerve

956.1 Femoral nerve

956.2 Posterior tibial nerve

956.3 Peroneal nerve

956.4 Cutaneous sensory nerve, lower limb

956.5 Other specified nerve(s) of pelvic girdle and lower limb

956.8 Multiple nerves of pelvic girdle and lower limb

956.9 Unspecified nerve of pelvic girdle and lower limb

957 Injury to other and unspecified nerves

957.0 Superficial nerves of head and neck

957.1 Other specified nerve(s)

957.8 Multiple nerves in several parts
Multiple nerve injury NOS

957.9 Unspecified site
Nerve injury NOS

CERTAIN TRAUMATIC COMPLICATIONS AND UNSPECIFIED INJURIES (958-959)

958 Certain early complications of trauma

Excludes: *adult respiratory distress syndrome (518.5)*
flail chest (807.4)
shock lung (518.5)
that occurring during or following medical procedures (996.0-999.9)

958.0 Air embolism
Pneumathemia

Excludes: *that complicating:*
abortion (634-638 with .6, 639.6)
ectopic or molar pregnancy (639.6)
pregnancy, childbirth, or the puerperium (673.0)

958.1 Fat embolism

Excludes: *that complicating:*
abortion (634-638 with .6, 639.6)
pregnancy, childbirth, or the puerperium (673.8)

958.2 Secondary and recurrent hemorrhage

958.3 Posttraumatic wound infection, not elsewhere classified

958.4 Traumatic shock
Shock (immediate) (delayed) following injury

Excludes: *shock:*
anaphylactic (995.0)
due to serum (999.4)
anesthetic (995.4)
electric (994.8)
following abortion (639.5)
lightning (994.0)
nontraumatic NOS (785.50)
obstetric (669.1)
postoperative (998.0)

958.5 Traumatic anuria
Crush syndrome
Renal failure following crushing

Excludes: *that due to a medical procedure (997.5)*

958.6 Volkmann's ischemic contracture
Posttraumatic muscle contracture

958.7 Traumatic subcutaneous emphysema

Excludes: *subcutaneous emphysema resulting from a procedure (998.81)*

958.8 Other early complications of trauma

● Code new to this edition ▲ Revision of existing code ④ ⑤ Fourth or fifth digit required

959 Injury, other and unspecified

Includes: injury NOS

Excludes: injury NOS of:
blood vessels (900.0-904.9)
eye (921.0-921.9)
head (854.0-854.1)
internal organs (860.0-869.1)
intracranial sites (854.1)
nerves (950.0-951.9, 953.0-957.9)
spinal cord (952.0-952.9)

959.0 Face and neck

Cheek
Ear
Eyebrow
Lip
Mouth
Nose
Throat

959.1 Trunk

Abdominal wall
Back
Breast
Buttock
Chest wall
External genital organs
Flank
Groin
Interscapular region
Perineum

Excludes: scapular region (959.2)

959.2 Shoulder and upper arm

Axilla
Scapular region

959.3 Elbow, forearm, and wrist

959.4 Hand, except finger

959.5 Finger

Fingernail
Thumb (nail)

959.6 Hip and thigh

Upper leg

959.7 Knee, leg, ankle, and foot

959.8 Other specified sites, including multiple

Excludes: multiple sites classifiable to the same four-digit category (959.0-959.7)

959.9 Unspecified site

POISONING BY DRUGS, MEDICINAL AND BIOLOGICAL SUBSTANCES (960-979)

Includes: overdose of these substances
wrong substances given or taken in error

Excludes: adverse effects ["hypersensitivity," "reaction," etc.] of correct substance properly administered. Such cases are to be classified according to the nature of the adverse effect, such as:
adverse effect NOS (995.2)
allergic lymphadenitis (289.3)
aspirin gastritis (535.4)
blood disorders (280.0-289.9)
dermatitis:
contact (692.0-692.9)
due to ingestion (693.0-693.9)
nephropathy (583.9)
[The drug giving rise to the adverse effect may be identified by use of categories E930-E949]
drug dependence (304.0-304.9)
drug reaction and poisoning affecting the newborn (760.0-779.9)
nondependent abuse of drugs (305.0-305.9)
pathological drug intoxication (292.2)

Use additional code to specify the effects of the poisoning

960 Poisoning by antibiotics

Excludes: antibiotics:
ear, nose, and throat (976.6)
eye (976.5)
local (976.0)

Add 4th or 5th digit | Nonspecific code | Unspecified code | Medicare secondary payer(MSP) alert

960.0 Penicillins
Ampicillin
Carbenicillin
Cloxacillin
Penicillin G

960.1 Antifungal antibiotics
Amphotericin B
Griseofulvin
Nystatin
Trichomycin

Excludes: *preparations intended for topical use (976.0-976.9)*

960.2 Chloramphenicol group
Chloramphenicol
Thiamphenicol

960.3 Erythromycin and other macrolides
Oleandomycin
Spiramycin

960.4 Tetracycline group
Doxycycline
Minocycline
Oxytetracycline

960.5 Cephalosporin group
Cephalexin
Cephaloglycin
Cephaloridine
Cephalothin

960.6 Antimycobacterial antibiotics
Cycloserine
Kanamycin
Rifampin
Streptomycin

960.7 Antineoplastic antibiotics
Actinomycin such as:
Cactinomycin
Dactinomycin
Bleomycin
Daunorubicin
Mitomycin

960.8 Other specified antibiotics

960.9 Unspecified antibiotic

961 Poisoning by other anti-infectives

Excludes: *anti-infectives:*
ear, nose, and throat (976.6)
eye (976.5)
local (976.0)

961.0 Sulfonamides
Sulfadiazine
Sulfafurazole
Sulfamethoxazole

961.1 Arsenical anti-infectives

961.2 Heavy metal anti-infectives
Compounds of:
antimony
bismuth
Compounds of:
lead
mercury

Excludes: *mercurial diuretics (974.0)*

961.3 Quinoline and hydroxyquinoline derivatives
Chiniofon
Diiodohydroxyquin

Excludes: *antimalarial drugs (961.4)*

961.4 Antimalarials and drugs acting on other blood protozoa
Chloroquine
Cycloguanil
Primaquine
Proguanil [chloroguanide]
Pyrimethamine
Quinine

961.5 Other antiprotozoal drugs
Emetine

961.6 Anthelmintics
Hexylresorcinol
Piperazine
Thiabendazole

961.7 Antiviral drugs
Methisazone

Excludes: *amantadine (966.4)*
cytarabine (963.1)
idoxuridine (976.5)

961.8 Other antimycobacterial drugs
Ethambutol
Ethionamide
Isoniazid
Para-aminosalicylic acid derivatives
Sulfones

961.9 Other and unspecified anti-infectives
Flucytosine
Nitrofuran derivatives

962 Poisoning by hormones and synthetic substitutes

Excludes: *oxytocic hormones (975.0)*

962.0 Adrenal cortical steroids
Cortisone derivatives
Desoxycorticosterone derivatives
Fluorinated corticosteroids

962.1 Androgens and anabolic congeners
Methandriol
Nandrolone
Oxymetholone
Testosterone

962.2 Ovarian hormones and synthetic substitutes
Contraceptives, oral
Estrogens
Estrogens and progestogens, combined
Progestogens

962.3 Insulins and antidiabetic agents
Acetohexamide
Biguanide derivatives, oral
Chlorpropamide
Glucagon
Insulin
Phenformin
Sulfonylurea derivatives, oral
Tolbutamide

962.4 Anterior pituitary hormones
Corticotropin
Gonadotropin
Somatotropin [growth hormone]

962.5 Posterior pituitary hormones
Vasopressin

Excludes: *oxytocic hormones (975.0)*

962.6 Parathyroid and parathyroid derivatives

962.7 Thyroid and thyroid derivatives
Dextrothyroxin
Levothyroxine sodium
Liothyronine
Thyroglobulin

962.8 Antithyroid agents
Iodides
Thiouracil
Thiourea

962.9 Other and unspecified hormones and synthetic substitutes

963 Poisoning by primarily systemic agents

963.0 Antiallergic and antiemetic drugs
Antihistamines
Chlorpheniramine
Diphenhydramine
Diphenylpyraline
Thonzylamine
Tripelennamine

Excludes: *phenothiazine-based tranquilizers (969.1)*

963.1 Antineoplastic and immunosuppressive drugs
Azathioprine
Busulfan
Chlorambucil
Cyclophosphamide
Cytarabine
Fluorouracil
Mercaptopurine
thio-TEPA

Excludes: *antineoplastic antibiotics (960.7)*

963.2 Acidifying agents

963.3 Alkalizing agents

963.4 Enzymes, not elsewhere classified
Penicillinase

963.5 Vitamins, not elsewhere classified
Vitamin A
Vitamin D

Excludes: *nicotinic acid (972.2)*
vitamin K (964.3)

963.8 Other specified systemic agents
Heavy metal antagonists

963.9 Unspecified systemic agent

964 Poisoning by agents primarily affecting blood constituents

964.0 Iron and its compounds
Ferric salts
Ferrous sulfate and other ferrous salts

964.1 Liver preparations and other antianemic agents
Folic acid

964.2 Anticoagulants
Coumarin
Heparin
Phenindione
Warfarin sodium

964.3 Vitamin K [phytonadione]

964.4 Fibrinolysis-affecting drugs
Aminocaproic acid
Streptodornase
Streptokinase
Urokinase

964.5 Anticoagulant antagonists and other coagulants
Hexadimethrine
Protamine sulfate

964.6 Gamma globulin

964.7 Natural blood and blood products
Blood plasma
Human fibrinogen
Packed red cells
Whole blood

Excludes: *transfusion reactions (999.4-999.8)*

964.8 Other specified agents affecting blood constituents
Macromolecular blood substitutes
Plasma expanders

964.9 Unspecified agent affecting blood constituents

965 Poisoning by analgesics, antipyretics, and antirheumatics

Excludes: *drug dependence (304.0-304.9)*
nondependent abuse (305.0-305.9)

965.0 Opiates and related narcotics

965.00 Opium (alkaloids), unspecified

965.01 Heroin
Diacetylmorphine

965.02 Methadone

965.09 Other
Codeine [methylmorphine]
Meperidine [pethidine]
Morphine

965.1 Salicylates
Acetylsalicylic acid [aspirin]
Salicylic acid salts

965.4 Aromatic analgesics, not elsewhere classified
Acetanilid
Paracetamol [acetaminophen]
Phenacetin [acetophenetidin]

965.5 Pyrazole derivatives
Aminophenazone [aminopyrine]
Phenylbutazone

965.6 Antirheumatics [antiphlogistics]
Gold salts
Indomethacin

Excludes: *salicylates (965.1)*
steroids (962.0-962.9)

965.7 Other non-narcotic analgesics
Pyrabital

965.8 Other specified analgesics and antipyretics
Pentazocine

965.9 Unspecified analgesic and antipyretic

966 Poisoning by anticonvulsants and anti-Parkinsonism drugs

966.0 Oxazolidine derivatives
Paramethadione
Trimethadione

966.1 Hydantoin derivatives
Phenytoin

● Code new to this edition
▲ Revision of existing code
④ ⑤ Fourth or fifth digit required

966.2 Succinimides
Ethosuximide
Phensuximide

966.3 Other and unspecified anticonvulsants
Primidone

Excludes: *barbiturates (967.0)*
sulfonamides (961.0)

966.4 Anti-Parkinsonism drugs
Amantadine
Ethopropazine [profenamine]
Levodopa [L-dopa]

967 Poisoning by sedatives and hypnotics

Excludes: *drug dependence (304.0-304.9)*
nondependent abuse (305.0-305.9)

967.0 Barbiturates
Amobarbital [amylobarbitone]
Barbital [barbitone]
Butabarbital [butabarbitone]
Pentobarbital [pentobarbitone]
Phenobarbital [phenobarbitone]
Secobarbital [quinalbarbitone]

Excludes: *thiobarbiturate anesthetics (968.3)*

967.1 Chloral hydrate group

967.2 Paraldehyde

967.3 Bromine compounds
Bromide
Carbromal (derivatives)

967.4 Methaqualone compounds

967.5 Glutethimide group

967.6 Mixed sedatives, not elsewhere classified

967.8 Other sedatives and hypnotics

967.9 Unspecified sedative or hypnotic
Sleeping:
drug } NOS
pill } NOS
tablet } NOS

968 Poisoning by other central nervous system depressants and anesthetics

Excludes: *drug dependence (304.0-304.9)*
nondependent abuse (305.0-305.9)

968.0 Central nervous system muscle-tone depressants
Chlorphenesin (carbamate)
Methocarbamol
Mephenesin

968.1 Halothane

968.2 Other gaseous anesthetics
Ether
Halogenated hydrocarbon derivatives, except halothane
Nitrous oxide

968.3 Intravenous anesthetics

Ketamine *Methohexital [methohexitone]*
Thiobarbiturates, such as thiopental sodium

968.4 Other and unspecified general anesthetics

968.5 Surface [topical] and infiltration anesthetics
Cocaine
Procaine
Lidocaine [lignocaine]
Tetracaine

968.6 Peripheral nerve and plexus-blocking anesthetics

968.7 Spinal anesthetics

968.9 Other and unspecified local anesthetics

969 Poisoning by psychotropic agents

Excludes: *drug dependence (304.0-304.9)*
nondependent abuse (305.0-305.9)

969.0 Antidepressants
Amitriptyline
Imipramine
Monoamine oxidase [MAO] inhibitors

969.1 Phenothiazine-based tranquilizers
Chlorpromazine
Fluphenazine
Prochlorperazine
Promazine

969.2 Butyrophenone-based tranquilizers
Haloperidol
Spiperone
Trifluperidol

969.3 Other antipsychotics, neuroleptics, and major tranquilizers

969.4 Benzodiazepine-based tranquilizers
Chlordiazepoxide
Diazepam
Flurazepam
Lorazepam
Medazepam
Nitrazepam

969.5 Other tranquilizers
Hydroxyzine
Meprobamate

969.6 Psychodysleptics [hallucinogens]
Cannabis (derivatives)
Lysergide [LSD]
Marihuana (derivatives)
Mescaline
Psilocin
Psilocybin

969.7 Psychostimulants
Amphetamine
Caffeine

Excludes: *central appetite depressants (977.0)*

969.8 Other specified psychotropic agents

969.9 Unspecified psychotropic agent

970 Poisoning by central nervous system stimulants

970.0 Analeptics
Lobeline
Nikethamide

970.1 Opiate antagonists
Levallorphan
Nalorphine
Naloxone

970.8 Other specified central nervous system stimulants

970.9 Unspecified central nervous system stimulant

971 Poisoning by drugs primarily affecting the autonomic nervous system

971.0 Parasympathomimetics [cholinergics]
Acetylcholine
Anticholinesterase:
  organophosphorus
  reversible
Pilocarpine

971.1 Parasympatholytics [anticholinergics and antimuscarinics] and spasmolytics
Atropine
Homatropine
Hyoscine [scopolamine]
Quaternary ammonium derivatives

Excludes: *papaverine (972.5)*

971.2 Sympathomimetics [adrenergics]
Epinephrine [adrenalin]
Levarterenol [noradrenalin]

971.3 Sympatholytics [antiadrenergics]
Phenoxybenzamine
Tolazoline hydrochloride

971.9 Unspecified drug primarily affecting autonomic nervous system

972 Poisoning by agents primarily affecting the cardiovascular system

972.0 Cardiac rhythm regulators
Practolol
Procainamide
Propranolol
Quinidine

Excludes: *lidocaine (968.5)*

972.1 Cardiotonic glycosides and drugs of similar action
Digitalis glycosides
Digoxin
Strophanthins

● Code new to this edition ▲ Revision of existing code ④ ⑤ Fourth or fifth digit required

972.2 Antilipemic and antiarteriosclerotic drugs
Clofibrate
Nicotinic acid derivatives

972.3 Ganglion-blocking agents
Pentamethonium bromide

972.4 Coronary vasodilators
Dipyridamole
Nitrates [nitroglycerin]
Nitrites

972.5 Other vasodilators
Cyclandelate
Diazoxide
Papaverine

Excludes: *nicotinic acid (972.2)*

972.6 Other antihypertensive agents
Clonidine
Guanethidine
Rauwolfia alkaloids
Reserpine

972.7 Antivaricose drugs, including sclerosing agents
Sodium morrhuate
Zinc salts

972.8 Capillary-active drugs
Adrenochrome derivatives
Metaraminol

972.9 Other and unspecified agents primarily affecting the cardiovascular system

973 Poisoning by agents primarily affecting the gastrointestinal system

973.0 Antacids and antigastric secretion drugs
Aluminum hydroxide
Magnesium trisilicate

973.1 Irritant cathartics
Bisacodyl
Castor oil
Phenolphthalein

973.2 Emollient cathartics
Dioctyl sulfosuccinates

973.3 Other cathartics, including intestinal atonia drugs
Magnesium sulfate

973.4 Digestants
Pancreatin
Papain
Pepsin

973.5 Antidiarrheal drugs
Kaolin
Pectin

Excludes: *anti-infectives (960.0-961.9)*

973.6 Emetics

973.8 Other specified agents primarily affecting the gastrointestinal system

973.9 Unspecified agent primarily affecting the gastrointestinal system

974 Poisoning by water, mineral, and uric acid metabolism drugs

974.0 Mercurial diuretics
Chlormerodrin
Mercaptomerin
Mersalyl

974.1 Purine derivative diuretics
Theobromine
Theophylline

Excludes: *aminophylline [theophylline ethylenediamine] (975.7)*
caffeine (969.7)

974.2 Carbonic acid anhydrase inhibitors
Acetazolamide

974.3 Saluretics
Benzothiadiazides
Chlorothiazide group

974.4 Other diuretics
Ethacrynic acid
Furosemide

974.5 Electrolytic, caloric, and water-balance agents

974.6 Other mineral salts, not elsewhere classified

974.7 Uric acid metabolism drugs
Allopurinol
Colchicine
Probenecid

Add 4th or 5th digit | Nonspecific code | Unspecified code | Medicare secondary payer(MSP) alert

975 Poisoning by agents primarily acting on the smooth and skeletal muscles and respiratory system

975.0 Oxytocic agents
Ergot alkaloids
Oxytocin
Prostaglandins

975.1 Smooth muscle relaxants
Adiphenine
Metaproterenol [orciprenaline]

Excludes: *papaverine (972.5)*

975.2 Skeletal muscle relaxants

975.3 Other and unspecified drugs acting on muscles

975.4 Antitussives
Dextromethorphan
Pipazethate

975.5 Expectorants
Acetylcysteine
Guaifenesin
Terpin hydrate

975.6 Anti-common cold drugs

975.7 Antiasthmatics
Aminophylline [theophylline ethylenediamine]

975.8 Other and unspecified respiratory drugs

976 Poisoning by agents primarily affecting skin and mucous membrane, ophthalmological, otorhinolaryngological, and dental drugs

976.0 Local anti-infectives and anti-inflammatory drugs

976.1 Antipruritics

976.2 Local astringents and local detergents

976.3 Emollients, demulcents, and protectants

976.4 Keratolytics, keratoplastics, other hair treatment drugs and preparations

976.5 Eye anti-infectives and other eye drugs
Idoxuridine

976.6 Anti-infectives and other drugs and preparations for ear, nose, and throat

976.7 Dental drugs topically applied

Excludes: *anti-infectives (976.0)*
local anesthetics (968.5)

976.8 Other agents primarily affecting skin and mucous membrane
Spermicides [vaginal contraceptives]

976.9 Unspecified agent primarily affecting skin and mucous membrane

977 Poisoning by other and unspecified drugs and medicinal substances

977.0 Dietetics
Central appetite depressants

977.1 Lipotropic drugs

977.2 Antidotes and chelating agents, not elsewhere classified

977.3 Alcohol deterrents

977.4 Pharmaceutical excipients
Pharmaceutical adjuncts

977.8 Other specified drugs and medicinal substances
Contrast media used for diagnostic x-ray procedures
Diagnostic agents and kits

977.9 Unspecified drug or medicinal substance

978 Poisoning by bacterial vaccines

978.0 BCG

978.1 Typhoid and paratyphoid

978.2 Cholera

978.3 Plague

978.4 Tetanus

978.5 Diphtheria

978.6 Pertussis vaccine, including combinations with a pertussis component

978.8 Other and unspecified bacterial vaccines

978.9 Mixed bacterial vaccines, except combinations with a pertussis component

979 Poisoning by other vaccines and biological substances

Excludes: *gamma globulin (964.6)*

979.0 Smallpox vaccine

979.1 Rabies vaccine

979.2 Typhus vaccine

979.3 Yellow fever vaccine

979.4 Measles vaccine

979.5 Poliomyelitis vaccine

979.6 Other and unspecified viral and rickettsial vaccines
Mumps vaccine

979.7 Mixed viral-rickettsial and bacterial vaccines, except combinations with a pertussis component

Excludes: *combinations with a pertussis component (978.6)*

979.9 Other and unspecified vaccines and biological substances

TOXIC EFFECTS OF SUBSTANCES CHIEFLY NONMEDICAL AS TO SOURCE (980-989)

Excludes: *burns from chemical agents (ingested) (947.0-947.9)*
localized toxic effects indexed elsewhere (001.0-799.9)
respiratory conditions due to external agents (506.0-508.9)

Use additional code to specify the nature of the toxic effect

980 Toxic effect of alcohol

980.0 Ethyl alcohol
Denatured alcohol
Ethanol
Grain alcohol

Excludes: *acute alcohol intoxication (305.0)*
in alcoholism (303.0)
drunkenness (simple) (305.0)
pathological (291.4)

980.1 Methyl alcohol
Methanol
Wood alcohol

980.2 Isopropyl alcohol
Dimethyl carbinol
Isopropanol
Rubbing alcohol

980.3 Fusel oil
Alcohol:
amyl
butyl
propyl

980.8 Other specified alcohols

980.9 Unspecified alcohol

981 Toxic effect of petroleum products
Benzine
Gasoline
Kerosene
Paraffin wax
Petroleum:
ether
naphtha
spirit

982 Toxic effect of solvents other than petroleum-based

982.0 Benzene and homologues

982.1 Carbon tetrachloride

982.2 Carbon disulfide
Carbon bisulfide

982.3 Other chlorinated hydrocarbon solvents
Tetrachloroethylene
Trichloroethylene

Excludes: *chlorinated hydrocarbon preparations other than solvents (989.2)*

982.4 Nitroglycol

982.8 Other nonpetroleum-based solvents
Acetone

983 Toxic effect of corrosive aromatics, acids, and caustic alkalis

983.0 Corrosive aromatics
Carbolic acid or phenol
Cresol

983.1 Acids
Acid:
hydrochloric
nitric
sulfuric

983.2 Caustic alkalis
Lye
Potassium hydroxide
Sodium hydroxide

983.9 Caustic, unspecified

984 Toxic effect of lead and its compounds (including fumes)
Includes: that from all sources except medicinal substances

984.0 Inorganic lead compounds
Lead dioxide
Lead salts

984.1 Organic lead compounds
Lead acetate
Tetraethyl lead

984.8 Other lead compounds

984.9 Unspecified lead compound

985 Toxic effect of other metals
Includes: that from all sources except medicinal substances

985.0 Mercury and its compounds
Minamata disease

985.1 Arsenic and its compounds

985.2 Manganese and its compounds

985.3 Beryllium and its compounds

985.4 Antimony and its compounds

985.5 Cadmium and its compounds

985.6 Chromium

985.8 Other specified metals
Brass fumes
Copper salts
Iron compounds
Nickel compounds

985.9 Unspecified metal

986 Toxic effect of carbon monoxide
Carbon monoxide from any source

987 Toxic effect of other gases, fumes, or vapors

987.0 Liquefied petroleum gases
Butane
Propane

987.1 Other hydrocarbon gas

987.2 Nitrogen oxides
Nitrogen dioxide
Nitrous fumes

987.3 Sulfur dioxide

987.4 Freon
Dichloromonofluoromethane

987.5 Lacrimogenic gas
Bromobenzyl cyanide
Chloroacetophenone
Ethyliodoacetate

987.6 Chlorine gas

987.7 Hydrocyanic acid gas

987.8 Other specified gases, fumes, or vapors
Phosgene
Polyester fumes

987.9 Unspecified gas, fume, or vapor

988 Toxic effect of noxious substances eaten as food

Excludes: *allergic reaction to food, such as:*
gastroenteritis (558.9)
rash (692.5, 693.1)
food poisoning (bacterial) (005.0-005.9)
toxic effects of food contaminants, such as:
aflatoxin and other mycotoxin (989.7)
mercury (985.0)

988.0 Fish and shellfish

988.1 Mushrooms

988.2 Berries and other plants

988.8 Other specified noxious substances eaten as food

988.9 Unspecified noxious substance eaten as food

989 Toxic effect of other substances, chiefly nonmedicinal as to source

989.0 Hydrocyanic acid and cyanides
Potassium cyanide
Sodium cyanide

Excludes: *gas and fumes (987.7)*

989.1 Strychnine and salts

989.2 Chlorinated hydrocarbons
Aldrin
Chlordane
DDT
Dieldrin

Excludes: *chlorinated hydrocarbon solvents (982.0-982.3)*

989.3 Organophosphate and carbamate
Carbaryl
Dichlorvos
Malathion
Parathion
Phorate
Phosdrin

989.4 Other pesticides, not elsewhere classified
Mixtures of insecticides

989.5 Venom
Bites of venomous snakes, lizards, and spiders
Tick paralysis

989.6 Soaps and detergents

989.7 Aflatoxin and other mycotoxin [food contaminants]

989.8 Other substances, chiefly nonmedicinal as to source

● **989.81 Asbestos**

● **989.82 Latex**

● **989.83 Silicone**

● **989.84 Tobacco**

● **989.89 Other**

989.9 Unspecified substance, chiefly nonmedicinal as to source

OTHER AND UNSPECIFIED EFFECTS OF EXTERNAL CAUSES (990-995)

990 Effects of radiation, unspecified
Complication of:
phototherapy
radiation therapy
Radiation sickness

Excludes: *specified adverse effects of radiation*
Such conditions are to be classified according to the nature of the adverse effect, as:
burns (940.0-949.5)
dermatitis (692.7-692.8)
leukemia (204.0-208.9)
pneumonia (508.0)
sunburn (692.71)
[The type of radiation giving rise to the adverse effect may be identified by use of the E codes.]

991 Effects of reduced temperature

991.0 Frostbite of face

991.1 Frostbite of hand

991.2 Frostbite of foot

991.3 Frostbite of other and unspecified sites

991.4 Immersion foot
Trench foot

991.5 Chilblains
Erythema pernio
Perniosis

991.6 Hypothermia
Hypothermia (accidental)

Excludes: *hypothermia following anesthesia (995.89)*
hypothermia not associated with low environmental temperature (780.9)

991.8 Other specified effects of reduced temperature

991.9 Unspecified effect of reduced temperature
Effects of freezing or excessive cold NOS

992 Effects of heat and light

Excludes: *burns (940.0-949.5)*
diseases of sweat glands due to heat (705.0-705.9)
malignant hyperpyrexia following anesthesia (995.89)
sunburn (692.71)

992.0 Heat stroke and sunstroke
Heat apoplexy
Heat pyrexia
Ictus solaris
Siriasis
Thermoplegia

992.1 Heat syncope
Heat collapse

992.2 Heat cramps

992.3 Heat exhaustion, anhydrotic
Heat prostration due to water depletion

Excludes: *that associated with salt depletion (992.4)*

992.4 Heat exhaustion due to salt depletion
Heat prostration due to salt (and water) depletion

992.5 Heat exhaustion, unspecified
Heat prostration NOS

992.6 Heat fatigue, transient

992.7 Heat edema

992.8 Other specified heat effects

992.9 Unspecified

993 Effects of air pressure

993.0 Barotrauma, otitic
Aero-otitis media
Effects of high altitude on ears

993.1 Barotrauma, sinus
Aerosinusitis
Effects of high altitude on sinuses

993.2 Other and unspecified effects of high altitude
Alpine sickness
Andes disease
Anoxia due to high altitude
Hypobaropathy
Mountain sickness

993.3 Caisson disease
Bends
Compressed-air disease
Decompression sickness
Divers' palsy or paralysis

993.4 Effects of air pressure caused by explosion

993.8 Other specified effects of air pressure

993.9 Unspecified effect of air pressure

994 Effects of other external causes

Excludes: *certain adverse effects not elsewhere classified (995.0-995.8)*

994.0 Effects of lightning
Shock from lightning
Struck by lightning NOS

Excludes: *burns (940.0-949.5)*

994.1 Drowning and nonfatal submersion
Bathing cramp
Immersion

994.2 Effects of hunger
Deprivation of food
Starvation

994.3 Effects of thirst
Deprivation of water

994.4 Exhaustion due to exposure

994.5 Exhaustion due to excessive exertion
Overexertion

994.6 Motion sickness
Air sickness
Seasickness
Travel sickness

994.7 Asphyxiation and strangulation
Suffocation (by):
- bedclothes
- cave-in
- constriction
- mechanical
- plastic bag
- pressure
- strangulation

Excludes: *asphyxia from:*
- *carbon monoxide (986)*
- *inhalation of food or foreign body (932-934.9)*
- *other gases, fumes, and vapors (987.0-987.9)*

994.8 Electrocution and nonfatal effects of electric current
Shock from electric current

Excludes: *electric burns (940.0-949.5)*

994.9 Other effects of external causes
Effects of:
- abnormal gravitational [G] forces or states
- weightlessness

995 Certain adverse effects not elsewhere classified

Note: This category is to be used to identify the effects not elsewhere classifiable of unknown, undetermined, or ill-defined causes. This category may also be used to provide an additional code to identify the effects of conditions classified elsewhere.

Excludes: *complications of surgical and medical care (996.0-999.9)*

995.0 Other anaphylactic shock
Code first any underlying condition such as:
- poisoning by drugs, medicinals and biologic substances (960-979)
- toxic effects of substances chiefly nonmedical as to source (980-989)

Use additional E code, if desired, to identify external cause, such as:
- adverse effects of correct medicinal substance properly administered (E930-E949)

Allergic shock, Anaphylactic reaction, Anaphylaxis — NOS or due to adverse effect of correct medicinal substance properly administered

Excludes: *anaphylactic reaction to serum (999.4)*
anaphylactic shock due to adverse food reaction (995.60-995.69)

995.1 Angioneurotic edema
Giant urticaria

Excludes: *Urticaria:*
- *due to serum (999.5)*
- *other specified (698.2, 708.0-708.9, 757.33)*

995.2 Unspecified adverse effect of drug, medicinal and biological substance
Adverse effect, Allergic reaction, Hypersensitivity, Idiosyncrasy — (due) to correct medicinal substance properly administered

Drug:
- hypersensitivity NOS
- reaction NOS

Excludes: *pathological drug intoxication (292.2)*

995.3 Allergy, unspecified
Allergic reaction NOS
Hypersensitivity NOS
Idiosyncrasy NOS

Excludes: *allergic reaction NOS to correct medicinal substance properly administered (995.2)*
specific types of allergic reaction, such as:
allergic diarrhea (558.9)
dermatitis (691.0-693.9)
hay fever (477.0-477.9)

995.4 Shock due to anesthesia
Shock due to anesthesia in which the correct substance was properly administered

Excludes: *complications of anesthesia in labor or delivery (668.0-668.9)*
overdose or wrong substance given (968.0-969.9)
postoperative shock NOS (998.0)
specified adverse effects of anesthesia classified elsewhere, such as:
anoxic brain damage (348.1)
hepatitis (070.0-070.9), etc.
unspecified adverse effect of anesthesia (995.2)

995.5 Child maltreatment syndrome
Battered baby or child syndrome NOS
Emotional and/or nutritional maltreatment of child

995.6 Anaphylactic shock due to adverse food reaction
Anaphylactic shock due to nonpoisonous foods

995.60 Due to unspecified food

995.61 Due to peanuts

995.62 Due to crustaceans

995.63 Due to fruits and vegetables

995.64 Due to tree nuts and seeds

995.65 Due to fish

995.66 Due to food additives

995.67 Due to milk products

995.68 Due to eggs

995.69 Due to other specified food

995.8 Other specified adverse effects, not elsewhere classified

995.81 Adult maltreatment syndrome
Abused person NEC
Battered:
person syndrome NEC
spouse
woman

995.89 Other
Malignant hyperpyrexia or hypothermia due to anesthesia

COMPLICATIONS OF SURGICAL AND MEDICAL CARE, NOT ELSEWHERE CLASSIFIED (996-999)

Excludes: *adverse effects of medicinal agents (001.0-799.9, 995.0-995.8)*
burns from local applications and irradiation (940.0-949.5)
complications of:
conditions for which the procedure was performed
surgical procedures during abortion, labor, and delivery (630-676.9)
poisoning and toxic effects of drugs and chemicals (960.0-989.9)
postoperative conditions in which no complications are present, such as:
artificial opening status (V44.0-V44.9)
closure of external stoma (V55.0-V55.9)
fitting of prosthetic device (V52.0-V52.9)
specified complications classified elsewhere
anesthetic shock (995.4)
electrolyte imbalance (276.0-276.9)
postlaminectomy syndrome (772.80-722.83)
postmastectomy lymphedema syndrome (457.0)
postoperative psychosis (293.0-293.9)
any other condition classified elsewhere in the Alphabetic Index when described as due to a procedure

996 Complications peculiar to certain specified procedures

Includes: complications, not elsewhere classified, in the use of artificial substitutes [e.g., Dacron, metal, Silastic, Teflon] or natural sources [e.g., bone] involving:
- anastomosis (internal)
- graft (bypass) (patch)
- implant
- internal device:
  - catheter
  - electronic
  - fixation
  - prosthetic
- reimplant
- transplant

Excludes: *accidental puncture or laceration during procedure (998.2)*
complications of internal anastomosis of:
- *gastrointestinal tract (997.4)*
- *urinary tract (997.5)*

other specified complications classified elsewhere, such as:
- *hemolytic anemia (283.1)*
- *functional cardiac disturbances (429.4)*
- *serum hepatitis (070.2-070.3)*

996.0 Mechanical complication of cardiac device, implant, and graft

Breakdown (mechanical)	Obstruction, mechanical
Displacement	Perforation
Leakage	Protrusion

996.00 Unspecified device, implant, and graft

996.01 Due to cardiac pacemaker (electrode)

996.02 Due to heart valve prosthesis

996.03 Due to coronary bypass graft

Excludes: *atherosclerosis of graft (414.02, 414.03)*
embolism [occlusion NOS] [thrombus] of graft (996.72)

996.04 Due to automatic implantable cardiac defibrillator

996.09 Other

996.1 Mechanical complication of other vascular device, implant, and graft

Mechanical complications involving:
- aortic (bifurcation) graft (replacement)
- arteriovenous: surgically created
  - fistula
  - shunt
- balloon (counterpulsation) device, intra-aortic
- carotid artery bypass graft
- dialysis catheter
- femoral-popliteal bypass graft
- umbrella device, vena cava

Excludes: *atherosclerosis of biological graft (440.30-440.32)*
embolism [occlusion NOS] [thrombus] of (biological) (synthetic) graft (996.74)

996.2 Mechanical complication of nervous system device, implant, and graft

Mechanical complications involving:
- dorsal column stimulator
- electrodes implanted in brain [brain "pacemaker"]
- peripheral nerve graft
- ventricular (communicating) shunt

996.3 Mechanical complication of genitourinary device, implant, and graft

996.30 Unspecified device, implant, and graft

996.31 Due to urethral [indwelling] catheter

996.32 Due to intrauterine contraceptive device

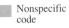

Add 4th or 5th digit | Nonspecific code | Unspecified code | Medicare secondary payer(MSP) alert

996.39 Other
Cystostomy catheter
Prosthetic reconstruction of vas deferens
Repair (graft) of ureter without mention of resection

Excludes: *complications due to:*
external stoma of urinary tract (997.5)
internal anastomosis of urinary tract (997.5)

996.4 Mechanical complication of internal orthopedic device, implant, and graft
Mechanical complications involving:
external (fixation) device utilizing internal screw(s), pin(s) or other methods of fixation
grafts of bone, cartilage, muscle, or tendon
internal (fixation) device such as nail, plate, rod, etc.

Excludes: *complications of external orthopedic device, such as:*
pressure ulcer due to cast (707.0)

996.5 Mechanical complication of other specified prosthetic device, implant, and graft
Mechanical complications involving:
prosthetic implant in:
bile duct
breast
chin
orbit of eye
nonabsorbable surgical material NOS
other graft, implant, and internal device, not elsewhere classified

996.51 Due to corneal graft

996.52 Due to graft of other tissue, not elsewhere classified
Skin graft failure or rejection

Excludes: *sloughing of temporary skin allografts or xenografts (pigskin)—omit code*

996.53 Due to ocular lens prosthesis

Excludes: *contact lenses—code to condition*

996.54 Due to breast prosthesis
Breast capsule (prosthesis)
Mammary implant

996.59 Due to other implant and internal device, not elsewhere classified
Nonabsorbable surgical material NOS
Prosthetic implant in:
bile duct
chin
orbit of eye

996.6 Infection and inflammatory reaction due to internal prosthetic device, implant, and graft
Infection (causing obstruction) } due to (presence of) any device, implant, and graft classifiable to 996.0-996.5
Inflammation } due to (presence of) any device, implant, and graft classifiable to 996.0-996.5

996.60 Due to unspecified device, implant, and graft

996.61 Due to cardiac device, implant, and graft
Cardiac pacemaker or defibrillator:
electrode(s), lead(s)
pulse generator
subcutaneous pocket
Coronary artery bypass graft
Heart valve prosthesis

996.62 Due to other vascular device, implant, and graft
Arterial graft
Arteriovenous fistula or shunt
Infusion pump
Vascular catheter (arterial) (dialysis) (venous)

996.63 Due to nervous system device, implant, and graft
Electrodes implanted in brain
Peripheral nerve graft
Spinal canal catheter
Ventricular (communicating) shunt (catheter)

996.64 Due to indwelling urinary catheter

996.65 Due to other genitourinary device, implant, and graft
Intrauterine contraceptive device

996.66 Due to internal joint prosthesis

996.67 Due to other internal orthopedic device, implant, and graft
Bone growth stimulator (electrode)
Internal fixation device (pin) (rod) (screw)

996.69 Due to other internal prosthetic device, implant, and graft
Breast prosthesis
Ocular lens prosthesis
Prosthetic orbital implant

996.7 Other complications of internal (biological) (synthetic) prosthetic device, implant, and graft

Complication NOS occlusion NOS Embolism Fibrosis Hemorrhage Pain Stenosis Thrombus	due to (presence of) any device, implant, and graft classifiable to 996.0-996.5

Excludes: *transplant rejection (996.8)*

996.70 Due to unspecified device, implant, and graft

996.71 Due to heart valve prosthesis

996.72 Due to other cardiac device, implant, and graft
Cardiac pacemaker or defibrillator:
electrode(s), lead(s)
subcutaneous pocket
Coronary artery bypass (graft)

Excludes: *occlusion due to atherosclerosis (414.02-414.03)*

996.73 Due to renal dialysis device, implant, and graft

996.74 Due to other vascular device, implant, and graft

Excludes: *occlusion of biological graft due to atherosclerosis (440.30-440.32)*

996.75 Due to nervous system device, implant, and graft

996.76 Due to genitourinary device, implant, and graft

996.77 Due to internal joint prosthesis

996.78 Due to other internal orthopedic device, implant, and graft

996.79 Due to other internal prosthetic device, implant, and graft

996.8 Complications of transplanted organ

Use additional code, if desired, to identify nature of complication, such as:
Cytomegalovirus (CMV) infection (078.5)
Transplant failure or rejection

996.80 Transplanted organ, unspecified

996.81 Kidney

996.82 Liver

996.83 Heart

996.84 Lung

996.85 Bone Marrow
Graft-versus-host disease (acute) (chronic)

996.86 Pancreas

996.89 Other specified transplanted organ
Intestines

996.9 Complications of reattached extremity or body part

996.90 Unspecified extremity

996.91 Forearm

996.92 Hand

996.93 Finger(s)

996.94 Upper extremity, other and unspecified

996.95 Foot and toe(s)

996.96 **Lower extremity, other and unspecified**

996.99 **Other specified body part**

997 **Complications affecting specified body systems, not elsewhere classified**

Excludes: *the listed conditions when specified as:*
causing shock (998.0)
complications of:
anesthesia:
adverse effect (001.0-799.9, 995.0-995.8)
in labor or delivery (668.0-668.9)
poisoning (968.0-969.9)
implanted device or graft (996.0-996.9)
obstetrical procedures (669.0-669.4)
reattached extremity (996.90-996.96)
transplanted organ (996.80-996.89)

Use additional code to identify complication

▲ **997.0** **Nervous system complications**

● **997.00** **Nervous system complication, unspecified**

● **997.01** **Central nervous system complication**
Anoxic brain damage
Cerebral hypoxia

Excludes: *cerebrovascular hemorrhage or infarction (997.02)*

● **997.02** **Iatrogenic cerebrovascular infarction or hemorrhage**
Postoperative stroke

● **997.09** **Other nervous system complications**

997.1 **Cardiac complications**

Cardiac: arrest insufficiency Cardiorespiratory failure Heart failure	during or resulting from a procedure

Excludes: *the listed conditions as long-term effects of cardiac surgery or due to the presence of cardiac prosthetic device (429.4)*

997.2 **Peripheral vascular complications**
Phlebitis or thrombophlebitis during or resulting from a procedure

Excludes: *the listed conditions due to:*
implant or catheter device (996.62)
infusion, perfusion, or transfusion (999.2)
complications affecting internal blood vessels, such as:
mesenteric artery (997.4)
renal artery (997.5)

997.3 **Respiratory complications**

Mendelson's syndrome Pneumonia (aspiration)	resulting from a procedure

Excludes: *iatrogenic [postoperative] pneumothorax (512.1)*
iatrogenic pulmonary embolism (415.11)
Mendelson's syndrome in labor and delivery (668.0)
specified complications classified elsewhere, such as:
adult respiratory distress syndrome (518.5)
pulmonary edema, postoperative (518.4)
respiratory insufficiency, acute, postoperative (518.5)
shock lung (518.5)
tracheostomy complication (519.0)

▲ **997.4 Digestive system complications**
Complications of intestinal (internal) anastomosis and bypass, not elsewhere classified, except that involving urinary tract
Hepatic failure } specified as due to a procedure
Hepatorenal syndrome } specified as due to a procedure
Intestinal obstruction NOS } specified as due to a procedure

Excludes: *specified gastrointestinal complications classified elsewhere, such as:*
blind loop syndrome (579.2)
colostomy or enterostomy complications (569.60-569.69)
gastrojejunal ulcer (534.0-534.9)
infection of external stoma (569.61)
pelvic peritoneal adhesions, female (614.6)
peritoneal adhesions (568.0)
peritoneal adhesions with obstruction (560.81)
postcholecystectomy syndrome (576.0)
postgastric surgery syndromes (564.2)

997.5 Urinary complications
Complications of:
external stoma of urinary tract
internal anastomosis and bypass of urinary tract, including that involving intestinal tract
Oliguria or anuria } specified as due to procedure
Renal: } specified as due to procedure
failure (acute) } specified as due to procedure
insufficiency (acute) } specified as due to procedure
Tubular necrosis (acute) } specified as due to procedure

Excludes: *specified complications classified elsewhere, such as:*
postoperative stricture of:
ureter (593.3)
urethra (598.2)

997.6 Late amputation stump complication
Excludes: *phantom limb (syndrome) (353.6)*
Use additional code to identify site (V49.60-V49.79)

997.60 Unspecified complication

997.61 Neuroma of amputation stump

997.62 Infection (chronic)

997.69 Other

997.9 Complications affecting other specified body systems, not elsewhere classified
Excludes: *specified complications classified elsewhere, such as:*
broad ligament laceration syndrome (620.6)
postartificial menopause syndrome (627.4)
postoperative stricture of vagina (623.2)

● **997.91 Hypertension**
Excludes: *essential hypertension (401.0-401.9)*

● **997.99 Other**
Vitreous touch syndrome

998 Other complications of procedures, not elsewhere classified

998.0 Postoperative shock
Collapse NOS } during or resulting from a surgical procedure
Shock (endotoxic) (hypovolemic) (septic) } during or resulting from a surgical procedure

Excludes: *shock:*
anaphylactic due to serum (999.4)
anesthetic (995.4)
electric (994.8)
following abortion (639.5)
obstetric (669.1)
traumatic (958.4)

998.1 Hemorrhage or hematoma complicating a procedure
Hemorrhage of any site resulting from a procedure
Excludes: *hemorrhage due to implanted device or graft (996.70-996.79)*
that complicating cesarean section or puerperal perineal wound (674.3)

Add 4th or 5th digit | Nonspecific code | Unspecified code | Medicare secondary payer(MSP) alert

998.2 Accidental puncture or laceration during a procedure
Accidental perforation by catheter or other instrument during a procedure on:
blood vessel
nerve
organ

Excludes: *iatrogenic [postoperative] pneumothorax (512.1)*
puncture or laceration caused by implanted device intentionally left in operation wound (996.0-996.5)
specified complications classified elsewhere, such as:
broad ligament laceration syndrome (620.6)
trauma from instruments during delivery (664.0-665.9)

998.3 Disruption of operation wound
Dehiscence } of operation wound
Rupture } of operation wound

Excludes: *disruption of:*
cesarean wound (674.1)
perineal wound, puerperal (674.2)

998.4 Foreign body accidentally left during a procedure
Adhesions } due to foreign body accidentally left in operative wound or body cavity during a procedure
Obstruction } due to foreign body accidentally left in operative wound or body cavity during a procedure
Perforation } due to foreign body accidentally left in operative wound or body cavity during a procedure

Excludes: *obstruction or perforation caused by implanted device intentionally left in body (996.0-996.5)*

998.5 Postoperative infection
Abscess: } postoperative
intra-abdominal } postoperative
stitch } postoperative
subphrenic } postoperative
wound } postoperative
Septicemia } postoperative

Excludes: *infection due to:*
implanted device (996.60-996.69)
infusion, perfusion, or transfusion (999.3)
postoperative obstetrical wound infection (674.3)

Use additional code to identify infection

998.6 Persistent postoperative fistula

998.7 Acute reaction to foreign substance accidentally left during a procedure
Peritonitis:
aseptic
chemical

998.8 Other specified complications of procedures, not elsewhere classified

998.81 Emphysema (subcutaneous) (surgical) resulting from a procedure

998.82 Cataract fragments in eye following cataract surgery

998.89 Other specified complications

998.9 Unspecified complication of procedure, not elsewhere classified
Postoperative complication NOS

Excludes: *complication NOS of obstetrical surgery or procedure (669.4)*

999 Complications of medical care, not elsewhere classified

Includes: complications, not elsewhere classified, of:
- dialysis (hemodialysis) (peritoneal) (renal)
- extracorporeal circulation
- hyperalimentation therapy
- immunization
- infusion
- inhalation therapy
- injection
- inoculation
- perfusion
- transfusion
- vaccination
- ventilation therapy

Excludes: *specified complications classified elsewhere such as:*
- *complications of implanted device (996.0-996.9)*
- *contact dermatitis due to drugs (692.3)*
- *dementia dialysis (294.8)*
  - *transient (293.9)*
- *dialysis disequilibrium syndrome (276.0-276.9)*
- *poisoning and toxic effects of drugs and chemicals (960.0-989.9)*
- *postvaccinal encephalitis (323.5)*
- *water and electrolyte imbalance (276.0-276.9)*

999.0 Generalized vaccinia

999.1 Air embolism

Air embolism to any site following infusion, perfusion, or transfusion

Excludes: *embolism specified as:*
- *complicating:*
  - *abortion (634-638 with .6, 639.6)*
  - *ectopic or molar pregnancy (639.6)*
  - *pregnancy, childbirth, or the puerperium (673.0)*
- *due to implanted device (996.7)*
- *traumatic (958.0)*

999.2 Other vascular complications

Phlebitis, Thromboembolism, Thrombophlebitis } following infusion, perfusion, or transfusion

Excludes: *the listed conditions when specified as:*
- *due to implanted device (996.61-996.62, 996.72-996.74)*
- *postoperative NOS (997.2)*

999.3 Other infection

Infection, Sepsis, Septicemia } following infusion, injection, transfusion, or vaccination

Excludes: *the listed conditions when specified as:*
- *due to implanted device (996.60-996.69)*
- *postoperative NOS (998.5)*

999.4 Anaphylactic shock due to serum

Excludes: *shock:*
- *allergic NOS (995.0)*
- *anaphylactic:*
  - *NOS (995.0)*
  - *due to drugs and chemicals (995.0)*

999.5 Other serum reaction

- Intoxication by serum
- Protein sickness
- Serum rash
- Serum sickness
- Urticaria due to serum

Excludes: *serum hepatitis (070.2-070.3)*

999.6 ABO incompatibility reaction

Incompatible blood transfusion
Reaction to blood group incompatibility in infusion or transfusion

999.7 Rh incompatibility reaction

Reactions due to Rh factor in infusion or transfusion

999.8 Other transfusion reaction
Septic shock due to transfusion
Transfusion reaction NOS

Excludes: *postoperative shock (998.0)*

999.9 Other and unspecified complications of medical care, not elsewhere classified
Complications, not elsewhere classified, of:
electroshock therapy
inhalation therapy
ultrasound therapy
ventilation therapy
Unspecified misadventure of medical care

Excludes: *unspecified complication of:*
phototherapy (990)
radiation therapy (990)

SUPPLEMENTARY CLASSIFICATION OF FACTORS INFLUENCING HEALTH STATUS AND CONTACT WITH HEALTH SERVICES (V01-V82)

This classification is provided to deal with occasions when circumstances other than a disease or injury classifiable to categories 001-999 (the main part of ICD)are recorded as "diagnoses" or "problems." This can arise mainly in three ways:

a) When a person who is not currently sick encounters the health services for some specific purpose, such as to act as a donor of an organ or tissue, to receive prophylactic vaccination, or to discuss a problem which is in itself not a disease or injury. This will be a fairly rare occurrence among hospital inpatients, but will be relatively more common among hospital outpatients and patients of family practitioners, health clinics, etc.

b) When a person with a known disease or injury, whether it is current or resolving, encounters the health care system for a specific treatment of that disease or injury (e.g., dialysis for renal disease; chemotherapy for malignancy; cast change).

c) When some circumstance or problem is present which influences the person's health status but is not in itself a current illness or injury. Such factors may be elicited during population surveys, when the person may or may not be currently sick, or be recorded as an additional factor to be borne in mind when the person is receiving care for some current illness or injury classifiable to categories 001-999.

In the latter circumstances the V code should be used only as a supplementary code and should not be the one selected for use in primary, single cause tabulations. Examples of these circumstances are a personal history of certain diseases, or a person with an artificial heart valve in situ.

PERSONS WITH POTENTIAL HEALTH HAZARDS RELATED TO COMMUNICABLE DISEASES (V01-V06)

Excludes: *family history of infectious and parasitic diseases (V18.8)*
personal history of infectious and parasitic diseases (V12.0)

V01 Contact with or exposure to communicable diseases

V01.0 Cholera
Conditions classifiable to 001

V01.1 Tuberculosis
Conditions classifiable to 010-018

V01.2 Poliomyelitis
Conditions classifiable to 045

V01.3 Smallpox
Conditions classifiable to 050

V01.4 Rubella
Conditions classifiable to 056

V01.5 Rabies
Conditions classifiable to 071

V01.6 Venereal diseases
Conditions classifiable to 090-099

V01.7 Other viral diseases
Conditions classifiable to 042-078, except as above

V01.8 Other communicable diseases
Conditions classifiable to 001-136, except as above

V01.9 Unspecified communicable disease

V02 Carrier or suspected carrier of infectious diseases

V02.0 Cholera

V02.1 Typhoid

V02.2 Amebiasis

V02.3 Other gastrointestinal pathogens

V02.4 Diphtheria

V02.5 Other specified bacterial diseases
Bacterial disease:
meningococcal
staphylococcal
streptococcal

V02.6 Viral hepatitis
Hepatitis Australian-antigen [HAA] [SH] carrier
Serum hepatitis carrier

V02.7 Gonorrhea

Add 4th or 5th digit | Nonspecific code | Unspecified code | Manifestation code

V02.8 Other venereal diseases

V02.9 Other specified infectious organism

V03 Need for prophylactic vaccination and inoculation against bacterial diseases

Excludes: *vaccination not carried out because of contraindication (V64.0)*
vaccines against combinations of diseases (V06.0-V06.9)

V03.0 Cholera alone

V03.1 Typhoid-paratyphoid alone [TAB]

V03.2 Tuberculosis [BCG]

V03.3 Plague

V03.4 Tularemia

V03.5 Diphtheria alone

V03.6 Pertussis alone

V03.7 Tetanus toxoid alone

V03.8 Other specified vaccinations against single bacterial diseases

V03.81 Hemophilus influenza, type B [Hib]

V03.82 Streptococcus pneumoniae [pneumococcus]

V03.89 Other specified vaccination

V03.9 Unspecified single bacterial disease

V04 Need for prophylactic vaccination and inoculation against certain viral diseases

Excludes: *vaccines against combinations of diseases (V06.0-V06.9)*

V04.0 Poliomyelitis

V04.1 Smallpox

V04.2 Measles alone

V04.3 Rubella alone

V04.4 Yellow fever

V04.5 Rabies

V04.6 Mumps alone

V04.7 Common cold

V04.8 Influenza

V05 Need for other prophylactic vaccination and inoculation against single diseases

Excludes: *vaccines against combinations of diseases (V06.0-V06.9)*

V05.0 Arthropod-borne viral encephalitis

V05.1 Other arthropod-borne viral diseases

V05.2 Leishmaniasis

V05.3 Viral hepatitis

V05.4 Varicella
Chickenpox

V05.8 Other specified disease

V05.9 Unspecified single disease

V06 Need for prophylactic vaccination and inoculation against combinations of diseases

Note: Use additional single vaccination codes from categories V03-V05 to identify any vaccinations not included in a combination code.

V06.0 Cholera with typhoid-paratyphoid [cholera + TAB]

V06.1 Diphtheria-tetanus-pertussis, combined [DTP]

V06.2 Diphtheria-tetanus-pertussis with typhoid-paratyphoid [DTP + TAB]

V06.3 Diphtheria-tetanus-pertussis with poliomyelitis [DTP + polio]

V06.4 Measles-mumps-rubella [MMR]

V06.5 Tetanus-diphtheria [Td]

V06.6 Streptococcus pneumoniae [pneumococcus] and influenza

V06.8 Other combinations

Excludes: *multiple single vaccination codes (V03.0-V05.9)*

V06.9 Unspecified combined vaccine

PERSONS WITH NEED FOR ISOLATION, OTHER POTENTIAL HEALTH HAZARDS AND PROPHYLACTIC MEASURES (V07-V09)

V07 Need for isolation and other prophylactic measures

Excludes: *prophylactic organ removal (V50.41-V50.49)*

V07.0 Isolation

Admission to protect the individual from his surroundings or for isolation of individual after contact with infectious diseases

V07.1 Desensitization to allergens

V07.2 Prophylactic immunotherapy

Administration of:
- antivenin
- immune sera [gamma globulin]
- RhoGAM
- tetanus antitoxin

V07.3 Other prophylactic chemotherapy

V07.31 Prophylactic fluoride administration

V07.39 Other prophylactic chemotherapy

Excludes: *maintenance chemotherapy following disease (V58.1)*

V07.4 Postmenopausal hormone replacement therapy

V07.8 Other specified prophylactic measure

V07.9 Unspecified prophylactic measure

V08 Asymptomatic human immunodeficiency virus [HIV] infection status

HIV positive NOS

Note: This code is ONLY to be used when NO HIV infection symptoms or conditions are present. If any HIV infection symptoms or conditions are present, see code 042.

Excludes: *AIDS (042)*
human immunodeficiency virus [HIV] disease (042)
exposure to HIV (V01.7)
nonspecific serologic evidence of HIV (795.71)
symptomatic human immunodeficiency virus [HIV] infection (042)

V09 Infection with drug-resistant microorganisms

Note: This category is intended for use as an additional code for infectious conditions classified elsewhere to indicate the presence of drug-resistance of the infectious organism.

V09.0 Infection with microorganisms resistant to penicillins

V09.1 Infection with microorganisms resistant to cephalosporins and other B-lactam antibiotics

V09.2 Infection with microorganisms resistant to macrolides

V09.3 Infection with microorganisms resistant to tetracyclines

V09.4 Infection with microorganisms resistant to aminoglycosides

V09.5 Infection with microorganisms resistant to quinolones and fluoroquinolones

V09.50 Without mention of resistance to multiple quinolones and fluoroquinolones

V09.51 With resistance to multiple quinolones and fluoroquinolones

V09.6 Infection with microorganisms resistant to sulfonamides

V09.7 Infection with microorganisms resistant to other specified antimycobacterial agents

Excludes: *Amikacin (V09.4)*
Kanamycin (V09.4)
Streptomycin [SM] (V09.4)

V09.70 Without mention of resistance to multiple antimycobacterial agents

V09.71 With resistance to multiple antimycobacterial agents

V09.8 Infection with microorganisms resistant to other specified drugs

V09.80 Without mention of resistance to multiple drugs

V09.81 With resistance to multiple drugs

V09.9 Infection with drug-resistant microorganisms, unspecified

Drug resistance NOS

V09.90 Without mention of multiple drug resistance

V09.91 With multiple drug resistance

Multiple drug resistance NOS

PERSONS WITH POTENTIAL HEALTH HAZARDS RELATED TO PERSONAL AND FAMILY HISTORY (V10-V19)

Excludes: *obstetric patients where the possibility that the fetus might be affected is the reason for observation or management during pregnancy (655.0-655.9)*

V10 Personal history of malignant neoplasm

V10.0 Gastrointestinal tract
History of conditions classifiable to 140-159

V10.00 Gastrointestinal tract, unspecified

V10.01 Tongue

V10.02 Other and unspecified oral cavity and pharynx

V10.03 Esophagus

V10.04 Stomach

V10.05 Large intestine

V10.06 Rectum, rectosigmoid junction, and anus

V10.07 Liver

V10.09 Other

V10.1 Trachea, bronchus, and lung
History of conditions classifiable to 162

V10.11 Bronchus and lung

V10.12 Trachea

V10.2 Other respiratory and intrathoracic organs
History of conditions classifiable to 160, 161, 163-165

V10.20 Respiratory organ, unspecified

V10.21 Larynx

V10.22 Nasal cavities, middle ear, and accessory sinuses

V10.29 Other

V10.3 Breast
History of conditions classifiable to 174 and 175

V10.4 Genital organs
History of conditions classifiable to 179-187

V10.40 Female genital organ, unspecified

V10.41 Cervix uteri

V10.42 Other parts of uterus

V10.43 Ovary

V10.44 Other female genital organs

V10.45 Male genital organ, unspecified

V10.46 Prostate

V10.47 Testis

V10.49 Other male genital organs

V10.5 Urinary organs
History of conditions classifiable to 188 and 189

V10.50 Urinary organ, unspecified

V10.51 Bladder

V10.52 Kidney

V10.59 Other

V10.6 Leukemia
Conditions classifiable to 204-208

Excludes: *leukemia in remission (204-208)*

V10.60 Leukemia, unspecified

V10.61 Lymphoid leukemia

V10.62 Myeloid leukemia

V10.63 Monocytic leukemia

V10.69 Other

V10.7 Other lymphatic and hematopoietic neoplasms

Conditions classifiable to 200-203

Excludes: *listed conditions in 200-203 in remission*

V10.71 Lymphosarcoma and reticulosarcoma

V10.72 Hodgkin's disease

V10.79 Other

V10.8 Personal history of malignant neoplasm of other sites
History of conditions classifiable to 170-173, 190-195

V10.81 Bone

V10.82 Malignant melanoma of skin

V10.83 Other malignant neoplasm of skin

V10.84 Eye

V10.85 Brain

V10.86 Other parts of nervous system

Excludes: *peripheral, sympathetic, and parasympathetic nerves (V10.89)*

V10.87 Thyroid

V10.88 Other endocrine glands and related structures

V10.89 Other

V10.9 Unspecified personal history of malignant neoplasm

V11 Personal history of mental disorder

V11.0 Schizophrenia

Excludes: *that in remission (295.0-295.9 with fifth-digit 5)*

V11.1 Affective disorders
Personal history of manic-depressive psychosis

Excludes: *that in remission (296.0-296.6 with fifth-digit 5, 6)*

V11.2 Neurosis

V11.3 Alcoholism

V11.8 Other mental disorders

V11.9 Unspecified mental disorder

V12 Personal history of certain other diseases

V12.0 Infectious and parasitic diseases

V12.00 Unspecified infectious and parasitic disease

V12.01 Tuberculosis

V12.02 Poliomyelitis

V12.03 Malaria

V12.09 Other

V12.1 Nutritional deficiency

V12.2 Endocrine, metabolic, and immunity disorders

Excludes: *history of allergy (V14.0-V14.9, V15.0)*

V12.3 Diseases of blood and blood-forming organs

V12.4 Disorders of nervous system and sense organs

V12.5 Diseases of circulatory system

Excludes: *old myocardial infarction (412)*
postmyocardial infarction syndrome (411.0)

● **V12.50 Unspecified circulatory disease**

● **V12.51 Venous thrombosis and embolism**
Pulmonary embolism

● **V12.52 Thrombophlebitis**

● **V12.59 Other**

V12.6 Diseases of respiratory system

V12.7 Diseases of digestive system

V12.70 Unspecified digestive disease

V12.71 **Peptic ulcer disease**

V12.72 **Colonic polyps**

V12.79 **Other**

V13 Personal history of other diseases

V13.0 Disorders of urinary system

V13.00 **Unspecified urinary disorder**

V13.01 **Urinary calculi**

V13.09 **Other**

V13.1 Trophoblastic disease

Excludes: *supervision during a current pregnancy (V23.1)*

V13.2 Other genital system and obstetric disorders

Excludes: *supervision during a current pregnancy of a woman with poor obstetric history (V23.0-V23.9)*
habitual aborter (646.3)
without current history (629.9)

V13.3 Diseases of skin and subcutaneous tissue

V13.4 Arthritis

V13.5 Other musculoskeletal disorders

V13.6 Congenital malformations

V13.7 Perinatal problems

V13.8 Other specified diseases

V13.9 Unspecified disease

V14 Personal history of allergy to medicinal agents

V14.0 Penicillin

V14.1 Other antibiotic agent

V14.2 Sulfonamides

V14.3 Other anti-infective agent

V14.4 Anesthetic agent

V14.5 Narcotic agent

V14.6 Analgesic agent

V14.7 Serum or vaccine

V14.8 Other specified medicinal agents

V14.9 Unspecified medicinal agent

V15 Other personal history presenting hazards to health

V15.0 Allergy, other than to medicinal agents

V15.1 Surgery to heart and great vessels

Excludes: *replacement by transplant or other means (V42.1-V42.2, V43.2-V43.4)*

V15.2 Surgery to other major organs

Excludes: *replacement by transplant or other means (V42.0-V43.8)*

V15.3 Irradiation

Previous exposure to therapeutic or other ionizing radiation

V15.4 Psychological trauma

Excludes: *history of condition classifiable to 290-316 (V11.0-V11.9)*

V15.5 Injury

V15.6 Poisoning

V15.7 Contraception

Excludes: *current contraceptive management (V25.0-V25.4)*
presence of intrauterine contraceptive device as incidental finding (V45.5)

V15.8 Other specified personal history presenting hazards to health

V15.81 **Noncompliance with medical treatment**

V15.82 **History of tobacco use**

Excludes: *tobacco dependence (305.1)*

● **V15.84 Exposure to asbestos**

● **V15.85 Exposure to potentially hazardous body fluids**

● **V15.86 Exposure to lead**

V15.89 Other

V15.9 Unspecified personal history presenting hazards to health

V16 Family history of malignant neoplasm

V16.0 Gastrointestinal tract
Family history of condition classifiable to 140-159

V16.1 Trachea, bronchus, and lung
Family history of condition classifiable to 162

V16.2 Other respiratory and intrathoracic organs
Family history of condition classifiable to 160-161, 163-165

V16.3 Breast
Family history of condition classifiable to 174

V16.4 Genital organs
Family history of condition classifiable to 179-187

V16.5 Urinary organs
Family history of condition classifiable to 189

V16.6 Leukemia
Family history of condition classifiable to 204-208

V16.7 Other lymphatic and hematopoietic neoplasms
Family history of condition classifiable to 200-203

V16.8 Other specified malignant neoplasm
Family history of other condition classifiable to 140-199

V16.9 Unspecified malignant neoplasm

V17 Family history of certain chronic disabling diseases

V17.0 Psychiatric condition

Excludes: *family history of mental retardation (V18.4)*

V17.1 Stroke (cerebrovascular)

V17.2 Other neurological diseases
Epilepsy
Huntington's chorea

V17.3 Ischemic heart disease

V17.4 Other cardiovascular diseases

V17.5 Asthma

V17.6 Other chronic respiratory conditions

V17.7 Arthritis

V17.8 Other musculoskeletal diseases

V18 Family history of certain other specific conditions

V18.0 Diabetes mellitus

V18.1 Other endocrine and metabolic diseases

V18.2 Anemia

V18.3 Other blood disorders

V18.4 Mental retardation

V18.5 Digestive disorders

V18.6 Kidney diseases

V18.7 Other genitourinary diseases

V18.8 Infectious and parasitic diseases

V19 Family history of other conditions

V19.0 Blindness or visual loss

V19.1 Other eye disorders

V19.2 Deafness or hearing loss

V19.3 Other ear disorders

V19.4 Skin conditions

V19.5 Congenital anomalies

V19.6 Allergic disorders

V19.7 Consanguinity

V19.8 Other condition

PERSONS ENCOUNTERING HEALTH SERVICES IN CIRCUMSTANCES RELATED TO REPRODUCTION AND DEVELOPMENT (V20-V29)

V20 Health supervision of infant or child

V20.0 Foundling

V20.1 Other healthy infant or child receiving care
Medical or nursing care supervision of healthy infant in cases of:
maternal illness, physical or psychiatric
socioeconomic adverse condition at home
too many children at home preventing or interfering with normal care

V20.2 Routine infant or child health check
Developmental testing of infant or child
Immunizations appropriate for age
Routine vision and hearing testing

Excludes: *special screening for developmental handicaps (V79.3)*

Use additional code(s) to identify:
Special screening examination(s) performed (V73.0-V82.9)

V21 Constitutional states in development

V21.0 Period of rapid growth in childhood

V21.1 Puberty

V21.2 Other adolescence

V21.8 Other specified constitutional states in development

V21.9 Unspecified constitutional state in development

V22 Normal pregnancy

Excludes: *pregnancy examination or test, pregnancy unconfirmed (V72.4)*

V22.0 Supervision of normal first pregnancy

V22.1 Supervision of other normal pregnancy

V22.2 Pregnant state, incidental
Pregnant state NOS

V23 Supervision of high-risk pregnancy

V23.0 Pregnancy with history of infertility

V23.1 Pregnancy with history of trophoblastic disease
Pregnancy with history of:
hydatidiform mole
vesicular mole

Excludes: *that without current pregnancy (V13.1)*

V23.2 Pregnancy with history of abortion
Pregnancy with history of conditions classifiable to 634-638

Excludes: *habitual aborter:*
care during pregnancy (646.3)
that without current pregnancy (629.9)

V23.3 Grand multiparity

Excludes: *care in relation to labor and delivery (659.4)*
that without current pregnancy (V61.5)

V23.4 Pregnancy with other poor obstetric history
Pregnancy with history of other conditions classifiable to 630-676

V23.5 Pregnancy with other poor reproductive history
Pregnancy with history of stillbirth or neonatal death

V23.7 Insufficient prenatal care
History of little or no prenatal care

V23.8 Other high-risk pregnancy

V23.9 Unspecified high-risk pregnancy

V24 Postpartum care and examination

V24.0 Immediately after delivery
Care and observation in uncomplicated cases

● Code new to this edition ▲ Revision of existing code ④ ⑤ Fourth or fifth digit required

V24.1 Lactating mother
Supervision of lactation

V24.2 Routine postpartum follow-up

V25 Encounter for contraceptive management

V25.0 General counseling and advice

V25.01 Prescription of oral contraceptives

V25.02 Initiation of other contraceptive measures
Fitting of diaphragm
Prescription of foams, creams, or other agents

V25.09 Other
Family planning advice

V25.1 Insertion of intrauterine contraceptive device

V25.2 Sterilization
Admission for interruption of fallopian tubes or vas deferens

V25.3 Menstrual extraction
Menstrual regulation

V25.4 Surveillance of previously prescribed contraceptive methods
Checking, reinsertion, or removal of contraceptive device
Repeat prescription for contraceptive method
Routine examination in connection with contraceptive maintenance

Excludes: *presence of intrauterine contraceptive device as incidental finding (V45.5)*

V25.40 Contraceptive surveillance, unspecified

V25.41 Contraceptive pill

V25.42 Intrauterine contraceptive device
Checking, reinsertion, or removal of intrauterine device

V25.43 Implantable subdermal contraceptive

V25.49 Other contraceptive method

V25.5 Insertion of implantable subdermal contraceptive

V25.8 Other specified contraceptive management
Postvasectomy sperm count

V25.9 Unspecified contraceptive management

V26 Procreative management

V26.0 Tuboplasty or vasoplasty after previous sterilization

V26.1 Artificial insemination

V26.2 Investigation and testing
Fallopian insufflation
Sperm counts

Excludes: *postvasectomy sperm count (V25.8)*

V26.3 Genetic counseling

V26.4 General counseling and advice

V26.8 Other specified procreative management

V26.9 Unspecified procreative management

V27 Outcome of delivery

Note: This category is intended for the coding of the outcome of delivery on the mother's record.

V27.0 Single liveborn

V27.1 Single stillborn

V27.2 Twins, both liveborn

V27.3 Twins, one liveborn and one stillborn

V27.4 Twins, both stillborn

V27.5 Other multiple birth, all liveborn

V27.6 Other multiple birth, some liveborn

V27.7 Other multiple birth, all stillborn

V27.9 Unspecified outcome of delivery
Single birth } outcome to infant unspecified
Multiple birth }

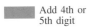

V28 Antenatal screening

Excludes: *routine prenatal care (V22.0-V23.9)*

V28.0 Screening for chromosomal anomalies by amniocentesis

V28.1 Screening for raised alpha-fetoprotein levels in amniotic fluid

V28.2 Other screening based on amniocentesis

V28.3 Screening for malformation using ultrasonics

V28.4 Screening for fetal growth retardation using ultrasonics

V28.5 Screening for isoimmunization

V28.8 Other specified antenatal screening

V28.9 Unspecified antenatal screening

V29 Observation and evaluation of newborns for suspected condition not found

Note: This category is to be used for newborns, within the neonatal period, (the first 28 days of life) who are suspected of having an abnormal condition resulting from exposure from the mother or the birth process, but without signs or symptoms, and, which after examination and observation, is found not to exist.

V29.0 Observation for suspected infectious condition

V29.1 Observation for suspected neurological condition

V29.2 Observation for suspected respiratory condition

V29.8 Observation for other specified suspected condition

V29.9 Observation for unspecified suspected condition

LIVEBORN INFANTS ACCORDING TO TYPE OF BIRTH (V30-V39)

Note: These categories are intended for the coding of liveborn infants who are consuming health care [e.g., crib or bassinet occupancy].

The following fourth-digit subdivisions are for use with categories V30-V39:

.0 Born in hospital

.1 Born before admission to hospital

.2 Born outside hospital and not hospitalized

The following two fifth-digits are for use with the fourth-digit .0, Born in hospital:

0 delivered without mention of cesarean delivery

1 delivered by cesarean delivery

④ **V30 Single liveborn**

④ **V31 Twin, mate liveborn**

④ **V32 Twin, mate stillborn**

④ **V33 Twin, unspecified**

④ **V34 Other multiple, mates all liveborn**

④ **V35 Other multiple, mates all stillborn**

④ **V36 Other multiple, mates live- and stillborn**

④ **V37 Other multiple, unspecified**

④ **V39 Unspecified**

PERSONS WITH A CONDITION INFLUENCING THEIR HEALTH STATUS (V40-V49)

Note: These categories are intended for use when these conditions are recorded as "diagnoses" or "problems."

V40 Mental and behavioral problems

V40.0 Problems with learning

V40.1 Problems with communication [including speech]

V40.2 Other mental problems

V40.3 Other behavioral problems

V40.9 Unspecified mental or behavioral problem

V41 Problems with special senses and other special functions

V41.0 Problems with sight

V41.1 Other eye problems

V41.2 Problems with hearing

V41.3 Other ear problems

V41.4 Problems with voice production

V41.5 Problems with smell and taste

V41.6 Problems with swallowing and mastication

V41.7 Problems with sexual function

Excludes: *marital problems (V61.1)*
psychosexual disorders (302.0-302.9)

V41.8 Other problems with special functions

V41.9 Unspecified problem with special functions

V42 Organ or tissue replaced by transplant
Includes: homologous or heterologous (animal) (human) transplant organ status

V42.0 Kidney

V42.1 Heart

V42.2 Heart valve

V42.3 Skin

V42.4 Bone

V42.5 Cornea

V42.6 Lung

V42.7 Liver

V42.8 Other specified organ or tissue
Intestine
Pancreas

V42.9 Unspecified organ or tissue

V43 Organ or tissue replaced by other means
Includes: replacement of organ by:
artificial device
mechanical device
prosthesis

Excludes: *cardiac pacemaker in situ (V45.01)*
fitting and adjustment of prosthetic device (V52.0-V52.9)
renal dialysis status (V45.1)

V43.0 Eye globe

V43.1 Lens
Pseudophakos

V43.2 Heart

V43.3 Heart valve

V43.4 Blood vessel

V43.5 Bladder

V43.6 Joint

V43.60 Unspecified joint

V43.61 Shoulder

V43.62 Elbow

V43.63 Wrist

V43.64 Hip

V43.65 Knee

V43.66 Ankle

V43.69 Other

V43.7 Limb

V43.8 Other organ or tissue

- ● **V43.81 Larynx**
- ● **V43.82 Breast**
- ● **V43.89 Other**

V44 Artificial opening status

Excludes: *artificial openings requiring attention or management (V55.0-V55.9)*

V44.0 Tracheostomy

V44.1 Gastrostomy

V44.2 Ileostomy

V44.3 Colostomy

V44.4 Other artificial opening of gastrointestinal tract

V44.5 Cystostomy

V44.6 Other artificial opening of urinary tract
Nephrostomy
Urethrostomy
Ureterostomy

V44.7 Artificial vagina

V44.8 Other artificial opening status

V44.9 Unspecified artificial opening status

V45 Other postsurgical states

Excludes: *aftercare management (V51-V58.9)*
malfunction or other complication—code to condition

V45.0 Cardiac device in situ

V45.00 Unspecified cardiac device

V45.01 Cardiac pacemaker

V45.02 Automatic implantable cardiac defibrillator

V45.09 Other specified cardiac device
Carotid sinus pacemaker in situ

V45.1 Renal dialysis status
Patient requiring intermittent renal dialysis
Presence of arterial-venous shunt (for dialysis)

Excludes: *admission for dialysis treatment, or session (V56.0)*

V45.2 Presence of cerebrospinal fluid drainage device
Cerebral ventricle (communicating) shunt, valve, or device in situ

Excludes: *malfunction (996.2)*

V45.3 Intestinal bypass or anastomosis status

V45.4 Arthrodesis status

V45.5 Presence of contraceptive device

Excludes: *checking, reinsertion, or removal of device (V25.42)*
complication from device (996.32)
insertion of device (V25.1)

V45.51 Intrauterine contraceptive device

V45.52 Subdermal contraceptive implant

V45.59 Other

V45.6 States following surgery of eye and adnexa
Cataract extraction
Filtering bleb
Surgical eyelid adhesion
} state following eye surgery

Excludes: *aphakia (379.31)*
artificial:
eye globe (V43.0)
lens (V43.1)

V45.8 Other postsurgical status

V45.81 Aortocoronary bypass status

V45.82 Percutaneous transluminal coronary angioplasty status

● **V45.83 Breast implant removal status**

V45.89 Other
Presence of neuropacemaker or other electronic device

Excludes: *artificial heart valve in situ (V43.3)*
vascular prosthesis in situ (V43.4)

V46 Other dependence on machines

V46.0 Aspirator

V46.1 Respirator
Iron lung

V46.8 Other enabling machines
Hyperbaric chamber

Possum [Patient-Operated-Selector-Mechanism]

Excludes: *cardiac pacemaker (V45.0)*
kidney dialysis machine (V45.1)

V46.9 Unspecified machine dependence

V47 Other problems with internal organs

V47.0 Deficiencies of internal organs

V47.1 Mechanical and motor problems with internal organs

V47.2 Other cardiorespiratory problems
Cardiovascular exercise intolerance with pain (with):
at rest
less than ordinary activity
ordinary activity

V47.3 Other digestive problems

V47.4 Other urinary problems

V47.5 Other genital problems

V47.9 Unspecified

V48 Problems with head, neck, and trunk

V48.0 Deficiencies of head

Excludes: *deficiencies of ears, eyelids, and nose (V48.8)*

V48.1 Deficiencies of neck and trunk

V48.2 Mechanical and motor problems with head

V48.3 Mechanical and motor problems with neck and trunk

V48.4 Sensory problem with head

V48.5 Sensory problem with neck and trunk

V48.6 Disfigurements of head

V48.7 Disfigurements of neck and trunk

V48.8 Other problems with head, neck, and trunk

V48.9 Unspecified problem with head, neck, or trunk

V49 Problems with limbs and other problems

V49.0 Deficiencies of limbs

V49.1 Mechanical problems with limbs

V49.2 Motor problems with limbs

V49.3 Sensory problems with limbs

V49.4 Disfigurements of limbs

V49.5 Other problems of limbs

V49.6 Upper limb amputation status

V49.60 Unspecified level

V49.61 Thumb

V49.62 Other finger(s)

V49.63 Hand

V49.64 Wrist
Disarticulation of wrist

V49.65 Below elbow

V49.66 Above elbow
Disarticulation of elbow

V49.67 Shoulder
Disarticulation of shoulder

V49.7 Lower limb amputation status

V49.70 Unspecified level

V49.71 Great toe

V49.72 Other toe(s)

V49.73 Foot

V49.74 Ankle
Disarticulation of ankle

V49.75 Below knee

V49.76 Above knee
Disarticulation of knee

V49.77 Hip
Disarticulation of hip

V49.8 Other specified problems influencing health status

V49.9 Unspecified

PERSONS ENCOUNTERING HEALTH SERVICES FOR SPECIFIC PROCEDURES AND AFTERCARE (V50-V59)

Note: Categories V51-V58 are intended for use to indicate a reason for care in patients who may have already been treated for some disease or injury not now present, but who are receiving care to consolidate the treatment, to deal with residual states, or to prevent recurrence.

Excludes: *follow-up examination for medical surveillance following treatment (V67.0-V67.9)*

V50 Elective surgery for purposes other than remedying health states

V50.0 Hair transplant

V50.1 Other plastic surgery for unacceptable cosmetic appearance
Breast augmentation or reduction
Face-lift

Excludes: *plastic surgery following healed injury or operation (V51)*

V50.2 Routine or ritual circumcision
Circumcision in the absence of significant medical indication

V50.3 Ear piercing

V50.4 Prophylactic organ removal

Excludes: *organ donations (V59.0-V59.9)*
therapeutic organ removal—code to condition

V50.41 Breast

V50.42 Ovary

V50.49 Other

V50.8 Other

V50.9 Unspecified

V51 Aftercare involving the use of plastic surgery
Plastic surgery following healed injury or operation
Repair of scarred tissue

Excludes: *cosmetic plastic surgery (V50.1)*
plastic surgery as treatment for current injury—code to condition

▲ **V52 Fitting and adjustment of prosthetic device and implant**
Includes: removal of device

Excludes: *malfunction or complication of prosthetic device (996.0-996.7)*
status only, without need for care (V43.0-V43.8)

V52.0 Artificial arm (complete) (partial)

V52.1 Artificial leg (complete) (partial)

V52.2 Artificial eye

V52.3 Dental prosthetic device

▲ **V52.4 Breast prosthesis and implant**

Excludes: *admission for implant insertion (V50.1)*

V52.8 Other specified prosthetic device

V52.9 Unspecified prosthetic device

V53 Fitting and adjustment of other device
Includes: removal of device
replacement of device

Excludes: *status only, without need for care (V45.0-V45.8)*

V53.0 Devices related to nervous system and special senses
Auditory substitution device
Visual substitution device

Neuropacemaker (brain) (peripheral nerve) (spinal cord)

V53.1 Spectacles and contact lenses

V53.2 Hearing aid

V53.3 Cardiac device
Reprogramming

V53.31 Cardiac pacemaker

Excludes: *mechanical complication of cardiac pacemaker (996.01)*

V53.32 Automatic implantable cardiac defibrillator

V53.39 Other cardiac device

V53.4 Orthodontic devices

▲ **V53.5 Other intestinal appliance**

Excludes: *colostomy (V55.3)*
ileostomy (V55.2)
other artificial opening of digestive tract (V55.4)

V53.6 Urinary devices
Urinary catheter

Excludes: *cystostomy (V55.5)*
nephrostomy (V55.6)
ureterostomy (V55.6)
urethrostomy (V55.6)

V53.7 Orthopedic devices
Orthopedic:
brace
cast

Orthopedic:
corset
shoes

Excludes: *other orthopedic aftercare (V54)*

V53.8 Wheelchair

V53.9 Other and unspecified device

V54 Other orthopedic aftercare

Excludes: *fitting and adjustment of orthopedic devices (V53.7)*
malfunction of internal orthopedic device (996.4)
other complication of nonmechanical nature (996.60-996.79)

V54.0 Aftercare involving removal of fracture plate or other internal fixation device
Removal of:
pins
plates

Removal of:
rods
screws

Excludes: *removal of external fixation device (V54.8)*

V54.8 Other orthopedic aftercare
Change, checking, or removal of:
Kirschner wire
plaster cast
splint, external
other external fixation or traction device

V54.9 Unspecified orthopedic aftercare

V55 Attention to artificial openings
Includes: closure
passage of sounds or bougies
reforming
removal or replacement of catheter
toilet or cleansing

Excludes: *complications of external stoma (519.0, 569.6, 997.4, 997.5)*
status only, without need for care (V44.0-V44.9)

V55.0 Tracheostomy

V55.1 Gastrostomy

V55.2 Ileostomy

V55.3 Colostomy

V55.4 Other artificial opening of digestive tract

V55.5 Cystostomy

V55.6 Other artificial opening of urinary tract
Nephrostomy
Urethrostomy
Ureterostomy

V55.7 Artificial vagina

V55.8 Other specified artificial opening

V55.9 Unspecified artificial opening

▲ **V56 Encounter for dialysis and dialysis catheter care**
Use additional code to identify the associated condition

Excludes: *dialysis preparation—code to condition*

V56.0 Extracorporeal dialysis
Dialysis (renal) NOS

Excludes: *dialysis status (V45.1)*

● **V56.1 Fitting and adjustment of dialysis (extracorporeal) (peritoneal) catheter**
Removal or replacement of catheter
Toilet or cleansing

V56.8 Other dialysis
Peritoneal dialysis

V57 Care involving use of rehabilitation procedures
Use additional code to identify underlying condition

V57.0 Breathing exercises

V57.1 Other physical therapy
Therapeutic and remedial exercises, except breathing

V57.2 Occupational therapy and vocational rehabilitation

V57.21 Encounter for occupational therapy

V57.22 Encounter for vocational therapy

V57.3 Speech therapy

V57.4 Orthoptic training

V57.8 Other specified rehabilitation procedure

V57.81 Orthotic training
Gait training in the use of artificial limbs

V57.89 Other
Multiple training or therapy

V57.9 Unspecified rehabilitation procedure

V58 Encounter for other and unspecified procedures and aftercare

Excludes: *convalescence (V66)*

V58.0 Radiotherapy
Encounter or admission for radiotherapy

Excludes: *encounter for radioactive implant—code to condition*

V58.1 Chemotherapy
Encounter or admission for chemotherapy

Excludes: *prophylactic chemotherapy against disease which has never been present (V03.0-V07.9)*

V58.2 Blood transfusion, without reported diagnosis

V58.3 Attention to surgical dressings and sutures
Change of dressings
Removal of sutures

V58.4 Other aftercare following surgery

Excludes: *attention to artificial openings (V55.0-V55.9)*
orthopedic aftercare (V54.0-V54.9)

V58.41 Encounter for planned postoperative wound closure

Excludes: *disruption of operative wound (998.3)*

V58.49 Other specified aftercare following surgery

V58.5 Orthodontics

Excludes: *fitting and adjustment of orthodontic device (V53.4)*

● **V58.6 Long-term (current) drug use**

● **V58.61 Long-term (current) use of anticoagulants**

● **V58.69 Long-term (current) use of other medications**
High-risk medications

▲ **V58.8 Other specified procedures and aftercare**

▲ **V58.81 Fitting and adjustment of vascular catheter**
Removal or replacement of catheter
Toilet or cleansing

Excludes: *complication of renal dialysis catheter (996.73)*
complication of vascular catheter (996.74)
dialysis preparation -- code to condition
encounter for dialysis (V56.0-V56.8)
fitting and adjustment of dialysis catheter (V56.1)

● **V58.82 Fitting and adjustment of non-vascular catheter NEC**
Removal or replacement of catheter
Toilet or cleansing

Excludes: *fitting and adjustment of peritoneal dialysis catheter (V56.1)*

V58.89 Other specified aftercare

V58.9 Unspecified aftercare

V59 Donors

Excludes: *examination of potential donor (V70.8)*
self-donation of organ or tissue -- code to condition

V59.0 Blood

● **V59.01 Whole blood**

● **V59.02 Stem cells**

● **V59.09 Other**

V59.1 Skin

V59.2 Bone

V59.3 Bone marrow

V59.4 Kidney

V59.5 Cornea

● **V59.6 Liver**

V59.8 Other specified organ or tissue

V59.9 Unspecified organ or tissue

PERSONS ENCOUNTERING HEALTH SERVICES IN OTHER CIRCUMSTANCES (V60-V68)

V60 Housing, household, and economic circumstances

V60.0 Lack of housing
Hobos
Social migrants
Tramps
Transients
Vagabonds

V60.1 Inadequate housing
Lack of heating
Restriction of space
Technical defects in home preventing adequate care

V60.2 Inadequate material resources
Economic problem
Poverty NOS

V60.3 Person living alone

V60.4 No other household member able to render care
Person requiring care (has) (is):
family member too handicapped, ill, or otherwise unsuited to render care
partner temporarily away from home
temporarily away from usual place of abode

Excludes: *holiday relief care (V60.5)*

V60.5 Holiday relief care
Provision of health care facilities to a person normally cared for at home, to enable relatives to take a vacation

V60.6 Person living in residential institution
Boarding school resident

V60.8 Other specified housing or economic circumstances

V60.9 Unspecified housing or economic circumstance

V61 Other family circumstances

Includes: when these circumstances or fear of them, affecting the person directly involved or others, are mentioned as the reason, justified or not, for seeking or receiving medical advice or care

V61.0 Family disruption

Divorce
Estrangement

V61.1 Marital problems

Marital conflict

Excludes: *problems related to:*
psychosexual disorders (302.0-302.9)
sexual function (V41.7)

V61.2 Parent-child problems

V61.20 Parent-child problem, unspecified

Concern about behavior of child
Parent-child conflict

V61.21 Child abuse

Child battering
Child neglect

Excludes: *effect of maltreatment on the child (995.5)*

V61.29 Other

Problem concerning adopted or foster child

V61.3 Problems with aged parents or in-laws

V61.4 Health problems within family

V61.41 Alcoholism in family

V61.49 Other

Care of } sick or handicapped person in family or household
Presence of } sick or handicapped person in family or household

V61.5 Multiparity

V61.6 Illegitimacy or illegitimate pregnancy

V61.7 Other unwanted pregnancy

V61.8 Other specified family circumstances

Problems with family members NEC

V61.9 Unspecified family circumstance

V62 Other psychosocial circumstances

Includes: those circumstances or fear of them, affecting the person directly involved or others, mentioned as the reason, justified or not, for seeking or receiving medical advice or care

Excludes: *previous psychological trauma (V15.4)*

V62.0 Unemployment

Excludes: *circumstances when main problem is economic inadequacy or poverty (V60.2)*

V62.1 Adverse effects of work environment

V62.2 Other occupational circumstances or maladjustment

Career choice problem
Dissatisfaction with employment

V62.3 Educational circumstances

Dissatisfaction with school environment
Educational handicap

V62.4 Social maladjustment

Cultural deprivation
Political, religious, or sex discrimination
Social:
isolation
persecution

V62.5 Legal circumstances

Imprisonment
Legal investigation
Litigation
Prosecution

V62.6 Refusal of treatment for reasons of religion or conscience

V62.8 Other psychological or physical stress, not elsewhere classified

V62.81 Interpersonal problems, not elsewhere classified

V62.82 Bereavement, uncomplicated

Excludes: *bereavement as adjustment reaction (309.0)*

V62.89 Other
Life circumstance problems
Phase of life problems

V62.9 Unspecified psychosocial circumstance

V63 Unavailability of other medical facilities for care

V63.0 Residence remote from hospital or other health care facility

V63.1 Medical services in home not available

Excludes: *no other household member able to render care (V60.4)*

V63.2 Person awaiting admission to adequate facility elsewhere

V63.8 Other specified reasons for unavailability of medical facilities
Person on waiting list undergoing social agency investigation

V63.9 Unspecified reason for unavailability of medical facilities

V64 Persons encountering health services for specific procedures, not carried out

V64.0 Vaccination not carried out because of contraindication

V64.1 Surgical or other procedure not carried out because of contraindication

V64.2 Surgical or other procedure not carried out because of patient's decision

V64.3 Procedure not carried out for other reasons

V65 Other persons seeking consultation without complaint or sickness

V65.0 Healthy person accompanying sick person
Boarder

V65.1 Person consulting on behalf of another person
Advice or treatment for nonattending third party

Excludes: *concern (normal) about sick person in family (V61.41-V61.49)*

V65.2 Person feigning illness
Malingerer
Peregrinating patient

V65.3 Dietary surveillance and counseling
Dietary surveillance and counseling (in):
- NOS
- colitis
- diabetes mellitus
- food allergies or intolerance
- gastritis
- hypercholesterolemia
- hypoglycemia
- obesity

V65.4 Other counseling, not elsewhere classified
Health:
- advice
- education
- instruction

Excludes: *counseling (for):*
- *contraception (V25.40-V25.49)*
- *genetic (V26.3)*
- *on behalf of third party (V65.1)*
- *procreative management (V26.4)*

V65.40 Counseling NOS

V65.41 Exercise counseling

V65.42 Counseling on substance use and abuse

V65.43 Counseling on injury prevention

V65.44 Human immunodeficiency virus [HIV] counseling

V65.45 Counseling on other sexually transmitted diseases

V65.49 Other specified counseling

V65.5 Person with feared complaint in whom no diagnosis was made
Feared condition not demonstrated
Problem was normal state
"Worried well"

V65.8 Other reasons for seeking consultation

Excludes: *specified symptoms*

V65.9 Unspecified reason for consultation

V66 Convalescence

V66.0 Following surgery

V66.1 Following radiotherapy

V66.2 Following chemotherapy

V66.3 Following psychotherapy and other treatment for mental disorder

V66.4 Following treatment of fracture

V66.5 Following other treatment

V66.6 Following combined treatment

V66.9 Unspecified convalescence

V67 Follow-up examination
Includes: surveillance only following completed treatment

Excludes: *surveillance of contraception (V25.40-V25.49)*

V67.0 Following surgery

V67.1 Following radiotherapy

V67.2 Following chemotherapy
Cancer chemotherapy follow-up

V67.3 Following psychotherapy and other treatment for mental disorder

V67.4 Following treatment of fracture

V67.5 Following other treatment

▲ **V67.51 Following completed treatment with high-risk medication, NEC**

Excludes: *long-term (current) drug use (V58.61-V58.69)*

V67.59 Other

V67.6 Following combined treatment

V67.9 Unspecified follow-up examination

V68 Encounters for administrative purposes

V68.0 Issue of medical certificates
Issue of medical certificate of: cause of death
fitness
incapacity

Excludes: *encounter for general medical examination (V70.0-V70.9)*

V68.1 Issue of repeat prescriptions
Issue of repeat prescription for: appliance
glasses
medications

Excludes: *repeat prescription for contraceptives (V25.41-V25.49)*

V68.2 Request for expert evidence

V68.8 Other specified administrative purpose

V68.81 Referral of patient without examination or treatment

V68.89 Other

V68.9 Unspecified administrative purpose

V69 Problems related to lifestyle

V69.0 Lack of physical exercise

V69.1 Inappropriate diet and eating habits

Excludes: *anorexia nervosa (307.1)*
bulimia (783.6)
malnutrition and other nutritional deficiencies (260-269.9)
other and unspecified eating disorders (307.50-307.59)

V69.2 High-risk sexual behavior

V69.3 Gambling and betting

Excludes: *pathological gambling (312.31)*

● Code new to this edition ▲ Revision of existing code ④ ⑤ Fourth or fifth digit required

V69.8 Other problems related to lifestyle
Self-damaging behavior

V69.9 Problem related to lifestyle, unspecified

PERSONS WITHOUT REPORTED DIAGNOSIS ENCOUNTERED DURING EXAMINATION AND INVESTIGATION OF INDIVIDUALS AND POPULATIONS (V70-V82)

Note: Nonspecific abnormal findings disclosed at the time of these examinations are classifiable to categories 790-796.

V70 General medical examination

Use additional code(s) to identify any special screening examination(s) performed (V73.0-V82.9)

V70.0 Routine general medical examination at a health care facility
Health checkup

Excludes: *health checkup of infant or child (V20.2)*

V70.1 General psychiatric examination, requested by the authority

V70.2 General psychiatric examination, other and unspecified

V70.3 Other medical examination for administrative purposes
General medical examination for:
admission to old age home
adoption
camp
driving license
immigration and naturalization
insurance certification
marriage
prison
school admission
sports competition

Excludes: *attendance for issue of medical certificates (V68.0)*
pre-employment screening (V70.5)

V70.4 Examination for medicolegal reasons
Blood-alcohol tests
Blood-drug tests

Excludes: *examination and observation following:*
accidents (V71.3, V71.4)
assault (V71.6)
rape (V71.5)

V70.5 Health examination of defined subpopulations
Armed forces personnel
Inhabitants of institutions
Occupational health examinations
Pre-employment screening
Preschool children
Prisoners
Prostitutes
Refugees
School children
Students

V70.6 Health examination in population surveys

Excludes: *special screening (V73.0-V82.9)*

V70.7 Examination for normal comparison or control in clinical research

V70.8 Other specified general medical examinations
Examination of potential donor of organ or tissue

V70.9 Unspecified general medical examination

V71 Observation and evaluation for suspected conditions not found

Note: This category is to be used when persons without a diagnosis are suspected of having an abnormal condition, without signs or symptoms, which requires study, but after examination and observation, is found not to exist. This category is also for use for administrative and legal observation status.

V71.0 Observation for suspected mental condition

V71.01 Adult antisocial behavior
Dyssocial behavior or gang activity in adult without manifest psychiatric disorder

V71.02 Childhood or adolescent antisocial behavior
Dyssocial behavior or gang activity in child or adolescent without manifest psychiatric disorder

V71.09 Other suspected mental condition

V71.1 Observation for suspected malignant neoplasm

V71.2 Observation for suspected tuberculosis

V71.3 Observation following accident at work

V71.4 Observation following other accident

Examination of individual involved in motor vehicle traffic accident

V71.5 Observation following alleged rape or seduction
Examination of victim or culprit

V71.6 Observation following other inflicted injury
Examination of victim or culprit

V71.7 Observation for suspected cardiovascular disease

V71.8 Observation for other specified suspected conditions

V71.9 Observation for unspecified suspected condition

V72 Special investigations and examinations
Includes: routine examination of specific system

Excludes: *general medical examination (V70.0-V70.4)*
general screening examination of defined population groups (V70.5, V70.6, V70.7)
routine examination of infant or child (V20.2)

Use additional code(s) to identify any special screening examination(s) performed (V73.0-V82.9)

V72.0 Examination of eyes and vision

V72.1 Examination of ears and hearing

V72.2 Dental examination

V72.3 Gynecological examination
Papanicolaou smear as part of general gynecological examination
Pelvic examination (annual) (periodic)

Excludes: *cervical Papanicolaou smear without general gynecological examination (V76.2)*
routine examination in contraceptive management (V25.40-V25.49)

V72.4 Pregnancy examination or test, pregnancy unconfirmed
Possible pregnancy, not (yet) confirmed

Excludes: *pregnancy examination with immediate confirmation (V22.0-V22.1)*

V72.5 Radiological examination, not elsewhere classified
Routine chest x-ray

Excludes: *examination for suspected tuberculosis (V71.2)*

V72.6 Laboratory examination

Excludes: *that for suspected disorder (V71.0-V71.9)*

V72.7 Diagnostic skin and sensitization tests
Allergy tests
Skin tests for hypersensitivity

Excludes: *diagnostic skin tests for bacterial diseases (V74.0-V74.9)*

V72.8 Other specified examinations

V72.81 Pre-operative cardiovascular examination

V72.82 Pre-operative respiratory examination

V72.83 Other specified pre-operative examination

V72.84 Pre-operative examination, unspecified

V72.85 Other specified examination

V72.9 Unspecified examination

V73 Special screening examination for viral and chlamydial diseases

V73.0 Poliomyelitis

V73.1 Smallpox

V73.2 Measles

V73.3 Rubella

V73.4 Yellow fever

V73.5 Other arthropod-borne viral diseases
Dengue fever
Hemorrhagic fever
Viral encephalitis:
 mosquito-borne
 tick-borne

V73.6 Trachoma

V73.8 Other specified viral and chlamydial diseases

V73.88 Other specified chlamydial diseases

V73.89 Other specified viral diseases

V73.9 Unspecified viral and chlamydial disease

V73.98 Unspecified chlamydial disease

V73.99 Unspecified viral disease

V74 Special screening examination for bacterial and spirochetal diseases

Includes: diagnostic skin tests for these diseases

V74.0 Cholera

V74.1 Pulmonary tuberculosis

V74.2 Leprosy [Hansen's disease]

V74.3 Diphtheria

V74.4 Bacterial conjunctivitis

V74.5 Venereal disease

V74.6 Yaws

V74.8 Other specified bacterial and spirochetal diseases

Brucellosis
Leptospirosis
Plague
Tetanus
Whooping cough

V74.9 Unspecified bacterial and spirochetal disease

V75 Special screening examination for other infectious diseases

V75.0 Rickettsial diseases

V75.1 Malaria

V75.2 Leishmaniasis

V75.3 Trypanosomiasis

Chagas' disease
Sleeping sickness

V75.4 Mycotic infections

V75.5 Schistosomiasis

V75.6 Filariasis

V75.7 Intestinal helminthiasis

V75.8 Other specified parasitic infections

V75.9 Unspecified infectious disease

V76 Special screening for malignant neoplasms

V76.0 Respiratory organs

V76.1 Breast

V76.2 Cervix

Routine cervical Papanicolaou smear

Excludes: *that as part of a general gynecological examination (V72.3)*

V76.3 Bladder

V76.4 Other sites

V76.41 Rectum

V76.42 Oral cavity

V76.43 Skin

V76.49 Other

V76.8 Other neoplasm

V76.9 Unspecified

V77 Special screening for endocrine, nutritional, metabolic, and immunity disorders

V77.0 Thyroid disorders

V77.1 Diabetes mellitus

V77.2 Malnutrition

V77.3 Phenylketonuria [PKU]

V77.4 Galactosemia

V77.5 Gout

V77.6 Cystic fibrosis

Screening for mucoviscidosis

V77.7 Other inborn errors of metabolism

V77.8 Obesity

V77.9 Other and unspecified endocrine, nutritional, metabolic, and immunity disorders

V78 Special screening for disorders of blood and blood-forming organs

V78.0 Iron deficiency anemia

V78.1 Other and unspecified deficiency anemia

V78.2 Sickle-cell disease or trait

V78.3 Other hemoglobinopathies

V78.8 Other disorders of blood and blood-forming organs

V78.9 Unspecified disorder of blood and blood-forming organs

V79 Special screening for mental disorders and developmental handicaps

V79.0 Depression

V79.1 Alcoholism

V79.2 Mental retardation

V79.3 Developmental handicaps in early childhood

V79.8 Other specified mental disorders and developmental handicaps

V79.9 Unspecified mental disorder and developmental handicap

V80 Special screening for neurological, eye, and ear diseases

V80.0 Neurological conditions

V80.1 Glaucoma

V80.2 Other eye conditions

Screening for:
- cataract
- congenital anomaly of eye
- senile macular lesions

Excludes: *general vision examination (V72.0)*

V80.3 Ear diseases

Excludes: *general hearing examination (V72.1)*

V81 Special screening for cardiovascular, respiratory, and genitourinary diseases

V81.0 Ischemic heart disease

V81.1 Hypertension

V81.2 Other and unspecified cardiovascular conditions

V81.3 Chronic bronchitis and emphysema

V81.4 Other and unspecified respiratory conditions

Excludes: *screening for:*
- *lung neoplasm (V76.0)*
- *pulmonary tuberculosis (V74.1)*

V81.5 Nephropathy

Screening for asymptomatic bacteriuria

V81.6 Other and unspecified genitourinary conditions

V82 Special screening for other conditions

V82.0 Skin conditions

V82.1 Rheumatoid arthritis

V82.2 Other rheumatic disorders

V82.3 Congenital dislocation of hip

V82.4 Postnatal screening for chromosomal anomalies

Excludes: *antenatal screening by amniocentesis (V28.0)*

V82.5 Chemical poisoning and other contamination

Screening for:
- heavy metal poisoning
- ingestion of radioactive substance
- poisoning from contaminated water supply
- radiation exposure

V82.6 Multiphasic screening

V82.8 Other specified conditions

V82.9 Unspecified condition

● Code new to this edition ▲ Revision of existing code ④ ⑤ Fourth or fifth digit required

SUPPLEMENTARY CLASSIFICATION OF EXTERNAL CAUSES OF INJURY AND POISONING (E800-E999)

This section is provided to permit the classification of environmental events, circumstances, and conditions as the cause of injury, poisoning, and other adverse effects. Where a code from this section is applicable, it is intended that it shall be used in addition to a code from one of the main chapters of *ICD-9-CM*, indicating the nature of the condition. Certain other conditions which may be stated to be due to external causes are classified in Chapters 1 to 16 of *ICD-9-CM*. For these, the "E" code classification should be used for more detailed analysis.

Machinery accidents [other than those connected with transport] are classifiable to category E919, in which the fourth-digit allows a broad classification of the type of machinery involved. If a more detailed classification of type of machinery is required, it is suggested that the "Classification of Industrial Accidents according to Agency," prepared by the International Labor Office, be used in addition. This is reproduced on page 571, for optional use.

Categories for "late effects" of accidents and other external causes are to be found at E929, E959, E969, E977, E989, and E999.

Definitions and examples related to transport accidents

(a) A **transport accident** (E800-E848) is any accident involving a device designed primarily for, or being used at the time primarily for, conveying persons or goods from one place to another.

Includes: accidents involving:
- aircraft and spacecraft (E840-E845)
- watercraft (E830-E838)
- motor vehicle (E810-E825)
- railway (E800-E807)
- other road vehicles (E826-E829)

In classifying accidents which involve more than one kind of transport, the above order of precedence of transport accidents should be used.

Accidents involving agriculture and construction machines, such as tractors, cranes, and bulldozers, are regarded as transport accidents only when these vehicles are under their own power on a highway [otherwise the vehicles are regarded as machinery]. Vehicles which can travel on land or water, such as hovercraft and other amphibious vehicles, are regarded as watercraft when on the water, as motor vehicles when on the highway, and as off-road motor vehicles when on land, but off the highway.

Excludes: *accidents:*
- *in sports which involve the use of transport but where the transport vehicle itself was not involved in the accident*
- *involving vehicles which are part of industrial equipment used entirely on industrial premises*
- *occurring during transportation but unrelated to the hazards associated with the means of transportation [e.g., injuries received in a fight on board ship; transport vehicle involved in a cataclysm such as an earthquake]*
- *to persons engaged in the maintenance or repair of transport equipment or vehicle not in motion, unless injured by another vehicle in motion*

(b) A **railway accident** is a transport accident involving a railway train or other railway vehicle operated on rails, whether in motion or not.

Excludes: *accidents:*
- *in repair shops*
- *in roundhouse or on turntable*
- *on railway premises but not involving a train or other railway vehicle*

(c) A **railway train** or **railway vehicle** is any device with or without cars coupled to it, designed for traffic on a railway.

Includes: interurban:
- electric car } (operated chiefly on its own right-of-way, not open to other traffic)
- streetcar }

railway train, any power [diesel] [electric] [steam]
- funicular
- monorail or two-rail
- subterranean or elevated

other vehicle designed to run on a railway track

Excludes: *interurban electric cars [streetcars] specified to be operating on a right-of-way that forms part of the public street or highway [definition (n)]*

(d) A **railway** or **railroad** is a right-of-way designed for traffic on rails, which is used by carriages or wagons transporting passengers or freight, and by other rolling stock, and which is not open to other public vehicular traffic.

E CODES

(e) A **motor vehicle accident** is a transport accident involving a motor vehicle. It is defined as a motor vehicle traffic accident or as a motor vehicle nontraffic accident according to whether the accident occurs on a public highway or elsewhere.

Excludes: *injury or damage due to cataclysm*
injury or damage while a motor vehicle, not under its own power, is being loaded on, or unloaded from, another conveyance

(f) A **motor vehicle traffic accident** is any motor vehicle accident occurring on a public highway [i.e., originating, terminating, or involving a vehicle partially on the highway]. A motor vehicle accident is assumed to have occurred on the highway unless another place is specified, except in the case of accidents involving only off-road motor vehicles which are classified as nontraffic accidents unless the contrary is stated.

(g) A **motor vehicle nontraffic accident** is any motor vehicle accident which occurs entirely in any place other than a public highway.

(h) A **public highway [trafficway]** or **street** is the entire width between property lines [or other boundary lines] of every way or place, of which any part is open to the use of the public for purposes of vehicular traffic as a matter of right or custom. A roadway is that part of the public highway designed, improved, and ordinarily used, for vehicular travel.

Includes: approaches (public) to:
docks
public building
station

Excludes: *driveway (private)*
parking lot
ramp
roads in:
airfield
farm
industrial premises
mine
private grounds
quarry

(i) A **motor vehicle** is any mechanically or electrically powered device, not operated on rails, upon which any person or property may be transported or drawn upon a highway. Any object such as a trailer, coaster, sled, or wagon being towed by a motor vehicle is considered a part of the motor vehicle.

Includes: automobile [any type]
bus
construction machinery, farm and industrial machinery, steam roller, tractor, army tank, highway grader, or similar vehicle on wheels or treads, while in transport under own power
fire engine (motorized)
motorcycle
motorized bicycle [moped] or scooter
trolley bus not operating on rails
truck
van

Excludes: *devices used solely to move persons or materials within the confines of a building and its premises, such as:*
building elevator
coal car in mine
electric baggage or mail truck used solely within a railroad station
electric truck used solely within an industrial plant
moving overhead crane

(j) A **motorcycle** is a two-wheeled motor vehicle having one or two riding saddles and sometimes having a third wheel for the support of a sidecar. The sidecar is considered part of the motorcycle.

Includes: motorized:
bicycle [moped]
scooter
tricycle

(k) An **off-road motor vehicle** is a motor vehicle of special design, to enable it to negotiate rough or soft terrain or snow. Examples of special design are high construction, special wheels and tires, driven by treads, or support on a cushion of air.

Includes: all terrain vehicle [ATV]
army tank
hovercraft, on land or swamp
snowmobile

(l) A **driver** of a motor vehicle is the occupant of the motor vehicle operating it or intending to operate it. A **motorcyclist** is the driver of a motorcycle. Other authorized occupants of a motor vehicle are **passengers**.

(m) An **other road vehicle** is any device, except a motor vehicle, in, on, or by which any person or property may be transported on a highway.

Includes: animal carrying a person or goods
animal-drawn vehicle
animal harnessed to conveyance
bicycle [pedal cycle]
streetcar
tricycle (pedal)

Excludes: *pedestrian conveyance [definition (q)]*

(n) A **streetcar** is a device designed and used primarily for transporting persons within a municipality, running on rails, usually subject to normal traffic control signals, and operated principally on a right-of-way that forms part of the traffic way. A trailer being towed by a streetcar is considered a part of the streetcar.

Includes: interurban or intraurban electric or streetcar, when specified to be operating on a street or public highway
tram (car)
trolley (car)

(o) A **pedal cycle** is any road transport vehicle operated solely by pedals.

Includes: bicycle
pedal cycle
tricycle

Excludes: *motorized bicycle [definition (i)]*

(p) A **pedal cyclist** is any person riding on a pedal cycle or in a sidecar attached to such a vehicle.

(q) A **pedestrian conveyance** is any human powered device by which a pedestrian may move other than by walking or by which a walking person may move another pedestrian.

Includes:

baby carriage
coaster wagon
ice skates
perambulator
pushcart
pushchair
roller skates
scooter
skateboard
skis
sled
wheelchair

(r) A **pedestrian** is any person involved in an accident who was not at the time of the accident riding in or on a motor vehicle, railroad train, streetcar, animal-drawn or other vehicle, or on a bicycle or animal.

Includes: person:
changing tire of vehicle
in or operating a pedestrian conveyance
making adjustment to motor of vehicle
on foot

(s) A **watercraft** is any device for transporting passengers or goods on the water.

(t) A **small boat** is any watercraft propelled by paddle, oars, or small motor, with a passenger capacity of less than ten.

Includes:

boat NOS
canoe
coble
dinghy
punt
raft
rowboat
rowing shell
scull
skiff
small motorboat

Excludes: *barge*
lifeboat (used after abandoning ship)
raft (anchored) being used as diving platform
yacht

(u) An **aircraft** is any device for transporting passengers or goods in the air.

Includes: airplane [any type]
balloon
bomber
dirigible
glider (hang)
military aircraft
parachute

(v) A **commercial transport aircraft** is any device for collective passenger or freight transportation by air, whether run on commercial lines for profit or by government authorities, with the exception of military craft.

RAILWAY ACCIDENTS (E800-E807)

Note: For definitions of railway accident and related terms see definitions (a) to (d).

Excludes: *accidents involving railway train and:*
aircraft (E840.0-E845.9)
motor vehicle (E810.0-E825.9)
watercraft (E830.0-E838.9)

The following fourth-digit subdivisions are for use with categories E800-E807 to identify the injured person:

.0 Railway employee
Any person who by virtue of his employment in connection with a railway, whether by the railway company or not, is at increased risk of involvement in a railway accident, such as:
catering staff of train
driver
guard
porter
postal staff on train
railway fireman
shunter
sleeping car attendant

.1 Passenger on railway
Any authorized person traveling on a train, except a railway employee.

Excludes: *intending passenger waiting at station (.8)*
unauthorized rider on railway vehicle (.8)

.2 Pedestrian
See definition (r)

.3 Pedal cyclist
See definition (p)

.8 Other specified person
Intending passenger or bystander waiting at station
Unauthorized rider on railway vehicle

.9 Unspecified person

④ **E800 Railway accident involving collision with rolling stock**
Includes: collision between railway trains or railway vehicles, any kind
collision NOS on railway
derailment with antecedent collision with rolling stock or NOS

④ **E801 Railway accident involving collision with other object**
Includes: collision of railway train with:
buffers
fallen tree on railway
gates
platform
rock on railway
streetcar
other nonmotor vehicle
other object

Excludes: *collision with:*
aircraft (E840.0-E842.9)
motor vehicle (E810.0-E810.9, E820.0-E822.9)

④ **E802 Railway accident involving derailment without antecedent collision**

④ **E803 Railway accident involving explosion, fire, or burning**

Excludes: *explosion or fire, with antecedent derailment (E802.0-E802.9)*
explosion or fire, with mention of antecedent collision (E800.0-E801.9)

④ **E804 Fall in, on, or from railway train**
Includes: fall while alighting from or boarding railway train

Excludes: *fall related to collision, derailment, or explosion of railway train (E800.0-E803.9)*

④ **E805** **Hit by rolling stock**

Includes:

crushed
injured
killed
knocked down
run over
} by railway train or part

Excludes: *pedestrian hit by object set in motion by railway train (E806.0-E806.9)*

④ **E806** **Other specified railway accident**

Includes: hit by object falling in railway train
injured by door or window on railway train
nonmotor road vehicle or pedestrian hit by object set in motion by railway train
railway train hit by falling:
earth NOS
rock
tree
other object

Excludes: *railway accident due to cataclysm (E908-E909)*

④ **E807** **Railway accident of unspecified nature**

Includes:

found dead
injured
} on railway right-of-way NOS

railway accident NOS

MOTOR VEHICLE TRAFFIC ACCIDENTS (E810-E819)

Note: For definitions of motor vehicle traffic accident, and related terms, see definitions (e) to (k).

Excludes: *accidents involving motor vehicle and aircraft (E840.0-E845.9)*

The following fourth-digit subdivisions are for use with categories E810-E819 to identify the injured person:

.0 Driver of motor vehicle other than motorcycle
See definition (l)

.1 Passenger in motor vehicle other than motorcycle
See definition (l)

.2 Motorcyclist
See definition (l)

.3 Passenger on motorcycle
See definition (l)

.4 Occupant of streetcar

.5 Rider of animal; occupant of animal-drawn vehicle

.6 Pedal cyclist
See definition (p)

.7 Pedestrian
See definition (r)

.8 Other specified person
Occupant of vehicle other than above
Person in railway train involved in accident
Unauthorized rider of motor vehicle

.9 Unspecified person

④ **E810** **Motor vehicle traffic accident involving collision with train**

Excludes: *motor vehicle collision with object set in motion by railway train (E815.0-E815.9)*
railway train hit by object set in motion by motor vehicle (E818.0-E818.9)

④ **E811** **Motor vehicle traffic accident involving re-entrant collision with another motor vehicle**

Includes: collision between motor vehicle which accidentally leaves the roadway then re-enters the same roadway, or the opposite roadway on a divided highway, and another motor vehicle

Excludes: *collision on the same roadway when none of the motor vehicles involved have left and re-entered the roadway (E812.0-E812.9)*

④ **E812** **Other motor vehicle traffic accident involving collision with motor vehicle**

Includes: collision with another motor vehicle parked, stopped, stalled, disabled, or abandoned on the highway
motor vehicle collision NOS

continued

Excludes: *collision with object set in motion by another motor vehicle (E815.0-E815.9)*
re-entrant collision with another motor vehicle (E811.0-E811.9)

④ **E813 Motor vehicle traffic accident involving collision with other vehicle**

Includes: collision between motor vehicle, any kind, and:
other road (nonmotor transport) vehicle, such as:
animal carrying a person
animal-drawn vehicle
pedal cycle
streetcar

Excludes: *collision with:*
object set in motion by nonmotor road vehicle (E815.0-E815.9)
pedestrian (E814.0-E814.9)
nonmotor road vehicle hit by object set in motion by motor vehicle (E818.0-E818.9)

④ **E814 Motor vehicle traffic accident involving collision with pedestrian**

Includes: collision between motor vehicle, any kind, and pedestrian
pedestrian dragged, hit, or run over by motor vehicle, any kind

Excludes: *pedestrian hit by object set in motion by motor vehicle (E818.0-E818.9)*

④ **E815 Other motor vehicle traffic accident involving collision on the highway**

Includes: collision (due to loss of control) (on highway) between motor vehicle, any kind, and:
abutment (bridge) (overpass)
animal (herded) (unattended)
fallen stone, traffic sign, tree, utility pole
guard rail or boundary fence
interhighway divider
landslide (not moving)
object set in motion by railway train or road vehicle (motor) (nonmotor)
object thrown in front of motor vehicle
safety island
temporary traffic sign or marker
wall of cut made for road
other object, fixed, movable, or moving

Excludes: *collision with:*
any object off the highway (resulting from loss of control) (E816.0-E816.9)
any object which normally would have been off the highway and is not stated to have been on it (E816.0-E816.9)
motor vehicle parked, stopped, stalled, disabled, or abandoned on highway (E812.0-E812.9)
moving landslide (E909)
motor vehicle hit by object:
set in motion by railway train or road vehicle (motor) (nonmotor) (E818.0-E818.9)
thrown into or on vehicle (E818.0-E818.9)

④ **E816 Motor vehicle traffic accident due to loss of control, without collision on the highway**

Includes: motor vehicle:
failing to make curve
going out of control (due to):
blowout
burst tire
driver falling asleep
driver inattention
excessive speed
failure of mechanical part
} and:
colliding with object off the highway
overturning
stopping abruptly off the highway

Excludes: *collision on highway following loss of control (E810.0-E815.9)*
loss of control of motor vehicle following collision on the highway (E810.0-E815.9)

④ **E817 Noncollision motor vehicle traffic accident while boarding or alighting**

Includes:
fall down stairs of motor bus
fall from car in street
injured by moving part of the vehicle
trapped by door of motor bus
} while boarding or alighting

④ **E818 Other noncollision motor vehicle traffic accident**

Includes:

accidental poisoning from exhaust gas generated by breakage of any part of explosion of any part of fall, jump, or being accidentally pushed from fire starting in hit by object thrown into or on injured by being thrown against some part of, or object in injury from moving part of object falling in or on object thrown on	motor vehicle while in motion

collision of railway train or road vehicle except motor vehicle, with object set in motion by motor vehicle
motor vehicle hit by object set in motion by railway train or road vehicle (motor) (nonmotor)
pedestrian, railway train, or road vehicle (motor) (nonmotor) hit by object set in motion by motor vehicle

Excludes: *collision between motor vehicle and:*
object set in motion by railway train or road vehicle (motor) (nonmotor) (E815.0-E815.9)
object thrown towards the motor vehicle (E815.0-E815.9)
person overcome by carbon monoxide generated by stationary motor vehicle off the roadway with motor running (E868.2)

④ **E819 Motor vehicle traffic accident of unspecified nature**

Includes: motor vehicle traffic accident NOS
traffic accident NOS

MOTOR VEHICLE NONTRAFFIC ACCIDENTS (E820-E825)

Note: For definitions of motor vehicle nontraffic accident and related terms see definitions (a) to (k).

Includes: accidents involving motor vehicles being used in recreational or sporting activities off the highway
collision and noncollision motor vehicle accidents occurring entirely off the highway

Excludes: *accidents involving motor vehicle and:*
aircraft (E840.0-E845.9)
watercraft (E830.0-E838.9)
accidents, not on the public highway, involving agricultural and construction machinery but not involving another motor vehicle (E919.0, E919.2, E919.7)

The following fourth-digit subdivisions are for use with categories E820-E825 to identify the injured person:

.0 Driver of motor vehicle other than motorcycle
See definition (l)

.1 Passenger in motor vehicle other than motorcycle
See definition (l)

.2 Motorcyclist
See definition (l)

.3 Passenger on motorcycle
See definition (l)

.4 Occupant of streetcar

.5 Rider of animal; occupant of animal-drawn vehicle

.6 Pedal cyclist
See definition (p)

.7 Pedestrian
See definition (r)

.8 Other specified person
Occupant of vehicle other than above
Person on railway train involved in accident
Unauthorized rider of motor vehicle

.9 Unspecified person

④ **E820 Nontraffic accident involving motor-driven snow vehicle**

Includes:

breakage of part of fall from hit by overturning of run over or dragged by	motor-driven snow vehicle (not on public highway)

collision of motor-driven snow vehicle with:
- animal (being ridden) (-drawn vehicle)
- another off-road motor vehicle
- other motor vehicle, not on public highway
- railway train
- other object, fixed or movable

injury caused by rough landing of motor-driven snow vehicle (after leaving ground on rough terrain)

Excludes: *accident on the public highway involving motor driven snow vehicle (E810.0-E819.9)*

④ **E821 Nontraffic accident involving other off-road motor vehicle**

Includes:

breakage of part of fall from hit by overturning of run over or dragged by thrown against some part of or object in	off-road motor vehicle, except snow vehicle (not on public highway)

collision with:
- animal (being ridden) (-drawn vehicle)
- another off-road motor vehicle, except snow vehicle
- other motor vehicle, not on public highway
- other object, fixed or movable

Excludes: *accident on public highway involving off-road motor vehicle (E810.0-E819.9)*
collision between motor driven snow vehicle and other off-road motor vehicle (E820.0-E820.9)
hovercraft accident on water (E830.0-E838.9)

④ **E822 Other motor vehicle nontraffic accident involving collision with moving object**

Includes: collision, not on public highway, between motor vehicle, except off-road motor vehicle and:
- animal
- nonmotor vehicle
- other motor vehicle, except off-road motor vehicle
- pedestrian
- railway train
- other moving object

Excludes: *collision with:*
- *motor-driven snow vehicle (E820.0-E820.9)*
- *other off-road motor vehicle (E821.0-E821.9)*

④ **E823 Other motor vehicle nontraffic accident involving collision with stationary object**

Includes: collision, not on public highway, between motor vehicle, except off-road motor vehicle, and any object, fixed or movable, but not in motion

④ **E824 Other motor vehicle nontraffic accident while boarding and alighting**

Includes:

fall injury from moving part of motor vehicle trapped by door of motor vehicle	while boarding or alighting from motor vehicle, except off-road motor vehicle, not on public highway

④ **E825 Other motor vehicle nontraffic accident of other and unspecified nature**

Includes:

accidental poisoning from carbon monoxide generated by breakage of any part of explosion of any part of fall, jump, or being accidentally pushed from fire starting in hit by object thrown into, towards, or on injured by being thrown against some part of, or object in injury from moving part of object falling in or on	motor vehicle while in motion, not on public highway

motor vehicle nontraffic accident NOS

Excludes: *fall from or in stationary motor vehicle (E884.9, E885)*
overcome by carbon monoxide or exhaust gas generated by stationary motor vehicle off the roadway with motor running (E868.2)
struck by falling object from or in stationary motor vehicle (E916)

OTHER ROAD VEHICLE ACCIDENTS (E826-E829)

Note: Other road vehicle accidents are transport accidents involving road vehicles other than motor vehicles. For definitions of other road vehicle and related terms see definitions (m) to (o).

Includes: accidents involving other road vehicles being used in recreational or sporting activities

Excludes: *collision of other road vehicle [any] with:*
aircraft (E840.0-E845.9)
motor vehicle (E813.0-E813.9, E820.0-E822.9)
railway train (E801.0-E801.9)

The following fourth-digit subdivisions are for use with categories E826-E829 to identify the injured person:

.0 Pedestrian
See definition (r)

.1 Pedal cyclist
See definition (p)

.2 Rider of animal

.3 Occupant of animal-drawn vehicle

.4 Occupant of streetcar

.8 Other specified person

.9 Unspecified person

④ **E826 Pedal cycle accident**
[0-9]

Includes: breakage of any part of pedal cycle
collision between pedal cycle and:
animal (being ridden) (herded) (unattended)
another pedal cycle
nonmotor road vehicle, any
pedestrian
other object, fixed, movable, or moving, not set in motion by motor vehicle, railway train, or aircraft
entanglement in wheel of pedal cycle
fall from pedal cycle
hit by object falling or thrown on the pedal cycle
pedal cycle accident NOS
pedal cycle overturned

Add 4th or 5th digit | Nonspecific code | Unspecified code | Manifestation code

④ **E827 Animal-drawn vehicle accident**

[0,2-4,8,9]

Includes breakage of any part of vehicle
collision between animal-drawn vehicle and:
animal (being ridden) (herded) (unattended)
nonmotor road vehicle, except pedal cycle
pedestrian, pedestrian conveyance, or pedestrian vehicle
other object, fixed, movable, or moving, not set in motion by motor vehicle, railway train, or aircraft

fall from
knocked down by
overturning of
run over by
thrown from
} animal-drawn vehicle

Excludes: *collision of animal-drawn vehicle with pedal cycle (E826.0-E826.9)*

④ **E828 Accident involving animal being ridden**

[0,2,4,8,9]

Includes: collision between animal being ridden and:
another animal
nonmotor road vehicle, except pedal cycle, and animal-drawn vehicle
pedestrian, pedestrian conveyance, or pedestrian vehicle
other object, fixed, movable, or moving, not set in motion by motor vehicle, railway train, or aircraft

fall from
knocked down by
thrown from
trampled by
} animal being ridden

ridden animal stumbled and fell

Excludes: *collision of animal being ridden with:*
animal-drawn vehicle (E827.0-E827.9)
pedal cycle (E826.0-E826.9)

④ **E829 Other road vehicle accidents**

[0,4,8,9]

Includes:

accident while boarding or alighting from
blow from object in
breakage of any part of
caught in door of
derailment of
fall in, on, or from
fire in
} streetcar nonmotor road vehicle not classifiable to E826-E828

collision between streetcar or nonmotor road vehicle, except as in E826-E828, and:
animal (not being ridden)
another nonmotor road vehicle not classifiable to E826-E828
pedestrian
other object, fixed, movable, or moving, not set in motion by motor vehicle, railway train, or aircraft
nonmotor road vehicle accident NOS
streetcar accident NOS

Excludes: *collision with:*
animal being ridden (E828.0-E828.9)
animal-drawn vehicle (E827.0-E827.9)
pedal cycle (E826.0-E826.9)

WATER TRANSPORT ACCIDENTS (E830-E838)

Note: For definitions of water transport accident and related terms see definitions (a), (s), and (t).

Includes: watercraft accidents in the course of recreational activities

Excludes: *accidents involving both aircraft, including objects set in motion by aircraft, and watercraft (E840.0-E845.9)*

The following fourth-digit subdivisions are for use with categories E830-E838 to identify the injured person:

.0 Occupant of small boat, unpowered

.1 Occupant of small boat, powered
See definition (t)

continued

Excludes: *water skier (.4)*

.2 Occupant of other watercraft—crew
Persons:
engaged in operation of watercraft
providing passenger services [cabin attendants, ship's physician, catering personnel]
working on ship during voyage in other capacity [musician in band, operators of shops and beauty parlors]

.3 Occupant of other watercraft—other than crew
Passenger
Occupant of lifeboat, other than crew, after abandoning ship

.4 Water skier

.5 Swimmer

.6 Dockers, stevedores
Longshoreman employed on the dock in loading and unloading ships

.8 Other specified person
Immigration and custom officials on board ship
Person:
accompanying passenger or member of crew
visiting boat
Pilot (guiding ship into port)

.9 Unspecified person

④ **E830 Accident to watercraft causing submersion**
Includes: submersion and drowning due to:
boat overturning
boat submerging
falling or jumping from burning ship
falling or jumping from crushed watercraft
ship sinking
other accident to watercraft

④ **E831 Accident to watercraft causing other injury**
Includes: any injury, except submersion and drowning, as a result of an accident to watercraft
burned while ship on fire
crushed between ships in collision
crushed by lifeboat after abandoning ship
fall due to collision or other accident to watercraft
hit by falling object due to accident to watercraft
injured in watercraft accident involving collision
struck by boat or part thereof after fall or jump from damaged boat

Excludes: *burns from localized fire or explosion on board ship (E837.0-E837.9)*

④ **E832 Other accidental submersion or drowning in water transport accident**
Includes: submersion or drowning as a result of an accident other than accident to the watercraft, such as:
fall:
from gangplank
from ship
overboard
thrown overboard by motion of ship
washed overboard

Excludes: *submersion or drowning of swimmer or diver who voluntarily jumps from boat not involved in an accident (E910.0-E910.9)*

④ **E833 Fall on stairs or ladders in water transport**

Excludes: *fall due to accident to watercraft (E831.0-E831.9)*

④ **E834 Other fall from one level to another in water transport**

Excludes: *fall due to accident to watercraft (E831.0-E831.9)*

④ **E835 Other and unspecified fall in water transport**

Excludes: *fall due to accident to watercraft (E831.0-E831.9)*

④ **E836 Machinery accident in water transport**

Includes: injuries in water transport caused by:
- deck, engine room, galley, laundry, loading } machinery

④ **E837 Explosion, fire, or burning in watercraft**

Includes: explosion of boiler on steamship
localized fire on ship

Excludes: *burning ship (due to collision or explosion) resulting in:*
submersion or drowning (E830.0-E830.9)
other injury (E831.0-E831.9)

④ **E838 Other and unspecified water transport accident**

Includes: accidental poisoning by gases or fumes on ship
atomic power plant malfunction in watercraft
crushed between ship and stationary object [wharf]
crushed between ships without accident to watercraft
crushed by falling object on ship or while loading or unloading
hit by boat while water skiing
struck by boat or part thereof (after fall from boat)
watercraft accident NOS

AIR AND SPACE TRANSPORT ACCIDENTS (E840-E845)

Note: For definition of aircraft and related terms see definitions (u) and (v).

The following fourth-digit subdivisions are for use with categories E840-E845 to identify the injured person:

.0 Occupant of spacecraft

.1 Occupant of military aircraft, any

Crew, Passenger (civilian) (military), Troops } in military aircraft [air force] [army] [national guard] [navy]

Excludes: *occupants of aircraft operated under jurisdiction of police departments (.5)*
parachutist (.7)

.2 Crew of commercial aircraft (powered) in surface to surface transport

.3 Other occupant of commercial aircraft (powered) in surface to surface transport

Flight personnel:
  not part of crew
  on familiarization flight
Passenger on aircraft (powered) NOS

.4 Occupant of commercial aircraft (powered) in surface to air transport

Occupant [crew] [passenger] of aircraft (powered) engaged in activities, such as:
  aerial spraying (crops) (fire retardants)
  air drops of emergency supplies
  air drops of parachutists, except from military craft
  crop dusting
  lowering of construction material [bridge or telephone pole]
  sky writing

.5 Occupant of other powered aircraft

Occupant [crew] [passenger] of aircraft [powered] engaged in activities, such as:
  aerobatic flying
  aircraft racing
  rescue operation
  storm surveillance
  traffic surveillance
Occupant of private plane NOS

.6 Occupant of unpowered aircraft, except parachutist

Occupant of aircraft classifiable to E842

.7 Parachutist (military) (other)

Person making voluntary descent

Excludes: *person making descent after accident to aircraft (.1-.6)*

.8 Ground crew, airline employee
Persons employed at airfields (civil) (military) or launching pads, not occupants of aircraft

.9 Other person

④ **E840 Accident to powered aircraft at takeoff or landing**
Includes:

collision of aircraft with any object, fixed, movable, or moving crash explosion on aircraft fire on aircraft forced landing	while taking off or landing

④ **E841 Accident to powered aircraft, other and unspecified**
Includes: aircraft accident NOS
aircraft crash or wreck NOS
any accident to powered aircraft while in transit or when not specified whether in transit, taking off, or landing
collision of aircraft with another aircraft, bird, or any object, while in transit
explosion on aircraft while in transit
fire on aircraft while in transit

④ **E842 Accident to unpowered aircraft**
[6-9]
Includes: any accident, except collision with powered aircraft, to:
balloon
glider
hang glider
kite carrying a person
hit by object falling from unpowered aircraft

④ **E843 Fall in, on, or from aircraft**
[0-9]
Includes: accident in boarding or alighting from aircraft, any kind
fall in, on, or from aircraft [any kind], while in transit, taking off, or landing, except when as a result of an accident to aircraft

④ **E844 Other specified air transport accidents**
[0-9]
Includes:

hit by: aircraft object falling from aircraft injury by or from: machinery on aircraft rotating propeller voluntary parachute descent poisoning by carbon monoxide from aircraft while in transit sucked into jet	without accident to aircraft

any accident involving other transport vehicle (motor) (nonmotor) due to being hit by object set in motion by aircraft (powered)

Excludes: *air sickness (E903)*
effects of:
high altitude (E902.0-E902.1)
pressure change (E902.0-E902.1)
injury in parachute descent due to accident to aircraft (840.0-E842.9)

④ **E845 Accident involving spacecraft**
[0,8,9]
Includes: launching pad accident

Excludes: *effects of weightlessness in spacecraft (E928.0)*

VEHICLE ACCIDENTS NOT ELSEWHERE CLASSIFIABLE (E846-E848)

E846 Accidents involving powered vehicles used solely within the buildings and premises of industrial or commercial establishment

Accident to, on, or involving:
- battery powered airport passenger vehicle
- battery powered trucks (baggage) (mail)
- coal car in mine
- logging car
- self propelled truck, industrial
- station baggage truck (powered)
- tram, truck, or tub (powered) in mine or quarry

Breakage of any part of vehicle

Collision with:
- pedestrian
- other vehicle or object within premises

Explosion of } powered vehicle, industrial or commercial
Fall from } powered vehicle, industrial or commercial
Overturning of } powered vehicle, industrial or commercial
Struck by } powered vehicle, industrial or commercial

Excludes: *accidental poisoning by exhaust gas from vehicle not elsewhere classifiable (E868.2)*
injury by crane, lift (fork), or elevator (E919.2)

E847 Accidents involving cable cars not running on rails

Accident to, on, or involving:
- cable car, not on rails
- ski chair-lift
- ski-lift with gondola
- téléférique

Breakage of cable

Caught or dragged by } cable car, not on rails
Fall or jump from } cable car, not on rails
Object thrown from or in } cable car, not on rails

E848 Accidents involving other vehicles, not elsewhere classifiable

Accident to, on, or involving:
- ice yacht
- land yacht
- nonmotor, nonroad vehicle NOS

□ ***E849 Place of occurrence***

The following category is for use with categories E850-E869 and E880-E928, to denote the place where the accident or poisoning occurred.

□ ***E849.0 Home***

Apartment
Boarding house
Farm house
Home premises
House (residential)
Noninstitutional place of residence
Private:
- *driveway*
- *garage*
- *garden*
- *home*
- *walk*

Swimming pool in private house or garden
Yard of home

Excludes: *home under construction but not yet occupied (E849.3)*
institutional place of residence (E849.7)

□ ***E849.1 Farm***

Farm:
- *buildings*
- *land under cultivation*

Excludes: *farm house and home premises of farm (E849.0)*

E849.2 Mine and quarry

Gravel pit
Sand pit
Tunnel under construction

● Code new to this edition ▲ Revision of existing code ④ ⑤ Fourth or fifth digit required

☐ ***E849.3*** ***Industrial place and premises***

Building under construction
Dockyard
Dry dock
Factory
  building
  premises
Garage (place of work)
Industrial yard
Loading platform (factory) (store)
Plant, industrial
Railway yard
Shop (place of work)
Warehouse
Workhouse

☐ ***E849.4*** ***Place for recreation and sport***

Amusement park
Baseball field
Basketball court
Beach resort
Cricket ground
Fives court
Football field
Golf course
Gymnasium
Hockey field
Holiday camp
Ice palace
Lake resort
Mountain resort
Playground, including school playground
Public park
Racecourse
Resort NOS
Riding school
Rifle range
Seashore resort
Skating rink
Sports ground
Sports palace
Stadium
Swimming pool, public
Tennis court
Vacation resort

Excludes: *that in private house or garden (E849.0)*

☐ ***E849.5*** ***Street and highway***

☐ ***E849.6*** ***Public building***

Building (including adjacent grounds) used by the general public or by a particular group of the public, such as:

airport
bank
café
casino
church
cinema
clubhouse
courthouse
dance hall
garage building (for car storage)
hotel
market (grocery or other commodity)
movie house
music hall
nightclub
office
office building
opera house
post office
public hall
radio broadcasting station
restaurant
school (state) (public) (private)
shop, commercial
station (bus) (railway)
store
theater

Excludes: *home garage (E849.0)*
industrial building or workplace (E849.3)

☐ ***E849.7*** ***Residential institution***

Children's home
Dormitory
Hospital
Jail
Old people's home
Orphanage
Prison
Reform school

☐ ***E849.8*** ***Other specified places***

Beach NOS
Canal
Caravan site NOS
Derelict house
Desert
Dock
Forest
Harbor
Hill
Lake NOS
Mountain
Parking lot
Parking place
Pond or pool (natural)
Prairie
Public place NOS
Railway line
Reservoir
River
Sea
Seashore NOS
Stream
Swamp
Trailer court
Woods

☐ ***E849.9*** ***Unspecified place***

ACCIDENTAL POISONING BY DRUGS, MEDICINAL SUBSTANCES, AND BIOLOGICALS (E850-E858)

Includes: accidental overdose of drug, wrong drug given or taken in error, and drug taken inadvertently
accidents in the use of drugs and biologicals in medical and surgical procedures

Excludes: *administration with suicidal or homicidal intent or intent to harm, or in circumstances classifiable to E980-E989 (E950.0-E950.5, E962.0, E980.0-E980.5)*
correct drug properly administered in therapeutic or prophylactic dosage, as the cause of adverse effect (E930.0-E949.9)

See Alphabetic Index for more complete list of specific drugs to be classified under the fourth-digit subdivisions. The American Hospital Formulary numbers can be used to classify new drugs listed by the American Hospital Formulary Service (AHFS). See appendix C.

E850 Accidental poisoning by analgesics, antipyretics, and antirheumatics

□ **E850.0 Heroin**
Diacetylmorphine

□ **E850.1 Methadone**

□ **E850.2 Other opiates and related narcotics**
Codeine [methylmorphine]
Meperidine [pethidine]
Morphine
Opium (alkaloids)

□ **E850.3 Salicylates**
Acetylsalicylic acid [aspirin]
Amino derivatives of salicylic acid
Salicylic acid salts

□ **E850.4 Aromatic analgesics, not elsewhere classified**
Acetanilid
Paracetamol [acetaminophen]
Phenacetin [acetophenetidin]

□ **E850.5 Pyrazole derivatives**
Aminophenazone [amidopyrine]
Phenylbutazone

□ **E850.6 Antirheumatics [antiphlogistics]**
Gold salts
Indomethacin

Excludes: *salicylates (E850.3)*
steroids (E858.0)

□ **E850.7 Other non-narcotic analgesics**
Pyrabital

E850.8 Other specified analgesics and antipyretics
Pentazocine

E850.9 Unspecified analgesic or antipyretic

E851 Accidental poisoning by barbiturates
Amobarbital [amylobarbitone]
Barbital [barbitone]
Butabarbital [butabarbitone]
Pentobarbital [pentobarbitone]
Phenobarbital [phenobarbitone]
Secobarbital [quinalbarbitone]

Excludes: *thiobarbiturates (E855.1)*

E852 Accidental poisoning by other sedatives and hypnotics

E852.0 Chloral hydrate group

E852.1 Paraldehyde

E852.2 Bromine compounds
Bromides
Carbromal (derivatives)

E852.3 Methaqualone compounds

E852.4 Glutethimide group

E852.5 Mixed sedatives, not elsewhere classified

E852.8 Other specified sedatives and hypnotics

E852.9 Unspecified sedative or hypnotic
Sleeping:
- drug, pill, tablet } NOS

E853 Accidental poisoning by tranquilizers

E853.0 Phenothiazine-based tranquilizers
Chlorpromazine
Fluphenazine
Prochlorperazine
Promazine

E853.1 Butyrophenone-based tranquilizers
Haloperidol
Spiperone
Trifluperidol

E853.2 Benzodiazepine-based tranquilizers
Chlordiazepoxide
Diazepam
Flurazepam
Lorazepam
Medazepam
Nitrazepam

E853.8 Other specified tranquilizers
Hydroxyzine
Meprobamate

E853.9 Unspecified tranquilizer

E854 Accidental poisoning by other psychotropic agents

E854.0 Antidepressants
Amitriptyline
Imipramine
Monoamine oxidase [MAO] inhibitors

E854.1 Psychodysleptics [hallucinogens]
Cannabis derivatives
Lysergide [LSD]
Marihuana (derivatives)
Mescaline
Psilocin
Psilocybin

E854.2 Psychostimulants
Amphetamine
Caffeine

Excludes: central appetite depressants (E858.8)

E854.3 Central nervous system stimulants
Analeptics
Opiate antagonists

● **E854.8 Other psychotropic agents**

E855 Accidental poisoning by other drugs acting on central and autonomic nervous system

E855.0 Anticonvulsant and anti-Parkinsonism drugs
Amantadine
Hydantoin derivatives
Levodopa [L-dopa]
Oxazolidine derivatives [paramethadione] [trimethadione]
Succinimides

E855.1 Other central nervous system depressants
Ether
Gaseous anesthetics
Halogenated hydrocarbon derivatives
Intravenous anesthetics
Thiobarbiturates, such as thiopental sodium

E855.2 Local anesthetics
Cocaine
Lidocaine [lignocaine]
Procaine
Tetracaine

E855.3 Parasympathomimetics [cholinergics]
Acetylcholine
Anticholinesterase:
- organophosphorus
- reversible

Pilocarpine

E855.4 Parasympatholytics [anticholinergics and antimuscarinics] and spasmolytics
Atropine
Homatropine
Hyoscine [scopolamine]
Quaternary ammonium derivatives

E855.5 Sympathomimetics [adrenergics]
Epinephrine [adrenalin]
Levarterenol [noradrenalin]

E855.6 Sympatholytics [antiadrenergics]
Phenoxybenzamine
Tolazoline hydrochloride

E855.8 Other specified drugs acting on central and autonomic nervous systems

E855.9 Unspecified drug acting on central and autonomic nervous systems

E856 Accidental poisoning by antibiotics

E857 Accidental poisoning by other anti-infectives

E858 Accidental poisoning by other drugs

E858.0 Hormones and synthetic substitutes

E858.1 Primarily systemic agents

E858.2 Agents primarily affecting blood constituents

E858.3 Agents primarily affecting cardiovascular system

E858.4 Agents primarily affecting gastrointestinal system

E858.5 Water, mineral, and uric acid metabolism drugs

E858.6 Agents primarily acting on the smooth and skeletal muscles and respiratory system

E858.7 Agents primarily affecting skin and mucous membrane, ophthalmological, otorhinolaryngological, and dental drugs

E858.8 Other specified drugs
Central appetite depressants

E858.9 Unspecified drug

ACCIDENTAL POISONING BY OTHER SOLID AND LIQUID SUBSTANCES, GASES, AND VAPORS (E860-E869)

Note: Categories in this section are intended primarily to indicate the external cause of poisoning states classifiable to 980-989. They may also be used to indicate external causes of localized effects classifiable to 001-799.

E860 Accidental poisoning by alcohol, not elsewhere classified

E860.0 Alcoholic beverages
Alcohol in preparations intended for consumption

E860.1 Other and unspecified ethyl alcohol and its products
Denatured alcohol
Ethanol NOS
Grain alcohol NOS
Methylated spirit

E860.2 Methyl alcohol
Methanol
Wood alcohol

E860.3 Isopropyl alcohol
Dimethyl carbinol
Isopropanol
Rubbing alcohol substitute
Secondary propyl alcohol

E860.4 Fusel oil
Alcohol:
- amyl
- butyl
- propyl

E860.8 Other specified alcohols

E860.9 Unspecified alcohol

E861 Accidental poisoning by cleansing and polishing agents, disinfectants, paints, and varnishes

E861.0 Synthetic detergents and shampoos

E861.1 Soap products

E861.2 Polishes

E861.3 Other cleansing and polishing agents
Scouring powders

E861.4 Disinfectants
Household and other disinfectants not ordinarily used on the person

Excludes: carbolic acid or phenol (E864.0)

E861.5 Lead paints

E861.6 Other paints and varnishes
Lacquers
Oil colors
Paints, other than lead
White washes

E861.9 Unspecified

E862 Accidental poisoning by petroleum products, other solvents and their vapors, not elsewhere classified

E862.0 Petroleum solvents

Petroleum:
  ether
  benzine
  naphtha

E862.1 Petroleum fuels and cleaners
Antiknock additives to petroleum fuels
Gas oils
Gasoline or petrol
Kerosene

Excludes: *kerosene insecticides (E863.4)*

E862.2 Lubricating oils

E862.3 Petroleum solids
Paraffin wax

E862.4 Other specified solvents
Benzene

E862.9 Unspecified solvent

E863 Accidental poisoning by agricultural and horticultural chemical and pharmaceutical preparations other than plant foods and fertilizers

Excludes: *plant foods and fertilizers (E866.5)*

E863.0 Insecticides of organochlorine compounds
Benzene hexachloride
Chlordane
DDT
Dieldrin
Endrine
Toxaphene

E863.1 Insecticides of organophosphorus compounds
Demeton
Diazinon
Dichlorvos
Malathion
Methyl parathion
Parathion
Phenylsulphthion
Phorate
Phosdrin

E863.2 Carbamates
Aldicarb
Carbaryl
Propoxur

E863.3 Mixtures of insecticides

E863.4 Other and unspecified insecticides
Kerosene insecticides

E863.5 Herbicides
2, 4-Dichlorophenoxyacetic acid [2, 4-D]
2, 4, 5-Trichlorophenoxyacetic acid [2, 4, 5-T]
Chlorates
Diquat
Mixtures of plant food and fertilizers with herbicides
Paraquat

E863.6 Fungicides
Organic mercurials (used in seed dressing)
Pentachlorophenols

E863.7 Rodenticides
Fluoroacetates
Squill and derivatives
Thallium
Warfarin
Zinc phosphide

E863.8 Fumigants
Cyanides
Methyl bromide
Phosphine

E863.9 Other and unspecified

E864 Accidental poisoning by corrosives and caustics, not elsewhere classified

Excludes: *those as components of disinfectants (E861.4)*

E864.0 Corrosive aromatics
Carbolic acid or phenol

E864.1 Acids
Acid:
  hydrochloric
  nitric
  sulfuric

E864.2 Caustic alkalis
Lye

E864.3 Other specified corrosives and caustics

E864.4 Unspecified corrosives and caustics

▲ **E865 Accidental poisoning from poisonous foodstuffs and poisonous plants**

Includes: any meat, fish, or shellfish
plants, berries, and fungi eaten as, or in mistake for, food, or by a child

Excludes: *anaphylactic shock due to adverse food reaction (995.6)*
food poisoning (bacterial) (005.0-005.9)
poisoning and toxic reactions to venomous plants (E905.6-E905.7)

E865.0 Meat

E865.1 Shellfish

E865.2 Other fish

E865.3 Berries and seeds

E865.4 Other specified plants

E865.5 Mushrooms and other fungi

E865.8 Other specified foods

E865.9 Unspecified foodstuff or poisonous plant

E866 Accidental poisoning by other and unspecified solid and liquid substances

Excludes: *these substances as a component of:*
medicines (E850.0-E858.9)
paints (E861.5-E861.6)
pesticides (E863.0-E863.9)
petroleum fuels (E862.1)

E866.0 Lead and its compounds and fumes

E866.1 Mercury and its compounds and fumes

E866.2 Antimony and its compounds and fumes

E866.3 Arsenic and its compounds and fumes

E866.4 Other metals and their compounds and fumes
Beryllium (compounds)
Brass fumes
Cadmium (compounds)
Copper salts
Iron (compounds)
Manganese (compounds)
Nickel (compounds)
Thallium (compounds)

E866.5 Plant foods and fertilizers

Excludes: *mixtures with herbicides (E863.5)*

E866.6 Glues and adhesives

E866.7 Cosmetics

E866.8 Other specified solid or liquid substances

E866.9 Unspecified solid or liquid substance

E867 Accidental poisoning by gas distributed by pipeline
Carbon monoxide from incomplete combustion of piped gas
Coal gas NOS
Liquefied petroleum gas distributed through pipes (pure or mixed with air)
Piped gas (natural) (manufactured)

E868 Accidental poisoning by other utility gas and other carbon monoxide

E868.0 Liquefied petroleum gas distributed in mobile containers
Butane
Liquefied hydrocarbon gas NOS
Propane
} or carbon monoxide from incomplete combustion of these gases

E868.1 Other and unspecified utility gas
Acetylene
Gas NOS used for lighting, heating, or cooking
Water gas
} or carbon monoxide from incomplete combustion of these gases

● Code new to this edition ▲ Revision of existing code ④ ⑤ Fourth or fifth digit required

E868.2 Motor vehicle exhaust gas
Exhaust gas from:
farm tractor, not in transit
gas engine
motor pump
motor vehicle, not in transit
any type of combustion engine not in watercraft

Excludes: *poisoning by carbon monoxide from:*
aircraft while in transit (E844.0-E844.9)
motor vehicle while in transit (E818.0-E818.9)
watercraft whether or not in transit (E838.0-E838.9)

E868.3 Carbon monoxide from incomplete combustion of other domestic fuels
Carbon monoxide from incomplete combustion of:
coal, coke, kerosene, wood } in domestic stove or fireplace

Excludes: *carbon monoxide from smoke and fumes due to conflagration (E890.0-E893.9)*

E868.8 Carbon monoxide from other sources
Carbon monoxide from:
blast furnace gas
incomplete combustion of fuels in industrial use
kiln vapor

E868.9 Unspecified carbon monoxide

E869 Accidental poisoning by other gases and vapors

Excludes: *effects of gases used as anesthetics (E855.1, E938.2)*
fumes from heavy metals (E866.0-E866.4)
smoke and fumes due to conflagration or explosion (E890.0-E899)

E869.0 Nitrogen oxides

E869.1 Sulfur dioxide

E869.2 Freon

E869.3 Lacrimogenic gas [tear gas]
Bromobenzyl cyanide
Chloroacetophenone
Ethyliodoacetate

E869.4 Second-hand tobacco smoke

E869.8 Other specified gases and vapors
Chlorine
Hydrocyanic acid gas

E869.9 Unspecified gases and vapors

MISADVENTURES TO PATIENTS DURING SURGICAL AND MEDICAL CARE (E870-E876)

Excludes: *accidental overdose of drug and wrong drug given in error (E850.0-E858.9)*
surgical and medical procedures as the cause of abnormal reaction by the patient, without mention of misadventure at the time of procedure (E878.0-E879.9)

E870 Accidental cut, puncture, perforation, or hemorrhage during medical care

E870.0 Surgical operation

E870.1 Infusion or transfusion

E870.2 Kidney dialysis or other perfusion

E870.3 Injection or vaccination

E870.4 Endoscopic examination

E870.5 Aspiration of fluid or tissue, puncture, and catheterization
Abdominal paracentesis
Aspirating needle biopsy
Blood sampling
Lumbar puncture
Thoracentesis

Excludes: *heart catheterization (E870.6)*

E870.6 Heart catheterization

E870.7 Administration of enema

E870.8 Other specified medical care

E870.9 Unspecified medical care

E871 Foreign object left in body during procedure

E871.0 Surgical operation

E871.1 Infusion or transfusion

E871.2 Kidney dialysis or other perfusion

E871.3 Injection or vaccination

E871.4 Endoscopic examination

E871.5 Aspiration of fluid or tissue, puncture, and catheterization
Abdominal paracentesis
Aspiration needle biopsy
Blood sampling
Lumbar puncture
Thoracentesis

Excludes: *heart catheterization (E871.6)*

E871.6 Heart catheterization

E871.7 Removal of catheter or packing

E871.8 Other specified procedures

E871.9 Unspecified procedure

E872 Failure of sterile precautions during procedure

E872.0 Surgical operation

E872.1 Infusion or transfusion

E872.2 Kidney dialysis and other perfusion

E872.3 Injection or vaccination

E872.4 Endoscopic examination

E872.5 Aspiration of fluid or tissue, puncture, and catheterization
Abdominal paracentesis
Aspirating needle biopsy
Blood sampling
Lumbar puncture
Thoracentesis

Excludes: *heart catheterization (E872.6)*

E872.6 Heart catheterization

E872.8 Other specified procedures

E872.9 Unspecified procedure

E873 Failure in dosage

Excludes: *accidental overdose of drug, medicinal or biological substance (E850.0-E858.9)*

E873.0 Excessive amount of blood or other fluid during transfusion or infusion

E873.1 Incorrect dilution of fluid during infusion

E873.2 Overdose of radiation in therapy

E873.3 Inadvertent exposure of patient to radiation during medical care

E873.4 Failure in dosage in electroshock or insulin-shock therapy

E873.5 Inappropriate [too hot or too cold] temperature in local application and packing

E873.6 Nonadministration of necessary drug or medicinal substance

E873.8 Other specified failure in dosage

E873.9 Unspecified failure in dosage

E874 Mechanical failure of instrument or apparatus during procedure

E874.0 Surgical operation

E874.1 Infusion and transfusion
Air in system

E874.2 Kidney dialysis and other perfusion

E874.3 Endoscopic examination

E874.4 Aspiration of fluid or tissue, puncture, and catheterization
Abdominal paracentesis
Aspirating needle biopsy
Blood sampling
Lumbar puncture
Thoracentesis

Excludes: *heart catheterization (E874.5)*

E874.5 Heart catheterization

E874.8 Other specified procedures

E874.9 Unspecified procedure

E875 Contaminated or infected blood, other fluid, drug, or biological substance

Includes: presence of:
bacterial pyrogens
endotoxin-producing bacteria
serum hepatitis-producing agent

E875.0 Contaminated substance transfused or infused

E875.1 Contaminated substance injected or used for vaccination

E875.2 Contaminated drug or biological substance administered by other means

E875.8 Other

E875.9 Unspecified

E876 Other and unspecified misadventures during medical care

E876.0 Mismatched blood in transfusion

E876.1 Wrong fluid in infusion

E876.2 Failure in suture and ligature during surgical operation

E876.3 Endotracheal tube wrongly placed during anesthetic procedure

E876.4 Failure to introduce or to remove other tube or instrument

Excludes: foreign object left in body during procedure (E871.0-E871.9)

E876.5 Performance of inappropriate operation

E876.8 Other specified misadventures during medical care

Performance of inappropriate treatment NEC

E876.9 Unspecified misadventure during medical care

SURGICAL AND MEDICAL PROCEDURES AS THE CAUSE OF ABNORMAL REACTION OF PATIENT OR LATER COMPLICATION, WITHOUT MENTION OF MISADVENTURE AT THE TIME OF PROCEDURE (E878-E879)

Includes: procedures as the cause of abnormal reaction, such as:
displacement or malfunction of prosthetic device
hepatorenal failure, postoperative
malfunction of external stoma
postoperative intestinal obstruction
rejection of transplanted organ

Excludes: anesthetic management properly carried out as the cause of adverse effect (E937.0-E938.9)
infusion and transfusion, without mention of misadventure in the technique of procedure (E930.0-E949.9)

E878 Surgical operation and other surgical procedures as the cause of abnormal reaction of patient, or of later complication, without mention of misadventure at the time of operation

E878.0 Surgical operation with transplant of whole organ

Transplantation of:
heart
kidney
liver

E878.1 Surgical operation with implant of artificial internal device

Cardiac pacemaker
Electrodes implanted in brain
Heart valve prosthesis
Internal orthopedic device

E878.2 Surgical operation with anastomosis, bypass, or graft, with natural or artificial tissues used as implant

Anastomosis:
arteriovenous
gastrojejunal
Graft of blood vessel, tendon, or skin

Excludes: external stoma (E878.3)

E878.3 Surgical operation with formation of external stoma

Colostomy
Cystostomy
Duodenostomy
Gastrostomy
Ureterostomy

E878.4 Other restorative surgery

E878.5 Amputation of limb(s)

E878.6 Removal of other organ (partial) (total)

E878.8 Other specified surgical operations and procedures

Add 4th or 5th digit | Nonspecific code | Unspecified code | Manifestation code

E878.9 Unspecified surgical operations and procedures

E879 Other procedures, without mention of misadventure at the time of procedure, as the cause of abnormal reaction of patient, or of later complication

E879.0 Cardiac catheterization

E879.1 Kidney dialysis

E879.2 Radiological procedure and radiotherapy

Excludes: *radio-opaque dyes for diagnostic x-ray procedures (E947.8)*

E879.3 Shock therapy

Electroshock therapy
Insulin-shock therapy

E879.4 Aspiration of fluid

Lumbar puncture
Thoracentesis

E879.5 Insertion of gastric or duodenal sound

E879.6 Urinary catheterization

E879.7 Blood sampling

E879.8 Other specified procedures

Blood transfusion

E879.9 Unspecified procedure

ACCIDENTAL FALLS (E880-E888)

Excludes: *falls (in or from):*
burning building (E890.8, E891.8)
into fire (E890.0-E899)
into water (with submersion or drowning) (E910.0-E910.9)
machinery (in operation) (E919.0-E919.9)
on edged, pointed, or sharp object (E920.0-E920.9)
transport vehicle (E800.0-E845.9)
vehicle not elsewhere classifiable (E846-E848)

E880 Fall on or from stairs or steps

E880.0 Escalator

● **E880.1 Fall on or from sidewalk curb**

Excludes: *fall from moving sidewalk (E885)*

E880.9 Other stairs or steps

E881 Fall on or from ladders or scaffolding

E881.0 Fall from ladder

E881.1 Fall from scaffolding

E882 Fall from or out of building or other structure

Fall from:
balcony
bridge
building
flagpole
tower

Fall from:
turret
viaduct
wall
window

Fall through roof

Excludes: *collapse of a building or structure (E916)*
fall or jump from burning building (E890.8, E891.8)

E883 Fall into hole or other opening in surface

Includes:
fall into:
cavity
dock
hole
pit
quarry

fall into:
shaft
swimming pool
tank
well

Excludes: *fall into water NOS (E910.9)*
that resulting in drowning or submersion without mention of injury (E910.0-E910.9)

E883.0 Accident from diving or jumping into water [swimming pool]

Strike or hit:
against bottom when jumping or diving into water
wall or board of swimming pool
water surface

Excludes: *diving with insufficient air supply (E913.2)*
effects of air pressure from diving (E902.2)

E883.1 Accidental fall into well

E883.2 Accidental fall into storm drain or manhole

E883.9 Fall into other hole or other opening in surface

E884 Other fall from one level to another

E884.0 Fall from playground equipment

Excludes: *recreational machinery (E919.8)*

E884.1 Fall from cliff

▲ **E884.2 Fall from chair**

● **E884.3 Fall from wheelchair**

● **E884.4 Fall from bed**

● **E884.5 Fall from other furniture**

● **E884.6 Fall from commode**
Toilet

E884.9 Other fall from one level to another
Fall from:
embankment
haystack
Fall from:
stationary vehicle
tree

E885 Fall on same level from slipping, tripping, or stumbling
Fall on moving sidewalk

E886 Fall on same level from collision, pushing, or shoving, by or with other person

Excludes: *crushed or pushed by a crowd or human stampede (E917.1)*

E886.0 In sports
Tackles in sports

Excludes: *kicked, stepped on, struck by object, in sports (E917.0)*

E886.9 Other and unspecified
Fall from collision of pedestrian (conveyance) with another pedestrian (conveyance)

E887 Fracture, cause unspecified

E888 Other and unspecified fall
Accidental fall NOS
Fall from bumping against object
Fall on same level NOS

ACCIDENTS CAUSED BY FIRE AND FLAMES (E890-E899)

Includes: asphyxia or poisoning due to conflagration or ignition
burning by fire
secondary fires resulting from explosion

Excludes: *arson (E968.0)*
fire in or on:
machinery (in operation) (E919.0-E919.9)
transport vehicle other than stationary vehicle (E800.0-E845.9)
vehicle not elsewhere classifiable (E846-E848)

E890 Conflagration in private dwelling
Includes: conflagration in:
apartment
boarding house
camping place
caravan
farmhouse
house
lodging house
mobile home
private garage
rooming house
tenement
conflagration originating from sources classifiable to E893-E898 in the above buildings

E890.0 Explosion caused by conflagration

Add 4th or 5th digit | Nonspecific code | Unspecified code | Manifestation code

E890.1 Fumes from combustion of polyvinylchloride [PVC] and similar material in conflagration

E890.2 Other smoke and fumes from conflagration

Carbon monoxide
Fumes NOS
Smoke NOS
} from conflagration in private building

E890.3 Burning caused by conflagration

E890.8 Other accident resulting from conflagration

Collapse of
Fall from
Hit by object falling from
Jump from
} burning private building

E890.9 Unspecified accident resulting from conflagration in private dwelling

E891 Conflagration in other and unspecified building or structure

Conflagration in:
- barn
- church
- convalescent and other residential home
- dormitory of educational institution
- factory

Conflagration in:
- farm outbuildings
- hospital
- hotel
- school
- store
- theater

Conflagration originating from sources classifiable to E893-E898, in the above buildings

E891.0 Explosion caused by conflagration

E891.1 Fumes from combustion of polyvinylchloride [PVC] and similar material in conflagration

E891.2 Other smoke and fumes from conflagration

Carbon monoxide
Fumes NOS
Smoke NOS
} from conflagration in building or structure

E891.3 Burning caused by conflagration

E891.8 Other accident resulting from conflagration

Collapse of
Fall from
Hit by object falling from
Jump from
} burning building or structure

E891.9 Unspecified accident resulting from conflagration of other and unspecified building or structure

E892 Conflagration not in building or structure

Fire (uncontrolled) (in) (of):
- forest
- grass
- hay
- lumber
- mine
- prairie
- transport vehicle [any], except while in transit
- tunnel

E893 Accident caused by ignition of clothing

Excludes: *ignition of clothing:*
from highly inflammable material (E894)
with conflagration (E890.0-E892)

E893.0 From controlled fire in private dwelling

Ignition of clothing from:
normal fire (charcoal) (coal) (electric) (gas) (wood) in:
- brazier
- fireplace
- furnace
- stove

} in private dwelling (as listed in E890)

E893.1 From controlled fire in other building or structure

Ignition of clothing from:
- normal fire (charcoal) (coal) (electric) (gas) (wood) in:
  - brazier
  - fireplace
  - furnace
  - stove

} in other building or structure (as listed in E891)

E893.2 From controlled fire not in building or structure

Ignition of clothing from:
- bonfire (controlled)
- brazier fire (controlled), not in building or structure
- trash fire (controlled)

Excludes: *conflagration not in building (E892)*
trash fire out of control (E892)

E893.8 From other specified sources

Ignition of clothing from:
- blowlamp
- blowtorch
- burning bedspread
- candle
- cigar

Ignition of clothing from:
- cigarette
- lighter
- matches
- pipe
- welding torch

E893.9 Unspecified source

Ignition of clothing (from controlled fire NOS) (in building NOS) NOS

E894 Ignition of highly inflammable material

Ignition of:
- benzine
- gasoline
- fat
- kerosene
- paraffin
- petrol

} (with ignition of clothing)

Excludes: *ignition of highly inflammable material with:*
conflagration (E890.0-E892)
explosion (E923.0-E923.9)

E895 Accident caused by controlled fire in private dwelling

Burning by (flame of) normal fire (charcoal) (coal) (electric) (gas) (wood) in:
- brazier
- fireplace
- furnace
- stove

} in private dwelling (as listed in E890)

Excludes: *burning by hot objects not producing fire or flames (E924.0-E924.9)*
ignition of clothing from these sources (E893.0)
poisoning by carbon monoxide from incomplete combustion of fuel (E867-E868.9)
that with conflagration (E890.0-E890.9)

E896 Accident caused by controlled fire in other and unspecified building or structure

Burning by (flame of) normal fire (charcoal) (coal) (electric) (gas) (wood) in:
- brazier
- fireplace
- furnace
- stove

} in other building or structure (as listed in E891)

Excludes: *burning by hot objects not producing fire or flames (E924.0-E924.9)*
ignition of clothing from these sources (E893.1)
poisoning by carbon monoxide from incomplete combustion of fuel (E867-E868.9)
that with conflagration (E891.0-E891.9)

E897 Accident caused by controlled fire not in building or structure

Burns from flame of:
- bonfire (controlled)
- brazier fire (controlled), not in building or structure
- trash fire (controlled)

continues

Excludes: *ignition of clothing from these sources (E893.2)*
trash fire out of control (E892)
that with conflagration (E892)

E898 Accident caused by other specified fire and flames

Excludes: *conflagration (E890.0-E892)*
that with ignition of:
clothing (E893.0-E893.9)
highly inflammable material (E894)

E898.0 Burning bedclothes
Bed set on fire NOS

E898.1 Other
Burning by:
blowlamp
blowtorch
candle
cigar
cigarette
fire in room NOS
Burning by:
lamp
lighter
matches
pipe
welding torch

E899 Accident caused by unspecified fire
Burning NOS

ACCIDENTS DUE TO NATURAL AND ENVIRONMENTAL FACTORS (E900-E909)

E900 Excessive heat

E900.0 Due to weather conditions
Excessive heat as the external cause of:
ictus solaris
siriasis
sunstroke

E900.1 Of man-made origin
Heat (in):
boiler room
drying room
factory
furnace room
Heat (in):
generated in transport vehicle
kitchen

E900.9 Of unspecified origin

E901 Excessive cold

E901.0 Due to weather conditions
Excessive cold as the cause of:
chilblains NOS
immersion foot

E901.1 Of man-made origin
Contact with or inhalation of:
dry ice
liquid air
liquid hydrogen
liquid nitrogen
Prolonged exposure in:
deep freeze unit
refrigerator

E901.8 Other specified origin

E901.9 Of unspecified origin

E902 High and low air pressure and changes in air pressure

E902.0 Residence or prolonged visit at high altitude
Residence or prolonged visit at high altitude as the cause of:
Acosta syndrome
Alpine sickness
altitude sickness
Andes disease
anoxia, hypoxia
barotitis, barodontalgia, barosinusitis, otitic barotrauma
hypobarism, hypobaropathy
mountain sickness
range disease

E902.1 In aircraft
Sudden change in air pressure in aircraft during ascent or descent as the cause of:
aeroneurosis
aviators' disease

E902.2 Due to diving
High air pressure from rapid descent in water
Reduction in atmospheric pressure while surfacing from deep water diving
} as the cause of:
caisson disease
divers' disease
divers' palsy or paralysis

E902.8 Due to other specified causes
Reduction in atmospheric pressure while surfacing from underground

E902.9 Unspecified cause

E903 Travel and motion

E904 Hunger, thirst, exposure, and neglect

Excludes: *any condition resulting from homicidal intent (E968.0-E968.9)*
hunger, thirst, and exposure resulting from accidents connected with transport (E800.0-E848)

E904.0 Abandonment or neglect of infants and helpless persons
Exposure to weather conditions
Hunger or thirst
} resulting from abandonment or neglect
Desertion of newborn
Inattention at or after birth
Lack of care (helpless person) (infant)

Excludes: *criminal [purposeful] neglect (E968.4)*

E904.1 Lack of food
Lack of food as the cause of:
inanition
insufficient nourishment
starvation

Excludes: *hunger resulting from abandonment or neglect (E904.0)*

E904.2 Lack of water
Lack of water as the cause of:
dehydration
inanition

Excludes: *dehydration due to acute fluid loss (276.5)*

E904.3 Exposure (to weather conditions), not elsewhere classifiable
Exposure NOS
Humidity
Struck by hailstones

Excludes: *struck by lightning (E907)*

E904.9 Privation, unqualified
Destitution

E905 Venomous animals and plants as the cause of poisoning and toxic reactions
Includes: chemical released by animal
insects
release of venom through fangs, hairs, spines, tentacles, and other venom apparatus

Excludes: *eating of poisonous animals or plants (E865.0-E865.9)*

E905.0 Venomous snakes and lizards
Cobra
Copperhead snake
Coral snake
Fer de lance
Gila monster
Krait
Mamba
Rattlesnake
Sea snake
Snake (venomous)
Viper
Water moccasin

Excludes: *bites of snakes and lizards known to be nonvenomous (E906.2)*

E905.1 Venomous spiders
Black widow spider
Brown spider
Tarantula (venomous)

E905.2 Scorpion

E905.3 Hornets, wasps, and bees
Yellow jacket

E905.4 Centipede and venomous millipede (tropical)

E905.5 Other venomous arthropods
Sting of:
ant
caterpillar

E905.6 Venomous marine animals and plants
Puncture by sea urchin spine
Sting of:
coral
jelly fish
Sting of:
nematocysts
sea anemone
sea cucumber
other marine animal or plant

Excludes: *bites and other injuries caused by nonvenomous marine animal (E906.2-E906.8)*
bite of sea snake (venomous) (E905.0)

E905.7 Poisoning and toxic reactions caused by other plants
Injection of poisons or toxins into or through skin by plant thorns, spines, or other mechanisms

Excludes: *puncture wound NOS by plant thorns or spines (E920.8)*

E905.8 Other specified

E905.9 Unspecified
Sting NOS
Venomous bite NOS

E906 Other injury caused by animals

Excludes: *poisoning and toxic reactions caused by venomous animals and insects (E905.0-E905.9)*
road vehicle accident involving animals (E827.0-E828.9)
tripping or falling over an animal (E885)

E906.0 Dog bite

E906.1 Rat bite

E906.2 Bite of nonvenomous snakes and lizards

E906.3 Bite of other animal except arthropod
Cats
Moray eel
Rodents, except rats
Shark

E906.4 Bite of nonvenomous arthropod
Insect bite NOS

● **E906.5 Bite by unspecified animal**
Animal bite NOS

E906.8 Other specified injury caused by animal
Butted by animal
Fallen on by horse or other animal, not being ridden
Gored by animal
Implantation of quills of porcupine
Pecked by bird
Run over by animal, not being ridden
Stepped on by animal, not being ridden

Excludes: *injury by animal being ridden (E828.0-E828.9)*

E906.9 Unspecified injury caused by animal

E907 Lightning

Excludes: *injury from:*
fall of tree or other object caused by lightning (E916)
fire caused by lightning (E890.0-E892)

E908 Cataclysmic storms, and floods resulting from storms

Excludes: *collapse of dam or man-made structure causing flood (E909.3)*
transport accident occurring after storm (E800.0-E848)

● **E908.0 Hurricane**
Storm surge
"Tidal wave" caused by storm action
Typhoon

● **E908.1 Tornado**
Cyclone
Twisters

● **E908.2 Floods**

Torrential rainfall
Flash flood

Excludes: *collapse of dam or man-made structure causing flood (909.3)*

● **E908.3 Blizzard (snow) (ice)**

● **E908.4 Dust storm**

● **E908.8 Other cataclysmic storms**

● **E908.9 Unspecified cataclysmic storms, and floods resulting from storms**
Storm NOS

E909 Cataclysmic earth surface movements and eruptions

Excludes: *"tidal wave" caused by storm action (E908.0)*
transport accident involving collision with avalanche or landslide not in motion (E800.0-E848)

● **E909.0 Earthquakes**

● **E909.1 Volcanic eruptions**
Burns from lava
Ash inhalation

● **E909.2 Avalanche, landslide, or mudslide**

● **E909.3 Collapse of dam or man-made structure**

● **E909.4 Tidal wave caused by earthquake**
Tidal wave NOS
Tsunami

Excludes: *tidal wave caused by tropical storm (E908.0)*

● **E909.8 Other cataclysmic earth surface movements and eruptions**

● **E909.9 Unspecified cataclysmic earth surface movements and eruptions**

ACCIDENTS CAUSED BY SUBMERSION, SUFFOCATION, AND FOREIGN BODIES (E910-E915)

E910 Accidental drowning and submersion
Includes: immersion
swimmers' cramp

Excludes: *diving accident (NOS) (resulting in injury except drowning) (E883.0)*
diving with insufficient air supply (E913.2)
drowning and submersion due to:
cataclysm (E908-E909)
machinery accident (E919.0-E919.9)
transport accident (E800.0-E845.9)
effect of high and low air pressure (E902.2)
injury from striking against objects while in running water (E917.2)

E910.0 While water-skiing
Fall from water skis with submersion or drowning

Excludes: *accident to water-skier involving a watercraft and resulting in submersion or other injury (E830.4, E831.4)*

E910.1 While engaged in other sport or recreational activity with diving equipment
Scuba diving NOS
Skin diving NOS
Underwater spear fishing NOS

E910.2 While engaged in other sport or recreational activity without diving equipment
Fishing or hunting, except from boat or with diving equipment
Ice skating
Playing in water
Surfboarding
Swimming NOS
Voluntarily jumping from boat, not involved in accident, for swim NOS
Wading in water

Excludes: *jumping into water to rescue another person (E910.3)*

E910.3 While swimming or diving for purposes other than recreation or sport
Marine salvage
Pearl diving
Placement of fishing nets
Rescue (attempt) of another person
Underwater construction or repairs
} (with diving equipment)

E910.4 In bathtub

E910.8 Other accidental drowning or submersion
Drowning in:
quenching tank
swimming pool

E910.9 Unspecified accidental drowning or submersion
Accidental fall into water NOS
Drowning NOS

E911 Inhalation and ingestion of food causing obstruction of respiratory tract or suffocation
Aspiration and inhalation of food [any] (into respiratory tract) NOS
Asphyxia by } food [including bone, seed in food, regurgitated food]
Choked on } food [including bone, seed in food, regurgitated food]
Suffocation by } food [including bone, seed in food, regurgitated food]
Compression of trachea } by food lodged in esophagus
Interruption of respiration } by food lodged in esophagus
Obstruction of respiration } by food lodged in esophagus
Obstruction of pharynx by food (bolus)

Excludes: *injury, except asphyxia and obstruction of respiratory passage, caused by food (E915)*
obstruction of esophagus by food without mention of asphyxia or obstruction of respiratory passage (E915)

E912 Inhalation and ingestion of other object causing obstruction of respiratory tract or suffocation
Aspiration and inhalation of foreign body except food (into respiratory tract) NOS
Foreign object [bean] [marble] in nose
Obstruction of pharynx by foreign body
Compression } by foreign body in esophagus
Interruption of respiration } by foreign body in esophagus
Obstruction of respiration } by foreign body in esophagus

Excludes: *injury, except asphyxia and obstruction of respiratory passage, caused by foreign body (E915)*
obstruction of esophagus by foreign body without mention of asphyxia or obstruction in respiratory passage (E915)

E913 Accidental mechanical suffocation

Excludes: *mechanical suffocation from or by:*
accidental inhalation or ingestion of:
food (E911)
foreign object (E912)
cataclysm (E908-E909)
explosion (E921.0-E921.9, E923.0-E923.9)
machinery accident (E919.0-E919.9)

E913.0 In bed or cradle

Excludes: *suffocation by plastic bag (E913.1)*

E913.1 By plastic bag

E913.2 Due to lack of air (in closed place)
Accidentally closed up in refrigerator or other airtight enclosed space
Diving with insufficient air supply

Excludes: *suffocation by plastic bag (E913.1)*

E913.3 By falling earth or other substance
Cave-in NOS

Excludes: *cave-in caused by cataclysmic earth surface movements and eruptions (E909)*
struck by cave-in without asphyxiation or suffocation (E916)

E913.8 Other specified means
Accidental hanging, except in bed or cradle

E913.9 Unspecified means
Asphyxia, mechanical NOS
Strangulation NOS
Suffocation NOS

E914 Foreign body accidentally entering eye and adnexa

Excludes: *corrosive liquid (E924.1)*

E915 Foreign body accidentally entering other orifice

Excludes: *aspiration and inhalation of foreign body, any, (into respiratory tract) NOS (E911-E912)*

OTHER ACCIDENTS (E916-E928)

E916 Struck accidentally by falling object

Collapse of building, except on fire
Falling:
- rock
- snowslide NOS
- stone
- tree

Object falling from:
- machine, not in operation
- stationary vehicle

Excludes: *collapse of building on fire (E890.0-E891.9)*
falling object in:
- *cataclysm (E908-E909)*
- *machinery accidents (E919.0-E919.9)*
- *transport accidents (E800.0-E845.9)*
- *vehicle accidents not elsewhere classifiable (E846-E848)*

object set in motion by:
- *explosion (E921.0-E921.9, E923.0-E923.9)*
- *firearm (E922.0-E922.9)*

projected object (E917.0-E917.9)

E917 Striking against or struck accidentally by objects or persons

Includes:

bumping into or against / colliding with / kicking against / stepping on / struck by } object (moving) (projected) (stationary); pedestrian conveyance; person

Excludes: *fall from:*
- *bumping into or against object (E888)*
- *collision with another person, except when caused by a crowd (E886.0-E886.9)*
- *stumbling over object (E885)*

injury caused by:
- *assault (E960.0-E960.1, E967.0-E967.9)*
- *cutting or piercing instrument (E920.0-E920.9)*
- *explosion (E921.0-E921.9, E923.0-E923.9)*
- *firearm (E922.0-E922.9)*
- *machinery (E919.0-E919.9)*
- *transport vehicle (E800.0-E845.9)*
- *vehicle not elsewhere classifiable (E846-E848)*

E917.0 In sports

Kicked or stepped on during game (football) (rugby)
Knocked down while boxing
Struck by hit or thrown ball
Struck by hockey stick or puck

E917.1 Caused by a crowd, by collective fear or panic

Crushed / Pushed / Stepped on } by crown or human stampede

E917.2 In running water

Excludes: *drowning or submersion (E910.0-E910.9)*
that in sports (E917.0)

E917.9 Other

Accident caused by air rifle [BB gun]

E918 Caught accidentally in or between objects

Caught, crushed, jammed, or pinched in or between moving or stationary objects, such as:
- escalator
- folding object
- hand tools, appliances, or implements
- sliding door and door frame
- under packing crate
- washing machine wringer

continued

Add 4th or 5th digit | Nonspecific code | Unspecified code | Manifestation code

Excludes: *injury caused by:*
cutting or piercing instrument (E920.0-E920.9)
machinery (E919.0-E919.9)
transport vehicle (E800.0-E845.9)
vehicle not elsewhere classifiable (E846-E848)
struck accidentally by:
falling object (E916)
object (moving) (projected) (E917.0-E917.9)

E919 Accidents caused by machinery

Includes:

burned by caught in (moving parts of) collapse of crushed by cut or pierced by drowning or submersion caused by explosion of, on, in fall from or into moving part of fire starting in or on mechanical suffocation caused by object falling from, on, in motion by overturning of pinned under run over by struck by thrown from	machinery (accident)

caught between machinery and other object
machinery accident NOS

Excludes: *accidents involving machinery, not in operation (E884.9, E916-E918)*
injury caused by:
electric current in connection with machinery (E925.0-E925.9)
escalator (E880.0, E918)
explosion of pressure vessel in connection with machinery (E921.0-E921.9)
moving sidewalk (E885)
powered hand tools, appliances, and implements (E916-E918, E920.0-E921.9, E923.0-E926.9)
transport vehicle accidents involving machinery (E800.0-E848.9)
poisoning by carbon monoxide generated by machine (E868.8)

E919.0 Agriculture machines

Animal-powered agricultural machine
Combine
Derrick, hay
Farm machinery NOS
Farm tractor
Harvester
Hay mower or rake
Reaper
Thresher

Excludes: *that in transport under own power on the highway (E810.0-E819.9)*
that being towed by another vehicle on the highway (E810.0-E819.9, E827.0-E827.9, E829.0-E829.9)
that involved in accident classifiable to E820-E829 (E820.0-E829.9)

E919.1 Mining and earth-drilling machinery

Bore or drill (land) (seabed)
Shaft hoist
Shaft lift
Under-cutter

Excludes: *coal car, tram, truck, and tub in mine (E846)*

E919.2 Lifting machines and appliances

Chain hoist Crane Derrick Elevator (building) (grain) Forklift truck Lift Pulley block Winch	except in agricultural or mining operations

Excludes: *that being towed by another vehicle on the highway (E810.0-E819.9, E827.0-E827.9, E829.0-E829.9)*
that in transport under own power on the highway (E810.0-E819.9)
that involved in accident classifiable to E820-E829 (E820.0-E829.9)

E919.3 Metalworking machines
Abrasive wheel
Forging machine
Lathe
Mechanical shears
Metal:
  drilling machine
  milling machine
  power press
  rolling-mill
  sawing machine

E919.4 Woodworking and forming machines
Band saw
Bench saw
Circular saw
Molding machine
Overhead plane
Powered saw
Radial saw
Sander

Excludes: *hand saw (E920.1)*

E919.5 Prime movers, except electrical motors
Gas turbine
Internal combustion engine
Steam engine
Water driven turbine

Excludes: *that being towed by other vehicle on the highway (E810.0-E819.9, E827.0-E827.9, E829.0-E829.9)*
that in transport under own power on the highway (E810.0-E819.9)

E919.6 Transmission machinery
Transmission:
  belt
  cable
  chain
  gear
  pinion
  pulley
  shaft

E919.7 Earth moving, scraping, and other excavating machines
Bulldozer
Road scraper
Steam shovel

Excludes: *that being towed by other vehicle on the highway (E810.0-E819.9, E827.0-E827.9, E829.0-E829.9)*
that in transport under own power on the highway (E810.0-E819.9)

E919.8 Other specified machinery
Machines for manufacture of:
  clothing
  foodstuffs and beverages
  paper
Printing machine
Recreational machinery
Spinning, weaving, and textile machines

E919.9 Unspecified machinery

E920 Accidents caused by cutting and piercing instruments or objects
Includes: accidental injury by fall on object:
  edged
  pointed
  sharp

E920.0 Powered lawn mower

E920.1 Other powered hand tools
Any powered hand tool [compressed air] [electric] [explosive cartridge] [hydraulic power], such as:
  drill
  hand saw
  hedge clipper
  rivet gun
  snow blower
  staple gun

Excludes: *band saw (E919.4)*
bench saw (E919.4)

E920.2 Powered household appliances and implements
Blender
Electric:
  beater or mixer
  can opener
  fan
  knife
  sewing machine
Garbage disposal appliance

E920.3 Knives, swords, and daggers

Add 4th or 5th digit | Nonspecific code | Unspecified code | Manifestation code

E920.4 Other hand tools and implements

Axe
Can opener NOS
Chisel
Fork
Hand saw
Hoe
Ice pick
Needle (sewing)
Paper cutter
Pitchfork
Rake
Scissors
Screwdriver
Sewing machine, not powered
Shovel

● **E920.5 Hypodermic needle**

Contaminated needle
Needle stick

E920.8 Other specified cutting and piercing instruments or objects

Arrow
Broken glass
Dart
Edge of stiff paper
Lathe turnings
Nail
Plant thorn
Splinter
Tin can lid

Excludes: *animal spines or quills (E906.8)*
flying glass due to explosion (E921.0-E923.9)

E920.9 Unspecified cutting and piercing instrument or object

E921 Accident caused by explosion of pressure vessel

Includes: accidental explosion of pressure vessels, whether or not part of machinery

Excludes: *explosion of pressure vessel on transport vehicle (E800.0-E845.9)*

E921.0 Boilers

E921.1 Gas cylinders

Air tank
Pressure gas tank

E921.8 Other specified pressure vessels

Aerosol can
Automobile tire
Pressure cooker

E921.9 Unspecified pressure vessel

E922 Accident caused by firearm missile

E922.0 Handgun

Pistol
Revolver

Excludes: *Verey pistol (E922.8)*

E922.1 Shotgun (automatic)

E922.2 Hunting rifle

Excludes: *air rifle [BB gun] (E917.9)*

E922.3 Military firearms

Army rifle
Machine gun

E922.8 Other specified firearm missile

Verey pistol [flare]

E922.9 Unspecified firearm missile

Gunshot wound NOS
Shot NOS

E923 Accident caused by explosive material

Includes: flash burns and other injuries resulting from explosion of explosive material
ignition of highly explosive material with explosion

Excludes: *explosion:*
in or on machinery (E919.0-E919.9)
on any transport vehicle, except stationary motor vehicle (E800.0-E848)
with conflagration (E890.0, E891.0, E892)
secondary fires resulting from explosion (E890.0-E899)

E923.0 Fireworks

E923.1 Blasting materials

Blasting cap
Detonator
Dynamite
Explosive [any] used in blasting operations

E923.2 Explosive gases

Acetylene
Butane
Coal gas
Explosion in mine NOS
Fire damp
Gasoline fumes
Methane
Propane

E923.8 Other explosive materials

Bomb
Explosive missile
Grenade
Mine
Shell
Torpedo
Explosion in munitions:
 dump
 factory

E923.9 Unspecified explosive material

Explosion NOS

E924 Accident caused by hot substance or object, caustic or corrosive material, and steam

Excludes: *burning NOS (E899)*
chemical burn resulting from swallowing a corrosive substance (E860.0-E864.4)
fire caused by these substances and objects (E890.0-E894)
radiation burns (E926.0-E926.9)
therapeutic misadventures (E870.0-E876.9)

E924.0 Hot liquids and vapors, including steam

Burning or scalding by:
 boiling water
 hot or boiling liquids not primarily caustic or corrosive
 liquid metal
 steam
 other hot vapor

Excludes: *hot (boiling) tap water (E924.2)*

E924.1 Caustic and corrosive substances

Burning by:
 acid [any kind]
 ammonia
 caustic oven cleaner or other substance
 corrosive substance
 lye
 vitriol

● **E924.2 Hot (boiling) tap water**

E924.8 Other

Burning by:
 heat from electric heating appliance
 hot object NOS
 light bulb
 steam pipe

E924.9 Unspecified

E925 Accident caused by electric current

Includes: electric current from exposed wire, faulty appliance, high voltage cable, live rail, or open electric socket as the cause of:
 burn
 cardiac fibrillation
 convulsion
 electric shock
 electrocution
 puncture wound
 respiratory paralysis

Excludes: *burn by heat from electrical appliance (E924.8)*
lightning (E907)

E925.0 Domestic wiring and appliances

E925.1 Electric power generating plants, distribution stations, transmission lines

Broken power line

E925.2 Industrial wiring, appliances, and electrical machinery

Conductors
Control apparatus
Electrical equipment and machinery
Transformers

E925.8 Other electric current

Wiring and appliances in or on:
- farm [not farmhouse]
- outdoors
- public building

Wiring and appliances in or on:
- residential institutions
- schools

E925.9 Unspecified electric current

Burns or other injury from electric current NOS
Electric shock NOS
Electrocution NOS

E926 Exposure to radiation

Excludes: *abnormal reaction to or complication of treatment without mention of misadventure (E879.2)*
atomic power plant malfunction in water transport (E838.0-E838.9)
misadventure to patient in surgical and medical procedures (E873.2-E873.3)
use of radiation in war operations (E996-E997.9)

E926.0 Radiofrequency radiation

Overexposure to:
- microwave radiation
- radar radiation
- radiofrequency
- radiofrequency radiation [any]

from:
- high-powered radio and television transmitters
- industrial radiofrequency induction heaters
- radar installations

E926.1 Infra-red heaters and lamps

Exposure to infra-red radiation from heaters and lamps as the cause of:
- blistering
- burning
- charring
- inflammatory change

Excludes: *physical contact with heater or lamp (E924.8)*

E926.2 Visible and ultraviolet light sources

Arc lamps
Black light sources
Electrical welding arc
Oxygas welding torch
Sun rays

Excludes: *excessive heat from these sources (E900.1-E900.9)*

E926.3 X-rays and other electromagnetic ionizing radiation

Gamma rays
X-rays (hard) (soft)

E926.4 Lasers

E926.5 Radioactive isotopes

Radiobiologicals
Radiopharmaceuticals

E926.8 Other specified radiation

Artificially accelerated beams of ionized particles generated by:
- betatrons
- synchrotrons

E926.9 Unspecified radiation

Radiation NOS

E927 Overexertion and strenuous movements

Excessive physical exercise
Overexertion (from):
- lifting
- pulling
- pushing

Strenuous movements in:
- recreational activities
- other activities

E928 Other and unspecified environmental and accidental causes

E928.0 Prolonged stay in weightless environment

Weightlessness in spacecraft (simulator)

E928.1 Exposure to noise

Noise (pollution)
Sound waves
Supersonic waves

E928.2 Vibration

E928.8 Other

E928.9 Unspecified accident

Accident NOS
Blow NOS

Casualty (not due to war) Decapitation Injury [any part of body, or unspecified] Killed Knocked down Mangled Wound	} stated as accidentally inflicted, but not otherwise specified

Excludes: *fracture, cause unspecified (E887)*
injuries undetermined whether accidentally or purposely inflicted (E980.0-E989)

LATE EFFECTS OF ACCIDENTAL INJURY (E929)

Note: This category is to be used to indicate accidental injury as the cause of death or disability from late effects, which are themselves classifiable elsewhere. The "late effects" include conditions reported as such or as sequelae which may occur at any time after the acute injury.

E929 Late effects of accidental injury

Excludes: *late effects of:*
surgical and medical procedures (E870.0-E879.9)
therapeutic use of drugs and medicines (E930.0-E949.9)

E929.0 Late effects of motor vehicle accident
Late effects of accidents classifiable to E810-E825

E929.1 Late effects of other transport accident
Late effects of accidents classifiable to E800-E807, E826-E838, E840-E848

E929.2 Late effects of accidental poisoning
Late effects of accidents classifiable to E850-E858, E860-E869

E929.3 Late effects of accidental fall
Late effects of accidents classifiable to E880-E888

E929.4 Late effects of accident caused by fire
Late effects of accidents classifiable to E890-E899

E929.5 Late effects of accident due to natural and environmental factors
Late effects of accidents classifiable to E900-E909

E929.8 Late effects of other accidents
Late effects of accidents classifiable to E910-E928.8

E929.9 Late effects of unspecified accident
Late effects of accidents classifiable to E928.9

DRUGS, MEDICINAL AND BIOLOGICAL SUBSTANCES CAUSING ADVERSE EFFECTS IN THERAPEUTIC USE (E930-E949)

Includes: correct drug properly administered in therapeutic or prophylactic dosage, as the cause of any adverse effect including allergic or hypersensitivity reactions

Excludes: *accidental overdose of drug and wrong drug given or taken in error (E850.0-E858.9)*
accidents in the technique of administration of drug or biological substance, such as accidental puncture during injection, or contamination of drug (E870.0-E876.9)
administration with suicidal or homicidal intent or intent to harm, or in circumstances classifiable to E980-E989 (E950.0-E950.5, E962.0, E980.0-E980.5)

See Alphabetic Index for more complete list of specific drugs to be classified under the fourth-digit subdivisions. The American Hospital Formulary numbers can be used to classify new drugs listed by the American Hospital Formulary Service (AHFS). See appendix C.

E930 Antibiotics

Excludes: *that used as eye, ear, nose, and throat [ENT], and local anti-infectives (E946.0-E946.9)*

E930.0 Penicillins
Natural
Synthetic
Semisynthetic, such as:
ampicillin
cloxacillin
nafcillin
oxacillin

E930.1 Antifungal antibiotics
Amphotericin B
Griseofulvin
Hachimycin [trichomycin]
Nystatin

Add 4th or 5th digit | Nonspecific code | Unspecified code | Manifestation code

E930.2 Chloramphenicol group
Chloramphenicol
Thiamphenicol

E930.3 Erythromycin and other macrolides
Oleandomycin
Spiramycin

E930.4 Tetracycline group
Doxycycline
Minocycline
Oxytetracycline

E930.5 Cephalosporin group
Cephalexin
Cephaloglycin
Cephaloridine
Cephalothin

E930.6 Antimycobacterial antibiotics
Cycloserine
Kanamycin
Rifampin
Streptomycin

E930.7 Antineoplastic antibiotics
Actinomycins, such as:
Cactinomycin
Dactinomycin
Bleomycin
Daunorubicin
Mitomycin

Excludes: *other antineoplastic drugs (E933.1)*

E930.8 Other specified antibiotics

E930.9 Unspecified antibiotic

E931 Other anti-infectives

Excludes: *ENT, and local anti-infectives (E946.0-E946.9)*

E931.0 Sulfonamides
Sulfadiazine
Sulfafurazole
Sulfamethoxazole

E931.1 Arsenical anti-infectives

E931.2 Heavy metal anti-infectives
Compounds of:
antimony
bismuth
Compounds of:
lead
mercury

Excludes: *mercurial diuretics (E944.0)*

E931.3 Quinoline and hydroxyquinoline derivatives
Chiniofon
Diiodohydroxyquin

Excludes: *antimalarial drugs (E931.4)*

E931.4 Antimalarials and drugs acting on other blood protozoa
Chloroquine phosphate
Cycloguanil
Primaquine
Proguanil [chloroguanide]
Pyrimethamine
Quinine (sulphate)

E931.5 Other antiprotozoal drugs
Emetine

E931.6 Anthelmintics
Hexylresorcinol
Male fern oleoresin
Piperazine
Thiabendazole

E931.7 Antiviral drugs
Methisazone

Excludes: *amantadine (E936.4)*
cytarabine (E933.1)
idoxuridine (E946.5)

E931.8 Other antimycobacterial drugs
Ethambutol
Ethionamide
Isoniazid
Para-aminosalicylic acid derivatives
Sulfones

E931.9 Other and unspecified anti-infectives
Flucytosine
Nitrofuran derivatives

E932 Hormones and synthetic substitutes

E932.0 Adrenal cortical steroids
Cortisone derivatives
Desoxycorticosterone derivatives
Fluorinated corticosteroids

E932.1 Androgens and anabolic congeners
Nandrolone phenpropionate
Oxymetholone
Testosterone and preparations

E932.2 Ovarian hormones and synthetic substitutes
Contraceptives, oral
Estrogens
Estrogens and progestogens combined
Progestogens

E932.3 Insulins and antidiabetic agents
Acetohexamide
Biguanide derivatives, oral
Chlorpropamide
Glucagon
Insulin
Phenformin
Sulfonylurea derivatives, oral
Tolbutamide

Excludes: *adverse effect of insulin administered for shock therapy (E879.3)*

E932.4 Anterior pituitary hormones
Corticotropin
Gonadotropin
Somatotropin [growth hormone]

E932.5 Posterior pituitary hormones
Vasopressin

Excludes: *oxytocic agents (E945.0)*

E932.6 Parathyroid and parathyroid derivatives

E932.7 Thyroid and thyroid derivatives
Dextrothyroxine
Levothyroxine sodium
Liothyronine
Thyroglobulin

E932.8 Antithyroid agents
Iodides
Thiouracil
Thiourea

E932.9 Other and unspecified hormones and synthetic substitutes

E933 Primarily systemic agents

E933.0 Antiallergic and antiemetic drugs
Antihistamines
Chlorpheniramine
Diphenhydramine
Diphenylpyraline
Thonzylamine
Tripelennamine

Excludes: *phenothiazine-based tranquilizers (E939.1)*

E933.1 Antineoplastic and immunosuppressive drugs
Azathioprine
Busulfan
Chlorambucil
Cyclophosphamide
Cytarabine
Fluorouracil
Mechlorethamine hydrochloride
Mercaptopurine
Triethylenethiophosphoramide [thio-TEPA]

Excludes: *antineoplastic antibiotics (E930.7)*

E933.2 Acidifying agents

E933.3 Alkalizing agents

E933.4 Enzymes, not elsewhere classified
Penicillinase

E933.5 Vitamins, not elsewhere classified
Vitamin A
Vitamin D

Excludes: *nicotinic acid (E942.2)*
vitamin K (E934.3)

E933.8 Other systemic agents, not elsewhere classified
Heavy metal antagonists

E933.9 Unspecified systemic agent

E934 Agents primarily affecting blood constituents

E934.0 Iron and its compounds
Ferric salts
Ferrous sulphate and other ferrous salts

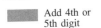

E934.1 Liver preparations and other antianemic agents
Folic acid

E934.2 Anticoagulants
Coumarin
Heparin
Phenindione
Prothrombin synthesis inhibitor
Warfarin sodium

E934.3 Vitamin K [phytonadione]

E934.4 Fibrinolysis-affecting drugs
Aminocaproic acid
Streptodornase
Streptokinase
Urokinase

E934.5 Anticoagulant antagonists and other coagulants
Hexadimethrine bromide
Protamine sulfate

E934.6 Gamma globulin

E934.7 Natural blood and blood products
Blood plasma
Human fibrinogen
Packed red cells
Whole blood

E934.8 Other agents affecting blood constituents
Macromolecular blood substitutes

E934.9 Unspecified agent affecting blood constituents

E935 Analgesics, antipyretics, and antirheumatics

E935.0 Heroin
Diacetylmorphine

□ **E935.1 Methadone**

□ **E935.2 Other opiates and related narcotics**
Codeine [methylmorphine]
Morphine
Opium (alkaloids)
Meperidine [pethidine]

□ **E935.3 Salicylates**
Acetylsalicylic acid [aspirin]
Amino derivatives of salicylic acid
Salicylic acid salts

□ **E935.4 Aromatic analgesics, not elsewhere classified**
Acetanilid
Paracetamol [acetaminophen]
Phenacetin [acetophenetidin]

□ **E935.5 Pyrazole derivatives**
Aminophenazone [aminopyrine]
Phenylbutazone

□ **E935.6 Antirheumatics [antiphlogistics]**
Gold salts
Indomethacin

Excludes: *salicylates (E935.3)*
steroids (E932.0)

□ **E935.7 Other non-narcotic analgesics**
Pyrabital

E935.8 Other specified analgesics and antipyretics
Pentazocine

E935.9 Unspecified analgesic and antipyretic

E936 Anticonvulsants and anti-Parkinsonism drugs

E936.0 Oxazolidine derivatives
Paramethadione
Trimethadione

E936.1 Hydantoin derivatives
Phenytoin

E936.2 Succinimides
Ethosuximide
Phensuximide

E936.3 Other and unspecified anticonvulsants
Beclamide
Primidone

E936.4 Anti-Parkinsonism drugs
Amantadine
Ethopropazine [profenamine]
Levodopa [L-dopa]

E937 Sedatives and hypnotics

E937.0 Barbiturates
Amobarbital [amylobarbitone]
Barbital [barbitone]

Butabarbital [butabarbitone]
Pentobarbital [pentobarbitone]
Phenobarbital [phenobarbitone]
Secobarbital [quinalbarbitone]

Excludes: *thiobarbiturates (E938.3)*

E937.1 Chloral hydrate group

E937.2 Paraldehyde

E937.3 Bromine compounds
Bromide
Carbromal (derivatives)

E937.4 Methaqualone compounds

E937.5 Glutethimide group

E937.6 Mixed sedatives, not elsewhere classified

E937.8 Other sedatives and hypnotics

E937.9 Unspecified
Sleeping:
drug, pill, tablet } NOS

E938 Other central nervous system depressants and anesthetics

E938.0 Central nervous system muscle-tone depressants
Chlorphenesin (carbamate)
Mephenesin
Methocarbamol

E938.1 Halothane

E938.2 Other gaseous anesthetics
Ether
Halogenated hydrocarbon derivatives, except halothane
Nitrous oxide

E938.3 Intravenous anesthetics
Ketamine
Methohexital [methohexitone]
Thiobarbiturates, such as thiopental sodium

E938.4 Other and unspecified general anesthetics

E938.5 Surface and infiltration anesthetics
Cocaine
Lidocaine [lignocaine]
Procaine
Tetracaine

E938.6 Peripheral nerve- and plexus-blocking anesthetics

E938.7 Spinal anesthetics

E938.9 Other and unspecified local anesthetics

E939 Psychotropic agents

E939.0 Antidepressants
Amitriptyline
Imipramine
Monoamine oxidase [MAO] inhibitors

E939.1 Phenothiazine-based tranquilizers
Chlorpromazine
Fluphenazine
Phenothiazine
Prochlorperazine
Promazine

E939.2 Butyrophenone-based tranquilizers
Haloperidol
Spiperone
Trifluperidol

E939.3 Other antipsychotics, neuroleptics, and major tranquilizers

E939.4 Benzodiazepine-based tranquilizers
Chlordiazepoxide
Diazepam
Flurazepam
Lorazepam
Medazepam
Nitrazepam

E939.5 Other tranquilizers
Hydroxyzine
Meprobamate

E939.6 Psychodysleptics [hallucinogens]
Cannabis (derivatives)
Lysergide [LSD]
Marihuana (derivatives)
Mescaline
Psilocin
Psilocybin

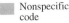

E939.7 Psychostimulants
Amphetamine
Caffeine

Excludes: *central appetite depressants (E947.0)*

E939.8 Other psychotropic agents

E939.9 Unspecified psychotropic agent

E940 Central nervous system stimulants

E940.0 Analeptics
Lobeline
Nikethamide

E940.1 Opiate antagonists
Levallorphan
Nalorphine
Naloxone

E940.8 Other specified central nervous system stimulants

E940.9 Unspecified central nervous system stimulant

E941 Drugs primarily affecting the autonomic nervous system

E941.0 Parasympathomimetics [cholinergics]
Acetylcholine
Anticholinesterase:
organophosphorus
reversible
Pilocarpine

E941.1 Parasympatholytics [anticholinergics and antimuscarinics] and spasmolytics
Atropine
Homatropine
Hyoscine [scopolamine]
Quaternary ammonium derivatives

Excludes: *papaverine (E942.5)*

E941.2 Sympathomimetics [adrenergics]
Epinephrine [adrenalin]
Levarterenol [noradrenalin]

E941.3 Sympatholytics [antiadrenergics]
Phenoxybenzamine
Tolazoline hydrochloride

E941.9 Unspecified drug primarily affecting the autonomic nervous system

E942 Agents primarily affecting the cardiovascular system

E942.0 Cardiac rhythm regulators
Practolol
Procainamide
Propranolol
Quinidine

E942.1 Cardiotonic glycosides and drugs of similar action
Digitalis glycosides
Digoxin
Strophanthins

E942.2 Antilipemic and antiarteriosclerotic drugs
Cholestyramine
Clofibrate
Nicotinic acid derivatives
Sitosterols

Excludes: *dextrothyroxine (E932.7)*

E942.3 Ganglion-blocking agents
Pentamethonium bromide

E942.4 Coronary vasodilators
Dipyridamole
Nitrates [nitroglycerin]
Nitrites
Prenylamine

E942.5 Other vasodilators
Cyclandelate
Diazoxide
Hydralazine
Papaverine

E942.6 Other antihypertensive agents
Clonidine
Guanethidine
Rauwolfia alkaloids
Reserpine

E942.7 Antivaricose drugs, including sclerosing agents
Monoethanolamine
Zinc salts

E942.8 Capillary-active drugs
Adrenochrome derivatives
Bioflavonoids
Metaraminol

E942.9 Other and unspecified agents primarily affecting the cardiovascular system

E943 Agents primarily affecting gastrointestinal system

E943.0 Antacids and antigastric secretion drugs
Aluminum hydroxide
Magnesium trisilicate

E943.1 Irritant cathartics
Bisacodyl
Castor oil
Phenolphthalein

E943.2 Emollient cathartics
Sodium dioctyl sulfosuccinate

E943.3 Other cathartics, including intestinal atonia drugs
Magnesium sulfate

E943.4 Digestants
Pancreatin
Papain
Pepsin

E943.5 Antidiarrheal drugs
Bismuth subcarbonate
Kaolin
Pectin

Excludes: *anti-infectives (E930.0-E931.9)*

E943.6 Emetics

E943.8 Other specified agents primarily affecting the gastrointestinal system

E943.9 Unspecified agent primarily affecting the gastrointestinal system

E944 Water, mineral, and uric acid metabolism drugs

E944.0 Mercurial diuretics
Chlormerodrin
Mercaptomerin
Mercurophylline
Mersalyl

E944.1 Purine derivative diuretics
Theobromine
Theophylline

Excludes: *aminophylline [theophylline ethylenediamine] (E945.7)*

E944.2 Carbonic acid anhydrase inhibitors
Acetazolamide

E944.3 Saluretics
Benzothiadiazides
Chlorothiazide group

E944.4 Other diuretics
Ethacrynic acid
Furosemide

E944.5 Electrolytic, caloric, and water-balance agents

E944.6 Other mineral salts, not elsewhere classified

E944.7 Uric acid metabolism drugs
Cinchophen and congeners
Colchicine
Phenoquin
Probenecid

E945 Agents primarily acting on the smooth and skeletal muscles and respiratory system

E945.0 Oxytocic agents
Ergot alkaloids
Prostaglandins

E945.1 Smooth muscle relaxants
Adiphenine
Metaproterenol [orciprenaline]

Excludes: *papaverine (E942.5)*

E945.2 Skeletal muscle relaxants
Alcuronium chloride
Suxamethonium chloride

E945.3 Other and unspecified drugs acting on muscles

E945.4 Antitussives
Dextromethorphan
Pipazethate hydrochloride

E945.5 Expectorants
Acetylcysteine
Cocillana
Guaifenesin [glyceryl guaiacolate]
Ipecacuanha
Terpin hydrate

E945.6 Anti-common cold drugs

E945.7 Antiasthmatics
Aminophylline [theophylline ethylenediamine]

E945.8 Other and unspecified respiratory drugs

E946 Agents primarily affecting skin and mucous membrane, ophthalmological, otorhinolaryngological, and dental drugs

E946.0 Local anti-infectives and anti-inflammatory drugs

Add 4th or 5th digit | Nonspecific code | Unspecified code | Manifestation code

E946.1 Antipruritics

E946.2 Local astringents and local detergents

E946.3 Emollients, demulcents, and protectants

E946.4 Keratolytics, keratoplastics, other hair treatment drugs and preparations

E946.5 Eye anti-infectives and other eye drugs
Idoxuridine

E946.6 Anti-infectives and other drugs and preparations for ear, nose, and throat

E946.7 Dental drugs topically applied

E946.8 Other agents primarily affecting skin and mucous membrane
Spermicides

E946.9 Unspecified agent primarily affecting skin and mucous membrane

E947 Other and unspecified drugs and medicinal substances

E947.0 Dietetics

E947.1 Lipotropic drugs

E947.2 Antidotes and chelating agents, not elsewhere classified

E947.3 Alcohol deterrents

E947.4 Pharmaceutical excipients

E947.8 Other drugs and medicinal substances
Contrast media used for diagnostic x-ray procedures
Diagnostic agents and kits

E947.9 Unspecified drug or medicinal substance

E948 Bacterial vaccines

E948.0 BCG vaccine

E948.1 Typhoid and paratyphoid

E948.2 Cholera

E948.3 Plague

E948.4 Tetanus

E948.5 Diphtheria

E948.6 Pertussis vaccine, including combinations with a pertussis component

E948.8 Other and unspecified bacterial vaccines

E948.9 Mixed bacterial vaccines, except combinations with a pertussis component

E949 Other vaccines and biological substances

Excludes: *gamma globulin (E934.6)*

E949.0 Smallpox vaccine

E949.1 Rabies vaccine

E949.2 Typhus vaccine

E949.3 Yellow fever vaccine

E949.4 Measles vaccine

E949.5 Poliomyelitis vaccine

E949.6 Other and unspecified viral and rickettsial vaccines
Mumps vaccine

E949.7 Mixed viral-rickettsial and bacterial vaccines, except combinations with a pertussis component

Excludes: *combinations with a pertussis component (E948.6)*

E949.9 Other and unspecified vaccines and biological substances

SUICIDE AND SELF-INFLICTED INJURY (E950-E959)

Includes: injuries in suicide and attempted suicide
self-inflicted injuries specified as intentional

E950 Suicide and self-inflicted poisoning by solid or liquid substances

E950.0 Analgesics, antipyretics, and antirheumatics

E950.1 Barbiturates

E950.2 Other sedatives and hypnotics

E950.3 Tranquilizers and other psychotropic agents

E950.4 Other specified drugs and medicinal substances

E950.5 Unspecified drug or medicinal substances

E950.6 Agricultural and horticultural chemical and pharmaceutical preparations other than plant foods and fertilizers

E950.7 Corrosive and caustic substances
Suicide and self-inflicted poisoning by substances classifiable to E864

E950.8 Arsenic and its compounds

E950.9 Other and unspecified solid and liquid substances

E951 Suicide and self-inflicted poisoning by gases in domestic use

E951.0 Gas distributed by pipeline

E951.1 Liquefied petroleum gas distributed in mobile containers

E951.8 Other utility gas

E952 Suicide and self-inflicted poisoning by other gases and vapors

E952.0 Motor vehicle exhaust gas

E952.1 Other carbon monoxide

E952.8 Other specified gases and vapors

E952.9 Unspecified gases and vapors

E953 Suicide and self-inflicted injury by hanging, strangulation, and suffocation

E953.0 Hanging

E953.1 Suffocation by plastic bag

E953.8 Other specified means

E953.9 Unspecified means

E954 Suicide and self-inflicted injury by submersion [drowning]

E955 Suicide and self-inflicted injury by firearms and explosives

E955.0 Handgun

E955.1 Shotgun

E955.2 Hunting rifle

E955.3 Military firearms

E955.4 Other and unspecified firearm
Gunshot NOS
Shot NOS

E955.5 Explosives

E955.9 Unspecified

E956 Suicide and self-inflicted injury by cutting and piercing instrument

E957 Suicide and self-inflicted injuries by jumping from high place

E957.0 Residential premises

E957.1 Other man-made structures

E957.2 Natural sites

E957.9 Unspecified

E958 Suicide and self-inflicted injury by other and unspecified means

E958.0 Jumping or lying before moving object

E958.1 Burns, fire

E958.2 Scald

E958.3 Extremes of cold

E958.4 Electrocution

E958.5 Crashing of motor vehicle

E958.6 Crashing of aircraft

E958.7 Caustic substances, except poisoning
Excludes: *poisoning by caustic substance (E950.7)*

E958.8 Other specified means

E958.9 Unspecified means

E959 Late effects of self-inflicted injury

Note: This category is to be used to indicate circumstances classifiable to E950-E958 as the cause of death or disability from late effects, which are themselves classifiable elsewhere. The "late effects" include conditions reported as such or as sequelae which may occur at any time after the attempted suicide or self-inflicted injury.

HOMICIDE AND INJURY PURPOSELY INFLICTED BY OTHER PERSONS (E960-E969)

Includes: injuries inflicted by another person with intent to injure or kill, by any means

Excludes: *injuries due to:*
legal intervention (E970-E978)
operations of war (E990-E999)

E960 Fight, brawl, rape

E960.0 Unarmed fight or brawl
Beatings NOS
Brawl or fight with hands, fists, feet
Injured or killed in fight NOS

Excludes: *homicidal:*
injury by weapons (E965.0-E966, E969)
strangulation (E963)
submersion (E964)

E960.1 Rape

E961 Assault by corrosive or caustic substance, except poisoning
Injury or death purposely caused by corrosive or caustic substance, such as:
acid [any]
corrosive substance
vitriol

Excludes: *burns from hot liquid (E968.3)*
chemical burns from swallowing a corrosive substance (E962.0-E962.9)

E962 Assault by poisoning

E962.0 Drugs and medicinal substances
Homicidal poisoning by any drug or medicinal substance

E962.1 Other solid and liquid substances

E962.2 Other gases and vapors

E962.9 Unspecified poisoning

E963 Assault by hanging and strangulation
Homicidal (attempt):
garrotting or ligature
hanging
strangulation
suffocation

E964 Assault by submersion [drowning]

E965 Assault by firearms and explosives

E965.0 Handgun
Pistol
Revolver

E965.1 Shotgun

E965.2 Hunting rifle

E965.3 Military firearms

E965.4 Other and unspecified firearm

E965.5 Antipersonnel bomb

E965.6 Gasoline bomb

E965.7 Letter bomb

E965.8 Other specified explosive
Bomb NOS (placed in):
car
house
Dynamite

E965.9 Unspecified explosive

E966 Assault by cutting and piercing instrument

Assassination (attempt), homicide (attempt) by any instrument classifiable under E920
Homicidal:
- cut, puncture, stab } any part of body
- Stabbed } any part of body

E967 Child battering and other maltreatment

E967.0 By parent

E967.1 By other specified person

E967.9 By unspecified person

E968 Assault by other and unspecified means

E968.0 Fire
Arson
Homicidal burns NOS

Excludes: *burns from hot liquid (E968.3)*

E968.1 Pushing from a high place

E968.2 Striking by blunt or thrown object

E968.3 Hot liquid
Homicidal burns by scalding

E968.4 Criminal neglect
Abandonment of child, infant, or other helpless person with intent to injure or kill

● **E968.5 Transport vehicle**
Being struck by other vehicle or run down with intent to injure
Pushed in front of, thrown from, or dragged by moving vehicle with intent to injure

E968.8 Other specified means
Bite of human being

E968.9 Unspecified means
Assassination (attempt) NOS
Homicidal (attempt):
- injury NOS
- wound NOS

Manslaughter (nonaccidental)
Murder (attempt) NOS
Violence, non-accidental

E969 Late effects of injury purposely inflicted by other person

Note: This category is to be used to indicate circumstances classifiable to E960-E968 as the cause of death or disability from late effects, which are themselves classifiable elsewhere. The "late effects" include conditions reported as such, or as sequelae which may occur at any time after the acute injury.

LEGAL INTERVENTION (E970-E978)

Includes: injuries inflicted by the police or other law-enforcing agents, including military on duty, in the course of arresting or attempting to arrest lawbreakers, suppressing disturbances, maintaining order, and other legal action
legal execution

Excludes: *injuries caused by civil insurrections (E990.0-E999)*

E970 Injury due to legal intervention by firearms
Gunshot wound
Injury by:
- machine gun
- revolver

Injury by:
- rifle pellet or rubber bullet
- shot NOS

E971 Injury due to legal intervention by explosives
Injury by:
- dynamite
- explosive shell
- grenade
- mortar bomb

E972 Injury due to legal intervention by gas
Asphyxiation by gas
Injury by tear gas
Poisoning by gas

E973 Injury due to legal intervention by blunt object
Hit, struck by:
- baton (nightstick)
- blunt object
- stave

E974 Injury due to legal intervention by cutting and piercing instrument
Cut
Injured by bayonet
Incised wound
Stab wound

E975 Injury due to legal intervention by other specified means
Blow
Manhandling

E976 Injury due to legal intervention by unspecified means

E977 Late effects of injuries due to legal intervention

Note: This category is to be used to indicate circumstances classifiable to E970-E976 as the cause of death or disability from late effects, which are themselves classifiable elsewhere. The "late effects" include conditions reported as such, or as sequelae which may occur at any time after the acute injury due to legal intervention.

E978 Legal execution

All executions performed at the behest of the judiciary or ruling authority [whether permanent or temporary] as:
asphyxiation by gas
beheading, decapitation (by guillotine)
capital punishment
electrocution
hanging
poisoning
shooting
other specified means

INJURY UNDETERMINED WHETHER ACCIDENTALLY OR PURPOSELY INFLICTED (E980-E989)

Note: Categories E980-E989 are for use when after a thorough investigation by the medical examiner, coroner, or other legal authority it cannot be determined whether the injuries are accidental, suicidal, or homicidal. They include self-inflicted injuries, but not poisoning, when not specified as accidental or as intentional.

E980 Poisoning by solid or liquid substances, undetermined whether accidentally or purposely inflicted

E980.0 Analgesics, antipyretics, and antirheumatics

E980.1 Barbiturates

E980.2 Other sedatives and hypnotics

E980.3 Tranquilizers and other psychotropic agents

E980.4 Other specified drugs and medicinal substances

E980.5 Unspecified drug or medicinal substance

E980.6 Corrosive and caustic substances
Poisoning, undetermined whether accidental or purposeful, by substances classifiable to E864

E980.7 Agricultural and horticultural chemical and pharmaceutical preparations other than plant foods and fertilizers

E980.8 Arsenic and its compounds

E980.9 Other and unspecified solid and liquid substances

E981 Poisoning by gases in domestic use, undetermined whether accidentally or purposely inflicted

E981.0 Gas distributed by pipeline

E981.1 Liquefied petroleum gas distributed in mobile containers

E981.8 Other utility gas

E982 Poisoning by other gases, undetermined whether accidentally or purposely inflicted

E982.0 Motor vehicle exhaust gas

E982.1 Other carbon monoxide

E982.8 Other specified gases and vapors

E982.9 Unspecified gases and vapors

E983 Hanging, strangulation, or suffocation, undetermined whether accidentally or purposely inflicted

E983.0 Hanging

E983.1 Suffocation by plastic bag

E983.8 Other specified means

E983.9 Unspecified means

E984 Submersion [drowning], undetermined whether accidentally or purposely inflicted

E985 Injury by firearms and explosives, undetermined whether accidentally or purposely inflicted

E985.0 Handgun

E985.1 Shotgun

E985.2 Hunting rifle

E985.3 Military firearms

E985.4 Other and unspecified firearm

E985.5 Explosives

E986 Injury by cutting and piercing instruments, undetermined whether accidentally or purposely inflicted

E987 Falling from high place, undetermined whether accidentally or purposely inflicted

E987.0 Residential premises

E987.1 Other man-made structures

E987.2 Natural sites

E987.9 Unspecified site

E988 Injury by other and unspecified means, undetermined whether accidentally or purposely inflicted

E988.0 Jumping or lying before moving object

E988.1 Burns, fire

E988.2 Scald

E988.3 Extremes of cold

E988.4 Electrocution

E988.5 Crashing of motor vehicle

E988.6 Crashing of aircraft

E988.7 Caustic substances, except poisoning

E988.8 Other specified means

E988.9 Unspecified means

E989 Late effects of injury, undetermined whether accidentally or purposely inflicted

Note: This category is to be used to indicate circumstances classifiable to E980-E988 as the cause of death or disability from late effects, which are themselves classifiable elsewhere. The "late effects" include conditions reported as such or as sequelae which may occur at any time after the acute injury, undetermined whether accidentally or purposely inflicted.

INJURY RESULTING FROM OPERATIONS OF WAR (E990-E999)

Includes: injuries to military personnel and civilians caused by war and civil insurrections and occurring during the time of war and insurrection

Excludes: *accidents during training of military personnel, manufacture of war material and transport, unless attributable to enemy action*

E990 Injury due to war operations by fires and conflagrations

Includes: asphyxia, burns, or other injury originating from fire caused by a fire-producing device or indirectly by any conventional weapon

E990.0 From gasoline bomb

E990.9 From other and unspecified source

E991 Injury due to war operations by bullets and fragments

E991.0 Rubber bullets (rifle)

E991.1 Pellets (rifle)

E991.2 Other bullets

Bullet [any, except rubber bullets and pellets]
- carbine
- machine gun
- pistol
- rifle
- shotgun

E991.3 Antipersonnel bomb (fragments)

E991.9 Other and unspecified fragments

Fragments from:
- artillery shell
- bombs, except antipersonnel
- grenade
- guided missile

Fragments from:
- land mine
- rockets
- shell

Shrapnel

E992 Injury due to war operations by explosion of marine weapons

Depth charge
Marine mines
Mine NOS, at sea or in harbor
Sea-based artillery shell
Torpedo
Underwater blast

E993 Injury due to war operations by other explosion

Accidental explosion of munitions being used in war
Accidental explosion of own weapons
Air blast NOS
Blast NOS
Explosion NOS

Explosion of:
- artillery shell
- breech block
- cannon block
- mortar bomb

Injury by weapon burst

E994 Injury due to war operations by destruction of aircraft

Airplane:
- burned
- exploded
- shot down

Crushed by falling airplane

E995 Injury due to war operations by other and unspecified forms of conventional warfare

Battle wounds
Bayonet injury
Drowned in war operations

E996 Injury due to war operations by nuclear weapons

Blast effects
Exposure to ionizing radiation from nuclear weapons
Fireball effects
Heat
Other direct and secondary effects of nuclear weapons

E997 Injury due to war operations by other forms of unconventional warfare

E997.0 Lasers

E997.1 Biological warfare

E997.2 Gases, fumes, and chemicals

E997.8 Other specified forms of unconventional warfare

E997.9 Unspecified form of unconventional warfare

E998 Injury due to war operations but occurring after cessation of hostilities

Injuries due to operations of war but occurring after cessation of hostilities by any means classifiable under E990-E997

Injuries by explosion of bombs or mines placed in the course of operations of war, if the explosion occurred after cessation of hostilities

E999 Late effect of injury due to war operations

Note: This category is to be used to indicate circumstances classifiable to E990-E998 as the cause of death or disability from late effects, which are themselves classifiable elsewhere. The "late effects" include conditions reported as such or as sequelae which may occur at any time after the acute injury, resulting from operations of war.

MORPHOLOGY OF NEOPLASMS

The World Health Organization has published an adaptation of the International Classification of Diseases for oncology (ICD-O). It contains a coded nomenclature for the morphology of neoplasms, which is reproduced here for those who wish to use it in conjunction with Chapter 2 of the *International Classification of Diseases, 9th Revision, Clinical Modification.*

The morphology code numbers consist of five digits; the first four identify the histological type of the neoplasm and the fifth indicates its behavior. The one-digit behavior code is as follows:

/0 Benign

/1 Uncertain whether benign or malignant
Borderline malignancy

/2 Carcinoma in situ
Intraepithelial
Noninfiltrating
Noninvasive

/3 Malignant, primary site

/6 Malignant, metastatic site
Secondary site

/9 Malignant, uncertain whether primary or metastatic site

In the nomenclature below, the morphology code numbers include the behavior code appropriate to the histological type of neoplasm, but this behavior code should be changed if other reported information makes this necessary. For example, "chordoma (M9370/3)" is assumed to be malignant; the term "benign chordoma" should be coded M9370/0. Similarly, "superficial spreading adenocarcinoma (M8143/3)" described as "noninvasive" should be coded M8143/2 and "melanoma (M8720/3)" described as "secondary" should be coded M8720/6.

The following table shows the correspondence between the morphology code and the different sections of Chapter 2:

Morphology code Histology/Behavior		**ICD-9-CM Chapter 2**	
Any	0	210-229	Benign neoplasms
M8000-M8004	1	239	Neoplasms of unspecified nature
M8010+	1	235-238	Neoplasms of uncertain behavior
Any	2	230-234	Carcinoma in situ
Any	3	140-195 200-208	Malignant neoplasms, stated or presumed to be primary
Any	6	196-198	Malignant neoplasms, stated or presumed to be secondary

The ICD-O behavior digit /9 is inapplicable in an ICD context, since all malignant neoplasms are presumed to be primary (/3) or secondary (/6) according to other information on the medical record.

Only the first-listed term of the full ICD-O morphology nomenclature appears against each code number in the list below. The ICD-9-CM Alphabetical Index (Volume 2), however, includes all the ICD-O synonyms as well as a number of other morphological names still likely to be encountered on medical records but omitted from ICD-O as outdated or otherwise undesirable.

A coding difficulty sometimes arises where a morphological diagnosis contains two qualifying adjectives that have different code numbers. An example is "transitional cell epidermoid carcinoma." "Transitional cell carcinoma NOS" is M8120/3 and "epidermoid carcinoma NOS" is M8070/3. In such circumstances, the higher number (M8120/3 in this example) should be used, as it is usually more specific.

CODED NOMENCLATURE FOR MORPHOLOGY OF NEOPLASMS

M800 **Neoplasms NOS**
M8000/0 *Neoplasm, benign*
M8000/1 *Neoplasm, uncertain whether benign or malignant*
M8000/3 *Neoplasm, malignant*
M8000/6 *Neoplasm, metastatic*
M8000/9 *Neoplasm, malignant, uncertain whether primary or metastatic*
M8001/0 *Tumor cells, benign*
M8001/1 *Tumor cells, uncertain whether benign or malignant*
M8001/3 *Tumor cells, malignant*
M8002/3 *Malignant tumor, small cell type*
M8003/3 *Malignant tumor, giant cell type*
M8004/3 *Malignant tumor, fusiform cell type*

M801-M804 **Epithelial neoplasms NOS**
M8010/0 *Epithelial tumor, benign*
M8010/2 *Carcinoma in situ NOS*
M8010/3 *Carcinoma NOS*
M8010/6 *Carcinoma, metastatic NOS*
M8010/9 *Carcinomatosis*
M8011/0 *Epithelioma, benign*
M8011/3 *Epithelioma, malignant*
M8012/3 *Large cell carcinoma NOS*
M8020/3 *Carcinoma, undifferentiated type NOS*
M8021/3 *Carcinoma, anaplastic type NOS*
M8022/3 *Pleomorphic carcinoma*
M8030/3 *Giant cell and spindle cell carcinoma*
M8031/3 *Giant cell carcinoma*
M8032/3 *Spindle cell carcinoma*
M8033/3 *Pseudosarcomatous carcinoma*
M8034/3 *Polygonal cell carcinoma*
M8035/3 *Spheroidal cell carcinoma*
M8040/1 *Tumorlet*
M8041/3 *Small cell carcinoma NOS*
M8042/3 *Oat cell carcinoma*
M8043/3 *Small cell carcinoma, fusiform cell type*

M805-M808 **Papillary and squamous cell neoplasms**
M8050/0 *Papilloma NOS (except Papilloma of urinary bladder M8120/1)*
M8050/2 *Papillary carcinoma in situ*
M8050/3 *Papillary carcinoma NOS*
M8051/0 *Verrucous papilloma*
M8051/3 *Verrucous carcinoma NOS*
M8052/0 *Squamous cell papilloma*
M8052/3 *Papillary squamous cell carcinoma*
M8053/0 *Inverted papilloma*
M8060/0 *Papillomatosis NOS*
M8070/2 *Squamous cell carcinoma in situ NOS*
M8070/3 *Squamous cell carcinoma NOS*
M8070/6 *Squamous cell carcinoma, metastatic NOS*
M8071/3 *Squamous cell carcinoma, keratinizing type NOS*
M8072/3 *Squamous cell carcinoma, large cell, nonkeratinizing type*
M8073/3 *Squamous cell carcinoma, small cell, nonkeratinizing type*
M8074/3 *Squamous cell carcinoma, spindle cell type*
M8075/3 *Adenoid squamous cell carcinoma*
M8076/2 *Squamous cell carcinoma in situ with questionable stromal invasion*
M8076/3 *Squamous cell carcinoma, microinvasive*
M8080/2 *Queyrat's erythroplasia*
M8081/2 *Bowen's disease*
M8082/3 *Lymphoepithelial carcinoma*

M809-M811 **Basal cell neoplasms**
M8090/1 *Basal cell tumor*
M8090/3 *Basal cell carcinoma NOS*
M8091/3 *Multicentric basal cell carcinoma*
M8092/3 *Basal cell carcinoma, morphea type*
M8093/3 *Basal cell carcinoma, fibroepithelial type*
M8094/3 *Basosquamous carcinoma*
M8095/3 *Metatypical carcinoma*
M8096/0 *Intraepidermal epithelioma of Jadassohn*
M8100/0 *Trichoepithelioma*
M8101/0 *Trichofolliculoma*

M8102/0 *Tricholemmoma*
M8110/0 *Pilomatrixoma*

M812-M813 Transitional cell papillomas and carcinomas
M8120/0 *Transitional cell papilloma NOS*
M8120/1 *Urothelial papilloma*
M8120/2 *Transitional cell carcinoma in situ*
M8120/3 *Transitional cell carcinoma NOS*
M8121/0 *Schneiderian papilloma*
M8121/1 *Transitional cell papilloma, inverted type*
M8121/3 *Schneiderian carcinoma*
M8122/3 *Transitional cell carcinoma, spindle cell type*
M8123/3 *Basaloid carcinoma*
M8124/3 *Cloacogenic carcinoma*
M8130/3 *Papillary transitional cell carcinoma*

M814-M838 Adenomas and adenocarcinomas
M8140/0 *Adenoma NOS*
M8140/1 *Bronchial adenoma NOS*
M8140/2 *Adenocarcinoma in situ*
M8140/3 *Adenocarcinoma NOS*
M8140/6 *Adenocarcinoma, metastatic NOS*
M8141/3 *Scirrhous adenocarcinoma*
M8142/3 *Linitis plastica*
M8143/3 *Superficial spreading adenocarcinoma*
M8144/3 *Adenocarcinoma, intestinal type*
M8145/3 *Carcinoma, diffuse type*
M8146/0 *Monomorphic adenoma*
M8147/0 *Basal cell adenoma*
M8150/0 *Islet cell adenoma*
M8150/3 *Islet cell carcinoma*
M8151/0 *Insulinoma NOS*
M8151/3 *Insulinoma, malignant*
M8152/0 *Glucagonoma NOS*
M8152/3 *Glucagonoma, malignant*
M8153/1 *Gastrinoma NOS*
M8153/3 *Gastrinoma, malignant*
M8154/3 *Mixed islet cell and exocrine adenocarcinoma*
M8160/0 *Bile duct adenoma*
M8160/3 *Cholangiocarcinoma*
M8161/0 *Bile duct cystadenoma*
M8161/3 *Bile duct cystadenocarcinoma*
M8170/0 *Liver cell adenoma*
M8170/3 *Hepatocellular carcinoma NOS*
M8180/0 *Hepatocholangioma, benign*
M8180/3 *Combined hepatocellular carcinoma and cholangiocarcinoma*
M8190/0 *Trabecular adenoma*
M8190/3 *Trabecular adenocarcinoma*
M8191/0 *Embryonal adenoma*
M8200/0 *Eccrine dermal cylindroma*
M8200/3 *Adenoid cystic carcinoma*
M8201/3 *Cribriform carcinoma*
M8210/0 *Adenomatous polyp NOS*
M8210/3 *Adenocarcinoma in adenomatous polyp*
M8211/0 *Tubular adenoma NOS*
M8211/3 *Tubular adenocarcinoma*
M8220/0 *Adenomatous polyposis coli*
M8220/3 *Adenocarcinoma in adenomatous polyposis coli*
M8221/0 *Multiple adenomatous polyps*
M8230/3 *Solid carcinoma NOS*
M8231/3 *Carcinoma simplex*
M8240/1 *Carcinoid tumor NOS*
M8240/3 *Carcinoid tumor, malignant*
M8241/1 *Carcinoid tumor, argentaffin NOS*
M8241/3 *Carcinoid tumor, argentaffin, malignant*
M8242/1 *Carcinoid tumor, nonargentaffin NOS*
M8242/3 *Carcinoid tumor, nonargentaffin, malignant*
M8243/3 *Mucocarcinoid tumor, malignant*
M8244/3 *Composite carcinoid*
M8250/1 *Pulmonary adenomatosis*
M8250/3 *Bronchiolo-alveolar adenocarcinoma*
M8251/0 *Alveolar adenoma*

M8251/3 *Alveolar adenocarcinoma*
M8260/0 *Papillary adenoma NOS*
M8260/3 *Papillary adenocarcinoma NOS*
M8261/1 *Villous adenoma NOS*
M8261/3 *Adenocarcinoma in villous adenoma*
M8262/3 *Villous adenocarcinoma*
M8263/0 *Tubulovillous adenoma*
M8270/0 *Chromophobe adenoma*
M8270/3 *Chromophobe carcinoma*
M8280/0 *Acidophil adenoma*
M8280/3 *Acidophil carcinoma*
M8281/0 *Mixed acidophil-basophil adenoma*
M8281/3 *Mixed acidophil-basophil carcinoma*
M8290/0 *Oxyphilic adenoma*
M8290/3 *Oxyphilic adenocarcinoma*
M8300/0 *Basophil adenoma*
M8300/3 *Basophil carcinoma*
M8310/0 *Clear cell adenoma*
M8310/3 *Clear cell adenocarcinoma NOS*
M8311/1 *Hypernephroid tumor*
M8312/3 *Renal cell carcinoma*
M8313/0 *Clear cell adenofibroma*
M8320/3 *Granular cell carcinoma*
M8321/0 *Chief cell adenoma*
M8322/0 *Water-clear cell adenoma*
M8322/3 *Water-clear cell adenocarcinoma*
M8323/0 *Mixed cell adenoma*
M8323/3 *Mixed cell adenocarcinoma*
M8324/0 *Lipoadenoma*
M8330/0 *Follicular adenoma*
M8330/3 *Follicular adenocarcinoma NOS*
M8331/3 *Follicular adenocarcinoma, well differentiated type*
M8332/3 *Follicular adenocarcinoma, trabecular type*
M8333/0 *Microfollicular adenoma*
M8334/0 *Macrofollicular adenoma*
M8340/3 *Papillary and follicular adenocarcinoma*
M8350/3 *Nonencapsulated sclerosing carcinoma*
M8360/1 *Multiple endocrine adenomas*
M8361/1 *Juxtaglomerular tumor*
M8370/0 *Adrenal cortical adenoma NOS*
M8370/3 *Adrenal cortical carcinoma*
M8371/0 *Adrenal cortical adenoma, compact cell type*
M8372/0 *Adrenal cortical adenoma, heavily pigmented variant*
M8373/0 *Adrenal cortical adenoma, clear cell type*
M8374/0 *Adrenal cortical adenoma, glomerulosa cell type*
M8375/0 *Adrenal cortical adenoma, mixed cell type*
M8380/0 *Endometrioid adenoma NOS*
M8380/1 *Endometrioid adenoma, borderline malignancy*
M8380/3 *Endometrioid carcinoma*
M8381/0 *Endometrioid adenofibroma NOS*
M8381/1 *Endometrioid adenofibroma, borderline malignancy*
M8381/3 *Endometrioid adenofibroma, malignant*

M839-M842 Adnexal and skin appendage neoplasms

M8390/0 *Skin appendage adenoma*
M8390/3 *Skin appendage carcinoma*
M8400/0 *Sweat gland adenoma*
M8400/1 *Sweat gland tumor NOS*
M8400/3 *Sweat gland adenocarcinoma*
M8401/0 *Apocrine adenoma*
M8401/3 *Apocrine adenocarcinoma*
M8402/0 *Eccrine acrospiroma*
M8403/0 *Eccrine spiradenoma*
M8404/0 *Hidrocystoma*
M8405/0 *Papillary hydradenoma*
M8406/0 *Papillary syringadenoma*
M8407/0 *Syringoma NOS*
M8410/0 *Sebaceous adenoma*
M8410/3 *Sebaceous adenocarcinoma*
M8420/0 *Ceruminous adenoma*
M8420/3 *Ceruminous adenocarcinoma*

M843 **Mucoepidermoid neoplasms**
M8430/1 *Mucoepidermoid tumor*
M8430/3 *Mucoepidermoid carcinoma*

M844-M849 **Cystic, mucinous, and serous neoplasms**
M8440/0 *Cystadenoma NOS*
M8440/3 *Cystadenocarcinoma NOS*
M8441/0 *Serous cystadenoma NOS*
M8441/1 *Serous cystadenoma, borderline malignancy*
M8441/3 *Serous cystadenocarcinoma NOS*
M8450/0 *Papillary cystadenoma NOS*
M8450/1 *Papillary cystadenoma, borderline malignancy*
M8450/3 *Papillary cystadenocarcinoma NOS*
M8460/0 *Papillary serous cystadenoma NOS*
M8460/1 *Papillary serous cystadenoma, borderline malignancy*
M8460/3 *Papillary serous cystadenocarcinoma*
M8461/0 *Serous surface papilloma NOS*
M8461/1 *Serous surface papilloma, borderline malignancy*
M8461/3 *Serous surface papillary carcinoma*
M8470/0 *Mucinous cystadenoma NOS*
M8470/1 *Mucinous cystadenoma, borderline malignancy*
M8470/3 *Mucinous cystadenocarcinoma NOS*
M8471/0 *Papillary mucinous cystadenoma NOS*
M8471/1 *Papillary mucinous cystadenoma, borderline malignancy*
M8471/3 *Papillary mucinous cystadenocarcinoma*
M8480/0 *Mucinous adenoma*
M8480/3 *Mucinous adenocarcinoma*
M8480/6 *Pseudomyxoma peritonei*
M8481/3 *Mucin-producing adenocarcinoma*
M8490/3 *Signet ring cell carcinoma*
M8490/6 *Metastatic signet ring cell carcinoma*

M850-M854 **Ductal, lobular, and medullary neoplasms**
M8500/2 *Intraductal carcinoma, noninfiltrating NOS*
M8500/3 *Infiltrating duct carcinoma*
M8501/2 *Comedocarcinoma, noninfiltrating*
M8501/3 *Comedocarcinoma NOS*
M8502/3 *Juvenile carcinoma of the breast*
M8503/0 *Intraductal papilloma*
M8503/2 *Noninfiltrating intraductal papillary adenocarcinoma*
M8504/0 *Intracystic papillary adenoma*
M8504/2 *Noninfiltrating intracystic carcinoma*
M8505/0 *Intraductal papillomatosis NOS*
M8506/0 *Subareolar duct papillomatosis*
M8510/3 *Medullary carcinoma NOS*
M8511/3 *Medullary carcinoma with amyloid stroma*
M8512/3 *Medullary carcinoma with lymphoid stroma*
M8520/2 *Lobular carcinoma in situ*
M8520/3 *Lobular carcinoma NOS*
M8521/3 *Infiltrating ductular carcinoma*
M8530/3 *Inflammatory carcinoma*
M8540/3 *Paget's disease, mammary*
M8541/3 *Paget's disease and infiltrating duct carcinoma of breast*
M8542/3 *Paget's disease, extramammary (except Paget's disease of bone)*

M855 **Acinar cell neoplasms**
M8550/0 *Acinar cell adenoma*
M8550/1 *Acinar cell tumor*
M8550/3 *Acinar cell carcinoma*

M856-M858 **Complex epithelial neoplasms**
M8560/3 *Adenosquamous carcinoma*
M8561/0 *Adenolymphoma*
M8570/3 *Adenocarcinoma with squamous metaplasia*
M8571/3 *Adenocarcinoma with cartilaginous and osseous metaplasia*
M8572/3 *Adenocarcinoma with spindle cell metaplasia*
M8573/3 *Adenocarcinoma with apocrine metaplasia*
M8580/0 *Thymoma, benign*
M8580/3 *Thymoma, malignant*

M859-M867 **Specialized gonadal neoplasms**
M8590/1 *Sex cord-stromal tumor*
M8600/0 *Thecoma NOS*
M8600/3 *Theca cell carcinoma*

M8610/0 *Luteoma NOS*
M8620/1 *Granulosa cell tumor NOS*
M8620/3 *Granulosa cell tumor, malignant*
M8621/1 *Granulosa cell-theca cell tumor*
M8630/0 *Androblastoma, benign*
M8630/1 *Androblastoma NOS*
M8630/3 *Androblastoma, malignant*
M8631/0 *Sertoli-Leydig cell tumor*
M8632/1 *Gynandroblastoma*
M8640/0 *Tubular androblastoma NOS*
M8640/3 *Sertoli cell carcinoma*
M8641/0 *Tubular androblastoma with lipid storage*
M8650/0 *Leydig cell tumor, benign*
M8650/1 *Leydig cell tumor NOS*
M8650/3 *Leydig cell tumor, malignant*
M8660/0 *Hilar cell tumor*
M8670/0 *Lipid cell tumor of ovary*
M8671/0 *Adrenal rest tumor*

M868-M871 Paragangliomas and glomus tumors
M8680/1 *Paraganglioma NOS*
M8680/3 *Paraganglioma, malignant*
M8681/1 *Sympathetic paraganglioma*
M8682/1 *Parasympathetic paraganglioma*
M8690/1 *Glomus jugulare tumor*
M8691/1 *Aortic body tumor*
M8692/1 *Carotid body tumor*
M8693/1 *Extra-adrenal paraganglioma NOS*
M8693/3 *Extra-adrenal paraganglioma, malignant*
M8700/0 *Pheochromocytoma NOS*
M8700/3 *Pheochromocytoma, malignant*
M8710/3 *Glomangiosarcoma*
M8711/0 *Glomus tumor*
M8712/0 *Glomangioma*

M872-M879 Nevi and melanomas
M8720/0 *Pigmented nevus NOS*
M8720/3 *Malignant melanoma NOS*
M8721/3 *Nodular melanoma*
M8722/0 *Balloon cell nevus*
M8722/3 *Balloon cell melanoma*
M8723/0 *Halo nevus*
M8724/0 *Fibrous papule of the nose*
M8725/0 *Neuronevus*
M8726/0 *Magnocellular nevus*
M8730/0 *Nonpigmented nevus*
M8730/3 *Amelanotic melanoma*
M8740/0 *Junctional nevus*
M8740/3 *Malignant melanoma in junctional nevus*
M8741/2 *Precancerous melanosis NOS*
M8741/3 *Malignant melanoma in precancerous melanosis*
M8742/2 *Hutchinson's melanotic freckle*
M8742/3 *Malignant melanoma in Hutchinson's melanotic freckle*
M8743/3 *Superficial spreading melanoma*
M8750/0 *Intradermal nevus*
M8760/0 *Compound nevus*
M8761/1 *Giant pigmented nevus*
M8761/3 *Malignant melanoma in giant pigmented nevus*
M8770/0 *Epithelioid and spindle cell nevus*
M8771/3 *Epithelioid cell melanoma*
M8772/3 *Spindle cell melanoma NOS*
M8773/3 *Spindle cell melanoma, type A*
M8774/3 *Spindle cell melanoma, type B*
M8775/3 *Mixed epithelioid and spindle cell melanoma*
M8780/0 *Blue nevus NOS*
M8780/3 *Blue nevus, malignant*
M8790/0 *Cellular blue nevus*

M880 Soft tissue tumors and sarcomas NOS
M8800/0 *Soft tissue tumor, benign*
M8800/3 *Sarcoma NOS*
M8800/9 *Sarcomatosis NOS*
M8801/3 *Spindle cell sarcoma*

M8802/3 *Giant cell sarcoma (except of bone M9250/3)*
M8803/3 *Small cell sarcoma*
M8804/3 *Epithelioid cell sarcoma*

M881-M883 Fibromatous neoplasms
M8810/0 *Fibroma NOS*
M8810/3 *Fibrosarcoma NOS*
M8811/0 *Fibromyxoma*
M8811/3 *Fibromyxosarcoma*
M8812/0 *Periosteal fibroma*
M8812/3 *Periosteal fibrosarcoma*
M8813/0 *Fascial fibroma*
M8813/3 *Fascial fibrosarcoma*
M8814/3 *Infantile fibrosarcoma*
M8820/0 *Elastofibroma*
M8821/1 *Aggressive fibromatosis*
M8822/1 *Abdominal fibromatosis*
M8823/1 *Desmoplastic fibroma*
M8830/0 *Fibrous histiocytoma NOS*
M8830/1 *Atypical fibrous histiocytoma*
M8830/3 *Fibrous histiocytoma, malignant*
M8831/0 *Fibroxanthoma NOS*
M8831/1 *Atypical fibroxanthoma*
M8831/3 *Fibroxanthoma, malignant*
M8832/0 *Dermatofibroma NOS*
M8832/1 *Dermatofibroma protuberans*
M8832/3 *Dermatofibrosarcoma NOS*

M884 Myxomatous neoplasms
M8840/0 *Myxoma NOS*
M8840/3 *Myxosarcoma*

M885-M888 Lipomatous neoplasms
M8850/0 *Lipoma NOS*
M8850/3 *Liposarcoma NOS*
M8851/0 *Fibrolipoma*
M8851/3 *Liposarcoma, well differentiated type*
M8852/0 *Fibromyxolipoma*
M8852/3 *Myxoid liposarcoma*
M8853/3 *Round cell liposarcoma*
M8854/3 *Pleomorphic liposarcoma*
M8855/3 *Mixed type liposarcoma*
M8856/0 *Intramuscular lipoma*
M8857/0 *Spindle cell lipoma*
M8860/0 *Angiomyolipoma*
M8860/3 *Angiomyoliposarcoma*
M8861/0 *Angiolipoma NOS*
M8861/1 *Angiolipoma, infiltrating*
M8870/0 *Myelolipoma*
M8880/0 *Hibernoma*
M8881/0 *Lipoblastomatosis*

M889-M892 Myomatous neoplasms
M8890/0 *Leiomyoma NOS*
M8890/1 *Intravascular leiomyomatosis*
M8890/3 *Leiomyosarcoma NOS*
M8891/1 *Epithelioid leiomyoma*
M8891/3 *Epithelioid leiomyosarcoma*
M8892/1 *Cellular leiomyoma*
M8893/0 *Bizarre leiomyoma*
M8894/0 *Angiomyoma*
M8894/3 *Angiomyosarcoma*
M8895/0 *Myoma*
M8895/3 *Myosarcoma*
M8900/0 *Rhabdomyoma NOS*
M8900/3 *Rhabdomyosarcoma NOS*
M8901/3 *Pleomorphic rhabdomyosarcoma*
M8902/3 *Mixed type rhabdomyosarcoma*
M8903/0 *Fetal rhabdomyoma*
M8904/0 *Adult rhabdomyoma*
M8910/3 *Embryonal rhabdomyosarcoma*
M8920/3 *Alveolar rhabdomyosarcoma*

M893-M899	**Complex mixed and stromal neoplasms**
M8930/3	*Endometrial stromal sarcoma*
M8931/1	*Endolymphatic stromal myosis*
M8932/0	*Adenomyoma*
M8940/0	*Pleomorphic adenoma*
M8940/3	*Mixed tumor, malignant NOS*
M8950/3	*Mullerian mixed tumor*
M8951/3	*Mesodermal mixed tumor*
M8960/1	*Mesoblastic nephroma*
M8960/3	*Nephroblastoma NOS*
M8961/3	*Epithelial nephroblastoma*
M8962/3	*Mesenchymal nephroblastoma*
M8970/3	*Hepatoblastoma*
M8980/3	*Carcinosarcoma NOS*
M8981/3	*Carcinosarcoma, embryonal type*
M8982/0	*Myoepithelioma*
M8990/0	*Mesenchymoma, benign*
M8990/1	*Mesenchymoma, NOS*
M8990/3	*Mesenchymoma, malignant*
M8991/3	*Embryonal sarcoma*
M900-M903	**Fibroepithelial neoplasms**
M9000/0	*Brenner tumor NOS*
M9000/1	*Brenner tumor, borderline malignancy*
M9000/3	*Brenner tumor, malignant*
M9010/0	*Fibroadenoma NOS*
M9011/0	*Intracanalicular fibroadenoma NOS*
M9012/0	*Pericanalicular fibroadenoma*
M9013/0	*Adenofibroma NOS*
M9014/0	*Serous adenofibroma*
M9015/0	*Mucinous adenofibroma*
M9020/0	*Cellular intracanalicular fibroadenoma*
M9020/1	*Cystosarcoma phyllodes NOS*
M9020/3	*Cystosarcoma phyllodes, malignant*
M9030/0	*Juvenile fibroadenoma*
M904	**Synovial neoplasms**
M9040/0	*Synovioma, benign*
M9040/3	*Synovial sarcoma NOS*
M9041/3	*Synovial sarcoma, spindle cell type*
M9042/3	*Synovial sarcoma, epithelioid cell type*
M9043/3	*Synovial sarcoma, biphasic type*
M9044/3	*Clear cell sarcoma of tendons and aponeuroses*
M905	**Mesothelial neoplasms**
M9050/0	*Mesothelioma, benign*
M9050/3	*Mesothelioma, malignant*
M9051/0	*Fibrous mesothelioma, benign*
M9051/3	*Fibrous mesothelioma, malignant*
M9052/0	*Epithelioid mesothelioma, benign*
M9052/3	*Epithelioid mesothelioma, malignant*
M9053/0	*Mesothelioma, biphasic type, benign*
M9053/3	*Mesothelioma, biphasic type, malignant*
M9054/0	*Adenomatoid tumor NOS*
M906-M909	**Germ cell neoplasms**
M9060/3	*Dysgerminoma*
M9061/3	*Seminoma NOS*
M9062/3	*Seminoma, anaplastic type*
M9063/3	*Spermatocytic seminoma*
M9064/3	*Germinoma*
M9070/3	*Embryonal carcinoma NOS*
M9071/3	*Endodermal sinus tumor*
M9072/3	*Polyembryoma*
M9073/1	*Gonadoblastoma*
M9080/0	*Teratoma, benign*
M9080/1	*Teratoma NOS*
M9080/3	*Teratoma, malignant NOS*
M9081/3	*Teratocarcinoma*
M9082/3	*Malignant teratoma, undifferentiated type*
M9083/3	*Malignant teratoma, intermediate type*
M9084/0	*Dermoid cyst*
M9084/3	*Dermoid cyst with malignant transformation*

M9090/0 *Struma ovarii NOS*
M9090/3 *Struma ovarii, malignant*
M9091/1 *Strumal carcinoid*

M910 Trophoblastic neoplasms
M9100/0 *Hydatidiform mole NOS*
M9100/1 *Invasive hydatidiform mole*
M9100/3 *Choriocarcinoma*
M9101/3 *Choriocarcinoma combined with teratoma*
M9102/3 *Malignant teratoma, trophoblastic*

M911 Mesonephromas
M9110/0 *Mesonephroma, benign*
M9110/1 *Mesonephric tumor*
M9110/3 *Mesonephroma, malignant*
M9111/1 *Endosalpingioma*

M912-M916 Blood vessel tumors
M9120/0 *Hemangioma NOS*
M9120/3 *Hemangiosarcoma*
M9121/0 *Cavernous hemangioma*
M9122/0 *Venous hemangioma*
M9123/0 *Racemose hemangioma*
M9124/3 *Kupffer cell sarcoma*
M9130/0 *Hemangioendothelioma, benign*
M9130/1 *Hemangioendothelioma NOS*
M9130/3 *Hemangioendothelioma, malignant*
M9131/0 *Capillary hemangioma*
M9132/0 *Intramuscular hemangioma*
M9140/3 *Kaposi's sarcoma*
M9141/0 *Angiokeratoma*
M9142/0 *Verrucous keratotic hemangioma*
M9150/0 *Hemangiopericytoma, benign*
M9150/1 *Hemangiopericytoma NOS*
M9150/3 *Hemangiopericytoma, malignant*
M9160/0 *Angiofibroma NOS*
M9161/1 *Hemangioblastoma*

M917 Lymphatic vessel tumors
M9170/0 *Lymphangioma NOS*
M9170/3 *Lymphangiosarcoma*
M9171/0 *Capillary lymphangioma*
M9172/0 *Cavernous lymphangioma*
M9173/0 *Cystic lymphangioma*
M9174/0 *Lymphangiomyoma*
M9174/1 *Lymphangiomyomatosis*
M9175/0 *Hemolymphangioma*

M918-M920 Osteomas and osteosarcomas
M9180/0 *Osteoma NOS*
M9180/3 *Osteosarcoma NOS*
M9181/3 *Chondroblastic osteosarcoma*
M9182/3 *Fibroblastic osteosarcoma*
M9183/3 *Telangiectatic osteosarcoma*
M9184/3 *Osteosarcoma in Paget's disease of bone*
M9190/3 *Juxtacortical osteosarcoma*
M9191/0 *Osteoid osteoma NOS*
M9200/0 *Osteoblastoma*

M921-M924 Chondromatous neoplasms
M9210/0 *Osteochondroma*
M9210/1 *Osteochondromatosis NOS*
M9220/0 *Chondroma NOS*
M9220/1 *Chondromatosis NOS*
M9220/3 *Chondrosarcoma NOS*
M9221/0 *Juxtacortical chondroma*
M9221/3 *Juxtacortical chondrosarcoma*
M9230/0 *Chondroblastoma NOS*
M9230/3 *Chondroblastoma, malignant*
M9240/3 *Mesenchymal chondrosarcoma*
M9241/0 *Chondromyxoid fibroma*

M925 Giant cell tumors
M9250/1 *Giant cell tumor of bone NOS*
M9250/3 *Giant cell tumor of bone, malignant*

M9251/1	*Giant cell tumor of soft parts NOS*
M9251/3	*Malignant giant cell tumor of soft parts*
M926	**Miscellaneous bone tumors**
M9260/3	*Ewing's sarcoma*
M9261/3	*Adamantinoma of long bones*
M9262/0	*Ossifying fibroma*
M927-M934	**Odontogenic tumors**
M9270/0	*Odontogenic tumor, benign*
M9270/1	*Odontogenic tumor NOS*
M9270/3	*Odontogenic tumor, malignant*
M9271/0	*Dentinoma*
M9272/0	*Cementoma NOS*
M9273/0	*Cementoblastoma, benign*
M9274/0	*Cementifying fibroma*
M9275/0	*Gigantiform cementoma*
M9280/0	*Odontoma NOS*
M9281/0	*Compound odontoma*
M9282/0	*Complex odontoma*
M9290/0	*Ameloblastic fibro-odontoma*
M9290/3	*Ameloblastic odontosarcoma*
M9300/0	*Adenomatoid odontogenic tumor*
M9301/0	*Calcifying odontogenic cyst*
M9310/0	*Ameloblastoma NOS*
M9310/3	*Ameloblastoma, malignant*
M9311/0	*Odontoameloblastoma*
M9312/0	*Squamous odontogenic tumor*
M9320/0	*Odontogenic myxoma*
M9321/0	*Odontogenic fibroma NOS*
M9330/0	*Ameloblastic fibroma*
M9330/3	*Ameloblastic fibrosarcoma*
M9340/0	*Calcifying epithelial odontogenic tumor*
M935-M937	**Miscellaneous tumors**
M9350/1	*Craniopharyngioma*
M9360/1	*Pinealoma*
M9361/1	*Pineocytoma*
M9362/3	*Pineoblastoma*
M9363/0	*Melanotic neuroectodermal tumor*
M9370/3	*Chordoma*
M938-M948	**Gliomas**
M9380/3	*Glioma, malignant*
M9381/3	*Gliomatosis cerebri*
M9382/3	*Mixed glioma*
M9383/1	*Subependymal glioma*
M9384/1	*Subependymal giant cell astrocytoma*
M9390/0	*Choroid plexus papilloma NOS*
M9390/3	*Choroid plexus papilloma, malignant*
M9391/3	*Ependymoma NOS*
M9392/3	*Ependymoma, anaplastic type*
M9393/1	*Papillary ependymoma*
M9394/1	*Myxopapillary ependymoma*
M9400/3	*Astrocytoma NOS*
M9401/3	*Astrocytoma, anaplastic type*
M9410/3	*Protoplasmic astrocytoma*
M9411/3	*Gemistocytic astrocytoma*
M9420/3	*Fibrillary astrocytoma*
M9421/3	*Pilocytic astrocytoma*
M9422/3	*Spongioblastoma NOS*
M9423/3	*Spongioblastoma polare*
M9430/3	*Astroblastoma*
M9440/3	*Glioblastoma NOS*
M9441/3	*Giant cell glioblastoma*
M9442/3	*Glioblastoma with sarcomatous component*
M9443/3	*Primitive polar spongioblastoma*
M9450/3	*Oligodendroglioma NOS*
M9451/3	*Oligodendroglioma, anaplastic type*
M9460/3	*Oligodendroblastoma*
M9470/3	*Medulloblastoma NOS*
M9471/3	*Desmoplastic medulloblastoma*
M9472/3	*Medullomyoblastoma*

M9480/3 *Cerebellar sarcoma NOS*
M9481/3 *Monstrocellular sarcoma*

M949-M952 Neuroepitheliomatous neoplasms
M9490/0 *Ganglioneuroma*
M9490/3 *Ganglioneuroblastoma*
M9491/0 *Ganglioneuromatosis*
M9500/3 *Neuroblastoma NOS*
M9501/3 *Medulloepithelioma NOS*
M9502/3 *Teratoid medulloepithelioma*
M9503/3 *Neuroepithelioma NOS*
M9504/3 *Spongioneuroblastoma*
M9505/1 *Ganglioglioma*
M9506/0 *Neurocytoma*
M9507/0 *Pacinian tumor*
M9510/3 *Retinoblastoma NOS*
M9511/3 *Retinoblastoma, differentiated type*
M9512/3 *Retinoblastoma, undifferentiated type*
M9520/3 *Olfactory neurogenic tumor*
M9521/3 *Esthesioneurocytoma*
M9522/3 *Esthesioneuroblastoma*
M9523/3 *Esthesioneuroepithelioma*

M953 Meningiomas
M9530/0 *Meningioma NOS*
M9530/1 *Meningiomatosis NOS*
M9530/3 *Meningioma, malignant*
M9531/0 *Meningotheliomatous meningioma*
M9532/0 *Fibrous meningioma*
M9533/0 *Psammomatous meningioma*
M9534/0 *Angiomatous meningioma*
M9535/0 *Hemangioblastic meningioma*
M9536/0 *Hemangiopericytic meningioma*
M9537/0 *Transitional meningioma*
M9538/1 *Papillary meningioma*
M9539/3 *Meningeal sarcomatosis*

M954-M957 Nerve sheath tumor
M9540/0 *Neurofibroma NOS*
M9540/1 *Neurofibromatosis NOS*
M9540/3 *Neurofibrosarcoma*
M9541/0 *Melanotic neurofibroma*
M9550/0 *Plexiform neurofibroma*
M9560/0 *Neurilemmoma NOS*
M9560/1 *Neurinomatosis*
M9560/3 *Neurilemmoma, malignant*
M9570/0 *Neuroma NOS*

M958 Granular cell tumors and alveolar soft part sarcoma
M9580/0 *Granular cell tumor NOS*
M9580/3 *Granular cell tumor, malignant*
M9581/3 *Alveolar soft part sarcoma*

M959-M963 Lymphomas, NOS or diffuse
M9590/0 *Lymphomatous tumor, benign*
M9590/3 *Malignant lymphoma NOS*
M9591/3 *Malignant lymphoma, non Hodgkin's type*
M9600/3 *Malignant lymphoma, undifferentiated cell type NOS*
M9601/3 *Malignant lymphoma, stem cell type*
M9602/3 *Malignant lymphoma, convoluted cell type NOS*
M9610/3 *Lymphosarcoma NOS*
M9611/3 *Malignant lymphoma, lymphoplasmacytoid type*
M9612/3 *Malignant lymphoma, immunoblastic type*
M9613/3 *Malignant lymphoma, mixed lymphocytic-histiocytic NOS*
M9614/3 *Malignant lymphoma, centroblastic-centrocytic, diffuse*
M9615/3 *Malignant lymphoma, follicular center cell NOS*
M9620/3 *Malignant lymphoma, lymphocytic, well differentiated NOS*
M9621/3 *Malignant lymphoma, lymphocytic, intermediate differentiation NOS*
M9622/3 *Malignant lymphoma, centrocytic*
M9623/3 *Malignant lymphoma, follicular center cell, cleaved NOS*
M9630/3 *Malignant lymphoma, lymphocytic, poorly differentiated NOS*
M9631/3 *Prolymphocytic lymphosarcoma*
M9632/3 *Malignant lymphoma, centroblastic type NOS*
M9633/3 *Malignant lymphoma, follicular center cell, noncleaved NOS*

M964 **Reticulosarcomas**
M9640/3 *Reticulosarcoma NOS*
M9641/3 *Reticulosarcoma, pleomorphic cell type*
M9642/3 *Reticulosarcoma, nodular*

M965-M966 **Hodgkin's disease**
M9650/3 *Hodgkin's disease NOS*
M9651/3 *Hodgkin's disease, lymphocytic predominance*
M9652/3 *Hodgkin's disease, mixed cellularity*
M9653/3 *Hodgkin's disease, lymphocytic depletion NOS*
M9654/3 *Hodgkin's disease, lymphocytic depletion, diffuse fibrosis*
M9655/3 *Hodgkin's disease, lymphocytic depletion, reticular type*
M9656/3 *Hodgkin's disease, nodular sclerosis NOS*
M9657/3 *Hodgkin's disease, nodular sclerosis, cellular phase*
M9660/3 *Hodgkin's paragranuloma*
M9661/3 *Hodgkin's granuloma*
M9662/3 *Hodgkin's sarcoma*

M969 **Lymphomas, nodular or follicular**
M9690/3 *Malignant lymphoma, nodular NOS*
M9691/3 *Malignant lymphoma, mixed lymphocytic-histiocytic, nodular*
M9692/3 *Malignant lymphoma, centroblastic-centrocytic, follicular*
M9693/3 *Malignant lymphoma, lymphocytic, well differentiated, nodular*
M9694/3 *Malignant lymphoma, lymphocytic, intermediate differentiation, nodular*
M9695/3 *Malignant lymphoma, follicular center cell, cleaved, follicular*
M9696/3 *Malignant lymphoma, lymphocytic, poorly differentiated, nodular*
M9697/3 *Malignant lymphoma, centroblastic type, follicular*
M9698/3 *Malignant lymphoma, follicular center cell, noncleaved, follicular*

M970 **Mycosis fungoides**
M9700/3 *Mycosis fungoides*
M9701/3 *Sezary's disease*

M971-M972 **Miscellaneous reticuloendothelial neoplasms**
M9710/3 *Microglioma*
M9720/3 *Malignant histiocytosis*
M9721/3 *Histiocytic medullary reticulosis*
M9722/3 *Letterer-Siwe's disease*

M973 **Plasma cell tumors**
M9730/3 *Plasma cell myeloma*
M9731/0 *Plasma cell tumor, benign*
M9731/1 *Plasmacytoma NOS*
M9731/3 *Plasma cell tumor, malignant*

M974 **Mast cell tumors**
M9740/1 *Mastocytoma NOS*
M9740/3 *Mast cell sarcoma*
M9741/3 *Malignant mastocytosis*

M975 **Burkitt's tumor**
M9750/3 *Burkitt's tumor*

M980-M994 **Leukemias**

M980 **Leukemias NOS**
M9800/3 *Leukemia NOS*
M9801/3 *Acute leukemia NOS*
M9802/3 *Subacute leukemia NOS*
M9803/3 *Chronic leukemia NOS*
M9804/3 *Aleukemic leukemia NOS*

M981 **Compound leukemias**
M9810/3 *Compound leukemia*

M982 **Lymphoid leukemias**
M9820/3 *Lymphoid leukemia NOS*
M9821/3 *Acute lymphoid leukemia*
M9822/3 *Subacute lymphoid leukemia*
M9823/3 *Chronic lymphoid leukemia*
M9824/3 *Aleukemic lymphoid leukemia*
M9825/3 *Prolymphocytic leukemia*

M983 **Plasma cell leukemias**
M9830/3 *Plasma cell leukemia*

M984 **Erythroleukemias**
M9840/3 *Erythroleukemia*
M9841/3 *Acute erythremia*

M9842/3	*Chronic erythremia*
M985	**Lymphosarcoma cell leukemias**
M9850/3	*Lymphosarcoma cell leukemia*
M986	**Myeloid leukemias**
M9860/3	*Myeloid leukemia NOS*
M9861/3	*Acute myeloid leukemia*
M9862/3	*Subacute myeloid leukemia*
M9863/3	*Chronic myeloid leukemia*
M9864/3	*Aleukemic myeloid leukemia*
M9865/3	*Neutrophilic leukemia*
M9866/3	*Acute promyelocytic leukemia*
M987	**Basophilic leukemias**
M9870/3	*Basophilic leukemia*
M988	**Eosinophilic leukemias**
M9880/3	*Eosinophilic leukemia*
M989	**Monocytic leukemias**
M9890/3	*Monocytic leukemia NOS*
M9891/3	*Acute monocytic leukemia*
M9892/3	*Subacute monocytic leukemia*
M9893/3	*Chronic monocytic leukemia*
M9894/3	*Aleukemic monocytic leukemia*
M990-M994	**Miscellaneous leukemias**
M9900/3	*Mast cell leukemia*
M9910/3	*Megakaryocytic leukemia*
M9920/3	*Megakaryocytic myelosis*
M9930/3	*Myeloid sarcoma*
M9940/3	*Hairy cell leukemia*
M995-M997	**Miscellaneous myeloproliferative and lymphoproliferative disorders**
M9950/1	*Polycythemia vera*
M9951/1	*Acute panmyelosis*
M9960/1	*Chronic myeloproliferative disease*
M9961/1	*Myelosclerosis with myeloid metaplasia*
M9962/1	*Idiopathic thrombocythemia*
M9970/1	*Chronic lymphoproliferative disease*

...ARY OF MENTAL DISORDERS

In... Stedma... in Chapter 5, "Mental Disorders," are listed here in alphabetic ...iptions originally appeared in the section on Mental Disorders in ...s, 9th Revision,[1] and others are included to define the psychiatric ...al definitions are based on material furnished by the American ...nclature and Statistics[2] and from A Psychiatric Glossary,[3] ...m Dorland's Illustrated Medical Dictionary[4] and from

1. Manual of th... ...s, Injuries, and Causes of Death, 9th Revision. World Health Org...
2. American Psychiatric ... ...lature and Statistics, Robert L. Spitzer, Chairman.
3. A *Psychiatric Glossary*, Fourth ... Association, Washington, D.C., 1975.
4. *Dorland's Illustrated Medical Dictio...* ... B. Saunders Company, Philadelphia, 1974.
5. *Stedman's Medical Dictionary*, Illustrated, Tw... ...ms and Wilkins, Baltimore, 1976.

Academic underachievement disorder: Failure to achieve in ...ks despite adequate intellectual capacity, a supportive and encouraging social environme... effort. The failure occurs in the absence of a demonstrable specific learning disability and is ...otional conflict not clearly associated with any other mental disorder.[2]

Adaptation reaction—*see* Adjustment reaction

Adjustment reaction or disorder: Mild or transient disorders lasting longer than acute stress reactions which occur in individuals of any age without any apparent pre-existing mental disorder. Such disorders are often relatively circumscribed or situation-specific, are generally reversible, and usually last only a few months. They are usually closely related in time and content to stresses such as bereavement, migration, or other experiences. Reactions to major stress that last longer than a few days are also included. In children such disorders are associated with no significant distortion of development.[1]

conduct disturbance: Mild or transient disorders in which the main disturbance predominantly involves a disturbance of conduct (e.g., an adolescent grief reaction resulting in aggressive or antisocial disorder).[1]

depressive reaction: States of depression, not specifiable as manic-depressive, psychotic, or neurotic.[1]

brief: Generally transient, in which the depressive symptoms are usually closely related in time and content to some stressful event.[1]

prolonged: Generally long-lasting, usually developing in association with prolonged exposure to a stressful situation.[1]

emotional disturbance: An adjustment disorder in which the main symptoms are emotional in type (e.g., anxiety, fear, worry) but not specifically depressive.[1]

mixed conduct and emotional disturbance: An adjustment reaction in which both emotional disturbance and disturbance of conduct are prominent features.[1]

Affective psychoses: Mental disorders, usually recurrent, in which there is a severe disturbance of mood (mostly compounded of depression and anxiety but also manifested as elation, and excitement) which is accompanied by one or more of the following: delusions, perplexity, disturbed attitude to self, disorder of perception and behavior; these are all in keeping with the individual's prevailing mood (as are hallucinations when they occur). There is a strong tendency to suicide. For practical reasons, mild disorders of mood may also be included here if the symptoms match closely the descriptions given; this applies particularly to mild hypomania.[1]

bipolar: A manic-depressive psychosis which has appeared in both the depressive and manic form, either alternating or separated by an interval of normality.[1]

atypical: An episode of affective psychosis with some, but not all, of the features of the one form of the disorder in individuals who have had a previous episode of the other form of the disorder.[2]

depressed: A manic-depressive psychosis, circular type, in which the depressive form is currently present.[1]

manic: A manic-depressive psychosis, circular type, in which the manic form is currently present.[1]

mixed: A manic-depressive psychosis, circular type, in which both manic and depressive symptoms are present at the same time.[1]

depressed type: A manic-depressive psychosis in which there is a widespread depressed mood of gloom and wretchedness with some degree of anxiety. There is often reduced activity but there may be restlessness and agitation. There is marked tendency to recurrence; in a few cases this may be at regular intervals.[1]

...ive
...stment
...itement out of
...ss (hypomania) to
...r ideas, distractibility,

...both the manic and depressed
...pecifically.[1]

...ually also physical, resulting from taking alcohol, ...hat always include a compulsion to take alcohol on ...erience its psychic effects, and sometimes to avoid the ... may not be present. A person may be dependent on alcohol ... diagnosis of drug dependence to identify the agent. If alcohol ...oholic psychosis or with physical complications, *both* diagnoses

Alcohol intoxica...

acute: A ...physical state resulting from alcohol ingestion characterized by slurred speech, unste... poor coordination, flushed facies, nystagmus, sluggish reflexes, fetor alcoholica, ...n, emotional instability (e.g., jollity followed by lugubriousness), excessive conviviality, lo...ity, and poorly inhibited sexual and aggressive behavior.[2]

id...ncratic: Acute psychotic episodes induced by relatively small amounts of alcohol. These are regarded as individual idiosyncratic reactions to alcohol, not due to excessive consumption and without conspicuous neurological signs of intoxication.[1]

pathological—*see* Alcohol intoxication, idiosyncratic

Alcoholic psychoses: Organic psychotic states due mainly to excessive consumption of alcohol; defects of nutrition are thought to play an important role.[1]

alcohol abstinence syndrome—*see* alcohol withdrawal syndrome below

alcohol amnestic syndrome: A syndrome of prominent and lasting reduction of memory span, including striking loss of recent memory, disordered time appreciation and confabulation, occurring in alcoholics as the sequel to an acute alcoholic psychosis (especially delirium tremens) or, more rarely, in the course of chronic alcoholism. It is usually accompanied by peripheral neuritis and may be associated with Wernicke's encephalopathy.[1]

alcohol withdrawal delirium [delirium tremens]: Acute or subacute organic psychotic states in alcoholics, characterized by clouded consciousness, disorientation, fear, illusions, delusions, hallucinations of any kind, notably visual and tactile, and restlessness, tremor and sometimes fever.[1]

alcohol withdrawal hallucinosis: A psychosis usually of less than six months' duration, with slight or no clouding of consciousness and much anxious restlessness in which auditory hallucinations, mostly of voices uttering insults and threats, predominate.[1]

alcohol withdrawal syndrome: Tremor of hands, tongue, and eyelids following cessation of prolonged heavy drinking of alcohol. Nausea and vomiting, dry mouth, headache, heavy perspiration, fitful sleep, acute anxiety attacks, mood depression, feelings of guilt and remorse, and irritability are associated features.[2]

alcohol delirium—*see* alcohol withdrawal delirium above

alcoholic dementia: Nonhallucinatory dementias occurring in association with alcoholism, but not characterized by the features of either alcohol withdrawal delirium [delirium tremens] or alcohol amnestic syndrome [Korsakoff's alcoholic psychosis].[1]

alcoholic hallucinosis—*see* alcohol withdrawal hallucinosis above

alcoholic jealousy: Chronic paranoid psychosis characterized by delusional jealousy and associated with alcoholism.[1]

alcoholic paranoia—*see* Alcoholic jealousy

alcoholic polyneuritic psychosis—*see* alcohol amnestic syndrome above

Alcoholism

acute—*see* Alcohol intoxication, acute

chronic—*see* Alcohol dependence syndrome

Alexia: Loss of a previously possessed reading facility that cannot be explained by defective visual acuity.[3]

Amnesia, psychogenic: A form of dissociative hysteria in which there is a temporary disturbance in the ability to recall important personal information which has already been registered and stored in memory. The sudden onset of this disturbance in the absence of an underlying organic mental disorder, and the extent of the disturbance being too great to be explained by ordinary forgetfulness, are the essential features.[2]

Amnestic syndrome: A syndrome of prominent and lasting reduction of memory span, including striking loss of recent memory, disordered time appreciation, and confabulation. The commonest causes are chronic alcoholism [alcohol amnestic syndrome; Korsakoff's alcoholic psychosis], chronic barbiturate dependence, and malnutrition. An amnestic syndrome may be the predominating disturbance in the early states of presenile and senile dementia, arteriosclerotic dementia, and in encephalitis and other inflammatory and degenerative diseases in which there is particular bilateral involvement of the temporal lobes, and certain temporal lobe tumors.[2]

alcoholic—*see* alcohol amnestic syndrome under Alcoholic psychoses

Amoral personality—*see* Personality disorder, antisocial type

Anancastic [anankastic] neurosis—*see* Neurotic disorder, obsessive-compulsive

Anancastic [anankastic] personality—*see* Personality disorder, compulsive type

Anorexia nervosa: A disorder in which the main features are persistent active refusal to eat and marked loss of weight. The level of activity and alertness is characteristically high in relation to the degree of emaciation. Typically the disorder begins in teenage girls but it may sometimes begin before puberty and rarely it occurs in males. Amenorrhea is usual and there may be a variety of other physiological changes including slow pulse and respiration, low body temperature, and dependent edema. Unusual eating habits and attitudes toward food are typical and sometimes starvation follows or alternates with periods of overeating. The accompanying psychiatric symptoms are diverse.[1]

Anxiety hysteria—*see* phobia under Neurotic disorders

Anxiety state (neurotic): Apprehension, tension, or uneasiness that stems from the anticipation of danger, the source of which is largely unknown or unrecognized.[3]

atypical: An anxiety disorder that does not fulfill the criteria of generalized or panic attack anxiety. An example might be an individual with a single morbid fear.[2]

generalized: A disorder of at least six months' duration in which the predominant feature is limited to diffuse and persistent anxiety without the specific symptoms that characterize phobic disorders, panic disorder, or obsessive-compulsive disorder.[2]

panic attack: An episodic and often chronic, recurrent disorder in which the predominant features are anxiety attacks and nervousness. The anxiety attacks are manifested by discrete periods of sudden onset of intense apprehension, fearfulness, or terror often associated with feelings of impending doom.[2]

Aphasia, developmental: A delay in the production of spoken language. Rarely, there is also a developmental delay in the comprehension of speech sounds.[1]

Arteriosclerotic dementia: Dementia attributable, because of physical signs (on examination of the central nervous system), to degenerative arterial disease of the brain. Symptoms suggesting a focal lesion in the brain are common. There may be a fluctuating or patchy intellectual defect with insight, and an intermittent course is common. Clinical differentiation from senile or presenile dementia, which may coexist with it, may be very difficult or impossible. The diagnosis of cerebral atherosclerosis should also be recorded.[1]

Asocial personality—*see* Personality disorder, antisocial type

Astasia-abasia, hysterical: A form of conversion hysteria in which the individual is unable to stand or walk although the legs are otherwise under control.[4]

Asthenia, psychogenic—*see* neurasthenia under Neurotic disorders

Asthenic personality—*see* Personality disorder, dependent type

Attention deficit disorder—*see* attention deficit disorder under Hyperkinetic syndrome of childhood.

Autism, infantile: A syndrome present from birth or beginning almost invariably in the first 30 months. Responses to auditory and sometimes to visual stimuli are abnormal, and there are usually severe problems in the understanding of spoken language. Speech is delayed and, if it develops, is characterized by echolalia, the reversal of pronouns, immature grammatical structure, and inability to use abstract terms. There is generally an impairment in the social use of both verbal and gestural language. Problems in social relationships are most severe before the age of five years and include an impairment in the development of eye-to-eye gaze, social attachments, and cooperative play. Ritualistic behavior is usual and may include abnormal routines, resistance to change, attachment to odd objects and stereotyped patterns of play. The capacity for abstract or symbolic thought and for imaginative play is diminished. Intelligence ranges from severely subnormal to normal or above. Performance is usually better on tasks involving rote memory or visuospatial skills than on those requiring symbolic or linguistic skills.[1]

Avoidant personality—*see* Personality disorder, avoidant type

"Bad trips": Acute intoxication from hallucinogen abuse, manifested by hallucinatory states lasting only a few days or less.[1]

Barbiturate abuse: Cases where an individual has taken the drug to the detriment of his health or social functioning, in doses above or for periods beyond those normally regarded as therapeutic.[1]

Bestiality—*see* Zoophilia

Bipolar disorder—*see* Affective psychosis, bipolar

atypical—*see* Affective psychosis, bipolar, atypical

Body-rocking—*see* Stereotyped repetitive movements

Borderline personality—*see* Personality disorder, borderline type

Borderline psychosis of childhood—*see* Psychosis, atypical childhood

Borderline schizophrenia—*see* Schizophrenia, latent

Bouffée délirante—*see* Paranoid reaction, acute

Briquet's disorder—*see* somatization disorder under Neurotic disorders

Bulimia: An episodic pattern of overeating [binge eating] accompanied by an awareness of the disordered eating pattern with a fear of not being able to stop eating voluntarily. Depressive moods and self-deprecating thoughts follow the episodes of binge eating.[2]

Catalepsy schizophrenia—*see* Schizophrenia, catatonic type

Catastrophic stress—*see* Gross stress reaction

Catatonia (schizophrenic)—*see* Schizophrenia, catatonic type

Character neurosis—*see* Personality disorders

Childhood autism—*see* Autism, infantile

Childhood type schizophrenia—*see* Psychosis, child

Chronic alcoholic brain syndrome—*see* alcoholic dementia under Alcoholic psychoses

Clay-eating—*see* Pica

Clumsiness syndrome—*see* coordination disorder under Developmental delay disorders, specific

Combat fatigue—*see* Posttraumatic disorder, acute

Compensation neurosis—*see* compensation neurosis under Neurotic disorders

Compulsive conduct disorder—*see* impulse control disorders under Conduct disorders

Compulsive neurosis—*see* Neurotic disorder, obsessive-compulsive

Compulsive personality—*see* Personality disorder, compulsive type

Concentration camp syndrome—*see* Posttraumatic stress disorder, prolonged

Conduct disorders: Disorders mainly involving aggressive and destructive behavior and disorders involving delinquency. It should be used for abnormal behavior, in individuals of any age, which gives rise to social disapproval but which is not part of any other psychiatric condition. Minor emotional disturbances may also be present. To be included, the behavior, as judged by its frequency, severity, and type of associations with other symptoms, must be abnormal in its context. Disturbances of conduct are distinguished from an adjustment reaction by a longer duration and by a lack of close relationship in time and content to some stress. They differ from a personality disorder by the absence of deeply ingrained maladaptive patterns of behavior present from adolescence or earlier.[1]

impulse control disorders: A failure to resist an impulse, drive, or temptation to perform some action which is harmful to the individual or to others. The impulse may or may not be consciously resisted, and the act may or may not be premeditated or planned. Prior to committing the act, there is an increasing sense of tension, and at the time of committing the act, there is an experience of either pleasure, gratification, or release. Immediately following the act, there may or may not be genuine regret, self-reproach, or guilt.[2] *See also* Intermittent explosive disorder, Isolated explosive disorder, Kleptomania, Pathological gambling, and Pyromania.

mixed disturbance of conduct and emotions: A disorder characterized by features of undersocialized and socialized disturbance of conduct, but in which there is also considerable emotional disturbance as shown, for example, by anxiety, misery, or obsessive manifestations.[1]

socialized conduct disorder: Conduct disorders in individuals who have acquired the values or behavior of a delinquent peer group to whom they are loyal and with whom they characteristically steal, play truant, and stay out late at night. There may also be sexual promiscuity.[1]

undersocialized conduct disturbance

aggressive type: A disorder characterized by a persistent pattern of disrespect for the feelings and well-being of others (bullying, physical aggression, cruel behavior, hostility, verbal abusiveness, impudence, defiance, negativism), aggressive antisocial behavior (destructiveness, stealing, persistent lying, frequent truancy, and vandalism), and failure to develop close and stable relationships with others.[2]

unaggressive type: A disorder in which there is a lack of concern for the rights and feelings of others to a degree which indicates a failure to establish a normal degree of affection, empathy, or bond with others. There are two patterns of behavior found. In one, the child is fearful and timid, lacking self-assertiveness, resorts to self-protective and manipulative lying, indulges in whining demandingness and temper tantrums, feels rejected and unfairly treated, and is mistrustful of others. In the other pattern of the disorder, the child approaches others strictly for his own gains and acts exclusively because of exploitative and extractive goals. The child lies brazenly and steals, appearing to feel no guilt, and forms no social bonds to other individuals.[2]

Confusion, psychogenic—*see* Psychosis, reactive confusion

Confusion, reactive—*see* Psychosis, reactive confusion

Confusional state

acute—*see* Delirium, acute

epileptic—*see* Delirium, acute

subacute—*see* Delirium, subacute

Conversion hysteria—*see* hysteria, conversion type under Neurotic disorders

Coordination disorder—*see* coordination disorder under Developmental delay disorders, specific

Culture shock: A form of stress reaction associated with an individual's assimilation into a new culture which is vastly different from that in which he was raised.[5]

Cyclic schizophrenia—*see* Schizophrenia, schizo-affective type

Cyclothymic personality or disorder—*see* Personality disorder, cyclothymic type

Delirium: Transient organic psychotic conditions with a short course in which there is a rapidly developing onset of disorganization of higher mental processes manifested by some degree of impairment of information processing, impaired or abnormal attention, perception, memory, and thinking. Clouded consciousness, confusion, disorientation, delusions, illusions, and often vivid hallucinations predominate in the clinical picture.[1,2]

acute: short-lived states, lasting hours or days, of the above type.[1]

subacute: states of the above type in which the symptoms, usually less florid, last for several weeks or longer, during which they may show marked fluctuations in intensity.[1]

Delirium tremens—*see* alcohol withdrawal delirium under Alcoholic psychoses

Delusions, systematized—*see* Paranoia

Dementia: A decrement in intellectual functioning of sufficient severity to interfere with occupational or social performance, or both. There is impairment of memory and abstract thinking, the ability to learn new skills, problem solving, and judgment. There is often also personality change or impairment in impulse control. Dementia in organic psychoses may be of a chronic or progressive nature, which if untreated are usually irreversible and terminal.[1,2]

alcoholic—*see* alcoholic dementia under Alcoholic psychoses

arteriosclerotic—*see* Arteriosclerotic dementia

multi-infarct—*see* Arteriosclerotic dementia

presenile—*see* Presenile dementia

repeated infarct—*see* Arteriosclerotic dementia

senile—*see* Senile dementia

Depersonalization syndrome—*see* depersonalization syndrome under Neurotic disorders

Depression: States of depression, usually of moderate but occasionally of marked intensity, which have no specifically manic-depressive or other psychotic depressive features, and which do not appear to be associated with stressful events or other features specified under neurotic depression.[1]

anxiety—*see* depression under Neurotic disorders

endogenous—*see* Affective psychosis, depressed type

monopolar—*see* Affective psychosis, depressed type

neurotic—*see* depression under Neurotic disorders

psychotic—*see* Affective psychosis, depressed type

psychotic reactive—*see* Psychosis, depressive

reactive—*see* depression under Neurotic disorders

reactive psychotic—*see* Psychosis, depressive

Depressive personality or character—*see* Personality disorder, chronic depressive type

Depressive reaction—*see* depressive reaction under Adjustment reaction

Depressive psychosis—*see* Affective psychosis, depressed type

Derealization (neurotic)—*see* depersonalization syndrome under Neurotic disorders

Developmental delay disorders, specific: A group of disorders in which a specific delay in development is the main feature. For many the delay is not explicable in terms of general intellectual retardation or of inadequate schooling. In each case development is related to biological maturation, but it is also influenced by nonbiological factors. A diagnosis of a specific developmental delay carries no etiological implications. A diagnosis of specific delay in development should not be made if it is due to a known neurological disorder.[1]

arithmetical disorder: Disorders in which the main feature is a serious impairment in the development of arithmetical skills.[1]

articulation disorder: A delay in the development of normal word-sound production resulting in defects of articulation. Omissions or substitutions of consonants are most frequent.[1]

coordination disorder: Disorders in which the main feature is a serious impairment in the development of motor coordination which is not explicable in terms of general intellectual retardation. The clumsiness is commonly associated with perceptual difficulties.[1]

mixed development disorder: A delay in the development of one specific skill (e.g., reading, arithmetic, speech, or coordination) is frequently associated with lesser delays in other skills. When this occurs the diagnosis should be made according to the skill most seriously impaired. The mixed category should be used only where the mixture of delayed skills is such that no one skill is preponderantly affected.[1]

motor retardation—*see* coordination disorder above

reading disorder or retardation: Disorders in which the main feature is a serious impairment in the development of reading or spelling skills which is not explicable in terms of general intellectual retardation or of inadequate schooling. Speech or language difficulties, impaired right-left differentiation, perceptuo-motor problems, and coding difficulties are frequently associated. Similar problems are often present in other members of the family. Adverse psychosocial factors may be present.[1]

speech or language disorder: Disorders in which the main feature is a serious impairment in the development of speech or language (syntax or semantic) which is not explicable in terms of general intellectual retardation. Most commonly there is a delay in the development of normal word-sound production resulting in defects of articulation. Omissions or substitutions of consonants are most frequent. There may also be a delay in the production of spoken language. Rarely, there is also a developmental delay in the comprehension of sounds. Includes cases in which delay is largely due to environmental privation.[1]

Dipsomania—*see* Alcohol dependence syndrome

Disorganized schizophrenia—*see* Schizophrenia, disorganized type

Dissociative hysteria—*see* hysteria, dissociative type under Neurotic disorders

Drug abuse: Includes cases where an individual, for whom no other diagnosis is possible, has come under medical care because of the maladaptive effect of a drug on which he is not dependent (*see* Drug dependence) and that he has taken on his own initiative to the detriment of his health or social functioning. When drug abuse is secondary to a psychiatric disorder, record the disorder as an additional diagnosis.[1]

Drug dependence: A state, psychic and sometimes also physical, resulting from taking a drug, characterized by behavioral and other responses that always include a compulsion to take a drug on a continuous or periodic basis in order to experience its psychic effects, and sometimes to avoid the discomfort of its absence. Tolerance may or may not be present. A person may be dependent on more than one drug.[1]

Drug psychoses: Organic mental syndromes which are due to consumption of drugs (notably amphetamines, barbiturates, and opiate and LSD groups) and solvents. Some of the syndromes in this group are not as severe as most conditions labeled "psychotic," but they are included here for practical reasons. The drug should be identified, and also a diagnosis of drug dependence should be recorded, if present.[1]

drug-induced hallucinosis: Hallucinatory states of more than a few days, but not more than a few months' duration, associated with large or prolonged intake of drugs, notably of the amphetamine and LSD groups. Auditory hallucinations usually predominate and there may be anxiety or restlessness. States following LSD or other hallucinogens lasting only a few days or less ["bad trips"] are not included.[1]

drug-induced organic delusional syndrome: Paranoid states of more than a few days, but not more than a few months' duration, associated with large or prolonged intake of drugs, notably of the amphetamine and LSD groups.[1]

drug withdrawal syndrome: States associated with drug withdrawal ranging from severe, as specified for alcohol withdrawal delirium [delirium tremens], to less severe states characterized by one or more symptoms such as convulsions, tremor, anxiety, restlessness, gastrointestinal and muscular complaints, and mild disorientation and memory disturbance.[1]

Drunkenness:

acute—*see* Alcohol intoxication, acute

pathologic—*see* Alcohol intoxication, idiosyncratic

simple: A state of inebriation due to alcohol consumption without conspicuous neurological signs of intoxication.[2]

sleep: An inability to fully arouse from the sleep state characterized by failure to attain full consciousness after arousal.[2]

Dyscalculia—*see* arithmetical disorder under Developmental delay disorders, specific

Dyslalia—*see* articulation disorder under Developmental delay disorders, specific

Dyslexia, developmental: A disorder in which the main feature is a serious impairment of reading skills which is not explicable in terms of general intellectual retardation or of inadequate schooling. Word-blindness and strephosymbolia (tendency to reverse letters and words in reading) are included.[1,3]

Dysmenorrhea, psychogenic: Painful menstruation due to disturbance of psychic control.[4]

Dyspareunia, functional—*see* functional dyspareunia under Psychosexual dysfunctions

Dyspraxia syndrome—*see* coordination disorder under Developmental delay disorders, specific

Dyssocial personality—*see* Personality disorder, antisocial type

Dysuria, psychogenic: Difficulty in passing urine due to psychic factors.[4]

Eating disorders: A group of disorders characterized by a conspicuous disturbance in eating behavior.[2] *See also* Bulimia, Pica, and Rumination, psychogenic.

Eccentric personality—*see* Personality disorder, eccentric type

Elective mutism: A pervasive and persistent refusal to speak in situations not attributable to a mental disorder. In some cases the behavior may manifest a form of withdrawal reaction to a specific stressful situation, or as a predominant feature in children exhibiting shyness or social withdrawal disorders.[2]

Emancipation disorder: An adjustment reaction in adolescents or young adults in which there is symptomatic expression (e.g., difficulty in making independent decisions, increased dependence on parental advice, adoption of values deliberately oppositional to parents) of a conflict over independence following the recent assumption of a status in which the individual is more independent of parental control or supervision.[2]

Emotional disturbances specific to childhood and adolescence: Less well-differentiated emotional disorders characteristic of the childhood period. When the emotional disorder takes the form of a neurosis, the appropriate diagnosis should be made. These disorders differ from adjustment reactions in terms of longer duration and by the lack of close relationship in time and content to some stress.[1] *See also* Academic underachievement disorder, Elective mutism, Identity disorder, Introverted disorder of childhood, Misery and unhappiness disorder, Oppositional disorder, Overanxious disorder, and Shyness disorder of childhood.

Encopresis: A disorder in which the main manifestation is the persistent voluntary or involuntary passage of formed stools of normal or near-normal consistency into places not intended for that purpose in the individual's own sociocultural setting. Sometimes the child has failed to gain bowel control, and sometimes he has gained control but then later again became encopretic. There may be a variety of associated psychiatric symptoms and there may be smearing of feces. The condition would not usually be diagnosed under the age of four years.[1]

Endogenous depression—*see* Affective psychosis, depressed type

Enuresis: A disorder in which the main manifestation is a persistent involuntary voiding of urine by day or night which is considered abnormal for the age of the individual. Sometimes the child will have failed to gain bladder control and in other cases he will have gained control and then lost it. Episodic or fluctuating enuresis should be included. The disorder would not usually be diagnosed under the age of four years.[1]

Epileptic confusional or twilight state—*see* Delirium, acute

Excitation

catatonic—*see* Schizophrenia, catatonic type

psychogenic—*see* Psychosis, excitative type

reactive—*see* Psychosis, excitative type

Exhaustion delirium—*see* Stress reaction, acute

Exhibitionism: Sexual deviation in which the main sexual pleasure and gratification is derived from exposure of the genitals to a person of the opposite sex.[1]

Explosive personality disorder—*see* Personality disorder, explosive type

Factitious illness: A form of hysterical neurosis in which there are physical or psychological symptoms that are not real, genuine, or natural, which are produced by the individual and are under his voluntary control.[2]

physical symptom type: The presentation of physical symptoms that may be total fabrication, self-inflicted, an exaggeration or exacerbation of a pre-existing physical condition, or any combination or variation of these.[2]

psychological symptom type: The voluntary production of symptoms suggestive of a mental disorder. Behavior may mimic psychosis or, rather, the individual's idea of psychosis.[2]

Fanatic personality—*see* Personality disorder, paranoid type

Fatigue neurosis—*see* neurasthenia under Neurotic disorders

Feeble-minded—*see* Mental retardation, mild

Fetishism: A sexual deviation in which nonliving objects are utilized as a preferred or exclusive method of stimulating erotic arousal.[2]

Finger-flicking—*see* Stereotyped repetitive movements

Folie à deux—*see* Shared paranoid disorder

Frigidity: A psychosexual dysfunction in which there is partial or complete failure to attain or maintain the lubrication-swelling response of sexual excitement until completion of the sexual act.[2]

Frontal lobe syndrome: Changes in behavior following damage to the frontal areas of the brain or following interference with the connections of those areas. There is a general diminution of self-control, foresight, creativity, and spontaneity, which may be manifest as increased irritability, selfishness, restlessness and lack of concern for others. Conscientiousness and powers of concentration are often diminished, but measurable deterioration of intellect or memory is not necessarily present. The overall picture is often one of emotional dullness, lack of drive, and slowness; but, particularly in persons previously with energetic, restless, or aggressive characteristics, there may be a change towards impulsiveness, boastfulness, temper outbursts, silly fatuous humor, and the development of unrealistic ambitions; the direction of change usually depends upon the previous personality. A considerable degree of recovery is possible and may continue over the course of several years.[1]

Fugue, psychogenic: A form of dissociative hysteria characterized by an episode of wandering with inability to recall one's prior identity. Both onset and recovery are rapid. Following recovery there is no recollection of events which took place during the fugue state.[2]

Ganser's syndrome (hysterical): A form of factitious illness in which the patient voluntarily produces symptoms suggestive of a mental disorder.[2]

Gender identity disorder—*see* gender identity disorder under Psychosexual identity disorders

Gilles de la Tourette's disorder or syndrome—*see* Gilles de la Tourette's disorder under Tics

Grief reaction—*see* depressive reaction, brief under Adjustment reaction

Gross stress reaction—*see* Stress reaction, acute

Group delinquency—*see* socialized conduct disorder under Conduct disorders

Habit spasm—*see* chronic motor tic disorder under Tics

Hangover (alcohol)—*see* Drunkenness, simple

Head-banging—*see* Stereotyped repetitive movements

Hebephrenia—*see* Schizophrenia, disorganized type

Heller's syndrome—*see* Psychosis, disintegrative

High grade defect—*see* Mental retardation, mild

Homosexuality: Exclusive or predominant sexual attraction for persons of the same sex with or without physical relationship. Record homosexuality as a diagnosis whether or not it is considered as a mental disorder.[1]

Hospital addiction syndrome—*see* Munchausen syndrome

Hospital hoboes—*see* Munchausen syndrome

Hospitalism: A mild or transient adjustment reaction characterized by withdrawal seen in hospitalized patients. In young children this may be manifested by elective mutism.[1]

Hyperkinetic syndrome of childhood: Disorders in which the essential features are short attention-span and distractibility. In early childhood the most striking symptom is disinhibited, poorly organized and poorly regulated extreme overactivity but in adolescence this may be replaced by underactivity. Impulsiveness, marked mood fluctuations, and aggression are also common symptoms. Delays in the development of specific skills are often present and disturbed, poor relationships are common. If the hyperkinesis is symptomatic of an underlying disorder, the diagnosis of the underlying disorder is recorded instead.[1]

attention deficit disorder: Cases of hyperkinetic syndrome in which short attention span, distractibility, and overactivity are the main manifestations without significant disturbance of conduct or delay in specific skills.[1]

hyperkinesis with developmental delay: Cases in which the hyperkinetic syndrome is associated with speech delay, clumsiness, reading difficulties, or other delays of specific skills.[1]

hyperkinetic conduct disorder: Cases in which the hyperkinetic syndrome is associated with marked conduct disturbance but not developmental delay.[1]

Hypersomnia: A disorder of initiating arousal from sleep or maintaining wakefulness.

persistent: Chronic difficulty in initiating arousal from sleep or maintaining wakefulness associated with major or minor depressive mental disorders.[2]

transient: Episodes of difficulty in arousal from sleep or maintaining wakefulness associated with acute or intermittent emotional reactions or conflicts.[2]

Hypochondriasis—*see* hypochondriasis under Neurotic disorders

Hypomania—*see* Affective psychosis, manic type

Hypomanic personality—*see* Personality disorder, chronic hypomanic type

Hyposomnia—*see* Insomnia

Hysteria—*see* hysteria under Neurotic disorders

anxiety—*see* phobia under Neurotic disorders

psychosis—*see* Psychosis, reactive

acute—*see* Psychosis, excitative type

Hysterical personality—*see* Personality disorder, histrionic type

Identity disorder: An emotional disorder caused by distress over the inability to reconcile aspects of the self into a relatively coherent and acceptable sense of self, not secondary to another mental disorder. The disturbance is manifested by intense subjective distress regarding uncertainty about a variety of issues relating to identity, including long-term goals, career choice, friendship patterns, values, and loyalties.[2]

Idiocy—*see* Mental retardation, profound

Imbecile—*see* Mental retardation, moderate

Impotence: A psychosexual dysfunction in which there is partial or complete failure to attain or maintain erection until completion of the sexual act.[2]

Impulse control disorder—*see* impulse control disorders under Conduct disorders

Inadequate personality—*see* Personality disorder, dependent type

Induced paranoid disorder—*see* Shared paranoid disorder

Inebriety—*see* Drunkenness, simple

Infantile autism—*see* Autism, infantile

Insomnia: A disorder of initiating or maintaining sleep.[2]

persistent: A chronic state of sleeplessness associated with chronic anxiety, major or minor depressive disorders, or psychoses.[2]

transient: Episodes of sleeplessness associated with acute or intermittent emotional reactions or conflicts.[2]

Intermittent explosive disorder: Recurrent episodes of sudden and significant loss of control of aggressive impulses, not accounted for by any other mental disorder, which results in serious assault or destruction of property. The magnitude of the behavior during an episode is grossly out of proportion to any psychosocial stressors which may have played a role in eliciting the episode of lack of control. Following each episode there is genuine regret or self-reproach at the consequences of the action and the inability to control the aggressive impulse.[2]

Introverted disorder of childhood: An emotional disturbance in children chiefly manifested by a lack of interest in social relationships and indifference to social praise or criticism.[2]

Introverted personality—*see* Personality disorder, introverted type

Involutional melancholia—*see* Affective psychosis, depressed type

Involutional paranoid state—*see* Paraphrenia

Isolated explosive disorder: A disorder of impulse control in which there is a single discrete episode characterized by failure to resist an impulse which leads to a single, violent externally- directed act, which has a catastrophic impact on others, and for which the available information does not justify the diagnosis of another mental disorder.[2]

Isolated phobia—*see* simple phobia under Phobia

Jet lag syndrome: A phase-shift disruption of the 24-hour sleep-wake cycle due to rapid time-zone changes experienced in long-distance travel.[2]

Kanner's syndrome—*see* Autism, infantile

Kleptomania: A disorder of impulse control characterized by a recurrent failure to resist impulses to steal objects not for immediate use or their monetary value. An increasing sense of tension is experienced prior to committing the act, with an intense experience of gratification at the time of committing the theft.[2]

Korsakoff's psychosis:

alcoholic—*see* alcohol amnestic syndrome under Alcoholic psychoses

nonalcoholic—*see* Amnestic syndrome

Latent schizophrenia—*see* Schizophrenia, latent

Lesbianism—*see* Homosexuality

Lobotomy syndrome—*see* Frontal lobe syndrome

LSD reaction: Acute intoxication from hallucinogen abuse, manifested by hallucinatory states lasting only a few days or less.[1]

Major depressive disorder—*see* Affective psychosis, depressed type

Malingering: A clinical picture in which the predominant feature is the presentation of fake or grossly exaggerated physical or psychiatric illness apparently under voluntary control. In contrast to factitious illness, the symptoms produced in malingering are in pursuit of a goal which, when known, is recognizable and obviously understandable in light of knowledge of the individual's circumstances. Examples of understandable goals include, but are not limited to, becoming a "patient" in order to avoid conscription or military duty, avoid work, obtain financial compensation, evade criminal prosecution, and obtain drugs.[2]

Mania (monopolar)—*see* Affective psychosis, manic type

Manic-depressive psychosis

circular type—*see* Affective psychosis, bipolar

depressed type—*see* Affective psychosis, depressed type

manic type—*see* Affective psychosis, manic type

mixed type—*see* Affective psychosis, mixed type

Manic disorder—*see* Affective psychosis, manic type

atypical—*see* Affective psychosis, manic type, atypical

Masochistic personality—*see* Personality disorder, masochistic type

Melancholia—*see* Affective psychoses

involutional—*see* Affective psychosis, depressed type

Mental retardation: A condition of arrested or incomplete development of mind which is especially characterized by subnormality of intelligence. The coding should be made on the individual's *current* level of functioning *without regard to its nature* or causation, such as psychosis, cultural deprivation, Down's syndrome, etc. Where there is a specific cognitive handicap—such as in speech—the diagnosis of mental retardation should be based on assessments of cognition *outside the area of specific handicap.* The assessment of intellectual level should be based on whatever information is available, including clinical evidence, adaptive behavior, and psychometric findings. The IQ levels given are based on a test with a mean of 100 and a standard deviation of 15, such as the Wechsler scales. They are provided only as a guide and should not be applied rigidly. Mental retardation often involves psychiatric disturbances and may often develop as a result of some physical disease or injury. In these cases, an additional diagnosis should be recorded to identify any associated condition, psychiatric or physical.[1]

mild mental retardation: IQ criteria 50-70. Individuals with this level of retardation are usually educable. During the pre-school period they can develop social and communication skills, have minimal retardation in sensorimotor areas, and often are not distinguished from normal children until a later age. During the school age period they can learn academic skills up to approximately the sixth-grade level. During the adult years, they can usually achieve social and vocational skills adequate for minimum self-support, but may need guidance and assistance when under social or economic stress.[2]

moderate mental retardation: IQ criteria 35-49. Individuals with this level of retardation are usually trainable. During the pre-school period they can talk or learn to communicate. They have poor social awareness and fair motor development. During the school age period they can profit from training in social and occupational skills, but they are unlikely to progress beyond the second-grade level in academic subjects. During their adult years they may achieve self-maintenance in unskilled or semi-skilled work under sheltered conditions. They need supervision and guidance when under mild social or economic stress.[2]

severe mental retardation: IQ criteria 20-34. Individuals with this level of retardation evidence poor motor development, minimal speech, and are generally unable to profit from training and self-help during the pre-school period. During the school age period they can talk or learn to communicate, can be trained in elementary health habits, and may profit from systematic habit training. During the adult years they may contribute partially to self-maintenance under complete supervision.[2]

profound mental retardation: IQ criteria under 20. Individuals with this level of retardation evidence minimal capacity for sensorimotor functioning and need nursing care during the pre-school period. During the school age period some further motor development may occur, and they may respond to minimal or limited training in self-help. During the adult years some motor and speech development may occur, and they may achieve very limited self-care and need nursing care.[2]

Merycism—*see* Rumination, psychogenic

Minimal brain dysfunction [MBD]—*see* Hyperkinetic syndrome of childhood

Misery and unhappiness disorder: An emotional disorder characteristic of childhood in which the main symptoms involve misery and unhappiness. There may also be eating and sleep disturbances.[1]

Mood swings (brief compensatory) (rebound): Mild disorders of mood (depression and anxiety or elation and excitement, occurring alternatingly or episodically) seen in affective psychosis.[1]

Motor tic disorders—*see* Tics

Motor-verbal tic disorder—*see* Gilles de la Tourette's disorder under Tics

Multi-infarct dementia or psychosis—*see* Arteriosclerotic dementia

Multiple operations syndrome—*see* Munchausen syndrome

Multiple personality: A form of dissociative hysteria in which there is the domination of the individual at any one time by one of two or more distinct personalities. Each personality is a full-integrated and complex unit with memories, behavior patterns, and social friendships which determine the nature of the individual's acts when uppermost in consciousness.[2]

Munchausen syndrome: A chronic form of factitious illness in which the individual demonstrates a plausible presentation of voluntarily produced physical symptomatology of such a degree that he is able to obtain and sustain multiple hospitalizations.[2]

Narcissistic personality—*see* Personality disorder, narcissistic type

Nervous debility—*see* neurasthenia under Neurotic disorders

Neurasthenia—*see* neurasthenia under Neurotic disorders

Neurotic delinquency—*see* mixed disturbance of conduct and emotions under Conduct disorders

Neurotic disorders: Neurotic disorders are mental disorders without any demonstrable organic basis in which the individual may have considerable insight and has unimpaired reality testing, in that he usually does not confuse his morbid subjective experiences and fantasies with external reality. Behavior may be greatly affected although usually remaining within socially acceptable limits, but personality is not disorganized. The principal manifestations include excessive anxiety, hysterical symptoms, phobias, obsessional and compulsive symptoms, and depression.[1]

anxiety states: Various combinations of physical and mental manifestations of anxiety, not attributable to real danger and occurring either in attacks [*see* Anxiety state, panic attacks] or as a persisting state [*see* Anxiety state, generalized]. The anxiety is usually diffuse and may extend to panic. Other neurotic features such as obsessional or hysterical symptoms may be present but do not dominate the clinical picture.[1]

compensation neurosis: Certain unconscious neurotic reactions in which features of secondary gain, such as a situational or financial advantage, are prominent.[3]

depersonalization: A neurotic disorder with an unpleasant state of disturbed perception in which external objects or parts of one's own body are experienced as changed in their quality, unreal, remote, or automatized. The patient is aware of the subjective nature of the change he experiences. If depersonalization occurs as a feature of anxiety, schizophrenia, or other mental disorder, the condition is classified according to the major psychiatric disorder.[1]

depression: A neurotic disorder characterized by disproportionate depression which has usually recognizably ensued on a distressing experience; it does not include among its features delusions or hallucinations, and there is often preoccupation with the psychic trauma which preceded the illness, e.g., loss of a cherished person or possession. Anxiety is also frequently present and mixed states of anxiety and depression should be included here. The distinction between depressive neurosis and psychosis should be made not only upon the degree of depression but also on the presence or absence of other neurotic and psychotic characteristics, and upon the degree of disturbance of the individual's behavior.[1]

hypochondriasis: A neurotic disorder in which the conspicuous features are excessive concern with one's health in general or the integrity and functioning of some part of one's body, or less frequently, one's mind. It is usually associated with anxiety and depression. It may occur as a feature of some other severe mental disorder (e.g., manic-depressive psychosis, depressed type, schizophrenia, hysteria) and in that case should be classified according to the corresponding major disorder.[1]

hysteria: A neurotic mental disorder in which motives, of which the patient seems unaware, produce either a restriction of the field of consciousness or disturbances of motor or sensory function which may seem to have psychological advantage or symbolic value.[1] There are three subtypes:

conversion type: The chief or only symptoms of the hysterical neurosis consist of psychogenic disturbance of function in some part of the body, e.g., paralysis, tremor, blindness, deafness, seizures.[1]

dissociative type: The most prominent feature of the hysterical neurosis is a narrowing of the field of consciousness which seems to serve an unconscious purpose and is commonly accompanied or followed by a selective amnesia. There may be dramatic but essentially superficial changes of personality [multiple personality], or sometimes the patient enters into a wandering state [fugue].[1]

factitious illness: Physical or psychological symptoms that are not real, genuine, or natural, which are produced by the individual and are under his voluntary control.[2]

neurasthenia: A neurotic disorder characterized by fatigue, irritability, headache, depression, insomnia, difficulty in concentration, and lack of capacity for enjoyment [anhedonia]. It may follow or accompany an infection or exhaustion, or arise from continued emotional stress. If neurasthenia is associated with a physical disorder, the latter should also be recorded as a diagnosis.[1]

obsessive-compulsive: States in which the outstanding symptom is a feeling of subjective compulsion, which must be resisted, to carry out some action, to dwell on an idea, to recall an experience, or to ruminate on an abstract topic. Unwanted thoughts which intrude, the insistency of words or ideas, ruminations or trains of thought are perceived by the individual to be inappropriate or nonsensical. The obsessional urge or idea is recognized as alien to the personality but as coming from within the self. Obsessional actions may be quasi-ritual performances designed to relieve anxiety, e.g., washing the hands to cope with contamination. Attempts to dispel the unwelcome thought or urges may lead to a severe inner struggle, with intense anxiety.[1]

occupational: A neurosis characterized by a functional disorder of a group of muscles used chiefly in one's occupation, marked by the occurrence of spasm, paresis, or incoordination on attempt to repeat the habitual movements (e.g., writers' cramp).[5]

phobic disorders: Neurotic states with abnormally intense dread of certain objects or specific situations which would not normally have that effect. If the anxiety tends to spread from a specified situation or object to a wider range of circumstances, it becomes akin to or identical with anxiety state and should be classified as such.[1] *See also* Phobia.

somatization disorder: A chronic, but fluctuating, neurotic disorder which begins early in life and is characterized by recurrent and multiple somatic complaints for which medical attention is sought but which are not apparently due to any physical illness. Complaints are presented in a dramatic, vague, or exaggerated way, or are part of a complicated medical history in which often many specific diagnoses have allegedly been made by other physicians. Complaints invariably refer to many organ systems (headache, fatigue, palpitations, fainting, nausea and vomiting, abdominal pains, bowel trouble, allergies, menstrual and sexual difficulties), and the individual frequently receives medical care from a number of physicians, sometimes simultaneously.[2]

Neurosis—*see* Neurotic disorders

Nightmares: Anxiety attacks occurring in dreams during REM sleep.[2]

Night terrors: A pathology of arousal from stage 4 sleep in which the individual experiences excessive terror and extreme panic (screaming, verbalizations), symptoms of autonomic activity, confusion, and poor recall for event.[2]

Nymphomania: Abnormal and excessive need or desire in the woman for sexual intercourse.[3]

Obsessional personality—*see* Personality disorder, compulsive type

Occupational neurosis—*see* Neurotic disorder, occupational

Oneirophrenia—*see* Schizophrenia, acute episode

Oppositional disorder of childhood or adolescence: A disorder characterized by pervasive opposition to all in authority regardless of self-interest, a continuous argumentativeness, and an unwillingness to respond to reasonable persuasion, not accounted for by a conduct disorder, adjustment disorder, or a psychosis of childhood. The oppositional behavior in this disorder is evoked by any demand, rule, suggestion, request, or admonishment placed on the individual.[2]

Organic affective syndrome: A clinical picture in which the predominating symptoms closely resemble those seen in either the depressive or manic affective disorders, occurring in the presence of evidence or history of a specific organic factor which is etiologically related to the disturbance, such as head trauma, endocranial tumors, and exocranial tumors secreting neurotoxic diatheses (e.g., pancreatic carcinoma). Excessive use of steroids, Cushing's syndrome, and other endocrine disorders may lead to an organic affective syndrome.[2]

Organic personality syndrome: Chronic, mild states of memory disturbance and intellectual deterioration, of nonpsychotic nature, often accompanied by increased irritability, querulousness, lassitude, and complaints of physical weakness. These states are often associated with old age, and may precede more severe states due to brain damage classifiable under senile or presenile dementia, dementia associated with other chronic organic psychotic brain syndromes, or delirium, delusions, hallucinosis, and depression in transient organic psychotic conditions.[1]

Organic psychosyndrome, focal (partial): A nonpsychotic organic mental disorder resembling the postconcussion syndrome associated with localized diseases of the brain or surrounding tissues.[1]

Organic psychotic conditions: Syndromes in which there is impairment of orientation, memory, comprehension, calculation, learning capacity, and judgment. These are the essential features but there may also be shallowness or lability of affect, or a more persistent disturbance of mood, lowering of ethical standards and exaggeration or emergence of personality traits, and diminished capacity for independent decision.[1] See also Alcohol psychoses, Arteriosclerotic dementia, Drug psychoses, Presenile dementia, and Senile dementia.

mixed paranoid and affective: Organic psychosis in which depressive and paranoid symptoms are the main features.[1]

transient: States characterized by clouded consciousness, confusion, disorientation, illusions, and often vivid hallucinations. They are usually due to some intra- or extracerebral toxic, infectious, metabolic or other systemic disturbance and are generally reversible. Depressive and paranoid symptoms may also be present but are not the main feature. The diagnosis of the associated physical or neurological condition should also be recorded.[1]

acute delirium: Short-lived states, lasting hours or days, of the above type.[1]

subacute delirium: States of the above type in which the symptoms, usually less florid, last for several weeks or longer during which they may show marked fluctuations in intensity.[1]

Organic reaction—*see* Organic psychotic conditions, transient

Overanxious disorder: An ill-defined emotional disorder characteristic of childhood in which the main symptoms involve anxiety and fearfulness.[1]

Panic disorder—*see* panic attack under Anxiety state

Paranoia: A rare chronic psychosis in which logically constructed systematized delusions have developed gradually without concomitant hallucinations or the schizophrenic type of disordered thinking. The delusions are mostly of grandeur (the paranoiac prophet or inventor), persecution, or somatic abnormality.[1]

alcoholic—*see* alcoholic jealousy under Alcoholic psychoses

querulans: A paranoid state which, though in many ways akin to schizophrenic or affective states, differs from other paranoid states and psychogenic paranoid psychosis.[1]

senile—*see* Paraphrenia

Paranoid personality—*see* Personality disorder, paranoid type

Paranoid reaction, acute: Paranoid states apparently provoked by some emotional stress. The stress is often misconstrued as an attack or threat. Such states are particularly prone to occur in prisoners or as acute reactions to a strange and threatening environment, e.g., in immigrants.[1]

Paranoid schizophrenia—*see* Schizophrenia, paranoid type

Paranoid state

involutional—*see* Paraphrenia

senile—*see* Paraphrenia

simple: A psychosis, acute or chronic, not classifiable as schizophrenia or affective psychosis, in which delusions, especially of being influenced, persecuted, or treated in some special way, are the main symptoms. The delusions are of a fairly fixed, elaborate, and systematized kind.[1]

Paranoid traits—*see* Personality disorder, paranoid type

Paraphilia—*see* Sexual deviations

Paraphrenia: Paranoid psychosis in which there are conspicuous hallucinations, often in several modalities. Affective symptoms and disordered thinking, if present, do not dominate the clinical picture, and the personality is well preserved.[1]

Paraphrenic schizophrenia—*see* Schizophrenia, paranoid type

Passive-aggressive personality — *see* Personality disorder, passive- aggressive type

Passive personality—*see* Personality disorder, dependent type

Pathological

alcohol intoxication—*see* Alcohol intoxication, idiosyncratic

drug intoxication: Individual idiosyncratic reactions to comparatively small quantities of a drug, which take the form of acute, brief psychotic states of any type.[1]

drunkenness—*see* Alcohol intoxication, idiosyncratic

gambling: A disorder of impulse control characterized by a chronic and progressive preoccupation with gambling and urge to gamble, with subsequent gambling behavior that compromises, disrupts, or damages personal, family, and vocational pursuits.[2]

personality—*see* Personality disorder

Pedophilia: Sexual deviations in which an adult engages in sexual activity with a child of the same or opposite sex.[1]

Peregrinating patient—*see* Malingering

Personality disorders: Deeply ingrained maladaptive patterns of behavior generally recognizable by the time of adolescence or earlier and continuing throughout most of adult life, although often becoming less obvious in middle or old age. The personality is abnormal either in the balance of its components, their quality and expression, or in its total aspect. Because of this deviation or psychopathy the patient suffers or others have to suffer, and there is an adverse effect upon the individual or on society. It includes what is sometimes called psychopathic personality, but if this is determined primarily by malfunctioning of the brain, it should be classified as one of the nonpsychotic organic brain syndromes. When the patient exhibits an anomaly of personality directly related to his neurosis or psychosis, e.g., schizoid personality and schizophrenia or anancastic personality and obsessive compulsive neurosis, the relevant neurosis or psychosis which is in evidence should be diagnosed in addition.[1]

affective type: A chronic personality disorder characterized by lifelong predominance of a pronounced mood. The illness does not have a clear onset, and there may be intermittent periods of disturbed mood separated by periods of normal mood.[1]

anancastic [anankastic] type—*see* Personality disorder, compulsive type

antisocial type: A personality disorder characterized by disregard for social obligations, lack of feeling for others, and impetuous violence or callous unconcern. There is a gross disparity between behavior and the prevailing social norms. Behavior is not readily modifiable by experience, including punishment. People with this personality are often affectively cold, and may be abnormally aggressive or irresponsible. Their tolerance to frustration is low; they blame others or offer plausible rationalizations for the behavior which brings them into conflict with society.[1]

asthenic type—*see* Personality disorder, dependent type

avoidant type: Individuals with this disorder exhibit excessive social inhibitions and shyness, a tendency to withdraw from opportunities for developing close relationships, and a fearful expectation that they will be belittled and humiliated. Desires for affection and acceptance are strong, but they are unwilling to enter relationships unless given unusually strong guarantees that they will be uncritically accepted. Therefore, they have few close relationships and suffer from feelings of loneliness and isolation.[2]

borderline type: Individuals with this disorder are characterized by instability in a variety of areas, including interpersonal relationships, behavior, mood, and self image. Interpersonal relationships are often intense and unstable with marked shifts of attitude over time. Frequently there is impulsive and unpredictable behavior which is potentially physically self-damaging. There may be problems tolerating being alone, and chronic feelings of emptiness or boredom.[2]

chronic depressive type: An affective personality disorder characterized by lifelong predominance of a chronic nonpsychotic disturbance involving either intermittent or sustained periods of depressed mood (marked by worry, pessimism, low output of energy, and a sense of futility).[2]

chronic hypomanic type: An affective personality disorder characterized by lifelong predominance of a chronic nonpsychotic disturbance involving either intermittent or sustained periods of abnormally elevated mood (unshakable optimism and an enhanced zest for life and activity).[2]

compulsive type: A personality disorder characterized by feelings of personal insecurity, doubt, and incompleteness leading to excessive conscientiousness, checking, stubbornness, and caution. There may be insistent and unwelcome thoughts or impulses which do not attain the severity of an obsessional neurosis. There is perfectionism and meticulous accuracy and a need to check repeatedly in an attempt to ensure this. Rigidity and excessive doubt may be conspicuous.[1]

cyclothymic type: A chronic nonpsychotic disturbance involving depressed and elevated mood, lasting at least two years, separated by periods of normal mood.[2]

dependent type: A personality disorder characterized by passive compliance with the wishes of elders and others and a weak inadequate response to the demands of daily life. Lack of vigor may show itself in the intellectual or emotional spheres; there is little capacity for enjoyment.[1]

eccentric type: A personality disorder characterized by oddities of behavior which do not conform to the clinical syndromes of personality disorders described elsewhere.[2]

explosive type: A personality disorder characterized by instability of mood with liability to intemperate outbursts of anger, hate, violence, or affection. Aggression may be expressed in words or in physical violence. The outbursts cannot readily be controlled by the affected persons, who are not otherwise prone to antisocial behavior.[1]

histrionic type: A personality disorder characterized by shallow, labile affectivity, dependence on others, craving for appreciation and attention, suggestibility, and theatricality. There is often sexual immaturity, e.g., frigidity and over-responsiveness to stimuli. Under stress hysterical symptoms [neurosis] may develop.[1]

hysterical type—*see* Personality disorder, histrionic type

inadequate type—*see* Personality disorder, dependent type

introverted type: A form of schizoid personality in which the essential features are a profound defect in the ability to form social relationships and to respond to the usual forms of social reinforcements. Such patients are characteristically "loners" who do not appear distressed by their social distance and are not interested in greater social involvements.[2]

masochistic type: A personality disorder in which the individual appears to arrange life situations so as to be defeated and humiliated.[2]

narcissistic type: A personality disorder in which interpersonal difficulties are caused by an inflated sense of self-worth, and indifference to the welfare of others. Achievement deficits and social irresponsibilities are justified and sustained by a boastful arrogance, expansive fantasies, facile rationalization, and frank prevarication.[2]

paranoid type: A personality disorder in which there is excessive sensitiveness to setbacks or to what are taken to be humiliations and rebuffs, a tendency to distort experience by misconstruing the neutral or friendly actions of others as hostile or contemptuous, and a combative and tenacious sense of personal rights. There may be a proneness to jealousy or excessive self-importance. Such persons may feel helplessly humiliated and put upon; others, likewise excessively sensitive, are aggressive and insistent. In all cases there is excessive self-reference.[1]

passive-aggressive type: A personality disorder characterized by aggressive behavior manifested in passive ways, such as obstructionism, pouting, procrastination, intentional inefficiency, or stubbornness. The *aggression* often arises from resentment at failing to find gratification in a relationship with an individual or institution upon which the individual is overdependent.[3]

passive type—*see* Personality disorder, dependent type

schizoid type: A personality disorder in which there is withdrawal from affectional, social, and other contacts with autistic preference for fantasy and introspective reserve. Behavior may be slightly eccentric or indicate avoidance of competitive situations. Apparent coolness and detachment may mask an incapacity to express feeling.

schizotypal type: A form of schizoid personality in which individuals with this disorder manifest various oddities of thinking, perception, communication, and behavior. The disturbance in thinking may be expressed as magical thinking, ideas of reference, or paranoid ideation. Perceptual disturbances may include recurrent illusions and derealization [depersonalization]. Frequently, but not invariably, the behavioral manifestations include social isolation and constricted or inappropriate affect which interferes with rapport in face-to-face interaction without any of the frank psychotic features which characterize schizophrenia.[2]

Phobia: Neurotic states with abnormally intense dread of certain objects or specific situations which would not normally have that effect. If the anxiety tends to spread from a specified situation or object to a wider range of circumstances, it becomes akin to or identical with anxiety state, and should be classified as such.[1]

acrophobia: Fear of heights[3]

agoraphobia: fear of leaving the familiar setting of the home, and is almost always preceded by a phase during which there are recurrent panic attacks. Because of the anticipatory fear of helplessness when having a panic attack, the patient is reluctant or refuses to be alone, travel or walk alone, or to be in situations where there is no ready access to help, such as in crowds, closed or open spaces, or crowded stores.[2]

ailurophobia: Fear of cats[3]

algophobia: Fear of pain[3]

claustrophobia: Fear of closed spaces[3]

isolated phobia—*see* simple phobia below

mysophobia: Fear of dirt or germs[3]

obsessional—*see* Neurotic disorder, obsessive-compulsive

panphobia: Fear of everything[3]

simple phobia: Fear of a discrete object or situation which is neither fear of leaving the familiar setting of the home [agoraphobia], or of being observed by others in certain situations [social phobia]. Examples of simple phobia are fear of animals, acrophobia, and claustrophobia.

social phobia: Fear of situations in which the subject is exposed to possible scrutiny by others, and the possibility exists that he may act in a fashion that will be considered shameful. The most common social phobias are fears of public speaking, blushing, eating in public, writing in front of others, or using public lavatories.[2]

xenophobia: Fear of strangers[3]

Pica: Perverted appetite of nonorganic origin in which there is persistent eating of non-nutritional substances. Typically, infants ingest paint, plaster, string, hair, or cloth. Older children may have access to animal droppings, sand, bugs, leaves, or pebbles. In the adult, eating of starch or clay-earth has been observed.[2]

Postconcussion syndrome: States occurring after generalized contusion of the brain, in which the symptom picture may resemble that of the frontal lobe syndrome or that of any of the neurotic disorders, but in which in addition, headache, giddiness, fatigue, insomnia, and a subjective feeling of impaired intellectual ability are usually prominent. Mood may fluctuate, and quite ordinary stress may produce exaggerated fear and apprehension. There may be marked intolerance of mental and physical exertion, undue sensitivity to noise, and hypochondriacal preoccupation. The symptoms are more common in persons who have previously suffered from neurotic or personality disorders, or when there is a possibility of compensation. This syndrome is particularly associated with the closed type of head injury when signs of localized brain damage are slight or absent, but it may also occur in other conditions.[1]

Postcontusion syndrome or encephalopathy—*see* Postconcussion syndrome

Postencephalitic syndrome: A nonpsychotic organic mental disorder resembling the postconcussion syndrome associated with central nervous system infections.[1]

Postleucotomy syndrome—*see* Frontal lobe syndrome

Posttraumatic brain syndrome, nonpsychotic—*see* Postconcussion syndrome

Posttraumatic organic psychosis—*see* Organic psychotic conditions, transient

Posttraumatic stress disorder: The development of characteristic symptoms (re-experiencing the traumatic event, numbing of responsiveness to or involvement with the external world, and a variety of other autonomic, dysphoric, or cognitive symptoms) after experiencing a psychologically traumatic event or events outside the normal range of human experience (e.g., rape or assault, military combat, natural catastrophes such as flood or earthquake, or other disaster, such as airplane crash, fires, bombings).[2]

acute: Brief, episodic, or recurrent disorders lasting less than six months' duration after the onset of trauma.[2]

prolonged: Chronic disorders of the above type lasting six months or more following the trauma.[2]

Premature ejaculation—*see* premature ejaculation under Psychosexual dysfunction.

Prepsychotic schizophrenia—*see* Schizophrenia, latent

Presbyophrenia—*see* Organic personality syndrome

Presenile dementia: Dementia occuring usually before the age of 65 in patients with the relatively rare forms of diffuse or lobar cerebral atrophy. The associated neurological condition (e.g., Alzheimer's disease, Pick's disease, Jakob-Creutzfeldt disease) should also be recorded as a diagnosis.[1]

Prodromal schizophrenia—*see* Schizophrenia, latent

Pseudoneurotic schizophrenia—*see* Schizophrenia, latent

Psychalgia: Pains of mental origin, e.g., headache or backache, for which a more precise medical or psychiatric diagnosis cannot be made.[1]

Psychasthenia: A functional neurosis marked by stages of pathological fear or anxiety, obsessions, fixed ideas, tics, feelings of inadequacy, self-accusation, and peculiar feelings of strangeness, unreality, and depersonalization.[4]

Psychic shock: A sudden disturbance of mental equilibrium produced by strong emotion in response to physical or mental stress.[4]

Psychic factors associated with physical diseases: Mental disturbances or psychic factors of any type thought to have played a major part in the etiology of physical conditions, usually involving tissue damage, classified elsewhere. The mental disturbance is usually mild and nonspecific, and the psychic factors (worry, fear, conflict, etc.) may be present without any overt psychiatric disorder. Examples of these conditions are asthma, dermatitis, eczema, duodenal ulcer, ulcerative colitis, and urticaria, specified as due to psychogenic factors.

Use an additional diagnosis to identify the physical condition. In the rare instance that an overt psychiatric disorder is thought to have caused the physical condition, the psychiatric diagnosis should be recorded in addition.[1]

Psychoneurosis—*see* Neurotic disorders

Psycho-organic syndrome—*see* Organic psychotic conditions, transient

Psychopathic constitutional state—*see* Personality disorders

Psychopathic personality—*see* Personality disorders

Psychophysiological disorders: A variety of physical symptoms or types of physiological malfunctions of mental origin, not involving tissue damage, and usually mediated through the autonomic nervous system. The disorders are classified according to the body system involved. If the physical symptom is secondary to a psychiatric disorder classifiable elsewhere, the physical symptom is not classified as a psychophysiological disorder. If tissue damage is involved, then the diagnosis is classified as a *Psychic factor associated with diseases classified elsewhere.*[1]

Psychosexual dysfunctions: A group of disorders in which there is recurrent and persistent dysfunction encountered during sexual activity. The dysfunction may be lifelong or acquired, generalized or situational, and total or partial.[2]

functional dyspareunia: Recurrent and persistent genital pain associated with coitus.[2]

functional vaginismus: A history of recurrent and persistent involuntary spasm of the musculature of the outer one-third of the vagina that interferes with sexual activity.[2]

inhibited female orgasm: Recurrent and persistent inhibition of the female orgasm as manifested by a delay or absence of orgasm following a normal sexual excitement phase during sexual activity.[2]

inhibited male orgasm: Recurrent and persistent inhibition of the male orgasm as manifested by a delay or absence of either the emission or ejaculation phases, or more usually, both following an adequate phase of sexual excitement.[2]

inhibited sexual desire: Persistent inhibition of desire for engaging in a particular form of sexual activity.[2]

inhibited sexual excitement: Recurrent and persistent inhibition of sexual excitement during sexual activity, manifested either by partial or complete failure to attain or maintain erection until completion of the sexual act [impotence], or partial or complete failure to attain or maintain the lubrication-swelling response of sexual excitement until completion of the sexual act [frigidity].[2]

premature ejaculation: Ejaculation occurs before the individual wishes it, because of recurrent and persistent absence of reasonable voluntary control of ejaculation and orgasm during sexual activity.[2]

Psychosexual gender identity disorders: Behavior occurring in preadolescents of immature psychosexuality, or in adults, in which there is an incongruence between the individual's anatomic sex and gender identity.[2]

gender identity disorder: In children or in adults a condition in which the individual would prefer to be of the other sex, and strongly prefers the clothes, toys, activities, and companionship of the other sex. Cross-dressing is intermittent, although it may be frequent. In children the commonest form is feminism in boys.[2]

trans-sexualism: A psychosexual identity disorder centered around fixed beliefs that the overt bodily sex is wrong. The resulting behavior is directed towards either changing the sexual organs by operation, or completely concealing the bodily sex by adopting both the dress and behavior of the opposite sex.[1]

Psychosomatic disorders—*see* Psychophysiological disorders

Psychosis: Mental disorders in which impairment of mental function has developed to a degree that interferes grossly with insight, ability to meet some ordinary demands of life or to maintain adequate contact with reality. It is not an exact or well defined term. Mental retardation is excluded.[1]

affective—*see* Affective psychoses

alcoholic—*see* Alcoholic psychoses

atypical childhood: A variety of atypical infantile psychoses which may show some, but not all, of the features of infantile autism. Symptoms may include stereotyped repetitive movements, hyperkinesis, self-injury, retarded speech development, echolalia, and impaired social relationships. Such disorders may occur in children of any level of intelligence but are particularly common in those with mental retardation.[1]

borderline, of childhood—*see* Psychosis, atypical childhood

child: A group of disorders in children, characterized by distortions in the timing, rate, and sequence of many psychological functions involving language development and social relations in which the severe qualitative abnormalities are not normal for any stage of development.[2] See also Autism, infantile, Psychosis, disintegrative, Psychosis, atypical childhood.

depressive—*see* Affective psychosis, depressed type

depressive type: A depressive psychosis which can be similar in its symptoms to manic-depressive psychosis, depressed type but is apparently provoked by saddening stress such as a bereavement, or a severe disappointment or frustration. There may be less diurnal variation of symptoms than in manic-depressive psychosis, depressed type, and the delusions are more often understandable in the context of the life experiences. There is usually a serious disturbance of behavior, e.g., major suicidal attempt.[1]

disintegrative: A disorder in which normal or near-normal development for the first few years is followed by a loss of social skills and of speech, together with a severe disorder of emotions, behavior, and relationships. Usually this loss of speech and of social competence takes place over a period of a few months and is accompanied by the emergence of overactivity and of stereotypies. In most cases there is intellectual impairment, but this is not a necessary part of the disorder. The condition may follow overt brain disease, such as measles encephalitis, but it may also occur in the absence of any known organic brain disease or damage. Any associated neurological disorder should also be recorded.[1]

epileptic: An organic psychotic condition associated with epilepsy.[1]

excitative type: An affective psychosis similar in its symptoms to manic-depressive psychosis, manic type, but apparently provoked by emotional stress.[1]

hypomanic—*see* Affective psychosis, manic type

hysterical—*see* Psychosis, reactive

acute—*see* Psychosis, excitative type

induced—*see* Shared paranoid disorder

infantile—*see* Autism, infantile

infective—*see* Organic psychotic conditions, transient

Korsakoff's:

alcoholic—*see* alcohol amnestic syndrome under Alcoholic psychoses

nonalcoholic—*see* Amnestic syndrome

manic-depressive—*see* Affective psychoses

multi-infarct—*see* Arteriosclerotic dementia

paranoid

chronic—*see* Paranoia

protracted reactive—*see* Psychosis, paranoid, psychogenic

psychogenic: Psychogenic or reactive paranoid psychosis of any type which is more protracted than the reactions described under paranoid reaction, acute.[1]

acute—*see* Paranoid reaction, acute

postpartum—*see* Psychosis, puerperal

psychogenic—*see* Psychosis, reactive

depressive—*see* Psychosis, depressive type

puerperal: Any psychosis occurring within a fixed period (approximately 90 days) after childbirth.[3] The diagnosis should be classified according to the predominant symptoms or characteristics, such as schizophrenia, affective psychosis, paranoid states, or other specified psychosis.

reactive: A psychotic condition which is largely or entirely attributable to a recent life experience. This diagnosis is not used for the wider range of psychoses in which environmental factors play some, but not the *major,* part in etiology.[1]

brief: A florid psychosis of at least a few hours' duration but lasting no more than two weeks, with sudden onset immediately following a severe environmental stress and eventually terminating in complete recovery to the pre-psychotic state.[2]

confusion: Mental disorders with clouded consciousness, disorientation (though less marked than in organic confusion), and diminished accessibility often accompanied by excessive activity and apparently provoked by emotional stress.[1]

depressive—*see* Psychosis, depressive type

schizo-affective—*see* Schizophrenia, schizo-affective type

schizophrenic—*see* Schizophrenia

schizophreniform—*see* Schizophrenia

affective type—*See* Schizophrenia, schizo-affective type

confusional type—*see* Schizophrenia, acute episode

senile—*see* Senile dementia, delusional type

Pyromania: A disorder of impulse control characterized by a recurrent failure to resist impulses to set fires without regard for the consequences, or with deliberate destructive intent. Invariably there is intense fascination with the setting of fires, seeing fires burn, and a satisfaction with the resultant destruction.[2]

Relationship problems of childhood: Emotional disorders characteristic of childhood in which the main symptoms involve relationship problems.[1]

Repeated infarct dementia—*see* Arteriosclerotic dementia

Residual schizophrenia—.*see* Schizophrenia, residual type

Restzustand (schizophrenia)—*see* Schizophrenia, residual type

Rumination:

obsessional: The constant preoccupation with certain thoughts, with inability to dismiss them from the mind.[4] *see* Neurotic disorder, obsessive-compulsive.

psychogenic: In children the regurgitation of food, with failure to thrive or weight loss developing after a period of normal functioning. Food is brought up without nausea, retching, or disgust. The food is then ejected from the mouth, or chewed and reswallowed.[2]

Sander's disease—*see* Paranoia

Satyriasis: Pathologic or exaggerated sexual desire or excitement in the man.[3]

Schizoid personality disorder—*see* Personality disorder, schizoid type

Schizophrenia: A group of psychoses in which there is a fundamental disturbance of personality, a characteristic distortion of thinking, often a sense of being controlled by alien forces, delusions which may be bizarre, disturbed perception, abnormal affect out of keeping with the real situation, and autism. Nevertheless, clear consciousness and intellectual capacity are usually maintained. The disturbance of personality involves its most basic functions which give the normal person his feeling of individuality, uniqueness, and self-direction. The most intimate thoughts, feelings, and acts are often felt to be known to or shared by others and explanatory delusions may develop, to the effect that natural or supernatural forces are at work to influence the schizophrenic person's thoughts and actions in ways that are often bizarre. He may see himself as the pivot of all that happens. Hallucinations, especially of hearing, are common and may comment on the patient or address him. Perception is frequently disturbed in other ways; there may be perplexity, irrelevant features may become all-important and accompanied by passivity feeling, may lead the patient to believe that everyday objects and situations possess a special, usually sinister, meaning intended for him. In the characteristic schizophrenic disturbance of thinking, peripheral and irrelevant features of a total concept, which are inhibited in normal directed mental activity, are brought to the forefront and utilized in place of the elements relevant and appropriate to the situation. Thus, thinking becomes vague, elliptical and obscure, and its expression in speech sometimes incomprehensible. Breaks and interpolations in the flow of consecutive thought are frequent, and the patient may be convinced that his thoughts are being withdrawn by some outside agency. Mood may be shallow, capricious, or incongruous. Ambivalence and disturbance of volition may appear as inertia, negativism, or stupor. Catatonia may be present. The diagnosis "schizophrenia" should not be made unless there is, or has been evident during the same illness, characteristic disturbance of thought, perception, mood, conduct, or personality—preferably in at least two of these areas. The diagnosis should not be restricted to conditions running a protracted, deteriorating, or chronic course. In addition to making the diagnosis on the criteria just given, effort should be made to specify one of the following subtypes of schizophrenia, according to the predominant symptoms.[1]

acute (undifferentiated): Schizophrenia of florid nature which cannot be classified as simple, catatonic, hebephrenic, paranoid, or any other types.[1]

acute episode: Schizophrenic disorders, other than simple, hebephrenic, catatonic, and paranoid, in which there is a dream-like state with slight clouding of consciousness and perplexity. External things, people, and events may become charged with personal significance for the patient. There may be ideas of reference and emotional turmoil. In many such cases remission occurs within a few weeks or months, even without treatment.[1]

atypical—*see* Schizophrenia, acute (undifferentiated)

borderline—*see* Schizophrenia, latent

catatonic type: Includes as an essential feature prominent psychomotor disturbances often alternating between extremes such as hyperkinesis and stupor, or automatic obedience and negativism. Constrained attitudes may be maintained for long periods: if the patient's limbs are put in some unnatural position they may be held there for some time after the external force has been removed. Severe excitement may be a striking feature of the condition. Depressive or hypomanic concomitants may be present.[1]

cenesthopathic—*see* Schizophrenia, acute (undifferentiated)

childhood type—*see* Psychosis, child

chronic undifferentiated—*see* Schizophrenia, residual

cyclic—*see* Schizophrenia, schizo-affective type

disorganized type: A form of schizophrenia in which affective changes are prominent, delusions and hallucinations fleeting and fragmentary, behavior irresponsible and unpredictable, and mannerisms common. The mood is shallow and inappropriate, accompanied by giggling or self-satisfied, self—absorbed smiling, or by a lofty manner, grimaces, mannerisms, pranks, hypochondriacal complaints, and reiterated phrases. Thought is disorganized. There is a tendency to remain solitary, and behavior seems empty of purpose and feeling. This form of schizophrenia usually starts between the ages of 15 and 25 years.[1]

hebephrenic type:—*see* Schizophrenia, disorganized type

latent: It has not been possible to produce a generally acceptable description for this condition. It is not recommended for general use, but a description is provided for those who believe it to be useful: a condition of eccentric or inconsequent behavior and anomalies of affect which give the impression of schizophrenia though no definite and characteristic schizophrenic anomalies, present or past, have been manifest.[1]

paranoid type: The form of schizophrenia in which relatively stable delusions, which may be accompanied by hallucinations, dominate the clinical picture. The delusions are frequently of persecution, but may take other forms (for example, of jealousy, exalted birth, Messianic mission, or bodily change). Hallucinations and erratic behavior may occur; in some cases conduct is seriously disturbed from the outset, thought disorder may be gross, and affective flattening with fragmentary delusions and hallucinations may develop.[1]

prepsychotic—*see* Schizophrenia, latent

prodromal—*see* Schizophrenia, latent

pseudoneurotic—*see* Schizophrenia, latent

residual: A chronic form of schizophrenia in which the symptoms that persist from the acute phase have mostly lost their sharpness. Emotional response is blunted and thought disorder, even when gross, does not prevent the accomplishment of routine work.[1]

schizo-affective type: A psychosis in which pronounced manic or depressive features are intermingled with schizophrenic features and which tends towards remission without permanent defect, but which is prone to recur. The diagnosis should be made only when both the affective and schizophrenic symptoms are pronounced.[1]

simple type: A psychosis in which there is insidious development of oddities of conduct, inability to meet the demands of society, and decline in total performance. Delusions and hallucinations are not in evidence and the condition is less obviously psychotic than are the hebephrenic, catatonic, and paranoid types of schizophrenia. With increasing social impoverishment vagrancy may ensue and the patient becomes self-absorbed, idle, and aimless. Because the schizophrenic symptoms are not clear-cut, diagnosis of this form should be made sparingly, if at all.[1]

simplex—*see* Schizophrenia, simple type

Schizophrenic syndrome of childhood—*see* Psychosis, child

Schizophreniform

attack—*see* Schizophrenia, acute episode

disorder—*see* Schizophrenia, acute episode

psychosis—*see* Schizophrenia

affective type—*see* Schizophrenia, schizo-affective type

confusional type—*see* Schizophrenia, acute episode

Schizotypal personality—Dementia occurring usually after the age of 65 in which any cerebral pathology other than that of senile atrophic change can be reasonably excluded.[1]

delirium: Senile dementia with a superimposed reversible episode of acute confusional state.[1]

delusional type: A type of senile dementia characterized by development in advanced old age, progressive in nature, in which delusions, varying from simple poorly formed paranoid delusions to highly formed paranoid delusional states, and hallucinations are also present.[1,2]

depressed type: A type of senile dementia characterized by development in advanced old age, progressive in nature, in which depressive features, ranging from mild to severe forms of manic-depressive affective psychosis, are also present. Disturbance of the sleep-waking cycle and preoccupation with dead people are often particularly prominent.[1,2]

paranoid type—*see* Senile dementia, delusional type

simple type—*see* Senile dementia

Sensitiver Beziehungswahn: A paranoid state which, though in many ways akin to schizophrenic or affective states, differs from paranoia, simple paranoid state, shared paranoid disorder, or psychogenic psychosis.[1]

Sensitivity reaction of childhood or adolescence—*see* Shyness disorder of childhood

Separation anxiety disorder: A clinical disorder in children in which the predominant disturbance is exaggerated distress at separation from parents, home, or other familial surroundings. When separation is instituted, the child may experience anxiety to the point of panic. In adults a similar disorder is seen in agoraphobic reactions.[2]

Sexual deviations: Abnormal sexual inclinations or behavior which are part of a referral problem. The limits and features of normal sexual behavior have not been stated absolutely in different societies and cultures, but are broadly such as serve approved social and biological purposes. The sexual activity of affected persons is directed primarily either towards people not of the opposite sex, or towards sexual acts not associated with coitus normally, or towards coitus performed under abnormal circumstances. If the anomalous behavior becomes manifest only during psychosis or other mental illness the condition should be classified under the major illness. It is common for more than one anomaly to occur together in the same individual; in that case the predominant deviation is classified. It is preferable not to diagnose sexual deviation in individuals who perform deviant sexual acts when normal sexual outlets are not available to them.[1] *see also* exhibitionism, Fetishism, Homosexuality, Nymphomania, Pedophilia, Satyriasis, Sexual masochism, Sexual sadism, Transvestism, Voyeurism, and Zoophilia.

Gender identity disorder and trans-sexualism are considered to be psychosexual gender identity disorders and are not included here.

Sexual masochism: A sexual deviation in which sexual arousal and pleasure is produced in an individual by his own physical or psychological suffering, and in which there are insistent and persistent fantasies wherein sexual excitement is produced as a result of suffering.[2]

Sexual sadism: A sexual deviation in which physical or psychological suffering inflicted on another person is utilized as a method of stimulating erotic excitement and orgasm, and in which there are insistent and persistent fantasies wherein sexual excitement is produced as a result of suffering inflicted on the partner.[2]

Shared paranoid disorder: Mainly delusional psychosis, usually chronic and often without florid features, which appears to have developed as a result of a close, if not dependent, relationship with another person who already has an established similar psychosis. The delusions are at least partly shared. The rare cases in which several persons are affected should also be included here.[1]

Shifting sleep-work schedule: A sleep disorder in which the phase- shift disruption of the 24-hour sleep-wake cycle occurs due to rapid changes in the individual's work schedule.[2]

Short sleeper: Individuals who typically need only 4-6 hours of sleep within the 24-hour cycle.[2]

Shyness disorder of childhood: A persistent and excessive shrinking from familiarity or contact with all strangers of sufficient severity as to interfere with peer functioning, yet there are warm and satisfying relationships with family members. A critical feature of this disorder is that the avoidant behavior with strangers persists even after prolonged exposure or contact.[2]

Sibling jealousy or rivalry: An emotional disorder related to competition between siblings for the love of a parent or for other recognition or gain.[3]

Simple phobia—*see* simple phobia under Phobia

Situational disturbance, acute—*see* Stress reaction, acute

Social phobia—*see* social phobia under Phobia

Social withdrawal of childhood—*see* Introverted disorder of childhood

Socialized conduct disorder—*see* socialized conduct disorder under Conduct disorders

Somatization disorder—*see* somatization disorder under Neurotic disorders

Somatoform disorder, atypical—*see* hypochondriasis under Neurotic disorders

Spasmus nutans—*see* Stereotyped repetitive movements

Specific academic or work inhibition: An adjustment reaction in which a specific academic or work inhibition occurs in an individual whose intellectual capacity, skills, and previous academic or work performance have been at least adequate, and in which the inhibition occurs despite apparent effort and is not due to any other mental disorder.[2]

Stammering—*see* Stuttering

Starch-eating—*see* Pica

Status postcommotio cerebri—*see* Postconcussion syndrome

Stereotyped repetitive movements: Disorders in which voluntary repetitive stereotyped movements, which are not due to any psychiatric or neurological condition, constitute the main feature. Includes head-banging, spasmus nutans, rocking, twirling, finger-flicking mannerisms, and eye poking. Such movements are particularly common in cases of mental retardation with sensory impairment or with environmental monotony.[1]

Stereotypies—*see* Stereotyped repetitive movements

Stress reaction

acute: Acute transient disorders of any severity and nature of emotions, consciousness, and psychomotor states (singly or in combination) which occur in individuals, without any apparent pre-existing mental disorder, in response to exceptional physical or mental stress, such as natural catastrophe or battle, and which usually subside within hours or days.[1]

chronic—*see* Adjustment reaction

Stupor

catatonic—*see* Schizophrenia, catatonic type

psychogenic—*see* Psychosis, reactive

Stuttering: Disorders in the rhythm of speech, in which the individual knows precisely what he wishes to say, but at the time is unable to say it because of an involuntary, repetitive prolongation or cessation of a sound.[1]

Subjective insomnia complaint: a complaint of insomnia made by the individual, which has not been investigated or proven.[2]

Systematized delusions—*see* Paranoia

Tension headache: Headache of mental origin for which a more precise medical or psychiatric diagnosis cannot be made.[1]

Tics: Disorders of no known organic origin in which the outstanding feature consists of quick, involuntary, apparently purposeless, and frequently repeated movements which are not due to any neurological condition. Any part of the body may be involved but the face is most frequently affected. Only one form of tic may be present, or there may be a combination of tics which are carried out simultaneously, alternatively, or consecutively.[1]

chronic motor tic disorder: A tic disorder starting in childhood and persisting into adult life. The tic is limited to no more than three motor areas, and rarely has a verbal component.[2]

Gilles de la Tourette's disorder [motor-verbal tic disorder]: a rare disorder occurring in individuals of any level of intelligence in which facial tics and tic-like throat noises become more marked and more generalized, and in which later whole words or short sentences (often with obscene content) are ejaculated spasmodically and involuntarily. There is some overlap with other varieties of tic.[1]

transient tic disorder of childhood: Facial or other tics beginning in childhood, but limited to one year in duration.[2]

Tobacco use disorder: Cases in which tobacco is used to the detriment of a person's health or social functioning or in which there is tobacco dependence. Dependence is included here rather than under drug dependence because tobacco differs from other drugs of dependence in its psychotoxic effects.[1]

Tranquilizer abuse: Cases where an individual has taken the drug to the detriment of his health or social functioning, in doses above or for periods beyond those normally regarded as therapeutic.[1]

Transient organic psychotic condition—*see* Organic psychotic conditions, transient

Trans-sexualism—*see* trans-sexualism under Psychosexual identity disorders

Transvestism: Sexual deviation in which there is recurrent and persistent dressing in clothes of the opposite sex, and initially in the early stage of the illness, for the purpose of sexual arousal.[2]

Twilight state

confusional—*see* Delirium, acute

psychogenic—*see* Psychosis, reactive confusion

Undersocialized conduct disorder—*see* undersocialized conduct disorder under Conduct disorders

Unsocialized aggressive disorder—*see* undersocialized conduct disorder, aggressive type under Conduct disorders

Vaginismus, functional—*see* functional vaginismus under Psychosexual dysfunctions

Vorbeireden: The symptom of the approximate answer or talking past the point, seen in the Ganser syndrome, a form of factitious illness.[2]

Voyeurism: A sexual deviation in which the individual repetitively seeks out situations in which he engages in looking at unsuspecting women who are either naked, in the act of disrobing, or engaging in sexual activity. The act of looking is accompanied by sexual excitement, frequently with orgasm. In its severe form, the act of peeping constitutes the preferred or exclusive sexual activity of the individual.[2]

Wernicke-Korsakoff syndrome—*see* alcohol amnestic syndrome under Alcoholic psychoses

Withdrawal reaction of childhood or adolescence—*see* Introverted disorder of childhood

Word-deafness: A developmental delay in the comprehension of speech sounds.[1]

Zoophilia: Sexual or anal intercourse with animals.[1]

1. Manual of the *International Classification of Diseases, Injuries, and Causes of Death.* 9th Revision. World Health Organization, Geneva, Switzerland, 1975.
2. American Psychiatric Association, Task Force on Nomenclature and Statistics, Robert L. Spitzer, Chairman.
3. *A Psychiatric Glossary*, Fourth Edition, American Psychiatric Association, Washington, D.C., 1975.
4. *Dorland's Illustrated Medical Dictionary.* Twenty-fifth Edition, W. B. Saunders Company, Philadelphia, 1974.
5. *Stedman's Medical Dictionary. Illustrated,* Twenty-third Edition, Williams and Wilkins, Baltimore, 1976.

CLASSIFICATION OF DRUGS BY AMERICAN HOSPITAL FORMULARY SERVICE LIST NUMBER AND THEIR ICD-9-CM EQUIVALENTS

The coding of adverse effects of drugs is keyed to the continually revised Hospital Formulary of the American Hospital Formulary Service (AHFS) published under the direction of the American Society of Hospital Pharmacists.

The following section gives the ICD-9-CM diagnosis code for each AHFS list.

	AHFS* LIST	ICD-9-CM Diagnosis Code
4:00	**ANTIHISTAMINE DRUGS**	963.0
8:00	**ANTI-INFECTIVE AGENTS**	
8:04	Amebacides	961.5
	hydroxyquinoline derivatives	961.3
	arsenical anti-infectives	961.1
8:08	Anthelmintics	961.6
	quinoline derivatives	961.3
8:12.04	Antifungal Antibiotics	960.1
	nonantibiotics	961.9
8:12.06	Cephalosporins	960.5
8:12.08	Chloramphenicol	960.2
8:12.12	The Erythromycins	960.3
8:12.16	The Penicillins	960.0
8:12.20	The Streptomycins	960.6
8:12.24	The Tetracyclines	960.4
8:12.28	Other Antibiotics	960.8
	antimycobacterial antibiotics	960.6
	macrolides	960.3
8:16	Antituberculars	961.8
	antibiotics	960.6
8:18	Antivirals	961.7
8:20	Plasmodicides (antimalarials)	961.4
8:24	Sulfonamides	961.0
8:26	The Sulfones	961.8
8:28	Treponemicides	961.2
8:32	Trichomonacides	961.5
	hydroxyquinoline derivatives	961.3
	nitrofuran derivatives	961.9
8:36	Urinary Germicides	961.9
	quinoline derivatives	961.3
8:40	Other Anti-Infectives	961.9
10:00	**ANTINEOPLASTIC AGENTS**	963.1
	antibiotics	960.7
	progestogens	962.2
12:00	**AUTONOMIC DRUGS**	
12:04	Parasympathomimetic (Cholinergic) Agents	971.0
12:08	Parasympatholytic (Cholinergic Blocking) Agents	971.1
12:12	Sympathomimetic (Adrenergic) Agents	971.2
12:16	Sympatholytic (Adrenergic Blocking) Agents	971.3
12:20	Skeletal Muscle Relaxants	975.2
	central nervous system muscle-tone depressants	968.0

	AHFS* LIST	ICD-9-CM Diagnosis Code
16:00	**BLOOD DERIVATIVES**	964.7
20:00	**BLOOD FORMATION AND COAGULATION**	
20:04	Antianemia Drugs	964.1
20:04.04	Iron Preparations	964.0
20:04.08	Liver and Stomach Preparations	964.1
20:12.04	Anticoagulants	964.2
20:12.08	Antiheparin agents	964.5
20:12.12	Coagulants	964.5
20:12.16	Hemostatics	964.5
	capillary-active drugs	972.8
	fibrinolysis-affecting agents	964.4
	natural products	964.7
24:00	**CARDIOVASCULAR DRUGS**	
24:04	Cardiac Drugs	972.9
	cardiotonic agents	972.1
	rhythm regulators	972.0
24:06	Antilipemic Agents	972.2
	thyroid derivatives	962.7
24:08	Hypotensive Agents	972.6
	adrenergic blocking agents	971.3
	ganglion-blocking agents	972.3
	vasodilators	972.5
24:12	Vasodilating Agents	972.5
	coronary	972.4
	nicotinic acid derivatives	972.2
24:16	Sclerosing Agents	972.7
28:00	**CENTRAL NERVOUS SYSTEM DRUGS**	
28:04	General Anesthetics	968.4
	gaseous anesthetics	968.2
	halothane	968.1
	intravenous anesthetics	968.3
28:08	Analgesics and Antipyretics	965.9
	antirheumatics	965.6
	aromatic analgesics	965.4
	non-narcotics NEC	965.7
	opium alkaloids	965.00
	heroin	965.01
	methadone	965.02
	specified type NEC	965.09
	pyrazole derivatives	965.5
	salicylates	965.1
	specified type NEC	965.8
28:10	Narcotic Antagonists	970.1
28:12	Anticonvulsants	966.3
	barbiturates	967.0
	benzodiazepine-based tranquilizers	969.4
	bromides	967.3
	hydantoin derivatives	966.1
	oxazolidine derivative	966.0
	succinimides	966.2
28:16.04	Antidepressants	969.0
28:16.08	Tranquilizers	969.5
	benzodiazepine-based	969.4
	butyrophenone-based	969.2
	major NEC	969.3
	phenothiazine-based	969.1

* American Hospital Formulary Service

	AHFS* LIST	ICD-9-CM Diagnosis Code
28:16.12	Other Psychotherapeutic Agents	969.8
28:20	Respiratory and Cerebral Stimulants	970.9
	analeptics	970.0
	anorexigenic agents	977.0
	psychostimulants	969.7
	specified type NEC	970.8
28:24	Sedatives and Hypnotics	967.9
	barbiturates	967.0
	benzodiazepine-based tranquilizers	969.4
	chloral hydrate group	967.1
	glutethamide group	967.5
	intravenous anesthetics	968.3
	methaqualone	967.4
	paraldehyde	967.2
	phenothiazine-based tranquilizers	969.1
	specified type NEC	967.8
	thiobarbiturates	968.3
	tranquilizer NEC	969.5
36:00	**DIAGNOSTIC AGENTS**	977.8
40:00	**ELECTROLYTE, CALORIC, AND WATER BALANCE AGENTS NEC**	974.5
40:04	Acidifying Agents	963.2
40:08	Alkalinizing Agents	963.3
40:10	Ammonia Detoxicants	974.5
40:12	Replacement Solutions NEC	974.5
	plasma volume expanders	964.8
40:16	Sodium-Removing Resins	974.5
40:18	Potassium-Removing Resins	974.5
40:20	Caloric Agents	974.5
40:24	Salt and Sugar Substitutes	974.5
40:28	Diuretics NEC	974.4
	carbonic acid anhydrase inhibitors	974.2
	mercurials	974.0
	purine derivatives	974.1
	saluretics	974.3
40:36	Irrigating Solutions	974.5
40:40	Uricosuric Agents	974.7
44:00	**ENZYMES NEC**	963.4
	fibrinolysis-affecting agents	964.4
	gastric agents	973.4
48:00	**EXPECTORANTS AND COUGH PREPARATIONS**	
	antihistamine agents	963.0
	antitussives	975.4
	codeine derivatives	965.09
	expectorants	975.5
	narcotic agents NEC	965.09
52:00	**EYE, EAR, NOSE, AND THROAT PREPARATIONS**	
52:04	Anti-Infectives	
	ENT	976.6
	ophthalmic	976.5
52:04.04	Antibiotics	
	ENT	976.6
	ophthalmic	976.5

	AHFS* LIST	ICD-9-CM Diagnosis Code
52:04.06	Antivirals	
	ENT	976.6
	ophthalmic	976.5
52:04.08	Sulfonamides	
	ENT	976.6
	ophthalmic	976.5
52:04.12	Miscellaneous Anti-Infectives	
	ENT	976.6
	ophthalmic	976.5
52:08	Anti-Inflammatory Agents	
	ENT	976.6
	ophthalmic	976.5
52:10	Carbonic Anhydrase Inhibitors	974.2
52:12	Contact Lens Solutions	976.5
52:16	Local Anesthetics	968.5
52:20	Miotics	971.0
52:24	Mydriatics	
	adrenergics	971.2
	anticholinergics	971.1
	antimuscarinics	971.1
	parasympatholytics	971.1
	spasmolytics	971.1
	sympathomimetics	971.2
52:28	Mouth Washes and Gargles	976.6
52:32	Vasoconstrictors	971.2
52:36	Unclassified Agents	
	ENT	976.6
	ophthalmic	976.5
56:00	**GASTROINTESTINAL DRUGS**	
56:04	Antacids and Absorbants	973.0
56:08	Anti-Diarrhea Agents	973.5
56:10	Antiflatulents	973.8
56:12	Cathartics NEC	973.3
	emollients	973.2
	irritants	973.1
56:16	Digestants	973.4
56:20	Emetics and Antiemetics	
	antiemetics	963.0
	emetics	973.6
56:24	Lipotropic Agents	977.1
60:00	**GOLD COMPOUNDS**	965.6
64:00	**HEAVY METAL ANTAGONISTS**	963.8
68:00	**HORMONES AND SYNTHETIC SUBSTITUTES**	
68:04	Adrenals	962.0
68:08	Androgens	962.1
68:12	Contraceptives	962.2
68:16	Estrogens	962.2
68:18	Gonadotropins	962.4
68:20	Insulins and Antidiabetic Agents	962.3
68:20.08	Insulins	962.3
68:24	Parathyroid	962.6

* American Hospital Formulary Service

	AHFS* LIST	ICD-9-CM Diagnosis Code
68:28	Pituitary	
	anterior	962.4
	posterior	962.5
68:32	Progestogens	962.2
68:34	Other Corpus Luteum Hormones	962.2
68:36	Thyroid and Antithyroid	
	antithyroid	962.8
	thyroid	962.7
72:00	**LOCAL ANESTHETICS NEC**	968.9
	topical (surface) agents	968.5
	infiltrating agents (intradermal) (subcutaneous) (submucosal)	968.5
	nerve blocking agents (peripheral) (plexus)(regional)	968.6
	spinal	968.7
76:00	**OXYTOCICS**	975.0
78:00	**RADIOACTIVE AGENTS**	990
80:00	**SERUMS, TOXOIDS, AND VACCINES**	
80:04	Serums	979.9
	immune globulin (gamma) (human)	964.6
80:08	Toxoids NEC	978.8
	diphtheria	978.5
	and tetanus	978.9
	with pertussis component	978.6
	tetanus	978.4
	and diphtheria	978.9
	with pertussis component	978.6
80:12	Vaccines NEC	979.9
	bacterial NEC	978.8
	with	
	other bacterial component	978.9
	pertussis component	978.6
	viral and rickettsial component	979.7
	rickettsial NEC	979.6
	with	
	bacterial component	979.7
	pertussis component	978.6
	viral component	979.7
	viral NEC	979.6
	with	
	bacterial component	979.7
	pertussis component	978.6
	rickettsial component	979.7
84:00	**SKIN AND MUCOUS MEMBRANE PREPARATIONS**	
84:04	Anti-Infectives	976.0
84:04.04	Antibiotics	976.0
84:04.08	Fungicides	976.0
84:04.12	Scabicides and Pediculicides	976.0
84:04.16	Miscellaneous Local Anti-Infectives	976.0
84:06	Anti-Inflammatory Agents	976.0
84:08	Antipruritics and Local Anesthetics	
	antipruritics	976.1
	local anesthetics	968.5
84:12	Astringents	976.2
84:16	Cell Stimulants and Proliferants	976.8
84:20	Detergents	976.2

	AHFS* LIST	ICD-9-CM Diagnosis Code
84:24	Emollients, Demulcents, and Protectants	976.3
84:28	Keratolytic Agents	976.4
84:32	Keratoplastic Agents	976.4
84:36	Miscellaneous Agents	976.8
86:00	**SPASMOLYTIC AGENTS**	975.1
	antiasthmatics	975.7
	papaverine	972.5
	theophyllin	974.1
88:00	**VITAMINS**	
88:04	Vitamin A	963.5
88:08	Vitamin B Complex	963.5
	hematopoietic vitamin	964.1
	nicotinic acid derivatives	972.2
88:12	Vitamin C	963.5
88:16	Vitamin D	963.5
88:20	Vitamin E	963.5
88:24	Vitamin K Activity	964.3
88:28	Multivitamin Preparations	963.5
92:00	**UNCLASSIFIED THERAPEUTIC AGENTS**	977.8

* American Hospital Formulary Service

CLASSIFICATION OF INDUSTRIAL ACCIDENTS ACCORDING TO AGENCY

Annex B to the Resolution concerning Statistics of Employment Injuries adopted by the Tenth International Conference of Labor Statisticians on 12 October 1962

1 MACHINES

11 Prime-Movers, except Electrical Motors
111 Steam engines
112 Internal combustion engines
119 Others

12 Transmission Machinery
121 Transmission shafts
122 Transmission belts, cables, pulleys, pinions, chains, gears
129 Others

13 Metalworking Machines
131 Power presses
132 Lathes
133 Milling machines
134 Abrasive wheels
135 Mechanical shears
136 Forging machines
137 Rolling-mills
139 Others

14 Wood and Assimilated Machines
141 Circular saws
142 Other saws
143 Molding machines
144 Overhand planes
149 Others

15 Agricultural Machines
151 Reapers (including combine reapers)
152 Threshers
159 Others

16 Mining Machinery
161 Under-cutters
169 Others

19 Other Machines Not Elsewhere Classified
191 Earth-moving machines, excavating and scraping machines, except means of transport
192 Spinning, weaving and other textile machines
193 Machines for the manufacture of foodstuffs and beverages
194 Machines for the manufacture of paper
195 Printing machines
199 Others

2 MEANS OF TRANSPORT AND LIFTING EQUIPMENT

21 Lifting Machines and Appliances
211 Cranes
212 Lifts and elevators
213 Winches
214 Pulley blocks
219 Others

22 Means of Rail Transport
221 Inter-urban railways
222 Rail transport in mines, tunnels, quarries, industrial establishments, docks, etc.
229 Others

23 Other Wheeled Means of Transport, Excluding Rail Transport
231 Tractors
232 Lorries
233 Trucks
234 Motor vehicles, not elsewhere classified
235 Animal-drawn vehicles

2 MEANS OF TRANSPORT AND LIFTING EQUIPMENT *continued*

236 Hand-drawn vehicles
239 Others

24 Means of Air Transport

25 Means of Water Transport
251 Motorized means of water transport
252 Non-motorized means of water transport

26 Other Means of Transport
261 Cable-cars
262 Mechanical conveyors, except cable-cars
269 Others

3 OTHER EQUIPMENT

31 Pressure Vessels
311 Boilers
312 Pressurized containers
313 Pressurized piping and accessories
314 Gas cylinders
315 Caissons, diving equipment
319 Others

32 Furnaces, Ovens, Kilns
321 Blast furnaces
322 Refining furnaces
323 Other furnaces
324 Kilns
325 Ovens

33 Refrigerating Plants

34 Electrical Installations, Including Electric Motors, but Excluding Electric Hand Tools
341 Rotating machines
342 Conductors
343 Transformers
344 Control apparatus
349 Others

35 Electric Hand Tools

36 Tools, Implements, and Appliances, Except Electric Hand Tools
361 Power-driven hand tools, except electric hand tools
362 Hand tools, not power-driven
369 Others

37 Ladders, Mobile Ramps

38 Scaffolding

39 Other Equipment, Not Elsewhere Classified

4 MATERIALS, SUBSTANCES AND RADIATIONS

41 Explosives

42 Dusts, Gases, Liquids and Chemicals, Excluding Explosives
421 Dusts
422 Gases, vapors, fumes
423 Liquids, not elsewhere classified
424 Chemicals, not elsewhere classified

43 Flying Fragments

44 Radiations
441 Ionizing radiations
449 Others

49 Other Materials and Substances Not Elsewhere Classified

5 WORKING ENVIRONMENT

51 Outdoor
511 Weather

5 WORKING ENVIRONMENT *continued*

512 Traffic and working surfaces
513 Water
519 Others

52 Indoor
521 Floors
522 Confined quarters
523 Stairs
524 Other traffic and working surfaces
525 Floor openings and wall openings
526 Environmental factors (lighting, ventilation, temperature, noise, etc.)
529 Others

53 Underground
531 Roofs and faces of mine roads and tunnels, etc.
532 Floors of mine roads and tunnels, etc.
533 Working-faces of mines, tunnels, etc.
534 Mine shafts
535 Fire
536 Water
539 Others

6 OTHER AGENCIES, NOT ELSEWHERE CLASSIFIED

61 Animals
611 Live animals
612 Animals products

69 Other Agencies, Not Elsewhere Classified

7 AGENCIES NOT CLASSIFIED FOR LACK OF SUFFICIENT DATA

LIST OF THREE-DIGIT CATEGORIES

1. INFECTIOUS AND PARASITIC DISEASES

Intestinal infectious diseases (001-009)

001 Cholera
002 Typhoid and paratyphoid fevers
003 Other salmonella infections
004 Shigellosis
005 Other food poisoning (bacterial)
006 Amebiasis
007 Other protozoal intestinal diseases
008 Intestinal infections due to other organisms
009 Ill-defined intestinal infections

Tuberculosis (010-018)

010 Primary tuberculous infection
011 Pulmonary tuberculosis
012 Other respiratory tuberculosis
013 Tuberculosis of meninges and central nervous system
014 Tuberculosis of intestines, peritoneum, and mesenteric glands
015 Tuberculosis of bones and joints
016 Tuberculosis of genitourinary system
017 Tuberculosis of other organs
018 Miliary tuberculosis

Zoonotic bacterial diseases (020-027)

020 Plague
021 Tularemia
022 Anthrax
023 Brucellosis
024 Glanders
025 Melioidosis
026 Rat-bite fever
027 Other zoonotic bacterial diseases

Other bacterial diseases (030-041)

030 Leprosy
031 Diseases due to other mycobacteria
032 Diphtheria
033 Whooping cough
034 Streptococcal sore throat and scarlatina
035 Erysipelas
036 Meningococcal infection
037 Tetanus
038 Septicemia
039 Actinomycotic infections
040 Other bacterial diseases
041 Bacterial infection in conditions classified elsewhere and of unspecified site

Human immunodeficiency virus (HIV) infection (042)

042 Human immunodeficiency virus (HIV) disease

Poliomyelitis and other non-arthropod-borne viral diseases of central nervous system (045-049)

045 Acute poliomyelitis
046 Slow virus infection of central nervous system
047 Meningitis due to enterovirus
048 Other enterovirus diseases of central nervous system
049 Other non-arthropod-borne viral diseases of central nervous system

Viral diseases accompanied by exanthem (050-057)

050 Smallpox
051 Cowpox and paravaccinia
052 Chickenpox
053 Herpes zoster
054 Herpes simplex
055 Measles
056 Rubella
057 Other viral exanthemata

1. INFECTIOUS AND PARASITIC DISEASES *continued*

Arthropod-borne viral diseases (060-066)

060 Yellow fever
061 Dengue
062 Mosquito-borne viral encephalitis
063 Tick-borne viral encephalitis
064 Viral encephalitis transmitted by other and unspecified arthropods
065 Arthropod-borne hemorrhagic fever
066 Other arthropod-borne viral diseases

Other diseases due to viruses and Chlamydiae (070-079)

070 Viral hepatitis
071 Rabies
072 Mumps
073 Ornithosis
074 Specific diseases due to Coxsackie virus
075 Infectious mononucleosis
076 Trachoma
077 Other diseases of conjunctiva due to viruses and Chlamydiae
078 Other diseases due to viruses and Chlamydiae
079 Viral and Chlamydial infection in conditions classified elsewhere and of unspecified site

Rickettsioses and other arthropod-borne diseases (080-088)

080 Louse-borne [epidemic] typhus
081 Other typhus
082 Tick-borne rickettsioses
083 Other rickettsioses
084 Malaria
085 Leishmaniasis
086 Trypanosomiasis
087 Relapsing fever
088 Other arthropod-borne diseases

Syphilis and other venereal diseases (090-099)

090 Congenital syphilis
091 Early syphilis, symptomatic
092 Early syphilis, latent
093 Cardiovascular syphilis
094 Neurosyphilis
095 Other forms of late syphilis, with symptoms
096 Late syphilis, latent
097 Other and unspecified syphilis
098 Gonococcal infections
099 Other venereal diseases

Other spirochetal diseases (100-104)

100 Leptospirosis
101 Vincent's angina
102 Yaws
103 Pinta
104 Other spirochetal infection

Mycoses (110-118)

110 Dermatophytosis
111 Dermatomycosis, other and unspecified
112 Candidiasis
114 Coccidioidomycosis
115 Histoplasmosis
116 Blastomycotic infection
117 Other mycoses
118 Opportunistic mycoses

Helminthiases (120-129)

120 Schistosomiasis [bilharziasis]
121 Other trematode infections
122 Echinococcosis
123 Other cestode infection
124 Trichinosis
125 Filarial infection and dracontiasis

1. INFECTIOUS AND PARASITIC DISEASES *continued*

126 Ancylostomiasis and necatoriasis
127 Other intestinal helminthiases
128 Other and unspecified helminthiases
129 Intestinal parasitism, unspecified

Other infectious and parasitic diseases (130-136)

130 Toxoplasmosis
131 Trichomoniasis
132 Pediculosis and phthirus infestation
133 Acariasis
134 Other infestation
135 Sarcoidosis
136 Other and unspecified infectious and parasitic diseases

Late effects of infectious and parasitic diseases (137-139)

137 Late effects of tuberculosis
138 Late effects of acute poliomyelitis
139 Late effects of other infectious and parasitic diseases

2. NEOPLASMS

Malignant neoplasm of lip, oral cavity, and pharynx (140-149)

140 Malignant neoplasm of lip
141 Malignant neoplasm of tongue
142 Malignant neoplasm of major salivary glands
143 Malignant neoplasm of gum
144 Malignant neoplasm of floor of mouth
145 Malignant neoplasm of other and unspecified parts of mouth
146 Malignant neoplasm of oropharynx
147 Malignant neoplasm of nasopharynx
148 Malignant neoplasm of hypopharynx
149 Malignant neoplasm of other and ill-defined sites within the lip, oral cavity, and pharynx

Malignant neoplasm of digestive organs and peritoneum (150-159)

150 Malignant neoplasm of esophagus
151 Malignant neoplasm of stomach
152 Malignant neoplasm of small intestine, including duodenum
153 Malignant neoplasm of colon
154 Malignant neoplasm of rectum, rectosigmoid junction, and anus
155 Malignant neoplasm of liver and intrahepatic bile ducts
156 Malignant neoplasm of gallbladder and extrahepatic bile ducts
157 Malignant neoplasm of pancreas
158 Malignant neoplasm of retroperitoneum and peritoneum
159 Malignant neoplasm of other and ill-defined sites within the digestive organs and peritoneum

Malignant neoplasm of respiratory and intrathoracic organs (160-165)

160 Malignant neoplasm of nasal cavities, middle ear, and accessory sinuses
161 Malignant neoplasm of larynx
162 Malignant neoplasm of trachea, bronchus, and lung
163 Malignant neoplasm of pleura
164 Malignant neoplasm of thymus, heart, and mediastinum
165 Malignant neoplasm of other and ill-defined sites within the respiratory system and intrathoracic organs

Malignant neoplasm of bone, connective tissue, skin, and breast (170-176)

170 Malignant neoplasm of bone and articular cartilage
171 Malignant neoplasm of connective and other soft tissue
172 Malignant melanoma of skin
173 Other malignant neoplasm of skin
174 Malignant neoplasm of female breast
175 Malignant neoplasm of male breast
176 Kaposi's sarcoma

Malignant neoplasm of genitourinary organs (179-189)

179 Malignant neoplasm of uterus, part unspecified
180 Malignant neoplasm of cervix uteri
181 Malignant neoplasm of placenta
182 Malignant neoplasm of body of uterus

2. NEOPLASMS *continued*

183 Malignant neoplasm of ovary and other uterine adnexa
184 Malignant neoplasm of other and unspecified female genital organs
185 Malignant neoplasm of prostate
186 Malignant neoplasm of testis
187 Malignant neoplasm of penis and other male genital organs
188 Malignant neoplasm of bladder
189 Malignant neoplasm of kidney and other and unspecified urinary organs

Malignant neoplasm of other and unspecified sites (190-199)

190 Malignant neoplasm of eye
191 Malignant neoplasm of brain
192 Malignant neoplasm of other and unspecified parts of nervous system
193 Malignant neoplasm of thyroid gland
194 Malignant neoplasm of other endocrine glands and related structures
195 Malignant neoplasm of other and ill-defined sites
196 Secondary and unspecified malignant neoplasm of lymph nodes
197 Secondary malignant neoplasm of respiratory and digestive systems
198 Secondary malignant neoplasm of other specified sites
199 Malignant neoplasm without specification of site

Malignant neoplasm of lymphatic and hematopoietic tissue (200-208)

200 Lymphosarcoma and reticulosarcoma
201 Hodgkin's disease
202 Other malignant neoplasm of lymphoid and histiocytic tissue
203 Multiple myeloma and immunoproliferative neoplasms
204 Lymphoid leukemia
205 Myeloid leukemia
206 Monocytic leukemia
207 Other specified leukemia
208 Leukemia of unspecified cell type

Benign neoplasms (210-229)

210 Benign neoplasm of lip, oral cavity, and pharynx
211 Benign neoplasm of other parts of digestive system
212 Benign neoplasm of respiratory and intrathoracic organs
213 Benign neoplasm of bone and articular cartilage
214 Lipoma
215 Other benign neoplasm of connective and other soft tissue
216 Benign neoplasm of skin
217 Benign neoplasm of breast
218 Uterine leiomyoma
219 Other benign neoplasm of uterus
220 Benign neoplasm of ovary
221 Benign neoplasm of other female genital organs
222 Benign neoplasm of male genital organs
223 Benign neoplasm of kidney and other urinary organs
224 Benign neoplasm of eye
225 Benign neoplasm of brain and other parts of nervous system
226 Benign neoplasm of thyroid gland
227 Benign neoplasm of other endocrine glands and related structures
228 Hemangioma and lymphangioma, any site
229 Benign neoplasm of other and unspecified sites

Carcinoma in situ (230-234)

230 Carcinoma in situ of digestive organs
231 Carcinoma in situ of respiratory system
232 Carcinoma in situ of skin
233 Carcinoma in situ of breast and genitourinary system
234 Carcinoma in situ of other and unspecified sites

Neoplasms of uncertain behavior (235-238)

235 Neoplasm of uncertain behavior of digestive and respiratory systems
236 Neoplasm of uncertain behavior of genitourinary organs
237 Neoplasm of uncertain behavior of endocrine glands and nervous system
238 Neoplasm of uncertain behavior of other and unspecified sites and tissues

Neoplasm of unspecified nature (239)

239 Neoplasm of unspecified nature

3. ENDOCRINE, NUTRITIONAL AND METABOLIC DISEASES, AND IMMUNITY DISORDERS

Disorders of thyroid gland (240-246)

240 Simple and unspecified goiter
241 Nontoxic nodular goiter
242 Thyrotoxicosis with or without goiter
243 Congenital hypothyroidism
244 Acquired hypothyroidism
245 Thyroiditis
246 Other disorders of thyroid

Diseases of other endocrine glands (250-259)

250 Diabetes mellitus
251 Other disorders of pancreatic internal secretion
252 Disorders of parathyroid gland
253 Disorders of the pituitary gland and its hypothalamic control
254 Diseases of thymus gland
255 Disorders of adrenal glands
256 Ovarian dysfunction
257 Testicular dysfunction
258 Polyglandular dysfunction and related disorders
259 Other endocrine disorders

Nutritional deficiencies (260-269)

260 Kwashiorkor
261 Nutritional marasmus
262 Other severe protein-calorie malnutrition
263 Other and unspecified protein-calorie malnutrition
264 Vitamin A deficiency
265 Thiamine and niacin deficiency states
266 Deficiency of B-complex components
267 Ascorbic acid deficiency
268 Vitamin D deficiency
269 Other nutritional deficiencies

Other metabolic disorders and immunity disorders (270-279)

270 Disorders of amino-acid transport and metabolism
271 Disorders of carbohydrate transport and metabolism
272 Disorders of lipoid metabolism
273 Disorders of plasma protein metabolism
274 Gout
275 Disorders of mineral metabolism
276 Disorders of fluid, electrolyte, and acid-base balance
277 Other and unspecified disorders of metabolism
278 Obesity and other hyperalimentation
279 Disorders involving the immune mechanism

4. DISEASES OF THE BLOOD AND BLOOD-FORMING ORGANS

Diseases of blood and blood-forming organs (280-289)

280 Iron deficiency anemias
281 Other deficiency anemias
282 Hereditary hemolytic anemias
283 Acquired hemolytic anemias
284 Aplastic anemia
285 Other and unspecified anemias
286 Coagulation defects
287 Purpura and other hemorrhagic conditions
288 Diseases of white blood cells
289 Other diseases of blood and blood-forming organs

5. MENTAL DISORDERS

Organic psychotic conditions (290-294)

290 Senile and presenile organic psychotic conditions
291 Alcoholic psychoses
292 Drug psychoses
293 Transient organic psychotic conditions
294 Other organic psychotic conditions (chronic)

5. MENTAL DISORDERS *continued*

Other psychoses (295-299)

295 Schizophrenic psychoses
296 Affective psychoses
297 Paranoid states
298 Other nonorganic psychoses
299 Psychoses with origin specific to childhood

Neurotic disorders, personality disorders, and other nonpsychotic mental disorders (300-316)

300 Neurotic disorders
301 Personality disorders
302 Sexual deviations and disorders
303 Alcohol dependence syndrome
304 Drug dependence
305 Nondependent abuse of drugs
306 Physiological malfunction arising from mental factors
307 Special symptoms or syndromes, not elsewhere classified
308 Acute reaction to stress
309 Adjustment reaction
310 Specific nonpsychotic mental disorders due to organic brain damage
311 Depressive disorder, not elsewhere classified
312 Disturbance of conduct, not elsewhere classified
313 Disturbance of emotions specific to childhood and adolescence
314 Hyperkinetic syndrome of childhood
315 Specific delays in development
316 Psychic factors associated with diseases classified elsewhere

Mental retardation (317-319)

317 Mild mental retardation
318 Other specified mental retardation
319 Unspecified mental retardation

6. DISEASES OF THE NERVOUS SYSTEM AND SENSE ORGANS

Inflammatory diseases of the central nervous system (320-326)

320 Bacterial meningitis
321 Meningitis due to other organisms
322 Meningitis of unspecified cause
323 Encephalitis, myelitis, and encephalomyelitis
324 Intracranial and intraspinal abscess
325 Phlebitis and thrombophlebitis of intracranial venous sinuses
326 Late effects of intracranial abscess or pyogenic infection

Hereditary and degenerative diseases of the central nervous system (330-337)

330 Cerebral degenerations usually manifest in childhood
331 Other cerebral degenerations
332 Parkinson's disease
333 Other extrapyramidal disease and abnormal movement disorders
334 Spinocerebellar disease
335 Anterior horn cell disease
336 Other diseases of spinal cord
337 Disorders of the autonomic nervous system

Other disorders of the central nervous system (340-349)

340 Multiple sclerosis
341 Other demyelinating diseases of central nervous system
342 Hemiplegia and hemiparesis
343 Infantile cerebral palsy
344 Other paralytic syndromes
345 Epilepsy
346 Migraine
347 Cataplexy and narcolepsy
348 Other conditions of brain
349 Other and unspecified disorders of the nervous system

Disorders of the peripheral nervous system (350-359)

350 Trigeminal nerve disorders
351 Facial nerve disorders
352 Disorders of other cranial nerves
353 Nerve root and plexus disorders

6. DISEASES OF THE NERVOUS SYSTEM AND SENSE ORGANS *continued*

354 Mononeuritis of upper limb and mononeuritis multiplex
355 Mononeuritis of lower limb and unspecified site
356 Hereditary and idiopathic peripheral neuropathy
357 Inflammatory and toxic neuropathy
358 Myoneural disorders
359 Muscular dystrophies and other myopathies

Disorders of the eye and adnexa (360-379)

360 Disorders of the globe
361 Retinal detachments and defects
362 Other retinal disorders
363 Chorioretinal inflammations and scars and other disorders of choroid
364 Disorders of iris and ciliary body
365 Glaucoma
366 Cataract
367 Disorders of refraction and accommodation
368 Visual disturbances
369 Blindness and low vision
370 Keratitis
371 Corneal opacity and other disorders of cornea
372 Disorders of conjunctiva
373 Inflammation of eyelids
374 Other disorders of eyelids
375 Disorders of lacrimal system
376 Disorders of the orbit
377 Disorders of optic nerve and visual pathways
378 Strabismus and other disorders of binocular eye movements
379 Other disorders of eye

Diseases of the ear and mastoid process (380-389)

380 Disorders of external ear
381 Nonsuppurative otitis media and Eustachian tube disorders
382 Suppurative and unspecified otitis media
383 Mastoiditis and related conditions
384 Other disorders of tympanic membrane
385 Other disorders of middle ear and mastoid
386 Vertiginous syndromes and other disorders of vestibular system
387 Otosclerosis
388 Other disorders of ear
389 Hearing loss

7. DISEASES OF THE CIRCULATORY SYSTEM

Acute rheumatic fever (390-392)

390 Rheumatic fever without mention of heart involvement
391 Rheumatic fever with heart involvement
392 Rheumatic chorea

Chronic rheumatic heart disease (393-398)

393 Chronic rheumatic pericarditis
394 Diseases of mitral valve
395 Diseases of aortic valve
396 Diseases of mitral and aortic valves
397 Diseases of other endocardial structures
398 Other rheumatic heart disease

Hypertensive disease (401-405)

401 Essential hypertension
402 Hypertensive heart disease
403 Hypertensive renal disease
404 Hypertensive heart and renal disease
405 Secondary hypertension

Ischemic heart disease (410-414)

410 Acute myocardial infarction
411 Other acute and subacute form of ischemic heart disease
412 Old myocardial infarction
413 Angina pectoris
414 Other forms of chronic ischemic heart disease

7. DISEASES OF THE CIRCULATORY SYSTEM *continued*

Diseases of pulmonary circulation (415-417)

415 Acute pulmonary heart disease
416 Chronic pulmonary heart disease
417 Other diseases of pulmonary circulation

Other forms of heart disease (420-429)

420 Acute pericarditis
421 Acute and subacute endocarditis
422 Acute myocarditis
423 Other diseases of pericardium
424 Other diseases of endocardium
425 Cardiomyopathy
426 Conduction disorders
427 Cardiac dysrhythmias
428 Heart failure
429 Ill-defined descriptions and complications of heart disease

Cerebrovascular disease (430-438)

430 Subarachnoid hemorrhage
431 Intracerebral hemorrhage
432 Other and unspecified intracranial hemorrhage
433 Occlusion and stenosis of precerebral arteries
434 Occlusion of cerebral arteries
435 Transient cerebral ischemia
436 Acute but ill-defined cerebrovascular disease
437 Other and ill-defined cerebrovascular disease
438 Late effects of cerebrovascular disease

Diseases of arteries, arterioles, and capillaries (440-448)

440 Atherosclerosis
441 Aortic aneurysm and dissection
442 Other aneurysm
443 Other peripheral vascular disease
444 Arterial embolism and thrombosis
446 Polyarteritis nodosa and allied conditions
447 Other disorders of arteries and arterioles
448 Diseases of capillaries

Diseases of veins and lymphatics, and other diseases of circulatory system (451-459)

451 Phlebitis and thrombophlebitis
452 Portal vein thrombosis
453 Other venous embolism and thrombosis
454 Varicose veins of lower extremities
455 Hemorrhoids
456 Varicose veins of other sites
457 Noninfective disorders of lymphatic channels
458 Hypotension
459 Other disorders of circulatory system

8. DISEASES OF THE RESPIRATORY SYSTEM

Acute respiratory infections (460-466)

460 Acute nasopharyngitis [common cold]
461 Acute sinusitis
462 Acute pharyngitis
463 Acute tonsillitis
464 Acute laryngitis and tracheitis
465 Acute upper respiratory infections of multiple or unspecified sites
466 Acute bronchitis and bronchiolitis

Other diseases of upper respiratory tract (470-478)

470 Deviated nasal septum
471 Nasal polyps
472 Chronic pharyngitis and nasopharyngitis
473 Chronic sinusitis
474 Chronic disease of tonsils and adenoids
475 Peritonsillar abscess
476 Chronic laryngitis and laryngotracheitis
477 Allergic rhinitis

8. DISEASES OF THE RESPIRATORY SYSTEM *continued*

478 Other diseases of upper respiratory tract

Pneumonia and influenza (480-487)

480 Viral pneumonia
481 Pneumococcal pneumonia
482 Other bacterial pneumonia
483 Pneumonia due to other specified organism
484 Pneumonia in infectious diseases classified elsewhere
485 Bronchopneumonia, organism unspecified
486 Pneumonia, organism unspecified
487 Influenza

Chronic obstructive pulmonary disease and allied conditions (490-496)

490 Bronchitis, not specified as acute or chronic
491 Chronic bronchitis
492 Emphysema
493 Asthma
494 Bronchiectasis
495 Extrinsic allergic alveolitis
496 Chronic airways obstruction, not elsewhere classified

Pneumoconioses and other lung diseases due to external agents (500-508)

500 Coalworkers' pneumoconiosis
501 Asbestosis
502 Pneumoconiosis due to other silica or silicates
503 Pneumoconiosis due to other inorganic dust
504 Pneumopathy due to inhalation of other dust
505 Pneumoconiosis, unspecified
506 Respiratory conditions due to chemical fumes and vapors
507 Pneumonitis due to solids and liquids
508 Respiratory conditions due to other and unspecified external agents

Other diseases of respiratory system (510-519)

510 Empyema
511 Pleurisy
512 Pneumothorax
513 Abscess of lung and mediastinum
514 Pulmonary congestion and hypostasis
515 Postinflammatory pulmonary fibrosis
516 Other alveolar and parietoalveolar pneumopathy
517 Lung involvement in conditions classified elsewhere
518 Other diseases of lung
519 Other diseases of respiratory system

9. DISEASES OF THE DIGESTIVE SYSTEM

Diseases of oral cavity, salivary glands, and jaws (520-529)

520 Disorders of tooth development and eruption
521 Diseases of hard tissues of teeth
522 Diseases of pulp and periapical tissues
523 Gingival and periodontal diseases
524 Dentofacial anomalies, including malocclusion
525 Other diseases and conditions of the teeth and supporting structures
526 Diseases of the jaws
527 Diseases of the salivary glands
528 Diseases of the oral soft tissues, excluding lesions specific for gingiva and tongue
529 Diseases and other conditions of the tongue

Diseases of esophagus, stomach, and duodenum (530-537)

530 Diseases of esophagus
531 Gastric ulcer
532 Duodenal ulcer
533 Peptic ulcer, site unspecified
534 Gastrojejunal ulcer
535 Gastritis and duodenitis
536 Disorders of function of stomach
537 Other disorders of stomach and duodenum

9. DISEASES OF THE DIGESTIVE SYSTEM *continued*

Appendicitis (540-543)

540 Acute appendicitis
541 Appendicitis, unqualified
542 Other appendicitis
543 Other diseases of appendix

Hernia of abdominal cavity (550-553)

550 Inguinal hernia
551 Other hernia of abdominal cavity, with gangrene
552 Other hernia of abdominal cavity, with obstruction, but without mention of gangrene
553 Other hernia of abdominal cavity without mention of obstruction or gangrene

Noninfectious enteritis and colitis (555-558)

555 Regional enteritis
556 Ulcerative colitis
557 Vascular insufficiency of intestine
558 Other noninfectious gastroenteritis and colitis

Other diseases of intestines and peritoneum (560-569)

560 Intestinal obstruction without mention of hernia
562 Diverticula of intestine
564 Functional digestive disorders, not elsewhere classified
565 Anal fissure and fistula
566 Abscess of anal and rectal regions
567 Peritonitis
568 Other disorders of peritoneum
569 Other disorders of intestine

Other diseases of digestive system (570-579)

570 Acute and subacute necrosis of liver
571 Chronic liver disease and cirrhosis
572 Liver abscess and sequelae of chronic liver disease
573 Other disorders of liver
574 Cholelithiasis
575 Other disorders of gallbladder
576 Other disorders of biliary tract
577 Diseases of pancreas
578 Gastrointestinal hemorrhage
579 Intestinal malabsorption

10. DISEASES OF THE GENITOURINARY SYSTEM

Nephritis, nephrotic syndrome, and nephrosis (580-589)

580 Acute glomerulonephritis
581 Nephrotic syndrome
582 Chronic glomerulonephritis
583 Nephritis and nephropathy, not specified as acute or chronic
584 Acute renal failure
585 Chronic renal failure
586 Renal failure, unspecified
587 Renal sclerosis, unspecified
588 Disorders resulting from impaired renal function
589 Small kidney of unknown cause

Other diseases of urinary system (590-599)

590 Infections of kidney
591 Hydronephrosis
592 Calculus of kidney and ureter
593 Other disorders of kidney and ureter
594 Calculus of lower urinary tract
595 Cystitis
596 Other disorders of bladder
597 Urethritis, not sexually transmitted, and urethral syndrome
598 Urethral stricture
599 Other disorders of urethra and urinary tract

Diseases of male genital organs (600-608)

600 Hyperplasia of prostate
601 Inflammatory diseases of prostate

10. DISEASES OF THE GENITOURINARY SYSTEM *continued*

602 Other disorders of prostate
603 Hydrocele
604 Orchitis and epididymitis
605 Redundant prepuce and phimosis
606 Infertility, male
607 Disorders of penis
608 Other disorders of male genital organs

Disorders of breast (610-611)

610 Benign mammary dysplasias
611 Other disorders of breast

Inflammatory disease of female pelvic organs (614-616)

614 Inflammatory disease of ovary, fallopian tube, pelvic cellular tissue, and peritoneum
615 Inflammatory diseases of uterus, except cervix
616 Inflammatory disease of cervix, vagina, and vulva

Other disorders of female genital tract (617-629)

617 Endometriosis
618 Genital prolapse
619 Fistula involving female genital tract
620 Noninflammatory disorders of ovary, fallopian tube, and broad ligament
621 Disorders of uterus, not elsewhere classified
622 Noninflammatory disorders of cervix
623 Noninflammatory disorders of vagina
624 Noninflammatory disorders of vulva and perineum
625 Pain and other symptoms associated with female genital organs
626 Disorders of menstruation and other abnormal bleeding from female genital tract
627 Menopausal and postmenopausal disorders
628 Infertility, female
629 Other disorders of female genital organs

11. COMPLICATIONS OF PREGNANCY, CHILDBIRTH AND THE PUERPERIUM

Ectopic and molar pregnancy (630-633)

630 Hydatidiform mole
631 Other abnormal product of conception
632 Missed abortion
633 Ectopic pregnancy

Other pregnancy with abortive outcome (634-639)

634 Abortion
635 Legally induced abortion
636 Illegally induced abortion
637 Unspecified abortion
638 Failed attempted abortion
639 Complications following abortion and ectopic and molar pregnancies

Complications mainly related to pregnancy (640-648)

640 Hemorrhage in early pregnancy
641 Antepartum hemorrhage, abruptio placentae, and placenta previa
642 Hypertension complicating pregnancy, childbirth, and the puerperium
643 Excessive vomiting in pregnancy
644 Early or threatened labor
645 Prolonged pregnancy
646 Other complications of pregnancy, not elsewhere classified
647 Infective and parasitic conditions in the mother classifiable elsewhere but complicating pregnancy, childbirth, and the puerperium
648 Other current conditions in the mother classifiable elsewhere but complicating pregnancy, childbirth, and the puerperium

Normal delivery, and other indications for care in pregnancy, labor, and delivery (650-659)

650 Normal delivery
651 Multiple gestation
652 Malposition and malpresentation of fetus
653 Disproportion
654 Abnormality of organs and soft tissues of pelvis
655 Known or suspected fetal abnormality affecting management of mother
656 Other fetal and placental problems affecting management of mother
657 Polyhydramnios

11. COMPLICATIONS OF PREGNANCY, CHILDBIRTH AND THE PUERPERIUM *continued*

658 Other problems associated with amniotic cavity and membranes
659 Other indications for care or intervention related to labor and delivery and not elsewhere classified

Complications occurring mainly in the course of labor and delivery (660-669)

660 Obstructed labor
661 Abnormality of forces of labor
662 Long labor
663 Umbilical cord complications
664 Trauma to perineum and vulva during delivery
665 Other obstetrical trauma
666 Postpartum hemorrhage
667 Retained placenta or membranes, without hemorrhage
668 Complications of the administration of anesthetic or other sedation in labor and delivery
669 Other complications of labor and delivery, not elsewhere classified

Complications of the puerperium (670-676)

670 Major puerperal infection
671 Venous complications in pregnancy and the puerperium
672 Pyrexia of unknown origin during the puerperium
673 Obstetrical pulmonary embolism
674 Other and unspecified complications of the puerperium, not elsewhere classified
675 Infections of the breast and nipple associated with childbirth
676 Other disorders of the breast associated with childbirth, and disorders of lactation
677 Late effects of complications of pregnancy, childbirth and the puerperium

12. DISEASES OF THE SKIN AND SUBCUTANEOUS TISSUE

Infections of skin and subcutaneous tissue (680-686)

680 Carbuncle and furuncle
681 Cellulitis and abscess of finger and toe
682 Other cellulitis and abscess
683 Acute lymphadenitis
684 Impetigo
685 Pilonidal cyst
686 Other local infections of skin and subcutaneous tissue

Other inflammatory conditions of skin and subcutaneous tissue (690-698)

690 Erythematosquamous dermatosis
691 Atopic dermatitis and related conditions
692 Contact dermatitis and other eczema
693 Dermatitis due to substances taken internally
694 Bullous dermatoses
695 Erythematous conditions
696 Psoriasis and similar disorders
697 Lichen
698 Pruritus and related conditions

Other diseases of skin and subcutaneous tissue (700-709)

700 Corns and callosities
701 Other hypertrophic and atrophic conditions of skin
702 Other dermatoses
703 Diseases of nail
704 Diseases of hair and hair follicles
705 Disorders of sweat glands
706 Diseases of sebaceous glands
707 Chronic ulcer of skin
708 Urticaria
709 Other disorders of skin and subcutaneous tissue

13. DISEASES OF THE MUSCULOSKELETAL SYSTEM AND CONNECTIVE TISSUE

Arthropathies and related disorders (710-719)

710 Diffuse diseases of connective tissue
711 Arthropathy associated with infections
712 Crystal arthropathies
713 Arthropathy associated with other disorders classified elsewhere
714 Rheumatoid arthritis and other inflammatory polyarthropathies
715 Osteoarthrosis and allied disorders

13. DISEASES OF THE MUSCULOSKELETAL SYSTEM AND CONNECTIVE TISSUE

continued

716 Other and unspecified arthropathies
717 Internal derangement of knee
718 Other derangement of joint
719 Other and unspecified disorder of joint

Dorsopathies (720-724)

720 Ankylosing spondylitis and other inflammatory spondylopathies
721 Spondylosis and allied disorders
722 Intervertebral disc disorders
723 Other disorders of cervical region
724 Other and unspecified disorders of back

Rheumatism, excluding the back (725-729)

725 Polymyalgia rheumatica
726 Peripheral enthesopathies and allied syndromes
727 Other disorders of synovium, tendon, and bursa
728 Disorders of muscle, ligament, and fascia
729 Other disorders of soft tissues

Osteopathies, chondropathies, and acquired musculoskeletal deformities (730-739)

730 Osteomyelitis, periostitis, and other infections involving bone
731 Osteitis deformans and osteopathies associated with other disorders classified elsewhere
732 Osteochondropathies
733 Other disorders of bone and cartilage
734 Flat foot
735 Acquired deformities of toe
736 Other acquired deformities of limbs
737 Curvature of spine
738 Other acquired deformity
739 Nonallopathic lesions, not elsewhere classified

14. CONGENITAL ANOMALIES

740 Anencephalus and similar anomalies
741 Spina bifida
742 Other congenital anomalies of nervous system
743 Congenital anomalies of eye
744 Congenital anomalies of ear, face, and neck
745 Bulbus cordis anomalies and anomalies of cardiac septal closure
746 Other congenital anomalies of heart
747 Other congenital anomalies of circulatory system
748 Congenital anomalies of respiratory system
749 Cleft palate and cleft lip
750 Other congenital anomalies of upper alimentary tract
751 Other congenital anomalies of digestive system
752 Congenital anomalies of genital organs
753 Congenital anomalies of urinary system
754 Certain congenital musculoskeletal deformities
755 Other congenital anomalies of limbs
756 Other congenital musculoskeletal anomalies
757 Congenital anomalies of the integument
758 Chromosomal anomalies
759 Other and unspecified congenital anomalies

15. CERTAIN CONDITIONS ORIGINATING IN THE PERINATAL PERIOD

Maternal causes of perinatal morbidity and mortality (760-763)

760 Fetus or newborn affected by maternal conditions which may be unrelated to present pregnancy
761 Fetus or newborn affected by maternal complications of pregnancy
762 Fetus or newborn affected by complications of placenta, cord, and membranes
763 Fetus or newborn affected by other complications of labor and delivery

Other conditions originating in the perinatal period (764-779)

764 Slow fetal growth and fetal malnutrition
765 Disorders relating to short gestation and unspecified low birthweight
766 Disorders relating to long gestation and high birthweight
767 Birth trauma

15. CERTAIN CONDITIONS ORIGINATING IN THE PERINATAL PERIOD *continued*

768 Intrauterine hypoxia and birth asphyxia
769 Respiratory distress syndrome
770 Other respiratory conditions of fetus and newborn
771 Infections specific to the perinatal period
772 Fetal and neonatal hemorrhage
773 Hemolytic disease of fetus or newborn, due to isoimmunization
774 Other perinatal jaundice
775 Endocrine and metabolic disturbances specific to the fetus and newborn
776 Hematological disorders of fetus and newborn
777 Perinatal disorders of digestive system
778 Conditions involving the integument and temperature regulation of fetus and newborn
779 Other and ill-defined conditions originating in the perinatal period

16. SYMPTOMS, SIGNS, AND ILL-DEFINED CONDITIONS

Symptoms (780-789)

780 General symptoms
781 Symptoms involving nervous and musculoskeletal systems
782 Symptoms involving skin and other integumentary tissue
783 Symptoms concerning nutrition, metabolism, and development
784 Symptoms involving head and neck
785 Symptoms involving cardiovascular system
786 Symptoms involving respiratory system and other chest symptoms
787 Symptoms involving digestive system
788 Symptoms involving urinary system
789 Other symptoms involving abdomen and pelvis

Nonspecific abnormal findings (790-796)

790 Nonspecific findings on examination of blood
791 Nonspecific findings on examination of urine
792 Nonspecific abnormal findings in other body substances
793 Nonspecific abnormal findings on radiological and other examination of body structure
794 Nonspecific abnormal results of function studies
795 Nonspecific abnormal histological and immunological findings
796 Other nonspecific abnormal findings

Ill-defined and unknown causes of morbidity and mortality (797-799)

797 Senility without mention of psychosis
798 Sudden death, cause unknown
799 Other ill-defined and unknown causes of morbidity and mortality

17. INJURY AND POISONING

Fracture of skull (800-804)

800 Fracture of vault of skull
801 Fracture of base of skull
802 Fracture of face bones
803 Other and unqualified skull fractures
804 Multiple fractures involving skull or face with other bones

Fracture of neck and trunk (805-809)

805 Fracture of vertebral column without mention of spinal cord injury
806 Fracture of vertebral column with spinal cord injury
807 Fracture of rib(s), sternum, larynx, and trachea
808 Fracture of pelvis
809 Ill-defined fractures of bones of trunk

Fracture of upper limb (810-819)

810 Fracture of clavicle
811 Fracture of scapula
812 Fracture of humerus
813 Fracture of radius and ulna
814 Fracture of carpal bone(s)
815 Fracture of metacarpal bone(s)
816 Fracture of one or more phalanges of hand
817 Multiple fractures of hand bones
818 Ill-defined fractures of upper limb
819 Multiple fractures involving both upper limbs, and upper limb with rib(s) and sternum

17. INJURY AND POISONING *continued*

Fracture of lower limb (820-829)

820 Fracture of neck of femur
821 Fracture of other and unspecified parts of femur
822 Fracture of patella
823 Fracture of tibia and fibula
824 Fracture of ankle
825 Fracture of one or more tarsal and metatarsal bones
826 Fracture of one or more phalanges of foot
827 Other, multiple, and ill-defined fractures of lower limb
828 Multiple fractures involving both lower limbs, lower with upper limb, and lower limb(s) with rib(s) and sternum
829 Fracture of unspecified bones

Dislocation (830-839)

830 Dislocation of jaw
831 Dislocation of shoulder
832 Dislocation of elbow
833 Dislocation of wrist
834 Dislocation of finger
835 Dislocation of hip
836 Dislocation of knee
837 Dislocation of ankle
838 Dislocation of foot
839 Other, multiple, and ill-defined dislocations

Sprains and strains of joints and adjacent muscles (840-848)

840 Sprains and strains of shoulder and upper arm
841 Sprains and strains of elbow and forearm
842 Sprains and strains of wrist and hand
843 Sprains and strains of hip and thigh
844 Sprains and strains of knee and leg
845 Sprains and strains of ankle and foot
846 Sprains and strains of sacroiliac region
847 Sprains and strains of other and unspecified parts of back
848 Other and ill-defined sprains and strains

Intracranial injury, excluding those with skull fracture (850-854)

850 Concussion
851 Cerebral laceration and contusion
852 Subarachnoid, subdural, and extradural hemorrhage, following injury
853 Other and unspecified intracranial hemorrhage following injury
854 Intracranial injury of other and unspecified nature

Internal injury of thorax, abdomen, and pelvis (860-869)

860 Traumatic pneumothorax and hemothorax
861 Injury to heart and lung
862 Injury to other and unspecified intrathoracic organs
863 Injury to gastrointestinal tract
864 Injury to liver
865 Injury to spleen
866 Injury to kidney
867 Injury to pelvic organs
868 Injury to other intra-abdominal organs
869 Internal injury to unspecified or ill-defined organs

Open wound of head, neck, and trunk (870-879)

870 Open wound of ocular adnexa
871 Open wound of eyeball
872 Open wound of ear
873 Other open wound of head
874 Open wound of neck
875 Open wound of chest (wall)
876 Open wound of back
877 Open wound of buttock
878 Open wound of genital organs (external), including traumatic amputation
879 Open wound of other and unspecified sites, except limbs

Open wound of upper limb (880-887)

880 Open wound of shoulder and upper arm

17. INJURY AND POISONING *continued*

881 Open wound of elbow, forearm, and wrist
882 Open wound of hand except finger(s) alone
883 Open wound of finger(s)
884 Multiple and unspecified open wound of upper limb
885 Traumatic amputation of thumb (complete) (partial)
886 Traumatic amputation of other finger(s) (complete) (partial)
887 Traumatic amputation of arm and hand (complete) (partial)

Open wound of lower limb (890-897)

890 Open wound of hip and thigh
891 Open wound of knee, leg [except thigh], and ankle
892 Open wound of foot except toe(s) alone
893 Open wound of toe(s)
894 Multiple and unspecified open wound of lower limb
895 Traumatic amputation of toe(s) (complete) (partial)
896 Traumatic amputation of foot (complete) (partial)
897 Traumatic amputation of leg(s) (complete) (partial)

Injury to blood vessels (900-904)

900 Injury to blood vessels of head and neck
901 Injury to blood vessels of thorax
902 Injury to blood vessels of abdomen and pelvis
903 Injury to blood vessels of upper extremity
904 Injury to blood vessels of lower extremity and unspecified sites

Late effects of injuries, poisonings, toxic effects, and other external causes (905-909)

905 Late effects of musculoskeletal and connective tissue injuries
906 Late effects of injuries to skin and subcutaneous tissues
907 Late effects of injuries to the nervous system
908 Late effects of other and unspecified injuries
909 Late effects of other and unspecified external causes

Superficial injury (910-919)

910 Superficial injury of face, neck, and scalp except eye
911 Superficial injury of trunk
912 Superficial injury of shoulder and upper arm
913 Superficial injury of elbow, forearm, and wrist
914 Superficial injury of hand(s) except finger(s) alone
915 Superficial injury of finger(s)
916 Superficial injury of hip, thigh, leg, and ankle
917 Superficial injury of foot and toe(s)
918 Superficial injury of eye and adnexa
919 Superficial injury of other, multiple, and unspecified sites

Contusion with intact skin surface (920-924)

920 Contusion of face, scalp, and neck except eye(s)
921 Contusion of eye and adnexa
922 Contusion of trunk
923 Contusion of upper limb
924 Contusion of lower limb and of other and unspecified sites

Crushing injury (925-929)

925 Crushing injury of face, scalp, and neck
926 Crushing injury of trunk
927 Crushing injury of upper limb
928 Crushing injury of lower limb
929 Crushing injury of multiple and unspecified sites

Effects of foreign body entering through orifice (930-939)

930 Foreign body on external eye
931 Foreign body in ear
932 Foreign body in nose
933 Foreign body in pharynx and larynx
934 Foreign body in trachea, bronchus, and lung
935 Foreign body in mouth, esophagus, and stomach
936 Foreign body in intestine and colon
937 Foreign body in anus and rectum
938 Foreign body in digestive system, unspecified
939 Foreign body in genitourinary tract

17. INJURY AND POISONING *continued*

Burns (940-949)

940 Burn confined to eye and adnexa
941 Burn of face, head, and neck
942 Burn of trunk
943 Burn of upper limb, except wrist and hand
944 Burn of wrist(s) and hand(s)
945 Burn of lower limb(s)
946 Burns of multiple specified sites
947 Burn of internal organs
948 Burns classified according to extent of body surface involved
949 Burn, unspecified

Injury to nerves and spinal cord (950-957)

950 Injury to optic nerve and pathways
951 Injury to other cranial nerve(s)
952 Spinal cord injury without evidence of spinal bone injury
953 Injury to nerve roots and spinal plexus
954 Injury to other nerve(s) of trunk excluding shoulder and pelvic girdles
955 Injury to peripheral nerve(s) of shoulder girdle and upper limb
956 Injury to peripheral nerve(s) of pelvic girdle and lower limb
957 Injury to other and unspecified nerves

Certain traumatic complications and unspecified injuries (958-959)

958 Certain early complications of trauma
959 Injury, other and unspecified

Poisoning by drugs, medicinal and biological substances (960-979)

960 Poisoning by antibiotics
961 Poisoning by other anti-infectives
962 Poisoning by hormones and synthetic substitutes
963 Poisoning by primarily systemic agents
964 Poisoning by agents primarily affecting blood constituents
965 Poisoning by analgesics, antipyretics, and antirheumatics
966 Poisoning by anticonvulsants and anti-Parkinsonism drugs
967 Poisoning by sedatives and hypnotics
968 Poisoning by other central nervous system depressants and anesthetics
969 Poisoning by psychotropic agents
970 Poisoning by central nervous system stimulants
971 Poisoning by drugs primarily affecting the autonomic nervous system
972 Poisoning by agents primarily affecting the cardiovascular system
973 Poisoning by agents primarily affecting the gastrointestinal system
974 Poisoning by water, mineral, and uric acid metabolism drugs
975 Poisoning by agents primarily acting on the smooth and skeletal muscles and respiratory system
976 Poisoning by agents primarily affecting skin and mucous membrane, ophthalmological, otorhinolaryngological, and dental drugs
977 Poisoning by other and unspecified drugs and medicinals
978 Poisoning by bacterial vaccines
979 Poisoning by other vaccines and biological substances

Toxic effects of substances chiefly nonmedicinal as to source (980-989)

980 Toxic effect of alcohol
981 Toxic effect of petroleum products
982 Toxic effect of solvents other than petroleum-based
983 Toxic effect of corrosive aromatics, acids, and caustic alkalis
984 Toxic effect of lead and its compounds (including fumes)
985 Toxic effect of other metals
986 Toxic effect of carbon monoxide
987 Toxic effect of other gases, fumes, or vapors
988 Toxic effect of noxious substances eaten as food
989 Toxic effect of other substances, chiefly nonmedicinal as to source

Other and unspecified effects of external causes (990-995)

990 Effects of radiation, unspecified
991 Effects of reduced temperature
992 Effects of heat and light
993 Effects of air pressure
994 Effects of other external causes

17. INJURY AND POISONING *continued*

995 Certain adverse effects, not elsewhere classified

Complications of surgical and medical care, not elsewhere classified (996-999)

996 Complications peculiar to certain specified procedures
997 Complications affecting specified body systems, not elsewhere classified
998 Other complications of procedures, not elsewhere classified
999 Complications of medical care, not elsewhere classified

SUPPLEMENTARY CLASSIFICATION OF FACTORS INFLUENCING HEALTH STATUS AND CONTACT WITH HEALTH SERVICES

Persons with potential health hazards related to communicable diseases (V01-V06)

V01 Contact with or exposure to communicable diseases
V02 Carrier or suspected carrier of infectious diseases
V03 Need for prophylactic vaccination and inoculation against bacterial diseases
V04 Need for prophylactic vaccination and inoculation against certain viral diseases
V05 Need for other prophylactic vaccination and inoculation against single diseases
V06 Need for prophylactic vaccination and inoculation against combinations of diseases

Persons with need for isolation, other potential health hazards and prophylactic measures (V07-V09)

V07 Need for isolation and other prophylactic measures
V08 Asymptomatic human immunodeficiency virus (HIV) infection status
V09 Infection with drug resistant microorganisms

Persons with potential health hazards related to personal and family history (V10-V19)

V10 Personal history of malignant neoplasm
V11 Personal history of mental disorder
V12 Personal history of certain other diseases
V13 Personal history of other diseases
V14 Personal history of allergy to medicinal agents
V15 Other personal history presenting hazards to health
V16 Family history of malignant neoplasm
V17 Family history of certain chronic disabling diseases
V18 Family history of certain other specific conditions
V19 Family history of other conditions

Persons encountering health services in circumstances related to reproduction and development (V20-V29)

V20 Health supervision of infant or child
V21 Constitutional states in development
V22 Normal pregnancy
V23 Supervision of high-risk pregnancy
V24 Postpartum care and examination
V25 Encounter for contraceptive management
V26 Procreative management
V27 Outcome of delivery
V28 Antenatal screening
V29 Observation and evaluation of newborns for suspected condition not found

Liveborn infants according to type of birth (V30-V39)

V30 Single liveborn
V31 Twin, mate liveborn
V32 Twin, mate stillborn
V33 Twin, unspecified
V34 Other multiple, mates all liveborn
V35 Other multiple, mates all stillborn
V36 Other multiple, mates live- and stillborn
V37 Other multiple, unspecified
V39 Unspecified

Persons with a condition influencing their health status (V40-V49)

V40 Mental and behavioral problems
V41 Problems with special senses and other special functions
V42 Organ or tissue replaced by transplant
V43 Organ or tissue replaced by other means
V44 Artificial opening status
V45 Other postsurgical states
V46 Other dependence on machines
V47 Other problems with internal organs
V48 Problems with head, neck, and trunk

SUPPLEMENTARY CLASSIFICATION...HEALTH STATUS/HEALTH SERVICES *continued*

V49 Problems with limbs and other problems

Persons encountering health services for specific procedures and aftercare (V50-V59)

V50 Elective surgery for purposes other than remedying health states
V51 Aftercare involving the use of plastic surgery
V52 Fitting and adjustment of prosthetic device and implant
V53 Fitting and adjustment of other device
V54 Other orthopedic aftercare
V55 Attention to artificial openings
V56 Encounter for dialysis and dialysis catheter care
V57 Care involving use of rehabilitation procedures
V58 Encounter for other and unspecified procedures and aftercare
V59 Donors

Persons encountering health services in other circumstances (V60-V68)

V60 Housing, household, and economic circumstances
V61 Other family circumstances
V62 Other psychosocial circumstances
V63 Unavailability of other medical facilities for care
V64 Persons encountering health services for specific procedures, not carried out
V65 Other persons seeking consultation without complaint or sickness
V66 Convalescence
V67 Follow-up examination
V68 Encounters for administrative purposes
V69 Encounters related to lifestyle

Persons without reported diagnosis encountered during examination and investigation of individuals and populations (V70-V82)

V70 General medical examination
V71 Observation and evaluation for suspected conditions not found
V72 Special investigations and examinations
V73 Special screening examination for and Chlamydial viral diseases
V74 Special screening examination for bacterial and spirochetal diseases
V75 Special screening examination for other infectious diseases
V76 Special screening for malignant neoplasms
V77 Special screening for endocrine, nutritional, metabolic, and immunity disorders
V78 Special screening for disorders of blood and blood-forming organs
V79 Special screening for mental disorders and developmental handicaps
V80 Special screening for neurological, eye, and ear diseases
V81 Special screening for cardiovascular, respiratory, and genitourinary diseases
V82 Special screening for other conditions

SUPPLEMENTARY CLASSIFICATION OF EXTERNAL CAUSES OF INJURY AND POISONING

Railway accidents (E800-E807)

E800 Railway accident involving collision with rolling stock
E801 Railway accident involving collision with other object
E802 Railway accident involving derailment without antecedent collision
E803 Railway accident involving explosion, fire, or burning
E804 Fall in, on, or from railway train
E805 Hit by rolling stock
E806 Other specified railway accident
E807 Railway accident of unspecified nature

Motor vehicle traffic accidents (E810-E819)

E810 Motor vehicle traffic accident involving collision with train
E811 Motor vehicle traffic accident involving re-entrant collision with another motor vehicle
E812 Other motor vehicle traffic accident involving collision with another motor vehicle
E813 Motor vehicle traffic accident involving collision with other vehicle
E814 Motor vehicle traffic accident involving collision with pedestrian
E815 Other motor vehicle traffic accident involving collision on the highway
E816 Motor vehicle traffic accident due to loss of control, without collision on the highway
E817 Noncollision motor vehicle traffic accident while boarding or alighting
E818 Other noncollision motor vehicle traffic accident
E819 Motor vehicle traffic accident of unspecified nature

Motor vehicle nontraffic accidents (E820-E825)

E820 Nontraffic accident involving motor-driven snow vehicle

SUPPLEMENTARY CLASSIFICATION...INJURY AND POISONING *continued*

E821 Nontraffic accident involving other off-road motor vehicle
E822 Other motor vehicle nontraffic accident involving collision with moving object
E823 Other motor vehicle nontraffic accident involving collision with stationary object
E824 Other motor vehicle nontraffic accident while boarding and alighting
E825 Other motor vehicle nontraffic accident of other and unspecified nature

Other road vehicle accidents (E826-E829)

E826 Pedal cycle accident
E827 Animal-drawn vehicle accident
E828 Accident involving animal being ridden
E829 Other road vehicle accidents

Water transport accidents (E830-E838)

E830 Accident to watercraft causing submersion
E831 Accident to watercraft causing other injury
E832 Other accidental submersion or drowning in water transport accident
E833 Fall on stairs or ladders in water transport
E834 Other fall from one level to another in water transport
E835 Other and unspecified fall in water transport
E836 Machinery accident in water transport
E837 Explosion, fire, or burning in watercraft
E838 Other and unspecified water transport accident

Air and space transport accidents (E840-E845)

E840 Accident to powered aircraft at takeoff or landing
E841 Accident to powered aircraft, other and unspecified
E842 Accident to unpowered aircraft
E843 Fall in, on, or from aircraft
E844 Other specified air transport accidents
E845 Accident involving spacecraft

Vehicle accidents, not elsewhere classifiable (E846-E849)

E846 Accidents involving powered vehicles used solely within the buildings and premises of an industrial or commercial establishment
E847 Accidents involving cable cars not running on rails
E848 Accidents involving other vehicles, not elsewhere classifiable
E849 Place of occurrence

Accidental poisoning by drugs, medicinal substances, and biologicals (E850-E858)

E850 Accidental poisoning by analgesics, antipyretics, and antirheumatics
E851 Accidental poisoning by barbiturates
E852 Accidental poisoning by other sedatives and hypnotics
E853 Accidental poisoning by tranquilizers
E854 Accidental poisoning by other psychotropic agents
E855 Accidental poisoning by other drugs acting on central and autonomic nervous systems
E856 Accidental poisoning by antibiotics
E857 Accidental poisoning by other anti-infectives
E858 Accidental poisoning by other drugs

Accidental poisoning by other solid and liquid substances, gases, and vapors (E860-E869)

E860 Accidental poisoning by alcohol, not elsewhere classified
E861 Accidental poisoning by cleansing and polishing agents, disinfectants, paints, and varnishes
E862 Accidental poisoning by petroleum products, other solvents and their vapors, not elsewhere classified
E863 Accidental poisoning by agricultural and horticultural chemical and pharmaceutical preparations other than plant foods and fertilizers
E864 Accidental poisoning by corrosives and caustics, not elsewhere classified
E865 Accidental poisoning from poisonous foodstuffs and poisonous plants
E866 Accidental poisoning by other and unspecified solid and liquid substances
E867 Accidental poisoning by gas distributed by pipeline
E868 Accidental poisoning by other utility gas and other carbon monoxide
E869 Accidental poisoning by other gases and vapors

Misadventures to patients during surgical and medical care (E870-E876)

E870 Accidental cut, puncture, perforation, or hemorrhage during medical care
E871 Foreign object left in body during procedure
E872 Failure of sterile precautions during procedure
E873 Failure in dosage
E874 Mechanical failure of instrument or apparatus during procedure

SUPPLEMENTARY CLASSIFICATION...INJURY AND POISONING *continued*

E875 Contaminated or infected blood, other fluid, drug, or biological substance
E876 Other and unspecified misadventures during medical care

Surgical and medical procedures as the cause of abnormal reaction of patient or later complication, without mention of misadventure at the time of procedure (E878-E879)

E878 Surgical operation and other surgical procedures as the cause of abnormal reaction of patient, or of later complication, without mention of misadventure at the time of operation
E879 Other procedures, without mention of misadventure at the time of procedure, as the cause of abnormal reaction of patient, or of later complication

Accidental falls (E880-E888)

E880 Fall on or from stairs or steps
E881 Fall on or from ladders or scaffolding
E882 Fall from or out of building or other structure
E883 Fall into hole or other opening in surface
E884 Other fall from one level to another
E885 Fall on same level from slipping, tripping, or stumbling
E886 Fall on same level from collision, pushing or shoving, by or with other person
E887 Fracture, cause unspecified
E888 Other and unspecified fall

Accidents caused by fire and flames (E890-E899)

E890 Conflagration in private dwelling
E891 Conflagration in other and unspecified building or structure
E892 Conflagration not in building or structure
E893 Accident caused by ignition of clothing
E894 Ignition of highly inflammable material
E895 Accident caused by controlled fire in private dwelling
E896 Accident caused by controlled fire in other and unspecified building or structure
E897 Accident caused by controlled fire not in building or structure
E898 Accident caused by other specified fire and flames
E899 Accident caused by unspecified fire

Accidents due to natural and environmental factors (E900-E909)

E900 Excessive heat
E901 Excessive cold
E902 High and low air pressure and changes in air pressure
E903 Travel and motion
E904 Hunger, thirst, exposure, and neglect
E905 Venomous animals and plants as the cause of poisoning and toxic reactions
E906 Other injury caused by animals
E907 Lightning
E908 Cataclysmic storms, and floods resulting from storms
E909 Cataclysmic earth surface movements and eruptions

Accidents caused by submersion, suffocation, and foreign bodies (E910-E915)

E910 Accidental drowning and submersion
E911 Inhalation and ingestion of food causing obstruction of respiratory tract or suffocation
E912 Inhalation and ingestion of other object causing obstruction of respiratory tract or suffocation
E913 Accidental mechanical suffocation
E914 Foreign body accidentally entering eye and adnexa
E915 Foreign body accidentally entering other orifice

Other accidents (E916-E928)

E916 Struck accidentally by falling object
E917 Striking against or struck accidentally by objects or persons
E918 Caught accidentally in or between objects
E919 Accidents caused by machinery
E920 Accidents caused by cutting and piercing instruments or objects
E921 Accident caused by explosion of pressure vessel
E922 Accident caused by firearm missile
E923 Accident caused by explosive material
E924 Accident caused by hot substance or object, caustic or corrosive material, and steam
E925 Accident caused by electric current
E926 Exposure to radiation
E927 Overexertion and strenuous movements

SUPPLEMENTARY CLASSIFICATION...INJURY AND POISONING *continued*

E928 Other and unspecified environmental and accidental causes

Late effects of accidental injury (E929)

E929 Late effects of accidental injury

Drugs, medicinal and biological substances causing adverse effects in therapeutic use (E930-E949)

E930 Antibiotics
E931 Other anti-infectives
E932 Hormones and synthetic substitutes
E933 Primarily systemic agents
E934 Agents primarily affecting blood constituents
E935 Analgesics, antipyretics, and antirheumatics
E936 Anticonvulsants and anti-Parkinsonism drugs
E937 Sedatives and hypnotics
E938 Other central nervous system depressants and anesthetics
E939 Psychotropic agents
E940 Central nervous system stimulants
E941 Drugs primarily affecting the autonomic nervous system
E942 Agents primarily affecting the cardiovascular system
E943 Agents primarily affecting gastrointestinal system
E944 Water, mineral, and uric acid metabolism drugs
E945 Agents primarily acting on the smooth and skeletal muscles and respiratory system
E946 Agents primarily affecting skin and mucous membrane, ophthalmological, otorhinolaryngological, and dental drugs
E947 Other and unspecified drugs and medicinal substances
E948 Bacterial vaccines
E949 Other vaccines and biological substances

Suicide and self-inflicted injury (E950-E959)

E950 Suicide and self-inflicted poisoning by solid or liquid substances
E951 Suicide and self-inflicted poisoning by gases in domestic use
E952 Suicide and self-inflicted poisoning by other gases and vapors
E953 Suicide and self inflicted injury by hanging, strangulation, and suffocation
E954 Suicide and self-inflicted injury by submersion [drowning]
E955 Suicide and self-inflicted injury by firearms and explosives
E956 Suicide and self-inflicted injury by cutting and piercing instruments
E957 Suicide and self-inflicted injuries by jumping from high place
E958 Suicide and self-inflicted injury by other and unspecified means
E959 Late effects of self-inflicted injury

Homicide and injury purposely inflicted by other persons (E960-E969)

E960 Fight, brawl, and rape
E961 Assault by corrosive or caustic substance, except poisoning
E962 Assault by poisoning
E963 Assault by hanging and strangulation
E964 Assault by submersion [drowning]
E965 Assault by firearms and explosives
E966 Assault by cutting and piercing instrument
E967 Child battering and other maltreatment
E968 Assault by other and unspecified means
E969 Late effects of injury purposely inflicted by other person

Legal intervention (E970-E978)

E970 Injury due to legal intervention by firearms
E971 Injury due to legal intervention by explosives
E972 Injury due to legal intervention by gas
E973 Injury due to legal intervention by blunt object
E974 Injury due to legal intervention by cutting and piercing instruments
E975 Injury due to legal intervention by other specified means
E976 Injury due to legal intervention by unspecified means
E977 Late effects of injuries due to legal intervention
E978 Legal execution

Injury undetermined whether accidentally or purposely inflicted (E980-E989)

E980 Poisoning by solid or liquid substances, undetermined whether accidentally or purposely inflicted
E981 Poisoning by gases in domestic use, undetermined whether accidentally or purposely inflicted

SUPPLEMENTARY CLASSIFICATION...INJURY AND POISONING *continued*

E982 Poisoning by other gases, undetermined whether accidentally or purposely inflicted
E983 Hanging, strangulation, or suffocation, undetermined whether accidentally or purposely inflicted
E984 Submersion [drowning], undetermined whether accidentally or purposely inflicted
E985 Injury by firearms and explosives, undetermined whether accidentally or purposely inflicted
E986 Injury by cutting and piercing instruments, undetermined whether accidentally or purposely inflicted
E987 Falling from high place, undetermined whether accidentally or purposely inflicted
E988 Injury by other and unspecified means, undetermined whether accidentally or purposely inflicted
E989 Late effects of injury, undetermined whether accidentally or purposely inflicted

Injury resulting from operations of war (E990-E999)

E990 Injury due to war operations by fires and conflagrations
E991 Injury due to war operations by bullets and fragments
E992 Injury due to war operations by explosion of marine weapons
E993 Injury due to war operations by other explosion
E994 Injury due to war operations by destruction of aircraft
E995 Injury due to war operations by other and unspecified forms of conventional warfare
E996 Injury due to war operations by nuclear weapons
E997 Injury due to war operations by other forms of unconventional warfare
E998 Injury due to war operations but occurring after cessation of hostilities
E999 Late effects of injury due to war operations

DISEASES: ALPHABETIC INDEX
VOLUME 2

A

AAV (disease) (illness) (infection)—*see* Human immunodeficiency virus (disease) (illness) (infection)
Abactio —*see* Abortion, induced
Abactus venter —*see* Abortion, induced
Abarognosis 781.9
Abasia (-astasia) 307.9
atactica 781.3
choreic 781.3
hysterical 300.11
paroxysmal trepidant 781.3
spastic 781.3
trembling 781.3
trepidans 781.3
Abderhalden-Kaufmann-Lignac syndrome (cystinosis) 270.0
Abdomen, abdominal —*see also* condition
accordion 306.4
acute 789.0
angina 557.1
burst 868.00
convulsive equivalent (*see also* Epilepsy) 345.5
heart 746.87
muscle deficiency syndrome 756.7
obstipum 756.7
Abdominalgia 789.0
periodic 277.3
Abduction contracture, hip or other joint —*see* Contraction, joint
Abercrombie's syndrome (amyloid degeneration) 277.3
Aberrant (congenital)—*see also* Malposition, congenital
adrenal gland 759.1
blood vessel NEC 747.60
arteriovenous NEC 747.60
cerebrovascular 747.81
gastrointestinal 747.61
lower limb 747.64
renal 747.62
spinal 747.82
upper limb 747.63
breast 757.6
endocrine gland NEC 759.2
gastrointestinal vessel (peripheral) 747.61
hepatic duct 751.69
lower limb vessel (peripheral) 747.64
pancreas 751.7
parathyroid gland 759.2
peripheral vascular vessel NEC 747.60
pituitary gland (pharyngeal) 759.2
renal blood vessel 747.62
sebaceous glands, mucous membrane, mouth 750.26
spinal vessel 747.82
spleen 759.0
testis (descent) 752.5
thymus gland 759.2
thyroid gland 759.2
upper limb vessel (peripheral) 747.63
Aberratio
lactis 757.6
testis 752.5
Aberration —*see also* Anomaly
chromosome—*see* Anomaly, chromosome(s)
distantial 368.9
mental (*see also* Disorder, mental, nonpsychotic) 300.9
Abetalipoproteinemia 272.5
Abionarce 780.7
Abiotrophy 799.8
Ablatio
placentae—*see* Placenta, ablatio
retinae (*see also* Detachment, retina) 361.9
Ablation
pituitary (gland) (with hypofunction) 253.7
placenta—*see* Placenta, ablatio
uterus 621.8
Ablepharia, ablepharon, ablephary 743.62
Ablepsia —*see* Blindness
Ablepsy —*see* Blindness
Ablutomania 300.3
Abnormal, abnormality, abnormalities —*see also* Anomaly
acid-base balance 276.4
fetus or newborn—*see* Distress, fetal
adaptation curve, dark 368.63
alveolar ridge 525.9
amnion 658.9
affecting fetus or newborn 762.9
anatomical relationship NEC 759.9
apertures, congenital, diaphragm 756.6
auditory perception NEC 388.40
autosomes NEC 758.5
13 758.1
18 758.2
21 or 22 758.0
D_1 758.1
E_3 758.2
G 758.0
ballistocardiogram 794.39
basal metabolic rate (BMR) 794.7
biosynthesis, testicular androgen 257.2
blood level (of)
cobalt 790.6
copper 790.6
iron 790.6
lithium 790.6
magnesium 790.6
mineral 790.6
zinc 790.6
blood pressure
elevated (without diagnosis of hypertension) 796.2
low (*see also* Hypotension) 458.9
reading (incidental) (isolated) (nonspecific) 796.3
bowel sounds 787.5
breathing behavior—*see* Respiration
caloric test 794.19
cervix (acquired) NEC 622.9
congenital 752.40
in pregnancy or childbirth 654.6
causing obstructed labor 660.2
affecting fetus or newborn 763.1
chemistry, blood NEC 790.6
chest sounds 786.7
chorion 658.9
affecting fetus or newborn 762.9
chromosomal NEC 758.9
analysis, nonspecific result 795.2
autosomes (*see also* Abnormal, autosomes NEC) 758.5
fetal, (suspected) affecting management of pregnancy 655.1
sex 758.8

VOL 2 ABC

Abnormal, abnormality . . .—*continued*
clinical findings NEC 796.4
communication—*see* Fistula
configuration of pupils 379.49
coronary
artery 746.85
vein 746.9
cortisol-binding globulin 255.8
course, Eustachian tube 744.24
dentofacial NEC 524.9
functional 524.5
specified type NEC 524.8
development, developmental NEC 759.9
bone 756.9
central nervous system 742.9
direction, teeth 524.3
Dynia (see also Defect, coagulation) 286.9
Ebstein 746.2
echocardiogram 793.2
echoencephalogram 794.01
echogram NEC—*see* Findings, abnormal, structure
electrocardiogram (ECG) (EKG) 794.31
electroencephalogram (EEG) 794.02
electromyogram (EMG) 794.17
ocular 794.14
electro-oculogram (EOG) 794.12
electroretinogram (ERG) 794.11
erythrocytes 289.9
congenital, with perinatal jaundice 282.9 *[774.0]*
Eustachian valve 746.9
excitability under minor stress 301.9
fat distribution 782.9
feces 787.7
fetal heart rate—*see* Distress, fetal
fetus NEC
affecting management of pregnancy—*see* Pregnancy, management affected by, fetal
causing disproportion 653.7
affecting fetus or newborn 763.1
causing obstructed labor 660.1
affecting fetus or newborn 763.1
findings without manifest disease—*see* Findings, abnormal
fluid
amniotic 792.3
cerebrospinal 792.0
peritoneal 792.9
pleural 792.9
synovial 792.9
vaginal 792.9
forces of labor NEC 661.9
affecting fetus or newborn 763.7
form, teeth 520.2
function studies
auditory 794.15
bladder 794.9
brain 794.00
cardiovascular 794.30
endocrine NEC 794.6
kidney 794.4
liver 794.8
nervous system
central 794.00
peripheral 794.19
oculomotor 794.14
pancreas 794.9
placenta 794.9
pulmonary 794.2

Abnormal, abnormality . . .—*continued*
retina 794.11
special senses 794.19
spleen 794.9
thyroid 794.5
vestibular 794.16
gait 781.2
hysterical 300.11
gastrin secretion 251.5
globulin
cortisol-binding 255.8
thyroid-binding 246.8
glucagon secretion 251.4
glucose tolerance test 790.2
in pregnancy, childbirth, or puerperium 648.8
fetus or newborn 775.0
gravitational (G) forces or states 994.9
hair NEC 704.2
hard tissue formation in pulp 522.3
head movement 781.0
heart
rate, fetus—see Distress, fetal
shadow 793.2
sounds NEC 785.3
hemoglobin (*see also* Disease, hemoglobin) 282.7
trait—*see* Trait, hemoglobin, abnormal
hemorrhage, uterus—*see* Hemorrhage, uterus
histology NEC 795.4
increase
in
appetite 783.6
development 783.9
involuntary movement 781.0
jaw closure 524.5
karyotype 795.2
knee jerk 796.1
labor NEC 661.9
affecting fetus or newborn 763.7
laboratory findings—*see* Findings, abnormal
length, organ or site, congenital—*see* Distortion
loss of weight 783.2
lung shadow 793.1
mammogram 793.8
Mantoux test 795.5
membranes (fetal)
affecting fetus or newborn 762.9
complicating pregnancy 658.8
menstruation—*see* Menstruation
metabolism (*see also* condition) 783.9
movement 781.0
disorder, NEC 333.90
specified, NEC 333.99
head 781.0
involuntary 781.0
specified type NEC 333.99
muscle contraction, localized 728.85
myoglobin (Aberdeen) (Annapolis) 289.9
narrowness, eyelid 743.62
optokinetic response 379.57
organs or tissues of pelvis NEC
in pregnancy or childbirth 654.9
affecting fetus or newborn 763.8
causing obstructed labor 660.2
affecting fetus or newborn 763.1
origin—*see* Malposition, congenital
palmar creases 757.2
Papanicolaou (smear)
cervix 795.0
other site 795.1

Abnormal, abnormality . . .—*continued*
parturition
affecting fetus or newborn 763.9
mother—*see* Delivery, complicated
pelvis (bony)—*see* Deformity, pelvis
percussion, chest 786.7
periods (grossly) (see also Menstruation) 626.9
phonocardiogram 794.39
placenta—*see* Placenta, abnormal
plantar reflex 796.1
plasma protein—*see* Deficiency, plasma, protein
pleural folds 748.8
position—*see also* Malposition
gravid uterus 654.4
causing obstructed labor 660.2
affecting fetus or newborn 763.1
posture NEC 781.9
presentation (fetus)—*see* Presentation, fetus, abnormal
product of conception NEC 631
puberty—*see* Puberty
pulmonary
artery 747.3
function, newborn 770.8
test results 794.2
ventilation, newborn 770.8
hyperventilation 786.01
pulsations in neck 785.1
pupil reflexes 379.40
quality of milk 676.8
radiological examination 793.9
abdomen NEC 793.6
biliary tract 793.3
breast 793.8
gastrointestinal tract 793.4
genitourinary organs 793.5
head 793.0
intrathoracic organ NEC 793.2
lung (field) 793.1
musculoskeletal system 793.7
retroperitoneum 793.6
skin and subcutaneous tissue 793.9
skull 793.0
red blood cells 790.0
morphology 790.0
volume 790.0
reflex NEC 796.1
renal function test 794.4
respiration signs—*see* Respiration
response to nerve stimulation 794.10
retinal correspondence 368.34
rhythm, heart—*see also* Arrhythmia fetus—*see* Distress, fetal
saliva 792.4
scan
brain 794.09
kidney 794.4
liver 794.8
lung 794.2
thyroid 794.5
secretion
gastrin 251.5
glucagon 251.4
semen 792.2
serum level (of)
acid phosphatase 790.5
alkaline phosphatase 790.5
amylase 790.5
enzymes NEC 790.5
lipase 790.5

Abnormal, abnormality . . .—*continued*
shape
cornea 743.41
gallbladder 751.69
gravid uterus 654.4
affecting fetus or newborn 763.8
causing obstructed labor 660.2
affecting fetus or newborn 763.1
head (see also Anomaly, skull) 756.0
organ or site, congenital NEC—*see* Distortion
sinus venosus 747.40
size
fetus, complicating delivery 653.5
causing obstructed labor 660.1
gallbladder 751.69
head (*see also* Anomaly, skull) 756.0
organ or site, congenital NEC—*see* Distortion
teeth 520.2
skin and appendages, congenital NEC 757.9
soft parts of pelvis—*see* Abnormal, organs or tissues of pelvis
spermatozoa 792.2
sputum (amount) (color) (excessive) (odor) (purulent) 786.4
stool NEC 787.7
bloody 578.1
occult 792.1
bulky 787.7
color (dark) (light) 792.1
content (fat) (mucus) (pus) 792.1
occult blood 792.1
synchondrosis 756.9
test results without manifest disease—*see* Findings, abnormal
thebesian valve 746.9
thermography—*see* Findings, abnormal, structure
threshold, cones or rods (eye) 368.63
thyroid-binding globulin 246.8
thyroid product 246.8
toxicology (findings) NEC 796.0
tracheal cartilage (congenital) 748.3
transport protein 273.8
ultrasound results—*see* Findings, abnormal, structure
umbilical cord
affecting fetus or newborn 762.6
complicating delivery 663.9
specified NEC 663.8
union
cricoid cartilage and thyroid cartilage 748.3
larynx and trachea 748.3
thyroid cartilage and hyoid bone 748.3
urination NEC 788.69
psychogenic 306.53
stream
intermittent 788.61
slowing 788.62
splitting 788.61
weak 788.62
urine (constituents) NEC 791.9
uterine hemorrhage (*see also* Hemorrhage, uterus) 626.9
climacteric 627.0
postmenopausal 627.1
vagina (acquired) (congenital)
in pregnancy or childbirth 654.7
affecting fetus or newborn 763.8
causing obstructed labor 660.2
affecting fetus or newborn 763.1
vascular sounds 785.9

Abnormal, abnormality . . .—*continued*
vectorcardiogram 794.39
visually evoked potential (VEP) 794.13
vulva (acquired) (congenital)
in pregnancy or childbirth 654.8
affecting fetus or newborn 763.8
causing obstructed labor 660.2
affecting fetus or newborn 763.1
weight
gain 783.1
of pregnancy 646.1
with hypertension—see Toxemia, of pregnancy
loss 783.2
x-ray examination—*see* Abnormal, radiological examination
Abnormally formed uterus —*see* Anomaly, uterus
Abnormity (any organ or part)—*see* Anomaly
ABO
hemolytic disease 773.1
incompatibility reaction 999.6
Abocclusion 524.2
Abolition, language 784.69
Aborter, habitual or recurrent NEC
without current pregnancy 629.9
current abortion (*see also* Abortion, spontaneous) 634.9
affecting fetus or newborn 761.8
observation in current pregnancy 646.3
Abortion (complete) (incomplete) (inevitable) (with retained products of conception) 637.9

Note—Use the following fifth-digit subclassification with categories 634-637:

0 unspecified
1 incomplete
2 complete

with
complication(s) (any) following previous abortion—*see* category 639
damage to pelvic organ (laceration) (rupture) (tear) 637.2
embolism (air) (amniotic fluid) (blood clot) (pulmonary) (pyemic) (septic) (soap) 637.6
genital tract and pelvic infection 637.0
hemorrhage, delayed or excessive 637.1
metabolic disorder 637.4
renal failure (acute) 637.3
sepsis (genital tract) (pelvic organ) 637.0
urinary tract 637.7
shock (postoperative) (septic) 637.5
specified complication NEC 637.7
toxemia 637.3
unspecified complication(s) 637.8
urinary tract infection 637.7
accidental—*see* Abortion, spontaneous
artificial—*see* Abortion, induced
attempted (failed)—*see* Abortion, failed
criminal—*see* Abortion, illegal
early—*see* Abortion, spontaneous
elective—*see* Abortion, legal
failed (legal) 638.9
with
damage to pelvic organ (laceration) (rupture) (tear) 638.2
embolism (air) (amniotic fluid) (blood clot) (pulmonary) (pyemic) (septic) (soap) 638.6
genital tract and pelvic infection 638.0

Abortion—*continued*
hemorrhage, delayed or excessive 638.1
metabolic disorder 638.4
renal failure (acute) 638.3
sepsis (genital tract) (pelvic organ) 638.0
urinary tract 638.7
shock (postoperative) (septic) 638.5
specified complication NEC 638.7
toxemia 638.3
unspecified complication(s) 638.8
urinary tract infection 638.7
fetal indication—*see* Abortion, legal
fetus 779.6
following threatened abortion—*see* Abortion, by type
habitual or recurrent (care during pregnancy) 646.3
with current abortion (*see also* Abortion, spontaneous) 634.9
affecting fetus or newborn 761.8
without current pregnancy 629.9
homicidal—*see* Abortion, illegal
illegal 636.9
with
damage to pelvic organ (laceration) (rupture) (tear) 636.2
embolism (air) (amniotic fluid) (blood clot) (pulmonary) (pyemic) (septic) (soap) 636.6
genital tract and pelvic infection 636.0
hemorrhage, delayed or excessive 636.1
metabolic disorder 636.4
renal failure 636.3
sepsis (genital tract) (pelvic organ) 636.0
urinary tract 636.7
shock (postoperative) (septic) 636.5
specified complication NEC 636.7
toxemia 636.3
unspecified complication(s) 636.8
urinary tract infection 636.7
fetus 779.6
induced 637.9
illegal—*see* Abortion, illegal
legal indications—*see* Abortion, legal
medical indications—*see* Abortion, legal
therapeutic—*see* Abortion, legal
late—*see* Abortion, spontaneous
legal (legal indication) (medical indication) (under medical supervision) 635.9
with
damage to pelvic organ (laceration) (rupture) (tear) 635.2
embolism (air) (amniotic fluid) (blood clot) (pulmonary) (pyemic) (septic) (soap) 635.6
genital tract and pelvic infection 635.0
hemorrhage, delayed or excessive 635.1
metabolic disorder 635.4
renal failure (acute) 635.3
sepsis (genital tract) (pelvic organ) 635.0
urinary tract 635.7
shock (postoperative) (septic) 635.5
specified complication NEC 635.7
toxemia 635.3
unspecified complication(s) 635.8
urinary tract infection 635.7
fetus 779.6
medical indication—*see* Abortion, legal
mental hygiene problem—*see* Abortion, legal
missed 632
operative—*see* Abortion, legal

Abortion—*continued*
psychiatric indication—*see* Abortion, legal
recurrent—*see* Abortion, spontaneous
self-induced—*see* Abortion, illegal
septic—*see* Abortion, by type, with sepsis
spontaneous 634.9
with
damage to pelvic organ (laceration) (rupture) (tear) 634.2
embolism (air) (amniotic fluid) (blood clot) (pulmonary) (pyemic) (septic) (soap) 634.6
genital tract and pelvic infection 634.0
hemorrhage, delayed or excessive 634.1
metabolic disorder 634.4
renal failure 634.3
sepsis (genital tract) (pelvic organ) 634.0
urinary tract 634.7
shock (postoperative) (septic) 634.5
specified complication NEC 634.7
toxemia 634.3
unspecified complication(s) 634.8
urinary tract infection 634.7
fetus 761.8
threatened 640.0
affecting fetus or newborn 762.1
surgical—*see* Abortion, legal
therapeutic—*see* Abortion, legal
threatened 640.0
affecting fetus or newborn 762.1
tubal—*see* Pregnancy, tubal
voluntary—*see* Abortion, legal
Abortus fever 023.9
Aboulomania 301.6
Abrachia 755.20
Abrachiatism 755.20
Abrachiocephalia 759.89
Abrachiocephalus 759.89
Abrami's disease (acquired hemolytic jaundice) 283.9
Abramov-Fiedler myocarditis (acute isolated myocarditis) 422.91
Abrasion —*see also* Injury, superficial, by site
dental 521.2
teeth, tooth (dentifrice) (habitual) (hard tissues) (occupational) (ritual) (traditional) (wedge defect) 521.2
Abrikossov's tumor (M9580/0)—*see also* Neoplasm, connective tissue, benign
malignant (M9580/3)—*see* Neoplasm, connective tissue, malignant
Abrism 988.8
Abruption, placenta —*see* Placenta, abruptio
Abruptio placentae —*see* Placenta, abruptio
Abscess (acute) (chronic) (infectional) (lymphangitic) (metastatic) (multiple) (pyogenic) (septic) (with lymphangitis) (*see also* Cellulitis) 682.9
abdomen, abdominal
cavity—*see* Abscess, peritoneum
wall 682.2
abdominopelvic—*see* Abscess, peritoneum
accessory sinus (chronic) (*see also* Sinusitis) 473.9
adrenal (capsule) (gland) 255.8
alveolar 522.5
with sinus 522.7
amebic 006.3
bladder 006.8
brain (with liver or lung abscess) 006.5

Abscess—*continued*
liver (without mention of brain or lung abscess) 006.3
with
brain abscess (and lung abscess) 006.5
lung abscess 006.4
lung (with liver abscess) 006.4
with brain abscess 006.5
seminal vesicle 006.8
specified site NEC 006.8
spleen 006.8
anaerobic 040.0
ankle 682.6
anorectal 566
antecubital space 682.3
antrum (chronic) (Highmore) (*see also* Sinusitis, maxillary) 473.0
anus 566
apical (tooth) 522.5
with sinus (alveolar) 522.7
appendix 540.1
areola (acute) (chronic) (nonpuerperal) 611.0
puerperal, postpartum 675.1
arm (any part, above wrist) 682.3
artery (wall) 447.2
atheromatous 447.2
auditory canal (external) 380.10
auricle (ear) (staphylococcal) (streptococcal) 380.10
axilla, axillary (region) 682.3
lymph gland or node 683
back (any part) 682.2
Bartholin's gland 616.3
with
abortion—*see* Abortion, by type, with sepsis
ectopic pregnancy (*see also* categories 633.0-633.9) 639.0
molar pregnancy (*see also* categories 630-632) 639.0
complicating pregnancy or puerperium 646.6
following
abortion 639.0
ectopic or molar pregnancy 639.0
bartholinian 616.3
Bezold's 383.01
bile, biliary, duct or tract (*see also* Cholecystitis) 576.8
bilharziasis 120.1
bladder (wall) 595.89
amebic 006.8
bone (subperiosteal) (*see also* Osteomyelitis) 730.0
accessory sinus (chronic) (*see also* Sinusitis) 473.9
acute 730.0
chronic or old 730.1
jaw (lower) (upper) 526.4
mastoid—*see* Mastoiditis, acute
petrous (*see also* Petrositis) 383.20
spinal (tuberculous) (*see also* Tuberculosis) 015.0 *[730.88]*
nontuberculous 730.08
bowel 569.5
brain (any part) 324.0
amebic (with liver or lung abscess) 006.5
cystic 324.0
late effect—*see* category 326
otogenic 324.0
tuberculous (*see also* Tuberculosis) 013.3
breast (acute) (chronic) (nonpuerperal) 611.0
newborn 771.5

Abscess—*continued*
  hepatic 572.0
    amebic (*see also* Abscess, liver, amebic) 006.3
    duct 576.8
  hip 682.6
    tuberculous (active) (*see also* Tuberculosis) 015.1
  ileocecal 540.1
  ileostomy (bud) 569.6
  iliac (region) 682.2
    fossa 540.1
  iliopsoas (tuberculous) (*see also* Tuberculosis) 015.0 *[730.88]*
    nontuberculous 728.89
  infraclavicular (fossa) 682.3
  inguinal (region) 682.2
    lymph gland or node 683
  intersphincteric (anus) 566
  intestine, intestinal 569.5
    rectal 566
  intra-abdominal (*see also* Abscess, peritoneum) 567.2
    postoperative 998.5
  intracranial 324.0
    late effect—*see* category 326
  intramammary—*see* Abscess, breast
  intramastoid (*see also* Mastoiditis, acute) 383.00
  intraorbital 376.01
  intraperitoneal—*see* Abscess, peritoneum
  intraspinal 324.1
    late effect—*see* category 326
  intratonsillar 475
  iris 364.3
  ischiorectal 566
  jaw (bone) (lower) (upper) 526.4
    skin 682.0
  joint (*see also* Arthritis, pyogenic) 711.0
    vertebral (tuberculous) (*see also* Tuberculosis) 015.0 *[730.88]*
      nontuberculous 724.8
  kidney 590.2
    with
      abortion—*see* Abortion, by type, with urinary tract infection
      calculus 592.0
      ectopic pregnancy (*see also* categories 633.0-633.9) 639.8
      molar pregnancy (*see also* categories 630-632) 639.8
    complicating pregnancy or puerperium 646.6
      affecting fetus or newborn 760.1
    following
      abortion 639.8
      ectopic or molar pregnancy 639.8
  knee 682.6
    joint 711.06
    tuberculous (active) (*see also* Tuberculosis) 015.2
  labium (majus) (minus) 616.4
    complicating pregnancy, childbirth, or puerperium 646.6
  lacrimal (passages) (sac) (*see also* Dacryocystitis) 375.30
    caruncle 375.30
    gland (*see also* Dacryoadenitis) 375.00
  lacunar 597.0
  larynx 478.79
  lateral (alveolar) 522.5
    with sinus 522.7
  leg, except foot 682.6
  lens 360.00

Abscess—*continued*
  lid 373.13
  lingual 529.0
    tonsil 475
  lip 528.5
  Littre's gland 597.0
  liver 572.0
    amebic 006.3
      with
        brain abscess (and lung abscess) 006.5
        lung abscess 006.4
    due to Entamoeba histolytica 006.3
    dysenteric (*see also* Abscess, liver, amebic) 006.3
    pyogenic 572.0
    tropical (*see also* Abscess, liver, amebic) 006.3
  loin (region) 682.2
  lumbar (tuberculous) (*see also* Tuberculosis) 015.0 *[730.88]*
    nontuberculous 682.2
  lung (miliary) (putrid) 513.0
    amebic (with liver abscess) 006.4
      with brain abscess 006.5
  lymph, lymphatic, gland or node (acute) 683
    any site, except mesenteric 683
    mesentery 289.2
  lymphangitic, acute—*see* Cellulitis
  malar 526.4
  mammary gland—*see* Abscess, breast
  marginal (anus) 566
  mastoid (process) (*see also* Mastoiditis, acute) 383.00
    subperiosteal 383.01
  maxilla, maxillary 526.4
    molar (tooth) 522.5
      with sinus 522.7
    premolar 522.5
    sinus (chronic) (*see also* Sinusitis, maxillary) 473.0
  mediastinum 513.1
  meibomian gland 373.12
  meninges (*see also* Meningitis) 320.9
  mesentery, mesenteric—*see* Abscess, peritoneum
  mesosalpinx (*see also* Salpingo-oophoritis) 614.2
  milk 675.1
  Monro's (psoriasis) 696.1
  mons pubis 682.2
  mouth (floor) 528.3
  multiple sites NEC 682.9
  mural 682.2
  muscle 728.89
  myocardium 422.92
  nabothian (follicle) (*see also* Cervicitis) 616.0
  nail (chronic) (with lymphangitis) 681.9
    finger 681.02
    toe 681.11
  nasal (fossa) (septum) 478.1
    sinus (chronic) (*see also* Sinusitis) 473.9
  nasopharyngeal 478.29
  nates 682.5
  navel 682.2
    newborn NEC 771.4
  neck (region) 682.1
    lymph gland or node 683
  nephritic (*see also* Abscess, kidney) 590.2
  nipple 611.0
    puerperal, postpartum 675.0
  nose (septum) 478.1
    external 682.0

Abscess—*continued*
omentum—*see* Abscess, peritoneum
operative wound 998.5
orbit, orbital 376.01
ossifluent—*see* Abscess, bone
ovary, ovarian (corpus luteum) (*see also* Salpingo-oophoritis) 614.2
oviduct (*see also* Salpingo-oophoritis) 614.2
palate (soft) 528.3
hard 526.4
palmar (space) 682.4
pancreas (duct) 577.0
paradental 523.3
parafrenal 607.2
parametric, parametrium (chronic) (*see also* Disease, pelvis, inflammatory) 614.4
acute 614.3
paranephric 590.2
parapancreatic 577.0
parapharyngeal 478.22
pararectal 566
parasinus (*see also* Sinusitis) 473.9
parauterine (*see also* Disease, pelvis, inflammatory) 614.4
acute 614.3
paravaginal (*see also* Vaginitis) 616.10
parietal region 682.8
parodontal 523.3
parotid (duct) (gland) 527.3
region 528.3
parumbilical 682.2
newborn 771.4
pectoral (region) 682.2
pelvirectal— *see* Abscess, peritoneum
pelvis, pelvic
female (chronic) (*see also* Disease, pelvis, inflammatory) 614.4
acute 614.3
male, peritoneal (cellular tissue)—*see* Abscess, peritoneum
tuberculous (*see also* Tuberculosis) 016.9
penis 607.2
gonococcal (acute) 098.0
chronic or duration of 2 months or over 098.2
perianal 566
periapical 522.5
with sinus (alveolar) 522.7
periappendiceal 540.1
pericardial 420.99
pericecal 540.1
pericemental 523.3
pericholecystic (*see also* Cholecystitis, acute) 575.0
pericoronal 523.3
peridental 523.3
perigastric 535.0
perimetric (*see also* Disease, pelvis, inflammatory) 614.4
acute 614.3
perinephric, perinephritic (*see also* Abscess, kidney) 590.2
perineum, perineal (superficial) 682.2
deep (with urethral involvement) 597.0
urethra 597.0
periodontal (parietal) 523.3
apical 522.5
periosteum, periosteal (*see also* Periostitis) 730.3
with osteomyelitis (*see also* Osteomyelitis) 730.2
acute or subacute 730.0

Abscess—*continued*
chronic or old 730.1
peripleuritic 510.9
with fistula 510.0
periproctic 566
periprostatic 601.2
perirectal (staphylococcal) 566
perirenal (tissue) (*see also* Abscess, kidney) 590.2
perisinuous (nose) (*see also* Sinusitis) 473.9
peritoneum, peritoneal (perforated) (ruptured) 567.2
with
abortion—*see* Abortion, by type, with sepsis
appendicitis 540.1
ectopic pregnancy (*see also* categories 633.0-633.9) 639.0
molar pregnancy (*see also* categories 630-632) 639.0
following
abortion 639.0
ectopic or molar pregnancy 639.0
pelvic, female (*see also* Disease, pelvis, inflammatory) 614.4
acute 614.3
postoperative 998.5
puerperal, postpartum, childbirth 670
tuberculous (*see also* Tuberculosis) 014.0
peritonsillar 475
perityphlic 540.1
periureteral 593.89
periurethral 597.0
gonococcal (acute) 098.0
chronic or duration of 2 months or over 098.2
periuterine (*see also* Disease, pelvis, inflammatory) 614.4
acute 614.3
perivesical 595.89
pernicious NEC 682.9
petrous bone—*see* Petrositis
phagedenic NEC 682.9
chancroid 099.0
pharynx, pharyngeal (lateral) 478.29
phlegmonous NEC 682.9
pilonidal 685.0
pituitary (gland) 253.8
pleura 510.9
with fistula 510.0
popliteal 682.6
postanal 566
postcecal 540.1
postlaryngeal 478.79
postnasal 478.1
postpharyngeal 478.24
posttonsillar 475
posttyphoid 002.0
Pott's (*see also* Tuberculosis) 015.0 *[730.88]*
pouch of Douglas (chronic) (*see also* Disease, pelvis, inflammatory) 614.4
premammary—*see* Abscess, breast
prepatellar 682.6
prostate (*see also* Prostatitis) 601.2
gonococcal (acute) 098.12
chronic or duration of 2 months or over 098.32
psoas (tuberculous) (*see also* Tuberculosis) 015.0 *[730.88]*
nontuberculous 728.89
pterygopalatine fossa 682.8
pubis 682.2

Abscess—*continued*
puerperal—Puerperal, abscess, by site
pulmonary—*see* Abscess, lung
pulp, pulpal (dental) 522.0
finger 681.01
toe 681.10
pyemic—*see* Septicemia
pyloric valve 535.0
rectovaginal septum 569.5
rectovesical 595.89
rectum 566
regional NEC 682.9
renal (*see also* Abscess, kidney) 590.2
retina 363.00
retrobulbar 376.01
retrocecal—*see* Abscess, peritoneum
retrolaryngeal 478.79
retromammary—*see* Abscess, breast
retroperineal 682.2
retroperitoneal—*see* Abscess, peritoneum
retropharyngeal 478.24
tuberculous (*see also* Tuberculosis) 012.8
retrorectal 566
retrouterine (*see also* Disease, pelvis, inflammatory) 614.4
acute 614.3
retrovesical 595.89
root, tooth 522.5
with sinus (alveolar) 522.7
round ligament (*see also* Disease, pelvis, inflammatory) 614.4
acute 614.3
rupture (spontaneous) NEC 682.9
sacrum (tuberculous) (*see also* Tuberculosis) 015.0 *[730.88]*
nontuberculous 730.08
salivary duct or gland 527.3
scalp (any part) 682.8
scapular 730.01
sclera 379.09
scrofulous (*see also* Tuberculosis) 017.2
scrotum 608.4
seminal vesicle 608.0
amebic 006.8
septal, dental 522.5
with sinus (alveolar) 522.7
septum (nasal) 478.1
serous (*see also* Periostitis) 730.3
shoulder 682.3
side 682.2
sigmoid 569.5
sinus (accessory) (chronic) (nasal) (*see also* Sinusitis) 473.9
intracranial venous (any) 324.0
late effect—*see* category 326
Skene's duct or gland 597.0
skin NEC 682.9
tuberculous (primary) (*see also* Tuberculosis) 017.0
sloughing NEC 682.9
specified site NEC 682.8
amebic 006.8
spermatic cord 608.4
sphenoidal (sinus) (*see also* Sinusitis, sphenoidal) 473.3
spinal
cord (any part) (staphylococcal) 324.1
tuberculous (*see also* Tuberculosis) 013.5
epidural 324.1
spine (column) (tuberculous) (*see also* Tuberculosis) 015.0 *[730.88]*

Abscess—*continued*
nontuberculous 730.08
spleen 289.59
amebic 006.8
staphylococcal NEC 682.9
stitch 998.5
stomach (wall) 535.0
strumous (tuberculous) (*see also* Tuberculosis) 017.2
subarachnoid 324.9
brain 324.0
cerebral 324.0
late effect—*see* category 326
spinal cord 324.1
subareolar—*see also* Abscess, breast
puerperal, postpartum 675.1
subcecal 540.1
subcutaneous NEC 682.9
subdiaphragmatic—*see* Abscess, peritoneum
subdorsal 682.2
subdural 324.9
brain 324.0
late effect—*see* category 326
spinal cord 324.1
subgaleal 682.8
subhepatic—*see* Abscess, peritoneum
sublingual 528.3
gland 527.3
submammary—*see* Abscess, breast
submandibular (region) (space) (triangle) 682.0
gland 527.3
submaxillary (region) 682.0
gland 527.3
submental (pyogenic) 682.0
gland 527.3
subpectoral 682.2
subperiosteal—*see* Abscess, bone
subperitoneal—*see* Abscess, peritoneum
subphrenic—*see also* Abscess, peritoneum
postoperative 998.5
subscapular 682.2
subungual 681.9
suburethral 597.0
sudoriparous 705.89
suppurative NEC 682.9
supraclavicular (fossa) 682.3
suprahepatic—*see* Abscess, peritoneum
suprapelvic (*see also* Disease, pelvis, inflammatory) 614.4
acute 614.3
suprapubic 682.2
suprarenal (capsule) (gland) 255.8
sweat gland 705.89
syphilitic 095.8
teeth, tooth (root) 522.5
with sinus (alveolar) 522.7
supporting structures NEC 523.3
temple 682.0
temporal region 682.0
temporosphenoidal 324.0
late effect—*see* category 326
tendon (sheath) 727.89
testicle—*see* Orchitis
thecal 728.89
thigh (acquired) 682.6
thorax 510.9
with fistula 510.0
throat 478.29
thumb (intrathecal) (periosteal) (subcutaneous) (subcuticular) 681.00
thymus (gland) 254.1

Abscess—*continued*
thyroid (gland) 245.0
toe (any) (intrathecal) (periosteal) (subcutaneous) (subcuticular) 681.10
tongue (staphylococcal) 529.0
tonsil(s) (lingual) 475
tonsillopharyngeal 475
tooth, teeth (root) 522.5
with sinus (alveolar) 522.7
supporting structure NEC 523.3
trachea 478.9
trunk 682.2
tubal (*see also* Salpingo-oophoritis) 614.2
tuberculous—*see* Tuberculosis, abscess
tubo-ovarian (*see also* Salpingo-oophoritis) 614.2
tunica vaginalis 608.4
umbilicus NEC 682.2
newborn 771.4
upper arm 682.3
upper respiratory 478.9
urachus 682.2
urethra (gland) 597.0
urinary 597.0
uterus, uterine (wall) (*see also* Endometritis) 615.9
ligament (*see also* Disease, pelvis, inflammatory) 614.4
acute 614.3
neck (*see also* Cervicitis) 616.0
uvula 528.3
vagina (wall) (*see also* Vaginitis) 616.10
vaginorectal (*see also* Vaginitis) 616.10
vas deferens 608.4
vermiform appendix 540.1
vertebra (column) (tuberculous) (*see also* Tuberculosis) 015.0 *[730.88]*
nontuberculous 730.0
vesical 595.89
vesicouterine pouch (*see also* Disease, pelvis, inflammatory) 614.4
vitreous (humor) (pneumococcal) 360.04
vocal cord 478.5
von Bezold's 383.01
vulva 616.4
complicating pregnancy, childbirth, or puerperium 646.6
vulvovaginal gland (*see also* Vaginitis) 616.3
web-space 682.4
wrist 682.4
Absence (organ or part) (complete or partial)
acoustic nerve 742.8
adrenal (gland) (congenital) 759.1
acquired 255.8
albumin (blood) 273.8
alimentary tract (complete) (congenital) (partial) 751.8
lower 751.5
upper 750.8
alpha-fucosidase 271.8
alveolar process (acquired) 525.8
congenital 750.26
anus, anal (canal) (congenital) 751.2
aorta (congenital) 747.22
aortic valve (congenital) 746.89
appendix, congenital 751.2
arm (acquired) V49.60
above elbow V49.66
below elbow V49.65
congenital (*see also* Deformity, reduction, upper limb) 755.20

Absence—*continued*
lower—*see* Absence, forearm, congenital
upper (complete) (partial) (with absence of distal elements, incomplete) 755.24
with
complete absence of distal elements 755.21
forearm (incomplete) 755.23
artery (congenital) (peripheral) NEC (*see also* Anomaly, peripheral vascular system) 747.60
brain 747.81
cerebral 747.81
coronary 746.85
pulmonary 747.3
umbilical 747.5
atrial septum 745.69
auditory canal (congenital) (external) 744.01
auricle (ear) (with stenosis or atresia of auditory canal), congenital 744.01
bile, biliary duct (common) or passage (congenital) 751.61
bladder (acquired) 596.8
congenital 753.8
bone (congenital) NEC 756.9
marrow 284.9
acquired (secondary) 284.8
congenital 284.0
hereditary 284.0
idiopathic 284.9
skull 756.0
bowel sounds 787.5
brain 740.0
specified part 742.2
breast(s) (acquired) 611.8
congenital 757.6
broad ligament (congenital) 752.19
bronchus (congenital) 748.3
calvarium, calvaria (skull) 756.0
canaliculus lacrimalis, congenital 743.65
carpal(s) (congenital) (complete) (partial) (with absence of distal elements, incomplete) (*see also* Deformity, reduction, upper limb) 755.28
with complete absence of distal elements 755.21
cartilage 756.9
caudal spine 756.13
cecum (acquired) (postoperative) (posttraumatic) 569.89
congenital 751.2
cementum 520.4
cerebellum (congenital) (vermis) 742.2
cervix (acquired) (uteri) 622.8
congenital 752.49
chin, congenital 744.89
cilia (congenital) 743.63
acquired 374.89
circulatory system, part NEC 747.89
clavicle 755.51
clitoris (congenital) 752.49
coccyx, congenital 756.13
cold sense (see also Disturbance, sensation) 782.0
colon (acquired) (postoperative) 569.89
congenital 751.2
congenital
lumen—see Atresia
organ or site NEC—*see* Agenesis
septum—*see* Imperfect, closure
corpus callosum (congenital) 742.2

Absence—*continued*
cricoid cartilage 748.3
diaphragm (congenital) (with hernia) 756.6
with obstruction 756.6
digestive organ(s) or tract, congenital (complete) (partial) 751.8
lower 751.5
upper 750.8
ductus arteriosus 747.89
duodenum (acquired) (postoperative) 564.2
congenital 751.1
ear, congenital 744.09
acquired 388.8
auricle 744.01
external 744.01
inner 744.05
lobe, lobule 744.21
middle, except ossicles 744.03
ossicles 744.04
ossicles 744.04
ejaculatory duct (congenital) 752.8
endocrine gland NEC (congenital) 759.2
epididymis (congenital) 752.8
acquired 608.89
epiglottis, congenital 748.3
epileptic (atonic) (typical) (*see also* Epilepsy) 345.0
erythrocyte 284.9
erythropoiesis 284.9
congenital 284.0
esophagus (congenital) 750.3
Eustachian tube (congenital) 744.24
extremity (acquired)
congenital (*see also* Deformity, reduction) 755.4
lower V49.70
upper V49.60
extrinsic muscle, eye 743.69
eye (acquired) 360.89
adnexa (congenital) 743.69
congenital 743.00
muscle (congenital) 743.69
eyelid (fold), congenital 743.62
acquired 374.89
face
bones NEC 756.0
specified part NEC 744.89
fallopian tube(s) (acquired) 620.8
congenital 752.19
femur, congenital (complete) (partial) (with absence of distal elements, incomplete) (*see also* Deformity, reduction, lower limb) 755.34
with
complete absence of distal elements 755.31
tibia and fibula (incomplete) 755.33
fibrin 790.92
fibrinogen (congenital) 286.3
acquired 286.6
fibula, congenital (complete) (partial) (with absence of distal elements, incomplete) (*see also* Deformity, reduction, lower limb) 755.37
with
complete absence of distal elements 755.31
tibia 755.35
with
complete absence of distal elements 755.31
femur (incomplete) 755.33

Absence—*continued*
with complete absence of distal elements 755.31
finger (acquired) V49.62
congenital (complete) (partial) (*see also* Deformity, reduction, upper limb) 755.29
meaning all fingers (complete) (partial) 755.21
transverse 755.21
fissures of lungs (congenital) 748.5
foot (acquired) V49.73
congenital (complete) 755.31
forearm (acquired) V49.65
congenital (complete) (partial) (with absence of distal elements, incomplete) (*see also* Deformity, reduction, upper limb) 755.25
with
complete absence of distal elements (hand and fingers) 755.21
humerus (incomplete) 755.23
fovea centralis 743.55
fucosidase 271.8
gallbladder (acquired) V45.89
congenital 751.69
gamma globulin (blood) 279.00
genital organs, congenital
female 752.8
external 752.49
internal NEC 752.8
male 752.8
genitourinary organs, congenital NEC 752.8
glottis 748.3
gonadal, congenital NEC 758.6
hair (congenital) 757.4
acquired—*see* Alopecia
hand (acquired) V49.63
congenital (complete) (*see also* Deformity, reduction, upper limb) 755.21
heart (congenital) 759.89
acquired—*see* Status, organ replacement
heat sense (*see also* Disturbance, sensation) 782.0
humerus, congenital (complete) (partial) (with absence of distal elements, incomplete) (*see also* Deformity, reduction, upper limb) 755.24
with
complete absence of distal elements 755.21
radius and ulna (incomplete) 755.23
hymen (congenital) 752.49
ileum (acquired) (postoperative) (posttraumatic) 569.89
congenital 751.1
immunoglobulin, isolated NEC 279.03
IgA 279.01
IgG 279.03
IgM 279.02
incus (acquired) 385.24
congenital 744.04
internal ear (congenital) 744.05
intestine (acquired) (small) 569.89
congenital 751.1
large 751.2
large 569.89
congenital 751.2
iris (congenital) 743.45
jaw—*see* Absence, mandible
jejunum (acquired) 569.89
congenital 751.1
joint, congenital NEC 755.8

Absence—*continued*
kidney(s) (acquired) 593.89
congenital 753.0
labium (congenital) (majus) (minus) 752.49
labyrinth, membranous 744.05
lacrimal apparatus (congenital) 743.65
larynx (congenital) 748.3
leg (acquired) V49.70
above knee V49.76
below knee V49.75
congenital (partial) (unilateral) (*see also* Deformity, reduction, lower limb) 755.31
lower (complete) (partial) (with absence of distal elements, incomplete) 755.35
with
complete absence of distal elements (foot and toes) 755.31
thigh (incomplete) 755.33
with complete absence of distal elements 755.31
upper—*see* Absence, femur
lens (congenital) 743.35
acquired 379.31
ligament, broad (congenital) 752.19
limb (acquired)
congenital (complete) (partial) (*see also* Deformity, reduction) 755.4
lower 755.30
complete 755.31
incomplete 755.32
longitudinal—*see* Deficiency, lower limb, longitudinal
transverse 755.31
upper 755.20
complete 755.21
incomplete 755.22
longitudinal—*see* Deficiency, upper limb, longitudinal
transverse 755.21
lower NEC V49.70
upper NEC V49.60
lip 750.26
liver (congenital) (lobe) 751.69
lumbar (congenital) (vertebra) 756.13
isthmus 756.11
pars articularis 756.11
lumen—*see* Atresia
lung (bilateral) (congenital) (fissure) (lobe) (unilateral) 748.5
acquired (any part) 518.89
mandible (congenital) 524.09
maxilla (congenital) 524.09
menstruation 626.0
metacarpal(s), congenital (complete) (partial) (with absence of distal elements, incomplete) (*see also* Deformity, reduction, upper limb) 755.28
with all fingers, complete 755.21
metatarsal(s), congenital (complete) (partial) (with absence of distal elements, incomplete) (*see also* Deformity, reduction, lower limb) 755.38
with complete absence of distal elements 755.31
muscle (congenital) (pectoral) 756.81
ocular 743.69
musculoskeletal system (congenital) NEC 756.9
nail(s) (congenital) 757.5
neck, part 744.89
nerve 742.8
nervous system, part NEC 742.8

Absence—*continued*
neutrophil 288.0
nipple (congenital) 757.6
nose (congenital) 748.1
acquired 738.0
nuclear 742.8
ocular muscle (congenital) 743.69
organ
of Corti (congenital) 744.05
or site, congenital NEC 759.89
osseous meatus (ear) 744.03
ovary (acquired) 620.8
congenital 752.0
oviduct (acquired) 620.8
congenital 752.19
pancreas (congenital) 751.7
acquired (postoperative) (posttraumatic) 577.8
parathyroid gland (congenital) 759.2
parotid gland(s) (congenital) 750.21
patella, congenital 755.64
pelvic girdle (congenital) 755.69
penis (congenital) 752.8
acquired 607.89
pericardium (congenital) 746.89
perineal body (congenital) 756.81
phalange(s), congenital 755.4
lower limb (complete) (intercalary) (partial) (terminal) (*see also* Deformity, reduction, lower limb) 755.39
meaning all toes (complete) (partial) 755.31
transverse 755.31
upper limb (complete) (intercalary) (partial) (terminal) (*see also* Deformity, reduction, upper limb) 755.29
meaning all digits (complete) (partial) 755.21
transverse 755.21
pituitary gland (congenital) 759.2
postoperative—*see* Absence, by site, acquired
prostate (congenital) 752.8
acquired 602.8
pulmonary
artery 747.3
trunk 747.3
valve (congenital) 746.01
vein 747.49
punctum lacrimale (congenital) 743.65
radius, congenital (complete) (partial) (with absence of distal elements, incomplete) 755.26
with
complete absence of distal elements 755.21
ulna 755.25
with
complete absence of distal elements 755.21
humerus (incomplete) 755.23
ray, congenital 755.4
lower limb (complete) (partial) (*see also* Deformity, reduction, lower limb) 755.38
meaning all rays 755.31
transverse 755.31
upper limb (complete) (partial) (*see also* Deformity, reduction, upper limb) 755.28
meaning all rays 755.21
transverse 755.21
rectum (congenital) 751.2
acquired 569.49
red cell 284.9
acquired (secondary) 284.8
congenital 284.0

Absence—*continued*
hereditary 284.0
idiopathic 284.9
respiratory organ (congenital) NEC 748.9
rib (acquired) 738.3
congenital 756.3
roof of orbit (congenital) 742.0
round ligament (congenital) 752.8
sacrum, congenital 756.13
salivary gland(s) (congenital) 750.21
scapula 755.59
scrotum, congenital 752.8
seminal tract or duct (congenital) 752.8
acquired 608.89
septum (congenital)—*see also* Imperfect, closure, septum
atrial 745.69
and ventricular 745.7
between aorta and pulmonary artery 745.0
ventricular 745.3
and atrial 745.7
sex chromosomes 758.8
shoulder girdle, congenital (complete) (partial) 755.59
skin (congenital) 757.39
skull bone 756.0
with
anencephalus 740.0
encephalocele 742.0
hydrocephalus 742.3
with spina bifida (*see also* Spina bifida) 741.0
microcephalus 742.1
spermatic cord (congenital) 752.8
spinal cord 742.59
spine, congenital 756.13
spleen (congenital) 759.0
acquired 289.59
sternum, congenital 756.3
stomach (acquired) (partial) (postoperative) 564.2
congenital 750.7
submaxillary gland(s) (congenital) 750.21
superior vena cava (congenital) 747.49
tarsal(s), congenital (complete) (partial) (with absence of distal elements, incomplete) (*see also* Deformity, reduction, lower limb) 755.38
teeth, tooth (congenital) 520.0
with abnormal spacing 524.3
acquired 525.1
with malocclusion 524.3
tendon (congenital) 756.81
testis (congenital) 752.8
acquired 608.89
thigh (acquired) 736.89
thumb (acquired) V49.61
congenital 755.29
thymus gland (congenital) 759.2
thyroid (gland) (surgical) 246.8
with hypothyroidism 244.0
cartilage, congenital 748.3
congenital 243
tibia, congenital (complete) (partial) (with absence of distal elements, incomplete) (*see also* Deformity, reduction, lower limb) 755.36
with
complete absence of distal elements 755.31
fibula 755.35
with

Absence—*continued*
complete absence of distal elements 755.31
femur (incomplete) 755.33
with complete absence of distal elements 755.31
toe (acquired) V49.72
congenital (complete) (partial) 755.39
meaning all toes 755.31
transverse 755.31
great V49.71
tongue (congenital) 750.11
tooth, teeth, (congenital) 520.0
with abnormal spacing 524.3
acquired 525.1
with malocclusion 524.3
trachea (cartilage) (congenital) (rings) 748.3
transverse aortic arch (congenital) 747.21
tricuspid valve 746.1
ulna, congenital (complete) (partial) (with absence of distal elements, incomplete) (*see also* Deformity, reduction, upper limb) 755.27
with
complete absence of distal elements 755.21
radius 755.25
with
complete absence of distal elements 755.21
humerus (incomplete) 755.23
umbilical artery (congenital) 747.5
ureter (congenital) 753.4
acquired 593.89
urethra, congenital 753.8
urinary system, part NEC 753.8
uterus (acquired) 621.8
congenital 752.3
uvula (congenital) 750.26
vagina, congenital 752.49
vas deferens (congenital) 752.8
acquired 608.89
vein (congenital) (peripheral) NEC (*see also* Anomaly, peripheral vascular system) 747.60
brain 747.81
great 747.49
portal 747.49
pulmonary 747.49
vena cava (congenital) (inferior) (superior) 747.49
ventral horn cell 742.59
ventricular septum 745.3
vermis of cerebellum 742.2
vertebra, congenital 756.13
vulva, congenital 752.49
Absentia epileptica (*see also* Epilepsy) 345.0
Absinthemia (*see also* Dependence) 304.6
Absinthism (*see also* Dependence) 304.6
Absorbent system disease 459.89
Absorption
alcohol, through placenta or breast milk 760.71
antibiotics, through placenta or breast milk 760.74
anti-infective, through placenta or breast milk 760.74
chemical NEC 989.9
specified chemical or substance—*see* Table of drugs and chemicals
through placenta or breast milk (fetus or newborn) 760.70
alcohol 760.71

Absorption—*continued*
anti-infective agents 760.74
cocaine 760.75
"crack" 760.75
diethylstilbestrol [DES] 760.76
hallucinogenic agents 760.73
medicinal agents NEC 760.79
narcotics 760.72
obstetric anesthetic or analgesic drug 763.5
specified agent NEC 760.79
suspected, affecting management of pregnancy 655.5
cocaine, through placenta or breast milk 760.75
drug NEC (*see also* Reaction, drug) 995.2
through placenta or breast milk (fetus or newborn) 760.70
alcohol 760.71
anti-infective agents 760.74
cocaine 760.75
"crack" 760.75
diethylstilbestrol [DES] 760.76
hallucinogenic agents 760.73
medicinal agents NEC 760.79
narcotics 760.72
obstetric anesthetic or analgesic drug 763.5
specified agent NEC 760.79
suspected, affecting management of pregnancy 655.5
fat, disturbance 579.8
hallucinogenic agents, through placenta or breast milk 760.73
immune sera, through placenta or breast milk 760.79
lactose defect 271.3
medicinal agents NEC, through placenta or breast milk 760.79
narcotics, through placenta or breast milk 760.72
noxious substance,—*see* Absorption, chemical
protein, disturbance 579.8
pus or septic, general—*see* Septicemia
quinine, through placenta or breast milk 760.74
toxic substance—*see* Absorption, chemical
uremic—*see* Uremia
Abstinence symptoms or syndrome
alcohol 291.8
drug 292.0
Abt-Letterer-Siwe syndrome (acute histiocytosis X) (M9722/3) 202.5
Abulia 799.8
Abulomania 301.6
Abuse
adult NEC 995.81
as reason for
couple seeking advice (including offender) V61.1
non-partner seeking advice (including offender) V62.81
alcohol (*see also* Alcoholism) 303.9
non-dependent 305.0
child NEC 995.5
affecting parent or family (including offender) V61.21
as reason for
family seeking advice (including offender) V61.21
non-family member seeking advice (including offender) V62.81
Abuse—*continued*
drugs, nondependent 305.9

Note—Use the following fifth-digit subclassification with category 305:

0 unspecified
1 continuous
2 episodic
3 in remission

amphetamine type 305.7
antidepressants 305.8
barbiturates 305.4
caffeine 305.9
cannabis 305.2
cocaine type 305.6
hallucinogens 305.3
hashish 305.2
LSD 305.3
marijuana 305.2
mixed 305.9
morphine type 305.5
opioid type 305.5
phencyclidine (PCP) 305.9
specified NEC 305.9
tranquilizers 305.4
specified person other than child 995.81
spouse 995.81
tobacco 305.1
Acalcerosis 275.4
Acalcicosis 275.4
Acalculia 784.69
developmental 315.1
Acanthocheilonemiasis 125.4
Acanthocytosis 272.5
Acanthokeratodermia 701.1
Acantholysis 701.8
bullosa 757.39
Acanthoma (benign) (M8070/0)—*see also* Neoplasm, by site, benign
malignant (M8070/3)—*see* Neoplasm, by site, malignant
Acanthosis (acquired) (nigricans) 701.2
adult 701.2
benign (congenital) 757.39
congenital 757.39
glycogenic
esophagus 530.8
juvenile 701.2
tongue 529.8
Acanthrocytosis 272.5
Acapnia 276.3
Acarbia 276.2
Acardia 759.89
Acardiacus amorphus 759.89
Acardiotrophia 429.1
Acardius 759.89
Acariasis 133.9
sarcoptic 133.0
Acaridiasis 133.9
Acarinosis 133.9
Acariosis 133.9
Acarodermatitis 133.9
urticarioides 133.9
Acarophobia 300.29
Acatalasemia 277.8
Acatalasia 277.8
Acatamathesia 784.69
Acataphasia 784.5
Acathisia 781.0
due to drugs 333.99

Acceleration, accelerated
atrioventricular conduction 426.7
idioventricular rhythm 427.89
Accessory (congenital)
adrenal gland 759.1
anus 751.5
appendix 751.5
atrioventricular conduction 426.7
auditory ossicles 744.04
auricle (ear) 744.1
autosome(s) NEC 758.5
21 or 22 758.0
biliary duct or passage 751.69
bladder 753.8
blood vessels (peripheral) (congenital) NEC (*see also* Anomaly, peripheral vascular system) 747.60
cerebral 747.81
coronary 746.85
bone NEC 756.9
foot 755.67
breast tissue, axilla 757.6
carpal bones 755.56
cecum 751.5
cervix 752.49
chromosome(s) NEC 758.9
13-15 758.1
16-18 758.2
21 or 22 758.0
autosome(s) NEC 758.5
D_1 758.1
E_3 758.2
G 758.0
sex 758.8
coronary artery 746.85
cusp(s), heart valve NEC 746.89
pulmonary 746.09
cystic duct 751.69
digits 755.00
ear (auricle) (lobe) 744.1
endocrine gland NEC 759.2
external os 752.49
eyelid 743.62
eye muscle 743.69
face bone(s) 756.0
fallopian tube (fimbria) (ostium) 752.19
fingers 755.01
foreskin 605
frontonasal process 756.0
gallbladder 751.69
genital organ(s)
female 752.8
external 752.49
internal NEC 752.8
male 752.8
genitourinary organs NEC 752.8
heart 746.89
valve NEC 746.89
pulmonary 746.09
hepatic ducts 751.69
hymen 752.49
intestine (large) (small) 751.5
kidney 753.3
lacrimal canal 743.65
leaflet, heart valve NEC 746.89
pulmonary 746.09
ligament, broad 752.19
liver (duct) 751.69
lobule (ear) 744.1
lung (lobe) 748.69
muscle 756.82
Accessory—*continued*
navicular of carpus 755.56
nervous system, part NEC 742.8
nipple 757.6
nose 748.1
organ or site NEC—*see* Anomaly, specified type NEC
ovary 752.0
oviduct 752.19
pancreas 751.7
parathyroid gland 759.2
parotid gland (and duct) 750.22
pituitary gland 759.2
placental lobe—*see* Placenta, abnormal
preauricular appendage 744.1
prepuce 605
renal arteries (multiple) 747.62
rib 756.3
cervical 756.2
roots (teeth) 520.2
salivary gland 750.22
sesamoids 755.8
sinus—*see* condition
skin tags 757.39
spleen 759.0
sternum 756.3
submaxillary gland 750.22
tarsal bones 755.67
teeth, tooth 520.1
causing crowding 524.3
tendon 756.89
thumb 755.01
thymus gland 759.2
thyroid gland 759.2
toes 755.02
tongue 750.13
tragus 744.1
ureter 753.4
urethra 753.8
urinary organ or tract NEC 753.8
uterus 752.2
vagina 752.49
valve, heart NEC 746.89
pulmonary 746.09
vertebra 756.19
vocal cords 748.3
vulva 752.49
Accident, accidental —*see also* condition
birth NEC 767.9
cardiovascular (*see also* Disease, cardiovascular) 429.2
cerebral (*see also* Disease, cerebrovascular, acute) 436
cerebrovascular (current) (CVA) (*see also* Disease, cerebrovascular, acute) 436
healed or old—*see also* category 438
without residuals V12.5
impending 435.9
late effect—*see* category 438
coronary (*see also* Infarct, myocardium) 410.9
craniovascular (*see also* Disease, cerebrovascular, acute) 436
during pregnancy, to mother
affecting fetus or newborn 760.5
heart, cardiac (*see also* Infarct, myocardium) 410.9
intrauterine 779.8
vascular—*see* Disease, cerebrovascular, acute
Accommodation
disorder of 367.51
drug-induced 367.89

Accommodation—*continued*
toxic 367.89
insufficiency of 367.4
paralysis of 367.51
hysterical 300.11
spasm of 367.53
Accouchement —*see* Delivery
Accreta placenta (without hemorrhage) 667.0
with hemorrhage 666.0
Accretio cordis (nonrheumatic) 423.1
Accretions on teeth 523.6
Accumulation secretion, prostate 602.8
Acephalia, acephalism, acephaly 740.0
Acephalic monster 740.0
Acephalobrachia monster 759.89
Acephalocardia 759.89
Acephalocardius 759.89
Acephalochiria 759.89
Acephalochirus monster 759.89
Acephalogaster 759.89
Acephalostomus monster 759.89
Acephalothorax 759.89
Acephalus 740.0
Acetonemia 790.6
diabetic 250.1
Acetonglycosuria 982.8
Acetonuria 791.6
Achalasia 530.0
cardia 530.0
digestive organs congenital NEC 751.8
esophagus 530.0
pelvirectal 751.3
psychogenic 306.4
pylorus 750.5
sphincteral NEC 564.8
Achard-Thiers syndrome (adrenogenital) 255.2
Ache (s)—*see* Pain
Acheilia 750.26
Acheiria 755.21
Achillobursitis 726.71
Achillodynia 726.71
Achlorhydria, achlorhydric 536.0
anemia 280.9
diarrhea 536.0
neurogenic 536.0
postvagotomy 564.2
psychogenic 306.4
secondary to vagotomy 564.2
Achloroblepsia 368.52
Achloropsia 368.52
Acholia 575.8
Acholuric jaundice (familial) (splenomegalic) (*see also* Spherocytosis) 282.0
acquired 283.9
Achondroplasia 756.4
Achrestic anemia 281.8
Achroacytosis, lacrimal gland 375.00
tuberculous (*see also* Tuberculosis) 017.3
Achroma, cutis 709.00
Achromate (congenital) 368.54
Achromatopia 368.54
Achromatopsia (congenital) 368.54
Achromia
congenital 270.2
parasitica 111.0
unguium 703.8
Achylia
gastrica 536.8
neurogenic 536.3
psychogenic 306.4
pancreatica 577.1
Achylosis 536.8
Acid
burn—*see also* Burn, by site
from swallowing acid—*see* Burn, internal organs
deficiency
amide nicotinic 265.2
amino 270.9
ascorbic 267
folic 266.2
nicotinic (amide) 265.2
pantothenic 266.2
intoxication 276.2
peptic disease 536.8
stomach 536.8
psychogenic 306.4
Acidemia 276.2
arginosuccinic 270.6
fetal—*see* Distress, fetal
pipecolic 270.7
Acidity, gastric (high) (low) 536.8
psychogenic 306.4
Acidocytopenia 288.0
Acidocytosis 288.3
Acidopenia 288.0
Acidosis 276.2
diabetic 250.1
fetal—*see also* Distress, fetal
affecting management of pregnancy 656.3
intrauterine—*see* Distress, fetal
kidney tubular 588.8
lactic 276.2
metabolic NEC 276.2
with respiratory acidosis 276.4
late, of newborn 775.7
renal
hyperchloremic 588.8
tubular (distal) (proximal) 588.8
respiratory 276.2
complicated by
metabolic acidosis 276.4
metabolic alkalosis 276.4
Aciduria 791.9
arginosuccinic 270.6
beta-aminoisobutyric (BAIB) 277.2
glycolic 271.8
organic 270.9
orotic (congenital) (hereditary) (pyrimidine deficiency) 281.4
Acladiosis 111.8
skin 111.8
Aclasis
diaphyseal 756.4
tarsoepiphyseal 756.59
Acleistocardia 745.5
Aclusion 524.4
Acmesthesia 782.0
Acne (pustular) (vulgaris) 706.1
agminata (*see also* Tuberculosis) 017.0
artificialis 706.1
atrophica 706.0
cachecticorum (Hebra) 706.1
conglobata 706.1
conjunctiva 706.1
cystic 706.1
decalvans 704.09
erythematosa 695.3
eyelid 706.1
frontalis 706.0
indurata 706.1
keloid 706.1
lupoid 706.0

Acne—*continued*
necrotic, necrotica 706.0
miliaris 704.8
nodular 706.1
occupational 706.1
papulosa 706.1
rodens 706.0
rosacea 695.3
scorbutica 267
scrofulosorum (Bazin) (*see also* Tuberculosis) 017.0
summer 692.72
tropical 706.1
varioliformis 706.0
Acneiform drug eruptions 692.3
Acnitis (primary) (*see also* Tuberculosis) 017.0
Acomia 704.00
Acontractile bladder 344.61
Aconuresis (*see also* Incontinence) 788.30
Acosta's disease 993.2
Acousma 780.1
Acoustic —*see* condition
Acousticophobia 300.29
Acquired —*see* condition
Acquired immunodeficiency syndrome —*see* Human immunodeficiency virus (disease) (illness) (infection)
Acragnosis 781.9
Acrania (monster) 740.0
Acroagnosis 781.9
Acroasphyxia, chronic 443.89
Acrobrachycephaly 756.0
Acrobystiolith 608.89
Acrobystitis 607.2
Acrocephalopolysyndactyly 755.55
Acrocephalosyndactyly 755.55
Acrocephaly 756.0
Acrochondrohyperplasia 759.82
Acrocyanosis 443.89
newborn 770.8
Acrodermatitis 686.8
atrophicans (chronica) 701.8
continua (Hallopeau) 696.1
enteropathica 686.8
Hallopeau's 696.1
perstans 696.1
pustulosa continua 696.1
recalcitrant pustular 696.1
Acrodynia 985.0
Acrodysplasia 755.55
Acrohyperhidrosis 780.8
Acrokeratosis verruciformis 757.39
Acromastitis 611.0
Acromegaly, acromegalia (skin) 253.0
Acromelalgia 443.89
Acromicria, acromikria 756.59
Acronyx 703.0
Acropachy, thyroid (*see also* Thyrotoxicosis) 242.9
Acropachyderma 757.39
Acroparesthesia 443.89
simple (Schultz's type) 443.89
vasomotor (Nothnagel's type) 443.89
Acropathy thyroid (*see also* Thyrotoxicosis) 242.9
Acrophobia 300.29
Acroposthitis 607.2
Acroscleriasis (*see also* Scleroderma) 710.1
Acroscleroderma (*see also* Scleroderma) 710.1
Acrosclerosis (*see also* Scleroderma) 710.1
Acrosphacelus 785.4
Acrosphenosyndactylia 755.55
Acrospiroma, eccrine (M8402/0)—*see* Neoplasm, skin, benign
Acrostealgia 732.9
Acrosyndactyly (*see also* Syndactylism) 755.10
Acrotrophodynia 991.4
Actinic —*see also* condition
cheilitis (due to sun) 692.72
chronic NEC 692.74
due to radiation, except from sun 692.82
conjunctivitis 370.24
dermatitis (due to sun) (*see also* Dermatitis, actinic) 692.70
due to
roentgen rays or radioactive substance 692.82
ultraviolet radiation, except from sun 692.82
sun NEC 692.70
elastosis solare 692.74
granuloma 692.73
keratitis 370.24
ophthalmia 370.24
reticuloid 692.73
Actinobacillosis, general 027.8
Actinobacillus
lignieresii 027.8
mallei 024
muris 026.1
Actinocutitis NEC (*see also* Dermatitis, actinic) 692.70
Actinodermatitis NEC (*see also* Dermatitis, actinic) 692.70
Actinomyces
israelii (infection)—*see* Actinomycosis
muris-ratti (infection) 026.1
Actinomycosis actinomycotic 039.9
with
pneumonia 039.1
abdominal 039.2
cervicofacial 039.3
cutaneous 039.0
pulmonary 039.1
specified site NEC 039.8
thoracic 039.1
Actinoneuritis 357.8
Action, heart
disorder 427.9
postoperative 997.1
irregular 427.9
postoperative 997.1
psychogenic 306.2
Active —*see* condition
Activity decrease, functional 780.9
Acute —*see also* condition
abdomen NEC 789.0
gallbladder (*see also* Cholecystitis, acute) 575.0
Acyanoblepsia 368.53
Acyanopsia 368.53
Acystia 753.8
Acystinervia —*see* Neurogenic, bladder
Acystineuria —*see* Neurogenic, bladder
Adactylia, adactyly (congenital) 755.4
lower limb (complete) (intercalary) (partial) (terminal) (*see also* Deformity, reduction, lower limb) 755.39
meaning all digits (complete) (partial) 755.31
transverse (complete) (partial) 755.31
upper limb (complete) (intercalary) (partial) (terminal) (*see also* Deformity, reduction, upper limb) 755.29
meaning all digits (complete) (partial) 755.21
transverse (complete) (partial) 755.21

Adair-Dighton syndrome (brittle bones and blue sclera, deafness) 756.51
Adamantinoblastoma (M9310/0)—*see* Ameloblastoma
Adamantinoma (M9310/0)—*see* Ameloblastoma
Adamantoblastoma (M9310/0)—*see* Ameloblastoma
Adams-Stokes (-Morgagni) disease or syndrome (syncope with heart block) 426.9
Adaptation reaction (*see also* Reaction, adjustment) 309.9
Addiction—*see also* **Dependence**
absinthe 304.6
alcoholic (ethyl) (methyl) (wood) 303.9
complicating pregnancy, childbirth, or puerperium 648.4
affecting fetus or newborn 760.71
suspected damage to fetus affecting management of pregnancy 655.4
drug (*see also* Dependence) 304.9
ethyl alcohol 303.9
heroin 304.0
hospital 301.51
methyl alcohol 303.9
methylated spirit 303.9
morphine (-like substances) 304.0
nicotine 305.1
opium 304.0
tobacco 305.1
wine 303.9
Addison's
anemia (pernicious) 281.0
disease (bronze) (primary adrenal insufficiency) 255.4
tuberculous (*see also* Tuberculosis) 017.6
keloid (morphea) 701.0
melanoderma (adrenal cortical hypofunction) 255.4
Addison-Biermer anemia (pernicious) 281.0
Addison-Gull disease —*see* Xanthoma
Addisonian crisis or melanosis (acute adrenocortical insufficiency) 255.4
Additional —*see also* Accessory
chromosome(s) 758.9
13-15 758.1
16-18 758.2
21 758.0
autosome(s) NEC 758.5
sex 758.8
Adduction contracture, hip or other joint —*see* Contraction, joint
Adenasthenia gastrica 536.0
Aden fever 061
Adenitis (*see also* Lymphadenitis) 289.3
acute, unspecified site 683
epidemic infectious 075
axillary 289.3
acute 683
chronic or subacute 289.1
Bartholin's gland 616.8
bulbourethral gland (*see also* Urethritis) 597.89
cervical 289.3
acute 683
chronic or subacute 289.1
chancroid (Ducrey's bacillus) 099.0
chronic (any lymph node, except mesenteric) 289.1
mesenteric 289.2
Cowper's gland (*see also* Urethritis) 597.89
epidemic, acute 075
gangrenous 683
Adenitis—*continued*
gonorrheal NEC 098.89
groin 289.3
acute 683
chronic or subacute 289.1
infectious 075
inguinal (region) 289.3
acute 683
chronic or subacute 289.1
lymph gland or node, except mesenteric 289.3
acute 683
chronic or subacute 289.1
mesenteric (acute) (chronic) (nonspecific) (subacute) 289.2
mesenteric (acute) (chronic) (nonspecific) (subacute) 289.2
due to Pasteurella multocida (P. septica) 027.2
parotid gland (suppurative) 527.2
phlegmonous 683
salivary duct or gland (any) (recurring) (suppurative) 527.2
scrofulous (*see also* Tuberculosis) 017.2
septic 289.3
Skene's duct or gland (*see also* Urethritis) 597.89
strumous, tuberculous (*see also* Tuberculosis) 017.2
subacute, unspecified site 289.1
sublingual gland (suppurative) 527.2
submandibular gland (suppurative) 527.2
submaxillary gland (suppurative) 527.2
suppurative 683
tuberculous—*see* Tuberculosis, lymph gland
urethral gland (*see also* Urethritis) 597.89
venereal NEC 099.8
Wharton's duct (suppurative) 527.2
Adenoacanthoma (M8570/3)—*see* Neoplasm, by site, malignant
Adenoameloblastoma (M9300/0) 213.1
upper jaw (bone) 213.0
Adenocarcinoma (M8140/3)—*see also* Neoplasm, by site, malignant

Note—The list of adjectival modifiers below is not exhaustive. A description of adenocarcinoma that does not appear in this list should be coded in the same manner as carcinoma with that description. Thus, "mixed acidophil-basophil adenocarcinoma," should be coded in the same manner as "mixed acidophil-basophil carcinoma," which appears in the list under "Carcinoma."

Except where otherwise indicated, the morphological varieties of adenocarcinoma in the list below should be coded by site as for "Neoplasm, malignant."

with
apocrine metaplasia (M8573/3)
cartilaginous (and osseous) metaplasia (M8571/3)
osseous (and cartilaginous) metaplasia (M8571/3)
spindle cell metaplasia (M8572/3)
squamous metaplasia (M8570/3)
acidophil (M8280/3)
specified site—*see* Neoplasm, by site, malignant
unspecified site 194.3
acinar (M8550/3)
acinic cell (M8550/3)

Adenocarcinoma—*continued*
adrenal cortical (M8370/3) 194.0
alveolar (M8251/3)
and
epidermoid carcinoma, mixed (M8560/3)
squamous cell carcinoma, mixed (M8560/3)
apocrine (M8401/3)
breast—*see* Neoplasm, breast, malignant
specified site NEC—*see* Neoplasm, skin, malignant
unspecified site 173.9
basophil (M8300/3)
specified site—*see* Neoplasm, by site, malignant
unspecified site 194.3
bile duct type (M8160/3)
liver 155.1
specified site NEC—*see* Neoplasm, by site, malignant
unspecified site 155.1
bronchiolar (M8250/3)—*see* Neoplasm, lung, malignant
ceruminous (M8420/3) 173.2
chromophobe (M8270/3)
specified site—*see* Neoplasm, by site, malignant
unspecified site 194.3
clear cell (mesonephroid type) (M8310/3)
colloid (M8480/3)
cylindroid type (M8200/3)
diffuse type (M8145/3)
specified site—*see* Neoplasm, by site, malignant
unspecified site 151.9
duct (infiltrating) (M8500/3)
with Paget's disease (M8541/3)—*see* Neoplasm, breast, malignant
specified site—*see* Neoplasm, by site, malignant
unspecified site 174.9
embryonal (M9070/3)
endometrioid (M8380/3)—*see* Neoplasm, by site, malignant
eosinophil (M8280/3)
specified site—*see* Neoplasm, by site, malignant
unspecified site 194.3
follicular (M8330/3)
and papillary (M8340/3) 193
moderately differentiated type (M8332/3) 193
pure follicle type (M8331/3) 193
specified site—*see* Neoplasm, by site, malignant
trabecular type (M8332/3) 193
unspecified type 193
well differentiated type (M8331/3) 193
gelatinous (M8480/3)
granular cell (M8320/3)
Hürthle cell (M8290/3) 193
in
adenomatous
polyp (M8210/3)
polyposis coli (M8220/3) 153.9
polypoid adenoma (M8210/3)
tubular adenoma (M8210/3)
villous adenoma (M8261/3)
infiltrating duct (M8500/3)
with Paget's disease (M8541/3)—*see* Neoplasm, breast, malignant
specified site—*see* Neoplasm, by site, malignant

Adenocarcinoma—*continued*
unspecified site 174.9
inflammatory (M8530/3)
specified site—*see* Neoplasm, by site, malignant
unspecified site 174.9
in situ (M8140/2)—*see* Neoplasm, by site, in situ
intestinal type (M8144/3)
specified site—*see* Neoplasm, by site, malignant
unspecified site 151.9
intraductal (noninfiltrating) (M8500/2)
papillary (M8503/2)
specified site—*see* Neoplasm, by site, in situ
unspecified site 233.0
specified site—*see* Neoplasm, by site, in situ
unspecified site 233.0
islet cell (M8150/3)
and exocrine, mixed (M8154/3)
specified site—*see* Neoplasm, by site, malignant
unspecified site 157.9
pancreas 157.4
specified site NEC—*see* Neoplasm, by site, malignant
unspecified site 157.4
lobular (M8520/3)
specified site—*see* Neoplasm, by site, malignant
unspecified site 174.9
medullary (M8510/3)
mesonephric (M9110/3)
mixed cell (M8323/3)
mucinous (M8480/3)
mucin-producing (M8481/3)
mucoid (M8480/3)—*see also* Neoplasm, by site, malignant
cell (M8300/3)
specified site—*see* Neoplasm, by site, malignant
unspecified site 194.3
nonencapsulated sclerosing (M8350/3) 193
oncocytic (M8290/3)
oxyphilic (M8290/3)
papillary (M8260/3)
and follicular (M8340/3) 193
intraductal (noninfiltrating) (M8503/2)
specified site—*see* Neoplasm, by site, in situ
unspecified site 233.0
serous (M8460/3)
specified site—*see* Neoplasm, by site, malignant
unspecified site 183.0
papillocystic (M8450/3)
specified site—*see* Neoplasm, by site, malignant
unspecified site 183.0
pseudomucinous (M8470/3)
specified site—*see* Neoplasm, by site, malignant
unspecified site 183.0
renal cell (M8312/3) 189.0
sebaceous (M8410/3)
serous (M8441/3)—*see also* Neoplasm, by site, malignant
papillary
specified site—*see* Neoplasm, by site, malignant
unspecified site 183.0
signet ring cell (M8490/3)

Adenocarcinoma—*continued*
superficial spreading (M8143/3)
sweat gland (M8400/3)—*see* Neoplasm, skin, malignant
trabecular (M8190/3)
tubular (M8211/3)
villous (M8262/3)
water-clear cell (M8322/3) 194.1
Adenofibroma (M9013/0)
clear cell (M8313/0)—*see* Neoplasm, by site, benign
endometrioid (M8381/0) 220
borderline malignancy (M8381/1) 236.2
malignant (M8381/3) 183.0
mucinous (M9015/0)
specified site—*see* Neoplasm, by site, benign
unspecified site 220
prostate 600
serous (M9014/0)
specified site—*see* Neoplasm, by site, benign
unspecified site 220
specified site—*see* Neoplasm, by site, benign
unspecified site 220
Adenofibrosis
breast 610.2
endometrioid 617.0
Adenoiditis 474.0
acute 463
Adenoids (congenital) (of nasal fossa) 474.9
hypertrophy 474.12
vegetations 474.2
Adenolipomatosis (symmetrical) 272.8
Adenolymphoma (M8561/0)
specified site—*see* Neoplasm, by site, benign
unspecified 210.2
Adenoma (sessile) (M8140/0)—*see also* Neoplasm, by site, benign

Note—Except where otherwise indicated, the morphological varieties of adenoma in the list below should be coded by site as for "Neoplasm, benign."

acidophil (M8280/0)
specified site—*see* Neoplasm, by site, benign
unspecified site 227.3
acinar (cell) (M8550/0)
acinic cell (M8550/0)
adrenal (cortex) (cortical) (functioning) (M8370/0) 227.0
clear cell type (M8373/0) 227.0
compact cell type (M8371/0) 227.0
glomerulosa cell type (M8374/0) 227.0
heavily pigmented variant (M8372/0) 227.0
mixed cell type (M8375/0) 227.0
alpha cell (M8152/0)
pancreas 211.7
specified site NEC—*see* Neoplasm, by site, benign
unspecified site 211.7
alveolar (M8251/0)
apocrine (M8401/0)
breast 217
specified site NEC—*see* Neoplasm, skin, benign
unspecified site 216.9
basal cell (M8147/0)
basophil (M8300/0)
specified site—*see* Neoplasm, by site, benign
unspecified site 227.3
beta cell (M8151/0)
pancreas 211.7

Adenoma—*continued*
specified site NEC—*see* Neoplasm, by site, benign
unspecified site 211.7
bile duct (M8160/0) 211.5
black (M8372/0) 227.0
bronchial (M8140/1) 235.7
carcinoid type (M8240/3)—*see* Neoplasm, lung, malignant
cylindroid type (M8200/3)—*see* Neoplasm, lung, malignant
ceruminous (M8420/0) 216.2
chief cell (M8321/0) 227.1
chromophobe (M8270/0)
(specified site—*see* Neoplasm, by site, benign
unspecified site 227.3
clear cell (M8310/0)
colloid (M8334/0)
specified site—*see* Neoplasm, by site, benign
unspecified site 226
cylindroid type, bronchus (M8200/3)—*see* Neoplasm, lung, malignant
duct (M8503/0)
embryonal (M8191/0)
endocrine, multiple (M8360/1)
single specified site—*see* Neoplasm, by site, uncertain behavior
two or more specified sites 237.4
unspecified site 237.4
endometrioid (M8380/0)—*see also* Neoplasm, by site, benign
borderline malignancy (M8380/1)—*see* Neoplasm, by site, uncertain behavior
eosinophil (M8280/0)
specified site—*see* Neoplasm, by site, benign
unspecified site 227.3
fetal (M8333/0)
specified site—*see* Neoplasm, by site, benign
unspecified site 226
follicular (M8330/0)
specified site—*see* Neoplasm, by site, benign
unspecified site 226
hepatocellular (M8170/0) 211.5
Hürthle cell (M8290/0) 226
intracystic papillary (M8504/0)
islet cell (functioning) (M8150/0)
pancreas 211.7
specified site NEC—*see* Neoplasm, by site, benign
unspecified site 211.7
liver cell (M8170/0) 211.5
macrofollicular (M8334/0)
specified site NEC—*see* Neoplasm, by site, benign
unspecified site 226
malignant, malignum (M8140/3)—*see* Neoplasm, by site, malignant
mesonephric (M9110/0)
microfollicular (M8333/0)
specified site—*see* Neoplasm, by site, benign
unspecified site 226
mixed cell (M8323/0)
monomorphic (M8146/0)
mucinous (M8480/0)
mucoid cell (M8300/0)
specified site—*see* Neoplasm, by site, benign
unspecified site 227.3
multiple endocrine (M8360/1)
single specified site—*see* Neoplasm, by site, uncertain behavior
two or more specified sites 237.4

Adenoma—*continued*
unspecified site 237.4
nipple (M8506/0) 217
oncocytic (M8290/0)
oxyphilic (M8290/0)
papillary (M8260/0)—*see also* Neoplasm, by site, benign
intracystic (M8504/0)
papillotubular (M8263/0)
Pick's tubular (M8640/0)
specified site—*see* Neoplasm, by site, benign
unspecified site
female 220
male 222.0
pleomorphic (M8940/0)
polypoid (M8210/0)
prostate (benign) 600
rete cell 222.0
sebaceous, sebaceum (gland) (senile) (M8410/0)—*see also* Neoplasm, skin, benign
disseminata 759.5
Sertoli cell (M8640/0)
specified site—*see* Neoplasm, by site, benign
unspecified site
female 220
male 222.0
skin appendage (M8390/0)—*see* Neoplasm, skin, benign
sudoriferous gland (M8400/0)—*see* Neoplasm, skin, benign
sweat gland or duct (M8400/0)—*see* Neoplasm, skin, benign
testicular (M8640/0)
specified site—*see* Neoplasm, by site, benign
unspecified site
female 220
male 222.0
thyroid 226
trabecular (M8190/0)
tubular (M8211/0)—*see also* Neoplasm, by site, benign
papillary (M8460/3)
Pick's (M8640/0)
specified site—*see* Neoplasm, by site, benign
unspecified site
female 220
male 222.0
tubulovillous (M8263/0)
villoglandular (M8263/0)
villous (M8261/1)—*see* Neoplasm, by site, uncertain behavior
water-clear cell (M8322/0) 227.1
wolffian duct (M9110/0)
Adenomatosis (M8220/0)
endocrine (multiple) (M8360/1)
single specified site—*see* Neoplasm, by site, uncertain behavior
two or more specified sites 237.4
unspecified site 237.4
erosive of nipple (M8506/0) 217
pluriendocrine—*see* Adenomatosis, endocrine
pulmonary (M8250/1) 235.7
malignant (M8250/3)—*see* Neoplasm, lung, malignant
specified site—*see* Neoplasm, by site, benign
unspecified site 211.3
Adenomatous
cyst, thyroid (gland)—*see* Goiter, nodular
Adenomatous—*continued*
goiter (nontoxic) (*see also* Goiter, nodular) 241.9
toxic or with hyperthyroidism 242.3
Adenomyoma (M8932/0)—*see also* Neoplasm, by site, benign
prostate 600
Adenomyometritis 617.0
Adenomyosis (uterus) (internal) 617.0
Adenopathy (lymph gland) 785.6
inguinal 785.6
mediastinal 785.6
mesentery 785.6
syphilitic (secondary) 091.4
tracheobronchial 785.6
tuberculous (*see also* Tuberculosis) 012.1
primary, progressive 010.8
tuberculous (*see also* Tuberculosis, lymph gland) 017.2
tracheobronchial 012.1
primary, progressive 010.8
Adenopharyngitis 462
Adenophlegmon 683
Adenosalpingitis 614.1
Adenosarcoma (M8960/3) 189.0
Adenosclerosis 289.3
Adenosis
breast (sclerosing) 610.2
vagina, congenital 752.49
Adentia (complete) (partial) (*see also* Absence, teeth) 520.0
Adherent
labium (minus) 624.4
pericardium (nonrheumatic) 423.1
rheumatic 393
placenta 667.0
with hemorrhage 666.0
prepuce 605
scar (skin) NEC 709.2
tendon in scar 709.2
Adhesion (s), adhesive (postinfectional)
abdominal (wall) (*see also* Adhesions, peritoneum) 568.0
amnion to fetus 658.8
affecting fetus or newborn 762.8
appendix 543.9
arachnoiditis—*see* Meningitis
auditory tube (Eustachian) 381.89
bands—*see also* Adhesions, peritoneum
cervix 622.3
uterus 621.5
bile duct (any) 576.8
bladder (sphincter) 596.8
bowel (*see also* Adhesions, peritoneum) 568.0
cardiac 423.1
rheumatic 398.99
cecum (*see also* Adhesions, peritoneum) 568.0
cervicovaginal 622.3
congenital 752.49
postpartal 674.8
old 622.3
cervix 622.3
clitoris 624.4
colon (*see also* Adhesions, peritoneum) 568.0
common duct 576.8
congenital—*see also* Anomaly, specified type NEC
fingers (*see also* Syndactylism, fingers) 755.11
labium (majus) (minus) 752.49
omental, anomalous 751.4
ovary 752.0

Adhesion—*continued*
peritoneal 751.4
toes (*see also* Syndactylism, toes) 755.13
tongue (to gum or roof of mouth) 750.12
conjunctiva (acquired) (localized) 372.62
congenital 743.63
extensive 372.63
cornea—*see* Opacity, cornea
cystic duct 575.8
diaphragm (*see also* Adhesions, peritoneum) 568.0
due to foreign body—*see* Foreign body
duodenum (*see also* Adhesions, peritoneum) 568.0
with obstruction 537.3
ear, middle—*see* Adhesions, middle ear
epididymis 608.89
epidural—*see* Adhesions, meninges
epiglottis 478.79
Eustachian tube 381.89
eyelid 374.46
postoperative 997.9
surgically created V45.6
gallbladder (*see also* Disease, gallbladder) 575.8
globe 360.89
heart 423.1
rheumatic 398.99
ileocecal (coil) (*see also* Adhesions, peritoneum) 568.0
ileum (*see also* Adhesions, peritoneum) 568.0
intestine (postoperative) (*see also* Adhesions, peritoneum) 568.0
with obstruction 560.81
with hernia—*see also* Hernia, by site, with obstruction
gangrenous—*see* Hernia, by site, with gangrene
intra-abdominal (*see also* Adhesions, peritoneum) 568.0
iris 364.70
to corneal graft 996.79
joint (*see also* Ankylosis) 718.5
kidney 593.89
labium (majus) (minus), congenital 752.49
liver 572.8
lung 511.0
mediastinum 519.3
meninges 349.2
cerebral (any) 349.2
congenital 742.4
congenital 742.8
spinal (any) 349.2
congenital 742.59
tuberculous (cerebral) (spinal) (*see also* Tuberculosis, meninges) 013.0
mesenteric (*see also* Adhesions, peritoneum) 568.0
middle ear (fibrous) 385.10
drum head 385.19
to
incus 385.11
promontorium 385.13
stapes 385.12
specified NEC 385.19
nasal (septum) (to turbinates) 478.1
nerve NEC 355.9
spinal 355.9
root 724.9
cervical NEC 723.4
lumbar NEC 724.4
lumbosacral 724.4

Adhesion—*continued*
thoracic 724.4
ocular muscle 378.60
omentum (*see also* Adhesions, peritoneum) 568.0
organ or site, congenital NEC—*see* Anomaly, specified type NEC
ovary 614.6
congenital (to cecum, kidney, or omentum) 752.0
parauterine 614.6
parovarian 614.6
pelvic (peritoneal)
female 614.6
male (*see also* Adhesions, peritoneum) 568.0
postpartal (old) 614.6
tuberculous (*see also* Tuberculosis) 016.9
penis to scrotum (congenital) 752.8
periappendiceal (*see also* Adhesions, peritoneum) 568.0
pericardium (nonrheumatic) 423.1
rheumatic 393
tuberculous (*see also* Tuberculosis) 017.9 *[420.0]*
pericholecystic 575.8
perigastric (*see also* Adhesions, peritoneum) 568.0
periovarian 614.6
periprostatic 602.8
perirectal (*see also* Adhesions, peritoneum) 568.0
perirenal 593.89
peritoneum, peritoneal (fibrous) (postoperative) 568.0
with obstruction (intestinal) 560.81
with hernia—*see also* Hernia, by site, with obstruction
gangrenous—*see* Hernia, by site, with gangrene
duodenum 537.3
congenital 751.4
pelvic, female 614.6
postpartal, pelvic 614.6
to uterus 614.6
peritubal 614.6
periureteral 593.89
periuterine 621.5
perivesical 596.8
perivesicular (seminal vesicle) 608.89
pleura, pleuritic 511.0
tuberculous (*see also* Tuberculosis, pleura) 012.0
pleuropericardial 511.0
postoperative (gastrointestinal tract) *(See also* Adhesions, peritoneum) 568.0
eyelid 997.9
surgically created V45.6
urethra 598.2
postpartal, old 624.4
preputial, prepuce 605
pulmonary 511.0
pylorus (*see also* Adhesions, peritoneum) 568.0
Rosenmüller's fossa 478.29
sciatic nerve 355.0
seminal vesicle 608.89
shoulder (joint) 726.0
sigmoid flexure (*see also* Adhesions, peritoneum) 568.0
spermatic cord (acquired) 608.89
congenital 752.8

Adhesion—*continued*
spinal canal 349.2
nerve 355.9
root 724.9
cervical NEC 723.4
lumbar NEC 724.4
lumbosacral 724.4
thoracic 724.4
stomach (*see also* Adhesions, peritoneum) 568.0
subscapular 726.2
tendonitis 726.90
shoulder 726.0
testicle 608.89
tongue (congenital) (to gum or roof of mouth) 750.12
acquired 529.8
trachea 519.1
tubo-ovarian 614.6
tunica vaginalis 608.89
ureter 593.89
uterus 621.5
to abdominal wall 621.5
in pregnancy or childbirth 654.4
affecting fetus or newborn 763.8
vagina (chronic) (postoperative) (postradiation) 623.2
vaginitis (congenital) 752.49
vesical 596.8
vitreous 379.29
Adie (-Holmes) syndrome (tonic pupillary reaction) 379.46
Adiponecrosis neonatorum 778.1
Adiposa dolorosa 272.8
Adiposalgia 272.8
Adiposis 278.0
cerebralis 253.8
dolorosa 272.8
tuberosa simplex 272.8
Adiposity 278.0
heart (*see also* Degeneration, myocardial) 429.1
localized 278.1
Adiposogenital dystrophy 253.8
Adjustment
prosthesis or other device—*see* Fitting of
reaction—*see* Reaction, adjustment
Administration, prophylactic
antibiotics V07.39
antitoxin, any V07.2
antivenin V07.2
chemotherapeutic agent NEC V07.39
chemotherapy NEC V07.39
diphtheria antitoxin V07.2
fluoride V07.31
gamma globulin V07.2
immune sera (gamma globulin) V07.2
passive immunization agent V07.2
RhoGAM V07.2
Admission (encounter)
as organ donor—*see* Donor
by mistake V68.9
for
adjustment (of)
artificial
arm (complete) (partial) V52.0
eye V52.2
leg (complete) (partial) V52.1
brain neuropacemaker V53.0
breast
implant V50.1
prosthesis V52.4

Admission—*continued*
cardiac device V53.39
defibrillator, automatic implantable V53.32
pacemaker V53.31
carotid sinus V53.39
catheter
non-vascular V58.82
vascular V58.81
colostomy belt V53.5
contact lenses V53.1
cystostomy device V53.6
dental prosthesis V52.3
device NEC V53.9
abdominal V53.5
cardiac V53.39
defibrillator, automatic implantable V53.32
pacemaker V53.31
carotid sinus V53.39
intrauterine contraceptive V25.1
nervous system V53.0
orthodontic V53.4
prosthetic V52.9
breast V52.4
dental V52.3
eye V52.2
specified type NEC V52.8
special senses V53.0
substitution
auditory V53.0
nervous system V53.0
visual V53.0
urinary V53.6
dialysis catheter (extracorporeal) (peritoneal) V56.1
diaphragm (contraceptive) V25.02
hearing aid V53.2
ileostomy device V53.5
intestinal appliance or device NEC V53.5
intrauterine contraceptive device V25.1
neuropacemaker (brain) (peripheral nerve) (spinal cord) V53.0
orthodontic device V53.4
orthopedic (device) V53.7
brace V53.7
cast V53.7
shoes V53.7
pacemaker
brain V53.0
cardiac V53.31
carotid sinus V53.39
peripheral nerve V53.0
spinal cord V53.0
prosthesis V52.9
arm (complete) (partial) V52.0
breast V52.4
dental V52.3
eye V52.2
leg (complete) (partial) V52.1
specified type NEC V52.8
spectacles V53.1
wheelchair V53.8
adoption referral or proceedings V68.89
aftercare (*see also* Aftercare) V58.9
cardiac pacemaker V53.31
chemotherapy V58.1
dialysis
extracorporeal (renal) V56.0
peritoneal V56.8
renal V56.0
fracture (*see also* Aftercare, fracture) V54.9

Admission—*continued*
specified type NEC V54.8
medical NEC V58.8
orthopedic V54.9
specified type NEC V54.8
pacemaker device
brain V53.0
cardiac V53.31
carotid sinus V53.39
nervous system V53.0
spinal cord V53.0
postoperative NEC V58.49
wound closure, planned V58.41
postpartum
immediately after delivery V24.0
routine follow-up V24.2
postradiation V58.0
radiation therapy V58.0
removal of
non-vascular catheter V58.82
vascular catheter V58.81
specified NEC V58.89
removal of vascular catheter V58.81
surgical NEC V58.49
wound closure, planned V58.41
artificial insemination V26.1
attention to artificial opening (of) V55.9
artificial vagina V55.7
colostomy V55.3
cystostomy V55.5
enterostomy V55.4
gastrostomy V55.1
ileostomy V55.2
jejunostomy V55.4
nephrostomy V55.6
specified site NEC V55.8
intestinal tract V55.4
urinary tract V55.6
tracheostomy V55.0
ureterostomy V55.6
urethrostomy V55.6
battery replacement
cardiac pacemaker V53.31
boarding V65.0
breast
augmentation or reduction V50.1
removal, prophylactic V50.41
change of
cardiac pacemaker (battery) V53.31
carotid sinus pacemaker V53.39
catheter in artificial opening—*see* Attention to, artificial, opening
dressing V58.3
fixation device
external V54.8
internal V54.0
Kirschner wire V54.8
neuropacemaker device (brain) (peripheral nerve) (spinal cord) V53.0
pacemaker device
brain V53.0
cardiac V53.31
carotid sinus V53.39
nervous system V53.0
plaster cast V54.8
splint, external V54.8
Steinmann pin V54.8
surgical dressing V58.3
traction device V54.8
checkup only V70.0
chemotherapy V58.1

Admission—*continued*
circumcision, ritual or routine (in absence of medical indication) V50.2
clinical research investigation V70.7
closure of artificial opening—*see* Attention to, artificial, opening
contraceptive
counseling V25.09
management V25.9
specified type NEC V25.8
convalescence following V66.9
chemotherapy V66.2
psychotherapy V66.3
radiotherapy V66.1
surgery V66.0
treatment (for) V66.5
combined V66.6
fracture V66.4
mental disorder NEC V66.3
specified condition NEC V66.5
cosmetic surgery NEC V50.1
following healed injury or operation V51
counseling (*see also* Counseling) V65.40
without complaint or sickness V65.49
contraceptive management V25.09
dietary V65.3
exercise V65.41
for nonattending third party V65.1
genetic V26.3
gonorrhea V65.45
HIV V65.44
human immunodeficiency virus V65.44
injury prevention V65.43
procreative management V26.4
sexually transmitted disease NEC V65.45
HIV V65.44
specified reason NEC V65.49
substance use and abuse V65.42
syphilis V65.45
desensitization to allergens V07.1
dialysis
catheter
fitting and adjustment V56.1
removal or replacement V56.1
extracorporeal (renal) V56.0
peritoneal V56.8
renal V56.0
dietary surveillance and counseling V65.3
ear piercing V50.3
elective surgery V50.9
breast
augmentation or reduction V50.1
removal, prophylactic V50.41
circumcision, ritual or routine (in absence of medical indication) V50.2
cosmetic NEC V50.1
following healed injury or operation V51
ear piercing V50.3
face-lift V50.1
hair transplant V50.0
plastic
cosmetic NEC V50.1
following healed injury or operation V51
prophylactic organ removal V50.49
breast V50.41
ovary V50.42
repair of scarred tissue (following healed injury or operation) V51
specified type NEC V50.8
examination (*see also* Examination) V70.9
administrative purpose NEC V70.3

Admission—*continued*
adoption V70.3
allergy V72.7
at health care facility V70.0
athletic team V70.3
camp V70.3
cardiovascular, preoperative V72.81
clinical research investigation V70.7
dental V72.2
developmental testing (child) (infant) V20.2
donor (potential) V70.8
driver's license V70.3
ear V72.1
employment V70.5
eye V72.0
follow-up (routine)—*see* Examination, follow-up
for admission to
old age home V70.3
school V70.3
general V70.9
specified reason NEC V70.8
gynecological V72.3
health supervision (child) (infant) V20.2
hearing V72.1
immigration V70.3
insurance certification V70.3
laboratory V72.6
marriage license V70.3
medical (general) (*see also* Examination, medical) V70.9
medicolegal reasons V70.4
naturalization V70.3
pelvic (annual) (periodic) V72.3
postpartum checkup V24.2
pregnancy (possible) (unconfirmed) V72.4
preoperative V72.84
cardiovascular V72.81
respiratory V72.82
specified NEC V72.83
prison V70.3
psychiatric (general) V70.2
requested by authority V70.1
radiological NEC V72.5
respiratory, preoperative V72.82
school V70.3
screening—*see* Screening
skin hypersensitivity V72.7
specified type NEC V72.85
sport competition V70.3
vision V72.0
well baby and child care V20.2
exercise therapy V57.1
face-lift, cosmetic reason V50.1
fitting (of)
artificial
arm (complete) (partial) V52.0
eye V52.2
leg (complete) (partial) V52.1
brain neuropacemaker V53.0
breast V52.4
implant V50.1
prosthesis V52.4
cardiac pacemaker V53.31
catheter
non-vascular V58.82
vascular V58.81
colostomy belt V53.5
contact lenses V53.1
cystostomy device V53.6
dental prosthesis V52.3

Admission—*continued*
device NEC V53.9
abdominal V53.5
intrauterine contraceptive V25.1
nervous system V53.0
orthodontic V53.4
prosthetic V52.9
breast V52.4
dental V52.3
eye V52.2
special senses V53.0
substitution
auditory V53.0
nervous system V53.0
visual V53.0
diaphragm (contraceptive) V25.02
hearing aid V53.2
ileostomy device V53.5
intestinal appliance or device NEC V53.5
intrauterine contraceptive device V25.1
neuropacemaker (brain) (peripheral nerve) (spinal cord) V53.0
orthodontic device V53.4
orthopedic (device) V53.7
brace V53.7
cast V53.7
shoes V53.7
pacemaker
brain V53.0
cardiac V53.31
carotid sinus V53.39
spinal cord V53.0
prosthesis V52.9
arm (complete) (partial) V52.0
breast V52.4
dental V52.3
eye V52.2
leg (complete) (partial) V52.1
specified type NEC V52.8
spectacles V53.1
wheelchair V53.8
follow-up examination (routine) (following) V67.9
cancer chemotherapy V67.2
chemotherapy V67.2
high-risk medication NEC V67.51
injury NEC V67.59
psychiatric V67.3
psychotherapy V67.3
radiotherapy V67.1
surgery V67.0
treatment (for) V67.9
combined V67.6
fracture V67.4
involving high-risk medication NEC V67.51
mental disorder V67.3
specified NEC V67.59
hair transplant, for cosmetic reason V50.0
health advice, education, or instruction V65.4
insertion (of)
subdermal implantable contraceptive V25.5
intrauterine device
insertion V25.1
management V25.42
investigation to determine further disposition V63.8
isolation V07.0
issue of
medical certificate NEC V68.0
repeat prescription NEC V68.1

Admission—*continued*
contraceptive device NEC V25.49
kidney dialysis V56.0
mental health evaluation V70.2
requested by authority V70.1
nonmedical reason NEC V68.89
nursing care evaluation V63.8
observation (without need for further medical care) (*see also* Observation) V71.9
accident V71.4
alleged rape or seduction V71.5
criminal assault V71.6
following accident V71.4
at work V71.3
foreign body ingestion V71.8
growth and development variations, childhood V21.0
inflicted injury NEC V71.6
ingestion of deleterious agent or foreign body V71.8
injury V71.6
malignant neoplasm V71.1
mental disorder V71.09
newborn—*see* Observation, suspected condition, newborn
rape V71.5
specified NEC V71.8
suspected disorder V71.9
accident V71.4
at work V71.3
benign neoplasm V71.8
cardiovascular V71.7
heart V71.7
inflicted injury NEC V71.6
malignant neoplasm V71.1
mental NEC V71.09
specified condition NEC V71.8
tuberculosis V71.2
tuberculosis V71.2
occupational therapy V57.21
organ transplant, donor—*see* Donor
ovary, ovarian removal, prophylactic V50.42
Papanicolaou smear, cervix V76.2
for suspected malignant neoplasm V76.2
no disease found V71.1
routine, as part of gynecological examination V72.3
passage of sounds or bougie in artificial opening—*see* Attention to, artificial, opening
peritoneal dialysis V56.8
physical therapy NEC V57.1
plastic surgery
cosmetic NEC V50.1
following healed injury or operation V51
postmenopausal hormone replacement therapy V07.4
postpartum observation
immediately after delivery V24.0
routine follow-up V24.2
poststerilization (for restoration) V26.0
procreative management V26.9
specified type NEC V26.8
prophylactic
administration of
antibiotics V07.39
antitoxin, any V07.2
antivenin V07.2
chemotherapeutic agent NEC V07.39
chemotherapy NEC V07.39
diphtheria antitoxin V07.2

Admission—*continued*
fluoride V07.31
gamma globulin V07.2
immune sera (gamma globulin) V07.2
RhoGAM V07.2
tetanus antitoxin V07.2
breathing exercises V57.0
chemotherapy NEC V07.39
fluoride V07.31
measure V07.9
specified type NEC V07.8
organ removal V50.49
breast V50.41
ovary V50.42
psychiatric examination (general) V70.2
requested by authority V70.1
radiation management V58.0
radiotherapy V58.0
reforming of artificial opening—*see* Attention to, artificial, opening
rehabilitation V57.9
multiple types V57.89
occupational V57.21
orthoptic V57.4
orthotic V57.81
physical NEC V57.1
specified type NEC V57.89
speech V57.3
vocational V57.22
removal of
cardiac pacemaker V53.31
cast (plaster) V54.8
catheter from artificial opening—*see* Attention to, artificial, opening
cystostomy catheter V55.5
device
fixation
external V54.8
internal V54.0
intrauterine contraceptive V25.42
traction, external V54.8
dressing V58.3
fixation device
external V54.8
internal V54.0
intrauterine contraceptive device V25.42
Kirschner wire V54.8
neuropacemaker (brain) (peripheral nerve) (spinal cord) V53.0
orthopedic fixation device
external V54.8
internal V54.0
pacemaker device
brain V53.0
cardiac V53.31
carotid sinus V53.39
nervous system V53.0
plaster cast V54.8
plate (fracture) V54.0
rod V54.0
screw (fracture) V54.0
splint, traction V54.8
Steinmann pin V54.8
subdermal implantable contraceptive V25.43
surgical dressing V58.3
sutures V58.3
traction device, external V54.8
ureteral stent V53.6
repair of scarred tissue (following healed injury or operation) V51
reprogramming of cardiac pacemaker V53.3

Admission—*continued*
restoration of organ continuity (poststerilization) (tuboplasty) (vasoplasty) V26.0
sensitivity test—*see also* Test, skin
allergy NEC V72.7
bacterial disease NEC V74.9
Dick V74.8
Kveim V82.8
Mantoux V74.1
mycotic infection NEC V75.4
parasitic disease NEC V75.8
Schick V74.3
Schultz-Charlton V74.8
social service (agency) referral or evaluation V63.8
speech therapy V57.3
sterilization V25.2
suspected disorder (ruled out) (without need for further care)—*see* Observation
tests only—*see* Test
therapy
blood transfusion, without reported diagnosis V58.2
breathing exercises V57.0
chemotherapy V58.1
prophylactic NEC V07.39
fluoride V07.31
dialysis (intermittent) (treatment)
extracorporeal V56.0
peritoneal V56.8
renal V56.0
specified type NEC V56.8
exercise (remedial) NEC V57.1
breathing V57.0
occupational V57.21
orthoptic V57.4
physical NEC V57.1
radiation V58.0
speech V57.3
vocational V57.22
toilet or cleaning
of artificial opening — *see* Attention to, artificial, opening
of non-vascular catheter V58.82
of vascular catheter V58.81
tubal ligation V25.2
tuboplasty for previous sterilization V26.0
vaccination, prophylactic (against)
arthropod-borne virus, viral NEC V05.1
disease NEC V05.1
encephalitis V05.0
Bacille Calmette Guérin (BCG) V03.2
BCG V03.2
chickenpox V05.4
cholera alone V03.0
with typhoid-paratyphoid (cholera + TAB) V06.0
common cold V04.7
dengue V05.1
diphtheria alone V03.5
diphtheria-tetanus [Td] without pertussis V06.5
diphtheria-tetanus-pertussis (DTP) V06.1
with
poliomyelitis (DTP + polio) V06.3
typhoid-paratyphoid (DTP + TAB) V06.2
disease (single) NEC V05.9
bacterial NEC V03.9
specified type NEC V03.89

Admission—*continued*
combinations NEC V06.9
specified type NEC V06.8
specified type NEC V05.8
encephalitis, viral, arthropod-borne V05.0
Hemophilus influenzae, type B [Hib] V03.81
hepatitis, viral V05.3
immune sera (gamma globulin) V07.2
influenza V04.8
with
Streptococcus pneumoniae [pneumococcus] V06.6
Leishmaniasis V05.2
measles alone V04.2
measles-mumps-rubella (MMR) V06.4
mumps alone V04.6
with measles and rubella (MMR) V06.4
not done because of contraindication V64.0
pertussis alone V03.6
plague V03.3
poliomyelitis V04.0
with diphtheria-tetanus-pertussis (DTP + polio) V06.3
rabies V04.5
rubella alone V04.3
with measles and mumps (MMR) V06.4
smallpox V04.1
specified type NEC V05.8
Streptococcus pneumoniae [pneumococcus] V03.82
with
influenza V06.6
tetanus toxoid alone V03.7
with diphtheria [Td] V06.5
and pertussis (DTP) V06.1
tuberculosis (BCG) V03.2
tularemia V03.4
typhoid alone V03.1
with diphtheria-tetanus-pertussis (TAB + DTP) V06.2
typhoid-paratyphoid alone (TAB) V03.1
typhus V05.8
varicella V05.4
viral encephalitis, arthropod-borne V05.0
viral hepatitis V05.3
yellow fever V04.4
vasectomy V25.2
vasoplasty for previous sterilization V26.0
vision examination V72.0
vocational therapy V57.22
waiting period for admission to other facility V63.2
undergoing social agency investigation V63.8
well baby and child care V20.2
x-ray of chest
for suspected tuberculosis V71.2
routine V72.5
Adnexitis (suppurative) (*see also* Salpingo-oophoritis) 614.2
Adolescence NEC V21.2
Adoption
agency referral V68.89
examination V70.3
held for V68.89
Adrenal gland —*see* condition
Adrenalism 255.9
tuberculous (*see also* Tuberculosis) 017.6
Adrenalitis, adrenitis 255.8
meningococcal hemorrhagic 036.3
Adrenarche, precocious 259.1
Adrenocortical syndrome 255.2

Adrenogenital syndrome (acquired) (congenital) 255.2
iatrogenic, fetus or newborn 760.79
Adventitious bursa —*see* Bursitis
Adynamia (episodica) (hereditary) (periodic) 359.3
Adynamic ileus or intestine (*see also* Ileus) 560.1
Aeration lung imperfect, newborn 770.5
Aerobullosis 993.3
Aerocele —*see* Embolism, air
Aerodermectasia
subcutaneous (traumatic) 958.7
surgical 998.81
surgical 998.81
Aerodontalgia 993.2
Aeroembolism 993.3
Aerogenes capsulatus infection (*see also* Gangrene, gas) 040.0
Aero-otitis media 993.0
Aerophagy, aerophagia 306.4
psychogenic 306.4
Aerosinusitis 993.1
Aerotitis 993.0
Affection, affections —*see also* Disease
sacroiliac (joint), old 724.6
shoulder region NEC 726.2
Afibrinogenemia 286.3
acquired 286.6
congenital 286.3
postpartum 666.3
African
sleeping sickness 086.5
tick fever 087.1
trypanosomiasis 086.5
Gambian 086.3
Rhodesian 086.4
Aftercare V58.9
artificial openings—*see* Attention to, artificial, opening
blood transfusion without reported diagnosis V58.2
breathing exercise V57.0
cardiac device V53.39
defibrillator, automatic implantable V53.32
pacemaker V53.31
carotid sinus V53.39
carotid sinus pacemaker V53.39
chemotherapy session (adjunctive) (maintenance) V58.1
defibrillator, automatic implantable cardiac V53.32
exercise (remedial) (therapeutic) V57.1
breathing V57.0
extracorporeal dialysis (intermittent) (treatment) V56.0
following surgery NEC V58.49
wound closure, planned V58.41
fracture V54.9
removal of
external fixation device V54.8
internal fixation device V54.0
specified care NEC V54.8
gait training V57.1
for use of artificial limb(s) V57.81
involving
dialysis (intermittent) (treatment)
extracorporeal V56.0
peritoneal V56.8
renal V56.0
gait training V57.1
Aftercare—*continued*
for use of artificial limb(s) V57.81
orthoptic training V57.4
orthotic training V57.81
radiotherapy session V58.0
removal of
dressings V58.3
fixation device
external V54.8
internal V54.0
fracture plate V54.0
pins V54.0
plaster cast V54.8
rods V54.0
screws V54.0
surgical dressings V58.3
sutures V58.3
traction device, external V54.8
neuropacemaker (brain) (peripheral nerve) (spinal cord) V53.0
occupational therapy V57.21
orthodontic V58.5
orthopedic V54.9
change of external fixation or traction device V54.8
removal of fixation device
external V54.8
internal V54.0
specified care NEC V54.8
orthoptic training V57.4
orthotic training V57.81
pacemaker
brain V53.0
cardiac V53.31
carotid sinus V53.39
peripheral nerve V53.0
spinal cord V53.0
peritoneal dialysis (intermittent) (treatment) V56.8
physical therapy NEC V57.1
breathing exercises V57.0
radiotherapy session V58.0
rehabilitation procedure V57.9
breathing exercises V57.0
multiple types V57.89
occupational V57.21
orthoptic V57.4
orthotic V57.81
physical therapy NEC V57.1
remedial exercises V57.1
specified type NEC V57.89
speech V57.3
therapeutic exercises V57.1
vocational V57.22
renal dialysis (intermittent) (treatment) V56.0
specified type NEC V58.89
removal of vascular catheter V58.81
speech therapy V57.3
vocational rehabilitation V57.22
After-cataract 366.50
obscuring vision 366.53
specified type, not obscuring vision 366.52
Agalactia 676.4
Agammaglobulinemia 279.00
with lymphopenia 279.2
acquired (primary) (secondary) 279.06
Bruton's X-linked 279.04
infantile sex-linked (Bruton's) (congenital) 279.04
Swiss-type 279.2
Aganglionosis (bowel) (colon) 751.3
Age (old) (*see also* Senile) 797

Agenesis —*see also* Absence, by site, congenital
acoustic nerve 742.8
adrenal (gland) 759.1
alimentary tract (complete) (partial) NEC 751.8
lower 751.2
upper 750.8
anus, anal (canal) 751.2
aorta 747.22
appendix 751.2
arm (complete) (partial) (*see also* Deformity, reduction, upper limb) 755.20
artery (peripheral) NEC (*see also* Anomaly, peripheral vascular system) 747.60
brain 747.81
coronary 746.85
pulmonary 747.3
umbilical 747.5
auditory (canal) (external) 744.01
auricle (ear) 744.01
bile, biliary duct or passage 751.61
bone NEC 756.9
brain 740.0
specified part 742.2
breast 757.6
bronchus 748.3
canaliculus lacrimalis 743.65
carpus NEC (*see also* Deformity, reduction, upper limb) 755.28
cartilage 756.9
cecum 751.2
cerebellum 742.2
cervix 752.49
chin 744.89
cilia 743.63
circulatory system, part NEC 747.89
clavicle 755.51
clitoris 752.49
coccyx 756.13
colon 751.2
corpus callosum 742.2
cricoid cartilage 748.3
diaphragm (with hernia) 756.6
digestive organ(s) or tract (complete) (partial) NEC 751.8
lower 751.2
upper 750.8
ductus arteriosus 747.89
duodenum 751.1
ear NEC 744.09
auricle 744.01
lobe 744.21
ejaculatory duct 752.8
endocrine (gland) NEC 759.2
epiglottis 748.3
esophagus 750.3
Eustachian tube 744.24
extrinsic muscle, eye 743.69
eye 743.00
adnexa 743.69
eyelid (fold) 743.62
face
bones NEC 756.0
specified part NEC 744.89
fallopian tube 752.19
femur NEC (*see also* Absence, femur, congenital) 755.34
fibula NEC (*see also* Absence, fibula, congenital) 755.37
finger NEC (*see also* Absence, finger, congenital) 755.29
foot (complete) (*see also* Deformity, reduction, lower limb) 755.31

Agenesis—*continued*
gallbladder 751.69
gastric 750.8
genitalia, genital (organ)
female 752.8
external 752.49
internal NEC 752.8
male 752.8
glottis 748.3
gonadal 758.6
hair 757.4
hand (complete) (*see also* Deformity, reduction, upper limb) 755.21
heart 746.89
valve NEC 746.89
aortic 746.89
mitral 746.89
pulmonary 746.01
hepatic 751.69
humerus NEC (*see also* Absence, humerus, congenital) 755.24
hymen 752.49
ileum 751.1
incus 744.04
intestine (small) 751.1
large 751.2
iris (dilator fibers) 743.45
jaw 524.09
jejunum 751.1
kidney(s) (partial) (unilateral) 753.0
labium (majus) (minus) 752.49
labyrinth, membranous 744.05
lacrimal apparatus (congenital) 743.65
larynx 748.3
leg NEC (*see also* Deformity, reduction, lower limb) 755.30
lens 743.35
limb (complete) (partial) (*see also* Deformity, reduction) 755.4
lower NEC 755.30
upper 755.20
lip 750.26
liver 751.69
lung (bilateral) (fissures) (lobe) (unilateral) 748.5
mandible 524.09
maxilla 524.09
metacarpus NEC 755.28
metatarsus NEC 755.38
muscle (any) 756.81
musculoskeletal system NEC 756.9
nail(s) 757.5
neck, part 744.89
nerve 742.8
nervous system, part NEC 742.8
nipple 757.6
nose 748.1
nuclear 742.8
organ
of Corti 744.05
or site not listed—*see* Anomaly, specified type NEC
osseous meatus (ear) 744.03
ovary 752.0
oviduct 752.19
pancreas 751.7
parathyroid (gland) 759.2
patella 755.64
pelvic girdle (complete) (partial) 755.69
penis 752.8
pericardium 746.89
perineal body 756.81

Agenesis—*continued*
pituitary (gland) 759.2
prostate 752.8
pulmonary
artery 747.3
trunk 747.3
vein 747.49
punctum lacrimale 743.65
radioulnar NEC (*see also* Absence, forearm, congenital) 755.25
radius NEC (*see also* Absence, radius, congenital) 755.26
rectum 751.2
renal 753.0
respiratory organ NEC 748.9
rib 756.3
roof of orbit 742.0
round ligament 752.8
sacrum 756.13
salivary gland 750.21
scapula 755.59
scrotum 752.8
seminal duct or tract 752.8
septum
atrial 745.69
between aorta and pulmonary artery 745.0
ventricular 745.3
shoulder girdle (complete) (partial) 755.59
skull (bone) 756.0
with
anencephalus 740.0
encephalocele 742.0
hydrocephalus 742.3
with spina bifida (*see also* Spina bifida) 741.0
microcephalus 742.1
spermatic cord 752.8
spinal cord 742.59
spine 756.13
lumbar 756.13
isthmus 756.11
pars articularis 756.11
spleen 759.0
sternum 756.3
stomach 750.7
tarsus NEC 755.38
tendon 756.81
testicular 752.8
testis 752.8
thymus (gland) 759.2
thyroid (gland) 243
cartilage 748.3
tibia NEC (*see also* Absence, tibia, congenital) 755.36
tibiofibular NEC 755.35
toe (complete) (partial) (*see also* Absence, toe, congenital) 755.39
tongue 750.11
trachea (cartilage) 748.3
ulna NEC (*see also* Absence, ulna, congenital) 755.27
ureter 753.4
urethra 753.8
urinary tract NEC 753.8
uterus 752.3
uvula 750.26
vagina 752.49
vas deferens 752.8
vein(s) (peripheral) NEC (*see also* Anomaly, peripheral vascular system) 747.60
brain 747.81
great 747.49

Agenesis—*continued*
portal 747.49
pulmonary 747.49
vena cava (inferior) (superior) 747.49
vermis of cerebellum 742.2
vertebra 756.13
lumbar 756.13
isthmus 756.11
pars articularis 756.11
vulva 752.49
Ageusia (*see also* Disturbance, sensation) 781.1
Aggressiveness 301.3
Aggressive outburst (*see also* Disturbance, conduct) 312.0
in children and adolescents 313.9
Aging skin 701.8
Agitated —*see* condition
Agitation 307.9
catatonic (*see also* Schizophrenia) 295.2
Aglossia (congenital) 750.11
Aglycogenosis 271.0
Agnail (finger) (with lymphangitis) 681.02
Agnosia (body image) (tactile) 784.69
verbal 784.69
auditory 784.69
secondary to organic lesion 784.69
developmental 315.8
secondary to organic lesion 784.69
visual 784.69
developmental 315.8
secondary to organic lesion 784.69
visual 368.16
developmental 315.31
Agoraphobia 300.22
with panic attacks 300.21
Agrammatism 784.69
Agranulocytopenia 288.0
Agranulocytosis (angina) (chronic) (cyclical) (genetic) (infantile) (periodic) (pernicious) 288.0
Agraphia (absolute) 784.69
with alexia 784.61
developmental 315.39
Agrypnia (*see also* Insomnia) 780.52
Ague (*see also* Malaria) 084.6
brass-founders' 985.8
dumb 084.6
tertian 084.1
Agyria 742.2
Ahumada-del Castillo syndrome (nonpuerperal galactorrhea and amenorrhea) 253.1
AIDS 042
AIDS-associated retrovirus (disease) (illness) 042
infection—*see* Human immunodeficiency virus, infection
AIDS-associated virus (disease) (illness) 042
infection—*see* Human immunodeficiency virus, infection
AIDS-like disease (illness) (syndrome) 042
AIDS-related complex 042
AIDS-related conditions 042
AIDS-related virus (disease) (illness) 042
infection—*see* Human immunodeficiency virus, infection
AIDS virus (disease) (illness) 042
infection—*see* Human immunodeficiency virus, infection
Ailment, heart —*see* Disease, heart
Ailurophobia 300.29
Ainhum (disease) 136.0

Air
anterior mediastinum 518.1
compressed, disease 993.3
embolism (any site) (artery) (cerebral) 958.0
with
abortion—*see* Abortion, by type, with embolism
ectopic pregnancy (*see also* categories 633.0-633.9) 639.6
molar pregnancy (*see also* categories 630-632) 639.6
due to implanted device—*see* Complications, due to (presence of) any device, implant, or graft classified to 996.0-996.5 NEC
following
abortion 639.6
ectopic or molar pregnancy 639.6
infusion, perfusion, or transfusion 999.1
in pregnancy, childbirth, or puerperium 673.0
traumatic 958.0
hunger 786.09
psychogenic 306.1
leak (lung) (pulmonary) (thorax) 512.8
iatrogenic 512.1
postoperative 512.1
rarefied, effects of—*see* Effect, adverse, high altitude
sickness 994.6
Airplane sickness 994.6
Akathisia, acathisia 781.0
due to drugs 333.99
Akinesia algeria 352.6
Akiyami 100.89
Akureyri disease (epidemic neuromyasthenia) 049.8
Alacrima (congenital) 743.65
Alactasia (hereditary) 271.3
Alalia 784.3
developmental 315.31
secondary to organic lesion 784.3
Alaninemia 270.8
Alastrim 050.1
Albarrán's disease (colibacilluria) 599.0
Albers-Schönberg's disease (marble bones) 756.52
Albert's disease 726.71
Albinism, albino (choroid) (cutaneous) (eye) (generalized) (isolated) (ocular) (oculocutaneous) (partial) 270.2
Albinismus 270.2
Albright (-Martin) (-Bantam) disease (pseudohypoparathyroidism) 275.4
Albright (-McCune) (-Sternberg) syndrome (osteitis fibrosa disseminata) 756.59
Albuminous —*see* condition
Albuminuria, albuminuric (acute) (chronic) (subacute) 791.0
Bence-Jones 791.0
cardiac 785.9
complicating pregnancy, childbirth, or puerperium 646.2
with hypertension—*see* Toxemia, of pregnancy
affecting fetus or newborn 760.1
cyclic 593.6
gestational 646.2
gravidarum 646.2
with hypertension—*see* Toxemia, of pregnancy
affecting fetus or newborn 760.1
heart 785.9
Albuminuria, albuminuric—*continued*
idiopathic 593.6
orthostatic 593.6
postural 593.6
pre-eclamptic (mild) 642.4
affecting fetus or newborn 760.0
severe 642.5
affecting fetus or newborn 760.0
recurrent physiologic 593.6
scarlatinal 034.1
Albumosuria 791.0
Bence-Jones 791.0
myelopathic (M9730/3) 203.0
Alcaptonuria 270.2
Alcohol, alcoholic
acute intoxication 305.0
with dependence 303.0
addiction (*see also* Alcoholism) 303.9
maternal
with suspected fetal damage affecting management of pregnancy 655.4
affecting fetus or newborn 760.71
amnestic disorder, persisting 291.1
anxiety 291.8
brain syndrome, chronic 291.2
cardiopathy 425.5
chronic (*see also* Alcoholism) 303.9
cirrhosis (liver) 571.2
delirium 291.0
acute 291.0
chronic 291.1
tremens 291.0
withdrawal 291.0
dementia NEC 291.2
deterioration 291.2
drunkenness (simple) 305.0
hallucinosis (acute) 291.3
insanity 291.9
intoxication (acute) 305.0
with dependence 303.0
pathological 291.4
jealousy 291.5
Korsakoff's, Korsakov's, Korsakow's 291.1
liver NEC 571.3
acute 571.1
chronic 571.2
mania (acute) (chronic) 291.9
mood 291.8
paranoia 291.5
paranoid (type) psychosis 291.5
pellagra 265.2
poisoning, accidental (acute) NEC 980.9
specified type of alcohol—*see* Table of drugs and chemicals
psychosis (*see also* Psychosis, alcoholic) 291.9
Korsakoff's, Korsakov's, Korsakow's 291.1
polyneuritic 291.1
with
delusions 291.5
hallucinations 291.3
withdrawal symptoms, syndrome NEC 291.8
delirium 291.0
hallucinosis 291.3

Alcoholism 303.9

> Note—Use the following fifth-digit subclassification with category 303:
>
> *0 unspecified*
> *1 continuous*
> *2 episodic*
> *3 in remission*

with psychosis (*see also* Psychosis, alcoholic) 291.9
acute 303.0
chronic 303.9
with psychosis 291.9
complicating pregnancy, childbirth, or puerperium 648.4
affecting fetus or newborn 760.71
history V11.3
Korsakoff's, Korsakov's, Korsakow's 291.1
suspected damage to fetus affecting management of pregnancy 655.4
Alder's anomaly or syndrome (leukocyte granulation anomaly) 288.2
Alder-Reilly anomaly (leukocyte granulation) 288.2
Aldosteronism (primary) (secondary) 255.1
congenital 255.1
Aldosteronoma (M8370/1) 237.2
Aldrich (-Wiskott) syndrome (eczema-thrombocytopenia) 279.12
Aleppo boil 085.1
Aleukemic —*see* condition
Aleukia
congenital 288.0
hemorrhagica 284.9
acquired (secondary) 284.8
congenital 284.0
idiopathic 284.9
splenica 289.4
Alexia (congenital) (developmental) 315.01
secondary to organic lesion 784.61
Algoneurodystrophy 733.7
Algophobia 300.29
Alibert's disease (mycosis fungoides) (M9700/3) 202.1
Alibert-Bazin disease (M9700/3) 202.1
Alice in Wonderland syndrome 293.89
Alienation, mental (*see also* Psychosis) 298.9
Alkalemia 276.3
Alkalosis 276.3
metabolic 276.3
with respiratory acidosis 276.4
respiratory 276.3
Alkaptonuria 270.2
Allen-Masters syndrome 620.6
Allergy, allergic (reaction) 995.3
air-borne substance (*see also* Fever, hay) 477.9
specified allergen NEC 477.8
alveolitis (extrinsic) 495.9
due to
Aspergillus clavatus 495.4
cryptostroma corticale 495.6
organisms (fungal, thermophilic actinomycete, other) growing in ventilation (air conditioning systems) 495.7
specified type NEC 495.8
anaphylactic shock 999.4
due to
food—*see* Anaphylactic shock, due to, food

Allergy, allergic—*continued*
angioneurotic edema 995.1
animal (dander) (epidermal) (hair) 477.8
arthritis (*see also* Arthritis, allergic) 716.2
asthma—*see* Asthma
bee sting (anaphylactic shock) 989.5
biological—*see* Allergy, drug
bronchial asthma—*see* Asthma
conjunctivitis (eczematous) 372.14
dander (animal) 477.8
dandruff 477.8
dermatitis (venenata)—*see* Dermatitis
diathesis V15.0
drug, medicinal substance, and biological (any) (correct medicinal substance properly administered) (external) (internal) 995.2
wrong substance given or taken NEC 977.9
specified drug or substance—*see* Table of drugs and chemicals
dust (house) (stock) 477.8
eczema—*see* Eczema
endophthalmitis 360.19
epidermal (animal) 477.8
feathers 477.8
food (any) (ingested) 693.1
atopic 691.8
in contact with skin 692.5
gastritis 535.4
gastroenteritis 558.9
gastrointestinal 558.9
grain 477.0
grass (pollen) 477.0
asthma (*see also* Asthma) 493.0
hay fever 477.0
hair (animal) 477.8
hay fever (grass) (pollen) (ragweed) (tree) (*see also* Fever, hay) 477.9
history (of) V15.0
horse serum—*see* Allergy, serum
inhalant 477.9
dust 477.8
pollen 477.0
specified allergen other than pollen 477.8
kapok 477.8
medicine—*see* Allergy, drug
migraine 346.2
pannus 370.62
pneumonia 518.3
pollen (any) (hay fever) 477.0
asthma (*see also* Asthma) 493.0
primrose 477.0
primula 477.0
purpura 287.0
ragweed (pollen) (Senecio jacobae) 477.0
asthma (*see also* Asthma) 493.0
hay fever 477.0
respiratory (*see also* Allergy, inhalant) 477.9
due to
drug—*see* Allergy, drug
food—*see* Allergy, food
rhinitis (*see also* Fever, hay) 477.9
rose 477.0
Senecio jacobae 477.0
serum (prophylactic) (therapeutic) 999.5
anaphylactic shock 999.4
shock (anaphylactic)
due to
adverse effect of correct medicinal substance properly administered 995.0
food—*see* Anaphylactic shock, due to, food

Allergy, allergic—*continued*
from serum or immunization 999.5
anaphylactic 999.4
sinusitis (*see also* Fever, hay) 477.9
skin reaction 692.9
specified substance—*see* Dermatitis, due to
tree (any) (hay fever) (pollen) 477.0
asthma (*see also* Asthma) 493.0
upper respiratory (*see also* Fever, hay) 477.9
urethritis 597.89
urticaria 708.0
vaccine—*see* Allergy, serum
Allescheriosis 117.6
Alligator skin disease (ichthyosis congenita) 757.1
acquired 701.1
Allocheiria, allochiria (*see also* Disturbance, sensation) 782.0
Almeida's disease (Brazilian blastomycosis) 116.1
Alopecia (atrophicans) (pregnancy) (premature) (senile) 704.00
adnata 757.4
areata 704.01
celsi 704.01
cicatrisata 704.09
circumscripta 704.01
congenital, congenitalis 757.4
disseminata 704.01
effluvium (telogen) 704.02
febrile 704.09
generalisata 704.09
hereditaria 704.09
marginalis 704.01
mucinosa 704.09
postinfectional 704.09
seborrheica 704.09
specific 091.82
syphilitic (secondary) 091.82
telogen effluvium 704.02
totalis 704.09
toxica 704.09
universalis 704.09
x-ray 704.09
Alper's disease 330.8
Alpha-lipoproteinemia 272.4
Alpha thalassemia 282.4
Alphos 696.1
Alpine sickness 993.2
Alport's syndrome (hereditary hematuria-nephropathy-deafness) 759.89
Alteration (of) altered
awareness 780.09
transient 780.02
consciousness 780.09
persistent vegetative state 780.03
transient 780.02
mental status 780.9
Alternaria (infection) 118
Alternating —*see* condition
Altitude, high (effects)—*see* Effect, adverse, high altitude
Aluminosis (of lung) 503
Alvarez syndrome (transient cerebral ischemia) 435.9
Alveolar capillary block syndrome 516.3
Alveolitis
allergic (extrinsic) 495.9

Alveolitis—*continued*
due to organisms (fungal, thermophilic actinomycete, other) growing in ventilation (air conditioning systems) 495.7
specified type NEC 495.8
due to
Aspergillus clavatus 495.4
Cryptostroma corticale 495.6
fibrosing (chronic) (cryptogenic) (lung) 516.3
idiopathic 516.3
rheumatoid 714.81
jaw 526.5
sicca dolorosa 526.5
Alveolus, alveolar —*see* condition
Alymphocytosis (pure) 279.2
Alymphoplasia, thymic 279.2
Alzheimer's
dementia (senile) 290.0
with
delirium 290.3
delusional features 290.20
depressive features 290.21
disease or sclerosis 331.0
with dementia—*see* Alzheimer's, demential
presenile 290.10
with
delirium 290.11
delusional features 290.12
depressive features 290.13
Amastia (*see also* Absence, breast) 611.8
Amaurosis (acquired) (congenital) (*see also* Blindness) 369.00
fugax 362.34
hysterical 300.11
Leber's (congenital) 362.76
tobacco 377.34
uremic—*see* Uremia
Amaurotic familial idiocy (infantile) (juvenile) (late) 330.1
Ambisexual 752.7
Amblyopia (acquired) (congenital) (partial) 368.00
color 368.59
acquired 368.55
deprivation 368.02
ex anopsia 368.00
hysterical 300.11
nocturnal 368.60
vitamin A deficiency 264.5
refractive 368.03
strabismic 368.01
suppression 368.01
tobacco 377.34
toxic NEC 377.34
uremic—*see* Uremia
Ameba, amebic (histolytica)-*see also* Amebiasis
abscess 006.3
bladder 006.8
brain (with liver and lung abscess) 006.5
liver 006.3
with
brain abscess (and lung abscess) 006.5
lung abscess 006.4
lung (with liver abscess) 006.4
with brain abscess 006.5
seminal vesicle 006.8
spleen 006.8
carrier (suspected of) V02.2
meningoencephalitis
due to Naegleria (gruberi) 136.2
primary 136.2

Amebiasis NEC 006.9
with
brain abscess (with liver or lung abscess) 006.5
liver abscess (without mention of brain or lung abscess) 006.3
lung abscess (with liver abscess) 006.4
with brain abscess 006.5
acute 006.0
bladder 006.8
chronic 006.1
cutaneous 006.6
cutis 006.6
due to organism other than Entamoeba histolytica 007.8
hepatic (*see also* Abscess, liver, amebic) 006.3
nondysenteric 006.2
seminal vesicle 006.8
specified
organism NEC 007.8
site NEC 006.8
Ameboma 006.8
Amelia 755.4
lower limb 755.31
upper limb 755.21
Ameloblastoma (M9310/0) 213.1
jaw (bone) (lower) 213.1
upper 213.0
long bones (M9261/3)—*see* Neoplasm, bone, malignant
malignant (M9310/3) 170.1
jaw (bone) (lower) 170.1
upper 170.0
mandible 213.1
tibial (M9261/3) 170.7
Amelogenesis imperfecta 520.5
nonhereditaria (segmentalis) 520.4
Amenorrhea (primary) (secondary) 626.0
due to ovarian dysfunction 256.8
hyperhormonal 256.8
Amentia (*see also* Retardation, mental) 319
Meynert's (nonalcoholic) 294.0
alcoholic 291.1
nevoid 759.6
American
leishmaniasis 085.5
mountain tick fever 066.1
trypanosomiasis—*see* Trypanosomiasis, American
Ametropia (*see also* Disorder, accommodation) 367.9
Amianthosis 501
Amimia 784.69
Amino acid
deficiency 270.9
anemia 281.4
metabolic disorder (*see also* Disorder, amino acid) 270.9
Aminoaciduria 270.9
imidazole 270.5
Amnesia (retrograde) 780.9
auditory 784.69
developmental 315.31
secondary to organic lesion 784.69
hysterical or dissociative type 300.12
psychogenic 300.12
transient global 437.7
Amnestic (confabulatory) syndrome 294.0
alcohol-induced 291.1
drug-induced 292.83
posttraumatic 294.0
Amniocentesis screening (for) V28.2
alpha-fetoprotein level, raised V28.1
chromosomal anomalies V28.0
Amnion, amniotic —*see also* condition
nodosum 658.8
Amnionitis (complicating pregnancy) 658.4
affecting fetus or newborn 762.7
Amoral trends 301.7
Amotio retinae (*see also* Detachment, retina) 361.9
Ampulla
lower esophagus 530.89
phrenic 530.89
Amputation
any part of fetus, to facilitate delivery 763.8
cervix (supravaginal) (uteri) 622.8
in pregnancy or childbirth 654.6
affecting fetus or newborn 763.8
clitoris—*see* Wound, open, clitoris
congenital
lower limb 755.31
upper limb 755.21
neuroma (traumatic)—*see also* Injury, nerve, by site
surgical complications (late) 997.61
penis—*see* Amputation, traumatic, penis
status (without complication)—*see* Absence, by site, acquired
stump (surgical)
abnormal, painful, or with complication (late) 997.60
healed or old NEC —*see also* Absence, by site, acquired
lower V49.70
upper V49.60
traumatic (complete) (partial)

> Note—"Complicated" includes traumatic amputation with delayed healing, delayed treatment, foreign body, or major infection.

arm 887.4
at or above elbow 887.2
complicated 887.3
below elbow 887.0
complicated 887.1
both (bilateral) (any level(s)) 887.6
complicated 887.7
complicated 887.5
finger(s) (one or both hands) 886.0
with thumb(s) 885.0
complicated 885.1
complicated 886.1
foot (except toe(s) only) 896.0
and other leg 897.6
complicated 897.7
both (bilateral) 896.2
complicated 896.3
complicated 896.1
toe(s) only (one or both feet) 895.0
complicated 895.1
genital organ(s) (external) NEC 878.8
complicated 878.9
hand (except finger(s) only) 887.0
and other arm 887.6
complicated 887.7
both (bilateral) 887.6
complicated 887.7
complicated 887.1

Amputation—*continued*
finger(s) (one or both hands) 886.0
with thumb(s) 885.0
complicated 885.1
complicated 886.1
thumb(s) (with fingers of either hand) 885.0
complicated 885.1
head 874.9
late effect—*see* Late, effects (of), amputation
leg 897.4
and other foot 897.6
complicated 897.7
at or above knee 897.2
complicated 897.3
below knee 897.0
complicated 897.1
both (bilateral) 897.6
complicated 897.7
complicated 897.5
lower limb(s) except toe(s)—*see* Amputation, traumatic, leg
nose—*see* Wound, open, nose
penis 878.0
complicated 878.1
sites other than limbs—*see* Wound, open, by site
thumb(s) (with finger(s) of either hand) 885.0
complicated 885.1
toe(s) (one or both feet) 895.0
complicated 895.1
upper limb(s)—*see* Amputation, traumatic, arm
Amputee (bilateral) (old) —*see* Absence, by site, acquired
Amusia 784.69
developmental 315.39
secondary to organic lesion 784.69
Amyelencephalus 740.0
Amyelia 742.59
Amygdalitis— *see* Tonsillitis
Amygdalolith 474.8
Amyloid disease or degeneration 277.3
heart 277.3 *[425.7]*
Amyloidosis (familial) (general) (generalized) (genetic) (primary) (secondary) 277.3
with lung involvement 277.3 *[517.8]*
heart 277.3 *[425.7]*
nephropathic 277.3 *[583.81]*
neuropathic (Portuguese) (Swiss) 277.3 *[357.4]*
pulmonary 277.3 *[517.8]*
systemic, inherited 277.3
Amylopectinosis (brancher enzyme deficiency) 271.0
Amylophagia 307.52
Amyoplasia, congenita 756.89
Amyotonia 728.2
congenita 358.8
Amyotrophia, amyotrophy, amyotrophic 728.2
congenita 756.89
diabetic 250.6 *[358.1]*
lateral sclerosis (syndrome) 335.20
neuralgic 353.5
sclerosis (lateral) 335.20
spinal progressive 335.21
Anacidity
gastric 536.0
psychogenic 306.4
Anaerosis of newborn 770.8
Analbuminemia 273.8
Analgesia (*see also* Anesthesia) 782.0
Analphalipoproteinemia 272.5
Anaphylactic shock or reaction (correct substance properly administered) 995.0
due to
food 995.60
additives 995.66
crustaceans 995.62
eggs 995.68
fish 995.65
fruits 995.63
milk products 995.67
nuts (tree) 995.64
peanuts 995.61
seeds 995.64
specified NEC 995.69
tree nuts 995.64
vegetables 995.63
immunization 999.4
overdose or wrong substance given or taken 977.9
specified drug—*see* Table of drugs and chemicals
serum 999.4
following sting(s) 989.5
purpura 287.0
serum 999.4
Anaphylactoid shock or reaction —*see* Anaphylactic shock
Anaphylaxis —*see* Anaphylactic shock
Anaplasia, cervix 622.1
Anarthria 784.5
Anarthritic rheumatoid disease 446.5
Anasarca 782.3
cardiac (*see also* Failure, heart, congestive) 428.0
fetus or newborn 778.0
lung 514
nutritional 262
pulmonary 514
renal (*see also* Nephrosis) 581.9
Anaspadias 752.6
Anastomosis
aneurysmal—*see* Aneurysm
arteriovenous, congenital NEC (*see also* Anomaly, arteriovenous) 747.60
ruptured, of brain (*see also* Hemorrhage, subarachnoid) 430
intestinal 569.89
complicated NEC 997.4
involving urinary tract 997.5
retinal and choroidal vessels 743.58
acquired 362.17
Anatomical narrow angle (glaucoma) 365.02
Ancylostoma (infection) (infestation) 126.9
americanus 126.1
braziliense 126.2
caninum 126.8
ceylanicum 126.3
duodenale 126.0
Necator americanus 126.1
Ancylostomiasis (intestinal) 126.9
Ancylostoma
americanus 126.1
caninum 126.8
ceylanicum 126.3
duodenale 126.0
braziliense 126.2
Necator americanus 126.1
Anders' disease or syndrome (adiposis tuberosa simplex) 272.8
Andersen's glycogen storage disease 271.0
Anderson's disease 272.7
Andes disease 993.2

Andrews' disease (bacterid) 686.8
Androblastoma (M8630/1)
benign (M8630/0)
specified site—*see* Neoplasm, by site, benign
unspecified site
female 220
male 222.0
malignant (M8630/3)
specified site—*see* Neoplasm, by site, malignant
unspecified site
female 183.0
male 186.9
specified site—*see* Neoplasm, by site, uncertain behavior
tubular (M8640/0)
with lipid storage (M8641/0)
specified site—*see* Neoplasm, by site, benign
unspecified site
female 220
male 222.0
specified site—*see* Neoplasm, by site, benign
unspecified site
female 220
male 222.0
unspecified site
female 236.2
male 236.4
Android pelvis 755.69
with disproportion (fetopelvic) 653.3
affecting fetus or newborn 763.1
causing obstructed labor 660.1
affecting fetus or newborn 763.1
Anectasis, pulmonary (newborn or fetus) 770.5
Anemia 285.9
with
disorder of
anaerobic glycolysis 282.3
pentose phosphate pathway 282.2
koilonychia 280.9
6-phosphogluconic dehydrogenase deficiency 282.2
achlorhydric 280.9
achrestic 281.8
Addison's (pernicious) 281.0
Addison-Biermer (pernicious) 281.0
agranulocytic 288.0
amino acid deficiency 281.4
aplastic 284.9
acquired (secondary) 284.8
congenital 284.0
constitutional 284.0
due to
chronic systemic disease 284.8
drugs 284.8
infection 284.8
radiation 284.8
idiopathic 284.9
myxedema 244.9
of or complicating pregnancy 648.2
red cell (acquired) (adult) (pure) (with thymoma) 284.8
congenital 284.0
specified type NEC 284.8
toxic (paralytic) 284.8
aregenerative 284.9
congenital 284.0
asiderotic 280.9
atypical (primary) 285.9

Anemia—*continued*
autohemolysis of Selwyn and Dacie (type I) 282.2
autoimmune hemolytic 283.0
Baghdad Spring 282.2
Balantidium coli 007.0
Biermer's (pernicious) 281.0
blood loss (chronic) 280.0
acute 285.1
bothriocephalus 123.4
brickmakers' (*see also* Ancylostomiasis) 126.9
cerebral 437.8
childhood 285.9
chlorotic 280.9
chronica congenita aregenerativa 284.0
chronic simple 281.9
combined system disease NEC 281.0 *[336.2]*
due to dietary deficiency 281.1 *[336.2]*
complicating pregnancy or childbirth 648.2
congenital (following fetal blood loss) 776.5
aplastic 284.0
due to isoimmunization NEC 773.2
Heinz-body 282.7
hereditary hemolytic NEC 282.9
nonspherocytic
Type I 282.2
Type II 282.3
pernicious 281.0
spherocytic (*see also* Spherocytosis) 282.0
Cooley's (erythroblastic) 282.4
crescent—*see* Disease, sickle-cell
cytogenic 281.0
Dacie's (nonspherocytic)
Type I 282.2
Type II 282.3
Davidson's (refractory) 284.9
deficiency 281.9
2, 3 diphosphoglycurate mutase 282.3
2, 3 PG 282.3
6-PGD 282.2
6-phosphogluronic dehydrogenase 282.2
amino acid 281.4
combined B_{12} and folate 281.3
enzyme, drug-induced (hemolytic) 282.2
erythrocytic glutathione 282.2
folate 281.2
dietary 281.2
drug-induced 281.2
folic acid 281.2
dietary 281.2
drug-induced 281.2
G-6-PD 282.2
GGS-R 282.2
glucose-6-phosphate dehydrogenase (G-6-PD) 282.2
glucose-phosphate isomerase 282.3
glutathione peroxidase 282.2
glutathione reductase 282.2
glyceraldehyde phosphate dehydrogenase 282.3
GPI 282.3
G SH 282.2
hexokinase 282.3
iron (Fe) 280.9
specified NEC 280.8
nutritional 281.9
with
poor iron absorption 280.9
specified deficiency NEC 281.8
due to inadequate dietary iron intake 280.1
specified type NEC 281.8

Anemia—*continued*
profound 285.9
progressive 285.9
malignant 281.0
pernicious 281.0
protein-deficiency 281.4
pseudoleukemica infantum 285.8
puerperal 648.2
pure red cell 284.8
congenital 284.0
pyridoxine-responsive (hypochromic) 285.0
pyruvate kinase (PK) deficiency 282.3
refractoria sideroblastica 285.0
refractory (primary) 284.9
with hemochromatosis 285.0
megaloblastic 281.3
sideroblastic 285.0
sideropenic 280.9
Rietti-Greppi-Micheli (thalassemia minor) 282.4
scorbutic 281.8
secondary (to) 285.9
blood loss (chronic) 280.0
acute 285.1
hemorrhage 280.0
acute 285.1
inadequate dietary iron intake 280.1
semiplastic 284.9
septic 285.9
sickle-cell (*see also* Disease, sickle-cell) 282.60
sideroachrestic 285.0
sideroblastic (acquired) (any type) (congenital) (drug-induced) (due to disease) (hereditary) (primary) (refractory) (secondary) (sex-linked hypochromic) (vitamin B_6 responsive) 285.0
sideropenic (refractory) 280.9
due to blood loss (chronic) 280.0
acute 285.1
simple chronic 281.9
specified type NEC 285.8
spherocytic (hereditary) (*see also* Spherocytosis) 282.0
splenic 285.8
familial (Gaucher's) 272.7
splenomegalic 285.8
stomatocytosis 282.8
syphilitic 095.8
target cell (oval) 282.4
thalassemia 282.4
thrombocytopenic (*see also* Thrombocytopenia) 287.5
toxic 284.8
triosephosphate isomerase deficiency 282.3
tropical, macrocytic 281.2
tuberculous (*see also* Tuberculosis) 017.9
vegan's 281.1
vitamin
B_6-responsive 285.0
B_{12} deficiency (dietary) 281.1
pernicious 281.0
von Jaksch's (pseudoleukemia infantum) 285.8
Witts' (achlorhydric anemia) 280.9
Zuelzer (-Ogden) (nutritional megaloblastic anemia) 281.2
Anencephalus, anencephaly 740.0
fetal, affecting management of pregnancy 655.0
Anergasia (*see also* Psychosis, organic) 294.9
senile 290.0
Anesthesia, anesthetic 782.0
complication or reaction NEC 995.2
due to
correct substance properly administered 995.2
overdose or wrong substance given 968.4
specified anesthetic—*see* Table of drugs and chemicals
cornea 371.81
death from
correct substance properly administered 995.4
during delivery 668.9
overdose or wrong substance given 968.4
specified anesthetic—*see* Table of drugs and chemicals
eye 371.81
functional 300.11
hyperesthetic, thalamic 348.8
hysterical 300.11
local skin lesion 782.0
olfactory 781.1
sexual (psychogenic) 302.72
shock
due to
correct substance properly administered 995.4
overdose or wrong substance given 968.4
specified anesthetic—*see* Table of drugs and chemicals
skin 782.0
tactile 782.0
testicular 608.9
thermal 782.0
Anetoderma (maculosum) 701.3
Aneuploidy NEC 758.5
Aneurin deficiency 265.1
Aneurysm (anastomotic) (artery) (cirsoid) (diffuse) (false) (fusiform) (multiple) (ruptured) (saccular) (varicose) 442.9
abdominal (aorta) 441.4
ruptured 441.3
syphilitic 093.0
aorta, aortic (nonsyphilitic) 441.9
abdominal 441.4
dissecting 441.02
ruptured 441.3
syphilitic 093.0
arch 441.2
ruptured 441.1
arteriosclerotic NEC 441.9
ruptured 441.5
ascending 441.2
ruptured 441.1
congenital 747.29
descending 441.9
abdominal 441.4
ruptured 441.3
ruptured 441.5
thoracic 441.2
ruptured 441.1
dissecting 441.00
abdominal 441.02
thoracic 441.01
thoracoabdominal 441.03
due to coarctation (aorta) 747.10
ruptured 441.5
sinus, right 747.29
syphilitic 093.0
thoracoabdominal 441.7
ruptured 441.6

Aneurysm—*continued*
thorax, thoracic (arch) (nonsyphilitic) 441.2
dissecting 441.01
ruptured 441.1
syphilitic 093.0
transverse 441.2
ruptured 441.1
valve (heart) (*see also* Endocarditis, aortic) 424.1
arteriosclerotic NEC 442.9
cerebral 437.3
ruptured (*see also* Hemorrhage, subarachnoid) 430
arteriovenous (congenital) (peripheral) NEC (*see also* Anomaly, arteriovenous) 747.60
acquired NEC 447.0
brain 437.3
ruptured (*see also* Hemorrhage, subarachnoid) 430
coronary 414.11
pulmonary 417.0
brain (cerebral) 747.81
ruptured (*see also* Hemorrhage, subarachnoid) 430
coronary 746.85
pulmonary 747.3
retina 743.58
specified site NEC 747.89
acquired 447.0
traumatic (*see also* Injury, blood vessel, by site) 904.9
basal—*see* Aneurysm, brain
berry (congenital) (ruptured) (*see also* Hemorrhage, subarachnoid) 430
brain 437.3
arteriosclerotic 437.3
ruptured (*see also* Hemorrhage, subarachnoid) 430
arteriovenous 747.81
acquired 437.3
ruptured (*see also* Hemorrhage, subarachnoid) 430
ruptured (*see also* Hemorrhage, subarachnoid) 430
berry (congenital) (ruptured) (*see also* Hemorrhage, subarachnoid) 430
congenital 747.81
ruptured (*see also* Hemorrhage, subarachnoid) 430
meninges 437.3
ruptured (*see also* Hemorrhage, subarachnoid) 430
miliary (congenital) (ruptured) (*see also* Hemorrhage, subarachnoid) 430
mycotic 421.0
ruptured (*see also* Hemorrhage, subarachnoid) 430
nonruptured 437.3
ruptured (*see also* Hemorrhage, subarachnoid) 430
syphilitic 094.87
syphilitic (hemorrhage) 094.87
traumatic—*see* Injury, intracranial
cardiac (false) (*see also* Aneurysm, heart) 414.10
carotid artery (common) (external) 442.81
internal 442.81
ruptured into brain (*see also* Hemorrhage, subarachnoid) 430
syphilitic 093.89
intracranial 094.87

Aneurysm—*continued*
cavernous sinus (*see also* Aneurysm, brain) 437.3
arteriovenous 747.81
ruptured (*see also* Hemorrhage, subarachnoid) 430
congenital 747.81
ruptured (*see also* Hemorrhage, subarachnoid) 430
celiac 442.84
central nervous system, syphilitic 094.89
cerebral—*see* Aneurysm, brain
chest—*see* Aneurysm, thorax
circle of Willis (*see also* Aneurysm, brain) 437.3
congenital 747.81
ruptured (*see also* Hemorrhage, subarachnoid) 430
ruptured (*see also* Hemorrhage, subarachnoid) 430
common iliac artery 442.2
congenital (peripheral) NEC 747.60
brain 747.81
ruptured (*see also* Hemorrhage, subarachnoid) 430
cerebral—*see* Aneurysm, brain, congenital
coronary 746.85
gastrointestinal 747.61
lower limb 747.64
pulmonary 747.3
renal 747.62
retina 743.58
specified site NEC 747.89
spinal 747.82
upper limb 747.63
conjunctiva 372.74
conus arteriosus (*see also* Aneurysm, heart) 414.10
coronary (arteriosclerotic) (artery) (vein) (*see also* Aneurysm, heart) 414.11
arteriovenous 746.85
congenital 746.85
syphilitic 093.89
cylindrical 441.9
ruptured 441.5
syphilitic 093.9
dissecting 442.9
aorta 441.00
abdominal 441.02
thoracic 441.01
thoracoabdominal 441.03
syphilitic 093.9
ductus arteriosus 747.0
embolic—*see* Embolism, artery
endocardial, infective (any valve) 421.0
femoral 442.3
gastroduodenal 442.84
gastroepiploic 442.84
heart (chronic or with a stated duration of over 8 weeks) (infectional) (wall) 414.10
acute or with a stated duration of 8 weeks or less (*see also* Infarct, myocardium) 410.9
congenital 746.89
valve—*see* Endocarditis
hepatic 442.84
iliac (common) 442.2
infective (any valve) 421.0
innominate (nonsyphilitic) 442.89
syphilitic 093.89
interauricular septum (*see also* Aneurysm, heart) 414.10

Aneurysm—*continued*
interventricular septum (*see also* Aneurysm, heart) 414.10
intracranial—*see* Aneurysm, brain
intrathoracic (nonsyphilitic) 441.2
ruptured 441.1
syphilitic 093.0
jugular vein 453.8
lower extremity 442.3
lung (pulmonary artery) 417.1
malignant 093.9
mediastinal (nonsyphilitic) 442.89
syphilitic 093.89
miliary (congenital) (ruptured) (*see also* Hemorrhage, subarachnoid) 430
mitral (heart) (valve) 424.0
mural (arteriovenous) (heart) (*see also* Aneurysm, heart) 414.10
mycotic, any site 421.0
ruptured, brain (*see also* Hemorrhage, subarachnoid) 430
myocardium (*see also* Aneurysm, heart) 414.10
neck 442.81
pancreaticoduodenal 442.84
patent ductus arteriosus 747.0
peripheral NEC 442.89
congenital NEC (*see also* Aneurysm, congenital) 747.60
popliteal 442.3
pulmonary 417.1
arteriovenous 747.3
acquired 417.0
syphilitic 093.89
valve (heart) (*see also* Endocarditis, pulmonary) 424.3
racemose 442.9
congenital (peripheral) NEC 747.60
radial 442.0
Rasmussen's (*see also* Tuberculosis) 011.2
renal 442.1
retinal (acquired) 362.17
congenital 743.58
diabetic 250.5 *[362.01]*
sinus, aortic (of Valsalva) 747.29
specified site NEC 442.89
spinal (cord) 442.89
congenital 747.82
syphilitic (hemorrhage) 094.89
spleen, splenic 442.83
subclavian 442.82
syphilitic 093.89
superior mesenteric 442.84
syphilitic 093.9
aorta 093.0
central nervous system 094.89
congenital 090.5
spine, spinal 094.89
thoracoabdominal 441.7
ruptured 441.6
thorax, thoracic (arch) (nonsyphilitic) 441.2
dissecting 441.01
ruptured 441.1
syphilitic 093.0
traumatic (complication) (early)—*see* Injury, blood vessel, by site
tricuspid (heart) (valve)—*see* Endocarditis, tricuspid
ulnar 442.0
upper extremity 442.0
valve, valvular—*see* Endocarditis

Aneurysm—*continued*
venous 456.8
congenital NEC (*see also* Aneurysm, congenital) 747.60
ventricle (arteriovenous) (*see also* Aneurysm, heart) 414.10
visceral artery NEC 442.84
Angiectasis 459.89
Angiectopia 459.9
Angiitis 447.6
allergic granulomatous 446.4
hypersensitivity 446.20
Goodpasture's syndrome 446.21
specified NEC 446.29
necrotizing 446.0
Wegener's (necrotizing respiratory granulomatosis) 446.4
Angina (attack) (cardiac) (chest) (effort) (heart) (pectoris) (syndrome) (vasomotor) 413.9
abdominal 557.1
agranulocytic 288.0
aphthous 074.0
catarrhal 462
crescendo 411.1
croupous 464.4
cruris 443.9
due to atherosclerosis NEC (*see also* Arteriosclerosis, extremities) 440.20
decubitus 413.0
diphtheritic (membranous) 032.0
erysipelatous 034.0
erythematous 462
exudative, chronic 476.0
faucium 478.29
gangrenous 462
diphtheritic 032.0
infectious 462
initial 411.1
intestinal 557.1
ludovici 528.3
Ludwig's 528.3
malignant 462
diphtheritic 032.0
membranous 464.4
diphtheritic 032.0
mesenteric 557.1
monocytic 075
nocturnal 413.0
phlegmonous 475
diphtheritic 032.0
preinfarctional 411.1
Prinzmetal's 413.1
progressive 411.1
pseudomembranous 101
psychogenic 306.2
pultaceous, diphtheritic 032.0
scarlatinal 034.1
septic 034.0
simple 462
stable NEC 413.9
staphylococcal 462
streptococcal 034.0
stridulous, diphtheritic 032.3
syphilitic 093.9
congenital 090.5
tonsil 475
trachealis 464.4
unstable 411.1
variant 413.1
Vincent's 101
Angioblastoma (M9161/1)—*see* Neoplasm, connective tissue, uncertain behavior

Angiocholecystitis (*see also* Cholecystitis, acute) 575.0
Angiocholitis (*see also* Cholecystitis, acute) 576.1
Angiodysgensis spinalis 336.1
Angiodysplasia (intestinalis) (intestine) 569.84
with hemorrhage 569.85
duodenum 537.82
with hemorrhage 537.83
stomach 537.82
with hemorrhage 537.83
Angioedema (allergic) (any site) (with urticaria) 995.1
hereditary 277.6
Angioendothelioma (M9130/1)—*see also* Neoplasm, by site, uncertain behavior
benign (M9130/0) (*see also* Hemangioma, by site) 228.00
bone (M9260/3)—*see* Neoplasm, bone, malignant
Ewing's (M9260/3)—*see* Neoplasm, bone, malignant
nervous system (M9130/0) 228.09
Angiofibroma (M9160/0)—*see also* Neoplasm, by site, benign
juvenile (M9160/0) 210.7
specified site—*see* Neoplasm, by site, benign
unspecified site 210.7
Angiohemophilia (A) (B) 286.4
Angioid streaks (choroid) (retina) 363.43
Angiokeratoma (M9141/0)—*see also* Neoplasm, skin, benign
corporis diffusum 272.7
Angiokeratosis
diffuse 272.7
Angioleiomyoma (M8894/0)—*see* Neoplasm, connective tissue, benign
Angioleucitis 683
Angiolipoma (M8861/0) (*see also* Lipoma, by site) 214.9
infiltrating (M8861/1)—*see* Neoplasm, connective tissue, uncertain behavior
Angioma (M9120/0) (*see also* Hemangioma, by site) 228.00
capillary 448.1
hemorrhagicum hereditaria 448.0
malignant (M9120/3)—*see* Neoplasm, connective tissue, malignant
pigmentosum et atrophicum 757.33
placenta—*see* Placenta, abnormal
plexiform (M9131/0)—*see* Hemangioma, by site
senile 448.1
serpiginosum 709.1
spider 448.1
stellate 448.1
Angiomatosis 757.32
bacillary 083.8
corporis diffusum universale 272.7
cutaneocerebral 759.6
encephalocutaneous 759.6
encephalofacial 759.6
encephalotrigeminal 759.6
hemorrhagic familial 448.0
hereditary familial 448.0
heredofamilial 448.0
meningo-oculofacial 759.6
multiple sites 228.09
neuro-oculocutaneous 759.6
retina (Hippel's disease) 759.6
retinocerebellosa 759.6
retinocerebral 759.6
systemic 228.09
Angiomyolipoma (M8860/0)
specified site—*see* Neoplasm, connective tissue, benign
unspecified site 223.0
Angiomyoliposarcoma (M8860/3)—*see* Neoplasm, connective tissue, malignant
Angiomyoma (M8894/0)—*see* Neoplasm, connective tissue, benign
Angiomyosarcoma (M8894/3)—*see* Neoplasm, connective tissue, malignant
Angioneurosis 306.2
Angioneurotic edema (allergic) (any site) (with urticaria) 995.1
hereditary 277.6
Angiopathia, angiopathy 459.9
diabetic (peripheral) 250.7 *[443.81]*
peripheral 443.9
diabetic 250.7 *[443.81]*
specified type NEC 443.89
retinae syphilitica 093.89
retinalis (juvenilis) 362.18
background 362.10
diabetic 250.5 *[362.01]*
proliferative 362.29
tuberculous (*see also* Tuberculosis) 017.3 *[362.18]*
Angiosarcoma (M9120/3)—*see* Neoplasm, connective tissue, malignant
Angiosclerosis —*see* Arteriosclerosis
Angioscotoma, enlarged 368.42
Angiospasm 443.9
brachial plexus 353.0
cerebral 435.9
cervical plexus 353.2
nerve
arm 354.9
axillary 353.0
median 354.1
ulnar 354.2
autonomic (*see also* Neuropathy, peripheral, autonomic) 337.9
axillary 353.0
leg 355.8
plantar 355.6
lower extremity—*see* Angiospasm, nerve, leg
median 354.1
peripheral NEC 355.9
spinal NEC 355.9
sympathetic (*see also* Neuropathy, peripheral, autonomic) 337.9
ulnar 354.2
upper extremity—*see* Angiospasm, nerve, arm
peripheral NEC 443.9
traumatic 443.9
foot 443.9
leg 443.9
vessel 443.9
Angiospastic disease or edema 443.9
Anguillulosis 127.2
Angulation
cecum (*see also* Obstruction, intestine) 560.9
coccyx (acquired) 738.6
congenital 756.19
femur (acquired) 736.39
congenital 755.69
intestine (large) (small) (*see also* Obstruction, intestine) 560.9
sacrum (acquired) 738.5
congenital 756.19
sigmoid (flexure) (*see also* Obstruction, intestine) 560.9

Angulation—*continued*
spine (*see also* Curvature, spine) 737.9
tibia (acquired) 736.89
congenital 755.69
ureter 593.3
wrist (acquired) 736.09
congenital 755.59
Angulus infectiosus 686.8
Anhedonia 302.72
Anhidrosis (lid) (neurogenic) (thermogenic) 705.0
Anhydration 276.5
with
hypernatremia 276.0
hyponatremia 276.1
Anhydremia 276.5
with
hypernatremia 276.0
hyponatremia 276.1
Anidrosis 705.0
Aniridia (congenital) 743.45
Anisakiasis (infection) (infestation) 127.1
Anisakis larva infestation 127.1
Aniseikonia 367.32
Anisocoria (pupil) 379.41
congenital 743.46
Anisocytosis 790.0
Anisometropia (congenital) 367.31
Ankle —*see* condition
Ankyloblepharon (acquired) (eyelid) 374.46
filiforme (adnatum) (congenital) 743.62
total 743.62
Ankylodactly (*see also* Syndactylism) 755.10
Ankyloglossia 750.0
Ankylosis (fibrous) (osseous) 718.50
ankle 718.57
any joint, produced by surgical fusion V45.4
cricoarytenoid (cartilage) (joint) (larynx) 478.79
dental 521.6
ear ossicle NEC 385.22
malleus 385.21
elbow 718.52
finger 718.54
hip 718.55
incostapedial joint (infectional) 385.22
joint, produced by surgical fusion NEC V45.4
knee 718.56
lumbosacral (joint) 724.6
malleus 385.21
multiple sites 718.59
postoperative (status) V45.4
sacroiliac (joint) 724.6
shoulder 718.51
specified site NEC 718.58
spine NEC 724.9
surgical V45.4
teeth, tooth (hard tissues) 521.6
temporomandibular joint 524.61
wrist 718.53
Ankylostoma— *see* Ancylostoma
Ankylostomiasis (intestinal)—*see* Ancylostomiasis
Ankylurethria (*see also* Stricture, urethra) 598.9
Annular —*see also* condition
detachment, cervix 622.8
organ or site, congenital NEC—*see* Distortion
pancreas (congenital) 751.7
Anodontia (complete) (partial) (vera) 520.0
with abnormal spacing 524.3
acquired 525.1
causing malocclusion 524.3
Anomaly, anomalous (congenital) (unspecified type) 759.9
abdomen 759.9
abdominal wall 756.7
acoustic nerve 742.9
adrenal (gland) 759.1
Alder (-Reilly) (leukocyte granulation) 288.2
alimentary tract 751.9
lower 751.5
specified type NEC 751.8
upper (any part, except tongue) 750.9
tongue 750.10
specified type NEC 750.19
alveolar ridge (process) 525.8
ankle (joint) 755.69
anus, anal (canal) 751.5
aorta, aortic 747.20
arch 747.21
coarctation (postductal) (preductal) 747.10
cusp or valve NEC 746.9
septum 745.0
specified type NEC 747.29
aorticopulmonary septum 745.0
apertures, diaphragm 756.6
appendix 751.5
aqueduct of Sylvius 742.3
with spina bifida (*see also* Spina bifida) 741.0
arm 755.50
reduction (*see also* Deformity, reduction, upper limb) 755.20
arteriovenous (congenital) (peripheral) NEC 747.60
brain 747.81
cerebral 747.81
coronary 746.85
gastrointestinal 747.61
lower limb 747.64
renal 747.62
specified site NEC 747.69
spinal 747.82
upper limb 747.63
artery (*see also* Anomaly, peripheral vascular system) NEC 747.60
brain 747.81
cerebral 747.81
coronary 746.85
eye 743.9
pulmonary 747.3
renal 747.62
retina 743.9
umbilical 747.5
arytenoepiglottic folds 748.3
atrial
bands 746.9
folds 746.9
septa 745.5
atrioventricular
canal 745.69
common 745.69
conduction 426.7
excitation 426.7
septum 745.4
atrium—*see* Anomaly, atrial
auditory canal 744.3
specified type NEC 744.29
with hearing impairment 744.02
auricle
ear 744.3
causing impairment of hearing 744.02
heart 746.9
septum 745.5

Anomaly, anomalous—*continued*
  autosomes, autosomal NEC 758.5
  Axenfeld's 743.44
  back 759.9
  band
    atrial 746.9
    heart 746.9
    ventricular 746.9
  Bartholin's duct 750.9
  biliary duct or passage 751.60
    atresia 751.61
  bladder (neck) (sphincter) (trigone) 753.9
    specified type NEC 753.8
  blood vessel 747.9
    artery—*see* Anomaly, artery
    peripheral vascular—*see* Anomaly, peripheral vascular system
    vein—*see* Anomaly, vein
  bone NEC 756.9
    ankle 755.69
    arm 755.50
    chest 756.3
    cranium 756.0
    face 756.0
    finger 755.50
    foot 755.67
    forearm 755.50
    frontal 756.0
    head 756.0
    hip 755.63
    leg 755.60
    lumbosacral 756.10
    nose 748.1
    pelvic girdle 755.60
    rachitic 756.4
    rib 756.3
    shoulder girdle 755.50
    skull 756.0
      with
        anencephalus 740.0
        encephalocele 742.0
        hydrocephalus 742.3
          with spina bifida (*see also* Spina bifida) 741.0
        microcephalus 742.1
    toe 755.66
  brain 742.9
    multiple 742.4
    reduction 742.2
    specified type NEC 742.4
    vessel 747.81
  branchial cleft NEC 744.49
    cyst 744.42
    fistula 744.41
    persistent 744.41
    sinus (external) (internal) 744.41
  breast 757.9
  broad ligament 752.10
    specified type NEC 752.19
  bronchus 748.3
  bulbar septum 745.0
  bulbus cordis 745.9
    persistent (in left ventricle) 745.8
  bursa 756.9
  canal of Nuck 752.9
  canthus 743.9
  capillary NEC (*see also* Anomaly, peripheral vascular system) 747.60
  cardiac 746.9
    septal closure 745.9
      acquired 429.71

Anomaly, amomalous—*continued*
      valve NEC 746.9
        pulmonary 746.00
        specified type NEC 746.89
  cardiovascular system 746.9
    complicating pregnancy, childbirth, or puerperium 648.5
  carpus 755.50
  cartilage, trachea 748.3
  cartilaginous 756.9
  caruncle, lacrimal, lachrymal 743.9
  cascade stomach 750.7
  cauda equina 742.59
  cecum 751.5
  cerebral—*see also* Anomaly, brain vessels 747.81
  cerebrovascular system 747.81
  cervix (uterus) 752.40
    with doubling of vagina and uterus 752.2
    in pregnancy or childbirth 654.6
      affecting fetus or newborn 763.8
      causing obstructed labor 660.2
        affecting fetus or newborn 763.1
  Chédiak-Higashi (-Steinbrinck) (congenital gigantism of peroxidase granules) 288.2
  cheek 744.9
  chest (wall) 756.3
  chin 744.9
    specified type NEC 744.89
  chordae tendineae 746.9
  choroid 743.9
    plexus 742.9
  chromosomes, chromosomal 758.9
    13 (13-15) 758.1
    18 (16-18) 758.2
    21 or 22 758.0
    autosomes NEC (*see also* Abnormality, autosomes) 758.5
      deletion 758.3
    Christchurch 758.3
    D_1 758.1
    E_3 758.2
    G 758.0
    mosaics 758.9
    sex 758.8
      complement, XO 758.6
      complement, XXX 758.8
      complement, XXY 758.7
      complement, XYY 758.8
      gonadal dysgenesis 758.6
      Klinefelter's 758.7
      Turner's 758.6
    trisomy 21 758.0
  cilia 743.9
  circulatory system 747.9
    specified type NEC 747.89
  clavicle 755.51
  clitoris 752.40
  coccyx 756.10
  colon 751.5
  common duct 751.60
  communication
    coronary artery 746.85
    left ventricle with right atrium 745.4
  concha (ear) 744.3
  connection
    renal vessels with kidney 747.62
    total pulmonary venous 747.41
  connective tissue 756.9
    specified type NEC 756.89

Anomaly, anomalous—*continued*
cornea 743.9
shape 743.41
size 743.41
specified type NEC 743.49
coronary
artery 746.85
vein 746.89
cranium—*see* Anomaly, skull
cricoid cartilage 748.3
cushion, endocardial 745.60
specified type NEC 745.69
cystic duct 751.60
dental arch relationship 524.2
dentition 520.6
dentofacial NEC 524.9
functional 524.5
specified type NEC 524.8
dermatoglyphic 757.2
Descemet's membrane 743.9
specified type NEC 743.49
development
cervix 752.40
vagina 752.40
vulva 752.40
diaphragm, diaphragmatic (apertures) NEC 756.6
digestive organ(s) or system 751.9
lower 751.5
specified type NEC 751.8
upper 750.9
distribution, coronary artery 746.85
ductus
arteriosus 747.0
Botalli 747.0
duodenum 751.5
dura 742.9
brain 742.4
spinal cord 742.59
ear 744.3
causing impairment of hearing 744.00
specified type NEC 744.09
external 744.3
causing impairment of hearing 744.02
specified type NEC 744.29
inner (causing impairment of hearing) 744.05
middle, except ossicles (causing impairment of hearing) 744.03
ossicles 744.04
ossicles 744.04
prominent auricle 744.29
specified type NEC 744.29
with hearing impairment 744.09
Ebstein's (heart) 746.2
tricuspid valve 746.2
ectodermal 757.9
Eisenmenger's (ventricular septal defect) 745.4
ejaculatory duct 752.9
specified type NEC 752.8
elbow (joint) 755.50
endocardial cushion 745.60
specified type NEC 745.69
endocrine gland NEC 759.2
epididymis 752.9
epiglottis 748.3
esophagus 750.9
specified type NEC 750.4
Eustachian tube 744.3
specified type NEC 744.24

Anomaly, anomalous—*continued*
eye (any part) 743.9
adnexa 743.9
specified type NEC 743.69
anophthalmos 743.00
anterior
chamber and related structures 743.9
angle 743.9
specified type NEC 743.44
specified type NEC 743.44
segment 743.9
combined 743.48
multiple 743.48
specified type NEC 743.49
cataract (*see also* Cataract) 743.30
glaucoma (*see also* Buphthalmia) 743.20
lid 743.9
specified type NEC 743.63
microphthalmos (*see also* Microphthalmos) 743.10
posterior segment 743.9
specified type NEC 743.59
vascular 743.58
vitreous 743.9
specified type NEC 743.51
ptosis (eyelid) 743.61
retina 743.9
specified type NEC 743.59
sclera 743.9
specified type NEC 743.47
specified type NEC 743.8
eyebrow 744.89
eyelid 743.9
specified type NEC 743.63
face (any part) 744.9
bone(s) 756.0
specified type NEC 744.89
fallopian tube 752.10
specified type NEC 752.19
fascia 756.9
specified type NEC 756.89
femur 755.60
fibula 755.60
finger 755.50
supernumerary 755.01
webbed (*see also* Syndactylism, fingers) 755.11
fixation, intestine 751.4
flexion (joint) 755.9
hip or thigh (*see also* Dislocation, hip, congenital) 754.30
folds, heart 746.9
foot 755.67
foramen
Botalli 745.5
ovale 745.5
forearm 755.50
forehead (*see also* Anomaly, skull) 756.0
form, teeth 520.2
fovea centralis 743.9
frontal bone (*see also* Anomaly, skull) 756.0
gallbladder 751.60
Gartner's duct 752.11
gastrointestinal tract 751.9
specified type NEC 751.8
vessel 747.61
genitalia, genital organ(s) or system
female 752.9
external 752.40
specified type NEC 752.49
internal NEC 752.9

Anomaly, anomalous—*continued*
male (external and internal) 752.9
epispadias 752.6
hydrocele, congenital 778.6
hypospadias 752.6
testis, undescended 752.5
specified type NEC 752.8
genitourinary NEC 752.9
Gerbode 745.4
globe (eye) 743.9
glottis 748.3
granulation or granulocyte, genetic 288.2
constitutional 288.2
leukocyte 288.2
gum 750.9
gyri 742.9
hair 757.9
specified type NEC 757.4
hand 755.50
hard tissue formation in pulp 522.3
head (*see also* Anomaly, skull) 756.0
heart 746.9
auricle 746.9
bands 746.9
fibroelastosis cordis 425.3
folds 746.9
malposition 746.87
maternal, affecting fetus or newborn 760.3
obstructive NEC 746.84
patent ductus arteriosus (Botalli) 747.0
septum 745.9
acquired 429.71
aortic 745.0
aorticopulmonary 745.0
atrial 745.5
auricular 745.5
between aorta and pulmonary artery 745.0
endocardial cushion type 745.60
specified type NEC 745.69
interatrial 745.5
interventricular 745.4
with pulmonary stenosis or atresia, dextraposition of aorta, and hypertrophy of right ventricle 745.2
acquired 429.71
specified type NEC 745.8
ventricular 745.4
with pulmonary stenosis or atresia, dextraposition of aorta, and hypertrophy of right ventricle 745.2
acquired 429.71
specified type NEC 746.89
tetralogy of Fallot 745.2
valve NEC 746.9
aortic 746.9
atresia 746.89
bicuspid valve 746.4
insufficiency 746.4
specified type NEC 746.89
stenosis 746.3
subaortic 746.81
supravalvular 747.22
mitral 746.9
atresia 746.89
insufficiency 746.6
specified type NEC 746.89
stenosis 746.5
pulmonary 746.00
atresia 746.01
insufficiency 746.09

Anomaly, anomalous—*continued*
stenosis 746.02
infundibular 746.83
subvalvular 746.83
tricuspid 746.9
atresia 746.1
stenosis 746.1
ventricle 746.9
heel 755.67
Hegglin's 288.2
hemianencephaly 740.0
hemicephaly 740.0
hemicrania 740.0
hepatic duct 751.60
hip (joint) 755.63
hourglass
bladder 753.8
gallbladder 751.69
stomach 750.7
humerus 755.50
hymen 752.40
hypersegmentation of neutrophils, hereditary 288.2
hypophyseal 759.2
ileocecal (coil) (valve) 751.5
ileum (intestine) 751.5
ilium 755.60
integument 757.9
specified type NEC 757.8
intervertebral cartilage or disc 756.10
intestine (large) (small) 751.5
fixational type 751.4
iris 743.9
specified type NEC 743.46
ischium 755.60
jaw NEC 524.9
closure 524.5
size NEC 524.00
specified type NEC 524.8
jaw-cranial base relationship 524.10
specified NEC 524.19
jejunum 751.5
joint 755.9
hip
dislocation (*see also* Dislocation, hip, congenital) 754.30
predislocation (*see also* Subluxation, congenital, hip) 754.32
preluxation (*see also* Subluxation, congenital, hip) 754.32
subluxation (*see also* Subluxation, congenital, hip) 754.32
lumbosacral 756.10
spondylolisthesis 756.12
spondylosis 756.11
multiple arthrogryposis 754.89
sacroiliac 755.69
Jordan's 288.2
kidney(s) (calyx) (pelvis) 753.9
vessel 747.62
Klippel-Feil (brevicollis) 756.16
knee (joint) 755.64
labium (majus) (minus) 752.40
labyrinth, membranous (causing impairment of hearing) 744.05
lacrimal
apparatus, duct or passage 743.9
specified type NEC 743.65
gland 743.9
specified type NEC 743.64
Langdon Down (mongolism) 758.0

Anomaly, anomalous—*continued*
larynx, laryngeal (muscle) 748.3
web, webbed 748.2
leg (lower) (upper) 755.60
reduction NEC (*see also* Deformity, reduction, lower limb) 755.30
lens 743.9
shape 743.36
specified type NEC 743.39
leukocytes, genetic 288.2
granulation (constitutional) 288.2
lid (fold) 743.9
ligament 756.9
broad 752.10
round 752.9
limb, except reduction deformity 755.9
lower 755.60
reduction deformity (*see also* Deformity, reduction, lower limb) 755.30
specified type NEC 755.69
upper 755.50
reduction deformity (*see also* Deformity, reduction, upper limb) 755.20
specified type NEC 755.59
lip 750.9
harelip (*see also* Cleft, lip) 749.10
specified type NEC 750.26
liver (duct) 751.60
atresia 751.69
lower extremity 755.60
vessel 747.64
lumbosacral (joint) (region) 756.10
lung (fissure) (lobe) NEC 748.60
agenesis 748.5
specified type NEC 748.69
lymphatic system 759.9
Madelung's (radius) 755.54
mandible 524.9
size NEC 524.00
maxilla 524.9
size NEC 524.00
May (-Hegglin) 288.2
meatus urinarius 753.9
specified type NEC 753.8
meningeal bands or folds, constriction of 742.8
meninges 742.9
brain 742.4
spinal 742.59
meningocele (*see also* Spina bifida) 741.9
mesentery 751.9
metacarpus 755.50
metatarsus 755.67
middle ear, except ossicles (causing impairment of hearing) 744.03
ossicles 744.04
mitral (leaflets) (valve) 746.9
atresia 746.89
insufficiency 746.6
specified type NEC 746.89
stenosis 746.5
mouth 750.9
specified type NEC 750.26
multiple NEC 759.7
specified type NEC 759.89
muscle 756.9
eye 743.9
specified type NEC 743.69
specified type NEC 756.89
musculoskeletal system, except limbs 756.9
specified type NEC 756.9

Anomaly, anomalous—*continued*
nail 757.9
specified type NEC 757.5
narrowness, eyelid 743.62
nasal sinus or septum 748.1
neck (any part) 744.9
specified type NEC 744.89
nerve 742.9
acoustic 742.9
specified type NEC 742.8
optic 742.9
specified type NEC 742.8
specified type NEC 742.8
nervous system NEC 742.9
brain 742.9
specified type NEC 742.4
specified type NEC 742.8
neurological 742.9
nipple 757.9
nonteratogenic NEC 754.89
nose, nasal (bone) (cartilage) (septum) (sinus) 748.1
ocular muscle 743.9
omphalomesenteric duct 751.0
opening, pulmonary veins 747.49
optic
disc 743.9
specified type NEC 743.57
nerve 742.9
opticociliary vessels 743.9
orbit (eye) 743.9
specified type NEC 743.66
organ
of Corti (causing impairment of hearing) 744.05
or site 759.9
specified type NEC 759.89
origin
both great arteries from same ventricle 745.11
coronary artery 746.85
innominate artery 747.69
left coronary artery from pulmonary artery 746.85
pulmonary artery 747.3
renal vessels 747.62
subclavian artery (left) (right) 747.21
osseous meatus (ear) 744.03
ovary 752.0
oviduct 752.10
palate (hard) (soft) 750.9
cleft (*see also* Cleft, palate) 749.00
pancreas (duct) 751.7
papillary muscles 746.9
parathyroid gland 759.2
paraurethral ducts 753.9
parotid (gland) 750.9
patella 755.64
Pelger-Huët (hereditary hyposegmentation) 288.2
pelvic girdle 755.60
specified type NEC 755.69
pelvis (bony) 755.60
complicating delivery 653.0
rachitic 268.1
fetal 756.4
penis (glans) 752.9
pericardium 746.89
peripheral vascular system NEC 747.60
gastrointestinal 747.61
lower limb 747.64

Anomaly, anomalous—*continued*
canal of Nuck 752.8
cardiac septal closure 745.8
carpus 755.59
cartilaginous 756.9
cecum 751.5
cervix 752.49
chest (wall) 756.3
chin 744.89
ciliary body 743.46
circulatory system 747.89
clavicle 755.51
clitoris 752.49
coccyx 756.19
colon 751.5
common duct 751.69
connective tissue 756.89
cricoid cartilage 748.3
cystic duct 751.69
diaphragm 756.6
digestive organ(s) or tract 751.8
lower 751.5
upper 750.8
duodenum 751.5
ear 744.29
auricle 744.29
causing impairment of hearing 744.02
causing impairment of hearing 744.09
inner (causing impairment of hearing) 744.05
middle, except ossicles 744.03
ossicles 744.04
ejaculatory duct 752.8
endocrine 759.2
epiglottis 748.3
esophagus 750.4
Eustachian tube 744.24
eye 743.8
lid 743.63
muscle 743.69
face 744.89
bone(s) 756.0
fallopian tube 752.19
fascia 756.89
femur 755.69
fibula 755.69
finger 755.59
foot 755.67
fovea centralis 743.55
gallbladder 751.69
Gartner's duct 752.8
gastrointestinal tract 751.8
genitalia, genital organ(s)
female 752.8
external 752.49
internal NEC 752.8
male 752.8
genitourinary tract NEC 752.8
glottis 748.3
hair 757.4
hand 755.59
heart 746.89
valve NEC 746.89
pulmonary 746.09
hepatic duct 751.69
hydatid of Morgagni 752.8
hymen 752.49
integument 757.8
intestine (large) (small) 751.5
fixational type 751.4
iris 743.46

Anomaly, anomalous—*continued*
jejunum 751.5
joint 755.8
kidney 753.3
knee 755.64
labium (majus) (minus) 752.49
labyrinth, membranous 744.05
larynx 748.3
leg 755.69
lens 743.39
limb, except reduction deformity 755.8
lower 755.69
reduction deformity (*see also* Deformity, reduction, lower limb) 755.30
upper 755.59
reduction deformity (*see also* Deformity, reduction, upper limb) 755.20
lip 750.26
liver 751.69
lung (fissure) (lobe) 748.69
meatus urinarius 753.8
metacarpus 755.59
mouth 750.26
muscle 756.89
eye 743.69
musculoskeletal system, except limbs 756.9
nail 757.5
neck 744.89
nerve 742.8
acoustic 742.8
optic 742.8
nervous system 742.8
nipple 757.6
nose 748.1
organ NEC 759.89
of Corti 744.05
osseous meatus (ear) 744.03
ovary 752.0
oviduct 752.19
pancreas 751.7
parathyroid 759.2
patella 755.64
pelvic girdle 755.69
penis 752.8
pericardium 746.89
peripheral vascular system NEC (*see also* Anomaly, peripheral vascular system) 747.60
pharynx 750.29
pituitary 759.2
prostate 752.8
radius 755.59
rectum 751.5
respiratory system 748.8
rib 756.3
round ligament 752.8
sacrum 756.19
salivary duct or gland 750.26
scapula 755.59
sclera 743.47
scrotum 752.8
seminal duct or tract 752.8
shoulder girdle 755.59
site NEC 759.89
skin 757.39
skull (bone(s)) 756.0
with
anencephalus 740.0
encephalocele 742.0

Anomaly, anomalous—*continued*
hydrocephalus 742.3
with spina bifida (*see also* Spina bifida) 741.0
microcephalus 742.1
specified organ or site NEC 759.89
spermatic cord 752.8
spinal cord 742.59
spine 756.19
spleen 759.0
sternum 756.3
stomach 750.7
tarsus 755.67
tendon 756.89
testis 752.8
thorax (wall) 756.3
thymus 759.2
thyroid (gland) 759.2
cartilage 748.3
tibia 755.69
toe 755.66
tongue 750.19
trachea (cartilage) 748.3
ulna 755.59
urachus 753.7
ureter 753.4
obstructive 753.2
urethra 753.8
obstructive 753.6
urinary tract 753.8
uterus 752.3
uvula 750.26
vagina 752.49
vascular NEC (*see also* Anomaly, peripheral vascular system) 747.60
brain 747.81
vas deferens 752.8
vein(s) (peripheral) NEC (*see also* Anomaly, peripheral vascular system) 747.60
brain 747.81
great 747.49
portal 747.49
pulmonary 747.49
vena cava (inferior) (superior) 747.49
vertebra 756.19
vulva 752.49
spermatic cord 752.9
spine, spinal 756.10
column 756.10
cord 742.9
meningocele (*see also* Spina bifida) 741.9
specified type NEC 742.59
spina bifida (*see also* Spina bifida) 741.9
vessel 747.82
meninges 742.59
nerve root 742.9
spleen 759.0
Sprengel's 755.52
sternum 756.3
stomach 750.9
specified type NEC 750.7
submaxillary gland 750.9
superior vena cava 747.40
talipes—*see* Talipes
tarsus 755.67
with complete absence of distal elements 755.31
teeth, tooth NEC 520.9
position 524.3
spacing 524.3

Anomaly, anomalous—*continued*
tendon 756.9
specified type NEC 756.89
termination
coronary artery 746.85
testis 752.9
thebesian valve 746.9
thigh 755.60
flexion (*see also* Subluxation, congenital, hip) 754.32
thorax (wall) 756.3
throat 750.9
thumb 755.50
supernumerary 755.01
thymus gland 759.2
thyroid (gland) 759.2
cartilage 748.3
tibia 755.60
saber 090.5
toe 755.66
supernumerary 755.02
webbed (*see also* Syndactylism, toes) 755.13
tongue 750.10
specified type NEC 750.19
trachea, tracheal 748.3
cartilage 748.3
rings 748.3
tragus 744.3
transverse aortic arch 747.21
trichromata 368.59
trichromatopsia 368.59
tricuspid (leaflet) (valve) 746.9
atresia 746.1
Ebstein's 746.2
specified type NEC 746.89
stenosis 746.1
trunk 759.9
Uhl's (hypoplasia of myocardium, right ventricle) 746.84
ulna 755.50
umbilicus 759.9
artery 747.5
union, trachea with larynx 748.3
unspecified site 759.9
upper extremity 755.50
vessel 747.63
urachus 753.7
specified type NEC 753.7
ureter 753.9
obstructive 753.2
specified type NEC 753.4
urethra (valve) 753.9
obstructive 753.6
specified type NEC 753.8
urinary tract or system (any part, except urachus) 753.9
specified type NEC 753.8
urachus 753.7
uterus 752.3
with only one functioning horn 752.3
in pregnancy or childbirth 654.0
affecting fetus or newborn 763.8
causing obstructed labor 660.2
affecting fetus or newborn 763.1
uvula 750.9
vagina 752.40
valleculae 748.3
valve (heart) NEC 746.9
formation, ureter 753.2
pulmonary 746.00
specified type NEC 746.89

Antibodies
maternal (blood group) (*see also* Incompatibility) 656.2
anti-D, cord blood 656.1
fetus or newborn 773.0
Antibody deficiency syndrome
agammaglobulinemic 279.00
congenital 279.04
hypogammaglobulinemic 279.00
Anticoagulant, circulating (*see also* Circulating anticoagulants) 286.5
Antimongolism syndrome 758.3
Antimonial cholera 985.4
Antisocial personality 301.7
Antithrombinemia (*see also* Circulating anticoagulants) 286.5
Antithromboplastinemia (*see also* Circulating anticoagulants) 286.5
Antithromboplastinogenemia (*see also* Circulating anticoagulants) 286.5
Antitoxin complication or reaction —*see* Complications, vaccination
Anton (-Babinski) syndrome (hemiasomatognosia) 307.9
Antritis (chronic) 473.0
acute 461.0
Antrum, antral —*see* condition
Anuria 788.5
with
abortion—*see* Abortion, by type, with renal failure
ectopic pregnancy (*see also* categories 633.0-633.9) 639.3
molar pregnancy (*see also* categories 630-632) 639.3
calculus (impacted) (recurrent) 592.9
kidney 592.0
ureter 592.1
congenital 753.3
due to a procedure 997.5
following
abortion 639.3
ectopic or molar pregnancy 639.3
newborn 753.3
postrenal 593.4
puerperal, postpartum, childbirth 669.3
specified as due to a procedure 997.5
sulfonamide
correct substance properly administered 788.5
overdose or wrong substance given or taken 961.0
traumatic (following crushing) 958.5
Anus, anal —*see* condition
Anusitis 569.49
Anxiety (neurosis) (reaction) (state) 300.00
alcohol-induced 291.8
depression 300.4
drug-induced 292.89
generalized 300.02
hysteria 300.20
in
acute stress reaction 308.0
transient adjustment reaction 309.24
panic type 300.01
separation, abnormal 309.21
Aorta, aortic —*see* condition
Aortectasia 441.9
Aortitis (nonsyphilitic) 447.6
arteriosclerotic 440.0
calcific 447.6
Döhle-Heller 093.1
Aortitis—*continued*
luetic 093.1
rheumatic (*see also* Endocarditis, acute, rheumatic) 391.1
rheumatoid—*see* Arthritis, rheumatoid
specific 093.1
syphilitic 093.1
congenital 090.5
Apathetic thyroid storm (*see also* Thyrotoxicosis) 242.9
Apepsia 536.8
achlorhydric 536.0
psychogenic 306.4
Aperistalsis, esophagus 530.0
Apert's syndrome (acrocephalosyndactyly) 755.55
Apert-Gallais syndrome (adrenogenital) 255.2
Apertognathia 524.2
Aphagia 783.0
psychogenic 307.1
Aphakia (acquired) (bilateral) (postoperative) (unilateral) 379.31
congenital 743.35
Aphalangia (congenital) 755.4
lower limb (complete) (intercalary) (partial) (terminal) 755.39
meaning all digits (complete) (partial) 755.31
transverse 755.31
upper limb (complete) (intercalary) (partial) (terminal) 755.29
meaning all digits (complete) (partial) 755.21
transverse 755.21
Aphasia (amnestic) (ataxic) (auditory) (Broca's) (choreatic) (classic) (expressive) (global) (ideational) (ideokinetic) (ideomotor) (jargon) (motor) (nominal) (receptive) (semantic) (sensory) (syntactic) (verbal) (visual) (Wernicke's) 784.3
developmental 315.31
syphilis, tertiary 094.89
uremic—*see* Uremia
Aphemia 784.3
uremic—*see* Uremia
Aphonia 784.41
clericorum 784.49
hysterical 300.11
organic 784.41
psychogenic 306.1
Aphthae, aphthous —*see also* condition
Bednar's 528.2
cachectic 529.0
epizootic 078.4
fever 078.4
oral 528.2
stomatitis 528.2
thrush 112.0
ulcer (oral) (recurrent) 528.2
genital organ(s) NEC
female 629.8
male 608.89
larynx 478.79
Apical —*see* condition
Aplasia —*see also* Agenesis
alveolar process (acquired) 525.8
congenital 750.26
aorta (congenital) 747.22
aortic valve (congenital) 746.89
axialis extracorticalis (congenital) 330.0
bone marrow (myeloid) 284.9
acquired (secondary) 284.8
congenital 284.0

Aplasia—*continued*
idiopathic 284.9
brain 740.0
specified part 742.2
breast 757.6
bronchus 748.3
cementum 520.4
cerebellar 742.2
congenital pure red cell 284.0
corpus callosum 742.2
erythrocyte 284.8
congenital 284.0
extracortical axial 330.0
eye (congenital) 743.00
fovea centralis (congenital) 743.55
germinal (cell) 606.0
iris 743.45
labyrinth, membranous 744.05
limb (congenital) 755.4
lower NEC 755.30
upper NEC 755.20
lung (bilateral) (congenital) (unilateral) 748.5
nervous system NEC 742.8
nuclear 742.8
ovary 752.0
Pelizaeus-Merzbacher 330.0
prostate (congenital) 752.8
red cell (pure) (with thymoma) 284.8
acquired (adult) (secondary) 284.8
congenital 284.0
hereditary 284.0
of infants 284.0
primary 284.0
round ligament (congenital) 752.8
salivary gland 750.21
skin (congenital) 757.39
spinal cord 742.59
spleen 759.0
testis (congenital) 752.8
thymic, with immunodeficiency 279.2
thyroid 243
uterus 752.3
ventral horn cell 742.59
Apleuria 756.3
Apnea, apneic (spells) 786.09
newborn, neonatorum 770.8
psychogenic 306.1
sleep NEC 780.57
with
hypersomnia 780.53
hyposomnia 780.51
insomnia 780.51
sleep disturbance NEC 780.57
Apneumatosis newborn 770.4
Apodia 755.31
Apophysitis (bone) (*see also* Osteochondrosis) 732.9
calcaneus 732.5
juvenile 732.6
Apoplectiform convulsions (*see also* Disease, cerebrovascular, acute) 436
Apoplexia, apoplexy, apoplectic (*see also* Disease, cerebrovascular, acute) 436
abdominal 569.89
adrenal 036.3
attack 436
basilar (*see also* Disease, cerebrovascular, acute) 436
brain (*see also* Disease, cerebrovascular, acute) 436

Apoplexia, apoplexy...—*continued*
bulbar (*see also* Disease, cerebrovascular, acute) 436
capillary (*see also* Disease, cerebrovascular, acute) 436
cardiac (*see also* Infarct, myocardium) 410.9
cerebral (*see also* Disease, cerebrovascular, acute) 436
chorea (*see also* Disease, cerebrovascular, acute) 436
congestive (*see also* Disease, cerebrovascular, acute) 436
newborn 767.4
embolic (*see also* Embolism, brain) 434.1
fetus 767.0
fit (*see also* Disease, cerebrovascular, acute) 436
healed or old—*see also* category 438
without residuals V12.59
heart (auricle) (ventricle) (*see also* Infarct, myocardium) 410.9
heat 992.0
hemiplegia (*see also* Disease, cerebrovascular, acute) 436
hemorrhagic (stroke) (*see also* Hemorrhage, brain) 432.9
ingravescent (*see also* Disease, cerebrovascular, acute) 436
late effect—*see* category 438
lung—*see* Embolism, pulmonary
meninges, hemorrhagic (*see also* Hemorrhage, subarachnoid) 430
neonatorum 767.0
newborn 767.0
pancreatitis 577.0
placenta 641.2
progressive (*see also* Disease, cerebrovascular, acute) 436
pulmonary (artery) (vein)—*see* Embolism, pulmonary
sanguineous (*see also* Disease, cerebrovascular, acute) 436
seizure (*see also* Disease, cerebrovascular, acute) 436
serous (*see also* Disease, cerebrovascular, acute) 436
spleen 289.59
stroke (*see also* Disease, cerebrovascular, acute) 436
thrombotic (*see also* Thrombosis, brain) 434.0
uremic—*see* Uremia
uteroplacental 641.2
Appendage
fallopian tube (cyst of Morgagni) 752.11
intestine (epiploic) 751.5
preauricular 744.1
testicular (organ of Morgagni) 752.8
Appendicitis 541
with
perforation, peritonitis (generalized), or rupture 540.0
with peritoneal abscess 540.1
peritoneal abscess 540.1
acute (catarrhal) (fulminating) (gangrenous) (inflammatory) (obstructive) (retrocecal) (suppurative) 540.9
with
perforation, peritonitis, or rupture 540.0
with peritoneal abscess 540.1
peritoneal abscess 540.1
amebic 006.8
chronic (recurrent) 542

Appendicitis—*continued*
exacerbation—*see* Appendicitis, acute
fulminating—*see* Appendicitis, acute
gangrenous—*see* Appendicitis, acute
healed (obliterative) 542
interval 542
neurogenic 542
obstructive 542
pneumococcal 541
recurrent 542
relapsing 542
retrocecal 541
subacute (adhesive) 542
subsiding 542
suppurative—*see* Appendicitis, acute
tuberculous (*see also* Tuberculosis) 014.8
Appendiclausis 543.9
Appendicolithiasis 543.9
Appendicopathia oxyurica 127.4
Appendix, appendicular —*see also* condition
Morgagni (male) 752.8
fallopian tube 752.11
Appetite
depraved 307.52
excessive 783.6
psychogenic 307.51
lack or loss (*see also* Anorexia) 783.0
nonorganic origin 307.59
perverted 307.52
hysterical 300.11
Apprehension, apprehensiveness (abnormal) (state) 300.00
specified type NEC 300.09
Approximal wear 521.1
Apraxia (classic) (ideational) (ideokinetic) (ideomotor) (motor) 784.69
oculomotor, congenital 379.51
verbal 784.69
Aptyalism 527.7
Arabicum elephantiasis (*see also* Infestation, filarial) 125.9
Arachnidism 989.5
Arachnitis —*see* Meningitis
Arachnodactyly 759.82
Arachnoidism 989.5
Arachnoiditis (acute) (adhesive) (basic) (brain) (cerebrospinal) (chiasmal) (chronic) (spinal) (*see also* Meningitis) 322.9
meningococcal (chronic) 036.0
syphilitic 094.2
tuberculous (*see also* Tuberculosis, meninges) 013.0
Araneism 989.5
Arboencephalitis, Australian 062.4
Arborization block (heart) 426.6
Arbor virus, arbovirus (infection) NEC 066.9
ARC 042
Arches —*see* condition
Arcuatus uterus 752.3
Arcus (cornea)
juvenilis 743.43
interfering with vision 743.42
senilis 371.41
Arc-welders' lung 503
Arc-welders' syndrome (photokeratitis) 370.24
Areflexia 796.1
Areola —*see* condition
Argentaffinoma (M8241/1)—*see also* Neoplasm, by site, uncertain behavior
benign (M8241/0)—*see* Neoplasm, by site, benign
malignant (M8241/3)—*see* Neoplasm, by site, malignant
syndrome 259.2
Argentinian hemorrhagic fever 078.7
Arginosuccinicaciduria 270.6
Argonz-Del Castillo syndrome (nonpuerperal galactorrhea and amenorrhea) 253.1
Argyll-Robertson phenomenon pupil, or syndrome (syphilitic) 094.89
atypical 379.45
nonluetic 379.45
nonsyphilitic 379.45
reversed 379.45
Argyria, argyriasis NEC 985.8
conjunctiva 372.55
cornea 371.16
from drug or medicinal agent
correct substance properly administered 709.09
overdose or wrong substance given or taken 961.2
Arhinencephaly 742.2
Arias-Stella phenomenon 621.3
Ariboflavinosis 266.0
Arizona enteritis 008.1
Arm —*see* condition
Armenian disease 277.3
Arnold-Chiari obstruction or syndrome (*see also* Spina bifida) 741.0
type I 348.4
type II (*see also* Spina bifida) 741.0
type III 742.0
type IV 742.2
Arrest, arrested
active phase of labor 661.1
affecting fetus or newborn 763.7
any plane in pelvis
complicating delivery 660.1
affecting fetus or newborn 763.1
bone marrow (*see also* Anemia, aplastic) 284.9
cardiac 427.5
with
abortion—*see* Abortion, by type, with specified complication NEC
ectopic pregnancy (*see also* categories 633.0-633.9) 639.8
molar pregnancy (*see also* categories 630-632) 639.8
complicating
anesthesia
correct substance properly administered 427.5
obstetric 668.1
overdose or wrong substance given 968.4
specified anesthetic—*see* Table of drugs and chemicals
delivery (cesarean) (instrumental) 669.4
ectopic or molar pregnancy 639.8
surgery (nontherapeutic) (therapeutic) 997.1
fetus or newborn 779.8
following
abortion 639.8
ectopic or molar pregnancy 639.8
postoperative (immediate) 997.1
long-term effect of cardiac surgery 429.4
cardiorespiratory (*see also* Arrest, cardiac) 427.5

Arrest, arrested—*continued*
deep transverse 660.3
affecting fetus or newborn 763.1
development or growth
bone 733.91
child 783.4
fetus 764.9
affecting management of pregnancy 656.5
tracheal rings 748.3
epiphyseal 733.91
granulopoiesis 288.0
heart—*see* Arrest, cardiac
respiratory 799.1
newborn 770.8
sinus 426.6
transverse (deep) 660.3
affecting fetus or newborn 763.1
Arrhenoblastoma (M8630.1)
benign (M8630/0)
specified site—*see* Neoplasm, by site, benign
unspecified site
female 220
male 222.0
malignant (M8630/3)
specified site— *see* Neoplasm, by site, malignant
unspecified site
female 183.0
male 186.9
specified site—*see* Neoplasm, by site, uncertain behavior
unspecified site
female 236.2
male 236.4
Arrhinencephaly 742.2
due to
trisomy 13 (13-15) 758.1
trisomy 18 (16-18) 758.2
Arrhythmia (auricle) (cardiac) (cordis) (gallop rhythm) (juvenile) (nodal) (reflex) (sinus) (supraventricular) (transitory) (ventricle) 427.9
bigeminal rhythm 427.89
block 426.9
bradycardia 427.89
contractions, premature 427.60
coronary sinus 427.89
ectopic 427.89
extrasystolic 427.60
postoperative 997.1
psychogenic 306.2
vagal 780.2
Arrillaga-Ayerza syndrome (pulmonary artery sclerosis with pulmonary hypertension) 416.0
Arsenical
dermatitis 692.4
keratosis 692.4
pigmentation 985.1
from drug or medicinal agent
correct substance properly administered 709.09
overdose or wrong substance given or taken 961.1
Arsenism 985.1
from drug or medicinal agent
correct substance properly administered 692.4
overdose or wrong substance given or taken 961.1
Arterial —*see* condition
Arteriectasis 447.8
Arteriofibrosis —*see* Arteriosclerosis
Arteriolar sclerosis —*see* Arteriosclerosis
Arteriolith —*see* Arteriosclerosis
Arteriolitis 447.6
necrotizing, kidney 447.5
renal—*see* Hypertension, kidney
Arteriolosclerosis —*see* Arteriosclerosis
Arterionephrosclerosis (*see also* Hypertension, kidney) 403.90
Arteriopathy 447.9
Arteriosclerosis, arteriosclerotic (artery) (deformans) (diffuse) (disease) (endarteritis) (general) (obliterans) (obliterative) (occlusive) (senile) (with calcification) 440.9
with
gangrene 440.24
psychosis (*see also* Psychosis, arteriosclerotic) 290.40
aorta 440.0
arteries of extremities NEC — *see* Arteriosclerosis, extremities
basilar (artery) (*see also* Occlusion, artery, basilar) 433.0
brain 437.0
bypass graft
coronary artery 414.02
autologous vein 414.02
nonautologous biological 414.03
extremity 440.30
autologous vein 440.31
nonautologous biological 440.32
cardiac — *see* Arteriosclerosis, coronary
cardiopathy — *see* Arteriosclerosis, coronary
cardiorenal (*see also* Hypertension, cardiorenal) 404.90
cardiovascular (*see also* Disease, cardiovascular) 429.2
carotid (artery) (common) (internal) (*see also* Occlusion, artery, carotid) 433.1
central nervous system 437.0
cerebral 437.0
late effect—*see* category 438
cerebrospinal 437.0
cerebrovascular 437.0
coronary (artery) 414.00
graft—*see* Arteriosclerosis, bypass graft
native artery 414.01
extremities (native artery) 440.20
bypass graft 440.30
autologous vein 440.31
nonautologous biological 440.32
claudication (intermittent) 440.21
and
gangrene 440.24
rest pain 440.22
and
gangrene 440.24
ulceration 440.23
and gangrene 440.24
ulceration 440.23
and gangrene 440.24
gangrene 440.24
rest pain 440.22
and
gangrene 440.24
ulceration 440.23
and gangrene 440.24
specified site NEC 440.29
ulceration 440.23
and gangrene 440.24
heart (disease) — *see also* Arteriosclerosis, coronary

Arteriosclerosis . . .—*continued*
valve 424.99
aortic 424.1
mitral 424.0
pulmonary 424.3
tricuspid 424.2
kidney (*see also* Hypertension, kidney) 403.90
labyrinth, labyrinthine 388.00
medial NEC 440.20
mesentery (artery) 557.1
Mönckeberg's 440.20
myocarditis 429.0
nephrosclerosis (*see also* Hypertension, kidney) 403.90
peripheral (of extremities) *see* Arteriosclerosis, extremities
precerebral 433.9
specified artery NEC 433.8
pulmonary (idiopathic) 416.0
renal (*see also* Hypertension, kidney) 403.90
arterioles (*see also* Hypertension, kidney) 403.90
artery 440.1
retinal (vascular) 440.8 *[362.13]*
specified artery NEC 440.8
with gangrene 440.8 *[785.4]*
spinal (cord) 437.0
vertebral (artery) (*see also* Occlusion, artery, vertebral) 433.2
Arteriospasm 443.9
Arteriovenous —*see* condition
Arteritis 447.6
allergic (*see also* Angiitis, hypersensitivity) 446.20
aorta (nonsyphilitic) 447.6
syphilitic 093.1
aortic arch 446.7
brachiocephalica 446.7
brain 437.4
syphilitic 094.89
branchial 446.7
cerebral 437.4
late effect—*see* category 438
syphilitic 094.89
coronary (artery) —*see also* Arteriosclerosis, coronary
rheumatic 391.9
chronic 398.99
syphilitic 093.89
cranial (left) (right) 446.5
deformans—*see* Arteriosclerosis
giant cell 446.5
necrosing or necrotizing 446.0
nodosa 446.0
obliterans—*see also* Arteriosclerosis
subclaviocarotica 446.7
pulmonary 417.8
retina 362.18
rheumatic—*see* Fever, rheumatic
senile—*see* Arteriosclerosis
suppurative 447.2
syphilitic (general) 093.89
brain 094.89
coronary 093.89
spinal 094.89
temporal 446.5
young female, syndrome 446.7
Artery, arterial —*see* condition
Arthralgia (*see also* Pain, joint) 719.4
allergic (*see also* Pain, joint) 719.4
in caisson disease 993.3
Arthralgia—*continued*
psychogenic 307.89
rubella 056.71
Salmonella 003.23
temporomandibular joint 524.62
Arthritis, arthritic (acute) (chronic) (subacute) 716.9

NOTE—Use the following fifth-digit subclassification with categories 711-712, 715-716:

0 site unspecified
1 shoulder region
2 upper arm
3 forearm
4 hand
5 pelvic region and thigh
6 lower leg
7 ankle and foot
8 other specified sites
9 multiple sites

allergic 716.2
ankylosing (crippling) (spine) 720.0
sites other than spine 716.9
atrophic 714.0
spine 720.9
back (*see also* Arthritis, spine) 721.90
Bechterew's (ankylosing spondylitis) 720.0
blennorrhagic 098.50
cervical, cervicodorsal (*see also* Spondylosis, cervical) 721.0
Charcot's 094.0 *[713.5]*
diabetic 250.6 *[713.5]*
syringomyelic 336.0 *[713.5]*
tabetic 094.0 *[713.5]*
chylous (*see also* Filariasis) 125.9 *[711.7]*
climacteric NEC 716.3
coccyx 721.8
cricoarytenoid 478.79
crystal (-induced)—*see* Arthritis, due to crystals
deformans (*see also* Osteoarthrosis) 715.9
spine 721.90
with myelopathy 721.91
degenerative (*see also* Osteoarthrosis) 715.9
idiopathic 715.09
polyarticular 715.09
spine 721.90
with myelopathy 721.91
dermatoarthritis, lipoid 272.8 *[713.0]*
due to or associated with
acromegaly 253.0 *[713.0]*
actinomycosis 039.8 *[711.4]*
amyloidosis 277.3 *[713.7]*
bacterial disease NEC 040.89 *[711.4]*
Behçet's syndrome 136.1 *[711.2]*
blastomycosis 116.0 *[711.6]*
brucellosis (*see also* Brucellosis) 023.9 *[711.4]*
caisson disease 993.3
coccidioidomycosis 114.3 *[711.6]*
coliform (Escherichia coli) 711.0
colitis, ulcerative (*see also* Colitis, ulcerative) 556.9 *[713.1]*
cowpox 051.0 *[711.5]*
crystals NEC 275.4 *[712.9]*
dicalcium phosphate 275.4 *[712.1]*
pyrophosphate 275.4 *[712.2]*
specified NEC 275.4 *[712.8]*
dermatoarthritis, lipoid 272.8 *[713.0]*
dermatological disorder NEC 709.9 *[713.3]*

Arthritis, arthritic—*continued*
diabetes 250.6 *[713.5]*
diphtheria 032.89 *[711.4]*
dracontiasis 125.7 *[711.7]*
dysentery 009.0 *[711.3]*
endocrine disorder NEC 259.9 *[713.0]*
enteritis NEC 009.1 *[711.3]*
infectious (*see also* Enteritis, infectious) 009.0 *[711.3]*
specified organism NEC 008.8 *[711.3]*
regional (*see also* Enteritis, regional) 555.9 *[713.1]*
specified organism NEC 008.8 *[711.3]*
epiphyseal slip, nontraumatic (old) 716.8
erysipelas 035 *[711.4]*
erythema
epidemic 026.1
multiforme 695.1 *[713.3]*
nodosum 695.2 *[713.3]*
Escherichia coli 711.0
filariasis NEC 125.9 *[711.7]*
gastrointestinal condition NEC 569.9 *[713.1]*
glanders 024 *[711.4]*
Gonococcus 098.50
gout 274.0
H. influenzae 711.0
helminthiasis NEC 128.9 *[711.7]*
hematological disorder NEC 289.9 *[713.2]*
hemochromatosis 275.0 *[713.0]*
hemoglobinopathy NEC (*see also* Disease, hemoglobin) 282.7 *[713.2]*
hemophilia (*see also* Hemophilia) 286.0 *[713.2]*
Hemophilus influenzae (H. influenzae) 711.0
Henoch (-Schönlein) purpura 287.0 *[713.6]*
histoplasmosis NEC (*see also* Histoplasmosis) 115.99 *[711.6]*
hyperparathyroidism 252.0 *[713.0]*
hypersensitivity reaction NEC 995.3 *[713.6]*
hypogammaglobulinemia (*see also* Hypogammaglobulinemia) 279.00 *[713.0]*
hypothyroidism NEC 244.9 *[713.0]*
infection (*see also* Arthritis, infectious) 711.9
infectious disease NEC 136.9 *[711.8]*
leprosy (*see also* Leprosy) 030.9 *[711.4]*
leukemia NEC (M9800/3) 208.9 *[713.2]*
lipoid dermatoarthritis 272.8 *[713.0]*
Lyme disease 088.81 *[711.8]*
meaning Osteoarthritis—*see* Osteoarthrosis
Mediterranean fever, familial 277.3 *[713.7]*
meningococcal infection 036.82
metabolic disorder NEC 277.9 *[713.0]*
multiple myelomatosis (M9730/3) 203.0 *[713.2]*
mumps 072.79 *[711.5]*
mycobacteria 031.8 *[711.4]*
mycosis NEC 117.9 *[711.6]*
neurological disorder NEC 349.9 *[713.5]*
ochronosis 270.2 *[713.0]*
O'Nyong Nyong 066.3 *[711.5]*
parasitic disease NEC 136.9 *[711.8]*
paratyphoid fever (*see also* Fever, paratyphoid) 002.9 *[711.3]*
Pneumococcus 711.0
poliomyelitis (*see also* Poliomyelitis) 045.9 *[711.5]*
Pseudomonas 711.0
psoriasis 696.0
pyogenic organism (E. coli) (H. influenzae) (Pseudomonas) (Streptococcus) 711.0
rat-bite fever 026.1 *[711.4]*

Arthritis, arthritic—*continued*
regional enteritis (*see also* Enteritis, regional) 555.9 *[713.1]*
Reiter's disease 099.3 *[711.1]*
respiratory disorder NEC 519.9 *[713.4]*
reticulosis, malignant (M9720/3) 202.3 *[713.2]*
rubella 056.71
salmonellosis 003.23
sarcoidosis 135 *[713.7]*
serum sickness 999.5 *[713.6]*
Staphylococcus 711.0
Streptococcus 711.0
syphilis (*see also* Syphilis) 094.0 *[711.4]*
syringomyelia 336.0 *[713.5]*
thalassemia 282.4 *[713.2]*
tuberculosis (*see also* Tuberculosis, arthritis) 015.9 *[711.4]*
typhoid fever 002.0 *[711.3]*
ulcerative colitis (*see also* Colitis, ulcerative) 556.9 *[713.1]*
urethritis
nongonococcal (*see also* Urethritis, nongonococcal) 099.40 *[711.1]*
nonspecific (*see also* Urethritis, nongonococcal) 099.40 *[711.1]*
Reiter's 099.3 *[711.1]*
viral disease NEC 079.99 *[711.5]*
erythema epidemic 026.1
gonococcal 098.50
gouty (acute) 274.0
hypertrophic (*see also* Osteoarthrosis) 715.9
spine 721.90
with myelopathy 721.91
idiopathic, blennorrheal 099.3
in caisson disease 993.3 *[713.8]*
infectious or infective (acute) (chronic) (subacute) NEC 711.9
nonpyogenic 711.9
spine 720.9
inflammatory NEC 714.9
juvenile rheumatoid (chronic) (polyarticular) 714.30
acute 714.31
monoarticular 714.33
pauciarticular 714.32
lumbar (*see also* Spondylosis, lumbar) 721.3
meningococcal 036.82
menopausal NEC 716.3
migratory—*see* Fever, rheumatic
neuropathic (Charcot's) 094.0 *[713.5]*
diabetic 250.6 *[713.5]*
nonsyphilitic NEC 349.9 *[713.5]*
syringomyelic 336.0 *[713.5]*
tabetic 094.0 *[713.5]*
nodosa (*see also* Osteoarthrosis) 715.9
spine 721.90
with myelopathy 721.91
nonpyogenic NEC 716.9
spine 721.90
with myelopathy 721.91
ochronotic 270.2 *[713.0]*
palindromic (*see also* Rheumatism, palindromic) 719.3
pneumococcal 711.0
postdysenteric 009.0 *[711.3]*
postrheumatic, chronic (Jaccoud's) 714.4
primary progressive 714.0
spine 720.9
proliferative 714.0
spine 720.0

NOTE—Use the following fifth-digit subclassification with categories 711-712, 716:

0 site unspecified
1 shoulder region
2 upper arm
3 forearm
4 hand
5 pelvic region and thigh
6 lower leg
7 ankle and foot
8 other specified sites
9 multiple sites

Asphyxia, asphyxiation—*continued*
pressure 994.7
reticularis 782.61
strangulation 994.7
submersion 994.1
traumatic NEC—*see* Injury, internal, intrathoracic organs
vomiting, vomitus—*see* Asphyxia, food or foreign body
Aspiration
acid pulmonary (syndrome) 997.3
obstetric 668.0
amniotic fluid 770.1
bronchitis 507.0
contents of birth canal 770.1
fetal pneumonitis 770.1
food, foreign body, or gasoline (with asphyxiation)—*see* Asphyxia, food or foreign body
meconium 770.1
mucus 933.1
into
bronchus (main) 934.1
lung 934.8
respiratory tract 934.9
specified part NEC 934.8
trachea 934.0
newborn 770.1
vaginal (fetus or newborn) 770.1
newborn 770.1
pneumonia 507.0
pneumonitis 507.0
fetus or newborn 770.1
obstetric 668.0
syndrome of newborn (massive) (meconium) 770.1
vernix caseosa 770.1
Asplenia 759.0
with mesocardia 746.87
Assam fever 085.0
Assimilation, pelvis
with disproportion 653.2
affecting fetus or newborn 763.1
causing obstructed labor 660.1
affecting fetus or newborn 763.1
Assmann's focus (*see also* Tuberculosis) 011.0
Astasia (-abasia) 307.9
hysterical 300.11
Asteatosis 706.8
cutis 706.8
Astereognosis 780.9
Asterixis 781.3
in liver disease 572.8
Asteroid hyalitis 379.22
Asthenia, asthenic 780.7
cardiac (*see also* Failure, heart) 428.9
psychogenic 306.2
cardiovascular (*see also* Failure, heart) 428.9
psychogenic 306.2
heart (*see also* Failure, heart) 428.9
psychogenic 306.2
hysterical 300.11
myocardial (*see also* Failure, heart) 428.9
psychogenic 306.2
nervous 300.5
neurocirculatory 306.2
neurotic 300.5
psychogenic 300.5
psychoneurotic 300.5
psychophysiologic 300.5
reaction, psychoneurotic 300.5
Asthenia, asthenic—*continued*
senile 797
Stiller's 780.7
tropical anhidrotic 705.1
Asthenopia 368.13
accommodative 367.4
hysterical (muscular) 300.11
psychogenic 306.7
Asthenospermia 792.2
Asthma, asthmatic (bronchial) (catarrh) (spasmodic) 493.9

NOTE—Use the following fifth-digit subclassification with category 493:

0 without mention of status asthmaticus
1 with status asthmaticus

with
chronic obstructive pulmonary disease (COPD) 493.2
hay fever 493.0
rhinitis, allergic 493.0
allergic 493.9
stated cause (external allergen) 493.0
atopic 493.0
cardiac (*see also* Failure, ventricular, left) 428.1
cardiobronchial (*see also* Failure, ventricular, left) 428.1
cardiorenal (*see also* Hypertension, cardiorenal) 404.90
childhood 493.0
colliers' 500
croup 493.9
detergent 507.8
due to
detergent 507.8
inhalation of fumes 506.3
internal immunological process 493.0
endogenous (intrinsic) 493.1
eosinophilic 518.3
exogenous (cosmetics) (dander or dust) (drugs) (dust) (feathers) (food) (hay) (platinum) (pollen) 493.0
extrinsic 493.0
grinders' 502
hay 493.0
heart (*see also* Failure, ventricular, left) 428.1
IgE 493.0
infective 493.1
intrinsic 493.1
Kopp's 254.8
late-onset 493.1
meat-wrappers' 506.9
Millar's (laryngismus stridulus) 478.75
millstone makers' 502
miners' 500
Monday morning 504
New Orleans (epidemic) 493.0
platinum 493.0
pneumoconiotic (occupational) NEC 505
potters' 502
psychogenic 316 *[493.9]*
pulmonary eosinophilic 518.3
red cedar 495.8
Rostan's (*see also* Failure, ventricular, left) 428.1
sandblasters' 502
sequoiosis 495.8
stonemasons' 502
thymic 254.8

Atheroma, atheromatous—*continued*
heart, cardiac —*see* Arteriosclerosis, coronary
mitral (valve) 424.0
myocardium, myocardial —*see* Arteriosclerosis, coronary
pulmonary valve (heart) (*see also* Endocarditis, pulmonary) 424.3
skin 706.2
tricuspid (heart) (valve) 424.2
valve, valvular—*see* Endocarditis
vertebral (artery) (*see also* Occlusion, artery, vertebral) 433.2
Atheromatosis —*see also* Arteriosclerosis
arterial, congenital 272.8
Atherosclerosis —*see* Arteriosclerosis
Athetosis (acquired) 781.0
bilateral 333.7
congenital (bilateral) 333.7
double 333.7
unilateral 781.0
Athlete's
foot 110.4
heart 429.3
Athletic team examination V70.3
Athrepsia 261
Athyrea (acquired) (*see also* Hypothyroidism) 244.9
congenital 243
Athyreosis (congenital) 243
acquired—*see* Hypothyroidism
Athyroidism (acquired) (*see also* Hypothyroidism) 244.9
congenital 243
Atmospheric pyrexia 992.0
Atonia, atony, atonic
abdominal wall 728.2
bladder (sphincter) 596.4
neurogenic NEC 596.54
with cauda equina syndrome 344.61
capillary 448.9
cecum 564.8
psychogenic 306.4
colon 564.8
psychogenic 306.4
congenital 779.8
dyspepsia 536.3
psychogenic 306.4
intestine 564.8
psychogenic 306.4
stomach 536.3
neurotic or psychogenic 306.4
psychogenic 306.4
uterus 661.2
affecting fetus or newborn 763.7
vesical 596.4
Atopy NEC V15.0
Atransferrinemia, congenital 273.8
Atresia, atretic (congenital) 759.89
alimentary organ or tract NEC 751.8
lower 751.2
upper 750.8
ani, anus, anal (canal) 751.2
aorta 747.22
with hypoplasia of ascending aorta and defective development of left ventricle (with mitral valve atresia) 746.7
arch 747.11
ring 747.21
aortic (orifice) (valve) 746.89
arch 747.11

Atresia, atretic—*continued*
aqueduct of Sylvius 742.3
with spina bifida (*see also* Spina bifida) 741.0
artery NEC (*see also* Atresia, blood vessel) 747.60
cerebral 747.81
coronary 746.85
eye 743.58
pulmonary 747.3
umbilical 747.5
auditory canal (external) 744.02
bile, biliary duct (common) or passage 751.61
acquired (*see also* Obstruction, biliary) 576.2
bladder (neck) 753.6
blood vessel (peripheral) NEC 747.60
cerebral 747.81
gastrointestinal 747.61
lower limb 747.64
pulmonary artery 747.3
renal 747.62
spinal 747.82
upper limb 747.63
bronchus 748.3
canal, ear 744.02
cardiac
valve 746.89
aortic 746.89
mitral 746.89
pulmonary 746.01
tricuspid 746.1
cecum 751.2
cervix (acquired) 622.4
congenital 752.49
in pregnancy or childbirth 654.6
affecting fetus or newborn 763.8
causing obstructed labor 660.2
affecting fetus or newborn 763.1
choana 748.0
colon 751.2
cystic duct 751.61
acquired 575.8
with obstruction (*see also* Obstruction, gallbladder) 575.2
digestive organs NEC 751.8
duodenum 751.1
ear canal 744.02
ejaculatory duct 752.8
epiglottis 748.3
esophagus 750.3
Eustachian tube 744.24
fallopian tube (acquired) 628.2
congenital 752.19
follicular cyst 620.0
foramen of
Luschka 742.3
with spina bifida (*see also* Spina bifida) 741.0
Magendie 742.3
with spina bifida (*see also* Spina bifida) 741.0
gallbladder 751.69
genital organ
external
female 752.49
male 752.8
internal
female 752.8
male 752.8
glottis 748.3
gullet 750.3

Atresia, atretic—*continued*
heart
valve NEC 746.89
aortic 746.89
mitral 746.89
pulmonary 746.01
tricuspid 746.1
hymen 752.42
acquired 623.3
postinfective 623.3
ileum 751.1
intestine (small) 751.1
large 751.2
iris, filtration angle (*see also* Buphthalmia) 743.20
jejunum 751.1
kidney 753.3
lacrimal, apparatus 743.65
acquired—*see* Stenosis, lacrimal
larynx 748.3
ligament, broad 752.19
lung 748.5
meatus urinarius 753.6
mitral valve 746.89
with atresia or hypoplasia of aortic orifice or valve, with hypoplasia of ascending aorta and defective development of left ventricle 746.7
nares (anterior) (posterior) 748.0
nasolacrimal duct 743.65
nasopharynx 748.8
nose, nostril 748.0
acquired 738.0
organ or site NEC—*see* Anomaly, specified type NEC
osseous meatus (ear) 744.03
oviduct (acquired) 628.2
congenital 752.19
parotid duct 750.23
acquired 527.8
pulmonary (artery) 747.3
valve 746.01
vein 747.49
pulmonic 746.01
pupil 743.46
rectum 751.2
salivary duct or gland 750.23
acquired 527.8
sublingual duct 750.23
acquired 527.8
submaxillary duct or gland 750.23
acquired 527.8
trachea 748.3
tricuspid valve 746.1
ureter 753.2
ureteropelvic junction 753.2
ureterovesical orifice 753.2
urethra (valvular) 753.6
urinary tract NEC 753.2
uterus 752.3
acquired 621.8
vagina (acquired) 623.2
congenital 752.49
postgonococcal (old) 098.2
postinfectional 623.2
senile 623.2
vascular NEC (*see also* Atresia, blood vessel) 747.60
cerebral 747.81
vas deferens 752.8

Atresia, atretic—*continued*
vein NEC (*see also* Atresia, blood vessel) 747.60
cardiac 746.89
great 747.49
portal 747.49
pulmonary 747.49
vena cava (inferior) (superior) 747.49
vesicourethral orifice 753.6
vulva 752.49
acquired 624.8
Atrichia, atrichosis 704.00
congenital (universal) 757.4
Atrioventricularis commune 745.69
Atrophia —*see also* Atrophy
alba 709.09
cutis 701.8
idiopathica progressiva 701.8
senilis 701.8
dermatological, diffuse (idiopathic) 701.8
flava hepatis (acuta) (subacuta) (*see also* Necrosis, liver) 570
gyrata of choroid and retina (central) 363.54
generalized 363.57
senilis 797
dermatological 701.8
unguium 703.8
congenita 757.5
Atrophoderma, atrophodermia 701.9
diffusum (idiopathic) 701.8
maculatum 701.3
et striatum 701.3
due to syphilis 095.8
syphilitic 091.3
neuriticum 701.8
pigmentosum 757.33
reticulatum symmetricum faciei 701.8
senile 701.8
symmetrical 701.8
vermiculata 701.8
Atrophy, atrophic
adrenal (autoimmune) (capsule) (cortex) (gland) 255.4
with hypofunction 255.4
alveolar process or ridge (edentulous) 525.2
appendix 543.9
Aran-Duchenne muscular 335.21
arm 728.2
arteriosclerotic—*see* Arteriosclerosis
arthritis 714.0
spine 720.9
bile duct (any) 576.8
bladder 596.8
blanche (of Milian) 701.3
bone (senile) 733.99
due to
disuse 733.7
infection 733.99
tabes dorsalis (neurogenic) 094.0
posttraumatic 733.99
brain (cortex) (progressive) 331.9
with dementia 290.10
Alzheimer's 331.0
with dementia—*see* Alzheimer's dementia
circumscribed (Pick's) 331.1
with dementia 290.10
congenital 742.4
hereditary 331.9
senile 331.2

Atrophy, atrophic—*continued*
breast 611.4
puerperal, postpartum 676.3
buccal cavity 528.9
cardiac (brown) (senile) (*see also* Degeneration, myocardial) 429.1
cartilage (infectional) (joint) 733.99
cast, plaster of Paris 728.2
cerebellar—*see* Atrophy, brain
cerebral—*see* Atrophy, brain
cervix (endometrium) (mucosa) (myometrium) (senile) (uteri) 622.8
menopausal 627.8
Charcot-Marie-Tooth 356.1
choroid 363.40
diffuse secondary 363.42
hereditary (*see also* Dystrophy, choroid) 363.50
gyrate
central 363.54
diffuse 363.57
generalized 363.57
senile 363.41
ciliary body 364.57
colloid, degenerative 701.3
conjunctiva (senile) 372.8
corpus cavernosum 607.89
cortical (*see also* Atrophy, brain) 331.9
Cruveilhier's 335.21
cystic duct 576.8
dacryosialadenopathy 710.2
degenerative
colloid 701.3
senile 701.3
Déjérine-Thomas 333.0
diffuse idiopathic, dermatological 701.8
disuse
bone 733.7
muscle 728.2
Duchenne-Aran 335.21
ear 388.9
edentulous alveolar ridge 525.2
emphysema, lung 492.8
endometrium (senile) 621.8
cervix 622.8
enteric 569.89
epididymis 608.3
eyeball, cause unknown 360.41
eyelid (senile) 374.50
facial (skin) 701.9
facioscapulohumeral (Landouzy-Déjérine) 359.1
fallopian tube (senile), acquired 620.3
fatty, thymus (gland) 254.8
gallbladder 575.8
gastric 537.89
gastritis (chronic) 535.1
gastrointestinal 569.89
genital organ, male 608.89
glandular 289.3
globe (phthisis bulbi) 360.41
gum 523.2
hair 704.2
heart (brown) (senile) (*see also* Degeneration, myocardial) 429.1
hemifacial 754.0
Romberg 349.89
hydronephrosis 591
infantile 261
paralysis, acute (*see also* Poliomyelitis, with paralysis) 045.1

Atrophy, atrophic—*continued*
intestine 569.89
iris (generalized) (postinfectional) (sector shaped) 364.59
essential 364.51
progressive 364.51
sphincter 364.54
kidney (senile) (*see also* Sclerosis, renal) 587
with hypertension (*see also* Hypertension, kidney) 403.90
congenital 753.0
hydronephrotic 591
infantile 753.0
lacrimal apparatus (primary) 375.13
secondary 375.14
Landouzy-Déjérine 359.1
laryngitis, infection 476.0
larynx 478.79
Leber's optic 377.16
lip 528.5
liver (acute) (subacute) (*see also* Necrosis, liver) 570
chronic (yellow) 571.8
yellow (congenital) 570
with
abortion—*see* Abortion, by type, with specified complication NEC
ectopic pregnancy (*see also* categories 633.0-633.9) 639.8
molar pregnancy (*see also* categories 630-632) 639.8
chronic 571.8
complicating pregnancy 646.7
following
abortion 639.8
ectopic or molar pregnancy 639.8
from injection, inoculation or transfusion (onset within 8 months after administration)—*see* Hepatitis, viral
healed 571.5
obstetric 646.7
postabortal 639.8
postimmunization—*see* Hepatitis, viral
posttransfusion—*see* Hepatitis, viral
puerperal, postpartum 674.8
lung (senile) 518.89
congenital 748.69
macular (dermatological) 701.3
syphilitic, skin 091.3
striated 095.8
muscle, muscular 728.2
disuse 728.2
Duchenne-Aran 335.21
extremity (lower) (upper) 728.2
familial spinal 335.11
general 728.2
idiopathic 728.2
infantile spinal 335.0
myelopathic (progressive) 335.10
myotonic 359.2
neuritic 356.1
neuropathic (peroneal) (progressive) 356.1
peroneal 356.1
primary (idiopathic) 728.2
progressive (familial) (hereditary) (pure) 335.21
adult (spinal) 335.19
infantile (spinal) 335.0
juvenile (spinal) 335.11

Atrophy, atrophic—*continued*
spinal 335.10
adult 335.19
hereditary or familial 335.11
infantile 335.0
pseudohypertrophic 359.1
spinal (progressive) 335.10
adult 335.19
Aran-Duchenne 335.10
familial 335.11
hereditary 335.11
infantile 335.0
juvenile 335.11
syphilitic 095.6
myocardium (*see also* Degeneration, myocardial) 429.1
myometrium (senile) 621.8
cervix 622.8
myotatic 728.2
myotonia 359.2
nail 703.8
congenital 757.5
nasopharynx 472.2
nerve—*see also* Disorder, nerve
abducens 378.54
accessory 352.4
acoustic or auditory 388.5
cranial 352.9
first (olfactory) 352.0
second (optic) (*see also* Atrophy, optic nerve) 377.10
third (oculomotor) (partial) 378.51
total 378.52
fourth (trochlear) 378.53
fifth (trigeminal) 350.8
sixth (abducens) 378.54
seventh (facial) 351.8
eighth (auditory) 388.5
ninth (glossopharyngeal) 352.2
tenth (pneumogastric) (vagus) 352.3
eleventh (accessory) 352.4
twelfth (hypoglossal) 352.5
facial 351.8
glossopharyngeal 352.2
hypoglossal 352.5
oculomotor (partial) 378.51
total 378.52
olfactory 352.0
peripheral 355.9
pneumogastric 352.3
trigeminal 350.8
trochlear 378.53
vagus (pneumogastric) 352.3
nervous system, congenital 742.8
neuritic (*see also* Disorder, nerve) 355.9
neurogenic NEC 355.9
bone
tabetic 094.0
nutritional 261
old age 797
olivopontocerebellar 333.0
optic nerve (ascending) (descending) (infectional) (nonfamilial) (papillomacular bundle) (postretinal) (secondary NEC) (simple) 377.10
associated with retinal dystrophy 377.13
dominant hereditary 377.16
glaucomatous 377.14
hereditary (dominant) (Leber's) 377.16
Leber's (hereditary) 377.16
partial 377.15

Atrophy, atrophic—*continued*
postinflammatory 377.12
primary 377.11
syphilitic 094.84
congenital 090.49
tabes dorsalis 094.0
orbit 376.45
ovary (senile), acquired 620.3
oviduct (senile), acquired 620.3
palsy, diffuse 335.20
pancreas (duct) (senile) 577.8
papillary muscle 429.81
paralysis 355.9
parotid gland 527.0
patches skin 701.3
senile 701.8
penis 607.89
pharyngitis 472.1
pharynx 478.29
pluriglandular 258.8
polyarthritis 714.0
prostate 602.2
pseudohypertrophic 359.1
renal (*see also* Sclerosis, renal) 587
reticulata 701.8
retina (*see also* Degeneration, retina) 362.60
hereditary (*see also* Dystrophy, retina) 362.70
rhinitis 472.0
salivary duct or gland 527.0
scar NEC 709.2
sclerosis, lobar (of brain) 331.0
with dementia 290.10
scrotum 608.89
seminal vesicle 608.89
senile 797
degenerative, of skin 701.3
skin (patches) (senile) 701.8
spermatic cord 608.89
spinal (cord) 336.8
acute 336.8
muscular (chronic) 335.10
adult 335.19
familial 335.11
juvenile 335.10
paralysis 335.10
acute (*see also* Poliomyelitis, with paralysis) 045.1
spine (column) 733.99
spleen (senile) 289.59
spots (skin) 701.3
senile 701.8
stomach 537.89
striate and macular 701.3
syphilitic 095.8
subcutaneous 701.9
due to injection 999.9
sublingual gland 527.0
submaxillary gland 527.0
Sudeck's 733.7
suprarenal (autoimmune) (capsule) (gland) 255.4
with hypofunction 255.4
tarso-orbital fascia, congenital 743.66
testis 608.3
thenar, partial 354.0
throat 478.29
thymus (fat) 254.8
thyroid (gland) 246.8
with
cretinism 243
myxedema 244.9
congenital 243

Atrophy, atrophic—*continued*
tongue (senile) 529.8
papillae 529.4
smooth 529.4
trachea 519.1
tunica vaginalis 608.89
turbinate 733.99
tympanic membrane (nonflaccid) 384.82
flaccid 384.81
ulcer (*see also* Ulcer, skin) 707.9
upper respiratory tract 478.9
uterus, uterine (acquired) (senile) 621.8
cervix 622.8
due to radiation (intended effect) 621.8
vagina (senile) 627.3
vascular 459.89
vas deferens 608.89
vertebra (senile) 733.99
vulva (primary) (senile) 624.1
Werdnig-Hoffmann 335.0
yellow (acute) (congenital) (liver) (subacute) (*see also* Necrosis, liver) 570
chronic 571.8
resulting from administration of blood, plasma, serum, or other biological substance (within 8 months of administration)—*see* Hepatitis, viral
Attack
akinetic (*see also* Epilepsy) 345.0
angina—*see* Angina
apoplectic (*see also* Disease, cerebrovascular, acute) 436
benign shuddering 333.93
bilious—*see* Vomiting
cataleptic 300.11
cerebral (*see also* Disease, cerebrovascular, acute) 436
coronary (*see also* Infarct, myocardium) 410.9
cyanotic, newborn 770.8
epileptic (*see also* Epilepsy) 345.9
epileptiform 780.3
heart (*see also* Infarct, myocardium) 410.9
hemiplegia (*see also* Disease, cerebrovascular, acute) 436
hysterical 300.11
jacksonian (*see also* Epilepsy) 345.5
myocardium, myocardial (*see also* Infarct, myocardium) 410.9
myoclonic (*see also* Epilepsy) 345.1
panic 300.01
paralysis (*see also* Disease, cerebrovascular, acute) 436
paroxysmal 780.3
psychomotor (*see also* Epilepsy) 345.4
salaam (*see also* Epilepsy) 345.6
schizophreniform (*see also* Schizophrenia) 295.4
sensory and motor 780.3
syncope 780.2
toxic, cerebral 780.3
transient ischemic (TIA) 435.9
unconsciousness 780.2
hysterical 300.11
vasomotor 780.2
vasovagal (idiopathic) (paroxysmal) 780.2
Attention to
artificial
opening (of) V55.9
digestive tract NEC V55.4
specified site NEC V55.8
urinary tract NEC V55.6
vagina V55.7
Attention to—*continued*
colostomy V55.3
cystostomy V55.5
gastrostomy V55.1
ileostomy V55.2
jejunostomy V55.4
nephrostomy V55.6
surgical dressings V58.3
sutures V58.3
tracheostomy V55.0
ureterostomy V55.6
urethrostomy V55.6
Attrition
gum 523.2
teeth (excessive) (hard tissues) 521.1
Atypical —*see also* condition
distribution, vessel (congenital) (peripheral) NEC 747.60
endometrium 621.9
kidney 593.89
Atypism, cervix 622.1
Audible tinnitus (*see also* Tinnitus) 388.30
Auditory —*see* condition
Audry's syndrome (acropachyderma) 757.39
Aujeszky's disease 078.89
Aura, jacksonian (*see also* Epilepsy) 345.5
Aurantiasis, cutis 278.3
Auricle, auricular —*see* condition
Auriculotemporal syndrome 350.8
Australian
Q fever 083.0
X disease 062.4
Autism, autistic (child) (infantile) 299.0
Autodigestion 799.8
Autoerythrocyte sensitization 287.2
Autographism 708.3
Autoimmune
cold sensitivity 283.0
disease NEC 279.4
hemolytic anemia 283.0
thyroiditis 245.2
Autoinfection, septic —*see* Septicemia
Autointoxication 799.8
Automatism 348.8
epileptic (*see also* Epilepsy) 345.4
paroxysmal, idiopathic (*see also* Epilepsy) 345.4
Autonomic, autonomous
bladder 596.54
neurogenic 596.54
with cauda equine 344.61
faciocephalalgia (*see also* Neuropathy, peripheral, autonomic) 337.9
hysterical seizure 300.11
imbalance (*see also* Neuropathy, peripheral, autonomic) 337.9
Autophony 388.40
Autosensitivity, erythrocyte 287.2
Autotopagnosia 780.9
Autotoxemia 799.8
Autumn —*see* condition
Avellis' syndrome 344.89
Aviators
disease or sickness (*see* also Effect, adverse, high altitude) 993.2
ear 993.0
effort syndrome 306.2
Avitaminosis (multiple NEC) (*see also* Deficiency, vitamin) 269.2
A 264.9

Avitaminosis—*continued*
B 266.9
with
beriberi 265.0
pellagra 265.2
B_1 265.1
B_2 266.0
B_6 266.1
B_{12} 266.2
C (with scurvy) 267
D 268.9
with
osteomalacia 268.2
rickets 268.0
E 269.1
G 266.0
H 269.1
K 269.0
multiple 269.2
nicotinic acid 265.2
P 269.1
Avulsion (traumatic) 879.8
blood vessel—*see* Injury, blood vessel, by site
cartilage—*see also* Dislocation, by site
knee, current (*see also* Tear, meniscus) 836.2
symphyseal (inner), complicating delivery 665.6
complicated 879.9
diaphragm—*see* Injury, internal, diaphragm
ear—*see* Wound, open, ear
epiphysis of bone—*see* Fracture, by site
external site other than limb—*see* Wound, open, by site
eye 871.3
fingernail—*see* Wound, open, finger
fracture—*see* Fracture, by site
genital organs, external—*see* Wound, open, genital organs
head (intracranial) NEC—*see also* Injury, intracranial, with open intracranial wound
complete 874.9
external site NEC 873.8
complicated 873.9
internal organ or site—*see* Injury, internal, by site
joint—*see also* Dislocation, by site
capsule—*see* Sprain, by site
ligament—*see* Sprain, by site
limb—*see also* Amputation, traumatic, by site
skin and subcutaneous tissue—*see* Wound, open, by site
muscle—*see* Sprain, by site
nerve (root)—*see* Injury, nerve, by site
scalp—*see* Wound, open, scalp
skin and subcutaneous tissue—*see* Wound, open, by site
symphyseal cartilage (inner), complicating delivery 665.6
tendon—*see also* Sprain, by site
with open wound—*see* Wound, open, by site
toenail—*see* Wound, open, toe(s)
tooth 873.63
complicated 873.73
Awareness of heart beat 785.1
Axe grinders' disease 502
Axenfeld's anomaly or syndrome 743.44
Axilla, axillary —*see also* condition
breast 757.6
Axonotmesis —*see* Injury, nerve, by site
Ayala's disease 756.89
Ayerza's disease or syndrome (pulmonary artery sclerosis with pulmonary hypertension) 416.0
Azoospermia 606.0
Azotemia 790.6
meaning uremia (*see also* Uremia) 586
Aztec ear 744.29
Azygos lobe, lung (fissure) 748.69

B

Baader's syndrome (erythema multiforme exudativum) 695.1
Baastrup's syndrome 721.5
Babesiasis 088.82
Babesiosis 088.82
Babington's disease (familial hemorrhagic telangiectasia) 448.0
Babinski's syndrome (cardiovascular syphilis) 093.89
Babinski-Fröhlich syndrome (adiposogenital dystrophy) 253.8
Babinski-Nageotte syndrome 344.89
Bacillary —*see* condition
Bacilluria 599.0
- asymptomatic, in pregnancy or puerperium 646.5
- tuberculous (*see also* Tuberculosis) 016.9

Bacillus—*see also* **Infection, bacillus**
- abortus infection 023.1
- anthracis infection 022.9
- coli
  - infection 041.4
    - generalized 038.42
    - intestinal 008.00
  - pyemia 038.42
  - septicemia 038.42
- Flexner's 004.1
- fusiformis infestation 101
- mallei infection 024
- Shiga's 004.0
- suipestifer infection (*see also* Infection, Salmonella) 003.9

Back —*see* condition
Backache (postural) 724.5
- psychogenic 307.89
- sacroiliac 724.6

Backflow (pyelovenous) (*see also* Disease, renal) 593.9
Backknee (*see also* Genu, recurvatum) 736.5
Bacteremia (*see also* Infection, bacillus) 790.7
- with
  - sepsis—*see* Septicemia
- during
  - labor 659.3
  - pregnancy 647.8
- newborn 771.8

Bacteria
- in blood (*see also* Bacteremia) 790.7
- in urine (*see also* Bacteriuria) 599.0

Bacterial —*see* condition
Bactericholia (*see also* Cholecystitis, acute) 575.0
Bacterid, bacteride (Andrews' pustular) 686.8
Bacteriuria, bacteruria 791.9
- with
  - urinary tract infection 599.0
- asymptomatic 791.9
  - in pregnancy or puerperium 646.5
    - affecting fetus or newborn 760.1

Bad
- breath 784.9
- heart—*see* Disease, heart
- trip (*see also* Abuse, drugs, nondependent) 305.3

Baehr-Schiffrin disease (thrombotic thrombocytopenic purpura) 446.6
Baelz's disease (cheilitis glandularis apostematosa) 528.5
Baerensprung's disease (eczema marginatum) 110.3
Bagassosis (occupational) 495.1
Baghdad boil 085.1
Bagratuni's syndrome (temporal arteritis) 446.5
Baker's
- cyst (knee) 727.51
  - tuberculous (*see also* Tuberculosis) 015.2
- itch 692.89

Bakwin-Krida syndrome (craniometaphyseal dysplasia) 756.89
Balanitis (circinata) (gangraenosa) (infectious) (vulgaris) 607.1
- amebic 006.8
- candidal 112.2
- chlamydial 099.53
- due to Ducrey's bacillus 099.0
- erosiva circinata et gangraenosa 607.1
- gangrenous 607.1
- gonococcal (acute) 098.0
  - chronic or duration of 2 months or over 098.2
- nongonococcal 607.1
- phagedenic 607.1
- venereal NEC 099.8
- xerotica obliterans 607.81

Balanoposthitis 607.1
- chlamydial 099.53
- gonococcal (acute) 098.0
  - chronic or duration of 2 months or over 098.2
- ulcerative NEC 099.8

Balanorrhagia —*see* Balanitis
Balantidiasis 007.0
Balantidiosis 007.0
Balbuties, balbutio 307.0
Bald
- patches on scalp 704.00
- tongue 529.4

Baldness (*see also* Alopecia) 704.00
Balfour's disease (chloroma) 205.3
Balint's syndrome (psychic paralysis of visual fixation) 368.16
Balkan grippe 083.0
Ball
- food 938
- hair 938

Ballantyne (-Runge) syndrome (postmaturity) 766.2
Balloon disease (*see also* Effect, adverse, high altitude) 993.2
Ballooning posterior leaflet syndrome 424.0
Baló's disease or concentric sclerosis 341.1
Bamberger's disease (hypertrophic pulmonary osteoarthropathy) 731.2
Bamberger-Marie disease (hypertrophic pulmonary osteoarthropathy) 731.2
Bamboo spine 720.0
Bancroft's filariasis 125.0
Band(s)
- adhesive (*see also* Adhesions, peritoneum) 568.0
- amniotic 658.8
  - affecting fetus or newborn 762.8
- anomalous or congenital—*see also* Anomaly, specified type NEC
  - atrial 746.9
  - heart 746.9
  - intestine 751.4
  - omentum 751.4
  - ventricular 746.9
- cervix 622.3
- gallbladder (congenital) 751.69

Band(s)—*continued*
intestinal (adhesive) (*see also* Adhesions, peritoneum) 568.0
congenital 751.4
obstructive (*see also* Obstruction, intestine) 560.81
periappendiceal (congenital) 751.4
peritoneal (adhesive) (*see also* Adhesions, peritoneum) 568.0
with intestinal obstruction 560.81
congenital 751.4
uterus 621.5
vagina 623.2
Bandl's ring (contraction)
complicating delivery 661.4
affecting fetus or newborn 763.7
Bang's disease (Brucella abortus) 023.1
Bangkok hemorrhagic fever 065.4
Bannister's disease 995.1
Bantam-Albright-Martin disease (pseudohypoparathyroidism) 275.4
Banti's disease or syndrome (with cirrhosis) (with portal hypertension)—*see* Cirrhosis, liver
Bar
calcaneocuboid 755.67
calcaneonavicular 755.67
cubonavicular 755.67
prostate 600
talocalcaneal 755.67
Baragnosis 780.9
Barasheh, barashek 266.2
Barcoo disease or rot (*see also* Ulcer, skin) 707.9
Bard-Pic syndrome (carcinoma, head of pancreas) 157.0
Bärensprung's disease (eczema marginatum) 110.3
Baritosis 503
Barium lung disease 503
Barlow's syndrome (meaning mitral valve prolapse) 424.0
Barlow (-Möller) disease or syndrome (meaning infantile scurvy) 267
Barodontalgia 993.2
Baron Münchausen syndrome 301.51
Barosinusitis 993.1
Barotitis 993.0
Barotrauma 993.2
odontalgia 993.2
otitic 993.0
sinus 993.1
Barraquer's disease or syndrome (progressive lipodystrophy) 272.6
Barré-Guillain syndrome 357.0
Barré-Liéou syndrome (posterior cervical sympathetic) 723.2
Barrel chest 738.3
Barrett's syndrome or ulcer (chronic peptic ulcer of esophagus) 530.2
Bársony-Polgár syndrome (corkscrew esophagus) 530.5
Bársony-Teschendorf syndrome (corkscrew esophagus) 530.5
Bartholin's
adenitis (*see also* Bartholinitis) 616.8
gland—*see* condition
Bartholinitis (suppurating) 616.8
gonococcal (acute) 098.0
chronic or duration of 2 months or over 098.2
Bartonellosis 088.0
Bartter's syndrome (secondary hyperaldosteronism with juxtaglomerular hyperplasia) 255.1
Basal—*see* condition
Basan's (hidrotic) ectodermal dysplasia 757.31
Baseball finger 842.13
Basedow's disease or syndrome (exophthalmic goiter) 242.0
Basic —*see* condition
Basilar —*see* condition
Bason's (hidrotic) ectodermal dysplasia 757.31
Basopenia 288.0
Basophilia 288.8
Basophilism (corticoadrenal) (Cushing's) (pituitary) (thymic) 255.0
Bassen-Kornzweig syndrome (abetalipoproteinemia) 272.5
Bat ear 744.29
Bateman's
disease 078.0
purpura (senile) 287.2
Bathing cramp 994.1
Bathophobia 300.23
Batten's disease, retina 330.1 *[362.71]*
Batten-Mayou disease 330.1 *[362.71]*
Batten-Steinert syndrome 359.2
Battered
adult (syndrome) 995.81
baby or child (syndrome) 995.5
affecting parent or family V61.21
as reason for family seeking advice V61.21
specified person other than child 995.81
spouse (syndrome) 995.81
Battey mycobacterium infection 031.0
Battledore placenta —*see* Placenta, abnormal
Battle exhaustion (*see also* Reaction, stress, acute) 308.9
Baumgarten-Cruveilhier (cirrhosis) disease, or syndrome 571.5
Bauxite
fibrosis (of lung) 503
workers' disease 503
Bayle's disease (dementia paralytica) 094.1
Bazin's disease (primary) (*see also* Tuberculosis) 017.1
Beach ear 380.12
Beaded hair (congenital) 757.4
Beard's disease (neurasthenia) 300.5
Bearn-Kunkel (-Slater) syndrome (lupoid hepatitis) 571.49
Beat
elbow 727.2
hand 727.2
knee 727.2
Beats
ectopic 427.60
escaped, heart 427.60
postoperative 997.1
premature (nodal) 427.60
atrial 427.61
auricular 427.61
postoperative 997.1
specified type NEC 427.69
supraventricular 427.61
ventricular 427.69
Beau's
disease or syndrome (*see also* Degeneration, myocardial) 429.1
lines (transverse furrows on fingernails) 703.8
Bechterew's disease (ankylosing spondylitis) 720.0

Bechterew-Strümpell-Marie syndrome (ankylosing spondylitis) 720.0
Beck's syndrome (anterior spinal artery occlusion) 433.8
Becker's
disease (idiopathic mural endomyocardial disease) 425.2
dystrophy 359.1
Beckwith (-Wiedemann) syndrome 759.89
Bedclothes, asphyxiation or suffocation by 994.7
Bednar's aphthae 528.2
Bedsore 707.0
with gangrene 707.0 *[785.4]*
Bedwetting (*see also* Enuresis) 788.36
Beer-drinkers' heart (disease) 425.5
Bee sting (with allergic or anaphylactic shock) 989.5
Begbie's disease (exophthalmic goiter) 242.0
Behavior disorder, disturbance *—see also* Disturbance, conduct
antisocial, without manifest psychiatric disorder
adolescent V71.02
adult V71.01
child V71.02
dyssocial, without manifest psychiatric disorder
adolescent V71.02
adult V71.01
child V71.02
high-risk—*see* Problem
Behçet's syndrome 136.1
Behr's disease 362.50
Beigel's disease or morbus (white piedra) 111.2
Bejel 104.0
Bekhterev's disease (ankylosing spondylitis) 720.0
Bekhterev-Strümpell-Marie syndrome (ankylosing spondylitis) 720.0
Belching (*see also* Eructation) 787.3
Bell's
disease (*see also* Psychosis, affective) 296.0
mania (*see also* Psychosis, affective) 296.0
palsy, paralysis 351.0
infant 767.5
newborn 767.5
syphilitic 094.89
spasm 351.0
Bence-Jones albuminuria, albuminosuria, or proteinuria 791.0
Bends 993.3
Benedikt's syndrome (paralysis) 344.89
Benign *—see also* condition
prostate
hyperplasia 600
neoplasm 222.2
Bennett's
disease (leukemia) 208.9
fracture (closed) 815.01
open 815.11
Benson's disease 379.22
Bent
back (hysterical) 300.11
nose 738.0
congenital 754.0
Bereavement V62.82
as adjustment reaction 309.0
Berger's paresthesia (lower limb) 782.0
Bergeron's disease (hysteroepilepsy) 300.11
Beriberi (acute) (atrophic) (chronic) (dry) (subacute) (wet) 265.0
with polyneuropathy 265.0 *[357.4]*
heart (disease) 265.0 *[425.7]*
Beriberi—*continued*
leprosy 030.1
neuritis 265.0 *[357.4]*
Berlin's disease or edema (traumatic) 921.3
Berloque dermatitis 692.72
Bernard-Horner syndrome (*see also* Neuropathy, peripheral, autonomic) 337.9
Bernard-Sergent syndrome (acute adrenocortical insufficiency) 255.4
Bernard-Soulier disease or thrombopathy 287.1
Bernhardt's disease or paresthesia 355.1
Bernhardt-Roth disease or syndrome (paresthesia) 355.1
Bernheim's syndrome (*see also* Failure, heart, congestive) 428.0
Bertielliasis 123.8
Bertolotti's syndrome (sacralization of fifth lumbar vertebra) 756.15
Beryllíosis (acute) (chronic) (lung) (occupational) 503
Besnier's
lupus pernio 135
prurigo (atopic dermatitis) (infantile eczema) 691.8
Besnier-Boeck disease or sarcoid 135
Besnier-Boeck-Schaumann disease (sarcoidosis) 135
Best's disease 362.76
Bestiality 302.1
Beta-adrenergic hyperdynamic circulatory state 429.82
Beta-aminoisobutyric aciduria 277.2
Beta-mercaptolactate-cysteine disulfiduria 270.0
Beta thalassemia (major) (minor) (mixed) 282.4
Beurmann's disease (sporotrichosis) 117.1
Bezoar 938
intestine 936
stomach 935.2
Bezold's abscess (*see also* Mastoiditis) 383.01
Bianchi's syndrome (aphasia-apraxia-alexia) 784.69
Bicornuate or bicornis uterus 752.3
in pregnancy or childbirth 654.0
with obstructed labor 660.2
affecting fetus or newborn 763.1
affecting fetus or newborn 763.8
Bicuspid aortic valve 746.4
Biedl-Bardet syndrome 759.89
Bielschowsky's disease 330.1
Bielschowsky-Jansky
amaurotic familial idiocy 330.1
disease 330.1
Biemond's syndrome (obesity, polydactyly, and mental retardation) 759.89
Biermer's anemia or disease (pernicious anemia) 281.0
Biett's disease 695.4
Bifid (congenital)—*see also* Imperfect, closure
apex, heart 746.89
clitoris 752.49
epiglottis 748.3
kidney 753.3
nose 748.1
patella 755.64
scrotum 752.8
toe 755.66
tongue 750.13
ureter 753.4

Bifid—*continued*
uterus 752.3
uvula 749.02
with cleft lip (*see also* Cleft, palate, with cleft lip) 749.20
Biforis uterus (suprasimplex) 752.3
Bifurcation (congenital)—*see also* Imperfect, closure
gallbladder 751.69
kidney pelvis 753.3
renal pelvis 753.3
rib 756.3
tongue 750.13
trachea 748.3
ureter 753.4
urethra 753.8
uvula 749.02
with cleft lip (*see also* Cleft, palate, with cleft lip) 749.20
vertebra 756.19
Bigeminal pulse 427.89
Bigeminy 427.89
Big spleen syndrome 289.4
Bilateral —*see* condition
Bile duct —*see* condition
Bile pigments in urine 791.4
Bilharziasis (*see also* Schistosomiasis) 120.9
chyluria 120.0
cutaneous 120.3
galacturia 120.0
hematochyluria 120.0
intestinal 120.1
lipemia 120.9
lipuria 120.0
Oriental 120.2
piarhemia 120.9
pulmonary 120.2
tropical hematuria 120.0
vesical 120.0
Biliary —*see* condition
Bilious (attack)—*see also* Vomiting
fever, hemoglobinuric 084.8
Bilirubinuria 791.4
Biliuria 791.4
Billroth's disease
meningocele (*see also* Spina bifida) 741.9
Bilobate placenta —*see* Placenta, abnormal
Bilocular
heart 745.7
stomach 536.8
Bing-Horton syndrome (histamine cephalgia) 346.2
Binswanger's disease or dementia 290.12
Biörck (-Thorson) syndrome (malignant carcinoid) 259.2
Biparta, bipartite —*see also* Imperfect, closure
carpal scaphoid 755.59
patella 755.64
placenta—*see* Placenta, abnormal
vagina 752.49
Bird
face 756.0
fanciers' lung or disease 495.2
Bird's disease (oxaluria) 271.8
Birth
abnormal fetus or newborn 763.9
accident, fetus or newborn—*see* Birth, injury
complications in mother—*see* Delivery, complicated
compression during NEC 767.9

Birth—*continued*
defect—*see* Anomaly
delayed, fetus 763.9
difficult NEC, affecting fetus or newborn 763.9
dry, affecting fetus or newborn 761.1
forced, NEC, affecting fetus or newborn 763.8
forceps, affecting fetus or newborn 763.2
hematoma of sternomastoid 767.8
immature 765.1
extremely 765.0
inattention, after or at 995.5
affecting parent or family V61.21
induced, affecting fetus or newborn 763.8
infant—*see* Newborn
injury NEC 767.9
adrenal gland 767.8
basal ganglia 767.0
brachial plexus (paralysis) 767.6
brain (compression) (pressure) 767.0
cerebellum 767.0
cerebral hemorrhage 767.0
conjunctiva 767.8
eye 767.8
fracture
bone, any except clavicle or spine 767.3
clavicle 767.2
femur 767.3
humerus 767.3
long bone 767.3
radius and ulna 767.3
skeleton NEC 767.3
skull 767.3
spine 767.4
tibia and fibula 767.3
hematoma 767.8
liver (subcapsular) 767.8
mastoid 767.8
skull 767.1
sternomastoid 767.8
testes 767.8
vulva 767.8
intracranial (edema) 767.0
laceration
brain 767.0
by scalpel 767.8
peripheral nerve 767.7
liver 767.8
meninges
brain 767.0
spinal cord 767.4
nerves (cranial, peripheral) 767.7
brachial plexus 767.6
facial 767.5
paralysis 767.7
brachial plexus 767.6
Erb (-Duchenne) 767.6
facial nerve 767.5
Klumpke (-Déjérine) 767.6
radial nerve 767.6
spinal (cord) (hemorrhage) (laceration) (rupture) 767.4
rupture
intracranial 767.0
liver 767.8
spinal cord 767.4
spleen 767.8
viscera 767.8
scalp 767.1
scalpel wound 767.8
skeleton NEC 767.3

Birth—*continued*
specified NEC 767.8
spinal cord 767.4
spleen 767.8
subdural hemorrhage 767.0
tentorial, tear 767.0
testes 767.8
vulva 767.8
instrumental, NEC, affecting fetus or newborn 763.2
lack of care, after or at 995.5
affecting parent or family V61.21
multiple
affected by maternal complications of pregnancy 761.5
healthy liveborn—*see* Newborn, multiple
neglect, after or at 995.5
affecting parent or family V61.21
newborn—*see* Newborn
palsy or paralysis NEC 767.7
precipitate, fetus or newborn 763.6
premature (infant) 765.1
prolonged, affecting fetus or newborn 763.9
retarded, fetus or newborn 763.9
shock, newborn 779.8
strangulation or suffocation
due to aspiration of amniotic fluid 770.1
mechanical 767.8
trauma NEC 767.9
triplet
affected by maternal complications of pregnancy 761.5
healthy liveborn—*see* Newborn, multiple
twin
affected by maternal complications of pregnancy 761.5
healthy liveborn—*see* Newborn, twin
ventouse, affecting fetus or newborn 763.3
Birthmark 757.32
Bisalbuminemia 273.8
Biskra button 085.1
Bite (s)
with intact skin surface—*see* Contusion
animal—*see* Wound, open, by site
intact skin surface—*see* Contusion
centipede 989.5
chigger 133.8
fire ant 989.5
flea—*see* Injury, superficial, by site
human (open wound)—*see also* Wound, open, by site
intact skin surface—*see* Contusion
insect
nonvenomous—*see* Injury, superficial, by site
venomous 989.5
mad dog (death from) 071
poisonous 989.5
red bug 133.8
reptile 989.5
nonvenomous—*see* Wound, open, by site
snake 989.5
nonvenomous—*see* Wound, open, by site
spider (venomous) 989.5
nonvenomous—*see* Injury, superficial, by site
venomous 989.5
Biting
cheek or lip 528.9
nail 307.9
Black
death 020.9
eye NEC 921.0
hairy tongue 529.3
lung disease 500
Blackfan-Diamond anemia or syndrome (congenital hypoplastic anemia) 284.0
Blackhead 706.1
Blackout 780.2
Blackwater fever 084.8
Bladder —*see* condition
Blast
blindness 921.3
concussion—*see* Blast, injury
injury 869.0
with open wound into cavity 869.1
abdomen or thorax—*see* Injury, internal, by site
brain (*see also* Concussion, brain) 850.9
with skull fracture—*see* Fracture, skull
ear (acoustic nerve trauma) 951.5
with perforation, tympanic membrane—*see* Wound, open, ear, drum
lung (*see also* Injury, internal, lung) 861.20
otitic (explosive) 388.11
Blastomycosis, blastomycotic (chronic) (cutaneous) (disseminated) (lung) (pulmonary) (systemic) 116.0
Brazilian 116.1
European 117.5
keloidal 116.2
North American 116.0
primary pulmonary 116.0
South American 116.1
Bleb(s) 709.8
emphysematous (bullous) (diffuse) (lung) (ruptured) (solitary) 492.0
filtering, eye (postglaucoma) (status) V45.6
with complication 997.99
postcataract extraction (complication) 997.99
lung (ruptured) 492.0
congenital 770.5
subpleural (emphysematous) 492.0
Bleeder (familial) (hereditary) (*see also* Defect, coagulation) 286.9
nonfamilial 286.9
Bleeding (*see also* Hemorrhage) 459.0
anal 569.3
anovulatory 628.0
atonic, following delivery 666.1
capillary 448.9
due to subinvolution 621.1
puerperal 666.2
ear 388.69
excessive, associated with menopausal onset 627.0
familial (*see also* Defect, coagulation) 286.9
following intercourse 626.7
gastrointestinal 578.9
gums 523.8
hemorrhoids—*see* Hemorrhoids, bleeding
intermenstrual
irregular 626.6
regular 626.5
intraoperative 998.1
irregular NEC 626.4
menopausal 627.0
mouth 528.9
nipple 611.79

Blindness—*continued*
night 368.60
acquired 368.62
congenital (Japanese) 368.61
hereditary 368.61
specified type NEC 368.69
vitamin A deficiency 264.5
nocturnal—*see* Blindness, night
one eye 369.60
with low vision of other eye 369.10
profound
both eyes 369.08
with impairment of lesser eye (specified as)
blind, not further specified 369.05
near-total 369.07
total 369.06
one eye 369.67
with vision of other eye (specified as)
near-normal 369.68
normal 369.69
psychic 784.69
severe
both eyes 369.22
with impairment of lesser eye (specified as)
blind, not further specified 369.11
low vision, not further specified 369.21
near-total 369.13
profound 369.14
total 369.12
one eye 369.71
with vision of other eye (specified as)
near-normal 369.72
normal 369.73
snow 370.24
sun 363.31
temporary 368.12
total
both eyes 369.01
one eye 369.61
with vision of other eye (specified as)
near-normal 369.62
normal 369.63
transient 368.12
traumatic NEC 950.9
word (developmental) 315.01
acquired 784.61
secondary to organic lesion 784.61
Blister —*see also* Injury, superficial, by site
beetle dermatitis 692.89
due to burn—*see* Burn, by site, second degree
fever 054.9
multiple, skin, nontraumatic 709.8
Bloating 787.3
Bloch-Siemens syndrome (incontinentia pigmenti) 757.33
Bloch-Stauffer dyshormonal dermatosis 757.33
Bloch-Sulzberger disease or syndrome (incontinentia pigmenti) (melanoblastosis) 757.33
Block
alveolar capillary 516.3
arborization (heart) 426.6
arrhythmic 426.9
atrioventricular (AV) (incomplete) (partial) 426.10
with
2:1 atrioventricular response block 426.13
atrioventricular dissociation 426.0
first degree (incomplete) 426.11
second degree (Mobitz type I) 426.13
Mobitz (type) II 426.12
Block—*continued*
third degree 426.0
complete 426.0
congenital 746.86
congenital 746.86
Mobitz (incomplete)
type I (Wenckebach's) 426.13
type II 426.12
partial 426.13
auriculoventricular (*see also* Block, atrioventricular) 426.10
complete 426.0
congenital 746.86
congenital 746.86
bifascicular (cardiac) 426.53
bundle branch (complete) (false) (incomplete) 426.50
bilateral 426.53
left (complete) (main stem) 426.3
with right bundle branch block 426.53
anterior fascicular 426.2
with
posterior fascicular block 426.3
right bundle branch block 426.52
hemiblock 426.2
incomplete 426.2
with right bundle branch block 426.53
posterior fascicular 426.2
with
anterior fascicular block 426.3
right bundle branch block 426.51
right 426.4
with
left bundle branch block (incomplete) (main stem) 426.53
left fascicular block 426.53
anterior 426.52
posterior 426.51
Wilson's type 426.4
cardiac 426.9
conduction 426.9
complete 426.0
Eustachian tube (*see also* Obstruction, Eustachian tube) 381.60
fascicular (left anterior) (left posterior) 426.2
foramen Magendie (acquired) 331.3
congenital 742.3
with spina bifida (*see also* Spina bifida) 741.0
heart 426.9
first degree (atrioventricular) 426.11
second degree (atrioventricular) 426.13
third degree (atrioventricular) 426.0
bundle branch (complete) (false) (incomplete) 426.50
bilateral 426.53
left (*see also* Block, bundle branch, left) 426.3
right (*see also* Block, bundle branch, right) 426.4
complete (atrioventricular) 426.0
congenital 746.86
incomplete 426.13
intra-atrial 426.6
intraventricular NEC 426.6
sinoatrial 426.6
specified type NEC 426.6
hepatic vein 453.0
intraventricular (diffuse) (myofibrillar) 426.6

Block—*continued*
bundle branch (complete) (false) (incomplete) 426.50
bilateral 426.53
left (*see also* Block, bundle branch, left) 426.3
right (*see also* Block, bundle branch, right) 426.4
kidney (*see also* Disease, renal) 593.9
postcystoscopic 997.5
myocardial (*see also* Block, heart) 426.9
nodal 426.10
optic nerve 377.49
organ or site (congenital) NEC—*see* Atresia
parietal 426.6
peri-infarction 426.6
portal (vein) 452
sinoatrial 426.6
sinoauricular 426.6
spinal cord 336.9
trifascicular 426.54
tubal 628.2
vein NEC 453.9
Blocq's disease or syndrome (astasia-abasia) 307.9
Blood
constituents, abnormal NEC 790.6
disease 289.9
specified NEC 289.8
donor V59.01
stem cells V59.02
dyscrasia 289.9
with
abortion—*see* Abortion, by type, with hemorrhage, delayed or excessive
ectopic pregnancy (*see also* categories 633.0-633.9) 639.1
molar pregnancy (*see also* categories 630-632) 639.1
fetus or newborn NEC 776.9
following
abortion 639.1
ectopic or molar pregnancy 639.1
puerperal, postpartum 666.3
flukes NEC (*see also* Infestation, Schistosoma) 120.9
in
feces (*see also* Melena) 578.1
occult 792.1
urine (*see also* Hematuria) 599.7
mole 631
occult 792.1
poisoning (*see also* Septicemia) 038.9
pressure
decreased, due to shock following injury 958.4
fluctuating 796.4
high (*see also* Hypertension) 401.9
incidental reading (isolated) (nonspecific), without diagnosis of hypertension 796.2
low (*see also* Hypotension) 458.9
incidental reading (isolated) (nonspecific), without diagnosis of hypotension 796.3
spitting (*see also* Hemoptysis) 786.3
staining cornea 371.12
transfusion
without reported diagnosis V58.2
donor V59.01
stem cells V59.02
reaction or complication—*see* Complications, transfusion
tumor—*see* Hematoma

Blood—*continued*
vessel rupture—*see* Hemorrhage
vomiting (*see also* Hematemesis) 578.0
Blood-forming organ disease 289.9
Bloodgood's disease 610.1
Bloodshot eye 379.93
Bloom (-Machacek) (-Torre) syndrome 757.39
Blotch, palpebral 372.55
Blount's disease (tibia vara) 732.4
Blount-Barber syndrome (tibia vara) 732.4
Blue
baby 746.9
bloater 491.20
with acute bronchitis or exacerbation 491.21
diaper syndrome 270.0
disease 746.9
dome cyst 610.0
drum syndrome 381.02
sclera 743.47
with fragility of bone and deafness 756.51
toe syndrome—*see* Atherosclerosis
Blueness (*see also* Cyanosis) 782.5
Blurring, visual 368.8
Blushing (abnormal) (excessive) 782.62
Boarder, hospital V65.0
infant V65.0
Bockhart's impetigo (superficial folliculitis) 704.8
Bodechtel-Guttmann disease (subacute sclerosing panencephalitis) 046.2
Boder-Sedgwick syndrome (ataxia-telangiectasia) 334.8
Body, bodies
Aschoff (*see also* Myocarditis, rheumatic) 398.0
asteroid, vitreous 379.22
choroid, colloid (degenerative) 362.57
hereditary 362.77
cytoid (retina) 362.82
drusen (retina) (*see also* Drusen) 362.57
optic disc 377.21
fibrin, pleura 511.0
foreign—*see* Foreign body
Hassall-Henle 371.41
loose
joint (*see also* Loose, body, joint) 718.1
knee 717.6
knee 717.6
sheath, tendon 727.82
Mallory's 034.1
Mooser 081.0
Negri 071
rice (joint) (*see also* Loose, body, joint) 718.1
knee 717.6
rocking 307.3
Boeck's
disease (sarcoidosis) 135
lupoid (miliary) 135
sarcoid 135
Boerhaave's syndrome (spontaneous esophageal rupture) 530.4
Boggy
cervix 622.8
uterus 621.8
Boil (*see also* Carbuncle) 680.9
abdominal wall 680.2
Aleppo 085.1
ankle 680.6
anus 680.5
arm (any part, above wrist) 680.3
auditory canal, external 680.0
axilla 680.3

Boil *—continued*
back (any part) 680.2
Baghdad 085.1
breast 680.2
buttock 680.5
chest wall 680.2
corpus cavernosum 607.2
Delhi 085.1
ear (any part) 680.0
eyelid 373.13
face (any part, except eye) 680.0
finger (any) 680.4
flank 680.2
foot (any part) 680.7
forearm 680.3
Gafsa 085.1
genital organ, male 608.4
gluteal (region) 680.5
groin 680.2
hand (any part) 680.4
head (any part, except face) 680.8
heel 680.7
hip 680.6
knee 680.6
labia 616.4
lacrimal (*see also* Dacryocystitis) 375.30
gland (*see also* Dacryoadenitis) 375.00
passages (duct) (sac) (*see also* Dacryocystitis) 375.30
leg, any part except foot 680.6
multiple sites 680.9
Natal 085.1
neck 680.1
nose (external) (septum) 680.0
orbit, orbital 376.01
partes posteriores 680.5
pectoral region 680.2
penis 607.2
perineum 680.2
pinna 680.0
scalp (any part) 680.8
scrotum 608.4
seminal vesicle 608.0
shoulder 680.3
skin NEC 680.9
specified site NEC 680.8
spermatic cord 608.4
temple (region) 680.0
testis 608.4
thigh 680.6
thumb 680.4
toe (any) 680.7
tropical 085.1
trunk 680.2
tunica vaginalis 608.4
umbilicus 680.2
upper arm 680.3
vas deferens 608.4
vulva 616.4
wrist 680.4
Bold hives (*see also* Urticaria) 708.9
Bolivian hemorrhagic fever 078.7
Bombé, iris 364.74
Bomford-Rhoads anemia (refractory) 284.9
Bone *—see* condition
Bonnevie-Ullrich syndrome 758.6
Bonnier's syndrome 386.19
Bonvale Dam fever 780.7
Bony block of joint 718.80
ankle 718.87
elbow 718.82
Bony block of joint*—continued*
foot 718.87
hand 718.84
hip 718.85
knee 718.86
multiple sites 718.89
pelvic region 718.85
shoulder (region) 718.81
specified site NEC 718.88
wrist 718.83
Borderline
intellectual functioning V62.89
pelvis 653.1
with obstruction during labor 660.1
affecting fetus or newborn 763.1
psychosis (*see also* Schizophrenia) 295.5
of childhood (*see also* Psychosis, childhood) 299.8
schizophrenia (*see also* Schizophrenia) 295.5
Borna disease 062.9
Bornholm disease (epidemic pleurodynia) 074.1
Borrelia vincentii (mouth) (pharynx) (tonsils) 101
Bostock's catarrh (*see also* Fever, hay) 477.9
Boston exanthem 048
Botalli, ductus (patent) (persistent) 747.0
Bothriocephalus latus infestation 123.4
Botulism 005.1
Bouba (*see also* Yaws) 102.9
Bouffée délirante 298.3
Bouillaud's disease or syndrome (rheumatic heart disease) 391.9
Bourneville's disease (tuberous sclerosis) 759.5
Boutonneuse fever 082.1
Boutonniere
deformity (finger) 736.21
hand (intrinsic) 736.21
Bouveret (-Hoffmann) disease or syndrome (paroxysmal tachycardia) 427.2
Bovine heart *—see* Hypertrophy, cardiac
Bowel *—see* condition
Bowen's
dermatosis (precancerous) (M8081/2)*—see* Neoplasm, skin, in situ
disease (M8081/2)*—see* Neoplasm, skin, in situ
epithelioma (M8081/2)*—see* Neoplasm, skin, in situ
type
epidermoid carcinoma in situ (M8081/2)*—see* Neoplasm, skin, in situ
intraepidermal squamous cell carcinoma (M8081/2)*-see* Neoplasm, skin, in situ
Bowing
femur 736.89
congenital 754.42
fibula 736.89
congenital 754.43
forearm 736.09
away from midline (cubitus valgus) 736.01
toward midline (cubitus varus) 736.02
leg(s), long bones, congenital 754.44
radius 736.09
away from midline (cubitus valgus) 736.01
toward midline (cubitus varus) 736.02
tibia 736.89
congenital 754.43
Bowleg (s) 736.42
congenital 754.44
rachitic 268.1
Boyd's dysentery 004.2
Brachial *—see* condition

Brodie's
abscess (localized) (chronic) (*see also* Osteomyelitis) 730.1
disease (joint) (*see also* Osteomyelitis) 730.1
Broken
arches 734
congenital 755.67
back—*see* Fracture, vertebra, by site
bone—*see* Fracture, by site
compensation—*see* Disease, heart
implant or internal device—*see* listing under Complications, mechanical
neck—*see* Fracture, vertebra, cervical
nose 802.0
open 802.1
tooth, teeth 873.63
complicated 873.73
Bromhidrosis 705.89
Bromidism, bromism
acute 967.3
correct substance properly administered 349.82
overdose or wrong substance given or taken 967.3
chronic (*see also* Dependence) 304.1
Bromidrosiphobia 300.23
Bromidrosis 705.89
Bronchi, bronchial —*see* condition
Bronchiectasis (cylindrical) (diffuse) (fusiform) (localized) (moniliform) (postinfectious) (recurrent) (saccular) 494
congenital 748.61
tuberculosis (*see also* Tuberculosis) 011.5
Bronchiolectasis —*see* Bronchiectasis
Bronchiolitis (acute) (infectious) (subacute) 466.1
with
bronchospasm or obstruction 466.1
influenza, flu, or grippe 487.1
catarrhal (acute) (subacute) 466.1
chemical 506.0
chronic 506.4
chronic (obliterative) 491.8
due to external agent—*see* Bronchitis, acute, due to
fibrosa obliterans 491.8
influenzal 487.1
obliterans 491.8
status post lung transplant 996.84
with organizing pneumonia (B.O.O.P.) 516.8
obliterative (chronic) (diffuse) (subacute) 491.8
due to fumes or vapors 506.4
vesicular—*see* Pneumonia, broncho-
Bronchitis (diffuse) (hypostatic) (infectious) (inflammatory) (simple) 490
with
emphysema—*see* Emphysema
influenza, flu, or grippe 487.1
obstruction airway, chronic 491.20
with acute exacerbation 491.21
tracheitis 490
acute or subacute 466.0
with bronchospasm or obstruction 466.0
chronic 491.8
acute or subacute 466.0
with
bronchospasm 466.0
chronic
bronchitis (obstructive) 491.21
obstructive pulmonary disease (COPD) 491.21
obstruction 466.0
tracheitis 466.0

Bronchitis—*continued*
chemical (due to fumes or vapors) 506.0
due to
fumes or vapors 506.0
radiation 508.8
allergic (acute) (*see also* Asthma) 493.9
arachidic 934.1
aspiration 507.0
due to fumes or vapors 506.0
asthmatic (acute) (*see also* Asthma) 493.9
chronic 491.20
with acute bronchitis or acute exacerbation 491.21
capillary 466.1
with bronchospasm or obstruction 466.1
chronic 491.8
caseous (*see also* Tuberculosis) 011.3
Castellani's 104.8
catarrhal 490
acute—*see* Bronchitis, acute
chronic 491.0
chemical (acute) (subacute) 506.0
chronic 506.4
due to fumes or vapors (acute) (subacute) 506.0
chronic 506.4
chronic 491.9
with
tracheitis (chronic) 491.8
asthmatic 491.20
with acute bronchitis or acute exacerbation 491.21
catarrhal 491.0
chemical (due to fumes and vapors) 506.4
due to
fumes or vapors (chemical) (inhalation) 506.4
radiation 508.8
tobacco smoking 491.0
mucopurulent 491.1
obstructive 491.20
with acute bronchitis or acute exacerbation 491.21
purulent 491.1
simple 491.0
specified type NEC 491.8
croupous 466.0
with bronchospasm or obstruction 466.0
due to fumes or vapors 506.0
emphysematous 491.20
with
acute bronchitis or acute exacerbation 491.21
exudative 466.0
fetid (chronic) (recurrent) 491.1
fibrinous, acute or subacute 466.0
with bronchospasm or obstruction 466.0
grippal 487.1
influenzal 487.1
membranous, acute or subacute 466.0
with bronchospasm or obstruction 466.0
moulders' 502
mucopurulent (chronic) (recurrent) 491.1
acute or subacute 466.0
non-obstructive 491.0
obliterans 491.8
obstructive (chronic) 491.20
with
acute bronchitis or acute exacerbation 491.21
acute 466.0
pituitous 491.1

Bronchitis—*continued*
plastic (inflammatory) 466.0
pneumococcal, acute or subacute 466.0
with bronchospasm or obstruction 466.0
pseudomembranous 466.0
purulent (chronic) (recurrent) 491.1
acute or subacute 466.0
with bronchospasm or obstruction 466.0
putrid 491.1
scrofulous (*see also* Tuberculosis) 011.3
senile 491.9
septic, acute or subacute 466.0
with bronchospasm or obstruction 466.0
smokers' 491.0
spirochetal 104.8
suffocative, acute or subacute 466.0
summer (*see also* Asthma) 493.9
suppurative (chronic) 491.1
acute or subacute 466.0
tuberculous (*see also* Tuberculosis) 011.3
ulcerative 491.8
Vincent's 101
Vincent's 101
viral, acute or subacute 466.0
with bronchospasm or obstruction 466.0
Bronchoalveolitis 485
Bronchoaspergillosis 117.3
Bronchocele
meaning
dilatation of bronchus 519.1
goiter 240.9
Bronchogenic carcinoma 162.9
Bronchohemisporosis 117.9
Broncholithiasis 518.89
tuberculous (*see also* Tuberculosis) 011.3
Bronchomoniliasis 112.89
Bronchomycosis 112.89
Bronchonocardiosis 039.1
Bronchopleuropneumonia —*see* Pneumonia, broncho-
Bronchopneumonia —*see* Pneumonia, broncho-
Bronchopneumonitis —*see* Pneumonia, broncho-
Bronchopulmonary —*see* condition
Bronchopulmonitis —*see* Pneumonia, broncho-
Bronchorrhagia 786.3
newborn 770.3
tuberculous (*see also* Tuberculosis) 011.3
Bronchorrhea (chronic) (purulent) 491.0
acute 466.0
Bronchospasm 519.1
with
asthma—*see* Asthma
bronchiolitis, acute 466.1
bronchitis—*see* Bronchitis
COPD 496
emphysema—*see* Emphysema
due to external agent—*see* Condition, respiratory, acute, due to
Bronchospirochetosis 104.8
Bronchostenosis 519.1
Bronchus —*see* condition
Bronze, bronzed
diabetes 275.0
disease (Addison's) (skin) 255.4
tuberculous (*see also* Tuberculosis) 017.6
Brooke's disease or tumor (M8100/0)—*see* Neoplasm, skin, benign
Brown's tendon sheath syndrome 378.61
Brown enamel of teeth (hereditary) 520.5
Brown-Séquard's paralysis (syndrome) 344.89
Brow presentation complicating delivery 652.4
causing obstructed labor 660.0
Brucella, brucellosis (infection) 023.9
abortus 023.1
canis 023.3
dermatitis, skin 023.9
melitensis 023.0
mixed 023.8
suis 023.2
Bruck's disease 733.99
Bruck-de Lange disease or syndrome (Amsterdam dwarf, mental retardation, and brachycephaly) 759.89
Brug's filariasis 125.1
Brugsch's syndrome (acropachyderma) 757.39
Bruhl's disease (splenic anemia with fever) 285.8
Bruise (skin surface intact)—*see also* Contusion
with
fracture—*see* Fracture, by site
open wound—*see* Wound, open, by site
internal organ (abdomen, chest, or pelvis)—*see* Injury, internal, by site
umbilical cord 663.6
affecting fetus or newborn 762.6
Bruit 785.9
arterial (abdominal) (carotid) 785.9
supraclavicular 785.9
Brushburn —*see* Injury, superficial, by site
Bruton's X-linked agammaglobulinemia 279.04
Bruxism 306.8
Bubbly lung syndrome 770.7
Bubo 289.3
blennorrhagic 098.89
chancroidal 099.0
climatic 099.1
due to Hemophilus ducreyi 099.0
gonococcal 098.89
indolent NEC 099.8
inguinal NEC 099.8
chancroidal 099.0
climatic 099.1
due to H. ducreyi 099.0
scrofulous (*see also* Tuberculosis) 017.2
soft chancre 099.0
suppurating 683
syphilitic 091.0
congenital 090.0
tropical 099.1
venereal NEC 099.8
virulent 099.0
Bubonic plague 020.0
Bubonocele —*see* Hernia, inguinal
Buccal —*see* condition
Buchanan's disease (juvenile osteochondrosis of iliac crest) 732.1
Buchem's syndrome (hyperostosis corticalis) 733.3
Buchman's disease (osteochondrosis, juvenile) 732.1
Bucket handle fracture (semilunar cartilage) (*see also* Tear, meniscus) 836.2
Budd-Chiari syndrome (hepatic vein thrombosis) 453.0
Budgerigar-fanciers' disease or lung 495.2
Büdinger-Ludloff-Läwen disease 717.89
Buerger's disease (thromboangiitis obliterans) 443.1
Bulbar —*see* condition
Bulbus cordis 745.9
persistent (in left ventricle) 745.8
Bulging fontanels (congenital) 756.0

Bulimia 783.6
nonorganic origin 307.51
Bulky uterus 621.2
Bulla(e) 709.8
lung (emphysematous) (solitary) 492.0
Bullet wound —*see also* Wound, open, by site
fracture—*see* Fracture, by site, open
internal organ (abdomen, chest, or pelvis)—*see* Injury, internal, by site, with open wound
intracranial—*see* Laceration, brain, with open wound
Bullis fever 082.8
Bullying (*see also* Disturbance, conduct) 312.0
Bundle
branch block (complete) (false) (incomplete) 426.50
bilateral 426.53
left (*see also* Block, bundle branch, left) 426.3
hemiblock 426.2
right (*see also* Block, bundle branch, right) 426.4
of His—*see* condition
of Kent syndrome (anomalous atrioventricular excitation) 426.7
Bungpagga 040.81
Bunion 727.1
Bunionette 727.1
Bunyamwera fever 066.3
Buphthalmia, buphthalmos (congenital) 743.20
associated with
keratoglobus, congenital 743.22
megalocornea 743.22
ocular anomalies NEC 743.22
isolated 743.21
simple 743.21
Bürger-Grütz disease or syndrome (essential familial hyperlipemia) 272.3
Buried roots 525.3
Burke's syndrome 577.8
Burkitt's
tumor (M9750/3) 200.2
type malignant, lymphoma, lymphoblastic, or undifferentiated (M9750/3) 200.2
Burn (acid) (cathode ray) (caustic) (chemical) (electric heating appliance) (electricity) (fire) (flame) (hot liquid or object) (irradiation) (lime) (radiation) (steam) (thermal) (x-ray) 949.0

Note—Use the following fifth-digit subclassification with category 948 to indicate the percent of body surface with third degree burn:

0 less than 10% or unspecified
1 10-19%
2 20-29%
3 30-39%
4 40-49%
5 50-59%
6 60-69%
7 70-79%
8 80-89%
9 90% or more of body surface

with
blisters—*see* Burn, by site, second degree
erythema—*see* Burn, by site, first degree

Burn—*continued*
skin loss (epidermal)—*see also* Burn, by site, second degree
full thickness—*see also* Burn, by site, third degree
with necrosis of underlying tissues—*see* Burn, by site, third degree, deep
first degree—*see* Burn, by site, first degree
second degree—*see* Burn, by site, second degree
third degree—*see also* Burn, by site, third degree
deep—*see* Burn, by site, third degree, deep
abdomen, abdominal (muscle) (wall) 942.03
with
other site(s), except trunk—*see* Burn, multiple, specified sites
trunk—*see* Burn, trunk, multiple sites
first degree 942.13
second degree 942.23
third degree 942.33
deep 942.43
with loss of body part 942.53
ankle 945.03
with
lower limb(s)–*see* Burn, leg, multiple sites
other site(s), except lower limb(s)—*see* Burn, multiple, specified sites
first degree 945.13
second degree 945.23
third degree 945.33
deep 945.43
with loss of body part 945.53
anus—*see* Burn, trunk, specified site NEC
arm(s) 943.00
with other site(s) (classifiable to more than one category in 940-945)—*see* Burn, multiple, specified sites
first degree 943.10
second degree 943.20
third degree 943.30
deep 943.40
with loss of body part 943.50
lower—*see* Burn, forearm(s)
multiple sites, except hand(s) or wrist(s) 943.09
first degree 943.19
second degree 943.29
third degree 943.39
deep 943.49
with loss of body part 943.59
upper 943.03
with other site(s) of upper limb(s), except hand(s) or wrist(s)—*see* Burn, arm(s), multiple sites
first degree 943.13
second degree 943.23
third degree 943.33
deep 943.43
with loss of body part 943.53
auditory canal (external)—*see* Burn, ear
auricle (ear)—*see* Burn, ear
axilla 943.04
with
hand(s) and wrist(s)—*see* Burn, multiple, specified sites
other site(s), except upper limb(s)—*see* Burn, multiple, specified sites
upper limb(s) except hand(s) or wrist(s)—*see* Burn, arm(s), multiple sites
first degree 943.14
second degree 943.24

Burn—*continued*
eyelid(s) 940.1
chemical 940.0
face—*see* Burn, head
finger (nail) (subungual) 944.01
with
hand(s)—*see* Burn, hand(s), multiple sites
other sites—*see* Burn, multiple, specified sites
thumb 944.04
first degree 944.14
second degree 944.24
third degree 944.34
deep 944.44
with loss of body part 944.54
first degree 944.11
second degree 944.21
third degree 944.31
deep 944.41
with loss of body part 944.51
multiple (digits) 944.03
with thumb—*see* Burn, finger, with thumb
first degree 944.13
second degree 944.23
third degree 944.33
deep 944.43
with loss of body part 944.53
flank—*see* Burn, abdomen
foot 945.02
with
lower limb(s)—*see* Burn, leg, multiple sites
other site(s), except lower limb(s)—*see* Burn, multiple, specified sites
first degree 945.12
second degree 945.22
third degree 945.32
deep 945.42
with loss of body part 945.52
forearm(s) 943.01
with
hand(s) and wrist(s)—*see* Burn, multiple, specified sites
other site(s), except upper limb(s)—*see* Burn, multiple, specified sites
upper limb(s) except hand(s) or wrist(s)—*see* Burn, arm(s), multiple sites
first degree 943.11
second degree 943.21
third degree 943.31
deep 943.41
with loss of body part 943.51
forehead 941.07
with
face or head—*see* Burn, head, multiple sites
other site(s), except face or head—*see* Burn, multiple, specified sites
first degree 941.17
second degree 941.27
third degree 941.37
deep 941.47
with loss of body part 941.57
fourth degree—*see* Burn, by site, third degree, deep
friction—*see* Injury, superficial, by site
from swallowing caustic or corrosive substance NEC—*see* Burn, internal organs
full thickness—*see* Burn, by site, third degree
gastrointestinal tract 947.3
genitourinary organs
external 942.05
with

Burn—*continued*
other site(s), except trunk—*see* Burn multiple, specified sites
trunk—*see* Burn, trunk, multiple sites
first degree 942.15
second degree 942.25
third degree 942.35
deep 942.45
with loss of body part 942.55
internal 947.8
globe (eye)—*see* Burn, eyeball
groin—*see* Burn, abdomen
gum 947.0
hand(s) (phalanges) (and wrist) 944.00
with other site(s) (classifiable to more than category in 940-945)—*see* Burn, multiple, specified sites
first degree 944.10
second degree 944.20
third degree 944.30
deep 944.40
with loss of body part 944.50
back (dorsal surface) 944.06
first degree 944.16
second degree 944.26
third degree 944.36
deep 944.46
with loss of body part 944.56
multiple sites 944.08
first degree 944.18
second degree 944.28
third degree 944.38
deep 944.48
with loss of body part 944.58
head (and face) 941.00
with other site(s) except face or neck—*see* Burn, multiple, specified sites
eye(s) only 940.9
specified part—*see* Burn, by site
first degree 941.10
second degree 941.20
third degree 941.30
deep 941.40
with loss of body part 941.50
multiple sites 941.09
with eyes—*see* Burn, eyes, with face, head, or neck
first degree 941.19
second degree 941.29
third degree 941.39
deep 941.49
with loss of body part 941.59
heel—*see* Burn, foot
hip—*see* Burn, trunk, specified site NEC
iliac region—*see* Burn, trunk, specified site NEC
infected 958.3
inhalation (*see also* Burn, internal organs) 947.9
internal organs 947.9
from caustic or corrosive substance (swallowing) NEC 947.9
specified NEC (*see also* Burn, by site) 947.8
interscapular region—*see* Burn, back
intestine (large) (small) 947.3
iris—*see* Burn, eyeball
knee 945.05
with
lower limb(s)—*see* Burn, leg, multiple sites
other site(s), except lower limb(s)—*see* Burn, multiple, specified sites

Burn—*continued*
first degree 945.15
second degree 945.25
third degree 945.35
deep 945.45
with loss of body part 945.55
labium (majus) (minus)—*see* Burn, genitourinary organs, external
lacrimal apparatus, duct, gland, or sac 940.1
chemical 940.0
larynx 947.1
late effect—*see* Late, effects (of), burn
leg 945.00
with other site(s) (classifiable to more than category in 940-945)—*see* Burn, multiple, specified sites
first degree 945.10
second degree 945.20
third degree 945.30
deep 945.40
with loss of body part 945.50
lower 945.04
with other part(s) of lower limb(s)—*see* Burn, leg, multiple sites
first degree 945.14
second degree 945.24
third degree 945.34
deep 945.44
with loss of body part 945.54
multiple sites 945.09
first degree 945.19
second degree 945.29
third degree 945.39
deep 945.49
with loss of body part 945.59
upper—*see* Burn, thigh
lightning—*see* Burn, by site
limb(s)
lower (including foot or toe(s))—*see* Burn, leg
upper (except wrist and hand)—*see* Burn, arm(s)
lip(s) 941.03
with
face or head—*see* Burn, head, multiple sites
other site(s), except face or head—*see* Burn, multiple, specified sites
first degree 941.13
second degree 941.23
third degree 941.33
deep 941.43
with loss of body part 941.53
lumbar region—*see* Burn, back
lung 947.1
malar region—*see* Burn, cheek
mastoid region—*see* Burn, scalp
membrane, tympanic—*see* Burn, ear
midthoracic region—*see* Burn, chest wall
mouth 947.0
multiple (*see also* Burn, unspecified) 949.0
specified sites (classifiable to more than one category in 940-945) 946.0
first degree 946.1
second degree 946.2
third degree 946.3
deep 946.4
with loss of body part 946.5
muscle, abdominal—*see* Burn, abdomen
nasal (septum)—*see* Burn, nose

Burn—*continued*
neck 941.08
with
face or head—*see* Burn, head, multiple sites
other site(s), except face or head—*see* Burn, multiple, specified sites
first degree 941.18
second degree 941.28
third degree 941.38
deep 941.48
with loss of body part 941.58
nose (septum) 941.05
with
face or head—*see* Burn, head, multiple sites
other site(s), except face or head—*see* Burn, multiple, specified sites
first degree 941.15
second degree 941.25
third degree 941.35
deep 941.45
with loss of body part 941.55
occipital region—*see* Burn, scalp
orbit region 940.1
chemical 940.0
oronasopharynx 947.0
palate 947.0
palm(s) 944.05
with
hand(s) and wrist(s)—*see* Burn, hand(s), multiple sites
other site(s), except hand(s) or wrist(s)—*see* Burn, multiple, specified sites
first degree 944.15
second degree 944.25
third degree 944.35
deep 944.45
with loss of a body part 944.55
parietal region—*see* Burn, scalp
penis–*see* Burn, genitourinary organs, external
perineum—*see* Burn, genitourinary organs, external
periocular area 940.1
chemical 940.0
pharynx 947.0
pleura 947.1
popliteal space—*see* Burn, knee
prepuce—*see* Burn, genitourinary organs, external
pubic region—*see* Burn, genitourinary organs, external
pudenda—*see* Burn, genitourinary organs, external
rectum 947.3
sac, lacrimal 940.1
chemical 940.0
sacral region—*see* Burn, back
salivary (ducts) (glands) 947.0
scalp 941.06
with
face or neck—*see* Burn, head, multiple sites
other site(s), except face or neck—*see* Burn, multiple, specified sites
first degree 941.16
second degree 941.26
third degree 941.36
deep 941.46
with loss of body part 941.56
scapular region 943.06
with
other site(s), except upper limb(s)—*see* Burn, multiple, specified sites

Burn—*continued*
upper limb(s), except hand(s) or wrist(s)—*see* Burn, arm(s), multiple sites
first degree 943.16
second degree 943.26
third degree 943.36
deep 943.46
with loss of body part 943.56
sclera—*see* Burn, eyeball
scrotum—*see* Burn, genitourinary organs, external
septum, nasal—*see* Burn, nose
shoulder(s) 943.05
with
hand(s) and wrist(s)—*see* Burn, multiple, specified sites
other site(s), except upper limb(s)—*see* Burn, multiple, specified sites
upper limb(s), except hand(s) or wrist(s)—*see* Burn, arm(s), multiple sites
first degree 943.15
second degree 943.25
third degree 943.35
deep 943.45
with loss of body part 943.55
skin NEC (*see also* Burn, unspecified) 949.0
skull—*see* Burn, head
small intestine 947.3
sternal region—*see* Burn, chest wall
stomach 947.3
subconjunctival—*see* Burn, conjunctiva
subcutaneous—*see* Burn, by site, third degree
submaxillary region—*see* Burn, head
submental region—*see* Burn, chin
supraclavicular fossa—*see* Burn, neck
supraorbital—*see* Burn, forehead
temple—*see* Burn, scalp
temporal region—*see* Burn, scalp
testicle—*see* Burn, genitourinary organs, external
testis—*see* Burn, genitourinary organs, external
thigh 945.06
with
lower limb(s)–*see* Burn, leg, multiple sites
other site(s), except lower limb(s)—*see* Burn, multiple, specified sites
first degree 945.16
second degree 945.26
third degree 945.36
deep 945.46
with loss of body part 945.56
thorax (external)—*see* Burn, chest wall
throat 947.0
thumb(s) (nail) (subungual) 944.02
with
finger(s)—*see* Burn, finger, with other sites, thumb
hand(s) and wrist(s)—*see* Burn, hand(s), multiple sites
other site(s), except hand(s) or wrist(s)—*see* Burn, multiple, specified sites
first degree 944.12
second degree 944.22
third degree 944.32
deep 944.42
with loss of body part 944.52
toe (nail) (subungual) 945.01
with
lower limb(s)—*see* Burn, leg, multiple sites
other site(s), except lower limb(s)—*see* Burn, multiple, specified sites

Burn—*continued*
first degree 945.11
second degree 945.21
third degree 945.31
deep 945.41
with loss of body part 945.51
tongue 947.0
tonsil 947.0
trachea 947.1
trunk 942.00
with other site(s) (classifiable to more than one category in 940-945)—*see* Burn, multiple, specified sites
first degree 942.10
second degree 942.20
third degree 942.30
deep 942.40
with loss of body part 942.50
multiple sites 942.09
first degree 942.19
second degree 942.29
third degree 942.39
deep 942.49
with loss of body part 942.59
specified site NEC 942.09
first degree 942.19
second degree 942.29
third degree 942.39
deep 942.49
with loss of body part 942.59
tunica vaginalis—*see* Burn, genitourinary organs, external
tympanic membrane—*see* Burn, ear
tympanum—*see* Burn, ear
unspecified site (multiple) 949.0
with extent of body surface involved specified
less than 10 percent 948.0
10-19 percent 948.1
20-29 percent 948.2
30-39 percent 948.3
40-49 percent 948.4
50-59 percent 948.5
60-69 percent 948.6
70-79 percent 948.7
80-89 percent 948.8
90 percent or more 948.9
first degree 949.1
second degree 949.2
third degree 949.3
deep 949.4
with loss of body part 949.5
uterus 947.4
uvula 947.0
vagina 947.4
vulva—*see* Burn, genitourinary organs, external
wrist(s) 944.07
with
hand(s)—*see* Burn, hand(s), multiple sites
other site(s), except hand(s)—*see* Burn, multiple, specified sites
first degree 944.17
second degree 944.27
third degree 944.37
deep 944.47
with loss of body part 944.57
Burnett's syndrome (milk-alkali) 999.9
Burnier's syndrome (hypophyseal dwarfism) 253.3
Burning
feet syndrome 266.2
sensation (*see also* Disturbance, sensation) 782.0
tongue 529.6

Burns' disease (osteochondrosis, lower ulna) 732.3
Bursa —*see also* condition
  pharynx 478.29
Bursitis NEC 727.3
  Achilles tendon 726.71
  adhesive 726.90
    shoulder 726.0
  ankle 726.79
  buttock 726.5
  calcaneal 726.79
  collateral ligament
    fibular 726.63
    tibial 726.62
  Duplay's 726.2
  elbow 726.33
  finger 726.8
  foot 726.79
  gonococcal 098.52
  hand 726.4
  hip 726.5
  infrapatellar 726.69
  ischiogluteal 726.5
  knee 726.60
  occupational NEC 727.2
  olecranon 726.33
  pes anserinus 726.61
  pharyngeal 478.29
  popliteal 727.51
  prepatellar 726.65
  radiohumeral 727.3
  scapulohumeral 726.19
    adhesive 726.0
  shoulder 726.10
    adhesive 726.0
  subacromial 726.19
    adhesive 726.0
  subcoracoid 726.19
  subdeltoid 726.19
    adhesive 726.0
  subpatellar 726.69
  syphilitic 095.7
  Thornwaldt's, Tornwaldt's (pharyngeal) 478.29
  toe 726.79
  trochanteric area 726.5
  wrist 726.4
Burst stitches or sutures (complication of surgery) 998.3
Buruli ulcer 031.1
Bury's disease (erythema elevatum diutinum) 695.89
Buschke's disease or scleredema (adultorum) 710.1
Busquet's disease (osteoperiostitis) (*see also* Osteomyelitis) 730.1
Busse-Buschke disease (cryptococcosis) 117.5
Buttock —*see* condition
Button
  Biskra 085.1
  Delhi 085.1
  oriental 085.1
Buttonhole hand (intrinsic) 736.21
Bwamba fever (encephalitis) 066.3
Byssinosis (occupational) 504
Bywaters' syndrome 958.5

C

Cacergasia 300.9
Cachexia 799.4
  cancerous (M8000/3) 199.1
  cardiac—*see* Disease, heart
  dehydration 276.5
    with
      hypernatremia 276.0
      hyponatremia 276.1
  due to malnutrition 261
  exophthalmic 242.0
  heart—*see* Disease, heart
  hypophyseal 253.2
  hypopituitary 253.2
  lead 984.9
    specified type of lead—*see* Table of drugs and chemicals
  malaria 084.9
  malignant (M8000/3) 199.1
  marsh 084.9
  nervous 300.5
  old age 797
  pachydermic—*see* Hypothyroidism
  paludal 084.9
  pituitary (postpartum) 253.2
  renal (*see also* Disease, renal) 593.9
  saturnine 984.9
    specified type of lead—*see* Table of drugs and chemicals
  senile 797
  Simmonds' (pituitary cachexia) 253.2
  splenica 289.59
  strumipriva (*see also* Hypothyroidism) 244.9
  tuberculous NEC (*see also* Tuberculosis) 011.9
café au lait spots 709.09
Caffey's disease or syndrome (infantile cortical hyperostosis) 756.59
Caisson disease 993.3
Caked breast (puerperal, postpartum) 676.2
Cake kidney 753.3
Calabar swelling 125.2
Calcaneal spur 726.73
Calcaneoapophysitis 732.5
Calcaneonavicular bar 755.67
Calcareous —*see* condition
Calcicosis (occupational) 502
Calciferol (vitamin D) deficiency 268.9
  with
    osteomalacia 268.2
    rickets (*see also* Rickets) 268.0
Calcification
  adrenal (capsule) (gland) 255.4
    tuberculous (*see also* Tuberculosis) 017.6
  aorta 440.0
  artery (annular)—*see* Arteriosclerosis
  auricle (ear) 380.89
  bladder 596.8
    due to S. hematobium 120.0
  brain (cortex)—*see* Calcification, cerebral
  bronchus 519.1
  bursa 727.82
  cardiac (*see also* Degeneration, myocardial) 429.1
  cartilage (postinfectional) 733.99
  cerebral (cortex) 348.8
    artery 437.0
  cervix (uteri) 622.8
  choroid plexus 349.2
  conjunctiva 372.54

Calcification—*continued*
  corpora cavernosa (penis) 607.89
  cortex (brain)—*see* Calcification, cerebral
  dental pulp (nodular) 522.2
  dentinal papilla 520.4
  disc, intervertebral 722.90
    cervical, cervicothoracic 722.91
    lumbar, lumbosacral 722.93
    thoracic, thoracolumbar 722.92
  fallopian tube 620.8
  falx cerebri—*see* Calcification, cerebral
  fascia 728.89
  gallbladder 575.8
  general 275.4
  heart (*see also* Degeneration, myocardial) 429.1
    valve—*see* Endocarditis
  intervertebral cartilage or disc (postinfectional) 722.90
    cervical, cervicothoracic 722.91
    lumbar, lumbosacral 722.93
    thoracic, thoracolumbar 722.92
  intracranial—*see* Calcification, cerebral
  intraspinal ligament 728.89
  joint 719.80
    ankle 719.87
    elbow 719.82
    foot 719.87
    hand 719.84
    hip 719.85
    knee 719.86
    multiple sites 719.89
    pelvic region 719.85
    shoulder (region) 719.81
    specified site NEC 719.88
    wrist 719.83
  kidney 593.89
    tuberculous (*see also* Tuberculosis) 016.0
  larynx (senile) 478.79
  lens 366.8
  ligament 728.89
    intraspinal 728.89
    knee (medial collateral) 717.89
  lung 518.89
    active 518.89
    postinfectional 518.89
    tuberculous (*see also* Tuberculosis, pulmonary) 011.9
  lymph gland or node (postinfectional) 289.3
    tuberculous (*see also* Tuberculosis, lymph gland) 017.2
  massive (paraplegic) 728.10
  medial NEC (*see also* Arteriosclerosis, extremities) 440.20
  meninges (cerebral) 349.2
  metastatic 275.4
  Mönckeberg's—*see* Arteriosclerosis
  muscle 728.10
    heterotopic, postoperative 728.13
  myocardium, myocardial (*see also* Degeneration, myocardial) 429.1
  ovary 620.8
  pancreas 577.8
  penis 607.99
  periarticular 728.89
  pericardium (*see also* Pericarditis) 423.8
  pineal gland 259.8
  pleura 511.0
    postinfectional 518.89

Calcification—*continued*
tuberculous (*see also* Tuberculosis, pleura) 012.0
pulp (dental) (nodular) 522.2
renal 593.89
rider's bone 733.99
sclera 379.16
semilunar cartilage 717.89
spleen 289.59
subcutaneous 709.3
suprarenal (capsule) (gland) 255.4
tendon (sheath) 727.82
with bursitis, synovitis or tenosynovitis 727.82
trachea 519.1
ureter 593.89
uterus 621.8
vitreous 379.29
Calcified —*see also* Calcification
hematoma NEC 959.9
Calcinosis (generalized) (interstitial) (tumoral) (universalis) 275.4
circumscripta 709.3
cutis 709.3
intervertebralis 275.4 (722.90)
Raynaud's
phenomenonsclerodactylytelangiectasis (CRST) 710.1
Calcium
blood
high (*see also* Hypercalcemia) 275.4
low (*see also* Hypocalcemia) 275.4
deposits—*see also* Calcification, by site
in bursa 727.82
in tendon (sheath) 727.82
with bursitis, synovitis or tenosynovitis 727.82
salts or soaps in vitreous 379.22
Calciuria 791.9
Calculi —*see* Calculus
Calculosis, intrahepatic —*see* Choledocholithiasis
Calculus, calculi, calculous 592.9
ampulla of Vater—*see* Choledocholithiasis
anuria (impacted) (recurrent) 592.0
appendix 543.9
bile duct (any)—*see* Choledocholithiasis
biliary—*see* Cholelithiasis
bilirubin, multiple—*see* Cholelithiasis
bladder (encysted) (impacted) (urinary) 594.1
diverticulum 594.0
bronchus 518.89
calyx (kidney) (renal) 592.0
congenital 753.3
cholesterol (pure) (solitary)—*see* Cholelithiasis
common duct (bile)—*see* Choledocholithiasis
conjunctiva 372.54
cystic 594.1
duct—*see* Cholelithiasis
dental 523.6
subgingival 523.6
supragingival 523.6
epididymis 608.89
gallbladder—*see also* Cholelithiasis
congenital 751.69
hepatic (duct)—*see* Choledocholithiasis
intestine (impaction) (obstruction) 560.39
kidney (impacted) (multiple) (pelvis) (recurrent) (staghorn) 592.0
congenital 753.3
lacrimal (passages) 375.57
liver (impacted)—*see* Choledocholithiasis
Calculus, calculi, calculous—*continued*
lung 518.89
nephritic (impacted) (recurrent) 592.0
nose 478.1
pancreas (duct) 577.8
parotid gland 527.5
pelvis, encysted 592.0
prostate 602.0
pulmonary 518.89
pyelitis (impacted) (recurrent) 592.9
pyelonephritis (impacted) (recurrent) 592.9
pyonephrosis (impacted) (recurrent) 592.9
renal (impacted) (recurrent) 592.0
congenital 753.3
salivary (duct) (gland) 527.5
seminal vesicle 608.89
staghorn 592.0
Stensen's duct 527.5
sublingual duct or gland 527.5
congenital 750.26
submaxillary duct, gland, or region 527.5
suburethral 594.8
tonsil 474.8
tooth, teeth 523.6
tunica vaginalis 608.89
ureter (impacted) (recurrent) 592.1
urethra (impacted) 594.2
urinary (duct) (impacted) (passage) (tract) 592.9
lower tract NEC 594.9
specified site 594.8
vagina 623.8
vesical (impacted) 594.1
Wharton's duct 527.5
Caliectasis 593.89
California
disease 114.0
encephalitis 062.5
Caligo cornea 371.03
Callositas, callosity (infected) 700
Callus (infected) 700
bone 726.91
excessive, following fracture—*see also* Late, effect (of), fracture
Calvé (-Perthes) disease (osteochondrosis, femoral capital) 732.1
Calvities (*see also* Alopecia) 704.00
Cameroon fever (*see also* Malaria) 084.6
Camptocormia 300.11
Camptodactyly (congenital) 755.59
Camurati-Engelmann disease (diaphyseal sclerosis) 756.59
Canal— *see* condition
Canaliculitis (lacrimal) (acute) 375.31
Actinomyces 039.8
chronic 375.41
Canavan's disease 330.0
Cancer (M8000/3)—*see also* Neoplasm, by site, malignant

Note—The term "cancer" when modified by an adjective or adjectival phrase indicating a morphological type should be coded in the same manner as "carcinoma" with that adjective or phrase. Thus, "squamous-cell cancer" should be coded in the same manner as "squamous-cell carcinoma," which appears in the list under "Carcinoma."

bile duct type (M8160/3), liver 155.1
hepatocellular (M8170/3) 155.0
Cancerous (M8000/3)—*see* Neoplasm, by site, malignant
Cancerphobia 300.29

Cancrum oris 528.1
Candidiasis, candidal 112.9
with pneumonia 112.4
balanitis 112.2
congenital 771.7
disseminated 112.5
endocarditis 112.81
esophagus 112.84
intertrigo 112.3
intestine 112.85
lung 112.4
meningitis 112.83
mouth 112.0
nails 112.3
neonatal 771.7
onychia 112.3
otitis externa 112.82
otomycosis 112.82
paronychia 112.3
perionyxis 112.3
pneumonia 112.4
pneumonitis 112.4
skin 112.3
specified site NEC 112.89
systemic 112.5
urogenital site NEC 112.2
vagina 112.1
vulva 112.1
vulvovaginitis 112.1
Candidiosis —*see* Candidiasis
Candiru infection or infestation 136.8
Canities (premature) 704.3
congenital 757.4
Canker (mouth) (sore) 528.2
rash 034.1
Cannabinosis 504
Canton fever 081.9
Cap
cradle 691.8
Capillariasis 127.5
Capillary —*see* condition
Caplan's syndrome 714.81
Caplan-Colinet syndrome 714.81
Capsule —*see* condition
Capsulitis (joint) 726.90
adhesive (shoulder) 726.0
labyrinthine 387.8
thyroid 245.9
Caput
crepitus 756.0
medusae 456.8
succedaneum 767.1
Carapata disease 087.1
Carate —*see* Pinta
Carboxyhemoglobinemia 986
Carbuncle 680.9
abdominal wall 680.2
ankle 680.6
anus 680.5
arm (any part, above wrist) 680.3
auditory canal, external 680.0
axilla 680.3
back (any part) 680.2
breast 680.2
buttock 680.5
chest wall 680.2
corpus cavernosum 607.2
ear (any part) (external) 680.0
eyelid 373.13
face (any part, except eye) 680.0
finger (any) 680.4

Carbuncle—*continued*
flank 680.2
foot (any part) 680.7
forearm 680.3
genital organ (male) 608.4
gluteal (region) 680.5
groin 680.2
hand (any part) 680.4
head (any part, except face) 680.8
heel 680.7
hip 680.6
kidney (*see also* Abscess, kidney) 590.2
knee 680.6
labia 616.4
lacrimal
gland (*see also* Dacryoadenitis) 375.00
passages (duct) (sac) (*see also* Dacryocystitis) 375.30
leg, any part except foot 680.6
lower extremity, any part except foot 680.6
malignant 022.0
multiple sites 680.9
neck 680.1
nose (external) (septum) 680.0
orbit, orbital 376.01
partes posteriores 680.5
pectoral region 680.2
penis 607.2
perineum 680.2
pinna 680.0
scalp (any part) 680.8
scrotum 608.4
seminal vesicle 608.0
shoulder 680.3
skin NEC 680.9
specified site NEC 680.8
spermatic cord 608.4
temple (region) 680.0
testis 608.4
thigh 680.6
thumb 680.4
toe (any) 680.7
trunk 680.2
tunica vaginalis 608.4
umbilicus 680.2
upper arm 680.3
urethra 597.0
vas deferens 608.4
vulva 616.4
wrist 680.4
Carbunculus (*see also* Carbuncle) 680.9
Carcinoid (tumor) (M8240/1)—*see also* Neoplasm, by site, uncertain behavior
and struma ovarii (M9091/1) 236.2
argentaffin (M8241/1)—*see* Neoplasm, by site uncertain behavior
malignant (M8241/3)—*see* Neoplasm, by site, malignant
benign (M9091/0) 220
composite (M8244/3)—*see* Neoplasm, by site, malignant
goblet cell (M8243/3)—*see* Neoplasm, by site, malignant
malignant (M8240/3)—*see* Neoplasm, by site, malignant
nonargentaffin (M8242/1)—*see also* Neoplasm, by site, uncertain behavior
malignant (M8242/3)—*see* Neoplasm, by site, malignant

Carcinoid—*continued*
strumal (M9091/1) 236.2
syndrome (intestinal) (metastatic) 259.2
type bronchial adenoma (M8240/3)—*see* Neoplasm, lung, malignant
Carcinoidosis 259.2
Carcinoma (M8010/3)—*see also* Neoplasm, by site, malignant

Note—Except where otherwise indicated, the morphological varieties of carcinoma in the list below should be coded by site as for "Neoplasm, malignant."

with
apocrine metaplasia (M8573/3)
cartilaginous (and osseous) metaplasia (M8571/3)
osseous (and cartilaginous) metaplasia (M8571/3)
productive fibrosis (M8141/3)
spindle cell metaplasia (M8572/3)
squamous metaplasia (M8570/3)
acidophil (M8280/3)
specified site—*see* Neoplasm, by site, malignant
unspecified site 194.3
acidophil-basophil, mixed (M8281/3)
specified site—*see* Neoplasm, by site, malignant
unspecified site 194.3
acinar (cell) (M8550/3)
acinic cell (M8550/3)
adenocystic (M8200/3)
adenoid
cystic (M8200/3)
squamous cell (M8075/3)
adenosquamous (M8560/3)
adnexal (skin) (M8390/3)—*see* Neoplasm, skin, malignant
adrenal cortical (M8370/3) 194.0
alveolar (M8251/3)
cell (M8250/3)—*see* Neoplasm, lung, malignant
anaplastic type (M8021/3)
apocrine (M8401/3)
breast—*see* Neoplasm, breast, malignant
specified site NEC—*see* Neoplasm, skin, malignant
unspecified site 173.9
basal cell (pigmented) (M8090/3)—*see also* Neoplasm, skin, malignant
fibro-epithelial type (M8093/3)—*see* Neoplasm, skin, malignant
morphea type (M8092/3)—*see* Neoplasm, skin, malignant
multicentric (M8091/3)—*see* Neoplasm, skin, malignant
basaloid (M8123/3)
basal-squamous cell, mixed (M8094/3)—*see* Neoplasm, skin, malignant
basophil (M8300/3)
specified site—*see* Neoplasm, by site, malignant
unspecified site 194.3
basophil-acidophil, mixed (M8281/3)
specified site—*see* Neoplasm, by site, malignant
unspecified site 194.3
basosquamous (M8094/3)—*see* Neoplasm, skin, malignant

Carcinoma—*continued*
bile duct type (M8160/3)
and hepatocellular, mixed (M8180/3) 155.0
liver 155.1
specified site NEC—*see* Neoplasm, by site, malignant
unspecified site 155.1
branchial or branchiogenic 146.8
bronchial or bronchogenic—*see* Neoplasm, lung, malignant
bronchiolar (terminal) (M8250/3)—*see* Neoplasm, lung, malignant
bronchiolo-alveolar (M8250/3)—*see* Neoplasm, lung, malignant
bronchogenic (epidermoid) 162.9
C cell (M8510/3)
specified site—*see* Neoplasm, by site, malignant
unspecified site 193
ceruminous (M8420/3) 173.2
chorionic (M9100/3)
specified site—*see* Neoplasm, by site, malignant
unspecified site
female 181
male 186.9
chromophobe (M8270/3)
specified site—*see* Neoplasm, by site, malignant
unspecified site 194.3
clear cell (mesonephroid type) (M8310/3)
cloacogenic (M8124/3)
specified site—*see* Neoplasm, by site, malignant
unspecified site 154.8
colloid (M8480/3)
cribriform (M8201/3)
cylindroid type (M8200/3)
diffuse type (M8145/3)
specified site—*see* Neoplasm, by site, malignant
unspecified site 151.9
duct (cell) (M8500/3)
with Paget's disease (M8541/3)—*see* Neoplasm, breast, malignant
infiltrating (M8500/3)
specified site—*see* Neoplasm, by site, malignant
unspecified site 174.9
ductal (M8500/3)
ductular, infiltrating (M8521/3)
embryonal (M9070/3)
and teratoma, mixed (M9081/3)
combined with choriocarcinoma (M9101/3)—*see* Neoplasm, by site, malignant
infantile type (M9071/3)
liver 155.0
polyembryonal type (M9072/3)
endometrioid (M8380/3)
eosinophil (M8280/3)
specified site—*see* Neoplasm, by site, malignant
unspecified site 194.3
epidermoid (M8070/3)—*see also* Carcinoma, squamous cell
and adenocarcinoma, mixed (M8560/3)
in situ, Bowen's type (M8081/2)—*see* Neoplasm, skin, in situ
intradermal—*see* Neoplasm, skin, in situ

Carcinoma—*continued*
fibroepithelial type basal cell (M8093/3)—*see* Neoplasm, skin, malignant
follicular (M8330/3)
and papillary (mixed) (M8340/3) 193
moderately differentiated type (M8332/3) 193
pure follicle type (M8331/3) 193
specified site—*see* Neoplasm, by site, malignant
trabecular type (M8332/3) 193
unspecified site 193
well differentiated type (M8331/3) 193
gelatinous (M8480/3)
giant cell (M8031/3)
and spindle cell (M8030/3)
granular cell (M8320/3)
granulosa cell (M8620/3) 183.0
hepatic cell (M8170/3) 155.0
hepatocellular (M8170/3) 155.0
and bile duct, mixed (M8180/3) 155.0
hepatocholangiolitic (M8180/3) 155.0
Hurthle cell (thyroid) 193
hypernephroid (M8311/3)
in
adenomatous
polyp (M8210/3)
polyposis coli (M8220/3) 153.9
pleomorphic adenoma (M8940/3)
polypoid adenoma (M8210/3)
situ (M8010/3)—*see* Carcinoma, in situ
tubular adenoma (M8210/3)
villous adenoma (M8261/3)
infiltrating duct (M8500/3)
with Paget's disease (M8541/3)—*see* Neoplasm, breast, malignant
specified site—*see* Neoplasm, by site, malignant
unspecified site 174.9
inflammatory (M8530/3)
specified site—*see* Neoplasm, by site, malignant
unspecified site 174.9
in situ (M8010/2)—*see also* Neoplasm, by site, in situ
epidermoid (M8070/2)—*see also* Neoplasm, by site, in situ
with questionable stromal invasion (M8076/2)
specified site—*see* Neoplasm, by site, in situ
unspecified site 233.1
Bowen's type (M8081/2)—*see* Neoplasm, skin, in situ
intraductal (M8500/2)
specified site—*see* Neoplasm, by site, in situ
unspecified site 233.0
lobular (M8520/2)
specified site—*see* Neoplasm, by site, in situ
unspecified site 233.0
papillary (M8050/2)—*see* Neoplasm, by site, in situ
squamous cell (M8070/2)—*see also* Neoplasm, by site, in situ
with questionable stromal invasion (M8076/2)
specified site—*see* Neoplasm, by site, in situ
unspecified site 233.1
transitional cell (M8120/2)—*see* Neoplasm, by site, in situ

Carcinoma—*continued*
intestinal type (M8144/3)
specified site—*see* Neoplasm, by site, malignant
unspecified site 151.9
intraductal (noninfiltrating) (M8500/2)
papillary (M8503/2)
specified site—*see* Neoplasm, by site, in situ
unspecified site 233.0
specified site—*see* Neoplasm, by site, in situ
unspecified site 233.0
intraepidermal (M8070/2)—*see also* Neoplasm, skin, in situ
squamous cell, Bowen's type (M8081/2)—*see* Neoplasm, skin, in situ
intraepithelial (M8010/2)—*see also* Neoplasm, by site, in situ
squamous cell (M8072/2)—*see* Neoplasm, by site, in situ
intraosseous (M9270/3) 170.1
upper jaw (bone) 170.0
islet cell (M8150/3)
and exocrine, mixed (M8154/3)
specified site—*see* Neoplasm, by site, malignant
unspecified site 157.9
pancreas 157.4
specified site NEC—*see* Neoplasm, by site, malignant
unspecified site 157.4
juvenile, breast (M8502/3)—*see* Neoplasm, breast, malignant
Kulchitsky's cell (carcinoid tumor of intestine) 259.2
large cell (M8012/3)
squamous cell, nonkeratinizing type (M8072/3)
Leydig cell (testis) (M8650/3)
specified site—*see* Neoplasm, by site, malignant
unspecified site 186.9
female 183.0
male 186.9
liver cell (M8170/3) 155.0
lobular (infiltrating) (M8520/3)
non-infiltrating (M8520/3)
specified site—*see* Neoplasm, by site, in situ
unspecified site 233.0
specified site—*see* Neoplasm, by site, malignant
unspecified site 174.9
lymphoepithelial (M8082/3)
medullary (M8510/3)
with
amyloid stroma (M8511/3)
specified site—*see* Neoplasm, by site, malignant
unspecified site 193
lymphoid stroma (M8512/3)
specified site—*see* Neoplasm, by site, malignant
unspecified site 174.9
mesometanephric (M9110/3)
mesonephric (M9110/3)
metastatic (M8010/6)—*see* Metastasis, cancer
metatypical (M8095/3)—*see* Neoplasm, skin, malignant
morphea type basal cell (M8092/3)—*see* Neoplasm, skin, malignant
mucinous (M8480/3)
mucin-producing (M8481/3)

Carcinoma—*continued*
mucin-secreting (M8481/3)
mucoepidermoid (M8430/3)
mucoid (M8480/3)
cell (M8300/3)
specified site—*see* Neoplasm, by site, malignant
unspecified site 194.3
mucous (M8480/3)
nonencapsulated sclerosing (M8350/3) 193
noninfiltrating
intracystic (M8504/2)—*see* Neoplasm, by site, in situ
intraductal (M8500/2)
papillary (M8503/2)
specified site—*see* Neoplasm, by site, in situ
unspecified site 233.0
specified site—*see* Neoplasm, by site, in situ
unspecified site 233.0
lobular (M8520/2)
specified site—*see* Neoplasm, by site, in situ
unspecified site 233.0
oat cell (M8042/3)
specified site—*see* Neoplasm, by site, malignant
unspecified site 162.9
odontogenic (M9270/3) 170.1
upper jaw (bone) 170.0
onocytic (M8290/3)
oxyphilic (M8290/3)
papillary (M8050/3)
and follicular (mixed) (M8340/3) 193
epidermoid (M8052/3)
intraductal (noninfiltrating) (M8503/2)
specified site—*see* Neoplasm, by site, in situ
unspecified site 233.0
serous (M8460/3)
specified site—*see* Neoplasm, by site, malignant
surface (M8461/3)
specified site—*see* Neoplasm, by site, malignant
unspecified site 183.0
unspecified site 183.0
squamous cell (M8052/3)
transitional cell (M8130/3)
papillocystic (M8450/3)
specified site—*see* Neoplasm, by site, malignant
unspecified site 183.0
parafollicular cell (M8510/3)
specified site—*see* Neoplasm, by site, malignant
unspecified site 193
pleomorphic (M8022/3)
polygonal cell (M8034/3)
prickle cell (M8070/3)
pseudoglandular, squamous cell (M8075/3)
pseudomucinous (M8470/3)
specified site—*see* Neoplasm, by site, malignant
unspecified site 183.0
pseudosarcomatous (M8033/3)
regaud type (M8082/3)—*see* Neoplasm, nasopharynx, malignant
renal cell (M8312/3) 189.0
reserve cell (M8041/3)
round cell (M8041/3)
Schmincke (M8082/3)—*see* Neoplasm, nasopharynx, malignant

Carcinoma—*continued*
Schneiderian (M8121/3)
specified site—*see* Neoplasm, by site, malignant
unspecified site 160.0
scirrhous (M8141/3)
sebaceous (M8410/3)—*see* Neoplasm, skin, malignant
secondary (M8010/6)—*see* Neoplasm, by site, malignant, secondary
secretory, breast (M8502/3)—*see* Neoplasm, breast, malignant
serous (M8441/3)
papillary (M8460/3)
specified site—*see* Neoplasm, by site, malignant
unspecified site 183.0
surface, papillary (M8461/3)
specified site—*see* Neoplasm, by site, malignant
unspecified site 183.0
Sertoli cell (M8640/3)
specified site—*see* Neoplasm, by site, malignant
unspecified site 186.9
signet ring cell (M8490/3)
metastatic (M8490/6)—*see* Neoplasm, by site, secondary
simplex (M8231/3)
skin appendage (M8390/3)—*see* Neoplasm, skin, malignant
small cell (M8041/3)
fusiform cell type (M8043/3)
squamous cell, non-keratinizing type (M8073/3)
solid (M8230/3)
with amyloid stroma (M8511/3)
specified site—*see* Neoplasm, by site, malignant
unspecified site 193
spheroidal cell (M8035/3)
spindle cell (M8032/3)
and giant cell (M8030/3)
spinous cell (M8070/3)
squamous (cell) (M8070/3)
adenoid type (M8075/3)
and adenocarcinoma, mixed (M8560/3)
intraepidermal, Bowen's type—*see* Neoplasm, skin, in situ
keratinizing type (large cell) (M8071/3)
large cell, non-keratinizing type (M8072/3)
microinvasive (M8076/3)
specified site—*see* Neoplasm, by site, malignant
unspecified site 180.9
non-keratinizing type (M8072/3)
papillary (M8052/3)
pseudoglandular (M8075/3)
small cell, non-keratinizing type (M8073/3)
spindle cell type (M8074/3)
verrucous (M8051/3)
superficial spreading (M8143/3)
sweat gland (M8400/3)—*see* Neoplasm, skin, malignant
theca cell (M8600/3) 183.0
thymic (M8580/3) 164.0
trabecular (M8190/3)
transitional (cell) (M8120/3)
papillary (M8130/3)
spindle cell type (M8122/3)

Care—*continued*
radiotherapy V66.1
surgery V66.0
surgical NEC V66.0
treatment (for) V66.5
combined V66.6
fracture V66.4
mental disorder NEC V66.3
specified type NEC V66.5
family member (handicapped) (sick)
creating problem for family V61.49
provided away from home for holiday relief V60.5
unavailable, due to
absence (person rendering care) (sufferer) V60.4
inability (any reason) of person rendering care V60.4
holiday relief V60.5
improper (at or after birth) (infant) (child) 995.5
affecting parent or family V61.21
as reason for family seeking advice V61.21
specified person other than child 995.81
lack of (at or after birth) (infant) (child) 995.5
affecting parent or family V61.21
as reason for family seeking advice V61.21
specified person other than child 995.81
lactation of mother V24.1
postpartum
immediately after delivery V24.0
routine follow-up V24.2
prenatal V22.1
first pregnancy V22.0
high risk pregnancy V23.9
specified problem NEC V23.8
unavailable, due to
absence of person rendering care V60.4
inability (any reason) of person rendering care V60.4
well baby V20.1
Caries (bone) (*see also* Tuberculosis, bone) 015.9 *[730.8]*
arrested 521.0
cementum 521.0
cerebrospinal (tuberculous) 015.0 *[730.88]*
dental (acute) (chronic) (incipient) (infected) (with pulp exposure) 521.0
dentin (acute) (chronic) 521.0
enamel (acute) (chronic) (incipient) 521.0
external meatus 380.89
hip (*see also* Tuberculosis) 015.1 *[730.85]*
knee 015.2 *[730.86]*
labyrinth 386.8
limb NEC 015.7 *[730.88]*
mastoid (chronic) (process) 383.1
middle ear 385.89
nose 015.7 *[730.88]*
orbit 015.7 *[730.88]*
ossicle 385.24
petrous bone 383.20
sacrum (tuberculous) 015.0 *[730.88]*
spine, spinal (column) (tuberculous) 015.0 *[730.88]*
syphilitic 095.5
congenital 090.0 *[730.8]*
teeth (internal) 521.0
vertebra (column) (tuberculous) 015.0 *[730.88]*
Carini's syndrome (ichthyosis congenita) 757.1
Carious teeth 521.0
Carneous mole 631
Carnosinemia 270.5
Carotid body or sinus syndrome 337.0
Carotidynia 337.0
Carotinemia (dietary) 278.3
Carotinosis (cutis) (skin) 278.3
Carpal tunnel syndrome 354.0
Carpenter's syndrome 759.89
Carpopedal spasm (*see also* Tetany) 781.7
Carpoptosis 736.05
Carrier (suspected) of
amebiasis V02.2
bacterial disease (meningococcal, staphylococcal, streptococcal) NEC V02.5
cholera V02.0
defective gene V19.8
diphtheria V02.4
dysentery (bacillary) V02.3
amebic V02.2
Endamoeba histolytica V02.2
gastrointestinal pathogens NEC V02.3
genetic defect V19.8
gonorrhea V02.7
HAA (hepatitis Australian-antigen) V02.6
hepatitis V02.6
Australian-antigen (HAA) V02.6
serum V02.6
viral V02.6
infective organism NEC V02.9
malaria V02.9
paratyphoid V02.3
Salmonella V02.3
typhosa V02.1
serum hepatitis V02.6
Shigella V02.3
staphylococcus NEC V02.5
typhoid V02.1
venereal disease NEC V02.8
Carrión's disease (Bartonellosis) 088.0
Car sickness 994.6
Carter's
relapsing fever (Asiatic) 087.0
Cartilage —*see* condition
Caruncle (inflamed)
abscess, lacrimal (*see also* Dacryocystitis) 375.30
conjunctiva 372.00
acute 372.00
eyelid 373.00
labium (majus) (minus) 616.8
lacrimal 375.30
urethra (benign) 599.3
vagina (wall) 616.8
Cascade stomach 537.6
Caseation lymphatic gland (*see also* Tuberculosis) 017.2
Caseous
bronchitis—*see* Tuberculosis, pulmonary
meningitis 013.0
pneumonia—*see* Tuberculosis, pulmonary
Cassidy (-Scholte) syndrome (malignant carcinoid) 259.2
Castellani's bronchitis 104.8
Castleman's tumor or lymphoma (mediastinal lymph node hyperplasia) 785.6
Castration, traumatic 878.2
complicated 878.3
Casts in urine 791.7
Cat's ear 744.29
Catalepsy 300.11
catatonic (acute) (*see also* Schizophrenia) 295.2

Catalepsy—*continued*
hysterical 300.11
schizophrenic (*see also* Schizophrenia) 295.2
Cataphasia 307.0
Cataplexy (idiopathic) 347
Cataract (anterior cortical) (anterior polar) (black) (capsular) (central) (cortical) (hypermature) (immature) (incipient) (mature) (nuclear) 366.9
anterior
and posterior axial embryonal 743.33
pyramidal 743.31
subcapsular polar
infantile, juvenile, or presenile 366.01
senile 366.13
associated with
calcinosis 275.4 *[366.42]*
craniofacial dysostosis 756.0 *[366.44]*
galactosemia 271.1 *[366.44]*
hypoparathyroidism 252.1 *[366.42]*
myotonic disorders 359.2 *[366.43]*
neovascularization 366.33
blue dot 743.39
cerulean 743.39
complicated NEC 366.30
congenital 743.30
capsular or subcapsular 743.31
cortical 743.32
nuclear 743.33
specified type NEC 743.39
total or subtotal 743.34
zonular 743.32
coronary (congenital) 743.39
acquired 366.12
cupuliform 366.14
diabetic 250.5 *[366.41]*
drug-induced 366.45
due to
chalcosis 360.24 *[366.34]*
chronic choroiditis (*see also* Choroiditis) 366.32 *[363.20]*
degenerative myopia 366.34 *[360.21]*
glaucoma (*see also* Glaucoma) 366.31 *[365.9]*
infection, intraocular NEC 366.32
inflammatory ocular disorder NEC 366.32
iridocyclitis, chronic 366.33 *[364.10]*
pigmentary retinal dystrophy 366.34 *[362.74]*
radiation 366.46
electric 366.46
glassblowers' 366.46
heat ray 366.46
heterochromic 366.33
in eye disease NEC 366.30
infantile (*see also* Cataract, juvenile) 366.00
intumescent 366.12
irradiational 366.46
juvenile 366.00
anterior subcapsular polar 366.01
combined forms 366.09
cortical 366.03
lamellar 366.03
nuclear 366.04
posterior subcapsular polar 366.02
specified NEC 366.09
zonular 366.03
lamellar 743.32
infantile, juvenile, or presenile 366.03
morgagnian 366.18
myotonic 359.2 *[366.43]*
myxedema 244.9 *[366.44]*
Cataract—*continued*
posterior, polar (capsular) 743.31
infantile, juvenile, or presenile 366.02
senile 366.14
presenile (*see also* Cataract, juvenile) 366.00
punctate
acquired 366.12
congenital 743.39
secondary (membrane) 366.50
obscuring vision 366.53
specified type, not obscuring vision 366.52
senile 366.10
anterior subcapsular polar 366.13
combined forms 366.19
cortical 366.15
hypermature 366.18
immature 366.12
incipient 366.12
mature 366.17
nuclear 366.16
posterior subcapsular polar 366.14
specified NEC 366.19
total or subtotal 366.17
snowflake 250.5 *[366.41]*
specified NEC 366.8
subtotal (senile) 366.17
congenital 743.34
sunflower 360.24 *[366.34]*
tetanic NEC 252.1 *[366.42]*
total (mature) (senile) 366.17
congenital 743.34
localized 366.21
traumatic 366.22
toxic 366.45
traumatic 366.20
partially resolved 366.23
total 366.22
zonular (perinuclear) 743.32
infantile, juvenile, or presenile 366.03
Cataracta 366.10
brunescens 366.16
cerulea 743.39
complicata 366.30
congenita 743.30
coralliformis 743.39
coronaria (congenital) 743.39
acquired 366.12
diabetic 250.5 *[366.41]*
floriformis 360.24 *[366.34]*
membranacea
accreta 366.50
congenita 743.39
nigra 366.16
Catarrh, catarrhal (inflammation) (*see also* condition) 460
acute 460
asthma, asthmatic (*see also* Asthma) 493.9
Bostock's (*see also* Fever, hay) 477.9
bowel—*see* Enteritis
bronchial 490
acute 466.0
chronic 491.0
subacute 466.0
cervix, cervical (canal) (uteri)—*see* Cervicitis
chest (*see also* Bronchitis) 490
chronic 472.0
congestion 472.0
conjunctivitis 372.03
due to syphilis 095.9
congenital 090.0
enteric—*see* Enteritis

Catarrh, catarrhal—*continued*
epidemic 487.1
Eustachian 381.50
eye (acute) (vernal) 372.03
fauces (*see also* Pharyngitis) 462
febrile 460
fibrinous acute 466.0
gastroenteric—*see* Enteritis
gastrointestinal—*see* Enteritis
gingivitis 523.0
hay (*see also* Fever, hay) 477.9
infectious 460
intestinal—*see* Enteritis
larynx (*see also* Laryngitis, chronic) 476.0
liver 070.1
with hepatic coma 070.0
lung (*see also* Bronchitis) 490
acute 466.0
chronic 491.0
middle ear (chronic)—*see* Otitis media, chronic
mouth 528.0
nasal (chronic) (*see also* Rhinitis) 472.0
acute 460
nasobronchial 472.2
nasopharyngeal (chronic) 472.2
acute 460
nose—*see* Catarrh, nasal
ophthalmia 372.03
pneumococcal, acute 466.0
pulmonary (*see also* Bronchitis) 490
acute 466.0
chronic 491.0
spring (eye) 372.13
suffocating (*see also* Asthma) 493.9
summer (hay) (*see also* Fever, hay) 477.9
throat 472.1
tracheitis 464.10
with obstruction 464.11
tubotympanal 381.4
acute (*see also* Otitis media, acute, nonsuppurative) 381.00
chronic 381.10
vasomotor (*see also* Fever, hay) 477.9
vesical (bladder)—*see* Cystitis
Catarrhus aestivus (*see also* Fever, hay) 477.9
Catastrophe, cerebral (*see also* Disease, cerebrovascular, acute) 436
Catatonia, catatonic (acute) 781.9
agitation 295.2
dementia (praecox) 295.2
excitation 295.2
excited type 295.2
schizophrenia 295.2
stupor 295.2
with
affective psychosis —*see* Psychosis, affective)
Cat-scratch —*see also* Injury, superficial
disease or fever 078.3
Cauda equina —*see also* condition syndrome 344.60
Cauliflower ear 738.7
Caul over face 768.9
Causalgia 355.9
lower limb 355.71
upper limb 354.4
Cause
external, general effects NEC 994.9
not stated 799.9
unknown 799.9
Caustic burn —*see also* Burn, by site
from swallowing caustic or corrosive substance—*see* Burn, internal organs
Cavare's disease (familial periodic paralysis) 359.3
Cave-in, injury
crushing (severe) (*see also* Crush, by site) 869.1
suffocation 994.7
Cavernitis (penis) 607.2
lymph vessel—*see* Lymphangioma
Cavernositis 607.2
Cavernous —*see* condition
Cavitation of lung (*see also* Tuberculosis) 011.2
nontuberculous 518.89
primary, progressive 010.8
Cavity
lung—*see* Cavitation of lung
optic papilla 743.57
pulmonary—*see* Cavitation of lung
teeth 521.0
vitreous (humor) 379.21
Cavovarus foot, congenital 754.59
Cavus foot (congenital) 754.71
acquired 736.73
Cazenave's
disease (pemphigus) NEC 694.4
lupus (erythematosus) 695.4
Cecitis —*see* Appendicitis
Cecocele —*see* Hernia
Cecum —*see* condition
Celiac
artery compression syndrome 447.4
disease 579.0
infantilism 579.0
Cell, cellular —*see also* condition
anterior chamber (eye) (positive aqueous ray) 364.04
Cellulitis (diffuse) (with lymphangitis) (*see also* Abscess) 682.9
abdominal wall 682.2
anaerobic (*see also* Gas gangrene) 040.0
ankle 682.6
anus 566
areola 611.0
arm (any part, above wrist) 682.3
artificial opening (external) 569.61
auditory canal (external) 380.10
axilla 682.3
back (any part) 682.2
breast 611.0
postpartum 675.1
broad ligament (*see also* Disease, pelvis, inflammatory) 614.4
acute 614.3
buttock 682.5
cervical (neck region) 682.1
cervix (uteri) (*see also* Cervicitis) 616.0
cheek, external 682.0
internal 528.3
chest wall 682.2
chronic NEC 682.9
colostomy 569.61
corpus cavernosum 607.2
digit 681.9
Douglas' cul-de-sac or pouch (chronic) (*see also* Disease, pelvis, inflammatory) 614.4
acute 614.3
drainage site (following operation) 998.5
ear, external 380.10
enterostomy 569.61
erysipelar (*see also* Erysipelas) 035
eyelid 373.13

Cellulitis—*continued*
face (any part, except eye) 682.0
finger (intrathecal) (periosteal) (subcutaneous) (subcuticular) 681.00
flank 682.2
foot (except toe) 682.7
forearm 682.3
gangrenous (*see also* Gangrene) 785.4
genital organ NEC
female—*see* Abscess, genital organ, female
male 608.4
glottis 478.71
gluteal (region) 682.5
gonococcal NEC 098.0
groin 682.2
hand (except finger or thumb) 682.4
head (except face) NEC 682.8
heel 682.7
hip 682.6
jaw (region) 682.0
knee 682.6
labium (majus) (minus) (*see also* Vulvitis) 616.10
larynx 478.71
leg, except foot 682.6
lip 528.5
mammary gland 611.0
mouth (floor) 528.3
multiple sites NEC 682.9
nasopharynx 478.21
navel 682.2
newborn NEC 771.4
neck (region) 682.1
nipple 611.0
nose 478.1
external 682.0
orbit, orbital 376.01
palate (soft) 528.3
pectoral (region) 682.2
pelvis, pelvic
with
abortion—*see* Abortion, by type, with sepsis
ectopic pregnancy (*see also* categories 633.0-633.9) 639.0
molar pregnancy (*see also* categories 630-632) 639.0
female (*see also* Disease, pelvis, inflammatory) 614.4
acute 614.3
following
abortion 639.0
ectopic or molar pregnancy 639.0
male (*see also* Abscess, peritoneum) 567.2
puerperal, postpartum, childbirth 670
penis 607.2
perineal, perineum 682.2
perirectal 566
peritonsillar 475
periurethral 597.0
periuterine (*see also* Disease, pelvis, inflammatory) 614.4
acute 614.3
pharynx 478.21
phlegmonous NEC 682.9
rectum 566
retromammary 611.0
retroperitoneal (*see also* Peritonitis) 567.2
round ligament (*see also* Disease, pelvis, inflammatory) 614.4
acute 614.3

Cellulitis—*continued*
scalp (any part) 682.8
dissecting 704.8
scrotum 608.4
seminal vesicle 608.0
septic NEC 682.9
shoulder 682.3
specified sites NEC 682.8
spermatic cord 608.4
submandibular (region) (space) (triangle) 682.0
gland 527.3
submaxillary 528.3
gland 527.3
submental (pyogenic) 682.0
gland 527.3
suppurative NEC 682.9
testis 608.4
thigh 682.6
thumb (intrathecal) (periosteal) (subcutaneous) (subcuticular) 681.00
toe (intrathecal) (periosteal) (subcutaneous) (subcuticular) 681.10
tonsil 475
trunk 682.2
tuberculous (primary) (*see also* Tuberculosis) 017.0
tunica vaginalis 608.4
umbilical 682.2
newborn NEC 771.4
vaccinal 999.3
vagina—*see* Vaginitis
vas deferens 608.4
vocal cords 478.5
vulva (*see also* Vulvitis) 616.10
wrist 682.4
Cementoblastoma, benign (M9273/0) 213.1
upper jaw (bone) 213.0
Cementoma (M9273/0) 213.1
gigantiform (M9276/0) 213.1
upper jaw (bone) 213.0
upper jaw (bone) 213.0
Cementoperiostitis 523.4
Cephalgia, cephalalgia (*see also* Headache) 784.0
histamine 346.2
nonorganic origin 307.81
psychogenic 307.81
tension 307.81
Cephalhematocele, cephalematocele
due to birth injury 767.1
fetus or newborn 767.1
traumatic (*see also* Contusion, head) 920
Cephalhematoma, cephalematoma (calcified)
due to birth injury 767.1
fetus or newborn 767.1
traumatic (*see also* Contusion, head) 920
Cephalic —*see* condition
Cephalitis —*see* Encephalitis
Cephalocele 742.0
Cephaloma —*see* Neoplasm, by site, malignant
Cephalomenia 625.8
Cephalopelvic —*see* condition
Cercomoniasis 007.3
Cerebellitis —*see* Encephalitis
Cerebellum (cerebellar)—*see* condition
Cerebral —*see* condition
Cerebritis —*see* Encephalitis
Cerebrohepatorenal syndrome 759.89
Cerebromacular degeneration 330.1
Cerebromalacia (*see also* Softening, brain) 434.9
Cerebrosidosis 272.7

Cerebrospasticity —*see* Palsy, cerebral
Cerebrospinal —*see* condition
Cerebrum —*see* condition
Ceroid storage disease 272.7
Cerumen (accumulation) (impacted) 380.4
Cervical —*see also* condition
  auricle 744.43
  rib 756.2
Cervicalgia 723.1
Cervicitis (acute) (chronic) (nonvenereal) (subacute) (with erosion or ectropion) 616.0
  with
    abortion—*see* Abortion, by type, with sepsis
    ectopic pregnancy (*see also* categories 633.0-633.9) 639.0
    molar pregnancy (*see also* categories 630-632) 639.0
    ulceration 616.0
  chlamydial 099.53
  complicating pregnancy or puerperium 646.6
    affecting fetus or newborn 760.8
  following
    abortion 639.0
    ectopic or molar pregnancy 639.0
  gonococcal (acute) 098.15
    chronic or duration of 2 months or more 098.35
  senile (atrophic) 616.0
  syphilitic 095.8
  trichomonal 131.09
  tuberculous (*see also* Tuberculosis) 016.7
Cervicoaural fistula 744.49
Cervicocolpitis (emphysematosa) (*see also* Cervicitis) 616.0
Cervix —*see* condition
Cesarean delivery, operation or section NEC 669.7
  affecting fetus or newborn 763.4
  post mortem, affecting fetus or newborn 761.6
  previous, affecting management of pregnancy 654.2
Céstan's syndrome 344.89
Céstan-Chenais paralysis 344.89
Céstan-Raymond syndrome 433.8
Cestode infestation NEC 123.9
  specified type NEC 123.8
Cestodiasis 123.9
Chaberts' disease 022.9
Chacaleh 266.2
Chafing 709.8
Chagas' disease (*see also* Trypanosomiasis, American) 086.2
  with heart involvement 086.0
Chagres fever 084.0
Chalasia (cardiac sphincter) 530.81
Chalazion 373.2
Chalazoderma 757.39
Chalcosis 360.24
  cornea 371.15
  crystalline lens 366.34 *[360.24]*
  retina 360.24.
Chalicosis (occupational) (pulmonum) 502
Chancre (any genital site) (hard) (indurated) (infecting) (primary) (recurrent) 091.0
  congenital 090.0
  conjunctiva 091.2
  Ducrey's 099.0
  extragenital 091.2
  eyelid 091.2
  Hunterian 091.0
  lip (syphilis) 091.2
Chancre—*continued*
  mixed 099.8
  nipple 091.2
  Nisbet's 099.0
  of
    carate 103.0
    pinta 103.0
    yaws 102.0
  palate, soft 091.2
  phagedenic 099.0
  Ricord's 091.0
  Rollet's (syphilitic) 091.0
  seronegative 091.0
  seropositive 091.0
  simple 099.0
  soft 099.0
    bubo 099.0
  urethra 091.0
  yaws 102.0
Chancriform syndrome 114.1
Chancroid 099.0
  anus 099.0
  penis (Ducrey's bacillus) 099.0
  perineum 099.0
  rectum 099.0
  scrotum 099.0
  urethra 099.0
  vulva 099.0
Chandipura fever 066.8
Chandler's disease (osteochondritis dissecans, hip) 732.7
Change (s) (of)—*see also* Removal of
  arteriosclerotic—*see* Arteriosclerosis
  battery
    cardiac pacemaker V53.31
  bone 733.90
    diabetic 250.8 *[731.8]*
    in disease, unknown cause 733.90
  bowel habits 787.99
  cardiorenal (vascular) (*see also* Hypertension, cardiorenal) 404.90
  cardiovascular—*see* Disease, cardiovascular
  circulatory 459.9
  cognitive or personality change of other type, nonpsychotic 310.1
  color, teeth, tooth
    during formation 520.8
    posteruptive 521.7
  contraceptive device V25.42
  cornea, corneal
    degenerative NEC 371.40
    membrane NEC 371.30
    senile 371.41
  coronary (*see also* Ischemia, heart) 414.9
  degenerative
    chamber angle (anterior) (iris) 364.56
    ciliary body 364.57
    spine or vertebra (*see also* Spondylosis) 721.90
  dental pulp, regressive 522.2
  dressing V58.3
  fixation device V54.8
    external V54.8
    internal V54.0
  heart—*see also* Disease, heart
  hip joint 718.95
  hyperplastic larynx 478.79
  hypertrophic
    nasal sinus (*see also* Sinusitis) 473.9
    turbinate, nasal 478.0
    upper respiratory tract 478.9

Change(s) (of)—*continued*
inflammatory—*see* Inflammation
joint (*see also* Derangement, joint) 718.90
sacroiliac 724.6
Kirschner wire V54.8
knee 717.9
macular, congenital 743.55
malignant (M——/3)—*see also* Neoplasm, by site, malignant

Note—for malignant change occurring in a neoplasm, use the appropriate M code with behavior digit /3 e.g., malignant change in uterine fibroid—M8890/3. For malignant change occurring in a nonneoplastic condition (e.g., gastric ulcer) use the M code M8000/3.

mental (status) NEC 780.9
due to or associated with physical condition—*see* Syndrome, brain
myocardium, myocardial—*see* Degeneration, myocardial
of life (*see also* Menopause) 627.2
pacemaker battery (cardiac) V53.31
peripheral nerve 355.9
personality (nonpsychotic) NEC 310.1
plaster cast V54.8
refractive, transient 367.81
regressive, dental pulp 522.2
retina 362.9
myopic (degenerative) (malignant) 360.21
vascular appearance 362.13
sacroiliac joint 724.6
scleral 379.19
degenerative 379.16
senile (*see also* Senility) 797
sensory (*see also* Disturbance, sensation) 782.0
skin texture 782.8
spinal cord 336.9
splint, external V54.8
subdermal implantable contraceptive V25.5
suture V58.3
traction device V54.8
trophic 355.9
arm NEC 354.9
leg NEC 355.8
lower extremity NEC 355.8
upper extremity NEC 354.9
vascular 459.9
vasomotor 443.9
voice 784.49
psychogenic 306.1
Changing sleep-work schedule, affecting sleep 307.45
Changuinola fever 066.0
Chapping skin 709.8
Character
depressive 301.12
Charcot's
arthropathy 094.0 *[713.5]*
cirrhosis—*see* Cirrhosis, biliary
disease 094.0
spinal cord 094.0
fever (biliary) (hepatic) (intermittent)—*see* Choledocholithiasis
joint (disease) 094.0 *[713.5]*
diabetic 250.6 *[713.5]*
syringomyelic 336.0 *[713.5]*
syndrome (intermittent claudication) 443.9
due to atherosclerosis 440.21
Charcot-Marie-Tooth disease, paralysis, or syndrome 356.1
Charleyhorse (quadriceps) 843.8
muscle, except quadriceps—*see* Sprain, by site
Charlouis' disease (*see also* Yaws) 102.9
Chauffeur's fracture —*see* Fracture, ulna, lower end
Cheadle (-Möller) (-Barlow) disease or syndrome (infantile scurvy) 267
Checking (of)
contraceptive device (intrauterine) V25.42
device
fixation V54.8
external V54.8
internal V54.0
traction V54.8
Kirschner wire V54.8
plaster cast V54.8
splint, external V54.8
Checkup
following treatment—*see* Examination
health V70.0
infant (not sick) V20.2
pregnancy (normal) V22.1
first V22.0
high risk pregnancy V23.9
specified problem NEC V23.8
Chédiak-Higashi (-Steinbrinck) anomaly, disease, or syndrome (congenital gigantism of peroxidase granules) 288.2
Cheek —*see also* condition
biting 528.9
Cheese itch 133.8
Cheese washers' lung 495.8
Cheilitis 528.5
actinic (due to sun) 692.72
chronic NEC 692.74
due to radiation, except from sun 692.82
due to radiation, except from sun 692.82
acute 528.5
angular 528.5
catarrhal 528.5
chronic 528.5
exfoliative 528.5
gangrenous 528.5
glandularis apostematosa 528.5
granulomatosa 351.8
infectional 528.5
membranous 528.5
Miescher's 351.8
suppurative 528.5
ulcerative 528.5
vesicular 528.5
Cheilodynia 528.5
Cheilopalatoschisis (*see also* Cleft, palate, with cleft lip) 749.20
Cheilophagia 528.9
Cheiloschisis (*see also* Cleft, lip) 749.10
Cheilosis 528.5
with pellagra 265.2
angular 528.5
due to
dietary deficiency 266.0
vitamin deficiency 266.0
Cheiromegaly 729.89
Cheiropompholyx 705.81
Cheloid (*see also* Keloid) 701.4
Chemical burn —*see also* Burn, by site
from swallowing chemical—*see* Burn, internal organs
Chemodectoma (M8693/1)—*see* Paraganglioma, nonchromaffin
Chemoprophylaxis NEC V07.39
Chemosis, conjunctiva 372.73

Chemotherapy
convalescence V66.2
encounter (for) V58.1
maintenance V58.1
prophylactic NEC V07.39
fluoride V07.31
Cherubism 526.89
Chest —*see* condition
Cheyne-Stokes respiration (periodic) 786.09
Chiari's
disease or syndrome (hepatic vein thrombosis) 453.0
malformation
type I 348.4
type II (*see also* Spina bifida) 741.0
type III 742.0
type IV 742.2
network 746.89
Chiari-Frommel syndrome 676.6
Chicago disease (North American blastomycosis) 116.0
Chickenpox (*see also* Varicella) 052.9
vaccination and inoculation (prophylactic) V05.4
Chiclero ulcer 085.4
Chiggers 133.8
Chignon 111.2
fetus or newborn (from vacuum extraction) 767.1
Chigoe disease 134.1
Chikungunya fever 066.3
Chilaiditi's syndrome (subphrenic displacement, colon) 751.4
Chilblains 991.5
lupus 991.5
Child
behavior causing concern V61.20
Childbed fever 670
Childbirth —*see also* Delivery
puerperal complications—*see* Puerperal
Childhood, period of rapid growth V21.0
Chill (s) 780.9
with fever 780.6
congestive 780.9
in malarial regions 084.6
septic—*see* Septicemia
urethral 599.84
Chilomastigiasis 007.8
Chin —*see* condition
Chinese dysentery 004.9
Chiropractic dislocation (*see also* Lesion, nonallopathic, by site) 739.9
Chitral fever 066.0
Chlamydia, chlamydial -*see* **condition**
Chloasma 709.09
cachecticorum 709.09
eyelid 374.52
congenital 757.33
hyperthyroid 242.0
gravidarum 646.8
idiopathic 709.09
skin 709.09
symptomatic 709.09
Chloroma (M9930/3) 205.3
Chlorosis 280.9
Egyptian (*see also* Ancylostomiasis) 126.9
miners' (*see also* Ancylostomiasis) 126.9
Chlorotic anemia 280.9
Chocolate cyst (ovary) 617.1
Choked
disk or disc—*see* Papilledema
on food, phlegm, or vomitus NEC (*see also* Asphyxia, food) 933.1
phlegm 933.1
while vomiting NEC (*see also* Asphyxia, food) 933.1
Chokes (resulting from bends) 993.3
Choking sensation 784.9
Cholangiectasis (*see also* Disease, gallbladder) 575.8
Cholangiocarcinoma (M8160/3)
and hepatocellular carcinoma, combined (M8180/3) 155.0
liver 155.1
specified site NEC—*see* Neoplasm, by site, malignant
unspecified site 155.1
Cholangiohepatitis 575.8
due to fluke infestation 121.1
Cholangiohepatoma (M8180/3) 155.0
Cholangiolitis (acute) (chronic) (extrahepatic) (gangrenous) 576.1
intrahepatic 575.8
paratyphoidal (*see also* Fever, paratyphoid) 002.9
typhoidal 002.0
Cholangioma (M8160/0) 211.5
malignant—*see* Cholangiocarcinoma
Cholangitis (acute) (ascending) (catarrhal) (chronic) (infective) (malignant) (primary) (recurrent) (sclerosing) (secondary) (stenosing) (suppurative) 576.1
chronic nonsuppurative destructive 571.6
nonsuppurative destructive (chronic) 571.6
Cholecystdocholithiasis —*see* Choledocholithiasis
Cholecystitis

Note—Use the following fifth-digit subclassification with category 574:

0 without mention of obstruction
1 with obstruction

with
calculus, stones in
bile duct (common) (hepatic) 574.4
gallbladder 574.1
choledocholithiasis 574.4
cholelithiasis 574.1
acute 575.0
with
calculus, stones in
bile duct (common) (hepatic) 574.3
gallbladder 574.0
choledocholithiasis 574.3
cholelithiasis 574.0
chronic 575.1
with
calculus, stones in
bile duct (common) (hepatic) 574.4
gallbladder 574.1
choledocholithiasis 574.4
cholelithiasis 574.1
emphysematous (acute) (*see also* Cholecystitis, acute) 575.0
gangrenous (*see also* Cholecystitis, acute) 575.0
paratyphoidal, current (*see also* Fever, paratyphoid) 002.9
suppurative (*see also* Cholecystitis, acute) 575.0
typhoidal 002.0

Choledochitis (suppurative) 576.1
Choledocholith —*see* Choledocholithiasis
Choledocholithiasis 574.5

Note—Use the following fifth-digit subclassification with category 574:

0 without mention of obstruction
1 with obstruction

with cholecystitis 574.4
acute 574.3
chronic 574.4
Cholelithiasis (impacted) (multiple) 574.2

Note—Use the following fifth-digit subclassification with category 574:

0 without mention of obstruction
1 with obstruction

with cholecystitis 574.1
acute 574.0
chronic 574.1
Cholemia (*see also* Jaundice) 782.4
familial 277.4
Gilbert's (familial nonhemolytic) 277.4
Cholemic gallstone —*see* Cholelithiasis
Choleperitoneum, choleperitonitis (*see also* Disease, gallbladder) 567.8
Cholera (algid) (Asiatic) (asphyctic) (epidemic) (gravis) (Indian) (malignant) (morbus) (pestilential) (spasmodic) 001.9
antimonial 985.4
carrier (suspected) of V02.0
classical 001.0
contact V01.0
due to
Vibrio
cholerae (Inaba, Ogawa, Hikojima serotypes) 001.0
El Tor 001.1
El Tor 001.1
exposure to V01.0
vaccination, prophylactic (against) V03.0
Cholerine (*see also* Cholera) 001.9
Cholestasis 576.8
Cholesteatoma (ear) 385.30
attic (primary) 385.31
diffuse 385.35
external ear (canal) 380.21
marginal (middle ear) 385.32
with involvement of mastoid cavity 385.33
secondary (with middle ear involvement) 385.33
mastoid cavity 385.30
middle ear (secondary) 385.32
with involvement of mastoid cavity 385.33
postmastoidectomy cavity (recurrent) 383.32
primary 385.31
recurrent, postmastoidectomy cavity 383.32
secondary (middle ear) 385.32
with involvement of mastoid cavity 385.33
Cholesteatosis (middle ear) (*see also* Cholesteatoma) 385.30
diffuse 385.35
Cholesteremia 272.0
Cholesterin
granuloma, middle ear 385.82
in vitreous 379.22
Cholesterol
deposit
retina 362.82
vitreous 379.22
imbibition of gallbladder (*see also* Disease, gallbladder) 575.6
Cholesterolemia 272.0
essential 272.0
familial 272.0
hereditary 272.0
Cholesterosis, cholesterolosis (gallbladder) 575.6
middle ear (*see also* Cholesteatoma) 385.30
with
cholecystitis—*see* Cholecystitis
cholelithiasis—*see* Cholelithiasis
Cholocolic fistula (*see also* Fistula, gallbladder) 575.5
Choluria 791.4
Chondritis (purulent) 733.99
costal 733.6
Tietze's 733.6
patella, posttraumatic 717.7
posttraumatica patellae 717.7
tuberculous (active) (*see also* Tuberculosis) 015.9
intervertebral 015.0 *[730.88]*
Chondroangiopathia calcarea seu punctate 756.59
Chondroblastoma (M9230/0)—*see also* Neoplasm, bone, benign
malignant (M9230/3)—*see* Neoplasm, bone, malignant
Chondrocalcinosis (articular) (crystal deposition) (dihydrate) (*see also* Arthritis, due to, crystals) 275.4 *[712.3]*
due to
calcium pyrophosphate 275.4 *[712.2]*
dicalcium phosphate crystals 275.4 *[712.1]*
pyrophosphate crystals 275.4 *[712.2]*
Chondrodermatitis nodularis helicis 380.00
Chondrodysplasia 756.4
angiomatose 756.4
calcificans congenita 756.59
epiphysialis punctata 756.59
hereditary deforming 756.4
Chondrodystrophia (fetalis) 756.4
calcarea 756.4
calcificans congenita 756.59
fetalis hypoplastica 756.59
hypoplastica calcinosa 756.59
punctata 756.59
tarda 277.5
Chondrodystrophy (familial) (hypoplastic) 756.4
Chondroectodermal dysplasia 756.55
Chondrolysis 733.99
Chondroma (M9220/0)—*see also* Neoplasm cartilage, benign
juxtacortical (M9221/0)—*see* Neoplasm, bone, benign
periosteal (M9221/0)—*see* Neoplasm, bone, benign
Chondromalacia 733.92
epiglottis (congenital) 748.3
generalized 733.92
knee 717.7
larynx (congenital) 748.3
localized, except patella 733.92
patella, patellae 717.7
systemic 733.92
tibial plateau 733.92
trachea (congenital) 748.3

Chondromatosis (M9220/1)—*see* Neoplasm, cartilage, uncertain behavior
Chondromyxosarcoma (M9220/3)—*see* Neoplasm, cartilage, malignant
Chondro-osteodysplasia (Morquio-Brailsford type) 277.5
Chondro-osteodystrophy 277.5
Chondro-osteoma (M9210/0)—*see* Neoplasm, bone, benign
Chondropathia tuberosa 733.6
Chondrosarcoma (M9220/3)—*see also* Neoplasm, cartilage, malignant
  juxtacortical (M9221/3)—*see* Neoplasm, bone, malignant
  mesenchymal (M9240/3)—*see* Neoplasm, connective tissue, malignant
Chordae tendineae rupture (chronic) 429.5
Chordee (nonvenereal) 607.89
  congenital 752.6
  gonococcal 098.2
Chorditis (fibrinous) (nodosa) (tuberosa) 478.5
Chordoma (M9370/3)—*see* Neoplasm, by site, malignant
Chorea (gravis) (minor) (spasmodic) 333.5
  with
    heart involvement—*see* Chorea with rheumatic heart disease
    rheumatic heart disease (chronic, inactive, or quiescent) (conditions classifiable to 393-398)—*see also* Rheumatic heart condition involved
      active or acute (conditions classifiable to 391) 392.0
  acute—*see* Chorea, Sydenham's
  apoplectic (*see also* Disease, cerebrovascular, acute) 436
  chronic 333.4
  electric 049.8
  gravidarum—*see* Eclampsia, pregnancy
  habit 307.22
  hereditary 333.4
  Huntington's 333.4
  posthemiplegic 344.89
  pregnancy—*see* Eclampsia, pregnancy
  progressive 333.4
    chronic 333.4
    hereditary 333.4
  rheumatic (chronic) 392.9
    with heart disease or involvement—*see* Chorea, with rheumatic heart disease
  senile 333.5
  Sydenham's 392.9
    with heart involvement—*see* Chorea, with rheumatic heart disease
    nonrheumatic 333.5
  variabilis 307.23
Choreoathetosis (paroxysmal) 333.5
Chorioadenoma (destruens) (M9100/1) 236.1
Chorioamnionitis 658.4
  affecting fetus or newborn 762.7
Chorioangioma (M9120/0) 219.8
Choriocarcinoma (M9100/3)
  combined with
    embryonal carcinoma (M9101/3)—*see* Neoplasm, by site, malignant
    teratoma (M9101/3)—*see* Neoplasm, by site, malignant
  specified site—*see* Neoplasm, by site, malignant
  unspecified site
    female 181
    male 186.9
Chorioencephalitis, lymphocytic (acute) (serous) 049.0
Chorioepithelioma (M9100/3)—*see* Choriocarcinoma
Choriomeningitis (acute) (benign) (lymphocytic) (serous) 049.0
Chorionepithelioma (M9100/3)—*see* Choriocarcinoma
Chorionitis (*see also* Scleroderma) 710.1
Chorioretinitis 363.20
  disseminated 363.10
    generalized 363.13
    in
      neurosyphilis 094.83
      secondary syphilis 091.51
    peripheral 363.12
    posterior pole 363.11
    tuberculous (*see also* Tuberculosis) 017.3 *[363.13]*
  due to
    histoplasmosis (*see also* Histoplasmosis) 115.92
    toxoplasmosis (acquired) 130.2
      congenital (active) 771.2
  focal 363.00
    juxtapapillary 363.01
    peripheral 363.04
    posterior pole NEC 363.03
  juxtapapillaris, juxtapapillary 363.01
  progressive myopia (degeneration) 360.21
  syphilitic (secondary) 091.51
    congenital (early) 090.0 *[363.13]*
      late 090.5 *[363.13]*
    late 095.8 *[363.13]*
  tuberculous (*see also* Tuberculosis) 017.3 *[363.13]*
Choristoma —*see* Neoplasm, by site, benign
Choroid —*see* condition
Choroideremia, choroidermia (initial stage) (late stage) (partial or total atrophy) 363.55
Choroiditis (*see also* Chorioretinitis) 363.20
  leprous 030.9 *[363.13]*
  senile guttate 363.41
  sympathetic 360.11
  syphilitic (secondary) 091.51
    congenital (early) 090.0 *[363.13]*
      late 090.5 *[363.13]*
    late 095.8 *[363.13]*
  Tay's 363.41
  tuberculous (*see also* Tuberculosis) 017.3 *[363.13]*
Choroidopathy NEC 363.9
  degenerative (*see also* Degeneration, choroid) 363.40
  hereditary (*see also* Dystrophy, choroid) 363.50
  specified type NEC 363.8
Choroidoretinitis —*see* Chorioretinitis
Choroidosis, central serous 362.41
Choroidretinopathy, serous 362.41
Christian's syndrome (chronic histiocytosis X) 277.8
Christian-Weber disease (nodular nonsuppurative panniculitis) 729.30
Christmas disease 286.1
Chromaffinoma (M8700/0)—*see also* Neoplasm, by site, benign
  malignant (M8700/3)—*see* Neoplasm, by site, malignant
Chromatopsia 368.59
Chromhidrosis, chromidrosis 705.89
Chromoblastomycosis 117.2
Chromomycosis 117.2

Chromophytosis 111.0
Chromotrichomycosis 111.8
Chronic —*see* condition
Chyle cyst, mesentery 457.8
Chylocele (nonfilarial) 457.8
  filarial (*see also* Infestation, filarial) 125.9
  tunica vaginalis (nonfilarial) 608.84
    filarial (*see also* Infestation, filarial) 125.9
Chylomicronemia (fasting) (with hyperprebetalipoproteinemia) 272.3
Chylopericardium (acute) 420.90
Chylothorax (nonfilarial) 457.8
  filarial (*see also* Infestation, filarial) 125.9
Chylous
  ascites 457.8
  cyst of peritoneum 457.8
  hydrocele 603.9
  hydrothorax (nonfilarial) 457.8
    filarial (*see also* Infestation, filarial) 125.9
Chyluria 791.1
  bilharziasis 120.0
  due to
    Brugia (malayi) 125.1
    Wuchereria (bancrofti) 125.0
      malayi 125.1
  filarial (*see also* Infestation, filarial) 125.9
  filariasis (*see also* Infestation, filarial) 125.9
  nonfilarial 791.1
Cicatricial (deformity)—*see* Cicatrix
Cicatrix (adherent) (contracted) (painful) (vicious) 709.2
  adenoid 474.8
  alveolar process 525.8
  anus 569.49
  auricle 380.89
  bile duct (*see also* Disease, biliary) 576.8
  bladder 596.8
  bone 733.99
  brain 348.8
  cervix (postoperative) (postpartal) 622.3
    in pregnancy or childbirth 654.6
      causing obstructed labor 660.2
  chorioretinal 363.30
    disseminated 363.35
    macular 363.32
    peripheral 363.34
    posterior pole NEC 363.33
  choroid—*see* Cicatrix, chorioretinal
  common duct (*see also* Disease, biliary) 576.8
  congenital 757.39
  conjunctiva 372.64
  cornea 371.00
    tuberculous (*see also* Tuberculosis) 017.3 *[371.05]*
  duodenum (bulb) 537.3
  esophagus 530.3
  eyelid 374.46
    with
      ectropion—*see* Ectropion
      entropion—*see* Entropion
  hypopharynx 478.29
  knee, semilunar cartilage 717.5
  lacrimal
    canaliculi 375.53
    duct
      acquired 375.56
      neonatal 375.55
    punctum 375.52
    sac 375.54
  larynx 478.79
  limbus (cystoid) 372.64
Cicatrix—*continued*
  lung 518.89
  macular 363.32
    disseminated 363.35
    peripheral 363.34
  middle ear 385.89
  mouth 528.9
  muscle 728.89
  nasolacrimal duct
    acquired 375.56
    neonatal 375.55
  nasopharynx 478.29
  palate (soft) 528.9
  penis 607.89
  prostate 602.8
  rectum 569.49
  retina 363.30
    disseminated 363.35
    macular 363.32
    peripheral 363.34
    posterior pole NEC 363.33
  semilunar cartilage—*see* Derangement, meniscus
  seminal vesicle 608.89
  skin 709.2
    infected 686.8
    postinfectional 709.2
    tuberculous (*see also* Tuberculosis) 017.0
  specified site NEC 709.2
  throat 478.29
  tongue 529.8
  tonsil (and adenoid) 474.8
  trachea 478.9
  tuberculous NEC (*see also* Tuberculosis) 011.9
  ureter 593.89
  urethra 599.84
  uterus 621.8
  vagina 623.4
    in pregnancy or childbirth 654.7
      causing obstructed labor 660.2
  vocal cord 478.5
  wrist, constricting (annular) 709.2
Cinchonism
  correct substance properly administered 386.9
  overdose or wrong substance given or taken 961.4
Circine herpes 110.5
Circle of Willis —*see* condition
Circular —*see also* condition
  hymen 752.49
Circulating anticoagulants 286.5
  following childbirth 666.3
  postpartum 666.3
Circulation
  collateral (venous), any site 459.89
  defective 459.9
    congenital 747.9
    lower extremity 459.89
  embryonic 747.9
  failure 799.8
    fetus or newborn 779.8
    peripheral 785.59
  fetal, persistence 747.9
  heart, incomplete 747.9
Circulatory system —*see* condition
Circulus senilis 371.41
Circumcision
  in absence of medical indication V50.2
  ritual V50.2
  routine V50.2
Circumscribed —*see* condition

Circumvallata placenta —*see* Placenta, abnormal
Cirrhosis, cirrhotic 571.5
with alcoholism 571.2
alcoholic (liver) 571.2
atrophic (of liver)—*see* Cirrhosis, portal
Baumgarten-Cruveilhier 571.5
biliary (cholangiolitic) (cholangitic) (cholestatic) (extrahepatic) (hypertrophic) (intrahepatic) (nonobstructive) (obstructive) (pericholangiolitic) (posthepatic) (primary) (secondary) (xanthomatous) 571.6
due to
clonorchiasis 121.1
flukes 121.3
brain 331.9
capsular—*see* Cirrhosis, portal
cardiac 571.5
alcoholic 571.2
central (liver)—*see* Cirrhosis, liver
Charcot's 571.6
cholangiolitic—*see* Cirrhosis, biliary
cholangitic—*see* Cirrhosis, biliary
cholestatic—*see* Cirrhosis, biliary
clitoris (hypertrophic) 624.2
coarsely nodular 571.5
congestive (liver)—*see* Cirrhosis, cardiac
Cruveilhier-Baumgarten 571.5
cryptogenic (of liver) 571.5
alcoholic 571.2
dietary (*see also* Cirrhosis, portal) 571.5
due to
bronzed diabetes 275.0
congestive hepatomegaly—*see* Cirrhosis, cardiac
cystic fibrosis 277.00
hemochromatosis 275.0
hepatolenticular degeneration 275.1
passive congestion (chronic)—*see* Cirrhosis, cardiac
Wilson's disease 275.1
xanthomatosis 272.2
extrahepatic (obstructive)—*see* Cirrhosis, biliary
fatty 571.8
alcoholic 571.0
florid 571.2
Glisson's—*see* Cirrhosis, portal
Hanot's (hypertrophic)—*see* Cirrhosis, biliary
hepatic—*see* Cirrhosis, liver
hepatolienal—*see* Cirrhosis, liver
hobnail—*see* Cirrhosis, portal
hypertrophic—*see also* Cirrhosis, liver
biliary—*see* Cirrhosis, biliary
Hanot's—*see* Cirrhosis, biliary
infectious NEC—*see* Cirrhosis, portal
insular—*see* Cirrhosis, portal
intrahepatic (obstructive) (primary) (secondary)—*see* Cirrhosis, biliary
juvenile (*see also* Cirrhosis, portal) 571.5
kidney (*see also* Sclerosis, renal) 587
Laennec's (of liver) 571.2
nonalcoholic 571.5
liver (chronic) (hepatolienal) (hypertrophic) (nodular) (splenomegalic) (unilobar) 571.5
with alcoholism 571.2
alcoholic 571.2
congenital (due to failure of obliteration of umbilical vein) 777.8
cryptogenic 571.5
alcoholic 571.2
Cirrhosis, cirrhotic—*continued*
fatty 571.8
alcoholic 571.0
macronodular 571.5
alcoholic 571.2
micronodular 571.5
alcoholic 571.2
nodular, diffuse 571.5
alcoholic 571.2
pigmentary 275.0
portal 571.5
alcoholic 571.2
postnecrotic 571.5
alcoholic 571.2
syphilitic 095.3
lung (chronic) (*see also* Fibrosis, lung) 515
macronodular (of liver) 571.5
alcoholic 571.2
malarial 084.9
metabolic NEC 571.5
micronodular (of liver) 571.5
alcoholic 571.2
monolobular—*see* Cirrhosis, portal
multilobular—*see* Cirrhosis, portal
nephritis (*see also* Sclerosis, renal) 587
nodular—*see* Cirrhosis, liver
nutritional (fatty) 571.5
obstructive (biliary) (extrahepatic) (intrahepatic)—*see* Cirrhosis, biliary
ovarian 620.8
paludal 084.9
pancreas (duct) 577.8
pericholangiolitic—*see* Cirrhosis, biliary
periportal—*see* Cirrhosis, portal
pigment, pigmentary (of liver) 275.0
portal (of liver) 571.5
alcoholic 571.2
posthepatitic (*see also* Cirrhosis, postnecrotic) 571.5
postnecrotic (of liver) 571.5
alcoholic 571.2
primary (intrahepatic)—*see* Cirrhosis, biliary
pulmonary (*see also* Fibrosis, lung) 515
renal (*see also* Sclerosis, renal) 587
septal (*see also* Cirrhosis, postnecrotic) 571.5
spleen 289.51
splenomegalic (of liver)—*see* Cirrhosis, liver
stasis (liver)—*see* Cirrhosis, liver
stomach 535.4
Todd's (*see also* Cirrhosis, biliary) 571.6
toxic (nodular)—*see* Cirrhosis, postnecrotic
trabecular—*see* Cirrhosis, postnecrotic
unilobar—*see* Cirrhosis, liver
vascular (of liver)—*see* Cirrhosis, liver
xanthomatous (biliary) (*see also* Cirrhosis, biliary) 571.6
due to xanthomatosis (familial) (metabolic) (primary) 272.2
Cistern, subarachnoid 793.0
Citrullinemia 270.6
Citrullinuria 270.6
Ciuffini-Pancoast tumor (M8010/3) (carcinoma, pulmonary apex) 162.3
Civatte's disease or poikiloderma 709.09
Clam diggers' itch 120.3
Clap —*see* Gonorrhea
Clark's paralysis 343.9
Clarke-Hadfield syndrome (pancreatic infantilism) 577.8
Clastothrix 704.2
Claude's syndrome 352.6

Claude Bernard-Horner syndrome (*see also* Neuropathy, peripheral, autonomic) 337.9
Claudication, intermittent 443.9
  cerebral (artery) (*see also* Ischemia, cerebral, transient) 435.9
  due to atherosclerosis 440.21
  spinal cord (arteriosclerotic) 435.1
    syphilitic 094.89
  spinalis 435.1
  venous (axillary) 453.8
Claudicatio venosa intermittens 453.8
Claustrophobia 300.29
Clavus (infected) 700
Claw foot (congenital) 754.71
  acquired 736.74
Claw hand (acquired) 736.06
  congenital 755.59
Clawtoe (congenital) 754.71
  acquired 735.5
Clay eating 307.52
Clay shovelers' fracture —*see* Fracture, vertebra, cervical
Cleansing of artificial opening (*see also* Attention to artificial opening) V55.9
Cleft (congenital)—*see also* Imperfect, closure
  alveolar process 525.8
  branchial (persistent) 744.41
    cyst 744.42
  clitoris 752.49
  cricoid cartilage, posterior 748.3
  facial (*see also* Cleft, lip) 749.10
  lip 749.10
    with cleft palate 749.20
      bilateral (lip and palate) 749.24
        with unilateral lip or palate 749.25
        complete 749.23
        incomplete 749.24
      unilateral (lip and palate) 749.22
        with bilateral lip or palate 749.25
        complete 749.21
        incomplete 749.22
    bilateral 749.14
      with cleft palate, unilateral 749.25
      complete 749.13
      incomplete 749.14
    unilateral 749.12
      with cleft palate, bilateral 749.25
      complete 749.11
      incomplete 749.12
  nose 748.1
  palate 749.00
    with cleft lip 749.20
      bilateral (lip and palate) 749.24
        with unilateral lip or palate 749.25
        complete 749.23
        incomplete 749.24
      unilateral (lip and palate) 749.22
        with bilateral lip or palate 749.25
        complete 749.21
        incomplete 749.22
    bilateral 749.04
      with cleft lip, unilateral 749.25
      complete 749.03
      incomplete 749.04
    unilateral 749.02
      with cleft lip, bilateral 749.25
      complete 749.01
      incomplete 749.02
  penis 752.8
  posterior, cricoid cartilage 748.3
  scrotum 752.8

Cleft—*continued*
  sternum (congenital) 756.3
  thyroid cartilage (congenital) 748.3
  tongue 750.13
  uvula 749.02
    with cleft lip (*see also* Cleft, lip, with cleft palate) 749.20
  water 366.12
Cleft hand (congenital) 755.58
Cleidocranial dysostosis 755.59
Cleidotomy, fetal 763.8
Cleptomania 312.32
Clérambault's syndrome 297.8
  erotomania 302.89
Clergyman's sore throat 784.49
Click, clicking
  systolic syndrome 785.2
Clifford's syndrome (postmaturity) 766.2
Climacteric (*see also* Menopause) 627.2
  arthritis NEC (*see also* Arthritis, climacteric) 716.3
  depression (*see also* Psychosis, affective) 296.2
  disease 627.2
    recurrent episode 296.3
    single episode 296.2
  female (symptoms) 627.2
  male (symptoms) (syndrome) 608.89
  melancholia (*see also* Psychosis, affective) 296.2
    recurrent episode 296.3
    single episode 296.2
  paranoid state 297.2
  paraphrenia 297.2
  polyarthritis NEC 716.39
    male 608.89
  symptoms (female) 627.2
Clinical research investigation V70.7
Clinodactyly 755.59
Clitoris —*see* condition
Cloaca, persistent 751.5
Clonorchiasis 121.1
Clonorchiosis 121.1
Clonorchis infection, liver 121.1
Clonus 781.0
Closed bite 524.2
Closure
  artificial opening (*see also* Attention to artificial opening) V55.9
  congenital, nose 748.0
  cranial sutures, premature 756.0
  defective or imperfect NEC—*see* Imperfect, closure
  fistula, delayed—*see* Fistula
  fontanelle, delayed 756.0
  foramen ovale, imperfect 745.5
  hymen 623.3
  interauricular septum, defective 745.5
  interventricular septum, defective 745.4
  lacrimal duct 375.56
    congenital 743.65
    neonatal 375.55
  nose (congenital) 748.0
    acquired 738.0
  vagina 623.2
  valve—*see* Endocarditis
  vulva 624.8
Clot (blood)
  artery (obstruction) (occlusion) (*see also* Embolism) 444.9
  bladder 596.7

Clot —*continued*
brain (extradural or intradural) (*see also* Thrombosis, brain) 434.0
late effects—*see* category 438
circulation 444.9
heart (*see also* Infarct, myocardium) 410.9
vein (*see also* Thrombosis) 453.9
Clotting defect NEC (*see also* Defect, coagulation) 286.9
Clouded state 780.09
epileptic (*see also* Epilepsy) 345.9
paroxysmal (idiopathic) (*see also* Epilepsy) 345.9
Clouding
corneal graft 996.51
Cloudy antrum, antra 473.0
Clouston's (hidrotic) ectodermal dysplasia 757.31
Clubbing of fingers 781.5
Clubfinger 736.29
acquired 736.29
congenital 754.89
Clubfoot (congenital) 754.70
acquired 736.71
equinovarus 754.51
paralytic 736.71
Club hand (congenital) 754.89
acquired 736.07
Clubnail (acquired) 703.8
congenital 757.5
Clump kidney 753.3
Clumsiness 781.3
syndrome 315.4
Cluttering 307.0
Clutton's joints 090.5
Coagulation, intravascular (diffuse) (disseminated) (*see also* Fibrinolysis) 286.6
newborn 776.2
Coagulopathy (*see also* Defect, coagulation) 286.9
consumption 286.6
intravascular (disseminated) NEC 286.6
newborn 776.2
Coalition
calcaneoscaphoid 755.67
calcaneus 755.67
tarsal 755.67
Coal miners'
elbow 727.2
lung 500
Coal workers' lung or pneumoconiosis 500
Coarctation
aorta (postductal) (preductal) 747.10
pulmonary artery 747.3
Coated tongue 529.3
Coats' disease 362.12
Cocainism (*see also* Dependence) 304.2
Coccidioidal granuloma 114.3
Coccidioidomycosis 114.9
with pneumonia 114.0
cutaneous (primary) 114.1
disseminated 114.3
extrapulmonary (primary) 114.1
lung 114.5
acute 114.0
chronic 114.4
primary 114.0
meninges 114.2
primary (pulmonary) 114.0
acute 114.0
prostate 114.3
Coccidioidomycosis—*continued*
pulmonary 114.5
acute 114.0
chronic 114.4
primary 114.0
specified site NEC 114.3
Coccidioidosis 114.9
lung 114.5
acute 114.0
chronic 114.4
primary 114.0
meninges 114.2
Coccidiosis (colitis) (diarrhea) (dysentery) 007.2
Cocciuria 599.0
Coccus in urine 599.0
Coccydynia 724.79
Coccygodynia 724.79
Coccyx —*see* condition
Cochin-China
diarrhea 579.1
anguilluliasis 127.2
ulcer 085.1
Cock's peculiar tumor 706.2
Cockayne's disease or syndrome (microcephaly and dwarfism) 759.89
Cockayne-Weber syndrome (epidermolysis bullosa) 757.39
Cocked-up toe 735.2
Codman's tumor (benign chondroblastoma) (M9230/0)—*see* Neoplasm, bone, benign
Coenurosis 123.8
Coffee workers' lung 495.8
Cogan's syndrome 370.52
congenital oculomotor apraxia 379.51
nonsyphilitic interstitial keratitis 370.52
Coiling, umbilical cord —*see* Complications, umbilical cord
Coitus, painful (female) 625.0
male 608.89
psychogenic 302.76
Cold 460
with influenza, flu, or grippe 487.1
abscess—*see also* Tuberculosis, abscess
articular—*see* Tuberculosis, joint
agglutinin
disease (chronic) or syndrome 283.0
hemoglobinuria 283.0
paroxysmal (cold) (nocturnal) 283.2
allergic (*see also* Fever, hay) 477.9
bronchus or chest—*see* Bronchitis
with grippe or influenza 487.1
common (head) 460
vaccination, prophylactic (against) V04.7
deep 464.10
effects of 991.9
specified effect NEC 991.8
excessive 991.9
specified effect NEC 991.8
exhaustion from 991.8
exposure to 991.9
specified effect NEC 991.8
grippy 487.1
head 460
injury syndrome (newborn) 778.2
on lung—*see* Bronchitis
rose 477.0
sensitivity, autoimmune 283.0
virus 460
Coldsore (*see also* Herpes, simplex) 054.9
Colibacillosis 041.4
generalized 038.42
Colibacilluria 599.0

Colic (recurrent) 789.0
abdomen 789.0
psychogenic 307.89
appendicular 543.9
appendix 543.9
bile duct—*see* Choledocholithiasis
biliary—*see* Cholelithiasis
bilious—*see* Cholelithiasis
common duct—*see* Choledocholithiasis
Devonshire NEC 984.9
specified type of lead—*see* Table of drugs and chemicals
flatulent 787.3
gallbladder or gallstone—*see* Cholelithiasis
gastric 536.8
hepatic (duct)—*see* Choledocholithiasis
hysterical 300.11
infantile 789.0
intestinal 789.0
kidney 788.0
lead NEC 984.9
specified type of lead—*see* Table of drugs and chemicals
liver (duct)—*see* Choledocholithiasis
mucous 564.1
psychogenic 316 *[564.1]*
nephritic 788.0
painter's NEC 984.9
pancreas 577.8
psychogenic 306.4
renal 788.0
saturnine NEC 984.9
specified type of lead—*see* Table of drugs and chemicals
spasmodic 789.0
ureter 788.0
urethral 599.84
due to calculus 594.2
uterus 625.8
menstrual 625.3
vermicular 543.9
virus 460
worm NEC 128.9
Colicystitis (*see also* Cystitis) 595.9
Colitis (acute) (catarrhal) (croupous) (cystica superficialis) (exudative) (hemorrhagic) (noninfectious) (phlegmonous) (presumed noninfectious) 558.9
adaptive 564.1
allergic 558.9
amebic (*see also* Amebiasis) 006.9
nondysenteric 006.2
anthrax 022.2
bacillary (*see also* Infection, Shigella) 004.9
balantidial 007.0
chronic 558.9
ulcerative (*see also* Colitis, ulcerative) 556.9
coccidial 007.2
dietetic 558.9
due to radiation 558.1
functional 558.9
gangrenous 009.0
giardial 007.1
granulomatous 555.1
gravis (*see also* Colitis, ulcerative) 556.9
infectious (*see also* Enteritis, due to, specific organism) 009.0
presumed 009.1
Colitis—*continued*
ischemic 557.9
acute 557.0
chronic 557.1
due to mesenteric artery insufficiency 557.1
membranous 564.1
psychogenic 316 *[564.1]*
mucous 564.1
psychogenic 316 *[564.1]*
necrotic 009.0
polyposa (*see also* Colitis, ulcerative) 556.9
protozoal NEC 007.9
pseudomembranous 008.45
pseudomucinous 564.1
regional 555.1
segmental 555.1
septic (*see also* Enteritis, due to, specific organism) 009.0
spastic 564.1
psychogenic 316 *[564.1]*
staphylococcus 008.41
food 005.0
thromboulcerative 557.0
toxic 558.2
transmural 555.1
trichomonal 007.3
tuberculous (ulcerative) 014.8
ulcerative (chronic) (idiopathic) (nonspecific) 556.9
entero- 556.0
fulminant 557.0
ileo- 556.1
left-sided 556.5
procto- 556.2
proctosigmoid 556.3
psychogenic 316 *[556]*
specified NEC 556.8
universal 556.6
Collagen disease NEC 710.9
nonvascular 710.9
vascular (allergic) (*see also* Angiitis, hypersensitivity) 446.20
Collagenosis (*see also* Collagen disease) 710.9
cardiovascular 425.4
mediastinal 519.3
Collapse 780.2
adrenal 255.8
cardiorenal (*see also* Hypertension, cardiorenal) 404.90
cardiorespiratory 785.51
fetus or newborn 779.8
cardiovascular (*see also* Disease, heart) 785.51
fetus or newborn 779.8
circulatory (peripheral) 785.59
with
abortion—*see* Abortion, by type, with shock
ectopic pregnancy (*see also* categories 633.0-633.9) 639.5
molar pregnancy (*see also* categories 630-632) 639.5
during or after labor and delivery 669.1
fetus or newborn 779.8
following
abortion 639.5
ectopic or molar pregnancy 639.5
during or after labor and delivery 669.1
fetus or newborn 779.8

Collapse—*continued*
external ear canal 380.50
secondary to
inflammation 380.53
surgery 380.52
trauma 380.51
general 780.2
heart—*see* Disease, heart
heat 992.1
hysterical 300.11
labyrinth, membranous (congenital) 744.05
lung (massive) (*see also* Atelectasis) 518.0
pressure, during labor 668.0
myocardial—*see* Disease, heart
nervous (*see also* Disorder, mental, nonpsychotic) 300.9
neurocirculatory 306.2
nose 738.0
postoperative (cardiovascular) 998.0
pulmonary (*see also* Atelectasis) 518.0
fetus or newborn 770.5
partial 770.5
primary 770.4
thorax 512.8
iatrogenic 512.1
postoperative 512.1
trachea 519.1
valvular—*see* Endocarditis
vascular (peripheral) 785.59
with
abortion—*see* Abortion, by type, with shock
ectopic pregnancy (*see also* categories 633.0-633.9) 639.5
molar pregnancy (*see also* categories 630-632) 639.5
cerebral (*see also* Disease, cerebrovascular, acute) 436
during or after labor and delivery 669.1
fetus or newborn 779.8
following
abortion 639.5
ectopic or molar pregnancy 639.5
vasomotor 785.59
vertebra 733.13
Collateral —*see also* condition
circulation (venous) 459.89
dilation, veins 459.89
Colles' fracture (closed) (reversed) (separation) 813.41
open 813.51
Collet's syndrome 352.6
Collet-Sicard syndrome 352.6
Colliculitis urethralis (*see also* Urethritis) 597.89
Colliers'
asthma 500
lung 500
phthisis (*see also* Tuberculosis) 011.4
Collodion baby (ichthyosis congenita) 757.1
Colloid milium 709.3
Coloboma NEC 743.49
choroid 743.59
fundus 743.52
iris 743.46
lens 743.36
lids 743.62
optic disc (congenital) 743.57
acquired 377.23
retina 743.56
sclera 743.47
Coloenteritis —*see* Enteritis
Colon —*see* condition
Coloptosis 569.89
Color
amblyopia NEC 368.59
acquired 368.55
blindness NEC (congenital) 368.59
acquired 368.55
Colostomy
attention to V55.3
fitting or adjustment V53.5
malfunctioning 569.69
status V44.3
Colpitis (*see also* Vaginitis) 616.10
Colpocele 618.6
Colpocystitis (*see also* Vaginitis) 616.10
Colporrhexis 665.4
Colpospasm 625.1
Column, spinal, vertebral —*see* condition
Coma 780.01
apoplectic (*see also* Disease, cerebrovascular, acute) 436
diabetic (with ketoacidosis) 250.3
hyperosmolar 250.2
eclamptic (*see also* Eclampsia) 780.3
epileptic 345.3
hepatic 572.2
hyperglycemic 250.2
hyperosmolar (diabetic) (nonketotic) 250.2
hypoglycemic 251.0
diabetic 250.3
insulin 250.3
hyperosmolar 250.2
non-diabetic 251.0
organic hyperinsulinism 251.0
Kussmaul's (diabetic) 250.3
liver 572.2
newborn 779.2
prediabetic 250.2
uremic—*see* Uremia
Combat fatigue (*see also* Reaction, stress, acute) 308.9
Combined —*see* condition
Comedo 706.1
Comedocarcinoma (M8501/3)—*see also* Neoplasm, breast, malignant
noninfiltrating (M8501/2)
specified site—*see* Neoplasm, by site, in situ
unspecified site 233.0
Comedomastitis 610.4
Comedones 706.1
lanugo 757.4
Comma bacillus, carrier (suspected) of V02.3
Comminuted fracture —*see* Fracture, by site
Common
aortopulmonary trunk 745.0
atrioventricular canal (defect) 745.69
atrium 745.69
cold (head) 460
vaccination, prophylactic (against) V04.7
truncus (arteriosus) 745.0
ventricle 745.3
Commotio (current)
cerebri (*see also* Concussion, brain) 850.9
with skull fracture—*see* Fracture, skull, by site
retinae 921.3
spinalis—*see* Injury, spinal, by site
Commotion (current)
brain (without skull fracture) (*see also* Concussion, brain) 850.9
with skull fracture—*see* Fracture, skull, by site
spinal cord—*see* Injury, spinal, by site

Communication
abnormal—*see also* Fistula
between
base of aorta and pulmonary artery 745.0
left ventricle and right atrium 745.4
pericardial sac and pleural sac 748.8
pulmonary artery and pulmonary vein 747.3
congenital, between uterus and anterior abdominal wall 752.3
bladder 752.3
intestine 752.3
rectum 752.3
left ventricular-right atrial 745.4
pulmonary artery-pulmonary vein 747.3
Compensation
broken—*see* Failure, heart, congestive
failure—*see* Failure, heart, congestive
neurosis, psychoneurosis 300.11
Complaint —*see also* Disease
bowel, functional 564.9
psychogenic 306.4
intestine, functional 564.9
psychogenic 306.4
kidney (*see also* Disease, renal) 593.9
liver 573.9
miners' 500
Complete —*see* condition
Complex
cardiorenal (*see also* Hypertension, cardiorenal) 404.90
castration 300.9
Costen's 524.60
ego-dystonic homosexuality 302.0
Eisenmenger's (ventricular septal defect) 745.4
homosexual, ego-dystonic 302.0
hypersexual 302.89
inferiority 301.9
jumped process
spine—*see* Dislocation, vertebra
primary, tuberculosis (*see also* Tuberculosis) 010.0
Taussig-Bing (transposition, aorta and overriding pulmonary artery) 745.11
Complications
abortion NEC—*see* categories 634-639
accidental puncture or laceration during a procedure 998.2
amputation stump (late) (surgical) 997.60
traumatic—*see* Amputation, traumatic
anastomosis (and bypass)—*see also* Complications, due to (presence of) any device, implant, or graft classified to 996.0-996.5 NEC
hemorrhage NEC 998.1
intestinal (internal) NEC 997.4
involving urinary tract 997.5
mechanical—*see* Complications, mechanical, graft
urinary tract (involving intestinal tract) 997.5
anesthesia, anesthetic NEC (*see also* Anesthesia, complication) 995.2
in labor and delivery 668.9
affecting fetus or newborn 763.5
cardiac 668.1
central nervous system 668.2
pulmonary 668.0
specified type NEC 668.8
aortocoronary (bypass) graft 996.03
atherosclerosis —*see* Arteriosclerosis, coronary
embolism 996.72

Complications—*continued*
occlusion NEC 996.72
thrombus 996.72
arthroplasty 996.4
artificial opening
cecostomy 569.60
colostomy 569.6
cystostomy 997.5
enterostomy 569.60
gastrostomy 997.4
ileostomy 569.60
jejunostomy 569.60
nephrostomy 997.5
tracheostomy 519.0
ureterostomy 997.5
urethrostomy 997.5
bile duct implant (prosthetic) NEC 996.79
infection or inflammation 996.69
mechanical 996.59
bleeding (intraoperative) (postoperative) 998.1
blood vessel graft 996.1
aortocoronary 996.03
atherosclerosis —*see* Arteriosclerosis, coronary
embolism 996.72
occlusion NEC 996.72
thrombus 996.72
atherosclerosis —*see* Arteriosclerosis, extremities
embolism 996.74
occlusion NEC 996.74
thrombus 996.74
bone growth stimulator NEC 996.78
infection or inflammation 996.67
bone marrow transplant 996.85
breast implant (prosthetic) NEC 996.79
infection or inflammation 996.69
mechanical 996.54
bypass—*see also* Complications, anastomosis
aortocoronary 996.03
atherosclerosis —*see* Arteriosclerosis, coronary
embolism 996.72
occlusion NEC 996.72
thrombus 996.72
carotid artery 996.1
atherosclerosis —*see* Arteriosclerosis, extremities
embolism 996.74
occlusion NEC 996.74
thrombus 996.74
cardiac (*see also* Disease, heart) 429.9
device, implant, or graft NEC 996.72
infection or inflammation 996.61
long-term effect 429.4
mechanical (*see also* Complications, mechanical, by type) 996.00
valve prosthesis 996.71
infection or inflammation 996.61
postoperative NEC 997.1
long-term effect 429.4
cardiorenal (*see also* Hypertension, cardiorenal) 404.90
carotid artery bypass graft 996.1
atherosclerosis —*see* Arteriosclerosis, extremities
embolism 996.74
occlusion NEC 996.74
thrombus 996.74

Complications—*continued*
cataract fragments in eye 998.82
catheter device—*see also* Complications, due to (presence of) any device, implant, or graft classified to 996.0-996.5 NEC
mechanical—*see* Complications, mechanical, catheter
cecostomy 569.60
cesarean section wound 674.3
chin implant (prosthetic) NEC 996.79
infection or inflammation 996.69
mechanical 996.59
colostomy (enterostomy) 569.60
contraceptive device, intrauterine NEC 996.76
infection 996.65
inflammation 996.65
mechanical 996.32
cord (umbilical)—*see* Complications, umbilical cord
cornea
due to
contact lens 371.82
coronary (artery) bypass (graft) NEC 996.03
atherosclerosis —*see* Arteriosclerosis, coronary
embolism 996.72
infection or inflammation 996.61
mechanical 996.03
occlusion NEC 996.72
specified type NEC 996.72
thrombus 996.72
cystostomy 997.5
delivery 669.9
procedure (instrumental) (manual) (surgical) 669.4
specified type NEC 669.8
dialysis (hemodialysis) (peritoneal) (renal) NEC 999.9
catheter—*see also* Complications, due to (presence of) any device, implant or graft classified to 996.0-996.5 NEC
infection or inflammation 996.62
peritoneal 996.69
mechanical 996.1
peritoneal 996.59
due to (presence of) any device, implant, or graft classified to 996.0-996.5
with infection or inflammation—*see* Complications, infection or inflammation, due to (presence of) any device, implant, or graft classified to 996.0-996.5 NEC
arterial NEC 996.74
coronary NEC 996.03
atherosclerosis —*see* Arteriosclerosis, coronary
embolism 996.72
occlusion NEC 996.72
specified type NEC 996.72
thrombus 996.72
renal dialysis 996.73
arteriovenous fistula or shunt NEC 996.74
bone growth stimulator 996.78
breast NEC 996.79
cardiac NEC 996.72
defibrillator 996.72
pacemaker 996.72
valve prosthesis 996.71

Complications—*continued*
catheter NEC 996.79
spinal 996.75
urinary, indwelling 996.76
vascular NEC 996.74
renal dialysis 996.73
ventricular shunt 996.75
coronary (artery) bypass (graft) NEC 996.03
atherosclerosis —*see* Arteriosclerosis, coronary
embolism 996.72
occlusion NEC 996.72
thrombus 996.72
electrodes
brain 996.75
heart 996.72
gastrointestinal NEC 996.79
genitourinary NEC 996.76
heart valve prosthesis NEC 996.71
infusion pump 996.74
internal
joint prosthesis 996.77
orthopedic NEC 996.78
specified type NEC 996.79
intrauterine contraceptive device NEC 996.76
joint prosthesis, internal NEC 996.77
mechanical—*see* Complications, mechanical
nervous system NEC 996.75
ocular lens NEC 996.79
orbital NEC 996.79
orthopedic NEC 996.78
joint, internal 996.77
renal dialysis 996.73
specified type NEC 996.79
urinary catheter, indwelling 996.76
vascular NEC 996.74
ventricular shunt 996.75
during dialysis NEC 999.9
ectopic or molar pregnancy NEC 639.9
electroshock therapy NEC 999.9
enterostomy 569.60
external (fixation) device with internal component(s) NEC 996.78
infection or inflammation 996.67
mechanical 996.4
extracorporeal circulation NEC 999.9
eye implant (prosthetic) NEC 996.79
infection or inflammation 996.69
mechanical
ocular lens 996.53
orbital globe 996.59
gastrointestinal, postoperative NEC (*see also* Complications, surgical procedures) 997.4
gastrostomy 997.4
genitourinary device, implant or graft NEC 996.76
infection or inflammation 996.65
urinary catheter, indwelling 996.64
mechanical (*see also* Complications, mechanical, by type) 996.30
specified NEC 996.39
graft (bypass) (patch)—*see also* Complications, due to (presence of) any device, implant, or graft classified to 996.0-996.5 NEC
bone marrow 996.85
corneal NEC 996.79
infection or inflammation 996.69
rejection or reaction 996.51
mechanical—*see* Complications, mechanical, graft

Complications—*continued*
organ (immune or nonimmune cause) (partial) (total) 996.80
bone marrow 996.85
heart 996.83
intestines 996.89
kidney 996.81
liver 996.82
lung 996.84
pancreas 996.86
specified NEC 996.89
skin NEC 996.79
infection or inflammation 996.69
rejection 996.52
heart—*see also* Disease, heart
transplant (immune or nonimmune cause) 996.83
hemorrhage (intraoperative) (postoperative) 998.1
hyperalimentation therapy NEC 999.9
immunization (procedure)—*see* Complications, vaccination
implant—*see also* Complications, due to (presence of) any device, implant, or graft classified to 996.0-996.5 NEC
mechanical—*see* Complications, mechanical, implant
infection and inflammation
due to (presence of) any device, implant, or graft classified to 996.0-996.5 NEC 996.60
arterial NEC 996.62
coronary 996.61
renal dialysis 996.62
arteriovenous fistula or shunt 996.62
bone growth stimulator 996.67
breast 996.69
cardiac 996.61
catheter NEC 996.69
peritoneal 996.69
spinal 996.63
urinary, indwelling 996.64
vascular NEC 996.62
ventricular shunt 996.63
coronary artery bypass 996.61
electrodes
brain 996.63
heart 996.61
gastrointestinal NEC 996.69
genitourinary NEC 996.65
indwelling urinary catheter 996.64
heart valve 996.61
infusion pump 996.62
intrauterine contraceptive device 996.65
joint prosthesis, internal 996.66
ocular lens 996.69
orbital (implant) 996.69
orthopedic NEC 996.67
joint, internal 996.66
specified type NEC 996.69
urinary catheter, indwelling 996.64
ventricular shunt 996.63
infusion (procedure) 999.9
blood—*see* Complications, transfusion
infection NEC 999.3
sepsis NEC 999.3
inhalation therapy NEC 999.9
injection (procedure) 999.9
drug reaction (*see also* Reaction, drug) 995.2
infection NEC 999.3
sepsis NEC 999.3

Complications—*continued*
serum (prophylactic) (therapeutic)—*see* Complications, vaccination
vaccine (any)—*see* Complications, vaccination
inoculation (any)—*see* Complications, vaccination
internal device (catheter) (electronic) (fixation) (prosthetic) NEC—*see also* Complications, due to (presence of) any device, implant, or graft classified to 996.0-996.5 NEC
mechanical—*see* Complications, mechanical
intestinal transplant (immune or nonimmune cause) 996.89
intraoperative bleeding or hemorrhage 998.1
intrauterine contraceptive device (*see also* Complications, contraceptive device) 996.76
infection or inflammation 996.65
with fetal damage affecting management of pregnancy 655.8
jejunostomy 569.60
kidney transplant (immune or nonimmune cause) 996.81
labor 669.9
specified condition NEC 669.8
liver transplant (immune or nonimmune cause) 996.82
lumbar puncture 349.0
mechanical
anastomosis—*see* Complications, mechanical, graft
bypass—*see* Complications, mechanical, graft
catheter NEC 996.59
cardiac 996.09
cystostomy 996.39
dialysis 996.1
during a procedure 998.2
urethral, indwelling 996.31
device NEC 996.59
balloon (counterpulsation), intra-aortic 996.1
cardiac 996.00
long-term effect 429.4
specified NEC 996.09
contraceptive, intrauterine 996.32
counterpulsation, intra-aortic 996.1
fixation, external, with internal components 996.4
fixation, internal (nail, rod, plate) 996.4
genitourinary 996.30
specified NEC 996.39
nervous system 996.2
orthopedic, internal 996.4
prosthetic NEC 996.59
umbrella, vena cava 996.1
vascular 996.1
dorsal column stimulator 996.2
electrode NEC 996.59
brain 996.2
cardiac 996.01
spinal column 996.2
fistula, arteriovenous, surgically created 996.1
graft NEC 996.52
aortic (bifurcation) 996.1
aortocoronary bypass 996.03
blood vessel NEC 996.1
bone 996.4
cardiac 996.00
carotid artery bypass 996.1
cartilage 996.4
corneal 996.51
coronary bypass 996.03

Complications—*continued*
reimplant—*see also* Complications, due to (presence of) any device, implant, or graft classified to 996.0-996.5 NEC
bone marrow 996.85
extremity (*see also* Complications, reattached, extremity) 996.90
due to infection 996.90
mechanical—*see* Complications, mechanical, reimplant
organ (immune or nonimmune cause) (partial) (total) (*see also* Complications, transplant, organ, by site) 996.80
renal allograft 996.81
renal dialysis—*see* Complications, dialysis
respiratory 519.9
device, implant or graft NEC 996.79
infection or inflammation 996.69
mechanical 996.59
distress syndrome, adult, following trauma or surgery 518.5
insufficiency, acute, postoperative 518.5
postoperative NEC 997.3
therapy NEC 999.9
sedation during labor and delivery 668.9
affecting fetus or newborn 763.5
cardiac 668.1
central nervous system 668.2
pulmonary 668.0
specified type NEC 668.8
shunt—*see also* Complications, due to (presence of) any device, implant, or graft classified to 996.0-996.5 NEC
mechanical—*see* Complications, mechanical, shunt
specified body system NEC
device, implant, or graft—*see* Complications, due to (presence of) any device, implant, or graft classified to 996.0-996.5 NEC
postoperative NEC 997.99
spinal puncture or tap 349.0
stoma, external
gastrointestinal tract NEC 997.4
urinary tract 997.5
surgical procedures 998.9
accidental puncture or laceration 998.2
amputation stump (late) 997.60
anastomosis—*see* Complications, anastomosis
burst stitches or sutures 998.3
cardiac 997.1
long-term effect following cardiac surgery 429.4
cataract fragments in eye 998.82
catheter device—*see* Complications, catheter device
cecostomy malfunction 569.69
colostomy malfunction 569.69
cystostomy malfunction 997.5
dehiscence (of incision) 998.3
dialysis NEC (*see also* Complications, dialysis) 999.9
disruption
anastomosis (internal)—*see* Complications, mechanical, graft
internal suture (line) 998.3
wound 998.3
dumping syndrome (postgastrectomy) 564.2
elephantiasis or lymphedema 997.99
postmastectomy 457.0
emphysema (surgical) 998.81
enterostomy malfunction 569.69

Complications—*continued*
evisceration 998.3
fistula (persistent postoperative) 998.6
foreign body inadvertently left in wound (sponge) (suture) (swab) 998.4
from nonabsorbable surgical material (Dacron) (mesh) (permanent suture) (reinforcing) (Teflon)—*see* Complications, due to (presence of) any device, implant, or graft classified to 996.0-996.5 NEC
gastrointestinal NEC 997.4
gastrostomy malfunction 997.4
hemorrhage or hematoma 998.1
ileostomy malfunction 569.69
internal prosthetic device NEC (*see also* Complications, internal device) 996.70
hemolytic anemia 283.19
infection or inflammation 996.60
malfunction—*see* Complications, mechanical
mechanical complication—*see* Complications, mechanical
thrombus 996.70
jejunostomy malfunction 569.69
malfunction of colostomy or enterostomy 569.69
nervous system NEC 997.00
obstruction, internal anastomosis—*see* Complications, mechanical, graft
other body system NEC 997.99
peripheral vascular NEC 997.2
postcardiotomy syndrome 429.4
postcholecystectomy syndrome 576.0
postcommissurotomy syndrome 429.4
postgastrectomy dumping syndrome 564.2
postmastectomy lymphedema syndrome 457.0
postmastoidectomy 383.30
cholesteatoma, recurrent 383.32
cyst, mucosal 383.31
granulation 383.33
inflammation, chronic 383.33
postvagotomy syndrome 564.2
postvalvulotomy syndrome 429.4
reattached extremity (infection) (rejection) (*see also* Complications, reattached, extremity) 996.90
respiratory NEC 997.3
shock (endotoxic) (hypovolemic) (septic) 998.0
shunt, prosthetic (thrombus)—*see also* Complications, due to (presence of) any device, implant, or graft classified to 996.0-996.5 NEC
hemolytic anemia 283.19
specified complication NEC 998.89
stitch abscess 998.5
transplant—*see* Complications, graft
ureterostomy malfunction 997.5
urethrostomy malfunction 997.5
urinary NEC 997.5
wound infection 998.5
therapeutic misadventure NEC 999.9
surgical treatment 998.9
tracheostomy 519.0
transfusion (blood) (lymphocytes) (plasma) NEC 999.8
atrophy, liver, yellow, subacute (within 8 months of administration)—*see* Hepatitis, viral
bone marrow 996.85

Concussion—*continued*
brain or cerebral (without skull fracture) 850.9
with
loss of consciousness 850.5
brief (less than one hour) 850.1
moderate (1-24 hours) 850.2
prolonged (more than 24 hours) (with complete recovery) (with return to pre-existing conscious level) 850.3
without return to pre-existing conscious level 850.4
mental confusion or disorientation (without loss of consciousness) 850.0
with loss of consciousness—*see* Concussion, brain, with, loss of consciousness
skull fracture—*see* Fracture, skull, by site
without loss of consciousness 850.0
cauda equina 952.4
cerebral—*see* Concussion, brain
conus medullaris (spine) 952.4
hydraulic—*see* Concussion, blast
internal organs—*see* Injury, internal, by site
labyrinth—*see* Injury, intracranial
ocular 921.3
osseous labyrinth—*see* Injury, intracranial
spinal (cord)—*see also* Injury, spinal, by site
due to
broken
back—*see* Fracture, vertebra, by site, with spinal cord injury
neck—*see* Fracture, vertebra, cervical, with spinal cord injury
fracture, fracture dislocation, or compression fracture of spine or vertebra—*see* Fracture, vertebra, by site, with spinal cord injury
syndrome 310.2
underwater blast—*see* Concussion, blast
Condition —*see also* Disease
psychiatric 298.9
respiratory NEC 519.9
acute or subacute NEC 519.9
due to
external agent 508.9
specified type NEC 508.8
fumes or vapors (chemical) (inhalation) 506.3
radiation 508.0
chronic NEC 519.9
due to
external agent 508.9
specified type NEC 508.8
fumes or vapors (chemical) (inhalation) 506.4
radiation 508.1
due to
external agent 508.9
specified type NEC 508.8
fumes or vapors (chemical) (inhalation) 506.9
Conduct disturbance (*see also* Disturbance, conduct) 312.9
adjustment reaction 309.3
hyperkinetic 314.2
Condyloma NEC 078.10
acuminatum 078.11
gonorrheal 098.0
latum 091.3
syphilitic 091.3
congenital 090.0
venereal, syphilitic 091.3
Confinement —*see* Delivery
Conflagration —*see also* Burn, by site
asphyxia (by inhalation of smoke, gases, fumes, or vapors) 987.9
specified agent—*see* Table of drugs and chemicals
Conflict
family V61.9
specified circumstance NEC V61.8
interpersonal NEC V62.81
marital V61.1
involving divorce or estrangement V61.0
parent-child V61.20
Confluent —*see* condition
Confusion, confused (mental) (state) (*see also* State, confusional) 298.9
acute 293.0
epileptic 293.0
postoperative 293.9
psychogenic 298.2
reactive (from emotional stress, psychological trauma) 298.2
subacute 293.1
Congelation 991.9
Congenital —*see also* condition
aortic septum 747.29
intrinsic factor deficiency 281.0
malformation—*see* Anomaly
Congestion, congestive (chronic) (passive)
asphyxia, newborn 768.9
bladder 596.8
bowel 569.89
brain (*see also* Disease, cerebrovascular NEC) 437.8
malarial 084.9
breast 611.79
bronchi 519.1
bronchial tube 519.1
catarrhal 472.0
cerebral—*see* Congestion, brain
cerebrospinal—*see* Congestion, brain
chest 514
chill 780.9
malarial (*see also* Malaria) 084.6
circulatory NEC 459.9
conjunctiva 372.71
due to disturbance of circulation 459.9
duodenum 537.3
enteritis—*see* Enteritis
eye 372.71
fibrosis syndrome (pelvic) 625.5
gastroenteritis—*see* Enteritis
general 799.8
glottis 476.0
heart (*see also* Failure, heart, congestive) 428.0
hepatic 573.0
hypostatic (lung) 514
intestine 569.89
intracranial—*see* Congestion, brain
kidney 593.89
labyrinth 386.50
larynx 476.0
liver 573.0
lung 514
active or acute (*see also* Pneumonia) 486
congenital 770.0
chronic 514
hypostatic 514
idiopathic, acute 518.5
passive 514

Congestion, congestive—*continued*
malaria, malarial (brain) (fever) (*see also* Malaria) 084.6
medulla—*see* Congestion, brain
nasal 478.1
orbit, orbital 376.33
inflammatory (chronic) 376.10
acute 376.00
ovary 620.8
pancreas 577.8
pelvic, female 625.5
pleural 511.0
prostate (active) 602.1
pulmonary—*see* Congestion, lung
renal 593.89
retina 362.89
seminal vesicle 608.89
spinal cord 336.1
spleen 289.51
chronic 289.51
stomach 537.89
trachea 464.11
urethra 599.84
uterus 625.5
with subinvolution 621.1
viscera 799.8
Congestive —*see* Congestion
Conical
cervix 622.6
cornea 371.60
teeth 520.2
Conjoined twins 759.4
causing disproportion (fetopelvic) 653.7
Conjugal maladjustment V61.1
involving divorce or estrangement V61.0
Conjunctiva —*see* condition
Conjunctivitis (exposure) (infectious) (nondiphtheritic) (pneumococcal) (pustular) (staphylococcal) (streptococcal) NEC 372.30
actinic 370.24
acute 372.00
atopic 372.05
contagious 372.03
follicular 372.02
hemorrhagic (viral) 077.4
adenoviral (acute) 077.3
allergic (chronic) 372.14
with hay fever 372.05
anaphylactic 372.05
angular 372.03
Apollo (viral) 077.4
atopic 372.05
blennorrhagic (neonatorum) 098.40
catarrhal 372.03
chemical 372.05
chlamydial 077.98
due to
Chlamydial trachomatis—*see* Trachoma
paratrachoma 077.0
chronic 372.10
allergic 372.14
follicular 372.12
simple 372.11
specified type NEC 372.14
vernal 372.13
diphtheritic 032.81
due to
dust 372.05
enterovirus type 70 077.4
erythema multiforme 695.1 *[372.33]*
filariasis (*see also* Filariasis) 125.9 *[372.15]*
Conjunctivitis—*continued*
mucocutaneous
disease NEC 372.33
leishmaniasis 085.5 *[372.15]*
Reiter's disease 099.3 *[372.33]*
syphilis 095.8 *[372.10]*
toxoplasmosis (acquired) 130.1
congenital (active) 771.2
trachoma—*see* Trachoma
dust 372.05
eczematous 370.31
epidemic 077.1
hemorrhagic 077.4
follicular (acute) 372.02
adenoviral (acute) 077.3
chronic 372.12
glare 370.24
gonococcal (neonatorum) 098.40
granular (trachomatous) 076.1
late effect 139.1
hemorrhagic (acute) (epidemic) 077.4
herpetic (simplex) 054.43
zoster 053.21
inclusion 077.0
infantile 771.6
influenzal 372.03
Koch-Weeks 372.03
light 372.05
medicamentosa 372.05
membranous 372.04
meningococcic 036.89
Morax-Axenfeld 372.02
mucopurulent NEC 372.03
neonatal 771.6
gonococcal 098.40
Newcastle's 077.8
nodosa 360.14
of Beal 077.3
parasitic 372.15
filariasis (*see also* Filariasis) 125.9 *[372.15]*
mucocutaneous leishmaniasis 085.5 *[372.15]*
Parinaud's 372.02
petrificans 372.39
phlyctenular 370.31
pseudomembranous 372.04
diphtheritic 032.81
purulent 372.03
Reiter's 099.3 *[372.33]*
rosacea 695.3 *[372.31]*
serous 372.01
viral 077.99
simple chronic 372.11
specified NEC 372.39
sunlamp 372.04
swimming pool 077.0
trachomatous (follicular) 076.1
acute 076.0
late effect 139.1
traumatic NEC 372.39
tuberculous (*see also* Tuberculosis) 017.3 *[370.31]*
tularemic 021.3
tularensis 021.3
vernal 372.13
limbar 372.13 *[370.32]*
viral 077.99
acute hemorrhagic 077.4
specified NEC 077.8
Conjunctoblepharitis —*see* Conjunctivitis
Conn (-Louis) syndrome (primary aldosteronism) 255.1
Connective tissue —*see* condition

Conradi (-Hünermann) syndrome or disease (chondrodysplasia calcificans congenita) 756.59
Consanguinity V19.7
Consecutive —*see* condition
Consolidated lung (base)—*see* Pneumonia, lobar
Constipation (atonic) (neurogenic) (simple) (spastic) 564.0
 drug induced
  correct substance properly administered 564.0
  overdose or wrong substance given or taken 977.9
   specified drug—*see* Table of drugs and chemicals
 neurogenic 564.0
 psychogenic 306.4
Constitutional —*see also* condition
 arterial hypotension (*see also* Hypotension) 458.9
 obesity 278.00
  morbid 278.01
 psychopathic state 301.9
 short stature 783.4
 state, developmental V21.9
  specified development NEC V21.8
 substandard 301.6
Constitutionally substandard 301.6
Constriction
 anomalous, meningeal bands or folds 742.8
 aortic arch (congenital) 747.10
 asphyxiation or suffocation by 994.7
 bronchus 519.1
 canal, ear (*see also* Stricture, ear canal, acquired) 380.50
 duodenum 537.3
 gallbladder (*see also* Obstruction, gallbladder) 575.2
  congenital 751.69
 intestine (*see also* Obstruction, intestine) 560.9
 larynx 478.74
  congenital 748.3
 meningeal bands or folds, anomalous 742.8
 organ or site, congenital NEC—*see* Atresia
 prepuce (congenital) 605
 pylorus 537.0
  adult hypertrophic 537.0
  congenital or infantile 750.5
  newborn 750.5
 ring (uterus) 661.4
  affecting fetus or newborn 763.7
 spastic—*see also* Spasm
  ureter 593.3
  urethra—*see* Stricture, urethra
 stomach 537.89
 ureter 593.3
 urethra—*see* Stricture, urethra
 visual field (functional) (peripheral) 368.45
Constrictive —*see* condition
Consultation V65.9
 medical—*see also* Counseling, medical
 specified reason NEC V65.8
 without complaint or sickness V65.9
  feared complaint unfounded V65.5
  specified reason NEC V65.8
Consumption —*see* Tuberculosis
Contact
 with
  AIDS virus V01.7
  cholera V01.0
  communicable disease V01.9
   specified type NEC V01.8
   viral NEC V01.7
Contact—*continued*
  German measles V01.4
  gonorrhea V01.6
  HIV V01.7
  human immunodeficiency virus V01.7
  parasitic disease NEC V01.8
  poliomyelitis V01.2
  rabies V01.5
  rubella V01.4
  smallpox V01.3
  syphilis V01.6
  tuberculosis V01.1
  venereal disease V01.6
  viral disease NEC V01.7
 dermatitis—*see* Dermatitis
Contamination, food (*see also* Poisoning, food) 005.9
Contraception, contraceptive
 advice NEC V25.09
  family planning V25.09
  fitting of diaphragm V25.02
  prescribing or use of
   oral contraceptive agent V25.01
   specified agent NEC V25.02
 counseling NEC V25.09
  family planning V25.09
  fitting of diaphragm V25.02
  prescribing or use of
   oral contraceptive agent V25.01
   specified agent NEC V25.02
 device (in situ) V45.59
  causing menorrhagia 996.76
  checking V25.42
  complications 996.32
  insertion V25.1
  intrauterine V45.51
  reinsertion V25.42
  removal V25.42
  subdermal V45.52
 fitting of diaphragm V25.02
 insertion
  intrauterine contraceptive device V25.1
  subdermal implantable V25.5
 maintenance V25.40
  examination V25.40
   intrauterine device V25.42
   oral contraceptive V25.41
   specified method NEC V25.49
   subdermal implantable V25.43
  intrauterine device V25.42
  oral contraceptive V25.41
  specified method NEC V25.49
  subdermal implantable V25.43
 management NEC V25.49
 prescription
  oral contraceptive agent V25.01
   repeat V25.41
  specified agent NEC V25.02
   repeat V25.49
 sterilization V25.2
 surveillance V25.40
  intrauterine device V25.42
  oral contraceptive agent V25.41
  specified method NEC V25.49
  subdermal implantable V25.43
Contraction, contracture, contracted
 Achilles tendon (*see also* Short, tendon, Achilles) 727.81
 anus 564.8
 axilla 729.9
 bile duct (*see also* Disease, biliary) 576.8

Contraction . . .—*continued*
bladder 596.8
neck or sphincter 596.0
bowel (*see also* Obstruction, intestine) 560.9
Braxton Hicks 644.1
bronchus 519.1
burn (old)—*see* Cicatrix
cecum (*see also* Obstruction, intestine) 560.9
cervix (*see also* Stricture, cervix) 622.4
congenital 752.49
cicatricial—*see* Cicatrix
colon (*see also* Obstruction, intestine) 560.9
conjunctiva trachomatous, active 076.1
late effect 139.1
Dupuytren's 728.6
eyelid 374.41
eye socket (after enucleation) 372.64
face 729.9
fascia (lata) (postural) 728.89
Dupuytren's 728.6
palmar 728.6
plantar 728.71
finger NEC 736.29
congenital 755.59
joint (*see also* Contraction, joint) 718.44
flaccid, paralytic
joint (*see also* Contraction, joint) 718.4
muscle 728.85
ocular 378.50
gallbladder (*see also* Obstruction, gallbladder) 575.2
hamstring 728.89
tendon 727.81
heart valve—*see* Endocarditis
Hicks' 644.1
hip (*see also* Contraction, joint) 718.4
hourglass
bladder 596.8
congenital 753.8
gallbladder (*see also* Obstruction, gallbladder) 575.2
congenital 751.69
stomach 536.8
congenital 750.7
psychogenic 306.4
uterus 661.4
affecting fetus or newborn 763.7
hysterical 300.11
infantile (*see also* Epilepsy) 345.6
internal os (*see also* Stricture, cervix) 622.4
intestine (*see also* Obstruction, intestine) 560.9
joint (abduction) (acquired) (adduction) (flexion) (rotation) 718.40
ankle 718.47
congenital NEC 755.8
generalized or multiple 754.89
lower limb joints 754.89
hip (*see also* Subluxation, congenital, hip) 754.32
lower limb (including pelvic girdle) not involving hip 754.89
upper limb (including shoulder girdle) 755.59
elbow 718.42
foot 718.47
hand 718.44
hip 718.45
hysterical 300.11
knee 718.46
multiple sites 718.49
pelvic region 718.45
shoulder (region) 718.41

Contraction . . .—*continued*
specified site NEC 718.48
wrist 718.43
kidney (granular) (secondary) (*see also* Sclerosis, renal) 587
congenital 753.3
hydronephritic 591
pyelonephritic (*see also* Pyelitis, chronic) 590.00
tuberculous (*see also* Tuberculosis) 016.0
ligament 728.89
congenital 756.89
liver—*see* Cirrhosis, liver
muscle (postinfectional) (postural) NEC 728.85
congenital 756.89
sternocleidomastoid 754.1
extraocular 378.60
eye (extrinsic) (*see also* Strabismus) 378.9
paralytic (*see also* Strabismus, paralytic) 378.50
flaccid 728.85
hysterical 300.11
ischemic (Volkmann's) 958.6
paralytic 728.85
posttraumatic 958.6
psychogenic 306.0
specified as conversion reaction 300.11
myotonic 728.85
neck (*see also* Torticollis) 723.5
congenital 754.1
psychogenic 306.0
ocular muscle (*see also* Strabismus) 378.9
paralytic (*see also* Strabismus, paralytic) 378.50
organ or site, congenital NEC—*see* Atresia
outlet (pelvis)—*see* Contraction, pelvis
palmar fascia 728.6
paralytic
joint (*see also* Contraction, joint) 718.4
muscle 728.85
ocular (*see also* Strabismus, paralytic) 378.50
pelvis (acquired) (general) 738.6
affecting fetus or newborn 763.1
complicating delivery 653.1
causing obstructed labor 660.1
generally contracted 653.1
causing obstructed labor 660.1
inlet 653.2
causing obstructed labor 660.1
midpelvic 653.8
causing obstructed labor 660.1
midplane 653.8
causing obstructed labor 660.1
outlet 653.3
causing obstructed labor 660.1
plantar fascia 728.71
premature
atrial 427.61
auricular 427.61
auriculoventricular 427.61
heart (junctional) (nodal) 427.60
supraventricular 427.61
ventricular 427.69
prostate 602.8
pylorus (*see also* Pylorospasm) 537.81
rectosigmoid (*see also* Obstruction, intestine) 560.9
rectum, rectal (sphincter) 564.8
psychogenic 306.4

Contraction . . .—*continued*
ring (Bandl's) 661.4
affecting fetus or newborn 763.7
scar—*see* Cicatrix
sigmoid (*see also* Obstruction, intestine) 560.9
socket, eye 372.64
spine (*see also* Curvature, spine) 737.9
stomach 536.8
hourglass 536.8
congenital 750.7
psychogenic 306.4
psychogenic 306.4
tendon (sheath) (*see also* Short, tendon) 727.81
toe 735.8
ureterovesical orifice (postinfectional) 593.3
urethra 599.84
uterus 621.8
abnormal 661.9
affecting fetus or newborn 763.7
clonic, hourglass or tetanic 661.4
affecting fetus or newborn 763.7
dyscoordinate 661.4
affecting fetus or newborn 763.7
hourglass 661.4
affecting fetus or newborn 763.7
hypotonic NEC 661.2
affecting fetus or newborn 763.7
incoordinate 661.4
affecting fetus or newborn 763.7
inefficient or poor 661.2
affecting fetus or newborn 763.7
irregular 661.2
affecting fetus or newborn 763.7
tetanic 661.4
affecting fetus or newborn 763.7
vagina (outlet) 623.2
vesical 596.8
neck or urethral orifice 596.0
visual field, generalized 368.45
Volkmann's (ischemic) 958.6
Contusion (skin surface intact) 924.9
with
crush injury—*see* Crush
dislocation—*see* Dislocation, by site
fracture—*see* Fracture, by site
internal injury—*see also* Injury, internal, by site
heart—*see* Contusion, cardiac
kidney—*see* Contusion, kidney
liver—*see* Contusion, liver
lung—*see* Contusion, lung
spleen—*see* Contusion, spleen
intracranial injury—*see* Injury, intracranial
nerve injury—*see* Injury, nerve
open wound—*see* Wound, open, by site
abdomen, abdominal (muscle) (wall) 922.2
organ(s) NEC 868.00
adnexa, eye NEC 921.9
ankle 924.21
with other parts of foot 924.20
arm 923.9
lower (with elbow) 923.10
upper 923.03
with shoulder or axillary region 923.09
auditory canal (external) (meatus) (and other part(s) of neck, scalp, or face, except eye) 920
auricle, ear (and other part(s) of neck, scalp, or face except eye) 920
axilla 923.02
with shoulder or upper arm 923.09

Contusion—*continued*
back 922.3
bone NEC 924.9
brain (cerebral) (membrane) (with hemorrhage) 851.8

Note—Use the following fifth-digit subclassification with categories 851-854:

0 unspecified state of consciousness
1 with no loss of consciousness
2 with brief [less than one hour] loss of consciousness
3 with moderate [1-24 hours] loss of consciousness
4 with prolonged [more than 24 hours] loss of consciousness and return to pre-existing conscious level
5 with prolonged [more than 24 hours] loss of consciousness, without return to pre-existing conscious level
6 with loss of consciousness of unspecified duration
9 with concussion, unspecified

with
open intracranial wound 851.9
skull fracture—*see* Fracture, skull, by site
cerebellum 851.4
with open intracranial wound 851.5
cortex 851.0
with open intracranial wound 851.1
occipital lobe 851.4
with open intracranial wound 851.5
stem 851.4
with open intracranial wound 851.5
breast 922.0
brow (and other part(s) of neck, scalp, or face, except eye) 920
buttock 922.3
canthus 921.1
cardiac 861.01
with open wound into thorax 861.11
cauda equina (spine) 952.4
cerebellum—*see* Contusion, brain, cerebellum
cerebral—*see* Contusion, brain
cheek(s) (and other part(s) of neck, scalp, or face, except eye) 920
chest (wall) 922.1
chin (and other part(s) of neck, scalp, or face, except eye) 920
clitoris 922.4
conjunctiva 921.1
conus medullaris (spine) 952.4
cornea 921.3
corpus cavernosum 922.4
cortex (brain) (cerebral)—*see* Contusion, brain, cortex
costal region 922.1
ear (and other part(s) of neck, scalp, or face except eye) 920
elbow 923.11
with forearm 923.10
epididymis 922.4
epigastric region 922.2
eye NEC 921.9
eyeball 921.3
eyelid(s) (and periocular area) 921.1
face (and neck, or scalp any part, except eye) 920
femoral triangle 922.2
fetus or newborn 772.6
finger(s) (nail) (subungual) 923.3

Contusion—*continued*
flank 922.2
foot (with ankle) (excluding toe(s)) 924.20
forearm (and elbow) 923.10
forehead (and other part(s) of neck, scalp, or face, except eye) 920
genital organs, external 922.4
globe (eye) 921.3
groin 922.2
gum(s) (and other part(s) of neck, scalp, or face, except eye) 920
hand(s) (except fingers alone) 923.20
head (any part, except eye) (and face) (and neck) 920
heart—*see* Contusion, cardiac
heel 924.20
hip 924.01
with thigh 924.00
iliac region 922.2
inguinal region 922.2
internal organs (abdomen, chest, or pelvis) NEC—*see* Injury, internal, by site
interscapular region 922.3
iris (eye) 921.3
kidney 866.01
with open wound into cavity 866.11
knee 924.11
with lower leg 924.10
labium (majus) (minus) 922.4
lacrimal apparatus, gland, or sac 921.1
larynx (and other part(s) of neck, scalp, or face, except eye) 920
late effect—*see* Late, effects (of), contusion
leg 924.5
lower (with knee) 924.10
lens 921.3
lingual (and other part(s) of neck, scalp, or face, except eye) 920
lip(s) (and other part(s) of neck, scalp, or face, except eye) 920
liver 864.01
with
laceration—*see* Laceration, liver
open wound into cavity 864.11
lower extremity 924.5
multiple sites 924.4
lumbar region 922.3
lung 861.21
with open wound into thorax 861.31
malar region (and other part(s) of neck, scalp, or face, except eye) 920
mandibular joint (and other part(s) of neck, scalp, or face, except eye) 920
mastoid region (and other part(s) of neck, scalp, or face, except eye) 920
membrane, brain—*see* Contusion, brain
midthoracic region 922.1
mouth (and other part(s) of neck, scalp, or face, except eye) 920
multiple sites (not classifiable to same three-digit category) 924.8
lower limb 924.4
trunk 922.8
upper limb 923.8
muscle NEC 924.9
myocardium—*see* Contusion, cardiac
nasal (septum) (and other part(s) of neck, scalp, or face, except eye) 920
neck (and scalp, or face any part, except eye) 920
nerve—*see* Injury, nerve, by site

Contusion—*continued*
nose (and other part(s) of neck, scalp, or face, except eye) 920
occipital region (scalp) (and neck or face, except eye) 920
lobe—*see* Contusion, brain, occipital lobe
orbit (region) (tissues) 921.2
palate (soft) (and other part(s) of neck, scalp, or face, except eye) 920
parietal region (scalp) (and neck, or face, except eye) 920
lobe—*see* Contusion, brain
penis 922.4
pericardium—*see* Contusion, cardiac
perineum 922.4
periocular area 921.1
pharynx (and other part(s) of neck, scalp, or face, except eye) 920
popliteal space (*see also* Contusion, knee) 924.11
prepuce 922.4
pubic region 922.4
pudenda 922.4
pulmonary—*see* Contusion, lung
quadriceps femoralis 924.00
rib cage 922.1
sacral region 922.3
salivary ducts or glands (and other part(s) of neck, scalp, or face, except eye) 920
scalp (and neck, or face any part, except eye) 920
scapular region 923.01
with shoulder or upper arm 923.09
sclera (eye) 921.3
scrotum 922.4
shoulder 923.00
with upper arm or axillar regions 923.09
skin NEC 924.9
skull 920
spermatic cord 922.4
spinal cord—*see also* Injury, spinal, by site
cauda equina 952.4
conus medullaris 952.4
spleen 865.01
with open wound into cavity 865.11
sternal region 922.1
stomach—*see* Injury, internal, stomach
subconjunctival 921.1
subcutaneous NEC 924.9
submaxillary region (and other part(s) of neck, scalp, or face, except eye) 920
submental region (and other part(s) of neck, scalp, or face, except eye) 920
subperiosteal NEC 924.9
supraclavicular fossa (and other part(s) of neck, scalp, or face, except eye) 920
supraorbital (and other part(s) of neck, scalp, or face, except eye) 920
temple (region) (and other part(s) of neck, scalp, or face, except eye) 920
testis 922.4
thigh (and hip) 924.00
thorax 922.1
organ—*see* Injury, internal, intrathoracic
throat (and other part(s) of neck, scalp, or face, except eye) 920
thumb(s) (nail) (subungual) 923.3
toe(s) (nail) (subungual) 924.3
tongue (and other part(s) of neck, scalp, or face, except eye) 920
trunk 922.9
multiple sites 922.8

Contusion—*continued*
specified site—*see* Contusion, by site
tunica vaginalis 922.4
tympanum (membrane) (and other part(s) of neck, scalp, or face, except eye) 920
upper extremity 923.9
multiple sites 923.8
uvula (and other part(s) of neck, scalp, or face, except eye) 920
vagina 922.4
vocal cord(s) (and other part(s) of neck, scalp, or face, except eye) 920
vulva 922.4
wrist 923.21
with hand(s), except finger(s) alone 923.20
Conus (any type) (congenital) 743.57
acquired 371.60
medullaris syndrome 336.8
Convalescence (following) V66.9
chemotherapy V66.2
medical NEC V66.5
psychotherapy V66.3
radiotherapy V66.1
surgery NEC V66.0
treatment (for) NEC V66.5
combined V66.6
fracture V66.4
mental disorder NEC V66.3
specified disorder NEC V66.5
Conversion
hysteria, hysterical, any type 300.11
neurosis, any 300.11
reaction, any 300.11
Converter, tuberculosis (test reaction) 795.5
Convulsions (idiopathic) 780.3
apoplectiform (*see also* Disease, cerebrovascular, acute) 436
brain 780.3
cerebral 780.3
cerebrospinal 780.3
due to trauma NEC—*see* Injury, intracranial
eclamptic (*see also* Eclampsia) 780.3
epileptic (*see also* Epilepsy) 345.9
epileptiform (*see also* Seizure, epileptiform) 780.3
epileptoid (*see also* Seizure, epileptiform) 780.3
ether
anesthetic
correct substance properly administered 780.3
overdose or wrong substance given 968.2
other specified type—*see* Table of drugs and chemicals
febrile 780.3
generalized 780.3
hysterical 300.11
infantile 780.3
epilepsy—*see* Epilepsy
internal 780.3
jacksonian (*see also* Epilepsy) 345.5
myoclonic 333.2
newborn 779.0
paretic 094.1
pregnancy (nephritic) (uremic)—*see* Eclampsia, pregnancy
psychomotor (*see also* Epilepsy) 345.4
puerperal, postpartum—*see* Eclampsia, pregnancy
recurrent 780.3
epileptic—*see* Epilepsy
reflex 781.0

Convulsions—*continued*
repetitive 780.3
epileptic—*see* Epilepsy
salaam (*see also* Epilepsy) 345.6
scarlatinal 034.1
spasmodic 780.3
tetanus, tetanic (*see also* Tetanus) 037
thymic 254.8
uncinate 780.3
uremic 586
Convulsive —*see also* Convulsions
disorder or state 780.3
epileptic—*see* Epilepsy
equivalent, abdominal (*see also* Epilepsy) 345.5
Cooke-Apert-Gallais syndrome (adrenogenital) 255.2
Cooley's anemia (erythroblastic) 282.4
Coolie itch 126.9
Cooper's
disease 610.1
hernia—*see* Hernia, Cooper's
Coordination disturbance 781.3
Copper wire arteries, retina 362.13
Copra itch 133.8
Coprolith 560.39
Coprophilia 302.89
Coproporphyria, hereditary 277.1
Coprostasis 560.39
with hernia—*see also* Hernia, by site, with obstruction
gangrenous—*see* Hernia, by site, with gangrene
Cor
biloculare 745.7
bovinum—*see* Hypertrophy, cardiac
bovis—*see also* Hypertrophy, cardiac
pulmonale (chronic) 416.9
acute 415.0
triatriatum, triatrium 746.82
triloculare 745.8
biatriatum 745.3
biventriculare 745.69
Corbus' disease 607.1
Cord— *see also* condition
around neck (tightly) (with compression)
affecting fetus or newborn 762.5
complicating delivery 663.1
without compression 663.3
affecting fetus or newborn 762.6
bladder NEC 344.61
tabetic 094.0
prolapse
affecting fetus or newborn 762.4
complicating delivery 663.0
Cord's angiopathy (*see also* Tuberculosis) 017.3 *[362.18]*
Cordis ectopia 746.87
Corditis (spermatic) 608.4
Corectopia 743.46
Cori type glycogen storage disease —*see* Disease, glycogen storage
Cork-handlers' disease or lung 495.3
Corkscrew esophagus 530.5
Corlett's pyosis (impetigo) 684
Corn (infected) 700
Cornea—*see also* **condition**
donor V59.5
guttata (dystrophy) 371.57
plana 743.41
Cornelia de Lange's syndrome (Amsterdam dwarf, mental retardation, and brachycephaly) 759.89

Cornual gestation or pregnancy —*see* Pregnancy, cornual
Cornu cutaneum 702.8
Coronary (artery)—*see also* condition
arising from aorta or pulmonary trunk 746.85
Corpora —*see also* condition
amylacea (prostate) 602.8
cavernosa—*see* condition
Corpulence (*see also* Obesity) 278.0
Corpus —*see* condition
Corrigan's disease —*see* Insufficiency, aortic
Corrosive burn —*see* Burn, by site
Corsican fever (*see also* Malaria) 084.6
Cortical —*see also* condition
blindness 377.75
necrosis, kidney (acute) (bilateral) 583.6
Corticoadrenal —*see* condition
Corticosexual syndrome 255.2
Coryza (acute) 460
with grippe or influenza 487.1
syphilitic 095.8
congenital (chronic) 090.0
Costen's syndrome or complex 524.60
Costiveness (*see also* Constipation) 564.0
Costochondritis 733.6
Cotard's syndrome (paranoia) 297.1
Cot death 798.0
Cotungo's disease 724.3
Cough 786.2
with hemorrhage (*see also* Hemoptysis) 786.3
affected 786.2
bronchial 786.2
with grippe or influenza 487.1
chronic 786.2
epidemic 786.2
functional 306.1
hemorrhagic 786.3
hysterical 300.11
laryngeal, spasmodic 786.2
nervous 786.2
psychogenic 306.1
smokers' 491.0
tea tasters' 112.89
Counseling V65.40
child abuse, maltreatment, or neglect V61.21
contraceptive NEC V25.09
device (intrauterine) V25.02
maintenance V25.40
intrauterine contraceptive device V25.42
oral contraceptive (pill) V25.41
specified type NEC V25.49
subdermal implantable V25.43
management NEC V25.9
oral contraceptive (pill) V25.01
prescription NEC V25.02
oral contraceptive (pill) V25.01
repeat prescription V25.41
repeat prescription V25.40
subdermal implantable V25.43
surveillance V25.40
dietary V65.3
exercise V65.41
explanation of
investigation finding NEC V65.49
medication NEC V65.49
family planning V25.09
for nonattending third party V65.1
genetic V26.3
gonorrhea V65.45
health (advice) (education) (instruction) NEC V65.49
Counseling—*continued*
HIV V65.44
human immunodeficiency virus V65.44
injury prevention V65.43
medical (for) V65.9
boarding school resident V60.6
condition not demonstrated V65.5
feared complaint and no disease found V65.5
institutional resident V60.1
on behalf of another V65.1
person living alone V60.3
parent-child conflict V61.20
specified problem NEC V61.29
procreative V65.49
sex NEC V65.49
transmitted disease NEC V65.45
HIV V65.44
specified reason NEC V65.49
substance use and abuse V65.42
syphilis V65.45
without complaint or sickness V65.49
Coupled rhythm 427.89
Couvelaire uterus (complicating delivery)—*see* Placenta, separation
Cowper's gland —*see* condition
Cowperitis (*see also* Urethritis) 597.89
gonorrheal (acute) 098.0
chronic or duration of 2 months or over 098.2
Cowpox (abortive) 051.0
due to vaccination 999.0
eyelid 051.0 *[373.5]*
postvaccination 999.0 *[373.5]*
Coxa
plana 732.1
valga (acquired) 736.31
congenital 755.61
late effect of rickets 268.1
vara (acquired) 736.32
congenital 755.62
late effect of rickets 268.1
Coxae malum senilis 715.25
Coxalgia (nontuberculous) 719.45
tuberculous (*see also* Tuberculosis) 015.1 *[730.85]*
Coxalgic pelvis 736.30
Coxitis 716.65
Coxsackie (infection) (virus) 079.2
central nervous system NEC 048
endocarditis 074.22
enteritis 008.67
meningitis (aseptic) 047.0
myocarditis 074.23
pericarditis 074.21
pharyngitis 074.0
pleurodynia 074.1
specific disease NEC 074.8
Crabs, meaning pubic lice 132.2
Crack baby 760.75
Cracked nipple 611.2
puerperal, postpartum 676.1
Cradle cap 690.11
Craft neurosis 300.89
Craigiasis 007.8
Cramp (s) 729.82
abdominal 789.0
bathing 994.1
colic 789.0
psychogenic 306.4
due to immersion 994.1
extremity (lower) (upper) NEC 729.82
fireman 992.2
heat 992.2

Cramp(s)—*continued*
hysterical 300.11
immersion 994.1
intestinal 789.0
psychogenic 306.4
linotypist's 300.89
organic 333.84
muscle (extremity) (general) 729.82
due to immersion 994.1
hysterical 300.11
occupational (hand) 300.89
organic 333.84
psychogenic 307.89
salt depletion 276.1
stoker 992.2
stomach 789.0
telegraphers' 308.9
organic 333.84
typists' 300.89
organic 333.84
uterus 625.8
menstrual 625.3
writers' 300.89
organic 333.84
Cranial —*see* condition
Cranioclasis, fetal 763.8
Craniocleidodysostosis 755.59
Craniofenestria (skull) 756.0
Craniolacunia (skull) 756.0
Craniopagus 759.4
Craniopathy, metabolic 733.3
Craniopharyngeal —*see* condition
Craniopharyngioma (M9350/1) 237.0
Craniorachischisis (totalis) 740.1
Cranioschisis 756.0
Craniostenosis 756.0
Craniosynostosis 756.0
Craniotabes (cause unknown) 733.3
rachitic 268.1
syphilitic 090.5
Craniotomy, fetal 763.8
Cranium —*see* condition
Craw-craw 125.3
Creaking joint 719.60
ankle 719.67
elbow 719.62
foot 719.67
hand 719.64
hip 719.65
knee 719.66
multiple sites 719.69
pelvic region 719.65
shoulder (region) 719.61
specified site NEC 719.68
wrist 719.63
Creeping
eruption 126.9
palsy 335.21
paralysis 335.21
Crenated tongue 529.8
Creotoxism 005.9
Crepitus
caput 756.0
joint 719.60
ankle 719.67
elbow 719.62
foot 719.67
hand 719.64
hip 719.65
knee 719.66
multiple sites 719.69

Crepitus—*continued*
pelvic region 719.65
shoulder (region) 719.61
specified site NEC 719.68
wrist 719.63
Crescent or conus choroid, congenital 743.57
Cretin, cretinism (athyrotic) (congenital) (endemic) (metabolic) (nongoitrous) (sporadic) 243
goitrous (sporadic) 246.1
pelvis (dwarf type) (male type) 243
with disproportion (fetopelvic) 653.1
affecting fetus or newborn 763.1
causing obstructed labor 660.1
affecting fetus or newborn 763.1
pituitary 253.3
Cretinoid degeneration 243
Creutzfeldt-Jakob disease (syndrome) 046.1
with dementia 290.10
Crib death 798.0
Cribriform hymen 752.49
Cri-du-chat syndrome 758.3
Crigler-Najjar disease or syndrome (congenital hyperbilirubinemia) 277.4
Crimean hemorrhagic fever 065.0
Criminalism 301.7
Crisis
abdomen 789.0
addisonian (acute adrenocortical insufficiency) 255.4
adrenal (cortical) 255.4
asthmatic—*see* Asthma
brain, cerebral (*see also* Disease, cerebrovascular, acute) 436
celiac 579.0
Dietl's 593.4
emotional NEC 309.29
acute reaction to stress 308.0
adjustment reaction 309.9
specific to childhood and adolescence 313.9
gastric (tabetic) 094.0
glaucomatocyclitic 364.22
heart (*see also* Failure, heart) 428.9
hypertensive—*see* Hypertension
nitritoid
correct substance properly administered 458.9
overdose or wrong substance given or taken 961.1
oculogyric 378.87
psychogenic 306.7
Pel's 094.0
psychosexual identity 302.6
rectum 094.0
renal 593.81
sickle cell 282.62
stomach (tabetic) 094.0
tabetic 094.0
thyroid (*see also* Thyrotoxicosis) 242.9
thyrotoxic (*see also* Thyrotoxicosis) 242.9
vascular—*see* Disease, cerebrovascular, acute
Crocq's disease (acrocyanosis) 443.89
Crohn's disease (*see also* Enteritis, regional) 555.9
Cronkhite-Canada syndrome 211.3
Crooked septum, nasal 470
Cross
birth (of fetus) complicating delivery 652.3
with successful version 652.1
causing obstructed labor 660.0
bite, anterior or posterior 524.2
eye (*see also* Esotropia) 378.00
Crossed ectopia of kidney 753.3

Crossfoot 754.50
Croup, croupus (acute) (angina) (catarrhal) (infective) (inflammatory) (laryngeal) (membranous) (nondiphtheritic) (pseudomembranous) 464.4
asthmatic (*see also* Asthma) 493.9
bronchial 466.0
diphtheritic (membranous) 032.3
false 478.75
spasmodic 478.75
diphtheritic 032.3
stridulous 478.75
diphtheritic 032.3
Crouzon's disease (craniofacial dysostosis) 756.0
Crowding, teeth 524.3
CRST syndrome (cutaneous systemic sclerosis) 710.1
Cruchet's disease (encephalitis lethargica) 049.8
Cruelty in children (*see also* Disturbance, conduct) 312.9
Crural ulcer (*see also* Ulcer, lower extremity) 707.1
Crush, crushed, crushing (injury) 929.9
with
fracture—*see* Fracture, by site
abdomen 926.19
internal—*see* Injury, internal, abdomen
ankle 928.21
with other parts of foot 928.20
arm 927.9
lower (and elbow) 927.10
upper 927.03
with shoulder or axillary region 927.09
axilla 927.02
with shoulder or upper arm 927.09
back 926.11
breast 926.19
buttock 926.12
cheek 925.1
chest—*see* Injury, internal, chest
ear 925.1
elbow 927.11
with forearm 927.10
face 925.1
finger(s) 927.3
with hand(s) 927.20
and wrist(s) 927.21
flank 926.19
foot, excluding toe(s) alone (with ankle) 928.20
forearm (and elbow) 927.10
genitalia, external (female) (male) 926.0
internal—*see* Injury, internal, genital organ NEC
hand, except finger(s) alone (and wrist) 927.20
head—*see* Fracture, skull, by site
heel 928.20
hip 928.01
with thigh 928.00
internal organ (abdomen, chest, or pelvis)—*see* Injury, internal, by site
knee 928.11
with leg, lower 928.10
labium (majus) (minus) 926.0
larynx 925.2
late effect—*see* Late, effects (of), crushing
leg 928.9
lower 928.10
and knee 928.11
upper 928.00
Crush, crushed, crushing—*continued*
limb
lower 928.9
multiple sites 928.8
upper 927.9
multiple sites 927.8
multiple sites NEC 929.0
neck 925.2
nerve—*see* Injury, nerve, by site
nose 802.0
open 802.1
penis 926.0
pharynx 925.2
scalp 925.2
scapular region 927.01
with shoulder or upper arm 927.09
scrotum 926.0
shoulder 927.00
with upper arm or axillary region 927.09
skull or cranium—*see* Fracture, skull, by site
spinal cord—*see* Injury, spinal, by site
syndrome (complication of trauma) 958.5
testis 926.0
thigh (with hip) 928.00
throat 925.2
thumb(s) (and fingers) 927.3
toe(s) 928.3
with foot 928.20
and ankle 928.21
tonsil 925.2
trunk 926.9
chest—*see* Injury, internal, intrathoracic organs NEC
internal organ—*see* Injury, internal, by site
multiple sites 926.8
specified site NEC 926.19
vulva 926.0
wrist 927.21
with hand(s), except fingers alone 927.20
Crusta lactea 691.8
Crusts 782.8
Crutch paralysis 953.4
Cruveilhier's disease 335.21
Cruveilhier-Baumgarten cirrhosis, disease, or syndrome 571.5
Cruz-Chagas disease (*see also* Trypanosomiasis) 086.2
Cryoglobulinemia (mixed) 273.2
Crypt (anal) (rectal) 569.49
Cryptitis (anal) (rectal) 569.49
Cryptococcosis (European) (pulmonary) (systemic) 117.5
Cryptococcus 117.5
epidermicus 117.5
neoformans, infection by 117.5
Cryptopapillitis (anus) 569.49
Cryptophthalmos (eyelid) 743.06
Cryptorchid, cryptorchism, cryptorchidism 752.5
Cryptosporidiosis 007.8
Cryptotia 744.29
Crystallopathy
calcium pyrophosphate (*see also* Arthritis) 275.4 *[712.2]*
dicalcium phosphate (*see also* Arthritis) 275.4 *[712.1]*
gouty 274.0
pyrophosphate NEC (*see also* Arthritis) 275.4 *[712.2]*
uric acid 274.0
Crystalluria 791.9

Csillag's disease (lichen sclerosus et atrophicus) 701.0
Cuban itch 050.1
Cubitus
valgus (acquired) 736.01
congenital 755.59
late effect of rickets 268.1
varus (acquired) 736.02
congenital 755.59
late effect of rickets 268.1
Cultural deprivation V62.4
Cupping of optic disc 377.14
Curling's ulcer —*see* Ulcer, duodenum
Curling esophagus 530.5
Curschmann (-Batten) (-Steinert) disease or syndrome 359.2
Curvature
organ or site, congenital NEC—*see* Distortion
penis (lateral) 752.8
Pott's (spinal) (*see also* Tuberculosis) 015.0 *[737.43]*
radius, idiopathic, progressive (congenital) 755.54
spine (acquired) (angular) (idiopathic) (incorrect) (postural) 737.9
congenital 754.2
due to or associated with
Charcot-Marie-Tooth disease 356.1 *[737.40]*
mucopolysaccharidosis 277.5 *[737.40]*
neurofibromatosis 237.71 *[737.40]*
osteitis
deformans 731.0 *[737.40]*
fibrosa cystica 252.0 *[737.40]*
osteoporosis (*see also* Osteoporosis) 733.00 *[737.40]*
poliomyelitis (*see also* Poliomyelitis) 138 *[737.40]*
tuberculosis (Pott's curvature) (*see also* Tuberculosis) 015.0 *[737.43]*
kyphoscoliotic (*see also* Kyphoscoliosis) 737.30
kyphotic (*see also* Kyphosis) 737.10
late effect of rickets 268.1 *[737.40]*
Pott's 015.0 *[737.40]*
scoliotic (*see also* Scoliosis) 737.30
specified NEC 737.8
tuberculous 015.0 *[737.40]*
Cushing's
basophilism, disease, or syndrome (iatrogenic) (idiopathic) (pituitary basophilism) (pituitary dependent) 255.0
ulcer—*see* Ulcer, peptic
Cushingoid due to steroid therapy
correct substance properly administered 255.0
overdose or wrong substance given or taken 962.0
Cut (external)—*see* Wound, open, by site
Cutaneous —*see also* condition
hemorrhage 782.7
horn (cheek) (eyelid) (mouth) 702.8
larva migrans 126.9
Cutis —*see also* condition
hyperelastic 756.83
acquired 701.8
laxa 756.83
senilis 701.8
marmorata 782.61
osteosis 709.3
pendula 756.83
acquired 701.8
rhomboidalis nuchae 701.8
Cutis—*continued*
verticis gyrata 757.39
acquired 701.8
Cyanopathy, newborn 770.8
Cyanosis 782.5
autotoxic 289.7
common atrioventricular canal 745.69
congenital 770.8
conjunctiva 372.71
due to
endocardial cushion defect 745.60
nonclosure, foramen botalli 745.5
patent foramen botalli 745.5
persistent foramen ovale 745.5
enterogenous 289.7
fetus or newborn 770.8
ostium primum defect 745.61
paroxysmal digital 443.0
retina, retinal 362.10
Cycle
anovulatory 628.0
menstrual, irregular 626.4
Cyclencephaly 759.89
Cyclical vomiting 536.2
psychogenic 306.4
Cyclitic membrane 364.74
Cyclitis (*see also* Iridocyclitis) 364.3
acute 364.00
primary 364.01
recurrent 364.02
chronic 364.10
in
sarcoidosis 135 *[364.11]*
tuberculosis (*see also* Tuberculosis) 017.3 *[364.11]*
Fuchs' heterochromic 364.21
granulomatous 364.10
lens induced 364.23
nongranulomatous 364.00
posterior 363.21
primary 364.01
recurrent 364.02
secondary (noninfectious) 364.04
infectious 364.03
subacute 364.00
primary 364.01
recurrent 364.02
Cyclokeratitis —*see* Keratitis
Cyclophoria 378.44
Cyclopia, cyclops 759.89
Cycloplegia 367.51
Cyclospasm 367.53
Cyclothymia 301.13
Cyclothymic personality 301.13
Cyclotropia 378.33
Cyesis —*see* Pregnancy
Cylindroma (M8200/3)—*see also* Neoplasm, by site, malignant
eccrine dermal (M8200/0)—*see* Neoplasm, skin, benign
skin (M8200/0)—*see* Neoplasm, skin, benign
Cylindruria 791.7
Cyllosoma 759.89
Cynanche
diphtheritic 032.3
tonsillaris 475
Cynorexia 783.6
Cyphosis —*see* Kyphosis
Cyprus fever (*see also* Brucellosis) 023.9
Cyriax's syndrome (slipping rib) 733.99

Cyst (mucus) (retention) (serous) (simple)

Note—In general, cysts are not neoplastic and are classified to the appropriate category for disease of the specified anatomical site. This generalization does not apply to certain types of cysts which are neoplastic in nature, for example, dermoid, nor does it apply to cysts of certain structures, for example, branchial cleft, which are classified as developmental anomalies. The following listing includes some of the most frequently reported sites of cysts as well as qualifiers which indicate the type of cyst. The latter qualifiers usually are not repeated under the anatomical sites. Since the code assignment for a given site may vary depending upon the type of cyst, the coder should refer to the listings under the specified type of cyst before consideration is given to the site.

accessory, fallopian tube 752.11
adenoid (infected) 474.8
adrenal gland 255.8
  congenital 759.1
air, lung 518.89
allantoic 753.7
alveolar process (jaw bone) 526.2
amnion, amniotic 658.8
anterior chamber (eye) 364.60
  exudative 364.62
  implantation (surgical) (traumatic) 364.61
  parasitic 360.13
anterior nasopalatine 526.1
antrum 478.1
anus 569.49
apical (periodontal) (tooth) 522.8
appendix 543.9
arachnoid, brain 348.0
arytenoid 478.79
auricle 706.2
Baker's (knee) 727.51
  tuberculous (*see also* Tuberculosis) 015.2
Bartholin's gland or duct 616.2
bile duct (*see also* Disease, biliary) 576.8
bladder (multiple) (trigone) 596.8
Blessig's 362.62
blood, endocardial (*see also* Endocarditis) 424.90
blue dome 610.0
bone (local) 733.20
  aneurysmal 733.22
  jaw 526.2
    developmental (odontogenic) 526.0
    fissural 526.1
    latent 526.89
  solitary 733.21
  unicameral 733.21
brain 348.0
  congenital 742.4
  hydatid (*see also* Echinococcus) 122.9
  third ventricle (colloid) 742.4
branchial (cleft) 744.42
branchiogenic 744.42
breast (benign) (blue dome) (pedunculated) (solitary) (traumatic) 610.0
  involution 610.4
  sebaceous 610.8
broad ligament (benign) 620.8
  embryonic 752.11

Cyst —*continued*
bronchogenic (mediastinal) (sequestration) 518.89
  congenital 748.4
buccal 528.4
bulbourethral gland (Cowper's) 599.89
bursa, bursal 727.49
  pharyngeal 478.26
calcifying odontogenic (M9301/0) 213.1
  upper jaw (bone) 213.0
canal of Nuck (acquired) (serous) 629.1
  congenital 752.41
canthus 372.75
carcinomatous (M8010/3)—*see* Neoplasm, by site, malignant
cartilage (joint)—*see* Derangement, joint
cauda equina 336.8
cavum septi pellucidi NEC 348.0
celomic (pericardium) 746.89
cerebellopontine (angle)—*see* Cyst, brain
cerebellum—*see* Cyst, brain
cerebral—*see* Cyst, brain
cervical lateral 744.42
cervix 622.8
  embryonal 752.41
  nabothian (gland) 616.0
chamber, anterior (eye) 364.60
  exudative 364.62
  implantation (surgical) (traumatic) 364.61
  parasitic 360.13
chiasmal, optic NEC (*see also* Lesion, chiasmal) 377.54
chocolate (ovary) 617.1
choledochal (congenital) 751.69
  acquired 576.8
choledochus 751.69
chorion 658.8
choroid plexus 348.0
chyle, mesentery 457.8
ciliary body 364.60
  exudative 364.64
  implantation 364.61
  primary 364.63
clitoris 624.8
coccyx (*see also* Cyst, bone) 733.20
colloid
  third ventricle (brain) 742.4
  thyroid gland—*see* Goiter
colon 569.89
common (bile) duct (*see also* Disease, biliary) 576.8
congenital NEC 759.89
  adrenal glands 759.1
  epiglottis 748.3
  esophagus 750.4
  fallopian tube 752.11
  kidney 753.10
    multiple 753.19
    single 753.11
  larynx 748.3
  liver 751.62
  lung 748.4
  mediastinum 748.8
  ovary 752.0
  oviduct 752.11
  pancreas 751.7
  periurethral (tissue) 753.8
  prepuce 752.8
  sublingual 750.26
  submaxillary gland 750.26
  thymus (gland) 759.2

Cyst —*continued*
tongue 750.19
ureterovesical orifice 753.4
vulva 752.41
conjunctiva 372.75
cornea 371.23
corpora quadrigemina 348.0
corpus
albicans (ovary) 620.2
luteum (ruptured) 620.1
Cowper's gland (benign) (infected) 599.89
cranial meninges 348.0
craniobuccal pouch 253.8
craniopharyngeal pouch 253.8
cystic duct (*see also* Disease, gallbladder) 575.8
Cysticercus (any site) 123.1
Dandy-Walker 742.3
with spina bifida (*see also* Spina bifida) 741.0
dental 522.8
developmental 526.0
eruption 526.0
lateral periodontal 526.0
primordial (keratocyst) 526.0
root 522.8
dentigerous 526.0
mandible 526.0
maxilla 526.0
dermoid (M9084/0)—*see also* Neoplasm, by site, benign
with malignant transformation (M9084/3) 183.0
implantation
external area or site (skin) NEC 709.8
iris 364.61
skin 709.8
vagina 623.8
vulva 624.8
mouth 528.4
oral soft tissue 528.4
sacrococcygeal 685.1
with abscess 685.0
developmental of ovary, ovarian 752.0
dura (cerebral) 348.0
spinal 349.2
ear (external) 706.2
echinococcal (*see also* Echinococcus) 122.9
embryonal
cervix uteri 752.41
genitalia, female external 752.41
uterus 752.3
vagina 752.41
endometrial 621.8
ectopic 617.9
endometrium (uterus) 621.8
ectopic—*see* Endometriosis
enteric 751.5
enterogenous 751.5
epidermal (inclusion) (*see also* Cyst, skin) 706.2
epidermoid (inclusion) (*see also* Cyst, skin) 706.2
mouth 528.4
not of skin—*see* Cyst, by site
oral soft tissue 528.4
epididymis 608.89
epiglottis 478.79
epiphysis cerebri 259.8
epithelial (inclusion) (*see also* Cyst, skin) 706.2
epoophoron 752.11
eruption 526.0
esophagus 530.89
ethmoid sinus 478.1

Cyst —*continued*
eye (retention) 379.8
congenital 743.03
posterior segment, congenital 743.54
eyebrow 706.2
eyelid (sebaceous) 374.84
infected 373.13
sweat glands or ducts 374.84
falciform ligament (inflammatory) 573.8
fallopian tube 620.8
female genital organs NEC 629.8
fimbrial (congenital) 752.11
fissural (oral region) 526.1
follicle (atretic) (graafian) (ovarian) 620.0
nabothian (gland) 616.0
follicular (atretic) (ovarian) 620.0
dentigerous 526.0
frontal sinus 478.1
gallbladder or duct 575.8
ganglion 727.43
Gartner's duct 752.11
gas, of mesentery 568.89
gingiva 523.8
gland of moll 374.84
globulomaxillary 526.1
graafian follicle 620.0
granulosal lutein 620.2
hemangiomatous (M9121/0) (*see also* Hemangioma) 228.00
hydatid (*see also* Echinococcus) 122.9
fallopian tube (Morgagni) 752.11
liver NEC 122.8
lung NEC 122.9
Morgagni 752.8
fallopian tube 752.11
specified site NEC 122.9
hymen 623.8
embryonal 752.41
hypopharynx 478.26
hypophysis, hypophyseal (duct) (recurrent) 253.8
cerebri 253.8
implantation (dermoid)
anterior chamber (eye) 364.61
external area or site (skin) NEC 709.8
iris 364.61
vagina 623.8
vulva 624.8
incisor, incisive canal 526.1
inclusion (epidermal) (epithelial) (epidermoid) (mucous) (squamous) (*see also* Cyst, skin) 706.2
not of skin—*see* Neoplasm, by site, benign
intestine (large) (small) 569.89
intracranial—*see* Cyst, brain
intraligamentous 728.89
knee 717.89
intrasellar 253.8
iris (idiopathic) 364.60
exudative 364.62
implantation (surgical) (traumatic) 364.61
miotic pupillary 364.55
parasitic 360.13
Iwanoff's 362.62
jaw (bone) (aneurysmal) (extravasation) (hemorrhagic) (traumatic) 526.2
developmental (odontogenic) 526.0
fissural 526.1
keratin 706.2
kidney (congenital) 753.10
acquired 593.2

Cyst —*continued*
calyceal (*see also* Hydronephrosis) 591
multiple 753.19
pyelogenic (*see also* Hydronephrosis) 591
simple 593.2
single 753.11
solitary (not congenital) 593.2
labium (majus) (minus) 624.8
sebaceous 624.8
lacrimal
apparatus 375.43
gland or sac 375.12
larynx 478.79
lens 379.39
congenital 743.39
lip (gland) 528.5
liver 573.8
congenital 751.62
hydatid (*see also* Echinococcus) 122.8
granulosis 122.0
multilocularis 122.5
lung 518.89
congenital 748.4
giant bullous 492.0
lutein 620.1
lymphangiomatous (M9173/0) 228.1
lymphoepithelial
mouth 528.4
oral soft tissue 528.4
macula 362.54
malignant (M8000/3)—*see* Neoplasm, by site, malignant
mammary gland (sweat gland) (*see also* Cyst, breast) 610.0
mandible 526.2
dentigerous 526.0
radicular 522.8
maxilla 526.2
dentigerous 526.0
radicular 522.8
median
anterior maxillary 526.1
palatal 526.1
mediastinum (congenital) 748.8
meibomian (gland) (retention) 373.2
infected 373.12
membrane, brain 348.0
meninges (cerebral) 348.0
spinal 349.2
meniscus knee 717.5
mesentery, mesenteric (gas) 568.89
chyle 457.8
gas 568.89
mesonephric duct 752.8
mesothelial
peritoneum 568.89
pleura (peritoneal) 568.89
milk 611.5
miotic pupillary (iris) 364.55
Morgagni (hydatid) 752.8
fallopian tube 752.11
mouth 528.4
mullerian duct 752.8
multilocular (ovary) (M8000/1) 239.5
myometrium 621.8
nabothian (follicle) (ruptured) 616.0
nasal sinus 478.1
nasoalveolar 528.4
nasolabial 528.4
nasopalatine (duct) 526.1
anterior 526.1

Cyst —*continued*
nasopharynx 478.26
neoplastic (M8000/1)—*see also* Neoplasm, by site, unspecified nature
benign (M8000/0)—*see* Neoplasm, by site, benign
uterus 621.8
nervous system—*see* Cyst, brain
neuroenteric 742.59
neuroepithelial ventricle 348.0
nipple 610.0
nose 478.1
skin of 706.2
odontogenic, developmental 526.0
omentum (lesser) 568.89
congenital 751.8
oral soft tissue (dermoid) (epidermoid) (lymphoepithelial) 528.4
ora serrata 361.19
orbit 376.81
ovary, ovarian (twisted) 620.2
adherent 620.2
chocolate 617.1
corpus
albicans 620.2
luteum 620.1
dermoid (M9084/0) 220
developmental 752.0
due to failure of involution NEC 620.2
endometrial 617.1
follicular (atretic) (graafian) (hemorrhagic) 620.0
hemorrhagic 620.2
in pregnancy or childbirth 654.4
affecting fetus or newborn 763.8
causing obstructed labor 660.2
affecting fetus or newborn 763.1
multilocular (M8000/1) 239.5
pseudomucinous (M8470/0) 220
retention 620.2
serous 620.2
theca lutein 620.2
tuberculous (*see also* Tuberculosis) 016.6
unspecified 620.2
oviduct 620.8
palatal papilla (jaw) 526.1
palate 526.1
fissural 526.1
median (fissural) 526.1
palatine, of papilla 526.1
pancreas, pancreatic 577.2
congenital 751.7
false 577.2
hemorrhagic 577.2
true 577.2
paranephric 593.2
para ovarian 752.11
paraphysis, cerebri 742.4
parasitic NEC 136.9
parathyroid (gland) 252.8
paratubal (fallopian) 620.8
paraurethral duct 599.89
paroophoron 752.11
parotid gland 527.6
mucous extravasation or retention 527.6
parovarian 752.11
pars planus 364.60
exudative 364.64
primary 364.63
pelvis, female
in pregnancy or childbirth 654.4

Cyst —*continued*
affecting fetus or newborn 763.8
causing obstructed labor 660.2
affecting fetus or newborn 763.1
penis (sebaceous) 607.89
periapical 522.8
pericardial (congenital) 746.89
acquired (secondary) 423.8
pericoronal 526.0
perineural (Tarlov's) 355.9
periodontal 522.8
lateral 526.0
peripancreatic 577.2
peripelvic (lymphatic) 593.2
peritoneum 568.89
chylous 457.8
pharynx (wall) 478.26
pilonidal (infected) (rectum) 685.1
with abscess 685.0
malignant (M9084/3) 173.5
pituitary (duct) (gland) 253.8
placenta (amniotic)—*see* Placenta, abnormal
pleura 519.8
popliteal 727.51
porencephalic 742.4
acquired 348.0
postanal (infected) 685.1
with abscess 685.0
posterior segment of eye, congenital 743.54
postmastoidectomy cavity 383.31
preauricular 744.47
prepuce 607.89
congenital 752.8
primordial (jaw) 526.0
prostate 600
pseudomucinous (ovary) (M8470/0) 220
pudenda (sweat glands) 624.8
pupillary, miotic 364.55
sebaceous 624.8
radicular (residual) 522.8
radiculodental 522.8
ranular 527.6
Rathke's pouch 253.8
rectum (epithelium) (mucous) 569.49
renal—*see* Cyst, kidney
residual (radicular) 522.8
retention (ovary) 620.2
retina 361.19
macular 362.54
parasitic 360.13
primary 361.13
secondary 361.14
retroperitoneal 568.89
sacrococcygeal (dermoid) 685.1
with abscess 685.0
salivary gland or duct 527.6
mucous extravasation or retention 527.6
Sampson's 617.1
sclera 379.19
scrotum (sebaceous) 706.2
sweat glands 706.2
sebaceous (duct) (gland) 706.2
breast 610.8
eyelid 374.84
genital organ NEC
female 629.8
male 608.89
scrotum 706.2
semilunar cartilage (knee) (multiple) 717.5
seminal vesicle 608.89

Cyst —*continued*
serous (ovary) 620.2
sinus (antral) (ethmoidal) (frontal) (maxillary) (nasal) (sphenoidal) 478.1
Skene's gland 599.89
skin (epidermal) (epidermoid, inclusion) (epithelial) (inclusion) (retention) (sebaceous) 706.2
breast 610.8
eyelid 374.84
genital organ NEC
female 629.8
male 608.89
neoplastic 216.3
scrotum 706.2
sweat gland or duct 705.89
solitary
bone 733.21
kidney 593.2
spermatic cord 608.89
sphenoid sinus 478.1
spinal meninges 349.2
spine (*see also* Cyst, bone) 733.20
spleen NEC 289.59
congenital 759.0
hydatid (*see also* Echinococcus) 122.9
spring water (pericardium) 746.89
subarachnoid 348.0
intrasellar 793.0
subdural (cerebral) 348.0
spinal cord 349.2
sublingual gland 527.6
mucous extravasation or retention 527.6
submaxillary gland 527.6
mucous extravasation or retention 527.6
suburethral 599.89
suprarenal gland 255.8
suprasellar—*see* Cyst, brain
sweat gland or duct 705.89
sympathetic nervous system 337.9
synovial 727.40
popliteal space 727.51
Tarlov's 355.9
tarsal 373.2
tendon (sheath) 727.42
testis 608.89
theca-lutein (ovary) 620.2
Thornwaldt's, Tornwaldt's 478.26
thymus (gland) 254.8
thyroglossal (duct) (infected) (persistent) 759.2
thyroid (gland) 246.2
adenomatous—*see* Goiter, nodular
colloid (*see also* Goiter) 240.9
thyrolingual duct (infected) (persistent) 759.2
tongue (mucous) 529.8
tonsil 474.8
tooth (dental root) 522.8
tubo-ovarian 620.8
inflammatory 614.1
tunica vaginalis 608.89
turbinate (nose) (*see also* Cyst, bone) 733.20
Tyson's gland (benign) (infected) 607.89
umbilicus 759.89
urachus 753.7
ureter 593.89
ureterovesical orifice 593.89
congenital 753.4
urethra 599.84
urethral gland (Cowper's) 599.89

Cyst —*continued*
- uterine
  - ligament 620.8
    - embryonic 752.11
  - tube 620.8
- uterus (body) (corpus) (recurrent) 621.8
  - embryonal 752.3
- utricle (ear) 386.8
  - prostatic 599.89
- utriculus masculinus 599.89
- vagina, vaginal (squamous cell) (wall) 623.8
  - embryonal 752.41
  - implantation 623.8
  - inclusion 623.8
- vallecula, vallecular 478.79
- ventricle, neuroepithelial 348.0
- verumontanum 599.89
- vesical (orifice) 596.8
- vitreous humor 379.29
- vulva (sweat glands) 624.8
  - congenital 752.41
  - implantation 624.8
  - inclusion 624.8
  - sebaceous gland 624.8
- vulvovaginal gland 624.8
- wolffian 752.8

Cystadenocarcinoma (M8440/3)—*see also* Neoplasm, by site, malignant
- bile duct type (M8161/3) 155.1
- endometrioid (M8380/3)—*see* Neoplasm, by site, malignant
- mucinous (M8470/3)
  - papillary (M8471/3)
    - specified site—*see* Neoplasm, by site, malignant
    - unspecified site 183.0
  - specified site—*see* Neoplasm, by site, malignant
  - unspecified site 183.0
- papillary (M8450/3)
  - mucinous (M8471/3)
    - specified site—*see* Neoplasm, by site, malignant
    - unspecified site 183.0
  - pseudomucinous (M8471/3)
    - specified site—*see* Neoplasm, by site, malignant
    - unspecified site 183.0
  - serous (M8460/3)
    - specified site—*see* Neoplasm, by site, malignant
    - unspecified site 183.0
  - specified site—*see* Neoplasm, by site, malignant
  - unspecified 183.0
- pseudomucinous (M8470/3)
  - papillary (M8471/3)
    - specified site—*see* Neoplasm, by site, malignant
    - unspecified site 183.0
  - specified site—*see* Neoplasm, by site, malignant
  - unspecified site 183.0
- serous (M8441/3)
  - papillary (M8460/3)
    - specified site—*see* Neoplasm, by site, malignant
    - unspecified site 183.0
  - specified site—*see* Neoplasm, by site, malignant
  - unspecified site 183.0

Cystadenofibroma (M9013/0)
- clear cell (M8313/0)—*see* Neoplasm, by site, benign
- endometrioid (M8381/0) 220
  - borderline malignancy (M8381/1) 236.2
  - malignant (M8381/3) 183.0
- mucinous (M9015/0)
  - specified site—*see* Neoplasm, by site, benign
  - unspecified site 220
- serous (M9014/0)
  - specified site—*see* Neoplasm, by site, benign
  - unspecified site 220
- specified site—*see* Neoplasm, by site, benign
- unspecified site 220

Cystadenoma (M8440/0)—*see also* Neoplasm, by site, benign
- bile duct (M8161/0) 211.5
- endometrioid (M8380/0)—*see also* Neoplasm, by site, benign
  - borderline malignancy (M8380/1)—*see* Neoplasm, by site, uncertain behavior
- malignant (M8440/3)—*see* Neoplasm, by site, malignant
- mucinous (M8470/0)
  - borderline malignancy (M8470/1)
    - specified site—*see* Neoplasm, uncertain behavior
    - unspecified site 236.2
  - papillary (M8471/0)
    - borderline malignancy (M8471/1)
      - specified site—*see* Neoplasm, by site, uncertain behavior
      - unspecified site 236.2
    - specified site—*see* Neoplasm, by site, benign
    - unspecified site 220
  - specified site—*see* Neoplasm, by site, benign
  - unspecified site 220
- papillary (M8450/0)
  - borderline malignancy (M8450/1)
    - specified site—*see* Neoplasm, by site, uncertain behavior
    - unspecified site 236.2
  - lymphomatosum (M8561/0) 210.2
  - mucinous (M8471/0)
    - borderline malignancy (M8471/1)
      - specified site—*see* Neoplasm, by site, uncertain behavior
      - unspecified site 236.2
    - specified site—*see* Neoplasm, by site, benign
    - unspecified site 220
  - pseudomucinous (M8471/0)
    - borderline malignancy (M8471/1)
      - specified site—*see* Neoplasm, by site, uncertain behavior
      - unspecified site 236.2
    - specified site—*see* Neoplasm, by site, benign
    - unspecified site 220
  - serous (M8460/0)
    - borderline malignancy (M8460/1)
      - specified site—*see* Neoplasm, by site, uncertain behavior
      - unspecified site 236.2
    - specified site—*see* Neoplasm, by site, benign
    - unspecified site 220
  - specified site—*see* Neoplasm, by site, benign
  - unspecified site 220

Cystocele (-rectocele)
female (without uterine prolapse) 618.0
with uterine prolapse 618.4
complete 618.3
incomplete 618.2
in pregnancy or childbirth 654.4
affecting fetus or newborn 763.8
causing obstructed labor 660.2
affecting fetus or newborn 763.1
male 596.8
Cystoid
cicatrix limbus 372.64
degeneration macula 362.53
Cystolithiasis 594.1
Cystoma (M8440/0)—*see also* Neoplasm, by site, benign
endometrial, ovary 617.1
mucinous (M8470/0)
specified site—*see* Neoplasm, by site, benign
unspecified site 220
serous (M8441/0)
specified site—*see* Neoplasm, by site, benign
unspecified site 220
simple (ovary) 620.2
Cystoplegia 596.53
Cystoptosis 596.8
Cystopyelitis (*see also* Pyelitis) 590.80
Cystorrhagia 596.8
Cystosarcoma phyllodes (M9020/1) 238.3
benign (M9020/0) 217
malignant (M9020/3)—*see* Neoplasm, breast, malignant
Cystostomy status V44.5
with complication 997.5
Cystourethritis (*see also* Urethritis) 597.89
Cystourethrocele (*see also* Cystocele)
female (without uterine prolapse) 618.0
with uterine prolapse 618.4
complete 618.3
incomplete 618.2
male 596.8
Cytomegalic inclusion disease 078.5
congenital 771.1
Cytomycosis, reticuloendothelial (*see also* Histoplasmosis, American) 115.00
Czerny's disease (periodic hydrarthrosis of the knee) 719.06

D

Daae (-Finsen) disease (epidemic pleurodynia) 074.1
Dabney's grip 074.1
Da Costa's syndrome (neurocirculatory asthenia) 306.2
Dacryoadenitis, dacryadenitis 375.00
  acute 375.01
  chronic 375.02
Dacryocystitis 375.30
  acute 375.32
  chronic 375.42
  neonatal 771.6
  phlegmonous 375.33
  syphilitic 095.8
    congenital 090.0
  trachomatous, active 076.1
    late effect 139.1
  tuberculous (*see also* Tuberculosis) 017.3
Dacryocystoblennorrhea 375.42
Dacryocystocele 375.43
Dacryolith, dacryolithiasis 375.57
Dacryoma 375.43
Dacryopericystitis (acute) (subacute) 375.32
  chronic 375.42
Dacryops 375.11
Dacryosialadenopathy, atrophic 710.2
Dacryostenosis 375.56
  congenital 743.65
Dactylitis 686.9
  bone (*see also* Osteomyelitis) 730.2
  sickle-cell 282.61
  syphilitic 095.5
  tuberculous (*see also* Tuberculosis) 015.5
Dactylolysis spontanea 136.0
Dactylosymphysis (*see also* Syndactylism) 755.10
Damage
  arteriosclerotic—*see* Arteriosclerosis
  brain 348.9
    anoxic, hypoxic 348.1
      during or resulting from a procedure 997.01
    child NEC 343.9
    due to birth injury 767.0
    minimal (child) (*see also* Hyperkinesia) 314.9
    newborn 767.0
  cardiac—*see also* Disease, heart
  cardiorenal (vascular) (*see also* Hypertension, cardiorenal) 404.90
  central nervous system—*see* Damage, brain
  cerebral NEC—*see* Damage, brain
  coccyx, complicating delivery 665.6
  coronary (*see also* Ischemia, heart) 414.9
  eye, birth injury 767.8
  heart—*see also* Disease, heart
    valve—*see* Endocarditis
  hypothalamus NEC 348.9
  liver 571.9
    alcoholic 571.3
  myocardium (*see also* Degeneration, myocardial) 429.1
  pelvic
    joint or ligament, during delivery 665.6
    organ NEC
      with
        abortion—*see* Abortion, by type, with damage to pelvic organs
        ectopic pregnancy (*see also* categories 633.0-633.9) 639.2
Damage—*continued*
        molar pregnancy (*see also* categories 630-632) 639.2
      during delivery 665.5
      following
        abortion 639.2
        ectopic or molar pregnancy 639.2
  renal (*see also* Disease, renal) 593.9
  skin, solar 692.79
    acute 692.72
    chronic 692.74
  subendocardium, subendocardial (*see also* Degeneration, myocardial) 429.1
  vascular 459.9
Dameshek's syndrome (erythroblastic anemia) 282.4
Dana-Putnam syndrome (subacute combined sclerosis with pernicious anemia) 281.0 *[336.2]*
Danbolt (-Closs) syndrome (acrodermatitis enteropathica) 686.8
Dandruff 690.18
Dandy fever 061
Dandy-Walker deformity or syndrome (atresia, foramen of Magendie) 742.3
  with spina bifida (*see also* Spina bifida) 741.0
Dangle foot 736.79
Danielssen's disease (anesthetic leprosy) 030.1
Danlos' syndrome 756.83
Darier's disease (congenital) (keratosis follicularis) 757.39
  due to vitamin A deficiency 264.8
  meaning erythema annulare centrifugum 695.0
Darier-Roussy sarcoid 135
Darling's
  disease (*see also* Histoplasmosis, American) 115.00
  histoplasmosis (*see also* Histoplasmosis, American) 115.00
Dartre 054.9
Darwin's tubercle 744.29
Davidson's anemia (refractory) 284.9
Davies' disease 425.0
Davies-Colley syndrome (slipping rib) 733.99
Dawson's encephalitis 046.2
Day blindness (*see also* Blindness, day) 368.60
Dead
  fetus
    retained (in utero) 656.4
      early pregnancy (death before 22 completed weeks gestation) 632
      late (death after 22 completed weeks gestation) 656.4
    syndrome 641.3
  labyrinth 386.50
  ovum, retained 631
Deaf and dumb NEC 389.7
Deaf mutism (acquired) (congenital) NEC 389.7
  endemic 243
  hysterical 300.11
  syphilitic, congenital 090.0

DEF

Deafness (acquired) (bilateral) (both ears) (complete) (congenital) (hereditary) (middle ear) (partial) (unilateral) 389.9
with blue sclera and fragility of bone 756.51
auditory fatigue 389.9
aviation 993.0
nerve injury 951.5
boilermakers' 951.5
central 389.14
with conductive hearing loss 389.2
conductive (air) 389.00
with sensorineural hearing loss 389.2
combined types 389.08
external ear 389.01
inner ear 389.04
middle ear 389.03
multiple types 389.08
tympanic membrane 389.02
emotional (complete) 300.11
functional (complete) 300.11
high frequency 389.8
hysterical (complete) 300.11
injury 951.5
low frequency 389.8
mental 784.69
mixed conductive and sensorineural 389.2
nerve 389.12
with conductive hearing loss 389.2
neural 389.12
with conductive hearing loss 389.2
noise-induced 388.12
nerve injury 951.5
nonspeaking 389.7
perceptive 389.10
with conductive hearing loss 389.2
central 389.14
combined types 389.18
multiple types 389.18
neural 389.12
sensory 389.11
psychogenic (complete) 306.7
sensorineural (*see also* Deafness, perceptive) 389.10
sensory 389.11
with conductive hearing loss 389.2
specified type NEC 389.8
sudden NEC 388.2
syphilitic 094.89
transient ischemic 388.02
transmission—*see* Deafness, conductive
traumatic 951.5
word (secondary to organic lesion) 784.69
developmental 315.31
Death
after delivery (cause not stated) (sudden) 674.9
anesthetic
due to
correct substance properly administered 995.4
overdose or wrong substance given 968.4
specified anesthetic—*see* Table of drugs and chemicals
during delivery 668.9
brain 348.8
cardiac—*see* Disease, heart
cause unknown 798.2
cot (infant) 798.0
crib (infant) 798.0
Death—*continued*
fetus, fetal (cause not stated) (intrauterine) 779.9
early, with retention (before 22 completed weeks gestation) 632
from asphyxia or anoxia (before labor) 768.0
during labor 768.1
late, affecting management of pregnancy (after 22 completed weeks gestation) 656.4
from pregnancy NEC 646.9
instantaneous 798.1
intrauterine (*see also* Death, fetus) 779.9
complicating pregnancy 656.4
maternal, affecting fetus or newborn 761.6
neonatal NEC 779.9
sudden (cause unknown) 798.1
during delivery 669.9
under anesthesia NEC 668.9
infant, syndrome (SIDS) 798.0
puerperal, during puerperium 674.9
unattended (cause unknown) 798.9
under anesthesia NEC
due to
correct substance properly administered 995.4
overdose or wrong substance given 968.4
specified anesthetic—*see* Table of drugs and chemicals
during delivery 668.9
violent 798.1
de Beurmann-Gougerot disease (sporotrichosis) 117.1
Debility (general) (infantile) (postinfectional) 799.3
with nutritional difficulty 269.9
congenital or neonatal NEC 779.9
nervous 300.5
old age 797
senile 797
Débove's disease (splenomegaly) 789.2
Decalcification
bone (*see also* Osteoporosis) 733.00
teeth 521.8
Decapitation 874.9
fetal (to facilitate delivery) 763.8
Decapsulation, kidney 593.89
Decay
dental 521.0
senile 797
tooth, teeth 521.0
Decensus, uterus —*see* Prolapse, uterus
Deciduitis (acute)
with
abortion—*see* Abortion, by type, with sepsis
ectopic pregnancy (*see also* categories 633.0-633.9) 639.0
molar pregnancy (*see also* categories 630-632) 639.0
affecting fetus or newborn 760.8
following
abortion 639.0
ectopic or molar pregnancy 639.0
in pregnancy 646.6
puerperal, postpartum 670
Deciduoma malignum (M9100/3) 181
Deciduous tooth (retained) 520.6
Decline (general) (*see also* Debility) 799.3

Defect, defective—*continued*
esophagus, congenital 750.9
extensor retinaculum 728.9
fibrin polymerization (*see also* Defect, coagulation) 286.3
filling
biliary tract 793.3
bladder 793.5
gallbladder 793.3
kidney 793.5
stomach 793.4
ureter 793.5
fossa ovalis 745.5
gene, carrier (suspected) of V19.8
Gerbode 745.4
glaucomatous, without elevated tension 365.89
Hageman (factor) (*see also* Defect, coagulation) 286.3
hearing (*see also* Deafness) 389.9
high grade 317
homogentisic acid 270.2
interatrial septal 745.5
acquired 429.71
interauricular septal 745.5
acquired 429.71
interventricular septal 745.4
with pulmonary stenosis or atresia, dextroposition of aorta, and hypertrophy of right ventricle 745.2
acquired 429.71
in tetralogy of Fallot 745.2
iodide trapping 246.1
iodotyrosine dehalogenase 246.1
kynureninase 270.2
learning, specific 315.2
mental (*see also* Retardation, mental) 319
osteochondral NEC 738.8
ostium
primum 745.61
secundum 745.5
pericardium 746.89
peroxidase-binding 246.1
placental blood supply—*see* Placenta, insufficiency
platelet (qualitative) 287.1
constitutional 286.4
postural, spine 737.9
protan 368.51
pulmonic cusps, congenital 746.00
renal pelvis 753.9
obstructive 753.2
specified type NEC 753.3
respiratory system, congenital 748.9
specified type NEC 748.8
retina, retinal 361.30
with detachment (*see also* Detachment, retina, with retinal defect) 361.00
multiple 361.33
with detachment 361.02
nerve fiber bundle 362.85
single 361.30
with detachment 361.01
septal (closure) (heart) NEC 745.9
acquired 429.71
atrial 745.5
specified type NEC 745.8
speech NEC 784.5
developmental 315.39
secondary to organic lesion 784.5
Taussig-Bing (transposition, aorta and overriding pulmonary artery) 745.11

Defect, defective—*continued*
teeth, wedge 521.2
thyroid hormone synthesis 246.1
tritan 368.53
ureter 753.9
obstructive 753.2
vascular (acquired) (local) 459.9
congenital (peripheral) NEC 747.60
gastrointestinal 747.61
lower limb 747.64
renal 747.62
specified NEC 747.69
spinal 747.82
upper limb 747.63
ventricular septal 745.4
with pulmonary stenosis or atresia, dextraposition of aorta, and hypertrophy of right ventricle 745.2
acquired 429.71
atrioventricular canal type 745.69
between infundibulum and anterior portion 745.4
in tetralogy of Fallot 745.2
isolated anterior 745.4
vision NEC 369.9
visual field 368.40
arcuate 368.43
heteronymous, bilateral 368.47
homonymous, bilateral 368.46
localized NEC 368.44
nasal step 368.44
peripheral 368.44
sector 368.43
voice 784.40
wedge, teeth (abrasion) 521.2
Defeminization syndrome 255.2
Deferentitis 608.4
gonorrheal (acute) 098.14
chronic or duration of 2 months or over 098.34
Defibrination syndrome (*see also* Fibrinolysis) 286.6
Deficiency, deficient
3-beta-hydroxysteroid dehydrogenase 255.2
6-phosphogluconic dehydrogenase (anemia) 282.2
11-beta-hydroxylase 255.2
17-alpha-hydroxylase 255.2
18-hydroxysteroid dehydrogenase 255.2
20-alpha-hydroxylase 255.2
21-hydroxylase 255.2
abdominal muscle syndrome 756.7
accelerator globulin (Ac G) (blood) (*see also* Defect, coagulation) 286.3
AC globulin (congenital) (*see also* Defect, coagulation) 286.3
acquired 286.7
activating factor (blood) (*see also* Defect, coagulation) 286.3
adenohypophyseal 253.2
adenosine deaminase 277.2
aldolase (hereditary) 271.2
alpha-1-antitrypsin 277.6
alpha-1-trypsin inhibitor 277.6
alpha-fucosidase 271.8
alpha-lipoprotein 272.5
alpha-mannosidase 271.8
amino acid 270.9
anemia—*see* Anemia, deficiency
aneurin 265.1
with beriberi 265.0

Deficiency, deficient—*continued*
glycogen synthetase 271.0
growth hormone 253.3
Hageman factor (congenital) (*see also* Defect, coagulation) 286.3
head V48.0
hemoglobin (*see also* Anemia) 285.9
hepatophosphorylase 271.0
hexose monophosphate (HMP) shunt 282.2
HGH (human growth hormone) 253.3
HG-PRT 277.2
homogentisic acid oxidase 270.2
hormone—*see also* Deficiency, by specific hormone
anterior pituitary (isolated) (partial) NEC 253.4
growth (human) 253.3
follicle-stimulating 253.4
growth (human) (isolated) 253.3
human growth 253.3
interstitial cell-stimulating 253.4
luteinizing 253.4
melanocyte-stimulating 253.4
testicular 257.2
human growth hormone 253.3
humoral 279.00
with
hyper-IgM 279.05
autosomal recessive 279.05
X-linked 279.05
increased IgM 279.05
congenital hypogammaglobulinemia 279.04
non-sex-linked 279.06
selective immunoglobulin NEC 279.03
IgA 279.01
IgG 279.03
IgM 279.02
increased 279.05
specified NEC 279.09
hydroxylase 255.2
hypoxanthine-guanine phosphoribosyltransferase (HG-PRT) 277.2
ICSH (interstitial cell-stimulating hormone) 253.4
immunity NEC 279.3
cell-mediated 279.10
with
hyperimmunoglobulinemia 279.2
thrombocytopenia and eczema 279.12
specified NEC 279.19
combined (severe) 279.2
syndrome 279.2
common variable 279.06
humoral NEC 279.00
IgA (secretory) 279.01
IgG 279.03
IgM 279.02
immunoglobulin, selective NEC 279.03
IgA 279.01
IgG 279.03
IgM 279.02
inositol (B complex) 266.2
interferon 279.4
internal organ V47.0
interstitial cell-stimulating hormone (ICSH) 253.4
intrinsic (urethral) sphincter (ISD) 599.82
intrinsic factor (Castle's) (congenital) 281.0
invertase 271.3
iodine 269.3
iron, anemia 280.9

Deficiency, deficient—*continued*
labile factor (congenital) (*see also* Defect, coagulation) 286.3
acquired 286.7
lacrimal fluid (acquired) 375.15
congenital 743.64
lactase 271.3
Laki-Lorand factor (*see also* Defect, coagulation) 286.3
lecithin-cholesterol acyltranferase 272.5
LH (luteinizing hormone) 253.4
limb V49.0
lower V49.0
congenital (*see also* Deficiency, lower limb, congenital) 755.30
upper V49.0
congenital (*see also* Deficiency, upper limb, congenital) 755.20
lipocaic 577.8
lipoid (high-density) 272.5
lipoprotein (familial) (high density) 272.5
liver phosphorylase 271.0
lower limb V49.0
congenital 755.30
with complete absence of distal elements 755.31
longitudinal (complete) (partial) (with distal deficiencies, incomplete) 755.32
with complete absence of distal elements 755.31
combined femoral, tibial, fibular (incomplete) 755.33
femoral 755.34
fibular 755.37
metatarsal(s) 755.38
phalange(s) 755.39
meaning all digits 755.31
tarsal(s) 755.38
tibia 755.36
tibiofibular 755.35
transverse 755.31
luteinizing hormone (LH) 253.4
lysosomal alpha-1, 4 glucosidase 271.0
magnesium 275.2
mannosidase 271.8
melanocyte-stimulating hormone (MSH) 253.4
menadione (vitamin K) 269.0
newborn 776.0
mental (familial) (hereditary) (*see also* Retardation, mental) 319
mineral NEC 269.3
molybdenum 269.3
moral 301.7
multiple, syndrome 260
myocardial (*see also* Insufficiency myocardial) 428.0
myophosphorylase 271.0
NADH (DPNH) -methemoglobin-reductase (congenital) 289.7
NADH diaphorase or reductase (congenital) 289.7
neck V48.1
niacin (amide) (-tryptophan) 265.2
nicotinamide 265.2
nicotinic acid (amide) 265.2
nose V48.8
number of teeth (*see also* Anodontia) 520.0
nutrition, nutritional 269.9
specified NEC 269.8

Deficiency, deficient—*continued*
C (ascorbic acid) (with scurvy) 267
D (calciferol) (ergosterol) 268.9
with
osteomalacia 268.2
rickets (*see also* Rickets) 268.0
E 269.1
folic acid 266.2
G 266.0
H 266.2
K 269.0
of newborn 776.0
nicotinic acid 265.2
P 269.1
PP 265.2
specified NEC 269.1
zinc 269.3
Deficient —*see also* Defic...
blink reflex 374.45
craniofacial axis 756.0
number of teeth (*see* ...ontia) 520.0
secretion of urine 78...
Deficit
neurologic NE... ...9
due to
cereb...vascular le...n (*see also* Disease,
...erebrovascu..., acute) 436
...ate effect—s... category 438
transient isch...nic attack 435.9
oxygen 799.0
Deflection
radius 736.09
septum (acquired) (nasal) (nose) 470
spine—*see* Curvature, spine
turbinate (nose) 470
Defluvium
capillorum (*see also* Alopecia) 704.00
ciliorum 374.55
unguium 703.8
Deformity 759.9
abdomen, congenital 759.9
abdominal wall
acquired 738.8
congenital 756.7
muscle deficiency syndrome 756.7
acquired (unspecified site) 738.9
specified site NEC 738.8
adrenal gland (congenital) 759.1
alimentary tract, congenital 751.9
lower 751.5
specified type NEC 751.8
upper (any part, except tongue) 750.9
specified type NEC 750.8
tongue 750.10
specified type NEC 750.19
ankle (joint) (acquired) 736.70
abduction 718.47
congenital 755.69
contraction 718.47
anus (congenital) 751.5
acquired 569.49
aorta (congenital) 747.20
acquired 447.8
arch 747.21
acquired 447.8
coarctation 747.10
...genital) 746.9
...also Endocarditis, aortic) 424.1
...1.5
...ired) 736.89
...genital 755.50
...riovenous (congenital) (peripheral) NEC 747.60
gastrointestinal 747.61
lower limb 747.64
renal 747.62
specified NEC 747.69
spinal 747.82
upper limb 747.63
artery (congenital) (peripheral) NEC (*see also* Deformity, vascular) 747.60
acquired 447.8
cerebral 747.81
coronary (congenital) 746.85
acquired (*see also* Ischemia, heart) 414.9
retinal 743.9
umbilical 747.5
atrial septal (congenital) (heart) 745.5
auditory canal (congenital) (external) (*see also* Deformity, ear) 744.3
acquired 380.50
auricle
ear (congenital) (*see also* Deformity, ear) 744.3
acquired 380.32
heart (congenital) 746.9
back (acquired)—*see* Deformity, spine
Bartholin's duct (congenital) 750.9
bile duct (congenital) 751.60
acquired 576.8
with calculus, choledocholithiasis, or stones—*see* Choledocholithiasis
biliary duct or passage (congenital) 751.60
acquired 576.8
with calculus, choledocholithiasis, or stones—*see* Choledocholithiasis
bladder (neck) (sphincter) (trigone) (acquired) 596.8
congenital 753.9
bone (acquired) NEC 738.9
congenital 756.9
turbinate 738.0
boutonniere (finger) 736.21
brain (congenital) 742.9
acquired 348.8
multiple 742.4
reduction 742.2
vessel (congenital) 747.81
breast (acquired) 611.8
congenital 757.9
bronchus (congenital) 748.3
acquired 519.1
bursa, congenital 756.9
canal of Nuck 752.9
canthus (congenital) 743.9
acquired 374.89
capillary (acquired) 448.9
congenital NEC (*see also* Deformity, vascular) 747.60
cardiac—*see* Deformity, heart
cardiovascular system (congenital) 746.9

Deformity—*continued*
caruncle, lacrimal (congenital) 743.9
acquired 375.69
cascade, stomach 537.6
cecum (congenital) 751.5
acquired 569.89
cerebral (congenital) 742.9
acquired 348.8
cervix (acquired) (uterus) 622.8
congenital 752.40
cheek (acquired) 738.19
congenital 744.9
chest (wall) (acquired) 738.3
congenital 754.89
late effect of rickets 268.1
chin (acquired) 738.19
congenital 744.9
choroid (congenital) 743.9
acquired 363.8
plexus (congenital) 742.9
acquired 349.2
cicatricial—*see* Cicatrix
cilia (congenital) 743.9
acquired 374.89
circulatory system (congenital) 747.9
clavicle (acquired) 738.8
congenital 755.51
clitoris (congenital) 752.40
acquired 624.8
clubfoot—*see* Clubfoot
coccyx (acquired) 738.6
congenital 756.10
colon (congenital) 751.5
acquired 569.89
concha (ear) (congenital) (*see also* Deformity, ear) 744.3
acquired 380.32
congenital, organ or site not listed (*see also* Anomaly) 759.9
cornea (congenital) 743.9
acquired 371.70
coronary artery (congenital) 746.85
acquired (*see also* Ischemia, heart) 414.9
cranium (acquired) 738.19
congenital (*see also* Deformity, skull, congenital) 756.0
cricoid cartilage (congenital) 748.3
acquired 478.79
cystic duct (congenital) 751.60
acquired 575.8
Dandy-Walker 742.3
with spina bifida (*see also* Spina bifida) 741.0
diaphragm (congenital) 756.6
acquired 738.8
digestive organ(s) or system (congenital) NEC 751.9
specified type NEC 751.8
ductus arteriosus 747.0
duodenal bulb 537.89
duodenum (congenital) 751.5
acquired 537.89
dura (congenital) 742.9
brain 742.4
acquired 349.2
spinal 742.59
acquired 349.2

Deformity—*continued*
ear (congenital) 744.3
acquired 380.32
auricle 744.3
causing impairment of hearing 744.02
causing impairment of hearing 744.00
external 744.3
causing impairment of hearing 744.02
internal 744.05
lobule 744.3
middle 744.03
ossicles 744.04
ossicles 744.04
ectodermal (congenital) NEC 757.9
specified type NEC 757.8
ejaculatory duct (congenital) 752.9
acquired 608.89
elbow (joint) (acquired) 736.00
congenital 755.50
contraction 718.42
endocrine gland NEC 759.2
epididymis (congenital) 752.9
acquired 608.89
torsion 608.2
epiglottis (congenital) 748.3
acquired 478.79
esophagus (congenital) 750.9
acquired 530.89
Eustachian tube (congenital) NEC 744.3
specified type NEC 744.24
extremity (acquired) 736.9
congenital, except reduction deformity 755.9
lower 755.60
upper 755.50
reduction—*see* Deformity, reduction
eye (congenital) 743.9
acquired 379.8
muscle 743.9
eyebrow (congenital) 744.89
eyelid (congenital) 743.9
acquired 374.89
specified type NEC 743.62
face (acquired) 738.19
congenital (any part) 744.9
due to intrauterine malposition and pressure 754.0
fallopian tube (congenital) 752.10
acquired 620.8
femur (acquired) 736.89
congenital 755.60
fetal
with fetopelvic disproportion 653.7
affecting fetus or newborn 763.1
causing obstructed labor 660.1
affecting fetus or newborn 763.1
known or suspected, affecting management of pregnancy 655.9
finger (acquired) 736.20
boutonniere type 736.21
congenital 755.50
flexion contracture 718.44
swan neck 736.22
flexion (joint) (acquired) 736.9
congenital NEC 755.9
hip or thigh (acquired) 736.39
congenital (*see also* Subluxation, congenital, hip) 754.32

Deformity—*continued*
foot (acquired) 736.70
cavovarus 736.75
congenital 754.59
congenital NEC 754.70
specified type NEC 754.79
valgus (acquired) 736.79
congenital 754.60
specified type NEC 754.69
varus (acquired) 736.79
congenital 754.50
specified type NEC 754.59
forearm (acquired) 736.00
congenital 755.50
forehead (acquired) 738.19
congenital (*see also* Deformity, skull, congenital) 756.0
frontal bone (acquired) 738.19
congenital (*see also* Deformity, skull, congenital) 756.0
gallbladder (congenital) 751.60
acquired 575.8
gastrointestinal tract (congenital) NEC 751.9
acquired 569.89
specified type NEC 751.8
genitalia, genital organ(s) or system NEC
congenital 752.9
female (congenital) 752.9
acquired 629.8
external 752.40
internal 752.9
male (congenital) 752.9
acquired 608.89
globe (eye) (congenital) 743.9
acquired 360.89
gum (congenital) 750.9
acquired 523.9
gunstock 736.02
hand (acquired) 736.00
claw 736.06
congenital 755.50
minus (and plus) (intrinsic) 736.09
pill roller (intrinsic) 736.09
plus (and minus) (intrinsic) 736.09
swan neck (intrinsic) 736.09
head (acquired) 738.10
congenital (*see also* Deformity, skull, congenital) 756.0
specified NEC 738.19
heart (congenital) 746.9
auricle (congenital) 746.9
septum 745.9
auricular 745.5
specified type NEC 745.8
ventricular 745.4
valve (congenital) NEC 746.9
acquired—*see* Endocarditis
pulmonary (congenital) 746.00
specified type NEC 746.89
ventricle (congenital) 746.9
heel (acquired) 736.76
congenital 755.67
hepatic duct (congenital) 751.60
acquired 576.8
with calculus, choledocholithiasis, or stones—*see* Choledocholithiasis
hip (joint) (acquired) 736.30
congenital NEC 755.63
flexion 718.45
congenital (*see also* Subluxation, congenital, hip) 754.32

Deformity—*continued*
hourglass—*see* Contraction, hourglass
humerus (acquired) 736.89
congenital 755.50
hymen (congenital) 752.40
hypophyseal (congenital) 759.2
ileocecal (coil) (valve) (congenital) 751.5
acquired 569.89
ileum (intestine) (congenital) 751.5
acquired 569.89
ilium (acquired) 738.6
congenital 755.60
integument (congenital) 757.9
intervertebral cartilage or disc (acquired)—*see also* Displacement, intervertebral disc
congenital 756.10
intestine (large) (small) (congenital) 751.5
acquired 569.89
iris (acquired) 364.75
congenital 743.9
prolapse 364.8
ischium (acquired) 738.6
congenital 755.60
jaw (acquired) (congenital) NEC 524.9
due to intrauterine malposition and pressure 754.0
joint (acquired) NEC 738.8
congenital 755.9
contraction (abduction) (adduction) (extension) (flexion)—*see* Contraction, joint
kidney(s) (calyx) (pelvis) (congenital) 753.9
acquired 593.89
vessel 747.62
acquired 459.9
Klippel-Feil (brevicollis) 756.16
knee (acquired) NEC 736.6
congenital 755.64
labium (majus) (minus) (congenital) 752.40
acquired 624.8
lacrimal apparatus or duct (congenital) 743.9
acquired 375.69
larynx (muscle) (congenital) 748.3
acquired 478.79
web (glottic) (subglottic) 748.2
leg (lower) (upper) (acquired) NEC 736.89
congenital 755.60
reduction—*see* Deformity, reduction, lower limb
lens (congenital) 743.9
acquired 379.39
lid (fold) (congenital) 743.9
acquired 374.89
ligament (acquired) 728.9
congenital 756.9
limb (acquired) 736.9
congenital, except reduction deformity 755.9
lower 755.60
reduction (*see also* Deformity, reduction, lower limb) 755.30
upper 755.50
reduction (*see also* Deformity, reduction, lower limb) 755.20
specified NEC 736.89
lip (congenital) NEC 750.9
acquired 528.5
specified type NEC 750.26

Deformity—*continued*
reduction (extremity) (limb) 755.4
brain 742.2
lower limb 755.30
with complete absence of distal elements 755.31
longitudinal (complete) (partial) (with distal deficiencies, incomplete) 755.32
with complete absence of distal elements 755.31
combined femoral, tibial, fibular (incomplete) 755.33
femoral 755.34
fibular 755.37
metatarsal(s) 755.38
phalange(s) 755.39
meaning all digits 755.31
tarsal(s) 755.38
tibia 755.36
tibiofibular 755.35
transverse 755.31
upper limb 755.20
with complete absence of distal elements 755.21
longitudinal (complete) (partial) (with distal deficiencies, incomplete) 755.22
with complete absence of distal elements 755.21
carpal(s) 755.28
combined humeral, radial, ulnar (incomplete) 755.23
humeral 755.24
metacarpal(s) 755.28
phalange(s) 755.29
meaning all digits 755.21
radial 755.26
radioulnar 755.25
ulnar 755.27
transverse (complete) (partial) 755.21
renal—*see* Deformity, kidney
respiratory system (congenital) 748.9
specified type NEC 748.8
rib (acquired) 738.3
congenital 756.3
cervical 756.2
rotation (joint) (acquired) 736.9
congenital 755.9
hip or thigh 736.39
congenital (*see also* Subluxation, congenital, hip) 754.32
sacroiliac joint (congenital) 755.69
acquired 738.5
sacrum (acquired) 738.5
congenital 756.10
saddle
back 737.8
nose 738.0
syphilitic 090.5
salivary gland or duct (congenital) 750.9
acquired 527.8
scapula (acquired) 736.89
congenital 755.50
scrotum (congenital) 752.9
acquired 608.89
sebaceous gland, acquired 706.8
seminal tract or duct (congenital) 752.9
acquired 608.89
septum (nasal) (acquired) 470
congenital 748.1

Deformity—*continued*
shoulder (joint) (acquired) 736.89
congenital 755.50
specified type NEC 755.59
contraction 718.41
sigmoid (flexure) (congenital) 751.5
acquired 569.89
sinus of Valsalva 747.29
skin (congenital) 757.9
acquired NEC 709.8
skull (acquired) 738.19
congenital 756.0
with
anencephalus 740.0
encephalocele 742.0
hydrocephalus 742.3
with spina bifida (*see also* Spina bifida) 741.0
microcephalus 742.1
due to intrauterine malposition and pressure 754.0
soft parts, organs or tissues (of pelvis)
in pregnancy or childbirth NEC 654.9
affecting fetus or newborn 763.8
causing obstructed labor 660.2
affecting fetus or newborn 763.1
spermatic cord (congenital) 752.9
acquired 608.89
torsion 608.2
spinal
column—*see* Deformity, spine
cord (congenital) 742.9
acquired 336.8
vessel (congenital) 747.82
nerve root (congenital) 742.9
acquired 724.9
vessel 747.82
spine (acquired) NEC 738.5
congenital 756.10
due to intrauterine malposition and pressure 754.2
kyphoscoliotic (*see also* Kyphoscoliosis) 737.30
kyphotic (*see also* Kyphosis) 737.10
lordotic (*see also* Lordosis) 737.20
rachitic 268.1
scoliotic (*see also* Scoliosis) 737.30
spleen
acquired 289.59
congenital 759.0
Sprengel's (congenital) 755.52
sternum (acquired) 738.3
congenital 756.3
stomach (congenital) 750.9
acquired 537.89
submaxillary gland (congenital) 750.9
acquired 527.8
swan neck (acquired)
finger 736.22
hand 736.09
talipes—*see* Talipes
teeth, tooth NEC 520.9
testis (congenital) 752.9
acquired 608.89
torsion 608.2
thigh (acquired) 736.89
congenital 755.60
thorax (acquired) (wall) 738.3
congenital 754.89
late effect of rickets 268.1

Degeneration, degenerative—*continued*
sphingolipidosis 272.7 *[330.2]*
vitamin B_{12} deficiency 266.2 *[331.7]*
motor centers 331.89
senile 331.2
specified type NEC 331.89
breast—*see* Disease, breast
Bruch's membrane 363.40
bundle of His 426.50
left 426.3
right 426.4
calcareous NEC 275.4
capillaries 448.9
amyloid 277.3
fatty 448.9
lardaceous 277.3
cardiac (brown) (calcareous) (fatty) (fibrous) (hyaline) (mural) (muscular) (pigmentary) (senile) (with arteriosclerosis) (*see also* Degeneration, myocardial) 429.1
valve, valvular—*see* Endocarditis
cardiorenal (*see also* Hypertension, cardiorenal) 404.90
cardiovascular (*see also* Disease, cardiovascular) 429.2
renal (*see also* Hypertension, cardiorenal) 404.90
cartilage (joint)—*see* Derangement, joint
cerebellar NEC 334.9
primary (hereditary) (sporadic) 334.2
cerebral—*see* Degeneration, brain
cerebromacular 330.1
cerebrovascular 437.1
due to hypertension 437.2
late effect—*see* category 438
cervical plexus 353.2
cervix 622.8
due to radiation (intended effect) 622.8
adverse effect or misadventure 622.8
changes, spine or vertebra (*see also* Spondylosis) 721.90
chitinous 277.3
chorioretinal 363.40
congenital 743.53
hereditary 363.50
choroid (colloid) (drusen) 363.40
hereditary 363.50
senile 363.41
diffuse secondary 363.42
cochlear 386.8
collateral ligament (knee) (medial) 717.82
lateral 717.81
combined (spinal cord) (subacute) 266.2 *[336.2]*
with anemia (pernicious) 281.0 *[336.2]*
due to dietary deficiency 281.1 *[336.2]*
due to vitamin B_{12} deficiency anemia (dietary) 281.1 *[336.2]*
conjunctiva 372.50
amyloid 277.3 *[372.50]*
cornea 371.40
calcerous 371.44
familial (hereditary) (*see also* Dystrophy, cornea) 371.50
macular 371.55
reticular 371.54
hyaline (of old scars) 371.41
marginal (Terrien's) 371.48
mosaic (shagreen) 371.41
nodular 371.46
peripheral 371.48
senile 371.41

Degeneration, degenerative—*continued*
cortical (cerebellar) (parenchymatous) 334.2
alcoholic 303.9 *[334.4]*
diffuse, due to arteriopathy 437.0
corticostriatal-spinal 334.8
cretinoid 243
cruciate ligament (knee) (posterior) 717.84
anterior 717.83
cutis 709.3
amyloid 277.3
dental pulp 522.2
disc disease—*see* Degeneration, intervertebral disc
dorsolateral (spinal cord)—*see* Degeneration, combined
endocardial 424.90
extrapyramidal NEC 333.90
eye NEC 360.40
macular (*see also* Degeneration, macula) 362.50
congenital 362.75
hereditary 362.76
fatty (diffuse) (general) 272.8
liver 571.8
alcoholic 571.0
localized site—*see* Degeneration, by site, fatty
placenta—*see* Placenta, abnormal
globe (eye) NEC 360.40
macular—*see* Degeneration, macula
grey matter 330.8
heart (brown) (calcareous) (fatty) (fibrous) (hyaline) (mural) (muscular) (pigmentary) (senile) (with arteriosclerosis) (*see also* Degeneration, myocardial) 429.1
amyloid 277.3 *[425.7]*
atheromatous —*see* Arteriosclerosis, coronary
gouty 274.82
hypertensive (*see also* Hypertension, heart) 402.90
ischemic 414.9
valve, valvular—*see* Endocarditis
hepatolenticular (Wilson's) 275.1
hepatorenal 572.4
heredofamilial
brain NEC 331.89
spinal cord NEC 336.8
hyaline (diffuse) (generalized) 728.9
localized—*see also* Degeneration, by site
cornea 371.41
keratitis 371.41
hypertensive vascular—*see* Hypertension
infrapatellar fat pad 729.31
internal semilunar cartilage 717.3
intervertebral disc 722.6
with myelopathy 722.70
cervical, cervicothoracic 722.4
with myelopathy 722.71
lumbar, lumbosacral 722.52
with myelopathy 722.73
thoracic, thoracolumbar 722.51
with myelopathy 722.72
intestine 569.89
amyloid 277.3
lardaceous 277.3
iris (generalized) (*see also* Atrophy, iris) 364.59
pigmentary 364.53
pupillary margin 364.54
ischemic—*see* Ischemia
joint disease (*see also* Osteoarthrosis) 715.9
multiple sites 715.09
spine (*see also* Spondylosis) 721.90

Degeneration, degenerative—*continued*
kidney (*see also* Sclerosis, renal) 587
amyloid 277.3 *[583.81]*
cyst, cystic (multiple) (solitary) 593.2
congenital (*see also* Cystic, disease, kidney) 753.10
fatty 593.89
fibrocystic (congenital) 753.19
lardaceous 277.3 *[583.81]*
polycystic (congenital) 753.12
adult type (APKD) 753.13
autosomal dominant 753.13
autosomal recessive 753.14
childhood type (CPKD) 753.14
infantile type 753.14
waxy 277.3 *[583.81]*
Kuhnt-Junius (retina) 362.52
labyrinth, osseous 386.8
lacrimal passages, cystic 375.12
lardaceous (any site) 277.3
lateral column (posterior), spinal cord (*see also* Degeneration, combined) 266.2 *[336.2]*
lattice 362.63
lens 366.9
infantile, juvenile, or presenile 366.00
senile 366.10
lenticular (familial) (progressive) (Wilson's) (with cirrhosis of liver) 275.1
striate artery 437.0
lethal ball, prosthetic heart valve 996.02
ligament
collateral (knee) (medial) 717.82
lateral 717.81
cruciate (knee) (posterior) 717.84
anterior 717.83
liver (diffuse) 572.8
amyloid 277.3
congenital (cystic) 751.62
cystic 572.8
congenital 751.62
fatty 571.8
alcoholic 571.0
hypertrophic 572.8
lardaceous 277.3
parenchymatous, acute or subacute (*see also* Necrosis, liver) 570
pigmentary 572.8
toxic (acute) 573.8
waxy 277.3
lung 518.8
lymph gland 289.3
hyaline 289.3
lardaceous 277.3
macula (acquired) (senile) 362.50
atrophic 362.51
Best's 362.76
congenital 362.75
cystic 362.54
cystoid 362.53
disciform 362.52
dry 362.51
exudative 362.52
familial pseudoinflammatory 362.77
hereditary 362.76
hole 362.54
juvenile (Stargardt's) 362.75
nonexudative 362.51
pseudohole 362.54
wet 362.52

Degeneration, degenerative—*continued*
medullary—*see* Degeneration, brain
membranous labyrinth, congenital (causing impairment of hearing) 744.05
meniscus—*see* Derangement, joint
microcystoid 362.62
mitral—*see* Insufficiency, mitral
Mönckeberg's (*see also* Arteriosclerosis, extremities) 440.20
moral 301.7
motor centers, senile 331.2
mural (*see also* Degeneration, myocardial) 429.1
heart, cardiac (*see also* Degeneration, myocardial) 429.1
myocardium, myocardial (*see also* Degeneration, myocardial) 429.1
muscle 728.9
fatty 728.9
fibrous 728.9
heart (*see also* Degeneration, myocardial) 429.1
hyaline 728.9
muscular progressive 728.2
myelin, central nervous system NEC 341.9
myocardium, myocardial (brown) (calcareous) (fatty) (fibrous) (hyaline) (mural) (muscular) (pigmentary) (senile) (with arteriosclerosis) 429.1
with rheumatic fever (conditions classifiable to 390) 398.0
active, acute, or subacute 391.2
with chorea 392.0
inactive or quiescent (with chorea) 398.0
amyloid 277.3 *[425.7]*
congenital 746.89
fetus or newborn 779.8
gouty 274.82
hypertensive (*see also* Hypertension, heart) 402.90
ischemic 414.8
rheumatic (*see also* Degeneration, myocardium, with rheumatic fever) 398.0
syphilitic 093.82
nasal sinus (mucosa) (*see also* Sinusitis) 473.9
frontal 473.1
maxillary 473.0
nerve—*see* Disorder, nerve
nervous system 349.89
amyloid 277.3 *[357.4]*
autonomic (*see also* Neuropathy, peripheral, autonomic) 337.9
fatty 349.89
peripheral autonomic NEC (*see also* Neuropathy, peripheral, autonomic) 337.9
nipple 611.9
nose 478.1
oculoacousticocerebral, congenital (progressive) 743.8
olivopontocerebellar (familial) (hereditary) 333.0
osseous labyrinth 386.8
ovary 620.8
cystic 620.2
microcystic 620.2
pallidal, pigmentary (progressive) 333.0
pancreas 577.8
tuberculous (*see also* Tuberculosis) 017.9
papillary muscle 429.81
paving stone 362.61
penis 607.89
peritoneum 568.89

Degeneration, degenerative—*continued*
pigmentary (diffuse) (general)
localized—*see* Degeneration, by site
pallidal (progressive) 333.0
secondary 362.65
pineal gland 259.8
pituitary (gland) 253.8
placenta (fatty) (fibrinoid) (fibroid)—*see* Placenta, abnormal
popliteal fat pad 729.31
posterolateral (spinal cord) (*see also* Degeneration, combined) 266.2 *[336.2]*
pulmonary valve (heart) (*see also* Endocarditis, pulmonary) 424.3
pulp (tooth) 522.2
pupillary margin 364.54
renal (*see also* Sclerosis, renal) 587
fibrocystic 753.19
polycystic 753.12
adult type (APKD) 753.13
autosomal dominant 753.13
autosomal recessive 753.14
childhood type (CPKD) 753.14
infantile type 753.14
reticuloendothelial system 289.8
retina (peripheral) 362.60
with retinal defect (*see also* Detachment, retina, with retinal defect) 361.00
cystic (senile) 362.50
cystoid 362.53
hereditary (*see also* Dystrophy, retina) 362.70
cerebroretinal 362.71
congenital 362.75
juvenile (Stargardt's) 362.75
macula 362.76
Kuhnt-Junius 362.52
lattice 362.63
macular (*see also* Degeneration, macula) 362.50
microcystoid 362.62
palisade 362.63
paving stone 362.61
pigmentary (primary) 362.74
secondary 362.65
posterior pole (*see also* Degeneration, macula) 362.50
secondary 362.66
senile 362.60
cystic 362.53
reticular 362.64
saccule, congenital (causing impairment of hearing) 744.05
sacculocochlear 386.8
senile 797
brain 331.2
cardiac, heart, or myocardium (*see also* Degeneration, myocardial) 429.1
motor centers 331.2
reticule 362.64
retina, cystic 362.50
vascular—*see* Arteriosclerosis
silicone rubber poppet (prosthetic valve) 996.02
sinus (cystic) (*see also* Sinusitis) 473.9
polypoid 471.1
skin 709.3
amyloid 277.3
colloid 709.3

Degeneration, degenerative—*continued*
spinal (cord) 336.8
amyloid 277.3
column 733.90
combined (subacute) (*see also* Degeneration, combined) 266.2 *[336.2]*
with anemia (pernicious) 281.0 *[336.2]*
dorsolateral (*see also* Degeneration, combined) 266.2 *[336.2]*
familial NEC 336.8
fatty 336.8
funicular (*see also* Degeneration, combined) 266.2 *[336.2]*
heredofamilial NEC 336.8
posterolateral (*see also* Degeneration, combined) 266.2 *[336.2]*
subacute combined—*see* Degeneration, combined
tuberculous (*see also* Tuberculosis) 013.8
spine 733.90
spleen 289.59
amyloid 277.3
lardaceous 277.3
stomach 537.89
lardaceous 277.3
strionigral 333.0
sudoriparous (cystic) 705.89
suprarenal (capsule) (gland) 255.8
with hypofunction 255.4
sweat gland 705.89
synovial membrane (pulpy) 727.9
tapetoretinal 362.74
adult or presenile form 362.50
testis (postinfectional) 608.89
thymus (gland) 254.8
fatty 254.8
lardaceous 277.3
thyroid (gland) 246.8
tricuspid (heart) (valve)—*see* Endocarditis, tricuspid
tuberculous NEC (*see also* Tuberculosis) 011.9
turbinate 733.90
uterus 621.8
cystic 621.8
vascular (senile)—*see also* Arteriosclerosis
hypertensive—*see* Hypertension
vitreoretinal (primary) 362.73
secondary 362.66
vitreous humor (with infiltration) 379.21
wallerian NEC—*see* Disorder, nerve
waxy (any site) 277.3
Wilson's hepatolenticular 275.1
Deglutition
paralysis 784.9
hysterical 300.11
pneumonia 507.0
Degos' disease or syndrome 447.8
Degradation disorder, branched-chain amino-acid 270.3
Dehiscence
anastomosis—*see* Complications, anastomosis
cesarean wound 674.1
episiotomy 674.2
operation wound 998.3
perineal wound (postpartum) 674.2
postoperative 998.3
abdomen 998.3
uterine wound 674.1

Dehydration (cachexia) 276.5
- hypertonic 276.0
- hypotonic 276.1
- newborn 775.5

Deiters' nucleus syndrome 386.19
Déjérine's disease 356.0
Déjérine-Klumpke paralysis 767.6
Déjérine-Roussy syndrome 348.8
Déjérine-Sottas disease or neuropathy (hypertrophic) 356.0
Déjérine-Thomas atrophy or syndrome 333.0
de Lange's syndrome (Amsterdam dwarf, mental retardation, and brachycephaly) 759.89
Delay, delayed
- adaptation, cones or rods 368.63
- any plane in pelvis
  - affecting fetus or newborn 763.1
  - complicating delivery 660.1
- birth or delivery NEC 662.1
  - affecting fetus or newborn 763.8
  - second twin, triplet, or multiple mate 662.3
- closure—*see also* Fistula
  - cranial suture 756.0
  - fontanel 756.0
- coagulation NEC 790.92
- conduction (cardiac) (ventricular) 426.9
- delivery NEC 662.1
  - second twin, triplet, etc. 662.3
    - affecting fetus or newborn 763.8
- development 783.4
  - intellectual NEC 315.9
  - learning NEC 315.2
  - physiological 783.4
  - reading 315.00
  - sexual 259.0
  - speech 315.39
    - associated with hyperkinesis 314.1
  - spelling 315.09
- gastric emptying 536.8
- menarche 256.3
  - due to pituitary hypofunction 253.4
- menstruation (cause unknown) 626.8
- milestone 783.4
- motility—*see* Hypomotility
- passage of meconium (newborn) 777.1
- primary respiration 768.9
- puberty 259.0
- sexual maturation, female 259.0

Del Castillo's syndrome (germinal aplasia) 606.0
Deleage's disease 359.8
Delhi (boil) (button) (sore) 085.1
Delinquency (juvenile) 312.9
- group (*see also* Disturbance, conduct) 312.2
- neurotic 312.4

Delirium, delirious 780.09
- acute (psychotic) 293.0
- alcoholic 291.0
  - acute 291.0
  - chronic 291.1
- alcoholicum 291.0
- chronic (*see also* Psychosis) 293.89
  - due to or associated with physical condition—*see* Psychosis, organic
- drug-induced 292.81
- eclamptic (*see also* Eclampsia) 780.3
- exhaustion (*see also* Reaction, stress, acute) 308.9
- hysterical 300.11

Delirium, delirious—*continued*
- in
  - presenile dementia 290.11
  - senile dementia 290.3
- induced by drug 292.81
- manic, maniacal (acute) (*see also* Psychosis, affective) 296.0
  - recurrent episode 296.1
  - single episode 296.0
- puerperal 293.9
- senile 290.3
- subacute (psychotic) 293.1
- thyroid (*see also* Thyrotoxicosis) 242.9
- traumatic—*see also* Injury, intracranial
  - with
    - lesion, spinal cord—*see* Injury, spinal, by site
    - shock, spinal—*see* Injury, spinal, by site
- tremens (impending) 291.0
- uremic—*see* Uremia
- withdrawal
  - alcoholic (acute) 291.0
    - chronic 291.1
  - drug 292.0

Delivery

Note—Use the following fifth-digit subclassification with categories 640-648, 651-676:

0 unspecified as to episode of care
1 delivered, with or without mention of
2 delivered, with mention of postpartum complication
3 antepartum condition or complication
4 postpartum condition or complication

- breech (assisted) (spontaneous) 652.2
  - affecting fetus or newborn 763.0
  - extraction NEC 669.6
- cesarean (for) 669.7
  - abnormal
    - cervix 654.6
    - pelvic organs or tissues 654.9
    - pelvis (bony) (major) NEC 653.0
    - presentation or position 652.9
      - in multiple gestation 652.6
    - size, fetus 653.5
    - soft parts (of pelvis) 654.9
    - uterus, congenital 654.0
    - vagina 654.7
    - vulva 654.8
  - abruptio placentae 641.2
  - acromion presentation 652.8
  - affecting fetus or newborn 763.4
  - anteversion, cervix or uterus 654.4
  - atony, uterus 661.2
  - bicornis or bicornuate uterus 654.0
  - breech presentation 652.2
  - brow presentation 652.4
  - cephalopelvic disproportion (normally formed fetus) 653.4
  - chin presentation 652.4
  - cicatrix of cervix 654.6
  - contracted pelvis (general) 653.1
    - inlet 653.2
    - outlet 653.3
  - cord presentation or prolapse 663.0
  - cystocele 654.4

Delivery—*continued*
deformity (acquired) (congenital)
pelvic organs or tissues NEC 654.9
pelvis (bony) NEC 653.0
displacement, uterus NEC 654.4
disproportion NEC 653.9
distress
fetal 656.3
maternal 669.0
eclampsia 642.6
face presentation 652.4
failed
forceps 660.7
trial of labor NEC 660.6
vacuum extraction 660.7
ventouse 660.7
fetal deformity 653.7
fetal-maternal hemorrhage 656.0
fetus, fetal
distress 656.3
prematurity 656.8
fibroid (tumor) (uterus) 654.1
hemorrhage (antepartum) (intrapartum) NEC 641.9
hydrocephalic fetus 653.6
incarceration of uterus 654.3
incoordinate uterine action 661.4
inertia, uterus 661.2
primary 661.0
secondary 661.1
lateroversion, uterus or cervix 654.4
mal lie 652.9
malposition
fetus 652.9
in multiple gestation 652.6
pelvic organs or tissues NEC 654.9
uterus NEC or cervix 654.4
malpresentation NEC 652.9
in multiple gestation 652.6
maternal
diabetes mellitus 648.0
heart disease NEC 648.6
meconium in liquor 656.3
without mention of fetal distress—omit code
staining only 792.3
oblique presentation 652.3
oversize fetus 653.5
pelvic tumor NEC 654.9
placental insufficiency 656.5
placenta previa 641.0
with hemorrhage 641.1
poor dilation, cervix 661.0
pre-eclampsia 642.4
severe 642.5
previous
cesarean delivery 654.2
surgery (to)
cervix 654.6
gynecological NEC 654.9
uterus NEC 654.9
from previous cesarean delivery 654.2
vagina 654.7
prolapse
arm or hand 652.7
uterus 654.4
prolonged labor 662.1
rectocele 654.4
retroversion, uterus or cervix 654.3
rigid
cervix 654.6
pelvic floor 654.4

Delivery—*continued*
perineum 654.8
vagina 654.7
vulva 654.8
sacculation, pregnant uterus 654.4
scar(s)
cervix 654.6
cesarean delivery 654.2
uterus NEC 654.9
due to previous cesarean delivery 654.2
Shirodkar suture in situ 654.5
shoulder presentation 652.8
stenosis or stricture, cervix 654.6
transverse presentation or lie 652.3
tumor, pelvic organs or tissues NEC 654.4
umbilical cord presentation or prolapse 663.0
completely normal case—*see category* 650
complicated (by) NEC 669.9
abdominal tumor, fetal 653.7
causing obstructed labor 660.1
abnormal, abnormality of
cervix 654.6
causing obstructed labor 660.2
forces of labor 661.9
formation of uterus 654.0
pelvic organs or tissues 654.9
causing obstructed labor 660.2
pelvis (bony) (major) NEC 653.0
causing obstructed labor 660.1
presentation or position NEC 652.9
causing obstructed labor 660.0
size, fetus 653.5
causing obstructed labor 660.1
soft parts (of pelvis) 654.9
causing obstructed labor 660.2
uterine contractions NEC 661.9
uterus (formation) 654.0
causing obstructed labor 660.2
vagina 654.7
causing obstructed labor 660.2
abnormally formed uterus (any type) (congenital) 654.0
causing obstructed labor 660.2
acromion presentation 652.8
causing obstructed labor 660.0
adherent placenta 667.0
with hemorrhage 666.0
adhesions, uterus (to abdominal wall) 654.4
advanced maternal age NEC 659.6
primigravida 659.5
air embolism 673.0
amnionitis 658.4
amniotic fluid embolism 673.1
anesthetic death 668.9
annular detachment, cervix 665.3
antepartum hemorrhage—*see* Delivery, complicated, hemorrhage
anteversion, cervix or uterus 654.4
causing obstructed labor 660.2
apoplexy 674.0
placenta 641.2
arrested active phase 661.1
asymmetrical pelvis bone 653.0
causing obstructed labor 660.1
atony, uterus (hypotonic) (inertia) 661.2
hypertonic 661.4
Bandl's ring 661.4
battledore placenta—*see* Placenta, abnormal
bicornis or bicornuate uterus 654.0
causing obstructed labor 660.2

Delivery—*continued*
birth injury to mother NEC 665.9
bleeding (*see also* Delivery, complicated, hemorrhage) 641.9
breech presentation (assisted) (spontaneous) 652.2
with successful version 652.1
causing obstructed labor 660.0
brow presentation 652.4
causing obstructed labor 660.0
cephalopelvic disproportion (normally formed fetus) 653.4
causing obstructed labor 660.1
cerebral hemorrhage 674.0
cervical dystocia 661.0
chin presentation 652.4
causing obstructed labor 660.0
cicatrix
cervix 654.6
causing obstructed labor 660.2
vagina 654.7
causing obstructed labor 660.2
colporrhexis 665.4
with perineal laceration 664.0
compound presentation 652.8
causing obstructed labor 660.0
compression of cord (umbilical) 663.2
around neck 663.1
cord prolapsed 663.0
contraction, contracted pelvis 653.1
causing obstructed labor 660.1
general 653.1
causing obstructed labor 660.1
inlet 653.2
causing obstructed labor 660.1
midpelvic 653.8
causing obstructed labor 660.1
midplane 653.8
causing obstructed labor 660.1
outlet 653.3
causing obstructed labor 660.1
contraction ring 661.4
cord (umbilical) 663.9
around neck, tightly or with compression 663.1
without compression 663.3
bruising 663.6
complication NEC 663.9
specified type NEC 663.8
compression NEC 663.2
entanglement NEC 663.3
with compression 663.2
forelying 663.0
hematoma 663.6
marginal attachment 663.8
presentation 663.0
prolapse (complete) (occult) (partial) 663.0
short 663.4
specified complication NEC 663.8
thrombosis (vessels) 663.6
vascular lesion 663.6
velamentous insertion 663.5
Couvelaire uterus 641.2
cretin pelvis (dwarf type) (male type) 653.1
causing obstructed labor 660.1
crossbirth 652.3
with successful version 652.1
causing obstructed labor 660.0
cyst (Gartner's duct) 654.7
cystocele 654.4
causing obstructed labor 660.2

Delivery—*continued*
death of fetus (near term) 656.4
early (before 22 completed weeks' gestation) 632
deformity (acquired) (congenital)
fetus 653.7
causing obstructed labor 660.1
pelvic organs or tissues NEC 654.9
causing obstructed labor 660.2
pelvis (bony) NEC 653.0
causing obstructed labor 660.1
delay, delayed
delivery in multiple pregnancy 662.3
due to locked mates 660.5
following rupture of membranes (spontaneous) 658.2
artificial 658.3
depressed fetal heart tones 656.3
diastasis recti 665.8
dilatation
bladder 654.4
causing obstructed labor 660.2
cervix, incomplete, poor or slow 661.0
diseased placenta 656.7
displacement uterus NEC 654.4
causing obstructed labor 660.2
disproportion NEC 653.9
causing obstructed labor 660.1
disruptio uteri—*see* Delivery, complicated, rupture, uterus
distress
fetal 656.3
maternal 669.0
double uterus (congenital) 654.0
causing obstructed labor 660.2
dropsy amnion 657
dysfunction, uterus 661.9
hypertonic 661.4
hypotonic 661.2
primary 661.0
secondary 661.1
incoordinate 661.4
dystocia
cervical 661.0
fetal—*see* Delivery, complicated, abnormal, presentation
maternal—*see* Delivery, complicated, prolonged labor
pelvic—*see* Delivery, complicated, contraction pelvis
positional 652.8
shoulder girdle 660.4
eclampsia 642.6
ectopic kidney 654.4
causing obstructed labor 660.2
edema, cervix 654.6
causing obstructed labor 660.2
effusion, amniotic fluid 658.1
elderly primigravida 659.5
embolism (pulmonary) 673.2
air 673.0
amniotic fluid 673.1
blood-clot 673.2
cerebral 674.0
fat 673.8
pyemic 673.3
septic 673.3
entanglement, umbilical cord 663.3
with compression 663.2
around neck (with compression) 663.1
eversion, cervix or uterus 665.2

Delivery—*continued*
excessive
fetal growth 653.5
causing obstructed labor 660.1
size of fetus 653.5
causing obstructed labor 660.1
face presentation 652.4
causing obstructed labor 660.0
to pubes 660.3
failure, fetal head to enter pelvic brim 652.5
causing obstructed labor 660.0
fetal
acid-base balance 656.3
death (near term) NEC 656.4
early (before 22 completed weeks' gestation) 632
deformity 653.7
causing obstructed labor 660.1
distress 656.3
heart-rate or rhythm 656.3
fetopelvic disproportion 653.4
causing obstructed labor 660.1
fever during labor 659.2
fibroid (tumor) (uterus) 654.1
causing obstructed labor 660.2
fibromyomata 654.1
causing obstructed labor 660.2
forelying umbilical cord 663.0
fracture of coccyx 665.6
hematoma 664.5
broad ligament 665.7
ischial spine 665.7
pelvic 665.7
perineum 664.5
soft tissues 665.7
subdural 674.0
umbilical cord 663.6
vagina 665.7
vulva or perineum 664.5
hemorrhage (uterine) (antepartum) (intrapartum) (pregnancy) 641.9
accidental 641.2
associated with
afibrinogenemia 641.3
coagulation defect 641.3
hyperfibrinolysis 641.3
hypofibrinogenemia 641.3
cerebral 674.0
due to
low-lying placenta 641.1
placenta previa 641.1
premature separation of placenta (normally implanted) 641.2
retained placenta 666.0
trauma 641.8
uterine leiomyoma 641.8
marginal sinus rupture 641.2
placenta NEC 641.9
postpartum (atonic) (immediate) (within 24 hours) 666.1
with retained or trapped placenta 666.0
third stage 666.0
delayed 666.2
secondary 666.2
hourglass contraction, uterus 661.4
hydramnios 657
hydrocephalic fetus 653.6
causing obstructed labor 660.1
hydrops fetalis 653.7
causing obstructed labor 660.1

Delivery—*continued*
hypertension—*see* Hypertension, complicating pregnancy
hypertonic uterine dysfunction 661.4
hypotonic uterine dysfunction 661.2
impacted shoulders 660.4
incarceration, uterus 654.3
causing obstructed labor 660.2
incomplete dilation (cervix) 661.0
incoordinate uterus 661.4
indication NEC 659.9
specified type NEC 659.8
inertia, uterus 661.2
hypertonic 661.4
hypotonic 661.2
primary 661.0
secondary 661.1
infantile
genitalia 654.4
causing obstructed labor 660.2
uterus (os) 654.4
causing obstructed labor 660.2
injury (to mother) NEC 665.9
intrauterine fetal death (near term) NEC 656.4
early (before 22 completed weeks' gestation) 632
inversion, uterus 665.2
kidney, ectopic 654.4
causing obstructed labor 660.2
knot (true), umbilical cord 663.2
labor, premature (before 37 completed weeks gestation) 644.2
laceration 664.9
anus (sphincter) 664.2
with mucosa 664.3
bladder (urinary) 665.5
bowel 665.5
central 664.4
cervix (uteri) 665.3
fourchette 664.0
hymen 664.0
labia (majora) (minora) 664.0
pelvic
floor 664.1
organ NEC 665.5
perineum, perineal 664.4
first degree 664.0
second degree 664.1
third degree 664.2
fourth degree 664.3
central 664.4
extensive NEC 664.4
muscles 664.1
skin 664.0
slight 664.0
peritoneum 665.5
periurethral tissue 665.5
rectovaginal (septum) (without perineal laceration) 665.4
with perineum 664.2
with anal or rectal mucosa 664.3
skin (perineum) 664.0
specified site or type NEC 664.8
sphincter ani 664.2
with mucosa 664.3
urethra 665.5
uterus 665.1
before labor 665.0
vagina, vaginal (deep) (high) (sulcus) (wall) (without perineal laceration) 665.4
with perineum 664.0

Delivery—*continued*
muscles, with perineum 664.1
vulva 664.0
lateroversion, uterus or cervix 654.4
causing obstructed labor 660.2
locked mates 660.5
low implantation of placenta—*see* Delivery, complicated, placenta, previa
mal lie 652.9
causing obstructed labor 660.0
malposition
fetus NEC 652.9
causing obstructed labor 660.0
pelvic organs or tissues NEC 654.9
causing obstructed labor 660.2
placenta 641.1
without hemorrhage 641.0
uterus NEC or cervix 654.4
causing obstructed labor 660.2
malpresentation 652.9
causing obstructed labor 660.0
marginal sinus (bleeding) (rupture) 641.2
maternal hypotension syndrome 669.2
meconium in liquor 656.3
membranes, retained—*see* Delivery, complicated, placenta, retained
mentum presentation 652.4
causing obstructed labor 660.0
metrorrhagia (myopathia)—*see* Delivery, complicated, hemorrhage
metrorrhexis—*see* Delivery, complicated, rupture, uterus
multiparity (grand) 659.4
myelomeningocele, fetus 653.7
causing obstructed labor 660.1
Nägele's pelvis 653.0
causing obstructed labor 660.1
nonengagement, fetal head 652.5
causing obstructed labor 660.0
oblique presentation 652.3
causing obstructed labor 660.0
obstetric
shock 669.1
trauma NEC 665.9
obstructed labor 660.9
due to
abnormality pelvic organs or tissues (conditions classifiable to 654.0-654.9) 660.2
deep transverse arrest 660.3
impacted shoulders 660.4
locked twins 660.5
malposition and malpresentation of fetus (conditions classifiable to 652.0-652.9) 660.0
persistent occipitoposterior 660.3
shoulder dystocia 660.4
occult prolapse of umbilical cord 663.0
oversize fetus 653.5
causing obstructed labor 660.1
pathological retraction ring, uterus 661.4
pelvic
arrest (deep) (high) (of fetal head) (transverse) 660.3
deformity (bone)—*see also* Deformity, pelvis, with disproportion
soft tissue 654.9
causing obstructed labor 660.2
tumor NEC 654.9

Delivery—*continued*
causing obstructed labor 660.2
penetration, pregnant uterus by instrument 665.1
perforation—*see* Delivery, complicated, laceration
persistent
hymen 654.8
causing obstructed labor 660.2
occipitoposterior 660.3
placenta, placental
ablatio 641.2
abnormality 656.7
with hemorrhage 641.2
abruptio 641.2
accreta 667.0
with hemorrhage 666.0
adherent (without hemorrhage) 667.0
with hemorrhage 666.0
apoplexy 641.2
battledore 663.8
detachment (premature) 641.2
disease 656.7
hemorrhage NEC 641.9
increta (without hemorrhage) 667.0
with hemorrhage 666.0
low (implantation) 641.1
without hemorrhage 641.0
malformation 656.7
with hemorrhage 641.2
malposition 641.1
without hemorrhage 641.0
marginal sinus rupture 641.2
percreta 667.0
with hemorrhage 666.0
premature separation 641.2
previa (central) (lateral) (marginal) (partial) 641.1
without hemorrhage 641.0
retained (with hemorrhage) 666.0
without hemorrhage 667.0
rupture of marginal sinus 641.2
separation (premature) 641.2
trapped 666.0
without hemorrhage 667.0
vicious insertion 641.1
polyhydramnios 657
polyp, cervix 654.6
causing obstructed labor 660.2
precipitate labor 661.3
premature
labor (before 37 completed weeks gestation) 644.2
rupture, membranes 658.1
delayed delivery following 658.2
presenting umbilical cord 663.0
previous
cesarean delivery 654.2
surgery
cervix 654.6
causing obstructed labor 660.2
gynecological NEC 654.9
causing obstructed labor 660.2
perineum 654.8
uterus NEC 654.9
due to previous cesarean delivery 654.2
vagina 654.7
causing obstructed labor 660.2
vulva 654.8
primary uterine inertia 661.0
primipara, elderly or old 659.5

Delivery—*continued*
prolapse
arm or hand 652.7
causing obstructed labor 660.0
cord (umbilical) 663.0
fetal extremity 652.8
foot or leg 652.8
causing obstructed labor 660.0
umbilical cord (complete) (occult) (partial) 663.0
uterus 654.4
causing obstructed labor 660.2
prolonged labor 662.1
first stage 662.0
second stage 662.2
active phase 661.2
due to
cervical dystocia 661.0
contraction ring 661.4
tetanic uterus 661.4
uterine inertia 661.2
primary 661.0
secondary 661.1
latent phase 661.0
pyrexia during labor 659.2
rachitic pelvis 653.2
causing obstructed labor 660.1
rectocele 654.4
causing obstructed labor 660.2
retained membranes or portions of placenta 666.2
without hemorrhage 667.1
retarded (prolonged) birth 662.1
retention secundines (with hemorrhage) 666.2
without hemorrhage 667.1
retroversion, uterus or cervix 654.3
causing obstructed labor 660.2
rigid
cervix 654.6
causing obstructed labor 660.2
pelvic floor 654.4
causing obstructed labor 660.2
perineum or vulva 654.8
causing obstructed labor 660.2
vagina 654.7
causing obstructed labor 660.2
Robert's pelvis 653.0
causing obstructed labor 660.1
rupture—*see also* Delivery, complicated, laceration
bladder (urinary) 665.5
cervix 665.3
marginal sinus 641.2
membranes, premature 658.1
pelvic organ NEC 665.5
perineum (without mention of other laceration)—*see* Delivery, complicated, laceration, perineum
peritoneum 665.5
urethra 665.5
uterus (during labor) 665.1
before labor 665.0
sacculation, pregnant uterus 654.4
sacral teratomas, fetal 653.7
causing obstructed labor 660.1
scar(s)
cervix 654.6
causing obstructed labor 660.2
cesarean delivery 654.2
causing obstructed labor 660.2

Delivery—*continued*
perineum 654.8
causing obstructed labor 660.2
uterus NEC 654.9
causing obstructed labor 660.2
due to previous cesarean delivery 654.2
vagina 654.7
causing obstructed labor 660.2
vulva 654.8
causing obstructed labor 660.2
scoliotic pelvis 653.0
causing obstructed labor 660.1
secondary uterine inertia 661.1
secundines, retained—*see* Delivery, complicated, placenta, retained
separation
placenta (premature) 641.2
pubic bone 665.6
symphysis pubis 665.6
septate vagina 654.7
causing obstructed labor 660.2
shock (birth) (obstetric) (puerperal) 669.1
short cord syndrome 663.4
shoulder
girdle dystocia 660.4
presentation 652.8
causing obstructed labor 660.0
Siamese twins 653.7
causing obstructed labor 660.1
slow slope active phase 661.2
spasm
cervix 661.4
uterus 661.4
spondylolisthesis, pelvis 653.3
causing obstructed labor 660.1
spondylolysis (lumbosacral) 653.3
causing obstructed labor 660.1
spondylosis 653.0
causing obstructed labor 660.1
stenosis or stricture
cervix 654.6
causing obstructed labor 660.2
vagina 654.7
causing obstructed labor 660.2
sudden death, unknown cause 669.9
tear (pelvic organ) (*see also* Delivery, complicated, laceration) 664.9
teratomas, sacral, fetal 653.7
causing obstructed labor 660.1
tetanic uterus 661.4
tipping pelvis 653.0
causing obstructed labor 660.1
transverse
arrest (deep) 660.3
presentation or lie 652.3
with successful version 652.1
causing obstructed labor 660.0
trauma (obstetrical) NEC 665.9
tumor
abdominal, fetal 653.7
causing obstructed labor 660.1
pelvic organs or tissues NEC 654.9
causing obstructed labor 660.2
umbilical cord (*see also* Delivery, complicated, cord) 663.9
around neck tightly, or with compression 663.1
entanglement NEC 663.3
with compression 663.2
prolapse (complete) (occult) (partial) 663.0

Dementia—*continued*
presenile 290.10
with
acute confusional state 290.11
delirium 290.11
delusional features 290.12
depressive features 290.13
depressed type 290.13
paranoid type 290.12
simple type 290.10
uncomplicated 290.10
primary (acute) (*see also* Schizophrenia) 295.0
progressive, syphilitic 094.1
puerperal—*see* Psychosis, puerperal
schizophrenic (*see also* Schizophrenia) 295.9
senile 290.0
with
acute confusional state 290.3
delirium 290.3
delusional features 290.20
depressive features 290.21
depressed type 290.21
exhaustion 290.0
paranoid type 290.20
simple type (acute) (*see also* Schizophrenia) 295.0
simplex (acute) (*see also* Schizophrenia) 295.0
syphilitic 094.1
uremic—*see* Uremia
Demerol dependence (*see also* Dependence) 304.0
Demineralization, ankle (*see also* Osteoporosis) 733.00
Demodex folliculorum (infestation) 133.8
de Morgan's spots (senile angiomas) 448.1
Demyelination, demyelinization
central nervous system 341.9
specified NEC 341.8
corpus callosum (central) 341.8
global 340
Dengue (fever) 061
sandfly 061
vaccination, prophylactic (against) V05.1
virus hemorrhagic fever 065.4
Dens
evaginatus 520.2
in dente 520.2
invaginatus 520.2
Density
increased, bone (disseminated) (generalized) (spotted) 733.99
lung (nodular) 518.89
Dental —*see also* condition
examination only V72.2
Dentia praecox 520.6
Denticles (in pulp) 522.2
Dentigerous cyst 526.0
Dentin
irregular (in pulp) 522.3
opalescent 520.5
secondary (in pulp) 522.3
sensitive 521.8
Dentinogenesis imperfecta 520.5
Dentinoma (M9271/0) 213.1
upper jaw (bone) 213.0
Dentition 520.7
abnormal 520.6
anomaly 520.6
delayed 520.6
difficult 520.7
disorder of 520.6
precocious 520.6
retarded 520.6
Denture sore (mouth) 528.9
Dependence

Note—Use the following fifth-digit subclassification with category 304:

0 unspecified
1 continuous
2 episodic
3 in remission

with
withdrawal symptoms
alcohol 291.8
drug 292.0
14-hydroxy-dihydromorphinone 304.0
absinthe 304.6
acemorphan 304.0
acetanilid(e) 304.6
acetophenetidin 304.6
acetorphine 304.0
acetyldihydrocodeine 304.0
acetyldihydrocodeinone 304.0
Adalin 304.1
Afghanistan black 304.3
agrypnal 304.1
alcohol, alcoholic (ethyl) (methyl) (wood) 303.9
maternal, with suspected fetal damage affecting management of pregnancy 655.4
allobarbitone 304.1
allonal 304.1
allylisopropylacetylurea 304.1
alphaprodine (hydrochloride) 304.0
Alurate 304.1
Alvodine 304.0
amethocaine 304.6
amidone 304.0
amidopyrine 304.6
aminopyrine 304.6
amobarbital 304.1
amphetamine(s) (type) (drugs classifiable to 969.7) 304.4
amylene hydrate 304.6
amylobarbitone 304.1
amylocaine 304.6
Amytal (sodium) 304.1
analgesic (drug) NEC 304.6
synthetic with morphine-like effect 304.0
anesthetic (agent) (drug) (gas) (general) (local) NEC 304.6
Angel dust 304.6
anileridine 304.0
antipyrine 304.6
aprobarbital 304.1
aprobarbitone 304.1
atropine 304.6
Avertin (bromide) 304.6
barbenyl 304.1
barbital(s) 304.1
barbitone 304.1
barbiturate(s) (compounds) (drugs classifiable to 967.0) 304.1
barbituric acid (and compounds) 304.1
benzedrine 304.4

Dependence—*continued*
benzylmorphine 304.0
Beta-chlor 304.1
bhang 304.3
blue velvet 304.0
Brevital 304.1
bromal (hydrate) 304.1
bromide(s) NEC 304.1
bromine compounds NEC 304.1
bromisovalum 304.1
bromoform 304.1
Bromo-seltzer 304.1
bromural 304.1
butabarbital (sodium) 304.1
butabarpal 304.1
butallylonal 304.1
butethal 304.1
buthalitone (sodium) 304.1
Butisol 304.1
butobarbitone 304.1
butyl chloral (hydrate) 304.1
caffeine 304.4
cannabis (indica) (sativa) (resin) (derivatives) (type) 304.3
carbamazepine 304.6
Carbrital 304.1
carbromal 304.1
carisoprodol 304.6
Catha (edulis) 304.4
chloral (betaine) (hydrate) 304.1
chloralamide 304.1
chloralformamide 304.1
chloralose 304.1
chlordiazepoxide 304.1
Chloretone 304.1
chlorobutanol 304.1
chlorodyne 304.1
chloroform 304.6
Cliradon 304.0
coca (leaf) and derivatives 304.2
cocaine 304.2
  hydrochloride 304.2
  salt (any) 304.2
codeine 304.0
combination of drugs (excluding morphine or opioid type drug) NEC 304.8
  morphine or opioid type drug with any other drug 304.7
croton-chloral 304.1
cyclobarbital 304.1
cyclobarbitone 304.1
dagga 304.3
Delvinal 304.1
Demerol 304.0
desocodeine 304.0
desomorphine 304.0
desoxyephedrine 304.4
DET 304.5
dexamphetamine 304.4
dexedrine 304.4
dextromethorphan 304.0
dextromoramide 304.0
dextronorpseudophedrine 304.4
dextrorphan 304.0
diacetylmorphine 304.0
Dial 304.1
diallylbarbituric acid 304.1
diamorphine 304.0
diazepam 304.1
dibucaine 304.6

Dependence—*continued*
dichloroethane 304.6
diethyl barbituric acid 304.1
diethylsulfone-diethylmethane 304.1
difencloxazine 304.0
dihydrocodeine 304.0
dihydrocodeinone 304.0
dihydrohydroxycodeinone 304.0
dihydroisocodeine 304.0
dihydromorphine 304.0
dihydromorphinone 304.0
dihydroxcodeinone 304.0
Dilaudid 304.0
dimenhydrinate 304.6
dimethylmeperidine 304.0
dimethyltriptamine 304.5
Dionin 304.0
diphenoxylate 304.6
dipipanone 304.0
d-lysergic acid diethylamide 304.5
DMT 304.5
Dolophine 304.0
DOM 304.2
Doriden 304.1
dormiral 304.1
Dormison 304.1
Dromoran 304.0
drug NEC 304.9
  analgesic NEC 304.6
  combination (excluding morphine or opioid type drug) NEC 304.8
    morphine or opioid type drug with any other drug 304.7
  complicating pregnancy, childbirth, or puerperium 648.3
    affecting fetus or newborn 779.5
  hallucinogenic 304.5
  hypnotic NEC 304.1
  narcotic NEC 304.9
  psychostimulant NEC 304.4
  sedative 304.1
  soporific NEC 304.1
  specified type NEC 304.6
  suspected damage to fetus affecting management of pregnancy 655.5
  synthetic, with morphine-like effect 304.0
  tranquilizing 304.1
duboisine 304.6
ectylurea 304.1
Endocaine 304.6
Equanil 304.1
Eskabarb 304.1
ethchlorvynol 304.1
ether (ethyl) (liquid) (vapor) (vinyl) 304.6
ethidene 304.6
ethinamate 304.1
ethoheptazine 304.6
ethyl
  alcohol 303.9
  bromide 304.6
  carbamate 304.6
  chloride 304.6
  morphine 304.0
ethylene (gas) 304.6
  dichloride 304.6
ethylidene chloride 304.6
etilfen 304.1
etorphine 304.0
etoval 304.1
eucodal 304.0

Dependence—*continued*
euneryl 304.1
Evipal 304.1
Evipan 304.1
fentanyl 304.0
ganja 304.3
gardenal 304.1
gardenpanyl 304.1
gelsemine 304.6
Gelsemium 304.6
Gemonil 304.1
glucochloral 304.1
glue (airplane) (sniffing) 304.6
glutethimide 304.1
hallucinogenics 304.5
hashish 304.3
headache powder NEC 304.6
Heavenly Blue 304.5
hedonal 304.1
hemp 304.3
heptabarbital 304.1
Heptalgin 304.0
heptobarbitone 304.1
heroin 304.0
salt (any) 304.0
hexethal (sodium) 304.1
hexobarbital 304.1
Hycodan 304.0
hydrocodone 304.0
hydromorphinol 304.0
hydromorphinone 304.0
hydromorphone 304.0
hydroxycodeine 304.0
hypnotic NEC 304.1
Indian hemp 304.3
intranarcon 304.1
Kemithal 304.1
ketobemidone 304.0
khat 304.4
kif 304.3
Lactuca (virosa) extract 304.1
lactucarium 304.1
laudanum 304.0
Lebanese red 304.3
Leritine 304.0
lettuce opium 304.1
Levanil 304.1
Levo-Dromoran 304.0
levo-iso-methadone 304.0
levorphanol 304.0
Librium 304.1
Lomotil 304.6
Lotusate 304.1
LSD (-25) (and derivatives) 304.5
Luminal 304.1
lysergic acid 304.5
amide 304.5
maconha 304.3
magic mushroom 304.5
marihuana 304.3
MDA (methylene dioxyamphetamine) 304.4
Mebaral 304.1
Medinal 304.1
Medomin 304.1
megahallucinogenics 304.5
meperidine 304.0
mephobarbital 304.1
meprobamate 304.1
mescaline 304.5
methadone 304.0

Dependence—*continued*
methamphetamine(s) 304.4
methaqualone 304.1
metharbital 304.1
methitural 304.1
methobarbitone 304.1
methohexital 304.1
methopholine 304.6
methyl
alcohol 303.9
bromide 304.6
morphine 304.0
sulfonal 304.1
methylated spirit 303.9
methylbutinol 304.6
methyldihydromorphinone 304.0
methylene
chloride 304.6
dichloride 304.6
dioxyamphetamine (MDA) 304.4
methylparafynol 304.1
methylphenidate 304.4
methyprylone 304.1
metopon 304.0
Miltown 304.1
morning glory seeds 304.5
morphinan(s) 304.0
morphine (sulfate) (sulfite) (type) (drugs classifiable to 965.00-965.09) 304.0
morphine or opioid type drug (drugs classifiable to 965.00-965.09) with any other drug 304.7
morphinol(s) 304.0
morphinon 304.0
morpholinylethylmorphine 304.0
mylomide 304.1
myristicin 304.5
narcotic (drug) NEC 304.9
nealbarbital 304.1
nealbarbitone 304.1
Nembutal 304.1
Neonal 304.1
Neraval 304.1
Neravan 304.1
neurobarb 304.1
nicotine 305.1
Nisentil 304.0
nitrous oxide 304.6
Noctec 304.1
Noludar 304.1
nonbarbiturate sedatives and tranquilizers with similar effect 304.1
noptil 304.1
normorphine 304.0
noscapine 304.0
Novocaine 304.6
Numorphan 304.0
nunol 304.1
Nupercaine 304.6
Oblivon 304.1
on
aspirator V46.0
hyperbaric chamber V46.8
iron lung V46.1
machine (enabling) V46.9
specified type NEC V46.8
Possum (Patient-Operated-Selector-Mechanism) V46.8
renal dialysis machine V45.1
respirator V46.1
opiate 304.0
opioids 304.0

Dependence—*continued*
opioid type drug 304.0
with any other drug 304.7
opium (alkaloids) (derivatives) (tincture) 304.0
ortal 304.1
Oxazepam 304.1
oxycodone 304.0
oxymorphone 304.0
Palfium 304.0
Panadol 304.6
pantopium 304.0
pantopon 304.0
papaverine 304.0
paracetamol 304.6
paracodin 304.0
paraldehyde 304.1
paregoric 304.0
Parzone 304.0
PCP (phencyclidine) 304.6
Pearly Gates 304.5
pentazocine 304.0
pentobarbital 304.1
pentobarbitone (sodium) 304.1
Pentothal 304.1
Percaine 304.6
Percodan 304.0
Perichlor 304.1
Pernocton 304.1
Pernoston 304.1
peronine 304.0
pethidine (hydrochloride) 304.0
petrichloral 304.1
peyote 304.5
Phanodorn 304.1
phenacetin 304.6
phenadoxone 304.0
phenaglycodol 304.1
phenazocine 304.0
phencyclidine 304.6
phenmetrazine 304.4
phenobal 304.1
phenobarbital 304.1
phenobarbitone 304.1
phenomorphan 304.0
phenonyl 304.1
phenoperidine 304.0
pholcodine 304.0
piminodine 304.0
Pipadone 304.0
Pitkin's solution 304.6
Placidyl 304.1
polysubstance 304.8
Pontocaine 304.6
pot 304.3
potassium bromide 304.1
Preludin 304.4
Prinadol 304.0
probarbital 304.1
procaine 304.6
propanal 304.1
propoxyphene 304.6
psilocibin 304.5
psilocin 304.5
psilocybin 304.5
psilocyline 304.5
psilocyn 304.5
psychedelic agents 304.5
psychostimulant NEC 304.4
psychotomimetic agents 304.5
pyrahexyl 304.3
Pyramidon 304.6

Dependence—*continued*
quinalbarbitone 304.1
racemoramide 304.0
racemorphan 304.0
Rela 304.6
scopolamine 304.6
secobarbital 304.1
Seconal 304.1
sedative NEC 304.1
nonbarbiturate with barbiturate effect 304.1
Sedormid 304.1
sernyl 304.1
sodium bromide 304.1
Soma 304.6
Somnal 304.1
Somnos 304.1
Soneryl 304.1
soporific (drug) NEC 304.1
specified drug NEC 304.6
speed 304.4
spinocaine 304.6
Stovaine 304.6
STP 304.5
stramonium 304.6
Sulfonal 304.1
sulfonethylmethane 304.1
sulfonmethane 304.1
Surital 304.1
synthetic drug with morphine-like effect 304.0
talbutal 304.1
tetracaine 304.6
tetrahydrocannabinol 304.3
tetronal 304.1
THC 304.3
thebacon 304.0
thebaine 304.0
thiamil 304.1
thiamylal 304.1
thiopental 304.1
tobacco 305.1
toluene, toluol 304.6
tranquilizer NEC 304.1
nonbarbiturate with barbiturate effect 304.1
tribromacetaldehyde 304.6
tribromethanol 304.6
tribromomethane 304.6
trichloroethanol 304.6
trichoroethyl phosphate 304.1
triclofos 304.1
Trional 304.1
Tuinal 304.1
Turkish Green 304.3
urethan(e) 304.6
Valium 304.1
Valmid 304.1
veganin 304.0
veramon 304.1
Veronal 304.1
versidyne 304.6
vinbarbital 304.1
vinbarbitone 304.1
vinyl bitone 304.1
vitamin B_6 266.1
wine 303.9
Zactane 304.6
Dependency
passive 301.6
reactions 301.6
Depersonalization (episode, in neurotic state) (neurotic) (syndrome) 300.6

Depletion
carbohydrates 271.9
complement factor 279.8
extracellular fluid 276.5
plasma 276.5
potassium 276.8
nephropathy 588.8
salt or sodium 276.1
causing heat exhaustion or prostration 992.4
nephropathy 593.9
volume 276.5
extracellular fluid 276.5
plasma 276.5
Deposit
argentous, cornea 371.16
bone, in Boeck's sarcoid 135
calcareous, calcium—*see* Calcification
cholesterol
retina 362.82
skin 709.3
vitreous (humor) 379.22
conjunctival 372.56
cornea, corneal NEC 371.10
argentous 371.16
in
cystinosis 270.0 *[371.15]*
mucopolysaccharidosis 277.5 *[371.15]*
crystalline, vitreous (humor) 379.22
hemosiderin, in old scars of cornea 371.11
metallic, in lens 366.45
skin 709.3
teeth, tooth (betel) (black) (green) (materia alba) (orange) (soft) (tobacco) 523.6
urate, in kidney (*see also* Disease, renal) 593.9
Depraved appetite 307.52
Depression 311
acute (*see also* Psychosis, affective) 296.2
recurrent episode 296.3
single episode 296.2
agitated (*see also* Psychosis, affective) 296.2
recurrent episode 296.3
single episode 296.2
anaclitic 309.21
anxiety 300.4
arches 734
congenital 754.61
autogenous (*see also* Psychosis, affective) 296.2
recurrent episode 296.3
single episode 296.2
basal metabolic rate (BMR) 794.7
bone marrow 289.9
central nervous system 799.1
newborn 779.2
cerebral 331.9
newborn 779.2
cerebrovascular 437.8
newborn 779.2
chest wall 738.3
endogenous (*see also* Psychosis, affective) 296.2
recurrent episode 296.3
single episode 296.2
functional activity 780.9
hysterical 300.11
involutional, climacteric, or menopausal (*see also* Psychosis, affective) 296.2
recurrent episode 296.3
single episode 296.2
manic (*see also* Psychosis, affective) 296.80
medullary 348.8
newborn 779.2
Depression—*continued*
mental 300.4
metatarsal heads—*see* Depression, arches
metatarsus—*see* Depression, arches
monopolar (*see also* Psychosis, affective) 296.2
recurrent episode 296.3
single episode 296.2
nervous 300.4
neurotic 300.4
nose 738.0
postpartum 648.4
psychogenic 300.4
reactive 298.0
psychoneurotic 300.4
psychotic (*see also* Psychosis, affective) 296.2
reactive 298.0
recurrent episode 296.3
single episode 296.2
reactive 300.4
neurotic 300.4
psychogenic 298.0
psychoneurotic 300.4
psychotic 298.0
recurrent 296.3
respiratory center 348.8
newborn 770.8
scapula 736.89
senile 290.21
situational (acute) (brief) 309.0
prolonged 309.1
skull 754.0
sternum 738.3
visual field 368.40
Depressive reaction —*see also* Reaction, depressive
acute (transient) 309.0
with anxiety 309.28
prolonged 309.1
situational (acute) 309.0
prolonged 309.1
Deprivation
cultural V62.4
emotional V62.89
affecting infant or child 995.5
as reason for family seeking advice V61.21
food 994.2
specific substance NEC 269.8
protein (familial) (kwashiorkor) 260
social V62.4
affecting infant or child 995.5
as reason for family seeking advice V61.21
symptoms, syndrome
alcohol 291.8
drug 292.0
vitamins (*see also* Deficiency, vitamin) 269.2
water 994.3
de Quervain's
disease (tendon sheath) 727.04
thyroiditis (subacute granulomatous thyroiditis) 245.1
Derangement
ankle (internal) 718.97
current injury (*see also* Dislocation, ankle) 837.0
recurrent 718.37
cartilage (articular) NEC (*see also* Disorder, cartilage, articular) 718.0
knee 717.9
recurrent 718.36
recurrent 718.3

Derangement—*continued*
collateral ligament (knee) (medial) (tibial) 717.82
current injury 844.1
lateral (fibular) 844.0
lateral (fibular) 717.81
current injury 844.0
cruciate ligament (knee) (posterior) 717.84
anterior 717.83
current injury 844.2
current injury 844.2
elbow (internal) 718.92
current injury (*see also* Dislocation, elbow) 832.00
recurrent 718.32
gastrointestinal 536.9
heart—*see* Disease, heart
hip (joint) (internal) (old) 718.95
current injury (*see also* Dislocation, hip) 835.00
recurrent 718.35
intervertebral disc—*see* Displacement, intervertebral disc
joint (internal) 718.90
ankle 718.97
current injury—*see also* Dislocation, by site
knee, meniscus or cartilage (*see also* Tear, meniscus) 836.2
elbow 718.92
foot 718.97
hand 718.94
hip 718.95
knee 717.9
multiple sites 718.99
pelvic region 718.95
recurrent 718.30
ankle 718.37
elbow 718.32
foot 718.37
hand 718.34
hip 718.35
knee 718.36
multiple sites 718.39
pelvic region 718.35
shoulder (region) 718.31
specified site NEC 718.38
temporomandibular (old) 524.69
wrist 718.33
shoulder (region) 718.91
specified site NEC 718.98
spine NEC 724.9
temporomandibular 524.69
wrist 718.93
knee (cartilage) (internal) 717.9
current injury (*see also* Tear, meniscus) 836.2
ligament 717.89
capsular 717.85
collateral—*see* Derangement, collateral ligament
cruciate—*see* Derangement, cruciate ligament
specified NEC 717.85
recurrent 718.36
low back NEC 724.9
meniscus NEC (knee) 717.5
current injury (*see also* Tear, meniscus) 836.2
lateral 717.40
anterior horn 717.42
posterior horn 717.43
specified NEC 717.49

Derangement—*continued*
medial 717.3
anterior horn 717.1
posterior horn 717.2
recurrent 718.3
site other than knee—*see* Disorder, cartilage, articular
mental (*see also* Psychosis) 298.9
rotator cuff (recurrent) (tear) 726.10
current 840.4
sacroiliac (old) 724.6
current—*see* Dislocation, sacroiliac
semilunar cartilage (knee) 717.5
current injury 836.2
lateral 836.1
medial 836.0
recurrent 718.3
shoulder (internal) 718.91
current injury (*see also* Dislocation, shoulder) 831.00
recurrent 718.31
spine (recurrent) NEC 724.9
current—*see* Dislocation, spine
temporomandibular (internal) (joint) (old) 524.69
current—*see* Dislocation, jaw
Dercum's disease or syndrome (adiposis dolorosa) 272.8
Derealization (neurotic) 300.6
Dermal —*see* condition
Dermaphytid —*see* Dermatophytosis
Dermatergosis —*see* Dermatitis
Dermatitis (allergic) (contact) (occupational) (venenata) 692.9
ab igne 692.82
acneiform 692.9
actinic (due to sun) 692.70
acute 692.72
chronic NEC 692.74
other than from sun NEC 692.82
ambustionis
due to
burn or scald—*see* Burn, by site
sunburn 692.71
amebic 006.6
ammonia 691.0
anaphylactoid NEC 692.9
arsenical 692.4
artefacta 698.4
psychogenic 316 *[698.4]*
asthmatic 691.8
atopic (allergic) (infantile) (intrinsic) 691.8
psychogenic 316 *[691.8]*
atrophicans 701.8
diffusa 701.8
maculosa 701.3
berlock, berloque 692.72
blastomycetic 116.0
blister beetle 692.89
Brucella NEC 023.9
bullosa 694.9
striata pratensis 692.6
bullous 694.9
mucosynechial, atrophic 694.60
with ocular involvement 694.61
seasonal 694.8
calorica
due to
burn or scald—*see* Burn, by site
cold 692.89
sunburn 692.71

Dermatitis—*continued*
  caterpillar 692.89
  cercarial 120.3
  combustionis
    due to
      burn or scald—*see* Burn, by site
      sunburn 692.71
  congelationis 991.5
  contusiformis 695.2
  diabetic 250.8
  diaper 691.0
  diphtheritica 032.85
  due to
    acetone 692.2
    acids 692.4
    adhesive plaster 692.4
    alcohol (skin contact) (substances classifiable to 980.0-980.9) 692.4
      taken internally 693.8
    alkalis 692.4
    allergy NEC 692.9
    ammonia (household) (liquid) 692.4
    arnica 692.3
    arsenic 692.4
      taken internally 693.8
    blister beetle 692.89
    cantharides 692.3
    carbon disulphide 692.2
    caterpillar 692.89
    caustics 692.4
    cereal (ingested) 693.1
      contact with skin 692.5
    chemical(s) NEC 692.4
      internal 693.8
      irritant NEC 692.4
      taken internally 693.8
    chlorocompounds 692.2
    coffee (ingested) 693.1
      contact with skin 692.5
    cold weather 692.89
    cosmetics 692.81
    cyclohexanes 692.2
    deodorant 692.81
    detergents 692.0
    dichromate 692.4
    drugs and medicinals (correct substance properly administered) (internal use) 693.0
      external (in contact with skin) 692.3
        wrong substance given or taken 976.9
          specified substance—*see* Table of drugs and chemicals
      wrong substance given or taken 977.9
        specified substance—*see* Table of drugs and chemicals
    dyes 692.89
      hair 692.89
    epidermophytosis—*see* Dermatophytosis
    esters 692.2
    external irritant NEC 692.9
      specified agent NEC 692.89
    eye shadow 692.81
    fish (ingested) 693.1
      contact with skin 692.5
    flour (ingested) 693.1
      contact with skin 692.5
    food (ingested) 693.1
      in contact with skin 692.5
    fruit (ingested) 693.1
      contact with skin 692.5
    fungicides 692.3
    furs 692.89

Dermatitis—*continued*
    glycols 692.2
    greases NEC 692.1
    hair dyes 692.89
    hot
      objects and materials—*see* Burn, by site
      weather or places 692.89
    hydrocarbons 692.2
    infrared rays, except from sun 692.82
      solar NEC (*see* also Dermatitis, due to, sun) 692.70
    ingested substance 693.9
      drugs and medicinals (*see also* Dermatitis, due to, drugs and medicinals) 693.0
      food 693.1
      specified substance NEC 693.8
    ingestion or injection of
      chemical 693.8
      drug (correct substance properly administered) 693.0
        wrong substance given or taken 977.9
          specified substance—*see* Table of drugs and chemicals
    insecticides 692.4
    internal agent 693.9
      drugs and medicinals (*see also* Dermatitis, due to, drugs and medicinals) 693.0
      food (ingested) 693.1
        in contact with skin 692.5
      specified agent NEC 693.8
    iodine 692.3
    iodoform 692.3
    irradiation 692.82
    jewelry 692.83
    keratolytics 692.3
    ketones 692.2
    lacquer tree (Rhus verniciflua) 692.6
    light (sun) NEC (*see also* Dermatitis, due to, sun) 692.70
      other 692.82
    low temperature 692.89
    mascara 692.81
    meat (ingested) 693.1
      contact with skin 692.5
    mercury, mercurials 692.3
    metals 692.83
    milk (ingested) 693.1
      contact with skin 692.5
    Neomycin 692.3
    nylon 692.4
    oils NEC 692.1
    paint solvent 692.2
    pediculocides 692.3
    petroleum products (substances classifiable to 981) 692.4
    phenol 692.3
    photosensitiveness, photosensitivity (sun) 692.72
      other light 692.82
    plants NEC 692.6
    plasters, medicated (any) 692.3
    plastic 692.4
    poison
      ivy (Rhus toxicodendron) 692.6
      oak (Rhus diversiloba) 692.6
      plant or vine 692.6
      sumac (Rhus venenata) 692.6
      vine (Rhus radicans) 692.6
    preservatives 692.89
    primrose (primula) 692.6

Dermatitis—*continued*
primula 692.6
radiation 692.82
sun NEC (*see also* Dermatitis, due to, sun) 692.70
radioactive substance 692.82
radium 692.82
ragweed (Senecio jacobae) 692.6
Rhus (diversiloba) (radicans) (toxicodendron) (venenata) (verniciflua) 692.6
rubber 692.4
scabicides 692.3
Senecio jacobae 692.6
solar radiation—*see* Dermatitis, due to, sun
solvents (any) (substances classifiable to 982.0-982.8) 692.2
chlorocompound group 692.2
cyclohexane group 692.2
ester group 692.2
glycol group 692.2
hydrocarbon group 692.2
ketone group 692.2
paint 692.2
specified agent NEC 692.89
sun 692.70
acute 692.72
chronic NEC 692.74
specified NEC 692.79
sunburn 692.71
sunshine NEC (*see also* Dermatitis, due to, sun) 692.70
tetrachlorethylene 692.2
toluene 692.2
topical medications 692.3
turpentine 692.2
ultraviolet rays, except from sun 692.82
sun NEC (*see also* Dermatitis, due to, sun) 692.70
vaccine or vaccination (correct substance properly administered) 693.0
wrong substance given or taken
bacterial vaccine 978.8
specified—*see* Table of drugs and chemicals
other vaccines NEC 979.9
specified—*see* Table of drugs and chemicals
varicose veins (*see also* Varicose, vein, inflamed or infected) 454.1
x-rays 692.82
dyshydrotic 705.81
dysmenorrheica 625.8
eczematoid NEC 692.9
infectious 690.8
eczematous NEC 692.9
epidemica 695.89
erysipelatosa 695.81
escharotica—*see* Burn, by site
exfoliativa, exfoliative 695.89
generalized 695.89
infantum 695.81
neonatorum 695.81

Dermatitis—*continued*
eyelid 373.31
allergic 373.32
contact 373.32
eczematous 373.31
herpes (zoster) 053.20
simplex 054.41
infective 373.5
due to
actinomycosis 039.3 *[373.5]*
herpes
simplex 054.41
zoster 053.20
impetigo 684 *[373.5]*
leprosy (*see also* Leprosy) 030.0 *[373.4]*
lupus vulgaris (tuberculous) (*see also* Tuberculosis) 017.0 *[373.4]*
mycotic dermatitis (*see also* Dermatomycosis) 111.9 *[373.5]*
vaccinia 051.0 *[373.5]*
postvaccination 999.0 *[373.5]*
yaws (*see also* Yaws) 102.9 *[373.4]*
facta, factitia 698.4
psychogenic 316 *[698.4]*
ficta 698.4
psychogenic 316 *[698.4]*
flexural 691.8
follicularis 704.8
friction 709.8
fungus 111.9
specified type NEC 111.8
gangrenosa, gangrenous (infantum) (*see also* Gangrene) 785.4
gestationis 646.8
gonococcal 098.89
gouty 274.89
harvest mite 133.8
heat 692.89
herpetiformis (bullous) (erythematous) (pustular) (vesicular) 694.0
juvenile 694.2
senile 694.5
hiemalis 692.89
hypostatic, hypostatica 454.1
with ulcer 454.2
impetiginous 684
infantile (acute) (chronic) (intertriginous) (intrinsic) (seborrheic) 691.8
infectiosa eczematoides 690.8
infectious (staphylococcal) (streptococcal) 686.9
eczematoid 690.8
infective eczematoid 690.8
Jacquet's (diaper dermatitis) 691.0
leptus 133.8
lichenified NEC 692.9
lichenoid, chronic 701.0
lichenoides purpurica pigmentosa 709.1
meadow 692.6
medicamentosa (correct substance properly administered) (internal use) (*see also* Dermatitis, due to, drugs or medicinals) 693.0
due to contact with skin 692.3
mite 133.8
multiformis 694.0
juvenile 694.2
senile 694.5
napkin 691.0
neuro 698.3
neurotica 694.0
nummular NEC 692.9

Dermatitis—*continued*
osteatosis, osteatotic 706.8
papillaris capillitii 706.1
pellagrous 265.2
perioral 695.3
perstans 696.1
photosensitivity (sun) 692.72
other light 692.82
pigmented purpuric lichenoid 709.1
polymorpha dolorosa 694.0
primary irritant 692.9
pruriginosa 694.0
pruritic NEC 692.9
psoriasiform nodularis 696.2
psychogenic 316
purulent 686.0
pustular contagious 051.2
pyococcal 686.0
pyocyaneus 686.0
pyogenica 686.0
radiation 692.82
repens 696.1
Ritter's (exfoliativa) 695.81
Schamberg's (progressive pigmentary dermatosis) 709.09
schistosome 120.3
seasonal bullous 694.8
seborrheic 690.10
infantile 690.12
sensitization NEC 692.9
septic 686.0
gonococcal 098.89
solar, solare NEC (*see also* Dermatitis, due to, sun) 692.70
stasis 459.81
due to
postphlebitic syndrome 459.1
varicose veins—*see* Varicose
ulcerated or with ulcer (varicose) 454.2
sunburn 692.71
suppurative 686.0
traumatic NEC 709.8
trophoneurotica 694.0
ultraviolet, except from sun 692.82
due to sun NEC (*see also* Dermatitis, due to, sun) 692.70
varicose 454.1
with ulcer 454.2
vegetans 686.8
verrucosa 117.2
xerotic 706.8
Dermatoarthritis, lipoid 272.8 *[713.0]*
Dermatochalasia, dermatochalasis 374.87
Dermatofibroma (lenticulare) (M8832/0)—*see also* Neoplasm, skin, benign
protuberans (M8832/1)—*see* Neoplasm, skin, uncertain behavior
Dermatofibrosarcoma (protuberans) (M8832/3) *see* Neoplasm, skin, malignant
Dermatographia 708.3
Dermatolysis (congenital) (exfoliativa) 757.39
acquired 701.8
eyelids 374.34
palpebrarum 374.34
senile 701.8
Dermatomegaly NEC 701.8
Dermatomucomyositis 710.3
Dermatomycosis 111.9
furfuracea 111.0
specified type NEC 111.8
Dermatomyositis (acute) (chronic) 710.3
Dermatoneuritis of children 985.0
Dermatophiliasis 134.1
Dermatophytide —*see* Dermatophytosis
Dermatophytosis (Epidermophyton) (infection) (microsporum) (tinea) (Trichophyton) 110.9
beard 110.0
body 110.5
deep seated 110.6
fingernails 110.1
foot 110.4
groin 110.3
hand 110.2
nail 110.1
perianal (area) 110.3
scalp 110.0
scrotal 110.8
specified site NEC 110.8
toenails 110.1
vulva 110.8
Dermatopolyneuritis 985.0
Dermatorrhexis 756.83
acquired 701.8
Dermatosclerosis (*see also* Scleroderma) 710.1
localized 701.0
Dermatosis 709.9
Andrews' 686.8
atopic 691.8
Bowen's (M8081/2)—*see* Neoplasm, skin, in situ
bullous 694.9
specified type NEC 694.8
erythematosquamous 690.8
exfoliativa 695.89
factitial 698.4
gonococcal 098.89
herpetiformis 694.0
juvenile 694.2
senile 694.5
hysterical 300.11
menstrual NEC 709.8
neutrophilic, acute febrile 695.89
occupational (*see also* Dermatitis) 692.9
papulosa nigra 709.8
pigmentary NEC 709.00
progressive 709.09
Schamberg's 709.09
Siemens-Bloch 757.33
progressive pigmentary 709.09
psychogenic 316
pustular subcorneal 694.1
Schamberg's (progressive pigmentary) 709.09
senile NEC 709.3
Unna's (seborrheic dermatitis) 690.18
Dermographia 708.3
Dermographism 708.3
Dermoid (cyst) (M9084/0)—*see also* Neoplasm, by site, benign
with malignant transformation (M9084/3) 183.0
Dermopathy
infiltrative, with thyrotoxicosis 242.0
senile NEC 709.3
Dermophytosis —*see* Dermatophytosis
Descemet's membrane —*see* condition
Descemetocele 371.72
Descending —*see* condition
Descensus uteri (complete) (incomplete) (partial) (without vaginal wall prolapse) 618.1
with mention of vaginal wall prolapse—*see* Prolapse, uterovaginal
Desensitization to allergens V07.1

Desert
rheumatism 114.0
sore (*see also* Ulcer, skin) 707.9
Desertion (child) (newborn) 995.5
specified person NEC 995.81
Desmoid (extra-abdominal) (tumor) (M8821/1)—*see also* Neoplasm, connective tissue, uncertain behavior
abdominal (M8822/1)—*see* Neoplasm, connective tissue, uncertain behavior
Despondency 300.4
Desquamative dermatitis NEC 695.89
Destruction
articular facet (*see also* Derangement, joint) 718.9
vertebra 724.9
bone 733.90
syphilitic 095.5
joint (*see also* Derangement, joint) 718.9
sacroiliac 724.6
kidney 593.89
live fetus to facilitate birth NEC 763.8
ossicles (ear) 385.24
rectal sphincter 569.49
septum (nasal) 478.1
tuberculous NEC (*see also* Tuberculosis) 011.9
tympanic membrane 384.82
tympanum 385.89
vertebral disc—*see* Degeneration, intervertebral disc
Destructiveness (*see also* Disturbance, conduct) 312.9
adjustment reaction 309.3
Detachment
cartilage—*see also* Sprain, by site
knee—*see* Tear, meniscus
cervix, annular 622.8
complicating delivery 665.3
choroid (old) (postinfectional) (simple) (spontaneous) 363.70
hemorrhagic 363.72
serous 363.71
knee, medial meniscus (old) 717.3
current injury 836.0
ligament—*see* Sprain, by site
placenta (premature)—*see* Placenta, separation
retina (recent) 361.9
with retinal defect (rhegmatogenous) 361.00
giant tear 361.03
multiple 361.02
partial
with
giant tear 361.03
multiple defects 361.02
retinal dialysis (juvenile) 361.04
single defect 361.01
retinal dialysis (juvenile) 361.04
single 361.01
subtotal 361.05
total 361.05
delimited (old) (partial) 361.06
old
delimited 361.06
partial 361.06
total or subtotal 361.07
pigment epithelium (RPE) (serous) 362.42
exudative 362.42
hemorrhagic 362.43
rhegmatogenous (*see also* Detachment, retina, with retinal defect) 361.00
serous (without retinal defect) 361.2

Detachment—*continued*
specified type NEC 361.89
traction (with vitreoretinal organization) 361.81
vitreous humor 379.21
Detergent asthma 507.8
Deterioration
epileptic 294.1
heart, cardiac (*see also* Degeneration, myocardial) 429.1
mental (*see also* Psychosis) 298.9
myocardium, myocardial (*see also* Degeneration, myocardial) 429.1
senile (simple) 797
transplanted organ—*see* Complications, transplant, organ, by site
de Toni-Fanconi syndrome (cystinosis) 270.0
Deuteranomaly 368.52
Deuteranopia (anomalous trichromat) (complete) (incomplete) 368.52
Deutschländer's disease —*see* Fracture, foot
Development
abnormal, bone 756.9
arrested 783.4
bone 733.91
child 783.4
due to malnutrition (protein-calorie) 263.2
fetus or newborn 764.9
tracheal rings (congenital) 748.3
defective, congenital—*see also* Anomaly
cauda equina 742.59
left ventricle 746.9
with atresia or hypoplasia of aortic orifice or valve with hypoplasia of ascending aorta 746.7
in hypoplastic left heart syndrome 746.7
delayed (*see also* Delay, development) 783.4
arithmetical skills 315.1
language (skills) 315.31
expressive 315.31
mixed receptive-expressive 315.31
learning skill, specified NEC 315.2
mixed skills 315.5
motor coordination 315.4
reading 315.00
specified
learning skill NEC 315.2
type NEC, except learning 315.8
speech 315.39
associated with hyperkinesia 314.1
phonological 315.39
spelling 315.09
written expression 315.2
imperfect, congenital—*see also* Anomaly
heart 746.9
lungs 748.60
improper (fetus or newborn) 764.9
incomplete (fetus or newborn) 764.9
affecting management of pregnancy 656.5
bronchial tree 748.3
organ or site not listed—*see* Hypoplasia
respiratory system 748.9
sexual, precocious NEC 259.1
tardy, mental (*see also* Retardation, mental) 319
Developmental —*see* condition
Devergie's disease (pityriasis rubra pilaris) 696.4

Deviation
conjugate (eye) 378.87
palsy 378.81
spasm, spastic 378.82
esophagus 530.89
eye, skew 378.87
midline (jaw) (teeth) 524.2
specified site NEC—*see* Malposition
organ or site, congenital NEC—*see* Malposition, congenital
septum (acquired) (nasal) 470
congenital 754.0
sexual 302.9
bestiality 302.1
coprophilia 302.89
ego-dystonic
homosexuality 302.0
lesbianism 302.0
erotomania 302.89
Clérambault's 297.8
exhibitionism (sexual) 302.4
fetishism 302.81
transvestic 302.3
frotteurism 302.89
homosexuality, ego-dystonic 302.0
pedophilic 302.2
lesbianism, ego-dystonic 302.0
masochism 302.83
narcissism 302.89
necrophilia 302.89
nymphomania 302.89
pederosis 302.2
pedophilia 302.2
sadism 302.84
sadomasochism 302.84
satyriasis 302.89
specified type NEC 302.89
transvestic fetishism 302.3
transvestism 302.3
voyeurism 302.82
zoophilia (erotica) 302.1
teeth, midline 524.2
trachea 519.1
ureter (congenital) 753.4
Devic's disease 341.0
Device
cerebral ventricle (communicating) in situ V45.2
contraceptive—*see* Contraceptive, device
drainage, cerebrospinal fluid V45.2
Devil's
grip 074.1
pinches (purpura simplex) 287.2
Devitalized tooth 522.9
Devonshire colic 984.9
specified type of lead—*see* Table of drugs and chemicals
Dextraposition, aorta 747.21
with ventricular septal defect, pulmonary stenosis or atresia, and hypertrophy of right ventricle 745.2
in tetralogy of Fallot 745.2
Dextratransposition, aorta 745.11
Dextrinosis, limit (debrancher enzyme deficiency) 271.0
Dextrocardia (corrected) (false) (isolated) (secondary) (true) 746.87
with
complete transposition of viscera 759.3
situs inversus 759.3
Dextroversion, kidney (left) 753.3
Dhobie itch 110.3
Diabetes, diabetic (brittle) (congenital) (familial) (mellitus) (severe) (slight) (without complication) 250.0

Note—Use the following fifth-digit subclassification with category 250:

0 *type II [non-insulin dependent type] [NIDDM type] [adult-onset type] or unspecified type, not stated as uncontrolled*
1 *type I [insulin dependent type] [IDDM] [juvenile type], not stated as uncontrolled*
2 *type II [non-insulin dependent type] [NIDDM type] [adult-onset type] or unspecified type, uncontrolled*
3 *type I [insulin dependent type] [IDDM] [juvenile type], uncontrolled*

with
coma (with ketoacidosis) 250.3
hyperosmolar (nonketotic) 250.2
complication NEC 250.9
specified NEC 250.8
gangrene 250.7 *[785.4]*
hyperosmolarity 250.2
ketosis, ketoacidosis 250.1
osteomyelitis 250.8 *[731.8]*
specified manifestations NEC 250.8
acetonemia 250.1
acidosis 250.1
amyotrophy 250.6 *[358.1]*
angiopathy, peripheral 250.7 *[443.81]*
asymptomatic 790.2
autonomic neuropathy (peripheral) 250.6 *[337.1]*
bone change 250.8 *[731.8]*
bronze, bronzed 275.0
cataract 250.5 *[366.41]*
chemical 790.2
complicating pregnancy, childbirth, or puerperium 648.8
coma (with ketoacidosis) 250.3
hyperglycemic 250.3
hyperosmolar (nonketotic) 250.2
hypoglycemic 250.3
insulin 250.3
complicating pregnancy, childbirth, or puerperium (maternal) 648.0
affecting fetus or newborn 775.0
complication NEC 250.9
specified NEC 250.8
dorsal sclerosis 250.6 *[340]*
dwarfism-obesity syndrome 258.1
gangrene 250.7 *[785.4]*
gastroparesis 250.6 *[536.3]*
gestational 648.8
complicating pregnancy, childbirth, or puerperium 648.8
glaucoma 240.5 *[365.44]*
glomerulosclerosis (intercapillary) 250.4 *[581.81]*
glycogenosis, secondary 250.8 *[259.8]*
hemochromatosis 275.0
hyperosmolar coma 250.2
hyperosmolarity 250.2
hypertension-nephrosis syndrome 250.4 *[581.81]*
hypoglycemia 250.8
hypoglycemic shock 250.8
insipidus 253.5
nephrogenic 588.1
pituitary 253.5

Diabetes, diabetic—*continued*
vasopressin-resistant 588.1
intercapillary glomerulosclerosis 250.4 *[581.81]*
iritis 250.5 *[364.42]*
ketosis, ketoacidosis 250.1
Kimmelstiel (-Wilson) disease or syndrome (intercapillary glomerulosclerosis) 250.4 *[581.81]*
Lancereaux's (diabetes mellitus with marked emaciation) 250.8 *[261]*
latent (chemical) 790.2
complicating pregnancy, childbirth, or puerperium 648.8
lipoidosis 250.8 *[272.7]*
macular edema 250.5 *[362.83]*
maternal
with manifest disease in the infant 775.1
affecting fetus or newborn 775.0
microaneurysms, retinal 250.5 *[362.01]*
mononeuropathy 250.6 *[355.9]*
neonatal, transient 775.1
nephropathy 250.4 *[583.81]*
nephrosis (syndrome) 250.4 *[581.81]*
neuralgia 250.6 *[357.2]*
neuritis 250.6 *[357.2]*
neurogenic arthropathy 250.6 *[713.5]*
neuropathy 250.6 *[357.2]*
nonclinical 790.2
osteomyelitis 250.8 *[731.8]*
peripheral autonomic neuropathy 250.6 *[337.1]*
phosphate 275.3
polyneuropathy 250.6 *[357.2]*
renal (true) 271.4
retinal
edema 250.5 *[362.83]*
hemorrhage 250.5 *[362.01]*
microaneurysms 250.5 *[362.01]*
retinitis 250.5 *[362.01]*
retinopathy 250.5 *[362.01]*
background 250.5 *[362.01]*
proliferative 250.5 *[362.02]*
steroid induced
correct substance properly administered 251.8
overdose or wrong substance given or taken 962.0
stress 790.2
subclinical 790.2
subliminal 790.2
sugar 250.0
ulcer (skin) 250.8 *[707.9]*
lower extremity 250.8 *[707.1]*
specified site NEC 250.8 *[707.8]*
xanthoma 250.8 *[272.2]*
Diacyclothrombopathia 287.1
Diagnosis deferred 799.9
Dialysis (intermittent) (treatment)
anterior retinal (juvenile) (with detachment) 361.04
extracorporeal V56.0
peritoneal V56.8
renal V56.0
status only V45.1
specified type NEC V56.8
Diamond-Blackfan anemia or syndrome (congenital hypoplastic anemia) 284.0
Diamond-Gardener syndrome (autoerythrocyte sensitization) 287.2
Diaper rash 691.0
Diaphoresis (excessive) NEC 780.8
Diaphragm —*see* condition
Diaphragmalgia 786.52
Diaphragmitis 519.4
Diaphyseal aclasis 756.4
Diaphysitis 733.99
Diarrhea, diarrheal (acute) (autumn) (bilious) (bloody) (catarrhal) (choleraic) (chronic) (gravis) (green) (infantile) (lienteric) (noninfectious) (presumed noninfectious) (putrefactive) (secondary) (sporadic) (summer) (symptomatic) (thermic) 787.91
achlorhydric 536.0
allergic 558.9
amebic (*see also* Amebiasis) 006.9
with abscess—*see* Abscess, amebic
acute 006.0
chronic 006.1
nondysenteric 006.2
bacillary—*see* Dysentery, bacillary
bacterial NEC 008.5
balantidial 007.0
bile salt-induced 579.8
cachectic NEC 558.9
chilomastix 007.8
choleriformis 001.1
chronic 558.9
ulcerative (*see also* Colitis, ulcerative) 556.9
coccidial 007.2
Cochin-China 579.1
anguilluliasis 127.2
psilosis 579.1
Dientamoeba 007.8
dietetic 558.9
due to
achylia gastrica 536.8
Aerobacter aerogenes 008.2
Bacillus coli—*see* Enteritis, E. coli
bacteria NEC 008.5
bile salts 579.8
Capillaria
hepatica 128.8
philippinensis 127.5
Clostridium perfringens (C) (F) 008.46
Enterobacter aerogenes 008.2
enterococci 008.49
Escherichia coli—*see* Enteritis, E. coli
Giardia lamblia 007.1
Heterophyes heterophyes 121.6
irritating foods 558.9
Metagonimus yokogawai 121.5
Necator americanus 126.1
Paracolobactrum arizonae 008.1
Paracolon bacillus NEC 008.47
Arizona 008.1
Proteus (bacillus) (mirabilis) (Morganii) 008.3
Pseudomonas aeruginosa 008.42
S. japonicum 120.2
specified organism NEC 008.8
bacterial 008.49
viral NEC 008.69
Staphylococcus 008.41
Streptococcus 008.49
anaerobic 008.46
Strongyloides stercoralis 127.2
Trichuris trichiuria 127.3
virus NEC (*see also* Enteritis, viral) 008.69
dysenteric 009.2
due to specified organism NEC 008.8
dyspeptic 558.9
endemic 009.3
epidemic 009.3
fermentative 558.9
flagellate 007.9

Diarrhea, diarrheal—*continued*
Flexner's (ulcerative) 004.1
functional 564.5
following gastrointestinal surgery 564.4
psychogenic 306.4
giardial 007.1
Giardia lamblia 007.1
hill 579.1
hyperperistalsis (nervous) 306.4
infectious 009.2
presumed 009.3
inflammatory 558.9
due to specified organism NEC 008.8
malarial (*see also* Malaria) 084.6
mite 133.8
mycotic 117.9
nervous 306.4
neurogenic 564.5
parenteral NEC 009.2
postgastrectomy 564.4
postvagotomy 564.4
prostaglandin induced 579.8
protozoal NEC 007.9
psychogenic 306.4
septic 009.2
due to specified organism NEC 008.8
specified organism NEC 008.8
bacterial 008.49
viral NEC 008.69
Staphylococcus 008.41
Streptococcus 008.49
anaerobic 088.46
toxic 558.2
travelers' 009.2
due to specified organism NEC 008.8
trichomonal 007.3
tropical 579.1
tuberculous 014.8
ulcerative (chronic) (*see also* Colitis, ulcerative) 556.9
viral (*see also* Enteritis, viral) 008.8
zymotic NEC 009.2
Diastasis
cranial bones 733.99
congenital 756.0
joint (traumatic)—*see* Dislocation, by site
muscle 728.84
congenital 756.89
recti (abdomen) 728.84
complicating delivery 665.8
congenital 756.7
Diastema, teeth, tooth 524.3
Diastematomyelia 742.51
Diataxia, cerebral, infantile 343.0
Diathesis
allergic V15.0
bleeding (familial) 287.9
cystine (familial) 270.0
gouty 274.9
hemorrhagic (familial) 287.9
newborn NEC 776.0
oxalic 271.8
scrofulous (*see also* Tuberculosis) 017.2
spasmophilic (*see also* Tetany) 781.7
ulcer 536.9
uric acid 274.9
Diaz's disease or osteochondrosis 732.5
Dibothriocephaliasis 123.4
larval 123.5
Dibothriocephalus (infection) (infestation) (latus) 123.4
larval 123.5
Dicephalus 759.4
Dichotomy, teeth 520.2
Dichromat, dichromata (congenital) 368.59
Dichromatopsia (congenital) 368.59
Dichuchwa 104.0
Dicroceliasis 121.8
Didelphys, didelphic (*see also* Double uterus) 752.2
Didymitis (*see also* Epididymitis) 604.90
Died —*see also* Death
without
medical attention (cause unknown) 798.9
sign of disease 798.2
Dientamoeba diarrhea 007.8
Dietary
inadequacy or deficiency 269.9
surveillance and counseling V65.3
Dietl's crisis 593.4
Dieulafoy's ulcer —*see* Ulcer, stomach
Difficult
birth, affecting fetus or newborn 763.9
delivery NEC 669.9
Difficulty
feeding 783.3
newborn 779.3
nonorganic (infant) NEC 307.59
mechanical, gastroduodenal stoma 537.89
reading 315.00
specific, spelling 315.09
swallowing (*see also* Dysphagia) 787.2
walking 719.7
Diffuse —*see* condition
Diffused ganglion 727.42
DiGeorge's syndrome (thymic hypoplasia) 279.11
Digestive —*see* condition
Di Guglielmo's disease or syndrome (M9841/3) 207.0
Diktyoma (M9051/3)—*see* Neoplasm, by site, malignant
Dilaceration, tooth 520.4
Dilatation
anus 564.8
venule—*see* Hemorrhoids
aorta (focal) (general) (*see also* Aneurysm, aorta) 441.9
congenital 747.29
infectional 093.0
ruptured 441.5
syphilitic 093.0
appendix (cystic) 543.9
artery 447.8
bile duct (common) (cystic) (congenital) 751.69
acquired 576.8
bladder (sphincter) 596.8
congenital 753.8
in pregnancy or childbirth 654.4
causing obstructed labor 660.2
affecting fetus or newborn 763.1
blood vessel 459.89
bronchus, bronchi 494
calyx (due to obstruction) 593.89
capillaries 448.9
cardiac (acute) (chronic) (*see also* Hypertrophy, cardiac) 429.3
congenital 746.89
valve NEC 746.89
pulmonary 746.09

Dilatation—*continued*
hypertensive (*see also* Hypertension, heart) 402.90
cavum septi pellucidi 742.4
cecum 564.8
psychogenic 306.4
cervix (uteri)—*see also* Incompetency, cervix
incomplete, poor, slow
affecting fetus or newborn 763.7
complicating delivery 661.0
affecting fetus or newborn 763.7
colon 564.7
congenital 751.3
due to mechanical obstruction 560.89
psychogenic 306.4
common bile duct (congenital) 751.69
acquired 576.8
with calculus, choledocholithiasis, or stones—*see* Choledocholithiasis
cystic duct 751.69
acquired (any bile duct) 575.8
duct, mammary 610.4
duodenum 564.8
esophagus 530.89
congenital 750.4
due to
achalasia 530.0
cardiospasm 530.0
Eustachian tube, congenital 744.24
fontanel 756.0
gallbladder 575.8
congenital 751.69
gastric 536.8
acute 536.1
psychogenic 306.4
heart (acute) (chronic) (*see also* Hypertrophy, cardiac) 429.3
congenital 746.89
hypertensive (*see also* Hypertension, heart) 402.90
valve—*see also* Endocarditis
congenital 746.89
ileum 564.8
psychogenic 306.4
inguinal rings—*see* Hernia, inguinal
jejunum 564.8
psychogenic 306.4
kidney (calyx) (collecting structures) (cystic) (parenchyma) (pelvis) 593.89
lacrimal passages 375.69
lymphatic vessel 457.1
mammary duct 610.4
Meckel's diverticulum (congenital) 751.0
meningeal vessels, congenital 742.8
myocardium (acute) (chronic) (*see also* Hypertrophy, cardiac) 429.3
organ or site, congenital NEC—*see* Distortion
pancreatic duct 577.8
pelvis, kidney 593.89
pericardium—*see* Pericarditis
pharynx 478.29
prostate 602.8
pulmonary
artery (idiopathic) 417.8
congenital 747.3
valve, congenital 746.09
pupil 379.43
rectum 564.8
renal 593.89
saccule vestibularis, congenital 744.05
salivary gland (duct) 527.8
sphincter ani 564.8

Dilatation—*continued*
stomach 536.8
acute 536.1
psychogenic 306.4
submaxillary duct 527.8
trachea, congenital 748.3
ureter (idiopathic) 593.89
congenital 753.2
due to obstruction 593.5
urethra (acquired) 599.84
vasomotor 443.9
vein 459.89
ventricular, ventricle (acute) (chronic) (*see also* Hypertrophy, cardiac) 429.3
cerebral, congenital 742.4
hypertensive (*see also* Hypertension, heart) 402.90
venule 459.89
anus—*see* Hemorrhoids
vesical orifice 596.8
Dilated, dilation —*see* Dilatation
Diminished
hearing (acuity) (*see also* Deafness) 389.9
pulse pressure 785.9
vision NEC 369.9
vital capacity 794.2
Diminuta taenia 123.6
Diminution, sense or sensation (cold) (heat) (tactile) (vibratory) (*see also* Disturbance, sensation) 782.0
Dimitri-Sturge-Weber disease (encephalocutaneous angiomatosis) 759.6
Dimple
parasacral 685.1
with abscess 685.0
pilonidal 685.1
with abscess 685.0
postanal 685.1
with abscess 685.0
Dioctophyma renale (infection) (infestation) 128.8
Dipetalonemiasis 125.4
Diphallus 752.8
Diphtheria, diphtheritic (gangrenous) (hemorrhagic) 032.9
carrier (suspected) of V02.4
cutaneous 032.85
cystitis 032.84
faucial 032.0
infection of wound 032.85
inoculation (anti) (not sick) V03.5
laryngeal 032.3
myocarditis 032.82
nasal anterior 032.2
nasopharyngeal 032.1
neurological complication 032.89
peritonitis 032.83
specified site NEC 032.89
Diphyllobothriasis (intestine) 123.4
larval 123.5
Diplacusis 388.41
Diplegia (upper limbs) 344.2
brain or cerebral 437.8
congenital 343.0
facial 351.0
congenital 352.6
infantile or congenital (cerebral) (spastic) (spinal) 343.0
lower limbs 344.1
syphilitic, congenital 090.49
Diplococcus, diplococcal —*see* condition
Diplomyelia 742.59

Diplopia 368.2
refractive 368.15
Dipsomania (*see also* Alcoholism) 303.9
with psychosis (*see also* Psychosis, alcoholic) 291.9
Dipylidiasis 123.8
intestine 123.8
Direction, teeth, abnormal 524.3
Dirt-eating child 307.52
Disability
heart—*see* Disease, heart
learning NEC 315.2
special spelling 315.09
Disarticulation (*see also* Derangement, joint) 718.9
meaning
amputation
status—*see* Absence, by site
traumatic —*see* Amputation, traumatic
dislocation, traumatic or congenital—*see* Dislocation
Disaster, cerebrovascular (*see also* Disease, cerebrovascular, acute) 436
Discharge
anal NEC 787.99
breast (female) (male) 611.79
conjunctiva 372.8
continued locomotor idiopathic (*see also* Epilepsy) 345.5
diencephalic autonomic idiopathic (*see also* Epilepsy) 345.5
ear 388.60
blood 388.69
cerebrospinal fluid 388.61
excessive urine 788.42
eye 379.93
nasal 478.1
nipple 611.79
patterned motor idiopathic (*see also* Epilepsy) 345.5
penile 788.7
postnasal—*see* Sinusitis
sinus, from mediastinum 510.0
umbilicus 789.9
urethral 788.7
bloody 599.84
vaginal 623.5
Discitis 722.90
cervical, cervicothoracic 722.91
lumbar, lumbosacral 722.93
thoracic, thoracolumbar 722.92
Discogenic syndrome —*see* Displacement, intervertebral disc
Discoid
kidney 753.3
meniscus, congenital 717.5
semilunar cartilage 717.5
Discoloration
mouth 528.9
nails 703.8
teeth 521.7
due to
drugs 521.7
metals (copper) (silver) 521.7
pulpal bleeding 521.7
during formation 520.8
posteruptive 521.7
Discomfort
chest 786.59
visual 368.13
Discomycosis —*see* Actinomycosis
Discontinuity, ossicles, ossicular chain 385.23
Discrepancy, leg length (acquired) 736.81
congenital 755.30
Discrimination
political V62.4
racial V62.4
religious V62.4
sex V62.4
Disease, diseased —*see also* Syndrome
Abrami's (acquired hemolytic jaundice) 283.9
absorbent system 459.89
accumulation—*see* Thesaurismosis
acid-peptic 536.8
Acosta's 993.2
Adams-Stokes (-Morgagni) (syncope with heart block) 426.9
Addison's (bronze) (primary adrenal insufficiency) 255.4
anemia (pernicious) 281.0
tuberculous (*see also* Tuberculosis) 017.6
Addison-Gull—*see* Xanthoma
adenoids (and tonsils) (chronic) 474.9
adrenal (gland) (capsule) (cortex) 255.9
hyperfunction 255.3
hypofunction 255.4
specified type NEC 255.8
ainhum (dactylolysis spontanea) 136.0
akamushi (scrub typhus) 081.2
Akureyri (epidemic neuromyasthenia) 049.8
Albarrán's (colibacilluria) 599.0
Albers-Schönberg's (marble bones) 756.52
Albert's 726.71
Albright (-Martin) (-Bantam) 275.4
Alibert's (mycosis fungoides) (M9700/3) 202.1
Alibert-Bazin (M9700/3) 202.1
alimentary canal 569.9
alligator skin (ichthyosis congenital) 757.1
acquired 701.1
Almeida's (Brazilian blastomycosis) 116.1
Alpers' 330.8
alpine 993.2
altitude 993.2
alveoli, teeth 525.9
Alzheimer's—*see* Alzheimer's
amyloid (any site) 277.3
anarthritic rheumatoid 446.5
Anders' (adiposis tuberosa simplex) 272.8
Andersen's (glycogenosis IV) 271.0
Anderson's (angiokeratoma corporis diffusum) 272.7
Andes 993.2
Andrews' (bacterid) 686.8
angiospastic, angiospasmodic 443.9
cerebral 435.9
with transient neurologic deficit 435.9
vein 459.89
anterior
chamber 364.9
horn cell 335.9
specified type NEC 335.8
antral (chronic) 473.0
acute 461.0
anus NEC 569.49
aorta (nonsyphilitic) 447.9
syphilitic NEC 093.89
aortic (heart) (valve) (*see also* Endocarditis, aortic) 424.1
apollo 077.4
aponeurosis 726.90
appendix 543.9
aqueous (chamber) 364.9

Disease, diseased—*continued*
arc-welders' lung 503
Armenian 277.3
Arnold-Chiari (*see also* Spina bifida) 741.0
arterial 447.9
occlusive (*see also* Occlusion, by site) 444.22
with embolus or thrombus—*see* Occlusion, by site
due to stricture or stenosis 447.1
specified type NEC 447.8
arteriocardiorenal (*see also* Hypertension, cardiorenal) 404.90
arteriolar (generalized) (obliterative) 447.9
specified type NEC 447.8
arteriorenal—*see* Hypertension, kidney
arteriosclerotic—*see also* Arteriosclerosis
cardiovascular 429.2
coronary —*see* Arteriosclerosis, coronary
heart —*see* Arteriosclerosis, coronary
vascular—*see* Arteriosclerosis
artery 447.9
cerebral 437.9
coronary —*see* Arteriosclerosis, coronary
specified type NEC 447.8
arthropod-borne NEC 088.9
specified type NEC 088.89
Asboe-Hansen's (incontinentia pigmenti) 757.33
atticoantral, chronic (with posterior or superior marginal perforation of ear drum) 382.2
auditory canal, ear 380.9
Aujeszky's 078.89
auricle, ear NEC 380.30
Australian X 062.4
autoimmune NEC 279.4
hemolytic (cold type) (warm type) 283.0
parathyroid 252.1
thyroid 245.2
aviators' (*see also* Effect, adverse, high altitude) 993.2
ax(e)-grinders' 502
Ayala's 756.89
Ayerza's (pulmonary artery sclerosis with pulmonary hypertension) 416.0
Babington's (familial hemorrhagic telangiectasia) 448.0
back bone NEC 733.90
bacterial NEC 040.89
zoonotic NEC 027.9
specified type NEC 027.8
Baehr-Schiffrin (thrombotic thrombocytopenic purpura) 446.6
Baelz's (cheilitis glandularis apostematosa) 528.5
Baerensprung's (eczema marginatum) 110.3
Balfour's (chloroma) 205.3
balloon (*see also* Effect, adverse, high altitude) 993.2
Baló's 341.1
Bamberger (-Marie) (hypertrophic pulmonary osteoarthropathy) 731.2
Bang's (Brucella abortus) 023.1
Bannister's 995.1
Banti's (with cirrhosis) (with portal hypertension)—*see* Cirrhosis, liver
Barcoo (*see also* Ulcer, skin) 707.9
barium lung 503
Barlow (-Möller) (infantile scurvy) 267
barometer makers' 985.0
Barraquer (-Simons) (progressive lipodystrophy) 272.6

Disease, diseased—*continued*
basal ganglia 333.90
degenerative NEC 333.0
specified NEC 333.89
Basedow's (exophthalmic goiter) 242.0
basement membrane NEC 583.89
with
pulmonary hemorrhage (Goodpasture's syndrome) 446.21 *[583.81]*
Bateman's 078.0
purpura (senile) 287.2
Batten's 330.1 *[362.71]*
Batten-Mayou (retina) 330.1 *[362.71]*
Batten-Steinert 359.2
Battey 031.0
Baumgarten-Cruveilhier (cirrhosis of liver) 571.5
bauxite-workers' 503
Bayle's (dementia paralytica) 094.1
Bazin's (primary) (*see also* Tuberculosis) 017.1
Beard's (neurasthenia) 300.5
Beau's (*see also* Degeneration, myocardial) 429.1
Bechterew's (ankylosing spondylitis) 720.0
Becker's (idiopathic mural endomyocardial disease) 425.2
Begbie's (exophthalmic goiter) 242.0
Behr's 362.50
Beigel's (white piedra) 111.2
Bekhterev's (ankylosing spondylitis) 720.0
Bell's (*see also* Psychosis, affective) 296.0
Bennett's (leukemia) 208.9
Benson's 379.22
Bergeron's (hysteroepilepsy) 300.11
Berlin's 921.3
Bernard-Soulier (thrombopathy) 287.1
Bernhardt (-Roth) 355.1
beryllium 503
Besnier-Boeck (-Schaumann) (sarcoidosis) 135
Best's 362.76
Beurmann's (sporotrichosis) 117.1
Bielschowsky (-Jansky) 330.1
Biermer's (pernicious anemia) 281.0
Biett's (discoid lupus erythematosus) 695.4
bile duct (*see also* Disease, biliary) 576.9
biliary (duct) (tract) 576.9
with calculus, choledocholithiasis, or stones—*see* Choledocholithiasis
Billroth's (meningocele) (*see also* Spina bifida) 741.9
Binswanger's 290.12
Bird's (oxaluria) 271.8
bird fanciers' 495.2
black lung 500
bladder 596.9
specified NEC 596.8
bleeder's 286.0
Bloch-Sulzberger (incontinentia pigmenti) 757.33
Blocq's (astasia-abasia) 307.9
blood (-forming organs) 289.9
specified NEC 289.8
vessel 459.9
Bloodgood's 610.1
Blount's (tibia vara) 732.4
blue 746.9
Bodechtel-Guttmann (subacute sclerosing panencephalitis) 046.2
Boeck's (sarcoidosis) 135

Disease, diseased—*continued*
cartilage NEC 733.90
specified NEC 733.99
Castellani's 104.8
cat-scratch 078.3
Cavare's (familial periodic paralysis) 359.3
Cazenave's (pemphigus) 694.4
cecum 569.9
celiac (adult) 579.0
infantile 579.0
cellular tissue NEC 709.9
central core 359.0
cerebellar, cerebellum—*see* Disease, brain
cerebral (*see also* Disease, brain) 348.9
arterial, artery 437.9
degenerative—*see* Degeneration, brain
cerebrospinal 349.9
cerebrovascular NEC 437.9
acute 436
embolic—*see* Embolism, brain
late effect—*see* category 438
puerperal, postpartum, childbirth 674.0
thrombotic—*see* Thrombosis, brain
arteriosclerotic 437.0
embolic—*see* Embolism, brain
ischemic, generalized NEC 437.1
late effect or sequela—*see* category 438
occlusive 437.1
puerperal, postpartum, childbirth 674.0
specified type NEC 437.8
thrombotic—*see* Thrombosis, brain
ceroid storage 272.7
cervix (uteri)
inflammatory 616.9
specified NEC 616.8
noninflammatory 622.9
specified NEC 622.8
Chabert's 022.9
Chagas' (*see also* Trypanosomiasis, American) 086.2
Chandler's (osteochondritis dissecans, hip) 732.7
Charcot's (joint) 094.0 *[713.5]*
spinal cord 094.0
Charcot-Marie-Tooth 356.1
Charlouis' (*see also* Yaws) 102.9
Cheadle (-Möller) (-Barlow) (infantile scurvy) 267
Chédiak-Steinbrinck (-Higashi) (congenital gigantism of peroxidase granules) 288.2
cheek, inner 528.9
chest 519.9
Chiari's (hepatic vein thrombosis) 453.0
Chicago (North American blastomycosis) 116.0
chignon (white piedra) 111.2
chigoe, chigo (jigger) 134.1
childhood granulomatous 288.1
Chinese liver fluke 121.1
chlamydial NEC 078.88
cholecystic (*see also* Disease, gallbladder) 575.9
choroid 363.9
degenerative (*see also* Degeneration, choroid) 363.40
hereditary (*see also* Dystrophy, choroid) 363.50
specified type NEC 363.8

Disease, diseased—*continued*
Christian's (chronic histiocytosis X) 277.8
Christian-Weber (nodular nonsuppurative panniculitis) 729.30
Christmas 286.1
ciliary body 364.9
circulatory (system) NEC 459.9
chronic, maternal, affecting fetus or newborn 760.3
specified NEC 459.89
syphilitic 093.9
congenital 090.5
Civatte's (poikiloderma) 709.09
climacteric 627.2
male 608.89
coagulation factor deficiency (congenital) (*see also* Defect, coagulation) 286.9
Coats' 362.12
coccidioidal pulmonary 114.5
acute 114.0
chronic 114.4
primary 114.0
residual 114.4
Cockayne's (microcephaly and dwarfism) 759.89
Cogan's 370.52
cold
agglutinin 283.0
or hemoglobinuria 283.0
paroxysmal (cold) (nocturnal) 283.2
hemagglutinin (chronic) 283.0
collagen NEC 710.9
nonvascular 710.9
specified NEC 710.8
vascular (allergic) (*see also* Angiitis, hypersensitivity) 446.20
colon 569.9
functional 564.9
congenital 751.3
ischemic 557.0
combined system (of spinal cord) 266.2 *[336.2]*
with anemia (pernicious) 281.0 *[336.2]*
compressed air 993.3
Concato's (pericardial polyserositis) 423.2
peritoneal 568.82
pleural—*see* Pleurisy
congenital NEC 799.8
conjunctiva 372.9
chlamydial 077.98
specified NEC 077.8
specified type NEC 372.8
viral 077.99
specified NEC 077.8
connective tissue, diffuse (*see also* Disease, collagen) 710.9
Conor and Bruch's (boutonneuse fever) 082.1
Conradi (-Hünermann) 756.59
Cooley's (erythroblastic anemia) 282.4
Cooper's 610.1
Corbus' 607.1
cork-handlers' 495.3
cornea (*see also* Keratopathy) 371.9
coronary (*see also* Ischemia, heart) 414.9
congenital 746.85
ostial, syphilitic 093.20
aortic 093.22
mitral 093.21
pulmonary 093.24
tricuspid 093.23

Disease, diseased—*continued*
Corrigan's—*see* Insufficiency, aortic
Cotugno's 724.3
Coxsackie (virus) NEC 074.8
cranial nerve NEC 352.9
Creutzfeldt-Jakob 046.1
with dementia 290.10
Crigler-Najjar (congenital hyperbilirubinemia) 277.4
Crocq's (acrocyanosis) 443.89
Crohn's (intestine) (*see also* Enteritis, regional) 555.9
Crouzon's (craniofacial dysostosis) 756.0
Cruchet's (encephalitis lethargica) 049.8
Cruveilhier's 335.21
Cruz-Chagas (*see also* Trypanosomiasis, American) 086.2
crystal deposition (*see also* Arthritis, due to, crystals) 712.9
Csillag's (lichen sclerosus et atrophicus) 701.0
Curschmann's 359.2
Cushing's (pituitary basophilism) 255.0
cystic
breast (chronic) 610.1
kidney, congenital (*see also* Cystic, disease, kidney) 753.10
liver, congenital 751.62
lung 518.89
congenital 748.4
pancreas 577.2
congenital 751.7
renal, congenital (*see also* Cystic, disease, kidney) 753.10
semilunar cartilage 717.5
cysticercus 123.1
cystine storage (with renal sclerosis) 270.0
cytomegalic inclusion (generalized) 078.5
with
pneumonia 078.5 *[484.1]*
congenital 771.1
Czerny's (periodic hydrarthrosis of the knee) 719.06
Daae (-Finsen) (epidemic pleurodynia) 074.1
dancing 297.8
Danielssen's (anesthetic leprosy) 030.1
Darier's (congenital) (keratosis follicularis) 757.39
erythema annulare centrifugum 695.0
vitamin A deficiency 264.8
Darling's (histoplasmosis) (*see also* Histoplasmosis, American) 115.00
Davies' 425.0
de Beurmann-Gougerot (sporotrichosis) 117.1
Débove's (splenomegaly) 789.2
deer fly (*see also* Tularemia) 021.9
deficiency 269.9
degenerative—*see also* Degeneration
disc—*see* Degeneration, intervertebral disc
Degos' 447.8
Déjérine (-Sottas) 356.0
Deleage's 359.8
demyelinating, demyelinizating (brain stem) (central nervous system) 341.9
multiple sclerosis 340
specified NEC 341.8
de Quervain's (tendon sheath) 727.04
thyroid (subacute granulomatous thyroiditis) 245.1

Disease, diseased—*continued*
Dercum's (adiposis dolorosa) 272.8
Deutschländer's—*see* Fracture, foot
Devergie's (pityriasis rubra pilaris) 696.4
Devic's 341.0
diaphorase deficiency 289.7
diaphragm 519.4
diarrheal, infectious 009.2
diatomaceous earth 502
Diaz's (osteochondrosis astragalus) 732.5
digestive system 569.9
Di Guglielmo's (erythemic myelosis) (M9841/3) 207.0
Dimitri-Sturge-Weber (encephalocutaneous angiomatosis) 759.6
disc, degenerative—*see* Degeneration, intervertebral disc
discogenic (*see also* Disease, intervertebral disc) 722.90
diverticular—*see* Diverticula
Down's (mongolism) 758.0
Dubini's (electric chorea) 049.8
Dubois' (thymus gland) 090.5
Duchenne's 094.0
locomotor ataxia 094.0
muscular dystrophy 359.1
paralysis 335.22
pseudohypertrophy, muscles 359.1
Duchenne-Griesinger 359.1
ductless glands 259.9
Duhring's (dermatitis herpetiformis) 694.0
Dukes (-Filatov) 057.8
duodenum NEC 537.9
specified NEC 537.89
Duplay's 726.2
Dupré's (meningism) 781.6
Dupuytren's (muscle contracture) 728.6
Durand-Nicolas-Favre (climatic bubo) 099.1
Duroziez's (congenital mitral stenosis) 746.5
Dutton's (trypanosomiasis) 086.9
Eales' 362.18
ear (chronic) (inner) NEC 388.9
middle 385.9
adhesive (*see also* Adhesions, middle ear) 385.10
specified NEC 385.89
Eberth's (typhoid fever) 002.0
Ebstein's
heart 746.2
meaning diabetes 250.4 *[581.81]*
Echinococcus (*see also* Echinococcus) 122.9
ECHO virus NEC 078.89
Economo's (encephalitis lethargica) 049.8
Eddowes' (brittle bones and blue sclera) 756.51
Edsall's 992.2
Eichstedt's (pityriasis versicolor) 111.0
Ellis-van Creveld (chondroectodermal dysplasia) 756.55
endocardium—*see* Endocarditis
endocrine glands or system NEC 259.9
specified NEC 259.8
endomyocardial, idiopathic mural 425.2
Engel-von Recklinghausen (osteitis fibrosa cystica) 252.0
Engelmann's (diaphyseal sclerosis) 756.59
English (rickets) 268.0
Engman's (infectious eczematoid dermatitis) 690.8
enteroviral, enterovirus NEC 078.89
central nervous system NEC 048

Disease, diseased—*continued*
glomerular
membranous, idiopathic 581.1
minimal change 581.3
glycogen storage (Andersen's) (Cori types 1-7) (Forbes') (McArdle-Schmid-Pearson) (Pompe's) (types I-VII) 271.0
cardiac 271.0 *[425.7]*
generalized 271.0
glucose-6-phosphatase deficiency 271.0
heart 271.0 *[425.7]*
hepatorenal 271.0
liver and kidneys 271.0
myocardium 271.0 *[425.7]*
von Gierke's (glycogenosis I) 271.0
Goldflam-Erb 358.0
Goldscheider's (epidermolysis bullosa) 757.39
Goldstein's (familial hemorrhagic telangiectasia) 448.0
gonococcal NEC 098.0
Goodall's (epidemic vomiting) 078.82
Gordon's (exudative enteropathy) 579.8
Gougerot's (trisymptomatic) 709.1
Gougerot-Carteaud (confluent reticulate papillomatosis) 701.8
Gougerot-Hailey-Hailey (benign familial chronic pemphigus) 757.39
graft-versus-host (bone marrow) 996.85
due to organ transplant NEC—*see* Complications, transplant, organ
grain-handlers' 495.8
Grancher's (splenopneumonia)—*see* Pneumonia
granulomatous (childhood) (chronic) 288.1
graphite lung 503
Graves' (exophthalmic goiter) 242.0
Greenfield's 330.0
green monkey 078.89
Griesinger's (*see also* Ancylostomiasis) 126.9
grinders' 502
Grisel's 723.5
Gruby's (tinea tonsurans) 110.0
Guertin's (electric chorea) 049.8
Guillain-Barré 357.0
Guinon's (motor-verbal tic) 307.23
Gull's (thyroid atrophy with myxedema) 244.8
Gull and Sutton's—*see* Hypertension, kidney
gum NEC 523.9
Günther's (congenital erythropoietic porphyria) 277.1
gynecological 629.9
specified NEC 629.8
H 270.0
Haas' 732.3
Habermann's (acute parapsoriasis varioliformis) 696.2
Haff 985.1
Hageman (congenital factor XII deficiency) (*see also* Defect, congenital) 286.3
Haglund's (osteochondrosis os tibiale externum) 732.5
Hagner's (hypertrophic pulmonary osteoarthropathy) 731.2
Hailey-Hailey (benign familial chronic pemphigus) 757.39
hair (follicles) NEC 704.9
specified type NEC 704.8
Hallervorden-Spatz 333.0

Disease, diseased—*continued*
Hallopeau's (lichen sclerosus et atrophicus) 701.0
Hamman's (spontaneous mediastinal emphysema) 518.1
hand, foot, and mouth 074.3
Hand-Schüller-Christian (chronic histiocytosis X) 277.8
Hanot's—*see* Cirrhosis, biliary
Hansen's (leprosy) 030.9
benign form 030.1
malignant form 030.0
Harada's 363.22
Harley's (intermittent hemoglobinuria) 283.2
Hart's (pellagra-cerebellar ataxia renal aminoaciduria) 270.0
Hartnup (pellagra-cerebellar ataxia-renal aminoaciduria) 270.0
Hashimoto's (struma lymphomatosa) 245.2
Hb—*see* Disease, hemoglobin
heart (organic) 429.9
with
acute pulmonary edema (*see also* Failure, ventricular, left) 428.1
hypertensive 402.91
with renal failure 404.92
benign 402.11
with renal failure 404.12
malignant 402.01
with renal failure 404.02
kidney disease—*see* Hypertension, cardiorenal
rheumatic fever (conditions classifiable to 390)
active 391.9
with chorea 392.0
inactive or quiescent (with chorea) 398.90
amyloid 277.3 *[425.7]*
aortic (valve) (*see also* Endocarditis, aortic) 424.1
arteriosclerotic or sclerotic (minimal) (senile)—*see* Arteriosclerosis, coronary
artery, arterial —*see* Arteriosclerosis, coronary
atherosclerotic —*see* Arteriosclerosis, coronary
beer drinkers' 425.5
beriberi 265.0 *[425.7]*
black 416.0
congenital NEC 746.9
cyanotic 746.9
maternal, affecting fetus or newborn 760.3
specified type NEC 746.89
congestive (*see also* Failure, heart, congestive) 428.0
coronary 414.9
cryptogenic 429.9
due to
amyloidosis 277.3 *[425.7]*
beriberi 265.0 *[425.7]*
cardiac glycogenosis 271.0 *[425.7]*
Friedreich's ataxia 334.0 *[425.8]*
gout 274.82
mucopolysaccharidosis 277.5 *[425.7]*
myotonia atrophica 359.2 *[425.8]*
progressive muscular dystrophy 359.1 *[425.8]*
sarcoidosis 135 *[425.8]*
fetal 746.9
inflammatory 746.89
fibroid (*see also* Myocarditis) 429.0

Disease, diseased—*continued*
functional 427.9
postoperative 997.1
psychogenic 306.2
glycogen storage 271.0 *[425.7]*
gonococcal NEC 098.85
gouty 274.82
hypertensive (*see also* Hypertension, heart) 402.90
benign 402.10
malignant 402.00
hyperthyroid (*see also* Hyperthyroidism) 242.9 *[425.7]*
incompletely diagnosed—*see* Disease, heart
ischemic (chronic) (*see also* Ischemia, heart) 414.9
acute (*see also* Infarct, myocardium) 410.9
without myocardial infarction 411.89
with coronary (artery) occlusion 411.81
asymptomatic 412
diagnosed on ECG or other special investigation but currently presenting no symptoms 412
kyphoscoliotic 416.1
mitral (*see also* Endocarditis, mitral) 394.9
muscular (*see also* Degeneration, myocardial) 429.1
postpartum 674.8
psychogenic (functional) 306.2
pulmonary (chronic) 416.9
acute 415.0
specified NEC 416.8
rheumatic (chronic) (inactive) (old) (quiescent) (with chorea) 398.90
active or acute 391.9
with chorea (active) (rheumatic) (Sydenham's) 392.0
specified type NEC 391.8
maternal, affecting fetus or newborn 760.3
rheumatoid—*see* Arthritis, rheumatoid
sclerotic —*see* Arteriosclerosis, coronary
senile (*see also* Myocarditis) 429.0
specified type NEC 429.89
syphilitic 093.89
aortic 093.1
aneurysm 093.0
asymptomatic 093.89
congenital 090.5
thyroid (gland) (*see also* Hyperthyroidism) 242.9 *[425.7]*
thyrotoxic (*see also* Thyrotoxicosis) 242.9 *[425.7]*
tuberculous (*see also* Tuberculosis) 017.9 *[425.8]*
valve, valvular (obstructive) (regurgitant)—*see also* Endocarditis
congenital NEC (*see also* Anomaly, heart, valve) 746.9
pulmonary 746.00
specified type NEC 746.89
vascular—*see* Disease, cardiovascular
heavy-chain (gamma G) 273.2
Heberden's 715.04
Hebra's
dermatitis exfoliativa 695.89
erythema multiforme exudativum 695.1
pityriasis
maculata et circinata 696.3
rubra 695.89
pilaris 696.4
prurigo 698.2

Disease, diseased—*continued*
Heerfordt's (uveoparotitis) 135
Heidenhain's 290.10
with dementia 290.10
Heilmeyer-Schöner (M9842/3) 207.1
Heine-Medin (*see also* Poliomyelitis) 045.9
Heller's (*see also* Psychosis, childhood) 299.1
Heller-Döhle (syphilitic aortitis) 093.1
hematopoietic organs 289.9
hemoglobin (Hb) 282.7
with thalassemia 282.4
abnormal (mixed) NEC 282.7
with thalassemia 282.4
AS genotype 282.5
Bart's 282.7
C (Hb-C) 282.7
with other abnormal hemoglobin NEC 282.7
elliptocytosis 282.7
Hb-S 282.63
sickle-cell 282.63
thalassemia 282.4
constant spring 282.7
D (Hb-D) 282.7
with other abnormal hemoglobin NEC 282.7
Hb-S 282.69
sickle-cell 282.69
thalassemia 282.4
E (Hb-E) 282.7
with other abnormal hemoglobin NEC 282.7
Hb-S 282.69
sickle-cell 282.69
thalassemia 282.4
elliptocytosis 282.7
F (Hb-F) 282.7
G (Hb-G) 282.7
H (Hb-H) 282.4
hereditary persistence, fetal (HPFH) ("Swiss variety") 282.7
high fetal gene 282.7
I thalassemia 282.4
M 289.7
S—*see* Disease, sickle-cell, Hb-S
spherocytosis 282.7
unstable, hemolytic 282.7
Zurich (Hb-Zurich) 282.7
hemolytic (fetus) (newborn) 773.2
autoimmune (cold type) (warm type) 283.0
due to or with
incompatibility
ABO (blood group) 773.1
blood (group) (Duffy) (Kell) (Kidd) (Lewis) (M) (S) NEC 773.2
Rh (blood group) (factor) 773.0
Rh negative mother 773.0
unstable hemoglobin 282.7
hemorrhagic 287.9
newborn 776.0
Henoch (-Schönlein) (purpura nervosa) 287.0
hepatic—*see* Disease, liver
hepatolenticular 275.1
heredodegenerative NEC
brain 331.89
spinal cord 336.8
Hers' (glycogenosis VI) 271.0
Herter (-Gee) (-Heubner) (nontropical sprue) 579.0
Herxheimer's (diffuse idiopathic cutaneous atrophy) 701.8
Heubner's 094.89
Heubner-Herter (nontropical sprue) 579.0

Disease, diseased—*continued*
high fetal gene or hemoglobin thalassemia 282.4
Hildenbrand's (typhus) 081.9
hip (joint) NEC 719.95
congenital 755.63
suppurative 711.05
tuberculous (*see also* Tuberculosis) 015.1 *[730.85]*
Hippel's (retinocerebral angiomatosis) 759.6
Hirschfeld's (acute diabetes mellitus) (*see also* Diabetes) 250.0
Hirschsprung's (congenital megacolon) 751.3
His (-Werner) (trench fever) 083.1
HIV 042
Hodgkin's (M9650/3) 201.9

Note—Use the following fifth-digit subclassification with categories 201:

0 unspecified site
1 lymph nodes of head, face, and neck
2 intrathoracic lymph nodes
3 intra-abdominal lymph nodes
4 lymph nodes of axilla and upper limb
5 lymph nodes of inguinal region and lower limb
6 intrapelvic lymph nodes
7 spleen
8 lymph nodes of multiple sites

lymphocytic
depletion (M9653/3) 201.7
diffuse fibrosis (M9654/3) 201.7
reticular type (M9655/3) 201.7
predominance (M9651/3) 201.4
lymphocytic-histiocytic predominance (M9651/3) 201.4
mixed cellularity (M9652/3) 201.6
nodular sclerosis (M9656/3) 201.5
cellular phase (M9657/3) 201.5
Hodgson's 441.9
ruptured 441.5
Hoffa (-Kastert) (liposynovitis prepatellaris) 272.8
Holla (*see also* Spherocytosis) 282.0
homozygous-Hb-S 282.61
hoof and mouth 078.4
hookworm (*see also* Ancylostomiasis) 126.9
Horton's (temporal arteritis) 446.5
host-versus-graft (immune or nonimmune cause) 996.80
bone marrow 996.85
heart 996.83
intestines 996.89
kidney 996.81
liver 996.82
lung 996.84
pancreas 996.86
specified NEC 996.89
HPFH (hereditary persistence of fetal hemoglobin) ("Swiss variety") 282.7
Huchard's (continued arterial hypertension) 401.9
Huguier's (uterine fibroma) 218.9
human immunodeficiency (virus) 042
hunger 251.1
Hunt's
dyssynergia cerebellaris myoclonica 334.2
herpetic geniculate ganglionitis 053.11
Huntington's 333.4
Huppert's (multiple myeloma) (M9730/3) 203.0

Disease, diseased—*continued*
Hurler's (mucopolysaccharidosis I) 277.5
Hutchinson's, meaning
angioma serpiginosum 709.1
cheiropompholyx 705.81
prurigo estivalis 692.72
Hutchinson-Boeck (sarcoidosis) 135
Hutchinson-Gilford (progeria) 259.8
hyaline (diffuse) (generalized) 728.9
membrane (lung) (newborn) 769
hydatid (*see also* Echinococcus) 122.9
Hyde's (prurigo nodularis) 698.3
hyperkinetic (*see also* Hyperkinesia) 314.9
heart 429.82
hypertensive (*see also* Hypertension) 401.9
hypophysis 253.9
hyperfunction 253.1
hypofunction 253.2
Iceland (epidemic neuromyasthenia) 049.8
I cell 272.7
ill-defined 799.8
immunologic NEC 279.9
immunoproliferative 203.8
inclusion 078.5
salivary gland 078.5
infancy, early NEC 779.9
infective NEC 136.9
inguinal gland 289.9
internal semilunar cartilage, cystic 717.5
intervertebral disc 722.90
with myelopathy 722.70
cervical, cervicothoracic 722.91
with myelopathy 722.71
lumbar, lumbosacral 722.93
with myelopathy 722.73
thoracic, thoracolumbar 722.92
with myelopathy 722.72
intestine 569.9
functional 564.9
congenital 751.3
psychogenic 306.4
lardaceous 277.3
organic 569.9
protozoal NEC 007.9
iris 364.9
iron
metabolism 275.0
storage 275.0
Isambert's (*see also* Tuberculosis, larynx) 012.3
Iselin's (osteochondrosis, fifth metatarsal) 732.5
Island (scrub typhus) 081.2
itai-itai 985.5
Jadassohn's (maculopapular erythroderma) 696.2
Jadassohn-Pellizari's (anetoderma) 701.3
Jakob-Creutzfeldt 046.1
with dementia 290.10
Jaksch (-Luzet) (pseudoleukemia infantum) 285.8
Janet's 300.89
Jansky-Bielschowsky 330.1
jaw NEC 526.9
fibrocystic 526.2
Jensen's 363.05
Jeune's (asphyxiating thoracic dystrophy) 756.4
jigger 134.1
Johnson-Stevens (erythema multiforme exudativum) 695.1

Disease, diseased—*continued*
joint NEC 719.9
ankle 719.97
Charcot 094.0 *[713.5]*
degenerative (*see also* Osteoarthrosis) 715.9
multiple 715.09
spine (*see also* Spondylosis) 721.90
elbow 719.92
foot 719.97
hand 719.94
hip 719.95
hypertrophic (chronic) (degenerative) (*see also* Osteoarthrosis) 715.9
spine (*see also* Spondylosis) 721.90
knee 719.96
Luschka 721.90
multiple sites 719.99
pelvic region 719.95
sacroiliac 724.6
shoulder (region) 719.91
specified site NEC 719.98
spine NEC 724.9
pseudarthrosis following fusion 733.82
sacroiliac 724.6
wrist 719.93
Jourdain's (acute gingivitis) 523.0
Jüngling's (sarcoidosis) 135
Kahler (-Bozzolo) (multiple myeloma) (M9730/3) 203.0
Kalischer's 759.6
Kaposi's 757.33
lichen ruber 697.8
acuminatus 696.4
moniliformis 697.8
xeroderma pigmentosum 757.33
Kaschin-Beck (endemic polyarthritis) 716.00
ankle 716.07
arm 716.02
lower (and wrist) 716.03
upper (and elbow) 716.02
foot (and ankle) 716.07
forearm (and wrist) 716.03
hand 716.04
leg 716.06
lower 716.06
upper 716.05
multiple sites 716.09
pelvic region (hip) (thigh) 716.05
shoulder region 716.01
specified site NEC 716.08
Katayama 120.2
Kawasaki 446.1
Kedani (scrub typhus) 081.2
kidney (functional) (pelvis) (*see also* Disease, renal) 593.9
cystic (congenital) 753.10
multiple 753.19
single 753.11
specified NEC 753.19
fibrocystic (congenital) 753.19
in gout 274.10
polycystic (congenital) 753.12
adult type (APKD) 753.13
autosomal dominant 753.13
autosomal recessive 753.14
childhood type (CPKD) 753.14
infantile type 753.14

Disease, diseased—*continued*
Kienböck's (carpal lunate) (wrist) 732.3
Kimmelstiel (-Wilson) (intercapillary glomerulosclerosis) 250.4 *[581.81]*
Kinnier Wilson's (hepatolenticular degeneration) 275.1
kissing 075
Kleb's (*see also* Nephritis) 583.9
Klinger's 446.4
Klippel's 723.8
Klippel-Feil (brevicollis) 756.16
knight's 911.1
Köbner's (epidermolysis bullosa) 757.39
Koenig-Wichmann (pemphigus) 694.4
Köhler's
first (osteoarthrosis juvenilis) 732.5
second (Freiberg's infraction, metatarsal head) 732.5
patellar 732.4
tarsal navicular (bone) (osteoarthrosis juvenilis) 732.5
Köhler-Freiberg (infraction, metatarsal head) 732.5
Köhler-Mouchet (osteoarthrosis juvenilis) 732.5
Köhler-Pellegrini-Stieda (calcification, knee joint) 726.62
König's (osteochondritis dissecans) 732.7
Korsakoff's (nonalcoholic) 294.0
alcoholic 291.1
Kostmann's (infantile genetic agranulocytosis) 288.0
Krabbe's 330.0
Kraepelin-Morel (*see also* Schizophrenia) 295.9
Kraft-Weber-Dimitri 759.6
Kufs' 330.1
Kugelberg-Welander 335.11
Kuhnt-Junius 362.52
Kümmell's (-Verneuil) (spondylitis) 721.7
Kundrat's (lymphosarcoma) 200.1
kuru 046.0
Kussmaul (-Meier) (polyarteritis nodosa) 446.0
Kyasanur Forest 065.2
Kyrle's (hyperkeratosis follicularis in cutem penetrans) 701.1
labia
inflammatory 616.9
specified NEC 616.8
noninflammatory 624.9
specified NEC 624.8
labyrinth, ear 386.8
lacrimal system (apparatus) (passages) 375.9
gland 375.00
specified NEC 375.89
Lafora's 333.2
Lagleyze-von Hippel (retinocerebral angiomatosis) 759.6
Lancereaux-Mathieu (leptospiral jaundice) 100.0
Landry's 357.0
Lane's 569.89
lardaceous (any site) 277.3
Larrey-Weil (leptospiral jaundice) 100.0
Larsen (-Johansson) (juvenile osteopathia patellae) 732.4
larynx 478.70
Lasègue's (persecution mania) 297.9
Leber's 377.16
Lederer's (acquired infectious hemolytic anemia) 283.19
Legg's (capital femoral osteochondrosis) 732.1

Disease, diseased—*continued*
Marfan's 090.49
congenital syphilis 090.49
meaning Marfan's syndrome 759.82
Marie-Bamberger (hypertrophic pulmonary osteoarthropathy) (secondary) 731.2
primary or idiopathic (acropachyderma) 757.39
pulmonary (hypertrophic osteoarthropathy) 731.2
Marie-Strümpell (ankylosing spondylitis) 720.0
Marion's (bladder neck obstruction) 596.0
Marsh's (exophthalmic goiter) 242.0
Martin's 715.27
mast cell 757.33
systemic (M9741/3) 202.6
mastoid (*see also* Mastoiditis) 383.9
process 385.9
maternal, unrelated to pregnancy NEC, affecting fetus or newborn 760.9
Mathieu's (leptospiral jaundice) 100.0
Mauclaire's 732.3
Mauriac's (erythema nodosum syphiliticum) 091.3
Maxcy's 081.0
McArdle (-Schmid-Pearson) (glycogenosis V) 271.0
mediastinum NEC 519.3
Medin's (*see also* Poliomyelitis) 045.9
Mediterranean (with hemoglobinopathy) 282.4
medullary center (idiopathic) (respiratory) 348.8
Meige's (chronic hereditary edema) 757.0
Meleda 757.39
Ménétrier's (hypertrophic gastritis) 535.2
Ménière's (active) 386.00
cochlear 386.02
cochleovestibular 386.01
inactive 386.04
in remission 386.04
vestibular 386.03
meningeal—*see* Meningitis
mental (*see also* Psychosis) 298.9
Merzbacher-Pelizaeus 330.0
mesenchymal 710.9
mesenteric embolic 557.0
metabolic NEC 277.9
metal polishers' 502
metastatic—*see* Metastasis
Mibelli's 757.39
microdrepanocytic 282.4
Miescher's 709.3
Mikulicz's (dryness of mouth, absent or decreased lacrimation) 527.1
Milkman (-Looser) (osteomalacia with pseudofractures) 268.2
Miller's (osteomalacia) 268.2
Mills' 335.29
Milroy's (chronic hereditary edema) 757.0
Minamata 985.0
Minor's 336.1
Minot's (hemorrhagic disease, newborn) 776.0
Minot-von Willebrand-Jürgens (angiohemophilia) 286.4
Mitchell's (erythromelalgia) 443.89
mitral—*see* Endocarditis, mitral
Mljet (mal de Meleda) 757.39
Möbius', Moebius' 346.8
Moeller's 267
Möller (-Barlow) (infantile scurvy) 267

Disease, diseased—*continued*
Mönckeberg's (*see also* arteriosclerosis, extremities) 440.20
Mondor's (thrombophlebitis of breast) 451.89
Monge's 993.2
Morel-Kraepelin (*see also* Schizophrenia) 295.9
Morgagni's (syndrome) (hyperostosis frontalis interna) 733.3
Morgagni-Adams-Stokes (syncope with heart block) 426.9
Morquio (-Brailsford) (-Ullrich) (mucopolysaccharidosis IV) 277.5
Morton's (with metatarsalgia) 355.6
Morvan's 336.0
motor neuron (bulbar) (mixed type) 335.20
Mouchet's (juvenile osteochondrosis, foot) 732.5
mouth 528.9
Moyamoya 437.5
Mucha's (acute parapsoriasis varioliformis) 696.2
mu-chain 273.2
mucolipidosis (I) (II) (III) 272.7
Münchmeyer's (exostosis luxurians) 728.11
Murri's (intermittent hemoglobinuria) 283.2
muscle 359.9
inflammatory 728.9
ocular 378.9
musculoskeletal system 729.9
mushroom workers' 495.5
Myà's (congenital dilation, colon) 751.3
mycotic 117.9
myeloproliferative (chronic) (M9960/1) 238.7
myocardium, myocardial (*see also* Degeneration, myocardial) 429.1
hypertensive (*see also* Hypertension, heart) 402.90
primary (idiopathic) 425.4
myoneural 358.9
Naegeli's 287.1
nail 703.9
specified type NEC 703.8
Nairobi sheep 066.1
nasal 478.1
cavity NEC 478.1
sinus (chronic)—*see* Sinusitis
navel (newborn) NEC 779.8
nemaline body 359.0
neoplastic, generalized (M8000/6) 199.0
nerve—*see* Disorder, nerve
nervous system (central) 349.9
autonomic, peripheral (*see also* Neuropathy, peripheral, autonomic) 337.9
congenital 742.9
inflammatory—*see* Encephalitis
parasympathetic (*see also* Neuropathy, peripheral, autonomic) 337.9
peripheral NEC 355.9
specified NEC 349.89
sympathetic (*see also* Neuropathy, peripheral, autonomic) 337.9
vegetative (*see also* Neuropathy, peripheral, autonomic) 337.9
Nettleship's (urticaria pigmentosa) 757.33
Neumann's (pemphigus vegetans) 694.4
neurologic (central) NEC (*see also* Disease, nervous system) 349.9
peripheral NEC 355.9

Disease, diseased—*continued*
neuromuscular system NEC 358.9
Newcastle 077.8
Nicolas (-Durand) -Favre (climatic bubo) 099.1
Niemann-Pick (lipid histiocytosis) 272.7
nipple 611.9
Paget's (M8540/3) 174.0
Nishimoto (-Takeuchi) 437.5
nonarthropod-borne NEC 078.89
central nervous system NEC 049.9
enterovirus NEC 078.89
non-autoimmune hemolytic NEC 283.10
Nonne-Milroy-Meige (chronic hereditary edema) 757.0
Norrie's (congenital progressive oculoacousticocerebral degeneration) 743.8
nose 478.1
nucleus pulposus—*see* Disease, intervertebral disc
nutritional 269.9
maternal, affecting fetus or newborn 760.4
oasthouse, urine 270.2
obliterative vascular 447.1
Odelberg's (juvenile osteochondrosis) 732.1
Oguchi's (retina) 368.61
Ohara's (*see also* Tularemia) 021.9
Ollier's (chondrodysplasia) 756.4
Opitz's (congestive splenomegaly) 289.51
Oppenheim's 358.8
Oppenheim-Urbach (necrobiosis lipoidica diabeticorum) 250.8 *[709.3]*
optic nerve NEC 377.49
orbit 376.9
specified NEC 376.89
Oriental liver fluke 121.1
Oriental lung fluke 121.2
Ormond's 593.4
Osgood's tibia (tubercle) 732.4
Osgood-Schlatter 732.4
Osler (-Vaquez) (polycythemia vera) (M9950/1) 238.4
Osler-Rendu (familial hemorrhagic telangiectasia) 448.0
osteofibrocystic 252.0
Otto's 715.35
outer ear 380.9
ovary (noninflammatory) NEC 620.9
cystic 620.2
polycystic 256.4
specified NEC 620.8
Owren's (congenital) (*see also* Defect, coagulation) 286.3
Paas' 756.59
Paget's (osteitis deformans) 731.0
with infiltrating duct carcinoma of the breast (M8541/3)—*see* Neoplasm, breast, malignant
bone 731.0
osteosarcoma in (M9184/3)—*see* Neoplasm, bone, malignant
breast (M8540/3) 174.0
extramammary (M8542/3)—*see also* Neoplasm, skin, malignant
anus 154.3
skin 173.5
malignant (M8540/3)
breast 174.0
specified site NEC (M8542/3)—*see* Neoplasm, skin, malignant
unspecified site 174.0

Disease, diseased—*continued*
mammary (M8540/3) 174.0
nipple (M8540/3) 174.0
palate (soft) 528.9
Paltauf-Sternberg 201.9
pancreas 577.9
cystic 577.2
congenital 751.7
fibrocystic 277.00
Panner's 732.3
capitellum humeri 732.3
head of humerus 732.3
tarsal navicular (bone) (osteochondrosis) 732.5
panvalvular—*see* Endocarditis, mitral
parametrium 629.9
parasitic NEC 136.9
cerebral NEC 123.9
intestinal NEC 129
mouth 112.0
skin NEC 134.9
specified type—*see* Infestation
tongue 112.0
parathyroid (gland) 252.9
specified NEC 252.8
Parkinson's 332.0
parodontal 523.9
Parrot's (syphilitic osteochondritis) 090.0
Parry's (exophthalmic goiter) 242.0
Parson's (exophthalmic goiter) 242.0
Pavy's 593.6
Paxton's (white piedra) 111.2
Payr's (splenic flexure syndrome) 569.89
pearl-workers' (chronic osteomyelitis) (*see also* Osteomyelitis) 730.1
Pel-Ebstein—*see* Disease, Hodgkin's
Pelizaeus-Merzbacher 330.0
with dementia 294.1
Pellegrini-Stieda (calcification, knee joint) 726.62
pelvis, pelvic
female NEC 629.9
specified NEC 629.8
gonococcal (acute) 098.19
chronic or duration of 2 months or over 098.39
infection (*see also* Disease, pelvis, inflammatory) 614.9
inflammatory (female) (PID) 614.9
with
abortion—*see* Abortion, by type, with sepsis
ectopic pregnancy (*see also* categories 633.0-633.9) 639.0
molar pregnancy (*see also* categories 630-632) 639.0
acute 614.3
chronic 614.4
complicating pregnancy 646.6
affecting fetus or newborn 760.8
following
abortion 639.0
ectopic or molar pregnancy 639.0
peritonitis (acute) 614.5
chronic NEC 614.7
puerperal, postpartum, childbirth 670
specified NEC 614.8
organ, female NEC 629.9
specified NEC 629.8
peritoneum, female NEC 629.9
specified NEC 629.8

Disease, diseased—*continued*
penis 607.9
inflammatory 607.2
peptic NEC 536.9
acid 536.8
periapical tissues NEC 522.9
pericardium 423.9
specified type NEC 423.8
perineum
female
inflammatory 616.9
specified NEC 616.8
noninflammatory 624.9
specified NEC 624.8
male (inflammatory) 682.2
periodic (familial) (Reimann's) NEC 277.3
paralysis 359.3
periodontal NEC 523.9
specified NEC 523.8
periosteum 733.90
peripheral
arterial 443.9
autonomic nervous system (*see also* Neuropathy, autonomic) 337.9
nerve NEC (*see also* Neuropathy) 356.9
multiple—*see* Polyneuropathy
vascular 443.9
specified type NEC 443.89
peritoneum 568.9
pelvic, female 629.9
specified NEC 629.8
Perrin-Ferraton (snapping hip) 719.65
persistent mucosal (middle ear) (with posterior or superior marginal perforation of ear drum) 382.2
Perthes' (capital femoral osteochondrosis) 732.1
Petit's (*see also* Hernia, lumbar) 553.8
Peutz-Jeghers 759.6
Peyronie's 607.89
Pfeiffer's (infectious mononucleosis) 075
pharynx 478.20
Phocas' 610.1
photochromogenic (acid-fast bacilli) (pulmonary) 031.0
nonpulmonary 031.9
Pick's
brain 331.1
with dementia 290.10
cerebral atrophy 331.1
with dementia 290.10
lipid histiocytosis 272.7
liver (pericardial pseudocirrhosis of liver) 423.2
pericardium (pericardial pseudocirrhosis of liver) 423.2
polyserositis (pericardial pseudocirrhosis of liver) 423.2
Pierson's (osteochondrosis) 732.1
pigeon fancier's or breeders' 495.2
pineal gland 259.8
pink 985.0
Pinkus' (lichen nitidus) 697.1
pinworm 127.4
pituitary (gland) 253.9
hyperfunction 253.1
hypofunction 253.2
pituitary snuff-takers' 495.8

Disease, diseased—*continued*
placenta
affecting fetus or newborn 762.2
complicating pregnancy or childbirth 656.7
pleura (cavity) (*see also* Pleurisy) 511.0
Plummer's (toxic nodular goiter) 242.3
pneumatic
drill 994.9
hammer 994.9
policeman's 729.2
Pollitzer's (hidradenitis suppurativa) 705.83
polycystic (congenital) 759.89
kidney or renal 753.12
adult type (APKD) 753.13
autosomal dominant 753.13
autosomal recessive 753.14
childhood type (CPKD) 753.14
infantile type 753.14
liver or hepatic 751.62
lung or pulmonary 518.89
congenital 748.4
ovary, ovaries 256.4
spleen 759.0
Pompe's (glycogenosis II) 271.0
Poncet's (tuberculous rheumatism) (*see also* Tuberculosis) 015.9
Posada-Wernicke 114.9
Potain's (pulmonary edema) 514
Pott's (*see also* Tuberculosis) 015.0 *[730.88]*
osteomyelitis 015.0 *[730.88]*
paraplegia 015.0 *[730.88]*
spinal curvature 015.0 *[737.43]*
spondylitis 015.0 *[720.81]*
Potter's 753.0
Poulet's 714.2
pregnancy NEC (*see also* Pregnancy) 646.9
Preiser's (osteoporosis) 733.09
Pringle's (tuberous sclerosis) 759.5
Profichet's 729.9
prostate 602.9
specified type NEC 602.8
protozoal NEC 136.8
intestine, intestinal NEC 007.9
pseudo-Hurler's (mucolipidosis III) 272.7
psychiatric (*see also* Psychosis) 298.9
psychotic (*see also* Psychosis) 298.9
Puente's (simple glandular cheilitis) 528.5
puerperal NEC (*see also* Puerperal) 674.9
pulmonary—*see also* Disease, lung
amyloid 277.3 *[517.8]*
artery 417.9
circulation, circulatory 417.9
specified NEC 417.8
diffuse obstructive (chronic) 496
with asthma (chronic) (obstructive) 493.2
heart (chronic) 416.9
specified NEC 416.8
hypertensive (vascular) 416.0
cardiovascular 416.0
obstructive diffuse (chronic) 496
with
acute exacerbation NEC 491.21
asthma (chronic) (obstructive) 493.2
valve (*see also* Endocarditis, pulmonary) 424.3

Disease, diseased—*continued*
pulp (dental) NEC 522.9
pulseless 446.7
Putnam's (subacute combined sclerosis with pernicious anemia) 281.0 *[336.2]*
Pyle (-Cohn) (craniometaphyseal dysplasia) 756.89
pyramidal tract 333.90
Quervain's
tendon sheath 727.04
thyroid (subacute granulomatous thyroiditis) 245.1
Quincke's—*see* Edema, angioneurotic
Quinquaud (acne decalvans) 704.09
rag sorters' 022.1
Raynaud's (Paroxysmal digital cyanosis) 443.0
reactive airway—*see* Asthma
Recklinghausen's (M9540/1) 237.71
bone (osteitis fibrosa cystica) 252.0
Recklinghausen-Applebaum (hemochromatosis) 275.0
Reclus' (cystic) 610.1
rectum NEC 569.49
Refsum's (heredopathia atactica polyneuritiformis) 356.3
Reichmann's (gastrosuccorrhea) 536.8
Reimann's (periodic) 277.3
Reiter's 099.3
renal (functional) (pelvis) 593.9
with
edema (*see also* Nephrosis) 581.9
exudative nephritis 583.89
lesion of interstitial nephritis 583.89
stated generalized cause—*see* Nephritis
acute—*see* Nephritis, acute
basement membrane NEC 583.89
with
pulmonary hemorrhage (Goodpasture's syndrome) 446.21 *[583.81]*
chronic—*see* Nephritis, chronic
complicating pregnancy or puerperium NEC 646.2
with hypertension—*see* Toxemia, of pregnancy
affecting fetus or newborn 760.1
cystic, congenital (*see also* Cystic, disease, kidney) 753.10
diabetic 250.4 *[583.81]*
due to
amyloidosis 277.3 *[583.81]*
diabetes mellitus 250.4 *[583.81]*
systemic lupus erythematosis 710.0 *[583.81]*
end-stage 585
exudative 583.89
fibrocystic (congenital) 753.19
gonococcal 098.19 *[583.81]*
gouty 274.10
hypertensive (*see also* Hypertension, kidney) 403.90
immune complex NEC 583.89
interstitial (diffuse) (focal) 583.89
lupus 710.0 *[583.81]*
maternal, affecting fetus or newborn 760.1
hypertensive 760.0
phosphate-losing (tubular) 588.0
polycystic (congenital) 753.12
adult type (APKD) 753.13
autosomal dominant 753.13
autosomal recessive 753.14
childhood type (CPKD) 753.14
infantile type 753.14

Disease, diseased—*continued*
specified lesion or cause NEC (*see also* Glomerulonephritis) 583.89
subacute 581.9
syphilitic 095.4
tuberculous (*see also* Tuberculosis) 016.0 *[583.81]*
tubular (*see also* Nephrosis, tubular) 584.5
Rendu-Olser-Weber (familial hemorrhagic telangiectasia) 448.0
renovascular (arteriosclerotic) (*see also* Hypertension, kidney) 403.90
respiratory (tract) 519.9
acute or subacute (upper) NEC 465.9
due to fumes or vapors 506.3
multiple sites NEC 465.8
noninfectious 478.9
streptococcal 034.0
chronic 519.9
arising in the perinatal period 770.7
due to fumes or vapors 506.4
due to
aspiration of liquids or solids 508.9
external agents NEC 508.9
specified NEC 508.8
fumes or vapors 506.9
acute or subacute NEC 506.3
chronic 506.4
fetus or newborn NEC 770.9
obstructive 496
specified type NEC 519.8
upper (acute) (infectious) NEC 465.9
multiple sites NEC 465.8
noninfectious NEC 478.9
streptococcal 034.0
retina, retinal NEC 362.9
Batten's or Batten-Mayou 330.1 *[362.71]*
degeneration 362.89
vascular lesion 362.17
rheumatic (*see also* Arthritis) 716.8
heart—*see* Disease, heart, rheumatic
rheumatoid (heart)—*see* Arthritis, rheumatoid
rickettsial NEC 083.9
specified type NEC 083.8
Riedel's (ligneous thyroiditis) 245.3
Riga (-Fede) (cachectic aphthae) 529.0
Riggs' (compound periodontitis) 523.4
Ritter's 695.81
Rivalta's (cervicofacial actinomycosis) 039.3
Robles' (onchocerciasis) 125.3 *[360.13]*
Roger's (congenital interventricular septal defect) 745.4
Rokitansky's (*see also* Necrosis, liver) 570
Romberg's 349.89
Rosenthal's (factor XI deficiency) 286.2
Rossbach's (hyperchlorhydria) 536.8
psychogenic 306.4
Roth (-Bernhardt) 355.1
Runeberg's (progressive pernicious anemia) 281.0
Rust's (tuberculous spondylitis) (*see also* Tuberculosis) 015.0 *[720.81]*
Rustitskii's (multiple myeloma) (M9730/3) 203.0
Ruysch's (Hirschsprung's disease) 751.3
Sachs (-Tay) 330.1
sacroiliac NEC 724.6
salivary gland or duct NEC 527.9
inclusion 078.5
streptococcal 034.0
virus 078.5

Disease, diseased—*continued*
Sander's (paranoia) 297.1
Sandhoff's 330.1
sandworm 126.9
Savill's (epidemic exfoliative dermatitis) 695.89
Schamberg's (progressive pigmentary dermatosis) 709.09
Schaumann's (sarcoidosis) 135
Schenck's (sporotrichosis) 117.1
Scheuermann's (osteochondrosis) 732.0
Schilder (-Flatau) 341.1
Schimmelbusch's 610.1
Schlatter's tibia (tubercle) 732.4
Schlatter-Osgood 732.4
Schmorl's 722.30
cervical 722.39
lumbar, lumbosacral 722.32
specified region NEC 722.39
thoracic, thoracolumbar 722.31
Scholz's 330.0
Schönlein (-Henoch) (purpura rheumatica) 287.0
Schottmüller's (*see also* Fever, paratyphoid) 002.9
Schüller-Christian (chronic histiocytosis X) 277.8
Schultz's (agranulocytosis) 288.0
Schwalbe-Ziehen-Oppenheimer 333.6
Schweninger-Buzzi (macular atrophy) 701.3
sclera 379.19
scrofulous (*see also* Tuberculosis) 017.2
scrotum 608.9
sebaceous glands NEC 706.9
Secretan's (posttraumatic edema) 782.3
semilunar cartilage, cystic 717.5
seminal vesicle 608.9
Senear-Usher (pemphigus erythematosus) 694.4
serum NEC 999.5
Sever's (osteochondrosis calcaneum) 732.5
Sézary's (reticulosis) (M9701/3) 202.2
Shaver's (bauxite pneumoconiosis) 503
Sheehan's (postpartum pituitary necrosis) 253.2
shimamushi (scrub typhus) 081.2
shipyard 077.1
sickle-cell 282.60
with
crisis 282.62
Hb-S disease 282.61
other abnormal hemoglobin (Hb-D) (Hb-E) (Hb-G) (Hb-J) (Hb-K) (Hb-O) (Hb-P) (high fetal gene) 282.69
elliptocytosis 282.60
Hb-C 282.63
Hb-S 282.61
with
crisis 282.62
Hb-C 282.63
other abnormal hemoglobin (Hb-D) (Hb-E) (Hb-G) (Hb-J) (Hb-K) (Hb-O) (Hb-P) (high fetal gene) 282.69
spherocytosis 282.60
thalassemia 282.4

Disease, diseased—*continued*
Siegal-Cattan-Mamou (periodic) 277.3
silo fillers' 506.9
Simian B 054.3
Simmonds' (pituitary cachexia) 253.2
Simons' (progressive lipodystrophy) 272.6
Sinding-Larsen (juvenile osteopathia patellae) 732.4
sinus—*see also* Sinusitis
brain 437.9
specified NEC 478.1
Sirkari's 085.0
sixth 057.8
Sjögren (-Gougerot) 710.2
with lung involvement 710.2 *[517.8]*
Skevas-Zerfus 989.5
skin NEC 709.9
due to metabolic disorder 277.9
specified type NEC 709.8
sleeping 347
meaning sleeping sickness (*see also* Trypanosomiasis) 086.5
small vessel 443.9
Smith-Strang (oasthouse urine) 270.2
Sneddon-Wilkinson (subcorneal pustular dermatosis) 694.1
South African creeping 133.8
specific NEC (*see also* Syphilis) 097.9
Spencer's (epidemic vomiting) 078.82
Spielmeyer-Stock 330.1
Spielmeyer-Vogt 330.1
spine, spinal 733.90
combined system (*see also* Degeneration, combined) 266.2 *[336.2]*
with pernicious anemia 281.0 *[336.2]*
cord NEC 336.9
congenital 742.9
demyelinating NEC 341.8
joint (*see also* Disease, joint, spine) 724.9
tuberculous 015.0 *[730.8]*
spinocerebellar 334.9
specified NEC 334.8
spleen (organic) (postinfectional) 289.50
amyloid 277.3
lardaceous 277.3
polycystic 759.0
specified NEC 289.59
sponge divers' 989.5
Stanton's (melioidosis) 025
Stargardt's 362.75
Steinert's 359.2
Sternberg's—*see* Disease, Hodgkin's
Stevens-Johnson (erythema multiforme exudativum) 695.1
Sticker's (erythema infectiosum) 057.0
Stieda's (calcification, knee joint) 726.62
Still's (juvenile rheumatoid arthritis) 714.30
Stiller's (asthenia) 780.7
Stokes' (exophthalmic goiter) 242.0
Stokes-Adams (syncope with heart block) 426.9
Stokvis (-Talma) (enterogenous cyanosis) 289.7
stomach NEC (organic) 537.9
functional 536.9
psychogenic 306.4
lardaceous 277.3
stonemasons' 502

Disease, diseased—*continued*
storage
glycogen (*see also* Disease, glycogen storage) 271.0
lipid 272.7
mucopolysaccharide 277.5
striatopallidal system 333.90
specified NEC 333.89
Strümpell-Marie (ankylosing spondylitis) 720.0
Stuart's (congenital factor X deficiency) (*see also* Defect, coagulation) 286.3
Stuart-Prower (congenital factor X deficiency) (*see also* Defect, coagulation) 286.3
Sturge (-Weber) (-Dimitri) (encephalocutaneous angiomatosis) 759.6
Stuttgart 100.89
Sudeck's 733.7
supporting structures of teeth NEC 525.9
suprarenal (gland) (capsule) 255.9
hyperfunction 255.3
hypofunction 255.4
Sutton's 709.09
Sutton and Gull's—*see* Hypertension, kidney
sweat glands NEC 705.9
specified type NEC 705.89
sweating 078.2
Sweeley-Klionsky 272.4
Swift (-Feer) 985.0
swimming pool (bacillus) 031.1
swineherd's 100.89
Sylvest's (epidemic pleurodynia) 074.1
Symmers (follicular lymphoma) (M9690/3) 202.0
sympathetic nervous system (*see also* Neuropathy, peripheral, autonomic) 337.9
synovium 727.9
syphilitic—*see* Syphilis
systemic tissue mast cell (M9741/3) 202.6
Taenzer's 757.4
Takayasu's (pulseless) 446.7
Talma's 728.85
Tangier (familial high-density lipoprotein deficiency) 272.5
Tarral-Besnier (pityriasis rubra pilaris) 696.4
Tay-Sachs 330.1
Taylor's 701.8
tear duct 375.69
teeth, tooth 525.9
hard tissues NEC 521.9
pulp NEC 522.9
tendon 727.9
inflammatory NEC 727.9
terminal vessel 443.9
testis 608.9
Thaysen-Gee (nontropical sprue) 579.0
Thomsen's 359.2
Thomson's (congenital poikiloderma) 757.33
Thornwaldt's, Tornwaldt's (pharyngeal bursitis) 478.29
throat 478.20
septic 034.0
thromboembolic (*see also* Embolism) 444.9
thymus (gland) 254.9
specified NEC 254.8
thyroid (gland) NEC 246.9
heart (*see also* Hyperthyroidism) 242.9 *[425.7]*
lardaceous 277.3
specified NEC 246.8
Tietze's 733.6

Disease, diseased—*continued*
Tommaselli's
correct substance properly administered 599.7
overdose or wrong substance given or taken 961.4
tongue 529.9
tonsils, tonsillar (and adenoids) (chronic) 474.9
specified NEC 474.8
tooth, teeth 525.9
hard tissues NEC 521.9
pulp NEC 522.9
Tornwaldt's (pharyngeal bursitis) 478.29
Tourette's 307.23
trachea 519.1
tricuspid—*see* Endocarditis, tricuspid
triglyceride-storage, type I, II, III 272.7
triple vessel (coronary arteries) —*see* Arteriosclerosis, coronary
trisymptomatic, Gougerot's 709.1
trophoblastic (*see also* Hydatidiform mole) 630
previous, affecting management of pregnancy V23.1
tsutsugamushi (scrub typhus) 081.2
tube (fallopian), noninflammatory 620.9
specified NEC 620.8
tuberculous NEC (*see also* Tuberculosis) 011.9
tubo-ovarian
inflammatory (*see also* Salpingo-oophoritis) 614.2
noninflammatory 620.9
specified NEC 620.8
tubotympanic, chronic (with anterior perforation of ear drum) 382.1
tympanum 385.9
Uhl's 746.84
umbilicus (newborn) NEC 779.8
Underwood's (sclerema neonatorum) 778.1
undiagnosed 799.9
Unna's (seborrheic dermatitis) 690.18
unstable hemoglobin hemolytic 282.7
Unverricht (-Lundborg) 333.2
Urbach-Oppenheim (necrobiosis lipoidica diabeticorum) 250.8 *[709.3]*
Urbach-Wiethe (lipoid proteinosis) 272.8
ureter 593.9
urethra 599.9
specified type NEC 599.84
urinary (tract) 599.9
bladder 596.9
specified NEC 596.8
maternal, affecting fetus or newborn 760.1
Usher-Senear (pemphigus erythematosus) 694.4
uterus (organic) 621.9
infective (*see also* Endometritis) 615.9
inflammatory (*see also* Endometritis) 615.9
noninflammatory 621.9
specified type NEC 621.8
uveal tract
anterior 364.9
posterior 363.9
vagabonds' 132.1
vagina, vaginal
inflammatory 616.9
specified NEC 616.8
noninflammatory 623.9
specified NEC 623.8
Valsuani's (progressive pernicious anemia, puerperal) 648.2
complicating pregnancy or puerperium 648.2

Disease, diseased—*continued*
valve, valvular—*see* Endocarditis
van Bogaert-Nijssen (-Peiffer) 330.0
van Creveld-von Gierke (glycogenosis I) 271.0
van den Bergh's (enterogenous cyanosis) 289.7
van Neck's (juvenile osteochondrosis) 732.1
Vaquez (-Osler) (polycythemia vera) (M9950/1) 238.4
vascular 459.9
arteriosclerotic—*see* Arteriosclerosis
hypertensive—*see* Hypertension
obliterative 447.1
peripheral 443.9
occlusive 459.9
peripheral (occlusive) 443.9
in diabetes mellitus 250.7 *[443.81]*
specified type NEC 443.89
vas deferens 608.9
vasomotor 443.9
vasospastic 443.9
vein 459.9
venereal 099.9
fifth 099.1
sixth 099.1
chlamydial NEC 099.50
anus 099.52
bladder 099.53
cervix 099.53
epididymis 099.54
genitourinary NEC 099.55
lower 099.53
specified NEC 099.54
pelvic inflammatory disease 099.54
perihepatic 099.56
peritoneum 099.56
pharynx 099.51
rectum 099.52
specified site NEC 099.59
testis 099.54
vagina 099.53
vulva 099.53
complicating pregnancy, childbirth, or puerperium 647.2
specified nature or type NEC 099.8
chlamydial—*see* Disease, venereal, chlamydial
Verneuil's (syphilitic bursitis) 095.7
Verse's (calcinosis intervertebralis) 275.4 *[722.90]*
vertebra, vertebral NEC 733.90
disc—*see* Disease, Intervertebral disc
vibration NEC 994.9
Vidal's (lichen simplex chronicus) 698.3
Vincent's (trench mouth) 101
Virchow's 733.99
virus (filterable) NEC 078.89
arbovirus NEC 066.9
arthropod-borne NEC 066.9
central nervous system NEC 049.9
specified type NEC 049.8
complicating pregnancy, childbirth, or puerperium 647.6
contact (with) V01.7
exposure to V01.7
Marburg 078.89
maternal
with fetal damage affecting management of pregnancy 655.3
nonarthropod-borne NEC 078.89
central nervous system NEC 049.9
specified NEC 049.8

Disease, diseased—*continued*
vitreous 379.29
vocal cords NEC 478.5
Vogt's (Cecile) 333.7
Vogt-Spielmeyer 330.1
Volhard-Fahr (malignant nephrosclerosis) 403.00
Volkmann's
acquired 958.6
von Bechterew's (ankylosing spondylitis) 720.0
von Economo's (encephalitis lethargica) 049.8
von Eulenburg's (congenital paramyotonia) 359.2
von Gierke's (glycogenosis I) 271.0
von Graefe's 378.72
von Hippel's (retinocerebral angiomatosis) 759.6
von Hippel-Lindau (angiomatosis retinocerebellosa) 759.6
von Jaksch's (pseudoleukemia infantum) 285.8
von Recklinghausen's (M9540/1) 237.71
bone (osteitis fibrosa cystica) 252.0
von Recklinghausen-Applebaum (hemochromatosis) 275.0
von Willebrand (-Jürgens) (angiohemophilia) 286.4
von Zambusch's (lichen sclerosus et atrophicus) 701.0
Voorhoeve's (dyschondroplasia) 756.4
Vrolik's (osteogenesis imperfecta) 756.51
vulva
noninflammatory 624.9
specified NEC 624.8
Wagner's (colloid milium) 709.3
Waldenström's (osteochondrosis capital femoral) 732.1
Wallgren's (obstruction of splenic vein with collateral circulation) 459.89
Wardrop's (with lymphangitis) 681.9
finger 681.02
toe 681.11
Wassilieff's (leptospiral jaundice) 100.0
wasting NEC 799.4
due to malnutrition 261
paralysis 335.21
Waterhouse-Friderichsen 036.3
waxy (any site) 277.3
Weber-Christian (nodular nonsuppurative panniculitis) 729.30
Wegner's (syphilitic osteochondritis) 090.0
Weil's (leptospiral jaundice) 100.0
of lung 100.0
Weir Mitchell's (erythromelalgia) 443.89
Werdnig-Hoffmann 335.0
Werlhof's (*see also* Purpura, thrombocytopenic) 287.3
Wermer's 258.0
Werner's (progeria adultorum) 259.8
Werner-His (trench fever) 083.1
Werner-Schultz (agranulocytosis) 288.0
Wernicke's (superior hemorrhagic polioencephalitis) 265.1
Wernicke-Posadas 114.9
Whipple's (intestinal lipodystrophy) 040.2
whipworm 127.3
white
blood cell 288.9
specified NEC 288.8
spot 701.0

Disease, diseased—*continued*
White's (congenital) (keratosis follicularis) 757.39
Whitmore's (melioidosis) 025
Widal-Abrami (acquired hemolytic jaundice) 283.9
Wilkie's 557.1
Wilkinson-Sneddon (subcorneal pustular dermatosis) 694.1
Willis' (diabetes mellitus) (*see also* Diabetes) 250.0
Wilson's (hepatolenticular degeneration) 275.1
Wilson-Brocq (dermatitis exfoliativa) 695.89
winter vomiting 078.82
Wise's 696.2
Wohlfart-Kugelberg-Welander 335.11
Woillez's (acute idiopathic pulmonary congestion) 518.5
Wolman's (primary familial xanthomatosis) 272.7
wool-sorters' 022.1
Zagari's (xerostomia) 527.7
Zahorsky's (exanthem subitum) 057.8
Ziehen-Oppenheim 333.6
zoonotic, bacterial NEC 027.9
specified type NEC 027.8
Disfigurement (due to scar) 709.2
head V48.6
limb V49.4
neck V48.7
trunk V48.7
Disgerminoma —*see* Dysgerminoma
Disinsertion, retina 361.04
Disintegration, complete, of the body 799.8
traumatic 869.1
Disk kidney 753.3
Dislocatable hip, congenita l (*see also* Dislocation, hip, congenital) 754.30
Dislocation (articulation) (closed) (displacement) (simple) (subluxation) 839.8

Note—"Closed" includes simple, complete, partial, uncomplicated, and unspecified dislocation. "Open" includes dislocation specified as infected or compound and dislocation with foreign body. "Chronic," "habitual," "old," or "recurrent" dislocations should be coded as indicated under the entry "Dislocation, recurrent"; and "pathological" as indicated under the entry "Dislocation, pathological." For late effect of dislocation see Late, effect, dislocation.

with fracture—*see* Fracture, by site
acromioclavicular (joint) (closed) 831.04
open 831.14
anatomical site (closed)
specified NEC 839.69
open 839.79
unspecified or ill-defined 839.8
open 839.9
ankle (scaphoid bone) (closed) 837.0
open 837.1
arm (closed) 839.8
open 839.9
astragalus (closed) 837.0
open 837.1
atlanto-axial (closed) 839.01
open 839.11
atlas (closed) 839.01
open 839.11

Dislocation—*continued*
axis (closed) 839.02
open 839.12
back (closed) 839.8
open 839.9
Bell-Daly 723.8
breast bone (closed) 839.61
open 839.71
capsule, joint—*see* Dislocation, by site
carpal (bone)—*see* Dislocation, wrist
carpometacarpal (joint) (closed) 833.04
open 833.14
cartilage (joint)—*see also* Dislocation, by site
knee—*see* Tear, meniscus
cervical, cervicodorsal, or cervicothoracic (spine) (vertebra)—*see* Dislocation, vertebra, cervical
chiropractic (*see also* Lesion, nonallopathic) 739.9
chondrocostal—*see* Dislocation, costochondral
chronic—*see* Dislocation, recurrent
clavicle (closed) 831.04
open 831.14
coccyx (closed) 839.41
open 839.51
collar bone (closed) 831.04
open 831.14
compound (open) NEC 839.9
congenital NEC 755.8
hip (*see also* Dislocation, hip, congenital) 754.30
lens 743.37
rib 756.3
sacroiliac 755.69
spine NEC 756.19
vertebra 756.19
coracoid (closed) 831.09
open 831.19
costal cartilage (closed) 839.69
open 839.79
costochondral (closed) 839.69
open 839.79
cricoarytenoid articulation (closed) 839.69
open 839.79
cricothyroid (cartilage) articulation (closed) 839.69
open 839.79
dorsal vertebrae (closed) 839.21
open 839.31
ear ossicle 385.23
elbow (closed) 832.00
anterior (closed) 832.01
open 832.11
congenital 754.89
divergent (closed) 832.09
open 832.19
lateral (closed) 832.04
open 832.14
medial (closed) 832.03
open 832.13
open 832.10
posterior (closed) 832.02
open 832.12
recurrent 718.32
specified type NEC 832.09
open 832.19
eye 360.81
lateral 376.36
eyeball 360.81
lateral 376.36

Dislocation—*continued*
femur
distal end (closed) 836.50
anterior 836.52
open 836.62
lateral 836.53
open 836.63
medial 836.54
open 836.64
open 836.60
posterior 836.51
open 836.61
proximal end (closed) 835.00
anterior (pubic) 835.03
open 835.13
obturator 835.02
open 835.12
open 835.10
posterior 835.01
open 835.11
fibula
distal end (closed) 837.0
open 837.1
proximal end (closed) 836.59
open 836.69
finger(s) (phalanx) (thumb) (closed) 834.00
interphalangeal (joint) 834.02
open 834.12
metacarpal (bone), distal end 834.01
open 834.11
metacarpophalangeal (joint) 834.01
open 834.11
open 834.10
recurrent 718.34
foot (closed) 838.00
open 838.10
recurrent 718.37
forearm (closed) 839.8
open 839.9
fracture—*see* Fracture, by site
glenoid (closed) 831.09
open 831.19
habitual—*see* Dislocation, recurrent
hand (closed) 839.8
open 839.9
hip (closed) 835.00
anterior 835.03
obturator 835.02
open 835.12
open 835.13
congenital (unilateral) 754.30
with subluxation of other hip 754.35
bilateral 754.31
open 835.10
posterior 835.01
open 835.11
recurrent 718.35
humerus (closed) 831.00
distal end (*see also* Dislocation, elbow) 832.00
open 831.10
proximal end (closed) 831.00
anterior (subclavicular) (subcoracoid) (subglenoid) (closed) 831.01
open 831.11
inferior (closed) 831.03
open 831.13
open 831.10
posterior (closed) 831.02
open 831.12

Dislocation—*continued*
implant—*see* Complications, mechanical
incus 385.23
infracoracoid (closed) 831.01
open 831.11
innominate (pubic junction) (sacral junction) (closed) 839.69
acetabulum (*see also* Dislocation, hip) 835.00
open 839.79
interphalangeal (joint)
finger or hand (closed) 834.02
open 834.12
foot or toe (closed) 838.06
open 838.16
jaw (cartilage) (meniscus) (closed) 830.0
open 830.1
recurrent 524.69
joint NEC (closed) 839.8
open 839.9
pathological—*see* Dislocation, pathological
recurrent—*see* Dislocation, recurrent
knee (closed) 836.50
anterior 836.51
open 836.61
congenital (with genu recurvatum) 754.41
habitual 718.36
lateral 836.54
open 836.64
medial 836.53
open 836.63
old 718.36
open 836.60
posterior 836.52
open 836.62
recurrent 718.36
rotatory 836.59
open 836.69
lacrimal gland 375.16
leg (closed) 839.8
open 839.9
lens (crystalline) (complete) (partial) 379.32
anterior 379.33
congenital 743.37
ocular implant 996.53
posterior 379.34
traumatic 921.3
ligament—*see* Dislocation, by site
lumbar (vertebrae) (closed) 839.20
open 839.30
lumbosacral (vertebrae) (closed) 839.20
congenital 756.19
open 839.30
mandible (closed) 830.0
open 830.1
maxilla (inferior) (closed) 830.0
open 830.1
meniscus (knee)—*see also* Tear, meniscus
other sites—*see* Dislocation, by site
metacarpal (bone)
distal end (closed) 834.01
open 834.11
proximal end (closed) 833.05
open 833.15
metacarpophalangeal (joint) (closed) 834.01
open 834.11
metatarsal (bone) (closed) 838.04
open 838.14
metatarsophalangeal (joint) (closed) 838.05
open 838.15

Dislocation—*continued*
midcarpal (joint) (closed) 833.03
open 833.13
midtarsal (joint) (closed) 838.02
open 838.12
Monteggia's—*see* Dislocation, hip
multiple locations (except fingers only or toes only) (closed) 839.8
open 839.9
navicular (bone) foot (closed) 837.0
open 837.1
neck (*see also* Dislocation, vertebra, cervical) 839.00
Nélaton's—*see* Dislocation, ankle
nontraumatic (joint)—*see* Dislocation, pathological
nose (closed) 839.69
open 839.79
not recurrent, not current injury—*see* Dislocation, pathological
occiput from atlas (closed) 839.01
open 839.11
old—*see* Dislocation, recurrent
open (compound) NEC 839.9
ossicle, ear 385.23
paralytic (flaccid) (spastic)—*see* Dislocation, pathological
patella (closed) 836.3
congenital 755.64
open 836.4
pathological NEC 718.20
ankle 718.27
elbow 718.22
foot 718.27
hand 718.24
hip 718.25
knee 718.26
lumbosacral joint 724.6
multiple sites 718.29
pelvic region 718.25
sacroiliac 724.6
shoulder (region) 718.21
specified site NEC 718.28
spine 724.8
sacroiliac 724.6
wrist 718.23
pelvis (closed) 839.69
acetabulum (*see also* Dislocation, hip) 835.00
open 839.79
phalanx
foot or toe (closed) 838.09
open 838.19
hand or finger (*see also* Dislocation, finger) 834.00
postpoliomyelitic—*see* Dislocation, pathological
prosthesis, internal—*see* Complications, mechanical
radiocarpal (joint) (closed) 833.02
open 833.12
radioulnar (joint)
distal end (closed) 833.01
open 833.11
proximal end (*see also* Dislocation, elbow) 832.00

Dislocation—*continued*
radius
distal end (closed) 833.00
open 833.10
proximal end (closed) 832.01
open 832.11
recurrent (*see also* Derangement, joint, recurrent) 718.3
elbow 718.32
hip 718.35
joint NEC 718.38
knee 718.36
lumbosacral (joint) 724.6
patella 718.36
sacroiliac 724.6
shoulder 718.31
temporomandibular 524.69
rib (cartilage) (closed) 839.69
congenital 756.3
open 839.79
sacrococcygeal (closed) 839.42
open 839.52
sacroiliac (joint) (ligament) (closed) 839.42
congenital 755.69
open 839.52
recurrent 724.6
sacrum (closed) 839.42
open 839.52
scaphoid (bone)
ankle or foot (closed) 837.0
open 837.1
wrist (closed) (*see also* Dislocation, wrist) 833.00
open 833.10
scapula (closed) 831.09
open 831.19
semilunar cartilage, knee—*see* Tear, meniscus
septal cartilage (nose) (closed) 839.69
open 839.79
septum (nasal) (old) 470
sesamoid bone—*see* Dislocation, by site
shoulder (blade) (ligament) (closed) 831.00
anterior (subclavicular) (subcoracoid) (subglenoid) (closed) 831.01
open 831.11
chronic 718.31
inferior 831.03
open 831.13
open 831.10
posterior (closed) 831.02
open 831.12
recurrent 718.31
skull—*see* Injury, intracranial
Smith's—*see* Dislocation, foot
spine (articular process) (*see also* Dislocation, vertebra) (closed) 839.40
atlanto-axial (closed) 839.01
open 839.11
recurrent 723.8
cervical, cervicodorsal, cervicothoracic (closed) (*see also* Dislocation, vertebrae, cervical) 839.00
open 839.10
recurrent 723.8
coccyx 839.41
open 839.51
congenital 756.19
due to birth trauma 767.4
open 839.50

Dislocation—*continued*
recurrent 724.9
sacroiliac 839.42
recurrent 724.6
sacrum (sacrococcygeal) (sacroiliac) 839.42
open 839.52
spontaneous—*see* Dislocation, pathological
sternoclavicular (joint) (closed) 839.61
open 839.71
sternum (closed) 839.61
open 839.71
subastragalar—*see* Dislocation, foot
subglenoid (closed) 831.01
open 831.11
symphysis
jaw (closed) 830.0
open 830.1
mandibular (closed) 830.0
open 830.1
pubis (closed) 839.69
open 839.79
tarsal (bone) (joint) 838.01
open 838.11
tarsometatarsal (joint) 838.03
open 838.13
temporomandibular (joint) (closed) 830.0
open 830.1
recurrent 524.69
thigh
distal end (*see also* Dislocation, femur, distal end) 836.50
proximal end (*see also* Dislocation, hip) 835.00
thoracic (vertebrae) (closed) 839.21
open 839.31
thumb(s) (*see also* Dislocation, finger) 834.00
thyroid cartilage (closed) 839.69
open 839.79
tibia
distal end (closed) 837.0
open 837.1
proximal end (closed) 836.50
anterior 836.51
open 836.61
lateral 836.54
open 836.64
medial 836.53
open 836.63
open 836.60
posterior 836.52
open 836.62
rotatory 836.59
open 836.69
tibiofibular
distal (closed) 837.0
open 837.1
superior (closed) 836.59
open 836.69
toe(s) (closed) 838.09
open 838.19
trachea (closed) 839.69
open 839.79
ulna
distal end (closed) 833.09
open 833.19
proximal end—*see* Dislocation, elbow

Dislocation—*continued*
vertebra (articular process) (body) (closed) 839.40
cervical, cervicodorsal or cervicothoracic (closed) 839.00
first (atlas) 839.01
open 839.11
second (axis) 839.02
open 839.12
third 839.03
open 839.13
fourth 839.04
open 839.14
fifth 839.05
open 839.15
sixth 839.06
open 839.16
seventh 839.07
open 839.17
congenital 756.19
multiple sites 839.08
open 839.18
open 839.10
congenital 756.19
dorsal 839.21
open 839.31
recurrent 724.9
lumbar, lumbosacral 839.20
open 839.30
open NEC 839.50
recurrent 724.9
specified region NEC 839.49
open 839.59
thoracic 839.21
open 839.31
wrist (carpal bone) (scaphoid) (semilunar) (closed) 833.00
carpometacarpal (joint) 833.04
open 833.14
metacarpal bone, proximal end 833.05
open 833.15
midcarpal (joint) 833.03
open 833.13
open 833.10
radiocarpal (joint) 833.02
open 833.12
radioulnar (joint) 833.01
open 833.11
recurrent 718.33
specified site NEC 833.09
open 833.19
xiphoid cartilage (closed) 839.61
open 839.71
Disobedience, hostile (covert) (overt) (*see also* Disturbance, conduct) 312.0
Disorder —*see also* Disease
academic underachievement, childhood and adolescence 313.83
accommodation 367.51
drug-induced 367.89
toxic 367.89
adjustment (*see also* Reaction, adjustment) 309.9
adrenal (capsule) (cortex) (gland) 255.9
specified type NEC 255.8
adrenogenital 255.2
affective (*see also* Psychosis, affective) 296.90
atypical 296.81
aggressive, unsocialized (*see also* Disturbance, conduct) 312.0

Disorder—*continued*
alcohol, alcoholic (*see also* Alcohol) 291.9
allergic—*see* Allergy
amino acid (metabolic) (*see also* Disturbance, metabolism, amino acid) 270.9
albinism 270.2
alkaptonuria 270.2
argininosuccinicaciduria 270.6
beta-amino-isobutyricaciduria 277.2
cystathioninuria 270.4
cystinosis 270.0
cystinuria 270.0
glycinuria 270.0
homocystinuria 270.4
imidazole 270.5
maple syrup (urine) disease 270.3
neonatal, transitory 775.8
oasthouse urine disease 270.2
ochronosis 270.2
phenylketonuria 270.1
phenylpyruvic oligophrenia 270.1
purine NEC 277.2
pyrimidine NEC 277.2
renal transport NEC 270.0
specified type NEC 270.8
transport NEC 270.0
renal 270.0
xanthinuria 277.2
amnestic (*see also* Amnestic syndrome) 294.0
anaerobic glycolysis with anemia 282.3
anxiety (*see also* Anxiety) 300.00
arteriole 447.9
specified type NEC 447.8
artery 447.9
specified type NEC 447.8
articulation—*see* Disorder, joint
Asperger's 299.8
attachment of infancy 313.89
attention deficit 314.00
with hyperactivity 314.01
predominantly
combined hyperactive/inattentive 314.01
hyperactive/impulsive 314.01
inattentive 314.00
residual type 314.8
autistic 299.0
autoimmune NEC 279.4
hemolytic (cold type) (warm type) 283.0
parathyroid 252.1
thyroid 245.2
avoidant, childhood or adolescence 313.21
balance
acid-base 276.9
mixed (with hypercapnia) 276.4
electrolyte 276.9
fluid 276.9
behavior NEC (*see also* Disturbance, conduct) 312.9
bilirubin excretion 277.4
bipolar (affective) (alternating) (Type I) (*see also* Psychosis, affective) 296.7
atypical 296.7
currently
depressed 296.5
hypomanic 296.4
manic 296.4
mixed 296.6
Type II (recurrent major depressive episodes with hypomania) 296.89

Disorder—*continued*
bladder 596.9
functional NEC 596.59
specified NEC 596.8
bone NEC 733.90
specified NEC 733.99
brachial plexus 353.0
branched-chain amino-acid degradation 270.3
breast 611.9
puerperal, postpartum 676.3
specified NEC 611.8
Briquet's 300.81
bursa 727.9
shoulder region 726.10
carbohydrate metabolism, congenital 271.9
cardiac, functional 427.9
postoperative 997.1
psychogenic 306.2
cardiovascular, psychogenic 306.2
cartilage NEC 733.90
articular 718.00
ankle 718.07
elbow 718.02
foot 718.07
hand 718.04
hip 718.05
knee 717.9
multiple sites 718.09
pelvic region 718.05
shoulder region 718.01
specified
site NEC 718.08
type NEC 733.99
wrist 718.03
cervical region NEC 723.9
cervical root (nerve) NEC 353.2
character NEC (*see also* Disorder, personality) 301.9
coagulation (factor) (*see also* Defect, coagulation) 286.9
factor VIII (congenital) (functional) 286.0
factor IX (congenital) (functional) 286.1
neonatal, transitory 776.3
coccyx 724.70
specified NEC 724.79
cognitive 294.9
colon 569.9
functional 564.9
congenital 751.3
conduct (*see also* Disturbance, conduct) 312.9
adjustment reaction 309.3
adolescent onset type 312.82
childhood onset type 312.81
compulsive 312.30
specified type NEC 312.39
hyperkinetic 314.2
socialized (type) 312.20
aggressive 312.23
unaggressive 312.21
specified NEC 312.89
conduction, heart 426.9
specified NEC 426.89
convulsive (secondary) (*see also* Convulsions) 780.3
due to injury at birth 767.0
idiopathic 780.3
coordination 781.3
cornea NEC 371.89
due to contact lens 371.82
corticosteroid metabolism NEC 255.2
cranial nerve—*see* Disorder, nerve, cranial

Disorder—*continued*
cyclothymic 301.13
degradation, branched-chain amino acid 270.3
dentition 520.6
depressive NEC 311
atypical 296.82
major (*see also* Psychosis, affective) 296.2
recurrent episode 296.3
single episode 296.2
development, specific 315.9
associated with hyperkinesia 314.1
language 315.31
learning 315.2
arithmetical 315.1
reading 315.00
mixed 315.5
motor coordination 315.4
specified type NEC 315.8
speech 315.39
diaphragm 519.4
digestive 536.9
fetus or newborn 777.9
specified NEC 777.8
psychogenic 306.4
disintegrative (childhood) 299.1
dissociative 300.14
identity 300.14
dysmorphic body 300.7
dysthymic 300.4
ear 388.9
degenerative NEC 388.00
external 380.9
specified 380.89
pinna 380.30
specified type NEC 388.8
vascular NEC 388.00
eating NEC 307.50
electrolyte NEC 276.9
with
abortion—*see* Abortion, by type, with metabolic disorder
ectopic pregnancy (*see also* categories 633.0-633.9) 639.4
molar pregnancy (*see also* categories 630-632) 639.4
acidosis 276.2
metabolic 276.2
respiratory 276.2
alkalosis 276.3
metabolic 276.3
respiratory 276.3
following
abortion 639.4
ectopic or molar pregnancy 639.4
neonatal, transitory NEC 775.5
emancipation as adjustment reaction 309.22
emotional (*see also* Disorder, mental, nonpsychotic) V40.9
endocrine 259.9
specified type NEC 259.8
esophagus 530.9
functional 530.5
psychogenic 306.4
explosive
intermittent 312.34
isolated 312.35
eye 379.90
globe—*see* Disorder, globe
ill-defined NEC 379.99
limited duction NEC 378.63
specified NEC 379.8

Disorder—*continued*
eyelid 374.9
degenerative 374.50
sensory 374.44
specified type NEC 374.89
vascular 374.85
factitious —*see* Illness, factitious
factor, coagulation (*see also* Defect, coagulation) 286.9
VIII (congenital) (functional) 286.0
IX (congenital) (functional) 286.1
fascia 728.9
feeding —*see* Feeding
female sexual arousal 302.72
fluid NEC 276.9
gastric (functional) 536.9
motility 536.8
psychogenic 306.4
secretion 536.8
gastrointestinal (functional) NEC 536.9
newborn (neonatal) 777.9
specified NEC 777.8
psychogenic 306.4
gender (child) 302.6
adult 302.85
gender identity (childhood) 302.6
adult-life 302.85
genitourinary system, psychogenic 306.50
globe 360.9
degenerative 360.20
specified NEC 360.29
specified type NEC 360.89
hearing—*see also* Deafness
conductive type (air) (*see also* Deafness, conductive) 389.00
mixed conductive and sensorineural 389.2
nerve 389.12
perceptive (*see also* Deafness, perceptive) 389.10
sensorineural type NEC (*see also* Deafness, perceptive) 389.10
heart action 427.9
postoperative 997.1
hematological, transient neonatal 776.9
specified type NEC 776.8
hematopoietic organs 289.9
hemorrhagic NEC 287.9
due to circulating anticoagulants 286.5
specified type NEC 287.8
hemostasis (*see also* Defect, coagulation) 286.9
homosexual conflict 302.0
hypomanic (chronic) 301.11
identity
childhood and adolescence 313.82
gender 302.6
gender 302.6
immune mechanism (immunity) 279.9
single complement (C_1-C_9) 279.8
specified type NEC 279.8
impulse control (*see also* Disturbance, conduct, compulsive) 312.30
integument, fetus or newborn 778.9
specified type NEC 778.8
interactional psychotic (childhood) (*see also* Psychosis, childhood) 299.1
intermittent explosive 312.34
intervertebral disc 722.90
cervical, cervicothoracic 722.91
lumbar, lumbosacral 722.93
thoracic, thoracolumbar 722.92

Disorder—*continued*
intestinal 569.9
functional NEC 564.9
congenital 751.3
postoperative 564.4
psychogenic 306.4
introverted, of childhood and adolescence 313.22
iron, metabolism 275.0
isolated explosive 312.35
joint NEC 719.90
ankle 719.97
elbow 719.92
foot 719.97
hand 719.94
hip 719.95
knee 719.96
multiple sites 719.99
pelvic region 719.95
psychogenic 306.0
shoulder (region) 719.91
specified site NEC 719.98
temporomandibular 524.60
specified NEC 524.69
wrist 719.93
kidney 593.9
functional 588.9
specified NEC 588.8
labyrinth, labyrinthine 386.9
specified type NEC 386.8
lactation 676.9
ligament 728.9
ligamentous attachments, peripheral—*see also* Enthesopathy
spine 720.1
limb NEC 729.9
psychogenic 306.0
lipid
metabolism, congenital 272.9
storage 272.7
lipoprotein deficiency (familial) 272.5
low back NEC 724.9
psychogenic 306.0
lumbosacral
plexus 353.1
root (nerve) NEC 353.4
lymphoproliferative (chronic) NEC (M9970/1) 238.7
major depressive (*see also* Psychosis, affective) 296.2
recurrent episode 296.3
single episode 296.2
male erectile 302.72
organic origin 607.84
manic (*see also* Psychosis, affective) 296.0
atypical 296.81
meniscus NEC (*see also* Disorder, cartilage, articular) 718.0
menopausal 627.9
specified NEC 627.8
menstrual 626.9
psychogenic 306.52
specified NEC 626.8
mental (nonpsychotic) 300.9
affecting management of pregnancy, childbirth, or puerperium 648.4
drug-induced 292.9
hallucinogen persistent perception 292.89
specified type NEC 292.89

Disorder—*continued*
due to or associated with
alcoholism 291.9
drug consumption NEC 292.9
specified type NEC 292.89
induced by drug 292.9
specified type NEC 292.89
neurotic (*see also* Neurosis) 300.9
presenile 310.1
psychotic NEC 290.10
previous, affecting management of pregnancy V23.8
psychoneurotic (*see also* Neurosis) 300.9
psychotic (*see also* Psychosis) 298.9
senile 290.20
specific, following organic brain damage 310.9
cognitive or personality change of other type 310.1
frontal lobe syndrome 310.0
postconcussional syndrome 310.2
specified type NEC 310.8
metabolism NEC 277.9
with
abortion—*see* Abortion, by type, with metabolic disorder
ectopic pregnancy (*see also* categories 633.0-633.9) 639.4
molar pregnancy (*see also* categories 630-632) 639.4
alkaptonuria 270.2
amino acid (*see also* Disorder, amino acid) 270.9
specified type NEC 270.8
ammonia 270.6
arginine 270.6
argininosuccinic acid 270.6
basal 794.7
bilirubin 277.4
calcium 275.4
carbohydrate 271.9
specified type NEC 271.8
cholesterol 272.9
citrulline 270.6
copper 275.1
corticosteroid 255.2
cystine storage 270.0
cystinuria 270.0
fat 272.9
following
abortion 639.4
ectopic or molar pregnancy 639.4
fructosemia 271.2
fructosuria 271.2
fucosidosis 271.8
galactose-1-phosphate uridyl transferase 271.1
glutamine 270.7
glycine 270.7
glycogen storage NEC 271.0
hepatorenal 271.0
hemochromatosis 275.0
in labor and delivery 669.0
iron 275.0
lactose 271.3
lipid 272.9
specified type NEC 272.8
storage 272.7
lipoprotein—*see also* Hyperlipemia
deficiency (familial) 272.5
lysine 270.7
magnesium 275.2

Disorder—*continued*
mannosidosis 271.8
mineral 275.9
specified type NEC 275.8
mucopolysaccharide 277.5
nitrogen 270.9
ornithine 270.6
oxalosis 271.8
pentosuria 271.8
phenylketonuria 270.1
phosphate 275.3
phosphorus 275.3
plasma protein 273.9
specified type NEC 273.8
porphyrin 277.1
purine 277.2
pyrimidine 277.2
serine 270.7
sodium 276.9
specified type NEC 277.8
steroid 255.2
threonine 270.7
urea cycle 270.6
xylose 271.8
micturition NEC 788.69
psychogenic 306.53
misery and unhappiness, of childhood and adolescence 313.1
motor tic 307.20
chronic 307.22
transient, childhood 307.21
movement NEC 333.90
hysterical 300.11
specified type NEC 333.99
stereotypic 307.3
mucopolysaccharide 277.5
muscle 728.9
psychogenic 306.0
specified type NEC 728.3
muscular attachments, peripheral—*see also* Enthesopathy
spine 720.1
musculoskeletal system NEC 729.9
psychogenic 306.0
myeloproliferative (chronic) NEC (M9960/1) 238.7
myoneural 358.9
due to lead 358.2
specified type NEC 358.8
toxic 358.2
myotonic 359.2
neck region NEC 723.9
nerve 349.9
abducens NEC 378.54
accessory 352.4
acoustic 388.5
auditory 388.5
auriculotemporal 350.8
axillary 353.0
cerebral—*see* Disorder, nerve, cranial
cranial 352.9
first 352.0
second 377.49
third
partial 378.51
total 378.52
fourth 378.53
fifth 350.9
sixth 378.54
seventh NEC 351.9

Disorder—*continued*
eighth 388.5
ninth 352.2
tenth 352.3
eleventh 352.4
twelfth 352.5
multiple 352.6
entrapment—*see* Neuropathy, entrapment
facial 351.9
specified NEC 351.8
femoral 355.2
glossopharyngeal NEC 352.2
hypoglossal 352.5
iliohypogastric 355.79
ilioinguinal 355.79
intercostal 353.8
lateral
cutaneous of thigh 355.1
popliteal 355.3
lower limb NEC 355.8
medial, popliteal 355.4
median NEC 354.1
obturator 355.79
oculomotor
partial 378.51
total 378.52
olfactory 352.0
optic 377.49
ischemic 377.41
nutritional 377.33
toxic 377.34
peroneal 355.3
phrenic 354.8
plantar 355.6
pneumogastric 352.3
posterior tibial 355.5
radial 354.3
recurrent laryngeal 352.3
root 353.9
specified NEC 353.8
saphenous 355.79
sciatic NEC 355.0
specified NEC 355.9
lower limb 355.79
upper limb 354.8
spinal 355.9
sympathetic NEC 337.9
trigeminal 350.9
specified NEC 350.8
trochlear 378.53
ulnar 354.2
upper limb NEC 354.9
vagus 352.3
nervous system NEC 349.9
autonomic (peripheral) (*see also* Neuropathy, peripheral, autonomic) 337.9
cranial 352.9
parasympathetic (*see also* Neuropathy, peripheral, autonomic) 337.9
specified type NEC 349.89
sympathetic (*see also* Neuropathy, peripheral, autonomic) 337.9
vegetative (*see also* Neuropathy, peripheral, autonomic) 337.9
neurohypophysis NEC 253.6
neurological NEC 781.9
peripheral NEC 355.9
neuromuscular NEC 358.9
hereditary NEC 359.1
specified NEC 358.8
toxic 358.2

Disorder—*continued*
neurotic 300.9
specified type NEC 300.89
neutrophil, polymorphonuclear (functional) 288.1
obsessive-compulsive 300.3
oppositional, childhood and adolescence 313.81
optic
chiasm 377.54
associated with
inflammatory disorders 377.54
neoplasm NEC 377.52
pituitary 377.51
pituitary disorders 377.51
vascular disorders 377.53
nerve 377.49
radiations 377.63
tracts 377.63
orbit 376.9
specified NEC 376.89
overanxious, of childhood and adolescence 313.0
pancreas, internal secretion (other than diabetes mellitus) 251.9
specified type NEC 251.8
panic 300.01
with agoraphobia 300.21
papillary muscle NEC 429.81
paranoid 297.9
induced 297.3
shared 297.3
parathyroid 252.9
specified type NEC 252.8
paroxysmal, mixed 780.3
pentose phosphate pathway with anemia 282.2
personality 301.9
affective 301.10
aggressive 301.3
amoral 301.7
anancastic, anankastic 301.4
antisocial 301.7
asocial 301.7
asthenic 301.6
borderline 301.83
compulsive 301.4
cyclothymic 301.13
dependent-passive 301.6
dyssocial 301.7
emotional instability 301.59
epileptoid 301.3
explosive 301.3
following organic brain damage 310.1
histrionic 301.50
hyperthymic 301.11
hypomanic (chronic) 301.11
hypothymic 301.12
hysterical 301.50
immature 301.89
inadequate 301.6
introverted 301.21
labile 301.59
moral deficiency 301.7
obsessional 301.4
obsessive (-compulsive) 301.4
overconscientious 301.4
paranoid 301.0
passive (-dependent) 301.6
passive-aggressive 301.84
pathological NEC 301.9
pseudosocial 301.7

Disorder—*continued*
psychopathic 301.9
schizoid 301.20
introverted 301.21
schizotypal 301.22
schizotypal 301.22
seductive 301.59
type A 301.4
unstable 301.59
pervasive developmental, childhood-onset 299.8
pigmentation, choroid (congenital) 743.53
pinna 380.30
specified type NEC 380.39
pituitary, thalamic 253.9
anterior NEC 253.4
iatrogenic 253.7
postablative 253.7
specified NEC 253.8
pityriasis-like NEC 696.8
platelets (blood) 287.1
polymorphonuclear neutrophils (functional) 288.1
porphyrin metabolism 277.1
postmenopausal 627.9
specified type NEC 627.8
posttraumatic stress 309.81
acute 308.3
brief 308.3
chronic 309.81
psoriatic-like NEC 696.8
psychic, with diseases classified elsewhere 316
psychogenic NEC (*see also* condition) 300.9
allergic NEC
respiratory 306.1
anxiety 300.00
atypical 300.00
generalized 300.02
appetite 307.50
articulation, joint 306.0
asthenic 300.5
blood 306.8
cardiovascular (system) 306.2
compulsive 300.3
cutaneous 306.3
depressive 300.4
digestive (system) 306.4
dysmenorrheic 306.52
dyspneic 306.1
eczematous 306.3
endocrine (system) 306.6
eye 306.7
feeding 307.59
functional NEC 306.9
gastric 306.4
gastrointestinal (system) 306.4
genitourinary (system) 306.50
heart (function) (rhythm) 306.2
hemic 306.8
hyperventilatory 306.1
hypochondriacal 300.7
hysterical 300.10
intestinal 306.4
joint 306.0
learning 315.2
limb 306.0
lymphatic (system) 306.8
menstrual 306.52
micturition 306.53
monoplegic NEC 306.0
motor 307.9
muscle 306.0

Disorder—*continued*
musculoskeletal 306.0
neurocirculatory 306.2
obsessive 300.3
occupational 300.89
organ or part of body NEC 306.9
organs of special sense 306.7
paralytic NEC 306.0
phobic 300.20
physical NEC 306.9
pruritic 306.3
rectal 306.4
respiratory (system) 306.1
rheumatic 306.0
sexual (function) 302.70
specified type NEC 302.79
skin (allergic) (eczematous) (pruritic) 306.3
sleep 307.40
initiation or maintenance 307.41
persistent 307.42
transient 307.41
specified type NEC 307.49
specified part of body NEC 306.8
stomach 306.4
psychomotor NEC 307.9
hysterical 300.11
psychoneurotic (*see also* Neurosis) 300.9
mixed NEC 300.89
psychophysiologic (*see also* Disorder, psychosomatic) 306.9
psychosexual identity (childhood) 302.6
adult-life 302.85
psychosomatic NEC 306.9
allergic NEC
respiratory 306.1
articulation, joint 306.0
cardiovascular (system) 306.2
cutaneous 306.3
digestive (system) 306.4
dysmenorrheic 306.52
dyspneic 306.1
endocrine (system) 306.6
eye 306.7
gastric 306.4
gastrointestinal (system) 306.4
genitourinary (system) 306.50
heart (functional) (rhythm) 306.2
hyperventilatory 306.1
intestinal 306.4
joint 306.0
limb 306.0
lymphatic (system) 306.8
menstrual 306.52
micturition 306.53
monoplegic NEC 306.0
muscle 306.0
musculoskeletal 306.0
neurocirculatory 306.2
organs of special sense 306.7
paralytic NEC 306.0
pruritic 306.3
rectal 306.4
respiratory (system) 306.1
rheumatic 306.0
sexual (function) 302.70
specified type NEC 302.79
skin 306.3
specified part of body NEC 306.8
stomach 306.4
purine metabolism NEC 277.2

Disorder—*continued*
pyrimidine metabolism NEC 277.2
reactive attachment (of infancy or early childhood) 313.89
reading, developmental 315.00
reflex 796.1
renal function, impaired 588.9
specified type NEC 588.8
renal transport NEC 588.8
respiration, respiratory NEC 519.9
due to
aspiration of liquids or solids 508.9
inhalation of fumes or vapors 506.9
psychogenic 306.1
retina 362.9
specified type NEC 362.89
sacroiliac joint NEC 724.6
sacrum 724.6
schizo-affective (*see also* Schizophrenia) 295.7
schizoid, childhood or adolescence 313.22
schizophreniform 295.4
schizotypal personality 301.22
secretion, thyrocalcitonin 246.0
seizure 780.3
recurrent 780.3
epileptic—*see* Epilepsy
sense of smell 781.1
psychogenic 306.7
separation anxiety 309.21
sexual (*see also* Deviation, sexual) 302.9
function, psychogenic 302.70
shyness, of childhood and adolescence 313.21
single complement (C_1-C_9) 279.8
skin NEC 709.9
fetus or newborn 778.9
specified type 778.8
psychogenic (allergic) (eczematous) (pruritic) 306.3
specified type NEC 709.8
vascular 709.1
sleep 780.50
circadian rhythm 307.45
initiation or maintenance (*see also* Insomnia) 780.52
nonorganic origin (transient) 307.41
persistent 307.42
nonorganic origin 307.40
specified type NEC 307.49
specified NEC 780.59
with apnea—*see* Apnea, sleep
social, of childhood and adolescence 313.22
specified NEC 780.59
soft tissue 729.9
somatization 300.81
somatoform 300.81
atypical 300.7
speech NEC 784.5
nonorganic origin 307.9
spine NEC 724.9
ligamentous or muscular attachments, peripheral 720.1
steroid metabolism NEC 255.2
stomach (functional) (*see also* Disorder, gastric) 536.9
psychogenic 306.4
storage, iron 275.0
stress (*see also* Reaction, stress, acute) 308.9
posttraumatic
acute 308.3
brief 308.3
chronic 309.81

Disorder—*continued*
substitution 300.11
suspected—*see* Observation
synovium 727.9
temperature regulation, fetus or newborn 778.4
temporomandibular joint NEC 524.60
specified NEC 524.69
tendon 727.9
shoulder region 726.10
thoracic root (nerve) NEC 353.3
thyrocalcitonin secretion 246.0
thyroid (gland) NEC 246.9
specified type NEC 246.8
tic 307.20
chronic (motor or vocal) 307.22
motor-verbal 307.23
organic origin 333.1
transient of childhood 307.21
tooth NEC 525.9
development NEC 520.9
specified type NEC 520.8
eruption 520.6
with abnormal position 524.3
specified type NEC 525.8
transport, carbohydrate 271.9
specified type NEC 271.8
tubular, phosphate-losing 588.0
tympanic membrane 384.9
unaggressive, unsocialized (*see also* Disturbance, conduct) 312.1
undersocialized, unsocialized—*see also* Disturbance, conduct
aggressive (type) 312.0
unaggressive (type) 312.1
vision, visual NEC 368.9
binocular NEC 368.30
cortex 377.73
associated with
inflammatory disorders 377.73
neoplasms 377.71
vascular disorders 377.72
pathway NEC 377.63
associated with
inflammatory disorders 377.63
neoplasms 377.61
vascular disorders 377.62
wakefulness (*see also* Hypersomnia) 780.54
nonorganic origin (transient) 307.43
persistent 307.44
Disorganized globe 360.29
Displacement, displaced

Note—For acquired displacement of bones,cartilage, joints, tendons, due to injury, see also Dislocation. Displacements at ages under one year should be considered congenital, provided there is no indication the condition was acquired after birth.

acquired traumatic of bond, cartilage, joint, tendon NEC (without fracture) (*see also* Dislocation) 839.8
with fracture—*see* Fracture, by site
adrenal gland (congenital) 759.1
appendix, retrocecal (congenital) 751.5
auricle (congenital) 744.29
bladder (acquired) 596.8
congenital 753.8
brachial plexus (congenital) 742.8
brain stem, caudal 742.4
canaliculus lacrimalis 743.65

Displacement, displaced—*continued*
cardia, through esophageal hiatus 750.6
cerebellum, caudal 742.4
cervix (*see also* Malposition, uterus) 621.6
colon (congenital) 751.4
device, implant, or graft—*see* Complications, mechanical
epithelium
columnar of cervix 622.1
cuboidal, beyond limits of external os (uterus) 752.49
esophageal mucosa into cardia of stomach, congenital 750.4
esophagus (acquired) 530.89
congenital 750.4
eyeball (acquired) (old) 376.36
congenital 743.8
current injury 871.3
lateral 376.36
fallopian tube (acquired) 620.4
congenital 752.19
opening (congenital) 752.19
gallbladder (congenital) 751.69
gastric mucosa 750.7
into
duodenum 750.7
esophagus 750.7
Meckel's diverticulum, congenital 750.7
globe (acquired) (lateral) (old) 376.36
current injury 871.3
heart (congenital) 746.87
acquired 429.89
hymen (congenital) (upward) 752.49
internal prosthesis NEC—*see* Complications, mechanical
intervertebral disc (with neuritis, radiculitis, sciatica, or other pain) 722.2
with myelopathy 722.70
cervical, cervicodorsal, cervicothoracic 722.0
with myelopathy 722.71
due to major trauma—*see* Dislocation, vertebra, cervical
due to major trauma—*see* Dislocation, vertebra
lumbar, lumbosacral 722.10
with myelopathy 722.73
due to major trauma—*see* Dislocation, vertebra, lumbar
thoracic, thoracolumbar 722.11
with myelopathy 722.72
due to major trauma—*see* Dislocation, vertebra, thoracic
intrauterine device 996.32
kidney (acquired) 593.0
congenital 753.3
lacrimal apparatus or duct (congenital) 743.65
macula (congenital) 743.55
Meckel's diverticulum (congenital) 751.0
nail (congenital) 757.5
acquired 703.8
opening of Wharton's duct in mouth 750.26
organ or site, congenital NEC—*see* Malposition, congenital
ovary (acquired) 620.4
congenital 752.0
free in peritoneal cavity (congenital) 752.0
into hernial sac 620.4
oviduct (acquired) 620.4
congenital 752.19

Distention—*continued*
  ureter 593.5
  uterus 621.8
Distichia, distichiasis (eyelid) 743.63
Distoma hepaticum infestation 121.3
Distomiasis 121.9
  bile passages 121.3
    due to Clonorchis sinensis 121.1
  hemic 120.9
  hepatic (liver) 121.3
    due to Clonorchis sinensis (clonorchiasis) 121.1
  intestinal 121.4
  liver 121.3
    due to Clonorchis sinensis 121.1
  lung 121.2
  pulmonary 121.2
Distomolar (fourth molar) 520.1
  causing crowding 524.3
Disto-occlusion 524.2
Distortion (congenital)
  adrenal (gland) 759.1
  ankle (joint) 755.69
  anus 751.5
  aorta 747.29
  appendix 751.5
  arm 755.59
  artery (peripheral) NEC (*see also* Distortion, peripheral vascular system) 747.60
    cerebral 747.81
    coronary 746.85
    pulmonary 747.3
    retinal 743.58
    umbilical 747.5
  auditory canal 744.29
    causing impairment of hearing 744.02
  bile duct or passage 751.69
  bladder 753.8
  brain 742.4
  bronchus 748.3
  cecum 751.5
  cervix (uteri) 752.49
  chest (wall) 756.3
  clavicle 755.51
  clitoris 752.49
  coccyx 756.19
  colon 751.5
  common duct 751.69
  cornea 743.41
  cricoid cartilage 748.3
  cystic duct 751.69
  duodenum 751.5
  ear 744.29
    auricle 744.29
      causing impairment of hearing 744.02
    causing impairment of hearing 744.09
    external 744.29
      causing impairment of hearing 744.02
    inner 744.05
    middle, except ossicles 744.03
      ossicles 744.04
    ossicles 744.04
  endocrine (gland) NEC 759.2
  epiglottis 748.3
  Eustachian tube 744.24
  eye 743.8
    adnexa 743.69
  face bone(s) 756.0
  fallopian tube 752.19
  femur 755.69

Distortion—*continued*
  fibula 755.69
  finger(s) 755.59
  foot 755.67
  gallbladder 751.69
  genitalia, genital organ(s)
    female 752.8
      external 752.49
      internal NEC 752.8
    male 752.8
  glottis 748.3
  gyri 742.4
  hand bone(s) 755.59
  heart (auricle) (ventricle) 746.89
    valve (cusp) 746.89
  hepatic duct 751.69
  humerus 755.59
  hymen 752.49
  ileum 751.5
  intestine (large) (small) 751.5
    with anomalous adhesions, fixation or malrotation 751.4
  jaw NEC 524.8
  jejunum 751.5
  kidney 753.3
  knee (joint) 755.64
  labium (majus) (minus) 752.49
  larynx 748.3
  leg 755.69
  lens 743.36
  liver 751.69
  lumbar spine 756.19
    with disproportion (fetopelvic) 653.0
      affecting fetus or newborn 763.1
      causing obstructed labor 660.1
  lumbosacral (joint) (region) 756.19
  lung (fissures) (lobe) 748.69
  nerve 742.8
  nose 748.1
  organ
    of Corti 744.05
    or site not listed—*see* Anomaly, specified type NEC
  ossicles, ear 744.04
  ovary 752.0
  oviduct 752.19
  pancreas 751.7
  parathyroid (gland) 759.2
  patella 755.64
  peripheral vascular system NEC 747.60
    gastrointestinal 747.61
    lower limb 747.64
    renal 747.62
    spinal 747.82
    upper limb 747.63
  pituitary (gland) 759.2
  radius 755.59
  rectum 751.5
  rib 756.3
  sacroiliac joint 755.69
  sacrum 756.19
  scapula 755.59
  shoulder girdle 755.59
  site not listed—*see* Anomaly, specified type NEC

Distortion—*continued*
skull bone(s) 756.0
with
anencephalus 740.0
encephalocele 742.0
hydrocephalus 742.3
with spina bifida (*see also* Spina bifida) 741.0
microcephalus 742.1
spinal cord 742.59
spine 756.19
spleen 759.0
sternum 756.3
thorax (wall) 756.3
thymus (gland) 759.2
thyroid (gland) 759.2
cartilage 748.3
tibia 755.69
toe(s) 755.66
tongue 750.19
trachea (cartilage) 748.3
ulna 755.59
ureter 753.4
causing obstruction 753.2
urethra 753.8
causing obstruction 753.6
uterus 752.3
vagina 752.49
vein (peripheral) NEC (*see also* Distortion, peripheral vascular system) 747.60
great 747.49
portal 747.49
pulmonary 747.49
vena cava (inferior) (superior) 747.49
vertebra 756.19
visual NEC 368.15
shape or size 368.14
vulva 752.49
wrist (bones) (joint) 755.59
Distress
abdomen 789.0
colon 789.0
emotional V40.9
epigastric 789.0
fetal (syndrome) 768.4
affecting management of pregnancy or childbirth 656.3
liveborn infant 768.4
first noted
before onset of labor 768.2
during labor or delivery 768.3
stillborn infant (death before onset of labor) 768.0
death during labor 768.1
gastrointestinal (functional) 536.9
psychogenic 306.4
intestinal (functional) NEC 564.9
psychogenic 306.4
intrauterine (*see also* Distress, fetal) 768.4
leg 729.5
maternal 669.0
mental V40.9
respiratory 786.09
acute (adult) 518.82
adult syndrome (following shock, surgery, or trauma) 518.5
specified NEC 518.82
fetus or newborn 770.8
syndrome (idiopathic) (newborn) 769
stomach 536.9
psychogenic 306.4
Distribution vessel, atypical NEC 747.60
coronary artery 746.85
spinal 747.82
Districhiasis 704.2
Disturbance —*see also* Disease
absorption NEC 579.9
calcium 269.3
carbohydrate 579.8
fat 579.8
protein 579.8
specified type NEC 579.8
vitamin (*see also* Deficiency, vitamin) 269.2
acid-base equilibrium 276.9
activity and attention, simple, with hyperkinesis 314.01
amino acid (metabolic) (*see also* Disorder, amino acid) 270.9
imidazole 270.5
maple syrup (urine) disease 270.3
transport 270.0
assimilation, food 579.9
attention, simple 314.00
with hyperactivity 314.01
auditory, nerve, except deafness 388.5
behavior (*see also* Disturbance, conduct) 312.9
blood clotting (hypoproteinemia) (mechanism) (*see also* Defect, coagulation) 286.9
central nervous system NEC 349.9
cerebral nerve NEC 352.9
circulatory 459.9
conduct 312.9

Note—Use the following fifth-digit subclassification with categories 312.0-312.2:

0 unspecified
1 mild
2 moderate
3 severe

adjustment reaction 309.3
adolescent onset type 312.82
childhood onset type 312.81
compulsive 312.30
intermittent explosive disorder 312.34
isolated explosive disorder 312.35
kleptomania 312.32
pathological gambling 312.31
pyromania 312.33
hyperkinetic 314.2
intermittent explosive 312.34
isolated explosive 312.35
mixed with emotions 312.4
socialized (type) 312.20
aggressive 312.23
unaggressive 312.21
specified type NEC 312.89
undersocialized, unsocialized
aggressive (type) 312.0
unaggressive (type) 312.1
coordination 781.3
cranial nerve NEC 352.9
deep sensibility—*see* Disturbance, sensation
digestive 536.9
psychogenic 306.4
electrolyte—*see* Imbalance, electrolyte

Disturbance—*continued*
emotions specific to childhood and adolescence 313.9
with
academic underachievement 313.83
anxiety and fearfulness 313.0
elective mutism 313.23
identity disorder 313.82
jealousy 313.3
misery and unhappiness 313.1
oppositional disorder 313.81
overanxiousness 313.0
sensitivity 313.21
shyness 313.21
social withdrawal 313.22
withdrawal reaction 313.22
involving relationship problems 313.3
mixed 313.89
specified type NEC 313.89
endocrine (gland) 259.9
neonatal, transitory 775.9
specified NEC 775.8
equilibrium 780.4
feeding (elderly) (infant) 783.3
newborn 779.3
nonorganic origin NEC 307.59
psychogenic NEC 307.59
fructose metabolism 271.2
gait 781.2
hysterical 300.11
gastric (functional) 536.9
motility 536.8
psychogenic 306.4
secretion 536.8
gastrointestinal (functional) 536.9
psychogenic 306.4
habit, child 307.9
hearing, except deafness 388.40
heart, functional (conditions classifiable to 426, 427, 428)
due to presence of (cardiac) prosthesis 429.4
postoperative (immediate) 997.1
long-term effect of cardiac surgery 429.4
psychogenic 306.2
hormone 259.9
innervation uterus, sympathetic, parasympathetic 621.8
keratinization NEC
gingiva 523.1
lip 528.5
oral (mucosa) (soft tissue) 528.7
tongue 528.7
labyrinth, labyrinthine (vestibule) 386.9
learning, specific NEC 315.2
memory (*see also* Amnesia) 780.9
mild, following organic brain damage 310.1
mental (*see also* Disorder, mental) 300.9
associated with diseases classified elsewhere 316
metabolism (acquired) (congenital) (*see also* Disorder, metabolism) 277.9
with
abortion—*see* Abortion, by type, with metabolic disorder
ectopic pregnancy (*see also* categories 633.0-633.9) 639.4
molar pregnancy (*see also* categories 630-632) 639.4

Disturbance—*continued*
amino acid (*see also* Disorder, amino acid) 270.9
aromatic NEC 270.2
branched-chain 270.3
specified type NEC 270.8
straight-chain NEC 270.7
sulfur-bearing 270.4
transport 270.0
ammonia 270.6
arginine 270.6
argininosuccinic acid 270.6
carbohydrate NEC 271.9
cholesterol 272.9
citrulline 270.6
cystathionine 270.4
fat 272.9
following
abortion 639.4
ectopic or molar pregnancy 639.4
general 277.9
carbohydrate 271.9
iron 275.0
phosphate 275.3
sodium 276.9
glutamine 270.7
glycine 270.7
histidine 270.5
homocystine 270.4
in labor or delivery 669.0
iron 275.0
isoleucine 270.3
leucine 270.3
lipoid 272.9
specified type NEC 272.8
lysine 270.7
methionine 270.4
neonatal, transitory 775.9
specified type NEC 775.8
nitrogen 788.9
ornithine 270.6
phosphate 275.3
phosphatides 272.7
serine 270.7
sodium NEC 276.9
threonine 270.7
tryptophan 270.2
tyrosine 270.2
urea cycle 270.6
valine 270.3
motor 796.1
nervous functional 799.2
neuromuscular mechanism (eye) due to syphilis 094.84
nutritional 269.9
nail 703.8
ocular motion 378.87
psychogenic 306.7
oculogyric 378.87
psychogenic 306.7
oculomotor NEC 378.87
psychogenic 306.7
olfactory nerve 781.1
optic nerve NEC 377.49
oral epithelium, including tongue 528.7
personality (pattern) (trait) (*see also* Disorder, personality) 301.9
following organic brain damage 310.1
polyglandular 258.9
psychomotor 307.9

Disturbance—*continued*
  pupillary 379.49
  reflex 796.1
  rhythm, heart 427.9
    postoperative (immediate) 997.1
      long-term effect of cardiac surgery 429.4
    psychogenic 306.2
  salivary secretion 527.7
  sensation (cold) (heat) (localization) (tactile discrimination localization) (texture) (vibratory) NEC 782.0
    hysterical 300.11
    skin 782.0
    smell 781.1
    taste 781.1
  sensory (*see also* Disturbance, sensation) 782.0
    innervation 782.0
  situational (transient) (*see also* Reaction, adjustment) 309.9
    acute 308.3
  sleep 780.50
    initiation or maintenance (*see also* Insomnia) 780.52
      nonorganic origin 307.41
    nonorganic origin 307.40
      specified type NEC 307.49
    specified NEC 780.59
      nonorganic origin 307.49
    wakefulness (*see also* Hypersomnia) 780.54
      nonorganic origin 307.43
    with apnea—*see* Apnea, sleep
  sociopathic 301.7
  speech NEC 784.5
    developmental 315.39
      associated with hyperkinesis 314.1
    secondary to organic lesion 784.5
  stomach (functional) (*see also* Disturbance, gastric) 536.9
  sympathetic (nerve) (*see also* Neuropathy, peripheral, autonomic) 337.9
  temperature sense 782.0
    hysterical 300.11
  tooth
    eruption 520.6
    formation 520.4
    structure, hereditary NEC 520.5
  touch (*see also* Disturbance, sensation) 782.0
  vascular 459.9
    arteriosclerotic—*see* Arteriosclerosis
  vasomotor 443.9
  vasospastic 443.9
  vestibular labyrinth 386.9
  vision, visual NEC 368.9
    psychophysical 368.16
    specified NEC 368.8
    subjective 368.10
  voice 784.40
  wakefulness (initiation or maintenance) (*see also* Hypersomnia) 780.54
    nonorganic origin 307.43
Disulfiduria, beta-mercaptolactate-cysteine 270.0
Disuse atrophy, bone 733.7
Ditthomska syndrome 307.81
Diuresis 788.42
Divers'
  palsy or paralysis 993.3
  squeeze 993.3
Diverticula, diverticulosis, diverticulum (acute) (multiple) (perforated) (ruptured) 562.10
  with diverticulitis 562.11
  aorta (Kommerell's) 747.21
  appendix (noninflammatory) 543.9
  bladder (acquired) (sphincter) 596.3
    congenital 753.8
  broad ligament 620.8
  bronchus (congenital) 748.3
    acquired 494
  calyx, calyceal (kidney) 593.89
  cardia (stomach) 537.1
  cecum 562.10
    with
      diverticulitis 562.11
        with hemorrhage 562.13
      hemorrhage 562.12
    congenital 751.5
  colon (acquired) 562.10
    with
      diverticulitis 562.11
        with hemorrhage 562.13
      hemorrhage 562.12
    congenital 751.5
  duodenum 562.00
    with
      diverticulitis 562.01
        with hemorrhage 562.03
      hemorrhage 562.02
    congenital 751.5
  epiphrenic (esophagus) 530.6
  esophagus (congenital) 750.4
    acquired 530.6
    epiphrenic 530.6
    pulsion 530.6
    traction 530.6
    Zenker's 530.6
  Eustachian tube 381.89
  fallopian tube 620.8
  gallbladder (congenital) 751.69
  gastric 537.1
  heart (congenital) 746.89
  ileum 562.00
    with
      diverticulitis 562.01
        with hemorrhage 562.03
      hemorrhage 562.02
  intestine (large) 562.10
    with
      diverticulitis 562.11
        with hemorrhage 562.13
      hemorrhage 562.12
    congenital 751.5
    small 562.00
      with
        diverticulitis 562.01
          with hemorrhage 562.03
        hemorrhage 562.02
      congenital 751.5
  jejunum 562.00
    with
      diverticulitis 562.01
        with hemorrhage 562.03
      hemorrhage 562.02
  kidney (calyx) (pelvis) 593.89
    with calculus 592.0
  Kommerell's 747.21
  laryngeal ventricle (congenital) 748.3
  Meckel's (displaced) (hypertrophic) 751.0
  midthoracic 530.6

Diverticula, diverticulosis . . .—*continued*
organ or site, congenital NEC—*see* Distortion
pericardium (congenital) (cyst) 746.89
acquired (true) 423.8
pharyngoesophageal (pulsion) 530.6
pharynx (congenital) 750.27
pulsion (esophagus) 530.6
rectosigmoid 562.10
with
diverticulitis 562.11
with hemorrhage 562.13
hemorrhage 562.12
congenital 751.5
rectum 562.10
with
diverticulitis 562.11
with hemorrhage 562.13
hemorrhage 562.12
renal (calyces) (pelvis) 593.89
with calculus 592.0
Rokitansky's 530.6
seminal vesicle 608.0
sigmoid 562.10
with
diverticulitis 562.11
with hemorrhage 562.13
hemorrhage 562.12
congenital 751.5
small intestine 562.00
with
diverticulitis 562.01
with hemorrhage 562.03
hemorrhage 562.02
stomach (cardia) (juxtacardia) (juxtapyloric) (acquired) 537.1
congenital 750.7
subdiaphragmatic 530.6
trachea (congenital) 748.3
acquired 519.1
traction (esophagus) 530.6
ureter (acquired) 593.89
congenital 753.4
ureterovesical orifice 593.89
urethra (acquired) 599.2
congenital 753.8
ventricle, left (congenital) 746.89
vesical (urinary) 596.3
congenital 753.8
Zenker's (esophagus) 530.6
Diverticulitis (acute) (*see also* Diverticula) 562.11
with hemorrhage 562.13
bladder (urinary) 596.3
cecum (perforated) 562.11
with hemorrhage 562.13
colon (perforated) 562.11
with hemorrhage 562.13
duodenum 562.01
with hemorrhage 562.03
esophagus 530.6
ileum (perforated) 562.01
with hemorrhage 562.03
intestine (large) (perforated) 562.11
with hemorrhage 562.13
small 562.01
with hemorrhage 562.03
jejunum (perforated) 562.01
with hemorrhage 562.03
Meckel's (perforated) 751.0
pharyngoesophageal 530.6
Diverticulitis—*continued*
rectosigmoid (perforated) 562.11
with hemorrhage 562.13
rectum 562.11
with hemorrhage 562.13
sigmoid (old) (perforated) 562.11
with hemorrhage 562.13
small intestine (perforated) 562.01
with hemorrhage 562.03
vesical (urinary) 596.3
Diverticulosis —*see* Diverticula
Division
cervix uteri 622.8
external os into two openings by frenum 752.49
external (cervical) into two openings by frenum 752.49
glans penis 752.8
hymen 752.49
labia minora (congenital) 752.49
ligament (partial or complete) (current)—*see also* Sprain, by site
with open wound—*see* Wound, open, by site
muscle (partial or complete) (current)—*see also* Sprain, by site
with open wound—*see* Wound, open, by site
nerve—*see* Injury, nerve, by site
penis glans 752.8
spinal cord—*see* Injury, spinal, by site
vein 459.9
traumatic—*see* Injury, vascular, by site
Divorce V61.0
Dix-Hallpike neurolabyrinthitis 386.12
Dizziness 780.4
hysterical 300.11
psychogenic 306.9
Doan-Wiseman syndrome (primary splenic neutropenia) 288.0
Dog bite —*see* Wound, open, by site
Döhle-Heller aortitis 093.1
Döhle body-panmyelopathic syndrome 288.2
Dolichocephaly, dolichocephalus 754.0
Dolichocolon 751.5
Dolichostenomelia 759.82
Donohue's syndrome (leprechaunism) 259.8
Donor
blood V59.01
bone V59.2
marrow V59.3
cornea V59.5
heart V59.8
kidney V59.4
liver V59.6
lung V59.8
lymphocyte V59.8
organ V59.9
specified NEC V59.8
potential, examination of V70.8
skin V59.1
specified organ or tissue NEC V59.8
stem cells V59.02
tissue V59.9
specified type NEC V59.8
Donovanosis (granuloma venereum) 099.2
DOPS (diffuse obstructive pulmonary syndrome) 496
Double
albumin 273.8
aortic arch 747.21
auditory canal 744.29
auricle (heart) 746.82

Double—*continued*
bladder 753.8
external (cervical) os 752.49
kidney with double pelvis (renal) 753.3
larynx 748.3
meatus urinarius 753.8
organ or site NEC—*see* Accessory
orifice
heart valve NEC 746.89
pulmonary 746.09
outlet, right ventricle 745.11
pelvis (renal) with double ureter 753.4
penis 752.8
tongue 750.13
ureter (one or both sides) 753.4
with double pelvis (renal) 753.4
urethra 753.8
urinary meatus 753.8
uterus (any degree) 752.2
with doubling of cervix and vagina 752.2
in pregnancy or childbirth 654.0
affecting fetus or newborn 763.8
vagina 752.49
with doubling of cervix and uterus 752.2
vision 368.2
vocal cords 748.3
vulva 752.49
whammy (syndrome) 360.81
Douglas' pouch, cul-de-sac —*see* condition
Down's disease or syndrome (mongolism) 758.0
Down-growth, epithelial (anterior chamber) 364.61
Dracontiasis 125.7
Dracunculiasis 125.7
Dracunculosis 125.7
Drainage
abscess (spontaneous)—*see* Abscess
anomalous pulmonary veins to hepatic veins or right atrium 747.41
stump (amputation) (surgical) 997.62
suprapubic, bladder 596.8
Dream state, hysterical 300.13
Drepanocytic anemia (*see also* Disease, sickle cell) 282.60
Dresbach's syndrome (elliptocytosis) 282.1
Dreschlera (infection) 118
hawaiiensis 117.8
Dressler's syndrome (postmyocardial infarction) 411.0
Dribbling (post-void) 788.35
Drift, ulnar 736.09
Drinking (alcohol)—*see also* Alcoholism
excessive, to excess NEC (*see also* Abuse, drugs, nondependent) 305.0
bouts, periodic 305.0
continual 303.9
episodic 305.0
habitual 303.9
periodic 305.0
Drip, postnasal (chronic)—*see* Sinusitis
Drivers' license examination V70.3
Droop, Cooper's 611.8
Drop
finger 736.29
foot 736.79
toe 735.8
wrist 736.05
Dropped
dead 798.1
heart beats 426.6
Dropsy, dropsical (*see also* Edema) 782.3
abdomen 789.5
amnion (*see also* Hydramnios) 657
brain—*see* Hydrocephalus
cardiac (*see also* Failure, heart, congestive) 428.0
cardiorenal (*see also* Hypertension, cardiorenal) 404.90
chest 511.9
fetus or newborn 778.0
due to isoimmunization 773.3
gangrenous (*see also* Gangrene) 785.4
heart (*see also* Failure, heart, congestive) 428.0
hepatic—*see* Cirrhosis, liver
infantile—*see* Hydrops, fetalis
kidney (*see also* Nephrosis) 581.9
liver—*see* Cirrhosis, liver
lung 514
malarial (*see also* Malaria) 084.9
neonatorum—*see* Hydrops, fetalis
nephritic 581.9
newborn—*see* Hydrops, fetalis
nutritional 269.9
ovary 620.8
pericardium (*see also* Pericarditis) 423.9
renal (*see also* Nephrosis) 581.9
uremic—*see* Uremia
Drowned, drowning 994.1
lung 518.5
Drowsiness 780.09
Drug —*see also* condition
addiction (*see also* listing under Dependence) 304.9
adverse effect NEC, correct substance properly administered 995.2
dependence (*see also* listing under Dependence) 304.9
habit (*see also* listing under Dependence) 304.9
overdose—*see* Table of drugs and chemicals
poisoning—*see* Table of drugs and chemicals
therapy (maintenance) status NEC V58.1
long-term (current) use V58.69
anticoagulant V58.61
wrong substance given or taken in error—*see* Table of drugs and chemicals
Drunkenness (*see also* Abuse, drugs, nondependent) 305.0
acute in alcoholism (*see also* Alcoholism) 303.0
chronic (*see also* Alcoholism) 303.9
pathologic 291.4
simple (acute) 305.0
in alcoholism 303.0
sleep 307.47
Drusen
optic disc or papilla 377.21
retina (colloid) (hyaloid degeneration) 362.57
hereditary 362.77
Drusenfieber 075
Dry, dryness —*see also* condition
eye 375.15
syndrome 375.15
larynx 478.79
mouth 527.7
nose 478.1
skin syndrome 701.1
socket (teeth) 526.5
throat 478.29
Duane's retraction syndrome 378.71
Duane-Stilling-Turk syndrome (ocular retraction syndrome) 378.71
Dubin-Johnson disease or syndrome 277.4

Dyschondroplasia (with hemangiomata) 756.4
Voorhoeve's 756.4
Dyschondrosteosis 756.59
Dyschromia 709.00
Dyscollagenosis 710.9
Dyscoria 743.41
Dyscraniopyophalangy 759.89
Dyscrasia
blood 289.9
with antepartum hemorrhage 641.3
fetus or newborn NEC 776.9
hemorrhage, subungual 287.8
puerperal, postpartum 666.3
ovary 256.8
plasma cell 273.9
pluriglandular 258.9
polyglandular 258.9
Dysdiadochokinesia 781.3
Dysectasia, vesical neck 596.8
Dysendocrinism 259.9
Dysentery, dysenteric (bilious) (catarrhal) (diarrhea) (epidemic) (gangrenous) (hemorrhagic) (infectious) (sporadic) (tropical) (ulcerative) 009.0
abscess, liver (*see also* Abscess, amebic) 006.3
amebic (*see also* Amebiasis) 006.9
with abscess—*see* Abscess, amebic
acute 006.0
carrier (suspected) of V02.2
chronic 006.1
arthritis (*see also* Arthritis, due to, dysentery) 009.0 *[711.3]*
bacillary 004.9 *[711.3]*
asylum 004.9
bacillary 004.9
arthritis 004.9 *[711.3]*
Boyd 004.2
Flexner 004.1
Schmitz (-Stutzer) 004.0
Shiga 004.0
Shigella 004.9
group A 004.0
group B 004.1
group C 004.2
group D 004.3
specified type NEC 004.8
Sonne 004.3
specified type NEC 004.8
bacterium 004.9
balantidial 007.0
Balantidium coli 007.0
Boyd's 004.2
Chilomastix 007.8
Chinese 004.9
choleriform 001.1
coccidial 007.2
Dientamoeba fragilis 007.8
due to specified organism NEC—*see* Enteritis, due to, by organism
Embadomonas 007.8
Endolimax nana—*see* Dysentery, amebic
Entamoba, entamebic—*see* Dysentery, amebic
Flexner's 004.1
Flexner-Boyd 004.2
giardial 007.1
Giardia lamblia 007.1
Hiss-Russell 004.1
lamblia 007.1
leishmanial 085.0
malarial (*see also* Malaria) 084.6

Dysentery, dysenteric—*continued*
metazoal 127.9
Monilia 112.89
protozoal NEC 007.9
Russell's 004.8
salmonella 003.0
schistosomal 120.1
Schmitz (-Stutzer) 004.0
Shiga 004.0
Shigella NEC (*see also* Dysentery, bacillary) 004.9
boydii 004.2
dysenteriae 004.0
Schmitz 004.0
Shiga 004.0
flexneri 004.1
Group A 004.0
Group B 004.1
Group C 004.2
Group D 004.3
Schmitz 004.0
Shiga 004.0
Sonnei 004.3
Sonne 004.3
strongyloidiasis 127.2
trichomonal 007.3
tuberculous (*see also* Tuberculosis) 014.8
viral (*see also* Enteritis, viral) 008.8
Dysequilibrium 780.4
Dysesthesia 782.0
hysterical 300.11
Dysfibrinogenemia (congenital) (*see also* Defect, coagulation) 286.3
Dysfunction
adrenal (cortical) 255.9
hyperfunction 255.3
hypofunction 255.4
associated with sleep stages or arousal from sleep 780.56
nonorganic origin 307.47
bladder NEC 596.59
bleeding, uterus 626.8
brain, minimal (*see also* Hyperkinesia) 314.9
cerebral 348.3
colon 564.9
psychogenic 306.4
colostomy or enterostomy 569.69
cystic duct 575.8
diastolic 429.9
with heart failure—*see* Failure, heart
due to
cardiomyopathy—*see* Cardiomyopathy
hypertension—*see* Hypertension, heart
endocrine NEC 259.9
endometrium 621.8
enteric stoma 569.69
enterostomy 569.69
Eustachian tube 381.81
gallbladder 575.8
gastrointestinal 536.9
gland, glandular NEC 259.9
heart 427.9
postoperative (immediate) 997.1
long-term effect of cardiac surgery 429.4
hemoglobin 288.8
hepatic 573.9
hepatocellular NEC 573.9

Dysfunction—*continued*
  hypophysis 253.9
    hyperfunction 253.1
    hypofunction 253.2
    posterior lobe 253.6
      hypofunction 253.5
  kidney (*see also* Disease, renal) 593.9
  labyrinthine 386.50
    specified NEC 386.58
  liver 573.9
    constitutional 277.4
  minimal brain (child) (*see also* Hyperkinesia) 314.9
  ovary, ovarian 256.9
    hyperfunction 256.1
      estrogen 256.0
    hypofunction 256.3
      postablative 256.2
    postablative 256.2
    specified NEC 256.8
  papillary muscle 429.81
    with myocardial infarction 410.8
  parathyroid 252.8
    hyperfunction 252.0
    hypofunction 252.1
  pineal gland 259.8
  pituitary (gland) 253.9
    hyperfunction 253.1
    hypofunction 253.2
    posterior 253.6
      hypofunction 253.5
  placental—*see* Placenta, insufficiency
  platelets (blood) 287.1
  polyglandular 258.9
    specified NEC 258.8
  psychosexual 302.70
    with
      dyspareunia (functional) (psychogenic) 302.76
      frigidity 302.72
      impotence 302.72
      inhibition
        orgasm
          female 302.73
          male 302.74
        sexual
          desire 302.71
          excitement 302.72
      premature ejaculation 302.75
      sexual aversion 302.79
      specified disorder NEC 302.79
      vaginismus 306.51
  pylorus 537.9
  rectum 564.9
    psychogenic 306.4
  segmental (*see also* Dysfunction, somatic) 739.9
  senile 797
  sinoatrial node 427.81
  somatic 739.9
    abdomen 739.9
    acromioclavicular 739.7
    cervical 739.1
    cervicothoracic 739.1
    costochondral 739.8
    costovertebral 739.8
    extremities
      lower 739.6
      upper 739.7
    head 739.0
    hip 739.5

Dysfunction—*continued*
    lumbar, lumbosacral 739.3
    occipitocervical 739.0
    pelvic 739.5
    pubic 739.5
    rib cage 739.8
    sacral 739.4
    sacrococcygeal 739.4
    sacroiliac 739.4
    specified site NEC 739.9
    sternochondral 739.8
    sternoclavicular 739.7
    temporomandibular 739.0
    thoracic, thoracolumbar 739.2
  stomach 536.9
    psychogenic 306.4
  suprarenal 255.9
    hyperfunction 255.3
    hypofunction 255.4
  symbolic NEC 784.60
    specified type NEC 784.69
  temporomandibular (joint) (joint-pain-syndrome) NEC 524.60
    specified NEC 524.69
  testicular 257.9
    hyperfunction 257.0
    hypofunction 257.2
    specified type NEC 257.8
  thymus 254.9
  thyroid 246.9
    complicating pregnancy, childbirth, or puerperium 648.1
    hyperfunction—*see* Hyperthyroidism
    hypofunction—*see* Hypothyroidism
  uterus, complicating delivery 661.9
    affecting fetus or newborn 763.7
    hypertonic 661.4
    hypotonic 661.2
      primary 661.0
      secondary 661.1
  velopharyngeal (acquired) 528.9
    congenital 750.29
  ventricular 429.9
    with congestive heart failure (*see also* Failure, heart, congestive) 428.0
    due to
      cardiomyopathy—*see* Cardiomyopathy
      hypertension—*see* Hypertension, heart
  vesicourethral NEC 596.59
  vestibular 386.50
    specified type NEC 386.58
Dysgammaglobulinemia 279.06
Dysgenesis
  gonadal (due to chromosomal anomaly) 758.6
    pure 752.7
  kidney(s) 753.0
  ovarian 758.6
  renal 753.0
  reticular 279.2
  seminiferous tubules 758.6
  tidal platelet 287.3
Dysgerminoma (M9060/3)
  specified site—*see* Neoplasm, by site, malignant
  unspecified site
    female 183.0
    male 186.9
Dysgeusia 781.1
Dysgraphia 781.3
Dyshidrosis 705.81
Dysidrosis 705.81
Dysinsulinism 251.8

Dyskaryotic cervical smear 795.0
Dyskeratosis (*see also* Keratosis) 701.1
bullosa hereditaria 757.39
cervix 622.1
congenital 757.39
follicularis 757.39
vitamin A deficiency 264.8
gingiva 523.8
oral soft tissue NEC 528.7
tongue 528.7
uterus NEC 621.8
Dyskinesia 781.3
biliary 575.8
esophagus 530.5
hysterical 300.11
intestinal 564.8
nonorganic origin 307.9
orofacial 333.82
psychogenic 307.9
tardive (oral) 333.82
Dyslalia 784.5
developmental 315.39
Dyslexia 784.61
developmental 315.02
secondary to organic lesion 784.61
Dysmaturity (*see also* Immaturity) 765.1
lung 770.4
pulmonary 770.4
Dysmenorrhea (essential) (exfoliative) (functional) (intrinsic) (membranous) (primary) (secondary) 625.3
psychogenic 306.52
Dysmetria 781.3
Dysmorodystrophia mesodermalis congenita 759.82
Dysnomia 784.3
Dysorexia 783.0
hysterical 300.11
Dysostosis
cleidocranial, cleidocranialis 755.59
craniofacial 756.0
Fairbank's (idiopathic familial generalized osteophytosis) 756.50
mandibularis 756.0
mandibulofacial, incomplete 756.0
multiplex 277.5
orodigitofacial 759.89
Dyspareunia (female) 625.0
male 608.89
psychogenic 302.76
Dyspepsia (allergic) (congenital) (fermentative) (flatulent) (functional) (gastric) (gastrointestinal) (neurogenic) (occupational) (reflex) 536.8
acid 536.8
atonic 536.3
psychogenic 306.4
diarrhea 558.9
psychogenic 306.4
intestinal 564.8
psychogenic 306.4
nervous 306.4
neurotic 306.4
psychogenic 306.4
Dysphagia 787.2
functional 300.11
hysterical 300.11
nervous 300.11
psychogenic 306.4
sideropenic 280.8
spastica 530.5
Dysphagocytosis, congenital 288.1
Dysphasia 784.5
Dysphonia 784.49
clericorum 784.49
functional 300.11
hysterical 300.11
psychogenic 306.1
spastica 478.79
Dyspigmentation —*see also* Pigmentation
eyelid (acquired) 374.52
Dyspituitarism 253.9
hyperfunction 253.1
hypofunction 253.2
posterior lobe 253.6
Dysplasia —*see also* Anomaly
artery
fibromuscular NEC 447.8
carotid 447.8
renal 447.3
bladder 596.8
bone (fibrous) NEC 733.29
diaphyseal, progressive 756.59
jaw 526.89
monostotic 733.29
polyostotic 756.54
solitary 733.29
brain 742.9
bronchopulmonary, fetus or newborn 770.7
cervix (uteri) 622.1
cervical intraepithelial neoplasia III [CIN III] 233.1
CIN III 233.1
chondroectodermal 756.55
chondromatose 756.4
craniocarpotarsal 759.89
craniometaphyseal 756.89
dentinal 520.5
diaphyseal, progressive 756.59
ectodermal (anhidrotic) (Bason) (Clouston's) (congenital) (Feinmesser) (hereditary) (hidrotic) (Marshall) (Robinson's) 757.31
epiphysealis 756.9
multiplex 756.56
punctata 756.59
epiphysis 756.9
multiple 756.56
epithelial
epiglottis 478.79
uterine cervix 622.1
erythroid NEC 289.8
eye (*see also* Microphthalmos) 743.10
familial metaphyseal 756.89
fibromuscular, artery NEC 447.8
carotid 447.8
renal 447.3
fibrous
bone NEC 733.29
diaphyseal, progressive 756.59
jaw 526.89
monostotic 733.29
polyostotic 756.54
solitary 733.29
hip (congenital) 755.63
with dislocation (*see also* Dislocation, hip, congenital) 754.30
hypohidrotic ectodermal 757.31
joint 755.8
kidney 753.15
leg 755.69
linguofacialis 759.89
lung 748.5

Dysplasia—*continued*
macular 743.55
mammary (benign) (gland) 610.9
cystic 610.1
specified type NEC 610.8
metaphyseal 756.9
familial 756.89
monostotic fibrous 733.29
muscle 756.89
myeloid NEC 289.8
nervous system (general) 742.9
neuroectodermal 759.6
oculoauriculovertebral 756.0
oculodentodigital 759.89
olfactogenital 253.4
osteo-onycho-arthro (hereditary) 756.89
periosteum 733.99
polyostotic fibrous 756.54
progressive diaphyseal 756.59
renal 753.15
renofacialis 753.0
retinal NEC 743.56
retrolental 362.21
spinal cord 742.9
thymic, with immunodeficiency 279.2
vagina 623.0
vocal cord 478.5
vulva 624.8
VIN III 233.3
Dyspnea (nocturnal) (paroxysmal) 786.09
asthmatic (bronchial) (*see also* Asthma) 493.9
with bronchitis (*see also* Asthma) 493.9
chronic 491.20
with acute exacerbation 491.21
cardiac (*see also* Failure, ventricular, left) 428.1
cardiac (*see also* Failure, ventricular, left) 428.1
functional 300.11
hyperventilation 786.01
hysterical 300.11
Monday morning 504
newborn 770.8
psychogenic 306.1
uremic—*see* Uremia
Dyspraxia 781.3
syndrome 315.4
Dysproteinemia 273.8
transient with copper deficiency 281.4
Dysprothrombinemia (constitutional) (*see also* Defect, coagulation) 286.3
Dysrhythmia
cardiac 427.9
postoperative (immediate) 997.1
long-term effect of cardiac surgery 429.4
specified type NEC 427.89
cerebral or cortical 348.3
Dyssecretosis, mucoserous 710.2
Dyssocial reaction without manifest psychiatric disorder
adolescent V71.02
adult V71.01
child V71.02
Dyssomnia NEC 780.56
nonorganic origin 307.47
Dyssplenism 289.4
Dyssynergia
biliary (*see also* Disease, biliary) 576.8
cerebellaris myoclonica 334.2
detrusor sphincter (bladder) 596.55
ventricular 429.89
Dystasia, hereditary areflexic 334.3
Dysthymia 300.4
Dysthymic disorder 300.4
Dysthyroidism 246.9
Dystocia 660.9
affecting fetus or newborn 763.1
cervical 661.0
affecting fetus or newborn 763.7
contraction ring 661.4
affecting fetus or newborn 763.7
fetal 660.9
abnormal size 653.5
affecting fetus or newborn 763.1
deformity 653.7
maternal 660.9
affecting fetus or newborn 763.1
positional 660.0
affecting fetus or newborn 763.1
shoulder (girdle) 660.4
affecting fetus or newborn 763.1
uterine NEC 661.4
affecting fetus or newborn 763.7
Dystonia
deformans progressiva 333.6
due to drugs 333.7
lenticularis 333.6
musculorum deformans 333.6
torsion (idiopathic) 333.6
fragments (of) 333.89
symptomatic 333.7
Dystonic
movements 781.0
Dystopia kidney 753.3
Dystrophy, dystrophia 783.9
adiposogenital 253.8
asphyxiating thoracic 756.4
Becker's type 359.1
brevicollis 756.16
Bruch's membrane 362.77
cervical (sympathetic) NEC 337.0
chondro-osseus with punctate epiphyseal dysplasia 756.59
choroid (hereditary) 363.50
central (areolar) (partial) 363.53
total (gyrate) 363.54
circinate 363.53
circumpapillary (partial) 363.51
total 363.52
diffuse
partial 363.56
total 363.57
generalized
partial 363.56
total 363.57
gyrate
central 363.54
generalized 363.57
helicoid 363.52
peripapillary—*see* Dystrophy, choroid, circumpapillary
serpiginous 363.54
cornea (hereditary) 371.50
anterior NEC 371.52
Cogan's 371.52
combined 371.57
crystalline 371.56
endothelial (Fuchs') 371.57
epithelial 371.50
juvenile 371.51
microscopic cystic 371.52
granular 371.53
lattice 371.54
macular 371.55
marginal (Terrien's) 371.48

Dystrophy, dystrophia—*continued*
Meesman's 371.51
microscopic cystic (epithelial) 371.52
nodular, Salzmann's 371.46
polymorphous 371.58
posterior NEC 371.58
ring-like 371.52
Salzmann's nodular 371.46
stromal NEC 371.56
dermatochondrocorneal 371.50
Duchenne's 359.1
due to malnutrition 263.9
Erb's 359.1
familial
hyperplastic periosteal 756.59
osseous 277.5
foveal 362.77
Fuchs', cornea 371.57
Gowers' muscular 359.1
hair 704.2
hereditary, progressive muscular 359.1
hypogenital, with diabetic tendency 759.81
Landouzy-Déjérine 359.1
Leyden-Möbius 359.1
mesodermalis congenita 759.82
muscular 359.1
congenital (hereditary) 359.0
myotonic 359.2
distal 359.1
Duchenne's 359.1
Erb's 359.1
fascioscapulohumeral 359.1
Gowers' 359.1
hereditary (progressive) 359.1
Landouzy-Déjérine 359.1
limb-girdle 359.1
myotonic 359.2
progressive (hereditary) 359.1
Charcot-Marie-Tooth 356.1
pseudohypertrophic (infantile) 359.1
myocardium, myocardial (*see also* Degeneration, myocardial) 429.1
myotonic 359.2
myotonica 359.2
nail 703.8
congenital 757.5
neurovascular (traumatic) (*see also* Neuropathy, peripheral, autonomic) 337.9
nutritional 263.9
ocular 359.1
oculocerebrorenal 270.8
oculopharyngeal 359.1
ovarian 620.8
papillary (and pigmentary) 701.1
pelvicrural atrophic 359.1
pigmentary (*see also* Acanthosis) 701.2
pituitary (gland) 253.8
polyglandular 258.8
posttraumatic sympathetic—*see* Dystrophy, sympathetic
progressive ophthalmoplegic 359.1

Dystrophy, dystrophia—*continued*
retina, retinal (hereditary) 362.70
albipunctate 362.74
Bruch's membrane 362.77
cone, progressive 362.75
hyaline 362.77
in
Bassen-Kornzweig syndrome 272.5 *[362.72]*
cerebroretinal lipidosis 330.1 *[362.71]*
Refsum's disease 356.3 *[362.72]*
systemic lipidosis 272.7 *[362.71]*
juvenile (Stargardt's) 362.75
pigmentary 362.74
pigment epithelium 362.76
progressive cone (-rod) 362.75
pseudoinflammatory foveal 362.77
rod, progressive 362.75
sensory 362.75
vitelliform 362.76
Salzmann's nodular 371.46
scapuloperoneal 359.1
skin NEC 709.9
sympathetic (posttraumatic) (reflex) 337.20
lower limb 337.22
specified NEC 337.29
upper limb 337.21
tapetoretinal NEC 362.74
thoracic asphyxiating 756.4
unguium 703.8
congenital 757.5
vitreoretinal (primary) 362.73
secondary 362.66
vulva 624.0
Dysuria 788.1
psychogenic 306.53

E

Eales' disease (syndrome) 362.18
Ear —*see also* condition
ache 388.70
otogenic 388.71
referred 388.72
lop 744.29
piercing V50.3
swimmers' acute 380.12
tank 380.12
tropical 111.8 *[380.15]*
wax 380.4
Earache 388.70
otogenic 388.71
referred 388.72
Eaton-Lambert syndrome (*see also* Neoplasm, by site, malignant) 199.1 *[358.1]*
Eberth's disease (typhoid fever) 002.0
Ebstein's
anomaly or syndrome (downward displacement, tricuspid valve into right ventricle) 746.2
disease (diabetes) 250.4 *[581.81]*
Eccentro-osteochondrodysplasia 277.5
Ecchondroma (M9210/0)—*see* Neoplasm, bone, benign
Ecchondrosis (M9210/1) 238.0
Ecchordosis physaliphora 756.0
Ecchymosis (multiple) 459.89
conjunctiva 372.72
eye (traumatic) 921.0
eyelids (traumatic) 921.1
newborn 772.6
spontaneous 782.7
traumatic—*see* Contusion
Echinococciasis —*see* Echinococcus
Echinococcosis —*see* Echinococcus
Echinococcus (infection) 122.9
granulosus 122.4
liver 122.0
lung 122.1
orbit 122.3 *[376.13]*
specified site NEC 122.3
thyroid 122.2
liver NEC 122.8
granulosus 122.0
multilocularis 122.5
lung NEC 122.9
granulosus 122.1
multilocularis 122.6
multilocularis 122.7
liver 122.5
specified site NEC 122.6
orbit 122.9 *[376.13]*
granulosus 122.3 *[376.13]*
multilocularis 122.6 *[376.13]*
specified site NEC 122.9
granulosus 122.3
multilocularis 122.6 *[376.13]*
thyroid NEC 122.9
granulosus 122.2
multilocularis 122.6
Echinorhynchiasis 127.7
Echinostomiasis 121.8
Echolalia 784.69
ECHO virus infection NEC 079.1
Eclampsia, eclamptic (coma) (convulsions) (delirium) 780.3
female, child-bearing age NEC—*see* Eclampsia, pregnancy
gravidarum—*see* Eclampsia, pregnancy
male 780.3
not associated with pregnancy or childbirth 780.3
pregnancy, childbirth or puerperium 642.6
with pre-existing hypertension 642.7
affecting fetus or newborn 760.0
uremic 586
Eclipse blindness (total) 363.31
Economic circumstance affecting care V60.9
specified type NEC V60.8
Economo's disease (encephalitis lethargica) 049.8
Ectasia, ectasis
aorta (*see also* Aneurysm, aorta) 441.9
ruptured 441.5
breast 610.4
capillary 448.9
cornea (marginal) (postinfectional) 371.71
duct (mammary) 610.4
kidney 593.89
mammary duct (gland) 610.4
papillary 448.9
renal 593.89
salivary gland (duct) 527.8
scar, cornea 371.71
sclera 379.11
Ecthyma 686.8
contagiosum 051.2
gangrenosum 686.0
infectiosum 051.2
Ectocardia 746.87
Ectodermal dysplasia, congenital 757.31
Ectodermosis erosiva pluriorificialis 695.1
Ectopic, ectopia (congenital) 759.89
abdominal viscera 751.8
due to defect in anterior abdominal wall 756.7
ACTH syndrome 255.0
adrenal gland 759.1
anus 751.5
auricular beats 427.61
beats 427.60
bladder 753.5
bone and cartilage in lung 748.69
brain 742.4
breast tissue 757.6
cardiac 746.87
cerebral 742.4
cordis 746.87
endometrium 617.9
gallbladder 751.69
gastric mucosa 750.7
gestation—*see* Pregnancy, ectopic
heart 746.87
hormone secretion NEC 259.3
hyperparathyroidism 259.3
kidney (crossed) (intrathoracic) (pelvis) 753.3
in pregnancy or childbirth 654.4
causing obstructed labor 660.2
lens 743.37
lentis 743.37
mole—*see* Pregnancy, ectopic

Ectopic, ectopia—*continued*
organ or site NEC—*see* Malposition, congenital
ovary 752.0
pancreas, pancreatic tissue 751.7
pregnancy—*see* Pregnancy, ectopic
pupil 364.75
renal 753.3
sebaceous glands of mouth 750.26
secretion
ACTH 255.0
adrenal hormone 259.3
adrenalin 259.3
adrenocorticotropin 255.0
antidiuretic hormone (ADH) 259.3
epinephrine 259.3
hormone NEC 259.3
norepinephrine 259.3
pituitary (posterior) 259.3
spleen 759.0
testis 752.5
thyroid 759.2
ureter 753.4
ventricular beats 427.69
vesicae 753.5
Ectrodactyly 755.4
finger (*see also* Absence, finger, congenital) 755.29
toe (*see also* Absence, toe, congenital) 755.39
Ectromelia 755.4
lower limb 755.30
upper limb 755.20
Ectropion 374.10
anus 569.49
cervix 622.0
with mention of cervicitis 616.0
cicatricial 374.14
congenital 743.62
eyelid 374.10
cicatricial 374.14
congenital 743.62
mechanical 374.12
paralytic 374.12
senile 374.11
spastic 374.13
iris (pigment epithelium) 364.54
lip (congenital) 750.26
acquired 528.5
mechanical 374.12
paralytic 374.12
rectum 569.49
senile 374.11
spastic 374.13
urethra 599.84
uvea 364.54
Eczema (acute) (allergic) (chronic) (erythematous) (fissum) (occupational) (rubrum) (squamous) 692.9
asteatotic 706.8
atopic 691.8
contact NEC 692.9
dermatitis NEC 692.9
due to specified cause—*see* Dermatitis, due to
dyshidrotic 705.81
external ear 380.22
flexural 691.8
gouty 274.89
herpeticum 054.0
hypertrophicum 701.8
hypostatic—*see* Varicose, vein
Eczema—*continued*
impetiginous 684
infantile (acute) (chronic) (due to any substance) (intertriginous) (seborrheic) 691.8
intertriginous NEC 692.9
infantile 691.8
intrinsic 691.8
lichenified NEC 692.9
marginatum 110.3
nummular 692.9
pustular 686.8
seborrheic 690.18
infantile 690.12
solare 692.72
stasis (lower extremity) 454.1
ulcerated 454.2
vaccination, vaccinatum 999.0
varicose (lower extremity)—*see* Varicose, vein
verrucosum callosum 698.3
Eczematoid, exudative 691.8
Eddowes' syndrome (brittle bones and blue sclera) 756.51
Edema, edematous 782.3
with nephritis (*see also* Nephrosis) 581.9
allergic 995.1
angioneurotic (allergic) (any site) (with urticaria) 995.1
hereditary 277.6
angiospastic 443.9
Berlin's (traumatic) 921.3
brain 348.5
due to birth injury 767.8
fetus or newborn 767.8
cardiac (*see also* Failure, heart, congestive) 428.0
cardiovascular (*see also* Failure, heart, congestive) 428.0
cerebral—*see* Edema, brain
cerebrospinal vessel—*see* Edema, brain
cervix (acute) (uteri) 622.8
puerperal, postpartum 674.8
chronic hereditary 757.0
circumscribed, acute 995.1
hereditary 277.6
complicating pregnancy (gestational) 646.1
with hypertension—*see* Toxemia, of pregnancy
conjunctiva 372.73
connective tissue 782.3
cornea 371.20
due to contact lenses 371.24
idiopathic 371.21
secondary 371.22
due to
lymphatic obstruction—*see* Edema, lymphatic
salt retention 276.0
epiglottis—*see* Edema, glottis
essential, acute 995.1
hereditary 277.6
extremities, lower—*see* Edema, legs
eyelid NEC 374.82
familial, hereditary (legs) 757.0
famine 262
fetus or newborn 778.5
genital organs
female 629.8
male 608.86

Edema, edematous—*continued*
gestational 646.1
with hypertension—*see* Toxemia, of pregnancy
glottis, glottic, glottides (obstructive) (passive) 478.6
allergic 995.1
hereditary 277.6
due to external agent—*see* Condition, respiratory, acute, due to specified agent
heart (*see also* Failure, heart, congestive) 428.0
newborn 779.8
heat 992.7
hereditary (legs) 757.0
inanition 262
infectious 782.3
intracranial 348.5
due to injury at birth 767.8
iris 364.8
joint (*see also* Effusion, joint) 719.0
larynx (*see also* Edema, glottis) 478.6
legs 782.3
due to venous obstruction 459.2
hereditary 757.0
localized 782.3
due to venous obstruction 459.2
lower extremity 459.2
lower extremities—*see* Edema, legs
lungs 514
acute 518.4
with heart disease or failure (*see also* Failure, ventricular, left) 428.1
congestive 428.0
chemical (due to fumes or vapors) 506.1
due to
external agent(s) NEC 508.9
specified NEC 508.8
fumes and vapors (chemical) (inhalation) 506.1
radiation 508.0
chemical (acute) 506.1
chronic 506.4
chronic 514
chemical (due to fumes or vapors) 506.4
due to
external agent(s) NEC 508.9
specified NEC 508.8
fumes or vapors (chemical) (inhalation) 506.4
radiation 508.1
due to
external agent 508.9
specified NEC 508.8
high altitude 993.2
near drowning 994.1
postoperative 518.4
terminal 514
lymphatic 457.1
due to mastectomy operation 457.0
macula 362.83
cystoid 362.53
diabetic 250.5 *[362.83]*
malignant (*see also* Gangrene, gas) 040.0
Milroy's 757.0
nasopharynx 478.25
neonatorum 778.5
nutritional (newborn) 262
with dyspigmentation, skin and hair 260
optic disc or nerve—*see* Papilledema

Edema, edematous—*continued*
orbit 376.33
circulatory 459.89
palate (soft) (hard) 528.9
pancreas 577.8
penis 607.83
periodic 995.1
hereditary 277.6
pharynx 478.25
pitting 782.3
pulmonary—*see* Edema, lung
Quincke's 995.1
hereditary 277.6
renal (*see also* Nephrosis) 581.9
retina (localized) (macular) (peripheral) 362.83
diabetic 250.5 *[362.83]*
salt 276.0
scrotum 608.86
seminal vesicle 608.86
spermatic cord 608.86
spinal cord 336.1
starvation 262
subconjunctival 372.73
subglottic (*see also* Edema, glottis) 478.6
supraglottic (*see also* Edema, glottis) 478.6
testis 608.86
toxic NEC 782.3
traumatic NEC 782.3
tunica vaginalis 608.86
vas deferens 608.86
vocal cord—*see* Edema, glottis
vulva (acute) 624.8
Edentia (complete) (partial) (*see also* Absence, tooth) 520.0
causing malocclusion 524.3
congenital (deficiency of tooth buds) 520.0
due to accident, extraction, or local periodontal disease 525.1
Edsall's disease 992.2
Educational handicap V62.3
Edwards' syndrome 758.2
Effect, adverse NEC
abnormal gravitational (G) forces or states 994.9
air pressure—*see* Effect, adverse, atmospheric pressure
altitude (high)—*see* Effect, adverse, high altitude
anesthetic
in labor and delivery NEC 668.9
affecting fetus or newborn 763.5
antitoxin—*see* Complications, vaccination
atmospheric pressure 993.9
due to explosion 993.4
high 993.3
low—*see* Effect, adverse, high altitude
specified effect NEC 993.8
biological, correct substance properly administered (*see also* Effect, adverse, drug) 995.2
blood (derivatives) (serum) (transfusion)—*see* Complications, transfusion
chemical substance NEC 989.9
specified—*see* Table of drugs and chemicals
cobalt, radioactive (*see also* Effect, adverse, radioactive substance) 990
cold (temperature) (weather) 991.9
chilblains 991.5
frostbite—*see* Frostbite
specified effect NEC 991.8

Effect, adverse—*continued*
drugs and medicinals NEC 995.2
correct substance properly administered 995.2
overdose or wrong substance given or taken 977.9
specified drug—*see* Table of drugs and chemicals
electric current (shock) 994.8
burn—*see* Burn, by site
electricity (electrocution) (shock) 994.8
burn—*see* Burn, by site
exertion (excessive) 994.5
exposure 994.9
exhaustion 994.4
external cause NEC 994.9
fallout (radioactive) NEC 990
fluoroscopy NEC 990
foodstuffs
allergic reaction (*see also* Allergy, food) 693.1
anaphylactic shock due to food NEC 995.60
noxious 988.9
specified type NEC (*see also* Poisoning, by name of noxious foodstuff) 988.8
gases, fumes, or vapors—*see* Table of drugs and chemicals
glue (airplane) sniffing 304.6
heat—*see* Heat
high altitude NEC 993.2
anoxia 993.2
on
fears 993.0
sinuses 993.1
polycythemia 289.0
hot weather—*see* Heat
hunger 994.2
immersion, foot 991.4
immunization—*see* Complications, vaccination
immunological agents—*see* Complications, vaccination
implantation (removable) of isotope or radium NEC 990
infrared (radiation) (rays) NEC 990
burn—*see* Burn, by site
dermatitis or eczema 692.82
infusion—*see* Complications, infusion
ingestion or injection of isotope (therapeutic) NEC 990
irradiation NEC (*see also* Effect, adverse, radiation) 990
isotope (radioactive) NEC 990
lack of care (child) (infant) (newborn) 995.5
specified person NEC 995.81
lightning 994.0
burn—*see* Burn, by site
Lirugin—*see* Complications, vaccination
medicinal substance, correct, properly administered (*see also* Effect, adverse, drugs) 995.2
mesothorium NEC 990
motion 994.6
noise, inner ear 388.10
overheated places—*see* Heat
polonium NEC 990
psychosocial, of work environment V62.1

Effect, adverse—*continued*
radiation (diagnostic) (fallout) (infrared) (natural source) (therapeutic) (tracer) (ultraviolet) (x-ray) NEC 990
with pulmonary manifestations
acute 508.0
chronic 508.1
dermatitis or eczema 692.82
due to sun NEC (*see also* Dermatitis, due to, sun) 692.70
fibrosis of lungs 508.1
maternal with suspected damage to fetus affecting management of pregnancy 655.6
pneumonitis 508.0
radioactive substance NEC 990
dermatitis or eczema 692.82
radioactivity NEC 990
radiotherapy NEC 990
dermatitis or eczema 692.82
radium NEC 990
reduced temperature 991.9
frostbite—*see* Frostbite
immersion, foot (hand) 991.4
specified effect NEC 991.8
roentgenography NEC 990
roentgenoscopy NEC 990
roentgen rays NEC 990
serum (prophylactic) (therapeutic) NEC 999.5
specified NEC 995.89
external cause NEC 994.9
strangulation 994.7
submersion 994.1
teletherapy NEC 990
thirst 994.3
transfusion—*see* Complications, transfusion
ultraviolet (radiation) (rays) NEC 990
burn—*see also* Burn, by site
from sun 692.71
dermatitis or eczema 692.82
due to sun NEC (*see also* Dermatitis, due to, sun) 692.70
uranium NEC 990
vaccine (any)—*see* Complications, vaccination
weightlessness 994.9
whole blood—*see also* Complications, transfusion
overdose or wrong substance given (*see also* Table of drugs and chemicals) 964.7
working environment V62.1
x-rays NEC 990
dermatitis or eczema 692.82
Effect, remote
of cancer, —*see* condition
Effects, late —*see* Late, effect (of)
Effluvium, telogen 704.02
Effort
intolerance 306.2
syndrome (aviators) (psychogenic) 306.2
Effusion
Amniotic fluid (*see also* Rupture, membranes, premature) 658.1
brain (serous) 348.5
bronchial (*see also* Bronchitis) 490
cerebral 348.5
cerebrospinal (*see also* Meningitis) 322.9
vessel 348.5
chest—*see* Effusion, pleura
intracranial 348.5

Effusion—*continued*
joint 719.00
ankle 719.07
elbow 719.02
foot 719.07
hand 719.04
hip 719.05
knee 719.06
multiple sites 719.09
pelvic region 719.05
shoulder (region) 719.01
specified site NEC 719.08
wrist 719.03
meninges (*see also* Meningitis) 322.9
pericardium, pericardial (*see also* Pericarditis) 423.9
acute 420.90
peritoneal (chronic) 568.82
pleura, pleurisy, pleuritic, pleuropericardial 511.9
bacterial, nontuberculous 511.1
fetus or newborn 511.9
malignant 197.2
nontuberculous 511.9
bacterial 511.1
pneumococcal 511.1
staphylococcal 511.1
streptococcal 511.1
tuberculous (*see also* Tuberculosis, pleura) 012.0
primary progressive 010.1
pulmonary—*see* Effusion, pleura
spinal (*see also* Meningitis) 322.9
thorax, thoracic—*see* Effusion, pleura
Eggshell nails 703.8
congenital 757.5
Ego-dystonic
homosexuality 302.0
lesbianism 302.0
Egyptian splenomegaly 120.1
Ehlers-Danlos syndrome 756.83
Eichstedt's disease (pityriasis versicolor) 111.0
Eisenmenger's complex or syndrome (ventricular septal defect) 745.4
Ejaculation, semen
painful 608.89
psychogenic 306.59
premature 302.75
Ekbom syndrome (restless legs) 333.99
Ekman's syndrome (brittle bones and blue sclera) 756.51
Elastic skin 756.83
acquired 701.8
Elastofibroma (M8820/0)—*see* Neoplasm, connective tissue, benign
Elastoidosis
cutanea nodularis 701.8
cutis cystica et comedonica 701.8
Elastoma 757.39
juvenile 757.39
Miescher's (elastosis perforans serpiginosa) 701.1
Elastomyofibrosis 425.3
Elastosis 701.8
atrophicans 701.8
perforans serpiginosa 701.1
reactive perforating 701.1
senilis 701.8
solar (actinic) 692.74
Elbow —*see* condition
Electric
current, electricity, effects (concussion) (fatal) (nonfatal) (shock) 994.8
burn—*see* Burn, by site
feet (foot) syndrome 266.2
Electrocution 994.8
Electrolyte imbalance 276.9
with
abortion—*see* Abortion, by type, with metabolic disorder
ectopic pregnancy (*see also* categories 633.0-633.9) 639.4
hyperemesis gravidarum (before 22 completed weeks gestation) 643.1
molar pregnancy (*see also* categories 630-632) 639.4
following
abortion 639.4
ectopic or molar pregnancy 639.4
Elephantiasis (nonfilarial) 457.1
arabicum (*see also* Infestation, filarial) 125.9
congenita hereditaria 757.0
congenital (any site) 757.0
due to
Brugia (malayi) 125.1
mastectomy operation 457.0
Wuchereria (bancrofti) 125.0
malayi 125.1
eyelid 374.83
filarial (*see also* Infestation, filarial) 125.9
filariensis (*see also* Infestation, filarial) 125.9
gingival 523.8
glandular 457.1
graecorum 030.9
lymphangiectatic 457.1
lymphatic vessel 457.1
due to mastectomy operation 457.0
neuromatosa 237.71
postmastectomy 457.0
scrotum 457.1
streptococcal 457.1
surgical 997.99
postmastectomy 457.0
telangiectodes 457.1
vulva (nonfilarial) 624.8
Elevated —*see* Elevation
Elevation
17-ketosteroids 791.9
acid phosphatase 790.5
alkaline phosphatase 790.5
amylase 790.5
antibody titers 795.79
basal metabolic rate (BMR) 794.7
blood pressure (*see also* Hypertension) 401.9
reading (incidental) (isolated) (nonspecific), no diagnosis of hypertension 796.2
body temperature (of unknown origin) (*see also* Pyrexia) 780.6
conjugate, eye 378.81
diaphragm, congenital 756.6
immunoglobulin level 795.79
indolacetic acid 791.9
lactic acid dehydrogenase (LDH) level 790.4
lipase 790.5
prostate specific antigen (PSA) 790.93
renin 790.99
in hypertension (*see also* Hypertension, renovascular) 405.91
Rh titer 999.7

Elevation—*continued*
scapula, congenital 755.52
sedimentation rate 790.1
SGOT 790.4
SGPT 790.4
transaminase 790.4
vanillylmandelic acid 791.9
venous pressure 459.89
VMA 791.9
Elliptocytosis (congenital) (hereditary) 282.1
Hb-C (disease) 282.7
hemoglobin disease 282.7
sickle-cell (disease) 282.60
trait 282.5
Ellis-van Creveld disease or syndrome (chondroectodermal dysplasia) 756.55
Ellison-Zollinger syndrome (gastric hypersecretion with pancreatic islet cell tumor) 251.5
Elongation, elongated (congenital)—*see also* Distortion
bone 756.9
cervix (uteri) 752.49
acquired 622.6
hypertrophic 622.6
colon 751.5
common bile duct 751.69
cystic duct 751.69
frenulum, penis 752.8
labia minora, acquired 624.8
ligamentum patellae 756.89
petiolus (epiglottidis) 748.3
styloid bone (process) 733.99
tooth, teeth 520.2
uvula 750.26
acquired 528.9
Elschnig bodies or pearls 366.51
El Tor cholera 001.1
Emaciation (due to malnutrition) 261
Emancipation disorder 309.22
Embadomoniasis 007.8
Embarrassment heart, cardiac —*see* Disease, heart
Embedded tooth, teeth 520.6
with abnormal position (same or adjacent tooth) 524.3
root only 525.3
Embolic —*see* condition
Embolism (septic) 444.9
with
abortion—*see* Abortion, by type, with embolism
ectopic pregnancy (*see also* categories 633.0-633.9) 639.6
molar pregnancy (*see also* categories 630-632) 639.6
air (any site) 958.0
with
abortion—*see* Abortion, by type, with embolism
ectopic pregnancy (*see also* categories 633.0-633.9) 639.6
molar pregnancy (*see also* categories 630-632) 639.6
due to implanted device—*see* Complications, due to (presence of) any device, implant, or graft classified to 996.0-996.5 NEC

Embolism—*continued*
following
abortion 639.6
ectopic or molar pregnancy 639.6
infusion, perfusion, or transfusion 999.1
in pregnancy, childbirth, or puerperium 673.0
traumatic 958.0
amniotic fluid (pulmonary) 673.1
with
abortion—*see* Abortion, by type, with embolism
ectopic pregnancy (*see also* categories 633.0-633.9) 639.6
molar pregnancy (*see also* categories 630-632) 639.6
following
abortion 639.6
ectopic or molar pregnancy 639.6
aorta, aortic 444.1
abdominal 444.0
bifurcation 444.0
saddle 444.0
thoracic 444.1
artery 444.9
auditory, internal 433.8
basilar (*see also* Occlusion, artery, basilar) 433.0
bladder 444.89
carotid (common) (internal) (*see also* Occlusion, artery, carotid) 433.1
cerebellar (anterior inferior) (posterior inferior) (superior) 433.8
cerebral (*see also* Embolism, brain) 434.1
choroidal (anterior) 433.8
communicating posterior 433.8
coronary (*see also* Infarct, myocardium) 410.9
without myocardial infarction 411.81
extremity 444.22
lower 444.22
upper 444.21
hypophyseal 433.8
mesenteric (with gangrene) 557.0
ophthalmic (*see also* Occlusion, retina) 362.30
peripheral 444.22
pontine 433.8
precerebral NEC—*see* Occlusion, artery, precerebral
pulmonary—*see* Embolism, pulmonary
renal 593.81
retinal (*see also* Occlusion, retina) 362.30
specified site NEC 444.89
vertebral (*see also* Occlusion, artery, vertebral) 433.2
auditory, internal 433.8
basilar (artery) (*see also* Occlusion, artery, basilar) 433.0
birth, mother—*see* Embolism, obstetrical
blood-clot
with
abortion—*see* Abortion, by type, with embolism
ectopic pregnancy (*see also* categories 633.0-633.9) 639.6
molar pregnancy (*see also* categories 630-632) 639.6
following
abortion 639.6
ectopic or molar pregnancy 639.6
in pregnancy, childbirth, or puerperium 673.2

Embolism—*continued*
brain 434.1
with
abortion—*see* Abortion, by type, with embolism
ectopic pregnancy (*see also* categories 633.0-633.9) 639.6
molar pregnancy (*see also* categories 630-632) 639.6
following
abortion 639.6
ectopic or molar pregnancy 639.6
late effect—*see* category 438
puerperal, postpartum, childbirth 674.0
capillary 448.9
cardiac (*see also* Infarct, myocardium) 410.9
carotid (artery) (common) (internal) (*see also* Occlusion, artery, carotid) 433.1
cavernous sinus (venous)—*see* Embolism, intracranial venous sinus
cerebral (*see also* Embolism, brain) 434.1
choroidal (anterior) (artery) 433.8
coronary (artery or vein) (systemic) (*see also* Infarct, myocardium) 410.9
without myocardial infarction 411.81
due to (presence of) any device, implant, or graft classifiable to 996.0-996.5 —*see* Complications, due to (presence of) any device, implant, or graft classified to 996.0-996.5 NEC
encephalomalacia (*see also* Embolism, brain) 434.1
extremities 444.22
lower 444.22
upper 444.21
eye 362.30
fat (cerebral) (pulmonary) (systemic) 958.1
with
abortion—*see* Abortion, by type, with embolism
ectopic pregnancy (*see also* categories 633.0-633.9) 639.6
molar pregnancy (*see also* categories 630-632) 639.6
complicating delivery or puerperium 673.8
following
abortion 639.6
ectopic or molar pregnancy 639.6
in pregnancy, childbirth, or the puerperium 673.8
femoral (artery) 444.22
vein 453.8
following
abortion 639.6
ectopic or molar pregnancy 639.6
infusion, perfusion, or transfusion
air 999.1
thrombus 999.2
heart (fatty) (*see also* Infarct, myocardium) 410.9
hepatic (vein) 453.0
iliac (artery) 444.81
iliofemoral 444.81
in pregnancy, childbirth, or puerperium (pulmonary)—*see* Embolism, obstetrical
intestine (artery) (vein) (with gangrene) 557.0
intracranial (*see also* Embolism, brain) 434.1
venous sinus (any) 325
late effect—*see* category 326
nonpyogenic 437.6
in pregnancy or puerperium 671.5

Embolism—*continued*
kidney (artery) 593.81
lateral sinus (venous)—*see* Embolism, intracranial venous sinus
longitudinal sinus (venous)—*see* Embolism, intracranial venous sinus
lower extremity 444.22
lung (massive)—*see* Embolism, pulmonary
meninges (*see also* Embolism, brain) 434.1
mesenteric (artery) (with gangrene) 557.0
multiple NEC 444.9
obstetrical (pulmonary) 673.2
air 673.0
amniotic fluid (pulmonary) 673.1
blood-clot 673.2
cardiac 674.8
fat 673.8
heart 674.8
pyemic 673.3
septic 673.3
specified NEC 674.8
ophthalmic (*see also* Occlusion, retina) 362.30
paradoxical NEC 444.9
penis 607.82
peripheral arteries NEC 444.22
lower 444.22
upper 444.21
pituitary 253.8
popliteal (artery) 444.22
portal (vein) 452
postoperative NEC 997.2
cerebral 997.02
peripheral vascular 997.2
pulmonary 997.3
precerebral artery (*see also* Occlusion, artery, precerebral) 433.9
puerperal—*see* Embolism, obstetrical
pulmonary (artery) (vein) 415.1
with
abortion—*see* Abortion, by type, with embolism
ectopic pregnancy (*see also* categories 633.0-633.9) 639.6
molar pregnancy (*see also* categories 630-632) 639.6
following
abortion 639.6
ectopic or molar pregnancy 639.6
iatrogenic 415.11
in pregnancy, childbirth, or puerperium—*see* Embolism, obstetrical
postoperative 415.11
pyemic (multiple) 038.9
with
abortion—*see* Abortion, by type, with embolism
ectopic pregnancy (*see also* categories 633.0-633.9) 639.6
molar pregnancy (*see also* categories 630-632) 639.6
Aerobacter aerogenes 038.49
enteric gram-negative bacilli 038.40
Enterobacter aerogenes 038.49
Escherichia coli 038.42
following
abortion 639.6
ectopic or molar pregnancy 639.6
Hemophilus influenzae 038.41
pneumococcal 038.2
Proteus vulgaris 038.49
Pseudomonas (aeruginosa) 038.43

Embolism—*continued*
puerperal, postpartum, childbirth (any organism) 673.3
Serratia 038.44
specified organism NEC 038.8
staphylococcal 038.1
streptococcal 038.0
renal (artery) 593.81
vein 453.3
retina, retinal (*see also* Occlusion, retina) 362.30
saddle (aorta) 444.0
septicemic—*see* Embolism, pyemic
sinus—*see* Embolism, intracranial venous sinus
soap
with
abortion—*see* Abortion, by type, with embolism
ectopic pregnancy (*see also* categories 633.0-633.9) 639.6
molar pregnancy (*see also* categories 630-632) 639.6
following
abortion 639.6
ectopic or molar pregnancy 639.6
spinal cord (nonpyogenic) 336.1
in pregnancy or puerperium 671.5
pyogenic origin 324.1
late effect—*see* category 326
spleen, splenic (artery) 444.89
thrombus (thromboembolism) following infusion, perfusion, or transfusion 999.2
upper extremity 444.21
vein 453.9
with inflammation or phlebitis—*see* Thrombophlebitis
cerebral (*see also* Embolism, brain) 434.1
coronary (*see also* Infarct, myocardium) 410.9
without myocardial infarction 411.81
hepatic 453.0
mesenteric (with gangrene) 557.0
portal 452
pulmonary—*see* Embolism, pulmonary
renal 453.3
specified NEC 453.8
with inflammation or phlebitis—*see* Thrombophlebitis
vena cava (inferior) (superior) 453.2
vessels of brain (*see also* Embolism, brain) 434.1
Embolization —*see* Embolism
Embolus —*see* Embolism
Embryoma (M9080/1)—*see also* Neoplasm, by site, uncertain behavior
benign (M9080/0)—*see* Neoplasm, by site, benign
kidney (M8960/3) 189.0
liver (M8970/3) 155.0
malignant (M9080/3)—*see also* Neoplasm, by site, malignant
kidney (M8960/3) 189.0
liver (M8970/3) 155.0
testis (M9070/3) 186.9
undescended 186.0
testis (M9070/3) 186.9
undescended 186.0
Embryonic
circulation 747.9
heart 747.9
vas deferens 752.8
Embryopathia NEC 759.9
Embryotomy, fetal 763.8
Embryotoxon 743.43
interfering with vision 743.42
Emesis —*see* also Vomiting
gravidarum—*see* Hyperemesis, gravidarum
Emissions, nocturnal (semen) 608.89
Emotional
crisis—*see* Crisis, emotional
disorder (*see also* Disorder, mental) 300.9
instability (excessive) 301.3
overlay—*see* Reaction, adjustment
upset 300.9
Emotionality, pathological 301.3
Emotogenic disease (*see also* Disorder, psychogenic) 306.9
Emphysema (atrophic) (centriacinar) (centrilobular) (chronic) (diffuse) (essential) (hypertrophic) (interlobular) (lung) (obstructive) (panlobular) (paracicatricial) (paracinar) (postural) (pulmonary) (senile) (subpleural) (traction) (unilateral) (unilobular) (vesicular) 492.8
with
bronchitis
acute and chronic 491.21
chronic 491.20
with acute bronchitis or acute exacerbation 491.21
bullous (giant) 492.0
cellular tissue 958.7
surgical 998.81
compensatory 518.2
congenital 770.2
conjunctiva 372.8
connective tissue 958.7
surgical 998.81
due to fumes or vapors 506.4
eye 376.89
eyelid 374.85
surgical 998.81
traumatic 958.7
fetus or newborn (interstitial) (mediastinal) (unilobular) 770.2
heart 416.9
interstitial 518.1
congenital 770.2
fetus or newborn 770.2
laminated tissue 958.7
surgical 998.81
mediastinal 518.1
fetus or newborn 770.2
newborn (interstitial) (mediastinal) (unilobular) 770.2
obstructive diffuse with fibrosis 492.8
orbit 376.89
subcutaneous 958.7
due to trauma 958.7
nontraumatic 518.1
surgical 998.81
surgical 998.81
thymus (gland) (congenital) 254.8
traumatic 958.7
tuberculous (*see also* Tuberculosis, pulmonary) 011.9
Employment examination (certification) V70.5
Empty sella (turcica) syndrome 253.8

Empyema (chest) (diaphragmatic) (double) (encapsulated) (general) (interlobar) (lung) (medial) (necessitatis) (perforating chest wall) (pleura) (pneumococcal) (residual) (sacculated) (streptococcal) (supradiaphragmatic) 510.9
with fistula 510.0
accessory sinus (chronic) (*see also* Sinusitis) 473.9
acute 510.9
with fistula 510.0
antrum (chronic) (*see also* Sinusitis, maxillary) 473.0
brain (any part) (*see also* Abscess, brain) 324.0
ethmoidal (sinus) (chronic) (*see also* Sinusitis, ethmoidal) 473.2
extradural (*see also* Abscess, extradural) 324.9
frontal (sinus) (chronic) (*see also* Sinusitis, frontal) 473.1
gallbladder (*see also* Cholecystitis, acute) 575.0
mastoid (process) (acute) (*see also* Mastoiditis, acute) 383.00
maxilla, maxillary 526.4
sinus (chronic) (*see also* Sinusitis, maxillary) 473.0
nasal sinus (chronic) (*see also* Sinusitis) 473.9
sinus (accessory) (nasal) (*see also* Sinusitis) 473.9
sphenoidal (chronic) (sinus) (*see also* Sinusitis, sphenoidal) 473.3
subarachnoid (*see also* Abscess, extradural) 324.9
subdural (*see also* Abscess, extradural) 324.9
tuberculous (*see also* Tuberculosis, pleura) 012.0
ureter (*see also* Ureteritis) 593.89
ventricular (*see also* Abscess, brain) 324.0
Enameloma 520.2
Encephalitis (bacterial) (chronic) (hemorrhagic) (idiopathic) (nonepidemic) (spurious) (subacute) 323.9
acute—*see also* Encephalitis, viral
disseminated (postinfectious) NEC 136.9 *[323.6]*
postimmunization or postvaccination 323.5
inclusional 049.8
inclusion body 049.8
necrotizing 049.8
arboviral, arbovirus NEC 064
arthropod-borne (*see also* Encephalitis, viral, arthropod-borne) 064
Australian X 062.4
Bwamba fever 066.3
California (virus) 062.5
Central European 063.2
Czechoslovakian 063.2
Dawson's (inclusion body) 046.2
diffuse sclerosing 046.2
due to
actinomycosis 039.8 *[323.4]*
cat-scratch disease 078.3 *[323.0]*
infectious mononucleosis 075 *[323.0]*
malaria (*see also* Malaria) 084.6 *[323.2]*
Negishi virus 064
ornithosis 073.7 *[323.0]*
prophylactic inoculation against smallpox 323.5
rickettsiosis (*see also* Rickettsiosis) 083.9 *[323.1]*

Encephalitis—*continued*
rubella 056.01
toxoplasmosis (acquired) 130.0
congenital (active) 771.2 *[323.4]*
typhus (fever) (*see also* Typhus) 081.9 *[323.1]*
vaccination (smallpox) 323.5
Eastern equine 062.2
endemic 049.8
epidemic 049.8
equine (acute) (infectious) (viral) 062.9
Eastern 062.2
Venezuelan 066.2
Western 062.1
Far Eastern 063.0
following vaccination or other immunization procedure 323.5
herpes 054.3
Ilheus (virus) 062.8
inclusion body 046.2
infectious (acute) (virus) NEC 049.8
influenzal 487.8 *[323.4]*
lethargic 049.8
Japanese (B type) 062.0
La Crosse 062.5
Langat 063.8
late effect—*see* Late, effect, encephalitis
lead 984.9 *[323.7]*
lethargic (acute) (infectious) (influenzal) 049.8
lethargica 049.8
louping ill 063.1
lupus 710.0
lymphatica 049.0
Mengo 049.8
meningococcal 036.1
mumps 072.2
Murray Valley 062.4
myoclonic 049.8
Negishi virus 064
otitic NEC 382.4 *[323.4]*
parasitic NEC 123.9 *[323.4]*
periaxialis (concentrica) (diffusa) 341.1
postchickenpox 052.0
postexanthematous NEC 057.9 *[323.6]*
postimmunization 323.5
postinfectious NEC 136.9 *[323.6]*
postmeasles 055.0
posttraumatic 323.8
postvaccinal (smallpox) 323.5
postvaricella 052.0
postviral NEC 079.99 *[323.6]*
postexanthematous 057.9 *[323.6]*
specified NEC 057.8 *[323.6]*
Powassan 063.8
progressive subcortical (Binswanger's) 290.12
Rio Bravo 049.8
rubella 056.01
Russian
autumnal 062.0
spring-summer type (taiga) 063.0
saturnine 984.9 *[323.7]*
Semliki Forest 062.8
serous 048
slow-acting virus NEC 046.8
specified cause NEC 323.8
St. Louis type 062.3
subacute sclerosing 046.2
subcorticalis chronica 290.12
summer 062.0
suppurative 324.0

Encephalitis—*continued*
syphilitic 094.81
congenital 090.41
tick-borne 063.9
torula, torular 117.5 *[323.4]*
toxic NEC 989.9 *[323.7]*
toxoplasmic (acquired) 130.0
congenital (active) 771.2 *[323.4]*
trichinosis 124 *[323.4]*
Trypanosomiasis (*see also* Trypanosomiasis) 086.9 *[323.2]*
tuberculous (*see also* Tuberculosis) 013.6
type B (Japanese) 062.0
type C 062.3
van Bogaert's 046.2
Venezuelan 066.2
Vienna type 049.8
viral, virus 049.9
arthropod-borne NEC 064
mosquito-borne 062.9
Australian X disease 062.4
California virus 062.5
Eastern equine 062.2
Ilheus virus 062.8
Japanese (B type) 062.0
Murray Valley 062.4
specified type NEC 062.8
St. Louis 062.3
type B 062.0
type C 062.3
Western equine 062.1
tick-borne 063.9
biundulant 063.2
Central European 063.2
Czechoslovakian 063.2
diphasic meningoencephalitis 063.2
Far Eastern 063.0
Langat 063.8
louping ill 063.1
Powassan 063.8
Russian spring-summer (taiga) 063.0
specified type NEC 063.8
vector unknown 064
slow acting NEC 046.8
specified type NEC 049.8
vaccination, prophylactic (against) V05.0
von Economo's 049.8
Western equine 062.1
West Nile type 066.3
Encephalocele 742.0
orbit 376.81
Encephalocystocele 742.0
Encephalomalacia (brain) (cerebellar) (cerebral) (cerebrospinal) (*see also* Softening, brain) 434.9
due to
hemorrhage (*see also* Hemorrhage, brain) 431
recurrent spasm of artery 435.9
embolic (cerebral) (*see also* Embolism, brain) 434.1
subcorticalis chronicus arteriosclerotica 290.12
thrombotic (*see also* Thrombosis, brain) 434.0
Encephalomeningitis —*see* Meningoencephalitis
Encephalomeningocele 742.0
Encephalomeningomyelitis —*see* Meningoencephalitis
Encephalomeningopathy (*see also* Meningoencephalitis) 349.9
Encephalomyelitis (chronic) (granulomatous) (hemorrhagic necrotizing, acute) (myalgic, benign) (*see also* Encephalitis) 323.9
abortive disseminated 049.8
acute disseminated (postinfectious) 136.9 *[323.6]*
postimmunization 323.5
due to or resulting from vaccination (any) 323.5
equine (acute) (infectious) 062.9
Eastern 062.2
Venezuelan 066.2
Western 062.1
funicularis infectiosa 049.8
late effect—*see* Late, effect, encephalitis
Munch-Peterson's 049.8
postchickenpox 052.0
postimmunization 323.5
postmeasles 055.0
postvaccinal (smallpox) 323.5
rubella 056.01
specified cause NEC 323.8
syphilitic 094.81
Encephalomyelocele 742.0
Encephalomyelomeningitis —*see* Meningoencephalitis
Encephalomyeloneuropathy 349.9
Encephalomyelopathy 349.9
subacute necrotizing (infantile) 330.8
Encephalomyeloradiculitis (acute) 357.0
Encephalomyeloradiculoneuritis (acute) 357.0
Encephalomyeloradiculopathy 349.9
Encephalomyocarditis 074.23
Encephalopathia hyperbilirubinemica newborn 774.7
due to isoimmunization (conditions classifiable to 773.0-773.2) 773.4
Encephalopathy (acute) 348.3
alcoholic 291.2
anoxic—*see* Damage, brain, anoxic
arteriosclerotic 437.0
late effect—*see* category 438
bilirubin, newborn 774.7
due to isoimmunization 773.4
congenital 742.9
demyelinating (callosal) 341.8
due to
birth injury (intracranial) 767.8
dialysis 294.8
transient 293.9
hyperinsulinism—*see* Hyperinsulinism
influenza (virus) 487.8
lack of vitamin (*see also* Deficiency, vitamin) 269.2
nicotinic acid deficiency 291.2
serum (nontherapeutic) (therapeutic) 999.5
syphilis 094.81
trauma (postconcussional) 310.2
current (*see also* Concussion, brain) 850.9
with skull fracture—*see* Fracture, skull, by site, with intracranial injury
vaccination 323.5
hepatic 572.2
hyperbilirubinemic, newborn 774.7
due to isoimmunization (conditions classifiable to 773.0-773.2) 773.4
hypertensive 437.2
hypoglycemic 251.2
hypoxic—*see* Damage, brain, anoxic
infantile cystic necrotizing (congenital) 341.8

- **Encephalopathy**—*continued*
  - lead 984.9 *[323.7]*
  - leukopolio 330.0
  - metabolic (toxic)—*see* Delirium
  - necrotizing, subacute 330.8
  - pellagrous 265.2
  - portal-systemic 572.2
  - postcontusional 310.2
  - posttraumatic 310.2
  - saturnine 984.9 *[323.7]*
  - spongioform, subacute (viral) 046.1
  - subacute
    - necrotizing 330.8
    - spongioform 046.1
    - viral, spongioform 046.1
  - subcortical progressive (Schilder) 341.1
    - chronic (Binswanger's) 290.12
  - toxic 349.82
    - metabolic—*see* Delirium
  - traumatic (postconcussional) 310.2
    - current (*see also* Concussion, brain) 850.9
      - with skull fracture—*see* Fracture, skull, by site, with intracranial injury
  - vitamin B deficiency NEC 266.9
  - Wernicke's (superior hemorrhagic polioencephalitis) 265.1
- **Enchephalorrhagia** (*see also* Hemorrhage, brain) 432.9
  - healed or old—*see also* category 438
    - without residuals V12.59
  - late effect—*see* category 438
- **Encephalosis, posttraumatic** 310.2
- **Enchondroma** (M9220/0)—*see also* Neoplasm, bone, benign
  - multiple, congenital 756.4
- **Enchondromatosis** (cartilaginous) (congenital) (multiple) 756.4
- **Enchondroses, multiple** (cartilaginous) (congenital) 756.4
- **Encopresis** (*see also* Incontinence, feces) 787.6
  - nonorganic origin 307.7
- **Encounter for** —*see also* Admission for
  - administrative purpose only V68.9
    - referral of patient without examination or treatment V68.81
    - specified purpose NEC V68.89
  - chemotherapy V58.1
  - radiotherapy V58.0
- **Encystment** —*see* Cyst
- **Endamebiasis** —*see* Amebiasis
- **Endamoeba** —*see* Amebiasis
- **Endarteritis** (bacterial, subacute) (infective) (septic) 447.6
  - brain, cerebral or cerebrospinal 437.4
    - late effect—*see* category 438
  - coronary (artery) —*see* Arteriosclerosis, coronary
  - deformans—*see* Arteriosclerosis
  - embolic (*see also* Embolism) 444.9
  - obliterans—*see also* Arteriosclerosis
    - pulmonary 417.8
  - pulmonary 417.8
  - retina 362.18
  - senile—*see* Arteriosclerosis
  - syphilitic 093.89
    - brain or cerebral 094.89
    - congenital 090.5
    - spinal 094.89
  - tuberculous (*see also* Tuberculosis) 017.9
- **Endemic** —*see* condition
- **Endocarditis** (chronic) (indeterminate) (interstitial) (marantis) (nonbacterial thrombotic) (residual) (sclerotic) (sclerous) (senile) (valvular) 424.90
  - with
    - rheumatic fever (conditions classifiable to 390)
      - active—*see* Endocarditis, acute, rheumatic
      - inactive or quiescent (with chorea) 397.9
  - acute or subacute 421.9
    - rheumatic (aortic) (mitral) (pulmonary) (tricuspid) 391.1
      - with chorea (acute) (rheumatic) (Sydenham's) 392.0
  - aortic (heart) (nonrheumatic) (valve) 424.1
    - with
      - mitral (valve) disease 396.9
        - active or acute 391.1
          - with chorea (acute) (rheumatic) (Sydenham's) 392.0
      - rheumatic fever (conditions classifiable to 390)
        - active—*see* Endocarditis, acute, rheumatic
        - inactive or quiescent (with chorea) 395.9
          - with mitral disease 396.9
    - acute or subacute 421.9
    - arteriosclerotic 424.1
    - congenital 746.89
    - hypertensive 424.1
    - rheumatic (chronic) (inactive) 395.9
      - with mitral (valve) disease 396.9
        - active or acute 391.1
          - with chorea (acute) (rheumatic) (Sydenham's) 392.0
      - active or acute 391.1
        - with chorea (acute) (rheumatic) (Sydenham's) 392.0
    - specified cause, except rheumatic 424.1
    - syphilitic 093.22
  - arteriosclerotic or due to arteriosclerosis 424.99
  - atypical verrucous (Libman-Sacks) 710.0 *[424.91]*
  - bacterial (acute) (any valve) (chronic) (subacute) 421.0
  - blastomycotic 116.0 *[421.1]*
  - candidal 112.81
  - congenital 425.3
  - constrictive 421.0
  - Coxsackie 074.22
  - due to
    - blastomycosis 116.0 *[421.1]*
    - candidiasis 112.81
    - Coxsackie (virus) 074.22
    - disseminated lupus erythematosus 710.0 *[424.91]*
    - histoplasmosis (*see also* Histoplasmosis) 115.94
    - hypertension (benign) 424.99
    - moniliasis 112.81
    - prosthetic cardiac valve 996.61
    - Q fever 083.0 *[421.1]*
    - serratia marcescens 421.0
    - typhoid (fever) 002.0 *[421.1]*
  - fetal 425.3
  - gonococcal 098.84
  - hypertensive 424.99
  - infectious or infective (acute) (any valve) (chronic) (subacute) 421.0
  - lenta (acute) (any valve) (chronic) (subacute) 421.0

Endocarditis—*continued*
Libman-Sacks 710.0 *[424.91]*
Loeffler's (parietal fibroplastic) 421.0
malignant (acute) (any valve) (chronic) (subacute) 421.0
meningococcal 036.42
mitral (chronic) (double) (fibroid) (heart) (inactive) (valve) (with chorea) 394.9
with
aortic (valve) disease 396.9
active or acute 391.1
with chorea (acute) (rheumatic) (Sydenham's) 392.0
rheumatic fever (conditions classifiable to 390)
active—*see* Endocarditis, acute, rheumatic
inactive or quiescent (with chorea) 394.9
with aortic valve disease 396.9
active or acute 391.1
bacterial 421.0
with chorea (acute) (rheumatic) (Sydenham's) 392.0
arteriosclerotic 424.0
congenital 746.89
hypertensive 424.0
nonrheumatic 424.0
acute or subacute 421.9
syphilitic 093.21
monilial 112.81
mycotic (acute) (any valve) (chronic) (subacute) 421.0
pneumococcic (acute) (any valve) (chronic) (subacute) 421.0
pulmonary (chronic) (heart) (valve) 424.3
with
rheumatic fever (conditions classifiable to 390)
active—*see* Endocarditis, acute, rheumatic
inactive or quiescent (with chorea) 397.1
acute or subacute 421.9
rheumatic 391.1
with chorea (acute) (rheumatic) (Sydenham's) 392.0
arteriosclerotic or due to arteriosclerosis 424.3
congenital 746.09
hypertensive or due to hypertension (benign) 424.3
rheumatic (chronic) (inactive) (with chorea) 397.1
active or acute 391.1
with chorea (acute) (rheumatic) (Sydenham's) 392.0
syphilitic 093.24
purulent (acute) (any valve) (chronic) (subacute) 421.0
rheumatic (chronic) (inactive) (with chorea) 397.9
active or acute (aortic) (mitral) (pulmonary) (tricuspid) 391.1
with chorea (acute) (rheumatic) (Sydenham's) 392.0
septic (acute) (any valve) (chronic) (subacute) 421.0
specified cause, except rheumatic 424.99
streptococcal (acute) (any valve) (chronic) (subacute) 421.0
subacute—*see* Endocarditis, acute

Endocarditis—*continued*
suppurative (any valve) (acute) (chronic) (subacute) 421.0
syphilitic NEC 093.20
toxic (*see also* Endocarditis, acute) 421.9
tricuspid (chronic) (heart) (inactive) (rheumatic) (valve) (with chorea) 397.0
with
rheumatic fever (conditions classifiable to 390)
active—*see* Endocarditis, acute, rheumatic
inactive or quiescent (with chorea) 397.0
active or acute 391.1
with chorea (acute) (rheumatic) (Sydenham's) 392.0
arteriosclerotic 424.2
congenital 746.89
hypertensive 424.2
nonrheumatic 424.2
acute or subacute 421.9
specified cause, except rheumatic 424.2
syphilitic 093.23
tuberculous (*see also* Tuberculosis) 017.9 *[424.91]*
typhoid 002.0 *[421.1]*
ulcerative (acute) (any valve) (chronic) (subacute) 421.0
vegetative (acute) (any valve) (chronic) (subacute) 421.0
verrucous (acute) (any valve) (chronic) (subacute) NEC 710.0 *[424.91]*
nonbacterial 710.0 *[424.91]*
nonrheumatic 710.0 *[424.91]*
Endocardium, endocardial —*see also* condition
cushion defect 745.60
specified type NEC 745.69
Endocervicitis (*see also* Cervicitis) 616.0
due to
intrauterine (contraceptive) device 996.65
gonorrheal (acute) 098.15
chronic or duration of 2 months or over 098.35
hyperplastic 616.0
syphilitic 095.8
trichomonal 131.09
tuberculous (*see also* Tuberculosis) 016.7
Endocrine —*see* condition
Endocrinopathy, pluriglandular 258.9
Endodontitis 522.0
Endomastoiditis (*see also* Mastoiditis) 383.9
Endometrioma 617.9
Endometriosis 617.9
appendix 617.5
bladder 617.8
bowel 617.5
broad ligament 617.3
cervix 617.0
colon 617.5
cul-de-sac (Douglas') 617.3
exocervix 617.0
fallopian tube 617.2
female genital organ NEC 617.8
gallbladder 617.8
in scar of skin 617.6
internal 617.0
intestine 617.5
lung 617.8
myometrium 617.0
ovary 617.1
parametrium 617.3

Endometriosis—*continued*
pelvic peritoneum 617.3
peritoneal (pelvic) 617.3
rectovaginal septum 617.4
rectum 617.5
round ligament 617.3
skin 617.6
specified site NEC 617.8
stromal (M8931/1) 236.0
umbilicus 617.8
uterus 617.0
internal 617.0
vagina 617.4
vulva 617.8
Endometritis (nonspecific) (purulent) (septic) (suppurative) 615.9
with
abortion—*see* Abortion, by type, with sepsis
ectopic pregnancy (*see also* categories 633.0-633.9) 639.0
molar pregnancy (*see also* categories 630-632) 639.0
acute 615.0
blennorrhagic 098.16
acute 098.16
chronic or duration of 2 months or over 098.36
cervix, cervical (*see also* Cervicitis) 616.0
hyperplastic 616.0
chronic 615.1
complicating pregnancy 646.6
affecting fetus or newborn 760.8
decidual 615.9
following
abortion 639.0
ectopic or molar pregnancy 639.0
gonorrheal (acute) 098.16
chronic or duration of 2 months or over 098.36
hyperplastic 621.3
cervix 616.0
polypoid—*see* Endometritis, hyperplastic
puerperal, postpartum, childbirth 670
senile (atrophic) 615.9
subacute 615.0
tuberculous (*see also* Tuberculosis) 016.7
Endometrium —*see* condition
Endomyocardiopathy, South African 425.2
Endomyocarditis —*see* Endocarditis
Endomyofibrosis 425.0
Endomyometritis (*see also* Endometritis) 615.9
Endopericarditis —*see* Endocarditis
Endoperineuritis —*see* Disorder, nerve
Endophlebitis (*see also* Phlebitis) 451.9
leg 451.2
deep (vessels) 451.19
superficial (vessels) 451.0
portal (vein) 572.1
retina 362.18
specified site NEC 451.89
syphilitic 093.89
Endophthalmia (*see also* Endophthalmitis) 360.00
gonorrheal 098.42
Endophthalmitis (globe) (infective) (metastatic) (purulent) (subacute) 360.00
acute 360.01
chronic 360.03
parasitic 360.13
phacoanaphylactic 360.19
specified type NEC 360.19
sympathetic 360.11
Endosalpingioma (M9111/1) 236.2
Endosteitis —*see* Osteomyelitis
Endothelioma, bone (M9260/3)—*see* Neoplasm, bone, malignant
Endotheliosis 287.8
hemorrhagic infectional 287.8
Endotoxic shock 785.59
Endotrachelitis (*see also* Cervicitis) 616.0
Enema rash 692.89
Engel-von Recklinghausen disease or syndrome (osteitis fibrosa cystica) 252.0
Engelmann's disease (diaphyseal sclerosis) 756.59
English disease (*see also* Rickets) 268.0
Engman's disease (infectious eczematoid dermatitis) 690.8
Engorgement
breast 611.79
newborn 778.7
puerperal, postpartum 676.2
liver 573.9
lung 514
pulmonary 514
retina, venous 362.37
stomach 536.8
venous, retina 362.37
Enlargement, enlarged —*see also* Hypertrophy
abdomen 789.3
adenoids 474.12
and tonsils 474.10
alveolar process or ridge 525.8
apertures of diaphragm (congenital) 756.6
blind spot, visual field 368.42
gingival 523.8
heart, cardiac (*see also* Hypertrophy, cardiac) 429.3
lacrimal gland, chronic 375.03
liver (*see also* Hypertrophy, liver) 789.1
lymph gland or node 785.6
orbit 376.46
organ or site, congenital NEC—*see* Anomaly, specified type NEC
parathyroid (gland) 252.0
pituitary fossa 793.0
prostate, simple 600
sella turcica 793.0
spleen (*see also* Splenomegaly) 789.2
congenital 759.0
thymus (congenital) (gland) 254.0
thyroid (gland) (*see also* Goiter) 240.9
tongue 529.8
tonsils 474.11
and adenoids 474.10
uterus 621.2
Enophthalmos 376.50
due to
atrophy of orbital tissue 376.51
surgery 376.52
trauma 376.52
Enostosis 526.89
Entamebiasis —*see* Amebiasis
Entamebic —*see* Amebiasis
Entanglement, umbilical cord (s) 663.3
with compression 663.2
affecting fetus or newborn 762.5
around neck with compression 663.1
twins in monoamniotic sac 663.2
Enteralgia 789.0
Enteric —*see* condition

Enteritis (acute) (catarrhal) (choleraic) (chronic) (congestive) (diarrheal) (exudative) (follicular) (hemorrhagic) (infantile) (lienteric) (noninfectious) (perforative) (phlegmonous) (presumed noninfectious) (pseudomembranous) 558.9
adaptive 564.1
aertrycke infection 003.0
allergic 558.9
amebic (*see also* Amebiasis) 006.9
with abscess—*see* Abscess, amebic
acute 006.0
with abscess—*see* Abscess, amebic
nondysenteric 006.2
chronic 006.1
with abscess—*see* Abscess, amebic
nondysenteric 006.2
nondysenteric 006.2
anaerobic (cocci) (gram-negative) (gram-positive) (mixed) NEC 008.46
bacillary NEC 004.9
bacterial NEC 008.5
specified NEC 008.49
Bacteroides (fragilis) (melaninogeniscus) (oralis) 008.46
Butyrivibrio (fibriosolvens) 008.46
Campylobacter 008.43
Candida 112.85
Chilomastix 007.8
choleriformis 001.1
chronic 558.9
ulcerative (*see also* Colitis, ulcerative) 556.9
cicatrizing (chronic) 555.0
Clostridium
botulinum 005.1
difficile 008.45
haemolyticum 008.46
novyi 008.46
perfringens (C) (F) 008.46
specified type NEC 008.46
coccidial 007.2
dietetic 558.9
due to
achylia gastrica 536.8
adenovirus 008.62
Aerobacter aerogenes 008.2
anaerobes—*see* Enteritis, anaerobic 008.46
Arizona (bacillus) 008.1
astrovirus 008.66
Bacillus coli—*see* Enteritis, E. coli 008.0
bacteria NEC 008.5
specified NEC 008.49
Bacteroides 008.46
Butyrivibrio (fibriosolvens) 008.46
Calcivirus 008.65
Campylobacter 008.43
Clostridium—*see* Enteritis, Clostridium
Cockle agent 008.64
Coxsackie (virus) 008.67
Ditchling agent 008.64
ECHO virus 008.67
Enterobacter aerogenes 008.2
enterococci 008.49
enterovirus NEC 008.67
Escherichia coli—*see* Enteritis, E. coli
Eubacterium 008.46
Fusobacterium (nucleatum) 008.46
gram-negative bacteria NEC 008.47
anaerobic NEC 008.46

Enteritis—*continued*
Hawaii agent 008.63
irritating foods 558.9
Klebsiella aerogenes 008.47
Marin County agent 008.66
Montgomery County agent 008.63
Norwalk-like agent 008.63
Norwalk virus 008.63
Otofuke agent 008.63
Paracolobactrum arizonae 008.1
paracolon bacillus NEC 008.47
Arizona 008.1
Paramatta agent 008.64
Peptococcus 008.46
Peptostreptococcus 008.46
Propionibacterium 008.46
Proteus (bacillus) (mirabilis) (morganii) 008.3
Pseudomonas aeruginosa 008.42
Rotavirus 008.61
Sapporo agent 008.63
small round virus (SRV) NEC 008.64
featureless NEC 008.63
structured NEC 008.63
Snow Mountain (SM) agent 008.63
specified
bacteria NEC 008.49
organism, nonbacterial NEC 008.8
virus NEC 008.69
Staphylococcus 008.41
Streptococcus 008.49
anaerobic 008.46
Taunton agent 008.63
Torovirus 008.69
Treponema 008.46
Veillonella 008.46
virus 008.8
specified type NEC 008.69
Wollan (W) agent 008.64
Yersinia enterocolitica 008.44
dysentery—*see* Dysentery
E. coli 008.00
enterohemorrhagic 008.04
enteroinvasive 008.03
enteropathogenic 008.01
enterotoxigenic 008.02
specified type NEC 008.09
el tor 001.1
embadomonial 007.8
epidemic 009.0
Eubacterium 008.46
fermentative 558.9
fulminant 557.0
Fusobacterium (nucleatum) 008.46
gangrenous (*see also* Enteritis, due to, by organism) 009.0
giardial 007.1
gram-negative bacteria NEC 008.47
anaerobic NEC 008.46
infectious NEC (*see also* Enteritis, due to, by organism) 009.0
presumed 009.1
influenzal 487.8
ischemic 557.9
acute 557.0
chronic 557.1
due to mesenteric artery insufficiency 557.1
membranous 564.1
mucous 564.1
myxomembranous 564.1

Enteritis—*continued*
necrotic (*see also* Enteritis, due to, by organism) 009.0
necroticans 005.2
necrotizing of fetus or newborn 777.5
neurogenic 564.1
newborn 777.8
necrotizing 777.5
parasitic NEC 129
paratyphoid (fever) (*see also* Fever, paratyphoid) 002.9
Peptococcus 008.46
Peptostreptococcus 008.46
Propionibacterium 008.46
protozoal NEC 007.9
regional (of) 555.9
intestine
large (bowel, colon, or rectum) 555.1
with small intestine 555.2
small (duodenum, ileum, or jejunum) 555.0
with large intestine 555.2
Salmonella infection 003.0
salmonellosis 003.0
segmental (*see also* Enteritis, regional) 555.9
septic (*see also* Enteritis, due to, by organism) 009.0
Shigella 004.9
simple 558.9
spasmodic 564.1
spastic 564.1
staphylococcal 008.41
due to food 005.0
streptococcal 008.49
anaerobic 008.46
toxic 558.2
Treponema (denticola) (macrodentium) 008.46
trichomonal 007.3
tuberculous (*see also* Tuberculosis) 014.8
typhosa 002.0
ulcerative (chronic) (*see also* Colitis, ulcerative) 556.9
Veillonella 008.46
viral 008.8
adenovirus 008.62
enterovirus 008.67
specified virus NEC 008.69
Yersinia enterocolitica 008.44
zymotic 009.0
Enteroarticular syndrome 099.3
Enterobiasis 127.4
Enterobius vermicularis 127.4
Enterocele (*see also* Hernia) 553.9
pelvis, pelvic (acquired) (congenital) 618.6
vagina, vaginal (acquired) (congenital) 618.6
Enterocolitis —*see also* Enteritis
fetus or newborn 777.8
necrotizing 777.5
fulminant 557.0
granulomatous 555.2
hemorrhagic (acute) 557.0
chronic 557.1
necrotizing (acute) (membranous) 557.0
primary necrotizing 777.5
pseudomembranous 008.45
radiation 558.1
newborn 777.5
ulcerative 556.0
Enterocystoma 751.5
Enterogastritis —*see* Enteritis
Enterogenous cyanosis 289.7
Enterolith, enterolithiasis (impaction) 560.39
with hernia—*see also* Hernia, by site, with obstruction
gangrenous—*see* Hernia, by site, with gangrene
Enteropathy 569.9
exudative (of Gordon) 579.8
gluten 579.0
hemorrhagic, terminal 557.0
protein-losing 579.8
Enteroperitonitis (*see also* Peritonitis) 567.9
Enteroptosis 569.89
Enterorrhagia 578.9
Enterospasm 564.1
psychogenic 306.4
Enterostenosis (*see also* Obstruction, intestine) 560.9
Enterostomy status V44.4
with complication 569.60
Enthesopathy 726.39
ankle and tarsus 726.70
elbow region 726.30
specified NEC 726.39
hip 726.5
knee 726.60
peripheral NEC 726.8
shoulder region 726.10
adhesive 726.0
spinal 720.1
wrist and carpus 726.4
Entrance, air into vein —*see* Embolism, air
Entrapment, nerve —*see* Neuropathy, entrapment
Entropion (eyelid) 374.00
cicatricial 374.04
congenital 743.62
late effect of trachoma (healed) 139.1
mechanical 374.02
paralytic 374.02
senile 374.01
spastic 374.03
Enucleation of eye (current) (traumatic) 871.3
Enuresis 788.30
habit disturbance 307.6
nocturnal 788.36
psychogenic 307.6
nonorganic origin 307.6
psychogenic 307.6
Enzymopathy 277.9
Eosinopenia 288.0
Eosinophilia 288.3
allergic 288.3
hereditary 288.3
idiopathic 288.3
infiltrative 518.3
Loeffler's 518.3
myalgia syndrome 710.5
pulmonary (tropical) 518.3
secondary 288.3
tropical 518.3
Eosinophilic —*see also* condition
fasciitis 728.89
granuloma (bone) 277.8
infiltration lung 518.3
Ependymitis (acute) (cerebral) (chronic) (granular) (*see also* Meningitis) 322.9
Ependymoblastoma (M9392/3)
specified site—*see* Neoplasm, by site, malignant
unspecified site 191.9

Note—use the following fifth-digit subclassification with categories 345.0, 345.1, 345.4-345.9

0 without mention of intractable epilepsy
1 with intractable epilepsy

Epilepsy, epileptic—*continued*
parasitic NEC 123.9
partial (focalized) 345.5
with
impairment of consciousness 345.4
memory and ideational disturbances 345.4
abdominal type 345.5
motor type 345.5
psychomotor type 345.4
psychosensory type 345.4
secondarily generalized 345.4
sensory type 345.5
somatomotor type 345.5
somatosensory type 345.5
temporal lobe type 345.4
visceral type 345.5
visual type 345.5
peripheral 345.9
petit mal 345.0
photokinetic 345.8
progressive myoclonic (familial) 333.2
psychic equivalent 345.5
psychomotor 345.4
psychosensory 345.4
reflex 345.1
seizure 345.9
senile 345.9
sensory-induced 345.5
sleep 347
somatomotor type 345.5
somatosensory 345.5
specified type NEC 345.8
status (grand mal) 345.3
focal motor 345.7
petit mal 345.2
psychomotor 345.7
temporal lobe 345.7
symptomatic 345.9
temporal lobe 345.4
tonic (-clonic) 345.1
traumatic (injury unspecified) 907.0
injury specified—*see* Late, effect (of) specified injury
twilight 293.0
uncinate (gyrus) 345.4
Unverricht (-Lundborg) (familial myoclonic) 333.2
visceral 345.5
visual 345.5
Epileptiform
convulsions 780.3
seizure 780.3
Epiloia 759.5
Epimenorrhea 626.2
Epipharyngitis (*see also* Nasopharyngitis) 460
Epiphora 375.20
due to
excess lacrimation 375.21
insufficient drainage 375.22
Epiphyseal arrest 733.91
femoral head 732.2
Epiphyseolysis, epiphysiolysis (*see also* Osteochondrosis) 732.9
Epiphysitis (*see also* Osteochondrosis) 732.9
juvenile 732.6
marginal (Scheuermann's) 732.0
os calcis 732.5
syphilitic (congenital) 090.0
vertebral (Scheuermann's) 732.0
Epiplocele (*see also* Hernia) 553.9
Epiploitis (*see also* Peritonitis) 567.9
Epiplosarcomphalocele (*see also* Hernia, umbilicus) 553.1
Episcleritis 379.00
gouty 274.89 *[379.09]*
nodular 379.02
periodica fugax 379.01
angioneurotic—*see* Edema, angioneurotic
specified NEC 379.09
staphylococcal 379.00
suppurative 379.00
syphilitic 095.0
tuberculous (*see also* Tuberculosis) 017.3 *[379.09]*
Episode
brain (*see also* Disease, cerebrovascular, acute) 436
cerebral (*see also* Disease, cerebrovascular, acute) 436
depersonalization (in neurotic state) 300.6
psychotic (*see also* Psychosis) 298.9
organic, transient 293.9
schizophrenic (acute) NEC (*see also* Schizophrenia) 295.4
Epispadias
female 753.8
male 752.6
Episplenitis 289.59
Epistaxis (multiple) 784.7
hereditary 448.0
vicarious menstruation 625.8
Epithelioma (malignant) (M8011/3)—*see also* Neoplasm, by site, malignant
adenoides cysticum (M8100/0)—*see* Neoplasm, skin, benign
basal cell (M8090/3)—*see* Neoplasm, skin, malignant
benign (M8011/0)—*see* Neoplasm, by site, benign
Bowen's (M8081/2)—*see* Neoplasm, skin, in situ
calcifying (benign) (Malherbe's) (M8110/0)—*see* Neoplasm, skin, benign
external site—*see* Neoplasm, skin, malignant
intraepidermal, Jadassohn (M8096/0)—*see* Neoplasm, skin, benign
squamous cell (M8070/3)—*see* Neoplasm, by site, malignant
Epitheliopathy
pigment, retina 363.15
posterior multifocal placoid (acute) 363.15
Epithelium, epithelial —*see* condition
Epituberculosis (allergic) (with atelectasis) (*see also* Tuberculosis) 010.8
Eponychia 757.5
Epstein's
nephrosis or syndrome (*see also* Nephrosis) 581.9
pearl (mouth) 528.4
Epstein-Barr infection (viral) 075
Epulis (giant cell) (gingiva) 523.8
Equinia 024
Equinovarus (congenital) 754.51
acquired 736.71
Equivalent
convulsive (abdominal) (*see also* Epilepsy) 345.5
epileptic (psychic) (*see also* Epilepsy) 345.5

Erb's
disease 359.1
palsy, paralysis (birth) (brachial) (newborn) 767.6
spinal (spastic) syphilitic 094.89
pseudohypertrophic muscular dystrophy 359.1
Erb (-Duchenne) paralysis (birth injury) (newborn) 767.6
Erb-Goldflam disease or syndrome 358.0
Erdheim's syndrome (acromegalic macrospondylitis) 253.0
Erection, painful (persistent) 607.3
Ergosterol deficiency (vitamin D) 268.9
with
osteomalacia 268.2
rickets (*see also* Rickets) 268.0
Ergotism (ergotized grain) 988.2
from ergot used as drug (migraine therapy)
correct substance properly administered 349.82
overdose or wrong substance given or taken 975.0
Erichsen's disease (railway spine) 300.16
Erlacher-Blount syndrome (tibia vara) 732.4
Erosio interdigitalis blastomycetica 112.3
Erosion
arteriosclerotic plaque—*see* Arteriosclerosis, by site
artery NEC 447.2
without rupture 447.8
bone 733.99
bronchus 519.1
cartilage (joint) 733.99
cervix (uteri) (acquired) (chronic) (congenital) 622.0
with mention of cervicitis 616.0
cornea (recurrent) (*see also* Keratitis) 371.42
traumatic 918.1
dental (idiopathic) (occupational) 521.3
duodenum, postpyloric—*see* Ulcer, duodenum
esophagus 530.89
gastric 535.4
intestine 569.89
lymphatic vessel 457.8
pylorus, pyloric (ulcer) 535,4
sclera 379.16
spine, aneurysmal 094.89
spleen 289.59
stomach 535.4
teeth (idiopathic) (occupational) 521.3
due to
medicine 521.3
persistent vomiting 521.3
urethra 599.84
uterus 621.8
vertebra 733.99
Erotomania 302.89
Clérambault's 297.8
Error
in diet 269.9
refractive 367.9
astigmatism (*see also* Astigmatism) 367.20
drug-induced 367.89
hypermetropia 367.0
hyperopia 367.0
myopia 367.1
presbyopia 367.4
toxic 367.89
Eructation 787.3
nervous 306.4
psychogenic 306.4
Eruption
creeping 126.9
drug—*see* Dermatitis, due to, drug
Hutchinson, summer 692.72
Kaposi's varicelliform 054.0
napkin (psoriasiform) 691.0
polymorphous
light (sun) 692.72
other source 692.82
psoriasiform, napkin 691.0
recalcitrant pustular 694.8
ringed 695.89
skin (*see also* Dermatitis) 782.1
creeping (meaning hookworm) 126.9
due to
chemical(s) NEC 692.4
internal use 693.8
drug—*see* Dermatitis, due to, drug
prophylactic inoculation or vaccination against disease—*see* Dermatitis, due to, vaccine
smallpox vaccination NEC—*see* Dermatitis, due to, vaccine
erysipeloid 027.1
feigned 698.4
Hutchinson, summer 692.72
Kaposi's, varicelliform 054.0
vaccinia 999.0
lichenoid, axilla 698.3
polymorphous, due to light 692.72
toxic NEC 695.0
vesicular 709.8
teeth, tooth
accelerated 520.6
delayed 520.6
difficult 520.6
disturbance of 520.6
in abnormal sequence 520.6
incomplete 520.6
late 520.6
natal 520.6
neonatal 520.6
obstructed 520.6
partial 520.6
persistent primary 520.6
premature 520.6
vesicular 709.8
Erysipelas (gangrenous) (infantile) (newborn) (phlegmonous) (suppurative) 035
external ear 035 *[380.13]*
puerperal, postpartum, childbirth 670
Erysipelatoid (Rosenbach's) 027.1
Erysipeloid (Rosenbach's) 027.1
Erythema, erythematous (generalized) 695.9
ab igne—*see* Burn, by site, first degree
annulare (centrifugum) (rheumaticum) 695.0
arthriticum epidemicum 026.1
brucellum (*see also* Brucellosis) 023.9
bullosum 695.1
caloricum—*see* Burn, by site, first degree
chronicum migrans 088.81
chronicum 088.81
circinatum 695.1
diaper 691.0
due to
chemical (contact) NEC 692.4
internal 693.8
drug (internal use) 693.0
contact 692.3

Erythema, erythematous—*continued*
elevatum diutinum 695.89
endemic 265.2
epidemic, arthritic 026.1
figuratum perstans 695.0
gluteal 691.0
gyratum (perstans) (repens) 695.1
heat—*see* Burn, by site, first degree
ichthyosiforme congenitum 757.1
induratum (primary) (scrofulosorum) (*see also* Tuberculosis) 017.1
nontuberculous 695.2
infantum febrile 057.8
infectional NEC 695.9
infectiosum 057.0
inflammation NEC 695.9
intertrigo 695.89
iris 695.1
lupus (discoid) (localized) (*see also* Lupus, erythematosus) 695.4
marginatum 695.0
rheumaticum—*see* Fever, rheumatic
medicamentosum—*see* Dermatitis, due to, drug
migrans 529.1
multiforme 695.1
bullosum 695.1
conjunctiva 695.1
exudativum (Hebra) 695.1
pemphigoides 694.5
napkin 691.0
neonatorum 778.8
nodosum 695.2
tuberculous (*see also* Tuberculosis) 017.1
nummular, nummulare 695.1
palmar 695.0
palmaris hereditarium 695.0
pernio 991.5
perstans solare 692.72
rash, newborn 778.8
scarlatiniform (exfoliative) (recurrent) 695.0
simplex marginatum 057.8
solare 692.71
streptogenes 696.5
toxic, toxicum NEC 695.0
newborn 778.8
tuberculous (primary) (*see also* Tuberculosis) 017.0
venenatum 695.0
Erythematosus —*see* condition
Erythematous —*see* condition
Erythermalgia (primary) 443.89
Erythralgia 443.89
Erythrasma 039.0
Erythredema 985.0
polyneuritica 985.0
polyneuropathy 985.0
Erythremia (acute) (M9841/3) 207.0
chronic (M9842/3) 207.1
secondary 289.0
Erythroblastopenia (acquired) 284.8
congenital 284.0
Erythroblastophthisis 284.0
Erythroblastosis (fetalis) (newborn) 773.2
due to
ABO
antibodies 773.1
incompatibility, maternal/fetal 773.1
isoimmunization 773.1
Rh
antibodies 773.0
incompatibility, maternal/fetal 773.0
isoimmunization 773.0
Erythrocyanosis (crurum) 443.89
Erythrocythemia —*see* Erythremia
Erythrocytosis (megalosplenic)
familial 289.6
oval, hereditary (*see also* Elliptocytosis) 282.1
secondary 289.0
stress 289.0
Erythroderma (*see also* Erythema) 695.9
desquamativa (in infants) 695.89
exfoliative 695.89
ichthyosiform, congenital 757.1
infantum 695.89
maculopapular 696.2
neonatorum 778.8
psoriaticum 696.1
secondary 695.9
Erythrogenesis imperfecta 284.0
Erythroleukemia (M9840/3) 207.0
Erythromelalgia 443.89
Erythromelia 701.8
Erythrophagocytosis 289.9
Erythrophobia 300.23
Erythroplakia
oral mucosa 528.7
tongue 528.7
Erythroplasia (Queyrat) (M8080/2)
specified site—*see* Neoplasm, skin, in situ
unspecified site 233.5
Erythropoiesis, idiopathic ineffective 285.0
Escaped beats, heart 427.60
postoperative 997.1
Esoenteritis —*see* Enteritis
Esophagalgia 530.89
Esophagectasis 530.89
due to cardiospasm 530.0
Esophagismus 530.5
Esophagitis (acute) (alkaline) (chemical) (chronic) (infectional) (necrotic) (peptic) (postoperative) (regurgitant) 530.10
candidal 112.84
reflux 530.11
specified NEC 530.19
tuberculous (*see also* Tuberculosis) 017.8
Esophagocele 530.6
Esophagodynia 530.89
Esophagomalacia 530.89
Esophagoptosis 530.89
Esophagospasm 530.5
Esophagostenosis 530.3
Esophagostomiasis 127.7
Esophagotracheal —*see* condition
Esophagus —*see* condition
Esophoria 378.41
convergence, excess 378.84
divergence, insufficiency 378.85
Esotropia (nonaccommodative) 378.00
accommodative 378.35
alternating 378.05
with
A pattern 378.06
specified noncomitancy NEC 378.08
V pattern 378.07
X pattern 378.08
Y pattern 378.08
intermittent 378.22
intermittent 378.20
alternating 378.22
monocular 378.21

Esotropia—*continued*
  monocular 378.01
    with
      A pattern 378.02
      specified noncomitancy NEC 378.04
      V pattern 378.03
      X pattern 378.04
      Y pattern 378.04
    intermittent 378.21
Espundia 085.5
Essential —*see* condition
Esterapenia 289.8
Esthesioneuroblastoma (M9522/3) 160.0
Esthesioneurocytoma (M9521/3) 160.0
Esthesioneuroepithelioma (M9523/3) 160.0
Esthiomene 099.1
Estivo-autumnal
  fever 084.0
  malaria 084.0
Estrangement V61.0
Estriasis 134.0
Ethanolaminuria 270.8
Ethanolism (*see also* Alcoholism) 303.9
Ether dependence, dependency (*see also* Dependence) 304.6
Etherism (*see also* Dependence) 304.6
Ethmoid, ethmoidal —*see* condition
Ethmoiditis (chronic) (nonpurulent) (purulent) (*see also* Sinusitis, ethmoidal) 473.2
  influenzal 487.1
  Woakes' 471.1
Ethylism (*see also* Alcoholism) 303.9
Eulenburg's disease (congenital paramyotonia) 359.2
Eunuchism 257.2
Eunuchoidism 257.2
  hypogonadotropic 257.2
European blastomycosis 117.5
Eustachian —*see* condition
Euthyroidism 244.9
Evaluation
  for suspected condition (*see also* Observation) V71.9
    newborn—*see* Observation, suspected, condition, newborn
    specified condition NEC V71.8
  mental health V70.2
    requested by authority V70.1
  nursing care V63.8
  social service V63.8
Evan's syndrome (thrombocytopenic purpura) 287.3
Eventration
  colon into chest—*see* Hernia, diaphragm
  diaphragm (congenital) 756.6
Eversion
  bladder 596.8
  cervix (uteri) 622.0
    with mention of cervicitis 616.0
  foot NEC 736.79
    congenital 755.67
  lacrimal punctum 375.51
  punctum lacrimale (postinfectional) (senile) 375.51
  ureter (meatus) 593.89
  urethra (meatus) 599.84
  uterus 618.1
    complicating delivery 665.2
      affecting fetus or newborn 763.8
    puerperal, postpartum 674.8
Evisceration
  birth injury 767.8
  bowel (congenital)—*see* Hernia, ventral
  congenital (*see also* Hernia, ventral) 553.29
  operative wound 998.3
  traumatic NEC 869.1
    eye 871.3
Evulsion —*see* Avulsion
Ewing's
  angioendothelioma (M9260/3)—*see* Neoplasm, bone, malignant
  sarcoma (M9260/3)—*see* Neoplasm, bone, malignant
  tumor (M9260/3)—*see* Neoplasm, bone, malignant
Exaggerated lumbosacral angle (with impinging spine) 756.12
Examination (general) (routine) (of) (for) V70.9
  allergy V72.7
  annual V70.0
  cardiovascular preoperative V72.81
  cervical Papanicolaou smear V76.2
    as a part of routine gynecological examination V72.3
  child care (routine) V20.2
  clinical research investigation (normal control patient) V70.7
  dental V72.2
  developmental testing (child) (infant) V20.2
  donor (potential) V70.8
  ear V72.1
  eye V72.0
  following
    accident (motor vehicle) V71.4
    alleged rape or seduction (victim or culprit) V71.5
    inflicted injury (victim or culprit) NEC V71.6
    rape or seduction, alleged (victim or culprit) V71.5
    treatment (for) V67.9
      combined V67.6
      fracture V67.4
      involving high-risk medication NEC V67.51
      mental disorder V67.3
      specified condition NEC V67.59
  follow-up (routine) (following) V67.9
    cancer chemotherapy V67.2
    chemotherapy V67.2
    disease NEC V67.59
    high-risk medication NEC V67.51
    injury NEC V67.59
    population survey V70.6
    postpartum V24.2
    psychiatric V67.3
    psychotherapy V67.3
    radiotherapy V67.1
    surgery V67.0
  gynecological V72.3
    for contraceptive maintenance V25.40
      intrauterine device V25.42
      pill V25.41
      specified method NEC V25.49
  health (of)
    armed forces personnel V70.5
    checkup V70.0
    child, routine V20.2
    defined subpopulation NEC V70.5
    inhabitants of institutions V70.5
    occupational V70.5
    pre-employment screening V70.5

Examination—*continued*
preschool children V70.5
for admission to school V70.3
prisoners V70.5
for entrance into prison V70.3
prostitutes V70.5
refugees V70.5
school children V70.5
students V70.5
hearing V72.1
infant V20.2
laboratory V72.6
lactating mother V24.1
medical (for) (of) V70.9
administrative purpose NEC V70.3
admission to
old age home V70.3
prison V70.3
school V70.3
adoption V70.3
armed forces personnel V70.5
at health care facility V70.0
camp V70.3
child, routine V20.2
clinical research, normal comparison in V70.7
control subject in clinical research V70.7
defined subpopulation NEC V70.5
donor (potential) V70.8
driving license V70.3
general V70.9
routine V70.0
specified reason NEC V70.8
immigration V70.3
inhabitants of institutions V70.5
insurance certification V70.3
marriage V70.3
medicolegal reasons V70.4
naturalization V70.3
occupational V70.5
population survey V70.6
pre-employment V70.5
preschool children V70.5
for admission to school V70.3
prison V70.3
prisoners V70.5
for entrance into prison V70.3
prostitutes V70.5
refugees V70.5
school children V70.5
specified reason NEC V70.8
sport competition V70.3
students V70.5
medicolegal reason V70.4
pelvic (annual) (periodic) V72.3
periodic (annual) (routine) V70.0
postpartum
immediately after delivery V24.0
routine follow-up V24.2
pregnancy (unconfirmed) (possible) V72.4
prenatal V22.1
first pregnancy V22.0
high-risk pregnancy V23.9
specified problem NEC V23.8
preoperative V72.84
cardiovascular V72.81
respiratory V72.82
specified NEC V72.83
psychiatric V70.2
follow-up not needing further care V67.3
requested by authority V70.1

Examination—*continued*
radiological NEC V72.5
respiratory preoperative V72.82
screening—*see* Screening
sensitization V72.7
skin V72.7
hypersensitivity V72.7
special V72.9
specified type or reason NEC V72.85
preoperative V72.83
specified NEC V72.83
teeth V72.2
victim or culprit following
alleged rape or seduction V71.5
inflicted injury NEC V71.6
vision V72.0
well baby V20.2
Exanthem, exanthema (*see also* Rash) 782.1
Boston 048
epidemic, with meningitis 048
lichenoid psoriasiform 696.2
subitum 057.8
viral, virus NEC 057.9
specified type NEC 057.8
Excess, excessive, excessively
alcohol level in blood 790.3
carbohydrate tissue, localized 278.1
carotene (dietary) 278.3
cold 991.9
specified effect NEC 991.8
convergence 378.84
development, breast 611.1
diaphoresis 780.8
divergence 378.85
drinking (alcohol) NEC (*see also* Abuse, drugs, nondependent) 305.0
continual (*see also* Alcoholism) 303.9
habitual (*see also* Alcoholism) 303.9
eating 783.6
eyelid fold (congenital) 743.62
fat 278.00
in heart (*see also* Degeneration, myocardial) 429.1
tissue, localized 278.1
foreskin 605
gas 787.3
gastrin 251.5
glucagon 251.4
heat (*see also* Heat) 992.9
large
colon 564.7
congenital 751.3
fetus or infant 766.0
with obstructed labor 660.1
affecting management of pregnancy 656.6
causing disproportion 653.5
newborn (weight of 4500 grams or more) 766.0
organ or site, congenital NEC—*see* Anomaly, specified type NEC
lid fold (congenital) 743.62
long
colon 751.5
organ or site, congenital NEC—*see* Anomaly, specified type NEC
umbilical cord (entangled)
affecting fetus or newborn 762.5
in pregnancy or childbirth 663.3
with compression 663.2

Excess, excessive, excessively—*continued*
menstruation 626.2
number of teeth 520.1
causing crowding 524.3
nutrients (dietary) NEC 783.6
potassium (K) 276.7
salivation (*see also* Ptyalism) 527.7
secretion—*see also* Hypersecretion
milk 676.6
sputum 786.4
sweat 780.8
short
organ or site, congenital NEC—*see* Anomaly, specified type NEC
umbilical cord
affecting fetus or newborn 762.6
in pregnancy or childbirth 663.4
skin NEC 701.9
eyelid 743.62
acquired 374.30
sodium (Na) 276.0
sputum 786.4
sweating 780.8
tearing (ducts) (eye) (*see also* Epiphora) 375.20
thirst 783.5
due to deprivation of water 994.3
vitamin
A (dietary) 278.2
administered as drug (chronic) (prolonged excessive intake) 278.2
reaction to sudden overdose 963.5
D (dietary) 278.4
administered as drug (chronic) (prolonged excessive intake) 278.4
reaction to sudden overdose 963.5
weight 278.00
gain 783.1
of pregnancy 646.1
loss 783.2
Excitability, abnormal , under minor stress 309.29
Excitation
catatonic (*see also* Schizophrenia) 295.2
psychogenic 298.1
reactive (from emotional stress, psychological trauma) 298.1
Excitement
manic (*see also* Psychosis, affective) 296.0
recurrent episode 296.1
single episode 296.0
mental, reactive (from emotional stress, psychological trauma) 298.1
state, reactive (from emotional stress, psychological trauma) 298.1
Excluded pupils 364.76
Excoriation (traumatic) (*see also* Injury, superficial, by site) 919.8
neurotic 698.4
Excyclophoria 378.44
Excyclotropia 378.33
Exencephalus, exencephaly 742.0
Exercise
breathing V57.0
remedial NEC V57.1
therapeutic NEC V57.1
Exfoliation, teeth due to systemic causes 525.0
Exfoliative —*see also* condition
dermatitis 695.89
Exhaustion, exhaustive (physical NEC) 780.7
battle (*see also* Reaction, stress, acute) 308.9
cardiac (*see also* Failure, heart) 428.9
delirium (*see also* Reaction, stress, acute) 308.9
due to
cold 991.8
excessive exertion 994.5
exposure 994.4
fetus or newborn 779.8
heart (*see also* Failure, heart) 428.9
heat 992.5
due to
salt depletion 992.4
water depletion 992.3
manic (*see also* Psychosis, affective) 296.0
recurrent episode 296.1
single episode 296.0
maternal, complicating delivery 669.8
affecting fetus or newborn 763.8
mental 300.5
myocardium, myocardial (*see also* Failure, heart) 428.9
nervous 300.5
old age 797
postinfectional NEC 780.7
psychogenic 300.5
psychosis (*see also* Reaction, stress, acute) 308.9
senile 797
dementia 290.0
Exhibitionism (sexual) 302.4
Exomphalos 756.7
Exophoria 378.42
convergence, insufficiency 378.83
divergence, excess 378.85
Exophthalmic
cachexia 242.0
goiter 242.0
ophthalmoplegia 242.0 *[376.22]*
Exophthalmos 376.30
congenital 743.66
constant 376.31
endocrine NEC 259.9 *[376.22]*
hyperthyroidism 242.0 *[376.21]*
intermittent NEC 376.34
malignant 242.0 *[376.21]*
pulsating 376.35
endocrine NEC 259.9 *[376.22]*
thyrotoxic 242.0 *[376.21]*
Exostosis 726.91
cartilaginous (M9210/0)—*see* Neoplasm, bone, benign
congenital 756.4
ear canal, external 380.81
gonococcal 098.89
hip 726.5
intracranial 733.3
jaw (bone) 526.81
luxurians 728.11
multiple (cancellous) (congenital) (hereditary) 756.4
nasal bones 726.91
orbit, orbital 376.42
osteocartilaginous (M9210/0)—*see* Neoplasm, bone, benign
spine 721.8
with spondylosis—*see* Spondylosis
syphilitic 095.5
wrist 726.4

Exotropia 378.10
alternating 378.15
with
A pattern 378.16
specified noncomitancy 378.18
V pattern 378.17
X pattern 378.18
Y pattern 378.18
intermittent 378.24
intermittent 378.20
alternating 378.24
monocular 378.23
monocular 378.11
with
A pattern 378.12
specified noncomitancy NEC 378.14
V pattern 378.13
X pattern 378.14
Y pattern 378.14
intermittent 378.23
Explanation of
investigation finding V65.4
medication V65.4
Exposure 994.9
cold 991.9
specified effect NEC 991.8
effects of 994.9
exhaustion due to 994.4
to
AIDS virus V01.7
asbestos V15.84
body fluids (hazardous) V15.85
cholera V01.0
communicable disease V01.9
specified type NEC V01.8
German measles V01.4
gonorrhea V01.6
hazardous body fluids V15.85
HIV V01.7
human immunodeficiency virus V01.7
lead V15.86
parasitic disease V01.8
poliomyelitis V01.2
potentially hazardous body fluids V15.85
rabies V01.5
rubella V01.4
smallpox V01.3
syphilis V01.6
tuberculosis V01.1
venereal disease V01.6
viral disease NEC V01.7
Exsanguination, fetal 772.0
Exstrophy
abdominal content 751.8
bladder (urinary) 753.5
Extensive —*see* condition
Extra —*see also* Accessory
rib 756.3
cervical 756.2
Extraction
with hook 763.8
breech NEC 669.6
affecting fetus or newborn 763.0
cataract postsurgical V45.6
manual NEC 669.8
affecting fetus or newborn 763.8
Extrasystole 427.60
atrial 427.61
postoperative 997.1
ventricular 427.69
Extrauterine gestation or pregnancy —*see* Pregnancy, ectopic
Extravasation
blood 459.0
lower extremity 459.0
chyle into mesentery 457.8
pelvicalyceal 593.4
pyelosinus 593.4
urine 788.8
from ureter 788.8
Extremity —*see* condition
Extrophy —*see* Exstrophy
Extroversion
bladder 753.5
uterus 618.1
complicating delivery 665.2
affecting fetus or newborn 763.8
postpartal (old) 618.1
Extrusion
breast implant (prosthetic) 996.54
device, implant, or graft—*see* Complications, mechanical
eye implant (ball) (globe) 996.59
intervertebral disc—*see* Displacement, intervertebral disc
lacrimal gland 375.43
mesh (reinforcing) 996.59
ocular lens implant 996.53
prosthetic device NEC—*see* Complications, mechanical
vitreous 379.26
Exudate, pleura —*see* Effusion, pleura
Exudates, retina 362.82
Exudative —*see* condition
Eye, eyeball, eyelid —*see* condition
Eyestrain 368.13
Eyeworm disease of Africa 125.2

F

Faber's anemia or syndrome (achlorhydric anemia) 280.9
Fabry's disease (angiokeratoma corporis diffusum) 272.7
Face, facial —*see* condition
Facet of cornea 371.44
Faciocephalalgia, autonomic (*see also* Neuropathy, peripheral, autonomic) 337.9
Facioscapulohumeral myopathy 359.1
Factitious disorder, illness —*see* Illness, factitious
Factor
  deficiency—*see* Deficiency, factor
  psychic, associated with diseases classified elsewhere 316
  risk—*see* Problem
Fahr-Volhard disease (malignant nephrosclerosis) 403.00
Failure, failed
  adenohypophyseal 253.2
  attempted abortion (legal) (*see also* Abortion, failed) 638.9
  bone marrow (anemia) 284.9
    acquired (secondary) 284.8
    congenital 284.0
    idiopathic 284.9
  cardiac (*see also* Failure, heart) 428.9
    newborn 779.8
  cardiorenal (chronic) 428.9
    hypertensive (*see also* Hypertension, cardiorenal) 404.93
  cardiorespiratory 799.1
    specified during or due to a procedure 997.1
      long-term effect of cardiac surgery 429.4
  cardiovascular (chronic) 428.9
  cerebrovascular 437.8
  cervical dilatation in labor 661.0
    affecting fetus or newborn 763.7
  circulation, circulatory 799.8
    fetus or newborn 779.8
    peripheral 785.50
  compensation—*see* Disease, heart
  congestive (*see also* Failure, heart, congestive) 428.0
  coronary (*see also* Insufficiency, coronary) 411.89
  descent of head (at term) 652.5
    affecting fetus or newborn 763.1
    in labor 660.0
      affecting fetus or newborn 763.1
  device, implant, or graft—*see* Complications, mechanical
  engagement of head NEC 652.5
    in labor 660.0
  extrarenal 788.9
  fetal head to enter pelvic brim 652.5
    affecting fetus or newborn 763.1
    in labor 660.0
      affecting fetus or newborn 763.1
  forceps NEC 660.7
    affecting fetus or newborn 763.1
  fusion (joint) (spinal) 996.4
  growth 783.4
  heart (acute) (sudden) 428.9
    with
      abortion—*see* Abortion, by type, with specified complication NEC
Failure, failed—*continued*
  heart—*continued*
      acute pulmonary edema (*see also* Failure, ventricular, left) 428.1
        with congestion 428.0
      decompensation (*see also* Failure, heart, congestive) 428.0
      dilation—*see* Disease, heart
      ectopic pregnancy (*see also* categories 633.0-633.9) 639.8
      molar pregnancy (*see also* categories 630-632) 639.8
    arteriosclerotic 440.9
    combined left-right sided 428.0
    compensated (*see also* Failure, heart, congestive) 428.0
    complicating
      abortion—*see* Abortion, by type, with specified complication NEC
      delivery (cesarean) (instrumental) 669.4
      ectopic pregnancy (*see also* categories 633.0-633.9) 639.8
      molar pregnancy (*see also* categories 630-632) 639.8
      obstetric anesthesia or sedation 668.1
      surgery 997.1
    congestive (compensated) (decompensated) 428.0
      with rheumatic fever (conditions classifiable to 390)
        active 391.8
        inactive or quiescent (with chorea) 398.91
      fetus or newborn 779.8
      hypertensive (*see also* Hypertension, heart) 402.91
        with renal disease (*see also* Hypertension, cardiorenal) 404.91
          with renal failure 404.93
        benign 402.11
        malignant 402.01
      rheumatic (chronic) (inactive) (with chorea) 398.91
        active or acute 391.8
          with chorea (Sydenham's) 392.0
    decompensated (*see also* Failure, heart, congestive) 428.0
    degenerative (*see also* Degeneration, myocardial) 429.1
    due to presence of (cardiac) prosthesis 429.4
    fetus or newborn 779.8
    following
      abortion 639.8
      cardiac surgery 429.4
      ectopic or molar pregnancy 639.8
    high output NEC 428.9
    hypertensive (*see also* Hypertension, heart) 402.91
      with renal disease (*see also* Hypertension, cardiorenal) 404.91
        with renal failure 404.93
      benign 402.11
      malignant 402.01
    left (ventricular) (*see also* Failure, ventricular, left) 428.1
      with right-sided failure 428.0
    low output (syndrome) NEC 428.9

Failure, failed—*continued*
organic—*see* Disease, heart
postoperative (immediate) 997.1
long term effect of cardiac surgery 429.4
rheumatic (chronic) (congestive) (inactive) 398.91
right (secondary to left heart failure, conditions classifiable to 428.1) (ventricular) (*see also* Failure, heart, congestive) 428.0
senile 797
specified during or due to a procedure 997.1
long-term effect of cardiac surgery 429.4
thyrotoxic (*see also* Thyrotoxicosis) 242.9 *[425.7]*
valvular—*see* Endocarditis
hepatic 572.8
acute 570
due to a procedure 997.4
hepatorenal 572.4
hypertensive heart (*see also* Hypertension, heart) 402.91
benign 402.11
malignant 402.01
induction (of labor) 659.1
abortion (legal) (*see also* Abortion, failed) 638.9
affecting fetus or newborn 763.8
by oxytocic drugs 659.1
instrumental 659.0
mechanical 659.0
medical 659.1
surgical 659.0
initial alveolar expansion, newborn 770.4
involution, thymus (gland) 254.8
kidney—*see* Failure, renal
lactation 676.4
Leydig's cell, adult 257.2
liver 572.8
acute 570
medullary 799.8
mitral—*see* Endocarditis, mitral
myocardium, myocardial (*see also* Failure, heart) 428.9
chronic (*see also* Failure, heart, congestive) 428.0
congestive (*see also* Failure, heart, congestive) 428.0
ovarian (primary) 256.3
iatrogenic 256.2
postablative 256.2
postirradiation 256.2
postsurgical 256.2
ovulation 628.0
prerenal 788.9
renal 586
with
abortion—*see* Abortion, by type, with renal failure
ectopic pregnancy (*see also* categories 633.0-633.9) 639.3
edema (*see also* Nephrosis) 581.9
hypertension (*see also* Hypertension, kidney) 403.91
hypertensive heart disease (conditions classifiable to 402) 404.92
with heart failure 404.93
benign 404.12
with heart failure 404.13

Failure, failed—*continued*
malignant 404.02
with heart failure 404.03
molar pregnancy (*see also* categories 630-632) 639.3
tubular necrosis (acute) 584.5
acute 584.9
with lesion of
necrosis
cortical (renal) 584.6
medullary (renal) (papillary) 584.7
tubular 584.5
specified pathology NEC 584.8
chronic 585
hypertensive or with hypertension (*see also* Hypertension, kidney) 403.91
due to a procedure 997.5
following
abortion 639.3
crushing 958.5
ectopic or molar pregnancy 639.3
labor and delivery (acute) 669.3
hypertensive (*see also* Hypertension, kidney) 403.91
puerperal, postpartum 669.3
respiration, respiratory 518.81
acute (acute-on-chronic) 518.81
center 348.8
newborn 770.8
chronic 518.81
due to trauma, surgery or shock 518.5
newborn 770.8
rotation
cecum 751.4
colon 751.4
intestine 751.4
kidney 753.3
segmentation—*see also* Fusion
fingers (*see also* Syndactylism, fingers) 755.11
toes (*see also* Syndactylism, toes) 755.13
seminiferous tubule, adult 257.2
senile (general) 797
with psychosis 290.20
testis, primary (seminal) 257.2
to thrive 783.4
transplant 996.80
bone marrow 996.85
organ (immune or nonimmune cause) 996.80
bone marrow 996.85
heart 996.83
intestines 996.89
kidney 996.81
liver 996.82
lung 996.84
pancreas 996.86
specified NEC 996.89
skin 996.52
temporary allograft or pigskin graft—*omit code*
trial of labor NEC 660.6
affecting fetus or newborn 763.1
urinary 586
vacuum extraction
abortion—*see* Abortion, failed
delivery NEC 660.7
affecting fetus or newborn 763.1
ventouse NEC 660.7
affecting fetus or newborn 763.1

Failure, failed—*continued*
ventricular (*see also* Failure, heart) 428.9
left 428.1
with rheumatic fever (conditions classifiable to 390)
active 391.8
with chorea 392.0
inactive or quiescent (with chorea) 398.91
hypertensive (*see also* Hypertension, heart) 402.91
benign 402.11
malignant 402.01
rheumatic (chronic) (inactive) (with chorea) 398.91
active or acute 391.8
with chorea 392.0
right (*see also* Failure, heart, congestive) 428.0
vital centers, fetus or newborn 779.8
weight gain 783.4
Fainting (fit) (spell) 780.2
Falciform hymen 752.49
Fall, maternal, affecting fetus or newborn 760.5
Fallen arches 734
Falling, any organ or part —*see* Prolapse
Fallopian
insufflation V26.2
tube—*see* condition
Fallot's
pentalogy 745.2
tetrad or tetralogy 745.2
triad or trilogy 746.09
Fallout, radioactive (adverse effect) NEC 990
False —*see also* condition
bundle branch block 426.50
bursa 727.89
croup 478.75
joint 733.82
labor (pains) 644.1
opening, urinary 752.8
passage, urethra (prostatic) 599.4
positive
serological test for syphilis 795.6
Wassermann reaction 795.6
pregnancy 300.11
Family, familial —*see also* condition
disruption V61.0
planning advice V25.09
problem V61.9
specified circumstance NEC V61.8
Famine 994.2
edema 262
Fanconi's anemia (congenital pancytopenia) 284.0
Fanconi (-de Toni) (-Debré) syndrome (cystinosis) 270.0
Farber (-Uzman) syndrome or disease (disseminated lipogranulomatosis) 272.8
Farcin 024
Farcy 024
Farmers '
lung 495.0
skin 692.74
Farsightedness 367.0
Fascia —*see* condition
Fasciculation 781.0
Fasciculitis optica 377.32
Fasciitis 729.4
eosinophilic 728.89
necrotizing 728.86
nodular 728.79
perirenal 593.4
plantar 728.71
pseudosarcomatous 728.79
traumatic (old) NEC 728.79
current—*see* Sprain, by site
Fasciola hepatica infestation 121.3
Fascioliasis 121.3
Fasciolopsiasis (small intestine) 121.4
Fasciolopsis (small intestine) 121.4
Fast pulse 785.0
Fat
embolism (cerebral) (pulmonary) (systemic) 958.1
with
abortion—*see* Abortion, by type, with embolism
ectopic pregnancy (*see also* categories 633.0-633.9) 639.6
molar pregnancy (*see also* categories 630-632) 639.6
complicating delivery or puerperium 673.8
following
abortion 639.6
ectopic or molar pregnancy 639.6
in pregnancy, childbirth, or the puerperium 673.8
excessive 278.00
in heart (*see also* Degeneration, myocardial) 429.1
general 278.00
hernia, herniation 729.30
eyelid 374.34
knee 729.31
orbit 374.34
retro-orbital 374.34
retropatellar 729.31
specified site NEC 729.39
indigestion 579.8
in stool 792.1
localized (pad) 278.1
heart (*see also* Degeneration, myocardial) 429.1
knee 729.31
retropatellar 729.31
necrosis—*see also* Fatty, degeneration
breast (aseptic) (segmental) 611.3
mesentery 567.8
omentum 567.8
pad 278.1
Fatal syncope 798.1
Fatigue 780.7
auditory deafness (*see also* Deafness) 389.9
chronic, syndrome 780.7
combat (*see also* Reaction, stress, acute) 308.9
during pregnancy 646.8
general 780.7
psychogenic 300.5
heat (transient) 992.6
muscle 729.89
myocardium (*see also* Failure, heart) 428.9
nervous 300.5
neurosis 300.5
operational 300.89
postural 729.89
posture 729.89
psychogenic (general) 300.5

Fatigue—*continued*
senile 797
syndrome NEC 300.5
chronic 780.7
undue 780.7
voice 784.49
Fatness 278.00
Fatty —*see also* condition
apron 278.1
degeneration (diffuse) (general) NEC 272.8
localized—*see* Degeneration, by site, fatty
placenta—*see* Placenta, abnormal
heart (enlarged) (*see also* Degeneration, myocardial) 429.1
infiltration (diffuse) (general) (*see also* Degeneration, by site, fatty) 272.8
heart (enlarged) (*see also* Degeneration, myocardial) 429.1
liver 571.8
alcoholic 571.0
necrosis—*see* Degeneration, fatty
phanerosis 272.8
Fauces —*see* condition
Fauchard's disease (periodontitis) 523.4
Faucitis 478.29
Faulty —*see also* condition
position of teeth 524.3
Favism (anemia) 282.2
Favre-Racouchot disease (elastoidosis cutanea nodularis) 701.8
Favus 110.9
beard 110.0
capitis 110.0
corporis 110.5
eyelid 110.8
foot 110.4
hand 110.2
scalp 110.0
specified site NEC 110.8
Fear, fearfulness (complex) (reaction) 300.20
child 313.0
of
animals 300.29
closed spaces 300.29
crowds 300.29
eating in public 300.23
heights 300.29
open spaces 300.22
with panic attacks 300.21
public speaking 300.23
streets 300.22
with panic attacks 300.21
travel 300.22
with panic attacks 300.21
washing in public 300.23
transient 308.0
Feared complaint unfounded V65.5
Febricula (continued) (simple) (*see also* Pyrexia) 780.6
Febrile (*see also* Pyrexia) 780.6
Febris (*see also* Fever) 780.6
aestiva (*see also* Fever, hay) 477.9
flava (*see also* Fever, yellow) 060.9
melitensis 023.0
pestis (*see also* Plague) 020.9
puerperalis 670
recurrens (*see also* Fever, relapsing) 087.9
pediculo vestimenti 087.0
rubra 034.1
typhoidea 002.0
typhosa 002.0
Fecal —*see* condition
Fecalith (impaction) 560.39
with hernia—*see also* Hernia, by site, with obstruction
gangrenous—*see* Hernia, by site, with gangrene
appendix 543.9
congenital 777.1
Fede's disease 529.0
Feeble-minded 317
Feeble rapid pulse due to shock following injury 958.4
Feeding
faulty (elderly) (infant) 783.3
newborn 779.3
formula check V20.2
improper (elderly) (infant) 783.3
newborn 779.3
problem (elderly) (infant) 783.3
newborn 779.3
nonorganic origin 307.59
Feer's disease 985.0
Feet —*see* condition
Feigned illness V65.2
Feil-Klippel syndrome (brevicollis) 756.16
Feinmesser's (hidrotic) ectodermal dysplasia 757.31
Felix's disease (juvenile osteochondrosis, hip) 732.1
Felon (any digit) (with lymphangitis) 681.01
herpetic 054.6
Felty's syndrome (rheumatoid arthritis with splenomegaly and leukopenia) 714.1
Feminism in boys 302.6
Feminization, testicular 257.8
with pseudohermaphroditism, male 257.8
Femoral hernia —*see* Hernia, femoral
Femora vara 736.32
Femur, femoral —*see* condition
Fenestrata placenta —*see* Placenta, abnormal
Fenestration, fenestrated —*see also* Imperfect, closure
aorta-pulmonary 745.0
aorticopulmonary 745.0
aortopulmonary 745.0
cusps, heart valve NEC 746.89
pulmonary 746.09
hymen 752.49
pulmonic cusps 746.09
Fenwick's disease 537.89
Fermentation (gastric) (gastrointestinal) (stomach) 536.8
intestine 564.8
psychogenic 306.4
psychogenic 306.4
Fernell's disease (aortic aneurysm) 441.9
Fertile eunuch syndrome 257.2
Fertility, meaning multiparity—*see* Multiparity
Fetal alcohol syndrome 760.71
Fetalis uterus 752.3
Fetid
breath 784.9
sweat 705.89
Fetishism 302.81
transvestic 302.3
Fetomaternal hemorrhage
affecting management of pregnancy 656.0
fetus or newborn 772.0
Fetus, fetal —*see also* condition
papyraceous 779.8
type lung tissue 770.4

Fever 780.6
with chills 780.6
in malarial regions (*see also* Malaria) 084.6
abortus NEC 023.9
Aden 061
African tick-borne 087.1
American
mountain tick 066.1
spotted 082.0
and ague (*see also* Malaria) 084.6
aphthous 078.4
arbovirus hemorrhagic 065.9
Assam 085.0
Australian A or Q 083.0
Bangkok hemorrhagic 065.4
biliary, Charcot's intermittent—*see* Choledocholithiasis
bilious, hemoglobinuric 084.8
blackwater 084.8
blister 054.9
Bonvale Dam 780.7
boutonneuse 082.1
brain 323.9
late effect—*see* category 326
breakbone 061
Bullis 082.8
Bunyamwera 066.3
Burdwan 085.0
Bwamba (encephalitis) 066.3
Cameroon (*see also* Malaria) 084.6
Canton 081.9
catarrhal (acute) 460
chronic 472.0
cat-scratch 078.3
cerebral 323.9
late effect—*see* category 326
cerebrospinal (meningococcal) (*see also* Meningitis, cerebrospinal) 036.0
Chagres 084.0
Chandipura 066.8
changuinola 066.0
Charcot's (biliary) (hepatic) (intermittent)—*see* Choledocholithiasis
Chikungunya (viral) 066.3
hemorrhagic 065.4
childbed 670
Chitral 066.0
Colombo (*see also* Fever, paratyphoid) 002.9
Colorado tick (virus) 066.1
congestive
malarial (*see also* Malaria) 084.6
remittent (*see also* Malaria) 084.6
Congo virus 065.0
continued 780.6
malarial 084.0
Corsican (*see also* Malaria) 084.6
Crimean hemorrhagic 065.0
Cyprus (*see also* Brucellosis) 023.9
dandy 061
deer fly (*see also* Tularemia) 021.9
dehydration, newborn 778.4
dengue (virus) 061
hemorrhagic 065.4
desert 114.0
due to heat 992.0
Dumdum 085.0
enteric 002.0
ephemeral (of unknown origin) (*see also* Pyrexia) 780.6
epidemic, hemorrhagic of the Far East 065.0

Fever—*continued*
erysipelatous (*see also* Erysipelas) 035
estivo-autumnal (malarial) 084.0
etiocholanolone 277.3
famine—*see also* Fever, relapsing
meaning typhus—*see* Typhus
Far Eastern hemorrhagic 065.0
five day 083.1
Fort Bragg 100.89
gastroenteric 002.0
gastromalarial (*see also* Malaria) 084.6
Gibraltar (*see also* Brucellosis) 023.9
glandular 075
Guama (viral) 066.3
Haverhill 026.1
hay (allergic) (with rhinitis) 477.9
with
asthma (bronchial) (*see also* Asthma) 493.0
due to
dander 477.8
dust 477.8
fowl 477.8
pollen, any plant or tree 477.0
specified allergen other than pollen 477.8
heat (effects) 992.0
hematuric, bilious 084.8
hemoglobinuric (malarial) 084.8
bilious 084.8
hemorrhagic (arthropod-borne) NEC 065.9
with renal syndrome 078.6
arenaviral 078.7
Argentine 078.7
Bangkok 065.4
Bolivian 078.7
Central Asian 065.0
chikungunya 065.4
Crimean 065.0
dengue (virus) 065.4
epidemic 078.6
of Far East 065.0
Far Eastern 065.0
Junin virus 078.7
Korean 078.6
Kyasanur forest 065.2
Machupo virus 078.7
mite-borne NEC 065.8
mosquito-borne 065.4
Omsk 065.1
Philippine 065.4
Russian (Yaroslav) 078.6
Singapore 065.4
Southeast Asia 065.4
Thailand 065.4
tick-borne NEC 065.3
hepatic (*see also* Cholecystitis) 575.8
intermittent (Charcot's)—*see* Choledocholithiasis
herpetic (*see also* Herpes) 054.9
Hyalomma tick 065.0
icterohemorrhagic 100.0
inanition 780.6
newborn 778.4
infective NEC 136.9
intermittent (bilious) (*see also* Malaria) 084.6
hepatic (Charcot)—*see* Choledocholithiasis
of unknown origin (*see also* Pyrexia) 780.6
pernicious 084.0
iodide
correct substance properly administered 780.6
overdose or wrong substance given or taken 975.5

Fever—*continued*
Japanese river 081.2
jungle yellow 060.0
Junin virus, hemorrhagic 078.7
Katayama 120.2
Kedani 081.2
Kenya 082.1
Korean hemorrhagic 078.6
Lassa 078.89
Lone Star 082.8
lung—*see* Pneumonia
Machupo virus, hemorrhagic 078.7
malaria, malarial (*see also* Malaria) 084.6
Malta (*see also* Brucellosis) 023.9
Marseilles 082.1
marsh (*see also* Malaria) 084.6
Mayaro (viral) 066.3
Mediterranean (*see also* Brucellosis) 023.9
familial 277.3
tick 082.1
meningeal—*see* Meningitis
metal fumes NEC 985.8
Meuse 083.1
Mexican—*see* Typhus, Mexican
Mianeh 087.1
miasmatic (*see also* Malaria) 084.6
miliary 078.2
milk, female 672
mill 504
mite-borne hemorrhagic 065.8
Monday 504
mosquito-borne NEC 066.3
hemorrhagic NEC 065.4
mountain 066.1
meaning
Rocky Mountain spotted 082.0
undulant fever (*see also* Brucellosis) 023.9
tick (American) 066.1
Mucambo (viral) 066.3
mud 100.89
Neapolitan (*see also* Brucellosis) 023.9
nine-mile 083.0
nonexanthematous tick 066.1
North Asian tick-borne typhus 082.2
Omsk hemorrhagic 065.1
O'nyong-nyong (viral) 066.3
Oropouche (viral) 066.3
Oroya 088.0
paludal (*see also* Malaria) 084.6
Panama 084.0
pappataci 066.0
paratyphoid 002.9
A 002.1
B (Schottmüller's) 002.2
C (Hirschfeld) 002.3
parrot 073.9
periodic 277.3
pernicious, acute 084.0
persistent (of unknown origin) (*see also* Pyrexia) 780.6
petechial 036.0
pharyngoconjunctival 077.2
adenoviral type 3 077.2
Philippine hemorrhagic 065.4
phlebotomus 066.0
Piry 066.8
Pixuna (viral) 066.3
Plasmodium ovale 084.3
pleural (*see also* Pleurisy) 511.0
pneumonic—*see* Pneumonia

Fever—*continued*
polymer fume 987.8
postoperative 998.89
due to infection 998.5
pretibial 100.89
puerperal, postpartum 670
putrid—*see* Septicemia
pyemic—*see* Septicemia
Q 083.0
with pneumonia 083.0 *[484.8]*
quadrilateral 083.0
quartan (malaria) 084.2
Queensland (coastal) 083.0
seven-day 100.89
Quintan (A) 083.1
quotidian 084.0
rabbit (*see also* Tularemia) 021.9
rat-bite 026.9
due to
Spirillum minor or minus 026.0
Spirochaeta morsus muris 026.0
Streptobacillus moniliformis 026.1
recurrent—*see* Fever, relapsing
relapsing 087.9
Carter's (Asiatic) 087.0
Dutton's (West African) 087.1
Koch's 087.9
louse-borne (epidemic) 087.0
Novy's (American) 087.1
Obermeyer's (European) 087.0
spirillum NEC 087.9
tick-borne (endemic) 087.1
remittent (bilious) (congestive) (gastric) (*see also* Malaria) 084.6
rheumatic (active) (acute) (chronic) (subacute) 390
with heart involvement 391.9
carditis 391.9
endocarditis (aortic) (mitral) (pulmonary) (tricuspid) 391.1
multiple sites 391.8
myocarditis 391.2
pancarditis, acute 391.8
pericarditis 391.0
specified type NEC 391.8
valvulitis 391.1
inactive or quiescent with cardiac hypertrophy 398.99
carditis 398.90
endocarditis 397.9
aortic (valve) 395.9
with mitral (valve) disease 396.9
mitral (valve) 394.9
with aortic (valve) disease 396.9
pulmonary (valve) 397.1
tricuspid (valve) 397.0
heart conditions (classifiable to 429.3, 429.6, 429.9) 398.99
failure (congestive) (conditions classifiable to 428.0, 428.9) 398.91
left ventricular failure (conditions classifiable to 428.1) 398.91
myocardial degeneration (conditions classifiable to 429.1) 398.0
myocarditis (conditions classifiable to 429.0) 398.0
pancarditis 398.99
pericarditis 393
Rift Valley (viral) 066.3
Rocky Mountain spotted 082.0

Fever—*continued*
rose 477.0
Ross river (viral) 066.3
Russian hemorrhagic 078.6
sandfly 066.0
San Joaquin (valley) 114.0
São Paulo 082.0
scarlet 034.1
septic—*see* Septicemia
seven-day 061
Japan 100.89
Queensland 100.89
shin bone 083.1
Singapore hemorrhagic 065.4
solar 061
sore 054.9
South African tick-bite 087.1
Southeast Asia hemorrhagic 065.4
spinal—*see* Meningitis
spirillary 026.0
splenic (*see also* Anthrax) 022.9
spotted (Rocky Mountain) 082.0
American 082.0
Brazilian 082.0
Colombian 082.0
meaning
cerebrospinal meningitis 036.0
typhus 082.9
spring 309.23
steroid
correct substance properly administered 780.6
overdose or wrong substance given or taken 962.0
streptobacillary 026.1
subtertian 084.0
Sumatran mite 081.2
sun 061
swamp 100.89
sweating 078.2
swine 003.8
sylvatic yellow 060.0
Tahyna 062.5
tertian—*see* Malaria, tertian
Thailand hemorrhagic 065.4
thermic 992.0
three day 066.0
with Coxsackie exanthem 074.8
tick
American mountain 066.1
Colorado 066.1
Kemerovo 066.1
Mediterranean 082.1
mountain 066.1
nonexanthematous 066.1
Quaranfil 066.1
tick-bite NEC 066.1
tick-borne NEC 066.1
hemorrhagic NEC 065.3
transitory of newborn 778.4
trench 083.1
tsutsugamushi 081.2
typhogastric 002.0
typhoid (abortive) (ambulant) (any site) (hemorrhagic) (infection) (intermittent) (malignant) (rheumatic) 002.0
typhomalarial (*see also* Malaria) 084.6
typhus—*see* Typhus
undulant (*see also* Brucellosis) 023.9
unknown origin (*see also* Pyrexia) 780.6
uremic—*see* Uremia

Fever—*continued*
uveoparotid 135
valley (Coccidioidomycosis) 114.0
Venezuelan equine 066.2
Volhynian 083.1
Wesselsbron (viral) 066.3
West
African 084.8
Nile (viral) 066.3
Whitmore's 025
Wolhynian 083.1
worm 128.9
Yaroslav hemorrhagic 078.6
yellow 060.9
jungle 060.0
sylvatic 060.0
urban 060.1
vaccination, prophylactic (against) V04.4
Zika (viral) 066.3
Fibrillation
atrial (established) (paroxysmal) 427.31
auricular (atrial) (established) 427.31
cardiac (ventricular) 427.41
coronary (*see also* Infarct, myocardium) 410.9
heart (ventricular) 427.41
muscular 728.9
postoperative 997.1
ventricular 427.41
Fibrin
ball or bodies, pleural (sac) 511.0
chamber, anterior (eye) (gelatinous exudate) 364.04
Fibrinogenolysis (hemorrhagic)—*see* Fibrinolysis
Fibrinogenopenia (congenital) (hereditary) (*see also* Defect, coagulation) 286.3
acquired 286.6
Fibrinolysis (acquired) (hemorrhagic) (pathologic) 286.6
with
abortion—*see* Abortion, by type, with hemorrhage, delayed or excessive
ectopic pregnancy (*see also* categories 633.0-633.9) 639.1
molar pregnancy (*see also* categories 630-632) 639.1
antepartum or intrapartum 641.3
affecting fetus or newborn 762.1
following
abortion 639.1
ectopic or molar pregnancy 639.1
newborn, transient 776.2
postpartum 666.3
Fibrinopenia (hereditary) (*see also* Defect, coagulation) 286.3
acquired 286.6
Fibrinopurulent —*see* condition
Fibrinous —*see* condition
Fibroadenoma (M9010/0)
cellular intracanalicular (M9020/0) 217
giant (intracanalicular) (M9020/0) 217
intracanalicular (M9011/0)
cellular (M9020/0) 217
giant (M9020/0) 217
specified site—*see* Neoplasm, by site, benign
unspecified site 217
juvenile (M9030/0) 217
pericanalicular (M9012/0)
specified site—*see* Neoplasm, by site, benign
unspecified site 217

Fibroadenoma—*continued*
phyllodes (M9020/0) 217
prostate 600
specified site—*see* Neoplasm, by site, benign
unspecified site 217
Fibroadenosis, breast (chronic) (cystic) (diffuse) (periodic) (segmental) 610.2
Fibroangioma (M9160/0)—*see also* Neoplasm, by site, benign
juvenile (M9160/0)
specified site—*see* Neoplasm, by site, benign
unspecified site 210.7
Fibrocellulitis progressiva ossificans 728.11
Fibrochondrosarcoma (M9220/3)—*see* Neoplasm, cartilage, malignant
Fibrocystic
disease 277.00
bone NEC 733.29
breast 610.1
jaw 526.2
kidney (congenital) 753.19
liver 751.62
lung 518.89
congenital 748.4
pancreas 277.00
kidney (congenital) 753.19
Fibrodysplasia ossificans multiplex (progressiva) 728.11
Fibroelastosis (cordis) (endocardial) (endomyocardial) 425.3
Fibroid (tumor) (M8890/0)—*see also* Neoplasm, connective tissue, benign
disease, lung (chronic) (*see also* Fibrosis, lung) 515
heart (disease) (*see also* Myocarditis) 429.0
induration, lung (chronic) (*see also* Fibrosis, lung) 515
in pregnancy or childbirth 654.1
affecting fetus or newborn 763.8
causing obstructed labor 660.2
affecting fetus or newborn 763.1
liver—*see* Cirrhosis, liver
lung (*see also* Fibrosis, lung) 515
pneumonia (chronic) (*see also* Fibrosis, lung) 515
uterus (M8890/0) (*see also* Leiomyoma, uterus) 218.9
Fibrolipoma (M8851/0) (*see also* Lipoma, by site) 214.9
Fibroliposarcoma (M8850/3)—*see* Neoplasm, connective tissue, malignant
Fibroma (M8810/0)—*see also* Neoplasm, connective tissue, benign
ameloblastic (M9330/0) 213.1
upper jaw (bone) 213.0
bone (nonossifying) 733.99
ossifying (M9262/0)—*see* Neoplasm, bone, benign
cementifying (M9274/0)—*see* Neoplasm, bone, benign
chondromyxoid (M9241/0)—*see* Neoplasm, bone, benign
desmoplastic (M8823/1)—*see* Neoplasm, connective tissue, uncertain behavior
facial (M8813/0)—*see* Neoplasm, connective tissue, benign
invasive (M8821/1)—*see* Neoplasm, connective tissue, uncertain behavior
Fibroma—*continued*
molle (M8851/0) (*see also* Lipoma, by site) 214.9
myxoid (M8811/0)—*see* Neoplasm, connective tissue, benign
nasopharynx, nasopharyngeal (juvenile) (M9160/0) 210.7
nonosteogenic (nonossifying)—*see* Dysplasia, fibrous
odontogenic (M9321/0) 213.1
upper jaw (bone) 213.0
ossifying (M9262/0)—*see* Neoplasm, bone, benign
periosteal (M8812/0)—*see* Neoplasm, bone, benign
prostate 600
soft (M8851/0) (*see also* Lipoma, by site) 214.9
Fibromatosis
abdominal (M8822/1)—*see* Neoplasm, connective tissue, uncertain behavior
aggressive (M8821/1)—*see* Neoplasm, connective tissue, uncertain behavior
Dupuytren's 728.6
gingival 523.8
plantar fascia 728.71
proliferative 728.79
pseudosarcomatous (proliferative) (subcutaneous) 728.79
subcutaneous pseudosarcomatous (proliferative) 728.79
Fibromyalgia 729.1
Fibromyoma (M8890/0)—*see also* Neoplasm, connective tissue, benign
uterus (corpus) (*see also* Leiomyoma, uterus) 218.9
in pregnancy or childbirth 654.1
affecting fetus or newborn 763.8
causing obstructed labor 660.2
affecting fetus or newborn 763.1
Fibromyositis (*see also* Myositis) 729.1
scapulohumeral 726.2
Fibromyxolipoma (M8852/0) (*see also* Lipoma, by site) 214.9
Fibromyxoma (M8811/0)—*see* Neoplasm, connective tissue, benign
Fibromyxosarcoma (M8811/3)—*see* Neoplasm, connective tissue, malignant
Fibro-odontoma, ameloblastic (M9290/0) 213.1
upper jaw (bone) 213.0
Fibro-osteoma (M9262/0)—*see* Neoplasm, bone, benign
Fibroplasia, retrolental 362.21
Fibropurulent —*see* condition
Fibrosarcoma (M8810/3)—*see also* Neoplasm, connective tissue, malignant
ameloblastic (M9330/3) 170.1
upper jaw (bone) 170.0
congenital (M8814/3)—*see* Neoplasm, connective tissue, malignant
fascial (M8813/3)—*see* Neoplasm, connective tissue, malignant
infantile (M8814/3)—*see* Neoplasm, connective tissue, malignant
odontogenic (M9330/3) 170.1
upper jaw (bone) 170.0
periosteal (M8812/3)—*see* Neoplasm, bone, malignant

Fibrosclerosis
breast 610.3
corpora cavernosa (penis) 607.89
familial multifocal NEC 710.8
multifocal (idiopathic) NEC 710.8
penis (corpora cavernosa) 607.89
Fibrosis, fibrotic
adrenal (gland) 255.8
alveolar (diffuse) 516.3
amnion 658.8
anal papillae 569.49
anus 569.49
appendix, appendiceal, noninflammatory 543.9
arteriocapillary—*see* Arteriosclerosis
bauxite (of lung) 503
biliary 576.8
due to Clonorchis sinensis 121.1
bladder 596.8
interstitial 595.1
localized submucosal 595.1
panmural 595.1
bone, diffuse 756.59
breast 610.3
capillary—*see also* Arteriosclerosis
lung (chronic) (*see also* Fibrosis, lung) 515
cardiac (*see also* Myocarditis) 429.0
cervix 622.8
chorion 658.8
corpus cavernosum 607.89
cystic (of pancreas) 277.00
due to (presence of) any device, implant, or graft—*see* Complications, due to (presence of) any device, implant, or graft classified to 996.0-996.5 NEC
ejaculatory duct 608.89
endocardium (*see also* Endocarditis) 424.90
endomyocardial (African) 425.0
epididymis 608.89
eye muscle 378.62
graphite (of lung) 503
heart (*see also* Myocarditis) 429.0
hepatic—*see also* Cirrhosis, liver
due to Clonorchis sinensis 121.1
hepatolienal—*see* Cirrhosis, liver
hepatosplenic—*see* Cirrhosis, liver
infrapatellar fat pad 729.31
interstitial pulmonary, newborn 770.7
intrascrotal 608.89
kidney (*see also* Sclerosis, renal) 587
liver—*see* Cirrhosis, liver
lung (atrophic) (capillary) (chronic) (confluent) (massive) (perialveolar) (peribronchial) 515
with
anthracosilicosis (occupational) 500
anthracosis (occupational) 500
asbestosis (occupational) 501
bagassosis (occupational) 495.1
bauxite 503
berylliosis (occupational) 503
byssinosis (occupational) 504
calcicosis (occupational) 502
chalicosis (occupational) 502
dust reticulation (occupational) 504
farmers' lung 495.0
gannister disease (occupational) 502
graphite 503
pneumonoconiosis (occupational) 505
pneumosiderosis (occupational) 503
siderosis (occupational) 503
silicosis (occupational) 502
tuberculosis (*see also* Tuberculosis) 011.4

Fibrosis, fibrotic—*continued*
diffuse (idiopathic) (interstitial) 516.3
due to
bauxite 503
fumes or vapors (chemical) (inhalation) 506.4
graphite 503
following radiation 508.1
postinflammatory 515
silicotic (massive) (occupational) 502
tuberculous (*see also* Tuberculosis) 011.4
lymphatic gland 289.3
median bar 600
mediastinum (idiopathic) 519.3
meninges 349.2
muscle NEC 728.2
iatrogenic (from injection) 999.9
myocardium, myocardial (*see also* Myocarditis) 429.0
oral submucous 528.8
ovary 620.8
oviduct 620.8
pancreas 577.8
cystic 277.00
penis 607.89
periappendiceal 543.9
periarticular (*see also* Ankylosis) 718.5
pericardium 423.1
perineum, in pregnancy or childbirth 654.8
affecting fetus or newborn 763.8
causing obstructed labor 660.2
affecting fetus or newborn 763.1
perineural NEC 355.9
foot 355.6
periureteral 593.89
placenta—*see* Placenta, abnormal
pleura 511.0
popliteal fat pad 729.31
preretinal 362.56
prostate (chronic) 600
pulmonary (chronic) (*see also* Fibrosis, lung) 515
alveolar capillary block 516.3
interstitial
diffuse (idiopathic) 516.3
newborn 770.7
radiation—*see* Effect, adverse, radiation
rectal sphincter 569.49
retroperitoneal, idiopathic 593.4
scrotum 608.89
seminal vesicle 608.89
senile 797
skin NEC 709.2
spermatic cord 608.89
spleen 289.59
bilharzial (*see also* Schistosomiasis) 120.9
subepidermal nodular (M8832/0)—*see* Neoplasm, skin, benign
submucous NEC 709.2
oral 528.8
tongue 528.8
syncytium—*see* Placenta, abnormal
testis 608.89
chronic, due to syphilis 095.8
thymus (gland) 254.8
tunica vaginalis 608.89
ureter 593.89
urethra 599.84
uterus (nonneoplastic) 621.8
bilharzial (*see also* Schistosomiasis) 120.9
neoplastic (*see also* Leiomyoma, uterus) 218.9

Fibrosis, fibrotic—*continued*
vagina 623.8
valve, heart (*see also* Endocarditis) 424.90
vas deferens 608.89
vein 459.89
lower extremities 459.89
vesical 595.1
Fibrositis (periarticular) (rheumatoid) 729.0
humeroscapular region 726.2
nodular, chronic
Jaccoud's 714.4
rheumatoid 714.4
ossificans 728.11
scapulohumeral 726.2
Fibrothorax 511.0
Fibrotic —*see* Fibrosis
Fibrous —*see* condition
Fibroxanthoma (M8831/0)—*see also* Neoplasm, connective tissue, benign
atypical (M8831/1)—*see* Neoplasm, connective tissue, uncertain behavior
malignant (M8831/3)—*see* Neoplasm, connective tissue, malignant
Fibroxanthosarcoma (M8831/3)—*see* Neoplasm, connective tissue, malignant
Fiedler's
disease (leptospiral jaundice) 100.0
myocarditis or syndrome (acute isolated myocarditis) 422.91
Fiessinger-Leroy (-Reiter) syndrome 099.3
Fiessinger-Rendu syndrome (erythema muliforme exudativum) 695.1
Fifth disease (eruptive) 057.0
venereal 099.1
Filaria, filarial —*see* Infestation, filarial
Filariasis (*see also* Infestation, filarial) 125.9
bancroftian 125.0
Brug's 125.1
due to
bancrofti 125.0
Brugia (Wuchereria) (malayi) 125.1
Loa loa 125.2
malayi 125.1
organism NEC 125.6
Wuchereria (bancrofti) 125.0
malayi 125.1
Malayan 125.1
ozzardi 125.5
specified type NEC 125.6
Filatoff's, Filatov's, Filatow's disease (infectious mononucleosis) 075
File-cutters' disease 984.9
specified type of lead—*see* Table of drugs and chemicals
Filling defect
biliary tract 793.3
bladder 793.5
duodenum 793.4
gallbladder 793.3
gastrointestinal tract 793.4
intestine 793.4
kidney 793.5
stomach 793.4
ureter 793.5
Filtering bleb, eye (postglaucoma) (status) V45.6
with complication or rupture 997.99
postcataract extraction (complication) 997.99
Fimbrial cyst (congenital) 752.11
Fimbriated hymen 752.49
Financial problem affecting care V60.2
Findings, abnormal, without diagnosis (examination) (laboratory test) 796.4
17-ketosteroids, elevated 791.9
acetonuria 791.6
acid phosphatase 790.5
albumin-globulin ratio 790.99
albuminuria 791.0
alcohol in blood 790.3
alkaline phosphatase 790.5
amniotic fluid 792.3
amylase 790.5
anisocytosis 790.0
antibody titers, elevated 795.79
antigen-antibody reaction 795.79
bacteriuria 791.9
ballistocardiogram 794.39
bicarbonate 276.9
bile in urine 791.4
bilirubin 277.4
bleeding time (prolonged) 790.92
blood culture, positive 790.7
blood gas level 790.91
blood sugar level 790.2
high 790.2
low 251.2
calcium 275.4
carbonate 276.9
casts, urine 791.7
catecholamines 791.9
cells, urine 791.7
cerebrospinal fluid (color) (content) (pressure) 792.0
chloride 276.9
cholesterol 272.9
chromosome analysis 795.2
chyluria 791.1
circulation time 794.39
cloudy urine 791.9
coagulation study 790.92
cobalt, blood 790.6
color of urine (unusual) NEC 791.9
copper, blood 790.6
crystals, urine 791.9
culture, positive NEC 795.3
blood 790.7
HIV V08
human immunodeficiency virus V08
nose 795.3
skin lesion NEC 795.3
spinal fluid 792.0
sputum 795.3
stool 792.1
throat 795.3
urine 791.9
viral
human immunodeficiency V08
wound 795.3
echocardiogram 793.2
echoencephalogram 794.01
echogram NEC—*see* Findings, abnormal, structure
electrocardiogram (ECG) (EKG) 794.31
electroencephalogram (EEG) 794.02
electrolyte level, urinary 791.9
electromyogram (EMG) 794.17
ocular 794.14
electro-oculogram (EOG) 794.12
electroretinogram (ERG) 794.11
enzymes, serum NEC 790.5
fibrinogen titer coagulation study 790.92

Findings, abnormal without diagnosis—*cont.*
filling defect—*see* Filling defect
function study NEC 794.9
auditory 794.15
bladder 794.9
brain 794.00
cardiac 794.30
endocrine NEC 794.6
thyroid 794.5
kidney 794.4
liver 794.8
nervous system
central 794.00
peripheral 794.19
oculomotor 794.14
pancreas 794.9
placenta 794.9
pulmonary 794.2
retina 794.11
special senses 794.19
spleen 794.9
vestibular 794.16
gallbladder, nonvisualization 793.3
glucose 790.2
tolerance test 790.2
glycosuria 791.5
heart
shadow 793.2
sounds 785.3
hematinuria 791.2
hematocrit
elevated 282.7
low 285.9
hematologic NEC 790.99
hematuria 599.7
hemoglobin
elevated 282.7
low 285.9
hemoglobinuria 791.2
histological NEC 795.4
hormones 259.9
immunoglobulins, elevated 795.79
indolacetic acid, elevated 791.9
iron 790.6
karyotype 795.2
ketonuria 791.6
lactic acid dehydrogenase (LDH) 790.4
lipase 790.5
lipids NEC 272.9
lithium, blood 790.6
lung field (coin lesion) (shadow) 793.1
magnesium, blood 790.6
mammogram 793.8
mediastinal shift 793.2
melanin, urine 791.9
microbiologic NEC 795.3
mineral, blood NEC 790.6
myoglobinuria 791.3
nitrogen derivatives, blood 790.6
nonvisualization of gallbladder 793.3
nose culture, positive 795.3
odor of urine (unusual) NEC 791.9
oxygen saturation 790.91
Papanicolaou (smear) 795.1
cervix (dyskaryotic) 795.0
other site 795.1
peritoneal fluid 792.9
phonocardiogram 794.39
phosphorus 275.3
pleural fluid 792.9
pneumoencephalogram 793.0

Findings, abnormal without diagnosis—*cont.*
PO_2-oxygen ratio 790.91
poikilocytosis 790.0
potassium
deficiency 276.8
excess 276.7
PPD 795.5
prostate specific antigen (PSA) 790.93
protein, serum NEC 790.99
proteinuria 791.0
prothrombin time (partial) (prolonged) (PT) (PTT) 790.92
pyuria 599.0
radiologic (x-ray) 793.9
abdomen 793.6
biliary tract 793.3
breast 793.8
gastrointestinal tract 793.4
genitourinary organs 793.5
head 793.0
intrathoracic organs NEC 793.2
lung 793.1
musculoskeletal 793.7
placenta 793.9
retroperitoneum 793.6
skin 793.9
skull 793.0
subcutaneous tissue 793.9
red blood cell 790.0
count 790.0
morphology 790.0
sickling 790.0
volume 790.0
saliva 792.4
scan NEC 794.9
bladder 794.9
bone 794.9
brain 794.09
kidney 794.4
liver 794.8
lung 794.2
pancreas 794.9
placental 794.9
spleen 794.9
thyroid 794.5
sedimentation rate, elevated 790.1
semen 792.2
serological (for)
human immunodeficiency virus (HIV)
inconclusive 795.71
positive V08
syphilis—*see* Findings, serology for syphilis
serology for syphilis
false positive 795.6
positive 097.1
false 795.6
follow-up of latent syphilis—*see* Syphilis, latent
only finding—*see* Syphilis, latent
serum 790.99
blood NEC 790.99
enzymes NEC 790.5
proteins 790.99
SGOT 790.4
SGPT 790.4
sickling of red blood cells 790.0
skin test, positive 795.79
tuberculin (without active tuberculosis) 795.5

Findings, abnormal without diagnosis—*cont.*
sodium 790.6
deficiency 276.1
excess 276.0
spermatozoa 792.2
spinal fluid 792.0
culture, positive 792.0
sputum culture, positive 795.3
for acid-fast bacilli 795.3
stool NEC 792.1
bloody 578.1
occult 792.1
color 792.1
culture, positive 792.1
occult blood 792.1
structure, body (echogram) (thermogram) (ultrasound) (x-ray) NEC 793.9
abdomen 793.6
breast 793.8
gastrointestinal tract 793.4
genitourinary organs 793.5
head 793.0
echogram (ultrasound) 794.01
intrathoracic organs NEC 793.2
lung 793.1
musculoskeletal 793.7
placenta 793.9
retroperitoneum 793.6
skin 793.9
subcutaneous tissue NEC 793.9
synovial fluid 792.9
thermogram—*see* Finding, abnormal, structure
throat culture, positive 795.3
thyroid (function) 794.5
metabolism (rate) 794.5
scan 794.5
uptake 794.5
total proteins 790.99
toxicology (drugs) (heavy metals) 796.0
transaminase (level) 790.4
triglycerides 272.9
tuberculin skin test (without active tuberculosis) 795.5
ultrasound—*see also* Finding, abnormal, structure
cardiogram 793.2
uric acid, blood 790.6
urine, urinary constituents 791.9
acetone 791.6
albumin 791.0
bacteria 791.9
bile 791.4
blood 599.7
casts or cells 791.7
chyle 791.1
culture, positive 791.9
glucose 791.5
hemoglobin 791.2
ketone 791.6
protein 791.0
pus 599.0
sugar 791.5
vaginal fluid 792.9
vanillylmandelic acid, elevated 791.9
vectorcardiogram (VCG) 793.2
ventriculogram (cerebral) 793.0
VMA, elevated 791.9

Findings, abnormal without diagnosis—*cont.*
Wassermann reaction
false positive 795.6
positive 097.1
follow-up of latent syphilis—*see* Syphilis, latent
only finding—*see* Syphilis, latent
white blood cell 288.9
count 288.9
elevated 288.8
low 288.0
differential 288.9
morphology 288.9
wound culture 795.3
xerography 793.8
zinc, blood 790.6
Finger —*see* condition
Fire, St. Anthony's (*see also* Erysipelas) 035
Fish
hook stomach 537.89
meal workers' lung 495.8
Fisher's syndrome 357.0
Fissure, fissured
abdominal wall (congenital) 756.7
anus, anal 565.0
congenital 751.5
buccal cavity 528.9
clitoris (congenital) 752.49
ear, lobule (congenital) 744.29
epiglottis (congenital) 748.3
larynx 478.79
congenital 748.3
lip 528.5
congenital (*see also* Cleft, lip) 749.10
nipple 611.2
puerperal, postpartum 676.1
palate (congenital) (*see also* Cleft, palate) 749.00
postanal 565.0
rectum 565.0
skin 709.8
streptococcal 686.9
spine (congenital) (*see also* Spina bifida) 741.9
sternum (congenital) 756.3
tongue (acquired) 529.5
congenital 750.13
Fistula (sinus) 686.9
abdomen (wall) 569.81
bladder 596.2
intestine 569.81
ureter 593.82
uterus 619.2
abdominorectal 569.81
abdominosigmoidal 569.81
abdominothoracic 510.0
abdominouterine 619.2
congenital 752.3
abdominovesical 596.2
accessory sinuses (*see also* Sinusitis) 473.9
actinomycotic—*see* Actinomycosis
alveolar
antrum (*see also* Sinusitis, maxillary) 473.0
process 522.7
anorectal 565.1
antrobuccal (*see also* Sinusitis, maxillary) 473.0
antrum (*see also* Sinusitis, maxillary) 473.0
anus, anal (infectional) (recurrent) 565.1
congenital 751.5
tuberculous (*see also* Tuberculosis) 014.8
aortic sinus 747.29
aortoduodenal 447.2

Fistula—*continued*
appendix, appendicular 543.9
arteriovenous (acquired) 447.0
brain 437.3
congenital 747.81
ruptured (*see also* Hemorrhage, subarachnoid) 430
ruptured (*see also* Hemorrhage, subarachnoid) 430
cerebral 437.3
congenital 747.81
congenital (peripheral) 747.60
brain—*see* Fistula, arteriovenous, brain, congenital
coronary 746.85
gastrointestinal 747.61
lower limb 747.64
pulmonary 747.3
renal 747.62
specified NEC 747.69
upper limb 747.63
coronary 414.19
congenital 746.85
heart 414.19
pulmonary (vessels) 417.0
congenital 747.3
surgically created (for dialysis) V45.1
complication NEC 996.73
atherosclerosis —*see* Arteriosclerosis, extremities
embolism 996.74
infection or inflammation 996.62
mechanical 996.1
occlusion NEC 996.74
thrombus 996.74
traumatic—*see* Injury, blood vessel, by site
artery 447.2
aural 383.81
congenital 744.49
auricle 383.81
congenital 744.49
Bartholin's gland 619.8
bile duct (*see also* Fistula, biliary) 576.4
biliary (duct) (tract) 576.4
congenital 751.69
bladder (neck) (sphincter) 596.2
into seminal vesicle 596.2
bone 733.99
brain 348.8
arteriovenous—*see* Fistula, arteriovenous, brain
branchial (cleft) 744.41
branchiogenous 744.41
breast 611.0
puerperal, postpartum 675.1
bronchial 510.0
bronchocutaneous, bronchomediastinal, bronchopleural, bronchopleuromediastinal (infective) 510.0
tuberculous (*see also* Tuberculosis) 011.3
bronchoesophageal 530.89
congenital 750.3
buccal cavity (infective) 528.3
canal, ear 380.89
carotid-cavernous
congenital 747.81
with hemorrhage 430
traumatic 900.82
with hemorrhage (see also Hemorrhage, brain, traumatic) 853.0
late effect 908.3

Fistula—*continued*
cecosigmoidal 569.81
cecum 569.81
cerebrospinal (fluid) 349.81
cervical, lateral (congenital) 744.41
cervicoaural (congenital) 744.49
cervicosigmoidal 619.1
cervicovesical 619.0
cervix 619.8
chest (wall) 510.0
cholecystocolic (*see also* Fistula, gallbladder) 575.5
cholecystocolonic (*see also* Fistula, gallbladder) 575.5
cholecystoduodenal (*see also* Fistula, gallbladder) 575.5
cholecystoenteric (*see also* Fistula, gallbladder) 575.5
cholecystogastric (*see also* Fistula, gallbladder) 575.5
cholecystointestinal (*see also* Fistula, gallbladder) 575.5
choledochoduodenal 576.4
cholocolic (*see also* Fistula, gallbladder) 575.5
coccyx 685.1
with abscess 685.0
colon 569.81
colostomy 569.69
colovaginal (acquired) 619.1
common duct (bile duct) 576.4
congenital, NEC—*see* Anomaly, specified type NEC
cornea, causing hypotony 360.32
coronary, arteriovenous 414.19
congenital 746.85
costal region 510.0
cul-de-sac, Douglas' 619.8
cutaneous 686.9
cystic duct (*see also* Fistula, gallbladder) 575.5
congenital 751.69
dental 522.7
diaphragm 510.0
bronchovisceral 510.0
pleuroperitoneal 510.0
pulmonoperitoneal 510.0
duodenum 537.4
ear (canal) (external) 380.89
enterocolic 569.81
enterocutaneous 569.81
enteroenteric 569.81
entero-uterine 619.1
congenital 752.3
enterovaginal 619.1
congenital 752.49
enterovesical 596.1
epididymis 608.89
tuberculous (*see also* Tuberculosis) 016.4
esophagobronchial 530.89
congenital 750.3
esophagocutaneous 530.89
esophagopleurocutaneous 530.89
esophagotracheal 530.84
congenital 750.3
esophagus 530.89
congenital 750.4
ethmoid (*see also* Sinusitis, ethmoidal) 473.2
eyeball (cornea) (sclera) 360.32
eyelid 373.11
fallopian tube (external) 619.2
fecal 569.81
congenital 751.5

Fistula—*continued*
from periapical lesion 522.7
frontal sinus (*see also* Sinusitis, frontal) 473.1
gallbladder 575.5
with calculus, cholelithiasis, stones (*see also* Cholelithiasis) 574.2
congenital 751.69
gastric 537.4
gastrocolic 537.4
congenital 750.7
tuberculous (*see also* Tuberculosis) 014.8
gastroenterocolic 537.4
gastroesophageal 537.4
gastrojejunal 537.4
gastrojejunocolic 537.4
genital
organs
female 619.9
specified site NEC 619.8
male 608.89
tract-skin (female) 619.2
hepatopleural 510.0
hepatopulmonary 510.0
horseshoe 565.1
ileorectal 569.81
ileosigmoidal 569.81
ileostomy 569.69
ileovesical 596.1
ileum 569.81
in ano 565.1
tuberculous (*see also* Tuberculosis) 014.8
inner ear (*see also* Fistula, labyrinth) 386.40
intestine 569.81
intestinocolonic (abdominal) 569.81
intestinoureteral 593.82
intestinouterine 619.1
intestinovaginal 619.1
congenital 752.49
intestinovesical 596.1
involving female genital tract 619.9
digestive-genital 619.1
genital tract-skin 619.2
specified site NEC 619.8
urinary-genital 619.0
ischiorectal (fossa) 566
jejunostomy 569.69
jejunum 569.81
joint 719.80
ankle 719.87
elbow 719.82
foot 719.87
hand 719.84
hip 719.85
knee 719.86
multiple sites 719.89
pelvic region 719.85
shoulder (region) 719.81
specified site NEC 719.88
tuberculous—*see* Tuberculosis, joint
wrist 719.83
kidney 593.89
labium (majus) (minus) 619.8
labyrinth, labyrinthine NEC 386.40
combined sites 386.48
multiple sites 386.48
oval window 386.42
round window 386.41
semicircular canal 386.43
lacrimal, lachrymal (duct) (gland) (sac) 375.61
lacrimonasal duct 375.61
laryngotracheal 748.3

Fistula—*continued*
larynx 478.79
lip 528.5
congenital 750.25
lumbar, tuberculous (*see also* Tuberculosis) 015.0 *[730.8]*
lung 510.0
lymphatic (node) (vessel) 457.8
mamillary 611.0
mammary (gland) 611.0
puerperal, postpartum 675.1
mastoid (process) (region) 383.1
maxillary (*see also* Sinusitis, maxillary) 473.0
mediastinal 510.0
mediastinobronchial 510.0
mediastinocutaneous 510.0
middle ear 385.89
mouth 528.3
nasal 478.1
sinus (*see also* Sinusitis) 473.9
nasopharynx 478.29
nipple—*see* Fistula, breast
nose 478.1
oral (cutaneous) 528.3
maxillary (*see also* Sinusitis, maxillary) 473.0
nasal (with cleft palate) (*see also* Cleft, palate) 749.00
orbit, orbital 376.10
oro-antral (*see also* Sinusitis, maxillary) 473.0
oval window (internal ear) 386.42
oviduct (external) 619.2
palate (hard) 526.89
soft 528.9
pancreatic 577.8
pancreaticoduodenal 577.8
parotid (gland) 527.4
region 528.3
pelvoabdominointestinal 569.81
penis 607.89
perianal 565.1
pericardium (pleura) (sac) (*see also* Pericarditis) 423.8
pericecal 569.81
perineal—*see* Fistula, perineum
perineorectal 569.81
perineosigmoidal 569.81
perineo-urethroscrotal 608.89
perineum, perineal (with urethral involvement) NEC 599.1
tuberculous (*see also* Tuberculosis) 017.9
ureter 593.82
perirectal 565.1
tuberculous (*see also* Tuberculosis) 014.8
peritoneum (*see also* Peritonitis) 567.2
periurethral 599.1
pharyngo-esophageal 478.29
pharynx 478.29
branchial cleft (congenital) 744.41
pilonidal (infected) (rectum) 685.1
with abscess 685.0
pleura, pleural, pleurocutaneous, pleuroperitoneal 510.0
stomach 510.0
tuberculous (*see also* Tuberculosis) 012.0
pleuropericardial 423.8
postauricular 383.81
postoperative, persistent 998.6
preauricular (congenital) 744.46
prostate 602.8

Fistula—*continued*
pulmonary 510.0
arteriovenous 417.0
congenital 747.3
tuberculous (*see also* Tuberculosis, pulmonary) 011.9
pulmonoperitoneal 510.0
rectolabial 619.1
rectosigmoid (intercommunicating) 569.81
rectoureteral 593.82
rectourethral 599.1
congenital 753.8
rectouterine 619.1
congenital 752.3
rectovaginal 619.1
congenital 752.49
old, postpartal 619.1
tuberculous (*see also* Tuberculosis) 014.8
rectovesical 596.1
congenital 753.8
rectovesicovaginal 619.1
rectovulvar 619.1
congenital 752.49
rectum (to skin) 565.1
tuberculous (*see also* Tuberculosis) 014.8
renal 593.89
retroauricular 383.81
round window (internal ear) 386.41
salivary duct or gland 527.4
congenital 750.24
sclera 360.32
scrotum (urinary) 608.89
tuberculous (*see also* Tuberculosis) 016.5
semicircular canals (internal ear) 386.43
sigmoid 569.81
vesicoabdominal 596.1
sigmoidovaginal 619.1
congenital 752.49
skin 686.9
ureter 593.82
vagina 619.2
sphenoidal sinus (*see also* Sinusitis, sphenoidal) 473.3
splenocolic 289.59
stercoral 569.81
stomach 537.4
sublingual gland 527.4
congenital 750.24
submaxillary
gland 527.4
congenital 750.24
region 528.3
thoracic 510.0
duct 457.8
thoracicoabdominal 510.0
thoracicogastric 510.0
thoracicointestinal 510.0
thoracoabdominal 510.0
thoracogastric 510.0
thorax 510.0
thyroglossal duct 759.2
thyroid 246.8
trachea (congenital) (external) (internal) 748.3
tracheoesophageal 530.84
congenital 750.3
following tracheostomy 519.0
traumatic
arteriovenous (*see also* Injury, blood vessel, by site) 904.9
brain—*see* Injury, intracranial

Fistula—*continued*
tuberculous—*see* Tuberculosis, by site
typhoid 002.0
umbilical 759.89
umbilico-urinary 753.8
urachal, urachus 753.7
ureter (persistent) 593.82
ureteroabdominal 593.82
ureterocervical 593.82
ureterorectal 593.82
ureterosigmoido-abdominal 593.82
ureterovaginal 619.0
ureterovesical 596.2
urethra 599.1
congenital 753.8
tuberculous (*see also* Tuberculosis) 016.3
urethroperineal 599.1
urethroperineovesical 596.2
urethrorectal 599.1
congenital 753.8
urethroscrotal 608.89
urethrovaginal 619.0
urethrovesical 596.2
urethrovesicovaginal 619.0
urinary (persistent) (recurrent) 599.1
uteroabdominal (anterior wall) 619.2
congenital 752.3
uteroenteric 619.1
uterofecal 619.1
uterointestinal 619.1
congenital 752.3
uterorectal 619.1
congenital 752.3
uteroureteric 619.0
uterovaginal 619.8
uterovesical 619.0
congenital 752.3
uterus 619.8
vagina (wall) 619.8
postpartal, old 619.8
vaginocutaneous (postpartal) 619.2
vaginoileal (acquired) 619.1
vaginoperineal 619.2
vesical NEC 596.2
vesicoabdominal 596.2
vesicocervicovaginal 619.0
vesicocolic 596.1
vesicocutaneous 596.2
vesicoenteric 596.1
vesicointestinal 596.1
vesicometrorectal 619.1
vesicoperineal 596.2
vesicorectal 596.1
congenital 753.8
vesicosigmoidal 596.1
vesicosigmoidovaginal 619.1
vesicoureteral 596.2
vesicoureterovaginal 619.0
vesicourethral 596.2
vesicourethrorectal 596.1
vesicouterine 619.0
congenital 752.3
vesicovaginal 619.0
vulvorectal 619.1
congenital 752.49
Fit 780.3
apoplectic (*see also* Disease, cerebrovascular, acute) 436
late effect—*see* category 438
epileptic (*see also* Epilepsy) 345.9

Fit *—continued*
fainting 780.2
hysterical 300.11
newborn 779.0
Fitting (of)
artificial
arm (complete) (partial) V52.0
breast V52.4
eye(s) V52.2
leg(s) (complete) (partial) V52.1
brain neuropacemaker V53.0
cardiac pacemaker V53.31
carotid sinus pacemaker V53.39
colostomy belt V53.5
contact lenses V53.1
cystostomy device V53.6
defibrillator, automatic implantable V53.32
dentures V52.3
device NEC V53.9
abdominal V53.5
cardiac
defibrillator, automatic implantable V53.32
pacemaker V53.31
specified NEC V53.39
intrauterine contraceptive V25.1
nervous system V53.0
orthodontic V53.4
orthoptic V53.1
prosthetic V52.9
breast V52.4
dental V52.3
eye V52.2
specified type NEC V52.8
special senses V53.0
substitution
auditory V53.0
nervous system V53.0
visual V53.0
urinary V53.6
diaphragm (contraceptive) V25.02
glasses (reading) V53.1
hearing aid V53.2
ileostomy device V53.5
intestinal appliance or device NEC V53.5
intrauterine contraceptive device V25.1
neuropacemaker (brain) (peripheral nerve) (spinal cord) V53.0
orthodontic device V53.4
orthopedic (device) V53.7
brace V53.7
cast V53.7
corset V53.7
shoes V53.7
pacemaker (cardiac) V53.31
brain V53.0
carotid sinus V53.39
peripheral nerve V53.0
spinal cord V53.0
prosthesis V52.9
arm (complete) (partial) V52.0
breast V52.4
dental V52.3
eye V52.2
leg (complete) (partial) V52.1
specified type NEC V52.8
spectacles V53.1
wheelchair V53.8
Fitz's syndrome (acute hemorrhagic pancreatitis) 577.0
Fitz-Hugh and Curtis syndrome (gonococcal peritonitis) 098.86
Fixation
joint—*see* Ankylosis
larynx 478.79
pupil 364.76
stapes 385.22
deafness (*see also* Deafness, conductive) 389.04
uterus (acquired)—*see* Malposition, uterus
vocal cord 478.5
Flaccid —*see* condition
foot 736.79
forearm 736.09
palate, congenital 750.26
Flail
chest 807.4
newborn 767.3
joint (paralytic) 718.80
ankle 718.87
elbow 718.82
foot 718.87
hand 718.84
hip 718.85
knee 718.86
multiple sites 718.89
pelvic region 718.85
shoulder (region) 718.81
specified site NEC 718.88
wrist 718.83
Flajani (-Basedow) syndrome or disease (exophthalmic goiter) 242.0
Flap, liver 572.8
Flare, anterior chamber (aqueous) (eye) 364.04
Flashback phenomena (drug) (hallucinogenic) 292.89
Flat
chamber (anterior) (eye) 360.34
chest, congenital 754.89
electroencephalogram (EEG) 348.8
foot (acquired) (fixed type) (painful) (postural) (spastic) 734
congenital 754.61
rocker bottom 754.61
vertical talus 754.61
rachitic 268.1
rocker bottom (congenital) 754.61
vertical talus, congenital 754.61
organ or site, congenital NEC—*see* Anomaly, specified type NEC
pelvis 738.6
with disproportion (fetopelvic) 653.2
affecting fetus or newborn 763.1
causing obstructed labor 660.1
affecting fetus or newborn 763.1
congenital 755.69
Flatau-Schilder disease 341.1
Flattening
head, femur 736.39
hip 736.39
lip (congenital) 744.89
nose (congenital) 754.0
acquired 738.0
Flatulence 787.3
Flatus 787.3
vaginalis 629.8
Flax dressers' disease 504
Flea bite —*see* Injury, superficial, by site
Fleischer (-Kayser) ring (corneal pigmentation) 275.1 *[371.14]*
Fleischner's disease 732.3
Fleshy mole 631
Flexibilitas cerea (*see also* Catalepsy) 300.11

Flexion
cervix (*see also* Malposition, uterus) 621.6
contracture, joint (*see also* Contraction, joint) 718.4
deformity, joint (*see also* Contraction, joint) 718.4
hip, congenital (*see also* Subluxation, congenital, hip) 754.32
uterus (*see also* Malposition, uterus) 621.6
Flexner's
bacillus 004.1
diarrhea (ulcerative) 004.1
dysentery 004.1
Flexner-Boyd dysentery 004.2
Flexure —*see* condition
Floater, vitreous 379.24
Floating
cartilage (joint) (*see also* Disorder, cartilage, articular) 718.0
knee 717.6
gallbladder (congenital) 751.69
kidney 593.0
congenital 753.3
liver (congenital) 751.69
rib 756.3
spleen 289.59
Flooding 626.2
Floor —*see* condition
Floppy
infant NEC 781.9
valve syndrome (mitral) 424.0
Flu —*see also* Influenza
gastric NEC 008.8
Fluctuating blood pressure 796.4
Fluid
abdomen 789.5
chest (*see also* Pleurisy, with effusion) 511.9
heart (*see also* Failure, heart, congestive) 428.0
joint (*see also* Effusion, joint) 719.0
loss (acute) 276.5
with
hypernatremia 276.0
hyponatremia 276.1
lung—*see also* Edema, lung
encysted 511.8
peritoneal cavity 789.5
pleural cavity (*see also* Pleurisy, with effusion) 511.9
retention 276.6
Flukes NEC (*see also* Infestation, fluke) 121.9
blood NEC (*see also* Infestation, Schistosoma) 120.9
liver 121.3
Fluor (albus) (vaginalis) 623.5
trichomonal (Trichomonas vaginalis) 131.00
Fluorosis (dental) (chronic) 520.3
Flushing 782.62
menopausal 627.2
Flush syndrome 259.2
Flutter
atrial or auricular 427.32
heart (ventricular) 427.42
atrial 427.32
impure 427.32
postoperative 997.1
ventricular 427.42
Flux (bloody) (serosanguineous) 009.0
Focal —*see* condition
Fochier's abscess —*see* Abscess, by site
Focus, Assmann's (*see also* Tuberculosis) 011.0
Fogo selvagem 694.4
Foix-Alajouanine syndrome 336.1
Folds, anomalous —*see also* Anomaly, specified type NEC
Bowman's membrane 371.31
Descemet's membrane 371.32
epicanthic 743.63
heart 746.89
posterior segment of eye, congenital 743.54
Folie à deux 297.3
Follicle
cervix (nabothian) (ruptured) 616.0
graafian, ruptured, with hemorrhage 620.0
nabothian 616.0
Folliclis (primary) (*see also* Tuberculosis) 017.0
Follicular —*see also* condition
cyst (atretic) 620.0
Folliculitis 704.8
abscedens et suffodiens 704.8
decalvans 704.09
gonorrheal (acute) 098.0
chronic or duration of 2 months or more 098.2
keloid, keloidalis 706.1
pustular 704.8
ulerythematosa reticulata 701.8
Folliculosis, conjunctival 372.02
Folling's disease (phenylketonuria) 270.1
Follow-up (examination) (routine) (following) V67.9
cancer chemotherapy V67.2
chemotherapy V67.2
fracture V67.4
high-risk medication V67.51
injury NEC V67.59
postpartum
immediately after delivery V24.0
routine V24.2
psychiatric V67.3
psychotherapy V67.3
radiotherapy V67.1
specified condition NEC V67.59
surgery V67.0
treatment V67.9
combined NEC V67.6
fracture V67.4
involving high-risk medication NEC V67.51
mental disorder V67.3
specified NEC V67.59
Fong's syndrome (hereditary osteoonychodysplasia) 756.89
Food
allergy 693.1
anaphylactic shock—*see* Anaphylactic shock, due to, food
asphyxia (from aspiration or inhalation) (*see also* Asphyxia, food) 933.1
choked on (*see also* Asphyxia, food) 933.1
deprivation 994.2
specified kind of food NEC 269.8
intoxication (*see also* Poisoning, food) 005.9
lack of 994.2
poisoning (*see also* Poisoning, food) 005.9
refusal or rejection NEC 307.59
strangulation or suffocation (*see also* Asphyxia, food) 933.1
toxemia (*see also* Poisoning, food) 005.9
Foot —*see also* condition
and mouth disease 078.4
process disease 581.3
Foramen ovale (nonclosure) (patent) (persistent) 745.5
Forbes' (glycogen storage) disease 271.0

Forbes-Albright syndrome (nonpuerperal amenorrhea and lactation associated with pituitary tumor) 253.1
Forced birth or delivery NEC 669.8
  affecting fetus or newborn NEC 763.8
Forceps
  delivery NEC 669.5
    affecting fetus or newborn 763.2
Fordyce's disease (ectopic sebaceous glands) (mouth) 750.26
Fordyce-Fox disease (apocrine miliaria) 705.82
Forearm —*see* condition
Foreign body

Note—For foreign body with open wound or other injury, see Wound, open, or the type of injury specified.

  accidentally left during a procedure 998.4
  anterior chamber (eye) 871.6
    magnetic 871.5
      retained or old 360.51
    retained or old 360.61
  ciliary body (eye) 871.6
    magnetic 871.5
      retained or old 360.52
    retained or old 360.62
  entering through orifice (current) (old)
    accessory sinus 932
    air passage (upper) 933.0
      lower 934.8
    alimentary canal 938
    alveolar process 935.0
    antrum (Highmore) 932
    anus 937
    appendix 936
    asphyxia due to (*see also* Asphyxia, food) 933.1
    auditory canal 931
    auricle 931
    bladder 939.0
    bronchioles 934.8
    bronchus (main) 934.1
    buccal cavity 935.0
    canthus (inner) 930.1
    cecum 936
    cervix (canal) uterine 939.1
    coil, ileocecal 936
    colon 936
    conjunctiva 930.1
    conjunctival sac 930.1
    cornea 930.0
    digestive organ or tract NEC 938
    duodenum 936
    ear (external) 931
    esophagus 935.1
    eye (external) 930.9
      combined sites 930.8
      intraocular—*see* Foreign body, by site
      specified site NEC 930.8
    eyeball 930.8
      intraocular—*see* Foreign body, intraocular
    eyelid 930.1
      retained or old 374.86
    frontal sinus 932
    gastrointestinal tract 938
    genitourinary tract 939.9
    globe 930.8
      penetrating 871.6
        magnetic 871.5
          retained or old 360.50
        retained or old 360.60

Foreign body—*continued*
    gum 935.0
    Highmore's antrum 932
    hypopharynx 933.0
    ileocecal coil 936
    ileum 936
    inspiration (of) 933.1
    intestine (large) (small) 936
    lacrimal apparatus, duct, gland, or sac 930.2
    larynx 933.1
    lung 934.8
    maxillary sinus 932
    mouth 935.0
    nasal sinus 932
    nasopharynx 933.0
    nose (passage) 932
    nostril 932
    oral cavity 935.0
    palate 935.0
    penis 939.3
    pharynx 933.0
    pyriform sinus 933.0
    rectosigmoid 937
      junction 937
    rectum 937
    respiratory tract 934.9
      specified part NEC 934.8
    sclera 930.1
    sinus 932
      accessory 932
      frontal 932
      maxillary 932
      nasal 932
      pyriform 933.0
    small intestine 936
    stomach (hairball) 935.2
    suffocation by (*see also* Asphyxia, food) 933.1
    swallowed 938
      tongue 933.0
    tear ducts or glands 930.2
    throat 933.0
    tongue 935.0
      swallowed 933.0
    tonsil, tonsillar 933.0
      fossa 933.0
    trachea 934.0
    ureter 939.0
    urethra 939.0
    uterus (any part) 939.1
    vagina 939.2
    vulva 939.2
    wind pipe 934.0
  granuloma (old) 728.82
    bone 733.99
    in operative wound (inadvertently left) 998.4
      due to surgical material intentionally left—*see* Complications, due to (presence of) any device, implant, or graft classified to 996.0-996.5 NEC
    muscle 728.82
    skin 709.4
    soft tissue NEC 728.82
    subcutaneous tissue 709.4
  in
    bone (residual) 733.99
    open wound—*see* Wound, open, by site complicated
    soft tissue (residual) 729.6
  inadvertently left in operation wound (causing adhesions, obstruction, or perforation) 998.4

Foreign body—*continued*
ingestion, ingested NEC 938
inhalation or inspiration (*see also* Asphyxia, food) 933.1
internal organ, not entering through an orifice—*see* Injury, internal, by site, with open wound
intraocular (nonmagnetic) 871.6
combined sites 871.6
magnetic 871.5
retained or old 360.59
retained or old 360.69
magnetic 871.5
retained or old 360.50
retained or old 360.60
specified site NEC 871.6
magnetic 871.5
retained or old 360.59
retained or old 360.69
iris (nonmagnetic) 871.6
magnetic 871.5
retained or old 360.52
retained or old 360.62
lens (nonmagnetic) 871.6
magnetic 871.5
retained or old 360.53
retained or old 360.63
lid, eye 930.1
ocular muscle 870.4
retained or old 376.6
old or residual
bone 733.99
eyelid 374.86
middle ear 385.83
muscle 729.6
ocular 376.6
retrobulbar 376.6
skin 709.4
soft tissue 729.6
subcutaneous tissue 709.4
operation wound, left accidentally 998.4
orbit 870.4
retained or old 376.6
posterior wall, eye 871.6
magnetic 871.5
retained or old 360.55
retained or old 360.65
respiratory tree 934.9
specified site NEC 934.8
retained (old) (nonmagnetic) (in)
anterior chamber (eye) 360.61
magnetic 360.51
ciliary body 360.62
magnetic 360.52
eyelid 374.86
globe 360.60
magnetic 360.50
intraocular 360.60
magnetic 360.50
specified site NEC 360.69
magnetic 360.59
iris 360.62
magnetic 360.52
lens 360.63
magnetic 360.53
muscle 729.6
orbit 376.6
posterior wall of globe 360.65
magnetic 360.55
retina 360.65
magnetic 360.55

Foreign body—*continued*
retrobulbar 376.6
soft tissue 729.6
vitreous 360.64
magnetic 360.54
retina 871.6
magnetic 871.5
retained or old 360.55
retained or old 360.65
superficial, without major open wound (*see also* Injury, superficial, by site) 919.6
swallowed NEC 938
vitreous (humor) 871.6
magnetic 871.5
retained or old 360.54
retained or old 360.64
Forking, aqueduct of Sylvius 742.3
with spina bifida (*see also* Spina bifida) 741.0
Formation
bone in scar tissue (skin) 709.3
connective tissue in vitreous 379.25
Elschnig pearls (postcataract extraction) 366.51
hyaline in cornea 371.49
sequestrum in bone (due to infection) (*see also* Osteomyelitis) 730.1
valve
colon, congenital 751.5
ureter (congenital) 753.2
Formication 782.0
Fort Bragg fever 100.89
Fossa —*see also* condition
pyriform—*see* condition
Foster-Kennedy syndrome 377.04
Fothergill's
disease, meaning scarlatina anginosa 034.1
neuralgia (*see also* Neuralgia, trigeminal) 350.1
Foul breath 784.9
Found dead (cause unknown) 798.9
Foundling V20.0
Fournier's disease (idiopathic gangrene) 608.83
Fourth
cranial nerve—*see* condition
disease 057.8
molar 520.1
Foville's syndrome 344.89
Fox's
disease (apocrine miliaria) 705.82
impetigo (contagiosa) 684
Fox-Fordyce disease (apocrine miliaria) 705.82

Fracture (abduction) (adduction) (avulsion) (compression) (crush) (dislocation) (oblique) (separation) (closed) 829.0

Note—For fracture of any of the following sites with fracture of other bones—see Fracture, multiple.

"Closed" includes the following descriptions of fractures, with or without delayed healing, unless they are specified as open or compound:

comminuted
depressed
elevated
fissured
greenstick
impacted
linear
march
simple
slipped epiphysis
spiral
unspecified

"Open" includes the following descriptions of fractures, with or without delayed healing:

compound
infected
missile
puncture
with foreign body

For late effect of fracture, see Late, effect, fracture, by site.

with
internal injuries in same region (conditions classifiable to 860-869)—*see also* Injury, internal, by site
pelvic region—*see* Fracture, pelvis
acetabulum (with visceral injury) (closed) 808.0
open 808.1
acromion (process) (closed) 811.01
open 811.11
alveolus (closed) 802.8
open 802.9
ankle (malleolus) (closed) 824.8
bimalleolar (Dupuytren's) (Pott's) 824.4
open 824.5
bone 825.21
open 825.31
lateral malleolus only (fibular) 824.2
open 824.3
medial malleolus only (tibial) 824.0
open 824.1
open 824.9
pathologic 733.16
talus 825.21
open 825.31
trimalleolar 824.6
open 824.7
antrum—*see* Fracture, skull, base
arm (closed) 818.0
and leg(s) (any bones) 828.0
open 828.1
both (any bones) (with rib(s)) (with sternum) 819.0
open 819.1
lower 813.80
open 813.90

Fracture—*continued*
open 818.1
upper—*see* Fracture, humerus
astragalus (closed) 825.21
open 825.31
atlas—*see* Fracture, vertebra, cervical, first
axis—*see* Fracture, vertebra, cervical, second
back—*see* Fracture, vertebra, by site
Barton's—*see* Fracture, radius, lower end
basal (skull)—*see* Fracture, skull, base
Bennett's (closed) 815.01
open 815.11
bimalleolar (closed) 824.4
open 824.5
bone (closed) NEC 829.0
birth injury NEC 767.3
open 829.1
pathologic NEC (*see also* Fracture, pathologic) 733.10
boot top—*see* Fracture, fibula
boxers'—*see* Fracture, metacarpal bone(s)
breast bone—*see* Fracture, sternum
bucket handle (semilunar cartilage)—*see* Tear, meniscus
bursting—*see* Fracture, phalanx, hand, distal
calcaneus (closed) 825.0
open 825.1
capitate (bone) (closed) 814.07
open 814.17
capitellum (humerus) (closed) 812.49
open 812.59
carpal bone(s) (wrist NEC) (closed) 814.00
open 814.10
specified site NEC 814.09
open 814.19
cartilage, knee (semilunar)—*see* Tear, meniscus
cervical—*see* Fracture, vertebra, cervical
chauffeur's—*see* Fracture, ulna, lower end
chisel—*see* Fracture, radius, upper end
clavicle (interligamentous part) (closed) 810.00
acromial end 810.03
open 810.13
due to birth trauma 767.2
open 810.10
shaft (middle third) 810.02
open 810.12
sternal end 810.01
open 810.11
clayshovelers'—*see* Fracture, vertebra, cervical
coccyx—*see also* Fracture, vertebra, coccyx
complicating delivery 665.6
collar bone—*see* Fracture, clavicle
Colles' (reversed) (closed) 813.41
open 813.51
comminuted—*see* Fracture, by site
compression—*see also* Fracture, by site
nontraumatic—*see* Fracture, pathologic
congenital 756.9
coracoid process (closed) 811.02
open 811.12
coronoid process (ulna) (closed) 813.02
mandible (closed) 802.23
open 802.33
open 813.12
costochondral junction—*see* Fracture, rib
costosternal junction—*see* Fracture, rib
cranium—*see* Fracture, skull, by site
cricoid cartilage (closed) 807.5
open 807.6
cuboid (ankle) (closed) 825.23
open 825.33

Fracture—*continued*
cuneiform
foot (closed) 825.24
open 825.34
wrist (closed) 814.03
open 814.13
due to
birth injury—*see* Birth injury, fracture
gunshot—*see* Fracture, by site, open
neoplasm—*see* Fracture, pathologic
osteoporosis—*see* Fracture, pathologic
Dupuytren's (ankle) (fibula) (closed) 824.4
open 824.5
radius 813.42
open 813.52
Duverney's—*see* Fracture, ilium
elbow—*see also* Fracture, humerus, lower end
olecranon (process) (closed) 813.01
open 813.11
supracondylar (closed) 812.41
open 812.51
ethmoid (bone) (sinus)—*see* Fracture, skull, base
face bone(s) (closed) NEC 802.8
with
other bone(s)—*see also* Fracture, multiple, skull
skull—*see also* Fracture, skull
involving other bones—*see* Fracture, multiple, skull
open 802.9
fatigue—*see* Fracture, march
femur, femoral (closed) 821.00
cervicotrochanteric 820.03
open 820.13
condyles, epicondyles 821.21
open 821.31
distal end—*see* Fracture, femur, lower end
epiphysis (separation)
capital 820.01
open 820.11
head 820.01
open 820.11
lower 821.22
open 821.32
trochanteric 820.01
open 820.11
upper 820.01
open 820.11
head 820.09
open 820.19
lower end or extremity (distal end) (closed) 821.20
condyles, epicondyles 821.21
open 821.31
epiphysis (separation) 821.22
open 821.32
multiple sites 821.29
open 821.39
open 821.30
specified site NEC 821.29
open 821.39
supracondylar 821.23
open 821.33
T-shaped 821.21
open 821.31
neck (closed) 820.8
base (cervicotrochanteric) 820.03
open 820.13
extracapsular 820.20
open 820.30

Fracture—*continued*
intertrochanteric (section) 820.21
open 820.31
intracapsular 820.00
open 820.10
intratrochanteric 820.21
open 821.31
midcervical 820.02
open 820.12
open 820.9
pathologic 733.14
specified part NEC 733.15
specified site NEC 820.09
open 820.19
transcervical 820.02
open 820.12
transtrochanteric 820.20
open 820.30
open 821.10
pathologic 733.14
specified part NEC 733.15
peritrochanteric (section) 820.20
open 820.30
shaft (lower third) (middle third) (upper third) 821.01
open 821.11
subcapital 820.09
open 820.19
subtrochanteric (region) (section) 820.22
open 820.32
supracondylar 821.23
open 821.33
transepiphyseal 820.01
open 820.11
trochanter (greater) (lesser) (*see also* Fracture, femur, neck, by site) 820.20
open 820.30
T-shaped, into knee joint 821.21
open 821.31
upper end 820.8
open 820.9
fibula (closed) 823.81
with tibia 823.82
open 823.92
distal end 824.8
open 824.9
epiphysis
lower 824.8
open 824.9
upper—*see* Fracture, fibula, upper end
head—*see* Fracture, fibula, upper end
involving ankle 824.2
open 824.3
lower end or extremity 824.8
open 824.9
malleolus (external) (lateral) 824.2
open 824.3
open NEC 823.91
pathologic 733.16
proximal end—*see* Fracture, fibula, upper end
shaft 823.21
with tibia 823.22
open 823.32
open 823.31
upper end or extremity (epiphysis) (head) (proximal end) (styloid) 823.01
with tibia 823.02
open 823.12
open 823.11

Fracture—*continued*
internal
ear—*see* Fracture, skull, base
semilunar cartilage, knee—*see* Tear, meniscus, medial
intertrochanteric—*see* Fracture, femur, neck, intertrochanteric
ischium (with visceral injury) (closed) 808.42
open 808.52
jaw (bone) (lower) (closed) (*see also* Fracture, mandible) 802.20
angle 802.25
open 802.35
open 802.30
upper—*see* Fracture, maxilla
knee
cap (closed) 822.0
open 822.1
cartilage (semilunar)—*see* Tear, meniscus
labyrinth (osseous)—*see* Fracture, skull, base
larynx (closed) 807.5
open 807.6
late effect—*see* Late, effects (of), fracture
Le Fort's—*see* Fracture, maxilla
leg (closed) 827.0
with rib(s) or sternum 828.0
open 828.1
both (any bones) 828.0
open 828.1
lower—*see* Fracture, tibia
open 827.1
upper—*see* Fracture, femur
limb
lower (multiple) (closed) NEC 827.0
open 827.1
upper (multiple) (closed) NEC 818.0
open 818.1
long bones, due to birth trauma—*see* Birth injury, fracture
lumbar—*see* Fracture, vertebra, lumbar
lunate bone (closed) 814.02
open 814.12
malar bone (closed) 802.4
open 802.5
Malgaigne's (closed) 808.43
open 808.53
malleolus (closed)0 824.8
bimalleolar 824.4
open 824.5
lateral 824.2
and medial—*see also* Fracture, malleolus, bimalleolar
with lip of tibia—*see* Fracture, malleolus, trimalleolar
open 824.3
medial (closed) 824.0
and lateral—*see also* Fracture, malleolus, bimalleolar
with lip of tibia—*see* Fracture, malleolus, trimalleolar
open 824.1
open 824.9
trimalleolar (closed) 824.6
open 824.7
malleus—*see* Fracture, skull, base
malunion 733.81

Fracture—*continued*
mandible (closed) 802.20
angle 802.25
open 802.35
body 802.28
alveolar border 802.27
open 802.37
open 802.38
symphysis 802.26
open 802.36
condylar process 802.21
open 802.31
coronoid process 802.23
open 802.33
multiple sites 802.29
open 802.39
open 802.30
ramus NEC 802.24
open 802.34
subcondylar 802.22
open 802.32
manubrium—*see* Fracture, sternum
march (closed) 825.20
open 825.30
maxilla, maxillary (superior) (upper jaw) (closed) 802.4
inferior—*see* Fracture, mandible
open 802.5
meniscus, knee—*see* Tear, meniscus
metacarpus, metacarpal (bone(s)), of one hand (closed) 815.00
with phalanx, phalanges, hand (finger(s)) (thumb) of same hand 817.0
open 817.1
base 815.02
first metacarpal 815.01
open 815.11
open 815.12
thumb 815.01
open 815.11
multiple sites 815.09
open 815.19
neck 815.04
open 815.14
open 815.10
shaft 815.03
open 815.13
metatarsus, metatarsal (bone(s)), of one foot (closed) 825.25
with tarsal bone(s) 825.29
open 825.39
open 825.35
Monteggia's (closed) 813.03
open 813.13
Moore's—*see* Fracture, radius, lower end
multangular bone (closed)
larger 814.05
open 814.15
smaller 814.06
open 814.16
multiple (closed) 829.0

Fracture—*continued*

Note—Multiple fractures of sites classifiable to the same three- or four-digit category are coded to that category, except for sites classifiable to 810-818 or 820-827 in different limbs.

Multiple fractures of sites classifiable to different fourth-digit subdivisions within the same three- digit category should be dealt with according to coding rules.

Multiple fractures of sites classifiable to different three-digit categories (identifiable from the listing under "Fracture"), and of sites classifiable to 810-818 or 820-827 in different limbs should be coded according to the following list, which should be referred to in the following priority order: skull or face bones, pelvis or vertebral column, legs, arms.

arm (multiple bones in same arm except in hand alone) (sites classifiable to 810-817 with sites classifiable to a different three-digit category in 810-817 in same arm) (closed) 818.0
open 818.1
arms, both or arm(s) with rib(s) or sternum (sites classifiable to 810-818 with sites classifiable to same range of categories in other limb or to 807) (closed) 819.0
open 819.1
bones of trunk NEC (closed) 809.0
open 809.1
hand, metacarpal bone(s) with phalanx or phalanges of same hand (sites classifiable to 815 with sites classifiable to 816 in same hand) (closed) 817.0
open 817.1
leg (multiple bones in same leg) (sites classifiable to 820-826 with sites classifiable to a different three-digit category in that range in same leg) (closed) 827.0
open 827.1
legs, both or leg(s) with arm(s), rib(s), or sternum (sites classifiable to 820-827 with sites classifiable to same range of categories in other leg or to 807 or 810-819) (closed) 828.0
open 828.1
open 829.1
pelvis with other bones except skull or face bones (sites classifiable to 808 with sites classifiable to 805-807 or 810-829) (closed) 809.0
open 809.1
skull, specified or unspecified bones, or face bone(s) with any other bone(s) (sites classifiable to 800-803 with sites classifiable to 805-829) (closed) 804.0

Fracture—*continued*

Note—Use the following fifth-digit subclassification with categories 800, 801, 803, and 804:

0 unspecified state of consciousness
1 with no loss of consciousness
2 with brief [less than one hour] loss of consciousness
3 with moderate [1-24 hours] loss of consciousness
4 with prolonged [more than 24 hours] loss of consciousness and return to pre-existing conscious level
5 with prolonged [more than 24 hours] loss of consciousness, without return to pre-existing conscious level
6 with loss of consciousness of unspecified duration
9 with concussion, unspecified

with
contusion, cerebral 804.1
epidural hemorrhage 804.2
extradural hemorrhage 804.2
hemorrhage (intracranial) NEC 804.3
intracranial injury NEC 804.4
laceration, cerebral 804.1
subarachnoid hemorrhage 804.2
subdural hemorrhage 804.2
open 804.5
with
contusion, cerebral 804.6
epidural hemorrhage 804.7
extradural hemorrhage 804.7
hemorrhage (intracranial) NEC 804.8
intracranial injury NEC 804.9
laceration, cerebral 804.6
subarachnoid hemorrhage 804.7
subdural hemorrhage 804.7
vertebral column with other bones, except skull or face bones (sites classifiable to 805 or 806 with sites classifiable to 807-808 or 810-829) (closed) 809.0
open 809.1
nasal (bone(s)) (closed) 802.0
open 802.1
sinus—Fracture, skull, base
navicular
carpal (wrist) (closed) 814.01
open 814.11
tarsal (ankle) (closed) 825.22
open 825.32
neck—*see* Fracture, vertebra, cervical
neural arch—*see* Fracture, vertebra, by site
nose, nasal, (bone) (septum) (closed) 802.0
open 802.1
occiput—*see* Fracture, skull, base
odontoid process—*see* Fracture, vertebra, cervical
olecranon (process) (ulna) (closed) 813.01
open 813.11
open 829.1
orbit, orbital (bone) (region) (closed) 802.8
floor (blow-out) 802.6
open 802.7
open 802.9
roof—*see* Fracture, skull, base
specified part NEC 802.8
open 802.9

Fracture—*continued*
os
calcis (closed) 825.0
open 825.1
magnum (closed) 814.07
open 814.17
pubis (with visceral injury) (closed) 808.2
open 808.3
triquetrum (closed) 814.03
open 814.13
osseous
auditory meatus—*see* Fracture, skull, base
labyrinth—*see* Fracture, skull, base
ossicles, auditory (incus) (malleus) (stapes)—*see* Fracture, skull, base
osteoporotic—*see* Fracture, pathologic
palate (closed) 802.8
open 802.9
paratrooper—*see* Fracture, tibia, lower end
parietal bone—*see* Fracture, skull, vault
parry—*see* Fracture, Monteggia's
patella (closed) 822.0
open 822.1
pathologic (cause unknown) 733.10
ankle 733.16
femur (neck) 733.14
specified NEC 733.15
fibula 733.16
hip 733.14
humerus 733.11
radius 733.12
specified site NEC 733.19
tibia 733.16
ulna 733.12
vertebrae (collapse) 733.13
wrist 733.12
pedicle (of vertebral arch)—*see* Fracture, vertebra, by site
pelvis, pelvic (bone(s)) (with visceral injury) (closed) 808.8
multiple (with disruption of pelvic circle) 808.43
open 808.53
open 808.9
rim (closed) 808.49
open 808.59
peritrochanteric (closed) 820.20
open 820.30
phalanx, phalanges, of one
foot (closed) 826.0
with bone(s) of same lower limb 827.0
open 827.1
open 826.1
hand (closed) 816.00
with metacarpal bone(s) of same hand 817.0
open 817.1
distal 816.02
open 816.12
middle 816.01
open 816.11
multiple sites NEC 816.03
open 816.13
open 816.10
proximal 816.01
open 816.11
pisiform (closed) 814.04
open 814.14
pond—Fracture, skull, vault
Pott's (closed) 824.4
open 824.5

Fracture—*continued*
prosthetic device, internal—*see* Complications, mechanical
pubis (with visceral injury) (closed) 808.2
open 808.3
Quervain's (closed) 814.01
open 814.11
radius (alone) (closed) 813.81
with ulna NEC 813.83
open 813.93
distal end—*see* Fracture, radius, lower end
epiphysis
lower—*see* Fracture, radius, lower end
upper—*see* Fracture, radius, upper end
head—*see* Fracture, radius, upper end
lower end or extremity (distal end) (lower epiphysis) 813.42
with ulna (lower end) 813.44
open 813.54
open 813.52
neck—*see* Fracture, radius, upper end
open NEC 813.91
pathologic 733.12
proximal end—*see* Fracture, radius, upper end
shaft (closed) 813.21
with ulna (shaft) 813.23
open 813.33
open 813.31
upper end 813.07
with ulna (upper end) 813.08
open 813.18
epiphysis 813.05
open 813.15
head 813.05
open 813.15
multiple sites 813.07
open 813.17
neck 813.06
open 813.16
open 813.17
specified site NEC 813.07
open 813.17
ramus
inferior or superior (with visceral injury) (closed) 808.2
open 808.3
ischium—*see* Fracture, ischium
mandible 802.24
open 802.34
rib(s) (closed) 807.0

Note—Use the following fifth-digit subclassification with categories 807.0-807.1:

0 rib(s), unspecified
1 one rib
2 two ribs
3 three ribs
4 four ribs
5 five ribs
6 six ribs
7 seven ribs
8 eight or more ribs
9 multiple ribs, unspecified

with flail chest (open) 807.4
open 807.1
root, tooth 873.63
complicated 873.73
sacrum—*see* Fracture, vertebra, sacrum

Fracture—*continued*
scaphoid
ankle (closed) 825.22
open 825.32
wrist (closed) 814.01
open 814.11
scapula (closed) 811.00
acromial, acromion (process) 811.01
open 811.11
body 811.09
open 811.19
coracoid process 811.02
open 811.12
glenoid (cavity) (fossa) 811.03
open 811.13
neck 811.03
open 811.13
open 811.10
semilunar
bone, wrist (closed) 814.02
open 814.12
cartilage (interior) (knee)—*see* Tear, meniscus
sesamoid bone—*see* Fracture, by site
Shepherd's (closed) 825.21
open 825.31
shoulder—*see also* Fracture, humerus, upper end
blade—*see* Fracture, scapula
silverfork—*see* Fracture, radius, lower end
sinus (ethmoid) (frontal) (maxillary) (nasal) (sphenoidal)—*see* Fracture, skull, base
maxillary—*see* Fracture, maxilla
Skillern's—*see* Fracture, radius, shaft
skull (multiple NEC) (with face bones) (closed) 803.0

Note—Use the following fifth-digit subclassification with categories 800, 801, 803, and 804:

0 unspecified state of consciousness
1 with no loss of consciousness
2 with brief [less than one hour] loss of consciousness
3 with moderate [1-24 hours] loss of consciousness
4 with prolonged [more than 24 hours] loss of consciousness and return to pre-existing conscious level
5 with prolonged [more than 24 hours] loss of consciousness, without return to pre-existing conscious level
6 with loss of consciousness of unspecified duration
9 with concussion, unspecified

with
contusion, cerebral 803.1
epidural hemorrhage 803.2
extradural hemorrhage 803.2
hemorrhage (intracranial) NEC 803.3
intracranial injury NEC 803.4
laceration, cerebral 803.1
other bones—*see* Fracture, multiple, skull
subarachnoid hemorrhage 803.2
subdural hemorrhage 803.2
base (antrum) (ethmoid bone) (fossa) (internal ear) (nasal sinus) (occiput) (sphenoid) (temporal bone) (closed) 801.0

Fracture—*continued*
with
contusion, cerebral 801.1
epidural hemorrhage 801.2
extradural hemorrhage 801.2
hemorrhage (intracranial) NEC 801.3
intracranial injury NEC 801.4
laceration, cerebral 801.1
subarachnoid hemorrhage 801.2
subdural hemorrhage 801.2
open 801.5
with
contusion, cerebral 801.6
epidural hemorrhage 801.7
extradural hemorrhage 801.7
hemorrhage (intracranial) NEC 801.8
intracranial injury NEC 801.9
laceration, cerebral 801.6
subarachnoid hemorrhage 801.7
subdural hemorrhage 801.7
birth injury 767.3
face bones—*see* Fracture, face bones
open 803.5
with
contusion, cerebral 803.6
epidural hemorrhage 803.7
extradural hemorrhage 803.7
hemorrhage (intracranial) NEC 803.8
intracranial injury NEC 803.9
laceration, cerebral 803.6
subarachnoid hemorrhage 803.7
subdural hemorrhage 803.7
vault (frontal bone) (parietal bone) (vertex) (closed) 800.0
with
contusion, cerebral 800.1
epidural hemorrhage 800.2
extradural hemorrhage 800.2
hemorrhage (intracranial) NEC 800.3
intracranial injury NEC 800.4
laceration, cerebral 800.1
subarachnoid hemorrhage 800.2
subdural hemorrhage 800.2
open 800.5
with
contusion, cerebral 800.6
epidural hemorrhage 800.7
extradural hemorrhage 800.7
hemorrhage (intracranial) NEC 800.8
intracranial injury NEC 800.9
laceration, cerebral 800.6
subarachnoid hemorrhage 800.7
subdural hemorrhage 800.7
Smith's 813.41
open 813.51
sphenoid (bone) (sinus)—*see* Fracture, skull, base
spine—*see also* Fracture, vertebra, by site
due to birth trauma 767.4
spinous process—*see* Fracture, vertebra, by site
spontaneous—*see* Fracture, pathologic
sprinters'—*see* Fracture, ilium
stapes—*see* Fracture, skull, base
stave—*see also* Fracture, metacarpus, metacarpal bone(s)
spine—*see* Fracture, tibia, upper end
sternum (closed) 807.2
with flail chest (open) 807.4
open 807.3
Stieda's—*see* Fracture, femur, lower end
stress—*see* Fracture, pathologic

Fracture—*continued*
styloid process
metacarpal (closed) 815.02
open 815.12
radius—*see* Fracture, radius, lower end
temporal bone—*see* Fracture, skull, base
ulna—*see* Fracture, ulna, lower end
supracondylar, elbow 812.41
open 812.51
symphysis pubis (with visceral injury) (closed) 808.2
open 808.3
talus (ankle bone) (closed) 825.21
open 825.31
tarsus, tarsal bone(s) (with metatarsus) of one foot (closed) NEC 825.29
open 825.39
temporal bone (styloid)—*see* Fracture, skull, base
tendon—*see* Sprain, by site
thigh—*see* Fracture, femur, shaft
thumb (and finger(s)) of one hand (closed) (*see also* Fracture, phalanx, hand) 816.00
with metacarpal bone(s) of same hand 817.0
open 817.1
metacarpal(s)—*see* Fracture, metacarpus
open 816.10
thyroid cartilage (closed) 807.5
open 807.6
tibia (closed) 823.80
with fibula 823.82
open 823.92
condyles—*see* Fracture, tibia, upper end
distal end 824.8
open 824.9
epiphysis
lower 824.8
open 824.9
upper—*see* Fracture, tibia, upper end
head (involving knee joint)—*see* Fracture, tibia, upper end
intercondyloid eminence—*see* Fracture, tibia, upper end
involving ankle 824.0
open 824.1
lower end or extremity (anterior lip) (posterior lip) 824.8
open 824.9
malleolus (internal) (medial) 824.0
open 824.1
open NEC 823.90
pathologic 733.16
proximal end—*see* Fracture, tibia, upper end
shaft 823.20
with fibula 823.22
open 823.32
open 823.30
spine—*see* Fracture, tibia, upper end
tuberosity—*see* Fracture, tibia, upper end
upper end or extremity (condyle) (epiphysis) (head) (spine) (proximal end) (tuberosity) 823.00
with fibula 823.02
open 823.12
open 823.10
toe(s), of one foot (closed) 826.0
with bone(s) of same lower limb 827.0
open 827.1
open 826.1
tooth (root) 873.63
complicated 873.73

Fracture—*continued*
trachea (closed) 807.5
open 807.6
transverse process—*see* Fracture, vertebra, by site
trapezium (closed) 814.05
open 814.15
trapezoid bone (closed) 814.06
open 814.16
trimalleolar (closed) 824.6
open 824.7
triquetral (bone) (closed) 814.03
open 814.13
trochanter (greater) (lesser) (closed) (*see also* Fracture, femur, neck, by site) 820.20
open 820.30
trunk (bones) (closed) 809.0
open 809.1
tuberosity (external)—*see* Fracture, by site
ulna (alone) (closed) 813.82
with radius NEC 813.83
open 813.93
coronoid process (closed) 813.02
open 813.12
distal end—*see* Fracture, ulna, lower end
epiphysis
lower—*see* Fracture, ulna, lower end
upper—*see* Fracture, ulna, upper, end
head—*see* Fracture, ulna, lower end
lower end (distal end) (head) (lower epiphysis) (styloid process) 813.43
with radius (lower end) 813.44
open 813.54
open 813.53
olecranon process (closed) 813.01
open 813.11
open NEC 813.92
pathologic 733.12
proximal end—*see* Fracture, ulna, upper end
shaft 813.22
with radius (shaft) 813.23
open 813.33
open 813.32
styloid process—*see* Fracture, ulna, lower end
transverse—*see* Fracture, ulna, by site
upper end (epiphysis) 813.04
with radius (upper end) 813.08
open 813.18
multiple sites 813.04
open 813.14
open 813.14
specified site NEC 813.04
open 813.14
unciform (closed) 814.08
open 814.18
vertebra, vertebral (back) (body) (column) (neural arch) (pedicle) (spine) (spinous process) (transverse process) (closed) 805.8
with
hematomyelia—*see* Fracture, vertebra, by site, with spinal cord injury
injury to
cauda equina—*see* Fracture, vertebra, sacrum, with spinal cord injury
nerve—*see* Fracture, vertebra, by site, with spinal cord injury
paralysis—*see* Fracture, vertebra, by site, with spinal cord injury
paraplegia—*see* Fracture, vertebra, by site, with spinal cord injury

Fracture—*continued*
quadriplegia—*see* Fracture, vertebra, by site, with spinal cord injury
spinal concussion—*see* Fracture, vertebra, by site, with spinal cord injury
spinal cord injury (closed) NEC 806.8

> Note—Use the following fifth-digit subclassification with categories 806.0-806.3:
>
> *C_1-C_4 or unspecified level and D_1-D_6 (T_1-T_6) or unspecified level with:*
>
> *0 unspecified spinal cord injury*
> *1 complete lesion of cord*
> *2 anterior cord syndrome*
> *3 central cord syndrome*
> *4 specified injury NEC*
>
> *C_5-C_7 level and D_7-D_{12} level with:*
>
> *5 unspecified spinal cord injury*
> *6 complete lesion of cord*
> *7 anterior cord syndrome*
> *8 central cord syndrome*
> *9 specified injury NEC*

cervical 806.0
open 806.1
dorsal, dorsolumbar 806.2
open 806.3
open 806.9
thoracic, thoracolumbar 806.2
open 806.3
atlanto-axial—*see* Fracture, vertebra, cervical
cervical (hangman) (teardrop) (closed) 805.00
with spinal cord injury—*see* Fracture, vertebra, with spinal cord injury, cervical
first (atlas) 805.01
open 805.11
second (axis) 805.02
open 805.12
third 805.03
open 805.13
fourth 805.04
open 805.14
fifth 805.05
open 805.15
sixth 805.06
open 805.16
seventh 805.07
open 805.17
multiple sites 805.08
open 805.18
open 805.10
coccyx (closed) 805.6
with spinal cord injury (closed) 806.60
cauda equina injury 806.62
complete lesion 806.61
open 806.71
open 806.72
open 806.70
specified type NEC 806.69
open 806.79
open 805.7
collapsed 733.13
compression, not due to trauma 733.13
dorsal (closed) 805.2
with spinal cord injury—*see* Fracture, vertebra, with spinal cord injury, dorsal
open 805.3

Fracture—*continued*
dorsolumbar (closed) 805.2
with spinal cord injury—*see* Fracture, vertebra, with spinal cord injury, dorsal
open 805.3
due to osteoporosis 733.13
fetus or newborn 767.4
lumbar (closed) 805.4
with spinal cord injury (closed) 806.4
open 806.5
open 805.5
nontraumatic 733.13
open NEC 805.9
pathologic 733.13
sacrum (closed) 805.6
with spinal cord injury 806.60
cauda equina injury 806.62
complete lesion 806.61
open 806.71
open 806.72
open 806.70
specified type NEC 806.69
open 806.79
open 805.7
site unspecified (closed) 805.8
with spinal cord injury (closed) 806.8
open 806.9
open 805.9
thoracic (closed) 805.2
with spinal cord injury—*see* Fracture, vertebra, with spinal cord injury, thoracic
open 805.3
vertex—*see* Fracture, skull, vault
vomer (bone) 802.0
open 802.1
Wagstaffe's—*see* Fracture, ankle
wrist (closed) 814.00
open 814.10
pathologic 733.12
xiphoid (process)—*see* Fracture, sternum
zygoma (zygomatic arch) (closed) 802.4
open 802.5

Fragile X syndrome 759.83

Fragilitas
crinium 704.2
hair 704.2
ossium 756.51
with blue sclera 756.51
unguium 703.8
congenital 757.5

Fragility
bone 756.51
with deafness and blue sclera 756.51
capillary (hereditary) 287.8
hair 704.2
nails 703.8

Fragmentation —*see* Fracture, by site

Frambesia, frambesial (tropica) (*see also* Yaws) 102.9
initial lesion or ulcer 102.0
primary 102.0

Frambeside
gummatous 102.4
of early yaws 102.2

Frambesioma 102.1

Franceschetti's syndrome (mandibulofacial dysostosis) 756.0

Francis' disease (*see also* Tularemia) 021.9

Frank's essential thrombocytopenia (*see also* Purpura, thrombocytopenic) 287.3

Franklin's disease (heavy chain) 273.2

Fraser's syndrome 759.89
Freckle 709.09
malignant melanoma in (M8742/3)—*see* Melanoma
melanotic (of Hutchinson) (M8742/2)—*see* Neoplasm, skin, in situ
Freeman-Sheldon syndrome 759.89
Freezing 991.9
specified effect NEC 991.8
Frei's disease (climatic bubo) 099.1
Freiberg's
disease (osteochondrosis, second metatarsal) 732.5
infraction of metatarsal head 732.5
osteochondrosis 732.5
Fremitus, friction, cardiac 785.3
Frenulum lingua 750.0
Frenum
external os 752.49
tongue 750.0
Frequency (urinary) NEC 788.41
micturition 788.41
nocturnal 788.43
psychogenic 306.53
Frey's syndrome (auriculotemporal syndrome) 350.8
Friction
burn (*see also* Injury, superficial, by site) 919.0
fremitus, cardiac 785.3
precordial 785.3
sounds, chest 786.7
Friderichsen-Waterhouse syndrome or disease 036.3
Friedländer's
B (bacillus) NEC (*see also* condition) 041.3
sepsis or septicemia 038.49
disease (endarteritis obliterans)—*see* Arteriosclerosis
Friedreich's
ataxia 334.0
combined systemic disease 334.0
disease 333.2
combined systemic 334.0
myoclonia 333.2
sclerosis (spinal cord) 334.0
Friedrich-Erb-Arnold syndrome (acropachyderma) 757.39
Frigidity 302.72
psychic or psychogenic 302.72
Fröhlich's disease or syndrome (adiposogenital dystrophy) 253.8
Froin's syndrome 336.8
Frommel's disease 676.6
Frommel-Chiari syndrome 676.6
Frontal —*see also* condition
lobe syndrome 310.0
Frostbite 991.3
face 991.0
foot 991.2
hand 991.1
specified site NEC 991.3
Frotteurism 302.89
Frozen 991.9
pelvis 620.8
shoulder 726.0
Fructosemia 271.2
Fructosuria (benign) (essential) 271.2
Fuchs'
black spot (myopic) 360.21
corneal dystrophy (endothelial) 371.57
heterochromic cyclitis 364.21
Fucosidosis 271.8
Fugue 780.9
hysterical (dissociative) 300.13
reaction to exceptional stress (transient) 308.1
Fuller Albright's syndrome (osteitis fibrosa disseminata) 756.59
Fuller's earth disease 502
Fulminant, fulminating —*see* condition
Functional —*see* condition
Fundus —*see also* condition
flavimaculatus 362.76
Fungemia 117.9
Fungus, fungous
cerebral 348.8
disease NEC 117.9
infection—*see* Infection, fungus
testis (*see also* Tuberculosis) 016.5 *[608.81]*
Funiculitis (acute) 608.4
chronic 608.4
endemic 608.4
gonococcal (acute) 098.14
chronic or duration of 2 months or over 098.34
tuberculous (*see also* Tuberculosis) 016.5
F.U.O. (*see also* Pyrexia) 780.6
Funnel
breast (acquired) 738.3
congenital 754.81
late effect of rickets 268.1
chest (acquired) 738.3
congenital 754.81
late effect of rickets 268.1
pelvis (acquired) 738.6
with disproportion (fetopelvic) 653.3
affecting fetus or newborn 763.1
causing obstructed labor 660.1
affecting fetus or newborn 763.1
congenital 755.69
tuberculous (*see also* Tuberculosis) 016.9
Furfur 690.18
microsporon 111.0
Furor, paroxysmal (idiopathic) (*see also* Epilepsy) 345.8
Furriers' lung 495.8
Furrowed tongue 529.5
congenital 750.13
Furrowing nail (s) (transverse) 703.8
congenital 757.5
Furuncle 680.9
abdominal wall 680.2
ankle 680.6
anus 680.5
arm (any part, above wrist) 680.3
auditory canal, external 680.0
axilla 680.3
back (any part) 680.2
breast 680.2
buttock 680.5
chest wall 680.2
corpus cavernosum 607.2
ear (any part) 680.0
eyelid 373.13
face (any part, except eye) 680.0
finger (any) 680.4
flank 680.2
foot (any part) 680.7
forearm 680.3
gluteal (region) 680.5
groin 680.2
hand (any part) 680.4
head (any part, except face) 680.8

G

Gafsa boil 085.1
Gain, weight (abnormal) (excessive) (*see also* Weight, gain) 783.1
Gaisböck's disease or syndrome (polycythemia hypertonica) 289.0
Gait
  abnormality 781.2
    hysterical 300.11
  ataxic 781.2
    hysterical 300.11
  disturbance 781.2
    hysterical 300.11
  paralytic 781.2
  scissor 781.2
  spastic 781.2
  staggering 781.2
    hysterical 300.11
Galactocele (breast) (infected) 611.5
  puerperal, postpartum 676.8
Galactophoritis 611.0
  puerperal, postpartum 675.2
Galactorrhea 676.6
  not associated with childbirth 611.6
Galactosemia (classic) (congenital) 271.1
Galactosuria 271.1
Galacturia 791.1
  bilharziasis 120.0
Galen's vein —*see* condition
Gallbladder —*see also* condition
  acute (*see also* Disease, gallbladder) 575.0
Gall duct —*see* condition
Gallop rhythm 427.89
Gallstone (cholemic) (colic) (impacted)—*see also* Cholelithiasis
  causing intestinal obstruction 560.31
Gambling, pathological 312.31
Gammaloidosis 277.3
Gammopathy 273.9
  macroglobulinemia 273.3
  monoclonal (benign) (essential) (idiopathic) (with lymphoplasmacytic dyscrasia) 273.1
Gamna's disease (siderotic splenomegaly) 289.51
Gampsodactylia (congenital) 754.71
Gamstorp's disease (adynamia episodica hereditaria) 359.3
Gandy-Nanta disease (siderotic splenomegaly) 289.51
Gang activity without manifest psychiatric disorder V71.09
  adolescent V71.02
  adult V71.01
  child V71.02
Gangliocytoma (M9490/0)—*see* Neoplasm, connective tissue, benign
Ganglioglioma (M9505/1)—*see* Neoplasm, by site, uncertain behavior
Ganglion 727.43
  joint 727.41
  of yaws (early) (late) 102.6
  periosteal (*see also* Periostitis) 730.3
  tendon sheath (compound) (diffuse) 727.42
  tuberculous (*see also* Tuberculosis) 015.9
Ganglioneuroblastoma (M9490/3)—*see* Neoplasm, connective tissue, malignant
Ganglioneuroma (M9490/0)—*see also* Neoplasm, connective tissue, benign
  malignant (M9490/3)—*see* Neoplasm, connective tissue, malignant
Ganglioneuromatosis (M9491/0)—*see* Neoplasm, connective tissue, benign
Ganglionitis
  fifth nerve (*see also* Neuralgia, trigeminal) 350.1
  gasserian 350.1
  geniculate 351.1
    herpetic 053.11
    newborn 767.5
  herpes zoster 053.11
  herpetic geniculate (Hunt's syndrome) 053.11
Gangliosidosis 330.1
Gangosa 102.5
Gangrene, gangrenous (anemia) (artery) (cellulitis) (dermatitis) (dry) (infective) (moist) (pemphigus) (septic) (skin) (stasis) (ulcer) 785.4
  with
    arteriosclerosis (native artery) 440.24
      bypass graft 440.30
        autologous vein 440.31
        nonautologous biological 440.32
    diabetes (mellitus) 250.7 *[785.4]*
  abdomen (wall) 785.4
    arteriosclerotic 440.29 *[785.4]*
  adenitis 683
  alveolar 526.5
  angina 462
    diphtheritic 032.0
  anus 569.49
  appendices epiploicae—*see* Gangrene, mesentery
  appendix—*see* Appendicitis, acute
  arteriosclerotic —*see* Arteriosclerosis, with, gangrene
  auricle 785.4
  Bacillus welchii (*see also* Gangrene, gas) 040.0
  bile duct (*see also* Cholangitis) 576.8
  bladder 595.89
  bowel—*see* Gangrene, intestine
  cecum—*see* Gangrene, intestine
  Clostridium perfringens or welchii (*see also* Gangrene, gas) 040.0
  colon—*see* Gangrene, intestine
  connective tissue 785.4
  cornea 371.40
  corpora cavernosa (infective) 607.2
    noninfective 607.89
  cutaneous, spreading 785.4
  decubital 707.0 *[785.4]*
  diabetic (any site) 250.7 *[785.4]*
  dropsical 785.4
  emphysematous (*see also* Gangrene, gas) 040.0
  epidemic (ergotized grain) 988.2
  epididymis (infectional) (*see also* Epididymitis) 604.99
  erysipelas (*see also* Erysipelas) 035
  extremity (lower) (upper) 785.4
  gallbladder or duct (*see also* Cholecystitis, acute) 575.0

Gangrene, gangrenous—*continued*
gas (bacillus) 040.0
with
abortion—*see* Abortion, by type, with sepsis
ectopic pregnancy (*see also* categories 633.0-633.9) 639.0
molar pregnancy (*see also* categories 630-632) 639.0
following
abortion 639.0
ectopic or molar pregnancy 639.0
puerperal, postpartum, childbirth 670
glossitis 529.0
gum 523.8
hernia—*see* Hernia, by site, with gangrene
hospital noma 528.1
intestine, intestinal (acute) (hemorrhagic) (massive) 557.0
with
hernia—*see* Hernia, by site, with gangrene
mesenteric embolism or infarction 557.0
obstruction (*see also* Obstruction, intestine) 560.9
laryngitis 464.0
liver 573.8
lung 513.0
spirochetal 104.8
lymphangitis 457.2
Meleney's (cutaneous) 686.0
mesentery 557.0
with
embolism or infarction 557.0
intestinal obstruction (*see also* Obstruction, intestine) 560.9
mouth 528.1
noma 528.1
orchitis 604.90
ovary (*see also* Salpingo-oophoritis) 614.2
pancreas 577.0
penis (infectional) 607.2
noninfective 607.89
perineum 785.4
pharynx 462
septic 034.0
pneumonia 513.0
Pott's 440.24
presenile 443.1
pulmonary 513.0
pulp, tooth 522.1
quinsy 475
Raynaud's (symmetric gangrene) 443.0 *[785.4]*
rectum 569.49
retropharyngeal 478.24
rupture—*see* Hernia, by site, with gangrene
scrotum 608.4
noninfective 608.83
senile 440.24
sore throat 462
spermatic cord 608.4
noninfective 608.89
spine 785.4
spirochetal NEC 104.8
spreading cutaneous 785.4
stomach 537.89
stomatitis 528.1
symmetrical 443.0 *[785.4]*
testis (infectional) (*see also* Orchitis) 604.99
noninfective 608.89
throat 462
diphtheritic 032.0
thyroid (gland) 246.8

Gangrene, gangrenous—*continued*
tonsillitis (acute) 463
tooth (pulp) 522.1
tuberculous NEC (*see also* Tuberculosis) 011.9
tunica vaginalis 608.4
noninfective 608.89
umbilicus 785.4
uterus (*see also* Endometritis) 615.9
uvulitis 528.3
vas deferens 608.4
noninfective 608.89
vulva (*see also* Vulvitis) 616.10
Gannister disease (occupational) 502
with tuberculosis—*see* Tuberculosis, pulmonary
Ganser's syndrome, hysterical 300.16
Gardner-Diamond syndrome (autoerythrocyte sensitization) 287.2
Gargoylism 277.5
Garré's
disease (*see also* Osteomyelitis) 730.1
osteitis (sclerosing) (*see also* Osteomyelitis) 730.1
osteomyelitis (*see also* Osteomyelitis) 730.1
Garrod's pads, knuckle 728.79
Gartner's duct
cyst 752.11
persistent 752.11
Gas
asphyxia, asphyxiation, inhalation, poisoning, suffocation NEC 987.9
specified gas—*see* Table of drugs and chemicals
bacillus gangrene or infection—*see* Gas, gangrene
cyst, mesentery 568.89
excessive 787.3
gangrene 040.0
with
abortion—*see* Abortion, by type, with sepsis
ectopic pregnancy (*see also* categories 633.0-633.9) 639.0
molar pregnancy (*see also* categories 630-632) 639.0
following
abortion 639.0
ectopic or molar pregnancy 639.0
puerperal, postpartum, childbirth 670
on stomach 787.3
pains 787.3
Gastradenitis 535.0
Gastralgia 536.8
psychogenic 307.89
Gastrectasis, gastrectasia 536.1
psychogenic 306.4
Gastric —*see* condition
Gastrinoma (M8153/1)
malignant (M8153/3)
pancreas 157.4
specified site NEC—*see* Neoplasm, by site, malignant
unspecified site 157.4
specified site—*see* Neoplasm, by site, uncertain behavior
unspecified site 235.5

Gastritis 535.5

> Note—Use the following fifth-digit subclassification for category 535:
>
> *0 without mention of hemorrhage*
> *1 with hemorrhage*

  acute 535.0
  alcoholic 535.3
  allergic 535.4
  antral 535.4
  atrophic 535.1
  atrophic-hyperplastic 535.1
  bile-induced 535.4
  catarrhal 535.0
  chronic (atrophic) 535.1
  cirrhotic 535.4
  corrosive (acute) 535.4
  dietetic 535.4
  due to diet deficiency 269.9 *[535.4]*
  eosinophilic 535.4
  erosive 535.4
  follicular 535.4
    chronic 535.1
  giant hypertrophic 535.2
  glandular 535.4
    chronic 535.1
  hypertrophic (mucosa) 535.2
    chronic giant 211.1
  irritant 535.4
  nervous 306.4
  phlegmonous 535.0
  psychogenic 306.4
  sclerotic 535.4
  spastic 536.8
  subacute 535.0
  superficial 535.4
  suppurative 535.0
  toxic 535.4
  tuberculous (*see also* Tuberculosis) 017.9
Gastrocarcinoma (M8010/3) 151.9
Gastrocolic —*see* condition
Gastrocolitis —*see* Enteritis
Gastrodisciasis 121.8
Gastroduodenitis (*see also* Gastritis) 535.5
  catarrhal 535.0
  infectional 535.0
  virus, viral 008.8
    specified type NEC 008.69
Gastrodynia 536.8
Gastroenteritis (acute) (catarrhal) (chronic) (congestive) (hemorrhagic) (noninfectious) (*see also* Enteritis) 558.9
  aertrycke infection 003.0
  allergic 558.9
  chronic 558.9
    ulcerative (*see also* Colitis, ulcerative) 556.9
  dietetic 558.9
  due to
    food poisoning (*see also* Poisoning, food) 005.9
    radiation 558.1
  epidemic 009.0
  functional 558.9
  infectious (*see also* Enteritis, due to, by organism) 009.0
    presumed 009.1
  salmonella 003.0
  septic (*see also* Enteritis, due to, by organism) 009.0
  toxic 558.2
Gastroenteritis—*continued*
  tuberculous (*see also* Tuberculosis) 014.8
  ulcerative (*see also* Colitis, ulcerative) 556.9
  viral NEC 008.8
    specified type NEC 008.69
  zymotic 009.0
Gastroenterocolitis —*see* Enteritis
Gastroenteropathy, protein-losing 579.8
Gastroenteroptosis 569.89
Gastroesophageal laceration-hemorrhage syndrome 530.7
Gastroesophagitis 530.19
Gastrohepatitis (*see also* Gastritis) 535.5
Gastrointestinal —*see* condition
Gastrojejunal —*see* condition
Gastrojejunitis (*see also* Gastritis) 535.5
Gastrojejunocolic —*see* condition
Gastroliths 537.89
Gastromalacia 537.89
Gastroparalysis 536.8
  diabetic 250.6 *[337.1]*
Gastroparesis 536.3
  diabetic 250.6 *[536.3]*
Gastropathy, exudative 579.8
Gastroptosis 537.5
Gastrorrhagia 578.0
Gastrorrhea 536.8
  psychogenic 306.4
Gastroschisis (congenital) 756.7
  acquired 569.89
Gastrospasm (neurogenic) (reflex) 536.8
  neurotic 306.4
  psychogenic 306.4
Gastrostaxis 578.0
Gastrostenosis 537.89
Gastrostomy status V44.1
  with complication 997.4
Gastrosuccorrhea (continuous) (intermittent) 536.8
  neurotic 306.4
  psychogenic 306.4
Gaucher's
  disease (adult) (cerebroside lipidosis) (infantile) 272.7
  hepatomegaly 272.7
  splenomegaly (cerebroside lipidosis) 272.7
Gayet's disease (superior hemorrhagic polioencephalitis) 265.1
Gayet-Wernicke's syndrome (superior hemorrhagic polioencephalitis) 265.1
Gee (-Herter) (-Heubner) (-Thaysen) disease or syndrome (nontropical sprue) 579.0
Gélineau's syndrome 347
Gemination, teeth 520.2
Gemistocytoma (M9411/3)
  specified site—*see* Neoplasm, by site, malignant
  unspecified site 191.9
General, generalized —*see* condition
Genital —*see* condition
Genito-anorectal syndrome 099.1
Genitourinary system —*see* condition
Genu
  congenital 755.64
  extrorsum (acquired) 736.42
    congenital 755.64
    late effects of rickets 268.1
  introrsum (acquired) 736.41
    congenital 755.64
    late effects of rickets 268.1
  rachitic (old) 268.1

Genu—*continued*
recurvatum (acquired) 736.5
congenital 754.40
with dislocation of knee 754.41
late effects of rickets 268.1
valgum (acquired) (knock-knee) 736.41
congenital 755.64
late effects of rickets 268.1
varum (acquired) (bowleg) 736.42
congenital 755.64
late effects of rickets 268.1
Geographic tongue 529.1
Geophagia 307.52
Geotrichosis 117.9
intestine 117.9
lung 117.9
mouth 117.9
Gephyrophobia 300.29
Gerbode defect 745.4
Gerhardt's
disease (erythromelalgia) 443.89
syndrome (vocal cord paralysis) 478.30
Gerlier's disease (epidemic vertigo) 078.81
German measles 056.9
exposure to V01.4
Germinoblastoma (diffuse) (M9614/3) 202.8
follicular (M9692/3) 202.0
Germinoma (M9064/3)—*see* Neoplasm, by site, malignant
Gerontoxon 371.41
Gerstmann's syndrome (finger agnosia) 784.69
Gestation (period)—*see also* Pregnancy
ectopic NEC (*see also* Pregnancy, ectopic) 633.9
Gestational proteinuria 646.2
with hypertension—*see* Toxemia, of pregnancy
Ghon tubercle primary infection (*see also* Tuberculosis) 010.0
Ghost
teeth 520.4
vessels, cornea 370.64
Ghoul hand 102.3
Giant
cell
epulis 523.8
peripheral (gingiva) 523.8
tumor, tendon sheath 727.02
colon (congenital) 751.3
esophagus (congenital) 750.4
kidney 753.3
urticaria 995.1
hereditary 277.6
Giardia lamblia infestation 007.1
Giardiasis 007.1
Gibert's disease (pityriasis rosea) 696.3
Gibraltar fever —*see* Brucellosis
Giddiness 780.4
hysterical 300.11
psychogenic 306.9
Gierke's disease (glycogenosis I) 271.0
Gigantism (cerebral) (hypophyseal) (pituitary) 253.0
Gilbert's disease or cholemia (familial nonhemolytic jaundice) 277.4
Gilchrist's disease (North American blastomycosis) 116.0
Gilford (-Hutchinson) disease or syndrome (progeria) 259.8
Gilles de la Tourette's disease (motor-verbal tic) 307.23
Gillespie's syndrome (dysplasia oculodentodigitalis) 759.89
Gingivitis 523.1
acute 523.0
necrotizing 101
catarrhal 523.0
chronic 523.1
desquamative 523.1
expulsiva 523.4
hyperplastic 523.1
marginal, simple 523.1
necrotizing, acute 101
pellagrous 265.2
ulcerative 523.1
acute necrotizing 101
Vincent's 101
Gingivoglossitis 529.0
Gingivopericementitis 523.4
Gingivosis 523.1
Gingivostomatitis 523.1
herpetic 054.2
Giovannini's disease 117.9
Gland, glandular —*see* condition
Glanders 024
Glanzmann (-Naegeli) disease or thrombasthenia 287.1
Glassblowers' disease 527.1
Glaucoma (capsular) (inflammatory) (noninflammatory) (primary) 365.9
with increased episcleral venous pressure 365.82
absolute 360.42
acute 365.22
narrow angle 365.22
secondary 365.60
angle closure 365.20
acute 365.22
chronic 365.23
intermittent 365.21
interval 365.21
residual stage 365.24
subacute 365.21
border line 365.00
chronic 365.11
noncongestive 365.11
open angle 365.11
simple 365.11
closed angle—*see* Glaucoma, angle closure
congenital 743.20
associated with other eye anomalies 743.22
simple 743.21
congestive—*see* Glaucoma, narrow angle
corticosteroid-induced (glaucomatous stage) 365.31
residual stage 365.32
hemorrhagic 365.60
hypersecretion 365.81
in or with
aniridia 743.45 *[365.42]*
Axenfeld's anomaly 743.44 *[365.41]*
concussion of globe 921.3 *[365.65]*
congenital syndromes NEC 759.89 *[365.44]*
dislocation of lens
anterior 379.33 *[365.59]*
posterior 379.34 *[365.59]*
disorder of lens NEC 365.59
epithelial down-growth 364.61 *[365.64]*
glaucomatocyclitic crisis 364.22 *[365.62]*
hypermature cataract 366.18 *[365.51]*
hyphema 364.41 *[365.63]*
inflammation, ocular 365.62
iridocyclitis 364.3 *[365.62]*

Glaucoma—*continued*
iris
anomalies NEC 743.46 *[365.42]*
atrophy, essential 364.51 *[365.42]*
bombé 364.74 *[365.61]*
rubeosis 364.42 *[365.63]*
microcornea 743.41 *[365.43]*
neurofibromatosis 237.71 *[365.44]*
ocular
cysts NEC 365.64
disorders NEC 365.60
trauma 365.65
tumors NEC 365.64
postdislocation of lens
anterior 379.33 *[365.59]*
posterior 379.34 *[365.59]*
pseudoexfoliation of capsule 366.11 *[365.52]*
pupillary block or seclusion 364.74 *[365.61]*
recession of chamber angle 364.77 *[365.65]*
retinal vein occlusion 362.35 *[365.63]*
Rieger's anomaly or syndrome 743.44 *[365.41]*
rubeosis of iris 364.42 *[365.63]*
seclusion of pupil 364.74 *[365.61]*
spherophakia 743.36 *[365.59]*
Sturge-Weber (-Dimitri) syndrome 759.6 *[365.44]*
systemic syndrome NEC 365.44
tumor of globe 365.64
vascular disorders NEC 365.63
infantile 365.14
congenital 743.20
associated with other eye anomalies 743.22
simple 743.21
juvenile 365.14
low tension 365.12
malignant 365.20
narrow angle (primary) 365.20
acute 365.22
chronic 365.23
intermittent 365.21
interval 365.21
residual stage 365.24
subacute 365.21
newborn 743.20
associated with other eye anomalies 743.22
simple 743.21
noncongestive (chronic) 365.11
nonobstructive (chronic) 365.11
obstructive 365.60
due to lens changes 365.59
open angle 365.10
with
borderline intraocular pressure 365.01
cupping of optic discs 365.01
primary 365.11
residual stage 365.15
phacolytic 365.51
with hypermature cataract 366.18 *[365.51]*
pigmentary 365.13
postinfectious 365.60
pseudoexfoliation 365.52
with pseudoexfoliation of capsule 366.11 *[365.52]*
secondary NEC 365.60
simple (chronic) 365.11
simplex 365.11
steroid responders 365.03
suspect 365.00
syphilitic 095.8

Glaucoma—*continued*
traumatic NEC 365.65
newborn 767.8
tuberculous (*see also* Tuberculosis) 017.3 *[365.62]*
wide angle (*see also* Glaucoma, open angle) 365.10
Glaucomatous flecks (subcapsular) 366.31
Glazed tongue 529.4
Gleet 098.2
Glénard's disease or syndrome (enteroptosis) 569.89
Glinski-Simmonds syndrome (pituitary cachexia) 253.2
Glioblastoma (multiforme) (M9440/3)
with sarcomatous component (M9442/3)
specified site—*see* Neoplasm, by site, malignant
unspecified site 191.9
giant cell (M9441/3)
specified site—*see* Neoplasm, by site, malignant
unspecified site 191.9
specified site—*see* Neoplasm, by site, malignant
unspecified site 191.9
Glioma (malignant) (M9380/3)
astrocytic (M9400/3)
specified site—*see* Neoplasm, by site, malignant
unspecified site 191.9
mixed (M9382/3)
specified site—*see* Neoplasm, by site, malignant
unspecified site 191.9
nose 748.1
specified site NEC—*see* Neoplasm, by site, malignant
subependymal (M9383/1) 237.5
unspecified site 191.9
Gliomatosis cerebri (M9381/3) 191.0
Glioneuroma (M9505/1)—*see* Neoplasm, by site, uncertain behavior
Gliosarcoma (M9380/3)
specified site—*see* Neoplasm, by site, malignant
unspecified site 191.9
Gliosis (cerebral) 349.89
spinal 336.0
Glisson's
cirrhosis—*see* Cirrhosis, portal
disease (*see also* Rickets) 268.0
Glissonitis 573.3
Globinuria 791.2
Globus 306.4
hystericus 300.11
Glomangioma (M8712/0) (*see also* Hemangioma) 228.00
Glomangiosarcoma (M8710/3)—*see* Neoplasm, connective tissue, malignant
Glomerular nephritis (*see also* Nephritis) 583.9
Glomerulitis (*see also* Nephritis) 583.9
Glomerulonephritis (*see also* Nephritis) 583.9
with
edema (*see also* Nephrosis) 581.9
lesion of
exudative nephritis 583.89
interstitial nephritis (diffuse) (focal) 583.89
necrotizing glomerulitis 583.4
acute 580.4
chronic 582.4

Glomerulonephritis—*continued*
renal necrosis 583.9
cortical 583.6
medullary 583.7
specified pathology NEC 583.89
acute 580.89
chronic 582.89
necrosis, renal 583.9
cortical 583.6
medullary (papillary) 583.7
specified pathology or lesion NEC 583.89
acute 580.9
with
exudative nephritis 580.89
interstitial nephritis (diffuse) (focal) 580.89
necrotizing glomerulitis 580.4
extracapillary with epithelial crescents 580.4
poststreptococcal 580.0
proliferative (diffuse) 580.0
rapidly progressive 580.4
specified pathology NEC 580.89
arteriolar (*see also* Hypertension, kidney) 403.90
arteriosclerotic (*see also* Hypertension, kidney) 403.90
ascending (*see also* Pyelitis) 590.80
basement membrane NEC 583.89
with
pulmonary hemorrhage (Goodpasture's syndrome) 446.21 *[583.81]*
chronic 582.9
with
exudative nephritis 582.89
interstitial nephritis (diffuse) (focal) 582.89
necrotizing glomerulitis 582.4
specified pathology or lesion NEC 582.89
endothelial 582.2
extracapillary with epithelial crescents 582.4
hypocomplementemic persistent 582.2
lobular 582.2
membranoproliferative 582.2
membranous 582.1
and proliferative (mixed) 582.2
sclerosing 582.1
mesangiocapillary 582.2
mixed membranous and proliferative 582.2
proliferative (diffuse) 582.0
rapidly progressive 582.4
sclerosing 582.1
cirrhotic—*see* Sclerosis, renal
desquamative—*see* Nephrosis
due to or associated with
amyloidosis 277.3 *[583.81]*
with nephrotic syndrome 277.3 *[581.81]*
chronic 277.3 *[582.81]*
diabetes mellitus 250.4 *[583.81]*
with nephrotic syndrome 250.4 *[581.81]*
diphtheria 032.89 *[580.81]*
gonococcal infection (acute) 098.19 *[583.81]*
chronic or duration or 2 months or over 098.39 *[583.81]*
infectious hepatitis 070.9 *[580.81]*
malaria (with nephrotic syndrome) 084.9 *[581.81]*
mumps 072.79 *[580.81]*
polyarteritis (nodosa) (with nephrotic syndrome) 446.0 *[581.81]*
specified pathology NEC 583.89
acute 580.89
chronic 582.89
streptotrichosis 039.8 *[583.81]*

Glomerulonephritis—*continued*
subacute bacterial endocarditis 421.0 *[580.81]*
syphilis (late) 095.4
congenital 090.5 *[583.81]*
early 091.69 *[583.81]*
systemic lupus erythematosus 710.0 *[583.81]*
with nephrotic syndrome 710.0 *[581.81]*
chronic 710.0 *[582.81]*
tuberculosis (*see also* Tuberculosis) 016.0 *[583.81]*
typhoid fever 002.0 *[580.81]*
extracapillary with epithelial crescents 583.4
acute 580.4
chronic 582.4
exudative 583.89
acute 580.89
chronic 582.89
focal (*see also* Nephritis) 583.9
embolic 580.4
granular 582.89
granulomatous 582.89
hydremic (*see also* Nephrosis) 581.9
hypocomplementemic persistent 583.2
with nephrotic syndrome 581.2
chronic 582.2
immune complex NEC 583.89
infective (*see also* Pyelitis) 590.80
interstitial (diffuse) (focal) 583.89
with nephrotic syndrome 581.89
acute 580.89
chronic 582.89
latent or quiescent 582.9
lobular 583.2
with nephrotic syndrome 581.2
chronic 582.2
membranoproliferative 583.2
with nephrotic syndrome 581.2
chronic 582.2
membranous 583.1
with nephrotic syndrome 581.1
and proliferative (mixed) 583.2
with nephrotic syndrome 581.2
chronic 582.2
chronic 582.1
sclerosing 582.1
with nephrotic syndrome 581.1
mesangiocapillary 583.2
with nephrotic syndrome 581.2
chronic 582.2
minimal change 581.3
mixed membranous and proliferative 583.2
with nephrotic syndrome 581.2
chronic 582.2
necrotizing 583.4
acute 580.4
chronic 582.4
nephrotic (*see also* Nephrosis) 581.9
old—*see* Glomerulonephritis, chronic
parenchymatous 581.89
poststreptococcal 580.0
proliferative (diffuse) 583.0
with nephrotic syndrome 581.0
acute 580.0
chronic 582.0
purulent (*see also* Pyelitis) 590.80
quiescent—*see* Nephritis, chronic
rapidly progressive 583.4
acute 580.4
chronic 582.4
sclerosing membranous (chronic) 582.1
with nephrotic syndrome 581.1

Glomerulonephritis—*continued*
septic (*see also* Pyelitis) 590.80
specified pathology or lesion NEC 583.89
with nephrotic syndrome 581.89
acute 580.89
chronic 582.89
suppurative (acute) (disseminated) (*see also* Pyelitis) 590.80
toxic—*see* Nephritis, acute
tubal, tubular—*see* Nephrosis, tubular
type II (Ellis)—*see* Nephrosis
vascular—*see* Hypertension, kidney
Glomerulosclerosis (*see also* Sclerosis, renal) 587
focal 582.1
with nephrotic syndrome 581.1
intercapillary (nodular) (with diabetes) 250.4 *[581.81]*
Glossagra 529.6
Glossalgia 529.6
Glossitis 529.0
areata exfoliativa 529.1
atrophic 529.4
benign migratory 529.1
gangrenous 529.0
Hunter's 529.4
median rhomboid 529.2
Moeller's 529.4
pellagrous 265.2
Glossocele 529.8
Glossodynia 529.6
exfoliativa 529.4
Glossoncus 529.8
Glossophytia 529.3
Glossoplegia 529.8
Glossoptosis 529.8
Glossopyrosis 529.6
Glossotrichia 529.3
Glossy skin 701.9
Glottis —*see* condition
Glottitis —*see* Glossitis
Glucagonoma (M8152/0)
malignant (M8152/3)
pancreas 157.4
specified site NEC—*see* Neoplasm, by site, malignant
unspecified site 157.4
pancreas 211.7
specified site NEC—*see* Neoplasm, by site, benign
unspecified site 211.7
Glucoglycinuria 270.7
Glue ear syndrome 381.20
Glue sniffing (airplane glue) (*see also* Dependence) 304.6
Glycinemia (with methylmalonic acidemia) 270.7
Glycinuria (renal) (with ketosis) 270.0
Glycogen
infiltration (*see also* Disease, glycogen storage) 271.0
storage disease (*see also* Disease, glycogen storage) 271.0
Glycogenosis (*see also* Disease, glycogen storage) 271.0
cardiac 271.0 *[425.7]*
Cori, types I-VII 271.0
diabetic, secondary 250.8 *[259.8]*
diffuse (with hepatic cirrhosis) 271.0
generalized 271.0
glucose-6-phosphatase deficiency 271.0
hepatophosphorylase deficiency 271.0
Glycogenosis—*continued*
hepatorenal 271.0
myophosphorylase deficiency 271.0
Glycopenia 251.2
Glycoprolinuria 270.8
Glycosuria 791.5
renal 271.4
Gnathostoma (spinigerum) (infection) (infestation) 128.1
wandering swellings from 128.1
Gnathostomiasis 128.1
Goiter (adolescent) (colloid) (diffuse) (dipping) (due to iodine deficiency) (endemic) (euthyroid) (heart) (hyperplastic) (internal) (intrathoracic) (juvenile) (mixed type) (nonendemic) (parenchymatous) (plunging) (sporadic) (subclavicular) (substernal) 240.9
with
hyperthyroidism (recurrent) (*see also* Goiter, toxic) 242.0
thyrotoxicosis (*see also* Goiter, toxic) 242.0
adenomatous (*see also* Goiter, nodular) 241.9
cancerous (M8000/3) 193
complicating pregnancy, childbirth, or puerperium 648.1
congenital 246.1
cystic (*see also* Goiter, nodular) 241.9
due to enzyme defect in synthesis of thyroid hormone (butane-insoluble iodine) (coupling) (deiodinase) (iodide trapping or organification) (iodotyrosine dehalogenase) (peroxidase) 246.1
dyshormonogenic 246.1
exophthalmic (*see also* Goiter, toxic) 242.0
familial (with deaf-mutism) 243
fibrous 245.3
lingual 759.2
lymphadenoid 245.2
malignant (M8000/3) 193
multinodular (nontoxic) 241.1
toxic or with hyperthyroidism (*see also* Goiter, toxic) 242.2
nodular (nontoxic) 241.9
with
hyperthyroidism (*see also* Goiter, toxic) 242.3
thyrotoxicosis (*see also* Goiter, toxic) 242.3
endemic 241.9
exophthalmic (diffuse) (*see also* Goiter, toxic) 242.0
multinodular (nontoxic) 241.1
sporadic 241.9
toxic (*see also* Goiter, toxic) 242.3
uninodular (nontoxic) 241.0
nontoxic (nodular) 241.9
multinodular 241.1
uninodular 241.0
pulsating (*see also* Goiter, toxic) 242.0
simple 240.0
toxic 242.0

Note—Use the following fifth-digit subclassification with category 242:

0 without mention of thyrotoxic crisis or storm
1 with mention of thyrotoxic crisis or storm

adenomatous 242.3
multinodular 242.2
uninodular 242.1
multinodular 242.2

Goiter—*continued*
nodular 242.3
multinodular 242.2
uninodular 242.1
uninodular 242.1
uninodular (nontoxic) 241.0
toxic or with hyperthyroidism (*see also* Goiter, toxic) 242.1
Goldberg (-Maxwell) (-Morris) syndrome (testicular feminization) 257.8
Goldblatt's
hypertension 440.1
kidney 440.1
Goldenhar's syndrome (oculoauriculovertebral dysplasia) 756.0
Goldflam-Erb disease or syndrome 358.0
Goldscheider's disease (epidermolysis bullosa) 757.39
Goldstein's disease (familial hemorrhagic telangiectasia) 448.0
Golfer's elbow 726.32
Goltz-Gorlin syndrome (dermal hypoplasia) 757.39
Gonadoblastoma (M9073/1)
specified site—*see* Neoplasm, by site uncertain behavior
unspecified site
female 236.2
male 236.4
Gonecystitis (*see also* Vesiculitis) 608.0
Gongylonemiasis 125.6
mouth 125.6
Goniosynechiae 364.73
Gonococcemia 098.89
Gonococcus, gonococcal (disease) (infection) (*see also* condition) 098.0
anus 098.7
bursa 098.52
chronic NEC 098.2
complicating pregnancy, childbirth, or puerperium 647.1
affecting fetus or newborn 760.2
conjunctiva, conjunctivitis (neonatorum) 098.40
dermatosis 098.89
endocardium 098.84
epididymo-orchitis 098.13
chronic or duration of 2 months or over 098.33
eye (newborn) 098.40
fallopian tube (chronic) 098.37
acute 098.17
genitourinary (acute) (organ) (system) (tract) (*see also* Gonorrhea) 098.0
lower 098.0
chronic 098.2
upper 098.10
chronic 098.30
heart NEC 098.85
joint 098.50
keratoderma 098.81
keratosis (blennorrhagica) 098.81
lymphatic (gland) (node) 098.89
meninges 098.82
orchitis (acute) 098.13
chronic or duration of 2 months or over 098.33
pelvis (acute) 098.19
chronic or duration of 2 months or over 098.39
pericarditis 098.83
peritonitis 098.86
pharyngitis 098.6
pharynx 098.6
Gonococcus, gonococcal—*continued*
proctitis 098.7
pyosalpinx (chronic) 098.37
acute 098.17
rectum 098.7
septicemia 098.89
skin 098.89
specified site NEC 098.89
synovitis 098.51
tendon sheath 098.51
throat 098.6
urethra (acute) 098.0
chronic of duration of 2 months or over 098.2
vulva (acute) 098.0
chronic or duration of 2 months or over 098.2
Gonocytoma (M9073/1)
specified site—*see* Neoplasm, by site, uncertain behavior
unspecified site
female 236.2
male 236.4
Gonorrhea 098.0
acute 098.0
Bartholin's gland (acute) 098.0
chronic or duration of 2 months or over 098.2
bladder (acute) 098.11
chronic or duration of 2 months or over 098.31
carrier (suspected of) V02.7
cervix (acute) 098.15
chronic or duration of 2 months or over 098.35
chronic 098.2
complicating pregnancy, childbirth, or puerperium 647.1
affecting fetus or newborn 760.2
conjunctiva, conjunctivitis (neonatorum) 098.40
contact V01.6
Cowper's gland (acute) 098.0
chronic or duration of 2 months or over 098.2
duration of two months or over 098.2
exposure to V01.6
fallopian tube (chronic) 098.37
acute 098.17
genitourinary (acute) (organ) (system) (tract) 098.0
chronic 098.2
duration of two months or over 098.2
kidney (acute) 098.19
chronic or duration of 2 months or over 098.39
ovary (acute) 098.19
chronic or duration of 2 months or over 098.39
pelvis (acute) 098.19
chronic or duration of 2 months or over 098.39
penis (acute) 098.0
chronic or duration of 2 months or over 098.2
prostate (acute) 098.12
chronic or duration of 2 months or over 098.32
seminal vesicle (acute) 098.14
chronic or duration of 2 months or over 098.34
specified site NEC—*see* Gonococcus
spermatic cord (acute) 098.14
chronic or duration of 2 months or over 098.34
urethra (acute) 098.0
chronic or duration of 2 months or over 098.2
vagina (acute) 098.0
chronic or duration of 2 months or over 098.2
vas deferens (acute) 098.14
chronic or duration of 2 months or over 098.34
vulva (acute) 098.0
chronic or duration of 2 months or over 098.2
Goodpasture's syndrome (pneumorenal) 446.21

Gopalan's syndrome (burning feet) 266.2
Gordon's disease (exudative enteropathy) 579.8
Gorlin-Chaudhry-Moss syndrome 759.89
Gougerot's syndrome (trisymptomatic) 709.1
Gougerot-Blum syndrome (pigmented purpuric lichenoid dermatitis) 709.1
Gougerot-Carteaud disease or syndrome (confluent reticulate papillomatosis) 701.8
Gougerot-Hailey-Hailey disease (benign familial chronic pemphigus) 757.39
Gougerot (-Houwer) -Sjögren syndrome (keratoconjunctivitis sicca) 710.2
Gouley's syndrome (constrictive pericarditis) 423.2
Goundou 102.6
Gout, gouty 274.9
  with specified manifestations NEC 274.89
  arthritis (acute) 274.0
  arthropathy 274.0
  degeneration, heart 274.82
  diathesis 274.9
  eczema 274.89
  episcleritis 274.89 *[379.09]*
  external ear (tophus) 274.81
  glomerulonephritis 274.10
  iritis 274.89 *[364.11]*
  joint 274.0
  kidney 274.10
  lead 984.9
    specified type of lead—*see* Table of drugs and chemicals
  nephritis 274.10
  neuritis 274.89 *[357.4]*
  phlebitis 274.89 *[451.9]*
  rheumatic 714.0
  saturnine 984.9
    specified type of lead—*see* Table of drugs and chemicals
  spondylitis 274.0
  synovitis 274.0
  syphilitic 095.8
  tophi 274.0
    ear 274.81
    heart 274.82
    specified site NEC 274.82
Gowers'
  muscular dystrophy 359.1
  syndrome (vasovagal attack) 780.2
Gowers-Paton-Kennedy syndrome 377.04
Gradenigo's syndrome 383.02
Graft-versus-host disease (bone marrow) 996.85
  due to organ transplant NEC—*see* Complications, transplant, organ
Graham Steell's murmur (pulmonic regurgitation) (*see also* Endocarditis, pulmonary) 424.3
Grain-handlers' disease or lung 495.8
Grain mite (itch) 133.8
Grand
  mal (idiopathic) (*see also* Epilepsy) 345.1
    hysteria of Charcot 300.11
    nonrecurrent or isolated 780.3
  multipara
    affecting management of labor and delivery 659.4
    status only (not pregnant) V61.5
Granite workers' lung 502
Granular —*see also* condition
  inflammation, pharynx 472.1
  kidney (contracting) (*see also* Sclerosis, renal) 587
  liver—*see* Cirrhosis, liver
  nephritis—*see* Nephritis
Granulation tissue, abnormal —*see also* Granuloma
  abnormal or excessive 701.5
  postmastoidectomy cavity 383.33
  postoperative 701.5
  skin 701.5
Granulocytopenia, granulocytopenic (primary) 288.0
  malignant 288.0
Granuloma NEC 686.1
  abdomen (wall) 568.89
    skin (pyogenicum) 686.1
      from residual foreign body 709.4
  annulare 695.89
  anus 569.49
  apical 522.6
  appendix 543.9
  aural 380.23
  beryllium (skin) 709.4
    lung 503
  bone (*see also* Osteomyelitis) 730.1
    eosinophilic 277.8
    from residual foreign body 733.99
  canaliculus lacrimalis 375.81
  cerebral 348.8
  cholesterin, middle ear 385.82
  coccidioidal (progressive) 114.3
    lung 114.4
    meninges 114.2
    primary (lung) 114.0
  colon 569.89
  conjunctiva 372.61
  dental 522.6
  ear, middle (cholesterin) 385.82
    with otitis media—*see* Otitis media
  eosinophilic 277.8
    bone 277.8
    lung 277.8
    oral mucosa 528.9
  exuberant 701.5
  eyelid 374.89
  facial
    lethal midline 446.3
    malignant 446.3
  fissuratum (gum) 523.8
  foot NEC 686.1
  foreign body (in soft tissue) NEC 728.82
    bone 733.99
    in operative wound 998.4
    muscle 728.82
    skin 709.4
    subcutaneous tissue 709.4
  fungoides 202.1
  gangraenescens 446.3
  giant cell (central) (jaw) (reparative) 526.3
    gingiva 523.8
    peripheral (gingiva) 523.8
  gland (lymph) 289.3
  Hodgkin's (M9661/3) 201.1
  ileum 569.89
  infectious NEC 136.9
  inguinale (Donovan) 099.2
    venereal 099.2
  intestine 569.89

Granuloma—*continued*
iridocyclitis 364.10
jaw (bone) 526.3
reparative giant cell 526.3
kidney (*see also* Infection, kidney) 590.9
lacrimal sac 375.81
larynx 478.79
lethal midline 446.3
lipid 277.8
lipoid 277.8
liver 572.8
lung (infectious) (*see also* Fibrosis, lung) 515
coccidioidal 114.4
eosinophilic 277.8
lymph gland 289.3
Majocchi's 110.6
malignant, face 446.3
mandible 526.3
mediastinum 519.3
midline 446.3
monilial 112.3
muscle 728.82
from residual foreign body 728.82
nasal sinus (*see also* Sinusitis) 473.9
operation wound 998.5
foreign body 998.4
stitch (external) 998.8
internal wound 996.7
talc 998.7
oral mucosa, eosinophilic or pyogenic 528.9
orbit, orbital 376.11
paracoccidioidal 116.1
penis, venereal 099.2
periapical 522.6
peritoneum 568.89
due to ova of helminths NEC (*see also* Helminthiasis) 128.9
postmastoidectomy cavity 383.33
postoperative–*see* Granuloma, operation wound
prostate 601.8
pudendi (ulcerating) 099.2
pudendorum (ulcerative) 099.2
pulp, internal (tooth) 521.4
pyogenic, pyogenicum (skin) 686.1
maxillary alveolar ridge 522.6
oral mucosa 528.9
rectum 569.49
reticulohistiocytic 277.8
rubrum nasi 705.89
sarcoid 135
Schistosoma 120.9
septic (skin) 686.1
silica (skin) 709.4
sinus (accessory) (infectional) (nasal) (*see also* Sinusitis) 473.9
skin (pyogenicum) 686.1
from foreign body or material 709.4
sperm 608.89
spine
syphilitic (epidural) 094.89
tuberculous (*see also* Tuberculosis) 015.0 *[730.88]*
stitch (postoperative) 998.8
internal wound 996.7
suppurative (skin) 686.1
suture (postoperative) 998.8
internal wound 996.7
swimming pool 031.1
talc 728.82
in operation wound 998.7

Granuloma—*continued*
telangiectaticum (skin) 686.1
trichophyticum 110.6
tropicum 102.4
umbilicus 686.1
newborn 771.4
urethra 599.84
uveitis 364.10
vagina 099.2
venereum 099.2
vocal cords 478.5
Wegener's (necrotizing respiratory granulomatosis) 446.4
Granulomatosis NEC 686.1
disciformis chronica et progressiva 709.3
infantiseptica 771.2
lipoid 277.8
lipophagic, intestinal 040.2
miliary 027.0
necrotizing, respiratory 446.4
progressive, septic 288.1
Wegener's (necrotizing respiratory) 446.4
Granulomatous tissue —*see* Granuloma
Granulosis rubra nasi 705.89
Graphite fibrosis (of lung) 503
Graphospasm 300.89
organic 333.84
Grating scapula 733.99
Gravel (urinary) (*see also* Calculus) 592.9
Graves' disease (exophthalmic goiter) (*see also* Goiter, toxic) 242.0
Gravis —*see* condition
Grawitz's tumor (hypernephroma) (M8312/3) 189.0
Grayness, hair (premature) 704.3
congenital 757.4
Gray or grey syndrome (chloramphenicol) (newborn) 779.4
Greenfield's disease 330.0
Green sickness 280.9
Greenstick fracture —*see* Fracture, by site
Greig's syndrome (hypertelorism) 756.0
Griesinger's disease (*see also* Ancylostomiasis) 126.9
Grinder's
asthma 502
lung 502
phthisis (*see also* Tuberculosis) 011.4
Grinding, teeth 306.8
Grip
Dabney's 074.1
devil's 074.1
Grippe, grippal —*see also* Influenza
Balkan 083.0
intestinal 487.8
summer 074.8
Grippy cold 487.1
Grisel's disease 723.5
Groin —*see* condition
Grooved
nails (transverse) 703.8
tongue 529.5
congenital 750.13
Ground itch 126.9
Growing pains, children 781.9

Growth (fungoid) (neoplastic) (new) (M8000/1)—*see also* Neoplasm, by site, unspecified nature
adenoid (vegetative) 474.12
benign (M8000/0)—*see* Neoplasm, by site, benign
fetal, poor 764.9
affecting management of pregnancy 656.5
malignant (M8000/3)—*see* Neoplasm, by site malignant
rapid, childhood V21.0
secondary (M8000/6)—*see* Neoplasm, by site, malignant, secondary
Gruber's hernia —*see* Hernia, Gruber's
Gruby's disease (tinea tonsurans) 110.0
G-trisomy 758.0
Guama fever 066.3
Gubler (-Millard) paralysis or syndrome 344.89
Guérin-Stern syndrome (arthrogryposis multiplex congenita) 754.89
Guertin's disease (electric chorea) 049.8
Guillain-Barré disease or syndrome 357.0
Guinea worms (infection) (infestation) 125.7
Guinon's disease (motor-verbal tic) 307.23
Gull's disease (thyroid atrophy with myxedema) 244.8
Gull and Sutton's disease —*see* Hypertension, kidney
Gum —*see* condition
Gumboil 522.7
Gumma (syphilitic) 095.9
artery 093.89
cerebral or spinal 094.89
bone 095.5
of yaws (late) 102.6
brain 094.89
cauda equina 094.89
central nervous system NEC 094.9
ciliary body 095.8 *[364.11]*
congenital 090.5
testis 090.5
eyelid 095.8 *[373.5]*
heart 093.89
intracranial 094.89
iris 095.8 *[364.11]*
kidney 095.4
larynx 095.8
leptomeninges 094.2
liver 095.3
meninges 094.2
myocardium 093.82
nasopharynx 095.8
neurosyphilitic 094.9
nose 095.8
orbit 095.8
palate (soft) 095.8
penis 095.8
pericardium 093.81
pharynx 095.8
pituitary 095.8
scrofulous (*see also* Tuberculosis) 017.0
skin 095.8
specified site NEC 095.8
spinal cord 094.89
tongue 095.8
tonsil 095.8
trachea 095.8
tuberculous (*see also* Tuberculosis) 017.0
Gumma—*continued*
ulcerative due to yaws 102.4
ureter 095.8
yaws 102.4
bone 102.6
Gunn's syndrome (jaw-winking syndrome) 742.8
Gunshot wound —*see also* Wound, open, by site
fracture—*see* Fracture, by site, open
internal organs (abdomen, chest, or pelvis)—*see* Injury, internal, by site, with open wound
intracranial—*see* Laceration, brain, with open intracranial wound
Günther's disease or syndrome (congenital erythropoietic porphyria) 277.1
Gustatory hallucination 780.1
Gynandrism 752.7
Gynandroblastoma (M8632/1)
specified site—*see* Neoplasm, by site, uncertain behavior
unspecified site
female 236.2
male 236.4
Gynandromorphism 752.7
Gynatresia (congenital) 752.49
Gynecoid pelvis, male 738.6
Gynecological examination V72.3
for contraceptive maintenance V25.40
Gynecomastia 611.1
Gynephobia 300.29
Gyrate scalp 757.39

H

Haas' disease (osteochondrosis head of humerus) 732.3
Habermann's disease (acute parapsoriasis varioliformis) 696.2
Habit, habituation
chorea 307.22
disturbance, child 307.9
drug (*see also* Dependence) 304.9
laxative (*see also* Abuse, drugs, nondependent) 305.9
spasm 307.20
chronic 307.22
transient of childhood 307.21
tic 307.20
chronic 307.22
transient of childhood 307.21
use of
nonprescribed drugs (*see also* Abuse, drugs, nondependent) 305.9
patent medicines (*see also* Abuse, drugs, nondependent) 305.9
vomiting 536.2
Hadfield-Clarke syndrome (pancreatic infantilism) 577.8
Haff disease 985.1
Hageman factor defect, deficiency, or disease (*see also* Defect, coagulation) 286.3
Haglund's disease (osteochondrosis os tibiale externum) 732.5
Haglund-Läwen-Fründ syndrome 717.89
Hagner's disease (hypertrophic pulmonary osteoarthropathy) 731.2
Hag teeth, tooth 524.3
Hailey-Hailey disease (benign familial chronic pemphigus) 757.39
Hair —*see also* condition
plucking 307.9
Hairball in stomach 935.2
Hairy black tongue 529.3
Half vertebra 756.14
Halitosis 784.9
Hallermann-Streiff syndrome 756.0
Hallervorden-Spatz disease or syndrome 333.0
Hallopeau's
acrodermatitis (continua) 696.1
disease (lichen sclerosis et atrophicus) 701.0
Hallucination (auditory) (gustatory) (olfactory) (tactile) 780.1
alcoholic 291.3
drug-induced 292.12
visual 368.16
Hallucinosis 298.9
alcoholic (acute) 291.3
drug-induced 292.12
Hallus —*see* Hallux
Hallux 735.9
malleus (acquired) 735.3
rigidus (acquired) 735.2
congenital 755.66
late effects of rickets 268.1
valgus (acquired) 735.0
congenital 755.66
varus (acquired) 735.1
congenital 755.66
Halo, visual 368.15
Hamartoblastoma 759.6
Hamartoma 759.6
epithelial (gingival), odontogenic, central, or peripheral (M9321/0) 213.1
upper jaw (bone) 213.0
vascular 757.32
Hamartosis, hamartoses NEC 759.6
Hamman's disease or syndrome (spontaneous mediastinal emphysema) 518.1
Hamman-Rich syndrome (diffuse interstitial pulmonary fibrosis) 516.3
Hammer toe (acquired) 735.4
congenital 755.66
late effects of rickets 268.1
Hand —*see* condition
Hand-Schüller-Christian disease or syndrome (chronic histiocytosis x) 277.8
Hand-foot syndrome 282.61
Hanging (asphyxia) (strangulation) (suffocation) 994.7
Hangnail (finger) (with lymphangitis) 681.02
Hangover (alcohol) (*see also* Abuse, drugs, nondependent) 305.0
Hanot's cirrhosis or disease —*see* Cirrhosis, biliary
Hanot-Chauffard (-Troisier) syndrome (bronze diabetes) 275.0
Hansen's disease (leprosy) 030.9
benign form 030.1
malignant form 030.0
Harada's disease or syndrome 363.22
Hard chancre 091.0
Hardening
artery—*see* Arteriosclerosis
brain 348.8
liver 571.8
Hare's syndrome (M8010/3) (carcinoma, pulmonary apex) 162.3
Harelip (*see also* Cleft, lip) 749.10
Harkavy's syndrome 446.0
Harlequin (fetus) 757.1
color change syndrome 779.8
Harley's disease (intermittent hemoglobinuria) 283.2
Harris'
lines 733.91
syndrome (organic hyperinsulinism) 251.1
Hart's disease or syndrome (pellagra-cerebellar ataxia-renal aminoaciduria) 270.0
Hartmann's pouch (abnormal sacculation of gallbladder neck) 575.8
Hartnup disease (pellagra-cerebellar ataxia-renal aminoaciduria) 270.0
Harvester lung 495.0
Hashimoto's disease or struma (struma lymphomatosa) 245.2
Hassall-Henle bodies (corneal warts) 371.41
Haut mal (*see also* Epilepsy) 345.1
Haverhill fever 026.1
Hawaiian wood rose dependence 304.5
Hawkins' keloid 701.4
Hay
asthma (*see also* Asthma) 493.0
fever (allergic) (with rhinitis) 477.9
with asthma (bronchial) (*see also* Asthma) 493.0

Hay —*continued*
allergic, due to grass, pollen, ragweed, or tree 477.0
conjunctivitis 372.05
due to
dander 477.8
dust 477.8
fowl 477.8
pollen 477.0
specified allergen other than pollen 477.8
Hayem-Faber syndrome (achlorhydric anemia) 280.9
Hayem-Widal syndrome (acquired hemolytic jaundice) 283.9
Haygarth's nodosities 715.04
Hazard-Crile tumor (M8350/3) 193
Hb (abnormal)
disease—*see* Disease, hemoglobin
trait—*see* Trait
H disease 270.0
Head —*see also* condition
banging 307.3
Headache 784.0
allergic 346.2
cluster 346.2
due to
loss, spinal fluid 349.0
lumbar puncture 349.0
saddle block 349.0
emotional 307.81
histamine 346.2
lumbar puncture 349.0
menopausal 627.2
migraine 346.9
nonorganic origin 307.81
postspinal 349.0
psychogenic 307.81
psychophysiologic 307.81
sick 346.1
spinal fluid loss 349.0
tension 307.81
vascular 784.0
migraine type 346.9
vasomotor 346.9
Health
advice V65.4
audit V70.0
checkup V70.0
education V65.4
hazard (*see also* History of) V15.9
specified cause NEC V15.89
instruction V65.4
services provided because (of)
boarding school residence V60.6
holiday relief for person providing home care V60.5
inadequate
housing V60.1
resources V60.2
lack of housing V60.0
no care available in home V60.4
person living alone V60.3
poverty V60.3
residence in institution V60.6
specified cause NEC V60.8
vacation relief for person providing home care V60.5
Healthy
donor (*see also* Donor) V59.9
infant or child
accompanying sick mother V65.0
receiving care V20.1
person
accompanying sick relative V65.0
admitted for sterilization V25.2
receiving prophylactic inoculation or vaccination (*see also* Vaccination, prophylactic) V05.9
Hearing examination V72.1
Heart —*see* condition
Heartburn 787.1
psychogenic 306.4
Heat (effects) 992.9
apoplexy 992.0
burn—*see also* Burn, by site
from sun 692.71
collapse 992.1
cramps 992.2
dermatitis or eczema 692.89
edema 992.7
erythema—*see* Burn, by site
excessive 992.9
specified effect NEC 992.8
exhaustion 992.5
anhydrotic 992.3
due to
salt (and water) depletion 992.4
water depletion 992.3
fatigue (transient) 992.6
fever 992.0
hyperpyrexia 992.0
prickly 705.1
prostration—*see* Heat, exhaustion
pyrexia 992.0
rash 705.1
specified effect NEC 992.8
stroke 992.0
sunburn 692.71
syncope 992.1
Heavy-chain disease 273.2
Heavy-for-dates (fetus or infant) 766.1
4500 grams or more 766.0
exceptionally 766.0
Hebephrenia, hebephrenic (acute) (*see also* Schizophrenia) 295.1
dementia (praecox) (*see also* Schizophrenia) 295.1
schizophrenia (*see also* Schizophrenia) 295.1
Heberden's
disease or nodes 715.04
syndrome (angina pectoris) 413.9
Hebra's disease
dermatitis exfoliativa 695.89
erythema multiforme exudativum 695.1
pityriasis 695.89
maculata et circinata 696.3
rubra 695.89
pilaris 696.4
prurigo 698.2
Hebra, nose 040.1
Hedinger's syndrome (malignant carcinoid) 259.2
Heel —*see* condition
Heerfordt's disease or syndrome (uveoparotitis) 135

Hegglin's anomaly or syndrome 288.2
Heidenhain's disease 290.10
with dementia 290.10
Heilmeyer-Schöner disease (M9842/3) 207.1
Heine-Medin disease (*see also* Poliomyelitis) 045.9
Heinz-body anemia, congenital 282.7
Heller's disease or syndrome (infantile psychosis) (*see also* Psychosis, childhood) 299.1
H.E.L.L.P. 642.5
Helminthiasis (*see also* Infestation, by specific parasite) 128.9
Ancylostoma (*see also* Ancylostoma) 126.9
intestinal 127.9
mixed types (types classifiable to more than one of the titles 120.0-127.7) 127.8
specified type 127.7
mixed types (intestinal) (types classifiable to more than one of the titles 120.0-127.7) 127.8
Necator americanus 126.1
specified type NEC 128.8
Trichinella 124
Heloma 700
Hemangioblastoma (M9161/1)—*see also* Neoplasm, connective tissue, uncertain behavior
malignant (M9161//3)—*see* Neoplasm, connective tissue, malignant
Hemangioblastomatosis, cerebelloretinal 759.6
Hemangioendothelioma (M9130/1)—*see also* Neoplasm, by site, uncertain behavior
benign (M9130/0) 228.00
bone (diffuse) (M9130/3)—*see* Neoplasm, bone, malignant
malignant (M9130/3)—*see* Neoplasm, connective tissue, malignant
nervous system (M9130/0) 228.09
Hemangioendotheliosarcoma (M9130/3)—*see* Neoplasm, connective tissue, malignant
Hemangiofibroma (M9160/0)—*see* Neoplasm, by site, benign
Hemangiolipoma (M8861/0)—*see* Lipoma
Hemangioma (M9120/0) 228.00
arteriovenous (M9123/0)—*see* Hemangioma, by site
brain 228.02
capillary (M9131/0)—*see* Hemangioma, by site
cavernous (M9121/0)—*see* Hemangioma, by site
central nervous system NEC 228.09
choroid 228.09
heart 228.09
infantile (M9131/0)—*see* Hemangioma, by site
intra-abdominal structures 228.04
intracranial structures 228.02
intramuscular (M9132/0)—*see* Hemangioma, by site
iris 228.09
juvenile (M9131/0)—*see* Hemangioma, by site
malignant (M9120/3)—*see* Neoplasm, connective tissue, malignant
meninges 228.09
brain 228.02
spinal cord 228.09
peritoneum 228.04
placenta—*see* Placenta, abnormal
plexiform (M9131/0)—*see* Hemangioma, by site
racemose (M9123/0)—*see* Hemangioma, by site
retina 228.03
retroperitoneal tissue 228.04
Hemangioma—*continued*
sclerosing (M8832/0)—*see* Neoplasm, skin, benign
simplex (M9131/0)—*see* Hemangioma, by site
skin and subcutaneous tissue 228.01
specified site NEC 228.09
spinal cord 228.09
venous (M9122/0)—*see* Hemangioma, by site
verrucous keratotic (M9142/0)—*see* Hemangioma, by site
Hemangiomatosis (systemic) 757.32
involving single site—*see* Hemangioma
Hemangiopericytoma (M9150/1)—*see also* Neoplasm, connective tissue, uncertain behavior
benign (M9150/0)—*see* Neoplasm, connective tissue, benign
malignant (M9150/3)—*see* Neoplasm, connective tissue, malignant
Hemangiosarcoma (M9120/3)—*see* Neoplasm, connective tissue, malignant
Hemarthrosis (nontraumatic) 719.0
ankle 719.17
elbow 719.12
foot 719.17
hand 719.14
hip 719.15
knee 719.16
multiple sites 719.19
pelvic region 719.15
shoulder (region) 719.11
specified site NEC 719.18
traumatic—*see* Sprain, by site
wrist 719.13
Hematemesis 578.0
with ulcer—*see* Ulcer, by site, with hemorrhage
due to S. japonicum 120.2
Goldstein's (familial hemorrhagic telangiectasia) 448.0
newborn 772.4
due to swallowed maternal blood 777.3
Hematidrosis 705.89
Hematinuria (*see also* Hemoglobinuria) 791.2
malarial 084.8
paroxysmal 283.2
Hematite miners' lung 503
Hematobilia 576.8
Hematocele (congenital) (diffuse) (idiopathic) 608.83
broad ligament 620.7
canal of Nuck 629.0
cord, male 608.83
fallopian tube 620.8
female NEC 629.0
ischiorectal 569.89
male NEC 608.83
ovary 629.0
pelvis, pelvic
female 629.0
with ectopic pregnancy (*see also* Pregnancy, ectopic) 633.9
male 608.83
periuterine 629.0
retrouterine 629.0
scrotum 608.83
spermatic cord (diffuse) 608.83
testis 608.84
traumatic—*see* Injury, internal, pelvis
tunica vaginalis 608.83
uterine ligament 629.0
uterus 621.4

Note—Hematomas are coded according to origin and the nature and site of the hematoma or the accompanying injury. Hematomas of unspecified origin are coded as injuries of the sites involved, except:
(a) *hematomas of genital organs which are coded as diseases of the organ involved unless they complicate pregnancy or delivery*
(b) *hematomas of the eye which are coded as diseases of the eye.*

For late effect of hematoma classifiable to 920-924 see Late, effect, contusion

Note—Use the following fifth-digit subclassification with categories 851-854:

0 *unspecified state of consciousness*
1 *with no loss of consciousness*
2 *with brief [less than one hour] loss of consciousness*
3 *with moderate [1-24 hours] loss of consciousness*
4 *with prolonged [more than 24 hours] loss of consciousness and return to pre-existing conscious level*
5 *with prolonged [more than 24 hours] loss of consciousness, without return to pre-existing conscious level*
6 *with loss of consciousness of unspecified duration*
9 *with concussion, unspecified*

Hematoma—*continued*
intracranial—*see* Hematoma, brain
kidney, cystic 593.81
traumatic 866.01
with open wound into cavity 866.11
labia (nontraumatic) 624.5
lingual (and other parts of neck, scalp, or face, except eye) 920
liver (subcapsular) 573.8
birth injury 767.8
fetus or newborn 767.8
traumatic NEC 864.01
with
laceration—*see* Laceration, liver
open wound into cavity 864.11
mediastinum—*see* Injury, internal, mediastinum
meninges, meningeal (brain)—*see also* Hematoma, brain, subarachnoid
spinal—*see* Injury, spinal, by site
mesosalpinx (nontraumatic) 620.8
traumatic—*see* Injury, internal, pelvis
muscle (traumatic)—*see* Contusion, by site
nasal (septum) (and other part(s) of neck, scalp, or face, except eye) 920
obstetrical surgical wound 674.3
orbit, orbital (nontraumatic) 376.32
traumatic 921.2
ovary (corpus luteum) (nontraumatic) 620.1
traumatic—*see* Injury, internal, ovary
pelvis (female) (nontraumatic) 629.8
complicating delivery 665.7
male 608.83
traumatic—*see also* Injury, internal, pelvis
specified organ NEC (*see also* Injury, internal, pelvis) 867.6
penis (nontraumatic) 607.82
pericranial (and neck, or face any part, except eye) 920
due to injury at birth 767.1
perineal wound (obstetrical) 674.3
complicating delivery 664.5
perirenal, cystic 593.81
pinna 380.31
placenta—*see* Placenta, abnormal
postoperative 998.1
retroperitoneal (nontraumatic) 568.81
traumatic—*see* Injury, internal, retroperitoneum
retropubic, male 568.81
scalp (and neck, or face any part, except eye) 920
fetus or newborn 767.1
scrotum (nontraumatic) 608.83
traumatic 922.4
seminal vesicle (nontraumatic) 608.83
traumatic—*see* Injury, internal, seminal vesicle
spermatic cord—*see also* Injury, internal, spermatic cord
nontraumatic 608.83
spinal (cord) (meninges)—*see also* Injury, spinal, by site
fetus or newborn 767.4
nontraumatic 336.1
spleen 865.01
with
laceration—*see* Laceration, spleen
open wound into cavity 865.11
sternocleidomastoid, birth injury 767.8

Hematoma—*continued*
sternomastoid, birth injury 767.8
subarachnoid—*see also* Hematoma, brain, subarachnoid
fetus or newborn 772.2
nontraumatic (*see also* Hemorrhage, subarachnoid) 430
newborn 772.2
subdural—*see also* Hematoma, brain, subdural
fetus or newborn (localized) 767.0
nontraumatic (*see also* Hemorrhage, subdural) 432.1
subperiosteal (syndrome) 267
traumatic—*see* Hematoma, by site
superficial, fetus or newborn 772.6
syncytium—*see* Placenta, abnormal
testis (nontraumatic) 608.83
birth injury 767.8
traumatic 922.4
tunica vaginalis (nontraumatic) 608.83
umbilical cord 663.6
affecting fetus or newborn 762.6
uterine ligament (nontraumatic) 620.7
traumatic—*see* Injury, internal, pelvis
uterus 621.4
traumatic—*see* Injury, internal, pelvis
vagina (nontraumatic) (ruptured) 623.6
complicating delivery 665.7
traumatic 922.4
vas deferens (nontraumatic) 608.83
traumatic—*see* Injury, internal, vas deferens
vitreous 379.23
vocal cord 920
vulva (nontraumatic) 624.5
complicating delivery 664.5
fetus or newborn 767.8
traumatic 922.4
Hematometra 621.4
Hematomyelia 336.1
with fracture of vertebra (*see also* Fracture, vertebra, by site, with spinal cord injury) 806.8
fetus or newborn 767.4
Hematomyelitis 323.9
late effect—*see* category 326
Hematoperitoneum (*see also* Hemoperitoneum) 568.81
Hematopneumothorax (*see also* Hemothorax) 511.8
Hematoporphyria (acquired) (congenital) 277.1
Hematoporphyrinuria (acquired) (congenital) 277.1
Hematorachis, hematorrhachis 336.1
fetus or newborn 767.4
Hematosalpinx 620.8
with
ectopic pregnancy (*see also* categories 633.0-633.9) 639.2
molar pregnancy (*see also* categories 630-632) 639.2
infectional (*see also* Salpingo-oophoritis) 614.2
Hematospermia 608.83
Hematothorax (*see also* Hemothorax) 511.8
Hematotympanum 381.03
Hematuria (benign) (essential) (idiopathic) 599.7
due to S. hematobium 120.0
endemic 120.0
intermittent 599.7
malarial 084.8
paroxysmal 599.7

Hematuria—*continued*
  sulfonamide
    correct substance properly administered 599.7
    overdose or wrong substance given or taken 961.0
  tropical (bilharziasis) 120.0
  tuberculous (*see also* Tuberculosis) 016.9
Hematuric bilious fever 084.8
Hemeralopia 368.60
  meaning day blindness 368.10
  vitamin A deficiency 264.5
Hemiabiotrophy 799.8
Hemi-akinesia 781.8
Hemianalgesia (*see also* Disturbance, sensation) 782.0
Hemianencephaly 740.0
Hemianesthesia (*see also* Disturbance, sensation) 782.0
Hemianopia, hemianopsia (altitudinal) (homonymous) 368.46
  binasal 368.47
  bitemporal 368.47
  heteronymous 368.47
  syphilitic 095.8
Hemiasomatognosia 307.9
Hemiathetosis 781.0
Hemiatrophy 799.8
  cerebellar 334.8
  face 349.89
    progressive 349.89
  fascia 728.9
  leg 728.2
  tongue 529.8
Hemiballism (us) 333.5
Hemiblock (cardiac) (heart) (left) 426.2
Hemicardia 746.89
Hemicephalus, hemicephaly 740.0
Hemichorea 333.5
Hemicrania 346.9
  congenital malformation 740.0
Hemidystrophy —*see* Hemiatrophy
Hemiectromelia 755.4
Hemihypalgesia (*see also* Disturbance, sensation) 782.0
Hemihypertrophy (congenital) 759.89
  cranial 756.0
Hemihypesthesia (*see also* Disturbance, sensation) 782.0
Hemi-inattention 781.8
Hemimelia 755.4
  lower limb 755.30
    paraxial (complete) (incomplete) (intercalary) (terminal) 755.32
      fibula 755.37
      tibia 755.36
    transverse (complete) (partial) 755.31
  upper limb 755.20
    paraxial (complete) (incomplete) (intercalary) (terminal) 755.22
      radial 755.26
      ulnar 755.27
    transverse (complete) (partial) 755.21
Hemiparalysis (*see also* Hemiplegia) 342.9
Hemiparesis (*see also* Hemiplegia) 342.9
Hemiparesthesia (*see also* Disturbance, sensation) 782.0
Hemiplegia 342.9
  acute (*see also* Disease, cerebrovascular, acute) 436
  alternans facialis 344.89
  apoplectic (*see also* Disease, cerebrovascular, acute) 436
    late effect or residual—*see* category 438
  arteriosclerotic 437.0
    late effect or residual—*see* category 438
  ascending (spinal) NEC 344.89
  attack (*see also* Disease, cerebrovascular, acute) 436
  brain, cerebral (current episode) 437.8
    congenital 343.1
  cerebral—*see* Hemiplegia, brain
  congenital (cerebral) (spastic) (spinal) 343.1
  conversion neurosis (hysterical) 300.11
  cortical—*see* Hemiplegia, brain
  due to
    arteriosclerosis 437.0
      late effect or residual—*see* category 438
    cerebrovascular lesion (*see also* Disease, cerebrovascular, acute) 436
      late effect—*see* category 438
  embolic (current) (*see also* Embolism, brain) 434.1
    late effect—*see* category 438
  flaccid 342.0
  hypertensive (current episode) 437.8
  infantile (postnatal) 343.4
  late effect
    birth injury, intracranial or spinal 343.4
    cerebrovascular lesion—*see* category 438
    viral encephalitis 139.0
  middle alternating NEC 344.89
  newborn NEC 767.0
  seizure (current episode) (*see also* Disease, cerebrovascular, acute) 436
  spastic 342.1
    congenital or infantile 343.1
  specified NEC 342.8
  thrombotic (current) (*see also* Thrombosis, brain) 434.0
    late effect—*see* category 438
Hemisection, spinal cord —*see* Fracture, vertebra, by site, with spinal cord injury
Hemispasm 781.0
  facial 781.0
Hemispatial neglect 781.8
Hemisporosis 117.9
Hemitremor 781.0
Hemivertebra 756.14
Hemobilia 576.8
Hemocholecyst 575.8
Hemochromatosis (acquired) (diabetic) (hereditary) (liver) (myocardium) (primary idiopathic) (secondary) 275.0
  with refractory anemia 285.0
Hemodialysis V56.0
Hemoglobin —*see also* condition
  abnormal (disease)—*see* Disease, hemoglobin
  AS genotype 282.5
  fetal, hereditary persistence 282.7
  high-oxygen-affinity 289.0
  low NEC 285.9
  S (Hb-S), heterozygous 282.5
Hemoglobinemia 283.2
  due to blood transfusion NEC 999.8
    bone marrow 996.85
  paroxysmal 283.2

Hemoglobinopathy (mixed) (*see also* Disease, hemoglobin) 282.7
with thalassemia 282.4
sickle-cell 282.60
with thalassemia 282.4
Hemoglobinuria, hemoglobinuric 791.2
with anemia, hemolytic, acquired (chronic) NEC 283.2
cold (agglutinin) (paroxysmal) (with Raynaud's syndrome) 283.2
due to
exertion 283.2
hemolysis (from external causes) NEC 283.2
exercise 283.2
fever (malaria) 084.8
infantile 791.2
intermittent 283.2
malarial 084.8
march 283.2
nocturnal (paroxysmal) 283.2
paroxysmal (cold) (nocturnal) 283.2
Hemolymphangioma (M9175/0) 228.1
Hemolysis
fetal—*see* Jaundice, fetus or newborn
intravascular (disseminated) NEC 286.6
with
abortion—*see* Abortion, by type, with hemorrhage, delayed or excessive
ectopic pregnancy (*see also* categories 633.0-633.9) 639.1
hemorrhage of pregnancy 641.3
affecting fetus or newborn 762.1
molar pregnancy (*see also* categories 630-632) 639.1
acute 283.2
following
abortion 639.1
ectopic or molar pregnancy 639.1
neonatal—*see* Jaundice, fetus or newborn
transfusion NEC 999.8
bone marrow 996.85
Hemolytic —*see also* condition
anemia—*see* Anemia, hemolytic
uremic syndrome 283.11
Hemometra 621.4
Hemopericardium (with effusion) 423.0
newborn 772.8
traumatic (*see also* Hemothorax, traumatic) 860.2
with open wound into thorax 860.3
Hemoperitoneum 568.81
infectional (*see also* Peritonitis) 567.2
traumatic—*see* Injury, internal, peritoneum
Hemophilia (familial) (hereditary) 286.0
A 286.0
B (Leyden) 286.1
B_m 286.1
C 286.2
calcipriva (*see also* Fibrinolysis) 286.7
classical 286.0
nonfamilial 286.7
vascular 286.4
Hemophilus influenzae NEC 041.5
arachnoiditis (basic) (brain) (spinal) 320.0
late effect—*see* category 326
bronchopneumonia 482.2
cerebral ventriculitis 320.0
late effect—*see* category 326
cerebrospinal inflammation 320.0
late effect—*see* category 326
Hemophilus influenzae—*continued*
infection NEC 041.5
leptomeningitis 320.0
late effect—*see* category 326
meningitis (cerebral) (cerebrospinal) (spinal) 320.0
late effect—*see* category 326
meningomyelitis 320.0
late effect—*see* category 326
pachymeningitis (adhesive) (fibrous) (hemorrhagic) (hypertrophic) (spinal) 320.0
late effect—*see* category 326
pneumonia (broncho-) 482.2
Hemophthalmos 360.43
Hemopneumothorax (*see also* Hemothorax) 511.8
traumatic 860.4
with open wound into thorax 860.5
Hemoptysis 786.3
due to Paragonimus (westermani) 121.2
newborn 770.3
tuberculous (*see also* Tuberculosis, pulmonary) 011.9
Hemorrhage, hemorrhagic (nontraumatic) 459.0
abdomen 459.0
accidental (antepartum) 641.2
affecting fetus or newborn 762.1
adenoid 474.8
adrenal (capsule) (gland) (medulla) 255.4
newborn 772.5
after labor—*see* Hemorrhage, postpartum
alveolar
lung, newborn 770.3
process 525.8
alveolus 525.8
amputation stump (surgical) 998.1
secondary, delayed 997.69
anemia (chronic) 280.0
acute 285.1
antepartum—*see* Hemorrhage, pregnancy
anus (sphincter) 569.3
apoplexy (stroke) 432.9
arachnoid—*see* Hemorrhage, subarachnoid
artery NEC 459.0
brain (*see also* Hemorrhage, brain) 431
middle meningeal—*see* Hemorrhage, subarachnoid
basilar (ganglion) (*see also* Hemorrhage, brain) 431
bladder 596.8
blood dyscrasia 289.9
bowel 578.9
newborn 772.4
brain (miliary) (nontraumatic) 431
with
birth injury 767.0
arachnoid—*see* Hemorrhage, subarachnoid
due to
birth injury 767.0
rupture of aneurysm (congenital) (*see also* Hemorrhage, subarachnoid) 430
mycotic 431
syphilis 094.89
epidural or extradural—*see* Hemorrhage, extradural
fetus or newborn (anoxic) (hypoxic) (due to birth trauma) (nontraumatic) 767.0
iatrogenic 997.02
postoperative 997.02
puerperal, postpartum, childbirth 674.0
stem 431

Hemorrhage, hemorrhagic—*continued*
subarachnoid, arachnoid or meningeal—*see* Hemorrhage, subarachnoid
subdural—*see* Hemorrhage, subdural
traumatic NEC 853.0

Note—Use the following fifth-digit subclassification with categories 851-854:

0 unspecified state of consciousness
1 with no loss of consciousness
2 with brief [less than one hour] loss of consciousness
3 with moderate [1-24 hours] loss of consciousness
4 with prolonged [more than 24 hours] loss of consciousness and return to pre-existing conscious level
5 with prolonged [more than 24 hours] loss of consciousness, without return to pre-existing conscious level
6 with loss of consciousness of unspecified duration
9 with concussion, unspecified

with
cerebral
contusion—*see* Contusion, brain
laceration—*see* Laceration, brain
open intracranial wound 853.1
skull fracture—*see* Fracture, skull, by site
extradural or epidural 852.4
with open intracranial wound 852.5
subarachnoid 852.0
with open intracranial wound 852.1
subdural 852.2
with open intracranial wound 852.3
breast 611.79
bronchial tube—*see* Hemorrhage, lung
bronchopulmonary—*see* Hemorrhage, lung
bronchus (cause unknown) (*see also* Hemorrhage, lung) 786.3
bulbar (*see also* Hemorrhage, brain) 431
bursa 727.89
capillary 448.9
primary 287.8
capsular—*see* Hemorrhage, brain
cardiovascular 429.89
cecum 578.9
cephalic (*see also* Hemorrhage, brain) 431
cerebellar (*see also* Hemorrhage, brain) 431
cerebellum (*see also* Hemorrhage, brain) 431
cerebral (*see also* Hemorrhage, brain) 431
fetus or newborn (anoxic) (traumatic) 767.0
cerebromeningeal (*see also* Hemorrhage, brain) 431
cerebrospinal (*see also* Hemorrhage, brain) 431
cerebrum (*see also* Hemorrhage, brain) 431
cervix (stump) (uteri) 622.8
cesarean section wound 674.3
chamber, anterior (eye) 364.41
childbirth—*see* Hemorrhage, complicating, delivery
choroid 363.61
expulsive 363.62
ciliary body 364.41
cochlea 386.8
colon—*see* Hemorrhage, intestine

Hemorrhage, hemorrhagic—*continued*
complicating
delivery 641.9
affecting fetus or newborn 762.1
associated with
afibrinogenemia 641.3
affecting fetus or newborn 763.8
coagulation defect 641.3
affecting fetus or newborn 763.8
hyperfibrinolysis 641.3
affecting fetus or newborn 763.8
hypofibrinogenemia 641.3
affecting fetus or newborn 763.8
due to
low-lying placenta 641.1
affecting fetus or newborn 762.0
placenta previa 641.1
affecting fetus or newborn 762.0
premature separation of placenta 641.2
affecting fetus or newborn 762.1
retained
placenta 666.0
secundines 666.2
trauma 641.8
affecting fetus or newborn 763.8
uterine leiomyoma 641.8
affecting fetus or newborn 763.8
surgical procedure 998.1
concealed NEC 459.0
congenital 772.9
conjunctiva 372.72
newborn 772.8
cord, newborn 772.0
slipped ligature 772.3
stump 772.3
corpus luteum (ruptured) 620.1
cortical (*see also* Hemorrhage, brain) 431
cranial 432.9
cutaneous 782.7
newborn 772.6
cyst, pancreas 577.2
cystitis—*see* Cystitis
delayed
with
abortion—*see* Abortion, by type, with hemorrhage, delayed or excessive
ectopic pregnancy (*see also* categories 633.0-633.9) 639.1
molar pregnancy (*see also* categories 630-632) 639.1
following
abortion 639.1
ectopic or molar pregnancy 639.1
postpartum 666.2
diathesis (familial) 287.9
newborn 776.0
disease 287.9
newborn 776.0
specified type NEC 287.8
disorder 287.9
due to circulating anticoagulants 286.5
specified type NEC 287.8
due to
any device, implant, or graft (presence of) classifiable to 996.0-996.5—*see* Complications, due to (presence of) any device, implant, or graft classified to 996.0—996.5 NEC
circulating anticoagulant 286.5
duodenum, duodenal 537.89
ulcer—*see* Ulcer, duodenum, with hemorrhage

Hemorrhage, hemorrhagic—*continued*
dura mater—*see* Hemorrhage, subdural
endotracheal—*see* Hemorrhage, lung
epidural—*see* Hemorrhage, extradural
episiotomy 674.3
esophagus 530.82
varix (*see also* Varix, esophagus, bleeding) 456.0
excessive
with
abortion—*see* Abortion, by type, with hemorrhage, delayed or excessive
ectopic pregnancy (*see also* categories 633.0-633.9) 639.1
molar pregnancy (*see also* categories 630-632) 639.1
following
abortion 639.1
ectopic or molar pregnancy 639.1
external 459.0
extradural (traumatic)—*see also* Hemorrhage, brain, traumatic, extradural
birth injury 767.0
fetus or newborn (anoxic) (traumatic) 767.0
nontraumatic 432.0
eye 360.43
chamber (anterior) (aqueous) 364.41
fundus 362.81
eyelid 374.81
fallopian tube 620.8
fetomaternal 772.0
affecting management of pregnancy or puerperium 656.0
fetus, fetal 772.0
from
cut end of co-twin's cord 772.0
placenta 772.0
ruptured cord 772.0
vasa previa 772.0
into
co-twin 772.0
mother's circulation 772.0
affecting management of pregnancy or puerperium 656.0
fever (*see also* Fever, hemorrhagic) 065.9
with renal syndrome 078.6
arthropod-borne NEC 065.9
Bangkok 065.4
Crimean 065.0
dengue virus 065.4
epidemic 078.6
Junin virus 078.7
Korean 078.6
Machupo virus 078.7
mite-borne 065.8
mosquito-borne 065.4
Philippine 065.4
Russian (Yaroslav) 078.6
Singapore 065.4
southeast Asia 065.4
Thailand 065.4
tick-borne NEC 065.3
fibrinogenolysis (*see also* Fibrinolysis) 286.6
fibrinolytic (acquired) (*see also* Fibrinolysis) 286.6
fontanel 767.1
from tracheostomy stoma 519.0
fundus, eye 362.81
funis
affecting fetus or newborn 772.0
complicating delivery 663.8

Hemorrhage, hemorrhagic—*continued*
gastric (*see also* Hemorrhage, stomach) 578.9
gastroenteric 578.9
newborn 772.4
gastrointestinal (tract) 578.9
newborn 772.4
genitourinary (tract) NEC 599.89
gingiva 523.8
globe 360.43
gravidarum—*see* Hemorrhage, pregnancy
gum 523.8
heart 429.89
hypopharyngeal (throat) 784.8
intermenstrual 626.8
irregular 626.6
regular 626.5
internal (organs) 459.0
capsule (*see also* Hemorrhage brain) 431
ear 386.8
newborn 772.8
intestine 578.9
congenital 772.4
newborn 772.4
into
bladder wall 596.7
bursa 727.89
corpus luysii (*see also* Hemorrhage, brain) 431
intra-abdominal 459.0
during or following surgery 998.1
intra-alveolar, newborn (lung) 770.3
intracerebral (*see also* Hemorrhage, brain) 431
intracranial NEC 432.9
puerperal, postpartum, childbirth 674.0
traumatic—*see* Hemorrhage, brain, traumatic
intramedullary NEC 336.1
intraocular 360.43
intraoperative 998.1
intrapartum—*see* Hemorrhage, complicating, delivery
intrapelvic
female 629.8
male 459.0
intraperitoneal 459.0
intrapontine (*see also* Hemorrhage, brain) 431
intrauterine 621.4
complicating delivery—*see* Hemorrhage, complicating, delivery
in pregnancy or childbirth—*see* Hemorrhage, pregnancy
postpartum (*see also* Hemorrhage, postpartum) 666.1
intraventricular (*see also* Hemorrhage, brain) 431
fetus or newborn (anoxic) (traumatic) 772.1
intravesical 596.7
iris (postinfectional) (postinflammatory) (toxic) 364.41
joint (nontraumatic) 719.10
ankle 719.17
elbow 719.12
foot 719.17
forearm 719.13
hand 719.14
hip 719.15
knee 719.16
lower leg 719.16
multiple sites 719.19
pelvic region 719.15
shoulder (region) 719.11
specified site NEC 719.18

Hemorrhage, hemorrhagic—*continued*
thigh 719.15
upper arm 719.12
wrist 719.13
kidney 593.81
knee (joint) 719.16
labyrinth 386.8
leg NEC 459.0
lenticular striate artery (*see also* Hemorrhage, brain) 431
ligature, vessel 998.1
liver 573.8
lower extremity NEC 459.0
lung 786.3
newborn 770.3
tuberculous (*see also* Tuberculosis, pulmonary) 011.9
malaria 084.8
marginal sinus 641.2
massive subaponeurotic, birth injury 767.1
maternal, affecting fetus or newborn 762.1
mediastinum 786.3
medulla (*see also* Hemorrhage, brain) 431
membrane (brain) (*see also* Hemorrhage, subarachnoid) 430
spinal cord—*see* Hemorrhage, spinal cord
meninges, meningeal (brain) (middle) (*see also* Hemorrhage, subarachnoid) 430
spinal cord—*see* Hemorrhage, spinal cord
mesentery 568.81
metritis 626.8
midbrain (*see also* Hemorrhage, brain) 431
mole 631
mouth 528.9
mucous membrane NEC 459.0
newborn 772.8
muscle 728.89
nail (subungual) 703.8
nasal turbinate 784.7
newborn 772.8
nasopharynx 478.29
navel, newborn 772.3
newborn 772.9
adrenal 772.5
alveolar (lung) 770.3
brain (anoxic) (hypoxic) (due to birth trauma) 767.0
cerebral (anoxic) (hypoxic) (due to birth trauma) 767.0
conjunctiva 772.8
cutaneous 772.6
diathesis 776.0
due to vitamin K deficiency 776.0
gastrointestinal 772.4
internal (organs) 772.8
intestines 772.4
intra-alveolar (lung) 770.3
intracranial (from any perinatal cause) 767.0
intraventricular (from any perinatal cause) 772.1
lung 770.3
pulmonary (massive) 770.3
spinal cord, traumatic 767.4
stomach 772.4
subaponeurotic (massive) 767.1
subarachnoid (from any perinatal cause) 772.2
subconjunctival 772.8
umbilicus 772.0
slipped ligature 772.3
vasa previa 772.0

Hemorrhage, hemorrhagic—*continued*
nipple 611.79
nose 784.7
newborn 772.8
obstetrical surgical wound 674.3
omentum 568.89
newborn 772.4
optic nerve (sheath) 377.42
orbit 376.32
ovary 620.1
oviduct 620.8
pancreas 577.8
parathyroid (gland) (spontaneous) 252.8
parturition—*see* Hemorrhage, complicating, delivery
penis 607.82
pericardium, pericarditis 423.0
perineal wound (obstetrical) 674.3
peritoneum, peritoneal 459.0
peritonsillar tissue 474.8
after operation on tonsils 998.1
due to infection 475
petechial 782.7
pituitary (gland) 253.8
placenta NEC 641.9
affecting fetus or newborn 762.1
from surgical or instrumental damage 641.8
affecting fetus or newborn 762.1
previa 641.1
affecting fetus or newborn 762.0
pleura—*see* Hemorrhage, lung
polioencephalitis, superior 265.1
polymyositis—*see* Polymyositis
pons (*see also* Hemorrhage, brain) 431
pontine (*see also* Hemorrhage, brain) 431
popliteal 459.0
postcoital 626.7
postextraction (dental) 998.1
postmenopausal 627.1
postnasal 784.7
postoperative 998.1
postpartum (atonic) (following delivery of placenta) 666.1
delayed or secondary (after 24 hours) 666.2
retained placenta 666.0
third stage 666.0
pregnancy (concealed) 641.9
accidental 641.2
affecting fetus or newborn 762.1
affecting fetus or newborn 762.1
before 22 completed weeks gestation 640.9
affecting fetus or newborn 762.1
due to
abruptio placenta 641.2
affecting fetus or newborn 762.1
afibrinogenemia or other coagulation defect (conditions classifiable to 286.0-286.9) 641.3
affecting fetus or newborn 762.1
coagulation defect 641.3
affecting fetus or newborn 762.1
hyperfibrinolysis 641.3
affecting fetus or newborn 762.1
hypofibrinogenemia 641.3
affecting fetus or newborn 762.1
leiomyoma, uterus 641.8
affecting fetus or newborn 762.1
low-lying placenta 641.1
affecting fetus or newborn 762.1
marginal sinus (rupture) 641.2
affecting fetus or newborn 762.1

Hemorrhage, hemorrhagic—*continued*
placenta previa 641.1
affecting fetus or newborn 762.0
premature separation of placenta (normally implanted) 641.2
affecting fetus or newborn 762.1
threatened abortion 640.0
affecting fetus or newborn 762.1
trauma 641.8
affecting fetus or newborn 762.1
early (before 22 completed weeks gestation) 640.9
affecting fetus or newborn 762.1
previous, affecting management of pregnancy or childbirth V23.4
unavoidable—*see* Hemorrhage, pregnancy, due to placenta previa
prepartum (mother)—*see* Hemorrhage, pregnancy
preretinal, cause unspecified 362.81
prostate 602.1
puerperal (*see also* Hemorrhage, postpartum) 666.1
pulmonary—*see also* Hemorrhage, lung
newborn (massive) 770.3
renal syndrome 446.21
purpura (primary) (*see also* Purpura, thrombocytopenic) 287.3
rectum (sphincter) 569.3
recurring, following initial hemorrhage at time of injury 958.2
renal 593.81
pulmonary syndrome 446.21
respiratory tract (*see also* Hemorrhage, lung) 786.3
retina, retinal (deep) (superficial) (vessels) 362.81
diabetic 250.5 *[362.01]*
due to birth injury 772.8
retrobulbar 376.89
retroperitoneal 459.0
retroplacental (*see also* Placenta, separation) 641.2
scalp 459.0
due to injury at birth 767.1
scrotum 608.83
secondary (nontraumatic) 459.0
following initial hemorrhage at time of injury 958.2
seminal vesicle 608.83
skin 782.7
newborn 772.6
spermatic cord 608.83
spinal (cord) 336.1
aneurysm (ruptured) 336.1
syphilitic 094.89
due to birth injury 767.4
fetus or newborn 767.4
spleen 289.59
spontaneous NEC 459.0
petechial 782.7
stomach 578.9
newborn 772.4
ulcer—*see* Ulcer, stomach, with hemorrhage
subaponeurotic, newborn 767.1
massive (birth injury) 767.1
subarachnoid (nontraumatic) 430
fetus or newborn (anoxic) (traumatic) 772.2
puerperal, postpartum, childbirth 674.0
traumatic—*see* Hemorrhage, brain, traumatic, subarachnoid

Hemorrhage, hemorrhagic—*continued*
subconjunctival 372.72
due to birth injury 772.8
newborn 772.8
subcortical (*see also* Hemorrhage, brain) 431
subcutaneous 782.7
subdiaphragmatic 459.0
subdural (nontraumatic) 432.1
due to birth injury 767.0
fetus or newborn (anoxic) (hypoxic) (due to birth trauma) 767.0
puerperal, postpartum, childbirth 674.0
spinal 336.1
traumatic—*see* Hemorrhage, brain, traumatic, subdural
subhyaloid 362.81
subperiosteal 733.99
subretinal 362.81
subtentorial (*see also* Hemorrhage, subdural) 432.1
subungual 703.8
due to blood dyscrasia 287.8
suprarenal (capsule) (gland) 255.4
fetus or newborn 772.5
tentorium (traumatic)—*see also* Hemorrhage, brain, traumatic
fetus or newborn 767.0
nontraumatic—*see* Hemorrhage, subdural
testis 608.83
thigh 459.0
third stage 666.0
thorax—*see* Hemorrhage, lung
throat 784.8
thrombocythemia 238.7
thymus (gland) 254.8
thyroid (gland) 246.3
cyst 246.3
tongue 529.8
tonsil 474.8
postoperative 998.1
tooth socket (postextraction) 998.1
trachea—*see* Hemorrhage, lung
traumatic—*see also* nature of injury
brain—*see* Hemorrhage, brain, traumatic
recurring or secondary (following initial hemorrhage at time of injury) 958.2
tuberculous NEC (*see also* Tuberculosis, pulmonary) 011.9
tunica vaginalis 608.83
ulcer—*see* Ulcer, by site, with hemorrhage
umbilicus, umbilical cord 772.0
after birth, newborn 772.3
complicating delivery 663.8
affecting fetus or newborn 772.0
slipped ligature 772.3
stump 772.3
unavoidable (due to placenta previa) 641.1
affecting fetus or newborn 762.0
upper extremity 459.0
urethra (idiopathic) 599.84
uterus, uterine (abnormal) 626.9
climacteric 627.0
complicating delivery—*see* Hemorrhage, complicating, delivery
due to
intrauterine contraceptive device 996.76
perforating uterus 996.32
functional or dysfunctional 626.8
in pregnancy—*see* Hemorrhage, pregnancy

Hemorrhage, hemorrhagic—*continued*
intermenstrual 626.8
irregular 626.6
regular 626.5
postmenopausal 627.1
postpartum (*see also* Hemorrhage, postpartum) 666.1
prepubertal 626.8
pubertal 626.3
puerperal (immediate) 666.1
vagina 623.8
vasa previa 663.5
affecting fetus or newborn 772.0
vas deferens 608.83
ventricular (*see also* Hemorrhage, brain) 431
vesical 596.8
viscera 459.0
newborn 772.8
vitreous (humor) (intraocular) 379.23
vocal cord 478.5
vulva 624.8
Hemorrhoids (anus) (rectum) (without complication) 455.6
bleeding, prolapsed, strangulated, or ulcerated NEC 455.8
external 455.5
internal 455.2
complicated NEC 455.8
complicating pregnancy and puerperium 671.8
external 455.3
with complication NEC 455.5
bleeding, prolapsed, strangulated, or ulcerated 455.5
thrombosed 455.4
internal 455.0
with complication NEC 455.2
bleeding, prolapsed, strangulated, or ulcerated 455.2
thrombosed 455.1
residual skin tag 455.9
sentinel pile 455.9
thrombosed NEC 455.7
external 455.4
internal 455.1
Hemosalpinx 620.8
Hemosiderosis 275.0
dietary 275.0
pulmonary (idiopathic) 275.0 *[516.1]*
transfusion NEC 999.8
bone marrow 996.85
Hemospermia 608.83
Hemothorax 511.8
bacterial, nontuberculous 511.1
newborn 772.8
nontuberculous 511.8
bacterial 511.1
pneumococcal 511.1
staphylococcal 511.1
streptococcal 511.1
traumatic 860.2
with
open wound into thorax 860.3
pneumothorax 860.4
with open wound into thorax 860.5
tuberculous (*see also* Tuberculosis, pleura) 012.0
Hemotympanum 385.89
Hench-Rosenberg syndrome (palindromic arthritis) (*see also* Rheumatism, palindromic) 719.3
Henle's warts 371.41
Henoch (-Schönlein)
disease or syndrome (allergic purpura) 287.0
purpura (allergic) 287.0
Henpue, henpuye 102.6
Heparitinuria 277.5
Hepar lobatum 095.3
Hepatalgia 573.8
Hepatic —*see also* condition
flexure syndrome 569.89
Hepatitis 573.3
acute (*see also* Necrosis, liver) 570
alcoholic 571.1
infective 070.1
with hepatic coma 070.0
alcoholic 571.1
amebic—*see* Abscess, liver, amebic
anicteric (acute)—*see* Hepatitis, viral
antigen-associated (HAA) *see* Hepatitis, viral, type B
Australian antigen (positive) *see* Hepatitis, viral, type B
catarrhal (acute) 070.1
with hepatic coma 070.0
chronic 571.40
newborn 070.1
with hepatic coma 070.0
chemical 573.3
cholangiolitic 573.8
cholestatic 573.8
chronic 571.40
active 571.49
viral—*see* Hepatitis, viral
aggressive 571.49
persistent 571.41
viral—*see* Hepatitis, viral
cytomegalic inclusion virus 078.5 *[573.1]*
diffuse 573.3
"dirty needle"—*see* Hepatitis, viral
with hepatic coma 070.2
drug-induced 573.3
due to
Coxsackie 074.8 *[573.1]*
cytomegalic inclusion virus 078.5 *[573.1]*
infectious mononucleosis 075 *[573.1]*
malaria 084.9 *[573.2]*
mumps 072.71
secondary syphilis 091.62
toxoplasmosis (acquired) 130.5
congenital (active) 771.2
epidemic—*see* Hepatitis, viral, type A
fetus or newborn 774.4
fibrous (chronic) 571.49
acute 570
from injection, inoculation, or transfusion (blood) (other substance) (plasma) (serum) (onset within 8 months after administration) *see* Hepatitis, viral
fulminant (viral) (*see also* Hepatitis, viral) 070.9
with hepatic coma 070.6
type A 070.1
with hepatic coma 070.0
type B—*see* Hepatitis, viral, Type B
giant cell (neonatal) 774.4
hemorrhagic 573.8
homologous serum—*see* Hepatitis, viral
hypertrophic (chronic) 571.49
acute 570
infectious, infective (acute) (chronic) (subacute) 070.1
with hepatic coma 070.0

Hepatitis—*continued*
inoculation—*see* Hepatitis, viral
interstitial (chronic) 571.49
acute 570
lupoid 571.49
malarial 084.9 *[573.2]*
malignant (*see also* Necrosis, liver) 570
neonatal (toxic) 774.4
newborn 774.4
parenchymatous (acute) (*see also* Necrosis, liver) 570
peliosis 573.3
persistent, chronic 571.41
plasma cell 571.49
postimmunization—*see* Hepatitis, viral
postnecrotic 571.49
posttransfusion—*see* Hepatitis, viral
recurrent 571.49
septic 573.3
serum—*see* Hepatitis, viral
carrier (suspected) of V02.6
subacute (*see also* Necrosis, liver) 570
suppurative (diffuse) 572.0
syphilitic (late) 095.3
congenital (early) 090.0 *[573.2]*
late 090.5 *[573.2]*
secondary 091.62
toxic (noninfectious) 573.3
fetus or newborn 774.4
tuberculous (*see also* Tuberculosis) 017.9
viral (acute) (anicteric) (cholangiolitic) (cholestatic) (chronic) (subacute) 070.9
with hepatic coma 070.6
AU-SH type virus—*see* Hepatitis, viral, type B
Australian antigen—*see* Hepatitis, viral, type B
B-antigen—*see* Hepatitis, viral, type B
Coxsackie 074.8 *[573.1]*
cytomegalic inclusion 078.5 *[573.1]*
IH (virus)—*see* Hepatitis, viral, type A
infectious hepatitis virus—*see* Hepatitis, viral, type A
serum hepatitis virus—*see* Hepatitis, viral, type B
SH—*see* Hepatitis, viral, type B
specified type NEC 070.59
with hepatic coma 070.49
type A 070.1
with hepatic coma 070.0
type B (acute) 070.30
with
hepatic coma 070.20
with hepatitis delta 070.21
hepatitis delta 070.31
with hepatic coma 070.21
chronic 070.32
with
hepatic coma 070.22
with hepatitis delta 070.23
hepatitis delta 070.33
with hepatic coma 070.23
type C (acute) 070.51
with hepatic coma 070.41
chronic 070.54
with hepatic coma 070.44
type delta (with hepatitis B carrier state) 070.52
with
active hepatitis B disease—*see* Hepatitis, viral, type B
hepatic coma 070.42

Hepatitis—*continued*
type E 070.53
with hepatic coma 070.43
vaccination and inoculation (prophylactic) V05.3
Waldenström's (lupoid hepatitis) 571.49
Hepatization, lung (acute)—*see also* Pneumonia, lobar
chronic (*see also* Fibrosis, lung) 515
Hepatoblastoma (M8970/3) 155.0
Hepatocarcinoma (M8170/3) 155.0
Hepatocholangiocarcinoma (M8180/3) 155.0
Hepatocholangioma, benign (M8180/0) 211.5
Hepatocholangitis 573.8
Hepatocystitis (*see also* Cholecystitis) 575.1
Hepatodystrophy 570
Hepatolenticular degeneration 275.1
Hepatolithiasis —*see* Choledocholithiasis
Hepatoma (malignant) (M8170/3) 155.0
benign (M8170/0) 211.5
congenital (M8970/3) 155.0
embryonal (M8970/3) 155.0
Hepatomegalia glycogenica diffusa 271.0
Hepatomegaly (*see also* Hypertrophy, liver) 789.1
congenital 751.69
syphilitic 090.0
due to Clonorchis sinensis 121.1
Gaucher's 272.7
syphilitic (congenital) 090.0
Hepatoptosis 573.8
Hepatorrhexis 573.8
Hepatosis, toxic 573.8
Hepatosplenomegaly 571.8
due to S. japonicum 120.2
hyperlipemic (Burger-Grutz type) 272.3
Herald patch 696.3
Hereditary —*see* condition
Heredodegeneration 330.9
macular 362.70
Heredopathia atactica polyneuritiformis 356.3
Heredosyphilis (*see also* Syphilis, congenital) 090.9
Hermaphroditism (true) 752.7
with specified chromosomal anomaly—*see* Anomaly, chromosomes, sex
Hernia, hernial (acquired) (recurrent) 553.9
with
gangrene (obstructed) NEC 551.9
obstruction NEC 552.9
and gangrene 551.9
abdomen (wall)—*see* Hernia, ventral
abdominal, specified site NEC 553.8
with
gangrene (obstructed) 551.8
obstruction 552.8
and gangrene 551.8
appendix 553.8
with
gangrene (obstructed) 551.8
obstruction 552.8
and gangrene 551.8
bilateral (inguinal)—*see* Hernia, inguinal
bladder (sphincter)
congenital (female) (male) 753.8
female 618.0
male 596.8
brain 348.4
congenital 742.0

Hernia, hernial—*continued*
broad ligament 553.8
cartilage, vertebral—*see* Displacement, intervertebral disc
cerebral 348.4
congenital 742.0
endaural 742.0
ciliary body 364.8
traumatic 871.1
colic 553.9
with
gangrene (obstructed) 551.9
obstruction 552.9
and gangrene 551.9
colon 553.9
with
gangrene (obstructed) 551.9
obstruction 552.9
and gangrene 551.9
colostomy (stoma) 569.69
Cooper's (retroperitoneal) 553.8
with
gangrene (obstructed) 551.8
obstruction 552.8
and gangrene 551.8
crural—*see* Hernia, femoral
diaphragm, diaphragmatic 553.3
with
gangrene (obstructed) 551.3
obstruction 552.3
and gangrene 551.3
congenital 756.6
due to gross defect of diaphragm 756.6
traumatic 862.0
with open wound into cavity 862.1
direct (inguinal)—*see* Hernia, inguinal
disc, intervertebral—*see* Displacement, intervertebral disc
diverticulum, intestine 553.9
with
gangrene (obstructed) 551.9
obstruction 552.9
and gangrene 551.9
double (inguinal)—*see* Hernia, inguinal
duodenojejunal 553.8
with
gangrene (obstructed) 551.8
obstruction 552.8
and gangrene 551.8
en glissade—*see* Hernia, inguinal
enterostomy (stoma) 569.69
epigastric 553.29
with
gangrene (obstruction) 551.29
obstruction 552.29
and gangrene 551.29
recurrent 553.21
with
gangrene (obstructed) 551.21
obstruction 552.21
and gangrene 551.21
esophageal hiatus (sliding) 553.3
with
gangrene (obstructed) 551.3
obstruction 552.3
and gangrene 551.3
congenital 750.6
external (inguinal)—*see* Hernia, inguinal
fallopian tube 620.4

Hernia, hernial—*continued*
fascia 728.89
fat 729.30
eyelid 374.34
orbital 374.34
pad 729.30
eye, eyelid 374.34
knee 729.31
orbit 374.34
popliteal (space) 729.31
specified site NEC 729.39
femoral (unilateral) 553.00
with
gangrene (obstructed) 551.00
obstruction 552.00
with gangrene 551.00
bilateral 553.02
gangrenous (obstructed) 551.02
obstructed 552.02
with gangrene 551.02
recurrent 553.03
gangrenous (obstructed) 551.03
obstructed 552.03
with gangrene 551.03
recurrent (unilateral) 553.01
bilateral 553.03
gangrenous (obstructed) 551.03
obstructed 552.03
with gangrene 551.03
gangrenous (obstructed) 551.01
obstructed 552.01
with gangrene 551.01
foramen
Bochdalek 553.3
with
gangrene (obstructed) 551.3
obstruction 552.3
and gangrene 551.3
congenital 756.6
magnum 348.4
Morgagni, morgagnian 553.3
with
gangrene 551.3
obstruction 552.3
and gangrene 551.3
congenital 756.6
funicular (umbilical) 553.1
with
gangrene (obstructed) 551.1
obstruction 552.1
and gangrene 551.1
spermatic cord—*see* Hernia, inguinal
gangrenous—*see* Hernia, by site, with gangrene
gastrointestinal tract 553.9
with
gangrene (obstructed) 551.9
obstruction 552.9
and gangrene 551.9
gluteal—*see* Hernia, femoral
Gruber's (internal mesogastric) 553.8
with
gangrene (obstructed) 551.8
obstruction 552.8
and gangrene 551.8
Hesselbach's 553.8
with
gangrene (obstructed) 551.8
obstruction 552.8
and gangrene 551.8

Hernia, hernial—*continued*
hiatal (esophageal) (sliding) 553.3
with
gangrene (obstructed) 551.3
obstruction 552.3
and gangrene 551.3
congenital 750.6
incarcerated (*see also* Hernia, by site, with obstruction) 552.9
gangrenous (*see also* Hernia, by site, with gangrene) 551.9
incisional 553.21
with
gangrene (obstructed) 551.21
obstruction 552.21
and gangrene 551.21
lumbar—*see* Hernia, lumbar
recurrent 553.21
with
gangrene (obstructed) 551.21
obstruction 552.21
and gangrene 551.21
indirect (inguinal)—*see* Hernia, inguinal
infantile—*see* Hernia, inguinal
infrapatellar fat pad 729.31
inguinal (direct) (double) (encysted) (external) (funicular) (indirect) (infantile) (internal) (interstitial) (oblique) (scrotal) (sliding) 550.9

Note—Use the following fifth-digit subclassification with category 550:

0 unilateral or unspecified (not specified as recurrent)
1 unilateral or unspecified, recurrent
2 bilateral (not specified as recurrent)
3 bilateral, recurrent

with
gangrene (obstructed) 550.0
obstruction 550.1
and gangrene 550.0
internal 553.8
with
gangrene (obstructed) 551.8
obstruction 552.8
and gangrene 551.8
inguinal—*see* Hernia, inguinal
interstitial 553.9
with
gangrene (obstructed) 551.9
obstruction 552.9
and gangrene 551.9
inguinal—*see* Hernia, inguinal
intervertebral cartilage or disc—*see* Displacement, intervertebral disc
intestine, intestinal 553.9
with
gangrene (obstructed) 551.9
obstruction 552.9
and gangrene 551.9
intra-abdominal 553.9
with
gangrene (obstructed) 551.9
obstruction 552.9
and gangrene 551.9
intraparietal 553.9
with
gangrene (obstructed) 551.9
obstruction 552.9
and gangrene 551.9

Hernia, hernial—*continued*
iris 364.8
traumatic 871.1
irreducible (*see also* Hernia, by site, with obstruction) 552.9
gangrenous (with obstruction) (*see also* Hernia, by site, with gangrene) 551.9
ischiatic 553.8
with
gangrene (obstructed) 551.8
obstruction 552.8
and gangrene 551.8
ischiorectal 553.8
with
gangrene (obstructed) 551.8
obstruction 552.8
and gangrene 551.8
lens 379.32
traumatic 871.1
linea
alba—*see* Hernia, epigastric
semilunaris—*see* Hernia, spigelian
Littre's (diverticular) 553.9
with
gangrene (obstructed) 551.9
obstruction 552.9
and gangrene 551.9
lumbar 553.8
with
gangrene (obstructed) 551.8
obstruction 552.8
and gangrene 551.8
intervertebral disc 722.10
lung (subcutaneous) 518.89
congenital 748.69
mediastinum 519.3
mesenteric (internal) 553.8
with
gangrene (obstructed) 551.8
obstruction 552.8
and gangrene 551.8
mesocolon 553.8
with
gangrene (obstructed) 551.8
obstruction 552.8
and gangrene 551.8
muscle (sheath) 728.89
nucleus pulposus—*see* Displacement, intervertebral disc
oblique (inguinal)—*see* Hernia, inguinal
obstructive (*see also* Hernia, by site, with obstruction) 552.9
gangrenous (with obstruction) (*see also* Hernia, by site, with gangrene) 551.9
obturator 553.8
with
gangrene (obstructed) 551.8
obstruction 552.8
and gangrene 551.8
omental 553.8
with
gangrene (obstructed) 551.8
obstruction 552.8
and gangrene 551.8
orbital fat (pad) 374.34
ovary 620.4
oviduct 620.4
paracolostomy (stoma) 569.69

Hernia, hernial—*continued*
paraduodenal 553.8
with
gangrene (obstructed) 551.8
obstruction 552.8
and gangrene 551.8
paraesophageal 553.3
with
gangrene (obstructed) 551.3
obstruction 552.3
and gangrene 551.3
congenital 750.6
parahiatal 553.3
with
gangrene (obstructed) 551.3
obstruction 552.3
and gangrene 551.3
paraumbilical 553.1
with
gangrene (obstructed) 551.1
obstruction 552.1
and gangrene 551.1
parietal 553.9
with
gangrene (obstructed) 551.9
obstruction 552.9
and gangrene 551.9
perineal 553.8
with
gangrene (obstructed) 551.8
obstruction 552.8
and gangrene 551.8
peritoneal sac, lesser 553.8
with
gangrene (obstructed) 551.8
obstruction 552.8
and gangrene 551.8
popliteal fat pad 729.31
postoperative 553.21
with
gangrene (obstructed) 551.21
obstruction 552.21
and gangrene 551.21
pregnant uterus 654.4
prevesical 596.8
properitoneal 553.8
with
gangrene (obstructed) 551.8
obstruction 552.8
and gangrene 551.8
pudendal 553.8
with
gangrene (obstructed) 551.8
obstruction 552.8
and gangrene 551.8
rectovaginal 618.6
retroperitoneal 553.8
with
gangrene (obstructed) 551.8
obstruction 552.8
and gangrene 551.8
Richter's (parietal) 553.9
with
gangrene (obstructed) 551.9
obstruction 552.9
and gangrene 551.9
Rieux's, Riex's (retrocecal) 553.8
with
gangrene (obstructed) 551.8
obstruction 552.8
and gangrene 551.8

Hernia, hernial—*continued*
sciatic 553.8
with
gangrene (obstructed) 551.8
obstruction 552.8
and gangrene 551.8
scrotum, scrotal—*see* Hernia, inguinal
sliding (inguinal)—*see also* Hernia, inguinal
hiatus—*see* Hernia, hiatal
spigelian 553.29
with
gangrene (obstructed) 551.29
obstruction 552.29
and gangrene 551.29
spinal (*see also* Spina bifida) 741.9
with hydrocephalus 741.0
strangulated (*see also* Hernia, by site, with obstruction) 552.9
gangrenous (with obstruction) (*see also* Hernia, by site, with gangrene) 551.9
supraumbilicus (linea alba)—*see* Hernia, epigastric
tendon 727.9
testis (nontraumatic) 095.8
Treitz's (fossa) 553.8
with
gangrene (obstructed) 551.8
obstruction 552.8
and gangrene 551.8
tunica
albuginea 608.89
vaginalis 752.8
umbilicus, umbilical 553.1
with
gangrene (obstructed) 551.1
obstruction 552.1
and gangrene 551.1
ureter 593.89
with obstruction 593.4
uterus 621.8
pregnant 654.4
vaginal (posterior) 618.6
Velpeau's (femoral) (*see also* Hernia, femoral) 553.00
ventral 553.20
with
gangrene (obstructed) 551.20
obstruction 552.20
and gangrene 551.20
recurrent 553.21
with
gangrene (obstructed) 551.21
obstruction 552.21
and gangrene 551.21
vesical
congenital (female) (male) 753.8
female 618.0
male 596.8
vitreous (into anterior chamber) 379.21
traumatic 871.1
Herniation —*see also* Hernia
brain (stem) 348.4
cerebral 348.4
gastric mucosa (into duodenal bulb) 537.89
mediastinum 519.3
nucleus pulposus—*see* Displacement, intervertebral disc
Herpangina 074.0

Herpes, herpetic 054.9
auricularis (zoster) 053.71
simplex 054.73
blepharitis (zoster) 053.20
simplex 054.41
circinate 110.5
circinatus 110.5
bullous 694.5
conjunctiva (simplex) 054.43
zoster 053.21
cornea (simplex) 054.43
disciform (simplex) 054.43
zoster 053.21
encephalitis 054.3
eye (zoster) 053.29
simplex 054.40
eyelid (zoster) 053.20
simplex 054.41
febrilis 054.9
fever 054.9
geniculate ganglionitis 053.11
genital, genitalis 054.10
specified site NEC 054.19
gestationis 646.8
gingivostomatitis 054.2
iridocyclitis (simplex) 054.44
zoster 053.22
iris (any site) 695.1
iritis (simplex) 054.44
keratitis (simplex) 054.43
dendritic 054.42
disciform 054.43
interstitial 054.43
zoster 053.21
keratoconjunctivitis (simplex) 054.43
zoster 053.21
labialis 054.9
meningococcal 036.89
lip 054.9
meningitis (simplex) 054.72
zoster 053.0
ophthalmicus (zoster) 053.20
simplex 054.40
otitis externa (zoster) 053.71
simplex 054.73
penis 054.13
perianal 054.10
pharyngitis 054.79
progenitalis 054.10
scrotum 054.19
septicemia 054.5
simplex 054.9
complicated 054.8
ophthalmic 054.40
specified NEC 054.49
specified NEC 054.79
congenital 771.2
external ear 054.73
keratitis 054.43
dendritic 054.42
meningitis 054.72
neuritis 054.79
specified complication NEC 054.79
ophthalmic 054.49
visceral 054.71
stomatitis 054.2
tonsurans 110.0
maculosus (of Hebra) 696.3
visceral 054.71
vulva 054.12
Herpes, herpetic—*continued*
vulvovaginitis 054.11
whitlow 054.6
zoster 053.9
auricularis 053.71
complicated 053.8
specified NEC 053.79
conjunctiva 053.21
cornea 053.21
ear 053.71
eye 053.29
geniculate 053.11
keratitis 053.21
interstitial 053.21
neuritis 053.10
ophthalmicus(a) 053.20
oticus 053.71
otitis externa 053.71
specified complication NEC 053.79
specified site NEC 053.9
zosteriform, intermediate type 053.9
Herrick's
anemia (hemoglobin S disease) 282.61
syndrome (hemoglobin S disease) 282.61
Hers' disease (glycogenosis VI) 271.0
Herter's infantilism (nontropical sprue) 579.0
Herter (-Gee) disease or syndrome (nontropical sprue) 579.0
Herxheimer's disease (diffuse idiopathic cutaneous atrophy) 701.8
Herxheimer's reaction 995.0
Hesselbach's hernia —*see* Hernia, Hesselbach's
Heterochromia (congenital) 743.46
acquired 364.53
cataract 366.33
cyclitis 364.21
hair 704.3
iritis 364.21
retained metallic foreign body 360.62
magnetic 360.52
uveitis 364.21
Heterophoria 378.40
alternating 378.45
vertical 378.43
Heterophyes, small intestine 121.6
Heterophyiasis 121.6
Heteropsia 368.8
Heterotopia, heterotopic —*see also* Malposition, congenital
cerebralis 742.4
pancreas, pancreatic 751.7
spinalis 742.59
Heterotropia 378.30
intermittent 378.20
vertical 378.31
vertical (constant) (intermittent) 378.31
Heubner's disease 094.89
Heubner-Herter disease or syndrome (nontropical sprue) 579.0
Hexadactylism 755.00
Heyd's syndrome (hepatorenal) 572.4
Hibernoma (M8880/0)—*see* Lipoma
Hiccough 786.8
epidemic 078.89
psychogenic 306.1
Hiccup (*see also* Hiccough) 786.8
Hicks (-Braxton) contractures 644.1
Hidradenitis (axillaris) (suppurative) 705.83

Hidradenoma (nodular) (M8400/0)—*see also* Neoplasm, skin, benign
clear cell (M8402/0)—*see* Neoplasm, skin, benign
papillary (M8405/0)—*see* Neoplasm, skin, benign
Hidrocystoma (M8404/0)—*see* Neoplasm, skin, benign
High
A_2 anemia 282.4
altitude effects 993.2
anoxia 993.2
on
ears 993.0
sinuses 993.1
polycythemia 289.0
arch
foot 755.67
palate 750.26
artery (arterial) tension (*see also* Hypertension) 401.9
without diagnosis of hypertension 796.2
basal metabolic rate (BMR) 794.7
blood pressure (*see also* Hypertension) 401.9
incidental reading (isolated) (nonspecific), no diagnosis of hypertension 796.2
compliance bladder 596.4
diaphragm (congenital) 756.6
frequency deafness (congenital) (regional) 389.8
head at term 652.5
affecting fetus or newborn 763.1
causing obstructed labor 660.0
affecting fetus or newborn 763.1
output failure (cardiac) (*see also* Failure, heart) 428.9
oxygen-affinity hemoglobin 289.0
palate 750.26
risk
behavior —*see* Problem
family situation V61.9
specified circumstance NEC V61.8
individual NEC V62.89
infant NEC V20.1
patient taking drugs (prescribed) V67.51
nonprescribed (*see also* Abuse, drugs, nondependent) 305.9
pregnancy V23.9
inadequate prenatal care V23.7
specified problem NEC V23.8
temperature (of unknown origin) (*see also* Pyrexia) 780.6
thoracic rib 756.3
Hildenbrand's disease (typhus) 081.9
Hilger's syndrome 337.0
Hill diarrhea 579.1
Hilliard's lupus (*see also* Tuberculosis) 017.0
Hilum —*see* condition
Hip —*see* condition
Hippel's disease (retinocerebral angiomatosis) 759.6
Hippus 379.49
Hirschfeld's disease (acute diabetes mellitus) (*see also* Diabetes) 250.0
Hirschsprung's disease or megacolon (congenital) 751.3
Hirsuties (*see also* Hypertrichosis) 704.1
Hirsutism (*see also* Hypertrichosis) 704.1
Hirudiniasis (external) (internal) 134.2
His-Werner disease (trench fever) 083.1
Hiss-Russell dysentery 004.1
Histamine cephalgia 346.2
Histidinemia 270.5
Histidinuria 270.5
Histiocytoma (M8832/0)—*see also* Neoplasm, skin, benign
fibrous (M8830/0)—*see also* Neoplasm, skin, benign
atypical (M8830/1)—*see* Neoplasm, connective tissue, uncertain behavior
malignant (M8830/0)—*see* Neoplasm, connective tissue, malignant
Histiocytosis (acute) (chronic) (subacute) 277.8
acute differentiated progressive (M9722/3) 202.5
cholesterol 277.8
essential 277.8
lipid, lipoid (essential) 272.7
lipochrome (familial) 288.1
malignant (M9720/3) 202.3
X (chronic) 277.8
acute (progressive) (M9722/3) 202.5
Histoplasmosis 115.90
with
endocarditis 115.94
meningitis 115.91
pericarditis 115.93
pneumonia 115.95
retinitis 115.92
specified manifestation NEC 115.99
African (due to Histoplasma duboisii) 115.10
with
endocarditis 115.14
meningitis 115.11
pericarditis 115.13
pneumonia 115.15
retinitis 115.12
specified manifestation NEC 115.19
American (due to Histoplasma capsulatum) 115.00
with
endocarditis 115.04
meningitis 115.01
pericarditis 115.03
pneumonia 115.05
retinitis 115.02
specified manifestation NEC 115.09
Darling's—*see* Histoplasmosis, American
large form (*see also* Histoplasmosis, African) 115.10
lung 115.05
small form (*see also* Histoplasmosis, American) 115.00
History (personal) of
affective psychosis V11.1
alcoholism V11.3
specified as drinking problem (*see also* Abuse, drugs, nondependent) 305.0
allergy to
analgesic agent NEC V14.6
anesthetic NEC V14.4
antibiotic agent NEC V14.1
penicillin V14.0
anti-infective agent NEC V14.3
diathesis V15.0
drug V14.9
specified type NEC V14.8
medicinal agents V14.9
specified type NEC V14.8
narcotic agent NEC V14.5
penicillin V14.0
radiographic dye V15.0
serum V14.7
specified nonmedicinal agents NEC V15.0
sulfa V14.2
sulfonamides V14.2

History—*continued*
therapeutic agent NEC V15.0
vaccine V14.7
anemia V12.3
arthritis V13.4
blood disease V12.3
calculi, urinary V13.01
cardiovascular disease V12.50
myocardial infarction 412
child abuse V61.21
cigarette smoking V15.82
circulatory system disease V12.50
myocardial infarction 412
congenital malformation V13.6
contraception V15.7
diathesis, allergic V15.0
digestive system disease V12.70
peptic ulcer V12.71
polyps, colonic V12.72
specified NEC V12.79
disease (of) V13.9
blood V12.3
blood-forming organs V12.3
cardiovascular system V12.50
circulatory system V12.50
digestive system V12.70
peptic ulcer V12.71
polyps, colonic V12.72
specified NEC V12.79
infectious V12.00
malaria V12.03
poliomyelitis V12.02
specified NEC V12.09
tuberculosis V12.01
parasitic V12.00
specified NEC V12.09
respiratory system V12.6
skin V13.3
specified site NEC V13.8
subcutaneous tissue V13.3
trophoblastic V13.1
affecting management of pregnancy V23.1
disorder (of) V13.9
endocrine V12.2
genital system V13.2
hematological V12.3
immunity V12.2
mental V11.9
affective type V11.1
manic-depressive V11.1
neurosis V11.2
schizophrenia V11.0
specified type NEC V11.8
metabolic V12.2
musculoskeletal NEC V13.5
nervous system V12.4
obstetric V13.2
affecting management of current pregnancy V23.4
sense organs V12.4
specified site NEC V13.8
urinary system V13.00
calculi V13.01
specified NEC V13.09
drug use
nonprescribed (*see also* Abuse, drugs, nondependent) 305.9
patent (*see also* Abuse, drugs, nondependent) 305.9

History—*continued*
effect NEC of external cause V15.89
embolism (pulmonary) V12.51
endocrine disorder V12.2
family
allergy V19.6
anemia V18.2
arteriosclerosis V17.4
arthritis V17.7
asthma V17.5
blindness V19.0
blood disorder NEC V18.3
cardiovascular disease V17.4
cerebrovascular disease V17.1
chronic respiratory condition NEC V17.6
congenital anomalies V19.5
consanguinity V19.7
coronary artery disease V17.3
cystic fibrosis V18.1
deafness V19.2
diabetes mellitus V18.0
digestive disorders V18.5
disease or disorder (of)
allergic V19.6
blood NEC V18.3
cardiovascular NEC V17.4
cerebrovascular V17.1
coronary artery V17.3
digestive V18.5
ear NEC V19.3
endocrine V18.1
eye NEC V19.1
genitourinary NEC V18.7
hypertensive V17.4
infectious V18.8
ischemic heart V17.3
kidney V18.6
mental V17.0
metabolic V18.1
musculoskeletal NEC V17.8
neurological NEC V17.2
parasitic V18.8
psychiatric condition V17.0
skin condition V19.4
ear disorder NEC V19.1
endocrine disease V18.1
epilepsy V17.2
eye disorder NEC V19.1
genitourinary disease NEC V18.7
glomerulonephritis V18.6
gout V18.1
hay fever V17.6
hearing loss V19.2
hematopoietic neoplasia V16.7
Hodgkin's disease V16.7
Huntington's chorea V17.2
hydrocephalus V19.5
hypertension V17.4
infectious disease V18.8
ischemic heart disease V17.3
kidney disease V18.6
leukemia V16.6
lymphatic malignant neoplasia NEC V16.7
malignant neoplasm (of) NEC V16.9
anorectal V16.0
anus V16.0
appendix V16.0
bladder V16.5
bone V16.8
brain V16.8
breast V16.3
male V16.8

History—*continued*
rectosigmoid junction V10.06
rectum V10.06
respiratory organs NEC V10.20
salivary gland V10.02
skin V10.83
melanoma V10.82
small intestine NEC V10.09
soft tissue NEC V10.89
specified site NEC V10.89
stomach V10.04
testis V10.47
thymus V10.29
thyroid V10.87
tongue V10.01
trachea V10.12
ureter V10.59
urethra V10.59
urinary organ V10.50
uterine adnexa V10.44
uterus V10.42
vagina V10.44
vulva V10.44
manic-depressive psychosis V11.1
mental disorder V11.9
affective type V11.1
manic-depressive V11.1
neurosis V11.2
schizophrenia V11.0
specified type NEC V11.8
metabolic disorder V12.2
musculoskeletal disorder NEC V13.5
myocardial infarction 412
nervous system disorder V12.4
neurosis V11.2
noncompliance with medical treatment V15.81
nutritional deficiency V12.1
obstetric disorder V13.2
affecting management of current pregnancy V23.4
parasitic disease V12.00
specified NEC V12.09
perinatal problems V13.7
poisoning V15.6
poliomyelitis V12.02
polyps, colonic V12.72
poor obstetric V23.4
psychiatric disorder V11.9
affective type V11.1
manic-depressive V11.1
neurosis V11.2
schizophrenia V11.0
specified type NEC V11.8
psychological trauma V15.4
psychoneurosis V11.2
radiation therapy V15.3
respiratory system disease V12.6
reticulosarcoma V10.71
schizophrenia V11.0
skin disease V13.3
smoking (tobacco) V15.82
subcutaneous tissue disease V13.3
surgery (major) to
great vessels V15.1
heart V15.1
major organs NEC V15.2
thrombophlebitis V12.52
thrombosis V12.51
tobacco use V15.82
trophoblastic disease V13.1
affecting management of pregnancy V23.1

History—*continued*
tuberculosis V12.01
ulcer, peptic V12.71
urinary system disorder V13.00
calculi V13.01
specified NEC V13.09
HIV infection (disease) (illness)—*see* Human immunodeficiency virus (disease) (illness) (infection)
Hives (bold) (*see also* Urticaria) 708.9
Hoarseness 784.49
Hobnail liver —*see* Cirrhosis, portal
Hobo, hoboism V60.0
Hodgkin's
disease (M9650/3) 201.9
lymphocytic
depletion (M9653/3) 201.7
diffuse fibrosis (M9654/3) 201.7
reticular type (M9655/3) 201.7
predominance (M9651/3) 201.4
lymphocytic-histiocytic predominance (M9651/3) 201.4
mixed cellularity (M9652/3) 201.6
nodular sclerosis (M9656/3) 201.5
cellular phase (M9657/3) 201.5
granuloma (M9661/3) 201.1
lymphogranulomatosis (M9650/3) 201.9
lymphoma (M9650/3) 201.9
lymphosarcoma (M9650/3) 201.9
paragranuloma (M9660/3) 201.0
sarcoma (M9662/3) 201.2
Hodgson's disease (aneurysmal dilatation of aorta) 441.9
ruptured 441.5
Hodi-potsy 111.0
Hoffa -(Kastert) disease or syndrome (liposynovitis prepatellaris) 272.8
Hoffmann's syndrome 244.9 *[359.5]*
Hoffmann-Bouveret syndrome (paroxysmal tachycardia) 427.2
Hole
macula 362.54
optic disc, crater-like 377.22
retina (macula) 362.54
round 361.31
with detachment 361.01
Holla disease (*see also* Spherocytosis) 282.0
Holländer-Simons syndrome (progressive lipodystrophy) 272.6
Hollow foot (congenital) 754.71
acquired 736.73
Holmes' syndrome (visual disorientation) 368.16
Holoprosencephaly 742.2
due to
trisomy 13 758.1
trisomy 18 758.2
Holthouse's hernia —*see* Hernia, inguinal
Homesickness 309.89
Homocystinemia 270.4
Homocystinuria 270.4
Homologous serum jaundice (prophylactic) (therapeutic)—*see* Hepatitis, viral
Homosexuality —*omit code*
ego-dystonic 302.0
pedophilic 302.2
problems with 302.0
Homozygous Hb-S disease 282.61
Honeycomb lung 518.89
congenital 748.4
Hong Kong ear 117.3
HOOD (hereditary osteo-onychodysplasia) 756.89

Hooded
clitoris 752.49
penis 752.8
Hookworm (anemia) (disease) (infestation)—*see* Ancylostomiasis
Hoppe-Goldflam syndrome 358.0
Hordeolum (external) (eyelid) 373.11
internal 373.12
Horn
cutaneous 702.8
cheek 702.8
eyelid 702.8
penis 702.8
iliac 756.89
nail 703.8
congenital 757.5
papillary 700
Horner's
syndrome (*see also* Neuropathy, peripheral, autonomic) 337.9
traumatic 954.0
teeth 520.4
Horseshoe kidney (congenital) 753.3
Horton's
disease (temporal arteritis) 446.5
headache or neuralgia 346.2
Hospitalism (in children) NEC 309.83
Hourglass contraction, contracture
bladder 596.8
gallbladder 575.2
congenital 751.69
stomach 536.8
congenital 750.7
psychogenic 306.4
uterus 661.4
affecting fetus or newborn 763.7
Household circumstance affecting care V60.9
specified type NEC V60.8
Housemaid's knee 727.2
Housing circumstance affecting care V60.9
specified type NEC V60.8
Huchard's disease (continued arterial hypertension) 401.9
Hudson-Stähli lines 371.11
Huguier's disease (uterine fibroma) 218.9
Hum, venous —*omit code*
Human bite (open wound)—*see also* Wound, open, by site
intact skin surface—*see* Contusion
Human immunovirus (disease) (illness) (infection)—*see* Human immunodeficiency virus (disease) (illness) (infection)
Human immunodeficiency virus (disease) (illness) 042
infection V08
with symptoms, symptomatic 042
Human immunodeficiency virus-2 infection 079.53
Human T-cell lymphotrophic virus I infection 079.51
Human T-cell lymphotrophic virus II infection 079.52
Human T-cell lymphotropic virus-III (disease) (illness) (infection)—*see* Human immunodeficiency virus (disease) (illness) (infection)
HTLV-I infection 079.51
HTLV-II infection 079.52
HTLV-III (disease) (illness) (infection)—*see* Human immunodeficiency virus (disease) (illness) (infection)
HTLV-III/LAV
(disease) (illness) (infection)—*see* Human immunodeficiency virus (disease) (illness) (infection)
Humpback (acquired) 737.9
congenital 756.19
Hunchback (acquired) 737.9
congenital 756.19
Hunger 994.2
air, psychogenic 306.1
disease 251.1
Hunner's ulcer (*see also* **Cystitis) 595.1**
Hunt's
neuralgia 053.11
syndrome (herpetic geniculate ganglionitis) 053.11
dyssynergia cerebellaris myoclonica 334.2
Hunter's glossitis 529.4
Hunter (-Hurler) syndrome (mucopolysaccharidosis II) 277.5
Hunterian chancre 091.0
Huntington's
chorea 333.4
disease 333.4
Huppert's disease (multiple myeloma) (M9730/3) 203.0
Hurler (-Hunter) disease or syndrome (mucopolysaccharidosis II) 277.5
Hürthle cell
adenocarcinoma (M8290/3) 193
adenoma (M8290/0) 226
carcinoma (M8290/3) 193
tumor (M8290/0) 226
Hutchinson's
disease meaning
angioma serpiginosum 709.1
cheiropompholyx 705.81
prurigo estivalis 692.72
summer eruption, or summer prurigo 692.72
incisors 090.5
melanotic freckle (M8742/2)—*see also* Neoplasm, skin, in situ
malignant melanoma in (M8742/3)—*see* Melanoma
teeth or incisors (congenital syphilis) 090.5
Hutchinson-Boeck disease or syndrome (sarcoidosis) 135
Hutchinson-Gilford disease or syndrome (progeria) 259.8
Hyaline
degeneration (diffuse) (generalized) 728.9
localized—*see* Degeneration, by site
membrane (disease) (lung) (newborn) 769
Hyalinosis cutis et mucosae 272.8
Hyalin plaque, sclera, senile 379.16
Hyalitis (asteroid) 379.22
syphilitic 095.8
Hydatid
cyst or tumor—*see also* Echinococcus
fallopian tube 752.11
mole—*see* Hydatidiform mole
Morgagni (congenital) 752.8
fallopian tube 752.11
Hydatidiform mole (benign) (complicating pregnancy) (delivered) (undelivered) 630
invasive (M9100/1) 236.1
malignant (M9100/1) 236.1
previous, affecting management of pregnancy V23.1
Hydatidosis —*see* Echinococcus
Hyde's disease (prurigo nodularis) 698.3

Hydradenitis 705.83
Hydradenoma (M8400/0)—*see* Hidradenoma
Hydralazine lupus or syndrome
correct substance properly administered 695.4
overdose or wrong substance given or taken 972.6
Hydramnios 657
affecting fetus or newborn 761.3
Hydrancephaly 742.3
with spina bifida (*see also* Spina bifida) 741.0
Hydranencephaly 742.3
with spina bifida (*see also* Spina bifida) 741.0
Hydrargyrism NEC 985.0
Hydrarthrosis (*see also* Effusion, joint) 719.0
gonococcal 098.50
intermittent (*see also* Rheumatism, palindromic) 719.3
of yaws (early) (late) 102.6
syphilitic 095.8
congenital 090.5
Hydremia 285.9
Hydrencephalocele (congenital) 742.0
Hydrencephalomeningocele (congenital) 742.0
Hydroa 694.0
aestivale 692.72
gestationis 646.8
herpetiformis 694.0
pruriginosa 694.0
vacciniforme 692.72
Hydroadenitis 705.83
Hydrocalycosis (*see also* Hydronephrosis) 591
congenital 753.2
Hydrocalyx (*see also* Hydronephrosis) 591
Hydrocele (calcified) (chylous) (idiopathic) (infantile) (inguinal canal) (recurrent) (senile) (spermatic cord) (testis) (tunica vaginalis) 603.9
canal of Nuck (female) 629.1
male 603.9
congenital 778.6
encysted 603.0
congenital 778.6
female NEC 629.8
infected 603.1
round ligament 629.8
specified type NEC 603.8
congenital 778.6
spinalis (*see also* Spina bifida) 741.9
vulva 624.8
Hydrocephalic fetus
affecting management of pregnancy 655.0
causing disproportion 653.6
with obstructed labor 660.1
affecting fetus or newborn 763.1
Hydrocephalus (acquired) (external) (internal) (malignant) (noncommunicating) (obstructive) (recurrent) 331.4
aqueduct of Sylvius stricture 742.3
with spina bifida (*see also* Spina bifida) 741.0
chronic 742.3
with spina bifida (*see also* Spina bifida) 741.0
communicating 331.3
congenital (external) (internal) 742.3
with spina bifida (*see also* Spina bifida) 741.0
due to
stricture of aqueduct of Sylvius 742.3
with spina bifida (*see also* Spina bifida) 741.0
toxoplasmosis (congenital) 771.2
fetal affecting management of pregnancy 655.0
Hydrocephalus—*continued*
foramen Magendie block (acquired) 331.3
congenital 742.3
with spina bifida (*see also* Spina bifida) 741.0
newborn 742.3
with spina bifida (*see also* Spina bifida) 741.0
otitic 331.4
syphilitic, congenital 090.49
tuberculous (*see also* Tuberculosis) 013.8
Hydrocolpos (congenital) 623.8
Hydrocystoma (M8404/0)—*see* Neoplasm, skin, benign
Hydroencephalocele (congenital) 742.0
Hydroencephalomeningocele (congenital) 742.0
Hydrohematopneumothorax (*see also* Hemothorax) 511.8
Hydromeningitis —*see* Meningitis
Hydromeningocele (spinal) (*see also* Spina bifida) 741.9
cranial 742.0
Hydrometra 621.8
Hydrometrocolpos 623.8
Hydromicrocephaly 742.1
Hydromphalus (congenital) (since birth) 757.39
Hydromyelia 742.53
Hydromyelocele (*see also* Spina bifida) 741.9
Hydronephrosis 591
atrophic 591
congenital 753.2
due to S. hematobium 120.0
early 591
functionless (infected) 591
infected 591
intermittent 591
primary 591
secondary 591
tuberculous (*see also* Tuberculosis) 016.0
Hydropericarditis (*see also* Pericarditis) 423.9
Hydropericardium (*see also* Pericarditis) 423.9
Hydroperitoneum 789.5
Hydrophobia 071
Hydrophthalmos (*see also* Buphthalmia) 743.20
Hydropneumohemothorax (*see also* Hemothorax) 511.8
Hydropneumopericarditis (*see also* Pericarditis) 423.9
Hydropneumopericardium (*see also* Pericarditis) 423.9
Hydropneumothorax 511.8
nontuberculous 511.8
bacterial 511.1
pneumococcal 511.1
staphylococcal 511.1
streptococcal 511.1
traumatic 860.0
with open wound into thorax 860.1
tuberculous (*see also* Tuberculosis, pleural) 012.0
Hydrops 782.3
abdominis 789.5
amnii (complicating pregnancy) (*see also* Hydramnios) 657
articulorum intermittens (*see also* Rheumatism, palindromic) 719.3
cardiac (*see also* Failure, heart, congestive) 428.0
congenital—*see* Hydrops, fetalis
endolymphatic (*see also* Disease, Ménière's) 386.00

Hydrops—*continued*
fetal(is) or newborn 778.0
due to isoimmunization 773.3
not due to isoimmunization 778.0
gallbladder 575.3
idiopathic (fetus or newborn) 778.0
joint (*see also* Effusion, joint) 719.0
labyrinth (*see also* Disease, Ménière's) 386.00
meningeal NEC 331.4
nutritional 262
pericardium—*see* Pericarditis
pleura (*see also* Hydrothorax) 511.8
renal (*see also* Nephrosis) 581.9
spermatic cord (*see also* Hydrocele) 603.9
Hydropyonephrosis (*see also* Pyelitis) 590.80
chronic 590.00
Hydrorachis 742.53
Hydrorrhea (nasal) 478.1
gravidarum 658.1
pregnancy 658.1
Hydrosadenitis 705.83
Hydrosalpinx (fallopian tube) (follicularis) 614.1
Hydrothorax (double) (pleural) 511.8
chylous (nonfilarial) 457.8
filaria (*see also* Infestation, filarial) 125.9
nontuberculous 511.8
bacterial 511.1
pneumococcal 511.1
staphylococcal 511.1
streptococcal 511.1
traumatic 862.29
with open wound into thorax 862.39
tuberculous (*see also* Tuberculosis, pleura) 012.0
Hydroureter 593.5
congenital 753.2
Hydroureteronephrosis (*see also* Hydronephrosis) 591
Hydrourethra 599.84
Hydroxykynureninuria 270.2
Hydroxyprolinemia 270.8
Hydroxyprolinuria 270.8
Hygroma (congenital) (cystic) (M9173/0) 228.1
prepatellar 727.3
subdural—*see* Hematoma, subdural
Hymen —*see* condition
Hymenolepiasis (diminuta) (infection) (infestation) (nana) 123.6
Hymenolepis (diminuta) (infection) (infestation) (nana) 123.6
Hypalgesia (*see also* Disturbance, sensation) 782.0
Hyperabduction syndrome 447.8
Hyperacidity, gastric 536.8
psychogenic 306.4
Hyperactive, hyperactivity
basal cell, uterine cervix 622.1
bladder 596.51
bowel (syndrome) 564.1
sounds 787.5
cervix epithelial (basal) 622.1
child 314.01
colon 564.1
gastrointestinal 536.8
psychogenic 306.4
intestine 564.1
labyrinth (unilateral) 386.51
with loss of labyrinthine reactivity 386.58
bilateral 386.52
nasal mucous membrane 478.1
stomach 536.8
thyroid (gland) (*see also* Thyrotoxicosis) 242.9
Hyperacusis 388.42
Hyperadrenalism (cortical) 255.3
medullary 255.6
Hyperadrenocorticism 255.3
congenital 255.2
iatrogenic
correct substance properly administered 255.3
overdose or wrong substance given or taken 962.0
Hyperaffectivity 301.11
Hyperaldosteronism (atypical) (hyperplastic) (normoaldosteronal) (normotensive) (primary) (secondary) 255.1
Hyperalgesia (*see also* Disturbance, sensation) 782.0
Hyperalimentation 783.6
carotene 278.3
specified NEC 278.8
vitamin A 278.2
vitamin D 278.4
Hyperaminoaciduria 270.9
arginine 270.6
citrulline 270.6
cystine 270.0
glycine 270.0
lysine 270.7
ornithine 270.6
renal (types I, II, III) 270.0
Hyperammonemia (congenital) 270.6
Hyperamnesia 780.9
Hyperamylasemia 790.5
Hyperaphia 782.0
Hyperazotemia 791.9
Hyperbetalipoproteinemia (acquired) (essential) (familial) (hereditary) (primary) (secondary) 272.0
with prebetalipoproteinemia 272.2
Hyperbilirubinemia 782.4
congenital 277.4
constitutional 277.4
neonatal (transient) (*see also* Jaundice, fetus or newborn) 774.6
of prematurity 774.2
Hyperbilirubinemica encephalopathia, newborn 774.7
due to isoimmunization 773.4
Hypercalcemia, hypercalcemic (idiopathic) 275.4
nephropathy 588.8
Hypercalcinuria 275.4
Hypercapnia 786.09
with mixed acid-base disorder 276.4
Hypercarotinemia 278.3
Hypercementosis 521.5
Hyperchloremia 276.9
Hyperchlorhydria 536.8
neurotic 306.4
psychogenic 306.4
Hypercholesterinemia —*see* Hypercholesterolemia
Hypercholesterolemia 272.0
with hyperglyceridemia, endogenous 272.2
essential 272.0
familial 272.0
hereditary 272.0
primary 272.0
pure 272.0
Hypercholesterolosis 272.0
Hyperchylia gastricsa 536.8
psychogenic 306.4
Hyperchylomicronemia (familial) (with hyperbetalipoproteinemia) 272.3

Hypercoagulation syndrome 289.8
Hypercorticosteronism
correct substance properly administered 255.3
overdose or wrong substance given or taken 962.0
Hypercortisonism
correct substance properly administered 255.3
overdose or wrong substance given or taken 962.0
Hyperdynamic beta-adrenergic state or syndrome (circulatory) 429.82
Hyperelectrolytemia 276.9
Hyperemesis 536.2
arising during pregnancy—*see* Hyperemesis, gravidarum
gravidarum (mild) (before 22 completed weeks gestation) 643.0
with
carbohydrate depletion 643.1
dehydration 643.1
electrolyte imbalance 643.1
metabolic disturbance 643.1
affecting fetus or newborn 761.8
severe (with metabolic disturbance) 643.1
psychogenic 306.4
Hyperemia (acute) 780.9
anal mucosa 569.49
bladder 596.7
cerebral 437.8
conjunctiva 372.71
ear, internal, acute 386.30
enteric 564.8
eye 372.71
eyelid (active) (passive) 374.82
intestine 564.8
iris 364.41
kidney 593.81
labyrinth 386.30
liver (active) (passive) 573.8
lung 514
ovary 620.8
passive 780.9
pulmonary 514
renal 593.81
retina 362.89
spleen 289.59
stomach 537.89
Hyperesthesia (body surface) (*see also* Disturbance, sensation) 782.0
larynx (reflex) 478.79
hysterical 300.11
pharynx (reflex) 478.29
Hyperestrinism 256.0
Hyperestrogenism 256.0
Hyperestrogenosis 256.0
Hyperextension, joint 718.80
ankle 718.87
elbow 718.82
foot 718.87
hand 718.84
hip 718.85
knee 718.86
multiple sites 718.89
pelvic region 718.85
shoulder (region) 718.81
specified site NEC 718.88
wrist 718.83
Hyperfibrinolysis —*see* Fibrinolysis
Hyperfolliculinism 256.0
Hyperfructosemia 271.2
Hyperfunction
adrenal (cortex) 255.3
androgenic, acquired benign 255.3
medulla 255.6
virilism 255.2
corticoadrenal NEC 255.3
labyrinth—*see* Hyperactive, labyrinth
medulloadrenal 255.6
ovary 256.1
estrogen 256.0
pancreas 577.8
parathyroid (gland) 252.0
pituitary (anterior) (gland) (lobe) 253.1
testicular 257.0
Hypergammaglobulinemia 289.8
monoclonal, benign (BMH) 273.1
polyclonal 273.0
Waldenström's 273.0
Hyperglobulinemia 273.8
Hyperglycemia 790.6
maternal
affecting fetus or newborn 775.0
manifest diabetes in infant 775.1
postpancreatectomy (complete) (partial) 251.3
Hyperglyceridemia 272.1
endogenous 272.1
essential 272.1
familial 272.1
hereditary 272.1
mixed 272.3
pure 272.1
Hyperglycinemia 270.7
Hypergonadism
ovarian 256.1
testicular (infantile) (primary) 257.0
Hyperheparinemia (*see also* Circulating anticoagulants) 286.5
Hyperhidrosis, hyperidrosis 780.8
psychogenic 306.3
Hyperhistidinemia 270.5
Hyperinsulinism (ectopic) (functional) (organic) NEC 251.1
iatrogenic 251.0
reactive 251.2
spontaneous 251.2
therapeutic misadventure (from administration of insulin) 962.3
Hyperiodemia 276.9
Hyperirritability (cerebral), in newborn 779.1
Hyperkalemia 276.7
Hyperkeratosis (*see also* Keratosis) 701.1
cervix 622.1
congenital 757.39
cornea 371.89
due to yaws (early) (late) (palmar or plantar) 102.3
eccentrica 757.39
figurata centrifuga atrophica 757.39
follicularis 757.39
in cutem penetrans 701.1
limbic (cornea) 371.89
palmoplantaris climacterica 701.1
pinta (carate) 103.1
senile (with pruritus) 702.0
tongue 528.7
universalis congenita 757.1
vagina 623.1
vocal cord 478.5
vulva 624.0

Hyperkinesia, hyperkinetic (disease) (reaction) (syndrome) 314.9
with
attention deficit —*see* Disorder, attention deficit
conduct disorder 314.2
developmental delay 314.1
simple disturbance of activity and attention 314.01
specified manifestation NEC 314.8
heart (disease) 429.82
of childhood or adolescence NEC 314.9
Hyperlacrimation (*see also* Epiphora) 375.20
Hyperlipemia (*see also* Hyperlipidemia) 272.4
Hyperlipidemia 272.4
carbohydrate-induced 272.1
combined 272.4
endogenous 272.1
exogenous 272.3
fat-induced 272.3
group
A 272.0
B 272.1
C 272.2
D 272.3
mixed 272.2
specified type NEC 272.4
Hyperlipidosis 272.7
hereditary 272.7
Hyperlipoproteinemia (acquired) (essential) (familial) (hereditary) (primary) (secondary) 272.4
Fredrickson type
I 272.3
IIa 272.0
IIb 272.2
III 272.2
IV 272.1
V 272.3
low-density-lipoid-type (LDL) 272.0
very-low-density-lipoid-type [VLDL] 272.1
Hyperlucent lung, unilateral 492.8
Hyperluteinization 256.1
Hyperlysinemia 270.7
Hypermagnesemia 275.2
neonatal 775.5
Hypermaturity (fetus or newborn) 766.2
Hypermenorrhea 626.2
Hypermetabolism 794.7
Hypermethioninemia 270.4
Hypermetropia (congenital) 367.0
Hypermobility
cecum 564.1
coccyx 724.71
colon 564.1
psychogenic 306.4
ileum 564.8
joint (acquired) 718.80
ankle 718.87
elbow 718.82
foot 718.87
hand 718.84
hip 718.85
knee 718.86
multiple sites 718.89
pelvic region 718.85
shoulder (region) 718.81
specified site NEC 718.88
wrist 718.83
Hypermobility—*continued*
kidney, congenital 753.3
meniscus (knee) 717.5
scapula 718.81
stomach 536.8
psychogenic 306.4
syndrome 728.5
testis, congenital 752.5
urethral 599.81
Hypermotility
gastrointestinal 536.8
intestine 564.1
psychogenic 306.4
stomach 536.8
Hypernasality 784.49
Hypernatremia 276.0
with water depletion 276.0
Hypernephroma (M8312/3) 189.0
Hyperopia 367.0
Hyperorexia 783.6
Hyperornithinemia 270.6
Hyperosmia (*see also* Disturbance, sensation) 781.1
Hyperosmolality 276.0
Hyperosteogenesis 733.99
Hyperostosis 733.99
calvarial 733.3
cortical 733.3
infantile 756.59
frontal, internal of skull 733.3
interna frontalis 733.3
monomelic 733.99
skull 733.3
congenital 756.0
vertebral 721.8
with spondylosis—*see* Spondylosis
ankylosing 721.6
Hyperovarianism 256.1
Hyperovarism, hyperovaria 256.1
Hyperoxaluria (primary) 271.8
Hyperoxia 987.8
Hyperparathyroidism 252.0
ectopic 259.3
secondary, of renal origin 588.8
Hyperpathia (*see also* Disturbance, sensation) 782.0
psychogenic 307.80
Hyperperistalsis 787.4
psychogenic 306.4
Hyperpermeability, capillary 448.9
Hyperphagia 783.6
Hyperphenylalaninemia 270.1
Hyperphoria 378.40
alternating 378.45
Hyperphosphatemia 275.3
Hyperpiesia (*see also* Hypertension) 401.9
Hyperpiesis (*see also* Hypertension) 401.9
Hyperpigmentation —*see* Pigmentation
Hyperpinealism 259.8
Hyperpipecolatemia 270.7
Hyperpituitarism 253.1
Hyperplasia, hyperplastic
adenoids (lymphoid tissue) 474.12
and tonsils 474.10
adrenal (capsule) (cortex) (gland) 255.8
with
sexual precocity (male) 255.2
virilism, adrenal 255.2
virilization (female) 255.2

Hyperplasia, hyperplastic—*continued*
congenital 255.2
due to excess ACTH (ectopic) (pituitary) 255.0
medulla 255.8
alpha cells (pancreatic)
with
gastrin excess 251.5
glucagon excess 251.4
appendix (lymphoid) 543.0
artery, fibromuscular NEC 447.8
carotid 447.8
renal 447.3
bone 733.99
marrow 289.9
breast (*see also* Hypertrophy, breast) 611.1
carotid artery 447.8
cementation, cementum (teeth) (tooth) 521.5
cervical gland 785.6
cervix (uteri) 622.1
basal cell 622.1
congenital 752.49
endometrium 622.1
polypoid 622.1
chin 524.05
clitoris, congenital 752.49
dentin 521.5
endocervicitis 616.0
endometrium, endometrial (adenomatous) (atypical) (cystic) (glandular) (polypoid) (uterus) 621.3
cervix 622.1
epithelial 709.8
focal, oral, including tongue 528.7
mouth (focal) 528.7
nipple 611.8
skin 709.8
tongue (focal) 528.7
vaginal wall 623.0
erythroid 289.9
fascialis ossificans (progressiva) 728.11
fibromuscular, artery NEC 447.8
carotid 447.8
renal 447.3
genital
female 629.8
male 608.89
gingiva 523.8
glandularis
cystica uteri 621.3
endometrium (uterus) 621.3
interstitialis uteri 621.3
granulocytic 288.8
gum 523.8
hymen, congenital 752.49
islands of Langerhans 251.1
islet cell (pancreatic) 251.9
alpha cells
with excess
gastrin 251.5
glucagon 251.4
beta cells 251.1
juxtaglomerular (complex) (kidney) 593.89
kidney (congenital) 753.3
liver (congenital) 751.69
lymph node (gland) 785.6
lymphoid (diffuse) (nodular) 785.6
appendix 543.0
intestine 569.89
mandibular 524.02
alveolar 524.72
unilateral condylar 526.89

Hyperplasia, hyperplastic—*continued*
Marchand multiple nodular (liver)—*see* Cirrhosis, postnecrotic
maxillary 524.01
alveolar 524.71
medulla, adrenal 255.8
myometrium, myometrial 621.2
nose (lymphoid) (polypoid) 478.1
oral soft tissue (inflammatory) (irritative) (mucosa) NEC 528.9
gingiva 523.8
tongue 529.8
organ or site, congenital NEC—*see* Anomaly, specified type NEC
ovary 620.8
palate, papillary 528.9
pancreatic islet cells 251.9
alpha
with excess
gastrin 251.5
glucagon 251.4
beta 251.1
parathyroid (gland) 252.0
persistent, vitreous (primary) 743.51
pharynx (lymphoid) 478.29
prostate (adenofibromatous) (nodular) 600
renal artery (fibromuscular) 447.3
reticuloendothelial (cell) 289.9
salivary gland (any) 527.1
Schimmelbusch's 610.1
suprarenal (capsule) (gland) 255.8
thymus (gland) (persistent) 254.0
thyroid (*see also* Goiter) 240.9
primary 242.0
secondary 242.2
tonsil (lymphoid tissue) 474.11
and adenoids 474.10
urethrovaginal 599.89
uterus, uterine (myometrium) 621.2
endometrium 621.3
vitreous (humor), primary persistent 743.51
vulva 624.3
zygoma 738.11
Hyperpnea (*see also* Hyperventilation) 786.01
Hyperpotassemia 276.7
Hyperprebetalipoproteinemia 272.1
with chylomicronemia 272.3
familial 272.1
Hyperprolactinemia 253.1
Hyperprolinemia 270.8
Hyperproteinemia 273.8
Hyperprothrombinemia 289.8
Hyperpselaphesia 782.0
Hyperpyrexia 780.6
heat (effects of) 992.0
malarial (*see also* Malaria) 084.6
malignant, due to anesthetic 995.89
rheumatic—*see* Fever, rheumatic
unknown origin (*see also* Pyrexia) 780.6
Hyperreactor, vascular 780.2
Hyperreflexia 796.1
bladder, autonomic 596.54
with cauda equina 344.61
detrusor 344.61
Hypersalivation (*see also* Ptyalism) 527.7
Hypersarcosinemia 270.8
Hypersecretion
ACTH 255.3
androgens (ovarian) 256.1
calcitonin 246.0

Hypersecretion—*continued*
corticoadrenal 255.3
cortisol 255.0
estrogen 256.0
gastric 536.8
psychogenic 306.4
gastrin 251.5
glucagon 251.4
hormone
ACTH 255.3
anterior pituitary 253.1
growth NEC 253.0
ovarian androgen 256.1
testicular 257.0
thyroid stimulating 242.8
insulin—*see* Hyperinsulinism
lacrimal glands (*see also* Epiphora) 375.20
medulloadrenal 255.6
milk 676.6
ovarian androgens 256.1
pituitary (anterior) 253.1
salivary gland (any) 527.7
testicular hormones 257.0
thyrocalcitonin 246.0
upper respiratory 478.9
Hypersegmentation, hereditary 288.2
eosinophils 288.2
neutrophil nuclei 288.2
Hypersensitive, hypersensitiveness hypersensitivity —*see also* Allergy
angiitis 446.20
specified NEC 446.29
carotid sinus 337.0
colon 564.1
psychogenic 306.4
DNA (deoxyribonucleic acid) NEC 287.2
drug (*see also* Allergy, drug) 995.2
esophagus 530.89
insect bites—*see* Injury, superficial, by site
labyrinth 386.58
pain (*see also* Disturbance, sensation) 782.0
pneumonitis NEC 495.9
reaction (*see also* Allergy) 995.3
upper respiratory tract NEC 478.8
stomach (allergic) (nonallergic) 536.8
psychogenic 306.4
Hypersomatotropism (classic) 253.0
Hypersomnia 780.54
with sleep apnea 780.53
nonorganic origin 307.43
persistent (primary) 307.44
transient 307.43
Hypersplenia 289.4
Hypersplenism 289.4
Hypersteatosis 706.3
Hypersuprarenalism 255.3
Hypersusceptibility —*see* Allergy
Hyper-TBG-nemia 246.8
Hypertelorism 756.0
orbit, orbital 376.41

"H" listing resumes after Hypertension table...

Hypertension, hypertensive

	Malignant	Benign	Unspecified
(arterial) (arteriolar) (crisis) (degeneration) (disease) (essential) (fluctuating) (idiopathic) (intermittent) (labile) (low renin) (orthostatic) (paroxysmal) (primary) (systemic) (uncontrolled) (vascular)	401.0	401.1	401.9
with			
heart involvement (conditions classifiable to 425.8, 428, 429.0-429.3, 429.8, 429.9 due to hypertension) (*see also* Hypertension, heart)	402.00	402.10	402.90
with kidney involvement—*see* Hypertension, cardiorenal			
renal involvement (only conditions classifiable to 585, 586, 587) (excludes conditions classifiable to 584) (*see also* Hypertension, kidney)	403.00	403.10	403.90
with heart involvement—*see* Hypertension, cardiorenal			
failure (and sclerosis) (*see also* Hypertension, kidney)	403.01	403.11	403.91
sclerosis without failure (*see also* Hypertension, kidney)	403.00	403.10	403.90
accelerated (*see also* Hypertension, by type, malignant)	401.0	—	—
antepartum—*see* Hypertension complicating pregnancy, childbirth, or the puerperium			
cardiorenal (disease)	404.00	404.10	404.90
with			
heart failure (congestive)	404.01	404.11	404.91
and renal failure	404.03	404.13	404.93
renal failure	404.02	404.12	404.92
and heart failure (congestive)	404.03	404.13	404.93
cardiovascular disease (arteriosclerotic) (sclerotic)	402.00	402.10	402.90
with			
heart failure (congestive)	402.01	402.11	402.91
renal involvement (conditions classifiable to 403) (*see also* Hypertension, cardiorenal)	404.00	404.10	404.90
cardiovascular renal (disease) (sclerosis) (*see also* Hypertension cardiorenal)	404.00	404.10	404.90
cerebrovascular disease NEC	437.2	437.2	437.2
complicating pregnancy, childbirth, or the puerperium	642.2	642.0	642.9
with			
albuminuria (and edema) (mild)	—	—	642.4
severe	—	—	642.5
edema (mild)	—	—	642.4
severe	—	—	642.5
heart disease	642.2	642.2	642.2
and renal disease	642.2	642.2	642.2
renal disease	642.2	642.2	642.2
and heart disease	642.2	642.2	642.2
chronic	642.2	642.0	642.0
with pre-eclampsia or eclampsia	642.7	642.7	642.7
fetus or newborn	760.0	760.0	760.0
essential	—	642.0	642.0
with pre-eclampsia or eclampsia	—	642.7	642.7
fetus or newborn	760.0	760.0	760.0
fetus or newborn	760.0	760.0	760.0
gestational	—	—	642.3
pre-existing	642.2	642.0	642.0
with pre-eclampsia or eclampsia	642.7	642.7	642.7
fetus or newborn	760.0	760.0	760.0
secondary to renal disease	642.1	642.1	642.1
with pre-eclampsia or eclampsia	642.7	642.7	642.7
fetus or newborn	760.0	760.0	760.0
transient	—	—	642.3
due to			
aldosteronism,primary	405.09	405.19	405.99
brain tumor	405.09	405.19	405.99
bulbar poliomyelitis	405.09	405.19	405.99
calculus			
kidney	405.09	405.19	405.99
ureter	405.09	405.19	405.99
coarctation, aorta	405.09	405.19	405.99
Cushing's disease	405.09	405.19	405.99
glomerulosclerosis (*see also* Hypertension, kidney)	403.00	403.10	403.90
periarteritis nodosa	405.09	405.19	405.99
pheochromocytoma	405.09	405.19	405.99
polycystic kidney(s)	405.09	405.19	405.99
polycythemia	405.09	405.19	405.99
porphyria	405.09	405.19	405.99
pyelonephritis	405.09	405.19	405.99

	Malignant	Benign	Unspecified
renal (artery)			
aneurysm	405.01	405.11	405.91
anomaly	405.01	405.11	405.91
embolism	405.01	405.11	405.91
fibromuscular hyperplasia	405.01	405.11	405.91
occlusion	405.01	405.11	405.91
stenosis	405.01	405.11	405.91
thrombosis	405.01	405.11	405.91
encephalopathy	437.2	437.2	437.2
gestational (transient) NEC	—	—	642.3
Goldblatt's	440.1	440.1	440.1
heart (disease) (conditions classifiable to 425.8, 428, 429.0-429.3, 429.8, 429.9 due to hypertension)	402.00	402.10	402.90
with			
heart failure	402.01	402.11	402.91
congestive	402.01	402.11	402.91
hypertensive kidney disease (conditions classifiable to 403) (*see also* Hypertension, cardiorenal)	404.00	404.10	404.90
renal sclerosis (*see also* Hypertension, cardiorenal)	404.00	404.10	404.90
intracranial, benign	—	348.2	—
intraocular	—	—	365.04
kidney	403.00	403.10	403.90
with			
heart involvement (conditions classifiable to 425.8, 428, 429.0-429.3, 429.8, 429.9 due to hypertension) (*see also* Hypertension cardiorenal)	404.00	404.10	404.90
hypertensive heart (disease) (conditions classifiable to 402) (*see also* Hypertension, cardiorenal)	404.00	404.10	404.90
lesser circulation	—	—	416.0
necrotizing	401.0	—	—
ocular	—	—	365.04
portal (due to chronic liver disease)	—	—	572.3
postoperative 997.91			
psychogenic	—	—	306.2
puerperal, postpartum—*see* Hypertension, complicating pregnancy, childbirth, or the puerperium			
pulmonary (artery) (idiopathic) (primary) (solitary)	—	—	416.0
with cor pulmonale (chronic)	—	—	416.8
acute	—	—	415.0
secondary	—	—	416.8
renal (disease) (*see also* Hypertension, kidney)	403.00	403.10	403.90
renovascular NEC	405.01	405.11	405.91
secondary NEC	405.09	405.19	405.99
due to			
aldosteronism, primary	405.09	405.19	405.99
brain tumor	405.09	405.19	405.99
bulbar poliomyelitis	405.09	405.19	405.99
calculus			
kidney	405.09	405.19	405.99
ureter	405.09	405.19	405.99
coarctation, aorta	405.09	405.19	405.99
Cushing's disease	405.09	405.19	405.99
glomerulosclerosis (*see also* Hypertension, kidney)	403.00	403.10	403.90
periarteritis nodosa	405.09	405.19	405.99
pheochromocytoma	405.09	405.19	405.99
polycystic kidney(s)	405.09	405.19	405.99
polycythemia	405.09	405.19	405.99
porphyria	405.09	405.19	405.99
pyelonephritis	405.09	405.19	405.99
renal (artery)			
aneurysm	405.01	405.11	405.91
anomaly	405.01	405.11	405.91
embolism	405.01	405.11	405.91
fibromuscular hyperplasia	405.01	405.11	405.91
occlusion	405.01	405.11	405.91
stenosis	405.01	405.11	405.91
thrombosis	405.01	405.11	405.91
transient	—	—	796.2
of pregnancy	—	—	642.3

Hyperthecosis, ovary 256.8
Hyperthermia (of unknown origin) (*see also* Pyrexia) 780.6
malignant (due to anesthesia) 995.89
newborn 778.4
Hyperthymergasia (*see also* Psychosis, affective) 296.0
reactive (from emotional stress, psychological trauma) 298.1
recurrent episode 296.1
single episode 296.0
Hyperthymism 254.8
Hyperthyroid (recurrent)—*see* Hyperthyroidism
Hyperthyroidism (latent) (preadult) (recurrent) (without goiter) 242.9

Note—Use the following fifth-digit subclassification with category 242:

0 without mention of thyrotoxic crisis or storm
1 with mention of thyrotoxic crisis or storm

with
goiter (diffuse) 242.0
adenomatous 242.3
multinodular 242.2
uninodular 242.1
nodular 242.3
multinodular 242.2
uninodular 242.1
thyroid nodule 242.1
complicating pregnancy, childbirth, or puerperium 648.1
neonatal (transient) 775.3
Hypertonia —Hypertonicity
Hypertonicity
bladder 596.51
fetus or newborn 779.8
gastrointestinal (tract) 536.8
infancy 779.8
due to electrolyte imbalance 779.8
muscle 728.85
stomach 536.8
psychogenic 306.4
uterus, uterine (contractions) 661.4
affecting fetus or newborn 763.7
Hypertony —*see* Hypertonicity
Hypertransaminemia 790.4
Hypertrichosis 704.1
congenital 757.4
eyelid 374.54
lanuginosa 757.4
acquired 704.1
Hypertriglyceridemia, essential 272.1
Hypertrophy, hypertrophic
adenoids (infectional) 474.12
and tonsils (faucial) (infective) (lingual) (lymphoid) 474.10
adrenal 255.8
alveolar process or ridge 525.8
anal papillae 569.49
apocrine gland 705.82
artery NEC 447.8
carotid 447.8
congenital (peripheral) NEC 747.60
gastrointestinal 747.61
lower limb 747.64
renal 747.62
specified NEC 747.69
spinal 747.82
upper limb 747.63

Hypertrophy, hypertrophic—*continued*
arthritis (chronic) (*see also* Osteoarthrosis) 715.9
spine (*see also* Spondylosis) 721.90
arytenoid 478.79
asymmetrical (heart) 429.9
auricular—*see* Hypertrophy, cardiac
Bartholin's gland 624.8
bile duct 576.8
bladder (sphincter) (trigone) 596.8
blind spot, visual field 368.42
bone 733.99
brain 348.8
breast 611.1
cystic 610.1
fetus or newborn 778.7
fibrocystic 610.1
massive pubertal 611.1
puerperal, postpartum 676.3
senile (parenchymatous) 611.1
cardiac (chronic) (idiopathic) 429.3
with
rheumatic fever (conditions classifiable to 390)
active 391.8
with chorea 392.0
inactive or quiescent (with chorea) 398.99
congenital NEC 746.89
fatty (*see also* Degeneration, myocardial) 429.1
hypertensive (*see also* Hypertension, heart) 402.90
rheumatic (with chorea) 398.99
active or acute 391.8
with chorea 392.0
valve (*see also* Endocarditis) 424.90
congenital NEC 746.89
cartilage 733.99
cecum 569.89
cervix (uteri) 622.6
congenital 752.49
elongation 622.6
clitoris (cirrhotic) 624.2
congenital 752.49
colon 569.89
congenital 751.3
conjunctiva, lymphoid 372.73
cornea 371.89
corpora cavernosa 607.89
duodenum 537.89
endometrium (uterus) 621.3
cervix 622.6
epididymis 608.89
esophageal hiatus (congenital) 756.6
with hernia—*see* Hernia, diaphragm
eyelid 374.30
falx, skull 733.99
fat pad 729.30
infrapatellar 729.31
knee 729.31
orbital 374.34
popliteal 729.31
prepatellar 729.31
retropatellar 729.31
specified site NEC 729.39
foot (congenital) 755.67
frenum, frenulum (tongue) 529.8
linguae 529.8
lip 528.5
gallbladder or cystic duct 575.8
gastric mucosa 535.2
gingiva 523.8

Hypertrophy, hypertrophic—*continued*
gland, glandular (general) NEC 785.6
gum (mucous membrane) 523.8
heart (idiopathic)—*see also* Hypertrophy, cardiac
valve—*see also* Endocarditis
congenital NEC 746.89
hemifacial 754.0
hepatic—*see* Hypertrophy, liver
hiatus (esophageal) 756.6
hilus gland 785.6
hymen, congenital 752.49
ileum 569.89
infrapatellar fat pad 729.31
intestine 569.89
jejunum 569.89
kidney (compensatory) 593.1
congenital 753.3
labial frenulum 528.5
labium (majus) (minus) 624.3
lacrimal gland, chronic 375.03
ligament 728.9
spinal 724.8
linguae frenulum 529.8
lingual tonsil (infectional) 474.11
lip (frenum) 528.5
congenital 744.81
liver 789.1
acute 573.8
cirrhotic—*see* Cirrhosis, liver
congenital 751.69
fatty—*see* Fatty, liver
lymph gland 785.6
tuberculous—*see* Tuberculosis, lymph gland
mammary gland—*see* Hypertrophy, breast
maxillary frenulum 528.5
Meckel's diverticulum (congenital) 751.0
medial meniscus, acquired 717.3
median bar 600
mediastinum 519.3
meibomian gland 373.2
meniscus, knee, congenital 755.64
metatarsal head 733.99
metatarsus 733.99
mouth 528.9
mucous membrane
alveolar process 523.8
nose 478.1
turbinate (nasal) 478.0
muscle 728.9
muscular coat, artery NEC 447.8
carotid 447.8
renal 447.3
myocardium (*see also* Hypertrophy, cardiac) 429.3
idiopathic 425.4
myometrium 621.2
nail 703.8
congenital 757.5
nasal 478.1
alae 478.1
bone 738.0
cartilage 478.1
mucous membrane (septum) 478.1
sinus (*see also* Sinusitis) 473.9
turbinate 478.0
nasopharynx, lymphoid (infectional) (tissue) (wall) 478.29
neck, uterus 622.6
nipple 611.1
normal aperture diaphragm (congenital) 756.6

Hypertrophy, hypertrophic—*continued*
nose (*see also* Hypertrophy, nasal) 478.1
orbit 376.46
organ or site, congenital NEC—*see* Anomaly, specified type NEC
osteoarthropathy (pulmonary) 731.2
ovary 620.8
palate (hard) 526.89
soft 528.9
pancreas (congenital) 751.7
papillae
anal 569.49
tongue 529.3
parathyroid (gland) 252.0
parotid gland 527.1
penis 607.89
phallus 607.89
female (clitoris) 624.2
pharyngeal tonsil 474.12
pharyngitis 472.1
pharynx 478.29
lymphoid (infectional) (tissue) (wall) 478.29
pituitary (fossa) (gland) 253.8
popliteal fat pad 729.31
preauricular (lymph) gland (Hampstead) 785.6
prepuce (congenital) 605
female 624.2
prostate (adenofibromatous) (asymptomatic) (benign) (early) (recurrent) 600
congenital 752.8
psuedoedematous hypodermal 757.0
pseudomuscular 359.1
pylorus (muscle) (sphincter) 537.0
congenital 750.5
infantile 750.5
rectal sphincter 569.49
rectum 569.49
renal 593.1
rhinitis (turbinate) 472.0
salivary duct or gland 527.1
congenital 750.26
scaphoid (tarsal) 733.99
scar 701.4
scrotum 608.89
sella turcica 253.8
seminal vesicle 608.89
sigmoid 569.89
skin condition NEC 701.9
spermatic cord 608.89
spinal ligament 728.9
spleen—*see* Splenomegaly
spondylitis (spine) (*see also* Spondylosis) 721.90
stomach 537.89
subaortic stenosis (idiopathic) 425.1
sublingual gland 527.1
congenital 750.26
submaxillary gland 527.1
suprarenal (gland) 255.8
tendon 727.9
testis 608.89
congenital 752.8
thymic, thymus (congenital) (gland) 254.0
thyroid (gland) (*see also* Goiter) 240.9
primary 242.0
secondary 242.2
toe (congenital) 755.65
acquired 735.8
tongue 529.8
congenital 750.15
frenum 529.8
papillae (foliate) 529.3

Hypertrophy, hypertrophic—*continued*
tonsil (faucial) (infective) (lingual) (lymphoid) 474.11
and adenoids 474.10
with tonsillitis 474.0
tunica vaginalis 608.89
turbinate (mucous membrane) 478.0
ureter 593.89
urethra 599.84
uterus 621.2
puerperal, postpartum 674.8
uvula 528.9
vagina 623.8
vas deferens 608.89
vein 459.89
ventricle, ventricular (heart) (left) (right)—*see also* Hypertrophy, cardiac
congenital 746.89
due to hypertension (left) (right) (*see also* Hypertension, heart) 402.90
benign 402.10
malignant 402.00
right with ventricular septal defect, pulmonary stenosis or atresia, and dextraposition of aorta 745.2
verumontanum 599.89
vesical 596.8
vocal cord 478.5
vulva 624.3
stasis (nonfilarial) 624.3
Hypertropia (intermittent) (periodic) 378.31
Hypertyrosinemia 270.2
Hyperuricemia 790.6
Hypervalinemia 270.3
Hyperventilation (tetany) 786.01
hysterical 300.11
psychogenic 306.1
syndrome 306.1
Hyperviscidosis 277.00
Hyperviscosity (of serum) (syndrome) NEC 273.3
polycythemic 289.0
sclerocythemic 282.8
Hypervitaminosis (dietary) NEC 278.8
A (dietary) 278.2
D (dietary) 278.4
from excessive administration or use of vitamin preparations (chronic) 278.8
reaction to sudden overdose 963.5
vitamin A 278.2
reaction to sudden overdose 963.5
vitamin D 278.4
reaction to sudden overdose 963.5
vitamin K
correct substance properly administered 278.8
overdose or wrong substance given or taken 964.3
Hypervolemia 276.6
Hypesthesia (*see also* Disturbance, sensation) 782.0
cornea 371.81
Hyphema (anterior chamber) (ciliary body) (iris) 364.41
traumatic 921.3
Hyphemia —*see* Hyphema
Hypoacidity, gastric 536.8
psychogenic 306.4
Hypoactive labyrinth (function)—*see* Hypofunction, labyrinth
Hypoadrenalism 255.4
tuberculous (*see also* Tuberculosis) 017.6
Hypoadrenocorticism 255.4
pituitary 253.4
Hypoalbuminemia 273.8
Hypoalphalipoproteinemia 272.5
Hypobarism 993.2
Hypobaropathy 993.2
Hypobetalipoproteinemia (familial) 272.5
Hypocalcemia 275.4
cow's milk 775.4
dietary 269.3
neonatal 775.4
phosphate-loading 775.4
Hypocalcification, teeth 520.4
Hypochloremia 276.9
Hypochlorhydria 536.8
neurotic 306.4
psychogenic 306.4
Hypocholesteremia 272.5
Hypochondria (reaction) 300.7
Hypochondriac 300.7
Hypochondriasis 300.7
Hypochromasia blood cells 280.9
Hypochromic anemia 280.9
due to blood loss (chronic) 280.0
acute 285.1
microcytic 280.9
Hypocoagulability (*see also* Defect, coagulation) 286.9
Hypocomplementemia 279.8
Hypocythemia (progressive) 284.9
Hypodontia (*see also* Anodontia) 520.0
Hypoeosinophilia 288.8
Hypoesthesia (*see also* Disturbance, sensation) 782.0
cornea 371.81
tactile 782.0
Hypoestrinism 256.3
Hypoestrogenism 256.3
Hypoferremia 280.9
due to blood loss (chronic) 280.0
Hypofertility
female 628.9
male 606.1
Hypofibrinogenemia) 286.3
acquired 286.6
congenital 286.3
Hypofunction
adrenal (gland) 255.4
cortex 255.4
medulla 255.5
specified NEC 255.5
cerebral 331.9
corticoadrenal NEC 255.4
intestinal 564.8
labyrinth (unilateral) 386.53
with loss of labyrinthine reactivity 386.55
bilateral 386.54
with loss of labyrinthine reactivity 386.56
Leydig cell 257.2
ovary 256.3
postablative 256.2
pituitary (anterior) (gland) (lobe) 253.2
posterior 253.5
testicular 257.2
iatrogenic 257.1
postablative 257.1
postirradiation 257.1
postsurgical 257.1

Hypogammaglobulinemia 279.00
acquired primary 279.06
non-sex-linked, congenital 279.06
sporadic 279.06
transient of infancy 279.09
Hypogenitalism (congenital) (female) (male) 752.8
Hypoglycemia (spontaneous) 251.2
coma 251.0
diabetic 250.3
diabetic 250.8
due to insulin 251.0
therapeutic misadventure 962.3
familial (idiopathic) 251.2
following gastrointestinal surgery 579.3
infantile (idiopathic) 251.2
in infant of diabetic mother 775.0
leucine-induced 270.3
neonatal 775.6
reactive 251.2
specified NEC 251.1
Hypoglycemic shock 251.0
diabetic 250.8
due to insulin 251.0
functional (syndrome) 251.1
Hypogonadism
female 256.3
gonadotrophic (isolated) 253.4
hypogonadotropic (isolated) (with anosmia) 253.4
isolated 253.4
male 257.2
ovarian (primary) 256.3
pituitary (secondary) 253.4
testicular (primary) (secondary) 257.2
Hypohidrosis 705.0
Hypohidrotic ectodermal dysplasia 757.31
Hypoidrosis 705.0
Hypoinsulinemia, postsurgical 251.3
postpancreatectomy (complete) (partial) 251.3
Hypokalemia 276.8
Hypokinesia 780.9
Hypoleukia splenica 289.4
Hypoleukocytosis 288.8
Hypolipidemia 272.5
Hypolipoproteinemia 272.5
Hypomagnesemia 275.2
neonatal 775.4
Hypomania, hypomanic reaction (*see also* Psychosis, affective) 296.0
recurrent episode 296.1
single episode 296.0
Hypomastia (congenital) 757.6
Hypomenorrhea 626.1
Hypometabolism 783.9
Hypomotility
gastrointestinal tract 536.8
psychogenic 306.4
intestine 564.8
psychogenic 306.4
stomach 536.8
psychogenic 306.4
Hyponasality 784.49
Hyponatremia 276.1
with water depletion 276.1
Hypo-ovarianism 256.3
Hypo-ovarism 256.3
Hypoparathyroidism (idiopathic) (surgically induced) 252.1
neonatal 775.4
Hypopharyngitis 462
Hypophoria 378.40
Hypophosphatasia 275.3
Hypophosphatemia (acquired) (congenital) (familial) 275.3
renal 275.3
Hypophyseal, hypophysis —*see also* condition
dwarfism 253.3
gigantism 253.0
syndrome 253.8
Hypophyseothalamic syndrome 253.8
Hypopiesis —*see* Hypotension
Hypopigmentation 709.00
eyelid 374.53
Hypopinealism 259.8
Hypopituitarism (juvenile) (syndrome) 253.2
due to
hormone therapy 253.7
hypophysectomy 253.7
radiotherapy 253.7
postablative 253.7
postpartum hemorrhage 253.2
Hypoplasia, hypoplasis 759.89
adrenal (gland) 759.1
alimentary tract 751.8
lower 751.2
upper 750.8
anus, anal (canal) 751.2
aorta 747.22
aortic
arch (tubular) 747.10
orifice or valve with hypoplasia of ascending aorta and defective development of left ventricle (with mitral valve atresia) 746.7
appendix 751.2
areola 757.6
arm (*see also* Absence, arm, congenital) 755.20
artery (congenital) (peripheral) NEC 747.60
brain 747.81
cerebral 747.81
coronary 746.85
gastrointestinal 747.61
lower limb 747.64
pulmonary 747.3
renal 747.62
retinal 743.58
specified NEC 747.69
spinal 747.82
umbilical 747.5
upper limb 747.63
auditory canal 744.29
causing impairment of hearing 744.02
biliary duct (common) or passage 751.61
bladder 753.8
bone NEC 756.9
face 756.0
malar 756.0
mandible 524.04
alveolar 524.74
marrow 284.9
acquired (secondary) 284.8
congenital 284.0
idiopathic 284.9
maxilla 524.03
alveolar 524.73
skull (*see also* Hypoplasia, skull) 756.0
brain 742.1
gyri 742.2
specified part 742.2
breast (areola) 757.6
bronchus (tree) 748.3

Hypoplasia, hypoplasis—*continued*
cardiac 746.89
valve—*see* Hypoplasia, heart, valve
vein 746.89
carpus (*see also* Absence, carpal, congenital) 755.28
cartilaginous 756.9
cecum 751.2
cementum 520.4
hereditary 520.5
cephalic 742.1
cerebellum 742.2
cervix (uteri) 752.49
chin 524.06
clavicle 755.51
coccyx 756.19
colon 751.2
corpus callosum 742.2
cricoid cartilage 748.3
dermal, focal (Goltz) 757.39
digestive organ(s) or tract NEC 751.8
lower 751.2
upper 750.8
ear 744.29
auricle 744.23
lobe 744.29
middle, except ossicles 744.03
ossicles 744.04
ossicles 744.04
enamel of teeth (neonatal) (postnatal) (prenatal) 520.4
hereditary 520.5
endocrine (gland) NEC 759.2
endometrium 621.8
epididymis 752.8
epiglottis 748.3
erythroid, congenital 284.0
erythropoietic, chronic acquired 284.8
esophagus 750.3
Eustachian tube 744.24
eye (*see also* Microphthalmos) 743.10
lid 743.62
face 744.89
bone(s) 756.0
fallopian tube 752.19
femur (*see also* Absence, femur, congenital) 755.34
fibula (*see also* Absence, fibula, congenital) 755.37
finger (*see also* Absence, finger, congenital) 755.29
focal dermal 757.39
foot 755.31
gallbladder 751.69
genitalia, genital organ(s)
female 752.8
external 752.49
internal NEC 752.8
in adiposogenital dystrophy 253.8
male 752.8
glottis 748.3
hair 757.4
hand 755.21
heart 746.89
left (complex) (syndrome) 746.7
valve NEC 746.89
pulmonary 746.01
humerus (*see also* Absence, humerus, congenital) 755.24
hymen 752.49

Hypoplasia, hypoplasis—*continued*
intestine (small) 751.1
large 751.2
iris 743.46
jaw 524.09
kidney(s) 753.0
labium (majus) (minus) 752.49
labyrinth, membranous 744.05
lacrimal duct (apparatus) 743.65
larynx 748.3
leg (*see also* Absence, limb, congenital, lower) 755.30
limb 755.4
lower (*see also* Absence, limb, congenital, lower) 755.30
upper (*see also* Absence, limb, congenital, upper) 755.20
liver 751.69
lung (lobe) 748.5
mammary (areolar) 757.6
mandibular 524.04
alveolar 524.74
unilateral condylar 526.89
maxillary 524.03
alveolar 524.73
medullary 284.9
megakaryocytic 287.3
metacarpus (*see also* Absence, metacarpal, congenital) 755.28
metatarsus (*see also* Absence, metatarsal, congenital) 755.38
muscle 756.89
eye 743.69
myocardium (congenital) (Uhl's anomaly) 746.84
nail(s) 757.5
nasolacrimal duct 743.65
nervous system NEC 742.8
neural 742.8
nose, nasal 748.1
ophthalmic (*see also* Microphthalmos) 743.10
organ
of Corti 744.05
or site NEC—*see* Anomaly, by site
osseous meatus (ear) 744.03
ovary 752.0
oviduct 752.19
pancreas 751.7
parathyroid (gland) 759.2
parotid gland 750.26
patella 755.64
pelvis, pelvic girdle 755.69
penis 752.8
peripheral vascular system (congenital) NEC 747.60
gastrointestinal 747.61
lower limb 747.64
renal 747.62
specified NEC 747.69
spinal 747.82
upper limb 747.63
pituitary (gland) 759.2
pulmonary 748.5
arteriovenous 747.3
artery 747.3
valve 746.01
punctum lacrimale 743.65
radioulnar (*see also* Absence, radius, congenital, with ulna) 755.25
radius (*see also* Absence, radius, congenital) 755.26

Hypoplasia, hypoplasis—*continued*
rectum 751.2
respiratory system NEC 748.9
rib 756.3
sacrum 756.19
scapula 755.59
shoulder girdle 755.59
skin 757.39
skull (bone) 756.0
with
anencephalus 740.0
encephalocele 742.0
hydrocephalus 742.3
with spina bifida (*see also* Spina bifida) 741.0
microcephalus 742.1
spinal (cord) (ventral horn cell) 742.59
vessel 747.82
spine 756.19
spleen 759.0
sternum 756.3
tarsus (*see also* Absence, tarsal, congenital) 755.38
testis, testicle 752.8
thymus (gland) 279.11
thyroid (gland) 243
cartilage 748.3
tibiofibular (*see also* Absence, tibia, congenital, with fibula) 755.35
toe (*see also* Absence, toe, congenital) 755.39
tongue 750.16
trachea (cartilage) (rings) 748.3
Turner's (tooth) 520.4
ulna (*see also* Absence, ulna, congenital) 755.27
umbilical artery 747.5
ureter 753.2
uterus 752.3
vagina 752.49
vascular (peripheral) NEC (*see also* Hypoplasia, peripheral vascular system) 747.60
brain 747.81
vein(s) (peripheral) NEC (*see also* Hypoplasia, peripheral vascular system 747.60
brain 747.81
cardiac 746.89
great 747.49
portal 747.49
pulmonary 747.49
vena cava (inferior) (superior) 747.49
vertebra 756.19
vulva 752.49
zonule (ciliary) 743.39
zygoma 738.12
Hypopotassemia 276.8
Hypoproaccelerinemia (*see also* Defect, coagulation) 286.3
Hypoproconvertinemia (congenital) (*see also* Defect, coagulation) 286.3
Hypoproteinemia (essential) (hypermetabolic) (idiopathic) 273.8
Hypoproteinosis 260
Hypoprothrombinemia (congenital) (hereditary) (idiopathic) (*see also* Defect, coagulation) 286.3
acquired 286.7
newborn 776.3
Hypopselaphesia 782.0
Hypopyon (anterior chamber) (eye) 364.05
iritis 364.05
ulcer (cornea) 370.04
Hypopyrexia 780.9
Hyporeflex 796.1
Hyporeninemia, extreme 790.99
in primary aldosteronism 255.1
Hyposecretion
ACTH 253.4
ovary 256.3
postablative 256.2
salivary gland (any) 527.7
Hyposegmentation of neutrophils, hereditary 288.2
Hyposiderinemia 280.9
Hyposmolality 276.1
syndrome 276.1
Hyposomatotropism 253.3
Hyposomnia (*see also* Insomnia) 780.52
Hypospadias (male) 752.6
female 753.8
Hypospermatogenesis 606.1
Hyposphagma 372.72
Hyposplenism 289.59
Hypostasis, pulmonary 514
Hypostatic —*see* condition
Hyposthenuria 593.89
Hyposuprarenalism 255.4
Hypo-TBG-nemia 246.8
Hypotension (arterial) (constitutional) 458.9
chronic 458.1
iatrogenic 458.2
maternal, syndrome (following labor and delivery) 669.2
orthostatic (chronic) 458.0
dysautonomic-dyskinetic syndrome 333.0
permanent idiopathic 458.1
postoperative 458.2
postural 458.0
transient 796.3
Hypothermia (accidental) 991.6
anesthetic 995.89
newborn NEC 778.3
not associated with low environmental temperature 780.9
Hypothymergasia (*see also* Psychosis, affective) 296.2
recurrent episode 296.3
single episode 296.2
Hypothyroidism (acquired) 244.9
complicating pregnancy, childbirth, or puerperium 648.1
congenital 243
due to
ablation 244.1
radioactive iodine 244.1
surgical 244.0
iodine (administration) (ingestion) 244.2
radioactive 244.1
irradiation therapy 244.1
p-aminosalicylic acid (PAS) 244.3
phenylbutazone 244.3
resorcinol 244.3
specified cause NEC 244.8
surgery 244.0
goitrous (sporadic) 246.1
iatrogenic NEC 244.3
iodine 244.2
pituitary 244.8
postablative NEC 244.1
postsurgical 244.0
primary 244.9
secondary NEC 244.8
specified cause NEC 244.8
sporadic goitrous 246.1

Hypotonia, hypotonicity, hypotony 781.3
benign congenital 358.8
bladder 596.4
congenital 779.8
benign 358.8
eye 360.30
due to
fistula 360.32
ocular disorder NEC 360.33
following loss of aqueous or vitreous 360.33
primary 360.31
infantile muscular (benign) 359.0
muscle 728.9
uterus, uterine (contractions)—*see* Inertia, uterus
Hypotrichosis 704.09
congenital 757.4
lid (congenital) 757.4
acquired 374.55
postinfectional NEC 704.09
Hypotropia 378.32
Hypoventilation 786.09
Hypovitaminosis (*see also* Deficiency, vitamin) 269.2
Hypovolemia 276.5
surgical shock 998.0
traumatic (shock) 958.4
Hypoxemia (*see also* Anoxia) 799.0
Hypoxia (*see also* Anoxia) 799.0
cerebral 348.1
during or resulting from a procedure 997.01
newborn 768.9
mild or moderate 768.6
severe 768.5
fetal—*see* Distress, fetal
intrauterine—*see* Distress, fetal
myocardial (*see also* Insufficiency, coronary) 411.89
arteriosclerotic —*see* Arteriosclerosis, coronary
newborn—*see* Asphyxia, newborn
Hypsarrhythmia (*see also* Epilepsy) 345.6
Hysteralgia, pregnant uterus 646.8
Hysteria, hysterical 300.10
anxiety 300.20
Charcot's gland 300.11
conversion (any manifestation) 300.11
dissociative type NEC 300.15
psychosis, acute 298.1
Hysteroepilepsy 300.11
Hysterotomy, affecting fetus or newborn 763.8

I

Iatrogenic syndrome of excess cortisol 255.0
Iceland disease (epidemic neuromyasthenia) 049.8
Ichthyosis (congenita) 757.1
acquired 701.1
fetalis gravior 757.1
follicularis 757.1
hystrix 757.39
lamellar 757.1
lingual 528.6
palmaris and plantaris 757.39
simplex 757.1
vera 757.1
vulgaris 757.1
Ichthyotoxism 988.0
bacterial (*see also* Poisoning, food) 005.9
Icteroanemia, hemolytic (acquired) 283.9
congenital (*see also* Spherocytosis) 282.0
Icterus (*see also* Jaundice) 782.4
catarrhal—*see* Icterus, infectious
conjunctiva 782.4
newborn 774.6
epidemic—*see* Icterus, infectious
febrilis—*see* Icterus, infectious
fetus or newborn—*see* Jaundice, fetus or newborn
gravis (*see also* Necrosis, liver) 570
complicating pregnancy 646.7
affecting fetus or newborn 760.8
fetus or newborn NEC 773.0
obstetrical 646.7
affecting fetus or newborn 760.8
hematogenous (acquired) 283.9
hemolytic (acquired) 283.9
congenital (*see also* Spherocytosis) 282.0
hemorrhagic (acute) 100.0
leptospiral 100.0
newborn 776.0
spirochetal 100.0
infectious 070.1
with hepatic coma 070.0
leptospiral 100.0
spirochetal 100.0
intermittens juvenilis 277.4
malignant (*see also* Necrosis, liver) 570
neonatorum (*see also* Jaundice, fetus or newborn) 774.6
pernicious (*see also* Necrosis, liver) 570
spirochetal 100.0
Ictus solaris, solis 992.0
Identity disorder 313.82
dissociative 300.14
gender role (child) 302.6
adult 302.85
psychosexual (child) 302.6
adult 302.85
Idioglossia 307.9
Idiopathic —*see* condition
Idiosyncrasy (*see also* Allergy) 995.3
drug, medicinal substance, and biological—*see* Allergy, drug
Idiot, idiocy (congenital) 318.2
amaurotic (Bielschowsky) (-Jansky) (family) (infantile (late)) (juvenile (late)) (Vogt-Spielmeyer) 330.1
microcephalic 742.1
Mongolian 758.0
oxycephalic 756.0
Id reaction (due to bacteria) 692.89
IgE asthma 493.0
Ileitis (chronic) (*see also* Enteritis) 558.9
infectious 009.0
noninfectious 558.9
regional (ulcerative) 555.0
with large intestine 555.2
segmental 555.0
with large intestine 555.2
terminal (ulcerative) 555.0
with large intestine 555.2
Ileocolitis (*see also* Enteritis) 558.9
infectious 009.0
regional 555.2
ulcerative 556.1
Ileostomy status V44.2
with complication 569.60
Ileotyphus 002.0
Ileum —*see* condition
Ileus (adynamic) (bowel) (colon) (inhibitory) (intestine) (neurogenic) (paralytic) 560.1
arteriomesenteric duodenal 537.2
due to gallstone (in intestine) 560.31
duodenal, chronic 537.2
following gastrointestinal surgery 997.4
gallstone 560.31
mechanical (*see also* Obstruction, intestine) 560.9
meconium 777.1
due to cystic fibrosis 277.01
myxedema 564.8
postoperative 997.4
transitory, newborn 777.4
Iliac —*see* condition
Ill, louping 063.1
Illegitimacy V61.6
Illness —*see also* Disease
factitious (with physical symptoms) 300.19
with psychological symptoms 300.16
chronic (with physical symptoms) 301.51
heart—*see* Disease, heart
manic-depressive (*see also* Psychosis, affective) 296.80
mental (*see also* Disorder, mental) 300.9
Imbalance 781.2
autonomic (*see also* Neuropathy, peripheral, autonomic) 337.9
electrolyte 276.9
with
abortion—*see* Abortion, by type, with metabolic disorder
ectopic pregnancy (*see also* categories 633.0-633.9) 639.4
hyperemesis gravidarum (before 22 completed weeks gestation) 643.1
molar pregnancy (*see also* categories 630-632) 639.4
following
abortion 639.4
ectopic or molar pregnancy 639.4
neonatal, transitory NEC 775.5
endocrine 259.9
eye muscle NEC 378.9
heterophoria—*see* Heterophoria
glomerulotubular NEC 593.89
hormone 259.9
hysterical (*see also* Hysteria) 300.10

Imbalance—*continued*
labyrinth NEC 386.50
posture 729.9
sympathetic (*see also* Neuropathy, peripheral, autonomic) 337.9
Imbecile, imbecility 318.0
moral 301.7
old age 290.9
senile 290.9
specified IQ—*see* IQ
unspecified IQ 318.0
Imbedding, intrauterine device 996.32
Imbibition, cholesterol (gallbladder) 575.6
Imerslund (-Gräsbeck) syndrome (anemia due to familial selective vitamin B_{12} malabsorption) 281.1
Iminoacidopathy 270.8
Iminoglycinuria, familial 270.8
Immature —*see also* Immaturity
personality 301.89
Immaturity 765.1
extreme 765.0
fetus or infant light-for-dates—*see* Light-for-dates
lung, fetus or newborn 770.4
organ or site NEC—*see* Hypoplasia
pulmonary, fetus or newborn 770.4
reaction 301.89
sexual (female) (male) 259.0
Immersion 994.1
foot 991.4
hand 991.4
Immobile, immobility
intestine 564.8
joint—*see* Ankylosis
syndrome (paraplegic) 728.3
Immunization
ABO
affecting management of pregnancy 656.2
fetus or newborn 773.1
complication—*see* Complications, vaccination
Rh factor
affecting management of pregnancy 656.1
fetus or newborn 773.0
from transfusion 999.7
Immunodeficiency 279.3
with
adenosine-deaminase deficiency 279.2
defect, predominant
B-cell 279.00
T-cell 279.10
hyperimmunoglobulinemia 279.2
lymphopenia, hereditary 279.2
thrombocytopenia and eczema 279.12
thymic
aplasia 279.2
dysplasia 279.2
autosomal recessive, Swiss-type 279.2
common variable 279.06
severe combined (SCID) 279.2
to Rh factor
affecting management of pregnancy 656.1
fetus or newborn 773.0
X-linked, with increased IgM 279.05
Immunotherapy, prophylactic V07.2
Impaction, impacted
bowel, colon, rectum 560.30
with hernia—*see also* Hernia, by site, with obstruction
gangrenous—*see* Hernia, by site, with gangrene

Impaction, impacted—*continued*
by
calculus 560.39
gallstone 560.31
fecal 560.39
specified type NEC 560.39
calculus—*see* Calculus
cerumen (ear) (external) 380.4
cuspid 520.6
with abnormal position (same or adjacent tooth) 524.3
dental 520.6
with abnormal position (same or adjacent tooth) 524.3
fecal, feces 560.39
with hernia—*see also* Hernia, by site, with obstruction
gangrenous—*see* Hernia, by site, with gangrene
fracture—*see* Fracture, by site
gallbladder—*see* Cholelithiasis
gallstone(s)—*see* Cholelithiasis
in intestine (any part) 560.31
intestine(s) 560.30
with hernia—*see also* Hernia, by site, with obstruction
gangrenous—*see* Hernia, by site, with gangrene
by
calculus 560.39
gallstone 560.31
fecal 560.39
specified type NEC 560.39
intrauterine device (IUD) 996.32
molar 520.6
with abnormal position (same or adjacent tooth) 524.3
shoulder 660.4
affecting fetus or newborn 763.1
tooth, teeth 520.6
with abnormal position (same or adjacent tooth) 524.3
turbinate 733.99
Impaired, impairment (function)
arm V49.1
movement, involving
musculoskeletal system V49.1
nervous system V49.2
auditory discrimination 388.43
back V48.3
body (entire) V49.8
hearing (*see also* Deafness) 389.9
heart—*see* Disease, heart
kidney (*see also* Disease, renal) 593.9
disorder resulting from 588.9
specified NEC 588.8
leg V49.1
movement, involving
musculoskeletal system V49.1
nervous system V49.2
limb V49.1
movement, involving
musculoskeletal system V49.1
nervous system V49.2
liver 573.8
mastication 524.9
mobility
ear ossicles NEC 385.22
incostapedial joint 385.22
malleus 385.21

Impaired, impairment—*continued*
myocardium, myocardial (*see also* Insufficiency, myocardial) 428.0
neuromusculoskeletal NEC V49.8
back V48.3
head V48.2
limb V49.2
neck V48.3
spine V48.3
trunk V48.3
rectal sphincter 787.99
renal (*see also* Disease, renal) 593.9
disorder resulting from 588.9
specified NEC 588.8
spine V48.3
vision NEC 369.9
both eyes NEC 369.3
moderate 369.74
both eyes 369.25
with impairment of lesser eye (specified as)
blind, not further specified 369.15
low vision, not further specified 369.23
near-total 369.17
profound 369.18
severe 369.24
total 369.16
one eye 369.74
with vision of other eye (specified as)
near-normal 369.75
normal 369.76
near-total 369.64
both eyes 369.04
with impairment of lesser eye (specified as)
blind, not further specified 369.02
total 369.03
one eye 369.64
with vision of other eye (specified as)
near-normal 369.65
normal 369.66
one eye 369.60
with low vision of other eye 369.10
profound 369.67
both eyes 369.08
with impairment of lesser eye (specified as)
blind, not further specified 369.05
near-total 369.07
total 369.06
one eye 369.67
with vision of other eye (specified as)
near-normal 369.68
normal 369.69
severe 369.71
both eyes 369.22
with impairment of lesser eye (specified as)
blind, not further specified 369.11
low vision, not further specified 369.21
near-total 369.13
profound 369.14
total 369.12
one eye 369.71
with vision of other eye (specified as)
near-normal 369.72
normal 369.73
total
both eyes 369.01

Impaired, impairment—*continued*
one eye 369.61
with vision of other eye (specified as)
near-normal 369.62
normal 369.63
Impaludism —*see* Malaria
Impediment, speech NEC 784.5
psychogenic 307.9
secondary to organic lesion 784.5
Impending
cerebrovascular accident or attack 435.9
coronary syndrome 411.1
delirium tremens 291.0
myocardial infarction 411.1
Imperception, auditory (acquired) (congenital) 389.9
Imperfect
aeration, lung (newborn) 770.5
closure (congenital)
alimentary tract NEC 751.8
lower 751.5
upper 750.8
atrioventricular ostium 745.69
atrium (secundum) 745.5
primum 745.61
branchial cleft or sinus 744.41
choroid 743.59
cricoid cartilage 748.3
cusps, heart valve NEC 746.89
pulmonary 746.09
ductus
arteriosus 747.0
Botalli 747.0
ear drum 744.29
causing impairment of hearing 744.03
endocardial cushion 745.60
epiglottis 748.3
esophagus with communication to bronchus or trachea 750.3
Eustachian valve 746.89
eyelid 743.62
face, facial (*see also* Cleft, lip) 749.10
foramen
Botalli 745.5
ovale 745.5
genitalia, genital organ(s) or system
female 752.8
external 752.49
internal NEC 752.8
uterus 752.3
male 752.8
glottis 748.3
heart valve (cusps) NEC 746.89
interatrial ostium or septum 745.5
interauricular ostium or septum 745.5
interventricular ostium or septum 745.4
iris 743.46
kidney 753.3
larynx 748.3
lens 743.36
lip (*see also* Cleft, lip) 749.10
nasal septum or sinus 748.1
nose 748.1
omphalomesenteric duct 751.0
optic nerve entry 743.57
organ or site NEC—*see* Anomaly, specified type, by site
ostium
interatrial 745.5
interauricular 745.5
interventricular 745.4

Imperfect—*continued*
palate (*see also* Cleft, palate) 749.00
preauricular sinus 744.46
retina 743.56
roof of orbit 742.0
sclera 743.47
septum
aortic 745.0
aorticopulmonary 745.0
atrial (secundum) 745.5
primum 745.61
between aorta and pulmonary artery 745.0
heart 745.9
interatrial (secundum) 745.5
primum 745.61
interauricular (secundum) 745.5
primum 745.61
interventricular 745.4
with pulmonary stenosis or atresia, dextraposition of aorta, and hypertrophy of right ventricle 745.2
in tetralogy of Fallot 745.2
nasal 748.1
ventricular 745.4
with pulmonary stenosis or atresia, dextraposition of aorta, and hypertrophy of right ventricle 745.2
in tetralogy of Fallot 745.2
skull 756.0
with
anencephalus 740.0
encephalocele 742.0
hydrocephalus 742.3
with spina bifida (*see also* Spina bifida) 741.0
microcephalus 742.1
spine (with meningocele) (*see also* Spina bifida) 741.90
thyroid cartilage 748.3
trachea 748.3
tympanic membrane 744.29
causing impairment of hearing 744.03
uterus (with communication to bladder, intestine, or rectum) 752.3
uvula 749.02
with cleft lip (*see also* Cleft, palate, with cleft lip) 749.20
vitelline duct 751.0
development—*see* Anomaly, by site
erection 607.84
fusion—*see* Imperfect, closure
inflation lung (newborn) 770.5
intestinal canal 751.5
poise 729.9
rotation—*see* Malrotation
septum, ventricular 745.4
Imperfectly descended testis 752.5
Imperforate (congenital)—*see also* Atresia
anus 751.2
bile duct 751.61
cervix (uteri) 752.49
esophagus 750.3
hymen 752.42
intestine (small) 751.1
large 751.2
jejunum 751.1
pharynx 750.29
rectum 751.2
salivary duct 750.23
ureter 753.2
Imperforate—*continued*
urethra 753.6
urinary meatus 753.6
vagina 752.49
Impervious (congenital)—*see also* Atresia
anus 751.2
bile duct 751.61
esophagus 750.3
intestine (small) 751.1
large 751.5
rectum 751.2
ureter 753.2
urethra 753.6
Impetiginization of other dermatoses 684
Impetigo (any organism) (any site) (bullous) (circinate) (contagiosa) (neonatorum) (simplex) 684
Bockhart's (superficial folliculitis) 704.8
external ear 684 *[380.13]*
eyelid 684 *[373.5]*
Fox's (contagiosa) 684
furfuracea 696.5
herpetiformis 694.3
nonobstetrical 694.3
staphylococcal infection 684
ulcerative 686.8
vulgaris 684
Impingement, soft tissue between teeth 524.2
Implant, endometrial 617.9
Implantation
anomalous—*see also* Anomaly, specified type, by site
ureter 753.4
cyst
external area or site (skin) NEC 709.8
iris 364.61
vagina 623.8
vulva 624.8
dermoid (cyst)
external area or site (skin) NEC 709.8
iris 364.61
vagina 623.8
vulva 624.8
placenta, low or marginal—*see* Placenta previa
Impotence (sexual) (psychogenic) 302.72
organic origin NEC 607.84
Impoverished blood 285.9
Impression, basilar 756.0
Imprisonment V62.5
Improper
care (child) (newborn) 995.5
affecting parent or family V61.21
as reason for family seeking advice V61.21
specified person other than child 995.81
development, infant 764.9
Improperly tied umbilical cord (causing hemorrhage) 772.3
Impulses, obsessional 300.3
Impulsive neurosis 300.3
Inaction, kidney (*see also* Disease, renal) 593.9
Inactive —*see* condition
Inadequate, inadequacy
biologic 301.6
cardiac and renal—*see* Hypertension, cardiorenal
constitutional 301.6
development
child 783.4
fetus 764.9
affecting management of pregnancy 656.5

Inadequate, inadequacy—*continued*
genitalia
after puberty NEC 259.0
congenital—*see* Hypoplasia, genitalia
lungs 748.5
organ or site NEC—*see* Hypoplasia, by site
dietary 269.9
education V62.3
environment
economic problem V60.2
household condition NEC V60.1
poverty V60.2
unemployment V62.0
functional 301.6
household care, due to
family member
handicapped or ill V60.4
temporarily away from home V60.4
on vacation V60.5
technical defects in home V60.1
temporary absence from home of person rendering care V60.4
housing (heating) (space) V60.1
material resources V60.2
mental (*see also* Retardation, mental) 319
nervous system 799.2
personality 301.6
prenatal care in current pregnancy V23.7
pulmonary
function 786.09
newborn 770.8
ventilation, newborn 770.8
respiration 786.09
newborn 770.8
social 301.6
Inanition 263.9
with edema 262
due to
deprivation of food 994.2
malnutrition 263.9
fever 780.6
Inappropriate secretion
ACTH 255.0
antidiuretic hormone (ADH) (excessive) 253.6
deficiency 253.5
ectopic hormone NEC 259.3
pituitary (posterior) 253.6
Inattention after or at birth 995.5
affecting parent or family V61.21
Inborn errors of metabolism —*see* Disorder, metabolism
Incarceration, incarcerated
bubonocele—*see also* Hernia, inguinal, with obstruction
gangrenous—*see* Hernia, inguinal, with gangrene
colon (by hernia)—*see also* Hernia, by site, with obstruction
gangrenous—*see* Hernia, by site, with gangrene
enterocele 552.9
gangrenous 551.9
epigastrocele 552.29
gangrenous 551.29
epiplocele 552.9
gangrenous 551.9
exomphalos 552.1
gangrenous 551.1
fallopian tube 620.8
hernia—*see also* Hernia, by site, with obstruction
Incarceration, incarcerated—*continued*
gangrenous—*see* Hernia, by site, with gangrene
iris, in wound 871.1
lens, in wound 871.1
merocele (*see also* Hernia, femoral, with obstruction) 552.00
Omentum (by hernia)—*see also* Hernia, by site, with obstruction
gangrenous—*see* Hernia, by site, with gangrene
omphalocele 756.7
rupture (meaning hernia) (*see also* Hernia, by site, with obstruction) 552.9
gangrenous (*see also* Hernia, by site, with gangrene) 551.9
sarcoepiplocele 552.9
gangrenous 551.9
sarcoepiplomphalocele 552.1
with gangrene 551.1
uterus 621.8
gravid 654.3
causing obstructed labor 660.2
affecting fetus or newborn 763.1
Incident, cerebrovascular (*see also* Disease, cerebrovascular, acute) 436
Incineration (entire body) (from fire, conflagration, electricity, or lightning)—*see* Burn, multiple, specified sites
Incised wound
external—*see* Wound, open, by site
internal organs (abdomen, chest, or pelvis)—*see* Injury, internal, by site, with open wound
Incision, incisional
hernia—*see* Hernia, incisional
surgical, complication—*see* Complications, surgical procedures
traumatic
external—*see* Wound, open, by site
internal organs (abdomen, chest or pelvis)—*see* Injury, internal, by site, with open wound
Inclusion
azurophilic leukocytic 288.2
blennorrhea (neonatal) (newborn) 771.6
cyst—*see* Cyst, skin
gallbladder in liver (congenital) 751.69
Incompatibility
ABO
affecting management of pregnancy 656.2
fetus or newborn 773.1
infusion or transfusion reaction 999.6
blood (group) (Duffy) (E) (K(ell)) (Kidd) (Lewis) (M) (N) (P) (S) NEC
affecting management of pregnancy 656.2
fetus or newborn 773.2
infusion or transfusion reaction 999.6
marital V61.1
involving divorce or estrangement V61.0
Rh (blood group) (factor)
affecting management of pregnancy 656.1
fetus or newborn 773.0
infusion or transfusion reaction 999.7
Rhesus—*see* Incompatibility, Rh
Incompetency, incompetence, incompetent
annular
aortic (valve) (*see also* Insufficiency, aortic) 424.1
mitral (valve)—(*see also* Insufficiency, mitral) 424.0

Incompetency, Incompetence . . .—*continued*
pulmonary valve (heart) (*see also* Endocarditis, pulmonary) 424.3
aortic (valve) (*see also* Insufficiency, aortic) 424.1
syphilitic 093.22
cardiac (orifice) 530.0
valve—*see* Endocarditis
cervix, cervical (os) 622.5
in pregnancy 654.5
affecting fetus or newborn 761.0
esophagogastric (junction) (sphincter) 530.0
heart valve, congenital 746.89
mitral (valve)—*see* Insufficiency, mitral
papillary muscle (heart) 429.81
pelvic fundus 618.8
pulmonary valve (heart) (*see also* Endocarditis, pulmonary) 424.3
congenital 746.09
tricuspid (annular) (rheumatic) (valve) (*see also* Endocarditis, tricuspid) 397.0
valvular—*see* Endocarditis
vein, venous (saphenous) (varicose) (*see also* Varicose, vein) 454.9
velopharyngeal (closure)
acquired 528.9
congenital 750.29
Incomplete —*see also* condition
bladder emptying 788.21
expansion lungs (newborn) 770.5
gestation (liveborn)—*see* Immaturity
rotation—*see* Malrotation
Incontinence 788.30
without sensory awareness 788.34
anal sphincter 787.6
continuous leakage 788.37
feces 787.6
due to hysteria 300.11
nonorganic origin 307.7
hysterical 300.11
mixed (male) (female) (urge and stress) 788.33
overflow 788.39
paradoxical 788.39
rectal 787.6
specified NEC 788.39
stress (female) 625.6
male NEC 788.32
urethral sphincter 599.84
urge 788.31
and stress (male) (female) 788.33
urine 788.30
active 788.30
male 788.30
stress 788.32
and urge 788.33
neurogenic 788.39
nonorganic origin 307.6
stress (female) 625.6
male NEC 788.32
urge 788.31
and stress 788.33
Incontinentia pigmenti 757.33
Incoordinate
uterus (action) (contractions) 661.4
affecting fetus or newborn 763.7
Incoordination
esophageal-pharyngeal (newborn) 787.2
muscular 781.3
papillary muscle 429.81
Increase, increased
abnormal, in development 783.9
androgens (ovarian) 256.1
anticoagulants (antithrombin) (anti-VIIIa) (anti-IXa) (anti-Xa) (anti-XIa) 286.5
postpartum 666.3
cold sense (*see also* Disturbance, sensation) 782.0
estrogen 256.0
function
adrenal (cortex) 255.3
medulla 255.6
pituitary (anterior) (gland) (lobe) 253.1
posterior 253.6
heat sense (*see also* Disturbance, sensation) 782.0
intracranial pressure 348.2
injury at birth 767.8
light reflex of retina 362.13
permeability, capillary 448.9
pressure
intracranial 348.2
injury at birth 767.8
intraocular 365.00
pulsations 785.9
pulse pressure 785.9
sphericity, lens 743.36
splenic activity 289.4
venous pressure 459.89
portal 572.3
Incrustation, cornea, lead or zinc 930.0
Incyclophoria 378.44
Incyclotropia 378.33
Indeterminate sex 752.7
India rubber skin 756.83
Indicanuria 270.2
Indigestion (bilious) (functional) 536.8
acid 536.8
catarrhal 536.8
due to decomposed food NEC 005.9
fat 579.8
nervous 306.4
psychogenic 306.4
Indirect —*see* condition
Indolent bubo NEC 099.8
Induced
abortion—*see* Abortion, induced
birth, affecting fetus or newborn 763.8
delivery—*see* Delivery
labor—*see* Delivery
Induration, indurated
brain 348.8
breast (fibrous) 611.79
puerperal, postpartum 676.3
broad ligament 620.8
chancre 091.0
anus 091.1
congenital 090.0
extragenital NEC 091.2
corpora cavernosa (penis) (plastic) 607.89
liver (chronic) 573.8
acute 573.8
lung (black) (brown) (chronic) (fibroid) (*see also* Fibrosis, lung) 515
essential brown 275.0 *[516.1]*
penile 607.89
phlebitic—*see* Phlebitis
skin 782.8
stomach 537.89
Induratio penis plastica 607.89
Industrial —*see* condition

Inebriety (*see also* Abuse, drugs, nondependent) 305.0
Inefficiency
kidney (*see also* Disease, renal) 593.9
thyroid (acquired) (gland) 244.9
Inelasticity, skin 782.8
Inequality, leg (acquired) (length) 736.81
congenital 755.30
Inertia
bladder 596.4
neurogenic 596.54
with cauda equina syndrome 344.61
stomach 536.8
psychogenic 306.4
uterus, uterine 661.2
affecting fetus or newborn 763.7
primary 661.0
secondary 661.1
vesical 596.4
neurogenic 596.54
with cauda equina 344.61
Infant —*see also* condition
held for adoption V68.89
newborn—*see* Newborn
syndrome of diabetic mother 775.0
"Infant Hercules" syndrome 255.2
Infantile —*see also* condition
genitalia, genitals 259.0
in pregnancy or childbirth NEC 654.4
affecting fetus or newborn 763.8
causing obstructed labor 660.2
affecting fetus or newborn 763.1
heart 746.9
kidney 753.3
lack of care 995.5
affecting parent or family V61.21
macula degeneration 362.75
melanodontia 521.0
os, uterus (*see also* Infantile, genitalia) 259.0
pelvis 738.6
with disproportion (fetopelvic) 653.1
affecting fetus or newborn 763.1
causing obstructed labor 660.1
affecting fetus or newborn 763.1
penis 259.0
testis 257.2
uterus (*see also* Infantile, genitalia) 259.0
vulva 752.49
Infantilism 259.9
with dwarfism (hypophyseal) 253.3
Brissaud's (infantile myxedema) 244.9
celiac 579.0
Herter's (nontropical sprue) 579.0
hypophyseal 253.3
hypothalamic (with obesity) 253.8
idiopathic 259.9
intestinal 579.0
pancreatic 577.8
pituitary 253.3
renal 588.0
sexual (with obesity) 259.0
Infants, healthy liveborn —*see* Newborn
Infarct, infarction
adrenal (capsule) (gland) 255.4
amnion 658.8
anterior (with contiguous portion of intraventricular septum) NEC (*see also* Infarct, myocardium) 410.1
appendices epiploicae 557.0
bowel 557.0
Infarct, infarction—*continued*
brain (stem) 434.91
embolic (*see also* Embolism, brain) 434.11
healed or old—*see also* category 438
without residuals V12.59
iatrogenic 997.02
postoperative 997.02
late effect—*see* category 438
puerperal, postpartum, childbirth 674.0
thrombotic (*see also* Thrombosis, brain) 434.01
breast 611.8
Brewer's (kidney) 593.81
cardiac (*see also* Infarct, myocardium) 410.9
cerebellar (*see also* Infarct, brain) 434.91
embolic (*see also* Embolism, brain) 434.11
cerebral (*see also* Infarct, brain) 434.91
embolic (*see also* Embolism, brain) 434.11
chorion 658.8
colon (acute) (agnogenic) (embolic) (hemorrhagic) (nonocclusive) (nonthrombotic) (occlusive) (segmental) (thrombotic) (with gangrene) 557.0
coronary artery (*see also* Infarct, myocardium) 410.9
embolic (*see also* Embolism) 444.9
fallopian tube 620.8
gallbladder 575.8
heart (*see also* Infarct, myocardium) 410.9
hepatic 573.4
hypophysis (anterior lobe) 253.8
impending (myocardium) 411.1
intestine (acute) (agnogenic) (embolic) (hemorrhagic) (nonocclusive) (nonthrombotic) (occlusive) (thrombotic) (with gangrene) 557.0
kidney 593.81
liver 573.4
lung (embolic) (thrombotic) 415.19
with
abortion—*see* Abortion, by type, with, embolism
ectopic pregnancy (*see also* categories 633.0-633.9) 639.6
molar pregnancy (*see also* categories 630-632) 639.6
following
abortion 639.6
ectopic or molar pregnancy 639.6
iatrogenic 415.11
in pregnancy, childbirth, or puerperium—*see* Embolism, obstetrical
postoperative 415.11
lymph node or vessel 457.8
medullary (brain)—*see* Infarct, brain
meibomian gland (eyelid) 374.85
mesentery, mesenteric (embolic) (thrombotic) (with gangrene) 557.0
midbrain—*see* Infarct, brain
myocardium, myocardial (acute or with a stated duration of 8 weeks or less) (with hypertension) 410.9

Note—use the following fifth-digit subclassification with category 410

0 episode unspecified
1 initial episode
2 subsequent episode without recurrence

Infarct, infarction—*continued*
with symptoms after 8 weeks from date of infarction 414.8
anterior (wall) (with contiguous portion of intraventricular septum) NEC 410.1
anteroapical (with contiguous portion of intraventricular septum) 410.1
anterolateral (wall) 410.0
anteroseptal (with contiguous portion of intraventricular septum) 410.1
apical-lateral 410.5
atrial 410.8
basal-lateral 410.5
chronic (with symptoms after 8 weeks from date of infarction) 414.8
diagnosed on ECG, but presenting no symptoms 412
diaphragmatic wall (with contiguous portion of intraventricular septum) 410.4
healed or old, currently presenting no symptoms 412
high lateral 410.5
impending 411.1
inferior (wall) (with contiguous portion of intraventricular septum) 410.4
inferolateral (wall) 410.2
inferoposterior wall 410.3
lateral wall 410.5
nontransmural 410.7
papillary muscle 410.8
past (diagnosed on ECG or other special investigation, but correctly presenting no symptoms) 412
with symptoms NEC 414.8
posterior (strictly) (true) (wall) 410.6
posterobasal 410.6
posteroinferior 410.3
posterolateral 410.5
previous, currently presenting no symptoms 412
septal 410.8
specified site NEC 410.8
subendocardial 410.7
syphilitic 093.82
nontransmural 410.7
omentum 557.0
ovary 620.8
pancreas 577.8
papillary muscle (*see also* Infarct, myocardium) 410.8
parathyroid gland 252.8
pituitary (gland) 253.8
placenta (complicating pregnancy) 656.7
affecting fetus or newborn 762.2
pontine—*see* Infarct, brain
posterior NEC (*see also* Infarct, myocardium) 410.6
prostate 602.8
pulmonary (artery) (hemorrhagic) (vein) 415.1
with
abortion—*see* Abortion, by type, with embolism
ectopic pregnancy (*see also* categories 633.0-633.9) 639.6
molar pregnancy (*see also* categories 630-632) 639.6
following
abortion 639.6
ectopic or molar pregnancy 639.6
iatrogenic 415.11

Infarct, infarction—*continued*
in pregnancy, childbirth, or puerperium—*see* Embolism, obstetrical
postoperative 415.11
renal 593.81
embolic or thrombotic 593.81
retina, retinal 362.84
with occlusion—*see* Occlusion, retina
spinal (acute) (cord) (embolic) (nonembolic) 336.1
spleen 289.59
embolic or thrombotic 444.89
subchorionic—*see* Infarct, placenta
subendocardial (*see also* Infarct, myocardium) 410.7
suprarenal (capsule) (gland) 255.4
syncytium—*see* Infarct, placenta
testis 608.83
thrombotic (*see also* Thrombosis) 453.9
artery, arterial—*see* Embolism
thyroid (gland) 246.3
ventricle (heart) (*see also* Infarct, myocardium) 410.9
Infecting —*see* condition
Infection, infected, infective (opportunistic) 136.9
with lymphangitis—*see* Lymphangitis
abortion—*see* Abortion, by type, with sepsis
abscess (skin)—*see* Abscess, by site
Absidia 117.7
Acanthocheilonema (perstans) 125.4
streptocerca 125.6
accessory sinus (chronic) (*see also* Sinusitis) 473.9
Achorion—*see* Dermatophytosis
Acremonium falciforme 117.4
acromioclavicular (joint) 711.91
actinobacillus
lignieresii 027.8
mallei 024
muris 026.1
actinomadura—*see* Actinomycosis
Actinomyces (israelii)—*see also* Actinomycosis
muris-ratti 026.1
Actinomycetales (actinomadura) (Actinomyces) (Nocardia) (Streptomyces)—*see* Actinomycosis
actinomycotic NEC (*see also* Actinomycosis) 039.9
adenoid (chronic) 474.0
acute 463
and tonsil (chronic) 474.0
acute or subacute 463
adenovirus NEC 079.0
in diseases classified elsewhere—*see* category 079
unspecified nature or site 079.0
Aerobacter aerogenes NEC 041.85
enteritis 008.2
aerogenes capsulatus (*see also* Gangrene, gas) 040.0
aertrycke (*see also* Infection, Salmonella) 003.9
ajellomyces dermatitidis 116.0
alimentary canal NEC (*see also* Enteritis, due to, by organism) 009.0
Allescheria boydii 117.6
Alternaria 118
alveolus, alveolar (process) (pulpal origin) 522.4
ameba, amebic (histolytica) (*see also* Amebiasis) 006.9
acute 006.0

Infection, infected, infective—*continued*
chronic 006.1
free-living 136.2
hartmanni 007.8
specified
site NEC 006.8
type NEC 007.8
amniotic fluid or cavity 658.4
affecting fetus or newborn 762.7
anaerobes (cocci) (gram-negative) (gram positive) (mixed) NEC 041.84
anal canal 569.49
Ancylostoma braziliense 126.2
Angiostrongylus cantonensis 128.8
anisakiasis 127.1
Anisakis larva 127.1
anthrax (*see also* Anthrax) 022.9
antrum (chronic) (*see also* Sinusitis, maxillary) 473.0
anus (papillae) (sphincter) 569.49
arbor virus NEC 066.9
arbovirus NEC 066.9
argentophil-rod 027.0
Ascaris lumbricoides 127.0
ascomycetes 117.4
Aspergillus (flavus) (fumigatus) (terreus) 117.3
atypical
acid-fast (bacilli) (*see also* Mycobacterium, atypical) 031.9
mycobacteria (*see also* Mycobacterium, atypical) 031.9
auditory meatus (circumscribed) (diffuse) (external) (*see also* Otitis, externa) 380.10
auricle (ear) (*see also* Otitis, externa) 380.10
axillary gland 683
Babesiasis 088.82
Babesiosis 088.82
Bacillus NEC 041.89
abortus 023.1
anthracis (*see also* Anthrax) 022.9
cereus (food poisoning) 005.89
coli—*see* Infection, Escherichia coli
coliform NEC 041.85
Ducrey's (any location) 099.0
Flexner's 004.1
fragilis NEC 041.82
Friedländer's NEC 041.3
fusiformis 101
gas (gangrene) (*see also* Gangrene, gas) 040.0
mallei 024
melitensis 023.0
paratyphoid, paratyphosus 002.9
A 002.1
B 002.2
C 002.3
Schmorl's 040.3
Shiga 004.0
suipestifer (*see also* Infection, Salmonella) 003.9
swimming pool 031.1
typhosa 002.0
welchii (*see also* Gangrene, gas) 040.0
Whitmore's 025
bacterial NEC 041.9
specified NEC 041.89
anaerobic NEC 041.84
gram-negative NEC 041.85
anaerobic NEC 041.84
Bacterium
paratyphosum 002.9
A 002.1

Infection, infected, infective—*continued*
B 002.2
C 002.3
typhosum 002.0
Bacteroides (fragilis) (melaninogenicus) (oralis) NEC 041.84
balantidium coli 007.0
Bartholin's gland 616.8
Basidiobolus 117.7
Bedsonia 079.98
specified NEC 079.88
bile duct 576.1
bladder (*see also* Cystitis) 595.9
Blastomyces, blastomycotic 116.0
brasiliensis 116.1
dermatitidis 116.0
European 117.5
Loboi 116.2
North American 116.0
South American 116.1
blood stream—*see* Septicemia
bone 730.9
specified—*see* Osteomyelitis
Bordetella 033.9
bronchiseptica 033.8
parapertussis 033.1
pertussis 033.0
Borrelia
bergdorfi 088.81
vincentii (mouth) (pharynx) (tonsil) 101
brain (*see also* Encephalitis) 323.9
late effect—*see* category 326
membranes—(*see also* Meningitis) 322.9
septic 324.0
late effect—*see* category 326
meninges (*see also* Meningitis) 320.9
branchial cyst 744.42
breast 611.0
puerperal, postpartum 675.2
with nipple 675.9
specified type NEC 675.8
nonpurulent 675.2
purulent 675.1
bronchus (*see also* Bronchitis) 490
fungus NEC 117.9
Brucella 023.9
abortus 023.1
canis 023.3
melitensis 023.0
mixed 023.8
suis 023.2
Brugia (Wuchereria) malayi 125.1
bursa—*see* Bursitis
buttocks (skin) 686.9
Candida (albicans) (tropicalis) (*see also* Candidiasis) 112.9
congenital 771.7
Candiru 136.8
Capillaria
hepatica 128.8
philippinensis 127.5
cartilage 733.99
cat liver fluke 121.0
cellulitis—*see* Cellulitis, by site
Cephalosporum falciforme 117.4
Cercomonas hominis (intestinal) 007.3
cerebrospinal (*see also* Meningitis) 322.9
late effect—*see* category 326
cervical gland 683
cervix (*see also* Cervicitis) 616.0
cesarean section wound 674.3
Chilomastix (intestinal) 007.8

Infection, infected, infective—*continued*
Chlamydia 079.98
specified NEC 079.88
Cholera (*see also* Cholera) 001.9
chorionic plate 658.8
Cladosporium
bantianum 117.8
carrionii 117.2
mansoni 111.1
trichoides 117.8
wernecki 111.1
Clonorchis (sinensis) (liver) 121.1
Clostridium (haemolyticum) (novyi) NEC 041.84
botulinum 005.1
congenital 771.8
histolyticum (*see also* Gangrene, gas) 040.0
oedematiens (*see also* Gangrene, gas) 040.0
perfringens 041.83
due to food 005.2
septicum (*see also* Gangrene, gas) 040.0
sordelii (*see also* Gangrene, gas) 040.0
welchii (*see also* Gangrene, gas) 040.0
due to food 005.2
Coccidioides (immitis) (*see also* Coccidioidomycosis) 114.9
coccus NEC 041.89
colon (*see also* Enteritis, due to, by organism) 009.0
bacillus—*see* Infection, Escherichia coli
colostomy or enterostomy 569.61
common duct 576.1
complicating pregnancy, childbirth, or puerperium NEC 647.9
affecting fetus or newborn 760.2
Condiobolus 117.7
congenital NEC 771.8
Candida albicans 771.7
chronic 771.2
clostridial 771.8
Cytomegalovirus 771.1
Escherichia coli 771.8
hepatitis, viral 771.2
Herpes simplex 771.2
listeriosis 771.2
malaria 771.2
poliomyelitis 771.2
rubella 771.0
Salmonella 771.8
streptococcal 771.8
toxoplasmosis 771.2
tuberculosis 771.2
urinary (tract) 771.8
vaccinia 771.2
corpus luteum (*see also* Salpingo-oophoritis) 614.2
Corynebacterium diphtheriae—*see* Diphtheria
Coxsackie (*see also* Coxsackie) 079.2
endocardium 074.22
heart NEC 074.20
in diseases classified elsewhere—*see* category 079
meninges 047.0
myocardium 074.23
pericardium 074.21
pharynx 074.0
specified disease NEC 074.8
unspecified nature or site 079.2
Cryptococcus neoformans 117.5
Cryptosporidia 007.8
Cunninghamella 117.7

Infection, infected, infective—*continued*
cyst—*see* Cyst
Cysticercus cellulosae 123.1
cytomegalovirus 078.5
congenital 771.1
dental (pulpal origin) 522.4
deuteromycetes 117.4
Dicrocoelium dendriticum 121.8
Dipetalonema (perstans) 125.4
streptocerca 125.6
diphtherial—*see* Diphtheria
Diphyllobothrium (adult) (latum) (pacificum) 123.4
larval 123.5
Diplogonoporus (grandis) 123.8
Dipylidium (caninum) 123.8
Dirofilaria 125.6
dog tapeworm 123.8
Dracunculus medinensis 125.7
Dreschlera 118
hawaiiensis 117.8
Ducrey's bacillus (any site) 099.0
due to or resulting from
device, implant, or graft (any) (presence of)—*see* Complications, infection and inflammation, due to (presence of) any device, implant, or graft classified to 996.0-996.5 NEC
injection, inoculation, infusion, transfusion, or vaccination (prophylactic) (therapeutic) 999.3
injury NEC—*see* Wound, open, by site, complicated
surgery 998.5
duodenum 535.6
ear—*see also* Otitis
external (*see also* Otitis, externa) 380.10
inner (*see also* Labyrinthitis) 386.30
middle —*see* Otitis, media
Eaton's agent NEC 041.81
Eberthella typhosa 002.0
echinococcosis 122.9
Echinococcus (*see also* Echinococcus) 122.9
Echinostoma 121.8
ECHO virus 079.1
in diseases classified elsewhere—*see* category 079
unspecified nature or site 079.1
Endamoeba—*see* Infection, ameba
endocardium (*see also* Endocarditis) 421.0
endocervix (*see also* Cervicitis) 616.0
Entamoeba—*see* Infection, ameba
enteric (*see also* Enteritis, due to, by organism) 009.0
Enterobacter aerogenes NEC 041.85
Enterobius vermicularis 127.4
Enterococcus NEC 041.00
enterovirus NEC 079.89
central nervous system NEC 048
enteritis 008.67
meningitis 047.9
Entomophthora 117.7
Epidermophyton—*see* Dermatophytosis
epidermophytosis—*see* Dermatophytosis
episiotomy 674.3
Epstein-Barr virus 075
erysipeloid 027.1
Erysipelothrix (insidiosa) (rhusiopathiae) 027.1
erythema infectiosum 057.0
Escherichia coli NEC 041.4
congenital 771.8

Infection, infected, infective—*continued*
enteritis—*see* Enteritis, E. coli
generalized 038.42
intestinal—*see* Enteritis, E. coli
ethmoidal (chronic) (sinus) (*see also* Sinusitis, ethmoidal) 473.2
Eubacterium 041.84
Eustachian tube (ear) 381.50
acute 381.51
chronic 381.52
exanthema subitum 057.8
external auditory canal (meatus) (*see also* Otitis, externa) 380.10
eye NEC 360.00
eyelid 373.9
specified NEC 373.8
fallopian tube (*see also* Salpingo-oophoritis) 614.2
fascia 728.89
Fasciola
gigantica 121.3
hepatica 121.3
Fasciolopsis (buski) 121.4
fetus (intra-amniotic)—*see* Infection, congenital
filarial—*see* Infestation, filarial
finger (skin) 686.9
abscess (with lymphangitis) 681.00
pulp 681.01
cellulitis (with lymphangitis) 681.00
distal closed space (with lymphangitis) 681.00
nail 681.02
fungus 110.1
fish tapeworm 123.4
larval 123.5
flagellate, intestinal 007.9
fluke—*see* Infestation, fluke
focal
teeth (pulpal origin) 522.4
tonsils 474.0
Fonsecaea
compactum 117.2
pedrosoi 117.2
food (*see also* Poisoning, food) 005.9
foot (skin) 686.9
fungus 110.4
Francisella tularensis (*see also* Tularemia) 021.9
frontal sinus (chronic) (*see also* Sinusitis, frontal) 473.1
fungus NEC 117.9
beard 110.0
body 110.5
dermatiacious NEC 117.8
foot 110.4
groin 110.3
hand 110.2
nail 110.1
pathogenic to compromised host only 118
perianal (area) 110.3
scalp 110.0
scrotum 110.8
skin 111.9
foot 110.4
hand 110.2
toenails 110.1
trachea 117.9
Fusarium 118
Fusobacterium 041.84
gallbladder (*see also* Cholecystitis, acute) 575.0
gas bacillus (*see also* Gas, gangrene) 040.0
gastric (*see also* Gastritis) 535.5
Gastrodiscoides hominis 121.8

Infection, infected, infective—*continued*
gastroenteric (*see also* Enteritis, due to, by organism) 009.0
gastrointestinal (*see also* Enteritis, due to, by organism) 009.0
generalized NEC (*see also* Septicemia) 038.9
genital organ or tract NEC
female 614.9
with
abortion—*see* Abortion, by type, with sepsis
ectopic pregnancy (*see also* categories 633.0-633.9) 639.0
molar pregnancy (*see also* categories 630-632) 639.0
complicating pregnancy 646.6
affecting fetus or newborn 760.8
following
abortion 639.0
ectopic or molar pregnancy 639.0
puerperal, postpartum, childbirth 670
minor or localized 646.6
affecting fetus or newborn 760.8
male 608.4
genitourinary tract NEC 599.0
Ghon tubercle, primary (*see also* Tuberculosis) 010.0
Giardia lamblia 007.1
gingival (chronic) 523.1
acute 523.0
Vincent's 101
glanders 024
Glenosporopsis amazonica 116.2
Gnathostoma spinigerum 128.1
Gongylonema 125.6
gonococcal NEC (*see also* Gonococcus) 098.0
gram-negative bacilli NEC 041.85
anaerobic 041.84
guinea worm 125.7
gum (*see also* Infection, gingival) 523.1
Hantavirus 079.81
heart 429.89
Helicobacter pylori (H. pylori) 041.86
helminths NEC 128.9
intestinal 127.9
mixed (types classifiable to more than one category in 120.0-127.7) 127.8
specified type NEC 127.7
specified type NEC 128.8
Hemophilus influenzae NEC 041.5
generalized 038.41
Herpes (simplex) (*see also* Herpes, simplex) 054.9
congenital 771.2
zoster (*see also* Herpes, zoster) 053.9
eye NEC 053.29
Heterophyes heterophyes 121.6
Histoplasma (*see also* Histoplasmosis) 115.90
capsulatum (*see also* Histoplasmosis, American) 115.00
duboisii (*see also* Histoplasmosis, African) 115.10
HIV V08
with symptoms, symptomatic 042
hookworm (*see also* Ancylostomiasis) 126.9
human immunodeficiency virus V08
with symptoms, symptomatic 042
human papilloma virus 079.4
hydrocele 603.1
hydronephrosis 591
Hymenolepis 123.6

Infection, infected, infective—*continued*
  hypopharynx 478.29
  inguinal glands 683
    due to soft chancre 099.0
  intestine, intestinal (*see also* Enteritis, due to, by organism) 009.0
  intrauterine (*see also* Endometritis) 615.9
    complicating delivery 646.6
      specified infection NEC in fetus or newborn 771.8
  isospora belli or hominis 007.2
  Japanese B encephalitis 062.0
  jaw (bone) (acute) (chronic) (lower) (subacute) (upper) 526.4
  joint—*see* Arthritis, infectious or infective
  kidney (cortex) (hematogenous) 590.9
    with
      abortion—*see* Abortion, by type, with urinary tract infection
      calculus 592.0
      ectopic pregnancy (*see also* categories 633.0-633.9) 639.8
      molar pregnancy (*see also* categories 630-632) 639.8
    complicating pregnancy or puerperium 646.6
      affecting fetus or newborn 760.1
    following
      abortion 639.8
      ectopic or molar pregnancy 639.8
    pelvis and ureter 590.3
  Klebsiella pneumoniae NEC 041.3
  knee (skin) NEC 686.9
    joint—*see* Arthritis, infectious
  Koch's (*see also* Tuberculosis, pulmonary) 011.9
  labia (majora) (minora) (*see also* Vulvitis) 616.10
  lacrimal
    gland (*see also* Dacryoadenitis) 375.00
    passages (duct) (sac) (*see also* Dacryocystitis) 375.30
  larynx NEC 478.79
  leg (skin) NEC 686.9
  Leishmania (*see also* Leishmaniasis) 085.9
    braziliensis 085.5
    donovani 085.0
    Ethiopica 085.3
    furunculosa 085.1
    infantum 085.0
    mexicana 085.4
    tropica (minor) 085.1
      major 085.2
  Leptosphaeria senegalensis 117.4
  leptospira (*see also* Leptospirosis) 100.9
    Australis 100.89
    Bataviae 100.89
    pyrogenes 100.89
    specified type NEC 100.89
  leptospirochetal NEC (*see also* Leptospirosis) 100.9
  Leptothrix—*see* Actinomycosis
  Listeria monocytogenes (listeriosis) 027.0
    congenital 771.2
  liver fluke—*see* Infestation, fluke, liver
  Loa loa 125.2
    eyelid 125.2 *[373.6]*
  Loboa loboi 116.2
  local, skin (staphylococcal) (streptococcal) NEC 686.9
    abscess—*see* Abscess, by site
    cellulitis—*see* Cellulitis, by site
    ulcer (*see also* Ulcer, skin) 707.9

Infection, infected, infective—*continued*
  Loefflerella
    mallei 024
    whitmori 025
  lung 518.89
    atypical Mycobacterium 031.0
      tuberculous (*see also* Tuberculosis, pulmonary) 011.9
    basilar 518.89
    chronic 518.89
    fungus NEC 117.9
    spirochetal 104.8
    virus—*see* Pneumonia, virus
  lymph gland (axillary) (cervical) (inguinal) 683
    mesenteric 289.2
  lymphoid tissue, base of tongue or posterior pharynx, NEC 474.0
  madurella
    grisea 117.4
    mycetomii 117.4
  major
    with
      abortion—*see* Abortion, by type, with sepsis
      ectopic pregnancy (*see also* categories 633.0-633.9) 639.0
      molar pregnancy (*see also* categories 630-632) 639.0
    following
      abortion 639.0
      ectopic or molar pregnancy 639.0
    puerperal, postpartum, childbirth 670
  malarial—*see* Malaria
  Malassezia furfur 111.0
  Malleomyces
    mallei 024
    pseudomallei 025
  mammary gland 611.0
    puerperal, postpartum 675.2
  Mansonella (ozzardi) 125.5
  mastoid (suppurative)—*see* Mastoiditis
  maxilla, maxillary 526.4
    sinus (chronic) (*see also* Sinusitis, maxillary) 473.0
  mediastinum 519.2
  medina 125.7
  meibomian
    cyst 373.12
    gland 373.12
  melioidosis 025
  meninges (*see also* Meningitis) 320.9
  meningococcal (*see also* condition) 036.9
    brain 036.1
    cerebrospinal 036.0
    endocardium 036.42
    generalized 036.2
    meninges 036.0
    meningococcemia 036.2
    specified site NEC 036.89
  mesenteric lymph nodes or glands NEC 289.2
  Metagonimus 121.5
  metatarsophalangeal 711.97
  microorganism resistant to drugs—*see* Resistance (to), drugs by microorganisms
  Microsporidia 136.8
  microsporum, microsporic—*see* Dermatophytosis
  Mima polymorpha NEC 041.85
  mixed flora NEC 041.89
  Monilia (*see also* Candidiasis) 112.9
    neonatal 771.7

Infection, infected, infective—*continued*
Monosporium apiospermum 117.6
mouth (focus) NEC 528.9
parasitic 112.0
Mucor 117.7
muscle NEC 728.89
mycelium NEC 117.9
mycetoma
actinomycotic NEC (*see also* Actinomycosis) 039.9
mycotic NEC 117.4
Mycobacterium, mycobacterial (*see also* Mycobacterium) 031.9
mycoplasma NEC 041.81
mycotic NEC 117.9
pathogenic to compromised host only 118
skin NEC 111.9
systemic 117.9
myocardium NEC 422.90
nail (chronic) (with lymphangitis) 681.9
finger 681.02
fungus 110.1
ingrowing 703.0
toe 681.11
fungus 110.1
nasal sinus (chronic) (*see also* Sinusitis) 473.9
nasopharynx (chronic) 478.29
acute 460
navel 686.9
newborn 771.4
Neisserian—*see* Gonococcus
Neotestudina rosatii 117.4
newborn, generalized 771.8
nipple 611.0
puerperal, postpartum 675.0
with breast 675.9
specified type NEC 675.8
Nocardia—*see* Actinomycosis
nose 478.1
nostril 478.1
obstetrical surgical wound 674.3
Oesophagostomum (apiostomum) 127.7
Oestrus ovis 134.0
Oidium albicans (*see also* Candidiasis) 112.9
Onchocerca (volvulus) 125.3
eye 125.3 *[360.13]*
eyelid 125.3 *[373.6]*
operation wound 998.5
Opisthorchis (felineus) (tenuicollis) (viverrini) 121.0
orbit 376.00
chronic 376.10
ovary (*see also* Salpingo-oophoritis) 614.2
Oxyuris vermicularis 127.4
pancreas 577.0
Paracoccidioides brasiliensis 116.1
Paragonimus (westermani) 121.2
parainfluenza virus 079.89
parameningococcus NEC 036.9
with meningitis 036.0
parasitic NEC 136.9
paratyphoid 002.9
Type A 002.1
Type B 002.2
Type C 002.3
paraurethral ducts 597.89
parotid gland 527.2

Infection, infected, infective—*continued*
Pasteurella NEC 027.2
multocida (cat-bite) (dog-bite) 027.2
pestis (*see also* Plague) 020.9
pseudotuberculosis 027.2
septica (cat-bite) (dog-bite) 027.2
tularensis (*see also* Tularemia) 021.9
pelvic, female (*see also* Disease, pelvis, inflammatory) 614.9
penis (glans) (retention) NEC 607.2
herpetic 054.13
Peptococcus 041.84
Peptostreptococcus 041.84
periapical (pulpal origin) 522.4
peridental 523.3
perineal wound (obstetrical) 674.3
periodontal 523.3
periorbital 376.00
chronic 376.10
perirectal 569.49
perirenal (*see also* Infection, kidney) 590.9
peritoneal (*see also* Peritonitis) 567.9
periureteral 593.89
periurethral 597.89
Petriellidium boydii 117.6
pharynx 478.29
Coxsackie virus 074.0
phlegmonous 462
posterior, lymphoid 474.0
Phialophora
gougerotii 117.8
jeanselmei 117.8
verrucosa 117.2
Piedraia hortai 111.3
pinna, acute 380.11
pinta 103.9
intermediate 103.1
late 103.2
mixed 103.3
primary 103.0
pinworm 127.4
pityrosporum furfur 111.0
pleuropneumonia-like organisms NEC (PPLO) 041.81
pneumococcal NEC 041.2
generalized (purulent) 038.2
Pneumococcus NEC 041.2
postoperative wound 998.5
posttraumatic NEC 958.3
postvaccinal 999.3
prepuce NEC 607.1
Propionibacterium 041.84
prostate (capsule) (*see also* Prostatitis) 601.9
Proteus (mirabilis) (morganii) (vulgaris) NEC 041.6
enteritis 008.3
protozoal NEC 136.8
intestinal NEC 007.9
Pseudomonas NEC 041.7
mallei 024
pneumonia 482.1
pseudomallei 025
psittacosis 073.9
puerperal, postpartum (major) 670
minor 646.6
pulmonary—*see* Infection, lung
purulent—*see* Abscess
putrid, generalized—*see* Septicemia
pyemic—*see* Septicemia
Pyrenochaeta romeroi 117.4

Infection, infected, infective—*continued*
Q fever 083.0
rabies 071
rectum (sphincter) 569.49
renal (*see also* Infection, kidney) 590.9
pelvis and ureter 590.3
resistant to drugs—*see* Resistance (to), drugs by microorganisms
respiratory 519.8
chronic 519.8
influenzal (acute) (upper) 487.1
lung 518.89
rhinovirus 460
upper (acute) (infectious) NEC 465.9
with flu, grippe, or influenza 487.1
influenzal 487.1
multiple sites NEC 465.8
streptococcal 034.0
viral NEC 465.9
resulting from presence of shunt or other internal prosthetic device—*see* Complications, infection and inflammation, due to (presence of) any device, implant, or graft classified to 996.0-996.5 NEC
retrovirus 079.50
human immunodeficiency virus type 2 [HIV-2] 079.53
human T-cell lymphotrophic virus type I [HTLV-I] 079.51
human T-cell lymphotrophic virus type II [HTLV-II] 079.52
specified NEC 079.59
Rhinocladium 117.1
Rhinosporidium (seeberi) 117.0
rhinovirus
in diseases classified elsewhere—*see* category 079
unspecified nature or site 079.3
Rhizopus 117.7
rickettsial 083.9
rickettsialpox 083.2
rubella (*see also* Rubella) 056.9
congenital 771.0
Saccharomyces (*see also* Candidiasis) 112.9
Saksenaea 117.7
salivary duct or gland (any) 527.2
Salmonella (aertrycke) (callinarum) (choleraesuis) (enteritidis) (suipestifer) (typhimurium) 003.9
with
arthritis 003.23
gastroenteritis 003.0
localized infection 003.20
specified type NEC 003.29
meningitis 003.21
osteomyelitis 003.24
pneumonia 003.22
septicemia 003.1
specified manifestation NEC 003.8
congenital 771.8
due to food (poisoning) (any serotype) (*see also* Poisoning, food, due to, Salmonella)
hirschfeldii 002.3
localized 003.20
specified type NEC 003.29
paratyphi 002.9
A 002.1
B 002.2
C 002.3
schottmuelleri 002.2

Infection, infected, infective—*continued*
specified type NEC 003.8
typhi 002.0
typhosa 002.0
saprophytic 136.8
Sarcocystis, lindemanni 136.5
scabies 133.0
Schistosoma—*see* Infestation, Schistosoma
Schmorl's bacillus 040.3
scratch or other superficial injury—*see* Injury, superficial, by site
scrotum (acute) NEC 608.4
secondary, burn or open wound (dislocation) (fracture) 958.3
seminal vesicle (*see also* Vesiculitis) 608.0
septic
generalized—*see* Septicemia
localized, skin (*see also* Abscess) 682.9
septicemic—*see* Septicemia
Serratia (marcescens) 041.85
generalized 038.44
sheep liver fluke 121.3
Shigella 004.9
boydii 004.2
dysenteriae 004.0
Flexneri 004.1
group
A 004.0
B 004.1
C 004.2
D 004.3
Schmitz (-Stutzer) 004.0
Schmitzii 004.0
Shiga 004.0
Sonnei 004.3
specified type NEC 004.8
sinus (*see also* Sinusitis) 473.9
pilonidal 685.1
with abscess 685.0
skin NEC 686.9
Skene's duct or gland (*see also* Urethritis) 597.89
skin (local) (staphylococcal) (streptococcal) NEC 686.9
abscess—*see* Abscess, by site
cellulitis—*see* Cellulitis, by site
due to fungus 111.9
specified type NEC 111.8
mycotic 111.9
specified type NEC 111.8
ulcer (*see also* Ulcer, skin) 707.9
slow virus 046.9
specified condition NEC 046.8
Sparganum (mansoni) (proliferum) 123.5
specific (*see also* Syphilis) 097.9
to perinatal period NEC 771.8
spermatic cord NEC 608.4
sphenoidal (chronic) (sinus) (*see also* Sinusitis, sphenoidal) 473.3
Spherophorus necrophorus 040.3
spinal cord NEC (*see also* Encephalitis) 323.9
abscess 324.1
late effect—*see* category 326
late effect—*see* category 326
meninges—*see* Meningitis
streptococcal 320.2
Spirillum
minus or minor 026.0
morsus muris 026.0
obermeieri 087.0

Infection, infected, infective—*continued*
spirochetal NEC 104.9
lung 104.8
specified nature or site NEC 104.8
spleen 289.59
Sporothrix schenckii 117.1
Sporotrichum (schenckii) 117.1
Sporozoa 136.8
staphylococcal NEC 041.10
aureus 041.11
food poisoning 005.0
generalized (purulent) 038.1
pneumonia 482.4
septicemia 038.1
specified NEC 041.19
steatoma 706.2
Stellantchasmus falcatus 121.6
Streptobacillus moniliformis 026.1
streptococcal NEC 041.00
congenital 771.8
generalized (purulent) 038.0
Group
A 041.01
B 041.02
C 041.03
D 041.04
G 041.05
pneumonia—*see* Pneumonia, streptococcal 482.3
septicemia 038.0
sore throat 034.0
specified NEC 041.09
Streptomyces—*see* Actinomycosis
streptotrichosis—*see* Actinomycosis
Strongyloides (stercoralis) 127.2
stump (amputation) (surgical) 997.62
traumatic—*see* Amputation, traumatic, by site, complicated
subcutaneous tissue, local NEC 686.9
submaxillary region 528.9
suipestifer (*see also* Infection, Salmonella) 003.9
swimming pool bacillus 031.1
syphilitic—*see* Syphilis
systemic—*see* Septicemia
Taenia—*see* Infestation, Taenia
Taeniarhynchus saginatus 123.2
tapeworm—*see* Infestation, tapeworm
tendon (sheath) 727.89
Ternidens diminutus 127.7
testis (*see also* Orchitis) 604.90
thigh (skin) 686.9
threadworm 127.4
throat 478.29
pneumococcal 462
staphylococcal 462
streptococcal 034.0
viral NEC (*see also* Pharyngitis) 462
thumb (skin) 686.9
abscess (with lymphangitis) 681.00
pulp 681.01
cellulitis (with lymphangitis) 681.00
nail 681.02
thyroglossal duct 529.8
toe (skin) 686.9
abscess (with lymphangitis) 681.10
cellulitis (with lymphangitis) 681.10
nail 681.11
fungus 110.1
tongue NEC 529.0
parasitic 112.0

Infection, infected, infective—*continued*
tonsil (and adenoid) (faucial) (lingual) (pharyngeal) 474.0
acute or subacute 463
tag 474.0
tooth, teeth 522.4
periapical (pulpal origin) 522.4
peridental 523.3
periodontal 523.3
pulp 522.0
socket 526.5
Torula histolytica 117.5
Toxocara (cani) (cati) (felis) 128.0
Toxoplasma gondii (*see also* Toxoplasmosis) 130.9
trachea, chronic 491.8
fungus 117.9
traumatic NEC 958.3
trematode NEC 121.9
trench fever 083.1
Treponema
denticola 041.84
macrodenticum 041.84
pallidum (*see also* Syphilis) 097.9
Trichinella (spiralis) 124
Trichomonas 131.9
bladder 131.09
cervix 131.09
hominis 007.3
intestine 007.3
prostate 131.03
specified site NEC 131.8
urethra 131.02
urogenitalis 131.00
vagina 131.01
vulva 131.01
Trichophyton, trichophytid—*see* Dermatophytosis
Trichosporon (beigelii) cutaneum 111.2
Trichostrongylus 127.6
Trichuris (trichiuria) 127.3
Trombicula (irritans) 133.8
Trypanosoma (*see also* Trypanosomiasis) 086.9
cruzi 086.2
tubal (*see also* Salpingo-oophoritis) 614.2
tuberculous NEC (*see also* Tuberculosis) 011.9
tubo-ovarian (*see also* Salpingo-oophoritis) 614.2
tunica vaginalis 608.4
tympanic membrane—*see* Myringitis
typhoid (abortive) (ambulant) (bacillus) 002.0
typhus 081.9
flea-borne (endemic) 081.0
louse-borne (epidemic) 080
mite-borne 081.2
recrudescent 081.1
tick-borne 082.9
African 082.1
North Asian 082.2
umbilicus (septic) 686.9
newborn NEC 771.4
ureter 593.89
urethra (*see also* Urethritis) 597.80
urinary (tract) NEC 599.0
with
abortion—*see* Abortion, by type, with urinary tract infection
ectopic pregnancy (*see also* categories 633.0-633.9) 639.8

Infection, infected, infective—*continued*
molar pregnancy (*see also* categories 630-632) 639.8
complicating pregnancy, childbirth, or puerperium 646.6
affecting fetus or newborn 760.1
asymptomatic 646.5
affecting fetus or newborn 760.1
diplococcal (acute) 098.0
chronic 098.2
due to Trichomonas (vaginalis) 131.00
following
abortion 639.8
ectopic or molar pregnancy 639.8
gonococcal (acute) 098.0
chronic or duration of 2 months or over 098.2
newborn 771.8
trichomonal 131.00
tuberculous (*see also* Tuberculosis) 016.3
uterus, uterine (*see also* Endometritis) 615.9
utriculus masculinus NEC 597.89
vaccination 999.3
vagina (granulation tissue) (wall) (*see also* Vaginitis) 616.10
varicella 052.9
varicose veins—*see* Varicose, veins
variola 050.9
major 050.0
minor 050.1
vas deferens NEC 608.4
Veillonella 041.84
verumontanum 597.89
vesical (*see also* Cystitis) 595.9
Vibrio
cholerae 001.0
El Tor 001.1
parahaemolyticus (food poisoning) 005.4
vulnificus 041.85
Vincent's (gums) (mouth) (tonsil) 101
virus, viral 079.99
adenovirus
in diseases classified elsewhere—*see* category 079
unspecified nature or site 079.0
central nervous system NEC 049.9
enterovirus 048
meningitis 047.9
specified type NEC 047.8
slow virus 046.9
specified condition NEC 046.8
chest 519.8
conjunctivitis 077.99
specified type NEC 077.8
Coxsackie (*see also* Infection, Coxsackie) 079.2
ECHO
in diseases classified elsewhere—*see* category 079
unspecified nature or site 079.1
encephalitis 049.9
arthropod-borne NEC 064
tick-borne 063.9
specified type NEC 063.8
enteritis NEC (*see also* Enteritis, viral) 008.8
exanthem NEC 057.9
Hantavirus 079.81
human papilloma 079.4
in diseases classified elsewhere—*see* category 079
intestine (*see also* Enteritis, viral) 008.8

Infection, infected, infective—*continued*
lung—*see* Pneumonia, viral
rhinovirus
in diseases classified elsewhere—*see* category 079
unspecified nature or site 079.3
salivary gland disease 078.5
slow 046.9
specified condition NEC 046.8
specified type NEC 079.89
in diseases classified elsewhere—*see* category 079
unspecified nature or site 079.99
warts 078.10
vulva (*see also* Vulvitis) 616.10
whipworm 127.3
Whitmore's bacillus 025
wound (local) (posttraumatic) NEC 958.3
with
dislocation—*see* Dislocation, by site, open
fracture—*see* Fracture, by site, open
open wound—*see* Wound, open, by site, complicated
postoperative 998.5
surgical 998.5
Wuchereria 125.0
bancrofti 125.0
malayi 125.1
yaws—*see* Yaws
yeast (*see also* Candidiasis) 112.9
yellow fever (*see also* Fever, yellow) 060.9
Yersinia pestis (*see also* Plague) 020.9
Zeis' gland 373.12
zoonotic bacterial NEC 027.9
Zopfia senegalensis 117.4
Infective, infectious —*see* condition
Inferiority complex 301.9
constitutional psychopathic 301.9
Infertility
female 628.9
associated with
adhesions, peritubal 614.6 *[628.2]*
anomaly
cervical mucus 628.4
congenital
cervix 628.4
fallopian tube 628.2
uterus 628.3
vagina 628.4
anovulation 628.0
dysmucorrhea 628.4
endometritis, tuberculous (*see also* Tuberculosis) 016.7 *[628.3]*
Stein-Leventhal syndrome 256.4 *[628.0]*
due to
adiposogenital dystrophy 253.8 *[628.1]*
anterior pituitary disorder NEC 253.4 *[628.1]*
hyperfunction 253.1 *[628.1]*
cervical anomaly 628.4
fallopian tube anomaly 628.2
ovarian failure 256.3 *[628.0]*
Stein-Leventhal syndrome 256.4 *[628.0]*
uterine anomaly 628.3
vaginal anomaly 628.4
nonimplantation 628.3
origin
cervical 628.4

Infertility—*continued*
pituitary-hypothalamus NEC 253.8 *[628.1]*
anterior pituitary NEC 253.4 *[628.1]*
hyperfunction NEC 253.1 *[628.1]*
dwarfism 253.3 *[628.1]*
panhypopituitarism 253.2 *[628.1]*
specified NEC 628.8
tubal (block) (occlusion) (stenosis) 628.2
adhesions 614.6 *[628.2]*
uterine 628.3
vaginal 628.4
previous, requiring supervision of pregnancy V23.0
male 606.9
absolute 606.0
due to
azoospermia 606.0
drug therapy 606.8
extratesticular cause NEC 606.8
germinal cell
aplasia 606.0
desquamation 606.1
hypospermatogenesis 606.1
infection 606.8
obstruction, afferent ducts 606.8
oligospermia 606.1
radiation 606.8
spermatogenic arrest (complete) 606.0
incomplete 606.1
systemic disease 606.8
Infestation 134.9
Acanthocheilonema (perstans) 125.4
streptocerca 125.6
Acariasis 133.9
demodex folliculorum 133.8
Sarcoptes scabiei 133.0
trombiculae 133.8
Agamofilaria streptocerca 125.6
Ancylostoma, Ankylostoma 126.9
americanum 126.1
braziliense 126.2
canium 126.8
ceylanicum 126.3
duodenale 126.0
new world 126.1
old world 126.0
Angiostrongylus cantonensis 128.8
anisakiasis 127.1
Anisakis larva 127.1
arthropod NEC 134.1
Ascaris lumbricoides 127.0
Bacillus fusiformis 101
Balantidium coli 007.0
beef tapeworm 123.2
Bothriocephalus (latus) 123.4
larval 123.5
broad tapeworm 123.4
larval 123.5
Brugia malayi 125.1
Candiru 136.8
Capillaria
hepatica 128.8
philippinensis 127.5
cat liver fluke 121.0
Cercomonas hominis (intestinal) 007.3
cestodes 123.9
specified type NEC 123.8
chigger 133.8
chigoe 134.1
Chilomastix 007.8
Infestation—*continued*
Clonorchis (sinensis) (liver) 121.1
coccidia 007.2
complicating pregnancy, childbirth, or puerperium 647.9
affecting fetus or newborn 760.8
Cysticercus cellulosae 123.1
Demodex folliculorum 133.8
Dermatobia (hominis) 134.0
Dibothriocephalus (latus) 123.4
larval 123.5
Dicrocoelium dendriticum 121.8
Diphyllobothrium (adult) (intestinal) (latum) (pacificum) 123.4
larval 123.5
Diplogonoporus (grandis) 123.8
Dipylidium (caninum) 123.8
Distoma hepaticum 121.3
dog tapeworm 123.8
Dracunculus medinensis 125.7
dragon worm 125.7
dwarf tapeworm 123.6
Echinococcus (*see also* Echinococcus) 122.9
Echinostoma ilocanum 121.8
Embadomonas 007.8
Endamoeba (histolytica)—*see* Infection, ameba
Entamoeba (histolytica)—*see* Infection, ameba
Enterobius vermicularis 127.4
Epidermophyton—*see* Dermatophytosis
eyeworm 125.2
Fasciola
gigantica 121.3
hepatica 121.3
Fasciolopsis (buski) (small intestine) 121.4
filarial 125.9
due to
Acanthocheilonema (perstans) 125.4
streptocerca 125.6
Brugia (Wuchereria) malayi 125.1
Dracunculus medinensis 125.7
guinea worms 125.7
Mansonella (ozzardi) 125.5
Onchocerca volvulus 125.3
eye 125.3 *[360.13]*
eyelid 125.3 *[373.6]*
Wuchereria (bancrofti) 125.0
malayi 125.1
specified type NEC 125.6
fish tapeworm 123.4
larval 123.5
fluke 121.9
blood NEC (*see also* Schistosomiasis) 120.9
cat liver 121.0
intestinal (giant) 121.4
liver (sheep) 121.3
cat 121.0
Chinese 121.1
clonorchiasis 121.1
fascioliasis 121.3
Oriental 121.1
lung (oriental) 121.2
sheep liver 121.3
fly larva 134.0
Gasterophilus (intestinalis) 134.0
Gastrodiscoides hominis 121.8
Giardia lamblia 007.1
Gnathostoma (spinigerum) 128.1
Gongylonema 125.6
guinea worm 125.7

Infestation—*continued*
helminth NEC 128.9
intestinal 127.9
mixed (types classifiable to more than one category in 120.0-127.7) 127.8
specified type NEC 127.7
specified type NEC 128.8
Heterophyes heterophyes (small intestine) 121.6
hookworm (*see also* Infestation, ancylostoma) 126.9
Hymenolepis (diminuta) (nana) 123.6
intestinal NEC 129
leeches (aquatic) (land) 134.2
Leishmania—*see* Leishmaniasis
lice (*see also* infestation, pediculus) 132.9
Linguatulidae, linguatula (pentastoma) (serrata) 134.1
Loa loa 125.2
eyelid 125.2 *[373.6]*
louse (*see also* Infestation, pediculus) 132.9
body 132.1
head 132.0
pubic 132.2
maggots 134.0
Mansonella (ozzardi) 125.5
medina 125.7
Metagonimus yokogawai (small intestine) 121.5
Microfilaria streptocerca 125.3
eye 125.3 *[360.13]*
eyelid 125.3 *[373.6]*
Microsporon furfur 111.0
microsporum—*see* Dermatophytosis
mites 133.9
scabic 133.0
specified type NEC 133.8
Monilia (albicans) (*see also* Candidiasis) 112.9
vagina 112.1
vulva 112.1
mouth 112.0
Necator americanus 126.1
nematode (intestinal) 127.9
Ancylostoma (*see also* Ancylostoma) 126.9
Ascaris lumbricoides 127.0
conjunctiva NEC 128.9
Dioctophyma 128.8
Enterobius vermicularis 127.4
Gnathostoma spinigerum 128.1
Oesophagostomum (apiostomum) 127.7
Physaloptera 127.4
specified type NEC 127.7
Strongyloides stercoralis 127.2
Ternidens diminutus 127.7
Trichinella spiralis 124
Trichostrongylus 127.6
Trichuris (trichiuria) 127.3
Oesophagostomum (apiostomum) 127.7
Oestrus ovis 134.0
Onchocerca (volvulus) 125.3
eye 125.3 *[360.13]*
eyelid 125.3 *[373.6]*
Opisthorchis (felineus) (tenuicollis) (viverrini) 121.0
Oxyuris vermicularis 127.4
Paragonimus (westermani) 121.2
parasite, parasitic NEC 136.9
eyelid 134.9 *[373.6]*
intestinal 129
mouth 112.0
orbit 376.13
skin 134.9
tongue 112.0

Infestation—*continued*
pediculus 132.9
capitis (humanus) (any site) 132.0
corporis (humanus) (any site) 132.1
eyelid 132.0 *[373.6]*
mixed (classifiable to more than one category in 132.0-132.2) 132.3
pubis (any site) 132.2
phthirus (pubis) (any site) 132.2
with any infestation classifiable to 132.0 and 132.1 132.3
pinworm 127.4
pork tapeworm (adult) 123.0
protozoal NEC 136.8
pubic louse 132.2
rat tapeworm 123.6
red bug 133.8
roundworm (large) NEC 127.0
sand flea 134.1
saprophytic NEC 136.8
Sarcoptes scabiei 133.0
scabies 133.0
Schistosoma 120.9
bovis 120.8
cercariae 120.3
hematobium 120.0
intercalatum 120.8
japonicum 120.2
mansoni 120.1
mattheii 120.8
specified
site—*see* Schistosomiasis
type NEC 120.8
spindale 120.8
screw worms 134.0
skin NEC 134.9
Sparganum (mansoni) (proliferum) 123.5
larval 123.5
specified type NEC 134.8
Spirometra larvae 123.5
Sporozoa NEC 136.8
Stellantchasmus falcatus 121.6
Strongyloides 127.2
Strongylus (gibsoni) 127.7
Taenia 123.3
diminuta 123.6
Echinococcus (*see also* Echinococcus) 122.9
mediocanellata 123.2
nana 123.6
saginata (mediocanellata) 123.2
solium (intestinal form) 123.0
larval form 123.1
Taeniarhynchus saginatus 123.2
tapeworm 123.9
beef 123.2
broad 123.4
larval 123.5
dog 123.8
dwarf 123.6
fish 123.4
larval 123.5
pork 123.0
rat 123.6
Ternidens diminutus 127.7
Tetranychus molestissimus 133.8
threadworm 127.4
tongue 112.0
Toxocara (cani) (cati) (felis) 128.0
trematode(s) NEC 121.9
Trichina spiralis 124

Infestation—*continued*
Trichinella spiralis 124
Trichocephalus 127.3
Trichomonas 131.9
bladder 131.09
cervix 131.09
intestine 007.3
prostate 131.03
specified site NEC 131.8
urethra (female) (male) 131.02
urogenital 131.00
vagina 131.01
vulva 131.01
Trichophyton—*see* Dermatophytosis
Trichostrongylus instabilis 127.6
Trichuris (trichiuria) 127.3
Trombicula (irritans) 133.8
Trypanosoma—*see* Trypanosomiasis
Tunga penetrans 134.1
Uncinaria americana 126.1
whipworm 127.3
worms NEC 128.9
intestinal 127.9
Wuchereria 125.0
bancrofti 125.0
malayi 125.1
Infiltrate, infiltration
with an iron compound 275.0
amyloid (any site) (generalized) 277.3
calcareous (muscle) NEC 275.4
localized—*see* Degeneration, by site
calcium salt (muscle) 275.4
corneal (*see also* Edema, cornea) 371.20
eyelid 373.9
fatty (diffuse) (generalized) 272.8
localized—*see* Degeneration, by site, fatty
glycogen, glycogenic (*see also* Disease, glycogen storage) 271.10
heart, cardiac
fatty (*see also* Degeneration, myocardial) 429.1
glycogenic 271.0 *[425.7]*
inflammatory in vitreous 379.29
kidney (*see also* Disease, renal) 593.9
leukemic (M9800/3)—*see* Leukemia
liver 573.8
fatty—*see* Fatty, liver
glycogen (*see also* Disease, glycogen storage) 271.0
lung (*see also* Infiltrate, pulmonary) 518.3
eosinophilic 518.3
x-ray finding only 793.1
lymphatic (*see also* Leukemia, lymphatic) 204.9
gland, pigmentary 289.3
muscle, fatty 728.9
myelogenous (*see also* Leukemia, myeloid) 205.9
myocardium, myocardial
fatty (*see also* Degeneration, myocardial) 429.1
glycogenic 271.0 *[425.7]*
pulmonary 518.3
with
eosinophilia 518.3
pneumonia—*see* Pneumonia, by type
x-ray finding only 793.1
Ranke's primary (*see also* Tuberculosis) 010.0
skin, lymphocyctic (benign) 709.8
thymus (gland) (fatty) 254.8
urine 788.8
vitreous humor 379.29
Infirmity 799.8
senile 797
Inflammation, inflamed, inflammatory (with exudation)
abducens (nerve) 378.54
accessory sinus (chronic) (*see also* Sinusitis) 473.9
adrenal (gland) 255.8
alimentary canal—*see* Enteritis
alveoli (teeth) 526.5
scorbutic 267
amnion—*see* Amnionitis
anal canal 569.49
antrum (chronic) (*see also* Sinusitis, maxillary) 473.0
anus 569.49
appendix (*see also* Appendicitis) 541
arachnoid—*see* Meningitis
areola 611.0
puerperal, postpartum 675.0
areolar tissue NEC 686.9
artery—*see* Arteritis
auditory meatus (external) (*see also* Otitis, externa) 380.10
Bartholin's gland 616.8
bile duct or passage 576.1
bladder (*see also* Cystitis) 595.9
bone—*see* Osteomyelitis
bowel (*see also* Enteritis) 558.9
brain (*see also* Encephalitis) 323.9
late effect—*see* category 326
membrane—*see* Meningitis
breast 611.0
puerperal, postpartum 675.2
broad ligament (*see also* Disease, pelvis, inflammatory) 614.4
acute 614.3
bronchus—*see* Bronchitis
bursa—*see* Bursitis
capsule
liver 573.3
spleen 289.59
catarrhal (*see also* Catarrh) 460
vagina 616.10
cecum (*see also* Appendicitis) 541
cerebral (*see also* Encephalitis) 323.9
late effect—*see* category 326
membrane—*see* Meningitis
cerebrospinal (*see also* Meningitis) 322.9
late effect—*see* category 326
meningococcal 036.0
tuberculous (*see also* Tuberculosis) 013.6
cervix (uteri) (*see also* Cervicitis) 616.0
chest 519.9
choroid NEC (*see also* Choroiditis) 363.20
cicatrix (tissue)—*see* Cicatrix
colon (*see also* Enteritis) 558.9
granulomatous 555.1
newborn 558.9
connective tissue (diffuse) NEC 728.9
cornea (*see also* Keratitis) 370.9
with ulcer (*see also* Ulcer, cornea) 370.00
corpora cavernosa (penis) 607.2
cranial nerve—*see* Disorder, nerve, cranial
diarrhea—*see* Diarrhea
disc (intervertebral) (space) 722.90
cervical, cervicothoracic 722.91
lumbar, lumbosacral 722.93
thoracic, thoracolumbar 722.93

Inflammation, inflamed, inflammatory—*cont.*
Douglas' cul-de-sac or pouch (chronic) (*see also* Disease, pelvis, inflammatory) 614.4
acute 614.3
due to (presence of) any device, implant, or graft classifiable to 996.0-996.5—*see* Complications, infection and inflammation, due to (presence of) any device, implant, or graft classified to 996.0-996.5 NEC
duodenum 535.6
dura mater—*see* Meningitis
ear—*see also* Otitis
external (*see also* Otitis, externa) 380.10
inner (*see also* Labyrinthitis) 386.30
middle—*see* Otitis media
esophagus 530.10
ethmoidal (chronic) (sinus) (*see also* Sinusitis, ethmoidal) 473.2
Eustachian tube (catarrhal) 381.50
acute 381.51
chronic 381.52
extrarectal 569.49
eye 379.99
eyelid 373.9
specified NEC 373.8
fallopian tube (*see also* Salpingo-oophoritis) 614.2
fascia 728.9
fetal membranes (acute) 658.4
affecting fetus or newborn 762.7
follicular, pharynx 472.1
frontal (chronic) (sinus) (*see also* Sinusitis, frontal) 473.1
gallbladder (*see also* Cholecystitis, acute) 575.0
gall duct (*see also* Cholecystitis) 575.1
gastrointestinal (*see also* Enteritis) 558.9
genital organ (diffuse) (internal)
female 614.9
with
abortion—*see* Abortion, by type, with sepsis
ectopic pregnancy (*see also* categories 633.0-633.9) 639.0
molar pregnancy (*see also* categories 630-632) 639.0
complicating pregnancy, childbirth, or puerperium 646.6
affecting fetus or newborn 760.8
following
abortion 639.0
ectopic or molar pregnancy 639.0
male 608.4
gland (lymph) (*see also* Lymphadenitis) 289.3
glottis (*see also* Laryngitis) 464.0
granular, pharynx 472.1
gum 523.1
heart (*see also* Carditis) 429.89
hepatic duct 576.8
hernial sac—*see* Hernia, by site
ileum (*see also* Enteritis) 558.9
terminal or regional 555.0
with large intestine 555.2
intervertebral disc 722.90
cervical, cervicothoracic 722.91
lumbar, lumbosacral 722.93
thoracic, thoracolumbar 722.92
intestine (*see also* Enteritis) 558.9
jaw (acute) (bone) (chronic) (lower) (suppurative) (upper) 526.4
jejunum—*see* Enteritis

Inflammation, inflamed, inflammatory—*cont.*
joint NEC (*see also* Arthritis) 716.9
sacroiliac 720.2
kidney (*see also* Nephritis) 583.9
knee (joint) 716.66
tuberculous (active) (*see also* Tuberculosis) 015.2
labium (majus) (minus) (*see also* Vulvitis) 616.10
lacrimal
gland (*see also* Dacryoadenitis) 375.00
passages (duct) (sac) (*see also* Dacryocystitis) 375.30
larynx (*see also* Laryngitis) 464.0
diphtheritic 032.3
leg NEC 686.9
lip 528.5
liver (capsule) (*see also* Hepatitis) 573.3
acute 570
chronic 571.40
suppurative 572.0
lung (acute) (*see also* Pneumonia) 486
chronic (interstitial) 518.89
lymphatic vessel (*see also* Lymphangitis) 457.2
lymph node or gland (*see also* Lymphadenitis) 289.3
mammary gland 611.0
puerperal, postpartum 675.2
maxilla, maxillary 526.4
sinus (chronic) (*see also* Sinusitis, maxillary) 473.0
membranes of brain or spinal cord—*see* Meningitis
meninges—*see* Meningitis
mouth 528.0
muscle 728.9
myocardium (*see also* Myocarditis) 429.0
nasal sinus (chronic) (*see also* Sinusitis) 473.9
nasopharynx—*see* Nasopharyngitis
navel 686.9
newborn NEC 771.4
nerve NEC 729.2
nipple 611.0
puerperal, postpartum 675.0
nose 478.1
suppurative 472.0
oculomotor nerve 378.51
optic nerve 377.30
orbit (chronic) 376.10
acute 376.00
chronic 376.10
ovary (*see also* Salpingo-oophoritis) 614.2
oviduct (*see also* Salpingo-oophoritis) 614.2
pancreas—*see* Pancreatitis
parametrium (chronic) (*see also* Disease, pelvis, inflammatory) 614.4
acute 614.3
parotid region 686.9
gland 527.2
pelvis, female (*see also* Disease, pelvis, inflammatory) 614.9
penis (corpora cavernosa) 607.2
perianal 569.49
pericardium (*see also* Pericarditis) 423.9
perineum (female) (male) 686.9
perirectal 569.49
peritoneum (*see also* Peritonitis) 567.9
periuterine (*see also* Disease, pelvis, inflammatory) 614.9
perivesical (*see also* Cystitis) 595.9
petrous bone (*see also* Petrositis) 383.20
pharynx (*see also* Pharyngitis) 462

Inflammation, inflamed, inflammatory—*cont.*
follicular 472.1
granular 472.1
pia mater—*see* Meningitis
pleura—*see* Pleurisy
postmastoidectomy cavity 383.30
chronic 383.33
prostate (*see also* Prostatitis) 601.9
rectosigmoid—*see* Rectosigmoiditis
rectum (*see also* Proctitis) 569.49
respiratory, upper (*see also* Infection, respiratory, upper) 465.9
chronic, due to external agent—*see* Condition, respiratory, chronic, due to, external agent
due to
fumes or vapors (chemical) (inhalation) 506.2
radiation 508.1
retina (*see also* Retinitis) 363.20
retrocecal (*see also* Appendicitis) 541
retroperitoneal (*see also* Peritonitis) 567.9
salivary duct or gland (any) (suppurative) 527.2
scorbutic, alveoli, teeth 267
scrotum 608.4
sigmoid—*see* Enteritis
sinus (*see also* Sinusitis) 473.9
Skene's duct or gland (*see also* Urethritis) 597.89
skin 686.9
spermatic cord 608.4
sphenoidal (sinus) (*see also* Sinusitis, sphenoidal) 473.3
spinal
cord (*see also* Encephalitis) 323.9
late effect—*see* category 326
membrane—*see* Meningitis
nerve—*see* Disorder, nerve
spine (*see also* Spondylitis) 720.9
spleen (capsule) 289.59
stomach—*see* Gastritis
stricture, rectum 569.49
subcutaneous tissue NEC 686.9
suprarenal (gland) 255.8
synovial (fringe) (membrane)—*see* Bursitis
tendon (sheath) NEC 727.9
testis (*see also* Orchitis) 604.90
thigh 686.9
throat (*see also* Sore throat) 462
thymus (gland) 254.8
thyroid (gland) (*see also* Thyroiditis) 245.9
tongue 529.0
tonsil—*see* Tonsillitis
trachea—*see* Tracheitis
trochlear nerve 378.53
tubal (*see also* Salpingo-oophoritis) 614.2
tuberculous NEC (*see also* Tuberculosis) 011.9
tubo-ovarian (*see also* Salpingo-oophoritis) 614.2
tunica vaginalis 608.4
tympanic membrane—*see* Myringitis
umbilicus, umbilical 686.9
newborn NEC 771.4
uterine ligament (*see also* Disease, pelvis, inflammatory) 614.4
acute 614.3
uterus (catarrhal) (*see also* Endometritis) 615.9
uveal tract (anterior) (*see also* Iridocyclitis) 364.3
posterior—*see* Chorioretinitis
sympathetic 360.11

Inflammation, inflamed, inflammatory—*cont.*
vagina (*see also* Vaginitis) 616.10
vas deferens 608.4
vein (*see also* Phlebitis) 451.9
thrombotic 451.9
cerebral (*see also* Thrombosis, brain) 434.0
leg 451.2
deep (vessels) NEC 451.19
superficial (vessels) 451.0
lower extremity 451.2
deep (vessels) NEC 451.19
superficial (vessels) 451.0
vocal cord 478.5
vulva (*see also* Vulvitis) 616.10
Inflation, lung imperfect (newborn) 770.5
Influenza, influenzal 487.1
with
bronchitis 487.1
bronchopneumonia 487.0
cold (any type) 487.1
digestive manifestations 487.8
hemoptysis 487.1
involvement of
gastrointestinal tract 487.8
nervous system 487.8
laryngitis 487.1
manifestations NEC 487.8
respiratory 487.1
pneumonia 487.0
pharyngitis 487.1
pneumonia (any form classifiable to 480-483, 485-486) 487.0
respiratory manifestations NEC 487.1
sinusitis 487.1
sore throat 487.1
tonsillitis 487.1
tracheitis 487.1
upper respiratory infection (acute) 487.1
abdominal 487.8
Asian 487.1
bronchial 487.1
bronchopneumonia 487.0
catarrhal 487.1
epidemic 487.1
gastric 487.8
intestinal 487.8
laryngitis 487.1
maternal affecting fetus or newborn 760.2
manifest influenza in infant 771.2
pharyngitis 487.1
pneumonia (any form) 487.0
respiratory (upper) 487.1
stomach 487.8
vaccination, prophylactic (against) V04.8
Influenza-like disease 487.1
Infraction, Freiberg's (metatarsal head) 732.5
Infusion complication, misadventure or reaction —*see* Complication, infusion
Ingestion
chemical—*see* Table of drugs and chemicals
drug or medicinal substance
correct substance properly administered 995.2
overdose or wrong substance given or taken 977.9
specified drug—*see* Table of drugs and chemicals
foreign body NEC (*see also* Foreign body) 938
Ingrowing
hair 704.8
nail (finger) (toe) (infected) 703.0

Inguinal —*see also* condition
testis 752.5
Inhalation
carbon monoxide 986
flame (asphyxia) (*see also* Burn, by site) 949.0
food or foreign body (*see also* Asphyxia, food or foreign body) 933.1
gas, fumes, or vapor (noxious) 987.9
specified agent—*see* Table of drugs and chemicals
liquid or vomitus (*see also* Asphyxia, food or foreign body) 933.1
lower respiratory tract NEC 934.9
meconium (fetus or newborn) 770.1
mucus (*see also* Asphyxia, mucus) 933.1
oil (causing suffocation) (*see also* Asphyxia, food or foreign body) 933.1
pneumonia—*see* Pneumonia, aspiration
smoke 987.9
steam 987.9
stomach contents or secretions (*see also* Asphyxia, food or foreign body) 933.1
in labor and deliver 668.0
Inhibition, inhibited
academic as adjustment reaction 309.23
orgasm
female 302.73
male 302.74
sexual
desire 302.71
excitement 302.72
work as adjustment reaction 309.23
Inhibitor, systemic lupus erythematosus (presence of) 286.5
Iniencephalus, iniencephaly 740.2
Injected eye 372.74
Injury 959.9

Note—For abrasion, insect bite (nonvenomous), blister, or scratch, *see* Injury, superficial. For laceration, traumatic rupture, tear, or penetrating wound of internal organs, such as heart, lung, liver, kidney, pelvic organs, whether or not accompanied by open wound in the same region, *see* Injury, internal. For nerve injury, see Injury, nerve. For late effect of injuries classifiable to 850-854, 860-869, 900-919, 950-959, *see* Late, effect, injury, by type.

abdomen, abdominal (viscera)—*see also* Injury, internal, abdomen
muscle or wall 959.1
acoustic, resulting in deafness 951.5
adenoid 959.0
adrenal (gland)—*see* Injury, internal, adrenal
alveolar (process) 959.0
ankle (and foot) (and knee) (and leg, except thigh) 959.7
anterior chamber, eye 921.3
anus 959.1
aorta (thoracic) 901.0
abdominal 902.0
appendix—*see* Injury, internal, appendix
arm, upper (and shoulder) 959.2
artery (complicating trauma) (*see also* Injury, blood vessel, by site) 904.9
cerebral or meningeal (*see also* Hemorrhage, brain, traumatic, subarachnoid) 852.0
auditory canal (external) (meatus) 959.0
auricle, auris, ear 959.0
axilla 959.2
Injury—*continued*
back 959.1
bile duct—*see* Injury, internal, bile duct
birth—*see also* Birth, injury
canal NEC, complicating delivery 665.9
bladder (sphincter)—*see* Injury, internal, bladder
blast (air) (hydraulic) (immersion) (underwater) NEC 869.0
with open wound into cavity NEC 869.1
abdomen or thorax—*see* Injury, internal, by site
brain—*see* Concussion, brain
ear (acoustic nerve trauma) 951.5
with perforation of tympanic membrane—*see* Wound, open, ear, drum
blood vessel NEC 904.9
abdomen 902.9
multiple 902.87
specified NEC 902.89
aorta (thoracic) 901.0
abdominal 902.0
arm NEC 903.9
axillary 903.00
artery 903.01
vein 903.02
azygos vein 901.89
basilic vein 903.1
brachial (artery) (vein) 903.1
bronchial 901.89
carotid artery 900.00
common 900.01
external 900.02
internal 900.03
celiac artery 902.20
specified branch NEC 902.24
cephalic vein (arm) 903.1
colica dextra 902.26
cystic
artery 902.24
vein 902.39
deep plantar 904.6
digital (artery) (vein) 903.5
due to accidental puncture or laceration during procedure 998.2
extremity
lower 904.8
multiple 904.7
specified NEC 904.7
upper 903.9
multiple 903.8
specified NEC 903.8
femoral
artery (superficial) 904.1
above profunda origin 904.0
common 904.0
vein 904.2
gastric
artery 902.21
vein 902.39
head 900.9
intracranial—*see* Injury, intracranial
multiple 900.82
specified NEC 900.89
hemiazygos vein 901.89
hepatic
artery 902.22
vein 902.11
hypogastric 902.59
artery 902.51
vein 902.52

Injury—*continued*
ileocolic
artery 902.26
vein 902.31
iliac 902.50
artery 902.53
specified branch NEC 902.59
vein 902.54
innominate
artery 901.1
vein 901.3
intercostal (artery) (vein) 901.81
jugular vein (external) 900.81
internal 900.1
leg NEC 904.8
mammary (artery) (vein) 901.82
mesenteric
artery 902.20
inferior 902.27
specified branch NEC 902.29
superior (trunk) 902.25
branches, primary 902.26
vein 902.39
inferior 902.32
superior (and primary subdivisions) 902.31
neck 900.9
multiple 900.82
specified NEC 900.89
ovarian 902.89
artery 902.81
vein 902.82
palmar artery 903.4
pelvis 902.9
multiple 902.87
specified NEC 902.89
plantar (deep) (artery) (vein) 904.6
popliteal 904.40
artery 904.41
vein 904.42
portal 902.33
pulmonary 901.40
artery 901.41
vein 901.42
radial (artery) (vein) 903.2
renal 902.40
artery 902.41
specified NEC 902.49
vein 902.42
saphenous
artery 904.7
vein (greater) (lesser) 904.3
splenic
artery 902.23
vein 902.34
subclavian
artery 901.1
vein 901.3
suprarenal 902.49
thoracic 901.9
multiple 901.83
specified NEC 901.89
tibial 904.50
artery 904.50
anterior 904.51
posterior 904.53
vein 904.50
anterior 904.52
posterior 904.54
ulnar (artery) (vein) 903.3

Injury—*continued*
uterine 902.59
artery 902.55
vein 902.56
vena cava
inferior 902.10
specified branches NEC 902.19
superior 901.2
brachial plexus 953.4
newborn 767.6
brain NEC (*see also* Injury, intracranial) 854.0
breast 959.1
broad ligament—*see* Injury, internal, broad ligament
bronchus, bronchi—*see* Injury, internal, bronchus
brow 959.0
buttock 959.1
canthus, eye 921.1
cathode ray 990
cauda equina 952.4
with fracture, vertebra—*see* Fracture, vertebra, sacrum
cavernous sinus (*see also* Injury, intracranial) 854.0
cecum—*see* Injury, internal, cecum
celiac ganglion or plexus 954.1
cerebellum (*see also* Injury, intracranial) 854.0
cervix (uteri)—*see* Injury, internal, cervix
cheek 959.0
chest—*see also* Injury, internal, chest wall 959.1
childbirth—*see also* Birth, injury
maternal NEC 665.9
chin 959.0
choroid (eye) 921.3
clitoris 959.1
coccyx 959.1
complicating delivery 665.6
colon—*see* Injury, internal, colon
common duct—*see* Injury, internal, common duct
conjunctiva 921.1
superficial 918.2
cord
spermatic—*see* Injury, internal, spermatic cord
spinal—*see* Injury, spinal, by site
cornea 921.3
abrasion 918.1
due to contact lens 371.82
penetrating—*see* Injury, eyeball, penetrating
superficial 918.1
due to contact lens 371.82
cortex (cerebral) (*see also* Injury, intracranial) 854.0
visual 950.3
costal region 959.1
costochondral 959.1
cranial
bones—*see* Fracture, skull, by site
cavity (*see also* Injury, intracranial) 854.0
nerve—*see* Injury, nerve, cranial
crushing—*see* Crush
cutaneous sensory nerve
lower limb 956.4
upper limb 955.5
delivery—*see also* Birth, injury
maternal NEC 665.9
Descemet's membrane—*see* Injury, eyeball, penetrating

Injury—*continued*
diaphragm—*see* Injury, internal, diaphragm
duodenum—*see* Injury, internal, duodenum
ear (auricle) (canal) (drum) (external) 959.0
elbow (and forearm) (and wrist) 959.3
epididymis 959.1
epigastric region 959.1
epiglottis 959.0
epiphyseal, current—*see* Fracture, by site
esophagus—*see* Injury, internal, esophagus
Eustachian tube 959.0
extremity (lower) (upper) NEC 959.8
eye 921.9
penetrating eyeball—*see* Injury, eyeball, penetrating
superficial 918.9
eyeball 921.3
penetrating 871.7
with
partial loss (of intraocular tissue) 871.12
prolapse or exposure (of intraocular tissue) 871.1
without prolapse 871.0
foreign body (nonmagnetic) 871.6
magnetic 871.5
superficial 918.9
eyebrow 959.0
eyelid(s) 921.1
laceration—*see* Laceration, eyelid
superficial 918.0
face (and neck) 959.0
fallopian tube—*see* Injury, internal, fallopian tube
finger(s) (nail) 959.5
flank 959.1
foot (and ankle) (and knee) (and leg except thigh) 959.7
forceps NEC 767.9
scalp 767.1
forearm (and elbow) (and wrist) 959.3
forehead 959.0
gallbladder—*see* Injury, internal, gallbladder
gasserian ganglion 951.2
gastrointestinal tract—*see* Injury, internal, gastrointestinal tract
genital organ(s)
with
abortion—*see* Abortion, by type, with, damage to pelvic organs
ectopic pregnancy (*see also* categories 633.0-633.9) 639.2
molar pregnancy (*see also* categories 630-632) 639.2
external 959.1
following
abortion 639.2
ectopic or molar pregnancy 639.2
internal—*see* Injury, internal, genital organs
obstetrical trauma NEC 665.9
affecting fetus or newborn 763.8
gland
lacrimal 921.1
laceration 870.8
parathyroid 959.0
salivary 959.0
thyroid 959.0
globe (eye) (*see also* Injury, eyeball) 921.3
grease gun—*see* Wound, open, by site, complicated
groin 959.1

Injury—*continued*
gum 959.0
hand(s) (except fingers) 959.4
head NEC (*see also* Injury, intracranial) 854.0
with
skull fracture—*see* Fracture, skull, by site
heart—*see* Injury, internal, heart
heel 959.7
hip (and thigh) 959.6
hymen 959.1
hyperextension (cervical) (vertebra) 847.0
ileum—*see* Injury, internal, ileum
iliac region 959.1
infrared rays NEC 990
instrumental (during surgery) 998.2
birth injury—*see* Birth, injury
nonsurgical (*see also* Injury, by site) 959.9
obstetrical 665.9
affecting fetus or newborn 763.8
bladder 665.5
cervix 665.3
high vaginal 665.4
perineal NEC 664.9
urethra 665.5
uterus 665.5
internal 869.0

Note—For injury of internal organ(s) by foreign body entering through a natural orifice (e.g., inhaled, ingested, or swallowed)—*see* Foreign body, entering through orifice.

For internal injury of any of the following sites with internal injury of any other of the sites—*see* Injury, internal, multiple.

with
fracture
pelvis—*see* Fracture, pelvis
specified site, except pelvis—*see* Injury, internal, by site
open wound into cavity 869.1
abdomen, abdominal (viscera) NEC 868.00
with
fracture, pelvis—*see* Fracture, pelvis
open wound into cavity 868.10
specified site NEC 868.09
with open wound into cavity 868.19
adrenal (gland) 868.01
with open wound into cavity 868.11
aorta (thoracic) 901.0
abdominal 902.0
appendix 863.85
with open wound into cavity 863.95
bile duct 868.02
with open wound into cavity 868.12
bladder (sphincter) 867.0
with
abortion—*see* Abortion, by type, with, damage to pelvic organs
ectopic pregnancy (*see also* categories 633.0-633.9) 639.2
molar pregnancy (*see also* categories 630-632) 639.2
open wound into cavity 867.1
following
abortion 639.2
ectopic or molar pregnancy 639.2
obstetrical trauma 665.5
affecting fetus or newborn 763.8
blood vessel—*see* Injury, blood vessel, by site

Injury—*continued*
broad ligament 867.6
with open wound into cavity 867.7
bronchus, bronchi 862.21
with open wound into cavity 862.31
cecum 863.89
with open wound into cavity 863.99
cervix (uteri) 867.4
with
abortion—*see* Abortion, by type, with damage to pelvic organs
ectopic pregnancy (*see also* categories 633.0-633.9) 639.2
molar pregnancy (*see also* categories 630-632) 639.2
open wound into cavity 867.5
following
abortion 639.2
ectopic or molar pregnancy 639.2
obstetrical trauma 665.3
affecting fetus or newborn 763.8
chest (*see also* Injury, internal, intrathoracic organs) 862.8
with open wound into cavity 862.9
colon 863.40
with
open wound into cavity 863.50
rectum 863.46
with open wound into cavity 863.56
ascending (right) 863.41
with open wound into cavity 863.51
descending (left) 863.43
with open wound into cavity 863.53
multiple sites 863.46
with open wound into cavity 863.56
sigmoid 863.44
with open wound into cavity 863.54
specified site NEC 863.49
with open wound into cavity 863.59
transverse 863.42
with open wound into cavity 863.52
common duct 868.02
with open wound into cavity 868.12
complicating delivery 665.9
affecting fetus or newborn 763.8
diaphragm 862.0
with open wound into cavity 862.1
duodenum 863.21
with open wound into cavity 863.31
esophagus (intrathoracic) 862.22
with open wound into cavity 862.32
cervical region 874.4
complicated 874.5
fallopian tube 867.6
with open wound into cavity 867.7
gallbladder 868.02
with open wound into cavity 868.12
gastrointestinal tract NEC 863.80
with open wound into cavity 863.90
genital organ NEC 867.6
with open wound into cavity 867.7
heart 861.00
with open wound into thorax 861.10
ileum 863.29
with open wound into cavity 863.39
intestine NEC 863.89
with open wound into cavity 863.99
large NEC 863.40
with open wound into cavity 863.50
small NEC 863.20
with open wound into cavity 863.30

Injury—*continued*
intra-abdominal (organ) 868.00
with open wound into cavity 868.10
multiple sites 868.09
with open wound into cavity 868.19
specified site NEC 868.09
with open wound into cavity 868.19
intrathoracic organs (multiple) 862.8
with open wound into cavity 862.9
diaphragm (only)—*see* Injury, internal, diaphragm
heart (only)—*see* Injury, internal, heart
lung (only)—*see* Injury, internal, lung
specified site NEC 862.29
with open wound into cavity 862.39
intrauterine (*see also* Injury, internal, uterus) 867.4
with open wound into cavity 867.5
jejunum 863.29
with open wound into cavity 863.39
kidney (subcapsular) 866.00
with
disruption of parenchyma (complete) 866.03
with open wound into cavity 866.13
hematoma (without rupture of capsule) 866.01
with open wound into cavity 866.11
laceration 866.02
with open wound into cavity 866.12
open wound into cavity 866.10
liver 864.00
with
contusion 864.01
with open wound into cavity 864.11
hematoma 864.01
with open wound into cavity 864.11
laceration 864.05
with open wound into cavity 864.15
major (disruption of hepatic parenchyma) 864.04
with open wound into cavity 864.14
minor (capsule only) 864.02
with open wound into cavity 864.12
moderate (involving parenchyma) 864.03
with open wound into cavity 864.13
multiple 864.04
stellate 864.04
with open wound in cavity 864.14
open wound into cavity 864.10
lung 861.20
with open wound into thorax 861.30
hemopneumothorax—*see* Hemopneumothorax, traumatic
hemothorax—*see* Hemothorax, traumatic
pneumohemothorax—*see* Pneumohemothorax, traumatic
pneumothorax—*see* Pneumothorax, traumatic
mediastinum 862.29
with open wound into cavity 862.39
mesentery 863.89
with open wound into cavity 863.99
mesosalpinx 867.6
with open wound into cavity 867.7

Injury—*continued*
multiple 869.0

Note—Multiple internal injuries of sites classifiable to the same three- or four- digit category should be classified to that category. Multiple injuries classifiable to different fourth-digit subdivisions of 861 (heart and lung injuries) should be dealt with according to coding rules.

with open wound into cavity 869.1
intra-abdominal organ (sites classifiable to 863-868)
with
intrathoracic organ(s) (sites classifiable to 861-862) 869.0
with open wound into cavity 869.1
other intra-abdominal organ(s) (sites classifiable to 863-868, except where classifiable to the same three-digit category) 868.09
with open wound into cavity 868.19
intrathoracic organ (sites classifiable to 861-862)
with
intra-abdominal organ(s) (sites classifiable to 863-868) 869.0
with open wound into cavity 869.1
other intrathoracic organ(s) (sites classifiable to 861-862, except where classifiable to the same three-digit category) 862.8
with open wound into cavity 862.9
myocardium—*see* Injury, internal, heart
ovary 867.6
with open wound into cavity 867.7
pancreas (multiple sites) 863.84
with open wound into cavity 863.94
body 863.82
with open wound into cavity 863.92
head 863.81
with open wound into cavity 863.91
tail 863.83
with open wound into cavity 863.93
pelvis, pelvic (organs) (viscera) 867.8
with
fracture, pelvis—*see* Fracture, pelvis
open wound into cavity 867.9
specified site NEC 867.6
with open wound into cavity 867.7
peritoneum 868.03
with open wound into cavity 868.13
pleura 862.29
with open wound into cavity 862.39
prostate 867.6
with open wound into cavity 867.7
rectum 863.45
with
colon 863.46
with open wound into cavity 863.56
open wound into cavity 863.55
retroperitoneum 868.04
with open wound into cavity 868.14
round ligament 867.6
with open wound into cavity 867.7
seminal vesicle 867.6
with open wound into cavity 867.7
spermatic cord 867.6
with open wound into cavity 867.7
scrotal—*see* Wound, open, spermatic cord

Injury—*continued*
spleen 865.00
with
disruption of parenchyma (massive) 865.04
with open wound into cavity 865.14
hematoma (without rupture of capsule) 865.01
with open wound into cavity 865.11
open wound into cavity 865.10
tear, capsular 865.02
with open wound into cavity 865.12
extending into parenchyma 865.03
with open wound into cavity 865.13
stomach 863.0
with open wound into cavity 863.1
suprarenal gland (multiple) 868.01
with open wound into cavity 868.11
thorax, thoracic (cavity) (organs) (multiple) (*see also* Injury, internal, intrathoracic organs) 862.8
with open wound into cavity 862.9
thymus (gland) 862.29
with open wound into cavity 862.39
trachea (intrathoracic) 862.29
with open wound into cavity 862.39
cervical region (*see also* Wound, open, trachea) 874.02
ureter 867.2
with open wound into cavity 867.3
urethra (sphincter) 867.0
with
abortion—*see* Abortion, by type, with, damage to pelvic organs
ectopic pregnancy (*see also* categories 633.0-633.9) 639.2
molar pregnancy (*see also* categories 630-632) 639.2
open wound into cavity 867.1
following
abortion 639.2
ectopic or molar pregnancy 639.2
obstetrical trauma 665.5
affecting fetus or newborn 763.8
uterus 867.4
with
abortion—*see* Abortion, by type, with, damage to pelvic organs
ectopic pregnancy (*see also* categories 633.0-633.9) 639.2
molar pregnancy (*see also* categories 630-632) 639.2
open wound into cavity 867.5
following
abortion 639.2
ectopic or molar pregnancy 639.2
obstetrical trauma NEC 665.5
affecting fetus or newborn 763.8
vas deferens 867.6
with open wound into cavity 867.7
vesical (sphincter) 867.0
with open wound into cavity 867.1
viscera (abdominal) (*see also* Injury, internal, multiple) 868.00
with
fracture, pelvis—*see* Fracture, pelvis
open wound into cavity 868.10
thoracic NEC (*see also* Injury, internal, intrathoracic organs) 862.8
with open wound into cavity 862.9

Injury—*continued*
interscapular region 959.1
intervertebral disc 959.1
intestine—*see* Injury, internal, intestine
intra-abdominal (organs) NEC—*see* Injury, internal, intra-abdominal
intracranial 854.0

Note—Use the following fifth-digit subclassification with categories 851-854:

0 unspecified state of consciousness
1 with no loss of consciousness
2 with brief [less than one hour] loss of consciousness
3 with moderate [1-24 hours] loss of consciousness
4 with prolonged [more than 24 hours] loss of consciousness and return to pre-existing conscious level
5 with prolonged [more than 24 hours] loss of consciousness, without return to pre-existing conscious level
6 with loss of consciousness of unspecified duration
9 with concussion, unspecified

with
open intracranial wound 854.1
skull fracture—*see* Fracture, skull, by site
contusion 851.8
with open intracranial wound 851.9
brain stem 851.4
with open intracranial wound 851.5
cerebellum 851.4
with open intracranial wound 851.5
cortex (cerebral) 851.0
with open intracranial wound 851.2
hematoma—*see* Injury, intracranial, hemorrhage
hemorrhage 853.0
with
laceration—*see* Injury, intracranial, laceration
open intracranial wound 853.1
extradural 852.4
with open intracranial wound 852.5
subarachnoid 852.0
with open intracranial wound 852.1
subdural 852.2
with open intracranial wound 852.3
laceration 851.8
with open intracranial wound 851.9
brain stem 851.6
with open intracranial wound 851.7
cerebellum 851.6
with open intracranial wound 851.7
cortex (cerebral) 851.2
with open intracranial wound 851.3
intraocular—*see* Injury, eyeball, penetrating
intrathoracic organs (multiple)—*see* Injury, internal, intrathoracic organs
intrauterine—*see* Injury, internal, intrauterine
iris 921.3
penetrating—*see* Injury, eyeball, penetrating
jaw 959.0
jejunum—*see* Injury, internal, jejunum

Injury—*continued*
joint NEC 959.9
old or residual 718.80
ankle 718.87
elbow 718.82
foot 718.87
hand 718.84
hip 718.85
knee 718.86
multiple sites 718.89
pelvic region 718.85
shoulder (region) 718.81
specified site NEC 718.88
wrist 718.83
kidney—*see* Injury, internal, kidney
knee (and ankle) (and foot) (and leg, except thigh) 959.7
labium (majus) (minus) 959.1
labyrinth, ear 959.0
lacrimal apparatus, gland, or sac 921.1
laceration 870.8
larynx 959.0
late effect—*see* Late, effects (of), injury
leg except thigh (and ankle) (and foot) (and knee) 959.7
upper or thigh 959.6
lens, eye 921.3
penetrating—*see* Injury, eyeball, penetrating
lid, eye—*see* Injury, eyelid
lip 959.0
liver—*see* Injury, internal, liver
lobe, parietal—*see* Injury, intracranial
lumbar (region) 959.1
plexus 953.5
lumbosacral (region) 959.1
plexus 953.5
lung—*see* Injury, internal, lung
malar region 959.0
mastoid region 959.0
maternal, during pregnancy, affecting fetus or newborn 760.5
maxilla 959.0
mediastinum—*see* Injury, internal, mediastinum
membrane
brain (*see also* Injury, intracranial) 854.0
tympanic 959.0
meningeal artery—*see* Hemorrhage, brain, traumatic, subarachnoid
meninges (cerebral)—*see* Injury, intracranial
mesenteric
artery—*see* Injury, blood vessel, mesenteric, artery
plexus, inferior 954.1
vein—*see* Injury, blood vessel, mesenteric, vein
mesentery—*see* Injury, internal, mesentery
mesosalpinx—*see* Injury, internal, mesosalpinx
middle ear 959.0
midthoracic region 959.1
mouth 959.0
multiple (sites not classifiable to the same four-digit category in 959.0-959.7) 959.8
internal 869.0
with open wound into cavity 869.1
musculocutaneous nerve 955.4
nail
finger 959.5
toe 959.7
nasal (septum) (sinus) 959.0
nasopharynx 959.0

Injury—*continued*
neck (and face) 959.0
nerve 957.9
abducens 951.3
abducent 951.3
accessory 951.6
acoustic 951.5
ankle and foot 956.9
anterior crural, femoral 956.1
arm (*see also* Injury, nerve, upper limb) 955.9
auditory 951.5
axillary 955.0
brachial plexus 953.4
cervical sympathetic 954.0
cranial 951.9
first or olfactory 951.8
second or optic 950.0
third or oculomotor 951.0
fourth or trochlear 951.1
fifth or trigeminal 951.2
sixth or abducens 951.3
seventh or facial 951.4
eighth, acoustic, or auditory 951.5
ninth or glossopharyngeal 951.8
tenth, pneumogastric, or vagus 951.8
eleventh or accessory 951.6
twelfth or hypoglossal 951.7
newborn 767.7
cutaneous sensory
lower limb 956.4
upper limb 955.5
digital (finger) 955.6
toe 956.5
facial 951.4
newborn 767.5
femoral 956.1
finger 955.9
foot and ankle 956.9
forearm 955.9
glossopharyngeal 951.8
hand and wrist 955.9
head and neck, superficial 957.0
hypoglossal 951.7
involving several parts of body 957.8
leg (*see also* Injury, nerve, lower limb) 956.9
lower limb 956.9
multiple 956.8
specified site NEC 956.5
lumbar plexus 953.5
lumbosacral plexus 953.5
median 955.1
forearm 955.1
wrist and hand 955.1
multiple (in several parts of body) (sites not classifiable to the same three-digit category) 957.8
musculocutaneous 955.4
musculospiral 955.3
upper arm 955.3
oculomotor 951.0
olfactory 951.8
optic 950.0
pelvic girdle 956.9
multiple sites 956.8
specified site NEC 956.5
peripheral 957.9
multiple (in several regions) (sites not classifiable to the same three-digit category) 957.8
specified site NEC 957.1

Injury—*continued*
peroneal 956.3
ankle and foot 956.3
lower leg 956.3
plantar 956.5
plexus 957.9
celiac 954.1
mesenteric, inferior 954.1
spinal 953.9
brachial 953.4
lumbosacral 953.5
multiple sites 953.8
sympathetic NEC 954.1
pneumogastric 951.8
radial 955.3
wrist and hand 955.3
sacral plexus 953.5
sciatic 956.0
thigh 956.0
shoulder girdle 955.9
multiple 955.8
specified site NEC 955.7
specified site NEC 957.1
spinal 953.9
plexus—*see* Injury, nerve, plexus, spinal
root 953.9
cervical 953.0
dorsal 953.1
lumbar 953.2
multiple sites 953.8
sacral 953.3
splanchnic 954.1
sympathetic NEC 954.1
cervical 954.0
thigh 956.9
tibial 956.5
ankle and foot 956.2
lower leg 956.5
posterior 956.2
toe 956.9
trigeminal 951.2
trochlear 951.1
trunk, excluding shoulder and pelvic girdles 954.9
specified site NEC 954.8
sympathetic NEC 954.1
ulnar 955.2
forearm 955.2
wrist (and hand) 955.2
upper limb 955.9
multiple 955.8
specified site NEC 955.7
vagus 951.8
wrist and hand 955.9
nervous system, diffuse 957.8
nose (septum) 959.0
obstetrical NEC 665.9
affecting fetus or newborn 763.8
occipital (region) (scalp) 959.0
lobe (*see also* Injury, intracranial) 854.0
optic 950.9
chiasm 950.1
cortex 950.3
nerve 950.0
pathways 950.2
orbit, orbital (region) 921.2
penetrating 870.3
with foreign body 870.4
ovary—*see* Injury, internal, ovary

Injury—*continued*
paint-gun—*see* Wound, open, by site, complicated
palate (soft) 959.0
pancreas—*see* Injury, internal, pancreas
parathyroid (gland) 959.0
parietal (region) (scalp) 959.0
lobe—*see* Injury, intracranial
pelvic
floor 959.1
complicating delivery 664.1
affecting fetus or newborn 763.8
joint or ligament, complicating delivery 665.6
affecting fetus or newborn 763.8
organs—*see also* Injury, internal, pelvis
with
abortion—*see* Abortion, by type, with damage to pelvic organs
ectopic pregnancy (*see also* categories 633.0-633.9) 639.2
molar pregnancy (*see also* categories 633.0-633.9) 639.2
following
abortion 639.2
ectopic or molar pregnancy 639.2
obstetrical trauma 665.5
affecting fetus or newborn 763.8
pelvis 959.1
penis 959.1
perineum 959.1
peritoneum—*see* Injury, internal, peritoneum
periurethral tissue
with
abortion—*see* Abortion, by type, with damage to pelvic organs
ectopic pregnancy (*see also* categories 633.0-633.9) 639.2
molar pregnancy (*see also* categories 630-632) 639.2
complicating delivery 665.5
affecting fetus or newborn 763.8
following
abortion 639.2
ectopic or molar pregnancy 639.2
phalanges
foot 959.7
hand 959.5
pharynx 959.0
pleura—*see* Injury, internal, pleura
popliteal space 959.7
prepuce 959.1
prostate—*see* Injury, internal, prostate
pubic region 959.1
pudenda 959.1
radiation NEC 990
radioactive substance or radium NEC 990
rectovaginal septum 959.1
rectum—*see* Injury, internal, rectum
retina 921.3
penetrating—*see* Injury, eyeball, penetrating
retroperitoneal—*see* Injury, internal, retroperitoneum
roentgen rays NEC 990
round ligament—*see* Injury, internal, round ligament
sacral (region) 959.1
plexus 953.5
sacroiliac ligament NEC 959.1
sacrum 959.1

Injury—*continued*
salivary ducts or glands 959.0
scalp 959.0
due to birth trauma 767.1
fetus or newborn 767.1
scapular region 959.2
sclera 921.3
penetrating—*see* Injury, eyeball, penetrating
superficial 918.2
scrotum 959.1
seminal vesicle—*see* Injury, internal, seminal vesicle
shoulder (and upper arm) 959.2
sinus
cavernous (*see also* Injury, intracranial) 854.0
nasal 959.0
skeleton NEC, birth injury 767.3
skin NEC 959.9
skull—*see* Fracture, skull, by site
soft tissue (of external sites) (severe)—*see* Wound, open, by site
specified site NEC 959.8
spermatic cord—*see* Injury, internal, spermatic cord
spinal (cord) 952.9
with fracture, vertebra—*see* Fracture, vertebra, by site, with spinal cord injury
cervical (C_1-C_4) 952.00
with
anterior cord syndrome 952.02
central cord syndrome 952.03
complete lesion of cord 952.01
incomplete lesion NEC 952.04
posterior cord syndrome 952.04
C_5-C_7 level 952.05
with
anterior cord syndrome 952.07
central cord syndrome 952.08
complete lesion of cord 952.06
incomplete lesion NEC 952.09
posterior cord syndrome 952.09
specified type NEC 952.09
specified type NEC 952.04
dorsal (D_1-D_6) (T_1-T_6) (thoracic) 952.10
with
anterior cord syndrome 952.12
central cord syndrome 952.13
complete lesion of cord 952.11
incomplete lesion NEC 952.14
posterior cord syndrome 952.14
D_7-D_{12} level (T_7-T_{12}) 952.15
with
anterior cord syndrome 952.17
central cord syndrome 952.18
complete lesion of cord 952.16
incomplete lesion NEC 952.19
posterior cord syndrome 952.19
specified type NEC 952.19
specified type NEC 952.14
lumbar 952.2
multiple sites 952.8
nerve (root) NEC—*see* Injury, nerve, spinal, root
plexus 953.9
brachial 953.4
lumbosacral 953.5
multiple sites 953.8
sacral 952.3
thoracic (*see also* Injury, spinal, dorsal) 952.10

Injury—*continued*
spleen—*see* Injury, internal, spleen
stellate ganglion 954.1
sternal region 959.1
stomach—*see* Injury, internal, stomach
subconjunctival 921.1
subcutaneous 959.9
subdural—*see* Injury, intracranial
submaxillary region 959.0
submental region 959.0
subungual
fingers 959.5
toes 959.7
superficial 919

Note—Use the following fourth-digit subdivisions with categories 910-919:

.0 Abrasion or friction burn without mention of infection
.1 Abrasion or friction burn, infected
.2 Blister without mention of infection
.3 Blister, infected
.4 Insect bite, nonvenomous, without mention of infection
.5 Insect bite, nonvenomous, infected
.6 Superficial foreign body (splinter) without major open wound and without mention of infection
.7 Superficial foreign body (splinter) without major open wound, infected
.8 Other and unspecified superficial injury without mention of infection
.9 Other and unspecified superficial injury, infected

For late effects of superficial injury, *see* category 906.2.

abdomen, abdominal (muscle) (wall) (and other part(s) of trunk) 911
ankle (and hip, knee, leg, or thigh) 916
anus (and other part(s) of trunk) 911
arm 913
upper (and shoulder) 912
auditory canal (external) (meatus) (and other part(s) of face, neck, or scalp, except eye) 910
axilla (and upper arm) 912
back (and other part(s) of trunk) 911
breast (and other part(s) of trunk) 911
brow (and other part(s) of face, neck or scalp, except eye) 910
buttock (and other part(s) of trunk) 911
canthus, eye 918.0
cheek(s) (and other part(s) of face, neck, or scalp, except eye) 910
chest wall (and other part(s) of trunk) 911
chin (and other part(s) of face, neck, or scalp, except eye) 910
clitoris (and other part(s) of trunk) 911
conjunctiva 918.2
cornea 918.1
due to contact lens 371.82
costal region (and other part(s) of trunk) 911
ear(s) (auricle) (canal) (drum) (external) (and other part(s) of face, neck, or scalp, except eye) 910
elbow (and forearm) (and wrist) 913
epididymis (and other part(s) of trunk) 911

Injury—*continued*
epigastric region (and other part(s) of trunk) 911
epiglottis (and other part(s) of face, neck, or scalp, except eye) 910
eye(s) (and adnexa) NEC 918.9
eyelid(s) (and periocular area) 918.0
face (any part(s), except eye) (and neck or scalp) 910
finger(s) (nail) (any) 915
flank (and other part(s) of trunk) 911
foot (phalanges) (and toe(s)) 917
forearm (and elbow) (and wrist) 913
forehead (and other part(s) of face, neck, or scalp, except eye) 910
globe (eye) 918.9
groin (and other part(s) of trunk) 911
gum(s) (and other part(s) of face, neck, or scalp, except eye) 910
hand(s) (except fingers alone) 914
head (and other part(s) of face, neck, or scalp, except eye) 910
heel (and foot or toe) 917
hip (and ankle, knee, leg, or thigh) 916
iliac region (and other part(s) of trunk) 911
interscapular region (and other part(s) of trunk) 911
iris 918.9
knee (and ankle, hip, leg, or thigh) 916
labium (majus) (minus) (and other part(s) of trunk) 911
lacrimal (apparatus) (gland) (sac) 918.0
leg (lower) (upper) (and ankle, hip, knee, or thigh) 916
lip(s) (and other part(s) of face, neck, or scalp, except eye) 910
lower extremity (except foot) 916
lumbar region (and other part(s) of trunk) 911
malar region (and other part(s) of face, neck, or scalp, except eye) 910
mastoid region (and other part(s) of face, neck, or scalp, except eye) 910
midthoracic region (and other part(s) of trunk) 911
mouth (and other part(s) of face, neck, or scalp, except eye) 910
multiple sites (not classifiable to the same three-digit category) 919
nasal (septum) (and other part(s) of face, neck, or scalp, except eye) 910
neck (and face or scalp, any part(s), except eye) 910
nose (septum) (and other part(s) of face, neck, or scalp, except eye) 910
occipital region (and other part(s) of face, neck, or scalp, except eye) 910
orbital region 918.0
palate (soft) (and other part(s) of face, neck, or scalp, except eye) 910
parietal region (and other part(s) of face, neck, or scalp, except eye) 910
penis (and other part(s) of trunk) 911
perineum (and other part(s) of trunk) 911
periocular area 918.0
pharynx (and other part(s) of face, neck, or scalp, except eye) 910
popliteal space (and ankle, hip, leg, or thigh) 916
prepuce (and other part(s) of trunk) 911
pubic region (and other part(s) of trunk) 911

Inspiration
food or foreign body (*see also* Asphyxia, food or foreign body) 933.1
mucus (*see also* Asphyxia, mucus) 933.1
Inspissated bile syndrome, newborn 774.4
Instability
detrusor 596.59
emotional (excessive) 301.3
joint (posttraumatic) 718.80
ankle 718.87
elbow 718.82
foot 718.87
hand 718.84
hip 718.85
knee 718.86
lumbosacral 724.6
multiple sites 718.89
pelvic region 718.85
sacroiliac 724.6
shoulder (region) 718.81
specified site NEC 718.88
wrist 718.83
lumbosacral 724.6
nervous 301.89
personality (emotional) 301.59
thyroid, paroxysmal 242.9
urethral 599.83
vasomotor 780.2
Insufficiency, insufficient
accommodation 367.4
adrenal (gland) (acute) (chronic) 255.4
medulla 255.5
primary 255.4
specified NEC 255.5
adrenocortical 255.4
anus 569.49
aortic (valve) 424.1
with
mitral (valve) disease 396.1
insufficiency, incompetence, or regurgitation 396.3
stenosis or obstruction 396.1
stenosis or obstruction 424.1
with mitral (valve) disease 396.8
congenital 746.4
rheumatic 395.1
with
mitral (valve) disease 396.1
insufficiency, incompetence, or regurgitation 396.3
stenosis or obstruction 396.1
stenosis or obstruction 395.2
with mitral (valve) disease 396.8
specified cause NEC 424.1
syphilitic 093.22
arterial 447.1
basilar artery 435.0
carotid artery 435.8
cerebral 437.1
coronary (acute or subacute) 411.89
mesenteric 557.1
peripheral 443.9
precerebral 435.9
vertebral artery 435.1
vertibrobasilar 435.3
arteriovenous 459.9
basilar artery 435.0
biliary 575.8
Insufficiency, insufficient—*continued*
cardiac (*see also* Insufficiency, myocardial) 428.0
complicating surgery 997.1
due to presence of (cardiac) prosthesis 429.4
postoperative 997.1
long-term effect of cardiac surgery 429.4
specified during or due to a procedure 997.1
long-term effect of cardiac surgery 429.4
cardiorenal (*see also* Hypertension, cardiorenal) 404.90
cardiovascular (*see also* Disease, cardiovascular) 429.2
renal (*see also* Hypertension, cardiorenal) 404.90
carotid artery 435.8
cerebral (vascular) 437.9
cerebrovascular 437.9
with transient focal neurological signs and symptoms 435.9
acute 437.1
with transient focal neurological signs and symptoms 435.9
circulatory NEC 459.9
fetus or newborn 779.8
convergence 378.83
coronary (acute or subacute) 411.89
chronic or with a stated duration of over 8 weeks 414.8
corticoadrenal 255.4
dietary 269.9
divergence 378.85
food 994.2
gastroesophageal 530.89
gonadal
ovary 256.3
testis 257.2
gonadotropic hormone secretion 253.4
heart—*see also* Insufficiency, myocardial
fetus or newborn 779.8
valve (*see also* Endocarditis) 424.90
congenital NEC 746.89
hepatic 573.8
idiopathic autonomic 333.0
kidney (*see also* Disease, renal) 593.9
labyrinth, labyrinthine (function) 386.53
bilateral 386.54
unilateral 386.53
lacrimal 375.15
liver 573.8
lung (acute) (*see also* Insufficiency, pulmonary) 518.82
following trauma, surgery, or shock 518.5
newborn 770.8
mental (congenital) (*see also* Retardation, mental) 319
mesenteric 557.1
mitral (valve) 424.0
with
aortic (valve) disease 396.3
insufficiency, incompetence, or regurgitation 396.3
stenosis or obstruction 396.2
obstruction or stenosis 394.2
with aortic valve disease 396.8
congenital 746.6

Insufficiency, insufficient—*continued*
rheumatic 394.1
with
aortic (valve) disease 396.3
insufficiency, incompetence, or regurgitation 396.3
stenosis or obstruction 396.2
obstruction or stenosis 394.2
with aortic valve disease 396.8
active or acute 391.1
with chorea, rheumatic (Sydenham's) 392.0
specified cause, except rheumatic 424.0
muscle
heart—*see* Insufficiency, myocardial
ocular (*see also* Strabismus) 378.9
myocardial, myocardium (with arteriosclerosis) 428.0
with rheumatic fever (conditions classifiable to 390)
active, acute, or subacute 391.2
with chorea 392.0
inactive or quiescent (with chorea) 398.0
congenital 746.89
due to presence of (cardiac) prosthesis 429.4
fetus or newborn 779.8
following cardiac surgery 429.4
hypertensive (*see also* Hypertension, heart) 402.91
benign 402.11
malignant 402.01
postoperative 997.1
long-term effect of cardiac surgery 429.4
rheumatic 398.0
active, acute, or subacute 391.2
with chorea (Sydenham's) 392.0
syphilitic 093.82
nourishment 994.2
organic 799.8
ovary 256.3
postablative 256.2
pancreatic 577.8
parathyroid (gland) 252.1
peripheral vascular (arterial) 443.9
pituitary (anterior) 253.2
posterior 253.5
placental—*see* Placenta, insufficiency
platelets 287.5
prenatal care in current pregnancy V23.7
progressive pluriglandular 258.9
pseudocholinesterase 289.8
pulmonary (acute) 518.82
following
shock 518.5
surgery 518.5
trauma 518.5
newborn 770.8
valve (*see also* Endocarditis, pulmonary) 424.3
congenital 746.09
pyloric 537.0
renal (acute) (chronic) (*see also* Disease, renal) 593.9
due to a procedure 997.5
respiratory 786.09
acute 518.82
following shock, surgery, or trauma 518.5
newborn 770.8
rotation—*see* Malrotation

Insufficiency, insufficient—*continued*
suprarenal 255.4
medulla 255.5
tarso-orbital fascia, congenital 743.66
tear film 375.15
testis 257.2
thyroid (gland) (acquired)—*see also* Hypothyroidism
congenital 243
tricuspid (*see also* Endocarditis, tricuspid) 397.0
congenital 746.89
syphilitic 093.23
urethral sphincter 599.84
valve, valvular (heart) (*see also* Endocarditis) 424.90
vascular 459.9
intestine NEC 557.9
mesenteric 557.1
peripheral 443.9
renal (*see also* Hypertension, kidney) 403.90
velopharyngeal
acquired 528.9
congenital 750.29
venous (peripheral) 459.81
ventricular—*see* Insufficiency, myocardial
vertebral artery 435.1
vertibrobasilar artery 435.3
weight gain during pregnancy 646.8
zinc 269.3
Insufflation
fallopian V26.2
meconium 770.1
Insular —*see* condition
Insulinoma (M8151/0)
malignant (M8151/3)
pancreas 157.4
specified site—*see* Neoplasm, by site, malignant
unspecified site 157.4
pancreas 211.7
specified site—*see* Neoplasm, by site, benign
unspecified site 211.7
Insuloma —*see* Insulinoma
Insult
brain 437.9
acute 436
cerebral 437.9
acute 436
cerebrovascular 437.9
acute 436
vascular NEC 437.9
acute 436
Insurance examination (certification) V70.3
Intemperance (*see also* Alcoholism) 303.9
Interception of pregnancy (menstrual extraction) V25.3
Intermenstrual
bleeding 626.4
irregular 626.6
regular 626.5
hemorrhage 626.4
irregular 626.6
regular 626.5
pain(s) 625.2
Intermittent— *see* condition
Internal —*see* condition
Interproximal wear 521.1
Interruption
aortic arch 747.11
bundle of His 426.50
fallopian tube (for sterilization) V25.2

Interruption—*continued*
phase-shift, sleep cycle 307.45
repeated REM-sleep 307.48
sleep
due to perceived environmental disturbances 307.48
phase-shift, of 24-hour sleep-wake cycle 307.45
repeated REM-sleep type 307.48
vas deferens (for sterilization) V25.2
Intersexuality 752.7
Interstitial —*see* condition
Intertrigo 695.89
labialis 528.5
Intervertebral disc —*see* condition
Intestine, intestinal —*see also* condition
flu 487.8
Intolerance
carbohydrate NEC 579.8
cardiovascular exercise, with pain (at rest) (with less than ordinary activity) (with ordinary activity) V47.2
disaccharide (hereditary) 271.3
drug
correct substance properly administered 995.2
wrong substance given or taken in error 977.9
specified drug—*see* Table of drugs and chemicals
effort 306.2
fat NEC 579.8
foods NEC 579.8
fructose (hereditary) 271.2
glucose (-galactose) (congenital) 271.3
gluten 579.0
lactose (hereditary) (infantile) 271.3
lysine (congenital) 270.7
milk NEC 579.8
protein (familial) 270.7
starch NEC 579.8
sucrose (-isomaltose) (congenital) 271.3
Intoxicated NEC (*see also* Alcoholism) 305.0
Intoxication
acid 276.2
acute
alcoholic 305.0
with alcoholism 303.0
hangover effects 305.0
caffeine 305.9
hallucinogenic (*see also* Abuse, drugs, nondependent) 305.3
alcohol (acute) 305.0
with alcoholism 303.0
hangover effects 305.0
idiosyncratic 291.4
pathological 291.4
alimentary canal 558.2
ammonia (hepatic) 572.2
chemical—*see also* Table of drugs and chemicals
via placenta or breast milk 760.70
alcohol 760.71
anti-infective agents 760.74
cocaine 760.75
"crack" 760.75
hallucinogenic agents NEC 760.73
medicinal agents NEC 760.79
narcotics 760.72
obstetric anesthetic or analgesic drug 763.5
specified agent NEC 760.79
suspected, affecting management of pregnancy 655.5
Intoxication—*continued*
cocaine, through placenta or breast milk 760.75
drug
correct substance properly administered (*see also* Allergy, drug) 995.2
newborn 779.4
obstetric anesthetic or sedation 668.9
affecting fetus or newborn 763.5
overdose or wrong substance given or taken—*see* Table of drugs and chemicals
pathologic 292.2
specific to newborn 779.4
via placenta or breast milk 760.70
alcohol 760.71
anti-infective agents 760.74
cocaine 760.75
"crack" 760.75
hallucinogenic agents 760.73
medicinal agents NEC 760.79
narcotics 760.72
obstetric anesthetic or analgesic drug 763.5
specified agent NEC 760.79
suspected, affecting management of pregnancy 655.5
enteric—*see* Intoxication, intestinal
fetus or newborn, via placenta or breast milk 760.70
alcohol 760.71
anti-infective agents 760.74
cocaine 760.75
"crack" 760.75
hallucinogenic agents 760.73
medicinal agents NEC 760.79
narcotics 760.72
obstetric anesthetic or analgesic drug 763.5
specified agent NEC 760.79
suspected, affecting management of pregnancy 655.5
food—*see* Poisoning, food
gastrointestinal 558.2
hallucinogenic (acute) 305.3
hepatocerebral 572.2
idiosyncratic alcohol 291.4
intestinal 569.89
due to putrefaction of food 005.9
methyl alcohol (*see also* Alcoholism) 305.0
with alcoholism 303.0
pathologic 291.4
drug 292.2
potassium (K) 276.7
septic
with
abortion—*see* Abortion, by type, with sepsis
ectopic pregnancy (*see also* categories 633.0-633.9) 639.0
molar pregnancy (*see also* categories 630-632) 639.0
during labor 659.3
following
abortion 639.0
ectopic or molar pregnancy 639.0
generalized—*see* Septicemia
puerperal, postpartum, childbirth 670
serum (prophylactic) (therapeutic) 999.5
uremic—*see* Uremia
water 276.6
Intracranial —*see* condition
Intrahepatic gallbladder 751.69
Intraligamentous —*see also* condition
pregnancy—*see* Pregnancy, cornual

Intraocular —*see also* condition
sepsis 360.00
Intrathoracic —*see also* condition
kidney 753.3
stomach—*see* Hernia, diaphragm
Intrauterine contraceptive device
checking V25.42
insertion V25.1
in situ V45.51
management V25.42
prescription V25.02
repeat V25.42
reinsertion V25.42
removal V25.42
Intraventricular —*see* condition
Intrinsic deformity —*see* Deformity
Intrusion, repetitive, of sleep (due to environmental disturbances) (with atypical polysomnographic features) 307.48
Intumescent, lens (eye) NEC 366.9
senile 366.12
Intussusception (colon) (enteric) (intestine) (rectum) 560.0
appendix 543.9
congenital 751.5
fallopian tube 620.8
ileocecal 560.0
ileocolic 560.0
ureter (with obstruction) 593.4
Invagination
basilar 756.0
colon or intestine 560.0
Invalid (since birth) 799.8
Invalidism (chronic) 799.8
Inversion
albumin-globulin (A-G) ratio 273.8
bladder 596.8
cecum (*see also* Intussusception) 560.0
cervix 622.8
nipple 611.79
congenital 757.6
puerperal, postpartum 676.3
optic papilla 743.57
organ or site, congenital NEC—*see* Anomaly, specified type NEC
sleep rhythm 780.55
nonorganic origin 307.45
testis (congenital) 752.5
uterus (postinfectional) (postpartal, old) 621.7
chronic 621.7
complicating delivery 665.2
affecting fetus or newborn 763.8
vagina—*see* Prolapse, vagina
Investigation
allergens V72.7
clinical research V70.7
Inviability —*see* Immaturity
Involuntary movement, abnormal 781.0
Involution, involutional —*see also* condition
breast, cystic or fibrocystic 610.1
depression (*see also* Psychosis, affective) 296.2
recurrent episode 296.3
single episode 296.2
melancholia (*see also* Psychosis, affective) 296.2
recurrent episode 296.3
single episode 296.2
ovary, senile 620.3
paranoid state (reaction) 297.2
paraphrenia (climacteric) (menopause) 297.2
psychosis 298.8
thymus failure 254.8
IQ
under 20 318.2
20-34 318.1
35-49 318.0
50-70 317
IRDS 769
Irideremia 743.45
Iridis rubeosis 364.42
diabetic 250.5 *[364.42]*
Iridochoroiditis (panuveitis) 360.12
Iridocyclitis NEC 364.3
acute 364.00
primary 364.01
recurrent 364.02
chronic 364.10
in
lepromatous leprosy 030.0 *[364.11]*
sarcoidosis 135 *[364.11]*
tuberculosis (*see also* Tuberculosis) 017.3 *[364.11]*
due to allergy 364.04
endogenous 364.01
gonococcal 098.41
granulomatous 364.10
herpetic (simplex) 054.44
zoster 053.22
hypopyon 364.05
lens induced 364.23
nongranulomatous 364.00
primary 364.01
recurrent 364.02
rheumatic 364.10
secondary 364.04
infectious 364.03
noninfectious 364.04
subacute 364.00
primary 364.01
recurrent 364.02
sympathetic 360.11
syphilitic (secondary) 091.52
tuberculous (chronic) (*see also* Tuberculosis) 017.3 *[364.11]*
Iridocyclochoroiditis (panuveitis) 360.12
Iridodialysis 364.76
Iridodonesis 364.8
Iridoplegia (complete) (partial) (reflex) 379.49
Iridoschisis 364.52
Iris —*see* condition
Iritis 364.3
acute 364.00
primary 364.01
recurrent 364.02
chronic 364.10
in
sarcoidosis 135 *[364.11]*
tuberculosis (*see also* Tuberculosis) 017.3 *[364.11]*
diabetic 250.5 *[364.42]*
due to
allergy 364.04
herpes simplex 054.44
leprosy 030.0 *[364.11]*
endogenous 364.01
gonococcal 098.41
gouty 274.89 *[364.11]*
granulomatous 364.10
hypopyon 364.05
lens induced 364.23
nongranulomatous 364.00
papulosa 095.8 *[364.11]*
primary 364.01

Iritis—*continued*
recurrent 364.02
rheumatic 364.10
secondary 364.04
infectious 364.03
noninfectious 364.04
subacute 364.00
primary 364.01
recurrent 364.02
sympathetic 360.11
syphilitic (secondary) 091.52
congenital 090.0 *[364.11]*
late 095.8 *[364.11]*
tuberculous (*see also* Tuberculosis) 017.3 *[364.11]*
uratic 274.89 *[364.11]*
Iron
deficiency anemia 280.9
metabolism disease 275.0
storage disease 275.0
Iron-miners' lung 503
Irradiated enamel (tooth, teeth) 521.8
Irradiation
burn—*see* Burn, by site
effects, adverse 990
Irreducible, irreducibility —*see* condition
Irregular, irregularity
action, heart 427.9
alveolar process 525.8
bleeding NEC 626.4
breathing 786.09
colon 569.89
contour of cornea 743.41
acquired 371.70
dentin in pulp 522.3
eye movements NEC 379.59
menstruation (cause unknown) 626.4
periods 626.4
prostate 602.9
pupil 364.75
respiratory 786.09
septum (nasal) 470
shape, organ or site, congenital NEC—*see* Distortion
sleep-wake rhythm (non-24-hour) 780.55
nonorganic origin 307.45
vertebra 733.99
Irritability (nervous) 799.2
bladder 596.8
neurogenic 596.54
with cauda equina syndrome 344.61
bowel (syndrome) 564.1
bronchial (*see also* Bronchitis) 490
cerebral, newborn 779.1
colon 564.1
psychogenic 306.4
duodenum 564.8
heart (psychogenic) 306.2
ileum 564.8
jejunum 564.8
myocardium 306.2
rectum 564.8
stomach 536.9
psychogenic 306.4
sympathetic (nervous system) (*see also* Neuropathy, peripheral, autonomic) 337.9
urethra 599.84
ventricular (heart) (psychogenic) 306.2
Irritable— *see* Irritability
Irritation
anus 569.49
axillary nerve 353.0
bladder 596.8
brachial plexus 353.0
brain (traumatic) (*see also* Injury, intracranial) 854.0
nontraumatic—*see* Encephalitis
bronchial (*see also* Bronchitis) 490
cerebral (traumatic) (*see also* Injury, intracranial) 854.0
nontraumatic—*see* Encephalitis
cervical plexus 353.2
cervix (*see also* Cervicitis) 616.0
choroid, sympathetic 360.11
cranial nerve—*see* Disorder, nerve, cranial
digestive tract 536.9
psychogenic 306.4
gastric 536.9
psychogenic 306.4
gastrointestinal (tract) 536.9
functional 536.9
psychogenic 306.4
globe, sympathetic 360.11
intestinal (bowel) 564.1
labyrinth 386.50
lumbosacral plexus 353.1
meninges (traumatic) (*see also* Injury, intracranial) 854.0
nontraumatic—*see* Meningitis
myocardium 306.2
nerve—*see* Disorder, nerve
nervous 799.2
nose 478.1
penis 607.89
perineum 709.9
peripheral
autonomic nervous system (*see also* Neuropathy, peripheral, autonomic) 337.9
nerve—*see* Disorder, nerve
peritoneum (*see also* Peritonitis) 567.9
pharynx 478.29
plantar nerve 355.6
spinal (cord) (traumatic)—*see also* Injury, spinal, by site
nerve—*see also* Disorder, nerve
root NEC 724.9
traumatic—*see* Injury, nerve, spinal
nontraumatic—*see* Myelitis
stomach 536.9
psychogenic 306.4
sympathetic nerve NEC (*see also* Neuropathy, peripheral, autonomic) 337.9
ulnar nerve 354.2
vagina 623.9
Isambert's disease 012.3
Ischemia, ischemic 459.9
basilar artery (with transient neurologic deficit) 435.0
bone NEC 733.40
bowel (transient) 557.9
acute 557.0
chronic 557.1
due to mesenteric artery insufficiency 557.1
brain—*see also* Ischemia, cerebral
recurrent focal 435.9
cardiac (*see also* Ischemia, heart) 414.9
cardiomyopathy 414.8
carotid artery (with transient neurologic deficit) 435.8

Ischemia, ischemic—*continued*
cerebral (chronic) (generalized) 437.1
arteriosclerotic 437.0
intermittent (with transient neurologic deficit) 435.9
puerperal, postpartum, childbirth 674.0
recurrent focal (with transient neurologic deficit) 435.9
transient (with transient neurologic deficit) 435.9
colon 557.9
acute 557.0
chronic 557.1
due to mesenteric artery insufficiency 557.1
coronary (chronic) (*see also* Ischemia, heart) 414.9
heart (chronic or with a stated duration of over 8 weeks) 414.9
acute or with a stated duration of 8 weeks or less (*see also* Infarct, myocardium) 410.9
without myocardial infarction 411.89
with coronary (artery) occlusion 411.81
subacute 411.89
intestine (transient) 557.9
acute 557.0
chronic 557.1
due to mesenteric artery insufficiency 557.1
kidney 593.81
labyrinth 386.50
muscles, leg 728.89
myocardium, myocardial (chronic or with a stated duration of over 8 weeks) 414.8
acute (*see also* Infarct, myocardium) 410.9
without myocardial infarction 411.89
with coronary (artery) occlusion 411.81
renal 593.81
retina, retinal 362.84
small bowel 557.9
acute 557.0
chronic 557.1
due to mesenteric artery insufficiency 557.1
spinal cord 336.1
subendocardial (*see also* Insufficiency, coronary) 411.89
vertebral artery (with transient neurologic deficit) 435.1
Ischialgia (*see also* Sciatica) 724.3
Ischiopagus 759.4
Ischium, ischial —*see* condition
Ischomenia 626.8
Ischuria 788.5
Iselin's disease or osteochondrosis 732.5
Islands of
parotid tissue in
lymph nodes 750.26
neck structures 750.26
submaxillary glands in
fascia 750.26
lymph nodes 750.26
neck muscles 750.26
Islet cell tumor, pancreas (M8150/0) 211.7
Isoimmunization NEC (*see also* Incompatibility) 656.2
fetus or newborn 773.2
ABO blood groups 773.1
Rhesus (Rh) factor 773.0
Isolation V07.0
social V62.4
Isosporosis 007.2
Issue
medical certificate NEC V68.0
cause of death V68.0
fitness V68.0
incapacity V68.0
repeat prescription NEC V68.1
appliance V68.1
contraceptive V25.40
device NEC V25.49
intrauterine V25.42
specified type NEC V25.49
pill V25.41
glasses V68.1
medicinal substance V68.1
Itch (*see also* Pruritus) 698.9
bakers' 692.89
barbers' 110.0
bricklayers' 692.89
cheese 133.8
clam diggers' 120.3
coolie 126.9
copra 133.8
Cuban 050.1
dew 126.9
dhobie 110.3
eye 379.99
filarial (*see also* Infestation, filarial) 125.9
grain 133.8
grocers' 133.8
ground 126.9
harvest 133.8
jock 110.3
Malabar 110.9
beard 110.0
foot 110.4
scalp 110.0
meaning scabies 133.0
Norwegian 133.0
perianal 698.0
poultrymen's 133.8
sarcoptic 133.0
scrub 134.1
seven year V61.1
meaning scabies 133.0
straw 133.8
swimmers' 120.3
washerwoman's 692.4
water 120.3
winter 698.8
Itsenko-Cushing syndrome (pituitary basophilism) 255.0
Ivemark's syndrome (asplenia with congenital heart disease) 759.0
Ivory bones 756.52
Ixodes 134.8
Ixodiasis 134.8

J

Jaccoud's nodular fibrositis, chronic (Jaccoud's syndrome) 714.4
Jackson's
membrane 751.4
paralysis or syndrome 344.89
veil 751.4
Jacksonian
epilepsy (*see also* Epilepsy) 345.5
seizures (focal) (*see also* Epilepsy) 345.5
Jacob's ulcer (M8090/3)—*see* Neoplasm, skin, malignant, by site
Jacquet's dermatitis (diaper dermatitis) 691.0
Jadassohn's
blue nevus (M8780/0)—*see* Neoplasm, skin, benign
disease (maculopapular erythroderma) 696.2
intraepidermal epithelioma (M8096/0)—*see* Neoplasm, skin, benign
Jadassohn-Lewandowski syndrome (pachyonychia congenita) 757.5
Jadassohn-Pellizari's disease (anetoderma) 701.3
Jadassohn-Tièche nevus (M8780/0)—*see* Neoplasm, skin, benign
Jaffe-Lichtenstein (-Uehlinger) syndrome 252.0
Jahnke's syndrome (encephalocutaneous angiomatosis) 759.6
Jakob-Creutzfeldt disease or syndrome 046.1
with dementia 290.10
Jaksch (-Luzet) disease or syndrome (pseudoleukemia infantum) 285.8
Jamaican
neuropathy 349.82
paraplegic tropical ataxic-spastic syndrome 349.82
Janet's disease (psychasthenia) 300.89
Janiceps 759.4
Jansky-Bielschowsky amaurotic familial idiocy 330.1
Japanese
B type encephalitis 062.0
river fever 081.2
seven-day fever 100.89
Jaundice (yellow) 782.4
acholuric (familial) (splenomegalic) (*see also* Spherocytosis) 282.0
acquired 283.9
breast milk 774.39
catarrhal (acute) 070.1
with hepatic coma 070.0
chronic 571.9
epidemic—*see* Jaundice, epidemic
cholestatic (benign) 782.4
chronic idiopathic 277.4
epidemic (catarrhal) 070.1
with hepatic coma 070.0
leptospiral 100.0
spirochetal 100.0
febrile (acute) 070.1
with hepatic coma 070.0
leptospiral 100.0
spirochetal 100.0
Jaundice—*continued*
fetus or newborn 774.6
due to or associated with
ABO
antibodies 773.1
incompatibility, maternal/fetal 773.1
isoimmunization 773.1
absence or deficiency of enzyme system for bilirubin conjugation (congenital) 774.39
blood group incompatibility NEC 773.2
breast milk inhibitors to conjugation 774.39
associated with preterm delivery 774.2
bruising 774.1
Crigler-Najjar syndrome 277.4 *[774.31]*
delayed conjugation 774.30
associated with preterm delivery 774.2
development 774.39
drugs or toxins transmitted from mother 774.1
G-6-PD deficiency 282.2 *[774.0]*
galactosemia 271.1 *[774.5]*
Gilbert's syndrome 277.4 *[774.31]*
hepatocellular damage 774.4
hereditary hemolytic anemia (*see also* Anemia, hemolytic) 282.9 *[774.0]*
hypothyroidism, congenital 243 *[774.31]*
incompatibility, maternal/fetal NEC 773.2
infection 774.1
inspissated bile syndrome 774.4
isoimmunization NEC 773.2
mucoviscidosis 277.01 *[774.5]*
obliteration of bile duct, congenital 751.61 *[774.5]*
polycythemia 774.1
preterm delivery 774.2
red cell defect 282.9 *[774.0]*
Rh
antibodies 773.0
incompatibility, maternal/fetal 773.0
isoimmunization 773.0
spherocytosis (congenital) 282.0 *[774.0]*
swallowed maternal blood 774.1
physiological NEC 774.6
from injection, inoculation, infusion, or transfusion (blood) (plasma) (serum) (other substance) (onset within 8 months after administration)—*see* Hepatitis, viral
Gilbert's (familial nonhemolytic) 277.4
hematogenous 283.9
hemolytic (acquired) 283.9
congenital (*see also* Spherocytosis) 282.0
hemorrhagic (acute) 100.0
leptospiral 100.0
newborn 776.0
spirochetal 100.0
hepatocellular 573.8
homologous (serum)—*see* Hepatitis, viral
idiopathic, chronic 277.4
infectious (acute) (subacute) 070.1
with hepatic coma 070.0
leptospiral 100.0
spirochetal 100.0
leptospiral 100.0
malignant (*see also* Necrosis, liver) 570
newborn (physiological) (*see also* Jaundice, fetus or newborn) 774.6

Jaundice—*continued*
nonhemolytic, congenital familial (Gilbert's) 277.4
nuclear, newborn (*see also* Kernicterus of newborn) 774.7
obstructive NEC (*see also* Obstruction, biliary) 576.8
postimmunization—*see* Hepatitis, viral
posttransfusion—*see* Hepatitis, viral
regurgitation (*see also* Obstruction, biliary) 576.8
serum (homologous) (prophylactic) (therapeutic)—*see* Hepatitis, viral
spirochetal (hemorrhagic) 100.0
symptomatic 782.4
newborn 774.6
Jaw —*see* condition
Jaw-blinking 374.43
congenital 742.8
Jaw-winking phenomenon or syndrome 742.8
Jealousy
alcoholic 291.5
childhood 313.3
sibling 313.3
Jejunitis (*see also* Enteritis) 558.9
Jejunostomy status V44.4
Jejunum, jejunal —*see* condition
Jensen's disease 363.05
Jericho boil 085.1
Jerks, myoclonic 333.2
Jeune's disease or syndrome (asphyxiating thoracic dystrophy) 756.4
Jigger disease 134.1
Job's syndrome (chronic granulomatous disease) 288.1
Jod-Basedow phenomenon 242.8
Johnson-Stevens disease (erythema multiforme exudativum) 695.1
Joint —*see also* condition
Charcot's 094.0 *[713.5]*
false 733.82
flail—*see* Flail, joint
mice—*see also* Loose, body, joint
knee 717.6
sinus to bone 730.9
von Gies' 095.8
Jordan's anomaly or syndrome 288.2
Josephs-Diamond-Blackfan anemia (congenital hypoplastic) 284.0
Jumpers' knee 727.2
Jungle yellow fever 060.0
Jüngling's disease (sarcoidosis) 135
Junin virus hemorrhagic fever 078.7
Juvenile —*see also* condition
delinquent 312.9
group (*see also* Disturbance, conduct) 312.2
neurotic 312.4

K

Kahler (-Bozzolo) disease (multiple myeloma) (M9730/3) 203.0
Kakergasia 300.9
Kakke 265.0
Kala-azar (Indian) (infantile) (Mediterranean) (Sudanese) 085.0
Kalischer's syndrome (encephalocutaneous angiomatosis) 759.6
Kallmann's syndrome (hypogonadotropic hypogonadism with anosmia) 253.4
Kanner's syndrome (autism) (*see also* Psychosis, childhood) 299.0
Kaolinosis 502
Kaposi's
disease 757.33
lichen ruber 696.4
acuminatus 696.4
moniliformis 697.8
xeroderma pigmentosum 757.33
sarcoma (M9140/3) 176.9
adipose tissue 176.1
aponeurosis 176.1
artery 176.1
blood vessel 176.1
bursa 176.1
connective tissue 176.1
external genitalia 176.8
fascia 176.1
fatty tissue 176.1
fibrous tissue 176.1
gastrointestinal tract NEC 176.3
ligament 176.1
lung 176.4
lymph
gland(s) 176.5
node(s) 176.5
lymphatic(s) NEC 176.1
muscle (skeletal) 176.1
oral cavity NEC 176.8
palate 176.2
scrotum 176.8
skin 176.0
soft tissue 176.1
specified site NEC 176.8
subcutaneous tissue 176.1
synovia 176.1
tendon (sheath) 176.1
vein 176.1
vessel 176.1
viscera NEC 176.9
vulva 176.8
varicelliform eruption 054.0
vaccinia 999.0
Kartagener's syndrome or triad (sinusitis, bronchiectasis, situs inversus) 759.3
Kasabach-Merritt syndrome (capillary hemangioma associated with thrombocytopenic purpura) 287.3
Kaschin-Beck disease (endemic polyarthritis)—*see* Disease, Kaschin-Beck
Kast's syndrome (dyschondroplasia with hemangiomas) 756.4
Katatonia (*see also* Schizophrenia) 295.2
Katayama disease or fever 120.2
Kathisophobia 781.0
Kawasaki disease 446.1
Kayser-Fleischer ring (cornea) (pseudosclerosis) 275.1 *[371.14]*
Kaznelson's syndrome (congenital hypoplastic anemia) 284.0
Kedani fever 081.2
Kelis 701.4
Kelly (-Patterson) syndrome (sideropenic dysphagia) 280.8
Keloid, cheloid 701.4
Addison's (morphea) 701.0
cornea 371.00
Hawkins' 701.4
scar 701.4
Keloma 701.4
Kenya fever 082.1
Keratectasia 371.71
congenital 743.41
Keratitis (nodular) (nonulcerative) (simple) (zonular) NEC 370.9
with ulceration (*see also* Ulcer, cornea) 370.00
actinic 370.24
arborescens 054.42
areolar 370.22
bullosa 370.8
deep—*see* Keratitis, interstitial
dendritic(a) 054.42
desiccation 370.34
diffuse interstitial 370.52
disciform(is) 054.43
varicella 052.7 *[370.44]*
epithelialis vernalis 372.13 *[370.32]*
exposure 370.34
filamentary 370.23
gonococcal (congenital) (prenatal) 098.43
herpes, herpetic (simplex) NEC 054.43
zoster 053.21
hypopyon 370.04
in
chickenpox 052.7 *[370.44]*
exanthema (*see also* Exanthem) 057.9 *[370.44]*
paravaccinia (*see also* Paravaccinia) 051.9 *[370.44]*
smallpox (*see also* Smallpox) 050.9 *[370.44]*
vernal conjunctivitis 372.13 *[370.32]*
interstitial (nonsyphilitic) 370.50
with ulcer (*see also* Ulcer, cornea) 370.00
diffuse 370.52
herpes, herpetic (simplex) 054.43
zoster 053.21
syphilitic (congenital) (hereditary) 090.3
tuberculous (*see also* Tuberculosis) 017.3 *[370.59]*
lagophthalmic 370.34
macular 370.22
neuroparalytic 370.35
neurotrophic 370.35
nummular 370.22
oyster-shuckers' 370.8
parenchymatous—*see* Keratitis, interstitial
petrificans 370.8
phlyctenular 370.31
postmeasles 055.71
punctata, punctate 370.21
leprosa 030.0 *[370.21]*
profunda 090.3
superficial (Thygeson's) 370.21
purulent 370.8
pustuliformis profunda 090.3

Keratitis—*continued*
rosacea 695.3 *[370.49]*
sclerosing 370.54
specified type NEC 370.8
stellate 370.22
striate 370.22
superficial 370.20
with conjunctivitis (*see also* Keratoconjunctivitis) 370.40
punctate (Thygeson's) 370.21
suppurative 370.8
syphilitic (congenital) (prenatal) 090.3
trachomatous 076.1
late effect 139.1
tuberculous (phlyctenular) (*see also* Tuberculosis) 017.3 *[370.31]*
ulcerated (*see also* Ulcer, cornea) 370.00
vesicular 370.8
welders' 370.24
xerotic (*see also* Keratomalacia) 371.45
vitamin A deficiency 264.4
Keratoacanthoma 238.2
Keratocele 371.72
Keratoconjunctivitis (*see also* Keratitis) 370.40
adenovirus type 8 077.1
epidemic 077.1
exposure 370.34
gonococcal 098.43
herpetic (simplex) 054.43
zoster 053.21
in
chickenpox 052.7 *[370.44]*
exanthema (*see also* Exanthem) 057.9 *[370.44]*
paravaccinia (*see also* Paravaccinia) 051.9 *[370.44]*
smallpox (*see also* Smallpox) 050.9 *[370.44]*
infectious 077.1
neurotrophic 370.35
phlyctenular 370.31
postmeasles 055.71
shipyard 077.1
sicca (Sjögren's syndrome) 710.2
not in Sjögren's syndrome 370.33
specified type NEC 370.49
tuberculous (phlyctenular) (*see also* Tuberculosis) 017.3 *[370.31]*
Keratoconus 371.60
acute hydrops 371.62
congenital 743.41
stable 371.61
Keratocyst (dental) 526.0
Keratoderma, keratodermia (congenital) (palmaris et plantaris) (symmetrical) 757.39
acquired 701.1
blennorrhagica 701.1
gonococcal 098.81
climacterium 701.1
eccentrica 757.39
gonorrheal 098.81
punctata 701.1
tylodes, progressive 701.1
Keratodermatocele 371.72
Keratoglobus 371.70
congenital 743.41
associated with buphthalmos 743.22
Keratohemia 371.12
Keratoiritis (*see also* Iridocyclitis) 364.3
syphilitic 090.3
tuberculous (*see also* Tuberculosis) 017.3 *[364.11]*
Keratolysis exfoliativa (congenital) 757.39
acquired 695.89
neonatorum 757.39
Keratoma 701.1
congenital 757.39
malignum congenitale 757.1
palmaris et plantaris hereditarium 757.39
senile 702.0
Keratomalacia 371.45
vitamin A deficiency 264.4
Keratomegaly 743.41
Keratomycosis 111.1
nigricans (palmaris) 111.1
Keratopathy 371.40
band (*see also* Keratitis) 371.43
bullous (*see also* Keratitis) 371.23
degenerative (*see also* Degeneration, cornea) 371.40
hereditary (*see also* Dystrophy, cornea) 371.50
discrete colliquative 371.49
Keratoscleritis, tuberculous (*see also* Tuberculosis) 017.3 *[370.31]*
Keratosis 701.1
actinic 702.0
arsenical 692.4
blennorrhagica 701.1
gonococcal 098.81
congenital (any type) 757.39
ear (middle) (*see also* Cholesteatoma) 385.30
female genital (external) 629.8
follicular, vitamin A deficiency 264.8
follicularis 757.39
acquired 701.1
congenital (acneiformis) (Siemens') 757.39
spinulosa (decalvans) 757.39
vitamin A deficiency 264.8
gonococcal 098.81
larynx, laryngeal 478.79
male genital (external) 608.89
middle ear (*see also* Cholesteatoma) 385.30
nigricans 701.2
congenital 757.39
obturans 380.21
palmaris et plantaris (symmetrical) 757.39
penile 607.89
pharyngeus 478.29
pilaris 757.39
acquired 701.1
punctata (palmaris et plantaris) 701.1
scrotal 608.89
seborrheic 702.19
inflamed 702.11
senilis 702.0
solar 702.0
suprafollicularis 757.39
tonsillaris 478.29
vagina 623.1
vegetans 757.39
vitamin A deficiency 264.8
Kerato-uveitis (*see also* Iridocyclitis) 364.3
Keraunoparalysis 994.0
Kerion (celsi) 110.0
Kernicterus of newborn (not due to isoimmunization) 774.7
due to isoimmunization (conditions classifiable to 773.0-773.2) 773.4
Ketoacidosis 276.2
diabetic 250.1
Ketonuria 791.6
branched-chain, intermittent 270.3
Ketosis 276.2
diabetic 250.1

Kidney —*see* condition
Kienböck's
disease 732.3
adult 732.8
osteochondrosis 732.3
Kimmelstiel (-Wilson) disease or syndrome (intercapillary glomerulosclerosis) 250.4 *[581.81]*
Kink, kinking
appendix 543.9
artery 447.1
cystic duct, congenital 751.61
hair (acquired) 704.2
ileum or intestine (*see also* Obstruction, intestine) 560.9
Lane's (*see also* Obstruction, intestine) 560.9
organ or site, congenital NEC—*see* Anomaly, specified type NEC, by site
ureter (pelvic junction) 593.3
congenital 753.2
vein(s) 459.2
caval 459.2
peripheral 459.2
Kinnier Wilson's disease (hepatolenticular degeneration) 275.1
Kissing
osteophytes 721.5
spine 721.5
vertebra 721.5
Klauder's syndrome (erythema multiforme exudativum) 695.1
Kleb's disease (*see also* Nephritis) 583.9
Klein-Waardenburg syndrome (ptosisepicanthus) 270.2
Kleine-Levin syndrome 349.89
Kleptomania 312.32
Klinefelter's syndrome 758.7
Klinger's disease 446.4
Klippel's disease 723.8
Klippel-Feil disease or syndrome (brevicollis) 756.16
Klippel-Trenaunay syndrome 759.89
Klumpke (-Déjérine) palsy, paralysis (birth) (newborn) 767.6
Klüver-Bucy (-Terzian) syndrome 310.0
Knee —*see* condition
Knifegrinders' rot (*see also* Tuberculosis) 011.4
Knock-knee (acquired) 736.41
congenital 755.64
Knot
intestinal, syndrome (volvulus) 560.2
umbilical cord (true) 663.2
affecting fetus or newborn 762.5
Knots, surfer 919.8
infected 919.9
Knotting (of)
hair 704.2
intestine 560.2
Knuckle pads (Garrod's) 728.79
Köbner's disease (epidermolysis bullosa) 757.39
Koch's
infection (*see also* Tuberculosis, pulmonary) 011.9
relapsing fever 087.9
Koch-Weeks conjunctivitis 372.03
Koenig-Wichman disease (pemphigus) 694.4
Köhler's disease (osteochondrosis) 732.5
first (osteochondrosis juvenilis) 732.5
second (Freiburg's infarction, metatarsal head) 732.5
patellar 732.4
tarsal navicular (bone) (osteoarthosis juvenilis) 732.5
Köhler-Mouchet disease (osteoarthrosis juvenilis) 732.5
Köhler-Pellegrini-Stieda disease or syndrome (calcification, knee joint) 726.62
Koilonychia 703.8
congenital 757.5
Kojevnikov's, Kojewnikoff's epilepsy (*see also* Epilepsy) 345.7
König's
disease (osteochondritis dissecans) 732.7
syndrome 564.8
Koniophthisis (*see also* Tuberculosis) 011.4
Koplik's spots 055.9
Kopp's asthma 254.8
Korean hemorrhagic fever 078.6
Korsakoff (-Wernicke) disease, psychosis, or syndrome (nonalcoholic) 294.0
alcoholic 291.1
Korsakov's disease —*see* Korsakoff's disease
Korsakow's disease —*see* Korsakoff's disease
Kostmann's disease or syndrome (infantile genetic agranulocytosis) 288.0
Krabbe's
disease (leukodystrophy) 330.0
syndrome
congenital muscle hypoplasia 756.89
cutaneocerebral angioma 759.6
Kraepelin-Morel disease (*see also* Schizophrenia) 295.9
Kraft-Weber-Dimitri disease 759.6
Kraurosis
ani 569.49
penis 607.0
vagina 623.8
vulva 624.0
Kreotoxism 005.9
Krukenberg's
spindle 371.13
tumor (M8490/6) 198.6
Kufs' disease 330.1
Kugelberg-Welander disease 335.11
Kuhnt-Junius degeneration or disease 362.52
Kulchitsky's cell carcinoma (carcinoid tumor of intestine) 259.2
Kümmell's disease or spondylitis 721.7
Kundrat's disease (lymphosarcoma) 200.1
Kunekune —*see* Dermatophytosis
Kunkel syndrome (lupoid hepatitis) 571.49
Kupffer cell sarcoma (M9124/3) 155.0
Kuru 046.0
Kussmaul's
coma (diabetic) 250.3
disease (polyarteritis nodosa) 446.0
respiration (air hunger) 786.09
Kwashiorkor (marasmus type) 260
Kyasanur Forest disease 065.2
Kyphoscoliosis, kyphoscoliotic (acquired) (*see also* Scoliosis) 737.30
congenital 756.19
due to radiation 737.33
heart (disease) 416.1

Kyphoscoliosis, kyphoscoliotic—*continued*
idiopathic 737.30
infantile
progressive 737.32
resolving 737.31
late effect of rickets 268.1 *[737.43]*
specified NEC 737.39
thoracogenic 737.34
tuberculous (*see also* Tuberculosis) 015.0 *[737.43]*
Kyphosis, kyphotic (acquired) (postural) 737.10
adolescent postural 737.0
congenital 756.19
dorsalis juvenilis 732.0
due to or associated with
Charcot-Marie-Tooth disease 356.1 *[737.41]*
mucopolysaccharidosis 277.5 *[737.41]*
neurofibromatosis 237.71 *[737.41]*
osteitis
deformans 731.0 *[737.41]*
fibrosa cystica 252.0 *[737.41]*
osteoporosis (*see also* Osteoporosis) 733.0 *[737.41]*
poliomyelitis (*see also* Poliomyelitis) 138 *[737.41]*
radiation 737.11
tuberculosis (*see also* Tuberculosis) 015.0 *[737.41]*
Kümmell's 721.7
late effect of rickets 268.1 *[737.41]*
Morquio-Brailsford type (spinal) 277.5 *[737.41]*
pelvis 738.6
postlaminectomy 737.12
specified cause NEC 737.19
syphilitic, congenital 090.5 *[737.41]*
tuberculous (*see also* Tuberculosis) 015.0 *[737.41]*
Kyrle's disease (hyperkeratosis follicularis in cutem penetrans) 701.1

L

Labia, labium —*see* condition
Labiated hymen 752.49
Labile
  blood pressure 796.4
  emotions, emotionality 301.3
  vasomotor system 443.9
Labioglossal paralysis 335.22
Labium leporinum (*see also* Cleft, lip) 749.10
Labor (*see also* Delivery)
  with complications—*see* Delivery, complicated
  abnormal NEC 661.9
    affecting fetus or newborn 763.7
  arrested active phase 661.1
    affecting fetus or newborn 763.7
  desultory 661.2
    affecting fetus or newborn 763.7
  dyscoordinate 661.4
    affecting fetus or newborn 763.7
  early onset (22-36 weeks gestation) 644.2
  failed
    induction 659.1
      mechanical 659.0
      medical 659.1
      surgical 659.0
    trial (vaginal delivery) 660.6
  false 644.1
  forced or induced, affecting fetus or newborn 763.8
  hypertonic 661.4
    affecting fetus or newborn 763.7
  hypotonic 661.2
    affecting fetus or newborn 763.7
    primary 661.0
      affecting fetus or newborn 763.7
    secondary 661.1
      affecting fetus or newborn 763.7
  incoordinate 661.4
    affecting fetus or newborn 763.7
  irregular 661.2
    affecting fetus or newborn 763.7
  long—*see* Labor, prolonged
  missed (at or near term) 656.4
  obstructed NEC 660.9
    affecting fetus or newborn 763.1
    specified cause NEC 660.8
      affecting fetus or newborn 763.1
  pains, spurious 644.1
  precipitate 661.3
    affecting fetus or newborn 763.6
  premature 644.2
    threatened 644.0
  prolonged or protracted 662.1
    first stage 662.0
      affecting fetus or newborn 763.8
    second stage 662.2
      affecting fetus or newborn 763.8
    affecting fetus or newborn 763.8
  threatened NEC 644.1
  undelivered 644.1
Labored breathing (*see also* Hyperventilation) 786.09
Labyrinthitis (inner ear) (destructive) (latent) 386.30
  circumscribed 386.32
  diffuse 386.31
  focal 386.32
  purulent 386.33
  serous 386.31
  suppurative 386.33
  syphilitic 095.8
  toxic 386.34
  viral 386.35
Laceration —*see also* Wound, open, by site
  accidental, complicating surgery 998.2
  Achilles tendon 845.09
    with open wound 892.2
  anus (sphincter) 863.89
    with
      abortion—*see* Abortion, by type, with damage to pelvic organs
      ectopic pregnancy (*see also* categories 633.0-633.9) 639.2
      molar pregnancy (*see also* categories 630-632) 639.2
    complicating delivery 664.2
      with laceration of anal or rectal mucosa 664.3
    following
      abortion 639.2
      ectopic or molar pregnancy 639.2
    nontraumatic, nonpuerperal 565.0
  bladder (urinary)
    with
      abortion—*see* Abortion, by type, with damage to pelvic organs
      ectopic pregnancy (*see also* categories 633.0-633.9) 639.2
      molar pregnancy (*see also* categories 630-632) 639.2
    following
      abortion 639.2
      ectopic or molar pregnancy 639.2
    obstetrical trauma 665.5
  blood vessel—*see* Injury, blood vessel, by site
  bowel
    with
      abortion—*see* Abortion, by type, with damage to pelvic organs
      ectopic pregnancy (*see also* categories 633.0-633.9) 639.2
      molar pregnancy (*see also* categories 630-632) 639.2
    following
      abortion 639.2
      ectopic or molar pregnancy 639.2
    obstetrical trauma 665.5

Laceration—*continued*
brain (with hemorrhage) (cerebral) (membrane) 851.8

Note—Use the following fifth-digit subclassification with categories 851-854:

0 unspecified state of consciousness
1 with no loss of consciousness
2 with brief [less than one hour] loss of consciousness
3 with moderate [1-24 hours] loss of consciousness
4 with prolonged [more than 24 hours] loss of consciousness and return to pre-existing conscious level
5 with prolonged [more than 24 hours] loss of consciousness, without return to pre-existing conscious level
6 with loss of consciousness of unspecified duration
9 with concussion, unspecified

with
open intracranial wound 851.9
skull fracture—see Fracture, skull, by site
cerebellum 851.6
with open intracranial wound 851.7
cortex 851.2
with open intracranial wound 851.3
during birth 767.0
stem 851.6
with open intracranial wound 851.7
broad ligament
with
abortion—*see* Abortion, by type, with damage to pelvic organs
ectopic pregnancy (*see also* categories 633.0-633.9) 639.2
molar pregnancy (*see also* categories 630-632) 639.2
following
abortion 639.2
ectopic or molar pregnancy 639.2
nontraumatic 620.6
obstetrical trauma 665.6
syndrome (nontraumatic) 620.6
capsule, joint—*see* Sprain, by site
cardiac—*see* Laceration, heart
causing eversion of cervix uteri (old) 622.0
central, complicating delivery 664.4
cerebellum—*see* Laceration, brain, cerebellum
cerebral—*see also* Laceration, brain
during birth 767.0
cervix (uteri)
with
abortion—*see* Abortion, by type, with damage to pelvic organs
ectopic pregnancy (*see also* categories 633.0-633.9) 639.2
molar pregnancy (*see also* categories 630-632) 639.2
following
abortion 639.2
ectopic or molar pregnancy 639.2
nonpuerperal, nontraumatic 622.3
obstetrical trauma (current) 665.3
old (postpartal) 622.3
traumatic—*see* Injury, internal, cervix
chordae heart 429.5
complicated 879.9

Laceration—*continued*
cornea—*see* Laceration, eyeball
cortex (cerebral)—*see* Laceration, brain, cortex
esophagus 530.89
eye(s)—*see* Laceration, ocular
eyeball NEC 871.4
with prolapse or exposure of intraocular tissue 871.1
penetrating—*see* Penetrating wound, eyeball
specified as without prolapse of intraocular tissue 871.0
eyelid NEC 870.8
full thickness 870.1
involving lacrimal passages 870.2
skin (and periocular area) 870.0
penetrating—*see* Penetrating wound, orbit
fourchette
with
abortion—*see* Abortion, by type, with damage to pelvic organs
ectopic pregnancy (*see also* categories 633.0-633.9) 639.2
molar pregnancy (*see also* categories 630-632) 639.2
complicating delivery 664.0
following
abortion 639.2
ectopic or molar pregnancy 639.2
heart (without penetration of heart chambers) 861.02
with
open wound into thorax 861.12
penetration of heart chambers 861.03
with open wound into thorax 861.13
hernial sac—*see* Hernia, by site
internal organ (abdomen) (chest) (pelvis) NEC—*see* Injury, internal, by site
kidney (parenchyma) 866.02
with
complete disruption of parenchyma (rupture) 866.03
with open wound into cavity 866.13
open wound into cavity 866.12
labia
complicating delivery 664.0
ligament—*see also* Sprain, by site
with open wound—*see* Wound, open, by site
liver 864.05
with open wound into cavity 864.15
major (disruption of hepatic parenchyma) 864.04
with open wound into cavity 864.14
minor (capsule only) 864.02
with open wound into cavity 864.12
moderate (involving parenchyma without major disruption) 864.03
with open wound into cavity 864.13
multiple 864.04
with open wound into cavity 864.14
stellate 864.04
with open wound into cavity 864.14
lung 861.22
with open wound into thorax 861.32
meninges—*see* Laceration, brain
meniscus (knee) (*see also* Tear, meniscus) 836.2
old 717.5
site other than knee—*see also* Sprain, by site
old NEC (*see also* Disorder, cartilage, articular) 718.0

Laceration—*continued*
muscle—*see also* Sprain, by site
with open wound—*see* Wound, open, by site
myocardium—*see* Laceration, heart
nerve—*see* Injury, nerve, by site
ocular NEC (*see also* Laceration, eyeball) 871.4
adnexa NEC 870.8
penetrating 870.3
with foreign body 870.4
orbit (eye) 870.8
penetrating 870.3
with foreign body 870.4
pelvic
floor (muscles)
with
abortion—*see* Abortion, by type, with damage to pelvic organs
ectopic pregnancy (*see also* categories 633.0-633.9) 639.2
molar pregnancy (*see also* categories 630-632) 639.2
complicating delivery 664.1
following
abortion 639.2
ectopic or molar pregnancy 639.2
nonpuerperal 618.7
old (postpartal) 618.7
organ NEC
with
abortion—*see* Abortion, by type, with damage to pelvic organs
ectopic pregnancy (*see also* categories 633.0-633.9) 639.2
molar pregnancy (*see also* categories 630-632) 639.2
complicating delivery 665.5
affecting fetus or newborn 763.8
following
abortion 639.2
ectopic or molar pregnancy 639.2
obstetrical trauma 665.5
perineum, perineal (old) (postpartal) 618.7
with
abortion—*see* Abortion, by type, with damage to pelvic floor
ectopic pregnancy (*see also* categories 633.0-633.9) 639.2
molar pregnancy (*see also* categories 630-632) 639.2
complicating delivery 664.4
first degree 664.0
second degree 664.1
third degree 664.2
fourth degree 664.3
central 664.4
involving
anal sphincter 664.2
fourchette 664.0
hymen 664.0
labia 664.0
pelvic floor 664.1
perineal muscles 664.1
rectovaginal septum 664.2
with anal mucosa 664.3
skin 664.0
sphincter (anal) 664.2
with anal mucosa 664.3
vagina 664.0
vaginal muscles 664.1
vulva 664.0
secondary 674.2

Laceration—*continued*
following
abortion 639.2
ectopic or molar pregnancy 639.2
male 879.6
complicated 879.7
muscles, complicating delivery 664.1
nonpuerperal, current injury 879.6
complicated 879.7
secondary (postpartal) 674.2
peritoneum
with
abortion—*see* Abortion, by type, with damage to pelvic organs
ectopic pregnancy (*see also* categories 633.0-633.9) 639.2
molar pregnancy (*see also* categories 630-632) 639.2
following
abortion 639.2
ectopic or molar pregnancy 639.2
obstetrical trauma 665.5
periurethral tissue
with
abortion—*see* Abortion, by type, with damage to pelvic organs
ectopic pregnancy (*see also* categories 633.0-633.9) 639.2
molar pregnancy (*see also* categories 630-632) 639.2
following
abortion 639.2
ectopic or molar pregnancy 639.2
obstetrical trauma 665.5
rectovaginal (septum)
with
abortion—*see* Abortion, by type, with damage to pelvic organs
ectopic pregnancy (*see also* categories 633.0-633.9) 639.2
molar pregnancy (*see also* categories 630-632) 639.2
complicating delivery 665.4
with perineum 664.2
involving anal or rectal mucosa 664.3
following
abortion 639.2
ectopic or molar pregnancy 639.2
nonpuerperal 623.4
old (postpartal) 623.4
spinal cord (meninges)—*see also* Injury, spinal, by site
due to injury at birth 767.4
fetus or newborn 767.4
spleen 865.09
with
disruption of parenchyma (massive) 865.04
with open wound into cavity 865.14
open wound into cavity 865.19
capsule (without disruption of parenchyma) 865.02
with open wound into cavity 865.12
parenchyma 865.03
with open wound into cavity 865.13
massive disruption (rupture) 865.04
with open wound into cavity 865.14

Laceration—*continued*
tendon 848.9
with open wound–*see* Wound, open, by site
Achilles 845.09
with open wound 892.2
lower limb NEC 844.9
with open wound NEC 894.2
upper limb NEC 840.9
with open wound NEC 884.2
tentorium cerebelli—*see* Laceration, brain, cerebellum
urethra
with
abortion—*see* Abortion, by type, with damage to pelvic organs
ectopic pregnancy (*see also* categories 633.0- 633.9) 639.2
molar pregnancy (*see also* categories 630-632) 639.2
following
abortion 639.2
ectopic or molar pregnancy 639.2
nonpuerperal, nontraumatic 599.84
obstetrical trauma 665.5
uterus
with
abortion—*see* Abortion, by type, with damage to pelvic organs
ectopic pregnancy (*see also* categories 633.0-633.9) 639.2
molar pregnancy (*see also* categories 630-632) 639.2
following
abortion 639.2
ectopic or molar pregnancy 639.2
nonpuerperal, nontraumatic 621.8
obstetrical trauma NEC 665.1
old (postpartal) 621.8
vagina
with
abortion—*see* Abortion, by type, with damage to pelvic organs
ectopic pregnancy (*see also* categories 633.0-633.9) 639.2
molar pregnancy (*see also* categories 630-632) 639.2
perineal involvement, complicating delivery 664.0
complicating delivery 665.4
first degree 664.0
second degree 664.1
third degree 664.2
fourth degree 664.3
high 665.4
muscles 664.1
sulcus 665.4
wall 665.4
following
abortion 639.2
ectopic or molar pregnancy 639.2
nonpuerperal, nontraumatic 623.4
old (postpartal) 623.4
valve, heart—*see* Endocarditis
vulva
with
abortion—*see* Abortion, by type, with damage to pelvic organs
ectopic pregnancy (*see also* categories 633.0-633.9) 639.2
molar pregnancy (*see also* categories 630-632) 639.2

Laceration—*continued*
complicating delivery 664.0
following
abortion 639.2
ectopic or molar pregnancy 639.2
nonpuerperal, nontraumatic 624.4
old (postpartal) 624.4
Lachrymal —*see* condition
Lachrymonasal duct —*see* condition
Lack of
appetite (*see also* Anorexia) 783.0
care
in home V60.4
of infant (at or after birth) 995.5
affecting parent or family V61.21
specified person NEC 995.81
coordination 781.3
development—*see also* Hypoplasia
physiological 783.4
education V62.3
energy 780.7
financial resources V60.2
food 994.2
in environment V60.8
growth 783.4
heating V60.1
housing (permanent) (temporary) V60.0
adequate V60.1
material resources V60.2
medical attention 799.8
memory (*see also* Amnesia) 780.9
mild, following organic brain damage 310.1
ovulation 628.0
person able to render necessary care V60.4
physical exercise V69.0
physiologic development 783.4
prenatal care in current pregnancy V23.7
shelter V60.0
water 994.3
Lacrimal —*see* condition
Lacrimation, abnormal (*see also* Epiphora) 375.20
Lacrimonasal duct —*see* condition
Lactation, lactating (breast) (puerperal) (postpartum)
defective 676.4
disorder 676.9
specified type NEC 676.8
excessive 676.6
failed 676.4
mastitis NEC 675.2
mother (care and/or examination) V24.1
nonpuerperal 611.6
suppressed 676.5
Lacticemia 271.3
excessive 276.2
Lactosuria 271.3
Lacunar skull 756.0
Laennec's cirrhosis (alcoholic) 571.2
nonalcoholic 571.5
Lafora's disease 333.2
Lag, lid (nervous) 374.41
Lagleyze-von Hippel disease (retinocerebral angiomatosis) 759.6
Lagophthalmos (eyelid) (nervous) 374.20
cicatricial 374.23
keratitis (*see also* Keratitis) 370.34
mechanical 374.22
paralytic 374.21

La grippe —*see* Influenza
Lahore sore 085.1
Lakes, venous (cerebral) 437.8
Laki-Lorand factor deficiency (*see also* Defect, coagulation) 286.3
Lalling 307.9
Lambliasis 007.1
Lame back 724.5
Lancereaux's diabetes (diabetes mellitus with marked emaciation) 250.8 *[261]*
Landouzy-Déjérine dystrophy (fascioscapulohumeral atrophy) 359.1
Landry's disease or paralysis 357.0
Landry-Guillain-Barré syndrome 357.0
Lane's
  band 751.4
  disease 569.89
  kink (*see also* Obstruction, intestine) 560.9
Langdon Down's syndrome (mongolism) 758.0
Language abolition 784.69
Lanugo (persistent) 757.4
Lardaceous
  degeneration (any site) 277.3
  disease 277.3
  kidney 277.3 *[583.81]*
  liver 277.3
Large
  baby (regardless of gestational age) 766.1
    exceptionally (weight of 4500 grams or more) 766.0
    of diabetic mother 775.0
  ear 744.22
  fetus—*see also* Oversize, fetus
    causing disproportion 653.5
      with obstructed labor 660.1
  for dates
    fetus or newborn (regardless of gestational age) 766.1
      affecting management of pregnancy 656.6
      exceptionally (weight of 4500 grams or more) 766.0
  physiological cup 743.57
  waxy liver 277.3
  white kidney—*see* Nephrosis
Larsen's syndrome (flattened facies and multiple congenital dislocations) 755.8
Larsen-Johansson disease (juvenile osteopathia patellae) 732.4
Larva migrans
  cutaneous NEC 126.9
    ancylostoma 126.9
  of Diptera in vitreous 128.0
  visceral NEC 128.0
Laryngeal —*see also* condition
  syncope 786.2
Laryngismus (acute) (infectious) (stridulous) 478.75
  congenital 748.3
  diphtheritic 032.3
Laryngitis (acute) (edematous) (fibrinous) (gangrenous) (infective) (infiltrative) (malignant) (membranous) (phlegmonous) (pneumococcal) (pseudomembranous) (septic) (subglottic) (suppurative) (ulcerative) (viral) 464.0
  with
    influenza, flu, or grippe 487.1
    tracheitis (*see also* Laryngotracheitis) 464.20
      with obstruction 464.21
      acute 464.20
        with obstruction 464.21
      chronic 476.1
  atrophic 476.0
  Borrelia vincentii 101
  catarrhal 476.0
  chronic 476.0
    with tracheitis (chronic) 476.1
    due to external agent—*see* Condition, respiratory, chronic, due to
  diphtheritic (membranous) 032.3
  due to external agent—*see* Inflammation, respiratory, upper, due to
  H. influenzae 464.0
  Hemophilus influenzae 464.0
  hypertrophic 476.0
  influenzal 487.1
  pachydermic 478.79
  sicca 476.0
  spasmodic 478.75
    acute 464.0
  streptococcal 034.0
  stridulous 478.75
  syphilitic 095.8
    congenital 090.5
  tuberculous (*see also* Tuberculosis, larynx) 012.3
  Vincent's 101
Laryngocele (congenital) (ventricular) 748.3
Laryngofissure 478.79
  congenital 748.3
Laryngomalacia (congenital) 748.3
Laryngopharyngitis (acute) 465.0
  chronic 478.9
    due to external agent—*see* Condition, respiratory, chronic, due to
  due to external agent—*see* Inflammation, respiratory, upper, due to
  septic 034.0
Laryngoplegia (*see also* Paralysis, vocal cord) 478.30
Laryngoptosis 478.79
Laryngospasm 478.75
  due to external agent—*see* Condition, respiratory, acute, due to
Laryngostenosis 478.74
  congenital 748.3
Laryngotracheitis (acute) (infectional) (viral) (*see also* Laryngitis) 464.20
  with obstruction 464.21
  atrophic 476.1
  Borrelia vincentii 101
  catarrhal 476.1
  chronic 476.1
    due to external agent—*see* Condition, respiratory, chronic, due to
  diphtheritic (membranous) 032.3
  due to external agent—*see* Inflammation, respiratory, upper, due to
  H. influenzae 464.20
    with obstruction 464.21
  hypertrophic 476.1
  influenzal 487.1
  pachydermic 478.75
  sicca 476.1
  spasmodic 478.75
    acute 464.20
      with obstruction 464.21

Laryngotracheitis—*continued*
streptococcal 034.0
stridulous 478.75
syphilitic 095.8
congenital 090.5
tuberculous (*see also* Tuberculosis, larynx) 012.3
Vincent's 101
Laryngotracheobronchitis (*see also* Bronchitis) 490
acute 466.0
chronic 491.8
viral 466.0
Laryngotracheobronchopneumonitis —*see* Pneumonia, broncho-
Larynx, laryngeal —*see* condition
Lasègue's disease (persecution mania) 297.9
Lassa fever 078.89
Lassitude (*see also* Weakness) 780.7
Late —*see also* condition
effect(s) (of)—*see also* condition
abscess
intracranial or intraspinal (conditions classifiable to 324)–*see* category 326
adverse effect of drug, medicinal or biological substance 909.5
allergic reaction 909.9
amputation
postoperative (late) 997.60
traumatic (injury classifiable to 885-887 and 895-897) 905.9
burn (injury classifiable to 948-949) 906.9
extremities NEC (injury classifiable to 943 or 945) 906.7
hand or wrist (injury classifiable to 944) 906.6
eye (injury classifiable to 940) 906.5
face, head, and neck (injury classifiable to 941) 906.5
specified site NEC (injury classifiable to 942 and 946-947) 906.8
cerebrovascular disease (conditions classifiable to 430-437)—*see* category 438
childbirth complication(s) 677
complication(s) of
childbirth 677
delivery 677
pregnancy 677
puerperium 677
surgical and medical care (conditions classifiable to 996-999) 909.3
trauma (conditions classifiable to 958) 908.6
contusion (injury classifiable to 920-924) 906.3
crushing (injury classifiable to 925-929) 906.4
delivery complication(s) 677
dislocation (injury classifiable to 830-839) 905.6
encephalitis or encephalomyelitis (conditions classifiable to 323)—*see* category 326
in infectious diseases 139.8
viral (conditions classifiable to 049.8, 049.9, 062-064) 139.0
external cause NEC (conditions classifiable to 995) 909.9
certain conditions classifiable to categories 991-994 909.4
foreign body in orifice (injury classifiable to 930-939) 908.5

Late —*continued*
fracture (multiple) (injury classifiable to 828-829) 905.5
extremity
lower (injury classifiable to 821-827) 905.4
neck of femur (injury classifiable to 820) 905.3
upper (injury classifiable to 810-819) 905.2
face and skull (injury classifiable to 800-804) 905.0
skull and face (injury classifiable to 800-804) 905.0
spine and trunk (injury classifiable to 805 and 807-809) 905.1
with spinal cord lesion (injury classifiable to 806) 907.2
infection
pyogenic, intracranial—*see* category 326
infectious diseases (conditions classifiable to 001-136) NEC 139.8
injury (injury classifiable to 959) 908.9
blood vessel 908.3
abdomen and pelvis (injury classifiable to 902) 908.4
extremity (injury classifiable to 903-904) 908.3
head and neck (injury classifiable to 900) 908.3
intracranial (injury classifiable to 850-854) 907.0
with skull fracture 905.0
thorax (injury classifiable to 901) 908.4
internal organ NEC (injury classifiable to 867 and 869) 908.2
abdomen (injury classifiable to 863-866 and 868) 908.1
thorax (injury classifiable to 860-862) 908.0
intracranial (injury classifiable to 850-854) 907.0
with skull fracture (injury classifiable to 800-801 and 803-804) 905.0
nerve NEC (injury classifiable to 957) 907.9
cranial (injury classifiable to 950-951) 907.1
peripheral NEC (injury classifiable to 957) 907.9
lower limb and pelvic girdle (injury classifiable to 956) 907.5
upper limb and shoulder girdle (injury classifiable to 955) 907.4
roots and plexus(es), spinal (injury classifiable to 953) 907.3
trunk (injury classifiable to 954) 907.3
pregnancy complication(s) 677
puerperal complication(s) 677
spinal
cord (injury classifiable to 806 and 952) 907.2
nerve root(s) and plexus(es) (injury classifiable to 953) 907.3
superficial (injury classifiable to 910-919) 906.2
tendon (tendon injury classifiable to 840-848, 880-884 with .2, and 890-894 with .2) 905.8

Late —*continued*
meningitis
bacterial (conditions classifiable to 320)—*see* category 326
unspecified cause (conditions classifiable to 322)—*see* category 326
myelitis (*see also* Late, effect(s) (of), encephalitis)—*see* category 326
parasitic diseases (conditions classifiable to 001-136 NEC) 139.8
phlebitis or thrombophlebitis of intracranial venous sinuses (conditions classifiable to 325)—*see* category 326
poisoning due to drug, medicinal or biological substance (conditions classifiable to 960-979) 909.0
poliomyelitis, acute (conditions classifiable to 045) 138
radiation (conditions classifiable to 990) 909.2
rickets 268.1
sprain and strain without mention of tendon injury (injury classifiable to 840-848, except tendon injury) 905.7
tendon involvement 905.8
toxic effect of
drug, medicinal or biological substance (conditions classifiable to 960-979) 909.0
nonmedical substance (conditions classifiable to 980-989) 909.1
trachoma (conditions classifiable to 076) 139.1
tuberculosis 137.0
bones and joints (conditions classifiable to 015) 137.3
central nervous system (conditions classifiable to 013) 137.1
genitourinary (conditions classifiable to 016) 137.2
pulmonary (conditions classifiable to 010-012) 137.0
specified organs NEC (conditions classifiable to 014, 017-018) 137.4
viral encephalitis (conditions classifiable to 049.8, 049.9, 062-064) 139.0
wound, open
extremity (injury classifiable to 880-884 and 890-894, except .2) 906.1
tendon (injury classifiable to 880-884 with .2 and 890-894 with .2) 905.8
head, neck, and trunk (injury classifiable to 870-879) 906.0
Latent —*see* condition
Lateral —*see* condition
Laterocession —*see* Lateroversion
Lateroflexion —*see* Lateroversion
Lateroversion
cervix—*see* Lateroversion, uterus
uterus, uterine (cervix) (postinfectional) (postpartal, old) 621.6
congenital 752.3
in pregnancy or childbirth 654.4
affecting fetus or newborn 763.8
Lathyrism 988.2
Launois' syndrome (pituitary gigantism) 253.0
Launois-Bensaude's lipomatosis 272.8
Launois-Cléret syndrome (adiposogenital dystrophy) 253.8
Laurence-Moon-Biedl syndrome (obesity, polydactyly, and mental retardation) 759.89
LAV (disease) (illness) (infection)—*see* Human immunodeficiency virus (disease) (illness) (infection)
LAV/HTLV-III (disease) (illness) (infection)—*see* Human immunodeficiency virus (disease) (illness) (infection)
Lawford's syndrome (encephalocutaneous angiomatosis) 759.6
Lax, laxity —*see also* Relaxation
ligament 728.4
skin (acquired) 701.8
congenital 756.83
Laxative habit (*see also* Abuse, drugs, nondependent) 305.9
Lazy leukocyte syndrome 288.0
Lead —*see also* condition
exposure to V15.86
incrustation of cornea 371.15
poisoning 984.9
specified type of lead—*see* Table of drugs and chemicals
Lead miner's lung 503
Leakage
amniotic fluid 658.1
with delayed delivery 658.2
affecting fetus or newborn 761.1
bile from drainage tube (T tube) 997.4
blood (microscopic), fetal, into maternal circulation 656.0
affecting management of pregnancy or puerperium 656.0
device, implant, or graft—*see* Complications, mechanical
spinal fluid at lumbar puncture site 997.09
urine, continuous 788.37
Leaky heart —*see* Endocarditis
Learning defect, specific NEC (strephosymbolia) 315.2
Leather bottle stomach (M8142/3) 151.9
Leber's
congenital amaurosis 362.76
optic atrophy (hereditary) 377.16
Lederer's anemia or disease (acquired infectious hemolytic anemia) 283.19
Lederer-Brill syndrome (acquired infectious hemolytic anemia) 283.19
Leeches (aquatic) (land) 134.2
Left-sided neglect 781.8
Leg —*see* condition
Legal investigation V62.5
Legg (-Calvé) -Perthes disease or syndrome (osteochondrosis, femoral capital) 732.1
Legionnaires' disease 482.83
Leigh's disease 330.8
Leiner's disease (exfoliative dermatitis) 695.89
Leiofibromyoma (M8890/0)—*see also* Leiomyoma
uterus (cervix) (corpus) (*see also* Leiomyoma, uterus) 218.9
Leiomyoblastoma (M8891/1)—*see* Neoplasm, connective tissue, uncertain behavior
Leiomyofibroma (M8890/0)—*see also* Neoplasm, connective tissue, benign
uterus (cervix) (corpus) (*see also* Leiomyoma, uterus) 218.9
Leiomyoma (M8890/0)—*see* Neoplasm, connective tissue, benign
bizarre (M8893/0)—*see* Neoplasm, connective tissue, benign

Leptus dermatitis 133.8
Léri's pleonosteosis 756.89
Léri-Weill syndrome 756.59
Leriche syndrome (aortic bifurcation occlusion) 444.0
Lermoyez's syndrome (*see also* Disease, Ménière's) 386.00
Lesbianism *—omit code*
egodystonic 302.0
problems with 302.0
Lesch-Nyhan syndrome (hypoxanthine-guanine-phosphoribosyltransferase deficiency) 277.2
Lesion
abducens nerve 378.54
alveolar process 525.8
anorectal 569.49
aortic (valve)—*see* Endocarditis, aortic
auditory nerve 388.5
basal ganglion 333.90
bile duct (*see also* Disease, biliary) 576.8
bladder 596.9
bone 733.90
brachial plexus 353.0
brain 348.8
congenital 742.9
vascular (*see also* Lesion, cerebrovascular) 437.9
degenerative 437.1
healed or old—*see also* category 438
without residuals V12.59
hypertensive 437.2
late effect—*see* category 438
buccal 528.9
calcified—*see* Calcification
canthus 373.9
carate—*see* Pinta, lesions
cardia 537.89
cardiac—*see also* Disease, heart congenital 746.9
valvular—*see* Endocarditis
cauda equina 344.60
with neurogenic bladder 344.61
cecum 569.89
cerebral—*see* Lesion, brain
cerebrovascular (*see also* Disease, cerebrovascular NEC) 437.9
degenerative 437.1
healed or old—*see also* category 438
without residuals V12.59
hypertensive 437.2
late effect—*see* category 438
specified type NEC 437.8
cervical root (nerve) NEC 353.2
chiasmal 377.54
associated with
inflammatory disorders 377.54
neoplasm NEC 377.52
pituitary 377.51
pituitary disorders 377.51
vascular disorders 377.53
chorda tympani 351.8
coin, lung 793.1
colon 569.89
congenital—*see* Anomaly
conjunctiva 372.9
coronary artery (*see also* Ischemia, heart) 414.9
cranial nerve 352.9
first 352.0
second 377.49
third
partial 378.51

Lesion—*continued*
total 378.52
fourth 378.53
fifth 350.9
sixth 378.54
seventh 351.9
eighth 388.5
ninth 352.2
tenth 352.3
eleventh 352.4
twelfth 352.5
cystic—*see* Cyst
degenerative—*see* Degeneration
dermal (skin) 709.9
duodenum 537.89
with obstruction 537.3
eyelid 373.9
gasserian ganglion 350.8
gastric 537.89
gastroduodenal 537.89
gastrointestinal 569.89
glossopharyngeal nerve 352.2
heart (organic)—*see also* Disease, heart
vascular—*see* Disease, cardiovascular
helix (ear) 709.9
hyperchromic, due to pinta (carate) 103.1
hyperkeratotic (*see also* Hyperkeratosis) 701.1
hypoglossal nerve 352.5
hypopharynx 478.29
hypothalamic 253.9
ileocecal coil 569.89
ileum 569.89
iliohypogastric nerve 355.79
ilioinguinal nerve 355.79
in continuity—*see* Injury, nerve, by site
inflammatory—*see* Inflammation
intestine 569.89
intracerebral—*see* Lesion, brain
intrachiasmal (optic) (*see also* Lesion, chiasmal) 377.54
intracranial, space-occupying NEC 784.2
joint 719.90
ankle 719.97
elbow 719.92
foot 719.97
hand 719.94
hip 719.95
knee 719.96
multiple sites 719.99
pelvic region 719.95
sacroiliac (old) 724.6
shoulder (region) 719.91
specified site NEC 719.98
wrist 719.93
keratotic (*see also* Keratosis) 701.1
kidney (*see also* Disease, renal) 593.9
laryngeal nerve (recurrent) 352.3
leonine 030.0
lip 528.5
liver 573.8
lumbosacral
plexus 353.1
root (nerve) NEC 353.4
lung 518.89
coin 793.1
maxillary sinus 473.0
mitral—*see* Endocarditis, mitral
motor cortex 348.8
nerve (*see also* Disorder, nerve) 355.9
nervous system 349.9
congenital 742.9

Lesion—*continued*
nonallopathic NEC 739.9
in region (of)
abdomen 739.9
acromioclavicular 739.7
cervical, cervicothoracic 739.1
costochondral 739.8
costovertebral 739.8
extremity
lower 739.6
upper 739.7
head 739.0
hip 739.5
lower extremity 739.6
lumbar, lumbosacral 739.3
occipitocervical 739.0
pelvic 739.5
pubic 739.5
rib cage 739.8
sacral, sacrococcygeal, sacroiliac 739.4
sternochondral 739.8
sternoclavicular 739.7
thoracic, thoracolumbar 739.2
upper extremity 739.7
nose (internal) 478.1
obstructive—*see* Obstruction
obturator nerve 355.79
occlusive
artery—*see* Embolism, artery
organ or site NEC—*see* Disease, by site
osteolytic 733.90
paramacular, of retina 363.32
peptic 537.89
periodontal, due to traumatic occlusion 523.8
perirectal 569.49
peritoneum (granulomatous) 568.89
pigmented (skin) 709.00
pinta—*see* Pinta, lesions
polypoid—*see* Polyp
prechiasmal (optic) (*see also* Lesion, chiasmal) 377.54
primary—*see also* Syphilis, primary
carate 103.0
pinta 103.0
yaws 102.0
pulmonary 518.89
valve (*see also* Endocarditis, pulmonary) 424.3
pylorus 537.89
radiation NEC 990
radium NEC 990
rectosigmoid 569.89
retina, retinal—*see also* Retinopathy
vascular 362.17
retroperitoneal 568.89
romanus 720.1
sacroiliac (joint) 724.6
salivary gland 527.8
benign lymphoepithelial 527.8
saphenous nerve 355.79
secondary—*see* Syphilis, secondary
sigmoid 569.89
sinus (accessory) (nasal) (*see also* Sinusitis) 473.9
skin 709.9
suppurative 686.0
space-occupying, intracranial NEC 784.2
spinal cord 336.9
congenital 742.9
traumatic (complete) (incomplete) (transverse)—*see also* Injury, spinal, by site

Lesion—*continued*
with
broken
back—*see* Fracture, vertebra, by site, with spinal cord injury
neck—*see* Fracture, vertebra, cervical, with spinal cord injury
fracture, vertebra—*see* Fracture, vertebra, by site, with spinal cord injury
spleen 289.50
stomach 537.89
syphilitic—*see* Syphilis
tertiary—*see* Syphilis, tertiary
thoracic root (nerve) 353.3
tonsillar fossa 474.9
tooth, teeth 525.8
white spot 521.0
traumatic NEC (*see also* nature and site of injury) 959.9
tricuspid (valve)—*see* Endocarditis, tricuspid
trigeminal nerve 350.9
ulcerated or ulcerative—*see* Ulcer
uterus NEC 621.9
vagus nerve 352.3
valvular—*see* Endocarditis
vascular 459.9
affecting central nervous system (*see also* Lesion, cerebrovascular) 437.9
following trauma (*see also* Injury, blood vessel, by site) 904.9
retina 362.17
traumatic—*see* Injury, blood vessel, by site
umbilical cord 663.6
affecting fetus or newborn 762.6
visual
cortex NEC (*see also* Disorder, visual, cortex) 377.73
pathway NEC (*see also* Disorder, visual, pathway) 377.63
warty—*see* Verruca
white spot, on teeth 521.0
x-ray NEC 990
Lethargic —*see* condition
Lethargy 780.7
Letterer-Siwe disease (acute histiocytosis X) (M9722/3) 202.5
Leucinosis 270.3
Leucocoria 360.44
Leucosarcoma (M9850/3) 207.8
Leukasmus 270.2
Leukemia, leukemic (congenital) (M9800/3) 208.9

Note—Use the following fifth-digit subclassification for categories 203-208:

0 without mention of remission
1 with remission

acute NEC (M9801/3) 208.0
aleukemic NEC (M9804/3) 208.8
granulocytic (M9864/3) 205.8
basophilic (M9870/3) 205.1
blast (cell) (M9801/3) 208.0
blastic (M9801/3) 208.0
granulocytic (M9861/3) 205.0
chronic NEC (M9803/3) 208.1
compound (M9810/3) 207.8
eosinophilic (M9880/3) 205.1
giant cell (M9910/3) 207.2
granulocytic (M9860/3) 205.9
acute (M9861/3) 205.0

Leukemia, leukemic—*continued*
aleukemic (M9864/3) 205.8
blastic (M9861/3) 205.0
chronic (M9863/3) 205.1
subacute (M9862/3) 205.2
subleukemic (M9864/3) 205.8
hairy cell (M9940/3) 202.4
hemoblastic (M9801/3) 208.0
histiocytic (M9890/3) 206.9
lymphatic (M9820/3) 204.9
acute (M9821/3) 204.0
aleukemic (M9824/3) 204.8
chronic (M9823/3) 204.1
subacute (M9822/3) 204.2
subleukemic (M9824/3) 204.8
lymphoblastic (M9821/3) 204.0
lymphocytic (M9820/3) 204.9
acute (M9821/3) 204.0
aleukemic (M9824/3) 204.8
chronic (M9823/3) 204.1
subacute (M9822/3) 204.2
subleukemic (M9824/3) 204.8
lymphogenous (M9820/3)—*see* Leukemia, lymphoid
lymphoid (M9820/3) 204.9
acute (M9821/3) 204.0
aleukemic (M9824/3) 204.8
blastic (M9821/3) 204.0
chronic (M9823/3) 204.1
subacute (M9822/3) 204.2
subleukemic (M9824/3) 204.8
lymphosarcoma cell (M9850/3) 207.8
mast cell (M9900/3) 207.8
megakaryocytic (M9910/3) 207.2
megakaryocytoid (M9910/3) 207.2
mixed (cell) (M9810/3) 207.8
monoblastic (M9891/3) 206.0
monocytic (Schilling-type) (M9890/3) 206.9
acute (M9891/3) 206.0
aleukemic (M9894/3) 206.8
chronic (M9893/3) 206.1
Naegeli-type (M9863/3) 205.1
subacute (M9892/3) 206.2
subleukemic (M9894/3) 206.8
monocytoid (M9890/3) 206.9
acute (M9891/3) 206.0
aleukemic (M9894/3) 206.8
chronic (M9893/3) 206.1
myelogenous (M9863/3) 205.1
subacute (M9892/3) 206.2
subleukemic (M9894/3) 206.8
monomyelocytic (M9860/3)—*see* Leukemia, myelomonocytic
myeloblastic (M9861/3) 205.0
myelocytic (M9863/3) 205.1
acute (M9861/3) 205.0
myelogenous (M9860/3) 205.9
acute (M9861/3) 205.0
aleukemic (M9864/3) 205.8
chronic (M9863/3) 205.1
monocytoid (M9863/3) 205.1
subacute (M9862/3) 205.2
subleukemic (M9864) 205.8
myeloid (M9860/3) 205.9
acute (M9861/3) 205.0
aleukemic (M9864/3) 205.8
chronic (M9863/3) 205.1
subacute (M9862/3) 205.2
subleukemic (M9864/3) 205.8
myelomonocytic (M9860/3) 205.9
acute (M9861/3) 205.0

Leukemia, leukemic—*continued*
chronic (M9863/3) 205.1
Naegeli-type monocytic (M9863/3) 205.1
neutrophilic (M9865/3) 205.1
plasma cell (M9830/3) 203.1
plasmacytic (M9830/3) 203.1
prolymphocytic (M9825/3)—*see* Leukemia, lymphoid
promyelocytic, acute (M9866/3) 205.0
Schilling-type monocytic (M9890/3)—*see* Leukemia, monocytic
stem cell (M9801/3) 208.0
subacute NEC (M9802/3) 208.2
subleukemic NEC (M9804/3) 208.8
thrombocytic (M9910/3) 207.2
undifferentiated (M9801/3) 208.0
Leukemoid reaction (lymphocytic) (monocytic) (myelocytic) 288.8
Leukocoria 360.44
Leukocythemia —*see* Leukemia
Leukocytosis 288.8
basophilic 288.8
eosinophilic 288.3
lymphocytic 288.8
monocytic 288.8
neutrophilic 288.8
Leukoderma 709.09
syphilitic 091.3
late 095.8
Leukodermia (*see also* Leukoderma) 709.09
Leukodystrophy (cerebral) (globoid cell) (metachromatic) (progressive) (sudanophilic) 330.0
Leukoedema, mouth or tongue 528.7
Leukoencephalitis
acute hemorrhagic (postinfectious) NEC 136.9 *[323.6]*
postimmunization or postvaccinal 323.5
subacute sclerosing 046.2
van Bogaert's 046.2
van Bogaert's (sclerosing) 046.2
Leukoencephalopathy (*see also* Encephalitis) 323.9
acute necrotizing hemorrhagic (postinfectious) 136.9 *[323.6]*
postimmunization or postvaccinal 323.5
metachromatic 330.0
multifocal (progressive) 046.3
progressive multifocal 046.3
Leukoerythroblastosis 289.0
Leukoerythrosis 289.0
Leukokeratosis (*see also* Leukoplakia) 702.8
mouth 528.6
nicotina palati 528.7
tongue 528.6
Leukokoria 360.44
Leukokoraurosis vulva, vulvae 624.0
Leukolymphosarcoma (M9850/3) 207.8
Leukoma (cornea) (interfering with central vision) 371.03
adherent 371.04
Leukomelanopathy, hereditary 288.2
Leukonychia (punctata) (striata) 703.8
congenital 757.5
Leukopathia
unguium 703.8
congenital 757.5
Leukopenia 288.0
cyclic 288.0
familial 288.0
malignant 288.0

Leukopenia—*continued*
periodic 288.0
transitory neonatal 776.7
Leukopenic —*see* condition
Leukoplakia 702.8
anus 569.49
bladder (postinfectional) 596.8
buccal 528.6
cervix (uteri) 622.2
esophagus 530.83
gingiva 528.6
kidney (pelvis) 593.89
larynx 478.79
lip 528.6
mouth 528.6
oral soft tissue (including tongue) (mucosa) 528.6
palate 528.6
pelvis (kidney) 593.89
penis (infectional) 607.0
rectum 569.49
syphilitic 095.8
tongue 528.6
tonsil 478.29
ureter (postinfectional) 593.89
urethra (postinfectional) 599.84
uterus 621.8
vagina 623.1
vesical 596.8
vocal cords 478.5
vulva 624.0
Leukopolioencephalopathy 330.0
Leukorrhea (vagina) 623.5
due to trichomonas (vaginalis) 131.00
trichomonal (Trichomonas vaginalis) 131.00
Leukosarcoma (M9850/3) 207.8
Leukosis (M9800/3)—*see* Leukemia
Lev's disease or syndrome (acquired complete heart block) 426.0
Levi's syndrome (pituitary dwarfism) 253.3
Levocardia (isolated) 746.87
with situs inversus 759.3
Levulosuria 271.2
Lewandowski's disease (primary) (*see also* Tuberculosis) 017.0
Lewandowski-Lutz disease (epidermodysplasia verruciformis) 078.19
Leyden's disease (periodic vomiting) 536.2
Leyden's-Möbius dystrophy 359.1
Leydig cell
carcinoma (M8650/3)
specified site—*see* Neoplasm, by site, malignant
unspecified site
female 183.0
male 186.9
tumor (M8650/1)
benign (M8650/0)
specified site—*see* Neoplasm, by site, benign
unspecified site
female 220
male 222.0
malignant (M8650/3)
specified site—*see* Neoplasm, by site, malignant
unspecified site
female 183.0
male 186.9
specified site—*see* Neoplasm, by site, uncertain behavior
Leydig cell—*continued*
unspecified site
female 236.2
male 236.4
Leydig-Sertoli cell tumor (M8631/0)
specified site—*see* Neoplasm, by site, benign
unspecified site
female 220
male 222.0
Liar, pathologic 301.7
Libman-Sacks disease or syndrome 710.0 *[424.91]*
Lice (infestation) 132.9
body (pediculus corporis) 132.1
crab 132.2
head (pediculus capitis) 132.0
mixed (classifiable to more than one of the categories 132.0-132.2) 132.3
pubic (pediculus pubis) 132.2
Lichen 697.9
albus 701.0
annularis 695.89
atrophicus 701.0
corneus obtusus 698.3
myxedematous 701.8
nitidus 697.1
pilaris 757.39
acquired 701.1
planopilaris 697.0
planus (acute) (chronicus) (hypertrophic) (verrucous) 697.0
morphoeicus 701.0
sclerosus (et atrophicus) 701.0
ruber 696.4
acuminatus 696.4
moniliformis 697.8
obtusus corneus 698.3
of Wilson 697.0
planus 697.0
sclerosus (et atrophicus) 701.0
scrofulosus (primary) (*see also* Tuberculosis) 017.0
simplex (Vidal's) 698.3
chronicus 698.3
circumscriptus 698.3
spinulosus 757.39
mycotic 117.9
striata 697.8
urticatus 698.2
Lichenification 698.3
nodular 698.3
Lichenoides tuberculosis (primary) (*see also* Tuberculosis) 017.0
Lichtheim's disease or syndrome (subacute combined sclerosis with pernicious anemia) 281.0 *[336.2]*
Lien migrans 289.59
Lientery (*see also* Diarrhea) 558.9
infectious 009.2
Life circumstance problem NEC V62.89
Ligament —*see* condition
Light-for-dates (infant) 764.0
with signs of fetal malnutrition 764.1
affecting management of pregnancy 656.5
Light-headedness 780.4
Lightning (effects) (shock) (stroke) (struck by) 994.0
burn—*see* Burn, by site
foot 266.2
Lightwood's disease or syndrome (renal tubular acidosis) 588.8
Lignac's disease (cystinosis) 270.0

Lignac (-de Toni) (-Fanconi) (-Debré) syndrome (cystinosis) 270.0
Lignac (-Fanconi) syndrome (cystinosis) 270.0
Ligneous thyroiditis 245.3
Likoff's syndrome (angina in menopausal women) 413.9
Limb —*see* condition
Limitation of joint motion (*see also* Stiffness, joint) 719.5
  sacroiliac 724.6
Limit dextrinosis 271.0
Limited
  cardiac reserve—*see* Disease, heart
  duction, eye NEC 378.63
Lindau's disease (retinocerebral angiomatosis) 759.6
Lindau (-von Hippel) disease (angiomatosis retinocerebellosa) 759.6
Linea corneae senilis 371.41
Lines
  Beau's (transverse furrows on fingernails) 703.8
  Harris' 733.91
  Hudson-Stähli 371.11
  Stähli's 371.11
Lingua
  geographical 529.1
  nigra (villosa) 529.3
  plicata 529.5
    congenital 750.13
  tylosis 528.6
Lingual (tongue)—*see also* condition
  thyroid 759.2
Linitis (gastric) 535.4
  plastica (M8142/3) 151.9
Lioderma essentialis (cum melanosis et telangiectasia) 757.33
Lip —*see also* condition
  biting 528.9
Lipalgia 272.8
Lipedema —*see* Edema
Lipemia (*see also* Hyperlipidemia) 272.4
  retina, retinalis 272.3
Lipidosis 272.7
  cephalin 272.7
  cerebral (infantile) (juvenile) (late) 330.1
  cerebroretinal 330.1 *[362.71]*
  cerebroside 272.7
  cerebrospinal 272.7
  chemically-induced 272.7
  cholesterol 272.7
  diabetic 250.8 *[272.7]*
  dystopic (hereditary) 272.7
  glycolipid 272.7
  hepatosplenomegalic 272.3
  hereditary, dystopic 272.7
  sulfatide 330.0
Lipoadenoma (M8324/0)—*see* Neoplasm, by site, benign
Lipoblastoma (M8881/0)—*see* Lipoma, by site
Lipoblastomatosis (M8881/0)—*see* Lipoma, by site
Lipochondrodystrophy 277.5
Lipochrome histiocytosis (familial) 288.1
Lipodystrophia progressiva 272.6
Lipodystrophy (progressive) 272.6
  insulin 272.6
  intestinal 040.2
Lipofibroma (M8851/0)—*see* Lipoma, by site
Lipoglycoproteinosis 272.8
Lipogranuloma, sclerosing 709.8
Lipogranulomatosis (disseminated) 272.8
  kidney 272.8
Lipoid —*see* condition
  histiocytosis 272.7
    essential 272.7
  nephrosis (*see also* Nephrosis) 581.3
  proteinosis of Urbach 272.8
Lipoidemia (*see also* Hyperlipidemia) 272.4
Lipoidosis (*see also* Lipidosis) 272.7
Lipoma (M8850/0) 214.9
  breast (skin) 214.1
  face 214.0
  fetal (M8881/0)—*see also* Lipoma, by site
    fat cell (M8880/0)—*see* Lipoma, by site
  infiltrating (M8856/0)—*see* Lipoma, by site
  intra-abdominal 214.3
  intramuscular (M8856/0)—*see* Lipoma, by site
  intrathoracic 214.2
  kidney 214.3
  mediastinum 214.2
  muscle 214.8
  peritoneum 214.3
  retroperitoneum 214.3
  skin 214.1
    face 214.0
  spermatic cord 214.4
  spindle cell (M8857/0)—*see* Lipoma, by site
  stomach 214.3
  subcutaneous tissue 214.1
    face 214.0
  thymus 214.2
  thyroid gland 214.2
Lipomatosis (dolorosa) 272.8
  fetal (M8881/0)—*see* Lipoma, by site
  Launois-Bensaude's 272.8
Lipomyohemangioma (M8860/0)
  specified site—*see* Neoplasm, connective tissue, benign
  unspecified site 223.0
Lipomyoma (M8860/0)
  specified site—*see* Neoplasm, connective tissue, benign
  unspecified site 223.0
Lipomyxoma (M8852/0)—*see* Lipoma, by site
Lipomyxosarcoma (M8852/3)—*see* Neoplasm, connective tissue, malignant
Lipophagocytosis 289.8
Lipoproteinemia (alpha) 272.4
  broad-beta 272.2
  floating-beta 272.2
  hyper-pre-beta 272.1
Lipoproteinosis (Rössle-Urbach-Wiethe) 272.8
Liposarcoma (M8850/3)—*see also* Neoplasm, connective tissue, malignant
  differentiated type (M8851/3)—*see* Neoplasm, connective tissue, malignant
  embryonal (M8852/3)—*see* Neoplasm, connective tissue, malignant
  mixed type (M8855/3)—*see* Neoplasm, connective tissue, malignant
  myxoid (M8852/3)—*see* Neoplasm, connective tissue, malignant
  pleomorphic (M8854/3)—*see* Neoplasm, connective tissue, malignant
  round cell (M8853/3)—*see* Neoplasm, connective tissue, malignant
  well differentiated type (M8851/3)—*see* Neoplasm, connective tissue, malignant
Liposynovitis prepatellaris 272.8
Lipping
  cervix 622.0
  spine (*see also* Spondylosis) 721.90
  vertebra (*see also* Spondylosis) 721.90
Lip pits (mucus), congenital 750.25

Lipschütz disease or ulcer 616.50
Lipuria 791.1
bilharziasis 120.0
Liquefaction, vitreous humor 379.21
Lisping 307.9
Lissauer's paralysis 094.1
Lissencephalia, lissencephaly 742.2
Listerellose 027.0
Listeriose 027.0
Listeriosis 027.0
congenital 771.2
fetal 771.2
suspected fetal damage affecting management of pregnancy 655.4
Listlessness 780.7
Lithemia 790.6
Lithiasis —*see also* Calculus
hepatic (duct)—*see* Choledocholithiasis
urinary 592.9
Lithopedion 779.9
affecting management of pregnancy 656.8
Lithosis (occupational) 502
with tuberculosis—*see* Tuberculosis, pulmonary
Lithuria 791.9
Litigation V62.5
Little
league elbow 718.82
stroke syndrome 435.9
Little's disease —*see* Palsy, cerebral
Littre's
gland—*see* condition
hernia—*see* Hernia, Littre's
Littritis (*see also* Urethritis) 597.89
Livedo 782.61
annularis 782.61
racemose 782.61
reticularis 782.61
Live flesh 781.0
Liver —*see also* condition
donor V59.8
Livida, asphyxia
newborn 768.6
Living
alone V60.3
with handicapped person V60.4
Lloyd's syndrome 258.1
Loa loa 125.2
Loasis 125.2
Lobe, lobar —*see* condition
Lobo's disease or blastomycosis 116.2
Lobomycosis 116.2
Lobotomy syndrome 310.0
Lobstein's disease (brittle bones and blue sclera) 756.51
Lobster-claw hand 755.58
Lobulation (congenital)—*see also* Anomaly, specified type NEC, by site
kidney, fetal 753.3
liver, abnormal 751.69
spleen 759.0
Lobule, lobular —*see* condition
Local, localized —*see* condition
Locked bowel or intestine (*see also* Obstruction, intestine) 560.9
Locked twins 660.5
affecting fetus or newborn 763.1
Locked-in state 344.81
Locking
joint (*see also* Derangement, joint) 718.90
knee 717.9
Lockjaw (*see also* Tetanus) 037
Locomotor ataxia (progressive) 094.0
Löffler's
endocarditis 421.0
eosinophilia or syndrome 518.3
pneumonia 518.3
syndrome (eosinophilic pneumonitis) 518.3
Löfgren's syndrome (sarcoidosis) 135
Loiasis 125.2
eyelid 125.2 *[373.6]*
Loneliness V62.89
Lone star fever 082.8
Long labor 662.1
affecting fetus or newborn 763.8
first stage 662.0
second stage 662.2
Long-term (current) drug use V58.69
anticoagulants V58.61
Longitudinal stripes or grooves, nails 703.8
congenital 757.5
Loop
intestine (*see also* Volvulus) 560.2
intrascleral nerve 379.29
vascular on papilla (optic) 743.57
Loose —*see also* condition
body
in tendon sheath 727.82
joint 718.10
ankle 718.17
elbow 718.12
foot 718.17
hand 718.14
hip 718.15
knee 717.6
multiple sites 718.19
pelvic region 718.15
prosthetic implant—*see* Complications, mechanical
shoulder (region) 718.11
specified site NEC 718.18
wrist 718.13
cartilage (joint) (*see also* Loose, body, joint) 718.1
knee 717.6
facet (vertebral) 724.9
prosthetic implant—*see* Complications, mechanical
sesamoid, joint (*see also* Loose, body, joint) 718.1
tooth, teeth 525.8
Loosening epiphysis 732.9
Looser (-Debray) -Milkman syndrome (osteomalacia with pseudofractures) 268.2
Lop ear (deformity) 744.29
Lorain's disease or syndrome (pituitary dwarfism) 253.3
Lorain-Levi syndrome (pituitary dwarfism) 253.3
Lordosis (acquired) (postural) 737.20
congenital 754.2
due to or associated with
Charcot-Marie-Tooth disease 356.1 *[737.42]*
mucopolysaccharidosis 277.5 *[737.42]*
neurofibromatosis 237.71 *[737.42]*
osteitis
deformans 731.0 *[737.42]*
fibrosa cystica 252.0 *[737.42]*
osteoporosis (*see also* Osteoporosis) 733.00 *[737.42]*
poliomyelitis (*see also* Poliomyelitis) 138 *[737.42]*
tuberculosis (*see also* Tuberculosis) 015.0 *[737.42]*
late effect of rickets 268.1 *[737.42]*

Lordosis—*continued*
postlaminectomy 737.21
postsurgical NEC 737.22
rachitic 268.1 *[737.42]*
specified NEC 737.29
tuberculous (*see also* Tuberculosis) 015.0 *[737.42]*
Loss
appetite 783.0
hysterical 300.11
nonorganic origin 307.59
psychogenic 307.59
blood—*see* Hemorrhage
central vision 368.41
consciousness 780.09
transient 780.2
control, sphincter, rectum 787.6
nonorganic origin 307.7
ear ossicle, partial 385.24
elasticity, skin 782.8
extremity or member, traumatic, current—*see* Amputation, traumatic
fluid (acute) 276.5
with
hypernatremia 276.0
hyponatremia 276.1
fetus or newborn 775.5
hair 704.00
hearing—*see also* Deafness
central 389.14
conductive (air) 389.00
with sensorineural hearing loss 389.2
combined types 389.08
external ear 389.01
inner ear 389.04
middle ear 389.03
multiple types 389.08
tympanic membrane 389.02
mixed type 389.2
nerve 389.12
neural 389.12
noise-induced 388.12
perceptive NEC (*see also* Loss, hearing, sensorineural) 389.10
sensorineural 389.10
with conductive hearing loss 389.2
central 389.14
combined types 389.18
multiple types 389.18
neural 389.12
sensory 389.11
sensory 389.11
specified type NEC 389.8
sudden NEC 388.2
labyrinthine reactivity (unilateral) 386.55
bilateral 386.56
memory (*see also* Amnesia) 780.9
mild, following organic brain damage 310.1
mind (*see also* Psychosis) 298.9
organ or part—*see* Absence, by site, acquired
sensation 782.0
sense of
smell (*see also* Disturbance, sensation) 781.1
taste (*see also* Disturbance, sensation) 781.1
touch (*see also* Disturbance, sensation) 781.1
sight (acquired) (complete) (congenital)—*see* Blindness
spinal fluid
headache 349.0
substance of
bone (*see also* Osteoporosis) 733.00
Loss —*continued*
cartilage 733.99
ear 380.32
vitreous (humor) 379.26
tooth, teeth, due to accident, extraction, or local periodontal disease 525.1
vision, visual (*see also* Blindness) 369.9
both eyes (*see also* Blindness, both eyes) 369.3
complete (*see also* Blindness, both eyes) 369.00
one eye 369.8
sudden 368.11
transient 368.12
vitreous 379.26
voice (*see also* Aphonia) 784.41
weight (cause unknown) 783.2
Louis-Bar syndrome (ataxia-telangiectasia) 334.8
Louping ill 063.1
Lousiness —*see* Lice
Low
back syndrome 724.2
basal metabolic rate (BMR) 794.7
birthweight 765.1
extreme (less than 1000 grams) 765.0
for gestational age 764.0
bladder compliance 596.52
blood pressure (*see also* Hypotension) 458.9
reading (incidental) (isolated) (nonspecific) 796.3
cardiac reserve—*see* Disease, heart
compliance bladder 596.52
frequency deafness—*see* Disorder, hearing
function—*see also* Hypofunction
kidney (*see also* Disease, renal) 593.9
liver 573.9
hemoglobin 285.9
implantation, placenta—*see* Placenta, previa
insertion, placenta—*see* Placenta, previa
lying
kidney 593.0
organ or site, congenital—*see* Malposition, congenital
placenta—*see* Placenta, previa
output syndrome (cardiac) (*see also* Failure, heart) 428.9
platelets (blood) (*see also* Thrombocytopenia) 287.5
reserve, kidney (*see also* Disease, renal) 593.9
salt syndrome 593.9
tension glaucoma 365.12
vision 369.9
both eyes 369.20
one eye 369.70
Lowe (-Terrey-MacLachlan) syndrome (oculocerebrorenal dystrophy) 270.8
Lower extremity —*see* condition
Lown (-Ganong)-Levine syndrome (short P-R interval, normal QRS complex, and paroxysmal supraventricular tachycardia) 426.81
LSD reaction (*see also* Abuse, drugs, nondependent) 305.3
L-shaped kidney 753.3
Lucas-Championnière disease (fibrinous bronchitis) 466.0
Lucey-Driscoll syndrome (jaundice due to delayed conjugation) 774.30
Ludwig's
angina 528.3
disease (submaxillary cellulitis) 528.3
Lues (venerea), luetic—*see* Syphilis

Luetscher's syndrome (dehydration) 276.5
Lumbago 724.2
  due to displacement, intervertebral disc 722.10
Lumbalgia 724.2
  due to displacement, intervertebral disc 722.10
Lumbar —*see* condition
Lumbarization, vertebra 756.15
Lumbermen's itch 133.8
Lump —*see also* Mass
  abdominal 789.3
  breast 611.72
  chest 786.6
  epigastric 789.3
  head 784.2
  kidney 753.3
  liver 789.1
  lung 786.6
  mediastinal 786.6
  neck 784.2
  nose or sinus 784.2
  pelvic 789.3
  skin 782.2
  substernal 786.6
  throat 784.2
  umbilicus 789.3
Lunacy (*see also* Psychosis) 298.9
Lunatomalacia 732.3
Lung —*see also* condition
  donor V59.8
  drug addict's 417.8
  mainliners' 417.8
  vanishing 492.0
Lupoid (miliary) of Boeck 135
Lupus 710.0
  Cazenave's (erythematosus) 695.4
  discoid (local) 695.4
  disseminated 710.0
  erythematodes (discoid) (local) 695.4
  erythematosus (discoid) (local) 695.4
    disseminated 710.0
    eyelid 373.34
    systemic 710.0
      with lung involvement 710.0 *[517.8]*
      inhibitor (presence of) 286.5
  exedens 017.0
  eyelid (*see also* Tuberculosis) 017.0 *[373.4]*
  Hilliard's 017.0
  hydralazine
    correct substance properly administered 695.4
    overdose or wrong substance given or taken 972.6
  miliaris disseminatus faciei 017.0
  nephritis 710.0 *[583.81]*
    acute 710.0 *[580.81]*
    chronic 710.0 *[582.81]*
  nontuberculous, not disseminated 695.4
  pernio (Besnier) 135
  tuberculous (*see also* Tuberculosis) 017.0
    eyelid (*see also* Tuberculosis) 017.0 *[373.4]*
  vulgaris 017.0
Luschka's joint disease 721.90
Luteinoma (M8610/0) 220
Lutembacher's disease or syndrome (atrial septal defect with mitral stenosis) 745.5
Luteoma (M8610/0) 220
Lutz-Miescher disease (elastosis perforans serpiginosa) 701.1
Lutz-Splendore-de Almeida disease (Brazilian blastomycosis) 116.1
Luxatio
  bulbi due to birth injury 767.8
Luxatio—*continued*
  coxae congenita (*see also* Dislocation, hip, congenital) 754.30
  erecta—*see* Dislocation, shoulder
  imperfecta—*see* Sprain, by site
  perinealis—*see* Dislocation, hip
Luxation —*see also* Dislocation, by site
  eyeball 360.81
    due to birth injury 767.8
    lateral 376.36
  genital organs (external) NEC—*see* Wound, open, genital organs
  globe (eye) 360.81
    lateral 376.36
  lacrimal gland (postinfectional) 375.16
  lens (old) (partial) 379.32
    congenital 743.37
      syphilitic 090.49 *[379.32]*
    Marfan's disease 090.49
    spontaneous 379.32
  penis—*see* Wound, open, penis
  scrotum—*see* Wound, open, scrotum
  testis—*see* Wound, open, testis
L-xyloketosuria 271.8
Lycanthropy (*see also* Psychosis) 298.9
Lyell's disease or syndrome (toxic epidermal necrolysis) 695.1
  due to drug
    correct substance properly administered 695.1
    overdose or wrong substance given or taken 977.9
      specified drug—*see* Table of drugs and chemicals
Lyme disease 088.81
Lymph
  gland or node—*see* condition
  scrotum (*see also* Infestation, filarial) 125.9
Lymphadenitis 289.3
  with
    abortion—*see* Abortion, by type, with sepsis
    ectopic pregnancy (*see also* categories 633.0-633.9) 639.0
    molar pregnancy (*see also* categories 630-632) 639.0
  acute 683
    mesenteric 289.2
  any site, except mesenteric 289.3
    acute 683
    chronic 289.1
    mesenteric (acute) (chronic) (nonspecific) (subacute) 289.2
    subacute 289.1
      mesenteric 289.2
  breast, puerperal, postpartum 675.2
  chancroidal (congenital) 099.0
  chronic 289.1
    mesenteric 289.2
  dermatopathic 695.89
  due to
    anthracosis (occupational) 500
    Brugia (Wuchereria) malayi 125.1
    diphtheria (toxin) 032.89
    lymphogranuloma venereum 099.1
    Wuchereria bancrofti 125.0
  following
    abortion 639.0
    ectopic or molar pregnancy 639.0
  generalized 289.3
  gonorrheal 098.89
  granulomatous 289.1
  infectional 683

Lymphadenitis—*continued*
mesenteric (acute) (chronic) (nonspecific) (subacute) 289.2
due to Bacillus typhi 002.0
tuberculous (*see also* Tuberculosis) 014.8
mycobacterial 031.8
purulent 683
pyogenic 683
regional 078.3
septic 683
streptococcal 683
subacute, unspecified site 289.1
suppurative 683
syphilitic (early) (secondary) 091.4
late 095.8
tuberculous—*see* Tuberculosis, lymph gland
venereal 099.1
Lymphadenoid goiter 245.2
Lymphadenopathy (general) 785.6
due to toxoplasmosis (acquired) 130.7
congenital (active) 771.2
Lymphadenopathy-associated virus (disease) (illness) (infection)—*see* Human Immunodeficiency virus (disease) (illness) (infection)
Lymphadenosis 785.6
acute 075
Lymphangiectasis 457.1
conjunctiva 372.8
postinfectional 457.1
scrotum 457.1
Lymphangiectatic elephantiasis, nonfilarial 457.1
Lymphangioendothelioma (M9170/0) 228.1
malignant (M9170/3)—*see* Neoplasm, connective tissue, malignant
Lymphangioma (M9170/0) 228.1
capillary (M9171/0) 228.1
cavernous (M9172/0) 228.1
cystic (M9173/0) 228.1
malignant (M9170/3)—*see* Neoplasm, connective tissue, malignant
Lymphangiomyoma (M9174/0) 228.1
Lymphangiomyomatosis (M9174/1)—*see* Neoplasm, connective tissue, uncertain behavior
Lymphangiosarcoma (M9170/3)—*see* Neoplasm, connective tissue, malignant
Lymphangitis 457.2
with
abortion—*see* Abortion, by type, with sepsis
abscess—*see* Abscess, by site
cellulitis—*see* Abscess, by site
ectopic pregnancy (*see also* categories 633.0-633.9) 639.0
molar pregnancy (*see also* categories 630-632) 639.0
acute (with abscess or cellulitis) 682.9
specified site—*see* Abscess, by site
breast, puerperal, postpartum 675.2
chancroidal 099.0
chronic (any site) 457.2
due to
Brugia (Wuchereria) malayi 125.1
Wuchereria bancrofti 125.0
following
abortion 639.0
ectopic or molar pregnancy 639.0
gangrenous 457.2
penis
acute 607.2

Lymphangitis—*continued*
gonococcal (acute) 098.0
chronic or duration of 2 months or more 098.2
puerperal, postpartum, childbirth 670
strumous, tuberculous (*see also* Tuberculosis) 017.2
subacute (any site) 457.2
tuberculous—*see* Tuberculosis, lymph gland
Lymphatic (vessel)—*see* condition
Lymphatism 254.8
scrofulous (*see also* Tuberculosis) 017.2
Lymphectasia 457.1
Lymphedema (*see also* Elephantiasis) 457.1
acquired (chronic) 457.1
chronic hereditary 757.0
congenital 757.0
idiopathic hereditary 757.0
praecox 457.1
secondary 457.1
surgical NEC 997.99
postmastectomy (syndrome) 457.0
Lymph-hemangioma (M9120/0)—*see* Hemangioma, by site
Lymphoblastic —*see* condition
Lymphoblastoma (diffuse) (M9630/3) 200.1
giant follicular (M9690/3) 202.0
macrofollicular (M9690/3) 202.0
Lymphoblastosis, acute benign 075
Lymphocele 457.8
Lymphocythemia 288.8
Lymphocytic —*see also* condition
chorioencephalitis (acute) (serous) 049.0
choriomeningitis (acute) (serous) 049.0
Lymphocytoma (diffuse) (malignant) (M9620/3) 200.1
Lymphocytomatosis (M9620/3) 200.1
Lymphocytopenia 288.8
Lymphocytosis (symptomatic) 288.8
infectious (acute) 078.89
Lymphoepithelioma (M8082/3)—*see* Neoplasm, by site, malignant
Lymphogranuloma (malignant) (M9650/3) 201.9
inguinale 099.1
venereal (any site) 099.1
with stricture of rectum 099.1
venereum 099.1
Lymphogranulomatosis (malignant) (M9650/3) 201.9
benign (Boeck's sarcoid) (Schaumann's) 135
Hodgkin's (M9650/3) 201.9
Lymphoid —*see* condition
Lympholeukoblastoma (M9850/3) 207.8
Lympholeukosarcoma (M9850/3) 207.8
Lymphoma (malignant) (M9590/3) 202.8

Note—Use the following fifth-digit subclassification with categories 200-202:

0 unspecified site
1 lymph nodes of head, face and neck
2 intrathoracic lymph nodes
3 intra-abdominal lymph nodes
4 lymph nodes of axilla and upper limb
5 lymph nodes of inguinal region and lower limb
6 intrapelvic lymph nodes
7 spleen
8 lymph nodes of multiple sites

benign (M9590/0)—*see* Neoplasm, by site, benign

M

Macacus ear 744.29
Maceration
  fetus (cause not stated) 779.9
  wet feet, tropical (syndrome) 991.4
Machupo virus hemorrhagic fever 078.7
Macleod's syndrome (abnormal transradiancy, one lung) 492.8
Macrocephalia, macrocephaly 756.0
Macrocheilia (congenital) 744.81
Macrochilia (congenital) 744.81
Macrocolon (congenital) 751.3
Macrocornea 743.41
  associated with buphthalmos 743.22
Macrocytic —*see* condition
Macrocytosis 289.8
Macrodactylia, macrodactylism (fingers) (thumbs) 755.57
  toes 755.65
Macrodontia 520.2
Macroencephaly 742.4
Macrogenia 524.05
Macrogenitosomia (female) (male) (praecox) 255.2
Macrogingivae 523.8
Macroglobulinemia (essential) (idiopathic) (monoclonal) (primary) (syndrome) (Waldenström's) 273.3
Macroglossia (congenital) 750.15
  acquired 529.8
Macrognathia, macrognathism (congenital) 524.00
  mandibular 524.02
    alveolar 524.72
  maxillary 524.01
    alveolar 524.71
Macrogyria (congenital) 742.4
Macrohydrocephalus (*see also* Hydrocephalus) 331.4
Macromastia (*see also* Hypertrophy, breast) 611.1
Macropsia 368.14
Macrosigmoid 564.7
  congenital 751.3
Macrospondylitis, acromegalic 253.0
Macrostomia (congenital) 744.83
Macrotia (external ear) (congenital) 744.22
Macula
  cornea, corneal
    congenital 743.43
      interfering with vision 743.42
    interfering with central vision 371.03
    not interfering with central vision 371.02
  degeneration (*see also* Degeneration, macula) 362.50
    hereditary (*see also* Dystrophy, retina) 362.70
  edema, cystoid 362.53
Maculae ceruleae 132.1
Macules and papules 709.8
Maculopathy, toxic 362.55
Madarosis 374.55
Madelung's
  deformity (radius) 755.54
  disease (lipomatosis) 272.8
  lipomatosis 272.8
Madness (*see also* Psychosis) 298.9
  myxedema (acute) 293.0
    subacute 293.1
Madura
  disease (actinomycotic) 039.9
    mycotic 117.4
  foot (actinomycotic) 039.4
    mycotic 117.4
Maduromycosis (actinomycotic) 039.9
  mycotic 117.4
Maffucci's syndrome (dyschondroplasia with hemangiomas) 756.4
Magenblase syndrome 306.4
Main en griffe (acquired) 736.06
  congenital 755.59
Maintenance
  chemotherapy regimen or treatment V58.1
  dialysis regimen or treatment
    extracorporeal (renal) V56.0
    peritoneal V56.8
    renal V56.0
  drug therapy or regimen V58.1
  external fixation NEC V54.8
  radiotherapy V58.0
  traction NEC V54.8
Majocchi's
  disease (purpura annularis telangiectodes) 709.1
  granuloma 110.6
Major —*see* condition
Mal
  cerebral (idiopathic) (*see also* Epilepsy) 345.9
  comital (*see also* Epilepsy) 345.9
  de los pintos (*see also* Pinta) 103.9
  de Meleda 757.39
  de mer 994.6
  lie—*see* Presentation, fetal
  perforant (*see also* Ulcer, lower extremity) 707.1
Malabar itch 110.9
  beard 110.0
  foot 110.4
  scalp 110.0
Malabsorption 579.9
  calcium 579.8
  carbohydrate 579.8
  disaccharide 271.3
  drug-induced 579.8
  due to bacterial overgrowth 579.8
  fat 579.8
  folate, congenital 281.2
  galactose 271.1
  glucose-galactose (congenital) 271.3
  intestinal 579.9
  isomaltose 271.3
  lactose (hereditary) 271.3
  methionine 270.4
  monosaccharide 271.8
  postgastrectomy 579.3
  postsurgical 579.3
  protein 579.8
  sucrose (-isomaltose) (congenital) 271.3
  syndrome 579.9
    postgastrectomy 579.3
    postsurgical 579.3
Malacia, bone 268.2
  juvenile (*see also* Rickets) 268.0
  Kienböck's (juvenile) (lunate) (wrist) 732.3
    adult 732.8

Malacoplakia
bladder 596.8
colon 569.89
pelvis (kidney) 593.89
ureter 593.89
urethra 599.84
Malacosteon 268.2
juvenile (*see also* Rickets) 268.0
Maladaptation —*see* Maladjustment
Maladie de Roger 745.4
Maladjustment
conjugal V61.1
involving divorce or estrangement V61.0
educational V62.3
family V61.9
specified circumstance NEC V61.8
marital V61.1
involving divorce or estrangement V61.0
occupational V62.2
simple, adult (*see also* Reaction, adjustment) 309.9
situational acute (*see also* Reaction, adjustment) 309.9
social V62.4
Malaise 780.7
Malakoplakia —*see* Malacoplakia
Malaria, malarial (fever) 084.6
algid 084.9
any type, with
algid malaria 084.9
blackwater fever 084.8
fever
blackwater 084.8
hemoglobinuric (bilious) 084.8
hemoglobinuria, malarial 084.8
hepatitis 084.9 *[573.2]*
nephrosis 084.9 *[581.81]*
pernicious complication NEC 084.9
cardiac 084.9
cerebral 084.9
cardiac 084.9
carrier (suspected) of V02.9
cerebral 084.9
complicating pregnancy, childbirth, or puerperium 647.4
congenital 771.2
congestion, congestive 084.6
brain 084.9
continued 084.0
estivo-autumnal 084.0
falciparum (malignant tertian) 084.0
hematinuria 084.8
hematuria 084.8
hemoglobinuria 084.8
hemorrhagic 084.6
induced (therapeutically) 084.7
accidental—*see* Malaria, by type
liver 084.9 *[573.2]*
malariae (quartan) 084.2
malignant (tertian) 084.0
mixed infections 084.5
monkey 084.4
ovale 084.3
pernicious, acute 084.0
Plasmodium, P.
falciparum 084.0
malariae 084.2
ovale 084.3
vivax 084.1
Malaria, malarial—*continued*
quartan 084.2
quotidian 084.0
recurrent 084.6
induced (therapeutically) 084.7
accidental—*see* Malaria, by type
remittent 084.6
specified types NEC 084.4
spleen 084.6
subtertian 084.0
tertian (benign) 084.1
malignant 084.0
tropical 084.0
typhoid 084.6
vivax (benign tertian) 084.1
Malassez's disease (testicular cyst) 608.89
Malassimilation 579.9
Maldescent, testis 752.5
Maldevelopment —*see also* Anomaly, by site
brain 742.9
colon 751.5
hip (joint) 755.63
congenital dislocation (*see also* Dislocation, hip, congenital) 754.30
mastoid process 756.0
middle ear, except ossicles 744.03
ossicles 744.04
newborn (not malformation) 764.9
ossicles, ear 744.04
spine 756.10
toe 755.66
Male type pelvis 755.69
with disproportion (fetopelvic) 653.2
affecting fetus or newborn 763.1
causing obstructed labor 660.1
affecting fetus or newborn 763.1
Malformation (congenital)—*see also* Anomaly
bone 756.9
bursa 756.9
Chiari
type I 348.4
type II (*see also* Spina bifida) 741.0
type III 742.0
type IV 742.2
circulatory system NEC 747.9
specified type NEC 747.89
cochlea 744.05
digestive system NEC 751.9
lower 751.5
specified type NEC 751.8
upper 750.9
eye 743.9
gum 750.9
heart NEC 746.9
specified type NEC 746.89
valve 746.9
internal ear 744.05
joint NEC 755.9
specified type NEC 755.8
Mondini's (congenital) (malformation, cochlea) 744.05
muscle 756.9
nervous system (central) 742.9
pelvic organs or tissues
in pregnancy or childbirth 654.9
affecting fetus or newborn 763.8
causing obstructed labor 660.2
affecting fetus or newborn 763.1
placenta (*see also* Placenta, abnormal) 656.7

Malformation—*continued*
respiratory organs 748.9
specified type NEC 748.8
Rieger's 743.44
sense organs NEC 742.9
specified type NEC 742.8
skin 757.9
specified type NEC 757.8
spinal cord 742.9
teeth, tooth NEC 520.9
tendon 756.9
throat 750.9
umbilical cord (complicating delivery) 663.9
affecting fetus or newborn 762.6
umbilicus 759.9
urinary system NEC 753.9
specified type NEC 753.8
Malfunction —*see also* Dysfunction
arterial graft 996.1
cardiac pacemaker 996.01
catheter device—*see* Complications, mechanical, catheter
colostomy 569.69
cystostomy 997.5
device, implant, or graft NEC—*see* Complications, mechanical
enteric stoma 569.69
enterostomy 569.69
gastroenteric 536.8
nephrostomy 997.5
pacemaker—*see* Complications, mechanical, pacemaker
prosthetic device, internal—*see* Complications, mechanical
tracheostomy 519.0
vascular graft or shunt 996.1
Malgaigne's fracture (closed) 808.43
open 808.53
Malherbe's
calcifying epithelioma (M8110/0)—*see* Neoplasm, skin, benign
tumor (M8110/0)—*see* Neoplasm, skin, benign
Malibu disease 919.8
infected 919.9
Malignancy (M8000/3)—*see* Neoplasm, by site, malignant
Malignant —*see* condition
Malingerer, malingering V65.2
Mallet, finger (acquired) 736.1
congenital 755.59
late effect of rickets 268.1
Malleus 024
Mallory's bodies 034.1
Mallory-Weiss syndrome 530.7
Malnutrition (calorie) 263.9
complicating pregnancy 648.9
degree
first 263.1
second 263.0
third 262
mild 263.1
moderate 263.0
severe 261
protein-calorie 262
fetus 764.2
"light-for-dates" 764.1
following gastrointestinal surgery 579.3
intrauterine or fetal 764.2
fetus or infant "light-for-dates" 764.1
Malnutrition—*continued*
lack of care, or neglect (child) (infant) 995.5
affecting parent or family V61.21
specified person NEC 995.81
malignant 260
mild 263.1
moderate 263.0
protein 260
protein-calorie 263.9
severe 262
specified type NEC 263.8
severe 261
protein-calorie NEC 262
Malocclusion (teeth) 524.4
due to
abnormal swallowing 524.5
accessory teeth (causing crowding) 524.3
dentofacial abnormality NEC 524.8
impacted teeth (causing crowding) 524.3
missing teeth 524.3
mouth breathing 524.5
supernumerary teeth (causing crowding) 524.3
thumb sucking 524.5
tongue, lip, or finger habits 524.5
temporomandibular (joint) 524.69
Malposition
cardiac apex (congenital) 746.87
cervix—*see* Malposition, uterus
congenital
adrenal (gland) 759.1
alimentary tract 751.8
lower 751.5
upper 750.8
aorta 747.21
appendix 751.5
arterial trunk 747.29
artery (peripheral) NEC (*see also* Malposition, congenital, peripheral vascular system) 747.60
coronary 746.85
pulmonary 747.3
auditory canal 744.29
causing impairment of hearing 744.02
auricle (ear) 744.29
causing impairment of hearing 744.02
cervical 744.43
biliary duct or passage 751.69
bladder (mucosa) 753.8
exteriorized or extroverted 753.5
brachial plexus 742.8
brain tissue 742.4
breast 757.6
bronchus 748.3
cardiac apex 746.87
cecum 751.5
clavicle 755.51
colon 751.5
digestive organ or tract NEC 751.8
lower 751.5
upper 750.8
ear (auricle) (external) 744.29
ossicles 744.04
endocrine (gland) NEC 759.2
epiglottis 748.3
Eustachian tube 744.24
eye 743.8
facial features 744.89
fallopian tube 752.19
finger(s) 755.59
supernumerary 755.01

Malposition—*continued*
foot 755.67
gallbladder 751.69
gastrointestinal tract 751.8
genitalia, genital organ(s) or tract
female 752.8
external 752.49
internal NEC 752.8
male 752.8
glottis 748.3
hand 755.59
heart 746.87
dextrocardia 746.87
with complete transposition of viscera 759.3
hepatic duct 751.69
hip (joint) (*see also* Dislocation, hip, congenital) 754.30
intestine (large) (small) 751.5
with anomalous adhesions, fixation, or malrotation 751.4
joint NEC 755.8
kidney 753.3
larynx 748.3
limb 755.8
lower 755.69
upper 755.59
liver 751.69
lung (lobe) 748.69
nail(s) 757.5
nerve 742.8
nervous system NEC 742.8
nose, nasal (septum) 748.1
organ or site NEC—*see* Anomaly, specified type NEC, by site
ovary 752.0
pancreas 751.7
parathyroid (gland) 759.2
patella 755.64
peripheral vascular system 747.60
gastrointestinal 747.61
lower limb 747.64
renal 747.62
specified NEC 747.69
spinal 747.82
upper limb 747.63
pituitary (gland) 759.2
respiratory organ or system NEC 748.9
rib (cage) 756.3
supernumerary in cervical region 756.2
scapula 755.59
shoulder 755.59
spinal cord 742.59
spine 756.19
spleen 759.0
sternum 756.3
stomach 750.7
symphysis pubis 755.69
testis (undescended) 752.5
thymus (gland) 759.2
thyroid (gland) (tissue) 759.2
cartilage 748.3
toe(s) 755.66
supernumerary 755.02
tongue 750.19
trachea 748.3
uterus 752.3

Malposition—*continued*
vein(s) (peripheral) NEC (*see also* Malposition, congenital, peripheral vascular system) 747.60
great 747.49
portal 747.49
pulmonary 747.49
vena cava (inferior) (superior) 747.49
device, implant, or graft—*see* Complications, mechanical
fetus NEC (*see also* Presentation, fetal) 652.9
with successful version 652.1
affecting fetus or newborn 763.1
before labor, affecting fetus or newborn 761.7
causing obstructed labor 660.0
in multiple gestation (one fetus or more) 652.6
with locking 660.5
causing obstructed labor 660.0
gallbladder (*see also* Disease, gallbladder) 575.8
gastrointestinal tract 569.89
congenital 751.8
heart (*see also* Malposition, congenital, heart) 746.87
intestine 569.89
congenital 751.5
pelvic organs or tissues
in pregnancy or childbirth 654.4
affecting fetus or newborn 763.8
causing obstructed labor 660.2
affecting fetus or newborn 763.1
placenta—*see* Placenta, previa
stomach 537.89
congenital 750.7
tooth, teeth (with impaction) 524.3
uterus or cervix (acquired) (acute) (adherent) (any degree) (asymptomatic) (postinfectional) (postpartal, old) 621.6
anteflexion or anteversion (*see also* Anteversion, uterus) 621.6
congenital 752.3
flexion 621.6
lateral (*see also* Lateroversion, uterus) 621.6
in pregnancy or childbirth 654.4
affecting fetus or newborn 763.8
causing obstructed labor 660.2
affecting fetus or newborn 763.1
inversion 621.6
lateral (flexion) (version) (*see also* Lateroversion, uterus) 621.6
lateroflexion (*see also* Lateroversion, uterus) 621.6
lateroversion (*see also* Lateroversion, uterus) 621.6
retroflexion or retroversion (*see also* Retroversion, uterus) 621.6
Malposture 729.9
Malpresentation, fetus (*see also* Presentation, fetal) 652.9
Malrotation
cecum 751.4
colon 751.4
intestine 751.4
kidney 753.3
Malta fever (*see also* Brucellosis) 023.9
Maltosuria 271.3
Maltreatment (of)
adult (emotional) 995.81
child (emotional) (nutritional) 995.5
affecting parent or family V61.21
specified person NEC 995.81
spouse (emotional) 995.81
Malt workers' lung 495.4

Malum coxae senilis 715.25
Malunion, fracture 733.81
Mammillitis (*see also* Mastitis) 611.0
puerperal, postpartum 675.2
Mammitis (*see also* Mastitis) 611.0
puerperal, postpartum 675.2
Mammoplasia 611.1
Management
contraceptive V25.9
specified type NEC V25.8
procreative V26.9
specified type NEC V26.8
Mangled NEC (*see also* nature and site of injury) 959.9
Mania (monopolar) (*see also* Psychosis, affective) 296.0
alcoholic (acute) (chronic) 291.9
Bell's—*see* Mania, chronic
chronic 296.0
recurrent episode 296.1
single episode 296.0
compulsive 300.3
delirious (acute) 296.0
recurrent episode 296.1
single episode 296.0
epileptic (*see also* Epilepsy) 345.4
hysterical 300.10
inhibited 296.89
puerperal (after delivery) 296.0
recurrent episode 296.1
single episode 296.0
recurrent episode 296.1
senile 290.8
single episode 296.0
stupor 296.89
stuporous 296.89
unproductive 296.89
Manic-depressive insanity, psychosis reaction, or syndrome (*see also* Psychosis, affective) 296.80
circular (alternating) 296.7
currently
depressed 296.5
episode unspecified 296.7
hypomanic, previously depressed 296.4
manic 296.4
mixed 296.6
depressed (type), depressive 296.2
atypical 296.82
recurrent episode 296.3
single episode 296.2
hypomanic 296.0
recurrent episode 296.1
single episode 296.0
manic 296.0
atypical 296.81
recurrent episode 296.1
single episode 296.0
mixed NEC 296.89
perplexed 296.89
stuporous 296.89
Manifestations, rheumatoid
lungs 714.81
pannus—*see* Arthritis, rheumatoid
subcutaneous nodules—*see* Arthritis, rheumatoid
Mankowsky's syndrome (familial dysplastic osteopathy) 731.2
Mannoheptulosuria 271.8
Mannosidosis 271.8
Manson's
disease (schistosomiasis) 120.1
pyosis (pemphigus contagiosus) 684
schistosomiasis 120.1
Mansonellosis 125.5
Manual —*see* condition
Maple bark disease 495.6
Maple bark-strippers' lung 495.6
Maple syrup (urine) disease or syndrome 270.3
Marable's syndrome (celiac artery compression) 447.4
Marasmus 261
brain 331.9
due to malnutrition 261
intestinal 569.89
nutritional 261
senile 797
tuberculous NEC (*see also* Tuberculosis) 011.9
Marble
bones 756.52
skin 782.61
Marburg disease (virus) 078.89
March
foot (closed) 825.20
open 825.30
hemoglobinuria 283.2
Marchand multiple nodular hyperplasia (liver) 571.5
Marchesani (-Weill) syndrome (brachymorphism and ectopia lentis) 759.89
Marchiafava (-Bignami) disease or syndrome 341.8
Marchiafava-Micheli syndrome (paroxysmal nocturnal hemoglobinuria) 283.2
Marcus Gunn's syndrome (jaw-winking syndrome) 742.8
Marfan's
congenital syphilis 090.49
disease 090.49
syndrome (arachnodactyly) 759.82
meaning congenital syphilis 090.49
with luxation of lens 090.49 *[379.32]*
Marginal
implantation, placenta—*see* Placenta, previa
placenta—*see* Placenta, previa
sinus (hemorrhage) (rupture) 641.2
affecting fetus or newborn 762.1
Marie's
cerebellar ataxia 334.2
syndrome (acromegaly) 253.0
Marie-Bamberger disease or syndrome (hypertrophic) (pulmonary) (secondary) 731.2
idiopathic (acropachyderma) 757.39
primary (acropachyderma) 757.39
Marie-Charcot-Tooth neuropathic atrophy, muscle 356.1
Marie-Strümpell arthritis or disease (ankylosing spondylitis) 720.0
Marihuana, marijuana
abuse (*see also* Abuse, drugs, nondependent) 305.2
dependence (*see also* Dependence) 304.3
Marion's disease (bladder neck obstruction) 596.0
Marital conflict V61.1
Mark
port wine 757.32
raspberry 757.32
strawberry 757.32
stretch 701.3
tattoo 709.09

Maroteaux-Lamy syndrome (mucopolysaccharidosis VI) 277.5
Marriage license examination V70.3
Marrow (bone)
arrest 284.9
megakaryocytic 287.3
poor function 289.9
Marseilles fever 082.1
Marsh's disease (exophthalmic goiter) 242.0
Marshall's (hidrotic) ectodermal dysplasia 757.31
Marsh fever (*see also* Malaria) 084.6
Martin's disease 715.27
Martin-Albright syndrome (pseudohypoparathyroidism) 275.4
Martorell-Fabre syndrome (pulseless disease) 446.7
Masculinization, female with adrenal hyperplasia 255.2
Masculinovoblastoma (M8670/0) 220
Masochism 302.83
Masons' lung 502
Mass
abdominal 789.3
anus 787.99
bone 733.90
breast 611.72
check 784.2
chest 786.6
cystic—*see* Cyst
ear 388.8
epigastric 789.3
eye 379.92
female genital organ 625.8
gum 784.2
head 784.2
intracranial 784.2
joint 719.60
ankle 719.67
elbow 719.62
foot 719.67
hand 719.64
hip 719.65
knee 719.66
multiple sites 719.69
pelvic region 719.65
shoulder (region) 719.61
specified site NEC 719.68
wrist 719.63
kidney (*see also* Disease, kidney) 593.9
lung 786.6
lymph node 785.6
malignant (M8000/3)—*see* Neoplasm, by site, malignant
mediastinal 786.6
mouth 784.2
muscle (limb) 729.89
neck 784.2
nose or sinus 784.2
palate 784.2
pelvis, pelvic 789.3
penis 607.89
perineum 625.8
rectum 787.99
scrotum 608.89
skin 782.2
specified organ NEC—*see* Disease of specified organ or site
splenic 789.2
substernal 786.6
thyroid (*see also* Goiter) 240.9
Mass—*continued*
superficial (localized) 782.2
testes 608.89
throat 784.2
tongue 784.2
umbilicus 789.3
uterus 625.8
vagina 625.8
vulva 625.8
Massive —*see* condition
Mastalgia 611.71
psychogenic 307.89
Mast cell
disease 757.33
systemic (M9741/3) 202.6
leukemia (M9900/3) 207.8
sarcoma (M9742/3) 202.6
tumor (M9740/1) 238.5
malignant (M9740/3) 202.6
Masters-Allen syndrome 620.6
Mastitis (acute) (adolescent) (diffuse) (interstitial) (lobular) (nonpuerperal) (nonsuppurative) (parenchymatous) (phlegmonous) (simple) (subacute) (suppurative) 611.0
chronic (cystic) (fibrocystic) 610.1
cystic 610.1
Schimmelbusch's type 610.1
fibrocystic 610.1
infective 611.0
lactational 675.2
lymphangitis 611.0
neonatal (noninfective) 778.7
infective 771.5
periductal 610.4
plasma cell 610.4
puerperal, postpartum, (interstitial) (nonpurulent) (parenchymatous) 675.2
purulent 675.1
stagnation 676.2
puerperalis 675.2
retromammary 611.0
puerperal, postpartum 675.1
submammary 611.0
puerperal, postpartum 675.1
Mastocytoma (M9740/1) 238.5
malignant (M9740/3) 202.6
Mastocytosis 757.33
malignant (M9741/3) 202.6
systemic (M9741/3) 202.6
Mastodynia 611.71
psychogenic 307.89
Mastoid —*see* condition
Mastoidalgia (*see also* Otalgia) 388.70
Mastoiditis (coalescent) (hemorrhagic) (pneumococcal) (streptococcal) (suppurative) 383.9
acute or subacute 383.00
with
Gradenigo's syndrome 383.02
petrositis 383.02
specified complication NEC 383.02
subperiosteal abscess 383.01
chronic (necrotic) (recurrent) 383.1
tuberculous (*see also* Tuberculosis) 015.6
Mastopathy, mastopathia 611.9
chronica cystica 610.1
diffuse cystic 610.1
estrogenic 611.8
ovarian origin 611.8
Mastoplasia 611.1
Masturbation 307.9

Maternal condition, affecting fetus or newborn
acute yellow atrophy of liver 760.8
albuminuria 760.1
anesthesia or analgesia 763.5
blood loss 762.1
chorioamnionitis 762.7
circulatory disease, chronic (conditions classifiable to 390-459, 745-747) 760.3
congenital heart disease (conditions classifiable to 745-746) 760.3
cortical necrosis of kidney 760.1
death 761.6
diabetes mellitus 775.0
manifest diabetes in the infant 775.1
disease NEC 760.9
circulatory system, chronic (conditions classifiable to 390-459, 745-747) 760.3
genitourinary system (conditions classifiable to 580-599) 760.1
respiratory (conditions classifiable to 490-519, 748) 760.3
eclampsia 760.0
hemorrhage NEC 762.1
hepatitis acute, malignant, or subacute 760.8
hyperemesis (gravidarum) 761.8
hypertension (arising during pregnancy) (conditions classifiable to 642) 760.0
infection
disease classifiable to 001-136 760.2
genital tract NEC 760.8
urinary tract 760.1
influenza 760.2
manifest influenza in the infant 771.2
injury (conditions classifiable to 800-996) 760.5
malaria 760.2
manifest malaria in infant or fetus 771.2
malnutrition 760.4
necrosis of liver 760.8
nephritis (conditions classifiable to 580-583) 760.1
nephrosis (conditions classifiable to 581) 760.1
noxious substance transmitted via breast milk or placenta 760.70
alcohol 760.71
anti-infective agents 760.74
cocaine 760.75
"crack" 760.75
diethylstilbestrol [DES] 760.76
hallucinogenic agents 760.73
medicinal agents NEC 760.79
narcotics 760.72
obstetric anesthetic or analgesic drug 760.72
specified agent NEC 760.79
nutritional disorder (conditions classifiable to 260-269) 760.4
operation unrelated to current delivery 760.6
pre-eclampsia 760.0
pyelitis or pyelonephritis, arising during pregnancy (conditions classifiable to 590) 760.1
renal disease or failure 760.1
respiratory disease, chronic (conditions classifiable to 490-519, 748) 760.3
rheumatic heart disease (chronic) (conditions classifiable to 393-398) 760.3
rubella (conditions classifiable to 056) 760.2
manifest rubella in the infant or fetus 771.0
surgery unrelated to current delivery 760.6
to uterus or pelvic organs 763.8

Maternal condition, affecting fetus. . .—*cont.*
syphilis (conditions classifiable to 090-097) 760.2
manifest syphilis in the infant or fetus 090.0
thrombophlebitis 760.3
toxemia (of pregnancy) 760.0
pre-eclamptic 760.0
toxoplasmosis (conditions classifiable to 130) 760.2
manifest toxoplasmosis in the infant or fetus 771.2
transmission of chemical substance through the placenta 760.70
alcohol 760.71
anti-infective 760.74
cocaine 760.75
"crack" 760.75
diethylstilbestrol [DES] 760.76
hallucinogenic agents 760.73
narcotics 760.72
specified substance NEC 760.79
uremia 760.1
urinary tract conditions (conditions classifiable to 580-599) 760.1
vomiting (pernicious) (persistent) (vicious) 761.8
Maternity —*see* Delivery
Matheiu's disease (leptospiral jaundice) 100.0
Mauclaire's disease or osteochondrosis 732.3
Maxcy's disease 081.0
Maxilla, maxillary —*see* condition
May (-Hegglin) anomaly or syndrome 288.2
Mayaro fever 066.3
Mazoplasia 610.8
MBD (minimal brain dysfunction), child (*see also* Hyperkinesia) 314.9
McArdle (-Schmid-Pearson) disease or syndrome (glycogenosis V) 271.0
McCune-Albright syndrome (osteitis fibrosa disseminata) 756.59
MCLS (mucocutaneous lymph node syndrome) 446.1
McQuarrie's syndrome (idiopathic familial hypoglycemia) 251.2
Measles (black) (hemorrhagic) (suppressed) 055.9
with
encephalitis 055.0
keratitis 055.71
keratoconjunctivitis 055.71
otitis media 055.2
pneumonia 055.1
complication 055.8
specified type NEC 055.79
encephalitis 055.0
French 056.9
German 056.9
keratitis 055.71
keratoconjunctivitis 055.71
liberty 056.9
otitis media 055.2
pneumonia 055.1
specified complications NEC 055.79
vaccination, prophylactic (against) V04.2
Meatitis, urethral (*see also* Urethritis) 597.89
Meat poisoning —*see* Poisoning, food
Meatus, meatal —*see* condition
Meat-wrappers' asthma 506.9
Meckel's
diverticulitis 751.0
diverticulum (displaced) (hypertrophic) 751.0

Meconium
aspiration 770.1
delayed passage in newborn 777.1
ileus 777.1
due to cystic fibrosis 277.01
in liquor 792.3
noted during delivery—*omit code*
insufflation 770.1
obstruction
fetus or newborn 777.1
in mucoviscidosis 277.01
passage of 792.3
noted during delivery—*omit code*
peritonitis 777.6
plug syndrome (newborn) NEC 777.1
Median —*see also* condition
arcuate ligament syndrome 447.4
bar (prostate) 600
vesical orifice 600
rhomboid glossitis 529.2
Mediastinal shift 793.2
Mediastinitis (acute) (chronic) 519.2
actinomycotic 039.8
syphilitic 095.8
tuberculous (*see also* Tuberculosis) 012.8
Mediastinopericarditis (*see also* Pericarditis) 423.9
acute 420.90
chronic 423.8
rheumatic 393
rheumatic, chronic 393
Mediastinum, mediastinal —*see* condition
Medical services provided for —*see* Health, services provided because (of)
Medicine poisoning (by overdose) (wrong substance given or taken in error) 977.9
specified drug or substance—*see* Table of drugs and chemicals
Medin's disease (poliomyelitis) 045.9
Mediterranean
anemia (with other hemoglobinopathy) 282.4
disease or syndrome (hemipathic) 282.4
fever (*see also* Brucellosis) 023.9
familial 277.3
kala-azar 085.0
leishmaniasis 085.0
tick fever 082.1
Medulla —*see* condition
Medullary
cystic kidney 753.16
sponge kidney 753.17
Medullated fibers
optic (nerve) 743.57
retina 362.85
Medulloblastoma (M9470/3)
desmoplastic (M9471/3) 191.6
specified site—*see* Neoplasm, by site, malignant
unspecified site 191.6
Medulloepithelioma (M9501/3)—*see also* Neoplasm, by site, malignant
teratoid (M9502/3)—*see* Neoplasm, by site, malignant
Medullomyoblastoma (M9472/3)
specified site—*see* Neoplasm, by site, malignant
unspecified site 191.6
Meekeren-Ehlers-Danlos syndrome 756.83
Megacaryocytic —*see* condition
Megacolon (acquired) (functional) (not Hirschsprung's disease) 564.7
aganglionic 751.3
Megacolon—*continued*
congenital, congenitum 751.3
Hirschsprung's (disease) 751.3
psychogenic 306.4
toxic (*see also* Colitis, ulcerative) 556.9
Megaduodenum 537.3
Megaesophagus (functional) 530.0
congenital 750.4
Megakaryocytic —*see* condition
Megalencephaly 742.4
Megalerythema (epidermicum) (infectiosum) 057.0
Megalia, cutis et ossium 757.39
Megaloappendix 751.5
Megalocephalus, megalocephaly NEC 756.0
Megalocornea 743.41
associated with buphthalmos 743.22
Megalocytic anemia 281.9
Megalodactylia (fingers) (thumbs) 755.57
toes 755.65
Megaloduodenum 751.5
Megaloesophagus (functional) 530.0
congenital 750.4
Megalogastria (congenital) 750.7
Megalomania 307.9
Megalophthalmos 743.8
Megalopsia 368.14
Megalosplenia (*see also* Splenomegaly) 789.2
Megaloureter 593.89
congenital 753.2
Megarectum 569.49
Megasigmoid 564.7
congenital 751.3
Megaureter 593.89
congenital 753.2
Megrim 346.9
Meibomian
cyst 373.2
infected 373.12
gland—*see* condition
infarct (eyelid) 374.85
stye 373.11
Meibomitis 373.12
Meige
-Milroy disease (chronic hereditary edema) 757.0
syndrome (blepharospasm-oromandibular dystonia) 333.82
Melalgia, nutritional 266.2
Melancholia (*see also* Psychosis, affective) 296.90
climacteric 296.2
recurrent episode 296.3
single episode 296.2
hypochondriac 300.7
intermittent 296.2
recurrent episode 296.3
single episode 296.2
involutional 296.2
recurrent episode 296.3
single episode 296.2
menopausal 296.2
recurrent episode 296.3
single episode 296.2
puerperal 296.2
reactive (from emotional stress, psychological trauma) 298.0
recurrent 296.3
senile 290.21
stuporous 296.2
recurrent episode 296.3
single episode 296.2

Melanemia 275.0
Melanoameloblastoma (M9363/0)—*see* Neoplasm, bone, benign
Melanoblastoma (M8720/3)—*see* Melanoma
Melanoblastosis
Block-Sulzberger 757.33
cutis linearis sive systematisata 757.33
Melanocarcinoma (M8720/3)—*see* Melanoma
Melanocytoma, eyeball (M8726/0) 224.0
Melanoderma, melanodermia 709.09
Addison's (primary adrenal insufficiency) 255.4
Melanodontia, infantile 521.0
Melanoepithelioma (M8720/3)—*see* Melanoma
Melanoma (malignant) (M8720/3) 172.9

Note—Except where otherwise indicated, the morphological varieties of melanoma in the list below should be coded by site as for "Melanoma (malignant)." Internal sites should be coded to malignant neoplasm of those sites.

abdominal wall 172.5
ala nasi 172.3
amelanotic (M8730/3)—*see* Melanoma, by site
ankle 172.7
anus, anal 154.3
canal 154.2
arm 172.6
auditory canal (external) 172.2
auricle (ear) 172.2
auricular canal (external) 172.2
axilla 172.5
axillary fold 172.5
back 172.5
balloon cell (M8722/3)—*see* Melanoma, by site
benign (M8720/0)—*see* Neoplasm, skin, benign
breast (female) (male) 172.5
brow 172.3
buttock 172.5
canthus (eye) 172.1
cheek (external) 172.3
chest wall 172.5
chin 172.3
choroid 190.6
conjunctiva 190.3
ear (external) 172.2
epithelioid cell (M8771/3)—*see also* Melanoma, by site
and spindle cell, mixed (M8775/3)—*see* Melanoma, by site
external meatus (ear) 172.2
eye 190.9
eyebrow 172.3
eyelid (lower) (upper) 172.1
face NEC 172.3
female genital organ (external) NEC 184.4
finger 172.6
flank 172.5
foot 172.7
forearm 172.6
forehead 172.3
foreskin 187.1
gluteal region 172.5
groin 172.5
hand 172.6
heel 172.7
helix 172.2
hip 172.7
in
giant pigmented nevus (M8761/3)—*see* Melanoma, by site
Melanoma—*continued*
Hutchinson's melanotic freckle (M8742/3)—*see* Melanoma, by site
junctional nevus (M8740/3)—*see* Melanoma, by site
precancerous melanosis (M8741/3)—*see* Melanoma, by site
interscapular region 172.5
iris 190.0
jaw 172.3
juvenile (M8770/0)—*see* Neoplasm, skin, benign
knee 172.7
labium
majus 184.1
minus 184.2
lacrimal gland 190.2
leg 172.7
lip (lower) (upper) 172.0
liver 197.7
lower limb NEC 172.7
male genital organ (external) NEC 187.9
meatus, acoustic (external) 172.2
meibomian gland 172.1
metastatic
of or from specified site—*see* Melanoma, by site
site not of skin—*see* Neoplasm, by site, malignant, secondary
to specified site—*see* Neoplasm, by site, malignant, secondary
unspecified site 172.9
nail 172.9
finger 172.6
toe 172.7
neck 172.4
nodular (M8721/3)—*see* Melanoma, by site
nose, external 172.3
orbit 190.1
penis 187.4
perianal skin 172.5
perineum 172.5
pinna 172.2
popliteal (fossa) (space) 172.7
prepuce 187.1
pubes 172.5
pudendum 184.4
retina 190.5
scalp 172.4
scrotum 187.7
septum nasal (skin) 172.3
shoulder 172.6
skin NEC 172.8
spindle cell (M8772/3)—*see also* Melanoma, by site
type A (M8773/3) 190.0
type B (M8774/3) 190.0
submammary fold 172.5
superficial spreading (M8743/3)—*see* Melanoma, by site
temple 172.3
thigh 172.7
toe 172.7
trunk NEC 172.5
umbilicus 172.5
upper limb NEC 172.6
vagina vault 184.0
vulva 184.4
Melanoplakia 528.9
Melanosarcoma (M8720/3)—*see also* Melanoma
epithelioid cell (M8771/3)—*see* Melanoma

Melanosis 709.09
addisonian (primary adrenal insufficiency) 255.4
tuberculous (*see also* Tuberculosis) 017.6
adrenal 255.4
colon 569.89
conjunctiva 372.55
congenital 743.49
corii degenerativa 757.33
cornea (presenile) (senile) 371.12
congenital 743.43
interfering with vision 743.42
prenatal 743.43
interfering with vision 743.42
eye 372.55
congenital 743.49
jute spinners' 709.09
lenticularis progressiva 757.33
liver 573.8
precancerous (M8741/2)—*see also* Neoplasm, skin, in situ
malignant melanoma in (M8741/3)—*see* Melanoma
Riehl's 709.09
sclera 379.19
congenital 743.47
suprarenal 255.4
tar 709.09
toxic 709.09
Melanuria 791.9
Melasma 709.09
adrenal (gland) 255.4
suprarenal (gland) 255.4
Melena 578.1
due to
swallowed maternal blood 777.3
ulcer—*see* Ulcer, by site, with hemorrhage
newborn 772.4
due to swallowed maternal blood 777.3
Meleney's
gangrene (cutaneous) 686.0
ulcer (chronic undermining) 686.0
Melioidosis 025
Melitensis, febris 023.0
Melitococcosis 023.0
Melkersson (-Rosenthal) syndrome 351.8
Mellitus, diabetes —*see* Diabetes
Melorheostosis (bone) (leri) 733.99
Meloschisis 744.83
Melotia 744.29
Membrana
capsularis lentis posterior 743.39
epipapillaris 743.57
Membranacea placenta —*see* Placenta, abnormal
Membranaceous uterus 621.8
Membrane, membranous —*see also* condition
folds, congenital—*see* Web
Jackson's 751.4
over face (causing asphyxia), fetus or newborn 768.9
premature rupture—*see* Rupture, membranes, premature
pupillary 364.74
persistent 743.46
retained (complicating delivery) (with hemorrhage) 666.2
without hemorrhage 667.1
secondary (eye) 366.50
unruptured (causing asphyxia) 768.9
vitreous humor 379.25
Membranitis, fetal 658.4
affecting fetus or newborn 762.7
Memory disturbance, loss or lack (*see also* Amnesia) 780.9
mild, following organic brain damage 310.1
Menadione (vitamin K) deficiency 269.0
Menarche, precocious 259.1
Mendacity, pathologic 301.7
Mende's syndrome (ptosis-epicanthus) 270.2
Mendelson's syndrome (resulting from a procedure) 997.3
obstetric 668.0
Ménétrier's disease or syndrome (hypertrophic gastritis) 535.2
Ménière's disease, syndrome, or vertigo 386.00
cochlear 386.02
cochleovestibular 386.01
inactive 386.04
in remission 386.04
vestibular 386.03
Meninges, meningeal —*see* condition
Meningioma (M9530/0)—*see also* Neoplasm, meninges, benign
angioblastic (M9535/0)—*see* Neoplasm, meninges, benign
angiomatous (M9534/0)—*see* Neoplasm, meninges, benign
endotheliomatous (M9531/0)—*see* Neoplasm, meninges, benign
fibroblastic (M9532/0)—*see* Neoplasm, meninges, benign
fibrous (M9532/0)—*see* Neoplasm, meninges, benign
hemangioblastic (M9535/0)—*see* Neoplasm, meninges, benign
hemangiopericytic (M9536/0)—*see* Neoplasm, meninges, benign
malignant (M9530/3)—*see* Neoplasm, meninges, malignant
meningiothelial (M9531/0)—*see* Neoplasm, meninges, benign
meningotheliomatous (M9531/0)—*see* Neoplasm, meninges, benign
mixed (M9537/0)—*see* Neoplasm, meninges, benign
multiple (M9530/1) 237.6
papillary (M9538/1) 237.6
psammomatous (M9533/0)—*see* Neoplasm, meninges, benign
syncytial (M9531/0)—*see* Neoplasm, meninges, benign
transitional (M9537/0)—*see* Neoplasm, meninges, benign
Meningiomatosis (diffuse) (M9530/1) 237.6
Meningism (*see also* Meningismus) 781.6
Meningismus (infectional) (pneumococcal) 781.6
due to serum or vaccine 997.09 *[321.8]*
influenzal NEC 487.8
Meningitis (basal) (basic) (basilar) (brain) (cerebral) (cervical) (congestive) (diffuse) (hemorrhagic) (infantile) (membranous) (metastatic) (nonspecific) (pontine) (progressive) (simple) (spinal) (subacute) (sympathetica) (toxic) 322.9
abacterial NEC (*see also* Meningitis, aseptic) 047.9
actinomycotic 039.8 *[320.7]*
adenoviral 049.1
Aerobacter aerogenes 320.82
anaerobes (cocci) (gram-negative) (gram-positive) (mixed) (NEC) 320.81
arbovirus NEC 066.9 *[321.2]*
specified type NEC 066.8 *[321.2]*

Meningitis—*continued*
syndrome 348.2
Serratia (marcescens) 320.82
specified organism NEC 320.89
sporadic cerebrospinal 036.0
sporotrichosis 117.1 *[321.1]*
staphylococcal 320.3
sterile 997.09
streptococcal (acute) 320.2
suppurative 320.9
specified organism NEC 320.89
syphilitic 094.2
acute 091.81
congenital 090.42
secondary 091.81
torula 117.5 *[321.0]*
traumatic (complication of injury) 958.8
Treponema (denticola) (macrodenticum) 320.81
trypanosomiasis 086.1 *[321.3]*
tuberculous (*see also* Tuberculosis, meninges) 013.0
typhoid 002.0 *[320.7]*
Veillonella 320.81
Vibrio vulnificus 320.82
viral, virus NEC (*see also* Meningitis, aseptic) 047.9
Wallgren's (*see also* Meningitis, aseptic) 047.9
Meningocele (congenital) (spinal) (*see also* Spina bifida) 741.9
acquired (traumatic) 349.2
cerebral 742.0
cranial 742.0
Meningocerebritis —*see* Meningoencephalitis
Meningococcemia (acute) (chronic) 036.2
Meningococcus, meningococcal (*see also* condition) 036.9
adrenalitis, hemorrhagic 036.3
carditis 036.40
carrier (suspected) of V02.5
cerebrospinal fever 036.0
encephalitis 036.1
endocarditis 036.42
infection NEC 036.9
meningitis (cerebrospinal) 036.0
myocarditis 036.43
optic neuritis 036.81
pericarditis 036.41
septicemia (chronic) 036.2
Meningoencephalitis (*see also* Encephalitis) 323.9
acute NEC 048
bacterial, purulent, pyogenic, or septic—*see* Meningitis
chronic NEC 094.1
diffuse NEC 094.1
diphasic 063.2
due to
actinomycosis 039.8 *[320.7]*
blastomycosis NEC (*see also* Blastomycosis) 116.0 *[323.4]*
free-living amebae 136.2
Listeria monocytogenes 027.0 *[320.7]*
Lyme disease 088.81 *[320.7]*
mumps 072.2
Naegleria (amebae) (gruberi) (organisms) 136.2
rubella 056.01
sporotrichosis 117.1 *[321.1]*
toxoplasmosis (acquired) 130.0
congenital (active) 771.2 *[323.4]*
Trypanosoma 086.1 *[323.2]*
Meningoencephalitis—*continued*
epidemic 036.0
herpes 054.3
herpetic 054.3
H. influenzae 320.0
infectious (acute) 048
influenzal 320.0
late effect—*see* category 326
Listeria monocytogenes 027.0 *[320.7]*
lymphocytic (serous) 049.0
mumps 072.2
parasitic NEC 123.9 *[323.4]*
pneumococcal 320.1
primary amebic 136.2
rubella 056.01
serous 048
lymphocytic 049.0
specific 094.2
staphylococcal 320.3
streptococcal 320.2
syphilitic 094.2
toxic NEC 989.9 *[323.7]*
due to
carbon tetrachloride 987.8 *[323.7]*
hydroxyquinoline derivatives poisoning 961.3 *[323.7]*
lead 984.9 *[323.7]*
mercury 985.0 *[323.7]*
thallium 985.8 *[323.7]*
toxoplasmosis (acquired) 130.0
trypanosomic 086.1 *[323.2]*
tuberculous (*see also* Tuberculosis, meninges) 013.0
virus NEC 048
Meningoencephalocele 742.0
syphilitic 094.89
congenital 090.49
Meningoencephalomyelitis (*see also* Meningoencephalitis) 323.9
acute NEC 048
disseminated (postinfectious) 136.9 *[323.6]*
postimmunization or postvaccination 323.5
due to
actinomycosis 039.8 *[320.7]*
torula 117.5 *[323.4]*
toxoplasma or toxoplasmosis (acquired) 130.0
congenital (active) 771.2 *[323.4]*
late effect—*see* category 326
Meningoencephalomyelopathy (*see also* Meningoencephalomyelitis) 349.9
Meningoencephalopathy (*see also* Meningoencephalitis) 348.3
Meningoencephalopoliomyelitis (*see also* Poliomyelitis, bulbar) 045.0
late effect 138
Meningomyelitis (*see also* Meningoencephalitis) 323.9
blastomycotic NEC (*see also* Blastomycosis) 116.0 *[323.4]*
due to
actinomycosis 039.8 *[320.7]*
blastomycosis (*see also* Blastomycosis) 116.0 *[323.4]*
Meningococcus 036.0
sporotrichosis 117.1 *[323.4]*
torula 117.5 *[323.4]*
late effect—*see* category 326
lethargic 049.8
meningococcal 036.0
syphilitic 094.2
tuberculous (*see also* Tuberculosis, meninges) 013.0

Meningomyelocele (*see also* Spina bifida) 741.9
syphilitic 094.89
Meningomyeloneuritis —*see* Meningoencephalitis
Meningoradiculitis —*see* Meningitis
Meningovascular —*see* condition
Meniscocytosis 282.60
Menkes' syndrome —*see* Syndrome, Menkes'
Menolipsis 626.0
Menometrorrhagia 626.2
Menopause, menopausal (symptoms) (syndrome) 627.2
arthritis (any site) NEC 716.3
artificial 627.4
bleeding 627.0
crisis 627.2
depression (*see also* Psychosis, affective) 296.2
agitated 296.2
recurrent episode 296.3
single episode 296.2
psychotic 296.2
recurrent episode 296.3
single episode 296.2
recurrent episode 296.3
single episode 296.2
melancholia (*see also* Psychosis, affective) 296.2
recurrent episode 296.3
single episode 296.2
paranoid state 297.2
paraphrenia 297.2
postsurgical 627.4
premature 256.3
postirradiation 256.2
postsurgical 256.2
psychoneurosis 627.2
psychosis NEC 298.8
surgical 627.4
toxic polyarthritis NEC 716.39
Menorrhagia (primary) 626.2
climacteric 627.0
menopausal 627.0
postclimacteric 627.1
postmenopausal 627.1
preclimacteric 627.0
premenopausal 627.0
puberty (menses retained) 626.3
Menorrhalgia 625.3
Menoschesis 626.8
Menostaxis 626.2
Menses, retention 626.8
Menstrual —*see* Menstruation
cycle, irregular 626.4
disorders NEC 626.9
extraction V25.3
fluid, retained 626.8
molimen 625.4
period, normal V65.5
regulation V25.3
Menstruation
absent 626.0
anovulatory 628.0
delayed 626.8
difficult 625.3
disorder 626.9
psychogenic 306.52
specified NEC 626.8
during pregnancy 640.8
excessive 626.2
frequent 626.2
infrequent 626.1
Menstruation—*continued*
irregular 626.4
latent 626.8
membranous 626.8
painful (primary) (secondary) 625.3
psychogenic 306.52
passage of clots 626.2
precocious 626.8
protracted 626.8
retained 626.8
retrograde 626.8
scanty 626.1
suppression 626.8
vicarious (nasal) 625.8
Mentagra (*see also* Sycosis) 704.8
Mental —*see also* condition
deficiency (*see also* Retardation, mental) 319
deterioration (*see also* Psychosis) 298.9
disorder (*see also* Disorder, mental) 300.9
exhaustion 300.5
insufficiency (congenital) (*see also* Retardation, mental) 319
observation without need for further medical care NEC V71.09
retardation (*see also* Retardation, mental) 319
subnormality (*see also* Retardation, mental) 319
mild 317
moderate 318.0
profound 318.2
severe 318.1
upset (*see also* Disorder, mental) 300.9
Meralgia paresthetica 355.1
Mercurial —*see* condition
Mercurialism NEC 985.0
Merergasia 300.9
Merocele (*see also* Hernia, femoral) 553.00
Meromelia 755.4
lower limb 755.30
intercalary 755.32
femur 755.34
tibiofibular (complete) (incomplete) 755.33
fibula 755.37
metatarsal(s) 755.38
tarsal(s) 755.38
tibia 755.36
tibiofibular 755.35
terminal (complete) (partial) (transverse) 755.31
longitudinal 755.32
metatarsal(s) 755.38
phalange(s) 755.39
tarsal(s) 755.38
transverse 755.31
upper limb 755.20
intercalary 755.22
carpal(s) 755.28
humeral 755.24
radioulnar (complete) (incomplete) 755.23
metacarpal(s) 755.28
phalange(s) 755.29
radial 755.26
radioulnar 755.25
ulnar 755.27
terminal (complete) (partial) (transverse) 755.21
longitudinal 755.22
carpal(s) 755.28
metacarpal(s) 755.28
phalange(s) 755.29
transverse 755.21
Merosmia 781.1

Merycism (*see also* Rumination)—*see also* Vomiting
  psychogenic 307.53
Merzbacher-Pelizaeus disease 330.0
Mesaortitis —*see* Aortitis
Mesarteritis —*see* Arteritis
Mesencephalitis (*see also* Encephalitis) 323.9
  late effect—*see* category 326
Mesenchymoma (M8990/1)—*see also* Neoplasm, connective tissue, uncertain behavior
  benign (M8990/0)—*see* Neoplasm, connective tissue, benign
  malignant (M8990/3)—*see* Neoplasm, connective tissue, malignant
Mesentery, mesenteric —*see* condition
Mesiodens, mesiodentes 520.1
  causing crowding 524.3
Mesio-occlusion 524.2
Mesocardia (with asplenia) 746.87
Mesocolon —*see* condition
Mesonephroma (malignant) (M9110/3)—*see also* Neoplasm, by site, malignant
  benign (M9110/0)—*see* Neoplasm, by site, benign
Mesophlebitis —*see* Phlebitis
Mesostromal dysgenesis 743.51
Mesothelioma (malignant) (M9050/3)—*see also* Neoplasm, by site, malignant
  benign (M9050/0)—*see* Neoplasm, by site, benign
  biphasic type (M9053/3)—*see also* Neoplasm, by site, malignant
    benign (M9053/0)—*see* Neoplasm, by site, benign
  epithelioid (M9052/3)—*see also* Neoplasm, by site, malignant
    benign (M9052/0)—*see* Neoplasm, by site, benign
  fibrous (M9051/3)—*see also* Neoplasm, by site, malignant
    benign (M9051/0)—*see* Neoplasm, by site, benign
Metabolism disorder 277.9
  specified type NEC 277.8
Metagonimiasis 121.5
Metagonimus infestation (small intestine) 121.5
Metal
  pigmentation (skin) 709.00
  polishers' disease 502
Metalliferous miners' lung 503
Metamorphopsia 368.14
Metaplasia
  bone, in skin 709.3
  breast 611.8
  cervix—*omit code*
  endometrium (squamous) 621.8
  intestinal, of gastric mucosa 537.89
  kidney (pelvis) (squamous) (*see also* Disease, renal) 593.89
  myelogenous 289.8
  myeloid (agnogenic) (megakaryocytic) 289.8
  spleen 289.59
  squamous cell
    amnion 658.8
    bladder 596.8
    cervix—*see* condition
    trachea 519.1
    tracheobronchial tree 519.1
    uterus 621.8
      cervix—*see* condition
Metastasis, metastatic
  abscess—*see* Abscess
  calcification 275.4
  cancer, neoplasm, or disease
    from specified site (M8000/3)—*see* Neoplasm, by site, malignant
    to specified site (M8000/6)—*see* Neoplasm, by site, secondary
  deposits (in) (M8000/6)—*see* Neoplasm, by site, secondary
  pneumonia 038.8 *[484.8]*
  spread (to) (M8000/6)—*see* Neoplasm, by site, secondary
Metatarsalgia 726.70
  anterior 355.6
  due to Freiberg's disease 732.5
  Morton's 355.6
Metatarsus, metatarsal —*see also* condition
  adductus (congenital)
    valgus 754.60
    varus 754.53
  primus varus 754.52
  valgus (adductus) (congenital) 754.60
  varus (adductus) (congenital) 754.53
    primus 754.52
Methemoglobinemia 289.7
  acquired (with sulfhemoglobinemia) 289.7
  congenital 289.7
  enzymatic 289.7
  Hb-M disease 289.7
  hereditary 289.7
  toxic 289.7
Methemoglobinuria (*see also* Hemoglobinuria) 791.2
Methioninemia 270.4
Metritis (catarrhal) (septic) (suppurative) (*see also* Endometritis) 615.9
  blennorrhagic 098.16
    chronic or duration of 2 months or over 098.36
  cervical (*see also* Cervicitis) 616.0
  gonococcal 098.16
    chronic or duration of 2 months or over 098.36
  hemorrhagic 626.8
  puerperal, postpartum, childbirth 670
  tuberculous (*see also* Tuberculosis) 016.7
Metropathia hemorrhagica 626.8
Metroperitonitis (*see also* Peritonitis, pelvic, female) 614.5
Metrorrhagia 626.6
  arising during pregnancy—*see* Hemorrhage, pregnancy
  postpartum NEC 666.2
  primary 626.6
  psychogenic 306.59
  puerperal 666.2
Metrorrhexis —*see* Rupture, uterus
Metrosalpingitis (*see also* Salpingo-oophoritis) 614.2
Metrostaxis 626.6
Metrovaginitis (*see also* Endometritis) 615.9
  gonococcal (acute) 098.16
    chronic or duration of 2 months or over 098.36
Mexican fever —*see* Typhus, Mexican
Meyenburg-Altherr-Uehlinger syndrome 733.99
Meyer-Schwickerath and Weyers syndrome (dysplasia oculodentodigitalis) 759.89
Meynert's amentia (nonalcoholic) 294.0
  alcoholic 291.1
Mibelli's disease 757.39
Mice, joint (*see also* Loose, body, joint) 718.1
  knee 717.6

Micheli-Rietti syndrome (thalassemia minor) 282.4
Michotte's syndrome 721.5
Micrencephalon, micrencephaly 742.1
Microaneurysm, retina 362.14
diabetic 250.5 *[362.01]*
Microangiopathy 443.9
diabetic (peripheral) 250.7 *[443.81]*
retinal 250.5 *[362.01]*
peripheral 443.9
diabetic 250.7 *[443.81]*
retinal 362.18
diabetic 250.5 *[362.01]*
thrombotic 446.6
Moschcowitz's (thrombotic thrombocytopenic purpura) 446.6
Microcephalus, microcephalic, microcephaly 742.1
due to toxoplasmosis (congenital) 771.2
Microcheilia 744.82
Microcolon (congenital) 751.5
Microcornea (congenital) 743.41
Microcytic —*see* condition
Microdontia 520.2
Microdrepanocytosis (thalassemia-Hb-S disease) 282.4
Microembolism, retina 362.33
Microencephalon 742.1
Microfilaria streptocerca infestation 125.3
Microgastria (congenital) 750.7
Microgenia 524.06
Microgenitalia (congenital) 752.8
Microglioma (M9710/3)
specified site—*see* Neoplasm, by site, malignant
unspecified site 191.9
Microglossia (congenital) 750.16
Micrognathia, micrognathism (congenital) 524.00
mandibular 524.04
alveolar 524.74
maxillary 524.03
alveolar 524.73
Microgyria (congenital) 742.2
Microinfarct, heart (*see also* Insufficiency, coronary) 411.89
Microlithiasis, alveolar, pulmonary 516.2
Micromyelia (congenital) 742.59
Microphakia (congenital) 743.36
Microphthalmia (congenital) (*see also* Microphthalmos) 743.10
Microphthalmos (congenital) 743.10
associated with eye and adnexal anomalies NEC 743.12
due to toxoplasmosis (congenital) 771.2
isolated 743.11
simple 743.11
syndrome 759.89
Micropsia 368.14
Microsporidiosis 136.8
Microsporon furfur infestation 111.0
Microsporosis (*see also* Dermatophytosis) 110.9
nigra 111.1
Microstomia (congenital) 744.84
Microthelia 757.6
Microthromboembolism —*see* Embolism
Microtia (congenital) (external ear) 744.23
Microtropia 378.34
Micturition
disorder NEC 788.69
psychogenic 306.53
Micturition—*continued*
frequency 788.41
psychogenic 306.53
nocturnal 788.43
painful 788.1
psychogenic 306.53
Middle
ear—*see* condition
lobe (right) syndrome 518.0
Midplane —*see* condition
Miescher's disease 709.3
cheilitis 351.8
granulomatosis disciformis 709.3
Miescher-Leder syndrome or granulomatosis 709.3
Mieten's syndrome 759.89
Migraine (idiopathic) 346.9
with aura 346.0
abdominal (syndrome) 346.2
allergic (histamine) 346.2
atypical 346.1
basilar 346.2
classical 346.0
common 346.1
hemiplegic 346.8
lower-half 346.2
menstrual 625.4
ophthalmic 346.8
ophthalmoplegic 346.8
retinal 346.2
variant 346.2
Migrant, social V60.0
Migratory, migrating —*see also* condition
person V60.0
testis, congenital 752.5
Mikulicz's disease or syndrome (dryness of mouth, absent or decreased lacrimation) 527.1
Milian atrophia blanche 701.3
Miliaria (crystallina) (rubra) (tropicalis) 705.1
apocrine 705.82
Miliary —*see* condition
Milium (*see also* Cyst, sebaceous) 706.2
colloid 709.3
eyelid 374.84
Milk
crust 691.8
excess secretion 676.6
fever, female 672
poisoning 988.8
retention 676.2
sickness 988.8
spots 423.1
Milkers' nodes 051.1
Milk-leg (deep vessels) 671.4
complicating pregnancy 671.3
nonpuerperal 451.19
puerperal, postpartum, childbirth 671.4
Milkman (-Looser) disease or syndrome (osteomalacia with pseudofractures) 268.2
Milky urine (*see also* Chyluria) 791.1
Millar's asthma (laryngismus stridulus) 478.75
Millard-Gubler paralysis or syndrome 344.89
Millard-Gubler-Foville paralysis 344.89
Miller's disease (osteomalacia) 268.2
Miller Fisher's syndrome 357.0
Milles' syndrome (encephalocutaneous angiomatosis) 759.6
Mills' disease 335.29
Millstone makers' asthma or lung 502
Milroy's disease (chronic hereditary edema) 757.0

Miners' —*see also* condition
asthma 500
elbow 727.2
knee 727.2
lung 500
nystagmus 300.89
phthisis (*see also* Tuberculosis) 011.4
tuberculosis (*see also* Tuberculosis) 011.4
Minkowski-Chauffard syndrome (*see also* Spherocytosis) 282.0
Minor —*see* condition
Minor's disease 336.1
Minot's disease (hemorrhagic disease, newborn) 776.0
Minot-von Willebrand (-Jürgens) disease or syndrome (angiohemophilia) 286.4
Minus (and plus) hand (intrinsic) 736.09
Miosis (persistent) (pupil) 379.42
Mirizzi's syndrome (hepatic duct stenosis) (*see also* Obstruction, biliary) 576.2
with calculus, cholelithiasis, or stones—*see* Choledocholithiasis
Mirror writing 315.09
secondary to organic lesion 784.69
Misadventure (prophylactic) (therapeutic) (*see also* Complications) 999.9
administration of insulin 962.3
infusion—*see* Complications, infusion
local applications (of fomentations, plasters, etc.) 999.9
burn or scald—*see* Burn, by site
medical care (early) (late) NEC 999.9
adverse effect of drugs or chemicals—*see* Table of drugs and chemicals
burn or scald—*see* Burn, by site
radiation NEC 990
radiotherapy NEC 990
surgical procedure (early) (late)—*see* Complications, surgical procedure
transfusion—*see* Complications, transfusion
vaccination or other immunological procedure—*see* Complications, vaccination
Misanthropy 301.7
Miscarriage —*see* Abortion, spontaneous
Mischief, malicious, child (*see also* Disturbance, conduct) 312.0
Mismanagement, feeding 783.3
Misplaced, misplacement
kidney (*see also* Disease, renal) 593.0
congenital 753.3
organ or site, congenital NEC—*see* Malposition, congenital
Missed
abortion 632
delivery (at or near term) 656.4
labor (at or near term) 656.4
Missing —*see also* Absence
teeth (acquired) 525.1
congenital (*see also* Anodontia) 520.0
vertebrae (congenital) 756.13
Misuse of drugs NEC (*see also* Abuse, drug, nondependent) 305.9
Mitchell's disease (erythromelalgia) 443.89
Mite (s)
diarrhea 133.8
grain (itch) 133.8
hair follicle (itch) 133.8
in sputum 133.8
Mitral —*see* condition
Mittelschmerz 625.2
Mixed —*see* condition
Mljet disease (mal de Meleda) 757.39
Mobile, mobility
cecum 751.4
coccyx 733.99
excessive—*see* Hypermobility
gallbladder 751.69
kidney 593.0
congenital 753.3
organ or site, congenital NEC—*see* Malposition, congenital
spleen 289.59
Mobitz heart block (atrioventricular) 426.10
type I (Wenckebach's) 426.13
type II 426.12
Möbius'
disease 346.8
syndrome
congenital oculofacial paralysis 352.6
ophthalmoplegic migraine 346.8
Moeller (-Barlow) disease (infantile scurvy) 267
glossitis 529.4
Mohr's syndrome (Types I and II) 759.89
Mola destruens (M9100/1) 236.1
Molarization, premolars 520.2
Molar pregnancy 631
hydatidiform (delivered) (undelivered) 630
Mold (s) in vitreous 117.9
Molding, head (during birth) 767.3
Mole (pigmented) (M8720/0)—*see also* Neoplasm, skin, benign
blood 631
Breus' 631
cancerous (M8720/3)—*see* Melanoma
carneous 631
destructive (M9100/1) 236.1
ectopic—*see* Pregnancy, ectopic
fleshy 631
hemorrhagic 631
hydatid, hydatidiform (benign) (complicating pregnancy) (delivered) (undelivered) (*see also* Hydatidiform mole) 630
invasive (M9100/1) 236.1
malignant (M9100/1) 236.1
previous, affecting management of pregnancy V23.1
invasive (hydatidiform) (M9100/1) 236.1
malignant
meaning
malignant hydatidiform mole (M9100/1) 236.1
melanoma (M8720/3)—*see* Melanoma
nonpigmented (M8730/0)—*see* Neoplasm, skin, benign
pregnancy NEC 631
skin (M8720/0)—*see* Neoplasm, skin, benign
tubal—*see* Pregnancy, tubal
vesicular (*see also* Hydatidiform mole) 630
Molimen, molimina (menstrual) 625.4
Mollaret's meningitis 047.9
Mollities (cerebellar) (cerebral) 437.8
ossium 268.2
Molluscum
contagiosum 078.0
epitheliale 078.0
fibrosum (M8851/0)—*see* Lipoma, by site
pendulum (M8851/0)—*see* Lipoma, by site
Mönckeberg's arteriosclerosis, degeneration disease, or sclerosis (*see also* Arteriosclerosis, extremities) 440.20
Monday fever 504
Monday morning dyspnea or asthma 504
Mondini's malformation (cochlea) 744.05

Mondor's disease (thrombophlebitis of breast) 451.89
Mongolian, mongolianism, mongolism mongoloid 758.0
spot 757.33
Monilethrix (congenital) 757.4
Monilia infestation —*see* Candidiasis
Moniliasis —*see also* Candidiasis
neonatal 771.7
vulvovaginitis 112.1
Monoarthritis 716.60
ankle 716.67
arm 716.62
lower (and wrist) 716.63
upper (and elbow) 716.62
foot (and ankle) 716.67
forearm (and wrist) 716.63
hand 716.64
leg 716.66
lower 716.66
upper 716.65
pelvic region (hip) (thigh) 716.65
shoulder (region) 716.61
specified site NEC 716.68
Monoblastic —*see* condition
Monochromatism (cone) (rod) 368.54
Monocytic —*see* condition
Monocytosis (symptomatic) 288.8
Monofixation syndrome 378.34
Monomania (*see also* Psychosis) 298.9
Mononeuritis 355.9
cranial nerve—*see* Disorder, nerve, cranial
femoral nerve 355.2
lateral
cutaneous nerve of thigh 355.1
popliteal nerve 355.3
lower limb 355.8
specified nerve NEC 355.79
medial popliteal nerve 355.4
median nerve 354.1
multiplex 354.5
plantar nerve 355.6
posterior tibial nerve 355.5
radial nerve 354.3
sciatic nerve 355.0
ulnar nerve 354.2
upper limb 354.9
specified nerve NEC 354.8
vestibular 388.5
Mononeuropathy (*see also* Mononeuritis) 355.9
diabetic NEC 250.6 *[355.9]*
lower limb 250.6 *[355.8]*
upper limb 250.6 *[354.9]*
iliohypogastric nerve 355.79
ilioinguinal nerve 355.79
obturator nerve 355.79
saphenous nerve 355.79
Mononucleosis, infectious 075
with hepatitis 075 *[573.1]*
Monoplegia 344.5
brain (current episode) (*see also* Paralysis, brain) 437.8
fetus or newborn 767.8
cerebral (current episode) (*see also* Paralysis, brain) 437.8
congenital or infantile (cerebral) (spastic) (spinal) 343.3
embolic (current) (*see also* Embolism, brain) 434.1
late effect—*see* category 438
infantile (cerebral) (spastic) (spinal) 343.3
Monoplegia—*continued*
lower limb 344.30
affecting
dominant side 344.31
nondominant side 344.32
newborn 767.8
psychogenic 306.0
specified as conversion reaction 300.11
thrombotic (current) (*see also* Thrombosis, brain) 434.0
late effect—*see* category 438
transient 781.4
upper limb 344.40
affecting
dominant side 344.41
nondominant side 344.42
Monorchism, monorchidism 752.8
Monster, monstrosity —*see* Anomaly
Monteggia's fracture (closed) 813.03
open 813.13
Mood swings
brief compensatory 296.99
rebound 296.99
Moore's syndrome (*see also* Epilepsy) 345.5
Mooren's ulcer (cornea) 370.07
Mooser-Neill reaction 081.0
Mooser bodies 081.0
Moral
deficiency 301.7
imbecility 301.7
Morax-Axenfeld conjunctivitis 372.03
Morbilli (*see also* Measles) 055.9
Morbus
anglicus, anglorum 268.0
Beigel 111.2
caducus (*see also* Epilepsy) 345.9
caeruleus 746.89
celiacus 579.0
comitialis (*see also* Epilepsy) 345.9
cordis—*see also* Disease, heart
valvulorum—*see* Endocarditis
coxae 719.95
tuberculous (*see also* Tuberculosis) 015.1
hemorrhagicus neonatorum 776.0
maculosus neonatorum 772.6
renum 593.0
senilis (*see also* Osteoarthrosis) 715.9
Morel-Kraepelin disease (*see also* Schizophrenia) 295.9
Morel-Moore syndrome (hyperostosis frontalis interna) 733.3
Morel-Morgagni syndrome (hyperostosis frontalis interna) 733.3
Morgagni
cyst, organ, hydatid, or appendage 752.8
fallopian tube 752.11
disease or syndrome (hyperostosis frontalis interna) 733.3
Morgagni-Adams-Stokes syndrome (syncope with heart block) 426.9
Morgagni-Stewart-Morel syndrome (hyperostosis frontalis interna) 733.3
Moria (*see also* Psychosis) 298.9
Morning sickness 643.0
Moron 317
Morphea (guttate) (linear) 701.0
Morphine dependence (*see also* Dependence) 304.0
Morphinism (*see also* Dependence) 304.0
Morphinomania (*see also* Dependence) 304.0
Morphoea 701.0

Morquio (-Brailsford) (-Ullrich) disease or syndrome (mucopolysaccharidosis IV) 277.5
kyphosis 277.5
Morris syndrome (testicular feminization) 257.8
Morsus humanus (open wound)—*see also* Wound, open, by site
skin surface intact—*see* Contusion
Mortification (dry) (moist) (*see also* Gangrene) 785.4
Morton's
disease 355.6
foot 355.6
metatarsalgia (syndrome) 355.6
neuralgia 355.6
neuroma 355.6
syndrome (metatarsalgia) (neuralgia) 355.6
toe 355.6
Morvan's disease 336.0
Mosaicism, mosaic (chromosomal) 758.9
autosomal 758.5
sex 758.8
Moschcowitz's syndrome (thrombotic thrombocytopenic purpura) 446.6
Mother yaw 102.0
Motion sickness (from travel, any vehicle) (from roundabouts or swings) 994.6
Mottled teeth (enamel) (endemic) (nonendemic) 520.3
Mottling enamel (endemic) (nonendemic) (teeth) 520.3
Mouchet's disease 732.5
Mould (s) (in vitreous) 117.9
Moulders'
bronchitis 502
tuberculosis (*see also* Tuberculosis) 011.4
Mounier-Kuhn syndrome 494
Mountain
fever—*see* Fever, mountain
sickness 993.2
with polycythemia, acquired 289.0
acute 289.0
tick fever 066.1
Mouse, joint (*see also* Loose, body, joint) 718.1
knee 717.6
Mouth —*see* condition
Movable
coccyx 724.71
kidney (*see also* Disease, renal) 593.0
congenital 753.3
organ or site, congenital NEC—*see* Malposition, congenital
spleen 289.59
Movement, abnormal (dystonic) (involuntary) 781.0
paradoxical facial 374.43
Moya Moya disease 437.5
Mozart's ear 744.29
Mucha's disease (acute parapsoriasis varioliformis) 696.2
Mucha-Haberman syndrome (acute parapsoriasis varioliformis) 696.2
Mu-chain disease 273.2
Mucinosis (cutaneous) (papular) 701.8
Mucocele
appendix 543.9
buccal cavity 528.9
gallbladder (*see also* Disease, gallbladder) 575.3
lacrimal sac 375.43
orbit (eye) 376.81
salivary gland (any) 527.6
sinus (accessory) (nasal) 478.1
Mucocele—*continued*
turbinate (bone) (middle) (nasal) 478.1
uterus 621.8
Mucocutaneous lymph node syndrome (acute) (febrile) (infantile) 446.1
Mucoenteritis 564.1
Mucolipidosis I, II, III 272.7
Mucopolysaccharidosis (types 1-6) 277.5
cardiopathy 277.5 *[425.7]*
Mucormycosis (lung) 117.7
Mucositis —*see also* Inflammation by site
necroticans agranulocytica 288.0
Mucous —*see also* condition
patches (syphilitic) 091.3
congenital 090.0
Mucoviscidosis 277.00
with meconium obstruction 277.01
Mucus
asphyxia or suffocation (*see also* Asphyxia, mucus) 933.1
newborn 770.1
in stool 792.1
plug (*see also* Asphyxia, mucus) 933.1
aspiration, of newborn 770.1
tracheobronchial 934.8
newborn 770.1
Muguet 112.0
Mulberry molars 090.5
Mullerian mixed tumor (M8950/3)—*see* Neoplasm, by site, malignant
Multicystic kidney 753.19
Multilobed placenta —*see* Placenta, abnormal
Multiparity V61.5
affecting
fetus or newborn 763.8
management of
labor and delivery 659.4
pregnancy V23.3
requiring contraceptive management (*see also* Contraception) V25.9
Multipartita placenta —*see* Placenta, abnormal
Multiple, multiplex —*see also* condition
birth
affecting fetus or newborn 761.5
healthy liveborn—*see* Newborn, multiple
digits (congenital) 755.00
fingers 755.01
toes 755.02
organ or site NEC—*see* Accessory
personality 300.14
renal arteries 747.62
Mumps 072.9
with complication 072.8
specified type NEC 072.79
encephalitis 072.2
hepatitis 072.71
meningitis (aseptic) 072.1
meningoencephalitis 072.2
oophoritis 072.79
orchitis 072.0
pancreatitis 072.3
polyneuropathy 072.72
vaccination, prophylactic (against) V04.6
Mumu (*see also* Infestation, filarial) 125.9
Münchausen syndrome 301.51
Münchmeyer's disease or syndrome (exostosis luxurians) 728.11
Mural —*see* condition
Murmur (cardiac) (heart) (nonorganic) (organic) 785.2
abdominal 787.5

Murmur—*continued*
aortic (valve) (*see also* Endocarditis, aortic) 424.1
benign—*omit code*
cardiorespiratory 785.2
diastolic—*see* condition
Flint (*see also* Endocarditis, aortic) 424.1
functional—*omit code*
Graham Steell (pulmonic regurgitation) (*see also* Endocarditis, pulmonary) 424.3
innocent—*omit code*
insignificant—*omit code*
midsystolic 785.2
mitral (valve)—*see* stenosis, mitral
physiologic—*see* condition
presystolic, mitral—*see* Insufficiency, mitral
pulmonic (valve) (*see also* Endocarditis, pulmonary) 424.3
Still's (vibratory)—*omit code*
systolic (valvular)—*see* condition
tricuspid (valve)—*see* Endocarditis, tricuspid
valvular—*see* condition
vibratory—*omit code*
undiagnosed 785.2
Murri's disease (intermittent hemoglobinuria) 283.2
Muscae volitantes 379.24
Muscle, muscular —*see* condition
Musculoneuralgia 729.1
Mushrooming hip 718.95
Mushroom workers' (pickers') lung 495.5
Mutism (*see also* Aphasia) 784.3
akinetic 784.3
deaf (acquired) (congenital) 389.7
elective (selective) 313.23
adjustment reaction 309.83
hysterical 300.11
Myà's disease (congenital dilation, colon) 751.3
Myalgia (intercostal) 729.1
eosinophilia syndrome 710.5
epidemic 074.1
cervical 078.89
psychogenic 307.89
traumatic NEC 959.9
Myasthenia, myasthenic 358.0
cordis—*see* Failure, heart
gravis 358.0
neonatal 775.2
pseudoparalytica 358.0
stomach 536.8
psychogenic 306.4
syndrome
in
botulism 005.1 *[358.1]*
diabetes mellitus 250.6 *[358.1]*
hypothyroidism (*see also* Hypothyroidism) 244.9 *[358.1]*
malignant neoplasm NEC 199.1 *[358.1]*
pernicious anemia 281.0 *[358.1]*
thyrotoxicosis (*see also* Thyrotoxicosis) 242.9 *[358.1]*
Mycelium infection NEC 117.9
Mycetismus 988.1
Mycetoma (actinomycotic) 039.9
bone 039.8
mycotic 117.4
foot 039.4
mycotic 117.4
madurae 039.9
mycotic 117.4
Mycetoma—*continued*
maduromycotic 039.9
mycotic 117.4
mycotic 117.4
nocardial 039.9
Mycobacteriosis —*see* Mycobacterium
Mycobacterium, mycobacterial (infection) 031.9
acid-fast (bacilli) 031.9
anonymous (*see also* Mycobacterium, atypical) 031.9
atypical (acid-fast bacilli) 031.9
cutaneous 031.1
pulmonary 031.0
tuberculous (*see also* Tuberculosis, pulmonary) 011.9
specified site NEC 031.8
avium 031.0
balnei 031.1
Battey 031.0
cutaneous 031.1
fortuitum 031.0
intracellulare (battey bacillus) 031.0
kakerifu 031.8
kansasii 031.0
kasongo 031.8
leprae—*see* Leprosy
luciflavum 031.0
marinum 031.1
pulmonary 031.0
tuberculous (*see also* Tuberculosis, pulmonary) 011.9
scrofulaceum 031.1
tuberculosis (human, bovine)—*see also* Tuberculosis
avian type 031.0
ulcerans 031.1
xenopi 031.0
Mycosis, mycotic 117.9
cutaneous NEC 111.9
ear 111.8 *[380.15]*
fungoides (M9700/3) 202.1
mouth 112.0
pharynx 117.9
skin NEC 111.9
stomatitis 112.0
systemic NEC 117.9
tonsil 117.9
vagina, vaginitis 112.1
Mydriasis (persistent) (pupil) 379.43
Myelatelia 742.59
Myelinoclasis, perivascular, acute (postinfectious) NEC 136.9 *[323.6]*
postimmunization or postvaccinal 323.5
Myelinosis, central pontine 341.8
Myelitis (acute) (ascending) (cerebellar) (childhood) (chronic) (descending) (diffuse) (disseminated) (pressure) (progressive) (spinal cord) (subacute) (transverse) (*see also* Encephalitis) 323.9
late effect—*see* category 326
optic neuritis in 341.0
postchickenpox 052.7
postvaccinal 323.5
syphilitic (transverse) 094.89
tuberculous (*see also* Tuberculosis) 013.6
virus 049.9
Myeloblastic —*see* condition
Myelocele (*see also* Spina bifida) 741.9
with hydrocephalus 741.0
Myelocystocele (*see also* Spina bifida) 741.9
Myelocytic —*see* condition

Myelocytoma 205.1
Myelodysplasia (spinal cord) 742.59
meaning myelodysplastic syndrome—*see* Syndrome, myelodysplastic
Myeloencephalitis —*see* Encephalitis
Myelofibrosis (osteosclerosis) 289.8
Myelogenous —*see* condition
Myeloid —*see* condition
Myelokathexis 288.0
Myeloleukodystrophy 330.0
Myelolipoma (M8870/0)—*see* Neoplasm, by site, benign
Myeloma (multiple) (plasma cell) (plasmacytic) (M9730/3) 203.0
monostotic (M9731/1) 238.6
solitary (M9731/1) 238.6
Myelomalacia 336.8
Myelomata, multiple (M9730/3) 203.0
Myelomatosis (M9730/3) 203.0
Myelomeningitis —*see* Meningoencephalitis
Myelomeningocele (spinal cord) (*see also* Spina bifida) 741.9
fetal, causing fetopelvic disproportion 653.7
Myelo-osteo-musculodysplasia hereditaria 756.89
Myelopathic —*see* condition
Myelopathy (spinal cord) 336.9
cervical 721.1
diabetic 250.6 *[336.3]*
drug-induced 336.8
due to or with
carbon tetrachloride 987.8 *[323.7]*
degeneration or displacement, intervertebral disc 722.70
cervical, cervicothoracic 722.71
lumbar, lumbosacral 722.73
thoracic, thoracolumbar 722.72
hydroxyquinoline derivatives 961.3 *[323.7]*
infection—*see* Encephalitis
intervertebral disc disorder 722.70
cervical, cervicothoracic 722.71
lumbar, lumbosacral 722.73
thoracic, thoracolumbar 722.72
lead 984.9 *[323.7]*
mercury 985.0 *[323.7]*
neoplastic disease (*see also* Neoplasm, by site) 239.9 *[336.3]*
pernicious anemia 281.0 *[336.3]*
spondylosis 721.91
cervical 721.1
lumbar, lumbosacral 721.42
thoracic 721.41
thallium 985.8 *[323.7]*
lumbar, lumbosacral 721.42
necrotic (subacute) 336.1
radiation-induced 336.8
spondylogenic NEC 721.91
cervical 721.1
lumbar, lumbosacral 721.42
thoracic 721.41
thoracic 721.41
toxic NEC 989.9 *[323.7]*
transverse (*see also* Encephalitis) 323.9
vascular 336.1
Myeloproliferative disease (M9960/1) 238.7
Myeloradiculitis (*see also* Polyneuropathy) 357.0
Myeloradiculodysplasia (spinal) 742.59
Myelosarcoma (M9930/3) 205.3
Myelosclerosis 289.8
with myeloid metaplasia (M9961/1) 238.7
disseminated, of nervous system 340
megakaryocytic (M9961/1) 238.7
Myelosis (M9860/3) (*see also* Leukemia, myeloid) 205.9
acute (M9861/3) 205.0
aleukemic (M9864/3) 205.8
chronic (M9863/3) 205.1
erythremic (M9840/3) 207.0
acute (M9841/3) 207.0
megakaryocytic (M9920/3) 207.2
nonleukemic (chronic) 288.8
subacute (M9862/3) 205.2
Myesthenia —*see* Myasthenia
Myiasis (cavernous) 134.0
orbit 134.0 *[376.13]*
Myoadenoma, prostate 600
Myoblastoma
granular cell (M9580/0)—*see also* Neoplasm, connective tissue, benign
malignant (M9580/3)—*see* Neoplasm, connective tissue, malignant
tongue (M9580/0) 210.1
Myocardial —*see* condition
Myocardiopathy (congestive) (constrictive) (familial) (hypertrophic nonobstructive) (idiopathic) (infiltrative) (obstructive) (primary) (restrictive) (sporadic) 425.4
alcoholic 425.5
amyloid 277.3 *[425.7]*
beriberi 265.0 *[425.7]*
cobalt-beer 425.5
due to
amyloidosis 277.3 *[425.7]*
beriberi 265.0 *[425.7]*
cardiac glycogenosis 271.0 *[425.7]*
Chagas' disease 086.0
Friedreich's ataxia 334.0 *[425.8]*
influenza 487.8 *[425.8]*
mucopolysaccharidosis 277.5 *[425.7]*
myotonia atrophica 359.2 *[425.8]*
progressive muscular dystrophy 359.1 *[425.8]*
sarcoidosis 135 *[425.8]*
glycogen storage 271.0 *[425.7]*
hypertrophic obstructive 425.1
metabolic NEC 277.9 *[425.7]*
nutritional 269.9 *[425.7]*
obscure (African) 425.2
postpartum 674.8
secondary 425.9
thyrotoxic (*see also* Thyrotoxicosis) 242.9 *[425.7]*
toxic NEC 425.9
Myocarditis (fibroid) (interstitial) (old) (progressive) (senile) (with arteriosclerosis) 429.0
with
rheumatic fever (conditions classifiable to 390) 398.0
active (*see also* Myocarditis, acute, rheumatic) 391.2
inactive or quiescent (with chorea) 398.0
active (nonrheumatic) 422.90
rheumatic 391.2
with chorea (acute) (rheumatic) (Sydenham's) 392.0
acute or subacute (interstitial) 422.90
due to Streptococcus (beta-hemolytic) 391.2
idiopathic 422.91
rheumatic 391.2
with chorea (acute) (rheumatic) (Sydenham's) 392.0
specified type NEC 422.99
aseptic of newborn 074.23

Myocarditis—*continued*
bacterial (acute) 422.92
chagasic 086.0
chronic (interstitial) 429.0
congenital 746.89
constrictive 425.4
Coxsackie (virus) 074.23
diphtheritic 032.82
due to or in
Coxsackie (virus) 074.23
diphtheria 032.82
epidemic louse-borne typhus 080 *[422.0]*
influenza 487.8 *[422.0]*
Lyme disease 088.81 *[422.0]*
scarlet fever 034.1 *[422.0]*
toxoplasmosis (acquired) 130.3
tuberculosis (*see also* Tuberculosis) 017.9 *[422.0]*
typhoid 002.0 *[422.0]*
typhus NEC 081.9 *[422.0]*
eosinophilic 422.91
epidemic of newborn 074.23
Fiedler's (acute) (isolated) (subacute) 422.91
giant cell (acute) (subacute) 422.91
gonococcal 098.85
granulomatous (idiopathic) (isolated) (nonspecific) 422.91
hypertensive (*see also* Hypertension, heart) 402.90
idiopathic 422.91
granulomatous 422.91
infective 422.92
influenzal 487.8 *[422.0]*
isolated (diffuse) (granulomatous) 422.91
malignant 422.99
meningococcal 036.43
nonrheumatic, active 422.90
parenchymatous 422.90
pneumococcal (acute) (subacute) 422.92
rheumatic (chronic) (inactive) (with chorea) 398.0
active or acute 391.2
with chorea (acute) (rheumatic) (Sydenham's) 392.0
septic 422.92
specific (giant cell) (productive) 422.91
staphylococcal (acute) (subacute) 422.92
suppurative 422.92
syphilitic (chronic) 093.82
toxic 422.93
rheumatic (*see also* Myocarditis, acute rheumatic) 391.2
tuberculous (*see also* Tuberculosis) 017.9 *[422.0]*
typhoid 002.0 *[422.0]*
valvular—*see* Endocarditis
viral, except Coxsackie 422.91
Coxsackie 074.23
of newborn (Coxsackie) 074.23
Myocardium, myocardial —*see* condition
Myocardosis (*see also* Cardiomyopathy) 425.4
Myoclonia (essential) 333.2
epileptica 333.2
Friedrich's 333.2
massive 333.2
Myoclonic
epilepsy, familial (progressive) 333.2
jerks 333.2
Myoclonus (familial essential) (multifocal) (simplex) 333.2
facial 351.8
Myoclonus—*continued*
massive (infantile) 333.2
pharyngeal 478.29
Myodiastasis 728.84
Myoendocarditis —*see also* Endocarditis
acute or subacute 421.9
Myoepithelioma (M8982/0)—*see* Neoplasm, by site, benign
Myofascitis (acute) 729.1
low back 724.2
Myofibroma (M8890/0)—*see also* Neoplasm, connective tissue, benign
uterus (cervix) (corpus) (*see also* Leiomyoma) 218.9
Myofibrosis 728.2
heart (*see also* Myocarditis) 429.0
humeroscapular region 726.2
scapulohumeral 726.2
Myofibrositis (*see also* Myositis) 729.1
scapulohumeral 726.2
Myogelosis (occupational) 728.89
Myoglobinuria 791.3
Myoglobulinuria, primary 791.3
Myokymia —*see also* Myoclonus
facial 351.8
Myolipoma (M8860/0)
specified site—*see* Neoplasm, connective tissue, benign
unspecified site 223.0
Myoma (M8895/0)—*see also* Neoplasm, connective tissue, benign
cervix (stump) (uterus) (*see also* Leiomyoma) 218.9
malignant (M8895/3)—*see* Neoplasm, connective tissue, malignant
prostate 600
uterus (cervix) (corpus) (*see also* Leiomyoma) 218.9
in pregnancy or childbirth 654.1
affecting fetus or newborn 763.8
causing obstructed labor 660.2
affecting fetus or newborn 763.1
Myomalacia 728.9
cordis, heart (*see also* Degeneration, myocardial) 429.1
Myometritis (*see also* Endometritis) 615.9
Myometrium —*see* condition
Myonecrosis, clostridial 040.0
Myopathy 359.9
alcoholic 359.4
amyloid 277.3 *[359.6]*
benign congenital 359.0
central core 359.0
centronuclear 359.0
congenital (benign) 359.0
distal 359.1
due to drugs 359.4
endocrine 259.9 *[359.5]*
specified type NEC 259.8 *[359.5]*
extraocular muscles 376.82
facioscapulohumeral 359.1
in
Addison's disease 255.4 *[359.5]*
amyloidosis 277.3 *[359.6]*
cretinism 243 *[359.5]*
Cushing's syndrome 255.0 *[359.5]*
disseminated lupus erythematosus 710.0 *[359.6]*
giant cell arteritis 446.5 *[359.6]*
hyperadrenocorticism NEC 255.3 *[359.5]*
hyperparathyroidism 252.0 *[359.5]*

Myopathy—*continued*
hypopituitarism 253.2 *[359.5]*
hypothyroidism (*see also* Hypothyroidism) 244.9 *[359.5]*
malignant neoplasm NEC (M8000/3) 199.1 *[359.6]*
myxedema (*see also* Myxedema) 244.9 *[359.5]*
polyarteritis nodosa 446.0 *[359.6]*
rheumatoid arthritis 714.0 *[359.6]*
sarcoidosis 135 *[359.6]*
scleroderma 710.1 *[359.6]*
Sjögren's disease 710.2 *[359.6]*
thyrotoxicosis (*see also* Thyrotoxicosis) 242.9 *[359.5]*
inflammatory 359.8
limb-girdle 359.1
myotubular 359.0
nemaline 359.0
ocular 359.1
oculopharyngeal 359.1
primary 359.8
progressive NEC 359.8
rod body 359.0
scapulohumeral 359.1
specified type NEC 359.8
toxic 359.4
Myopericarditis (*see also* Pericarditis) 423.9
Myopia (axial) (congenital) (increased curvature or refraction, nucleus of lens) 367.1
degenerative, malignant 360.21
malignant 360.21
progressive high (degenerative) 360.21
Myosarcoma (M8895/3)—*see* Neoplasm, connective tissue, malignant
Myosis (persistent) 379.42
stromal (endolymphatic) (M8931/1) 236.0
Myositis 729.1
clostridial 040.0
due to posture 729.1
epidemic 074.1
fibrosa or fibrous (chronic) 728.2
Volkmann's (complicating trauma) 958.6
infective 728.0
interstitial 728.81
multiple—*see* Polymyositis
occupational 729.1
orbital, chronic 376.12
ossificans 728.12
circumscribed 728.12
progressive 728.11
traumatic 728.12
progressive fibrosing 728.11
purulent 728.0
rheumatic 729.1
rheumatoid 729.1
suppurative 728.0
syphilitic 095.6
traumatic (old) 729.1
Myospasia impulsiva 307.23
Myotonia (acquisita) (intermittens) 728.85
atrophica 359.2
congenita 359.2
dystrophica 359.2
Myotonic pupil 379.46
Myriapodiasis 134.1
Myringitis
with otitis media—*see* Otitis media
acute 384.00
specified type NEC 384.09
bullosa hemorrhagica 384.01
Myringitis—*continued*
bullous 384.01
chronic 384.1
Mysophobia 300.29
Mytilotoxism 988.0
Myxadenitis labialis 528.5
Myxedema (adult) (idiocy) (infantile) (juvenile) (thyroid gland) (*see also* Hypothyroidism) 244.9
circumscribed 242.9
congenital 243
cutis 701.8
localized (pretibial) 242.9
madness (acute) 293.0
subacute 293.1
papular 701.8
pituitary 244.8
postpartum 674.8
pretibial 242.9
primary 244.9
Myxochondrosarcoma (M9220/3)—*see* Neoplasm, cartilage, malignant
Myxofibroma (M8811/0)—*see also* Neoplasm, connective tissue, benign
odontogenic (M9320/0) 213.1
upper jaw (bone) 213.0
Myxofibrosarcoma (M8811/3)—*see* Neoplasm, connective tissue, malignant
Myxolipoma (M8852/0) (*see also* Lipoma, by site) 214.9
Myxoliposarcoma (M8852/3)—*see* Neoplasm, connective tissue, malignant
Myxoma (M8840/0)—*see also* Neoplasm, connective tissue, benign
odontogenic (M9320/0) 213.1
upper jaw (bone) 213.0
Myxosarcoma (M8840/3)—*see* Neoplasm, connective tissue, malignant

N

Naegeli's
disease (hereditary hemorrhagic thrombasthenia) 287.1
leukemia, monocytic (M9863/3) 205.1
syndrome (incontinentia pigmenti) 757.33
Naffziger's syndrome 353.0
Naga sore (*see also* Ulcer, skin) 707.9
Nägele's pelvis 738.6
with disproportion (fetopelvic) 653.0
affecting fetus or newborn 763.1
causing obstructed labor 660.1
affecting fetus or newborn 763.1
Nager-de Reynier syndrome (dysostosis mandibularis) 756.0
Nail —*see also* condition
biting 307.9
patella syndrome (hereditary osteo-onychodysplasia) 756.89
Nanism, nanosomia (*see also* Dwarfism) 259.4
hypophyseal 253.3
pituitary 253.3
renis, renalis 588.0
Nanukayami 100.89
Napkin rash 691.0
Narcissism 301.81
Narcolepsy 347
Narcosis
carbon dioxide (respiratory) 786.09
due to drug
correct substance properly administered 780.09
overdose or wrong substance given or taken 977.9
specified drug—*see* Table of drugs and chemicals
Narcotism (chronic) (*see also* listing under Dependence) 304.9
acute
correct substance properly administered 349.82
overdose or wrong substance given or taken 967.8
specified drug—*see* Table of drugs and chemicals
Narrow
anterior chamber angle 365.02
pelvis (inlet) (outlet)—*see* Contraction, pelvis
Narrowing
artery NEC 447.1
auditory, internal 433.8
basilar 433.0
with other precerebral artery 433.3
bilateral 433.3
carotid 433.1
with other precerebral artery 433.3
bilateral 433.3
cerebellar 433.8
choroidal 433.8
communicating posterior 433.8
coronary —*see also* Arteriosclerosis, coronary
congenital 746.85
due to syphilis 090.5
hypophyseal 433.8
pontine 433.8
precerebral NEC 433.9
multiple or bilateral 433.3
specified NEC 433.8
Narrowing—*continued*
vertebral 433.2
with other precerebral artery 433.3
bilateral 433.3
auditory canal (external) (*see also* Stricture, ear canal, acquired) 380.50
cerebral arteries 437.0
cicatricial—*see* Cicatrix
congenital—*see* Anomaly, congenital
coronary artery—*see* Narrowing, artery, coronary
ear, middle 385.22
Eustachian tube (*see also* Obstruction, Eustachian tube) 381.60
eyelid 374.46
congenital 743.62
intervertebral disc or space NEC—*see* Degeneration, intervertebral disc
joint space, hip 719.85
larynx 478.74
lids 374.46
congenital 743.62
mesenteric artery (with gangrene) 557.0
palate 524.8
palpebral fissure 374.46
retinal artery 362.13
ureter 593.3
urethra (*see also* Stricture, urethra) 598.9
Narrowness, abnormal, eyelid 743.62
Nasal —*see* condition
Nasolacrimal —*see* condition
Nasopharyngeal —*see also* condition
bursa 478.29
pituitary gland 759.2
torticollis 723.5
Nasopharyngitis (acute) (infective) (subacute) 460
chronic 472.2
due to external agent—*see* Condition, respiratory, chronic, due to
due to external agent—*see* Condition, respiratory, due to
septic 034.0
streptococcal 034.0
suppurative (chronic) 472.2
ulcerative (chronic) 472.2
Nasopharynx, nasopharyngeal —*see* condition
Natal tooth, teeth 520.6
Nausea (*see also* Vomiting) 787.02
epidemic 078.82
gravidarum—*see* Hyperemesis, gravidarum
marina 994.6
with vomiting 787.01
Naval —*see* condition
Neapolitan fever (*see also* Brucellosis) 023.9
Nearsightedness 367.1
Near-syncope 780.2
Nebécourt's syndrome 253.3
Nebula, cornea (eye) 371.01
congenital 743.43
interfering with vision 743.42
Necator americanus infestation 126.1
Necatoriasis 126.1
Neck —*see* condition
Necrencephalus (*see also* Softening, brain) 437.8
Necrobacillosis 040.3

Necrobiosis 799.8
brain or cerebral (*see also* Softening, brain) 437.8
lipoidica 709.3
diabeticorum 250.8 *[709.3]*
Necrodermolysis 695.1
Necrolysis, toxic epidermal 695.1
due to drug
correct substance properly administered 695.1
overdose or wrong substance given or taken 977.9
specified drug—*see* Table of drugs and chemicals
Necrophilia 302.89
Necrosis, necrotic
adrenal (capsule) (gland) 255.8
antrum, nasal sinus 478.1
aorta (hyaline) (*see also* Aneurysm, aorta) 441.9
cystic medial 441.00
abdominal 441.02
thoracic 441.01
thoracoabdominal 441.03
ruptured 441.5
arteritis 446.0
artery 447.5
aseptic, bone 733.40
femur (head) (neck) 733.42
medial condyle 733.43
humoral head 733.41
medial femoral condyle 733.43
specified site NEC 733.49
talus 733.44
avascular, bone NEC (*see also* Necrosis, aseptic, bone) 733.40
bladder (aseptic) (sphincter) 596.8
bone (*see also* Osteomyelitis) 730.1
acute 730.0
aseptic or avascular 733.40
femur (head) (neck) 733.42
medial condyle 733.43
humoral head 733.41
medial femoral condyle 733.43
specified site NEC 733.49
talus 733.44
ethmoid 478.1
ischemic 733.40
jaw 526.4
marrow 289.8
Paget's (osteitis deformans) 731.0
tuberculous—*see* Tuberculosis, bone
brain (softening) (*see also* Softening, brain) 437.8
breast (aseptic) (fat) (segmental) 611.3
bronchus, bronchi 519.1
central nervous system NEC (*see also* Softening, brain) 437.8
cerebellar (*see also* Softening, brain) 437.8
cerebral (softening) (*see also* Softening, brain) 437.8
cerebrospinal (softening) (*see also* Softening, brain) 437.8
cornea (*see also* Keratitis) 371.40
cortical, kidney 583.6
cystic medial (aorta) 441.00
abdominal 441.02
thoracic 441.01
thoracoabdominal 441.03
dental 521.0
pulp 522.1

Necrosis, necrotic—*continued*
due to swallowing corrosive substance—*see* Burn, by site
ear (ossicle) 385.24
esophagus 530.89
ethmoid (bone) 478.1
eyelid 374.50
fat, fatty (generalized) (*see also* Degeneration, fatty) 272.8
breast (aseptic) (segmental) 611.3
intestine 569.89
localized—*see* Degeneration, by site, fatty
mesentery 567.8
omentum 567.8
pancreas 577.8
peritoneum 567.8
skin (subcutaneous) 709.3
newborn 778.1
femur (aseptic) (avascular) 733.42
head 733.42
medial condyle 733.43
neck 733.42
gallbladder (*see also* Cholecystitis, acute) 575.0
gangrenous 785.4
gastric 537.89
glottis 478.79
heart (myocardium)—*see* Infarct, myocardium
hepatic (*see also* Necrosis, liver) 570
hip (aseptic) (avascular) 733.42
intestine (acute) (hemorrhagic) (massive) 557.0
ischemic 785.4
jaw 526.4
kidney (bilateral) 583.9
acute 584.9
cortical 583.6
acute 584.6
with
abortion—*see* Abortion, by type, with renal failure
ectopic pregnancy (*see also* categories 633.0-633.9) 639.3
molar pregnancy (*see also* categories 630-632) 639.3
complicating pregnancy 646.2
affecting fetus or newborn 760.1
following labor and delivery 669.3
medullary (papillary) (*see also* Pyelitis) 590.80
in
acute renal failure 584.7
nephritis, nephropathy 583.7
papillary (*see also* Pyelitis) 590.80
in
acute renal failure 584.7
nephritis, nephropathy 583.7
tubular 584.5
with
abortion—*see* Abortion, by type, with renal failure
ectopic pregnancy (*see also* categories 633.0-633.9) 639.3
molar pregnancy (*see also* categories 630-632) 639.3
complicating
abortion 639.3
ectopic or molar pregnancy 639.3
pregnancy 646.2
affecting fetus or newborn 760.1
following labor and delivery 669.3
traumatic 958.5
larynx 478.79

Necrosis, necrotic—*continued*
liver (acute) (congenital) (diffuse) (massive) (subacute) 570
with
abortion—*see* Abortion, by type, with specified complication NEC
ectopic pregnancy (*see also* categories 633.0-633.9) 639.8
molar pregnancy (*see also* categories 630-632) 639.8
complicating pregnancy 646.7
affecting fetus or newborn 760.8
following
abortion 639.8
ectopic or molar pregnancy 639.8
obstetrical 646.7
postabortal 639.8
puerperal, postpartum 674.8
toxic 573.3
lung 513.0
lymphatic gland 683
mammary gland 611.3
mastoid (chronic) 383.1
mesentery 557.0
fat 567.8
mitral valve—*see* Insufficiency, mitral
myocardium, myocardial—*see* Infarct, myocardium
nose (septum) 478.1
omentum 557.0
with mesenteric infarction 557.0
fat 567.8
orbit, orbital 376.10
ossicles, ear (aseptic) 385.24
ovary (*see also* Salpingo-oophoritis) 614.2
pancreas (aseptic) (duct) (fat) 577.8
acute 577.0
infective 577.0
papillary, kidney (*see also* Pyelitis) 590.80
peritoneum 557.0
with mesenteric infarction 557.0
fat 567.8
pharynx 462
in granulocytopenia 288.0
phosphorus 983.9
pituitary (gland) (postpartum) (Sheehan) 253.2
placenta (*see also* Placenta, abnormal) 656.7
pneumonia 513.0
pulmonary 513.0
pulp (dental) 522.1
pylorus 537.89
radiation—*see* Necrosis, by site
radium—*see* Necrosis, by site
renal—*see* Necrosis, kidney
sclera 379.19
scrotum 608.89
skin or subcutaneous tissue 709.8
due to burn—*see* Burn, by site
gangrenous 785.4
spine, spinal (column) 730.18
acute 730.18
cord 336.1
spleen 289.59
stomach 537.89
stomatitis 528.1
subcutaneous fat 709.3
fetus or newborn 778.1
subendocardial—*see* Infarct, myocardium
suprarenal (capsule) (gland) 255.8

Necrosis, necrotic—*continued*
teeth, tooth 521.0
testis 608.89
thymus (gland) 254.8
tonsil 474.8
trachea 519.1
tuberculous NEC—*see* Tuberculosis
tubular (acute) (anoxic) (toxic) 584.5
due to a procedure 997.5
umbilical cord, affecting fetus or newborn 762.6
vagina 623.8
vertebra (lumbar) 730.18
acute 730.18
tuberculous (*see also* Tuberculosis) 015.0 *[730.8]*
vesical (aseptic) (bladder) 596.8
x-ray—*see* Necrosis, by site
Necrospermia 606.0
Necrotizing angiitis 446.0
Negativism 301.7
Neglect (child) (newborn) NEC 995.5
affecting parent or family V61.21
after or at birth 995.5
affecting parent or family V61.21
hemispatial 781.8
left-sided 781.8
sensory 781.8
specified person other than child 995.81
visuospatial 781.8
Negri bodies 071
Neill-Dingwall syndrome (microcephaly and dwarfism) 759.89
Neisserian infection NEC—*see* Gonococcus
Nematodiasis NEC (*see also* Infestation, Nematode) 127.9
ancylostoma (*see also* Ancylostomiasis) 126.9
Neoformans cryptococcus infection 117.5
Neonatal —*see also* condition
teeth, tooth 520.6
Neonatorum —*see* condition

"N" listing resumes after "Neoplasm, neoplastic" table…

	Malignant — Primary	Malignant — Secondary	Malignant — Ca in situ	Benign	Uncertain Behavior	Unspecified
Neoplasm, neoplastic	**199.1**	**199.1**	**234.9**	**229.9**	**238.9**	**239.9**

Note—1. The list below gives the code numbers for neoplasms by anatomical site. For each site there are six possible code numbers according to whether the neoplasm in question is malignant, benign, in situ, of uncertain behavior, or of unspecified nature. The description of the neoplasm will often indicate which of the six columns is appropriate; e.g., malignant melanoma of skin, benign fibroadenoma of breast, carcinoma in situ of cervix uteri.

Where such descriptors are not present, the remainder of the Index should be consulted where guidance is given to the appropriate column for each morphological (histological) variety listed; e.g., Mesonephroma—see Neoplasm, malignant; Embryoma—see also Neoplasm, uncertain behavior; Disease, Bowen's—see Neoplasm, skin, in situ. However, the guidance in the Index can be overridden if one of the descriptors mentioned above is present; e.g., malignant adenoma of colon is coded to 153.9 and not to 211.3 as the adjective "malignant" overrides the Index entry "Adenoma—see also Neoplasm, benign."

Note—2. Sites marked with the sign * (e.g., face NEC*) should be classified to malignant neoplasm of skin of these sites if the variety of neoplasm is a squamous cell carcinoma or an epidermoid carcinoma and to benign neoplasm of skin of these sites if the variety of neoplasm is a papilloma (any type).

	Primary	Secondary	Ca in situ	Benign	Uncertain Behavior	Unspecified
abdomen, abdominal	195.2	198.89	234.8	229.8	238.8	239.8
cavity	195.2	198.89	234.8	229.8	238.8	239.8
organ	195.2	198.89	234.8	229.8	238.8	239.8
viscera	195.2	198.89	234.8	229.8	238.8	239.8
wall	173.5	198.2	232.5	216.5	238.2	239.2
connective tissue	171.5	198.89	—	215.5	238.1	239.2
abdominopelvic	195.8	198.89	234.8	229.8	238.8	239.8
accessory sinus—*see* Neoplasm, sinus						
acoustic nerve	192.0	198.4	—	225.1	237.9	239.7
acromion (process)	170.4	198.5	—	213.4	238.0	239.2
adenoid (pharynx) (tissue)	147.1	198.89	230.0	210.7	235.1	239.0
adipose tissue *(see also* Neoplasm, connective tissue)	171.9	198.89	—	215.9	238.1	239.2
adnexa (uterine)	183.9	198.82	233.3	221.8	236.3	239.5
adrenal (cortex) (gland) (medulla)	194.0	198.7	234.8	227.0	237.2	239.7
ala nasi (external)	173.3	198.2	232.3	216.3	238.2	239.2
alimentary canal or tract NEC	159.9	197.8	230.9	211.9	235.5	239.0
alveolar	143.9	198.89	230.0	210.4	235.1	239.0
mucosa	143.9	198.89	230.0	210.4	235.1	239.0
lower	143.1	198.89	230.0	210.4	235.1	239.0
upper	143.0	198.89	230.0	210.4	235.1	239.0
ridge or process	170.1	198.5	—	213.1	238.0	239.2
carcinoma	143.9	—	—	—	—	—
lower	143.1	—	—	—	—	—
upper	143.0	—	—	—	—	—
lower	170.1	198.5	—	213.1	238.0	239.2
mucosa	143.9	198.89	230.0	210.4	235.1	239.0
lower	143.1	198.89	230.0	210.4	235.1	239.0
upper	143.0	198.89	230.0	210.4	235.1	239.0
upper	170.0	198.5	—	213.0	238.0	239.2
sulcus	145.1	198.89	230.0	210.4	235.1	239.0
alveolus	143.9	198.89	230.0	210.4	235.1	239.0
lower	143.1	198.89	230.0	210.4	235.1	239.0
upper	143.0	198.89	230.0	210.4	235.1	239.0
ampulla of Vater	156.2	197.8	230.8	211.5	235.3	239.0
ankle NEC*	195.5	198.89	232.7	229.8	238.8	239.8
anorectum, anorectal (junction)	154.8	197.5	230.7	211.4	235.2	239.0
antecubital fossa or space*	195.4	198.89	232.6	229.8	238.8	239.8
antrum (Highmore) (maxillary)	160.2	197.3	231.8	212.0	235.9	239.1
pyloric	151.2	197.8	230.2	211.1	235.2	239.0
tympanicum	160.1	197.3	231.8	212.0	235.9	239.1
anus, anal	154.3	197.5	230.6	211.4	235.5	239.0
canal	154.2	197.5	230.5	211.4	235.5	239.0

	Malignant					
	Primary	Secondary	Ca in situ	Benign	Uncertain Behavior	Unspecified
anus, anal—*continued*						
contiguous sites with rectosigmoid junction or rectum	154.8	—	—	—	—	—
margin	173.5	198.2	232.5	216.5	238.2	239.2
skin	173.5	198.2	232.5	216.5	238.2	239.2
sphincter	154.2	197.5	230.5	211.4	235.5	239.0
aorta (thoracic)	171.4	198.89	—	215.4	238.1	239.2
abdominal	171.5	198.89	—	215.5	238.1	239.2
aortic body	194.6	198.89	—	227.6	237.3	239.7
aponeurosis	171.9	198.89	—	215.9	238.1	239.2
palmar	171.2	198.89	—	215.2	238.1	239.2
plantar	171.3	198.89	—	215.3	238.1	239.2
appendix	153.5	197.5	230.3	211.3	235.2	239.0
arachnoid (cerebral)	192.1	198.4	—	225.2	237.6	239.7
spinal	192.3	198.4	—	225.4	237.6	239.7
areola (female)	174.0	198.81	233.0	217	238.3	239.3
male	175.0	198.81	233.0	217	238.3	239.3
arm NEC*	195.4	198.89	232.6	229.8	238.8	239.8
artery—*see* Neoplasm, connective tissue						
aryepiglottic fold	148.2	198.89	230.0	210.8	235.1	239.0
hypopharyngeal aspect	148.2	198.89	230.0	210.8	235.1	239.0
laryngeal aspect	161.1	197.3	231.0	212.1	235.6	239.1
marginal zone	148.2	198.89	230.0	210.8	235.1	239.0
arytenoid (cartilage)	161.3	197.3	231.0	212.1	235.6	239.1
fold—*see* Neoplasm, aryepiglottic						
atlas	170.2	198.5	—	213.2	238.0	239.2
atrium, cardiac	164.1	198.89	—	212.7	238.8	239.8
auditory						
canal (external) (skin)	173.2	198.2	232.2	216.2	238.2	239.2
internal	160.1	197.3	231.8	212.0	235.9	239.1
nerve	192.0	198.4	—	225.1	237.9	239.7
tube	160.1	197.3	231.8	212.0	235.9	239.1
opening	147.2	198.89	230.0	210.7	235.1	239.0
auricle, ear	173.2	198.2	232.2	216.2	238.2	239.2
cartilage	171.0	198.89	—	215.0	238.1	239.2
auricular canal (external)	173.2	198.2	232.2	216.2	238.2	239.2
internal	160.1	197.3	231.8	212.0	235.9	239.1
autonomic nerve or nervous system NEC	171.9	198.89	—	215.9	238.1	239.2
axilla, axillary	195.1	198.89	234.8	229.8	238.8	239.8
fold	173.5	198.2	232.5	216.5	238.2	239.2
back NEC*	195.8	198.89	232.5	229.8	238.8	239.8
Bartholin's gland	184.1	198.82	233.3	221.2	236.3	239.5
basal ganglia	191.0	198.3	—	225.0	237.5	239.6
basis pedunculi	191.7	198.3	—	225.0	237.5	239.6
bile or biliary (tract)	156.9	197.8	230.8	211.5	235.3	239.0
canaliculi (biliferi) (intrahepatic)	155.1	197.8	230.8	211.5	235.3	239.0
canals, interlobular	155.1	197.8	230.8	211.5	235.3	239.0
contiguous sites	156.8	—	—	—	—	—
duct or passage (common) (cyst) (extrahepatic)	156.1	197.8	230.8	211.5	235.3	239.0
contiguous sites with gallbladder	156.8	—	—	—	—	—
interlobular	155.1	197.8	230.8	211.5	235.3	239.0
intrahepatic	155.1	197.8	230.8	211.5	235.3	239.0
and extrahepatic	156.9	197.8	230.8	211.5	235.3	239.0
bladder (urinary)	188.9	198.1	233.7	223.3	236.7	239.4
contiguous sites	188.8	—	—	—	—	—
dome	188.1	198.1	233.7	223.3	236.7	239.4
neck	188.5	198.1	233.7	223.3	236.7	239.4
orifice	188.9	198.1	233.7	223.3	236.7	239.4
ureteric	188.6	198.1	233.7	223.3	236.7	239.4
urethral	188.5	198.1	233.7	223.3	236.7	239.4
sphincter	188.8	198.1	233.7	223.3	236.7	239.4
trigone	188.0	198.1	233.7	223.3	236.7	239.4

	Malignant Primary	Malignant Secondary	Malignant Ca in situ	Benign	Uncertain Behavior	Unspecified
urachus	188.7	—	233.7	223.3	236.7	239.4
wall	188.9	198.1	233.7	223.3	236.7	239.4
anterior	188.3	198.1	233.7	223.3	236.7	239.4
lateral	188.2	198.1	233.7	223.3	236.7	239.4
posterior	188.4	198.1	233.7	223.3	236.7	239.4
blood vessel—*see* Neoplasm, connective tissue						

Note—Carcinomas and adenocarcinomas, of any type other than intraosseous or odontogenic, of the sites listed under "Neoplasm, bone" should be considered as constituting metastatic spread from an unspecified primary site and coded to 198.5 for morbidity coding and to 199.1 for underlying cause of death coding.

	Malignant Primary	Malignant Secondary	Malignant Ca in situ	Benign	Uncertain Behavior	Unspecified
bone (periosteum)	170.9	198.5	—	213.9	238.0	239.2
acetabulum	170.6	198.5	—	213.6	238.0	239.2
acromion (process)	170.4	198.5	—	213.4	238.0	239.2
ankle	170.8	198.5	—	213.8	238.0	239.2
arm NEC	170.4	198.5	—	213.4	238.0	239.2
astragalus	170.8	198.5	—	213.8	238.0	239.2
atlas	170.2	198.5	—	213.2	238.0	239.2
axis	170.2	198.5	—	213.2	238.0	239.2
back NEC	170.2	198.5	—	213.2	238.0	239.2
calcaneus	170.8	198.5	—	213.8	238.0	239.2
calvarium	170.0	198.5	—	213.0	238.0	239.2
carpus (any)	170.5	198.5	—	213.5	238.0	239.2
cartilage NEC	170.9	198.5	—	213.9	238.0	239.2
clavicle	170.3	198.5	—	213.3	238.0	239.2
clivus	170.0	198.5	—	213.0	238.0	239.2
coccygeal vertebra	170.6	198.5	—	213.6	238.0	239.2
coccyx	170.6	198.5	—	213.6	238.0	239.2
costal cartilage	170.3	198.5	—	213.3	238.0	239.2
costovertebral joint	170.3	198.5	—	213.3	238.0	239.2
cranial	170.0	198.5	—	213.0	238.0	239.2
cuboid	170.8	198.5	—	213.8	238.0	239.2
cuneiform	170.9	198.5	—	213.9	238.0	239.2
ankle	170.8	198.5	—	213.8	238.0	239.2
wrist	170.5	198.5	—	213.5	238.0	239.2
digital	170.9	198.5	—	213.9	238.0	239.2
finger	170.5	198.5	—	213.5	238.0	239.2
toe	170.8	198.5	—	213.8	238.0	239.2
elbow	170.4	198.5	—	213.4	238.0	239.2
ethmoid (labyrinth)	170.0	198.5	—	213.0	238.0	239.2
face	170.0	198.5	—	213.0	238.0	239.2
lower jaw	170.1	198.5	—	213.1	238.0	239.2
femur (any part)	170.7	198.5	—	213.7	238.0	239.2
fibula (any part)	170.7	198.5	—	213.7	238.0	239.2
finger (any)	170.5	198.5	—	213.5	238.0	239.2
foot	170.8	198.5	—	213.8	238.0	239.2
forearm	170.4	198.5	—	213.4	238.0	239.2
frontal	170.0	198.5	—	213.0	238.0	239.2
hand	170.5	198.5	—	213.5	238.0	239.2
heel	170.8	198.5	—	213.8	238.0	239.2
hip	170.6	198.5	—	213.6	238.0	239.2
humerus (any part)	170.4	198.5	—	213.4	238.0	239.2
hyoid	170.0	198.5	—	213.0	238.0	239.2
ilium	170.6	198.5	—	213.6	238.0	239.2
innominate	170.6	198.5	—	213.6	238.0	239.2
intervertebral cartilage or disc	170.2	198.5	—	213.2	238.0	239.2
ischium	170.6	198.5	—	213.6	238.0	239.2
jaw (lower)	170.1	198.5	—	213.1	238.0	239.2
upper	170.0	198.5	—	213.0	238.0	239.2
knee	170.7	198.5	—	213.7	238.0	239.2
leg NEC	170.7	198.5	—	213.7	238.0	239.2
limb NEC	170.9	198.5	—	213.9	238.0	239.2
lower (long bones)	170.7	198.5	—	213.7	238.0	239.2

	Malignant: Primary	Malignant: Secondary	Malignant: Ca in situ	Benign	Uncertain Behavior	Unspecified
bone—*continued*						
short bones	170.8	198.5	—	213.8	238.0	239.2
upper (long bones)	170.4	198.5	—	213.4	238.0	239.2
short bones	170.5	198.5	—	213.5	238.0	239.2
long	170.9	198.5	—	213.9	238.0	239.2
lower limbs NEC	170.7	198.5	—	213.7	238.0	239.2
upper limbs NEC	170.4	198.5	—	213.4	238.0	239.2
malar	170.0	198.5	—	213.0	238.0	239.2
mandible	170.1	198.5	—	213.1	238.0	239.2
marrow NEC	202.9	198.5	—	—	—	238.7
mastoid	170.0	198.5	—	213.0	238.0	239.2
maxilla, maxillary (superior)	170.0	198.5	—	213.0	238.0	239.2
inferior	170.1	198.5	—	213.1	238.0	239.2
metacarpus (any)	170.5	198.5	—	213.5	238.0	239.2
metatarsus (any)	170.8	198.5	—	213.8	238.0	239.2
navicular (ankle)	170.8	198.5	—	213.8	238.0	239.2
hand	170.5	198.5	—	213.5	238.0	239.2
nose, nasal	170.0	198.5	—	213.0	238.0	239.2
occipital	170.0	198.5	—	213.0	238.0	239.2
orbit	170.0	198.5	—	213.0	238.0	239.2
parietal	170.0	198.5	—	213.0	238.0	239.2
patella	170.8	198.5	—	213.8	238.0	239.2
pelvic	170.6	198.5	—	213.6	238.0	239.2
phalanges	170.9	198.5	—	213.9	238.0	239.2
foot	170.8	198.5	—	213.8	238.0	239.2
hand	170.5	198.5	—	213.5	238.0	239.2
pubic	170.6	198.5	—	213.6	238.0	239.2
radius (any part)	170.4	198.5	—	213.4	238.0	239.2
rib	170.3	198.5	—	213.3	238.0	239.2
sacral vertebra	170.6	198.5	—	213.6	238.0	239.2
sacrum	170.6	198.5	—	213.6	238.0	239.2
scaphoid (of hand)	170.5	198.5	—	213.5	238.0	239.2
of ankle	170.8	198.5	—	213.8	238.0	239.2
scapula (any part)	170.4	198.5	—	213.4	238.0	239.2
sella turcica	170.0	198.5	—	213.0	238.0	239.2
short	170.9	198.5	—	213.9	238.0	239.2
lower limb	170.8	198.5	—	213.8	238.0	239.2
upper limb	170.5	198.5	—	213.5	238.0	239.2
shoulder	170.4	198.5	—	213.4	238.0	239.2
skeleton, skeletal NEC	170.9	198.5	—	213.9	238.0	239.2
skull	170.0	198.5	—	213.0	238.0	239.2
sphenoid	170.0	198.5	—	213.0	238.0	239.2
spine, spinal (column)	170.2	198.5	—	213.2	238.0	239.2
coccyx	170.6	198.5	—	213.6	238.0	239.2
sacrum	170.6	198.5	—	213.6	238.0	239.2
sternum	170.3	198.5	—	213.3	238.0	239.2
tarsus (any)	170.8	198.5	—	213.8	238.0	239.2
temporal	170.0	198.5	—	213.0	238.0	239.2
thumb	170.5	198.5	—	213.5	238.0	239.2
tibia (any part)	170.7	198.5	—	213.7	238.0	239.2
toe (any)	170.8	198.5	—	213.8	238.0	239.2
trapezium	170.5	198.5	—	213.5	238.0	239.2
trapezoid	170.5	198.5	—	213.5	238.0	239.2
turbinate	170.0	198.5	—	213.0	238.0	239.2
ulna (any part)	170.4	198.5	—	213.4	238.0	239.2
unciform	170.5	198.5	—	213.5	238.0	239.2
vertebra (column)	170.2	198.5	—	213.2	238.0	239.2
coccyx	170.6	198.5	—	213.6	238.0	239.2
sacrum	170.6	198.5	—	213.6	238.0	239.2
vomer	170.0	198.5	—	213.0	238.0	239.2
wrist	170.5	198.5	—	213.5	238.0	239.2
xiphoid process	170.3	198.5	—	213.3	238.0	239.2
zygomatic	170.0	198.5	—	213.0	238.0	239.2

	Malignant Primary	Malignant Secondary	Malignant Ca in situ	Benign	Uncertain Behavior	Unspecified
book-leaf (mouth)	145.8	198.89	230.0	210.4	235.1	239.0
bowel—*see* Neoplasm, intestine						
brachial plexus	171.2	198.89	—	215.2	238.1	239.2
brain NEC	191.9	198.3	—	225.0	237.5	239.6
basal ganglia	191.0	198.3	—	225.0	237.5	239.6
cerebellopontine angle	191.6	198.3	—	225.0	237.5	239.6
cerebellum NOS	191.6	198.3	—	225.0	237.5	239.6
cerebrum	191.0	198.3	—	225.0	237.5	239.6
choroid plexus	191.5	198.3	—	225.0	237.5	239.6
contiguous sites	191.8	—	—	—	—	—
corpus callosum	191.8	198.3	—	225.0	237.5	239.6
corpus striatum	191.0	198.3	—	225.0	237.5	239.6
cortex (cerebral)	191.0	198.3	—	225.0	237.5	239.6
frontal lobe	191.1	198.3	—	225.0	237.5	239.6
globus pallidus	191.0	198.3	—	225.0	237.5	239.6
hippocampus	191.2	198.3	—	225.0	237.5	239.6
hypothalamus	191.0	198.3	—	225.0	237.5	239.6
internal capsule	191.0	198.3	—	225.0	237.5	239.6
medulla oblongata	191.7	198.3	—	225.0	237.5	239.6
meninges	192.1	198.4	—	225.2	237.6	239.7
midbrain	191.7	198.3	—	225.0	237.5	239.6
occipital lobe	191.4	198.3	—	225.0	237.5	239.6
parietal lobe	191.3	198.3	—	225.0	237.5	239.6
peduncle	191.7	198.3	—	225.0	237.5	239.6
pons	191.7	198.3	—	225.0	237.5	239.6
stem	191.7	198.3	—	225.0	237.5	239.6
tapetum	191.8	198.3	—	225.0	237.5	239.6
temporal lobe	191.2	198.3	—	225.0	237.5	239.6
thalamus	191.0	198.3	—	225.0	237.5	239.6
uncus	191.2	198.3	—	225.0	237.5	239.6
ventricle (floor)	191.5	198.3	—	225.0	237.5	239.6
branchial (cleft) (vestiges)	146.8	198.89	230.0	210.6	235.1	239.0
breast (connective tissue) (female) (glandular tissue) (soft parts)	174.9	198.81	233.0	217	238.3	239.3
areola	174.0	198.81	233.0	217	238.3	239.3
male	175.0	198.81	233.0	217	238.3	239.3
axillary tail	174.6	198.81	233.0	217	238.3	239.3
central portion	174.1	198.81	233.0	217	238.3	239.3
contiguous sites	174.8	—	—	—	—	—
ectopic sites	174.8	198.81	233.0	217	238.3	239.3
inner	174.8	198.81	233.0	217	238.3	239.3
lower	174.8	198.81	233.0	217	238.3	239.3
lower-inner quadrant	174.3	198.81	233.0	217	238.3	239.3
lower-outer quadrant	174.5	198.81	233.0	217	238.3	239.3
male	175.9	198.81	233.0	217	238.3	239.3
areola	175.0	198.81	233.0	217	238.3	239.3
ectopic tissue	175.9	198.81	233.0	217	238.3	239.3
nipple	175.0	198.81	233.0	217	238.3	239.3
mastectomy site (skin)	173.5	198.2	—	—	—	—
specified as breast tissue	174.8	198.81	—	—	—	—
midline	174.8	198.81	233.0	217	238.3	239.3
nipple	174.0	198.81	233.0	217	238.3	239.3
male	175.0	198.81	233.0	217	238.3	239.3
outer	174.8	198.81	233.0	217	238.3	239.3
skin	173.5	198.2	232.5	216.5	238.2	239.2
tail (axillary)	174.6	198.81	233.0	217	238.3	239.3
upper	174.8	198.81	233.0	217	238.3	239.3
upper-inner quadrant	174.2	198.81	233.0	217	238.3	239.3
upper-outer quadrant	174.4	198.81	233.0	217	238.3	239.3
broad ligament	183.3	198.82	233.3	221.0	236.3	239.5
bronchiogenic, bronchogenic (lung)	162.9	197.0	231.2	212.3	235.7	239.1
bronchiole	162.9	197.0	231.2	212.3	235.7	239.1

	Malignant					
	Primary	Secondary	Ca in situ	Benign	Uncertain Behavior	Unspecified
bronchus	162.9	197.0	231.2	212.3	235.7	239.1
carina	162.2	197.0	231.2	212.3	235.7	239.1
contiguous sites with lung or trachea	162.8	—	—	—	—	—
lower lobe of lung	162.5	197.0	231.2	212.3	235.7	239.1
main	162.2	197.0	231.2	212.3	235.7	239.1
middle lobe of lung	162.4	197.0	231.2	212.3	235.7	239.1
upper lobe of lung	162.3	197.0	231.2	212.3	235.7	239.1
brow	173.3	198.2	232.3	216.3	238.2	239.2
buccal (cavity)	145.9	198.89	230.0	210.4	235.1	239.0
commissure	145.0	198.89	230.0	210.4	235.1	239.0
groove (lower) (upper)	145.1	198.89	230.0	210.4	235.1	239.0
mucosa	145.0	198.89	230.0	210.4	235.1	239.0
sulcus (lower) (upper)	145.1	198.89	230.0	210.4	235.1	239.0
bulbourethral gland	189.3	198.1	233.9	223.81	236.99	239.5
bursa—*see* Neoplasm, connective tissue						
buttock NEC*	195.3	198.89	232.5	229.8	238.8	239.8
calf*	195.5	198.89	232.7	229.8	238.8	239.8
calvarium	170.0	198.5	—	213.0	238.0	239.2
calyx, renal	189.1	198.0	233.9	223.1	236.91	239.5
canal						
anal	154.2	197.5	230.5	211.4	235.5	239.0
auditory (external)	173.2	198.2	232.2	216.2	238.2	239.2
auricular (external)	173.2	198.2	232.2	216.2	238.2	239.2
canaliculi, biliary (biliferi) (intrahepatic)	155.1	197.8	230.8	211.5	235.3	239.0
canthus (eye) (inner) (outer)	173.1	198.2	232.1	216.1	238.2	239.2
capillary—*see* Neoplasm, connective tissue						
caput coli	153.4	197.5	230.3	211.3	235.2	239.0
cardia (gastric)	151.0	197.8	230.2	211.1	235.2	239.0
cardiac orifice (stomach)	151.0	197.8	230.2	211.1	235.2	239.0
cardio-esophageal junction	151.0	197.8	230.2	211.1	235.2	239.0
cardio-esophagus	151.0	197.8	230.2	211.1	235.2	239.0
carina (bronchus)	162.2	197.0	231.2	212.3	235.7	239.1
carotid (artery)	171.0	198.89	—	215.0	238.1	239.2
body	194.5	198.89	—	227.5	237.3	239.7
carpus (any bone)	170.5	198.5	—	213.5	238.0	239.2
cartilage (articular) (joint) NEC—*see also* Neoplasm, bone	170.9	198.5	—	213.9	238.0	239.2
arytenoid	161.3	197.3	231.0	212.1	235.6	239.1
auricular	171.0	198.89	—	215.0	238.1	239.2
bronchi	162.2	197.3	—	212.3	235.7	239.1
connective tissue—*see* Neoplasm, connective tissue						
costal	170.3	198.5	—	213.3	238.0	239.2
cricoid	161.3	197.3	231.0	212.1	235.6	239.1
cuneiform	161.3	197.3	231.0	212.1	235.6	239.1
ear (external)	171.0	198.89	—	215.0	238.1	239.2
ensiform	170.3	198.5	—	213.3	238.0	239.2
epiglottis	161.1	197.3	231.0	212.1	235.6	239.1
anterior surface	146.4	198.89	230.0	210.6	235.1	239.0
eyelid	171.0	198.89	—	215.0	238.1	239.2
intervertebral	170.2	198.5	—	213.2	238.0	239.2
larynx, laryngeal	161.3	197.3	231.0	212.1	235.6	239.1
nose, nasal	160.0	197.3	231.8	212.0	235.9	239.1
pinna	171.0	198.89	—	215.0	238.1	239.2
rib	170.3	198.5	—	213.3	238.0	239.2
semilunar (knee)	170.7	198.5	—	213.7	238.0	239.2
thyroid	161.3	197.3	231.0	212.1	235.6	239.1
trachea	162.0	197.3	231.1	212.2	235.7	239.1
cauda equina	192.2	198.3	—	225.3	237.5	239.7
cavity						
buccal	145.9	198.89	230.0	210.4	235.1	239.0
nasal	160.0	197.3	231.8	212.0	235.9	239.1
oral	145.9	198.89	230.0	210.4	235.1	239.0

	Malignant					
	Primary	Secondary	Ca in situ	Benign	Uncertain Behavior	Unspecified
cavity—*continued*						
peritoneal	158.9	197.6	—	211.8	235.4	239.0
tympanic	160.1	197.3	231.8	212.0	235.9	239.1
cecum	153.4	197.5	230.3	211.3	235.2	239.0
central						
nervous system—*see* Neoplasm, nervous system						
white matter	191.0	198.3	—	225.0	237.5	239.6
cerebellopontine (angle)	191.6	198.3	—	225.0	237.5	239.6
cerebellum, cerebellar	191.6	198.3	—	225.0	237.5	239.6
cerebrum, cerebral (cortex) (hemisphere) (white matter)	191.0	198.3	—	225.0	237.5	239.6
meninges	192.1	198.4	—	225.2	237.6	239.7
peduncle	191.7	198.3	—	225.0	237.5	239.6
ventricle (any)	191.5	198.3	—	225.0	237.5	239.6
cervical region	195.0	198.89	234.8	229.8	238.8	239.8
cervix (cervical) (uteri) (uterus)	180.9	198.82	233.1	219.0	236.0	239.5
canal	180.0	198.82	233.1	219.0	236.0	239.5
contiguous sites	180.8	—	—	—	—	—
endocervix (canal) (gland)	180.0	198.82	233.1	219.0	236.0	239.5
exocervix	180.1	198.82	233.1	219.0	236.0	239.5
external os	180.1	198.82	233.1	219.0	236.0	239.5
internal os	180.0	198.82	233.1	219.0	236.0	239.5
nabothian gland	180.0	198.82	233.1	219.0	236.0	239.5
squamocolumnar junction	180.8	198.82	233.1	219.0	236.0	239.5
stump	180.8	198.82	233.1	219.0	236.0	239.5
cheek	195.0	198.89	234.8	229.8	238.8	239.8
external	173.3	198.2	232.3	216.3	238.2	239.2
inner aspect	145.0	198.89	230.0	210.4	235.1	239.0
internal	145.0	198.89	230.0	210.4	235.1	239.0
mucosa	145.0	198.89	230.0	210.4	235.1	239.0
chest (wall) NEC	195.1	198.89	234.8	229.8	238.8	239.8
chiasma opticum	192.0	198.4	—	225.1	237.9	239.7
chin	173.3	198.2	232.3	216.3	238.2	239.2
choana	147.3	198.89	230.0	210.7	235.1	239.0
cholangiole	155.1	197.8	230.8	211.5	235.3	239.0
choledochal duct	156.1	197.8	230.8	211.5	235.3	239.0
choroid	190.6	198.4	234.0	224.6	238.8	239.8
plexus	191.5	198.3	—	225.0	237.5	239.6
ciliary body	190.0	198.4	234.0	224.0	238.8	239.8
clavicle	170.3	198.5	—	213.3	238.0	239.2
clitoris	184.3	198.82	233.3	221.2	236.3	239.5
clivus	170.0	198.5	—	213.0	238.0	239.2
cloacogenic zone	154.8	197.5	230.7	211.4	235.5	239.0
coccygeal						
body or glomus	194.6	198.89	—	227.6	237.3	239.7
vertebra	170.6	198.5	—	213.6	238.0	239.2
coccyx	170.6	198.5	—	213.6	238.0	239.2
colon—*see also* Neoplasm, intestine, large and rectum	154.0	197.5	230.4	211.4	235.2	239.0
column, spinal—*see* Neoplasm, spine						
columnella	173.3	198.2	232.3	216.3	238.2	239.2
commissure						
labial, lip	140.6	198.89	230.0	210.4	235.1	239.0
laryngeal	161.0	197.3	231.0	212.1	235.6	239.1
common (bile) duct	156.1	197.8	230.8	211.5	235.3	239.0
concha	173.2	198.2	232.2	216.2	238.2	239.2
nose	160.0	197.3	231.8	212.0	235.9	239.1
conjunctiva	190.3	198.4	234.0	224.3	238.8	239.8

	Malignant					
	Primary	Secondary	Ca in situ	Benign	Uncertain Behavior	Unspecified
connective tissue NEC	171.9	198.89	—	215.9	238.1	239.2

Note—For neoplasms of connective tissue (blood vessel, bursa, fasica, ligament, muscle, peripheral nerves, sympathetic and parasympathetic nerves, and ganglia, synovia, tendon, etc.) or of morphological types that indicate connective tissue, code according to the list under "Neoplasm, connective tissue;" for sites that do not appear in this list, code to neoplasm of that site; e.g.: liposarcoma, shoulder 171.2; leiomyosarcoma,stomach 151.9; neurofibroma,chest wall 215.4.

Morphological types that indicate connective tissue appear in their proper place in the alphabetic index with the instruction "see Neoplasm, connective tissue..."

	Primary	Secondary	Ca in situ	Benign	Uncertain Behavior	Unspecified
abdomen	171.5	198.89	—	215.5	238.1	239.2
abdominal wall	171.5	198.89	—	215.5	238.1	239.2
ankle	171.3	198.89	—	215.3	238.1	239.2
antecubital fossa or space	171.2	198.89	—	215.2	238.1	239.2
arm	171.2	198.89	—	215.2	238.1	239.2
auricle (ear)	171.0	198.89	—	215.0	238.1	239.2
axilla	171.4	198.89	—	215.4	238.1	239.2
back	171.7	198.89	—	215.7	238.1	239.2
breast (female) *(see also* Neoplasm, breast)	174.9	198.81	233.0	217	238.3	239.3
male	175.9	198.81	233.0	217	238.3	239.3
buttock	171.6	198.89	—	215.6	238.1	239.2
calf	171.3	198.89	—	215.3	238.1	239.2
cervical region	171.0	198.89	—	215.0	238.1	239.2
cheek	171.0	198.89	—	215.0	238.1	239.2
chest (wall)	171.4	198.89	—	215.4	238.1	239.2
chin	171.0	198.89	—	215.0	238.1	239.2
contiguous sites	171.8	—	—	—	—	—
diaphragm	171.4	198.89	—	215.4	238.1	239.2
ear (external)	171.0	198.89	—	215.0	238.1	239.2
elbow	171.2	198.89	—	215.2	238.1	239.2
extrarectal	171.6	198.89	—	215.6	238.1	239.2
extremity	171.8	198.89	—	215.8	238.1	239.2
lower	171.3	198.89	—	215.3	238.1	239.2
upper	171.2	198.89	—	215.2	238.1	239.2
eyelid	171.0	198.89	—	215.0	238.1	239.2
face	171.0	198.89	—	215.0	238.1	239.2
finger	171.2	198.89	—	215.2	238.1	239.2
flank	171.7	198.89	—	215.7	238.1	239.2
foot	171.3	198.89	—	215.3	238.1	239.2
forearm	171.2	198.89	—	215.2	238.1	239.2
forehead	171.0	198.89	—	215.0	238.1	239.2
gluteal region	171.6	198.89	—	215.6	238.1	239.2
great vessels NEC	171.4	198.89	—	215.4	238.1	239.2
groin	171.6	198.89	—	215.6	238.1	239.2
hand	171.2	198.89	—	215.2	238.1	239.2
head	171.0	198.89	—	215.0	238.1	239.2
heel	171.3	198.89	—	215.3	238.1	239.2
hip	171.3	198.89	—	215.3	238.1	239.2
hypochondrium	171.5	198.89	—	215.5	238.1	239.2
iliopsoas muscle	171.6	198.89	—	215.5	238.1	239.2
infraclavicular region	171.4	198.89	—	215.4	238.1	239.2
inguinal (canal) (region)	171.6	198.89	—	215.6	238.1	239.2
intrathoracic	171.4	198.89	—	215.4	238.1	239.2
ischorectal fossa	171.6	198.89	—	215.6	238.1	239.2
jaw	143.9	198.89	230.0	210.4	235.1	239.0
knee	171.3	198.89	—	215.3	238.1	239.2
leg	171.3	198.89	—	215.3	238.1	239.2

	Malignant Primary	Malignant Secondary	Malignant Ca in situ	Benign	Uncertain Behavior	Unspecified
connective tissue—*continued*						
limb NEC	171.9	198.89	—	215.8	238.1	239.2
lower	171.3	198.89	—	215.3	238.1	239.2
upper	171.2	198.89	—	215.2	238.1	239.2
nates	171.6	198.89	—	215.6	238.1	239.2
neck	171.0	198.89	—	215.0	238.1	239.2
orbit	190.1	198.4	234.0	224.1	238.8	239.8
pararectal	171.6	198.89	—	215.6	238.1	239.2
para-urethral	171.6	198.89	—	215.6	238.1	239.2
paravaginal	171.6	198.89	—	215.6	238.1	239.2
pelvis (floor)	171.6	198.89	—	215.6	238.1	239.2
pelvo-abdominal	171.8	198.89	—	215.8	238.1	239.2
perineum	171.6	198.89	—	215.6	238.1	239.2
perirectal (tissue)	171.6	198.89	—	215.6	238.1	239.2
periurethral (tissue)	171.6	198.89	—	215.6	238.1	239.2
popliteal fossa or space	171.3	198.89	—	215.3	238.1	239.2
presacral	171.6	198.89	—	215.6	238.1	239.2
psoas muscle	171.5	198.89	—	215.5	238.1	239.2
pterygoid fossa	171.0	198.89	—	215.0	238.1	239.2
rectovaginal septum or wall	171.6	198.89	—	215.6	238.1	239.2
rectovesical	171.6	198.89	—	215.6	238.1	239.2
retroperitoneum	158.0	197.6	—	211.8	235.4	239.0
sacrococcygeal region	171.6	198.89	—	215.6	238.1	239.2
scalp	171.0	198.89	—	215.0	238.1	239.2
scapular region	171.4	198.89	—	215.4	238.1	239.2
shoulder	171.2	198.89	—	215.2	238.1	239.2
skin (dermis) NEC	173.9	198.2	232.9	216.9	238.2	239.2
submental	171.0	198.89	—	215.0	238.1	239.2
supraclavicular region	171.0	198.89	—	215.0	238.1	239.2
temple	171.0	198.89	—	215.0	238.1	239.2
temporal region	171.0	198.89	—	215.0	238.1	239.2
thigh	171.3	198.89	—	215.3	238.1	239.2
thoracic (duct) (wall)	171.4	198.89	—	215.4	238.1	239.2
thorax	171.4	198.89	—	215.4	238.1	239.2
thumb	171.2	198.89	—	215.2	238.1	239.2
toe	171.3	198.89	—	215.3	238.1	239.2
trunk	171.7	198.89	—	215.7	238.1	239.2
umbilicus	171.5	198.89	—	215.5	238.1	239.2
vesicorectal	171.6	198.89	—	215.6	238.1	239.2
wrist	171.2	198.89	—	215.2	238.1	239.2
conus medullaris	192.2	198.3	—	225.3	237.5	239.7
cord (true) (vocal)	161.0	197.3	231.0	212.1	235.6	239.1
false	161.1	197.3	231.0	212.1	235.6	239.1
spermatic	187.6	198.82	233.6	222.8	236.6	239.5
spinal (cervical) (lumbar) (thoracic)	192.2	198.3	—	225.3	237.5	239.7
cornea (limbus)	190.4	198.4	234.0	224.4	238.8	239.8
corpus						
albicans	183.0	198.6	233.3	220	236.2	239.5
callosum, brain	191.8	198.3	—	225.0	237.5	239.6
cavernosum	187.3	198.82	233.5	222.1	236.6	239.5
gastric	151.4	197.8	230.2	211.1	235.2	239.0
penis	187.3	198.82	233.5	222.1	236.6	239.5
striatum, cerebrum	191.0	198.3	—	225.0	237.5	239.6
uteri	182.0	198.82	233.2	219.1	236.0	239.5
isthmus	182.1	198.82	233.2	219.1	236.0	239.5
cortex						
adrenal	194.0	198.7	234.8	227.0	237.2	239.7
cerebral	191.0	198.3	—	225.0	237.5	239.6
costal cartilage	170.3	198.5	—	213.3	238.0	239.2
costovertebral joint	170.3	198.5	—	213.3	238.0	239.2

	Malignant					
	Primary	Secondary	Ca in situ	Benign	Uncertain Behavior	Unspecified
Cowper's gland	189.3	198.1	233.9	223.81	236.99	239.5
cranial (fossa, any)	191.9	198.3	—	225.0	237.5	239.6
meninges	192.1	198.4	—	225.2	237.6	239.7
nerve (any)	192.0	198.4	—	225.1	237.9	239.7
craniobuccal pouch	194.3	198.89	234.8	227.3	237.0	239.7
craniopharyngeal (duct) (pouch)	194.3	198.89	234.8	227.3	237.0	239.7
cricoid	148.0	198.89	230.0	210.8	235.1	239.0
cartilage	161.3	197.3	231.0	212.1	235.6	239.1
cricopharynx	148.0	198.89	230.0	210.8	235.1	239.0
crypt of Morgagni	154.8	197.5	230.7	211.4	235.2	239.0
crystalline lens	190.0	198.4	234.0	224.0	238.8	239.8
cul-de-sac (Douglas')	158.8	197.6	—	211.8	235.4	239.0
cuneiform cartilage	161.3	197.3	231.0	212.1	235.6	239.1
cutaneous—*see* Neoplasm, skin						
cutis—*see* Neoplasm, skin						
cystic (bile) duct (common)	156.1	197.8	230.8	211.5	235.3	239.0
dermis—*see* Neoplasm, skin						
diaphragm	171.4	198.89	—	215.4	238.1	239.2
digestive organs, system, tube, tract NEC	159.9	197.8	230.9	211.9	235.5	239.0
contiguous sites with peritoneum	159.8	—	—	—	—	—
disc, intervertebral	170.2	198.5	—	213.2	238.0	239.2
disease, generalized	199.0	199.0	234.9	229.9	238.9	199.0
disseminated	199.0	199.0	234.9	229.9	238.9	199.0
Douglas' cul-de-sac or pouch	158.8	197.6	—	211.8	235.4	239.0
duodenojejunal junction	152.8	197.4	230.7	211.2	235.2	239.0
duodenum	152.0	197.4	230.7	211.2	235.2	239.0
dura (cranial) (mater)	192.1	198.4	—	225.2	237.6	239.7
cerebral	192.1	198.4	—	225.2	237.6	239.7
spinal	192.3	198.4	—	225.4	237.6	239.7
ear (external)	173.2	198.2	232.2	216.2	238.2	239.2
auricle or auris	173.2	198.2	232.2	216.2	238.2	239.2
canal, external	173.2	198.2	232.2	216.2	238.2	239.2
cartilage	171.0	198.89	—	215.0	238.1	239.2
external meatus	173.2	198.2	232.2	216.2	238.2	239.2
inner	160.1	197.3	231.8	212.0	235.9	239.1
lobule	173.2	198.2	232.2	216.2	238.2	239.2
middle	160.1	197.3	231.8	212.0	235.9	239.1
contiguous sites with accessory sinuses or nasal cavities	160.8	—	—	—	—	—
skin	173.2	198.2	232.2	216.2	238.2	239.2
earlobe	173.2	198.2	232.2	216.2	238.2	239.2
ejaculatory duct	187.8	198.82	233.6	222.8	236.6	239.5
elbow NEC*	195.4	198.89	232.6	229.8	238.8	239.8
endocardium	164.1	198.89	—	212.7	238.8	239.8
endocervix (canal) (gland)	180.0	198.82	233.1	219.0	236.0	239.5
endocrine gland NEC	194.9	198.89	—	227.9	237.4	239.7
pluriglandular NEC	194.8	198.89	234.8	227.8	237.4	239.7
endometrium (gland) (stroma)	182.0	198.82	233.2	219.1	236.0	239.5
ensiform cartilage	170.3	198.5	—	213.3	238.0	239.2
enteric—*see* Neoplasm, intestine						
ependyma (brain)	191.5	198.3	—	225.0	237.5	239.6
epicardium	164.1	198.89	—	212.7	238.8	239.8
epididymis	187.5	198.82	233.6	222.3	236.6	239.5
epidural	192.9	198.4	—	225.9	237.9	239.7
epiglottis	161.1	197.3	231.0	212.1	235.6	239.1
anterior aspect or surface	146.4	198.89	230.0	210.6	235.1	239.0
cartilage	161.3	197.3	231.0	212.1	235.6	239.1
free border (margin)	146.4	198.89	230.0	210.6	235.1	239.0
junctional region	146.5	198.89	230.0	210.6	235.1	239.0
posterior (laryngeal) surface	161.1	197.3	231.0	212.1	235.6	239.1
suprahyoid portion	161.1	197.3	231.0	212.1	235.6	239.1

	Malignant					
	Primary	Secondary	Ca in situ	Benign	Uncertain Behavior	Unspecified
esophagogastric junction	151.0	197.8	230.2	211.1	235.2	239.0
esophagus	150.9	197.8	230.1	211.0	235.5	239.0
abdominal	150.2	197.8	230.1	211.0	235.5	239.0
cervical	150.0	197.8	230.1	211.0	235.5	239.0
contiguous sites	150.8	—	—	—	—	—
distal (third)	150.5	197.8	230.1	211.0	235.5	239.0
lower (third)	150.5	197.8	230.1	211.0	235.5	239.0
middle (third)	150.4	197.8	230.1	211.0	235.5	239.0
proximal (third)	150.3	197.8	230.1	211.0	235.5	239.0
specified part NEC	150.8	197.8	230.1	211.0	235.5	239.0
thoracic	150.1	197.8	230.1	211.0	235.5	239.0
upper (third)	150.3	197.8	230.1	211.0	235.5	239.0
ethmoid (sinus)	160.3	197.3	231.8	212.0	235.9	239.1
bone or labyrinth	170.0	198.5	—	213.0	238.0	239.2
Eustachian tube	160.1	197.3	231.8	212.0	235.9	239.1
exocervix	180.1	198.82	233.1	219.0	236.0	239.5
external						
meatus (ear)	173.2	198.2	232.2	216.2	238.2	239.2
os, cervix uteri	180.1	198.82	233.1	219.0	236.0	239.5
extradural	192.9	198.4	—	225.9	237.9	239.7
extrahepatic (bile) duct	156.1	197.8	230.8	211.5	235.3	239.0
contiguous sites with gallbladder	156.8	—	—	—	—	—
extraocular muscle	190.1	198.4	234.0	224.1	238.8	239.8
extrarectal	195.3	198.89	234.8	229.8	238.8	239.8
extremity*	195.8	198.89	232.8	229.8	238.8	239.8
lower*	195.5	198.89	232.7	229.8	238.8	239.8
upper*	195.4	198.89	232.6	229.8	238.8	239.8
eye NEC	190.9	198.4	234.0	224.9	238.8	239.8
contiguous sites	190.8	—	—	—	—	—
specified sites NEC	190.8	198.4	234.0	224.8	238.8	239.8
eyeball	190.0	198.4	234.0	224.0	238.8	239.8
eyebrow	173.3	198.2	232.3	216.3	238.2	239.2
eyelid (lower) (skin) (upper)	173.1	198.2	232.1	216.1	238.2	239.2
cartilage	171.0	198.89	—	215.0	238.1	239.2
face NEC*	195.0	198.89	232.3	229.8	238.8	239.8
fallopian tube (accessory)	183.2	198.82	233.3	221.0	236.3	239.5
falx (cerebelli) (cerebri)	192.1	198.4	—	225.2	237.6	239.7
fascia—*see also* Neoplasm, connective tissue						
palmar	171.2	198.89	—	215.2	238.1	239.2
plantar	171.3	198.89	—	215.3	238.1	239.2
fatty tissue—*see* Neoplasm, connective tissue						
fauces, faucial NEC	146.9	198.89	230.0	210.6	235.1	239.0
pillars	146.2	198.89	230.0	210.6	235.1	239.0
tonsil	146.0	198.89	230.0	210.5	235.1	239.0
femur (any part)	170.7	198.5	—	213.7	238.0	239.2
fetal membrane	181	198.82	233.2	219.8	236.1	239.5
fibrous tissue—*see* Neoplasm, connective tissue						
fibula (any part)	170.7	198.5	—	213.7	238.0	239.2
filum terminale	192.2	198.3	—	225.3	237.5	239.7
finger NEC*	195.4	198.89	232.6	229.8	238.8	239.8
flank NEC*	195.8	198.89	232.5	229.8	238.8	239.8
follicle, nabothian	180.0	198.82	233.1	219.0	236.0	239.5
foot NEC*	195.5	198.89	232.7	229.8	238.8	239.8
forearm NEC*	195.4	198.89	232.6	229.8	238.8	239.8
forehead (skin)	173.3	198.2	232.3	216.3	238.2	239.2
foreskin	187.1	198.82	233.5	222.1	236.6	239.5

	Malignant					
	Primary	Secondary	Ca in situ	Benign	Uncertain Behavior	Unspecified
fornix						
pharyngeal	147.3	198.89	230.0	210.7	235.1	239.0
vagina	184.0	198.82	233.3	221.1	236.3	239.5
fossa (of)						
anterior (cranial)	191.9	198.3	—	225.0	237.5	239.6
cranial	191.9	198.3	—	225.0	237.5	239.6
ischiorectal	195.3	198.89	234.8	229.8	238.8	239.8
middle (cranial)	191.9	198.3	—	225.0	237.5	239.6
pituitary	194.3	198.89	234.8	227.3	237.0	239.7
posterior (cranial)	191.9	198.3	—	225.0	237.5	239.6
pterygoid	171.0	198.89	—	215.0	238.1	239.2
pyriform	148.1	198.89	230.0	210.8	235.1	239.0
Rosenmüller	147.2	198.89	230.0	210.7	235.1	239.0
tonsillar	146.1	198.89	230.0	210.6	235.1	239.0
fourchette	184.4	198.82	233.3	221.2	236.3	239.5
frenulum						
labii—*see* Neoplasm, lip, internal						
linguae	141.3	198.89	230.0	210.1	235.1	239.0
frontal						
bone	170.0	198.5	—	213.0	238.0	239.2
lobe, brain	191.1	198.3	—	225.0	237.5	239.6
meninges	192.1	198.4	—	225.2	237.6	239.7
pole	191.1	198.3	—	225.0	237.5	239.6
sinus	160.4	197.3	231.8	212.0	235.9	239.1
fundus						
stomach	151.3	197.8	230.2	211.1	235.2	239.0
uterus	182.0	198.82	233.2	219.1	236.0	239.5
gall duct (extrahepatic)	156.1	197.8	230.8	211.5	235.3	239.0
intrahepatic	155.1	197.8	230.8	211.5	235.3	239.0
gallbladder	156.0	197.8	230.8	211.5	235.3	239.0
contiguous sites with extrahepatic bile ducts	156.8	—	—	—	—	—
ganglia (*see also* Neoplasm, connective tissue)	171.9	198.89	—	215.9	238.1	239.2
basal	191.0	198.3	—	225.0	237.5	239.6
ganglion (*see also* Neoplasm, connective tissue)	171.9	198.89	—	215.9	238.1	239.2
cranial nerve	192.0	198.4	—	225.1	237.9	239.7
Gartner's duct	184.0	198.82	233.3	221.1	236.3	239.5
gastric—*see* Neoplasm, stomach						
gastrocolic	159.8	197.8	230.9	211.9	235.5	239.0
gastroesophageal junction	151.0	197.8	230.2	211.1	235.2	239.0
gastrointestinal (tract) NEC	159.9	197.8	230.9	211.9	235.5	239.0
generalized	199.0	199.0	234.9	229.9	238.9	199.0
genital organ or tract						
female NEC	184.9	198.82	233.3	221.9	236.3	239.5
contiguous sites	184.8	—	—	—	—	—
specified site NEC	184.8	198.82	233.3	221.8	236.3	239.5
male NEC	187.9	198.82	233.6	222.9	236.6	239.5
contiguous sites	187.8	—	—	—	—	—
specified site NEC	187.8	198.82	233.6	222.8	236.6	239.5
genitourinary tract						
female	184.9	198.82	233.3	221.9	236.3	239.5
male	187.9	198.82	233.6	222.9	236.6	239.5
gingiva (alveolar) (marginal)	143.9	198.89	230.0	210.4	235.1	239.0
lower	143.1	198.89	230.0	210.4	235.1	239.0
mandibular	143.1	198.89	230.0	210.4	235.1	239.0
maxillary	143.0	198.89	230.0	210.4	235.1	239.0
upper	143.0	198.89	230.0	210.4	235.1	239.0

	Malignant					
	Primary	Secondary	Ca in situ	Benign	Uncertain Behavior	Unspecified
gland, glandular (lymphatic) (system)—*see also* Neoplasm, lymph gland						
endocrine NEC	194.9	198.89	—	227.9	237.4	239.7
salivary—*see* Neoplasm, salivary, gland						
glans penis	187.2	198.82	233.5	222.1	236.6	239.5
globus pallidus	191.0	198.3	—	225.0	237.5	239.6
glomus						
coccygeal	194.6	198.89	—	227.6	237.3	239.7
jugularis	194.6	198.89	—	227.6	237.3	239.7
glosso-epiglottic fold(s)	146.4	198.89	230.0	210.6	235.1	239.0
glossopalatine fold	146.2	198.89	230.0	210.6	235.1	239.0
glossopharyngeal sulcus	146.1	198.89	230.0	210.6	235.1	239.0
glottis	161.0	197.3	231.0	212.1	235.6	239.1
gluteal region*	195.3	198.89	232.5	229.8	238.8	239.8
great vessels NEC	171.4	198.89	—	215.4	238.1	239.2
groin NEC*	195.3	198.89	232.5	229.8	238.8	239.8
gum	143.9	198.89	230.0	210.4	235.1	239.0
contiguous sites	143.8	—	—	—	—	—
lower	143.1	198.89	230.0	210.4	235.1	239.0
upper	143.0	198.89	230.0	210.4	235.1	239.0
hand NEC*	195.4	198.89	232.6	229.8	238.8	239.8
head NEC*	195.0	198.89	232.4	229.8	238.8	239.8
heart	164.1	198.89	—	212.7	238.8	239.8
contiguous sites with mediastinum or thymus	164.8	—	—	—	—	—
heel NEC*	195.5	198.89	232.7	229.8	238.8	239.8
helix	173.2	198.2	232.2	216.2	238.2	239.2
hematopoietic, hemopoietic tissue NEC	202.8	198.89	—	—	—	238.7
hemisphere, cerebral	191.0	198.3	—	225.0	237.5	239.6
hemorrhoidal zone	154.2	197.5	230.5	211.4	235.5	239.0
hepatic	155.2	197.7	230.8	211.5	235.3	239.0
duct (bile)	156.1	197.8	230.8	211.5	235.3	239.0
flexure (colon)	153.0	197.5	230.3	211.3	235.2	239.0
primary	155.0	—	—	—	—	—
hilus of lung	162.2	197.0	231.2	212.3	235.7	239.1
hip NEC*	195.5	198.89	232.7	229.8	238.8	239.8
hippocampus, brain	191.2	198.3	—	225.0	237.5	239.6
humerus (any part)	170.4	198.5	—	213.4	238.0	239.2
hymen	184.0	198.82	233.3	221.1	236.3	239.5
hypopharynx, hypopharyngeal NEC	148.9	198.89	230.0	210.8	235.1	239.0
contiguous sites	148.8	—	—	—	—	—
postcricoid region	148.0	198.89	230.0	210.8	235.1	239.0
posterior wall	148.3	198.89	230.0	210.8	235.1	239.0
pyriform fossa (sinus)	148.1	198.89	230.0	210.8	235.1	239.0
specified site NEC	148.8	198.89	230.0	210.8	235.1	239.0
wall	148.9	198.89	230.0	210.8	235.1	239.0
posterior	148.3	198.89	230.0	210.8	235.1	239.0
hypophysis	194.3	198.89	234.8	227.3	237.0	239.7
hypothalamus	191.0	198.3	—	225.0	237.5	239.6
ileocecum, ileocecal (coil, junction, valve)	153.4	197.5	230.3	211.3	235.2	239.0
ileum	152.2	197.4	230.7	211.2	235.2	239.0
ilium	170.6	198.5	—	213.6	238.0	239.2
immunoproliferative NEC	203.8	—	—	—	—	—
infraclavicular (region)*	195.1	198.89	232.5	229.8	238.8	239.8
inguinal (region)*	195.3	198.89	232.5	229.8	238.8	239.8
insula	191.0	198.3	—	225.0	237.5	239.6
insular tissue (pancreas)	157.4	197.8	230.9	211.7	235.5	239.0
brain	191.0	198.3	—	225.0	237.5	239.6

	Malignant					
	Primary	Secondary	Ca in situ	Benign	Uncertain Behavior	Unspecified
interarytenoid fold	148.2	198.89	230.0	210.8	235.1	239.0
hypopharyngeal aspect	148.2	198.89	230.0	210.8	235.1	239.0
laryngeal aspect	161.1	197.3	231.0	212.1	235.6	239.1
marginal zone	148.2	198.89	230.0	210.8	235.1	239.0
interdental papillae	143.9	198.89	230.0	210.4	235.1	239.0
lower	143.1	198.89	230.0	210.4	235.1	239.0
upper	143.0	198.89	230.0	210.4	235.1	239.0
internal						
capsule	191.0	198.3	—	225.0	237.5	239.6
os (cervix)	180.0	198.82	233.1	219.0	236.0	239.5
intervertebral cartilage or disc	170.2	198.5	—	213.2	238.0	239.2
intestine, intestinal	159.0	197.8	230.7	211.9	235.2	239.0
large	153.9	197.5	230.3	211.3	235.2	239.0
appendix	153.5	197.5	230.3	211.3	235.2	239.0
caput coli	153.4	197.5	230.3	211.3	235.2	239.0
cecum	153.4	197.5	230.3	211.3	235.2	239.0
colon	153.9	197.5	230.3	211.3	235.2	239.0
and rectum	154.0	197.5	230.4	211.4	235.2	239.0
ascending	153.6	197.5	230.3	211.3	235.2	239.0
caput	153.4	197.5	230.3	211.3	235.2	239.0
contiguous sites	153.8	—	—	—	—	—
descending	153.2	197.5	230.3	211.3	235.2	239.0
distal	153.2	197.5	230.3	211.3	235.2	239.0
left	153.2	197.5	230.3	211.3	235.2	239.0
pelvic	153.3	197.5	230.3	211.3	235.2	239.0
right	153.6	197.5	230.3	211.3	235.2	239.0
sigmoid (flexure)	153.3	197.5	230.3	211.3	235.2	239.0
transverse	153.1	197.5	230.3	211.3	235.2	239.0
contiguous sites	153.8	—	—	—	—	—
hepatic flexure	153.0	197.5	230.3	211.3	235.2	239.0
ileocecum,ileocecal (coil, valve)	153.4	197.5	230.3	211.3	235.2	239.0
sigmoid flexure (lower) (upper)	153.3	197.5	230.3	211.3	235.2	239.0
splenic flexure	153.7	197.5	230.3	211.3	235.2	239.0
small	152.9	197.4	230.7	211.2	235.2	239.0
contiguous sites	152.8	—	—	—	—	—
duodenum	152.0	197.4	230.7	211.2	235.2	239.0
ileum	152.2	197.4	230.7	211.2	235.2	239.0
jejunum	152.1	197.4	230.7	211.2	235.2	239.0
tract NEC	159.0	197.8	230.7	211.9	235.2	239.0
intra-abdominal	195.2	198.89	234.8	229.8	238.8	239.8
intracranial NEC	191.9	198.3	—	225.0	237.5	239.6
intrahepatic (bile) duct	155.1	197.8	230.8	211.5	235.3	239.0
intraocular	190.0	198.4	234.0	224.0	238.8	239.8
intraorbital	190.1	198.4	234.0	224.1	238.8	239.8
intrasellar	194.3	198.89	234.8	227.3	237.0	239.7
intrathoracic (cavity) (organs NEC)	195.1	198.89	234.8	229.8	238.8	239.8
contiguous sites with respiratory organs	165.8	—	—	—	—	—
iris	190.0	198.4	234.0	224.0	238.8	239.8
ischiorectal (fossa)	195.3	198.89	234.8	229.8	238.8	239.8
ischium	170.6	198.5	—	213.6	238.0	239.2
island of Reil	191.0	198.3	—	225.0	237.5	239.6
islands or islets of Langerhans	157.4	197.8	230.9	211.7	235.5	239.0
isthmus uteri	182.1	198.82	233.2	219.1	236.0	239.5
jaw	195.0	198.89	234.8	229.8	238.8	239.8
bone	170.1	198.5	—	213.1	238.0	239.2
carcinoma	143.9	—	—	—	—	—
lower	143.1	—	—	—	—	—
upper	143.0	—	—	—	—	—
lower	170.1	198.5	—	213.1	238.0	239.2
upper	170.0	198.5	—	213.0	238.0	239.2

	Malignant					
	Primary	Secondary	Ca in situ	Benign	Uncertain Behavior	Unspecified
jaw—*continued*						
carcinoma (any type) (lower) (upper)	195.0	—	—	—	—	—
skin	173.3	198.2	232.3	216.3	238.2	239.2
soft tissues	143.9	198.89	230.0	210.4	235.1	239.0
lower	143.1	198.89	230.0	210.4	235.1	239.0
upper	143.0	198.89	230.0	210.4	235.1	239.0
jejunum	152.1	197.4	230.7	211.2	235.2	239.0
joint NEC *(see also* Neoplasm, bone)	170.9	198.5	—	213.9	238.0	239.2
acromioclavicular	170.4	198.5	—	213.4	238.0	239.2
bursa or synovial membrane—*see* Neoplasm, connective tissue						
costovertebral	170.3	198.5	—	213.3	238.0	239.2
sternocostal	170.3	198.5	—	213.3	238.0	239.2
temporomandibular	170.1	198.5	—	213.1	238.0	239.2
junction						
anorectal	154.8	197.5	230.7	211.4	235.5	239.0
cardioesophageal	151.0	197.8	230.2	211.1	235.2	239.0
esophagogastric	151.0	197.8	230.2	211.1	235.2	239.0
gastroesophageal	151.0	197.8	230.2	211.1	235.2	239.0
hard and soft palate	145.5	198.89	230.0	210.4	235.1	239.0
ileocecal	153.4	197.5	230.3	211.3	235.2	239.0
pelvirectal	154.0	197.5	230.4	211.4	235.2	239.0
pelviureteric	189.1	198.0	233.9	223.1	236.91	239.5
rectosigmoid	154.0	197.5	230.4	211.4	235.2	239.0
squamocolumnar, of cervix	180.8	198.82	233.1	219.0	236.0	239.5
kidney (parenchyma)	189.0	198.0	233.9	223.0	236.91	239.5
calyx	189.1	198.0	233.9	223.1	236.91	239.5
hilus	189.1	198.0	233.9	223.1	236.91	239.5
pelvis	189.1	198.0	233.9	223.1	236.91	239.5
knee NEC*	195.5	198.89	232.7	229.8	238.8	239.8
labia (skin)	184.4	198.82	233.3	221.2	236.3	239.5
majora	184.1	198.82	233.3	221.2	236.3	239.5
minora	184.2	198.82	233.3	221.2	236.3	239.5
labial—*see also* Neoplasm, lip						
sulcus (lower) (upper)	145.1	198.89	230.0	210.4	235.1	239.0
labium (skin)	184.4	198.82	233.3	221.2	236.3	239.5
majus	184.1	198.82	233.3	221.2	236.3	239.5
minus	184.2	198.82	233.3	221.2	236.3	239.5
lacrimal						
canaliculi	190.7	198.4	234.0	224.7	238.8	239.8
duct (nasal)	190.7	198.4	234.0	224.7	238.8	239.8
gland	190.2	198.4	234.0	224.2	238.8	239.8
punctum	190.7	198.4	234.0	224.7	238.8	239.8
sac	190.7	198.4	234.0	224.7	238.8	239.8
Langerhans, islands or islets	157.4	197.8	230.9	211.7	235.5	239.0
laryngopharynx	148.9	198.89	230.0	210.8	235.1	239.0
larynx, laryngeal NEC	161.9	197.3	231.0	212.1	235.6	239.1
aryepiglottic fold	161.1	197.3	231.0	212.1	235.6	239.1
cartilage (arytenoid) (cricoid) (cuneiform) (thyroid)	161.3	197.3	231.0	212.1	235.6	239.1
commissure (anterior) (posterior)	161.0	197.3	231.0	212.1	235.6	239.1
contiguous sites	161.8	—	—	—	—	—
extrinsic NEC	161.1	197.3	231.0	212.1	235.6	239.1
meaning hypopharynx	148.9	198.89	230.0	210.8	235.1	239.0
interarytenoid fold	161.1	197.3	231.0	212.1	235.6	239.1
intrinsic	161.0	197.3	231.0	212.1	235.6	239.1
ventricular band	161.1	197.3	231.0	212.1	235.6	239.1
leg NEC*	195.5	198.89	232.7	229.8	238.8	239.8
lens, crystalline	190.0	198.4	234.0	224.0	238.8	239.8

	Malignant Primary	Malignant Secondary	Malignant Ca in situ	Benign	Uncertain Behavior	Unspecified
lid (lower) (upper)	173.1	198.2	232.1	216.1	238.2	239.2
ligament—*see also* Neoplasm, connective tissue						
broad	183.3	198.82	233.3	221.0	236.3	239.5
Mackenrodt's	183.8	198.82	233.3	221.8	236.3	239.5
non-uterine—*see* Neoplasm, connective tissue						
round	183.5	198.82	—	221.0	236.3	239.5
sacro-uterine	183.4	198.82	—	221.0	236.3	239.5
uterine	183.4	198.82	—	221.0	236.3	239.5
utero-ovarian	183.8	198.82	233.3	221.8	236.3	239.5
uterosacral	183.4	198.82	—	221.0	236.3	239.5
limb*	195.8	198.89	232.8	229.8	238.8	239.8
lower*	195.5	198.89	232.7	229.8	238.8	239.8
upper*	195.4	198.89	232.6	229.8	238.8	239.8
limbus of cornea	190.4	198.4	234.0	224.4	238.8	239.8
lingual NEC *(see also* Neoplasm, tongue)	141.9	198.89	230.0	210.1	235.1	239.0
lingula, lung	162.3	197.0	231.2	212.3	235.7	239.1
lip (external) (lipstick area) (vermillion border)	140.9	198.89	230.0	210.0	235.1	239.0
buccal aspect—*see* Neoplasm, lip, internal						
commissure	140.6	198.89	230.0	210.4	235.1	239.0
contiguous sites	140.8	—	—	—	—	—
with oral cavity or pharynx	149.8	—	—	—	—	—
frenulum—*see* Neoplasm, lip, internal						
inner aspect—*see* Neoplasm, lip, internal						
internal (buccal) (frenulum) (mucosa) (oral)	140.5	198.89	230.0	210.0	235.1	239.0
lower	140.4	198.89	230.0	210.0	235.1	239.0
upper	140.3	198.89	230.0	210.0	235.1	239.0
lower	140.1	198.89	230.0	210.0	235.1	239.0
internal (buccal) (frenulum) (mucosa) (oral)	140.4	198.89	230.0	210.0	235.1	239.0
mucosa—*see* Neoplasm, lip, internal						
oral aspect—*see* Neoplasm, lip, internal						
skin (commissure) (lower) (upper)	173.0	198.2	232.0	216.0	238.2	239.2
upper	140.0	198.89	230.0	210.0	235.1	239.0
internal (buccal) (frenulum) (mucosa) (oral)	140.3	198.89	230.0	210.0	235.1	239.0
liver	155.2	197.7	230.8	211.5	235.3	239.0
primary	155.0	—	—	—	—	—
lobe						
azygos	162.3	197.0	231.2	212.3	235.7	239.1
frontal	191.1	198.3	—	225.0	237.5	239.6
lower	162.5	197.0	231.2	212.3	235.7	239.1
middle	162.4	197.0	231.2	212.3	235.7	239.1
occipital	191.4	198.3	—	225.0	237.5	239.6
parietal	191.3	198.3	—	225.0	237.5	239.6
temporal	191.2	198.3	—	225.0	237.5	239.6
upper	162.3	197.0	231.2	212.3	235.7	239.1
lumbosacral plexus	171.6	198.4	—	215.6	238.1	239.2
lung	162.9	197.0	231.2	212.3	235.7	239.1
azygos lobe	162.3	197.0	231.2	212.3	235.7	239.1
carina	162.2	197.0	231.2	212.3	235.7	239.1
contiguous sites with bronchus or trachea	162.8	—	—	—	—	—
hilus	162.2	197.0	231.2	212.3	235.7	239.1

	Malignant					
	Primary	Secondary	Ca in situ	Benign	Uncertain Behavior	Unspecified
lung—*continued*						
lingula	162.3	197.0	231.2	212.3	235.7	239.1
lobe NEC	162.9	197.0	231.2	212.3	235.7	239.1
lower lobe	162.5	197.0	231.2	212.3	235.7	239.1
main bronchus	162.2	197.0	231.2	212.3	235.7	239.1
middle lobe	162.4	197.0	231.2	212.3	235.7	239.1
upper lobe	162.3	197.0	231.2	212.3	235.7	239.1
lymph, lymphatic						
channel NEC (*see also* Neoplasm, connective tissue)	171.9	198.89	—	215.9	238.1	239.2
gland (secondary)	—	196.9	—	229.0	238.8	239.8
abdominal	—	196.2	—	229.0	238.8	239.8
aortic	—	196.2	—	229.0	238.8	239.8
arm	—	196.3	—	229.0	238.8	239.8
auricular (anterior) (posterior)	—	196.0	—	229.0	238.8	239.8
axilla, axillary	—	196.3	—	229.0	238.8	239.8
brachial	—	196.3	—	229.0	238.8	239.8
bronchial	—	196.1	—	229.0	238.8	239.8
bronchopulmonary	—	196.1	—	229.0	238.8	239.8
celiac	—	196.2	—	229.0	238.8	239.8
cervical	—	196.0	—	229.0	238.8	239.8
cervicofacial	—	196.0	—	229.0	238.8	239.8
Cloquet	—	196.5	—	229.0	238.8	239.8
colic	—	196.2	—	229.0	238.8	239.8
common duct	—	196.2	—	229.0	238.8	239.8
cubital	—	196.3	—	229.0	238.8	239.8
diaphragmatic	—	196.1	—	229.0	238.8	239.8
epigastric, inferior	—	196.6	—	229.0	238.8	239.8
epitrochlear	—	196.3	—	229.0	238.8	239.8
esophageal	—	196.1	—	229.0	238.8	239.8
face	—	196.0	—	229.0	238.8	239.8
femoral	—	196.5	—	229.0	238.8	239.8
gastric	—	196.2	—	229.0	238.8	239.8
groin	—	196.5	—	229.0	238.8	239.8
head	—	196.0	—	229.0	238.8	239.8
hepatic	—	196.2	—	229.0	238.8	239.8
hilar (pulmonary)	—	196.1	—	229.0	238.8	239.8
splenic	—	196.2	—	229.0	238.8	239.8
hypogastric	—	196.6	—	229.0	238.8	239.8
ileocolic	—	196.2	—	229.0	238.8	239.8
iliac	—	196.6	—	229.0	238.8	239.8
infraclavicular	—	196.3	—	229.0	238.8	239.8
inguina, inguinal	—	196.5	—	229.0	238.8	239.8
innominate	—	196.1	—	229.0	238.8	239.8
intercostal	—	196.1	—	229.0	238.8	239.8
intestinal	—	196.2	—	229.0	238.8	239.8
intrabdominal	—	196.2	—	229.0	238.8	239.8
intrapelvic	—	196.6	—	229.0	238.8	239.8
intrathoracic	—	196.1	—	229.0	238.8	239.9
jugular	—	196.0	—	229.0	238.8	239.8
leg	—	196.5	—	229.0	238.8	239.8
limb						
lower	—	196.5	—	229.0	238.8	239.8
upper	—	196.3	—	229.0	238.8	239.8
lower limb	—	196.5	—	229.0	238.8	238.9
lumbar	—	196.2	—	229.0	238.8	239.8
mandibular	—	196.0	—	229.0	238.8	239.8
mediastinal	—	196.1	—	229.0	238.8	239.8
mesenteric (inferior) (superior)	—	196.2	—	229.0	238.8	239.8
midcolic	—	196.2	—	229.0	238.8	239.8

	Malignant					
	Primary	Secondary	Ca in situ	Benign	Uncertain Behavior	Unspecified
lymph, lymphatic—*continued*						
multiple sites in categories 196.0-196.6	—	196.8	—	229.0	238.8	239.8
neck	—	196.0	—	229.0	238.8	239.8
obturator	—	196.6	—	229.0	238.8	239.8
occipital	—	196.0	—	229.0	238.8	239.8
pancreatic	—	196.2	—	229.0	238.8	239.8
para-aortic	—	196.2	—	229.0	238.8	239.8
paracervical	—	196.6	—	229.0	238.8	239.8
parametrial	—	196.6	—	229.0	238.8	239.8
parasternal	—	196.1	—	229.0	238.8	239.8
parotid	—	196.0	—	229.0	238.8	239.8
pectoral	—	196.3	—	229.0	238.8	239.8
pelvic	—	196.6	—	229.0	238.8	239.8
peri-aortic	—	196.2	—	229.0	238.8	239.8
peripancreatic	—	196.2	—	229.0	238.8	239.8
popliteal	—	196.5	—	229.0	238.8	239.8
porta hepatis	—	196.2	—	229.0	238.8	239.8
portal	—	196.2	—	229.0	238.8	239.8
preauricular	—	196.0	—	229.0	238.8	239.8
prelaryngeal	—	196.0	—	229.0	238.8	239.8
presymphysial	—	196.6	—	229.0	238.8	239.8
pretracheal	—	196.0	—	229.0	238.8	239.8
primary (any site) NEC	202.9	—	—	—	—	—
pulmonary (hiler)	—	196.1	—	229.0	238.8	239.8
pyloric	—	196.2	—	229.0	238.8	239.8
retroperitoneal	—	196.2	—	229.0	238.8	239.8
retropharyngeal	—	196.0	—	229.0	238.8	239.8
Rosenmüller's	—	196.5	—	229.0	238.8	239.8
sacral	—	196.6	—	229.0	238.8	239.8
scalene	—	196.0	—	229.0	238.8	239.8
site NEC	—	196.9	—	229.0	238.8	239.8
splenic (hilar)	—	196.2	—	229.0	238.8	239.8
subclavicular	—	196.3	—	229.0	238.8	239.8
subinguinal	—	196.5	—	229.0	238.8	239.8
sublingual	—	196.0	—	229.0	238.8	239.8
submandibular	—	196.0	—	229.0	238.8	239.8
submaxillary	—	196.0	—	229.0	238.8	239.8
submental	—	196.0	—	229.0	238.8	239.8
subscapular	—	196.3	—	229.0	238.8	239.8
supraclavicular	—	196.0	—	229.0	238.8	239.8
thoracic	—	196.1	—	229.0	238.8	239.8
tibial	—	196.5	—	229.0	238.8	239.8
tracheal	—	196.1	—	229.0	238.8	239.8
tracheobronchial	—	196.1	—	229.0	238.8	239.8
upper limb	—	196.3	—	229.0	238.8	239.8
Virchow's	—	196.0	—	229.0	238.8	239.8
node—*see also* Neoplasm, lymph gland						
primary NEC	202.9	—	—	—	—	—
vessel (*see also* Neoplasm, connective tissue)	171.9	198.89	—	215.9	238.1	239.2
Mackenrodt's ligament	183.8	198.82	233.3	221.8	236.3	239.5
malar	170.0	198.5	—	213.0	238.0	239.2
region—*see* Neoplasm, cheek						
mammary gland—*see* Neoplasm, breast						
mandible	170.1	198.5	—	213.1	238.0	239.2
alveolar						
mucose	143.1	198.89	230.0	210.4	235.1	239.0
ridge or process	170.1	198.5	—	213.1	238.0	239.2
carcinoma	143.1	—	—	—	—	—
carcinoma	143.1	—	—	—	—	—

	Malignant					
	Primary	Secondary	Ca in situ	Benign	Uncertain Behavior	Unspecified
marrow (bone) NEC	202.9	198.5	—	—	—	238.7
mastectomy site (skin)	173.5	198.2	—	—	—	—
specified as breast tissue	174.8	198.81	—	—	—	—
mastoid (air cells) (antrum) (cavity)	160.1	197.3	231.8	212.0	235.9	239.1
bone or process	170.0	198.5	—	213.0	238.0	239.2
maxilla, maxillary (superior)	170.0	198.5	—	213.0	238.0	239.2
alveolar						
mucosa	143.0	198.89	230.0	210.4	235.1	239.0
ridge or process	170.0	198.5	—	213.0	238.0	239.2
carcinoma	143.0	—	—	—	—	—
antrum	160.2	197.3	231.8	212.0	235.9	239.1
carcinoma	143.0	—	—	—	—	—
inferior—*see* Neoplasm, mandible						
sinus	160.2	197.3	231.8	212.0	235.9	239.1
meatus						
external (ear)	173.2	198.2	232.2	216.2	238.2	239.2
Meckel's diverticulum	152.3	197.4	230.7	211.2	235.2	239.0
mediastinum, mediastinal	164.9	197.1	—	212.5	235.8	239.8
anterior	164.2	197.1	—	212.5	235.8	239.8
contiguous sites with heart and thymus	164.8	—	—	—	—	—
posterior	164.3	197.1	—	212.5	235.8	239.8
medulla						
adrenal	194.0	198.7	234.8	227.0	237.2	239.7
oblongata	191.7	198.3	—	225.0	237.5	239.6
meibomian gland	173.1	198.2	232.1	216.1	238.2	239.2
melanoma —*see* Melanoma						
meninges (brain) (cerebral) (cranial) (intracranial)	192.1	198.4	—	225.2	237.6	239.7
spinal (cord)	192.3	198.4	—	225.4	237.6	239.7
meniscus, knee joint (lateral) (medial)	170.7	198.5	—	213.7	238.0	239.2
mesentery, mesenteric	158.8	197.6	—	211.8	235.4	239.0
mesoappendix	158.8	197.6	—	211.8	235.4	239.0
mesocolon	158.8	197.6	—	211.8	235.4	239.0
mesopharynx—*see* Neoplasm, oropharynx						
mesosalpinx	183.3	198.82	233.3	221.0	236.3	239.5
mesovarium	183.3	198.82	233.3	221.0	236.3	239.5
metacarpus (any bone)	170.5	198.5	—	213.5	238.0	239.2
metastatic NEC—*see also* Neoplasm, by site, secondary	—	199.1	—	—	—	—
metatarsus (any bone)	170.8	198.5	—	213.8	238.0	239.2
midbrain	191.7	198.3	—	225.0	237.5	239.6
milk duct—*see* Neoplasm, breast						
mons						
pubis	184.4	198.82	233.3	221.2	236.3	239.5
veneris	184.4	198.82	233.3	221.2	236.3	239.5
motor tract	192.9	198.4	—	225.9	237.9	239.7
brain	191.9	198.3	—	225.0	237.5	239.6
spinal	192.2	198.3	—	225.3	237.5	239.7
mouth	145.9	198.89	230.0	210.4	235.1	239.0
contiguous sites	145.8	—	—	—	—	—
floor	144.9	198.89	230.0	210.3	235.1	239.0
anterior portion	144.0	198.89	230.0	210.3	235.1	239.0
contiguous sites	144.8	—	—	—	—	—
lateral portion	144.1	198.89	230.0	210.3	235.1	239.0
roof	145.5	198.89	230.0	210.4	235.1	239.0
specified part NEC	145.8	198.89	230.0	210.4	235.1	239.0
vestibule	145.1	198.89	230.0	210.4	235.1	239.0
mucosa						
alveolar (ridge or process)	143.9	198.89	230.0	210.4	235.1	239.0
lower	143.1	198.89	230.0	210.4	235.1	239.0
upper	143.0	198.89	230.0	210.4	235.1	239.0

	Malignant — Primary	Malignant — Secondary	Malignant — Ca in situ	Benign	Uncertain Behavior	Unspecified
mucosa—*continued*						
buccal	145.0	198.89	230.0	210.4	235.1	239.0
cheek	145.0	198.89	230.0	210.4	235.1	239.0
lip—*see* Neoplasm, lip, internal						
nasal	160.0	197.3	231.8	212.0	235.9	239.1
oral	145.0	198.89	230.0	210.4	235.1	239.0
Müllerian duct						
female	184.8	198.82	233.3	221.8	236.3	239.5
male	187.8	198.82	233.6	222.8	236.6	239.5
multiple sites NEC	199.0	199.0	234.9	229.9	238.9	199.0
muscle—*see also* Neoplasm, connective tissue						
extraocular	190.1	198.4	234.0	224.1	238.8	239.8
myocardium	164.1	198.89	—	212.7	238.8	239.8
myometrium	182.0	198.82	233.2	219.1	236.0	239.5
myopericardium	164.1	198.89	—	212.7	238.8	239.8
nabothian gland (follicle)	180.0	198.82	233.1	219.0	236.0	239.5
nail	173.9	198.2	232.9	216.9	238.2	239.2
finger	173.6	198.2	232.6	216.6	238.2	239.2
toe	173.7	198.2	232.7	216.7	238.2	239.2
nares, naris (anterior) (posterior)	160.0	197.3	231.8	212.0	235.9	239.1
nasal—*see* Neoplasm, nose						
nasolabial groove	173.3	198.2	232.3	216.3	238.2	239.2
nasolacrimal duct	190.7	198.4	234.0	224.7	238.8	239.8
nasopharynx, nasopharyngeal	147.9	198.89	230.0	210.7	235.1	239.0
contiguous sites	147.8	—	—	—	—	—
floor	147.3	198.89	230.0	210.7	235.1	239.0
roof	147.0	198.89	230.0	210.7	235.1	239.0
specified site NEC	147.8	198.89	230.0	210.7	235.1	239.0
wall	147.9	198.89	230.0	210.7	235.1	239.0
anterior	147.3	198.89	230.0	210.7	235.1	239.0
lateral	147.2	198.89	230.0	210.7	235.1	239.0
posterior	147.1	198.89	230.0	210.7	235.1	239.0
superior	147.0	198.89	230.0	210.7	235.1	239.0
nates	173.5	198.2	232.5	216.5	238.2	239.2
neck NEC*	195.0	198.89	234.8	229.8	238.8	239.8
nerve (autonomic) (ganglion) (parasympathetic) (peripheral) (sympathetic)—*see also* Neoplasm, connective tissue						
abducens	192.0	198.4	—	225.1	237.9	239.7
accessory (spinal)	192.0	198.4	—	225.1	237.9	239.7
acoustic	192.0	198.4	—	225.1	237.9	239.7
auditory	192.0	198.4	—	225.1	237.9	239.7
brachial	171.2	198.89	—	215.2	238.1	239.2
cranial (any)	192.0	198.4	—	225.1	237.9	239.7
facial	192.0	198.4	—	225.1	237.9	239.7
femoral	171.3	198.89	—	215.3	238.1	239.2
glossopharyngeal	192.0	198.4	—	225.1	237.9	239.7
hypoglossal	192.0	198.4	—	225.1	237.9	239.7
intercostal	171.4	198.89	—	215.4	238.1	239.2
lumbar	171.7	198.89	—	215.7	238.1	239.2
median	171.2	198.89	—	215.2	238.1	239.2
obturator	171.3	198.89	—	215.3	238.1	239.2
oculomotor	192.0	198.4	—	225.1	237.9	239.7
olfactory	192.0	198.4	—	225.1	237.9	239.7
optic	192.0	198.4	—	225.1	237.9	239.7
peripheral NEC	171.9	198.89	—	215.9	238.1	239.2
radial	171.2	198.89	—	215.2	238.1	239.2
sacral	171.6	198.89	—	215.6	238.1	239.2
sciatic	171.3	198.89	—	215.3	238.1	239.2
spinal NEC	171.9	198.89	—	215.9	238.1	239.2

	Malignant					
	Primary	Secondary	Ca in situ	Benign	Uncertain Behavior	Unspecified
nerve—*continued*						
trigeminal	192.0	198.4	—	225.1	237.9	239.7
trochlear	192.0	198.4	—	225.1	237.9	239.7
ulnar	171.2	198.89	—	215.2	238.1	239.2
vagus	192.0	198.4	—	225.1	237.9	239.7
nervous system (central) NEC	192.9	198.4	—	225.9	237.9	239.7
autonomic NEC	171.9	198.89	—	215.9	238.1	239.2
brain—*see also* Neoplasm, brain						
membrane or meninges	192.1	198.4	—	225.2	237.6	239.7
contiguous sites	192.8	—	—	—	—	—
parasympathetic NEC	171.9	198.89	—	215.9	238.1	239.2
sympathetic NEC	171.9	198.89	—	215.9	238.1	239.2
nipple (female)	174.0	198.81	233.0	217	238.3	239.3
male	175.0	198.81	233.0	217	238.3	239.3
nose, nasal	195.0	198.89	234.8	229.8	238.8	239.8
ala (external)	173.3	198.2	232.3	216.3	238.2	239.2
bone	170.0	198.5	—	213.0	238.0	239.2
cartilage	160.0	197.3	231.8	212.0	235.9	239.1
cavity	160.0	197.3	231.8	212.0	235.9	239.1
contiguous sites with accessory sinuses or middle ear	160.8	—	—	—	—	—
choana	147.3	198.89	230.0	210.7	235.1	239.0
external (skin)	173.3	198.2	232.3	216.3	238.2	239.2
fossa	160.0	197.3	231.8	212.0	235.9	239.1
internal	160.0	197.3	231.8	212.0	235.9	239.1
mucosa	160.0	197.3	231.8	212.0	235.9	239.1
septum	160.0	197.3	231.8	212.0	235.9	239.1
posterior margin	147.3	198.89	230.0	210.7	235.1	239.0
sinus—*see* Neoplasm, sinus						
skin	173.3	198.2	232.3	216.3	238.2	239.2
turbinate (mucosa)	160.0	197.3	231.8	212.0	235.9	239.1
bone	170.0	198.5	—	213.0	238.0	239.2
vestibule	160.0	197.3	231.8	212.0	235.9	239.1
nostril	160.0	197.3	231.8	212.0	235.9	239.1
nucleus pulposus	170.2	198.5	—	213.2	238.0	239.2
occipital						
bone	170.0	198.5	—	213.0	238.0	239.2
lobe or pole, brain	191.4	198.3	—	225.0	237.5	239.6
odontogenic—*see* Neoplasm, jaw bone						
oesophagus—*see* Neoplasm, esophagus						
olfactory nerve or bulb	192.0	198.4	—	225.1	237.9	239.7
olive (brain)	191.7	198.3	—	225.0	237.5	239.6
omentum	158.8	197.6	—	211.8	235.4	239.0
operculum (brain)	191.0	198.3	—	225.0	237.5	239.6
optic nerve, chiasm, or tract	192.0	198.4	—	225.1	237.9	239.7
oral (cavity)	145.9	198.89	230.0	210.4	235.1	239.0
contiguous sites with lip or pharynx	149.8	—	—	—	—	—
ill-defined	149.9	198.89	230.0	210.4	235.1	239.0
mucosa	145.9	198.89	230.0	210.4	235.1	239.0
orbit	190.1	198.4	234.0	224.1	238.8	239.8
bone	170.0	198.5	—	213.0	238.0	239.2
eye	190.1	198.4	234.0	224.1	238.8	239.8
soft parts	190.1	198.4	234.0	224.1	238.8	239.8
organ of Zuckerkandl	194.6	198.89	—	227.6	237.3	239.7
oropharynx	146.9	198.89	230.0	210.6	235.1	239.0
branchial cleft (vestige)	146.8	198.89	230.0	210.6	235.1	239.0
contiguous sites	146.8	—	—	—	—	—
junctional region	146.5	198.89	230.0	210.6	235.1	239.0
lateral wall	146.6	198.89	230.0	210.6	235.1	239.0
pillars of fauces	146.2	198.89	230.0	210.6	235.1	239.0

	Malignant Primary	Malignant Secondary	Malignant Ca in situ	Benign	Uncertain Behavior	Unspecified
oropharynx—*continued*						
posterior wall	146.7	198.89	230.0	210.6	235.1	239.0
specified part NEC	146.8	198.89	230.0	210.6	235.1	239.0
vallecula	146.3	198.89	230.0	210.6	235.1	239.0
os						
external	180.1	198.82	233.1	219.0	236.0	239.5
internal	180.0	198.82	233.1	219.0	236.0	239.5
ovary	183.0	198.6	233.3	220	236.2	239.5
oviduct	183.2	198.82	233.3	221.0	236.3	239.5
palate	145.5	198.89	230.0	210.4	235.1	239.0
hard	145.2	198.89	230.0	210.4	235.1	239.0
junction of hard and soft palate	145.5	198.89	230.0	210.4	235.1	239.0
soft	145.3	198.89	230.0	210.4	235.1	239.0
nasopharyngeal surface	147.3	198.89	230.0	210.7	235.1	239.0
posterior surface	147.3	198.89	230.0	210.7	235.1	239.0
superior surface	147.3	198.89	230.0	210.7	235.1	239.0
palatoglossal arch	146.2	198.89	230.0	210.6	235.1	239.0
palatopharyngeal arch	146.2	198.89	230.0	210.6	235.1	239.0
pallium	191.0	198.3	—	225.0	237.5	239.6
palpebra	173.1	198.2	232.1	216.1	238.2	239.2
pancreas	157.9	197.8	230.9	211.6	235.5	239.0
body	157.1	197.8	230.9	211.6	235.5	239.0
contiguous sites	157.8	—	—	—	—	—
duct (of Santorini) (of Wirsung)	157.3	197.8	230.9	211.6	235.5	239.0
ectopic tissue	157.8	197.8	230.9	211.6	235.5	239.0
head	157.0	197.8	230.9	211.6	235.5	239.0
islet cells	157.4	197.8	230.9	211.7	235.5	239.0
neck	157.8	197.8	230.9	211.6	235.5	239.0
tail	157.2	197.8	230.9	211.6	235.5	239.0
para-aortic body	194.6	198.89	—	227.6	237.3	239.7
paraganglion NEC	194.6	198.89	—	227.6	237.3	239.7
parametrium	183.4	198.82	—	221.0	236.3	239.5
paranephric	158.0	197.6	—	211.8	235.4	239.0
pararectal	195.3	198.89	—	229.8	238.8	239.8
parasagittal (region)	195.0	198.89	234.8	229.8	238.8	239.8
parasellar	192.9	198.4	—	225.9	237.9	239.7
parathyroid (gland)	194.1	198.89	234.8	227.1	237.4	239.7
paraurethral	195.3	198.89	—	229.8	238.8	239.8
gland	189.4	198.1	233.9	223.89	236.99	239.5
paravaginal	195.3	198.89	—	229.8	238.8	239.8
parenchyma, kidney	189.0	198.0	233.9	223.0	236.91	239.5
parietal						
bone	170.0	198.5	—	213.0	238.0	239.2
lobe, brain	191.3	198.3	—	225.0	237.5	239.6
paroophoron	183.3	198.82	233.3	221.0	236.3	239.5
parotid (duct) (gland)	142.0	198.89	230.0	210.2	235.0	239.0
parovarium	183.3	198.82	233.3	221.0	236.3	239.5
patella	170.8	198.5	—	213.8	238.0	239.2
peduncle, cerebral	191.7	198.3	—	225.0	237.5	239.6
pelvirectal junction	154.0	197.5	230.4	211.4	235.2	239.0
pelvis, pelvic	195.3	198.89	234.8	229.8	238.8	239.8
bone	170.6	198.5	—	213.6	238.0	239.2
floor	195.3	198.89	234.8	229.8	238.8	239.8
renal	189.1	198.0	233.9	223.1	236.91	239.5
viscera	195.3	198.89	234.8	229.8	238.8	239.8
wall	195.3	198.89	234.8	229.8	238.8	239.8
pelvo-abdominal	195.8	198.89	234.8	229.8	238.8	239.8
penis	187.4	198.82	233.5	222.1	236.6	239.5
body	187.3	198.82	233.5	222.1	236.6	239.5
corpus (cavernosum)	187.3	198.82	233.5	222.1	236.6	239.5
glans	187.2	198.82	233.5	222.1	236.6	239.5
skin NEC	187.4	198.82	233.5	222.1	236.6	239.5

	Malignant					
	Primary	Secondary	Ca in situ	Benign	Uncertain Behavior	Unspecified
periadrenal (tissue)	158.0	197.6	—	211.8	235.4	239.0
perianal (skin)	173.5	198.2	232.5	216.5	238.2	239.2
pericardium	164.1	198.89	—	212.7	238.8	239.8
perinephric	158.0	197.6	—	211.8	235.4	239.0
perineum	195.3	198.89	234.8	229.8	238.8	239.8
periodontal tissue NEC	143.9	198.89	230.0	210.4	235.1	239.0
periosteum—*see* Neoplasm, bone						
peripancreatic	158.0	197.6	—	211.8	235.4	239.0
peripheral nerve NEC	171.9	198.89	—	215.9	238.1	239.2
perirectal (tissue)	195.3	198.89	—	229.8	238.8	239.8
perirenal (tissue)	158.0	197.6	—	211.8	235.4	239.0
peritoneum, peritoneal (cavity)	158.9	197.6	—	211.8	235.4	239.0
contiguous sites	158.8	—	—	—	—	—
with digestive organs	159.8	—	—	—	—	—
parietal	158.8	197.6	—	211.8	235.4	239.0
pelvic	158.8	197.6	—	211.8	235.4	239.0
specified part NEC	158.8	197.6	—	211.8	235.4	239.0
peritonsillar (tissue)	195.0	198.89	234.8	229.8	238.8	239.8
periurethral tissue	195.3	198.89	—	229.8	238.8	239.8
phalanges	170.9	198.5	—	213.9	238.0	239.2
foot	170.8	198.5	—	213.8	238.0	239.2
hand	170.5	198.5	—	213.5	238.0	239.2
pharynx, pharyngeal	149.0	198.89	230.0	210.9	235.1	239.0
bursa	147.1	198.89	230.0	210.7	235.1	239.0
fornix	147.3	198.89	230.0	210.7	235.1	239.0
recess	147.2	198.89	230.0	210.7	235.1	239.0
region	149.0	198.89	230.0	210.9	235.1	239.0
tonsil	147.1	198.89	230.0	210.7	235.1	239.0
wall (lateral) (posterior)	149.0	198.89	230.0	210.9	235.1	239.0
pia mater (cerebral) (cranial)	192.1	198.4	—	225.2	237.6	239.7
spinal	192.3	198.4	—	225.4	237.6	239.7
pillars of fauces	146.2	198.89	230.0	210.6	235.1	239.0
pineal (body) (gland)	194.4	198.89	234.8	227.4	237.1	239.7
pinna (ear) NEC	173.2	198.2	232.2	216.2	238.2	239.2
cartilage	171.0	198.89	—	215.0	238.1	239.2
piriform fossa or sinus	148.1	198.89	230.0	210.8	235.1	239.0
pituitary (body) (fossa) (gland) (lobe)	194.3	198.89	234.8	227.3	237.0	239.7
placenta	181	198.82	233.2	219.8	236.1	239.5
pleura, pleural (cavity)	163.9	197.2	—	212.4	235.8	239.1
contiguous sites	163.8	—	—	—	—	—
parietal	163.0	197.2	—	212.4	235.8	239.1
visceral	163.1	197.2	—	212.4	235.8	239.1
plexus						
brachial	171.2	198.89	—	215.2	238.1	239.2
cervical	171.0	198.89	—	215.0	238.1	239.2
choroid	191.5	198.3	—	225.0	237.5	239.6
lumbosacral	171.6	198.89	—	215.6	238.1	239.2
sacral	171.6	198.89	—	215.6	238.1	239.2
pluri-endocrine	194.8	198.89	234.8	227.8	237.4	239.7
pole						
frontal	191.1	198.3	—	225.0	237.5	239.6
occipital	191.4	198.3	—	225.0	237.5	239.6
pons (varolii)	191.7	198.3	—	225.0	237.5	239.6
popliteal fossa or space*	195.5	198.89	234.8	229.8	238.8	239.8
postcricoid (region)	148.0	198.89	230.0	210.8	235.1	239.0
posterior fossa (cranial)	191.6	198.3	—	225.0	237.5	239.6
postnasal space	147.9	198.89	230.0	210.7	235.1	239.0
prepuce	187.1	198.82	233.5	222.1	236.6	239.5
prepylorus	151.1	197.8	230.2	211.1	235.2	239.0
presacral (region)	195.3	198.89	—	229.8	238.8	239.8

	Malignant					
	Primary	Secondary	Ca in situ	Benign	Uncertain Behavior	Unspecified
prostate (gland)	185	198.82	233.4	222.2	236.5	239.5
utricle	189.3	198.1	233.9	223.81	236.99	239.5
pterygoid fossa	171.0	198.89	—	215.0	238.1	239.2
pubic bone	170.6	198.5	—	213.6	238.0	239.2
pudenda, pudendum (female)	184.4	198.82	233.3	221.2	236.3	239.5
pulmonary	162.9	197.0	231.2	212.3	235.7	239.1
putamen	191.0	198.3	—	225.0	237.5	239.6
pyloric						
antrum	151.2	197.8	230.2	211.1	235.2	239.0
canal	151.1	197.8	230.2	211.1	235.2	239.0
pylorus	151.1	197.8	230.2	211.1	235.2	239.0
pyramid (brain)	191.7	198.3	—	225.0	237.5	239.6
pyriform fossa or sinus	148.1	198.89	230.0	210.8	235.1	239.0
radius (any part)	170.4	198.5	—	213.4	238.0	239.2
Rathke's pouch	194.3	198.89	234.8	227.3	237.0	239.7
rectosigmoid (colon) (junction)	154.0	197.5	230.4	211.4	235.2	239.0
contiguous sites with anus or rectum	154.8	—	—	—	—	—
rectouterine pouch	158.8	197.6	—	211.8	235.4	239.0
rectovaginal septum or wall	195.3	198.89	234.8	229.8	238.8	239.8
rectovesical septum	195.3	198.89	234.8	229.8	238.8	239.8
rectum (ampulla)	154.1	197.5	230.4	211.4	235.2	239.0
and colon	154.0	197.5	230.4	211.4	235.2	239.0
contiguous sites with anus or rectosigmoid junction	154.8	—	—	—	—	—
renal	189.0	198.0	233.9	223.0	236.91	239.5
calyx	189.1	198.0	233.9	223.1	236.91	239.5
hilus	189.1	198.0	233.9	223.1	236.91	239.5
parenchyma	189.0	198.0	233.9	223.0	236.91	239.5
pelvis	189.1	198.0	233.9	223.1	236.91	239.5
respiratory						
organs or system NEC	165.9	197.3	231.9	212.9	235.9	239.1
contiguous sites with intrathoracic						
organs	165.8	—	—	—	—	—
specified sites NEC	165.8	197.3	231.8	212.8	235.9	239.1
tract NEC	165.9	197.3	231.9	212.9	235.9	239.1
upper	165.0	197.3	231.9	212.9	235.9	239.1
retina	190.5	198.4	234.0	224.5	238.8	239.8
retrobulbar	190.1	198.4	—	224.1	238.8	239.8
retrocecal	158.0	197.6	—	211.8	235.4	239.0
retromolar (area) (triangle) (trigone)	145.6	198.89	230.0	210.4	235.1	239.0
retro-orbital	195.0	198.89	234.8	229.8	238.8	239.8
retroperitoneal (space) (tissue)	158.0	197.6	—	211.8	235.4	239.0
contiguous sites	158.8	—	—	—	—	—
retroperitoneum	158.0	197.6	—	211.8	235.4	239.0
contiguous sites	158.8	—	—	—	—	—
retropharyngeal	149.0	198.89	230.0	210.9	235.1	239.0
retrovesical (septum)	195.3	198.89	234.8	229.8	238.8	239.8
rhinencephalon	191.0	198.3	—	225.0	237.5	239.6
rib	170.3	198.5	—	213.3	238.0	239.2
Rosenmüller's fossa	147.2	198.89	230.0	210.7	235.1	239.0
round ligament	183.5	198.82	—	221.0	236.3	239.5
sacrococcyx, sacrococcygeal	170.6	198.5	—	213.6	238.0	239.2
region	195.3	198.89	234.8	229.8	238.8	239.8
sacrouterine ligament	183.4	198.82	—	221.0	236.3	239.5
sacrum, sacral (vertebra)	170.6	198.5	—	213.6	238.0	239.2
salivary gland or duct (major)	142.9	198.89	230.0	210.2	235.0	239.0
contiguous sites	142.8	—	—	—	—	—
minor NEC	145.9	198.89	230.0	210.4	235.1	239.0
parotid	142.0	198.89	230.0	210.2	235.0	239.0
pluriglandular	142.8	198.89	230.0	210.2	235.0	239.0

	Malignant					
	Primary	Secondary	Ca in situ	Benign	Uncertain Behavior	Unspecified
salivary gland or duct (major)—*continued*						
sublingual	142.2	198.89	230.0	210.2	235.0	239.0
submandibular	142.1	198.89	230.0	210.2	235.0	239.0
submaxillary	142.1	198.89	230.0	210.2	235.0	239.0
salpinx (uterine)	183.2	198.82	233.3	221.0	236.3	239.5
Santorini's duct	157.3	197.8	230.9	211.6	235.5	239.0
scalp	173.4	198.2	232.4	216.4	238.2	239.2
scapula (any part)	170.4	198.5	—	213.4	238.0	239.2
scapular region	195.1	198.89	234.8	229.8	238.8	239.8
scar NEC (*see also* Neoplasm, skin)	173.9	198.2	232.9	216.9	238.2	239.2
sciatic nerve	171.3	198.89	—	215.3	238.1	239.2
sclera	190.0	198.4	234.0	224.0	238.8	239.8
scrotum (skin)	187.7	198.82	233.6	222.4	236.6	239.5
sebaceous gland—*see* Neoplasm, skin						
sella turcica	194.3	198.89	234.8	227.3	237.0	239.7
bone	170.0	198.5	—	213.0	238.0	239.2
semilunar cartilage (knee)	170.7	198.5	—	213.7	238.0	239.2
seminal vesicle	187.8	198.82	233.6	222.8	236.6	239.5
septum						
nasal	160.0	197.3	231.8	212.0	235.9	239.1
posterior margin	147.3	198.89	230.0	210.7	235.1	239.0
rectovaginal	195.3	198.89	234.8	229.8	238.8	239.8
rectovesical	195.3	198.89	234.8	229.8	238.8	239.8
urethrovaginal	184.9	198.82	233.3	221.9	236.3	239.5
vesicovaginal	184.9	198.82	233.3	221.9	236.3	239.5
shoulder NEC*	195.4	198.89	232.6	229.8	238.8	239.8
sigmoid flexure (lower) (upper)	153.3	197.5	230.3	211.3	235.2	239.0
sinus (accessory)	160.9	197.3	231.8	212.0	235.9	239.1
bone (any)	170.0	198.5	—	213.0	238.0	239.2
contiguous sites with middle ear or nasal cavities	160.8	—	—	—	—	—
ethmoidal	160.3	197.3	231.8	212.0	235.9	239.1
frontal	160.4	197.3	231.8	212.0	235.9	239.1
maxillary	160.2	197.3	231.8	212.0	235.9	239.1
nasal, paranasal NEC	160.9	197.3	231.8	212.0	235.9	239.1
pyriform	148.1	198.89	230.0	210.8	235.1	239.0
sphenoidal	160.5	197.3	231.8	212.0	235.9	239.1
skeleton, skeletal NEC	170.9	198.5	—	213.9	238.0	239.2
Skene's gland	189.4	198.1	233.9	223.89	236.99	239.5
skin NEC	173.9	198.2	232.9	216.9	238.2	239.2
abdominal wall	173.5	198.2	232.5	216.5	238.2	239.2
ala nasi	173.3	198.2	232.3	216.3	238.2	239.2
ankle	173.7	198.2	232.7	216.7	238.2	239.2
antecubital space	173.6	198.2	232.6	216.6	238.2	239.2
anus	173.5	198.2	232.5	216.5	238.2	239.2
arm	173.6	198.2	232.6	216.6	238.2	239.2
auditory canal (external)	173.2	198.2	232.2	216.2	238.2	239.2
auricle (ear)	173.2	198.2	232.2	216.2	238.2	239.2
auricular canal (external)	173.2	198.2	232.2	216.2	238.2	239.2
axilla, axillary fold	173.5	198.2	232.5	216.5	238.2	239.2
back	173.5	198.2	232.5	216.5	238.2	239.2
breast	173.5	198.2	232.5	216.5	238.2	239.2
brow	173.3	198.2	232.3	216.3	238.2	239.2
buttock	173.5	198.2	232.5	216.5	238.2	239.2
calf	173.7	198.2	232.7	216.7	238.2	239.2
canthus (eye) (inner) (outer)	173.1	198.2	232.1	216.1	238.2	239.2
cervical region	173.4	198.2	232.4	216.4	238.2	239.2
cheek (external)	173.3	198.2	232.3	216.3	238.2	239.2
chest (wall)	173.5	198.2	232.5	216.5	238.2	239.2
chin	173.3	198.2	232.3	216.3	238.2	239.2

	Malignant					
	Primary	Secondary	Ca in situ	Benign	Uncertain Behavior	Unspecified
skin NEC—*continued*						
clavicular area	173.5	198.2	232.5	216.5	238.2	239.2
clitoris	184.3	198.82	233.3	221.2	236.3	239.5
columnella	173.3	198.2	232.3	216.3	238.2	239.2
concha	173.2	198.2	232.2	216.2	238.2	239.2
contiguous sites	173.8	—	—	—	—	—
ear (external)	173.2	198.2	232.2	216.2	238.2	239.2
elbow	173.6	198.2	232.6	216.6	238.2	239.2
eyebrow	173.3	198.2	232.3	216.3	238.2	239.2
eyelid	173.1	198.2	232.1	216.1	238.2	239.2
face NEC	173.3	198.2	232.3	216.3	238.2	239.2
female genital organs (external)	184.4	198.82	233.3	221.2	236.3	239.5
clitoris	184.3	198.82	233.3	221.2	236.3	239.5
labium NEC	184.4	198.82	233.3	221.2	236.3	239.5
majus	184.1	198.82	233.3	221.2	236.3	239.5
minus	184.2	198.82	233.3	221.2	236.3	239.5
pudendum	184.4	198.82	233.3	221.2	236.3	239.5
vulva	184.4	198.82	233.3	221.2	236.3	239.5
finger	173.6	198.2	232.6	216.6	238.2	239.2
flank	173.5	198.2	232.5	216.5	238.2	239.2
foot	173.7	198.2	232.7	216.7	238.2	239.2
forearm	173.6	198.2	232.6	216.6	238.2	239.2
forehead	173.3	198.2	232.3	216.3	238.2	239.2
glabella	173.3	198.2	232.3	216.3	238.2	239.2
gluteal region	173.5	198.2	232.5	216.5	238.2	239.2
groin	173.5	198.2	232.5	216.5	238.2	239.2
hand	173.6	198.2	232.6	216.6	238.2	239.2
head NEC	173.4	198.2	232.4	216.4	238.2	239.2
heel	173.7	198.2	232.7	216.7	238.2	239.2
helix	173.2	198.2	232.2	216.2	238.2	239.2
hip	173.7	198.2	232.7	216.7	238.2	239.2
infraclavicular region	173.5	198.2	232.5	216.5	238.2	239.2
inguinal region	173.5	198.2	232.5	216.5	238.2	239.2
jaw	173.3	198.2	232.3	216.3	238.2	239.2
knee	173.7	198.2	232.7	216.7	238.2	239.2
labia						
majora	184.1	198.82	233.3	221.2	236.3	239.5
minora	184.2	198.82	233.3	221.2	236.3	239.5
leg	173.7	198.2	232.7	216.7	238.2	239.2
lid (lower) (upper)	173.1	198.2	232.1	216.1	238.2	239.2
limb NEC	173.9	198.2	232.9	216.9	238.2	239.5
lower	173.7	198.2	232.7	216.7	238.2	239.2
upper	173.6	198.2	232.6	216.6	238.2	239.2
lip (lower) (upper)	173.0	198.2	232.0	216.0	238.2	239.2
male genital organs	187.9	198.82	233.6	222.9	236.6	239.5
penis	187.4	198.82	233.5	222.1	236.6	239.5
prepuce	187.1	198.82	233.5	222.1	236.6	239.5
scrotum	187.7	198.82	233.6	222.4	236.6	239.5
mastectomy site	173.5	198.2	—	—	—	—
specified as breast tissue	174.8	198.81	—	—	—	
meatus, acoustic (external)	173.2	198.2	232.2	216.2	238.2	239.2
melanoma —*see* Melanoma						
nates	173.5	198.2	232.5	216.5	238.2	239.2
neck	173.4	198.2	232.4	216.4	238.2	239.2
nose (external)	173.3	198.2	232.3	216.3	238.2	239.2
palm	173.6	198.2	232.6	216.6	238.2	239.2
palpebra	173.1	198.2	232.1	216.1	238.2	239.2
penis NEC	187.4	198.82	233.5	222.1	236.6	239.5
perianal	173.5	198.2	232.5	216.5	238.2	239.2
perineum	173.5	198.2	232.5	216.5	238.2	239.2

	Malignant					
	Primary	Secondary	Ca in situ	Benign	Uncertain Behavior	Unspecified
skin NEC—*continued*						
pinna	173.2	198.2	232.2	216.2	238.2	239.2
plantar	173.7	198.2	232.7	216.7	238.2	239.2
popliteal fossa or space	173.7	198.2	232.7	216.7	238.2	239.2
prepuce	187.1	198.82	233.5	222.1	236.6	239.5
pubes	173.5	198.2	232.5	216.5	238.2	239.2
sacrococcygeal region	173.5	198.2	232.5	216.5	238.2	239.2
scalp	173.4	198.2	232.4	216.4	238.2	239.2
scapular region	173.5	198.2	232.5	216.5	238.2	239.2
scrotum	187.7	198.82	233.6	222.4	236.6	239.5
shoulder	173.6	198.2	232.6	216.6	238.2	239.2
sole (foot)	173.7	198.2	232.7	216.7	238.2	239.2
specified sites NEC	173.8	198.2	232.8	216.8	232.8	239.2
submammary fold	173.5	198.2	232.5	216.5	238.2	239.2
supraclavicular region	173.4	198.2	232.4	216.4	238.2	239.2
temple	173.3	198.2	232.3	216.3	238.2	239.2
thigh	173.7	198.2	232.7	216.7	238.2	239.2
thoracic wall	173.5	198.2	232.5	216.5	238.2	239.2
thumb	173.6	198.2	232.6	216.6	238.2	239.2
toe	173.7	198.2	232.7	216.7	238.2	239.2
tragus	173.2	198.2	232.2	216.2	238.2	239.2
trunk	173.5	198.2	232.5	216.5	238.2	239.2
umbilicus	173.5	198.2	232.5	216.5	238.2	239.2
vulva	184.4	198.82	233.3	221.2	236.3	239.5
wrist	173.6	198.2	232.6	216.6	238.2	239.2
skull	170.0	198.5	—	213.0	238.0	239.2
soft parts or tissues—*see* Neoplasm, connective tissue						
specified site NEC	195.8	198.89	234.8	229.8	238.8	239.8
spermatic cord	187.6	198.82	233.6	222.8	236.6	239.5
sphenoid	160.5	197.3	231.8	212.0	235.9	239.1
bone	170.0	198.5	—	213.0	238.0	239.2
sinus	160.5	197.3	231.8	212.0	235.9	239.1
sphincter						
anal	154.2	197.5	230.5	211.4	235.5	239.0
of Oddi	156.1	197.8	230.8	211.5	235.3	239.0
spine, spinal (column)	170.2	198.5	—	213.2	238.0	239.2
bulb	191.7	198.3	—	225.0	237.5	239.6
coccyx	170.6	198.5	—	213.6	238.0	239.2
cord (cervical) (lumbar) (sacral) (thoracic)	192.2	198.3	—	225.3	237.5	239.7
dura mater	192.3	198.4	—	225.4	237.6	239.7
lumbosacral	170.2	198.5	—	213.2	238.0	239.2
membrane	192.3	198.4	—	225.4	237.6	239.7
meninges	192.3	198.4	—	225.4	237.6	239.7
nerve (root)	171.9	198.89	—	215.9	238.1	239.2
pia mater	192.3	198.4	—	225.4	237.6	239.7
root	171.9	198.89	—	215.9	238.1	239.2
sacrum	170.6	198.5	—	213.6	238.0	239.2
spleen, splenic NEC	159.1	197.8	230.9	211.9	235.5	239.0
flexure (colon)	153.7	197.5	230.3	211.3	235.2	239.0
stem, brain	191.7	198.3	—	225.0	237.5	239.6
Stensen's duct	142.0	198.89	230.0	210.2	235.0	239.0
sternum	170.3	198.5	—	213.3	238.0	239.2
stomach	151.9	197.8	230.2	211.1	235.2	239.0
antrum (pyloric)	151.2	197.8	230.2	211.1	235.2	239.0
body	151.4	197.8	230.2	211.1	235.2	239.0
cardia	151.0	197.8	230.2	211.1	235.2	239.0
cardiac orifice	151.0	197.8	230.2	211.1	235.2	239.0
contiguous sites	151.8	—	—	—	—	—
corpus	151.4	197.8	230.2	211.1	235.2	239.0

	Malignant					
	Primary	Secondary	Ca in situ	Benign	Uncertain Behavior	Unspecified
stomach—*continued*						
fundus	151.3	197.8	230.2	211.1	235.2	239.0
greater curvature NEC	151.6	197.8	230.2	211.1	235.2	239.0
lesser curvature NEC	151.5	197.8	230.2	211.1	235.2	239.0
prepylorus	151.1	197.8	230.2	211.1	235.2	239.0
pylorus	151.1	197.8	230.2	211.1	235.2	239.0
wall NEC	151.9	197.8	230.2	211.1	235.2	239.0
anterior NEC	151.8	197.8	230.2	211.1	235.2	239.0
posterior NEC	151.8	197.8	230.2	211.1	235.2	239.0
stroma, endometrial	182.0	198.82	233.2	219.1	236.0	239.5
stump, cervical	180.8	198.82	233.1	219.0	236.0	239.5
subcutaneous (nodule) (tissue) NEC—*see* Neoplasm, connective tissue						
subdural	192.1	198.4	—	225.2	237.6	239.7
subglottis, subglottic	161.2	197.3	231.0	212.1	235.6	239.1
sublingual	144.9	198.89	230.0	210.3	235.1	239.0
gland or duct	142.2	198.89	230.0	210.2	235.0	239.0
submandibular gland	142.1	198.89	230.0	210.2	235.0	239.0
submaxillary gland or duct	142.1	198.89	230.0	210.2	235.0	239.0
submental	195.0	198.89	234.8	229.8	238.8	239.8
subpleural	162.9	197.0	—	212.3	235.7	239.1
substernal	164.2	197.1	—	212.5	235.8	239.8
sudoriferous, sudoriparous gland, site unspecified	173.9	198.2	232.9	216.9	238.2	239.2
specified site—*see* Neoplasm, skin						
supraclavicular region	195.0	198.89	234.8	229.8	238.8	239.8
supraglottis	161.1	197.3	231.0	212.1	235.6	239.1
suprarenal (capsule) (cortex) (gland) (medulla)	194.0	198.7	234.8	227.0	237.2	239.7
suprasellar (region)	191.9	198.3	—	225.0	237.5	239.6
sweat gland (apocrine) (eccrine), site unspecified	173.9	198.2	232.9	216.9	238.2	239.2
specified site—*see* Neoplasm, skin						
sympathetic nerve or nervous system NEC	171.9	198.89	—	215.9	238.1	239.2
symphysis pubis	170.6	198.5	—	213.6	238.0	239.2
synovial membrane—*see* Neoplasm, connective tissue						
tapetum, brain	191.8	198.3	—	225.0	237.5	239.6
tarsus (any bone)	170.8	198.5	—	213.8	238.0	239.2
temple (skin)	173.3	198.2	232.3	216.3	238.2	239.2
temporal						
bone	170.0	198.5	—	213.0	238.0	239.2
lobe or pole	191.2	198.3	—	225.0	237.5	239.6
region	195.0	198.89	234.8	229.8	238.8	239.8
skin	173.3	198.2	232.3	216.3	238.2	239.2
tendon (sheath)—*see* Neoplasm, connective tissue						
tentorium (cerebelli)	192.1	198.4	—	225.2	237.6	239.7
testis, testes (descended) (scrotal)	186.9	198.82	233.6	222.0	236.4	239.5
ectopic	186.0	198.82	233.6	222.0	236.4	239.5
retained	186.0	198.82	233.6	222.0	236.4	239.5
undescended	186.0	198.82	233.6	222.0	236.4	239.5
thalamus	191.0	198.3	—	225.0	237.5	239.6
thigh NEC*	195.5	198.89	234.8	229.8	238.8	239.8
thorax, thoracic (cavity) (organs NEC)	195.1	198.89	234.8	229.8	238.8	239.8
duct	171.4	198.89	—	215.4	238.1	239.2
wall NEC	195.1	198.89	234.8	229.8	238.8	239.8
throat	149.0	198.89	230.0	210.9	235.1	239.0
thumb NEC*	195.4	198.89	232.6	229.8	238.8	239.8

	Malignant					
	Primary	Secondary	Ca in situ	Benign	Uncertain Behavior	Unspecified
thymus (gland)	164.0	198.89	—	212.6	235.8	239.8
contiguous sites with heart and mediastinum	164.8	—	—	—	—	—
thyroglossal duct	193	198.89	234.8	226	237.4	239.7
thyroid (gland)	193	198.89	234.8	226	237.4	239.7
cartilage	161.3	197.3	231.0	212.1	235.6	239.1
tibia (any part)	170.7	198.5	—	213.7	238.0	239.2
toe NEC*	195.5	198.89	232.7	229.8	238.8	239.8
tongue	141.9	198.89	230.0	210.1	235.1	239.0
anterior (two-thirds) NEC	141.4	198.89	230.0	210.1	235.1	239.0
dorsal surface	141.1	198.89	230.0	210.1	235.1	239.0
ventral surface	141.3	198.89	230.0	210.1	235.1	239.0
base (dorsal surface)	141.0	198.89	230.0	210.1	235.1	239.0
border (lateral)	141.2	198.89	230.0	210.1	235.1	239.0
contiguous sites	141.8	—	—	—	—	—
dorsal surface NEC	141.1	198.89	230.0	210.1	235.1	239.0
fixed part NEC	141.0	198.89	230.0	210.1	235.1	239.0
foramen cecum	141.1	198.89	230.0	210.1	235.1	239.0
frenulum linguae	141.3	198.89	230.0	210.1	235.1	239.0
junctional zone	141.5	198.89	230.0	210.1	235.1	239.0
margin (lateral)	141.2	198.89	230.0	210.1	235.1	239.0
midline NEC	141.1	198.89	230.0	210.1	235.1	239.0
mobile part NEC	141.4	198.89	230.0	210.1	235.1	239.0
posterior (third)	141.0	198.89	230.0	210.1	235.1	239.0
root	141.0	198.89	230.0	210.1	235.1	239.0
surface (dorsal)	141.1	198.89	230.0	210.1	235.1	239.0
base	141.0	198.89	230.0	210.1	235.1	239.0
ventral	141.3	198.89	230.0	210.1	235.1	239.0
tip	141.2	198.89	230.0	210.1	235.1	239.0
tonsil	141.6	198.89	230.0	210.1	235.1	239.0
tonsil	146.0	198.89	230.0	210.5	235.1	239.0
fauces, faucial	146.0	198.89	230.0	210.5	235.1	239.0
lingual	141.6	198.89	230.0	210.1	235.1	239.0
palatine	146.0	198.89	230.0	210.5	235.1	239.0
pharyngeal	147.1	198.89	230.0	210.7	235.1	239.0
pillar (anterior) (posterior)	146.2	198.89	230.0	210.6	235.1	239.0
tonsillar fossa	146.1	198.89	230.0	210.6	235.1	239.0
tooth socket NEC	143.9	198.89	230.0	210.4	235.1	239.0
trachea (cartilage) (mucosa)	162.0	197.3	231.1	212.2	235.7	239.1
contiguous sites with bronchus or lung	162.8	—	—	—	—	—
tracheobronchial	162.8	197.3	231.1	212.2	235.7	239.1
contiguous sites with lung	162.8	—	—	—	—	—
tragus	173.2	198.2	232.2	216.2	238.2	239.2
trunk NEC*	195.8	198.89	232.5	229.8	238.8	239.8
tubo-ovarian	183.8	198.82	233.3	221.8	236.3	239.5
tunica vaginalis	187.8	198.82	233.6	222.8	236.6	239.5
turbinate (bone)	170.0	198.5	—	213.0	238.0	239.2
nasal	160.0	197.3	231.8	212.0	235.9	239.1
tympanic cavity	160.1	197.3	231.8	212.0	235.9	239.1
ulna (any part)	170.4	198.5	—	213.4	238.0	239.2
umbilicus, umbilical	173.5	198.2	232.5	216.5	238.2	239.2
uncus, brain	191.2	198.3	—	225.0	237.5	239.6
unknown site or unspecified	199.1	199.1	234.9	229.9	238.9	239.9
urachus	188.7	198.1	233.7	223.3	236.7	239.4
ureter, ureteral	189.2	198.1	233.9	223.2	236.91	239.5
orifice (bladder)	188.6	198.1	233.7	223.3	236.7	239.4
ureter-bladder (junction)	188.6	198.1	233.7	223.3	236.7	239.4
urethra, urethral (gland)	189.3	198.1	233.9	223.81	236.99	239.5
orifice, internal	188.5	198.1	233.7	223.3	236.7	239.4
urethrovaginal (septum)	184.9	198.82	233.3	221.9	236.3	239.5

	Malignant Primary	Malignant Secondary	Malignant Ca in situ	Benign	Uncertain Behavior	Unspecified
urinary organ or system NEC	189.9	198.1	233.9	223.9	236.99	239.5
bladder—*see* Neoplasm, bladder						
contiguous sites	189.8	—	—	—	—	—
specified sites NEC	189.8	198.1	233.9	223.89	236.99	239.5
utero-ovarian	183.8	198.82	233.3	221.8	236.3	239.5
ligament	183.3	198.82	—	221.0	236.3	239.5
uterosacral ligament	183.4	198.82	—	221.0	236.3	239.5
uterus, uteri, uterine	179	198.82	233.2	219.9	236.0	239.5
adnexa NEC	183.9	198.82	233.3	221.8	236.3	239.5
contiguous sites	183.8	—	—	—	—	—
body	182.0	198.82	233.2	219.1	236.0	239.5
contiguous sites	182.8	—	—	—	—	—
cervix	180.9	198.82	233.1	219.0	236.0	239.5
cornu	182.0	198.82	233.2	219.1	236.0	239.5
corpus	182.0	198.82	233.2	219.1	236.0	239.5
endocervix (canal) (gland)	180.0	198.82	233.1	219.0	236.0	239.5
endometrium	182.0	198.82	233.2	219.1	236.0	239.5
exocervix	180.1	198.82	233.1	219.0	236.0	239.5
external os	180.1	198.82	233.1	219.0	236.0	239.5
fundus	182.0	198.82	233.2	219.1	236.0	239.5
internal os	180.0	198.82	233.1	219.0	236.0	239.5
isthmus	182.1	198.82	233.2	219.1	236.0	239.5
ligament	183.4	198.82	—	221.0	236.3	239.5
broad	183.3	198.82	233.3	221.0	236.3	239.5
round	183.5	198.82	—	221.0	236.3	239.5
lower segment	182.1	198.82	233.2	219.1	236.0	239.5
myometrium	182.0	198.82	233.2	219.1	236.0	239.5
squamocolumnar junction	180.8	198.82	233.1	219.0	236.0	239.5
tube	183.2	198.82	233.3	221.0	236.3	239.5
utricle, prostatic	189.3	198.1	233.9	223.81	236.99	239.5
uveal tract	190.0	198.4	234.0	224.0	238.8	239.8
uvula	145.4	198.89	230.0	210.4	235.1	239.0
vagina, vaginal (fornix) (vault) (wall)	184.0	198.82	233.3	221.1	236.3	239.5
vaginovesical	184.9	198.82	233.3	221.9	236.3	239.5
septum	194.9	198.82	233.3	221.9	236.3	239.5
vallecula (epiglottis)	146.3	198.89	230.0	210.6	235.1	239.0
vascular—*see* Neoplasm, connective tissue						
vas deferens	187.6	198.82	233.6	222.8	236.6	239.5
Vater's ampulla	156.2	197.8	230.8	211.5	235.3	239.0
vein, venous—*see* Neoplasm, connective tissue						
vena cava (abdominal) (inferior)	171.5	198.89	—	215.5	238.1	239.2
superior	171.4	198.89	—	215.4	238.1	239.2
ventricle (cerebral) (floor) (fourth) (lateral) (third)	191.5	198.3	—	225.0	237.5	239.6
cardiac (left) (right)	164.1	198.89	—	212.7	238.8	239.8
ventricular band of larynx	161.1	197.3	231.0	212.1	235.6	239.1
ventriculus—*see* Neoplasm, stomach						
vermillion border—*see* Neoplasm, lip						
vermis, cerebellum	191.6	198.3	—	225.0	237.5	239.6
vertebra (column)	170.2	198.5	—	213.2	238.0	239.2
coccyx	170.6	198.5	—	213.6	238.0	239.2
sacrum	170.6	198.5	—	213.6	238.0	239.2
vesical—*see* Neoplasm, bladder						
vesicle, seminal	187.8	198.82	233.6	222.8	236.6	239.5
vesicocervical tissue	184.9	198.82	233.3	221.9	236.3	239.5
vesicorectal	195.3	198.89	234.8	229.8	238.8	239.8
vesicovaginal	184.9	198.82	233.3	221.9	236.3	239.5
septum	184.9	198.82	233.3	221.9	236.3	239.5
vessel (blood)—*see* Neoplasm, connective tissue						

	Malignant					
	Primary	Secondary	Ca in situ	Benign	Uncertain Behavior	Unspecified
vestibular gland, greater	184.1	198.82	233.3	221.2	236.3	239.5
vestibule						
mouth	145.1	198.89	230.0	210.4	235.1	239.0
nose	160.0	197.3	231.8	212.0	235.9	239.1
Virchow's gland	—	196.0	—	229.0	238.8	239.8
viscera NEC	195.8	198.89	234.8	229.8	238.8	239.8
vocal cords (true)	161.0	197.3	231.0	212.1	235.6	239.1
false	161.1	197.3	231.0	212.1	235.6	239.1
vomer	170.0	198.5	—	213.0	238.0	239.2
vulva	184.4	198.82	233.3	221.2	236.3	239.5
vulvovaginal gland	184.4	198.82	233.3	221.2	236.3	239.5
Waldeyer's ring	149.1	198.89	230.0	210.9	235.1	239.0
Wharton's duct	142.1	198.89	230.0	210.2	235.0	239.0
white matter (central) (cerebral)	191.0	198.3	—	225.0	237.5	239.6
windpipe	162.0	197.3	231.1	212.2	235.7	239.1
Wirsung's duct	157.3	197.8	230.9	211.6	235.5	239.0
wolffian (body) (duct)						
female	184.8	198.82	233.3	221.8	236.3	239.5
male	187.8	198.82	233.6	222.8	236.6	239.5
womb—*see* Neoplasm, uterus						
wrist NEC*	195.4	198.89	232.6	229.8	238.8	239.8
xiphoid process	170.3	198.5	—	213.3	238.0	239.2
Zuckerkandl's organ	194.6	198.89	—	227.6	237.3	239.7

Neovascularization
choroid 362.16
ciliary body 364.42
cornea 370.60
deep 370.63
localized 370.61
iris 364.42
retina 362.16
subretinal 362.16
Nephralgia 788.0
Nephritis, nephritic (albuminuric) (azotemic) (congenital) (degenerative) (diffuse) (disseminated) (epithelial) (familial) (focal) (granulomatous) (hemorrhagic) (infantile) (nonsuppurative, excretory) (uremic) 583.9
with
edema—*see* Nephrosis
lesion of
glomerulonephritis
hypocomplementemic persistent 583.2
with nephrotic syndrome 581.2
chronic 582.2
lobular 583.2
with nephrotic syndrome 581.2
chronic 582.2
membranoproliferative 583.2
with nephrotic syndrome 581.2
chronic 582.2
membranous 583.1
with nephrotic syndrome 581.1
chronic 582.1
mesangiocapillary 583.2
with nephrotic syndrome 581.2
chronic 582.2
mixed membranous and proliferative 583.2
with nephrotic syndrome 581.2
chronic 582.2
proliferative (diffuse) 583.0
with nephrotic syndrome 581.0
acute 580.0
chronic 582.0
rapidly progressive 583.4
acute 580.4
chronic 582.4
interstitial nephritis (diffuse) (focal) 583.89
with nephrotic syndrome 581.89
acute 580.89
chronic 582.89
necrotizing glomerulitis 583.4
acute 580.4
chronic 582.4
renal necrosis 583.9
cortical 583.6
medullary 583.7
specified pathology NEC 583.89
with nephrotic syndrome 581.89
acute 580.89
chronic 582.89
necrosis, renal 583.9
cortical 583.6
medullary (papillary) 583.7
nephrotic syndrome (*see also* Nephrosis) 581.9
papillary necrosis 583.7
specified pathology NEC 583.89
acute 580.9
extracapillary with epithelial crescents 580.4
hypertensive (*see also* Hypertension, kidney) 403.90
necrotizing 580.4
poststreptococcal 580.0
proliferative (diffuse) 580.0
Nephritis, nephritic—*continued*
rapidly progressive 580.4
specified pathology NEC 580.89
amyloid 277.3 *[583.81]*
chronic 277.3 *[582.81]*
arteriolar (*see also* Hypertension, kidney) 403.90
arteriosclerotic (*see also* Hypertension, kidney) 403.90
ascending (*see also* Pyelitis) 590.80
atrophic 582.9
basement membrane NEC 583.89
with
pulmonary hemorrhage (Goodpasture's syndrome) 446.21 *[583.81]*
calculous, calculus 592.0
cardiac (*see also* Hypertension, kidney) 403.90
cardiovascular (*see also* Hypertension, kidney) 403.90
chronic 582.9
arteriosclerotic (*see also* Hypertension, kidney) 403.90
hypertensive (*see also* Hypertension, kidney) 403.90
cirrhotic (*see also* Sclerosis, renal) 587
complicating pregnancy, childbirth, or puerperium 646.2
with hypertension 642.1
affecting fetus or newborn 760.0
affecting fetus or newborn 760.1
croupous 580.9
desquamative—*see* Nephrosis
due to
amyloidosis 277.3 *[583.81]*
chronic 277.3 *[582.81]*
arteriosclerosis (*see also* Hypertension, kidney) 403.90
diabetes mellitus 250.4 *[583.81]*
with nephrotic syndrome 250.4 *[581.81]*
diphtheria 032.89 *[580.81]*
gonococcal infection (acute) 098.19 *[583.81]*
chronic or duration of 2 months or over 098.39 *[583.81]*
gout 274.10
infectious hepatitis 070.9 *[580.81]*
mumps 072.79 *[580.81]*
specified kidney pathology NEC 583.89
acute 580.89
chronic 582.89
streptotrichosis 039.8 *[583.81]*
subacute bacterial endocarditis 421.0 *[580.81]*
systemic lupus erythematosus 710.0 *[583.81]*
chronic 710.0 *[582.81]*
typhoid fever 002.0 *[580.81]*
endothelial 582.2
end stage (chronic) (terminal) NEC 585
epimembranous 581.1
exudative 583.89
with nephrotic syndrome 581.89
acute 580.89
chronic 582.89
gonococcal (acute) 098.19 *[583.81]*
chronic or duration of 2 months or over 098.39 *[583.81]*
gouty 274.10
hereditary (Alport's syndrome) 759.89
hydremic—*see* Nephrosis
hypertensive (*see also* Hypertension, kidney) 403.90
hypocomplementemic persistent 583.2
with nephrotic syndrome 581.2
chronic 582.2

Nephritis, nephritic—*continued*
immune complex NEC 583.89
infective (*see also* Pyelitis) 590.80
interstitial (diffuse) (focal) 583.89
with nephrotic syndrome 581.89
acute 580.89
chronic 582.89
latent or quiescent—*see* Nephritis, chronic
lead 984.9
specified type of lead—*see* Table of drugs and chemicals
lobular 583.2
with nephrotic syndrome 581.2
chronic 582.2
lupus 710.0 *[583.81]*
acute 710.0 *[580.81]*
chronic 710.0 *[582.81]*
membranoproliferative 583.2
with nephrotic syndrome 581.2
chronic 582.2
membranous 583.1
with nephrotic syndrome 581.1
chronic 582.1
mesangiocapillary 583.2
with nephrotic syndrome 581.2
chronic 582.2
minimal change 581.3
mixed membranous and proliferative 583.2
with nephrotic syndrome 581.2
chronic 582.2
necrotic, necrotizing 583.4
acute 580.4
chronic 582.4
nephrotic—*see* Nephrosis
old—*see* Nephritis, chronic
parenchymatous 581.89
polycystic 753.12
adult type (APKD) 753.13
autosomal dominant 753.13
autosomal recessive 753.14
childhood type (CPKD) 753.14
infantile type 753.14
poststreptococcal 580.0
pregnancy—*see* Nephritis, complicating pregnancy
proliferative 583.0
with nephrotic syndrome 581.0
acute 580.0
chronic 582.0
purulent (*see also* Pyelitis) 590.80
rapidly progressive 583.4
acute 580.4
chronic 582.4
salt-losing or salt-wasting (*see also* Disease, renal) 593.9
saturnine 984.9
specified type of lead—*see* Table of drugs and chemicals
septic (*see also* Pyelitis) 590.80
specified pathology NEC 583.89
acute 580.89
chronic 582.89
staphylococcal (*see also* Pyelitis) 590.80
streptotrichosis 039.8 *[583.81]*
subacute (*see also* Nephrosis) 581.9
suppurative (*see also* Pyelitis) 590.80
syphilitic (late) 095.4
congenital 090.5 *[583.81]*
early 091.69 *[583.81]*
terminal (chronic) (end-stage) NEC 585
toxic—*see* Nephritis, acute

Nephritis, nephritic—*continued*
tubal, tubular—*see* Nephrosis, tubular
tuberculous (*see also* Tuberculosis) 016.0 *[583.81]*
type II (Ellis)—*see* Nephrosis
vascular—*see* Hypertension, kidney
war 580.9
Nephroblastoma (M8960/3) 189.0
epithelial (M8961/3) 189.0
mesenchymal (M8962/3) 189.0
Nephrocalcinosis 275.4
Nephrocystitis, pustular (*see also* Pyelitis) 590.80
Nephrolithiasis (congenital) (pelvis) (recurrent) 592.0
uric acid 274.11
Nephroma (M8960/3) 189.0
mesoblastic (M8960/1) 236.9
Nephronephritis (*see also* Nephrosis) 581.9
Nephronopthisis 753.16
Nephropathy (*see also* Nephritis) 583.9
with
exudative nephritis 583.89
interstitial nephritis (diffuse) (focal) 583.89
medullary necrosis 583.7
necrosis 583.9
cortical 583.6
medullary or papillary 583.7
papillary necrosis 583.7
specified lesion or cause NEC 583.89
analgesic 583.89
with medullary necrosis, acute 584.7
arteriolar (*see also* Hypertension, kidney) 403.90
arteriosclerotic (*see also* Hypertension, kidney) 403.90
complicating pregnancy 646.2
diabetic 250.4 *[583.81]*
gouty 274.10
specified type NEC 274.19
hypercalcemic 588.8
hypertensive (*see also* Hypertension, kidney) 403.90
hypokalemic (vacuolar) 588.8
obstructive 593.89
congenital 753.2
phenacetin 584.7
phosphate-losing 588.0
potassium depletion 588.8
proliferative (*see also* Nephritis, proliferative) 583.0
protein-losing 588.8
salt-losing or salt-wasting (*see also* Disease, renal) 593.9
sickle-cell (*see also* Disease, sickle-cell) 282.60 *[583.81]*
toxic 584.5
vasomotor 584.5
water-losing 588.8
Nephroptosis (*see also* Disease, renal) 593.0
congenital (displaced) 753.3
Nephropyosis (*see also* Abscess, kidney) 590.2
Nephrorrhagia 593.81
Nephrosclerosis (arteriolar) (arteriosclerotic) (chronic) (hyaline) (*see also* Hypertension, kidney) 403.90
gouty 274.10
hyperplastic (arteriolar) (*see also* Hypertension, kidney) 403.90
senile (*see also* Sclerosis, renal) 587

Nephrosis, nephrotic (Epstein's) (syndrome) 581.9
 with
  lesion of
   focal glomerulosclerosis 581.1
   glomerulonephritis
    endothelial 581.2
    hypocomplementemic persistent 581.2
    lobular 581.2
    membranoproliferative 581.2
    membranous 581.1
    mesangiocapillary 581.2
    minimal change 581.3
    mixed membranous and proliferative 581.2
    proliferative 581.0
   segmental hyalinosis 581.1
   specified pathology NEC 581.89
 acute—*see* Nephrosis, tubular
 anoxic—*see* Nephrosis, tubular
 arteriosclerotic (*see also* Hypertension, kidney) 403.90
 chemical—*see* Nephrosis, tubular
 cholemic 572.4
 complicating pregnancy, childbirth, or puerperium—*see* Nephritis, complicating pregnancy
 diabetic 250.4 *[581.81]*
 hemoglobinuric—*see* Nephrosis, tubular
 in
  amyloidosis 277.3 *[581.81]*
  diabetes mellitus 250.4 *[581.81]*
  epidemic hemorrhagic fever 078.6
  malaria 084.9 *[581.81]*
  polyarteritis 446.0 *[581.81]*
  systemic lupus erythematosus 710.0 *[581.81]*
 ischemic—*see* Nephrosis, tubular
 lipoid 581.3
 lower nephron—*see* Nephrosis, tubular
 lupoid 710.0 *[581.81]*
 lupus 710.0 *[581.81]*
 malarial 084.9 *[581.81]*
 minimal change 581.3
 necrotizing—*see* Nephrosis, tubular
 osmotic (sucrose) 588.8
 polyarteritic 446.0 *[581.81]*
 radiation 581.9
 specified lesion or cause NEC 581.89
 syphilitic 095.4
 toxic—*see* Nephrosis, tubular
 tubular (acute) 584.5
  due to a procedure 997.5
  radiation 581.9
Nephrosonephritis hemorrhagic (endemic) 078.6
Nephrostomy status V44.6
 with complication 997.5
Nerve —*see* condition
Nerves 799.2
Nervous (*see also* condition) 799.2
 breakdown 300.9
 heart 306.2
 stomach 306.4
 tension 799.2
Nervousness 799.2
Nesidioblastoma (M8150/0)
 pancreas 211.7
 specified site NEC—*see* Neoplasm, by site, benign
 unspecified site 211.7
Netherton's syndrome (ichthyosiform erythroderma) 757.1
Nettle rash 708.8
Nettleship's disease (urticaria pigmentosa) 757.33
Neumann's disease (pemphigus vegetans) 694.4
Neuralgia, neuralgic (acute) (*see also* Neuritis) 729.2
 accessory (nerve) 352.4
 acoustic (nerve) 388.5
 ankle 355.8
 anterior crural 355.8
 anus 787.99
 arm 723.4
 auditory (nerve) 388.5
 axilla 353.0
 bladder 788.1
 brachial 723.4
 brain—*see* Disorder, nerve, cranial
 broad ligament 625.9
 cerebral—*see* Disorder, nerve, cranial
 ciliary 346.2
 cranial nerve—*see also* Disorder, nerve, cranial
  fifth or trigeminal (*see also* Neuralgia, trigeminal) 350.1
 ear 388.71
  middle 352.1
 facial 351.8
 finger 354.9
 flank 355.8
 foot 355.8
 forearm 354.9
 Fothergill's (*see also* Neuralgia, trigeminal) 350.1
  postherpetic 053.12
 glossopharyngeal (nerve) 352.1
 groin 355.8
 hand 354.9
 heel 355.8
 Horton's 346.2
 Hunt's 053.11
 hypoglossal (nerve) 352.5
 iliac region 355.8
 infraorbital (*see also* Neuralgia, trigeminal) 350.1
 inguinal 355.8
 intercostal (nerve) 353.8
  postherpetic 053.19
 jaw 352.1
 kidney 788.0
 knee 355.8
 loin 355.8
 malarial (*see also* Malaria) 084.6
 mastoid 385.89
 maxilla 352.1
 median thenar 354.1
 metatarsal 355.6
 middle ear 352.1
 migrainous 346.2
 Morton's 355.6
 nerve, cranial—*see* Disorder, nerve, cranial
 nose 352.0
 olfactory (nerve) 352.0
 ophthalmic 377.30
  postherpetic 053.19
 optic (nerve) 377.30
 penis 607.9
 perineum 355.8
 pleura 511.0
 postherpetic NEC 053.19
  geniculate ganglion 053.11
  ophthalmic 053.19
  trifacial 053.12
  trigeminal 053.12

Neuralgia, neuralgic—*continued*
pubic region 355.8
radial (nerve) 723.4
rectum 787.99
sacroiliac joint 724.3
sciatic (nerve) 724.3
scrotum 608.9
seminal vesicle 608.9
shoulder 354.9
Sluder's 337.0
specified nerve NEC—*see* Disorder, nerve
spermatic cord 608.9
sphenopalatine (ganglion) 337.0
subscapular (nerve) 723.4
suprascapular (nerve) 723.4
testis 608.89
thenar (median) 354.1
thigh 355.8
tongue 352.5
trifacial (nerve) (*see also* Neuralgia, trigeminal) 350.1
trigeminal (nerve) 350.1
postherpetic 053.12
tympanic plexus 388.71
ulnar (nerve) 723.4
vagus (nerve) 352.3
wrist 354.9
writers' 300.89
organic 333.84
Neurapraxia —*see* Injury, nerve
Neurasthenia 300.5
cardiac 306.2
gastric 306.4
heart 306.2
postfebrile 780.7
postviral 780.7
Neurilemmoma (M9560/0)—*see also* Neoplasm, connective tissue, benign
acoustic (nerve) 225.1
malignant (M9560/3)—*see also* Neoplasm, connective tissue, malignant
acoustic (nerve) 192.0
Neurilemmosarcoma (M9560/3)—*see* Neoplasm, connective tissue, malignant
Neurilemoma —*see* Neurilemmoma
Neurinoma (M9560/0)—*see* Neurilemmoma
Neurinomatosis (M9560/1)—*see also* Neoplasm, connective tissue, uncertain behavior
centralis 759.5
Neuritis (*see also* Neuralgia) 729.2
abducens (nerve) 378.54
accessory (nerve) 352.4
acoustic (nerve) 388.5
syphilitic 094.86
alcoholic 357.5
with psychosis 291.1
amyloid, any site 277.3 *[357.4]*
anterior crural 355.8
arising during pregnancy 646.4
arm 723.4
ascending 355.2
auditory (nerve) 388.5
brachial (nerve) NEC 723.4
due to displacement, intervertebral disc 722.0
cervical 723.4
chest (wall) 353.8
costal region 353.8

Neuritis—*continued*
cranial nerve—*see also* Disorder, nerve, cranial
first or olfactory 352.0
second or optic 377.30
third or oculomotor 378.52
fourth or trochlear 378.53
fifth or trigeminal (*see also* Neuralgia, trigeminal) 350.1
sixth or abducens 378.54
seventh or facial 351.8
newborn 767.5
eighth or acoustic 388.5
ninth or glossopharyngeal 352.1
tenth or vagus 352.3
eleventh or accessory 352.4
twelfth or hypoglossal 352.5
Déjérine-Sottas 356.0
diabetic 250.6 *[357.2]*
diphtheritic 032.89 *[357.4]*
due to
beriberi 265.0 *[357.4]*
displacement, prolapse, protrusion, or rupture of intervertebral disc 722.2
cervical 722.0
lumbar, lumbosacral 722.10
thoracic, thoracolumbar 722.11
herniation, nucleus pulposus 722.2
cervical 722.0
lumbar, lumbosacral 722.10
thoracic, thoracolumbar 722.11
endemic 265.0 *[357.4]*
facial (nerve) 351.8
newborn 767.5
general—*see* Polyneuropathy
geniculate ganglion 351.1
due to herpes 053.11
glossopharyngeal (nerve) 352.1
gouty 274.89 *[357.4]*
hypoglossal (nerve) 352.5
ilioinguinal (nerve) 355.8
in diseases classified elsewhere—*see* Polyneuropathy, in
infectious (multiple) 357.0
intercostal (nerve) 353.8
interstitial hypertrophic progressive NEC 356.9
leg 355.8
lumbosacral NEC 724.4
median (nerve) 354.1
thenar 354.1
multiple (acute) (infective) 356.9
endemic 265.0 *[357.4]*
multiplex endemica 265.0 *[357.4]*
nerve root (*see also* Radiculitis) 729.2
oculomotor (nerve) 378.52
olfactory (nerve) 352.0
optic (nerve) 377.30
in myelitis 341.0
meningococcal 036.81
pelvic 355.8
peripheral (nerve)—*see also* Neuropathy, peripheral
complicating pregnancy or puerperium 646.4
specified nerve NEC—*see* Mononeuritis
pneumogastric (nerve) 352.3
postchickenpox 052.7
postherpetic 053.19
progressive hypertrophic interstitial NEC 356.9
puerperal, postpartum 646.4
radial (nerve) 723.4
retrobulbar 377.32
syphilitic 094.85

Neuritis—*continued*
rheumatic (chronic) 729.2
sacral region 355.8
sciatic (nerve) 724.3
due to displacement of intervertebral disc 722.10
serum 999.5
specified nerve NEC—*see* Disorder, nerve
spinal (nerve) 355.9
root (*see also* Radiculitis) 729.2
subscapular (nerve) 723.4
suprascapular (nerve) 723.4
syphilitic 095.8
thenar (median) 354.1
thoracic NEC 724.4
toxic NEC 357.7
trochlear (nerve) 378.53
ulnar (nerve) 723.4
vagus (nerve) 352.3
Neuroangiomatosis, encephalofacial 759.6
Neuroastrocytoma (M9505/1)—*see* Neoplasm, by site, uncertain behavior
Neuro-avitaminosis 269.2
Neuroblastoma (M9500/3)
olfactory (M9522/3) 160.0
specified site—*see* Neoplasm, by site, malignant
unspecified site 194.0
Neurochorioretinitis (*see also* Chorioretinitis) 363.20
Neurocirculatory asthenia 306.2
Neurocytoma (M9506/0)—*see* Neoplasm, by site, benign
Neurodermatitis (circumscribed) (circumscripta) (local) 698.3
atopic 691.8
diffuse (Brocq) 691.8
disseminated 691.8
nodulosa 698.3
Neuroencephalomyelopathy, optic 341.0
Neuroepithelioma (M9503/3)—*see also* Neoplasm, by site, malignant
olfactory (M9521/3) 160.0
Neurofibroma (M9540/0)—*see also* Neoplasm, connective tissue, benign
melanotic (M9541/0)—*see* Neoplasm, connective tissue, benign
multiple (M9540/1) 237.70
Type 1 237.71
Type 2 237.72
plexiform (M9550/0)—*see* Neoplasm, connective tissue, benign
Neurofibromatosis (multiple) (M9540/1) 237.70
acoustic 237.72
malignant (M9540/3)—*see* Neoplasm, connective tissue, malignant
Type 1 237.71
Type 2 237.72
von Recklinghausen's 237.71
Neurofibrosarcoma (M9540/3)—*see* Neoplasm, connective tissue, malignant
Neurogenic —*see also* condition
bladder (atonic) (automatic) (autonomic) (flaccid) (hypertonic) (hypotonic) (inertia) (infranuclear) (irritable) (motor) (nonreflex) (nuclear) (paralysis) (reflex) (sensory) (spastic) (supranuclear) (uninhibited) 596.54
with cauda equina syndrome 344.61
heart 306.2
Neuroglioma (M9505/1)—*see* Neoplasm, by site, uncertain behavior
Neurolabyrinthitis (of Dix and Hallpike) 386.12
Neurolathyrism 988.2
Neuroleprosy 030.1
Neuroleptic malignant syndrome 333.92
Neurolipomatosis 272.8
Neuroma (M9570/0)—*see also* Neoplasm, connective tissue, benign
acoustic (nerve) (M9560/0) 225.1
amputation (traumatic)—*see also* Injury, nerve, by site
surgical complication (late) 997.61
appendix 211.3
auditory nerve 225.1
digital 355.6
toe 355.6
interdigital (toe) 355.6
intermetatarsal 355.6
Morton's 355.6
multiple 237.70
Type 1 237.71
Type 2 237.72
nonneoplastic 355.9
arm NEC 354.9
leg NEC 355.8
lower extremity NEC 355.8
specified site NEC—*see* Mononeuritis, by site
upper extremity NEC 354.9
optic (nerve) 225.1
plantar 355.6
plexiform (M9550/0)—*see* Neoplasm, connective tissue, benign
surgical (nonneoplastic) 355.9
arm NEC 354.9
leg NEC 355.8
lower extremity NEC 355.8
upper extremity NEC 354.9
traumatic—*see also* Injury, nerve, by site
old—*see* Neuroma, nonneoplastic
Neuromyalgia 729.1
Neuromyasthenia (epidemic) 049.8
Neuromyelitis 341.8
ascending 357.0
optica 341.0
Neuromyopathy NEC 358.9
Neuromyositis 729.1
Neuronevus (M8725/0)—*see* Neoplasm, skin, benign
Neuronitis 357.0
ascending (acute) 355.2
vestibular 386.12
Neuroparalytic —*see* condition
Neuropathy, neuropathic (*see also* Disorder, nerve) 355.9
alcoholic 357.5
with psychosis 291.1
arm NEC 354.9
autonomic (peripheral)—*see* Neuropathy, peripheral, autonomic
axillary nerve 353.0
brachial plexus 353.0
cervical plexus 353.2
chronic
progressive segmentally demyelinating 357.8
relapsing demyelinating 357.8
congenital sensory 356.2
Déjérine-Sottas 356.0
diabetic 250.6 *[357.2]*
entrapment 355.9
iliohypogastric nerve 355.79
ilioinguinal nerve 355.79
lateral cutaneous nerve of thigh 355.1
median nerve 354.0
obturator nerve 355.79

Neuropathy, neuropathic—*continued*
peroneal nerve 355.3
posterior tibial nerve 355.5
saphenous nerve 355.79
ulnar nerve 354.2
facial nerve 351.9
hereditary 356.9
peripheral 356.0
sensory (radicular) 356.2
hypertrophic
Charcot-Marie-Tooth 356.1
Déjérine-Sottas 356.0
interstitial 356.9
Refsum 356.3
intercostal nerve 354.8
ischemic—*see* Disorder, nerve
Jamaican (ginger) 357.7
leg NEC 355.8
lower extremity NEC 355.8
lumbar plexus 353.1
median nerve 354.1
multiple (acute) (chronic) (*see also* Polyneuropathy) 356.9
optic 377.39
ischemic 377.41
nutritional 377.33
toxic 377.34
peripheral (nerve) (*see also* Polyneuropathy) 356.9
arm NEC 354.9
autonomic 337.9
amyloid 277.3 *[337.1]*
idiopathic 337.0
in
amyloidosis 277.3 *[337.1]*
diabetes (mellitus) 250.6 *[337.1]*
diseases classified elsewhere 337.1
gout 274.89 *[337.1]*
hyperthyroidism 242.9 *[337.1]*
due to
antitetanus serum 357.6
arsenic 357.7
drugs 357.6
lead 357.7
organophosphate compounds 357.7
toxic agent NEC 357.7
hereditary 356.0
idiopathic 356.9
progressive 356.4
specified type NEC 356.8
in diseases classified elsewhere—*see* Polyneuropathy, in
leg NEC 355.8
lower extremity NEC 355.8
upper extremity NEC 354.9
plantar nerves 355.6
progressive hypertrophic interstitial 356.9
radicular NEC 729.2
brachial 723.4
cervical NEC 723.4
hereditary sensory 356.2
lumbar 724.4
lumbosacral 724.4
thoracic NEC 724.4
sacral plexus 353.1
sciatic 355.0
spinal nerve NEC 355.9
root (*see also* Radiculitis) 729.2
toxic 357.7
trigeminal sensory 350.8
ulnar nerve 354.2

Neuropathy, neuropathic—*continued*
upper extremity NEC 354.9
uremic 585 *[357.4]*
vitamin B_{12} 266.2 *[357.4]*
with anemia (pernicious) 281.0 *[357.4]*
due to dietary deficiency 281.1 *[357.4]*
Neurophthisis —*see also* Disorder, nerve
peripheral 356.9
diabetic 250.6 *[357.2]*
Neuropraxia —*see* Injury,nerve
Neuroretinitis 363.05
syphilitic 094.85
Neurosarcoma (M9540/3)—*see* Neoplasm, connective tissue, malignant
Neurosclerosis —*see* Disorder, nerve
Neurosis, neurotic 300.9
accident 300.16
anancastic, anankastic 300.3
anxiety (state) 300.00
generalized 300.02
panic type 300.01
asthenic 300.5
bladder 306.53
cardiac (reflex) 306.2
cardiovascular 306.2
climacteric, unspecified type 627.2
colon 306.4
compensation 300.16
compulsive, compulsion 300.3
conversion 300.11
craft 300.89
cutaneous 306.3
depersonalization 300.6
depressive (reaction) (type) 300.4
endocrine 306.6
environmental 300.89
fatigue 300.5
functional (*see also* Disorder, psychosomatic) 306.9
gastric 306.4
gastrointestinal 306.4
genitourinary 306.50
heart 306.2
hypochondriacal 300.7
hysterical 300.10
conversion type 300.11
dissociative type 300.15
impulsive 300.3
incoordination 306.0
larynx 306.1
vocal cord 306.1
intestine 306.4
larynx 306.1
hysterical 300.11
sensory 306.1
menopause, unspecified type 627.2
mixed NEC 300.89
musculoskeletal 306.0
obsessional 300.3
phobia 300.3
obsessive-compulsive 300.3
occupational 300.89
ocular 306.7
oral 307.0
organ (*see also* Disorder, psychosomatic) 306.9
pharynx 306.1
phobic 300.20
posttraumatic (acute) (situational) 308.3
chronic 309.81
psychasthenic (type) 300.89

Neurosis, neurotic—*continued*
railroad 300.16
rectum 306.4
respiratory 306.1
rumination 306.4
senile 300.89
sexual 302.70
situational 300.89
specified type NEC 300.89
state 300.9
with depersonalization episode 300.6
stomach 306.4
vasomotor 306.2
visceral 306.4
war 300.16
Neurospongioblastosis diffusa 759.5
Neurosyphilis (arrested) (early) (inactive) (late) (latent) (recurrent) 094.9
with ataxia (cerebellar) (locomotor) (spastic) (spinal) 094.0
acute meningitis 094.2
aneurysm 094.89
arachnoid (adhesive) 094.2
arteritis (any artery) 094.89
asymptomatic 094.3
congenital 090.40
dura (mater) 094.89
general paresis 094.1
gumma 094.9
hemorrhagic 094.9
juvenile (asymptomatic) (meningeal) 090.40
leptomeninges (aseptic) 094.2
meningeal 094.2
meninges (adhesive) 094.2
meningovascular (diffuse) 094.2
optic atrophy 094.84
parenchymatous (degenerative) 094.1
paresis (*see also* Paresis, general) 094.1
paretic (*see also* Paresis, general) 094.1
relapse 094.9
remission in (sustained) 094.9
serological 094.3
specified nature or site NEC 094.89
tabes (dorsalis) 094.0
juvenile 090.40
tabetic 094.0
juvenile 090.40
taboparesis 094.1
juvenile 090.40
thrombosis 094.89
vascular 094.89
Neurotic (*see also* Neurosis) 300.9
excoriation 698.4
psychogenic 306.3
Neurotmesis —*see* Injury, nerve, by site
Neurotoxemia —*see* Toxemia
Neutroclusion 524.2
Neutropenia, neutropenic (chronic) (cyclic) (drug-induced) (genetic) (idiopathic) (immune) (infantile) (malignant) (periodic) (pernicious) (primary) (splenic) (splenomegaly) (toxic) 288.0
chronic hypoplastic 288.0
congenital (nontransient) 288.0
neonatal, transitory (isoimmune) (maternal transfer) 776.7
Neutrophilia, hereditary giant 288.2
Nevocarcinoma (M8720/3)—*see* Melanoma
Nevus (M8720/0)—*see also* Neoplasm, skin, benign

Note—Except where otherwise indicated, the varieties of nevus in the list below that are followed by a morphology code number (M----/0) should be coded by site as for "Neoplasm, skin, benign."

acanthotic 702.8
achromic (M8730/0)
amelanotic (M8730/0)
anemic, anemicus 709.09
angiomatous (M9120/0) (*see also* Hemangioma) 228.00
araneus 448.1
avasculosus 709.09
balloon cell (M8722/0)
bathing trunk (M8761/1) 238.2
blue (M8780/0)
cellular (M8790/0)
giant (M8790/0)
Jadassohn's (M8780/0)
malignant (M8780/3)—*see* Melanoma
capillary (M9131/0) (*see also* Hemangioma) 228.00
cavernous (M9121/0) (*see also* Hemangioma) 228.00
cellular (M8720/0)
blue (M8790/0)
comedonicus 757.33
compound (M8760/0)
conjunctiva (M8720/0) 224.3
dermal (M8750/0)
and epidermal (M8760/0)
epithelioid cell (and spindle cell) (M8770/0)
flammeus 757.32
osteohypertrophic 759.89
hairy (M8720/0)
halo (M8723/0)
hemangiomatous (M9120/0) (*see also* Hemangioma) 228.00
intradermal (M8750/0)
intraepidermal (M8740/0)
involuting (M8724/0)
Jadassohn's (blue) (M8780/0)
junction, junctional (M8740/0)
malignant melanoma in (M8740/3)—*see* Melanoma
juvenile (M8770/0)
lymphatic (M9170/0) 228.1
magnocellular (M8726/0)
specified site—*see* Neoplasm, by site, benign
unspecified site 224.0
malignant (M8720/3)—*see* Melanoma
meaning hemangioma (M9120/0) (*see also* Hemangioma) 228.00
melanotic (pigmented) (M8720/0)
multiplex 759.5
nonneoplastic 448.1
nonpigmented (M8730/0)
nonvascular (M8720/0)
oral mucosa, white sponge 750.26
osteohypertrophic, flammeus 759.89
papillaris (M8720/0)
papillomatosus (M8720/0)
pigmented (M8720/0)
giant (M8761/1)—*see also* Neoplasm, skin, uncertain behavior
malignant melanoma in (M8761/3)—*see* Melanoma
systematicus 757.33

Nevus—*continued*
pilosus (M8720/0)
port wine 757.32
sanguineous 757.32
sebaceous (senile) 702.8
senile 448.1
spider 448.1
spindle cell (and epithelioid cell) (M8770/0)
stellar 448.1
strawberry 757.32
syringocystadenomatous papilliferous (M8406/0)
unius lateris 757.33
Unna's 757.32
vascular 757.32
verrucous 757.33
white sponge (oral mucosa) 750.26
Newborn (infant) (liveborn)
multiple NEC
born in hospital (without mention of cesarean delivery or section) V37.00
with cesarean delivery or section V37.01
born outside hospital
hospitalized V37.1
not hospitalized V37.2
mates all liveborn
born in hospital (without mention of cesarean delivery or section) V34.00
with cesarean delivery or section V34.01
born outside hospital
hospitalized V34.1
not hospitalized V34.2
mates all stillborn
born in hospital (without mention of cesarean delivery or section) V35.00
with cesarean delivery or section V35.01
born outside hospital
hospitalized V35.1
not hospitalized V35.2
mates liveborn and stillborn
born in hospital (without mention of cesarean delivery or section) V36.00
with cesarean delivery or section V36.01
born outside hospital
hospitalized V36.1
not hospitalized V36.2
single
born in hospital (without mention of cesarean delivery or section) V30.00
with cesarean delivery or section V30.01
born outside hospital
hospitalized V30.1
not hospitalized V30.2
twin NEC
born in hospital (without mention of cesarean delivery or section) V33.00
with cesarean delivery or section V33.01
born outside hospital
hospitalized V33.1
not hospitalized V33.2
mate liveborn
born in hospital V31.0
born outside hospital
hospitalized V31.1
not hospitalized V31.2
mate stillborn
born in hospital V32.0
born outside hospital
hospitalized V32.1
not hospitalized V32.2
Newborn—*continued*
unspecified as to single or multiple birth
born in hospital (without mention of cesarean delivery or section) V39.00
with cesarean delivery or section V39.01
born outside hospital
hospitalized V39.1
not hospitalized V39.2
Newcastle's conjunctivitis or disease 077.8
Nezelof's syndrome (pure alymphocytosis) 279.13
Niacin (amide) deficiency 265.2
Nicolas-Durand-Favre disease (climatic bubo) 099.1
Nicolas-Favre disease (climatic bubo) 099.1
Nicotinic acid (amide) deficiency 265.2
Niemann-Pick disease (lipid histiocytosis) (splenomegaly) 272.7
Night
blindness (*see also* Blindness, night) 368.60
congenital 368.61
vitamin A deficiency 264.5
cramps 729.82
sweats 780.8
terrors, child 307.46
Nightmare 307.47
REM-sleep type 307.47
Nipple —*see* condition
Nisbet's chancre 099.0
Nishimoto (-Takeuchi) disease 437.5
Nitritoid crisis or reaction —*see* Crisis, nitritoid
Nitrogen retention, extrarenal 788.9
Nitrosohemoglobinemia 289.8
Njovera 104.0
No
diagnosis 799.9
disease (found) V71.9
room at the inn V65.0
Nocardiasis —*see* Nocardiosis
Nocardiosis 039.9
with pneumonia 039.1
lung 039.1
specified type NEC 039.8
Nocturia 788.43
psychogenic 306.53
Nocturnal —*see also* condition
dyspnea (paroxysmal) 786.09
emissions 608.89
enuresis 788.36
psychogenic 307.6
frequency (micturition) 788.43
psychogenic 306.53
Nodal rhythm disorder 427.89
Nodding of head 781.0
Node (s)—*see also* Nodule
Heberden's 715.04
larynx 478.79
lymph—*see* condition
milkers' 051.1
Osler's 421.0
rheumatic 729.89
Schmorl's 722.30
lumbar, lumbosacral 722.32
specified region NEC 722.39
thoracic, thoracolumbar 722.31
singers' 478.5
skin NEC 782.2
tuberculous—*see* Tuberculosis, lymph gland
vocal cords 478.5
Nodosities, Haygarth's 715.04

Nodule (s), nodular
actinomycotic (*see also* Actinomycosis) 039.9
arthritic—*see* Arthritis, nodosa
cutaneous 782.2
Haygarth's 715.04
inflammatory—*see* Inflammation
juxta-articular 102.7
syphilitic 095.7
yaws 102.7
larynx 478.79
lung, solitary 518.89
emphysematous 492.8
milkers' 051.1
prostate 600
rheumatic 729.89
rheumatoid—*see* Arthritis rheumatoid
scrotum (inflammatory) 608.4
singers' 478.5
skin NEC 782.2
solitary, lung 518.89
emphysematous 492.8
subcutaneous 782.2
thyroid (gland) (nontoxic) (uninodular) 241.0
with
hyperthyroidism 242.1
thyrotoxicosis 242.1
toxic or with hyperthyroidism 242.1
vocal cords 478.5
Noma (gangrenous) (hospital) (infective) 528.1
auricle (*see also* Gangrene) 785.4
mouth 528.1
pudendi (*see also* Vulvitis) 616.10
vulvae (*see also* Vulvitis) 616.10
Nomadism V60.0
Non-autoimmune hemolytic anemia NEC 283.10
Nonclosure —*see also* Imperfect, closure
ductus
arteriosus 747.0
Botalli 747.0
Eustachian valve 746.89
foramen
Botalli 745.5
ovale 745.5
Nondescent (congenital)—*see also* Malposition, congenital
cecum 751.4
colon 751.4
testis 752.5
Nondevelopment
brain 742.1
specified part 742.2
heart 746.89
organ or site, congenital NEC—*see* Hypoplasia
Nonengagement
head NEC 652.5
in labor 660.1
affecting fetus or newborn 763.1
Nonexanthematous tick fever 066.1
Nonexpansion, lung (newborn) NEC 770.4
Nonfunctioning
cystic duct (*see also* Disease, gallbladder) 575.8
gallbladder (*see also* Disease, gallbladder) 575.8
kidney (*see also* Disease, renal) 593.9
labyrinth 386.58
Nonhealing stump (surgical) 997.60
Nonimplantation of ovum, causing infertility 628.3
Noninsufflation, fallopian tube 628.2
Nonne-Milroy-Meige syndrome (chronic hereditary edema) 757.0
Nonovulation 628.0
Nonpatent fallopian tube 628.2
Nonpneumatization, lung NEC 770.4
Nonreflex bladder 596.54
with cauda equina 344.61
Nonretention of food —*see also* Vomiting
Nonrotation —*see* Malrotation
Nonsecretion, urine (*see also* Anuria) 788.5
newborn 753.3
Nonunion
fracture 733.82
organ or site, congenital NEC—*see* Imperfect, closure
symphysis pubis, congenital 755.69
top sacrum, congenital 756.19
Nonviability 765.0
Nonvisualization, gallbladder 793.3
Nonvitalized tooth 522.9
Normal
delivery—*see* category 650
menses V65.5
state (feared complaint unfounded) V65.5
Normoblastosis 289.8
Normocytic anemia (infectional) 285.9
due to blood loss (chronic) 280.0
acute 285.1
Norrie's disease (congenital) (progressive oculoacousticocerebral degeneration) 743.8
North American blastomycosis 116.0
Norwegian itch 133.0
Nose, nasal —*see* condition
Nosebleed 784.7
Nosomania 298.9
Nosophobia 300.29
Nostalgia 309.89
Notch of iris 743.46
Notched lip, congenital (*see also* Cleft, lip) 749.10
Notching nose, congenital (tip) 748.1
Nothnagel's
syndrome 378.52
vasomotor acroparesthesia 443.89
Novy's relapsing fever (American) 087.1
Noxious
foodstuffs, poisoning by
fish 988.0
fungi 988.1
mushrooms 988.1
plants (food) 988.2
shellfish 988.0
specified type NEC 988.8
toadstool 988.1
substances transmitted through placenta or breast milk 760.70
alcohol 760.71
anti-infective agents 760.74
cocaine 760.75
"crack" 760.75
hallucinogenic agents NEC 760.73
medicinal agents NEC 760.79
narcotics 760.72
obstetric anesthetic or analgesic 763.5
specified agent NEC 760.79
suspected, affecting management of pregnancy 655.5
Nuchal hitch (arm) 652.8
Nucleus pulposus —*see* condition
Numbness 782.0
Nuns' knee 727.2
Nursemaid's
elbow 832.0
shoulder 831.0
Nutmeg liver 573.8

Nutrition, deficient or insufficient (particular kind of food) 269.9
due to
insufficient food 994.2
lack of
care 995.5
food 994.2
Nyctalopia (*see also* Blindness, night) 368.60
vitamin A deficiency 264.5
Nycturia 788.43
psychogenic 306.53
Nymphomania 302.89
Nystagmus 379.50
associated with vestibular system disorders 379.54
benign paroxysmal positional 386.11
central positional 386.2
congenital 379.51
deprivation 379.53
dissociated 379.55
latent 379.52
miners' 300.89
positional
benign paroxysmal 386.11
central 386.2
specified NEC 379.56
vestibular 379.54
visual deprivation 379.53

O

Oasthouse urine disease 270.2
Obermeyer's relapsing fever (European) 087.0
Obesity (constitutional) (exogenous) (familial) (nutritional) (simple) 278.00
adrenal 255.8
due to hyperalimentation 278.00
endocrine NEC 259.9
endogenous 259.9
Fröhlich's (adiposogenital dystrophy) 253.8
glandular NEC 259.9
hypothyroid (*see also* Hypothyroidism) 244.9
morbid 278.01
of pregnancy 646.1
pituitary 253.8
thyroid (*see also* Hypothyroidism) 244.9
Oblique —*see also* condition
lie before labor, affecting fetus or newborn 761.7
Obliquity, pelvis 738.6
Obliteration
abdominal aorta 446.7
appendix (lumen) 543.9
artery 447.1
ascending aorta 446.7
bile ducts 576.8
with calculus, choledocholithiasis, or stones—*see* Choledocholithiasis
congenital 751.61
jaundice from 751.61 *[774.5]*
common duct 576.8
with calculus, choledocholithiasis, or stones—*see* Choledocholithiasis
congenital 751.61
cystic duct 575.8
with calculus, choledocholithiasis, or stones—*see* Choledocholithiasis
disease, arteriolar 447.1
endometrium 621.8
eye, anterior chamber 360.34
fallopian tube 628.2
lymphatic vessel 457.1
postmastectomy 457.0
organ or site, congenital NEC—*see* Atresia
placental blood vessels—*see* Placenta, abnormal
supra-aortic branches 446.7
ureter 593.89
urethra 599.84
vein 459.9
vestibule (oral) 525.8
Observation (for) V71.9
without need for further medical care V71.9
accident NEC V71.4
at work V71.3
criminal assault V71.6
deleterious agent ingestion V71.8
disease V71.9
cardiovascular V71.7
heart V71.7
mental V71.09
specified condition NEC V71.8
foreign body ingestion V71.8
growth and development variations V21.8
injuries (accidental) V71.4
inflicted NEC V71.6
during alleged rape or seduction V71.5
malignant neoplasm, suspected V71.1
postpartum
immediately after delivery V24.0
routine follow-up V24.2
Observation—*continued*
pregnancy
high-risk V23.9
specified problem NEC V23.8
normal (without complication) V22.1
with nonobstetric complication V22.2
first V22.0
rape or seduction, alleged V71.5
injury during V71.5
suicide attempt, alleged V71.8
suspected (undiagnosed) (unproven)
cardiovascular disease V71.7
child or wife battering victim V71.6
concussion (cerebral) V71.6
condition NEC V71.8
infant—*see* Observation, suspected, condition, newborn
newborn V29.9
cardiovascular disease V29.8
congenital anomaly V29.8
infectious V29.0
ingestion foreign object V29.8
injury V29.8
neoplasm V29.8
neurological V29.1
poison, poisoning V29.8
respiratory V29.2
specified NEC V29.8
infectious disease not requiring isolation V71.8
malignant neoplasm V71.1
mental disorder V71.09
neoplasm
benign V71.8
malignant V71.1
specified condition NEC V71.8
tuberculosis V71.2
tuberculosis, suspected V71.2
Obsession, obsessional 300.3
ideas and mental images 300.3
impulses 300.3
neurosis 300.3
phobia 300.3
psychasthenia 300.3
ruminations 300.3
state 300.3
syndrome 300.3
Obsessive-compulsive 300.3
neurosis 300.3
reaction 300.3
Obstetrical trauma NEC (complicating delivery) 665.9
with
abortion—*see* Abortion, by type, with damage to pelvic organs
ectopic pregnancy (*see also* categories 633.0-633.9) 639.2
molar pregnancy (*see also* categories 630-632) 639.2
affecting fetus or newborn 763.8
following
abortion 639.2
ectopic or molar pregnancy 639.2
Obstipation (*see also* Constipation) 564.0
psychogenic 306.4

Obstruction, . . . obstructive—*continued*
internal anastomosis—*see* Complications, mechanical, graft
intestine (mechanical) (neurogenic) (paroxysmal) (postinfectional) (reflex) 560.9
with
adhesions (intestinal) (peritoneal) 560.81
hernia—*see also* Hernia, by site, with obstruction
gangrenous—*see* Hernia, by site, with gangrene
adynamic (*see also* Ileus) 560.1
by gallstone 560.31
congenital or infantile (small) 751.1
large 751.2
due to
Ascaris lumbricoides 127.0
mural thickening 560.89
procedure 997.4
involving urinary tract 997.5
impaction 560.39
infantile—*see* Obstruction, intestine, congenital
newborn
due to
fecaliths 777.1
inspissated milk 777.2
meconium (plug) 777.1
in mucoviscidosis 277.01
transitory 777.4
specified cause NEC 560.89
transitory, newborn 777.4
volvulus 560.2
intracardiac ball valve prosthesis 996.02
jaundice (*see also* Obstruction, biliary) 576.8
congenital 751.61
jejunum (*see also* Obstruction, intestine) 560.9
kidney 593.89
labor 660.9
affecting fetus or newborn 763.1
by
bony pelvis (conditions classifiable to 653.0-653.9) 660.1
deep transverse arrest 660.3
impacted shoulder 660.4
locked twins 660.5
malposition (fetus) (conditions classifiable to 652.0-652.9) 660.0
head during labor 660.3
persistent occipitoposterior position 660.3
soft tissue, pelvic (conditions classifiable to 654.0-654.9) 660.2
lacrimal
canaliculi 375.53
congenital 743.65
punctum 375.52
sac 375.54
lacrimonasal duct 375.56
congenital 743.65
neonatal 375.55
lacteal, with steatorrhea 579.2
laryngitis (*see also* Laryngitis) 464.0
larynx 478.79
congenital 748.3
liver 573.8
cirrhotic (*see also* Cirrhosis, liver) 571.5
lung 518.89
with
asthma—*see* Asthma
bronchitis (chronic) 491.2
emphysema NEC 492.8

Obstruction, . . . obstructive—*continued*
airway, chronic 496
chronic NEC 496
with
asthma (chronic) (obstructive) 493.2
disease, chronic 496
with
asthma (chronic) (obstructive) 493.2
emphysematous 492.8
lymphatic 457.1
meconium
fetus or newborn 777.1
in mucoviscidosis 277.01
newborn due to fecaliths 777.1
mediastinum 519.3
mitral (rheumatic)—*see* Stenosis, mitral
nasal 478.1
duct 375.56
neonatal 375.55
sinus—*see* Sinusitis
nasolacrimal duct 375.56
congenital 743.65
neonatal 375.55
nasopharynx 478.29
nose 478.1
organ or site, congenital NEC—*see* Atresia
pancreatic duct 577.8
parotid gland 527.8
pelviureteral junction (*see also* Obstruction, ureter) 593.4
pharynx 478.29
portal (circulation) (vein) 452
prostate 600
valve (urinary) 596.0
pulmonary
valve (heart) (*see also* Endocarditis, pulmonary) 424.3
vein, isolated 747.49
pyemic—*see* Septicemia
pylorus (acquired) 537.0
congenital 750.5
infantile 750.5
rectosigmoid (*see also* Obstruction, intestine) 560.9
rectum 569.49
renal 593.89
respiratory 519.8
chronic 496
retinal (artery) (vein) (central) (*see also* Occlusion, retina) 362.30
salivary duct (any) 527.8
with calculus 527.5
sigmoid (*see also* Obstruction, intestine) 560.9
sinus (accessory) (nasal) (*see also* Sinusitis) 473.9
Stensen's duct 527.8
stomach 537.89
acute 536.1
congenital 750.7
submaxillary gland 527.8
with calculus 527.5
thoracic duct 457.1
thrombotic—*see* Thrombosis
tooth eruption 520.6
trachea 519.1
tracheostomy airway 519.0
tricuspid—*see* Endocarditis, tricuspid
upper respiratory, congenital 748.8
ureter (pelvic juncture) (functional) 593.4
congenital 753.2
due to calculus 592.1

Occlusion—*continued*
precerebral artery—*see* Occlusion, artery, precerebral NEC
puncta lacrimalia 375.52
pupil 364.74
pylorus (*see also* Stricture, pylorus) 537.0
renal artery 593.81
retina, retinal (vascular) 362.30
artery, arterial 362.30
branch 362.32
central (total) 362.31
partial 362.33
transient 362.34
tributary 362.32
vein 362.30
branch 362.36
central (total) 362.35
incipient 362.37
partial 362.37
tributary 362.36
spinal artery 433.8
teeth (mandibular) (posterior lingual) 524.2
thoracic duct 457.1
tubal 628.2
ureter (complete) (partial) 593.4
congenital 753.2
urethra (*see also* Stricture, urethra) 598.9
congenital 753.6
uterus 621.8
vagina 623.2
vascular NEC 459.9
vein—*see* Thrombosis
vena cava (inferior) (superior) 453.2
ventricle (brain) NEC 331.4
vertebral (artery)—*see* Occlusion, artery, vertebral
vessel (blood) NEC 459.9
vulva 624.8
Occlusio pupillae 364.74
Occupational
problems NEC V62.2
therapy V57.21
Ochlophobia 300.29
Ochronosis (alkaptonuric) (congenital) (endogenous) 270.2
with chloasma of eyelid 270.2
Ocular muscle —*see also* condition
myopathy 359.1
Oculoauriculovertebral dysplasia 756.0
Oculogyric
crisis or disturbance 378.87
psychogenic 306.7
Oculomotor syndrome 378.81
Oddi's sphincter spasm 576.5
Odelberg's disease (juvenile osteochondrosis) 732.1
Odontalgia 525.9
Odontoameloblastoma (M9311/0) 213.1
upper jaw (bone) 213.0
Odontoclasia 521.0
Odontoclasis 873.63
complicated 873.73
Odontodysplasia, regional 520.4
Odontogenesis imperfecta 520.5
Odontoma (M9280/0) 213.1
ameloblastic (M9311/0) 213.1
upper jaw (bone) 213.0
calcified (M9280/0) 213.1
upper jaw (bone) 213.0
complex (M9282/0) 213.1
upper jaw (bone) 213.0
Odontoma—*continued*
compound (M9281/0) 213.1
upper jaw (bone) 213.0
fibroameloblastic (M9290/0) 213.1
upper jaw (bone) 213.0
follicular 526.0
upper jaw (bone) 213.0
Odontomyelitis (closed) (open) 522.0
Odontonecrosis 521.0
Odontorrhagia 525.8
Odontosarcoma, ameloblastic (M9290/3) 170.1
upper jaw (bone) 170.0
Oesophagostomiasis 127.7
Oesophagostomum infestation 127.7
Oestriasis 134.0
Ogilvie's syndrome (sympathicotonic colon obstruction) 560.89
Oguchi's disease (retina) 368.61
Ohara's disease (*see also* Tularemia) 021.9
Oidiomycosis (*see also* Candidiasis) 112.9
Oidiomycotic meningitis 112.83
Oidium albicans infection (*see also* Candidiasis) 112.9
Old age 797
dementia (of) 290.0
Olfactory —*see* condition
Oligemia 285.9
Oligergasia (*see also* Retardation, mental) 319
Oligoamnios 658.0
affecting fetus or newborn 761.2
Oligoastrocytoma, mixed (M9382/3)
specified site—*see* Neoplasm, by site, malignant
unspecified site 191.9
Oligocythemia 285.9
Oligodendroblastoma (M9460/3)
specified site—*see* Neoplasm, by site, malignant
unspecified site 191.9
Oligodendroglioma (M9450/3)
anaplastic type (M9451/3)
specified site—*see* Neoplasm, by site, malignant
unspecified site 191.9
specified site—*see* Neoplasm, by site, malignant
unspecified site 191.9
Oligodendroma —*see* Oligodendroglioma
Oligodontia (*see also* Anodontia) 520.0
Oligoencephalon 742.1
Oligohydramnios 658.0
affecting fetus or newborn 761.2
due to premature rupture of membranes 658.1
affecting fetus or newborn 761.2
Oligohydrosis 705.0
Oligomenorrhea 626.1
Oligophrenia (*see also* Retardation, mental) 319
phenylpyruvic 270.1
Oligospermia 606.1
Oligotrichia 704.09
congenita 757.4
Oliguria 788.5
with
abortion—*see* Abortion, by type, with renal failure
ectopic pregnancy (*see also* categories 633.0-633.9) 639.3
molar pregnancy (*see also* categories 630-632) 639.3
complicating
abortion 639.3
ectopic or molar pregnancy 639.3

Oliguria—*continued*
pregnancy 646.2
with hypertension—*see* Toxemia, of pregnancy
due to a procedure 997.5
following labor and delivery 669.3
heart or cardiac—*see* Failure, heart, congestive
puerperal, postpartum 669.3
specified due to a procedure 997.5
Ollier's disease (chondrodysplasia) 756.4
Omentitis (*see also* Peritonitis) 567.9
Omentocele (*see also* Hernia, omental) 553.8
Omentum, omental —*see* condition
Omphalitis (congenital) (newborn) 771.4
not of newborn 686.9
tetanus 771.3
Omphalocele 756.7
Omphalomesenteric duct, persistent 751.0
Omphalorrhagia, newborn 772.3
Omsk hemorrhagic fever 065.1
Onanism 307.9
Onchocerciasis 125.3
eye 125.3 *[360.13]*
Onchocercosis 125.3
Oncocytoma (M8290/0)—*see* Neoplasm, by site, benign
Ondine's curse 348.8
Oneirophrenia (*see also* Schizophrenia) 295.4
Onychauxis 703.8
congenital 757.5
Onychia (with lymphangitis) 681.9
dermatophytic 110.1
finger 681.02
toe 681.11
Onychitis (with lymphangitis) 681.9
finger 681.02
toe 681.11
Onychocryptosis 703.0
Onychodystrophy 703.8
congenital 757.5
Onychogryphosis 703.8
Onychogryposis 703.8
Onycholysis 703.8
Onychomadesis 703.8
Onychomalacia 703.8
Onychomycosis 110.1
finger 110.1
toe 110.1
Onycho-osteodysplasia 756.89
Onychophagy 307.9
Onychoptosis 703.8
Onychorrhexis 703.8
congenital 757.5
Onychoschizia 703.8
Onychotrophia (*see also* Atrophy, nail) 703.8
O'nyong-nyong fever 066.3
Onyxis (finger) (toe) 703.0
Onyxitis (with lymphangitis) 681.9
finger 681.02
toe 681.11
Oophoritis (cystic) (infectional) (interstitial) (*see also* Salpingo-oophoritis) 614.2
complicating pregnancy 646.6
fetal (acute) 752.0
gonococcal (acute) 098.19
chronic or duration of 2 months or over 098.39
tuberculous (*see also* Tuberculosis) 016.6
Opacity, opacities
cornea 371.00
central 371.03
Opacity, opacities—*continued*
congenital 743.43
interfering with vision 743.42
degenerative (*see also* Degeneration, cornea) 371.40
hereditary (*see also* Dystrophy, cornea) 371.50
inflammatory (*see also* Keratitis) 370.9
late effect of trachoma (healed) 139.1
minor 371.01
peripheral 371.02
enamel (fluoride) (nonfluoride) (teeth) 520.3
lens (*see also* Cataract) 366.9
snowball 379.22
vitreous (humor) 379.24
congenital 743.51
Opalescent dentin (hereditary) 520.5
Open, opening
abnormal, organ or site, congenital—*see* Imperfect, closure
angle with
borderline intraocular pressure 365.01
cupping of discs 365.01
bite (anterior) (posterior) 524.2
false—*see* Imperfect, closure
wound—*see* Wound, open, by site
Operation
causing mutilation of fetus 763.8
destructive, on live fetus, to facilitate birth 763.8
for delivery, fetus or newborn 763.8
maternal, unrelated to current delivery, affecting fetus or newborn 760.6
Operational fatigue 300.89
Operative —*see* condition
Operculitis (chronic) 523.4
acute 523.3
Operculum, retina 361.32
with detachment 361.01
Ophiasis 704.01
Ophthalmia (*see also* Conjunctivitis) 372.30
actinic rays 370.24
allergic (acute) 372.05
chronic 372.14
blennorrhagic (neonatorum) 098.40
catarrhal 372.03
diphtheritic 032.81
Egyptian 076.1
electric, electrica 370.24
gonococcal (neonatorum) 098.40
metastatic 360.11
migraine 346.8
neonatorum, newborn 771.6
gonococcal 098.40
nodosa 360.14
phlyctenular 370.31
with ulcer (*see also* Ulcer, cornea) 370.00
sympathetic 360.11
Ophthalmitis —*see* Ophthalmia
Ophthalmocele (congenital) 743.66
Ophthalmoneuromyelitis 341.0
Ophthalmopathy, infiltrative with thyrotoxicosis 242.0
Ophthalmoplegia (*see also* Strabismus) 378.9
anterior internuclear 378.86
ataxia-areflexia syndrome 357.0
bilateral 378.9
diabetic 250.5 *[378.86]*
exophthalmic 242.0 *[376.22]*
external 378.55
progressive 378.72
total 378.56

Ophthalmoplegia—*continued*
interna(l) (complete) (total) 367.52
internuclear 378.86
migraine 346.8
painful 378.55
Parinaud's 378.81
progressive external 378.72
supranuclear, progressive 333.0
total (external) 378.56
internal 367.52
unilateral 378.9
Opisthognathism 524.00
Opisthorchiasis (felineus) (tenuicollis) (viverrini) 121.0
Opisthotonos, opisthotonus 781.0
Opitz's disease (congestive splenomegaly) 289.51
Opiumism (*see also* Dependence) 304.0
Oppenheim's disease 358.8
Oppenheim-Urbach disease or syndrome (necrobiosis lipoidica diabeticorum) 250.8 *[709.3]*
Opsoclonia 379.59
Optic nerve —*see* condition
Orbit —*see* condition
Orchioblastoma (M9071/3) 186.9
Orchitis (nonspecific) (septic) 604.90
with abscess 604.0
blennorrhagic (acute) 098.13
chronic or duration of 2 months or over 098.33
diphtheritic 032.89 *[604.91]*
filarial 125.9 *[604.91]*
gangrenous 604.99
gonococcal (acute) 098.13
chronic or duration of 2 months or over 098.33
mumps 072.0
parotidea 072.0
suppurative 604.99
syphilitic 095.8 *[604.91]*
tuberculous (*see also* Tuberculosis) 016.5 *[608.81]*
Orf 051.2
Organic —*see also* condition
heart—*see* Disease, heart
insufficiency 799.8
Oriental
bilharziasis 120.2
schistosomiasis 120.2
sore 085.1
Orifice —*see* condition
Origin, both great vessels from right ventricle 745.11
Ormond's disease or syndrome 593.4
Ornithosis 073.9
with
complication 073.8
specified NEC 073.7
pneumonia 073.0
pneumonitis (lobular) 073.0
Orodigitofacial dysostosis 759.89
Oropouche fever 066.3
Orotaciduria, oroticaciduria (congenital) (hereditary) (pyrimidine deficiency) 281.4
Oroya fever 088.0
Orthodontics V58.5
adjustment V53.4
aftercare V58.5
fitting V53.4
Orthopnea 786.02
Orthoptic training V57.4
Os, uterus —*see* condition
Osgood-Schlatter
disease 732.4
osteochondrosis 732.4
Osler's
disease (M9950/1) (polycythemia vera) 238.4
nodes 421.0
Osler-Rendu disease (familial hemorrhagic telangiectasia) 448.0
Osler-Vaquez disease (M9950/1) (polycythemia vera) 238.4
Osler-Weber-Rendu syndrome (familial hemorrhagic telangiectasia) 448.0
Osmidrosis 705.89
Osseous —*see* condition
Ossification
artery—*see* Arteriosclerosis
auricle (ear) 380.39
bronchus 519.1
cardiac (*see also* Degeneration, myocardial) 429.1
cartilage (senile) 733.99
coronary —*see* Arteriosclerosis, coronary
diaphragm 728.10
ear 380.39
middle (*see also* Otosclerosis) 387.9
falx cerebri 349.2
fascia 728.10
fontanel
defective or delayed 756.0
premature 756.0
heart (*see also* Degeneration, myocardial) 429.1
valve—*see* Endocarditis
larynx 478.79
ligament
posterior longitudinal 724.8
cervical 723.7
meninges (cerebral) 349.2
spinal 336.8
multiple, eccentric centers 733.99
muscle 728.10
heterotopic, postoperative 728.13
myocardium, myocardial (*see also* Degeneration, myocardial) 429.1
penis 607.81
periarticular 728.89
sclera 379.16
tendon 727.82
trachea 519.1
tympanic membrane (*see also* Tympanosclerosis) 385.00
vitreous (humor) 360.44
Osteitis (*see also* Osteomyelitis) 730.2
acute 730.0
alveolar 526.5
chronic 730.1
condensans (ilii) 733.5
deformans (Paget's) 731.0
due to or associated with malignant neoplasm (*see also* Neoplasm, bone, malignant) 170.9 *[731.1]*
due to yaws 102.6
fibrosa NEC 733.29
cystica (generalisata) 252.0
disseminata 756.59
osteoplastica 252.0
fragilitans 756.51
Garré's (sclerosing) 730.1
infectious (acute) (subacute) 730.0
chronic or old 730.1
jaw (acute) (chronic) (lower) (neonatal) (suppurative) (upper) 526.4

Osteitis—*continued*
parathyroid 252.0
petrous bone (*see also* Petrositis) 383.20
pubis 733.5
sclerotic, nonsuppurative 730.1
syphilitic 095.5
tuberculosa
cystica (of Jüngling) 135
multiplex cystoides 135
Osteoarthritica spondylitis (spine) (*see also* Spondylosis) 721.90
Osteoarthritis (*see also* Osteoarthrosis) 715.9
distal interphalangeal 715.9
hyperplastic 731.2
interspinalis (*see also* Spondylosis) 721.90
spine, spinal NEC (*see also* Spondylosis) 721.90
Osteoarthropathy (*see also* Osteoarthrosis) 715.9
chronic idiopathic hypertrophic 757.39
familial idiopathic 757.39
hypertrophic pulmonary 731.2
secondary 731.2
idiopathic hypertrophic 757.39
primary hypertrophic 731.2
pulmonary hypertrophic 731.2
secondary hypertrophic 731.2
Osteoarthrosis (degenerative) (hypertrophic) (rheumatoid) 715.9

Note—Use the following fifth-digit subclassification with category 715:

0 site unspecified
1 shoulder region
2 upper arm
3 forearm
4 hand
5 pelvic region and thigh
6 lower leg
7 ankle and foot
8 other specified sites except spine
9 multiple sites

deformans alkaptonurica 270.2
generalized 715.09
juvenilis (Köhler's) 732.5
localized 715.3
idiopathic 715.1
primary 715.1
secondary 715.2
multiple sites, not specified as generalized 715.89
polyarticular 715.09
spine (*see also* Spondylosis) 721.90
Osteoblastoma (M9200/0)—*see* Neoplasm, bone, benign
Osteochondritis (*see also* Osteochondrosis) 732.9
dissecans 732.7
hip 732.7
ischiopubica 732.1
multiple 756.59
syphilitic (congenital) 090.0
Osteochondrodermodysplasia 756.59
Osteochondrodystrophy 277.5
deformans 277.5
familial 277.5
fetalis 756.4
Osteochondrolysis 732.7
Osteochondroma (M9210/0)—*see also* Neoplasm, bone, benign
multiple, congenital 756.4
Osteochondromatosis (M9210/1) 238.0
synovial 727.82
Osteochondromyxosarcoma (M9180/3)—*see* Neoplasm, bone, malignant
Osteochondropathy NEC 732.9
Osteochondrosarcoma (M9180/3)—*see* Neoplasm, bone, malignant
Osteochondrosis 732.9
acetabulum 732.1
adult spine 732.8
astragalus 732.5
Blount's 732.4
Buchanan's (juvenile osteochondrosis of iliac crest) 732.1
Buchman's (juvenile osteochondrosis) 732.1
Burns' 732.3
calcaneus 732.5
capitular epiphysis (femur) 732.1
carpal
lunate (wrist) 732.3
scaphoid 732.3
coxae juvenilis 732.1
deformans juvenilis (coxae) (hip) 732.1
Scheuermann's 732.0
spine 732.0
tibia 732.4
vertebra 732.0
Diaz's (astragalus) 732.5
dissecans (knee) (shoulder) 732.7
femoral capital epiphysis 732.1
femur (head) (juvenile) 732.1
foot (juvenile) 732.5
Freiberg's (disease) (second metatarsal) 732.5
Haas' 732.3
Haglund's (os tibiale externum) 732.5
hand (juvenile) 732.3
head of
femur 732.1
humerus (juvenile) 732.3
hip (juvenile) 732.1
humerus (juvenile) 732.3
iliac crest (juvenile) 732.1
ilium (juvenile) 732.1
ischiopubic synchondrosis 732.1
Iselin's (osteochondrosis fifth metatarsal) 732.5
juvenile, juvenilis 732.6
arm 732.3
capital femoral epiphysis 732.1
capitellum humeri 732.3
capitular epiphysis 732.1
carpal scaphoid 732.3
clavicle, sternal epiphysis 732.6
coxae 732.1
deformans 732.1
foot 732.5
hand 732.3
hip and pelvis 732.1
lower extremity, except foot 732.4
lunate, wrist 732.3
medial cuneiform bone 732.5
metatarsal (head) 732.5
metatarsophalangeal 732.5
navicular, ankle 732.5
patella 732.4
primary patellar center (of Köhler) 732.4
specified site NEC 732.6
spine 732.0
tarsal scaphoid 732.5
tibia (epiphysis) (tuberosity) 732.4
upper extremity 732.3

Osteochondrosis—*continued*
vertebra (body) (Calvé) 732.0
epiphyseal plates (of Scheuermann) 732.0
Kienböck's (disease) 732.3
Köhler's (disease) (navicular, ankle) 732.5
patellar 732.4
tarsal navicular 732.5
Legg-Calvé-Perthes (disease) 732.1
lower extremity (juvenile) 732.4
lunate bone 732.3
Mauclaire's 732.3
metacarpal heads (of Mauclaire) 732.3
metatarsal (fifth) (head) (second) 732.5
navicular, ankle 732.5
os calcis 732.5
Osgood-Schlatter 732.4
os tibiale externum 732.5
Panner's 732.3
patella (juvenile) 732.4
patellar center
primary (of Köhler) 732.4
secondary (of Sinding-Larsen) 732.4
pelvis (juvenile) 732.1
Pierson's 732.1
radial head (juvenile) 732.3
Scheuermann's 732.0
Sever's (calcaneum) 732.5
Sinding-Larsen (secondary patellar center) 732.4
spine (juvenile) 732.0
adult 732.8
symphysis pubis (of Pierson) (juvenile) 732.1
syphilitic (congenital) 090.0
tarsal (navicular) (scaphoid) 732.5
tibia (proximal) (tubercle) 732.4
tuberculous—*see* Tuberculosis, bone
ulna 732.3
upper extremity (juvenile) 732.3
van Neck's (juvenile osteochondrosis) 732.1
vertebral (juvenile) 732.0
adult 732.8
Osteoclastoma (M9250/1) 238.0
malignant (M9250/3)—*see* Neoplasm, bone, malignant
Osteocopic pain 733.90
Osteodynia 733.90
Osteodystrophy
azotemic 588.0
chronica deformans hypertrophica 731.0
congenital 756.50
specified type NEC 756.59
deformans 731.0
fibrosa localisata 731.0
parathyroid 252.0
renal 588.0
Osteofibroma (M9262/0)—*see* Neoplasm, bone, benign
Osteofibrosarcoma (M9182/3)—*see* Neoplasm, bone, malignant
Osteogenesis imperfecta 756.51
Osteogenic —*see* condition
Osteoma (M9180/0)—*see also* Neoplasm, bone, benign
osteoid (M9191/0)—*see also* Neoplasm, bone, benign
giant (M9200/0)—*see* Neoplasm, bone, benign
Osteomalacia 268.2
chronica deformans hypertrophica 731.0
due to vitamin D deficiency 268.2
infantile (*see also* Rickets) 268.0
juvenile (*see also* Rickets) 268.0
pelvis 268.2
vitamin D-resistant 275.3
Osteomalacic bone 268.2
Osteomalacosis 268.2
Osteomyelitis (general) (infective) (localized) (neonatal) (purulent) (pyogenic) (septic) (staphylococcal) (streptococcal) (suppurative) (with periostitis) 730.2

Note—Use the following fifth-digit subclassification with category 730:

0 site unspecified
1 shoulder region
2 upper arm
3 forearm
4 hand
5 pelvic region and thigh
6 lower leg
7 ankle and foot
8 other specified sites
9 multiple sites

acute or subacute 730.0
chronic or old 730.1
due to or associated with
diabetes mellitus 250.8 *[731.8]*
tuberculosis (*see also* Tuberculosis, bone) 015.9 *[730.8]*
limb bones 015.5 *[730.8]*
specified bones NEC 015.7 *[730.8]*
spine 015.0 *[730.8]*
typhoid 002.0 *[730.8]*
Garré's 730.1
jaw (acute) (chronic) (lower) (neonatal) (suppurative) (upper) 526.4
nonsuppurating 730.1
orbital 376.03
petrous bone (*see also* Petrositis) 383.20
Salmonella 003.24
sclerosing, nonsuppurative 730.1
sicca 730.1
syphilitic 095.5
congenital 090.0 *[730.8]*
tuberculous—*see* Tuberculosis, bone
typhoid 002.0 *[730.8]*
Osteomyelofibrosis 289.8
Osteomyelosclerosis 289.8
Osteonecrosis (*see also* Osteomyelitis) 730.1
Osteo-onycho-arthro dysplasia 756.89
Osteo-onychodysplasia, hereditary 756.89
Osteopathia
condensans disseminata 756.53
hyperostotica multiplex infantilis 756.59
hypertrophica toxica 731.2
striata 756.4
Osteopathy resulting from poliomyelitis (*see also* Poliomyelitis) 045.9 *[730.7]*
familial dysplastic 731.2
Osteopecilia 756.53
Osteopenia 733.90
Osteoperiostitis (*see also* Osteomyelitis) 730.2
ossificans toxica 731.2
toxica ossificans 731.2
Osteopetrosis (familial) 756.52
Osteophyte —*see* Exostosis
Osteophytosis —*see* Exostosis
Osteopoikilosis 756.53
Osteoporosis (generalized) 733.00
circumscripta 731.0
disuse 733.03
drug-induced 733.09
idiopathic 733.02
postmenopausal 733.01

Osteoporosis—*continued*
posttraumatic 733.7
senile 733.01
specified type NEC 733.09
Osteoporosis-osteomalacia syndrome 268.2
Osteopsathyrosis 756.51
Osteoradionecrosis, jaw 526.89
Osteosarcoma (M9180/3)—*see also* Neoplasm, bone, malignant
chondroblastic (M9181/3)—*see* Neoplasm, bone, malignant
fibroblastic (M9182/3)—*see* Neoplasm, bone, malignant
in Paget's disease of bone (M9184/3)—*see* Neoplasm, bone, malignant
juxtacortical (M9190/3)—*see* Neoplasm, bone, malignant
parosteal (M9190/3)—*see* Neoplasm, bone, malignant
telangiectatic (M9183/3)—*see* Neoplasm, bone, malignant
Osteosclerosis 756.52
fragilis (generalisata) 756.52
myelofibrosis 289.8
Osteosclerotic anemia 289.8
Osteosis
acromegaloid 757.39
cutis 709.3
parathyroid 252.0
renal fibrocystic 588.0
Österreicher-Turner syndrome 756.89
Ostium
atrioventriculare commune 745.69
primum (arteriosum) (defect) (persistent) 745.61
secundum (arteriosum) (defect) (patent) (persistent) 745.5
Ostrum-Furst syndrome 756.59
Otalgia 388.70
otogenic 388.71
referred 388.72
Othematoma 380.31
Otitic hydrocephalus 348.2
Otitis 382.9
with effusion 381.4
purulent 382.4
secretory 381.4
serous 381.4
suppurative 382.4
acute 382.9
adhesive (*see also* Adhesions, middle ear) 385.10
chronic 382.9
with effusion 381.3
mucoid, mucous (simple) 381.20
purulent 382.3
secretory 381.3
serous 381.10
suppurative 382.3
diffuse parasitic 136.8
externa (acute) (diffuse) (hemorrhagica) 380.10
actinic 380.22
candidal 112.82
chemical 380.22
chronic 380.23
mycotic—*see* Otitis, externa, mycotic
specified type NEC 380.23
circumscribed 380.10
contact 380.22

Otitis—*continued*
due to
erysipelas 035 *[380.13]*
impetigo 684 *[380.13]*
seborrheic dermatitis 690.10 *[380.13]*
eczematoid 380.22
furuncular 680.0 *[380.13]*
infective 380.10
chronic 380.16
malignant 380.14
mycotic (chronic) 380.15
due to
aspergillosis 117.3 *[380.15]*
moniliasis 112.82
otomycosis 111.8 *[380.15]*
reactive 380.22
specified type NEC 380.22
tropical 111.8 *[380.15]*
insidiosa (*see also* Otosclerosis) 387.9
interna (*see also* Labyrinthitis) 386.30
media (hemorrhagic) (staphylococcal) (streptococcal) 382.9
acute 382.9
with effusion 381.00
allergic 381.04
mucoid 381.05
sanguineous 381.06
serous 381.04
catarrhal 381.00
exudative 381.00
mucoid 381.02
allergic 381.05
necrotizing 382.00
with spontaneous rupture of ear drum 382.01
in
influenza 487.8 *[382.02]*
measles 055.2
scarlet fever 034.1 *[382.02]*
nonsuppurative 381.00
purulent 382.00
with spontaneous rupture of ear drum 382.01
sanguineous 381.03
allergic 381.06
secretory 381.01
seromucinous 381.02
serous 381.01
allergic 381.04
suppurative 382.00
with spontaneous rupture of ear drum 382.01
due to
influenza 487.8 *[382.02]*
scarlet fever 034.1 *[382.02]*
transudative 381.00
adhesive (*see also* Adhesions, middle ear) 385.10
allergic 381.4
acute 381.04
mucoid 381.05
sanguineous 381.06
serous 381.04
chronic 381.3
catarrhal 381.4
acute 381.00
chronic (simple) 381.10
chronic 382.9
with effusion 381.3
adhesive (*see also* Adhesions, middle ear) 385.10

Otitis—*continued*
allergic 381.3
atticoantral, suppurative (with posterior or superior marginal perforation of ear drum) 382.2
benign suppurative (with anterior perforation of ear drum) 382.1
catarrhal 381.10
exudative 381.3
mucinous 381.20
mucoid, mucous (simple) 381.20
mucosanguineous 381.29
nonsuppurative 381.3
purulent 382.3
secretory 381.3
seromucinous 381.3
serosanguineous 381.19
serous (simple) 381.10
suppurative 382.3
atticoantral (with posterior or superior marginal perforation of ear drum) 382.2
benign (with anterior perforation of ear drum) 382.1
tuberculous (*see also* Tuberculosis) 017.4
tubotympanic 382.1
transudative 381.3
exudative 381.4
acute 381.00
chronic 381.3
fibrotic (*see also* Adhesions, middle ear) 385.10
mucoid, mucous 381.4
acute 381.02
chronic (simple) 381.20
mucosanguineous, chronic 381.29
nonsuppurative 381.4
acute 381.00
chronic 381.3
postmeasles 055.2
purulent 382.4
acute 382.00
with spontaneous rupture of ear drum 382.01
chronic 382.3
sanguineous, acute 381.03
allergic 381.06
secretory 381.4
acute or subacute 381.01
chronic 381.3
seromucinous 381.4
acute or subacute 381.02
chronic 381.3
serosanguineous, chronic 381.19
serous 381.4
acute or subacute 381.01
chronic (simple) 381.10
subacute—*see* Otitis, media, acute
suppurative 382.4
acute 382.00
with spontaneous rupture of ear drum 382.01
chronic 382.3
atticoantral 382.2
benign 382.1
tuberculous (*see also* Tuberculosis) 017.4
tubotympanic 382.1
transudative 381.4
acute 381.00
chronic 381.3
tuberculous (*see also* Tuberculosis) 017.4
postmeasles 055.2

Otoconia 386.8
Otolith syndrome 386.19
Otomycosis 111.8 *[380.15]*
in
aspergillosis 117.3 *[380.15]*
moniliasis 112.82
Otopathy 388.9
Otoporosis (*see also* Otosclerosis) 387.9
Otorrhagia 388.69
traumatic—*see* nature of injury
Otorrhea 388.60
blood 388.69
cerebrospinal (fluid) 388.61
Otosclerosis (general) 387.9
cochlear (endosteal) 387.2
involving
otic capsule 387.2
oval window
nonobliterative 387.0
obliterative 387.1
round window 387.2
nonobliterative 387.0
obliterative 387.1
specified type NEC 387.8
Otospongiosis (*see also* Otosclerosis) 387.9
Otto's disease or pelvis 715.35
Outburst, aggressive (*see also* Disturbance, conduct) 312.0
in children and adolescents 313.9
Outcome of delivery
multiple birth NEC V27.9
all liveborn V27.5
all stillborn V27.7
some liveborn V27.6
unspecified V27.9
single V27.9
liveborn V27.0
stillborn V27.1
twins V27.9
both liveborn V27.2
both stillborn V27.4
one liveborn, one stillborn V27.3
Outlet —*see also* condition
syndrome (thoracic) 353.0
Outstanding ears (bilateral) 744.29
Ovalocytosis (congenital) (hereditary) (*see also* Elliptocytosis) 282.1
Ovarian —*see also* condition
pregnancy—*see* Pregnancy, ovarian
vein syndrome 593.4
Ovaritis (cystic) (*see also* Salpingo-oophoritis) 614.2
Ovary, ovarian —*see* condition
Overactive —*see also* Hyperfunction
eye muscle (*see also* Strabismus) 378.9
hypothalamus 253.8
thyroid (*see also* Thyrotoxicosis) 242.9
Overactivity, child 314.01
Overbite (deep) (excessive) (horizontal) (vertical) 524.2
Overbreathing (*see also* Hyperventilation) 786.01
Overconscientious personality 301.4
Overdevelopment —*see also* Hypertrophy
breast (female) (male) 611.1
nasal bones 738.0
prostate, congenital 752.8
Overdistention —*see* Distention
Overdose overdosage (drug) 977.9
specified drug or substance—*see* Table of drugs and chemicals

Overeating 783.6
with obesity 278.0
nonorganic origin 307.51
Overexertion (effects) (exhaustion) 994.5
Overexposure (effects) 994.9
exhaustion 994.4
Overfeeding (*see also* Overeating) 783.6
Overgrowth, bone NEC 733.99
Overheated (effects) (places)—*see* Heat
Overinhibited child 313.0
Overjet 524.2
Overlaid, overlying (suffocation) 994.7
Overlapping toe (acquired) 735.8
congenital (fifth toe) 755.66
Overload
fluid 276.6
potassium (K) 276.7
sodium (Na) 276.0
Overnutrition (*see also* Hyperalimentation) 783.6
Overproduction —*see also* Hypersecretion
ACTH 255.3
cortisol 255.0
growth hormone 253.0
thyroid-stimulating hormone (TSH) 242.8
Overriding
aorta 747.21
finger (acquired) 736.29
congenital 755.59
toe (acquired) 735.8
congenital 755.66
Oversize
fetus (weight of 4500 grams or more) 766.0
affecting management of pregnancy 656.6
causing disproportion 653.5
with obstructed labor 660.1
affecting fetus or newborn 763.1
Overstrained 780.7
heart—*see* Hypertrophy, cardiac
Overweight (*see also* Obesity) 278.00
Overwork 780.7
Oviduct —*see* condition
Ovotestis 752.7
Ovulation (cycle)
failure or lack of 628.0
pain 625.2
Ovum
blighted 631
dropsical 631
pathologic 631
Owren's disease or syndrome (parahemophilia) (*see also* Defect, coagulation) 286.3
Oxalosis 271.8
Oxaluria 271.8
Ox heart —*see* Hypertrophy, cardiac
OX syndrome 758.6
Oxycephaly, oxycephalic 756.0
syphilitic, congenital 090.0
Oxyuriasis 127.4
Oxyuris vermicularis (infestation) 127.4
Ozena 472.0

P

Pacemaker syndrome 429.4
Pachyderma, pachydermia 701.8
  laryngis 478.5
  laryngitis 478.79
  larynx (verrucosa) 478.79
Pachydermatitis 701.8
Pachydermatocele (congenital) 757.39
  acquired 701.8
Pachydermatosis 701.8
Pachydermoperiostitis
  secondary 731.2
Pachydermoperiostosis
  primary idiopathic 757.39
  secondary 731.2
Pachymeningitis (adhesive) (basal) (brain) (cerebral) (cervical) (chronic) (circumscribed) (external) (fibrous) (hemorrhagic) (hypertrophic) (internal) (purulent) (spinal) (suppurative) (*see also* Meningitis) 322.9
  gonococcal 098.82
Pachyonychia (congenital) 757.5
  acquired 703.8
Pachyperiosteodermia
  primary or idiopathic 757.39
  secondary 731.2
Pachyperiostosis
  primary or idiopathic 757.39
  secondary 731.2
Pacinian tumor (M9507/0)—*see* Neoplasm, skin, benign
Pads, knuckle or Garrod's 728.79
Paget's disease (osteitis deformans) 731.0
  with infiltrating duct carcinoma of the breast (M8541/3)—*see* Neoplasm, breast, malignant
  bone 731.0
    osteosarcoma in (M9184/3)—*see* Neoplasm, bone, malignant
  breast (M8540/3) 174.0
  extramammary (M8542/3)—*see also* Neoplasm, skin, malignant
    anus 154.3
      skin 173.5
  malignant (M8540/3)
    breast 174.0
    specified site NEC (M8542/3)—*see* Neoplasm, skin, malignant
    unspecified site 174.0
  mammary (M8540/3) 174.0
  necrosis of bone 731.0
  nipple (M8540/3) 174.0
  osteitis deformans 731.0
Paget-Schroetter syndrome (intermittent venous claudication) 453.8
Pain (s)
  abdominal 789.0
  adnexa (uteri) 625.9
  alimentary, due to vascular insufficiency 557.9
  anginoid (*see also* Pain, precordial) 786.51
  anus 569.42
  arch 729.5
  arm 729.5
  back (postural) 724.5
    low 724.2
    psychogenic 307.89
  bile duct 576.9
  bladder 788.9
Pain —*continued*
  bone 733.90
  breast 611.71
    psychogenic 307.89
  broad ligament 625.9
  cartilage NEC 733.90
  cecum 789.0
  cervicobrachial 723.3
  chest (central) 786.50
    wall (anterior) 786.52
  coccyx 724.79
  colon 789.0
  common duct 576.9
  coronary—*see* Angina
  costochondral 786.52
  diaphragm 786.52
  due to (presence of) any device, implant, or graft classifiable to 996.0-996.5—*see* Complications, due to (presence of) any device, implant, or graft classified to 996.0-996.5 NEC
  ear (*see also* Otalgia) 388.70
  epigastric, epigastrium 789.0
  extremity (lower) (upper) 729.5
  eye 379.91
  face, facial 784.0
    atypical 350.2
    nerve 351.8
  false (labor) 644.1
  female genital organ NEC 625.9
    psychogenic 307.89
  finger 729.5
  flank 789.0
  foot 729.5
  gallbladder 575.9
  gas (intestinal) 787.3
  gastric 536.8
  generalized 780.9
  genital organ
    female 625.9
    male 608.9
    psychogenic 307.89
  groin 789.0
  growing 781.9
  hand 729.5
  head (*see also* Headache) 784.0
  heart (*see also* Pain, precordial) 786.51
  infraorbital (*see also* Neuralgia, trigeminal) 350.1
  intermenstrual 625.2
  jaw 526.9
  joint 719.40
    ankle 719.47
    elbow 719.42
    foot 719.47
    hand 719.44
    hip 719.45
    knee 719.46
    multiple sites 719.49
    pelvic region 719.45
    psychogenic 307.89
    shoulder (region) 719.41
    specified site NEC 719.48
    wrist 719.43
  kidney 788.0
  labor, false or spurious 644.1
  laryngeal 784.1

Pain —*continued*
leg 729.5
limb 729.5
low back 724.2
lumbar region 724.2
mastoid (*see also* Otalgia) 388.70
maxilla 526.9
metacarpophalangeal (joint) 719.44
metatarsophalangeal (joint) 719.47
mouth 528.9
muscle 729.1
intercostal 786.52
nasal 478.1
nasopharynx 478.29
neck NEC 723.1
psychogenic 307.89
nerve NEC 729.2
neuromuscular 729.1
nose 478.1
ocular 379.91
ophthalmic 379.91
orbital region 379.91
osteocopic 733.90
ovary 625.9
psychogenic 307.89
over heart (*see also* Pain, precordial) 786.51
ovulation 625.2
pelvic (female) 625.9
male NEC 789.0
psychogenic 307.89
psychogenic 307.89
penis 607.9
psychogenic 307.89
pericardial (*see also* Pain, precordial) 786.51
perineum
female 625.9
male 608.9
pharynx 478.29
pleura, pleural, pleuritic 786.52
post-operative —*see* Pain, by site
preauricular 388.70
precordial (region) 786.51
psychogenic 307.89
psychogenic 307.80
cardiovascular system 307.89
gastrointestinal system 307.89
genitourinary system 307.89
heart 307.89
musculoskeletal system 307.89
respiratory system 307.89
skin 306.3
radicular (spinal) (*see also* Radiculitis) 729.2
rectum 569.42
respiration 786.52
retrosternal 786.51
rheumatic NEC 729.0
muscular 729.1
rib 786.50
root (spinal) (*see also* Radiculitis) 729.2
round ligament (stretch) 625.9
sacroiliac 724.6
sciatic 724.3
scrotum 608.9
psychogenic 307.89
seminal vesicle 608.9
sinus 478.1
skin 782.0
spermatic cord 608.9
spinal root (*see also* Radiculitis) 729.2

Pain —*continued*
stomach 536.8
psychogenic 307.89
substernal 786.51
temporomandibular (joint) 524.62
temporomaxillary joint 524.62
testis 608.9
psychogenic 307.89
thoracic spine 724.1
with radicular and visceral pain 724.4
throat 784.1
tibia 733.90
toe 729.5
tongue 529.6
tooth 525.9
trigeminal (*see also* Neuralgia, trigeminal) 350.1
umbilicus 789.0
ureter 788.0
urinary (organ) (system) 788.0
uterus 625.9
psychogenic 307.89
vagina 625.9
vertebrogenic (syndrome) 724.5
vesical 788.9
vulva 625.9
xiphoid 733.90
Painful —*see also* Pain
arc syndrome 726.19
coitus
female 625.0
male 608.89
psychogenic 302.76
ejaculation (semen) 608.89
psychogenic 302.79
erection 607.3
feet syndrome 266.2
menstruation 625.3
psychogenic 306.52
micturition 788.1
ophthalmoplegia 378.55
respiration 786.52
scar NEC 709.2
urination 788.1
wire sutures 998.89
Painters' colic 984.9
specified type of lead—*see* Table of drugs and chemicals
Palate —*see* condition
Palatoplegia 528.9
Palatoschisis (*see also* Cleft, palate) 749.00
Palilalia 784.69
Palindromic arthritis (*see also* Rheumatism, palindromic) 719.3
Pallor 782.61
temporal, optic disc 377.15
Palmar —*see also* condition
fascia—*see* condition
Palpable
cecum 569.89
kidney 593.89
liver 573.9
lymph nodes 785.6
ovary 620.8
prostate 602.9
spleen (*see also* Splenomegaly) 789.2
uterus 625.8
Palpitation (heart) 785.1
psychogenic 306.2

Palsy (*see also* Paralysis) 344.9
atrophic diffuse 335.20
Bell's 351.0
newborn 767.5
birth 767.7
brachial plexus 353.0
fetus or newborn 767.6
brain—*see also* Palsy, cerebral
noncongenital or noninfantile 344.89
due to vascular lesion—*see* category 438
syphilitic 094.89
congenital 090.49
bulbar (chronic) (progressive) 335.22
pseudo NEC 335.23
supranuclear NEC 344.89
cerebral (congenital) (infantile) (spastic) 343.9
athetoid 333.7
diplegic 343.0
due to previous vascular lesion—*see* category 438
hemiplegic 343.1
monoplegic 343.3
noncongenital or noninfantile 437.8
due to previous vascular lesion—*see* category 438
paraplegic 343.0
quadriplegic 343.2
spastic, not congenital or infantile 344.89
syphilitic 094.89
congenital 090.49
tetraplegic 343.2
cranial nerve—*see also* Disorder, nerve, cranial
multiple 352.6
creeping 335.21
divers' 993.3
Erb's (birth injury) 767.6
facial 351.0
newborn 767.5
glossopharyngeal 352.2
Klumpke (-Déjérine) 767.6
lead 984.9
specified type of lead—*see* Table of drugs and chemicals
median nerve (tardy) 354.0
peroneal nerve (acute) (tardy) 355.3
pseudobulbar NEC 335.23
radial nerve (acute) 354.3
seventh nerve 351.0
newborn 767.5
shaking (*see also* Parkinsonism) 332.0
spastic (cerebral) (spinal) 343.9
hemiplegic 343.1
specified nerve NEC—*see* Disorder, nerve
supranuclear NEC 356.8
ulnar nerve (tardy) 354.2
wasting 335.21
Paltauf-Sternberg disease 201.9
Paludism —*see* Malaria
Panama fever 084.0
Panaris (with lymphangitis) 681.9
finger 681.02
toe 681.11
Panaritium (with lymphangitis) 681.9
finger 681.02
toe 681.11
Panarteritis (nodosa) 446.0
brain or cerebral 437.4
Pancake heart 793.2
with cor pulmonale (chronic) 416.9
Pancarditis (acute) (chronic) 429.89
with
rheumatic
fever (active) (acute) (chronic) (subacute) 391.8
inactive or quiescent 398.99
rheumatic, acute 391.8
chronic or inactive 398.99
Pancoast's syndrome or tumor (carcinoma, pulmonary apex) (M8010/3) 162.3
Pancoast-Tobias syndrome (M8010/3) (carcinoma, pulmonary apex) 162.3
Pancolitis 556.6
Pancreas, pancreatic —*see* condition
Pancreatitis 577.0
acute (edematous) (hemorrhagic) (recurrent) 577.0
annular 577.0
apoplectic 577.0
calcereous 577.0
chronic (infectious) 577.1
recurrent 577.1
cystic 577.2
fibrous 577.8
gangrenous 577.0
hemorrhagic (acute) 577.0
interstitial (chronic) 577.1
acute 577.0
malignant 577.0
mumps 072.3
painless 577.1
recurrent 577.1
relapsing 577.1
subacute 577.0
suppurative 577.0
syphilitic 095.8
Pancreatolithiasis 577.8
Pancytolysis 289.9
Pancytopenia (acquired) 284.8
with malformations 284.0
congenital 284.0
Panencephalitis —*see also* Encephalitis
subacute, sclerosing 046.2
Panhematopenia 284.8
congenital 284.0
constitutional 284.0
splenic, primary 289.4
Panhemocytopenia 284.8
congenital 284.0
constitutional 284.0
Panhypogonadism 257.2
Panhypopituitarism 253.2
prepubertal 253.3
Panic (attack) (state) 300.01
reaction to exceptional stress (transient) 308.0
Panmyelopathy, familial constitutional 284.0
Panmyelophthisis 284.9
acquired (secondary) 284.8
congenital 284.0
idiopathic 284.9
Panmyelosis (acute) (M9951/1) 238.7
Panner's disease 732.3
capitellum humeri 732.3
head of humerus 732.3
tarsal navicular (bone) (osteochondrosis) 732.5
Panneuritis endemica 265.0 *[357.4]*

Note—Except where otherwise indicated, the morphological varieties of papilloma in the list below should be coded by site as for "Neoplasm, benign."

Paraganglioma (M8680/1)
adrenal (M8700/0) 227.0
malignant (M8700/3) 194.0
aortic body (M8691/1) 237.3
malignant (M8691/3) 194.6
carotid body (M8692/1) 237.3
malignant (M8692/3) 194.5
chromaffin (M8700/0)—*see also* Neoplasm, by site, benign
malignant (M8700/3)—*see* Neoplasm, by site, malignant
extra-adrenal (M8693/1)
malignant (M8693/3)
specified site—*see* Neoplasm, by site, malignant
unspecified site 194.6
specified site—*see* Neoplasm, by site, uncertain behavior
unspecified site 237.3
glomus jugulare (M8690/1) 237.3
malignant (M8690/3) 194.6
jugular (M8690/1) 237.3
malignant (M8680/3)
specified site—*see* Neoplasm, by site, malignant
unspecified site 194.6
nonchromaffin (M8693/1)
malignant (M8693/3)
specified site—*see* Neoplasm, by site, malignant
unspecified site 194.6
specified site—*see* Neoplasm, by site, uncertain behavior
unspecified site 237.3
parasympathetic (M8682/1)
specified site—*see* Neoplasm, by site, uncertain behavior
unspecified site 237.3
specified site—*see* Neoplasm, by site, uncertain behavior
sympathetic (M8681/1)
specified site—*see* Neoplasm, by site, uncertain behavior
unspecified site 237.3
unspecified site 237.3
Parageusia 781.1
psychogenic 306.7
Paragonimiasis 121.2
Paragranuloma, Hodgkin's (M9660/3) 201.0
Parahemophilia (*see also* Defect, coagulation) 286.3
Parakeratosis 690
psoriasiformis 696.2
variegata 696.2
Paralysis, paralytic (complete) (incomplete) 344.9
with
broken
back—*see* Fracture, vertebra, by site, with spinal cord injury
neck—*see* Fracture, vertebra, cervical, with spinal cord injury
fracture, vertebra—*see* Fracture, vertebra, by site, with spinal cord injury
syphilis 094.89
abdomen and back muscles 355.9
abdominal muscles 355.9
abducens (nerve) 378.54
abductor 355.9
lower extremity 355.8
upper extremity 354.9
Paralysis, paralytic—*continued*
accessory nerve 352.4
accommodation 367.51
hysterical 300.11
acoustic nerve 388.5
agitans 332.0
arteriosclerotic 332.0
alternating 344.89
oculomotor 344.89
amyotrophic 335.20
ankle 355.8
anterior serratus 355.9
anus (sphincter) 569.49
apoplectic (current episode) (*see also* Disease, cerebrovascular, acute) 436
late effect—*see* category 438
arm 344.40
affecting
dominant side 344.41
nondominant side 344.42
both 344.2
due to old CVA—*see* category 438
hysterical 300.11
psychogenic 306.0
transient 781.4
traumatic NEC (*see also* Injury, nerve, upper limb) 955.9
arteriosclerotic (current episode) 437.0
late effect—*see* category 438
ascending (spinal), acute 357.0
associated, nuclear 344.89
asthenic bulbar 358.0
ataxic NEC 334.9
general 094.1
athetoid 333.7
atrophic 356.9
infantile, acute (*see also* Poliomyelitis, with paralysis) 045.1
muscle NEC 355.9
progressive 335.21
spinal (acute) (*see also* Poliomyelitis, with paralysis) 045.1
attack (*see also* Disease, cerebrovascular, acute) 436
axillary 353.0
Babinski-Nageotte's 344.89
Bell's 351.0
newborn 767.5
Benedikt's 344.89
birth (injury) 767.7
brain 767.0
intracranial 767.0
spinal cord 767.4
bladder (sphincter) 596.53
neurogenic 596.54
with cauda equina syndrome 344.61
puerperal, postpartum, childbirth 665.5
sensory 596.54
with cauda equina 344.61
spastic 596.54
with cauda equina 344.61
bowel, colon, or intestine (*see also* Ileus) 560.1
brachial plexus 353.0
due to birth injury 767.6
newborn 767.6
brain
congenital—*see* Palsy, cerebral
current episode 437.8
diplegia 344.2

Paralysis, paralytic—*continued*
due to previous vascular lesion—*see* category 438
hemiplegia 342.9
due to previous vascular lesion—*see* category 438
infantile—*see* Palsy, cerebral
monoplegia—*see also* Monoplegia
due to previous vascular lesion—*see* category 438
paraplegia 344.1
quadriplegia —*see* Quadriplegia
syphilitic, congenital 090.49
triplegia 344.89
bronchi 519.1
Brown-Séquard's 344.89
bulbar (chronic) (progressive) 335.22
infantile (*see also* Poliomyelitis, bulbar) 045.0
poliomyelitic (*see also* Poliomyelitis, bulbar) 045.0
pseudo 335.23
supranuclear 344.89
bulbospinal 358.0
cardiac (*see also* Failure, heart) 428.9
cerebral
current episode 437.8
spastic, infantile—*see* Palsy, cerebral
cerebrocerebellar 437.8
diplegic infantile 343.0
cervical
plexus 353.2
sympathetic NEC 337.0
Céstan-Chenais 344.89
Charcot-Marie-Tooth type 356.1
childhood—*see* Palsy, cerebral
Clark's 343.9
colon (*see also* Ileus) 560.1
compressed air 993.3
compression
arm NEC 354.9
cerebral—*see* Paralysis, brain
leg NEC 355.8
lower extremity NEC 355.8
upper extremity NEC 354.9
congenital (cerebral) (spastic) (spinal)—*see* Palsy, cerebral
conjugate movement (of eye) 378.81
cortical (nuclear) (supranuclear) 378.81
convergence 378.83
cordis (*see also* Failure, heart) 428.9
cortical (*see also* Paralysis, brain) 437.8
cranial or cerebral nerve (*see also* Disorder, nerve, cranial) 352.9
creeping 335.21
crossed leg 344.89
crutch 953.4
deglutition 784.9
hysterical 300.11
dementia 094.1
descending (spinal) NEC 335.9
diaphragm (flaccid) 519.4
due to accidental section of phrenic nerve during procedure 998.2
digestive organs NEC 564.8
diplegic—*see* Diplegia
divergence (nuclear) 378.85
divers' 993.3
Duchenne's 335.22
due to intracranial or spinal birth injury—*see* Palsy, cerebral

Paralysis, paralytic—*continued*
embolic (current episode) (*see also* Embolism, brain) 434.1
late effect or old—*see* category 438
enteric (*see also* Ileus) 560.1
with hernia—*see* Hernia, by site, with obstruction
Erb's syphilitic spastic spinal 094.89
Erb (-Duchenne) (birth) (newborn) 767.6
esophagus 530.89
essential, infancy (*see also* Poliomyelitis) 045.9
extremity
lower —*see* Paralysis, leg
spastic (hereditary) 343.3
noncongenital or noninfantile 344.1
transient (cause unknown) 781.4
upper —*see* Paralysis, arm
eye muscle (extrinsic) 378.55
intrinsic 367.51
facial (nerve) 351.0
birth injury 767.5
congenital 767.5
following operation NEC 998.2
newborn 767.5
familial 359.3
periodic 359.3
spastic 334.1
fauces 478.29
finger NEC 354.9
foot NEC 355.8
gait 781.2
gastric nerve 352.3
gaze 378.81
general 094.1
ataxic 094.1
insane 094.1
juvenile 090.40
progressive 094.1
tabetic 094.1
glossopharyngeal (nerve) 352.2
glottis (*see also* Paralysis, vocal cord) 478.30
gluteal 353.4
Gubler (-Millard) 344.89
hand 354.9
hysterical 300.11
psychogenic 306.0
heart (*see also* Failure, heart) 428.9
hemifacial, progressive 349.89
hemiplegic—*see* Hemiplegia
hyperkalemic periodic (familial) 359.3
hypertensive (current episode) 437.8
hypoglossal (nerve) 352.5
hypokalemic periodic 359.3
Hyrtl's sphincter (rectum) 569.49
hysterical 300.11
ileus (*see also* Ileus) 560.1
infantile (*see also* Poliomyelitis) 045.9
atrophic acute 045.1
bulbar 045.0
cerebral—*see* Palsy, cerebral
paralytic 045.1
progressive acute 045.9
spastic—*see* Palsy, cerebral
spinal 045.9
infective (*see also* Poliomyelitis) 045.9
inferior nuclear 344.9
insane, general or progressive 094.1
internuclear 378.86
interosseous 355.9
intestine (*see also* Ileus) 560.1

Paralysis, paralytic—*continued*
- intracranial (current episode) (*see also* Paralysis, brain) 437.8
  - due to birth injury 767.0
- iris 379.49
  - due to diphtheria (toxin) 032.81 *[379.49]*
- ischemic, Volkmann's (complicating trauma) 958.6
- Jackson's 344.89
- jake 357.7
- Jamaica ginger (jake) 357.7
- juvenile general 090.40
- Klumpke (-Déjérine) (birth) (newborn) 767.6
- labioglossal (laryngeal) (pharyngeal) 335.22
- Landry's 357.0
- laryngeal nerve (recurrent) (superior) (*see also* Paralysis, vocal cord) 478.30
- larynx (*see also* Paralysis, vocal cord) 478.30
  - due to diphtheria (toxin) 032.3
- late effect
  - due to
    - birth injury, brain or spinal (cord)—*see* Palsy, cerebral
    - edema, brain or cerebral—*see* Paralysis, brain
    - lesion
      - cerebrovascular—*see* category 438
      - spinal (cord)—*see* Paralysis, spinal
- lateral 335.24
- lead 984.9
  - specified type of lead—*see* Table of drugs and chemicals
- left side—*see* Hemiplegia
- leg 344.30
  - affecting
    - dominant side 344.31
    - nondominant side 344.32
  - both (*see also* Paraplegia) 344.1
  - crossed 344.89
  - hysterical 300.11
  - psychogenic 306.0
  - transient or transitory 781.4
    - traumatic NEC (*see also* Injury, nerve, lower limb) 956.9
- levator palpebrae superioris 374.31
- limb NEC 344.5
  - all four—*see* Quadriplegia
  - quadriplegia—*see* Quadriplegia
- lip 528.5
- Lissauer's 094.1
- local 355.9
- lower limb—*see also* Paralysis, leg
  - both (*see also* Paraplegia) 344.1
- lung 518.89
  - newborn 770.8
- median nerve 354.1
- medullary (tegmental) 344.89
- mesencephalic NEC 344.89
  - tegmental 344.89
- middle alternating 344.89
- Millard-Gubler-Foville 344.89
- monoplegic—*see* Monoplegia
- motor NEC 344.9
  - cerebral—*see* Paralysis, brain
  - spinal—*see* Paralysis, spinal
- multiple
  - cerebral—*see* Paralysis, brain
  - spinal—*see* Paralysis, spinal

Paralysis, paralytic—*continued*
- muscle (flaccid) 359.9
  - due to nerve lesion NEC 355.9
  - eye (extrinsic) 378.55
    - intrinsic 367.51
    - oblique 378.51
  - iris sphincter 364.8
  - ischemic (complicating trauma) (Volkmann's) 958.6
  - pseudohypertrophic 359.1
- muscular (atrophic) 359.9
  - progressive 335.21
- musculocutaneous nerve 354.9
- musculospiral 354.9
- nerve—*see also* Disorder, nerve
  - third or oculomotor (partial) 378.51
    - total 378.52
  - fourth or trochlear 378.53
  - sixth or abducens 378.54
  - seventh or facial 351.0
    - birth injury 767.5
    - due to
      - injection NEC 999.9
      - operation NEC 997.09
    - newborn 767.5
  - accessory 352.4
  - auditory 388.5
  - birth injury 767.7
  - cranial or cerebral (*see also* Disorder, nerve, cranial) 352.9
  - facial 351.0
    - birth injury 767.5
    - newborn 767.5
  - laryngeal (*see also* Paralysis, vocal cord) 478.30
  - newborn 767.7
  - phrenic 354.8
    - newborn 767.7
  - radial 354.3
    - birth injury 767.6
    - newborn 767.6
  - syphilitic 094.89
  - traumatic NEC (*see also* Injury, nerve, by site) 957.9
  - trigeminal 350.9
  - ulnar 354.2
- newborn NEC 767.0
- normokalemic periodic 359.3
- obstetrical, newborn 767.7
- ocular 378.9
- oculofacial, congenital 352.6
- oculomotor (nerve) (partial) 378.51
  - alternating 344.89
  - external bilateral 378.55
  - total 378.52
- olfactory nerve 352.0
- palate 528.9
- palatopharyngolaryngeal 352.6
- paratrigeminal 350.9
- periodic (familial) (hyperkalemic) (hypokalemic) (normokalemic) (secondary) 359.3
- peripheral
  - autonomic nervous system—*see* Neuropathy, peripheral, autonomic
  - nerve NEC 355.9
- peroneal (nerve) 355.3
- pharynx 478.29
- phrenic nerve 354.8
- plantar nerves 355.6
- pneumogastric nerve 352.3

Paralysis, paralytic—*continued*
poliomyelitis (current) (*see also* Poliomyelitis, with paralysis) 045.1
bulbar 045.0
popliteal nerve 355.3
pressure (*see also* Neuropathy, entrapment) 355.9
progressive 335.21
atrophic 335.21
bulbar 335.22
general 094.1
hemifacial 349.89
infantile, acute (*see also* Poliomyelitis) 045.9
multiple 335.20
pseudobulbar 335.23
pseudohypertrophic 359.1
muscle 359.1
psychogenic 306.0
pupil, pupillary 379.49
quadriceps 355.8
quadriplegic (*see also* Quadriplegia) 344.0
radial nerve 354.3
birth injury 767.6
rectum (sphincter) 569.49
rectus muscle (eye) 378.55
recurrent laryngeal nerve (*see also* Paralysis, vocal cord) 478.30
respiratory (muscle) (system) (tract) 786.09
center NEC 344.89
fetus or newborn 770.8
congenital 768.9
newborn 768.9
right side—*see* Hemiplegia
Saturday night 354.3
saturnine 984.9
specified type of lead—*see* Table of drugs and chemicals
sciatic nerve 355.0
secondary—*see* Paralysis, late effect
seizure (cerebral) (current episode) (*see also* Disease, cerebrovascular, acute) 436
late effect—*see* category 438
senile NEC 344.9
serratus magnus 355.9
shaking (*see also* Parkinsonism) 332.0
shock (*see also* Disease, cerebrovascular, acute) 436
late effect—*see* category 438
shoulder 354.9
soft palate 528.9
spasmodic—*see* Paralysis, spastic
spastic 344.9
cerebral infantile—*see* Palsy, cerebral
congenital (cerebral)—*see* Palsy, cerebral
familial 334.1
hereditary 334.1
infantile 343.9
noncongenital or noninfantile, cerebral 344.9
syphilitic 094.0
spinal 094.89
sphincter, bladder (*see also* Paralysis, bladder) 596.53
spinal (cord) NEC 344.1
accessory nerve 352.4
acute (*see also* Poliomyelitis) 045.9
ascending acute 357.0
atrophic (acute) (*see also* Poliomyelitis, with paralysis) 045.1
spastic, syphilitic 094.89
congenital NEC 343.9

Paralysis, paralytic—*continued*
hemiplegic —*see* Hemiplegia
hereditary 336.8
infantile (*see also* Poliomyelitis) 045.9
late effect NEC 344.89
monoplegic—*see* Monoplegia
nerve 355.9
progressive 335.10
quadriplegic —*see* Quadriplegia
spastic NEC 343.9
traumatic—*see* Injury, spinal, by site
sternomastoid 352.4
stomach 536.3
nerve 352.3
stroke (current episode) (*see also* Disease, cerebrovascular, acute) 436
late effect—*see* category 438
subscapularis 354.8
superior nuclear NEC 334.9
supranuclear 356.8
sympathetic
cervical NEC 337.0
nerve NEC (*see also* Neuropathy, peripheral, autonomic) 337.9
nervous system—*see* Neuropathy, peripheral, autonomic
syndrome 344.9
specified NEC 344.89
syphilitic spastic spinal (Erb's) 094.89
tabetic general 094.1
thigh 355.8
throat 478.29
diphtheritic 032.0
muscle 478.29
thrombotic (current episode) (*see also* Thrombosis, brain) 434.0
old—*see* category 438
thumb NEC 354.9
tick (-bite) 989.5
Todd's (postepileptic transitory paralysis) 344.89
toe 355.6
tongue 529.8
transient
arm or leg NEC 781.4
traumatic NEC (*see also* Injury, nerve, by site) 957.9
trapezius 352.4
traumatic, transient NEC (*see also* Injury, nerve, by site) 957.9
trembling (*see also* Parkinsonism) 332.0
triceps brachii 354.9
trigeminal nerve 350.9
trochlear nerve 378.53
ulnar nerve 354.2
upper limb —*see also* Paralysis, arm
both (*see also* Diplegia) 344.2
uremic—*see* Uremia
uveoparotitic 135
uvula 528.9
hysterical 300.11
postdiphtheritic 032.0
vagus nerve 352.3
vasomotor NEC 337.9
velum palati 528.9
vesical (*see also* Paralysis, bladder) 596.53
vestibular nerve 388.5
visual field, psychic 368.16

Paralysis, paralytic—*continued*
vocal cord 478.30
bilateral (partial) 478.33
complete 478.34
complete (bilateral) 478.34
unilateral (partial) 478.31
complete 478.32
Volkmann's (complicating trauma) 958.6
wasting 335.21
Weber's 344.89
wrist NEC 354.9
Paramedial orifice, urethrovesical 753.8
Paramenia 626.9
Parametritis (chronic) (*see also* Disease, pelvis, inflammatory) 614.4
acute 614.3
puerperal, postpartum, childbirth 670
Parametrium, parametric —*see* condition
Paramnesia (*see also* Amnesia) 780.9
Paramolar 520.1
causing crowding 524.3
Paramyloidosis 277.3
Paramyoclonus multiplex 333.2
Paramyotonia 359.2
congenita 359.2
Paraneoplastic syndrome —*see* condition
Parangi (*see also* Yaws) 102.9
Paranoia 297.1
alcoholic 291.5
querulans 297.8
senile 290.20
Paranoid
dementia (*see also* Schizophrenia) 295.3
praecox (acute) 295.3
senile 290.20
personality 301.0
psychosis 297.9
alcoholic 291.5
climacteric 297.2
drug-induced 292.11
involutional 297.2
menopausal 297.2
protracted reactive 298.4
psychogenic 298.4
acute 298.3
senile 290.20
reaction (chronic) 297.9
acute 298.3
schizophrenia (acute) (*see also* Schizophrenia) 295.3
state 297.9
alcohol-induced 291.5
climacteric 297.2
drug-induced 292.11
due to or associated with
arteriosclerosis (cerebrovascular) 290.42
presenile brain disease 290.12
senile brain disease 290.20
involutional 297.2
menopausal 297.2
senile 290.20
simple 297.0
specified type NEC 297.8
tendencies 301.0
traits 301.0
trends 301.0
type, psychopathic personality 301.0
Paraparesis (*see also* Paralysis) 344.9
Paraphasia 784.3
Paraphilia (***see also*** Deviation, sexual) 302.9
Paraphimosis (congenital) 605
chancroidal 099.0
Paraphrenia, paraphrenic (late) 297.2
climacteric 297.2
dementia (*see also* Schizophrenia) 295.3
involutional 297.2
menopausal 297.2
schizophrenia (acute) (*see also* Schizophrenia) 295.3
Paraplegia 344.1
with
broken back—*see* Fracture, vertebra, by site, with spinal cord injury
fracture, vertebra—*see* Fracture, vertebra, by site, with spinal cord injury
ataxic—*see* Degeneration, combined, spinal cord
brain (current episode) (*see also* Paralysis, brain) 437.8
cerebral (current episode) (*see also* Paralysis, brain) 437.8
congenital or infantile (cerebral) (spastic) (spinal) 343.0
cortical—*see* Paralysis, brain
familial spastic 334.1
functional (hysterical) 300.11
hysterical 300.11
infantile 343.0
late effect 344.1
Pott's (*see also* Tuberculosis) 015.0 *[730.88]*
psychogenic 306.0
spastic
Erb's spinal 094.89
hereditary 334.1
not infantile or congenital 344.1
spinal (cord)
traumatic NEC—*see* Injury, spinal, by site
syphilitic (spastic) 094.89
traumatic NEC—*see* Injury, spinal, by site
Paraproteinemia 273.2
benign (familial) 273.1
monoclonal 273.1
secondary to malignant or inflammatory disease 273.1
Parapsoriasis 696.2
en plaques 696.2
guttata 696.2
lichenoides chronica 696.2
retiformis 696.2
varioliformis (acuta) 696.2
Parascarlatina 057.8
Parasitic —*see also* condition
disease NEC (*see also* Infestation, parasitic) 136.9
contact V01.8
exposure to V01.8
intestinal NEC 129
skin NEC 134.9
stomatitis 112.0
sycosis 110.0
beard 110.0
scalp 110.0
twin 759.4
Parasitism NEC 136.9
intestinal NEC 129
skin NEC 134.9
specified—*see* Infestation
Parasitophobia 300.29
Parasomnia 780.59
nonorganic origin 307.47
Paraspadias 752.8
Paraspasm facialis 351.8
Parathyroid gland —*see* condition
Parathyroiditis (autoimmune) 252.1
Parathyroprival tetany 252.1

Paratrachoma 077.0
Paratyphilitis (*see also* Appendicitis) 541
Paratyphoid (fever)—*see* Fever, paratyphoid
Paratyphus —*see* Fever, paratyphoid
Paraurethral duct 753.8
Para-urethritis 597.89
  gonococcal (acute) 098.0
    chronic or duration of 2 months or over 098.2
Paravaccinia NEC 051.9
  milkers' node 051.1
Paravaginitis (*see also* Vaginitis) 616.10
Parencephalitis (*see also* Encephalitis) 323.9
  late effect—*see* category 326
Parergasia 298.9
Paresis (*see also* Paralysis) 344.9
  accommodation 367.51
  bladder (spastic) (sphincter) (*see also* Paralysis, bladder) 596.53
    tabetic 094.0
  bowel, colon, or intestine (*see also* Ileus) 560.1
  brain or cerebral—*see* Paralysis, brain
  extrinsic muscle, eye 378.55
  general 094.1
    arrested 094.1
    brain 094.1
    cerebral 094.1
    insane 094.1
    juvenile 090.40
      remission 090.49
    progressive 094.1
    remission (sustained) 094.1
    tabetic 094.1
  heart (*see also* Failure, heart) 428.9
  infantile (*see also* Poliomyelitis) 045.9
  insane 094.1
  juvenile 090.40
  late effect—*see* Paralysis, late effect
  luetic (general) 094.1
  peripheral progressive 356.9
  pseudohypertrophic 359.1
  senile NEC 344.9
  stomach 536.3
  syphilitic (general) 094.1
    congenital 090.40
  transient, limb 781.4
  vesical (sphincter) NEC 596.53
Paresthesia (*see also* Disturbance, sensation) 782.0
  Berger's (paresthesia of lower limb) 782.0
  Bernhardt 355.1
  Magnan's 782.0
Paretic —*see* condition
Parinaud's
  conjunctivitis 372.02
  oculoglandular syndrome 372.02
  ophthalmoplegia 378.81
  syndrome (paralysis of conjugate upward gaze) 378.81
Parkes Weber and Dimitri syndrome (encephalocutaneous angiomatosis) 759.6
Parkinson's disease, syndrome, or tremor —*see* Parkinsonism
Parkinsonism (arteriosclerotic) (idiopathic) (primary) 332.0
  associated with orthostatic hypotension (idiopathic) (symptomatic) 333.0
  due to drugs 332.1
  secondary 332.1
  syphilitic 094.82
Parodontitis 523.4
Parodontosis 523.5
Paronychia (with lymphangitis) 681.9
  candidal (chronic) 112.3
  chronic 681.9
    candidal 112.3
    finger 681.02
    toe 681.11
  finger 681.02
  toe 681.11
  tuberculous (primary) (*see also* Tuberculosis) 017.0
Parorexia NEC 307.52
  hysterical 300.11
Parosmia 781.1
  psychogenic 306.7
Parotid gland —*see* condition
Parotiditis (*see also* Parotitis) 527.2
  epidemic 072.9
  infectious 072.9
Parotitis 527.2
  allergic 527.2
  chronic 527.2
  epidemic (*see also* Mumps) 072.9
  infectious (*see also* Mumps) 072.9
  noninfectious 527.2
  nonspecific toxic 527.2
  not mumps 527.2
  postoperative 527.2
  purulent 527.2
  septic 527.2
  suppurative (acute) 527.2
  surgical 527.2
  toxic 527.2
Paroxysmal —*see also* condition
  dyspnea (nocturnal) 786.09
Parrot's disease (syphilitic osteochondritis) 090.0
Parrot fever 073.9
Parry's disease or syndrome (exophthalmic goiter) 242.0
Parry-Romberg syndrome 349.89
Parson's disease (exophthalmic goiter) 242.0
Parsonage-Aldren-Turner syndrome 353.5
Parsonage-Turner syndrome 353.5
Pars planitis 363.21
Particolored infant 757.39
Parturition —*see* Delivery
Passage
  false, urethra 599.4
  of sounds or bougies (*see also* Attention to artificial opening) V55.9
Passive —*see* condition
Pasteurella septica 027.2
Pasteurellosis (*see also* Infection, Pasteurella) 027.2
PAT (paroxysmal atrial tachycardia) 427.0
Patau's syndrome (trisomy D_1) 758.1
Patch
  herald 696.3
Patches
  mucous (syphilitic) 091.3
    congenital 090.0
  smokers' (mouth) 528.6
Patellar —*see* condition
Patent —*see also* Imperfect closure
  atrioventricular ostium 745.69
  canal of Nuck 752.41
  cervix 622.5
    complicating pregnancy 654.5
      affecting fetus or newborn 761.0
  ductus arteriosus or Botalli 747.0

Patent—*continued*
Eustachian
tube 381.7
valve 746.89
foramen
Botalli 745.5
ovale 745.5
interauricular septum 745.5
interventricular septum 745.4
omphalomesenteric duct 751.0
os (uteri)—*see* Patent, cervix
ostium secundum 745.5
urachus 753.7
vitelline duct 751.0
Paterson's syndrome (sideropenic dysphagia) 280.8
Paterson (-Brown) (-Kelly) syndrome (sideropenic dysphagia) 280.8
Paterson-Kelly syndrome or web (sideropenic dysphagia) 280.8
Pathologic, pathological —*see also* condition
asphyxia 799.0
drunkenness 291.4
emotionality 301.3
liar 301.7
personality 301.9
resorption, tooth 521.4
sexuality (*see also* Deviation, sexual) 302.9
Pathology (of)—*see* Disease
Patterned motor discharges, idiopathic (*see also* Epilepsy) 345.5
Patulous —*see also* Patent
anus 569.49
Eustachian tube 381.7
Pause, sinoatrial 427.81
Pavor nocturnus 307.46
Pavy's disease 593.6
Paxton's disease (white piedra) 111.2
Payr's disease or syndrome (splenic flexure syndrome) 569.89
Pearls
Elschnig 366.51
enamel 520.2
Pearl-workers' disease (chronic osteomyelitis) (*see also* Osteomyelitis) 730.1
Pectenitis 569.49
Pectenosis 569.49
Pectoral —*see* condition
Pectus
carinatum (congenital) 754.82
acquired 738.3
rachitic (*see also* Rickets) 268.0
excavatum (congenital) 754.81
acquired 738.3
rachitic (*see also* Rickets) 268.0
recurvatum (congenital) 754.81
acquired 738.3
Pedatrophia 261
Pederosis 302.2
Pediculosis (infestation) 132.9
capitis (head louse) (any site) 132.0
corporis (body louse) (any site) 132.1
eyelid 132.0 *[373.6]*
mixed (classifiable to more than one category in 132.0-132.2) 132.3
pubis (pubic louse) (any site) 132.2
vestimenti 132.1
vulvae 132.2
Pediculus (infestation)—*see* Pediculosis
Pedophilia 302.2
Peg-shaped teeth 520.2
Pel's crisis 094.0
Pel-Ebstein disease —*see* Disease, Hodgkin's
Pelade 704.01
Pelger-Huët anomaly or syndrome (hereditary hyposegmentation) 288.2
Peliosis (rheumatica) 287.0
Pelizaeus-Merzbacher
disease 330.0
sclerosis, diffuse cerebral 330.0
Pellagra (alcoholic or with alcoholism) 265.2
with polyneuropathy 265.2 *[357.4]*
Pellagra-cerebellar-ataxia-renal aminoaciduria syndrome 270.0
Pellegrini's disease (calcification, knee joint) 726.62
Pellegrini (-Stieda) disease or syndrome (calcification, knee joint) 726.62
Pellizzi's syndrome (pineal) 259.8
Pelvic —*see also* condition
congestion-fibrosis syndrome 625.5
kidney 753.3
Pelvioectasis 591
Pelviolithiasis 592.0
Pelviperitonitis
female (*see also* Peritonitis, pelvic, female) 614.5
male (*see also* Peritonitis) 567.2
Pelvis, pelvic —*see also* condition or type
infantile 738.6
Nägele's 738.6
obliquity 738.6
Robert's 755.69
Pemphigoid 694.5
benign, mucous membrane 694.60
with ocular involvement 694.61
bullous 694.5
cicatricial 694.60
with ocular involvement 694.61
juvenile 694.2
Pemphigus 694.4
benign 694.5
chronic familial 757.39
Brazilian 694.4
circinatus 694.0
congenital, traumatic 757.39
conjunctiva 694.61
contagiosus 684
erythematodes 694.4
erythematosus 694.4
foliaceus 694.4
frambesiodes 694.4
gangrenous (*see also* Gangrene) 785.4
malignant 694.4
neonatorum, newborn 684
ocular 694.61
papillaris 694.4
seborrheic 694.4
South American 694.4
syphilitic (congenital) 090.0
vegetans 694.4
vulgaris 694.4
wildfire 694.4
Pendred's syndrome (familial goiter with deaf-mutism) 243
Pendulous
abdomen 701.9
in pregnancy or childbirth 654.4
affecting fetus or newborn 763.8
breast 611.8

Penetrating wound —*see also* Wound, open, by site
with internal injury—*see* Injury, internal, by site, with open wound
eyeball 871.7
with foreign body (nonmagnetic) 871.6
magnetic 871.5
ocular (*see also* Penetrating wound, eyeball) 871.7
adnexa 870.3
with foreign body 870.4
orbit 870.3
with foreign body 870.4
Penetration, pregnant uterus by instrument
with
abortion—*see* Abortion, by type, with damage to pelvic organs
ectopic pregnancy (*see also* categories 633.0-633.9) 639.2
molar pregnancy (*see also* categories 630-632) 639.2
complication of delivery 665.1
affecting fetus or newborn 763.8
following
abortion 639.2
ectopic or molar pregnancy 639.2
Penfield's syndrome (*see also* Epilepsy) 345.5
Penicilliosis of lung 117.3
Penis —*see* condition
Penitis 607.2
Penta X syndrome 758.8
Pentalogy (of Fallot) 745.2
Pentosuria (benign) (essential) 271.8
Peptic acid disease 536.8
Peregrinating patient V65.2
Perforated —*see* Perforation
Perforation, perforative (nontraumatic)
antrum (*see also* Sinusitis, maxillary) 473.0
appendix 540.0
with peritoneal abscess 540.1
atrial septum, multiple 745.5
attic, ear 384.22
healed 384.81
bile duct, except cystic (*see also* Disease, biliary) 576.3
cystic 575.4
bladder (urinary)—*see also* Injury, internal, bladder
with
abortion—*see* Abortion, by type, with damage to pelvic organs
ectopic pregnancy (*see also* categories 633.0-633.9) 639.2
molar pregnancy (*see also* categories 630-632) 639.2
following
abortion 639.2
ectopic or molar pregnancy 639.2
obstetrical trauma 665.5
bowel 569.83
with
abortion—*see* Abortion, by type, with damage to pelvic organs
ectopic pregnancy (*see also* categories 633.0-633.9) 639.2
molar pregnancy (*see also* categories 630-632) 639.2
fetus or newborn 777.6
following
abortion 639.2
ectopic or molar pregnancy 639.2
Perforation, perforative—*continued*
obstetrical trauma 665.5
broad ligament
with
abortion—*see* Abortion, by type, with damage to pelvic organs
ectopic pregnancy (*see also* categories 633.0-633.9) 639.2
molar pregnancy (*see also* categories 630-632) 639.2
following
abortion 639.2
ectopic or molar pregnancy 639.2
obstetrical trauma 665.6
by
device, implant, or graft—*see* Complications, mechanical
foreign body left accidentally in operation wound 998.4
instrument (any) during a procedure, accidental 998.2
cecum 540.0
with peritoneal abscess 540.1
cervix (uteri)—*see also* Injury, internal, cervix
with
abortion—*see* Abortion, by type, with damage to pelvic organs
ectopic pregnancy (*see also* categories 633.0-633.9) 639.2
molar pregnancy (*see also* categories 630-632) 639.2
following
abortion 639.2
ectopic or molar pregnancy 639.2
obstetrical trauma 665.3
colon 569.83
common duct (bile) 576.3
cornea (*see also* Ulcer, cornea) 370.00
due to ulceration 370.06
cystic duct 575.4
diverticulum (*see also* Diverticula) 562.10
small intestine 562.00
duodenum, duodenal (ulcer)—*see* Ulcer, duodenum, with perforation
ear drum—*see* Perforation, tympanum
enteritis—*see* Enteritis
esophagus 530.4
ethmoidal sinus (*see also* Sinusitis, ethmoidal) 473.2
foreign body (external site)—*see also* Wound, open, by site, complicated
internal site, by ingested object—*see* Foreign body
frontal sinus (*see also* Sinusitis, frontal) 473.1
gallbladder or duct (*see also* Disease, gallbladder) 575.4
gastric (ulcer)—*see* Ulcer, stomach, with perforation
heart valve—*see* Endocarditis
ileum 569.83
instrumental
external—*see* Wound, open, by site
pregnant uterus, complicating delivery 665.9
surgical (accidental) (blood vessel) (nerve) (organ) 998.2
intestine 569.83
with
abortion—*see* Abortion, by type, with damage to pelvic organs
ectopic pregnancy (*see also* categories 633.0-633.9) 639.2

Perforation, perforative—*continued*
molar pregnancy (*see also* categories 630-632) 639.2
fetus or newborn 777.6
obstetrical trauma 665.5
ulcerative NEC 569.83
jejunum, jejunal 569.83
ulcer—*see* Ulcer, gastrojejunal, with perforation
mastoid (antrum) (cell) 383.89
maxillary sinus (*see also* Sinusitis, maxillary) 473.0
membrana tympani—*see* Perforation, tympanum
nasal
septum 478.1
congenital 748.1
syphilitic 095.8
sinus (*see also* Sinusitis) 473.9
congenital 748.1
palate (hard) 526.89
soft 528.9
syphilitic 095.8
syphilitic 095.8
palatine vault 526.89
syphilitic 095.8
congenital 090.5
pelvic
floor
with
abortion—*see* Abortion, by type, with damage to pelvic organs
ectopic pregnancy (*see also* categories 633.0-633.9) 639.2
molar pregnancy (*see also* categories 630-632) 639.2
obstetrical trauma 664.1
organ
with
abortion—*see* Abortion, by type, with damage to pelvic organs
ectopic pregnancy (*see also* categories 633.0-633.9) 639.2
molar pregnancy (*see also* categories 630-632) 639.2
following
abortion 639.2
ectopic or molar pregnancy 639.2
obstetrical trauma 665.5
perineum—*see* Laceration, perineum
periurethral tissue
with
abortion—*see* Abortion, by type, with damage to pelvic organs
ectopic pregnancy (*see also* categories 630-632) 639.2
molar pregnancy (*see also* categories 630-632) 639.2
pharynx 478.29
pylorus, pyloric (ulcer)—*see* Ulcer, stomach, with perforation
rectum 569.49
sigmoid 569.83
sinus (accessory) (chronic) (nasal) (*see also* Sinusitis) 473.9
sphenoidal sinus (*see also* Sinusitis, sphenoidal) 473.3
stomach (due to ulcer)—*see* Ulcer, stomach, with perforation
surgical (accidental) (by instrument) (blood vessel) (nerve) (organ) 998.2

Perforation, perforative—*continued*
traumatic
external—*see* Wound, open, by site
eye (*see also* Penetrating wound, ocular) 871.7
internal organ—*see* Injury, internal, by site
tympanum (membrane) (persistent posttraumatic) (postinflammatory) 384.20
attic 384.22
central 384.21
healed 384.81
marginal NEC 384.23
multiple 384.24
pars flaccida 384.22
total 384.25
traumatic—*see* Wound, open, ear, drum
typhoid, gastrointestinal 002.0
ulcer—*see* Ulcer, by site, with perforation
ureter 593.89
urethra
with
abortion—*see* Abortion, by type, with damage to pelvic organs
ectopic pregnancy (*see also* categories 633.0-633.9) 639.2
molar pregnancy (*see also* categories 630-632) 639.2
following
abortion 639.2
ectopic or molar pregnancy 639.2
obstetrical trauma 665.5
uterus—*see also* Injury, internal, uterus
with
abortion—*see* Abortion, by type, with damage to pelvic organs
ectopic pregnancy (*see also* categories 633.0-633.9) 639.2
molar pregnancy (*see also* categories 630-632) 639.2
by intrauterine contraceptive device 996.32
following
abortion 639.2
ectopic or molar pregnancy 639.2
obstetrical trauma—*see* Injury, internal, uterus, obstetrical trauma
uvula 528.9
syphilitic 095.8
vagina—*see* Laceration, vagina
viscus NEC 799.8
traumatic 868.00
with open wound into cavity 868.10
Periadenitis mucosa necrotica recurrens 528.2
Periangiitis 446.0
Periantritis 535.4
Periappendicitis (acute) (*see also* Appendicitis) 541
Periarteritis (disseminated) (infectious) (necrotizing) (nodosa) 446.0
Periarthritis (joint) 726.90
Duplay's 726.2
gonococcal 098.50
humeroscapularis 726.2
scapulohumeral 726.2
shoulder 726.2
wrist 726.4
Periarthrosis (angioneural)—*see* Periarthritis
Peribronchitis 491.9
tuberculous (*see also* Tuberculosis) 011.3
Pericapsulitis, adhesive (shoulder) 726.0

Pericarditis (granular) (with decompensation) (with effusion) 423.9
with
rheumatic fever (conditions classifiable to 390)
active (*see also* Pericarditis, rheumatic) 391.0
inactive or quiescent 393
actinomycotic 039.8 *[420.0]*
acute (nonrheumatic) 420.90
with chorea (acute) (rheumatic) (Sydenham's) 392.0
bacterial 420.99
benign 420.91
hemorrhagic 420.90
idiopathic 420.91
infective 420.90
nonspecific 420.91
rheumatic 391.0
with chorea (acute) (rheumatic) (Sydenham's) 392.0
sicca 420.90
viral 420.91
adhesive or adherent (external) (internal) 423.1
acute—*see* Pericarditis, acute
rheumatic (external) (internal) 393
amebic 006.8 *[420.0]*
bacterial (acute) (subacute) (with serous or seropurulent effusion) 420.99
calcareous 423.2
cholesterol (chronic) 423.8
acute 420.90
chronic (nonrheumatic) 423.8
rheumatic 393
constrictive 423.2
Coxsackie 074.21
due to
actinomycosis 039.8 *[420.0]*
amebiasis 006.8 *[420.0]*
Coxsackie (virus) 074.21
histoplasmosis (*see also* Histoplasmosis) 115.93
nocardiosis 039.8 *[420.0]*
tuberculosis (*see also* Tuberculosis) 017.9 *[420.0]*
fibrinocaseous (*see also* Tuberculosis) 017.9 *[420.0]*
fibrinopurulent 420.99
fibrinous—*see* Pericarditis, rheumatic
fibropurulent 420.99
fibrous 423.1
gonococcal 098.83
hemorrhagic 423.0
idiopathic (acute) 420.91
infective (acute) 420.90
meningococcal 036.41
neoplastic (chronic) 423.8
acute 420.90
nonspecific 420.91
obliterans, obliterating 423.1
plastic 423.1
pneumococcal (acute) 420.99
postinfarction 411.0
purulent (acute) 420.99
rheumatic (active) (acute) (with effusion) (with pneumonia) 391.0
with chorea (acute) (rheumatic) (Sydenham's) 392.0
chronic or inactive (with chorea) 393
septic (acute) 420.99
serofibrinous—*see* Pericarditis, rheumatic
staphylococcal (acute) 420.99

Pericarditis—*continued*
streptococcal (acute) 420.99
suppurative (acute) 420.99
syphilitic 093.81
tuberculous (acute) (chronic) (*see also* Tuberculosis) 017.9 *[420.0]*
uremic 585 *[420.0]*
viral (acute) 420.91
Pericardium, pericardial —*see* condition
Pericellulitis (*see also* Cellulitis) 682.9
Pericementitis 523.4
acute 523.3
chronic (suppurative) 523.4
Pericholecystitis (*see also* Cholecystitis) 575.1
Perichondritis
auricle 380.00
acute 380.01
chronic 380.02
bronchus 491.9
ear (external) 380.00
acute 380.01
chronic 380.02
larynx 478.71
syphilitic 095.8
typhoid 002.0 *[478.71]*
nose 478.1
pinna 380.00
acute 380.01
chronic 380.02
trachea 478.9
Periclasia 523.5
Pericolitis 569.89
Pericoronitis (chronic) 523.4
acute 523.3
Pericystitis (*see also* Cystitis) 595.9
Pericytoma (M9150/1)—*see also* Neoplasm, connective tissue, uncertain behavior
benign (M9150/0)—*see* Neoplasm, connective tissue, benign
malignant (M9150/3)—*see* Neoplasm, connective tissue, malignant
Peridacryocystitis, acute 375.32
Peridiverticulitis (*see also* Diverticulitis) 562.11
Periduodenitis 535.6
Periendocarditis (*see also* Endocarditis) 424.90
acute or subacute 421.9
Periepididymitis (*see also* Epididymitis) 604.90
Perifolliculitis (abscedens) 704.8
capitis, abscedens et suffodiens 704.8
dissecting, scalp 704.8
scalp 704.8
superficial pustular 704.8
Perigastritis (acute) 535.0
Perigastrojejunitis (acute) 535.0
Perihepatitis (acute) 573.3
chlamydial 099.56
gonococcal 098.86
Peri-ileitis (subacute) 569.89
Perilabyrinthitis (acute)—*see* Labyrinthitis
Perimeningitis —*see* Meningitis
Perimetritis (*see also* Endometritis) 615.9
Perimetrosalpingitis (*see also* Salpingo-oophoritis) 614.2
Perinephric —*see* condition
Perinephritic —*see* condition
Perinephritis (*see also* Infection, kidney) 590.9
purulent (*see also* Abscess, kidney) 590.2
Perineum, perineal —*see* condition
Perineuritis NEC 729.2

Periodic —*see also* condition
disease (familial) 277.3
edema 995.1
hereditary 277.6
fever 277.3
paralysis (familial) 359.3
peritonitis 277.3
polyserositis 277.3
somnolence 347
Periodontal
cyst 522.8
pocket 523.8
Periodontitis (chronic) (complex) (compound) (local) (simplex) 523.4
acute 523.3
apical 522.6
acute (pulpal origin) 522.4
Periodontoclasia 523.5
Periodontosis 523.5
Periods —*see also* Menstruation
heavy 626.2
irregular 626.4
Perionychia (with lymphangitis) 681.9
finger 681.02
toe 681.11
Perioophoritis (*see also* Salpingo-oophoritis) 614.2
Periorchitis (*see also* Orchitis) 604.90
Periosteum, periosteal —*see* condition
Periostitis (circumscribed) (diffuse) (infective) 730.3

Note—Use the following fifth-digit subclassification with category 730:

0 site unspecified
1 shoulder region
2 upper arm
3 forearm
4 hand
5 pelvic region and thigh
6 lower leg
7 ankle and foot
8 other specified sites
9 multiple sites

with osteomyelitis (*see also* Osteomyelitis) 730.2
acute or subacute 730.0
chronic or old 730.1
albuminosa, albuminosus 730.3
alveolar 526.5
alveolodental 526.5
dental 526.5
gonorrheal 098.89
hyperplastica, generalized 731.2
jaw (lower) (upper) 526.4
monomelic 733.99
orbital 376.02
syphilitic 095.5
congenital 090.0 *[730.8]*
secondary 091.61
tuberculous (*see also* Tuberculosis, bone) 015.9 *[730.8]*
yaws (early) (hypertrophic) (late) 102.6
Periostosis (*see also* Periostitis) 730.3
with osteomyelitis (*see also* Osteomyelitis) 730.2
acute or subacute 730.0
chronic or old 730.1
hyperplastic 756.59
Periphlebitis (*see also* Phlebitis) 451.9
lower extremity 451.2
deep (vessels) 451.19
superficial (vessels) 451.0
portal 572.1
retina 362.18
superficial (vessels) 451.0
tuberculous (*see also* Tuberculosis) 017.9
retina 017.3 *[362.18]*
Peripneumonia —*see* Pneumonia
Periproctitis 569.49
Periprostatitis (*see also* Prostatitis) 601.9
Perirectal —*see* condition
Perirenal —*see* condition
Perisalpingitis (*see also* Salpingo-oophoritis) 614.2
Perisigmoiditis 569.89
Perisplenitis (infectional) 289.59
Perispondylitis —*see* Spondylitis
Peristalsis reversed or visible 787.4
Peritendinitis (*see also* Tenosynovitis) 726.90
adhesive (shoulder) 726.0
Perithelioma (M9150/1)—*see* Pericytoma
Peritoneum, peritoneal —*see* condition
Peritonitis (acute) (adhesive) (fibrinous) (hemorrhagic) (idiopathic) (localized) (perforative) (primary) (with adhesions) (with effusion) 567.9
with or following
abortion—*see* Abortion, by type, with sepsis
abscess 567.2
appendicitis 540.0
with peritoneal abscess 540.1
ectopic pregnancy (*see also* categories 633.0-633.9) 639.0
molar pregnancy (*see also* categories 630-632) 639.0
aseptic 998.7
bacterial 567.2
bile, biliary 567.8
chemical 998.7
chlamydial 099.56
chronic proliferative 567.8
congenital NEC 777.6
diaphragmatic 567.2
diffuse NEC 567.2
diphtheritic 032.83
disseminated NEC 567.2
due to
bile 567.8
foreign
body or object accidentally left during a procedure (instrument) (sponge) (swab) 998.4
substance accidentally left during a procedure (chemical) (powder) (talc) 998.7
talc 998.7
urine 567.8
fibrinopurulent 567.2
fibrinous 567.2
fibrocaseous (*see also* Tuberculosis) 014.0
fibropurulent 567.2
general, generalized (acute) 567.2
gonococcal 098.86
in infective disease NEC 136.9 *[567.0]*
meconium (newborn) 777.6
pancreatic 577.8
paroxysmal, benign 277.3

Peritonitis—*continued*
pelvic
female (acute) 614.5
chronic NEC 614.7
with adhesions 614.6
puerperal, postpartum, childbirth 670
male (acute) 567.2
periodic (familial) 277.3
phlegmonous 567.2
pneumococcal 567.1
postabortal 639.0
proliferative, chronic 567.8
puerperal, postpartum, childbirth 670
purulent 567.2
septic 567.2
staphylococcal 567.2
streptococcal 567.2
subdiaphragmatic 567.2
subphrenic 567.2
suppurative 567.2
syphilitic 095.2
congenital 090.0 *[567.0]*
talc 998.7
tuberculous (*see also* Tuberculosis) 014.0
urine 567.8
Peritonsillar —*see* condition
Peritonsillitis 475
Perityphlitis (*see also* Appendicitis) 541
Periureteritis 593.89
Periurethral —*see* condition
Periurethritis (gangrenous) 597.89
Periuterine —*see* condition
Perivaginitis (*see also* Vaginitis) 616.10
Perivasculitis, retinal 362.18
Perivasitis (chronic) 608.4
Perivesiculitis (seminal) (*see also* Vesiculitis) 608.0
Perlèche 686.8
due to
moniliasis 112.0
riboflavin deficiency 266.0
Pernicious —*see* condition
Pernio, perniosis 991.5
Persecution
delusion 297.9
social V62.4
Perseveration (tonic) 784.69
Persistence, persistent (congenital) 759.89
anal membrane 751.2
arteria stapedia 744.04
atrioventricular canal 745.69
bloody ejaculate 792.2
branchial cleft 744.41
bulbus cordis in left ventricle 745.8
canal of Cloquet 743.51
capsule (opaque) 743.51
cilioretinal artery or vein 743.51
cloaca 751.5
communication—*see* Fistula, congenital
convolutions
aortic arch 747.21
fallopian tube 752.19
oviduct 752.19
uterine tube 752.19
double aortic arch 747.21
ductus
arteriosus 747.0
Botalli 747.0

Persistence, persistent—*continued*
fetal
circulation 747.9
form of cervix (uteri) 752.49
hemoglobin (hereditary) ("Swiss variety") 282.7
foramen
Botalli 745.5
ovale 745.5
Gartner's duct 752.11
hemoglobin, fetal (hereditary) (HPFH) 282.7
hyaloid
artery (generally incomplete) 743.51
system 743.51
hymen (tag)
in pregnancy or childbirth 654.8
causing obstructed labor 660.2
lanugo 757.4
left
posterior cardinal vein 747.49
root with right arch of aorta 747.21
superior vena cava 747.49
Meckel's diverticulum 751.0
mesonephric duct 752.8
fallopian tube 752.11
mucosal disease (middle ear) (with posterior or superior marginal perforation of ear drum) 382.2
nail(s), anomalous 757.5
occiput, anterior or posterior 660.3
fetus or newborn 763.1
omphalomesenteric duct 751.0
organ or site NEC—*see* Anomaly, specified type NEC
ostium
atrioventriculare commune 745.69
primum 745.61
secundum 745.5
ovarian rests in fallopian tube 752.19
pancreatic tissue in intestinal tract 751.5
primary (deciduous)
teeth 520.6
vitreous hyperplasia 743.51
pupillary membrane 743.46
iris 743.46
Rhesus (Rh) titer 999.7
right aortic arch 747.21
sinus
urogenitalis 752.8
venosus with imperfect incorporation in right auricle 747.49
thymus (gland) 254.8
hyperplasia 254.0
thyroglossal duct 759.2
thyrolingual duct 759.2
truncus arteriosus or communis 745.0
tunica vasculosa lentis 743.39
umbilical sinus 753.7
urachus 753.7
vegetative state 780.03
vitelline duct 751.0
wolffian duct 752.8
Person (with)
admitted for clinical research, as control subject V70.7
awaiting admission to adequate facility elsewhere V63.2
undergoing social agency investigation V63.8
concern (normal) about sick person in family V61.49
consulting on behalf of another V65.1

Person—*continued*
feared
complaint in whom no diagnosis was made V65.5
condition not demonstrated V65.5
feigning illness V65.2
healthy, accompanying sick person V65.0
living (in)
alone V60.3
boarding school V60.6
residence remote from hospital or medical care facility V63.0
residential institution V60.6
without
adequate
financial resources V60.2
housing (heating) (space) V60.1
housing (permanent) (temporary) V60.0
material resources V60.2
person able to render necessary care V60.4
shelter V60.0
medical services in home not available V63.1
on waiting list V63.2
undergoing social agency investigation V63.8
sick or handicapped in family V61.49
"worried well" V65.5
Personality
affective 301.10
aggressive 301.3
amoral 301.7
anancastic, anankastic 301.4
antisocial 301.7
asocial 301.7
asthenic 301.6
avoidant 301.82
borderline 301.83
change 310.1
compulsive 301.4
cycloid 301.13
cyclothymic 301.13
dependent 301.6
depressive (chronic) 301.12
disorder, disturbance NEC 301.9
with
antisocial disturbance 301.7
pattern disturbance NEC 301.9
sociopathic disturbance 301.7
trait disturbance 301.9
dual 300.14
dyssocial 301.7
eccentric 301.89
"haltlose" type 301.89
emotionally unstable 301.59
epileptoid 301.3
explosive 301.3
fanatic 301.0
histrionic 301.50
hyperthymic 301.11
hypomanic 301.11
hypothymic 301.12
hysterical 301.50
immature 301.89
inadequate 301.6
labile 301.59
masochistic 301.89
morally defective 301.7
multiple 300.14
narcissistic 301.81
obsessional 301.4
obsessive (-compulsive) 301.4
overconscientious 301.4
paranoid 301.0
Personality—*continued*
passive (-dependent) 301.6
passive-aggressive 301.84
pathologic NEC 301.9
pattern defect or disturbance 301.9
pseudosocial 301.7
psychoinfantile 301.59
psychoneurotic NEC 301.89
psychopathic 301.9
with
amoral trend 301.7
antisocial trend 301.7
asocial trend 301.7
pathologic sexuality (*see also* Deviation, sexual) 302.9
mixed types 301.9
schizoid 301.20
introverted 301.21
schizotypal 301.22
with sexual deviation (*see also* Deviation, sexual) 302.9
antisocial 301.7
dyssocial 301.7
type A 301.4
unstable (emotional) 301.59
Perthes' disease (capital femoral osteochondrosis) 732.1
Pertussis (*see also* Whooping cough) 033.9
vaccination, prophylactic (against) V03.6
Peruvian wart 088.0
Perversion, perverted
appetite 307.52
hysterical 300.11
function
pineal gland 259.8
pituitary gland 253.9
anterior lobe
deficient 253.2
excessive 253.1
posterior lobe 253.6
placenta—*see* Placenta, abnormal
sense of smell or taste 781.1
psychogenic 306.7
sexual (*see also* Deviation, sexual) 302.9
Pervious, congenital —*see also* Imperfect, closure
ductus arteriosus 747.0
Pes (congenital) (*see also* Talipes) 754.70
abductus (congenital) 754.60
acquired 736.79
acquired NEC 736.79
planus 734
adductus (congenital) 754.79
acquired 736.79
cavus 754.71
acquired 736.73
planovalgus (congenital) 754.69
acquired 736.79
planus (acquired) (any degree) 734
congenital 754.61
rachitic 268.1
valgus (congenital) 754.61
acquired 736.79
varus (congenital) 754.50
acquired 736.79
Pest (*see also* Plague) 020.9
Pestis (*see also* Plague) 020.9
bubonica 020.0
fulminans 020.0
minor 020.8
pneumonica—*see* Plague, pneumonic

Petechia, petechiae 782.7
fetus or newborn 772.6
Petechial
fever 036.0
typhus 081.9
Petges-Cléjat or Petges-Clégat syndrome (poikilodermatomyositis) 710.3
Petit's
disease (*see also* Hernia, lumbar) 553.8
Petit mal (idiopathic) (*see also* Epilepsy) 345.0
status 345.2
Petrellidosis 117.6
Petrositis 383.20
acute 383.21
chronic 383.22
Peutz-Jeghers disease or syndrome 759.6
Peyronie's disease 607.89
Pfeiffer's disease 075
Phacentocele 379.32
traumatic 921.3
Phacoanaphylaxis 360.19
Phacocele (old) 379.32
traumatic 921.3
Phaehyphomycosis 117.8
Phagedena (dry) (moist) (*see also* Gangrene) 785.4
arteriosclerotic 440.24
geometric 686.0
penis 607.89
senile 440.24
sloughing 785.4
tropical (*see also* Ulcer, skin) 707.9
vulva 616.50
Phagedenic —*see also* condition
abscess—*see also* Abscess
chancroid 099.0
bubo NEC 099.8
chancre 099.0
ulcer (tropical) (*see also* Ulcer, skin) 707.9
Phagomania 307.52
Phakoma 362.89
Phantom limb (syndrome) 353.6
Pharyngeal —*see also* condition
arch remnant 744.41
pouch syndrome 279.11
Pharyngitis (acute) (catarrhal) (gangrenous) (infective) (malignant) (membranous) (phlegmonous) (pneumococcal) (pseudomembranous) (simple) (staphylococcal) (subacute) (suppurative) (ulcerative) (viral) 462
with influenza, flu, or grippe 487.1
aphthous 074.0
atrophic 472.1
chlamydial 099.51
chronic 472.1
Coxsackie virus 074.0
diphtheritic (membranous) 032.0
follicular 472.1
fusospirochetal 101
gonococcal 098.6
granular (chronic) 472.1
herpetic 054.79
hypertrophic 472.1
infectional, chronic 472.1
influenzal 487.1
lymphonodular, acute 074.8
septic 034.0
streptococcal 034.0
tuberculous (*see also* Tuberculosis) 012.8
vesicular 074.0
Pharyngoconjunctival fever 077.2
Pharyngoconjunctivitis, viral 077.2
Pharyngolaryngitis (acute) 465.0
chronic 478.9
septic 034.0
Pharyngoplegia 478.29
Pharyngotonsillitis 465.8
tuberculous 012.8
Pharyngotracheitis (acute) 465.8
chronic 478.9
Pharynx, pharyngeal —*see* condition
Phase of life problem NEC V62.89
Phenomenon
Arthus'—*see* Arthus' phenomenon
flashback (drug) 292.89
jaw-winking 742.8
Jod-Basedow 242.8
L. E. cell 710.0
lupus erythematosus cell 710.0
Pelger-Huët (hereditary hyposegmentation) 288.2
Raynaud's (paroxysmal digital cyanosis) (secondary) 443.0
Reilly's (*see also* Neuropathy, peripheral, autonomic) 337.9
vasomotor 780.2
vasospastic 443.9
vasovagal 780.2
Wenckebach's, heart block (second degree) 426.13
Phenylketonuria (PKU) 270.1
Phenylpyruvicaciduria 270.1
Pheochromoblastoma (M8700/3)
specified site—*see* Neoplasm, by site, malignant
unspecified site 194.0
Pheochromocytoma (M8700/0)
malignant (M8700/3)
specified site—*see* Neoplasm, by site, malignant
unspecified site 194.0
specified site—*see* Neoplasm, by site, benign
unspecified site 227.0
Phimosis (congenital) 605
chancroidal 099.0
due to infection 605
Phlebectasia (*see also* Varicose, vein) 454.9
congenital NEC 747.60
esophagus (*see also* Varix, esophagus) 456.1
with hemorrhage (*see also* Varix, esophagus, bleeding) 456.0
Phlebitis (infective) (pyemic) (septic) (suppurative) 451.9
antecubital vein 451.82
arm NEC 451.84
axillary vein 451.89
basilic vein 451.82
deep 451.83
superficial 451.82
basilic vein 451.82
blue 451.19
brachial vein 451.83
breast, superficial 451.89
cavernous (venous) sinus—*see* Phlebitis, intracranial sinus
cephalic vein 451.82
cerebral (venous) sinus—*see* Phlebitis, intracranial sinus
chest wall, superficial 451.89
complicating pregnancy or puerperium 671.9
affecting fetus or newborn 760.3
cranial (venous) sinus—*see* Phlebitis, intracranial sinus

Phlebitis—*continued*
deep (vessels) 451.19
femoral vein 451.11
specified vessel NEC 451.19
due to implanted device—*see* Complications, due to (presence of) any device, implant, or graft classified to 996.0-996.5 NEC
during or resulting from a procedure 997.2
femoral vein (deep) (superficial) 451.11
femoropopliteal 451.19
following infusion, perfusion, or transfusion 999.2
gouty 274.89 *[451.9]*
hepatic veins 451.89
iliac vein 451.81
iliofemoral 451.11
intracranial sinus (any) (venous) 325
late effect—*see* category 326
nonpyogenic 437.6
in pregnancy or puerperium 671.5
jugular vein 451.89
lateral (venous) sinus—*see* Phlebitis, intracranial sinus
leg 451.2
deep (vessels) 451.19
femoral vein 451.11
specified vessel NEC 451.19
superficial (vessels) 451.0
femoral vein 451.11
longitudinal sinus—*see* Phlebitis, intracranial sinus
lower extremity 451.2
deep (vessels) 451.19
femoral vein 451.11
specified vessel NEC 451.19
superficial (vessels) 451.0
femoral vein 451.11
migrans, migrating (superficial) 453.1
pelvic
with
abortion—*see* Abortion, by type, with sepsis
ectopic pregnancy (*see also* categories 633.0-633.9) 639.0
molar pregnancy (*see also* categories 630-632) 639.0
following
abortion 639.0
ectopic or molar pregnancy 639.0
puerperal, postpartum 671.4
popliteal vein 451.19
portal (vein) 572.1
postoperative 997.2
pregnancy 671.9
deep 671.3
specified type NEC 671.5
superficial 671.2
puerperal, postpartum, childbirth 671.9
deep 671.4
lower extremities 671.2
pelvis 671.4
specified site NEC 671.5
superficial 671.2
radial vein 451.83
retina 362.18
saphenous (great) (long) 451.0
accessory or small 451.0
sinus (meninges)—*see* Phlebitis, intracranial sinus
specified site NEC 451.89
subclavian vein 451.89
syphilitic 093.89

Phlebitis—*continued*
tibial vein 451.19
ulcer, ulcerative 451.9
leg 451.2
deep (vessels) 451.19
femoral vein 451.11
specified vessel NEC 451.19
superficial (vessels) 451.0
femoral vein 451.11
lower extremity 451.2
deep (vessels) 451.19
femoral vein 451.11
specified vessel NEC 451.19
superficial (vessels) 451.0
ulnar vein 451.83
umbilicus 451.89
upper extremity—*see* Phlebitis, arm
uterus (septic) (*see also* Endometritis) 615.9
varicose (leg) (lower extremity) (*see also* Varicose, vein) 454.1
Phlebofibrosis 459.89
Phleboliths 459.89
Phlebosclerosis 459.89
Phlebothrombosis —*see* Thrombosis
Phlebotomus fever 066.0
Phlegm, choked on 933.1
Phlegmasia
alba dolens (deep vessels) 451.19
complicating pregnancy 671.3
nonpuerperal 451.19
puerperal, postpartum, childbirth 671.4
cerulea dolens 451.19
Phlegmon (*see also* Abscess) 682.9
erysipelatous (*see also* Erysipelas) 035
iliac 682.2
fossa 540.1
throat 478.29
Phlegmonous —*see* condition
Phlyctenulosis (allergic) (keratoconjunctivitis) (nontuberculous) 370.31
cornea 370.31
with ulcer (*see also* Ulcer, cornea) 370.00
tuberculous (*see also* Tuberculosis) 017.3 *[370.31]*
Phobia, phobic (reaction) 300.20
animal 300.29
isolated NEC 300.29
obsessional 300.3
simple NEC 300.29
social 300.23
specified NEC 300.29
state 300.20
Phocas' disease 610.1
Phocomelia 755.4
lower limb 755.32
complete 755.33
distal 755.35
proximal 755.34
upper limb 755.22
complete 755.23
distal 755.25
proximal 755.24
Phoria (*see also* Heterophoria) 378.40
Phosphate-losing tubular disorder 588.0
Phosphatemia 275.3
Phosphaturia 275.3
Photoallergic response 692.72
Photocoproporphyria 277.1
Photodermatitis (sun) 692.72
light other than sun 692.82
Photokeratitis 370.24
Photo-ophthalmia 370.24

Photophobia 368.13
Photopsia 368.15
Photoretinitis 363.31
Photoretinopathy 363.31
Photosensitiveness (sun) 692.72
light other than sun 692.82
Photosensitization (sun) skin 692.72
light other than sun 692.82
Phototoxic response 692.72
Phrenitis 323.9
Phrynoderma 264.8
Phthiriasis (pubis) (any site) 132.2
with any infestation classifiable to 132.0 and 132.1 132.3
Phthirus infestation —*see* Phthiriasis
Phthisis (*see also* Tuberculosis) 011.9
bulbi (infectional) 360.41
colliers' 011.4
cornea 371.05
eyeball (due to infection) 360.41
millstone makers' 011.4
miners' 011.4
potters' 011.4
sandblasters' 011.4
stonemasons' 011.4
Phycomycosis 117.7
Physalopteriasis 127.7
Physical therapy NEC V57.1
breathing exercises V57.0
Physiological cup, optic papilla
borderline, glaucoma suspect 365.00
enlarged 377.14
glaucomatous 377.14
Phytobezoar 938
intestine 936
stomach 935.2
Pian (*see also* Yaws) 102.9
Pianoma 102.1
Piarhemia, piarrhemia (*see also* Hyperlipemia) 272.4
bilharziasis 120.9
Pica 307.52
hysterical 300.11
Pick's
cerebral atrophy 331.1
with dementia 290.10
disease
brain 331.1
dementia in 290.10
lipid histiocytosis 272.7
liver (pericardial pseudocirrhosis of liver) 423.2
pericardium (pericardial pseudocirrhosis of liver) 423.2
polyserositis (pericardial pseudocirrhosis of liver) 423.2
syndrome
heart (pericardial pseudocirrhosis of liver) 423.2
liver (pericardial pseudocirrhosis of liver) 423.2
tubular adenoma (M8640/0)
specified site—*see* Neoplasm, by site, benign
unspecified site
female 220
male 222.0
Pick-Herxheimer syndrome (diffuse idiopathic cutaneous atrophy) 701.8
Pick-Niemann disease (lipid histiocytosis) 272.7
Pickwickian syndrome (cardiopulmonary obesity) 278.8
Piebaldism, classic 709.09
Piedra 111.2
beard 111.2
black 111.3
white 111.2
black 111.3
scalp 111.3
black 111.3
white 111.2
white 111.2
Pierre Marie's syndrome (pulmonary hypertrophic osteoarthropathy) 731.2
Pierre Marie-Bamberger syndrome (hypertrophic pulmonary osteoarthropathy) 731.2
Pierre Mauriac's syndrome (diabetes-dwarfism-obesity) 258.1
Pierre Robin deformity or syndrome (congenital) 756.0
Pierson's disease or osteochondrosis 732.1
Pigeon
breast or chest (acquired) 738.3
congenital 754.82
rachitic (*see also* Rickets) 268.0
breeders' disease or lung 495.2
fanciers' disease or lung 495.2
toe 735.8
Pigmentation (abnormal) 709.00
anomaly 709.00
congenital 757.33
specified NEC 709.09
conjunctiva 372.55
cornea 371.10
anterior 371.11
posterior 371.13
stromal 371.12
lids (congenital) 757.33
acquired 374.52
limbus corneae 371.10
metals 709.00
optic papilla, congenital 743.57
retina (congenital) (grouped) (nevoid) 743.53
acquired 362.74
scrotum, congenital 757.33
Piles —*see* Hemorrhoids
Pili
annulati or torti (congenital) 757.4
incarnati 704.8
Pill roller hand (intrinsic) 736.09
Pilomatrixoma (M8110/0)—*see* Neoplasm, skin, benign
Pilonidal —*see* condition
Pimple 709.8
Pinched nerve —*see* Neuropathy, entrapment
Pineal body or gland —*see* condition
Pinealoblastoma (M9362/3) 194.4
Pinealoma (M9360/1) 237.1
malignant (M9360/3) 194.4
Pineoblastoma (M9362/3) 194.4
Pineocytoma (M9361/1) 237.1
Pinguecula 372.51
Pinhole meatus (*see also* Stricture, urethra) 598.9
Pink
disease 985.0
eye 372.03
puffer 492.8
Pinkus' disease (lichen nitidus) 697.1
Pinpoint
meatus (*see also* Stricture, urethra) 598.9
os (uteri) (*see also* Stricture, cervix) 622.4
Pinselhaare (congenital) 757.4

Pinta 103.9
cardiovascular lesions 103.2
chancre (primary) 103.0
erythematous plaques 103.1
hyperchromic lesions 103.1
hyperkeratosis 103.1
lesions 103.9
cardiovascular 103.2
hyperchromic 103.1
intermediate 103.1
late 103.2
mixed 103.3
primary 103.0
skin (achromic) (cicatricial) (dyschromic) 103.2
hyperchromic 103.1
mixed (achromic and hyperchromic) 103.3
papule (primary) 103.0
skin lesions (achromic) (cicatricial) (dyschromic) 103.2
hyperchromic 103.1
mixed (achromic and hyperchromic) 103.3
vitiligo 103.2
Pintid 103.0
Pinworms (disease) (infection) (infestation) 127.4
Piry fever 066.8
Pistol wound —*see* Gunshot wound
Pit, lip (mucus), congenital 750.25
Pitchers' elbow 718.82
Pithecoid pelvis 755.69
with disproportion (fetopelvic) 653.2
affecting fetus or newborn 763.1
causing obstructed labor 660.1
Pithiatism 300.11
Pitted —*see also* Pitting
teeth 520.4
Pitting (edema) (*see also* Edema) 782.3
lip 782.3
nail 703.8
congenital 757.5
Pituitary gland —*see* condition
Pituitary snuff-takers' disease 495.8
Pityriasis 696.5
alba 696.5
capitis 690.11
circinata (et maculata) 696.3
Hebra's (exfoliative dermatitis) 695.89
lichenoides et varioliformis 696.2
maculata (et circinata) 696.3
nigra 111.1
pilaris 757.39
acquired 701.1
Hebra's 696.4
rosea 696.3
rotunda 696.3
rubra (Hebra) 695.89
pilaris 696.4
sicca 690.18
simplex 690.18
specified type NEC 696.5
streptogenes 696.5
versicolor 111.0
scrotal 111.0
Placenta, placental
ablatio 641.2
affecting fetus or newborn 762.1
abnormal, abnormality 656.7
with hemorrhage 641.8
affecting fetus or newborn 762.1
affecting fetus or newborn 762.2

Placenta, placental—*continued*
abruptio 641.2
affecting fetus or newborn 762.1
accessory lobe—*see* Placenta, abnormal
accreta (without hemorrhage) 667.0
with hemorrhage 666.0
adherent (without hemorrhage) 667.0
with hemorrhage 666.0
apoplexy—*see* Placenta, separation
battledore—*see* Placenta, abnormal
bilobate—*see* Placenta, abnormal
bipartita—*see* Placenta, abnormal
carneous mole 631
centralis—*see* Placenta, previa
circumvallata—*see* Placenta, abnormal
cyst (amniotic)—*see* Placenta, abnormal
deficiency—*see* Placenta insufficiency
degeneration—*see* Placenta, insufficiency
detachment (partial) (premature) (with hemorrhage) 641.2
affecting fetus or newborn 762.1
dimidiata—*see* Placenta, abnormal
disease 656.7
affecting fetus or newborn 762.2
duplex—*see* Placenta, abnormal
dysfunction—*see* Placenta, insufficiency
fenestrata—*see* Placenta, abnormal
fibrosis—*see* Placenta, abnormal
fleshy mole 631
hematoma—*see* Placenta, abnormal
hemorrhage NEC—*see* Placenta, separation
hormone disturbance or malfunction—*see* Placenta, abnormal
hyperplasia—*see* Placenta, abnormal
increta (without hemorrhage) 667.0
with hemorrhage 666.0
infarction 656.7
affecting fetus or newborn 762.2
insertion, vicious—*see* Placenta, previa
insufficiency
affecting
fetus or newborn 762.2
management of pregnancy 656.5
lateral—*see* Placenta, previa
low implantation or insertion—*see* Placenta, previa
low-lying—*see* Placenta, previa
malformation—*see* Placenta, abnormal
malposition—*see* Placenta, previa
marginalis, marginata—*see* Placenta, previa
marginal sinus (hemorrhage) (rupture) 641.2
affecting fetus or newborn 762.1
membranacea—*see* Placenta, abnormal
multilobed—*see* Placenta, abnormal
multipartita—*see* Placenta, abnormal
necrosis—*see* Placenta, abnormal
percreta (without hemorrhage) 667.0
with hemorrhage 666.0
polyp 674.4
previa (central) (centralis) (complete) (lateral) (marginal) (marginalis) (partial) (partialis) (total) (with hemorrhage) 641.1
affecting fetus or newborn 762.0
noted
before labor, without hemorrhage (with cesarean delivery) 641.0
during pregnancy (without hemorrhage) 641.0
without hemorrhage (before labor and delivery) (during pregnancy) 641.0

Placenta, placental—*continued*
retention (with hemorrhage) 666.0
fragments, complicating puerperium (delayed hemorrhage) 666.2
without hemorrhage 667.1
postpartum, puerperal 666.2
without hemorrhage 667.0
separation (normally implanted) (partial) (premature) (with hemorrhage) 641.2
affecting fetus or newborn 762.1
septuplex—*see* Placenta, abnormal
small—*see* Placenta, insufficiency
softening (premature)—*see* Placenta, abnormal
spuria—*see* Placenta, abnormal
succenturiata—*see* Placenta, abnormal
syphilitic 095.8
transfusion syndromes 762.3
transmission of chemical substance—*see* Absorption, chemical, through placenta
trapped (with hemorrhage) 666.0
without hemorrhage 667.0
trilobate—*see* Placenta, abnormal
tripartita—*see* Placenta, abnormal
triplex—*see* Placenta, abnormal
varicose vessel—*see* Placenta, abnormal
vicious insertion—*see* Placenta, previa
Placentitis
affecting fetus or newborn 762.7
complicating pregnancy 658.4
Plagiocephaly (skull) 754.0
Plague 020.9
abortive 020.8
ambulatory 020.8
bubonic 020.0
cellulocutaneous 020.1
lymphatic gland 020.0
pneumonic 020.5
primary 020.3
secondary 020.4
pulmonary—*see* Plague, pneumonic
pulmonic—*see* Plague, pneumonic
septicemic 020.2
tonsillar 020.9
septicemic 020.2
vaccination, prophylactic (against) V03.3
Planning, family V25.09
contraception V25.9
procreation V26.4
Plaque
artery, arterial—*see* Arteriosclerosis
calcareous—*see* Calcification
Hollenhorst's (retinal) 362.33
tongue 528.6
Plasma cell myeloma 203.0
Plasmacytoma, plasmocytoma (solitary) (M9731/1) 238.6
benign (M9731/0)—*see* Neoplasm, by site, benign
malignant (M9731/3) 203.8
Plasmacytosis 288.8
Plaster ulcer (*see also* Decubitus) 707.0
Platybasia 756.0
Platyonychia (congenital) 757.5
acquired 703.8
Platypelloid pelvis 738.6
with disproportion (fetopelvic) 653.2
affecting fetus or newborn 763.1
causing obstructed labor 660.1
affecting fetus or newborn 763.1
congenital 755.69
Platyspondylia 756.19
Plethora 782.62
newborn 776.4
Pleura, pleural —*see* condition
Pleuralgia 786.52
Pleurisy (acute) (adhesive) (chronic) (costal) (diaphragmatic) (double) (dry) (fetid) (fibrinous) (fibrous) (interlobar) (latent) (lung) (old) (plastic) (primary) (residual) (sicca) (sterile) (subacute) (unresolved) (with adherent pleura) 511.0
with
effusion (without mention of cause) 511.9
bacterial, nontuberculous 511.1
nontuberculous NEC 511.9
bacterial 511.1
pneumococcal 511.1
specified type NEC 511.8
staphylococcal 511.1
streptococcal 511.1
tuberculous (*see also* Tuberculosis, pleura) 012.0
primary, progressive 010.1
influenza, flu, or grippe 487.1
tuberculosis—*see* Pleurisy, tuberculous
encysted 511.8
exudative (*see also* Pleurisy, with effusion) 511.9
bacterial, nontuberculous 511.1
fibrinopurulent 510.9
with fistula 510.0
fibropurulent 510.9
with fistula 510.0
hemorrhagic 511.8
influenzal 487.1
pneumococcal 511.0
with effusion 511.1
purulent 510.9
with fistula 510.0
septic 510.9
with fistula 510.0
serofibrinous (*see also* Pleurisy, with effusion) 511.9
bacterial, nontuberculous 511.1
seropurulent 510.9
with fistula 510.0
serous (*see also* Pleurisy, with effusion) 511.9
bacterial, nontuberculous 511.1
staphylococcal 511.0
with effusion 511.1
streptococcal 511.0
with effusion 511.1
suppurative 510.9
with fistula 510.0
traumatic (post) (current) 862.29
with open wound into cavity 862.39
tuberculous (with effusion) (*see also* Tuberculosis, pleura) 012.0
primary, progressive 010.1
Pleuritis sicca —*see* Pleurisy
Pleurobronchopneumonia (*see also* Pneumonia, broncho-) 485
Pleurodynia 786.52
epidemic 074.1
viral 074.1
Pleurohepatitis 573.8
Pleuropericarditis (*see also* Pericarditis) 423.9
acute 420.90
Pleuropneumonia (acute) (bilateral) (double) (septic) (*see also* Pneumonia) 486
chronic (*see also* Fibrosis, lung) 515
Pleurorrhea (*see also* Hydrothorax) 511.8
Plexitis, brachial 353.0

Plica
polonica 132.0
tonsil 474.8
Plicae dysphonia ventricularis 784.49
Plicated tongue 529.5
congenital 750.13
Plug
bronchus NEC 519.1
meconium (newborn) NEC 777.1
mucus—*see* Mucus, plug
Plumbism 984.9
specified type of lead—*see* Table of drugs and chemicals
Plummer's disease (toxic nodular goiter) 242.3
Plummer-Vinson syndrome (sideropenic dysphagia) 280.8
Pluricarential syndrome of infancy 260
Plurideficiency syndrome of infancy 260
Plus (and minus) hand (intrinsic) 736.09
Pneumathemia —*see* Air, embolism, by type
Pneumatic drill or hammer disease 994.9
Pneumatocele (lung) 518.89
intracranial 348.8
tension 492.0
Pneumatosis
cystoides intestinalis 569.89
peritonei 568.89
pulmonum 492.8
Pneumaturia 599.84
Pneumoblastoma (M8981/3)—*see* Neoplasm, lung, malignant
Pneumocephalus 348.8
Pneumococcemia 038.2
Pneumococcus, pneumococcal —*see* condition
Pneumoconiosis (due to) (inhalation of) 505
aluminum 503
asbestos 501
bagasse 495.1
bauxite 503
beryllium 503
carbon electrode makers' 503
coal
miners' (simple) 500
workers' (simple) 500
cotton dust 504
diatomite fibrosis 502
dust NEC 504
inorganic 503
lime 502
marble 502
organic NEC 504
fumes or vapors (from silo) 506.9
graphite 503
hard metal 503
mica 502
moldy hay 495.0
rheumatoid 714.81
silica NEC 502
and carbon 500
silicate NEC 502
talc 502
Pneumocystis carinii pneumonia 136.3
Pneumocystosis 136.3
with pneumonia 136.3
Pneumoenteritis 025
Pneumohemopericardium (*see also* Pericarditis) 423.9
Pneumohemothorax (*see also* Hemothorax) 511.8
traumatic 860.4
with open wound into thorax 860.5
Pneumohydropericardium (*see also* Pericarditis) 423.9
Pneumohydrothorax (*see also* Hydrothorax) 511.8
Pneumomediastinum 518.1
congenital 770.2
fetus or newborn 770.2
Pneumomycosis 117.9
Pneumonia (acute) (Alpenstich) (benign) (bilateral) (brain) (cerebral) (circumscribed) (congestive) (creeping) (delayed resolution) (double) (epidemic) (fever) (flash) (fulminant) (fungoid) (granulomatous) (hemorrhagic) (incipient) (infantile) (infectious) (infiltration) (insular) (intermittent) (latent) (lobe) (migratory) (newborn) (organized) (overwhelming) (primary) (progressive) (pseudolobar) (purulent) (resolved) (secondary) (senile) (septic) (suppurative) (terminal) (true) (unresolved) (vesicular) 486
with influenza, flu, or grippe 487.0
adenoviral 480.0
adynamic 514
alba 090.0
allergic 518.3
alveolar—*see* Pneumonia, lobar
anaerobes 482.81
anthrax 022.1 *[484.5]*
apex, apical—*see* Pneumonia, lobar
ascaris 127.0 *[484.8]*
aspiration 507.0
due to
aspiration of microorganisms
bacterial 482.9
specified type NEC 482.89
specified organism NEC 483.8
bacterial NEC 482.89
viral 480.9
specified type NEC 480.8
food (regurgitated) 507.0
gastric secretions 507.0
milk 507.0
oils, essences 507.1
solids, liquids NEC 507.8
vomitus 507.0
newborn 770.1
asthenic 514
atypical (disseminated, focal) (primary) 486
with influenza 487.0
bacillus 482.9
specified type NEC 482.89
bacterial 482.9
specified type NEC 482.89
Bacteroides (fragilis) (oralis) (melaninogenicus) 482.81
basal, basic, basilar—*see* Pneumonia, lobar
broncho-, bronchial (confluent) (croupous) (diffuse) (disseminated) (hemorrhagic) (involving lobes) (lobar) (terminal) 485
with influenza 487.0
allergic 518.3
aspiration (*see also* Pneumonia, aspiration) 507.0
bacterial 482.9
specified type NEC 482.89
capillary 466.1
with bronchospasm or obstruction 466.1
chronic (*see also* Fibrosis, lung) 515
congenital (infective) 770.0
diplococcal 481
Eaton's agent 483.0
Escherichia coli (E. coli) 482.82

Pneumonia—*continued*
    Friedländer's bacillus 482.0
    Hemophilus influenzae 482.2
    hiberno-vernal 083.0 *[484.8]*
    hypostatic 514
    influenzal 487.0
    inhalation (*see also* Pneumonia, aspiration) 507.0
      due to fumes or vapors (chemical) 506.0
    Klebsiella 482.0
    lipid 507.1
      endogenous 516.8
    Mycoplasma (pneumoniae) 483.0
    ornithosis 073.0
    pleuropneumonia-like organisms (PPLO) 483.0
    pneumococcal 481
    Proteus 482.83
    pseudomonas 482.1
    specified organism NEC 483.8
      bacterial NEC 482.89
    staphylococcal 482.4
    streptococcal—*see* Pneumonia, streptococcal
    typhoid 002.0 *[484.8]*
    viral, virus (*see also* Pneumonia, viral) 480.9
  Butyrivibrio (fibriosolvens) 482.81
  Candida 112.4
  capillary 466.1
    with bronchospasm or obstruction 466.1
  caseous (*see also* Tuberculosis) 011.6
  catarrhal—*see* Pneumonia, broncho-
  central—*see* Pneumonia, lobar
  Chlamydia, chlamydial 078.88 *[484.8]*
    pneumoniae 078.88 *[484.8]*
    psittaci 073.0
    specified type NEC 078.88 *[484.8]*
    trachomatis 078.88 *[484.8]*
  cholesterol 516.8
  chronic (*see also* Fibrosis, lung) 515
  cirrhotic (chronic) (*see also* Fibrosis, lung) 515
  Clostridium (haemolyticum) (novyi) NEC 482.81
  confluent—*see* Pneumonia, broncho-
  congenital (infective) 770.0
    aspiration 770.1
  croupous—*see* Pneumonia, lobar
  cytomegalic inclusion 078.5 *[484.1]*
  deglutition (*see also* Pneumonia, aspiration) 507.0
  desquamative interstitial 516.8
  diffuse—*see* Pneumonia, broncho-
  diplococcal, diplococcus (broncho-) (lobar) 481
  disseminated (focal)—*see* Pneumonia, broncho-
  due to
    adenovirus 480.0
    Bacterium anitratum 482.83
    Chlamydia, chlamydial 078.88 *[484.8]*
      pneumoniae 078.88 *[484.8]*
      psittaci 073.0
      specified type NEC 078.88 *[484.8]*
      trachomatis 078.88 *[484.8]*
    coccidioidomycosis 114.0
    Diplococcus (pneumoniae) 481
    Eaton's agent 483.0
    Escherichia coli (E. coli) 482.82
    Friedländer's bacillus 482.0
    fumes or vapors (chemical) (inhalation) 506.0
    fungus NEC 117.9 *[484.7]*
      coccidioidomycosis 114.0
    Hemophilus influenzae (H. influenzae) 482.2

Pneumonia—*continued*
    Herellea 482.83
    influenza 487.0
    Klebsiella pneumoniae 482.0
    Mycoplasma (pneumoniae) 483.0
    parainfluenza virus 480.2
    pleuropneumonia-like organism (PPLO) 483.0
    Pneumococcus 481
    Pneumocystis carinii 136.3
    Proteus 482.83
    pseudomonas 482.1
    respiratory syncytial virus 480.1
    rickettsia 083.9 *[484.8]*
    specified
      bacteria NEC 482.89
      organism NEC 483.8
      virus NEC 480.8
    Staphylococcus 482.4
    Streptococcus—*see also* Pneumonia, streptococcal
      pneumoniae 481
    virus (*see also* Pneumonia, viral) 480.9
  Eaton's agent 483.0
  embolic, embolism (*see also* Embolism, pulmonary) 415.1
  eosinophilic 518.3
  Escherichia coli (E. coli) 482.82
  Eubacterium 482.81
  fibrinous—*see* Pneumonia, lobar
  fibroid (chronic) (*see also* Fibrosis, lung) 515
  fibrous (*see also* Fibrosis, lung) 515
  Friedländer's bacillus 482.0
  Fusobacterium (nucleatum) 482.81
  gangrenous 513.0
  giant cell (*see also* Pneumonia, viral) 480.9
  gram-negative bacteria NEC 482.83
    anaerobic 482.81
  grippal 487.0
  Hemophilus influenzae (bronchial) (lobar) 482.2
  hypostatic (broncho-) (lobar) 514
  in
    actinomycosis 039.1
    anthrax 022.1 *[484.5]*
    aspergillosis 117.3 *[484.6]*
    candidiasis 112.4
    coccidioidomycosis 114.0
    cytomegalic inclusion disease 078.5 *[484.1]*
    histoplasmosis (*see also* Histoplasmosis) 115.95
    infectious disease NEC 136.9 *[484.8]*
    measles 055.1
    mycosis, systemic NEC 117.9 *[484.7]*
    nocardiasis, nocardiosis 039.1
    ornithosis 073.0
    pneumocystosis 136.3
    psittacosis 073.0
    Q fever 083.0 *[484.8]*
    salmonellosis 003.22
    toxoplasmosis 130.4
    tularemia 021.2
    typhoid (fever) 002.0 *[484.8]*
    varicella 052.1
    whooping cough (*see also* Whooping cough) 033.9 *[484.3]*
  infective, acquired prenatally 770.0
  influenzal (broncho) (lobar) (virus) 487.0
  inhalation (*see also* Pneumonia, aspiration) 507.0
    fumes or vapors (chemical) 506.0

Pneumonia—*continued*
interstitial 516.8
with influenzal 487.0
acute 136.3
chronic (*see also* Fibrosis, lung) 515
desquamative 516.8
hypostatic 514
lipoid 507.1
lymphoid 516.8
plasma cell 136.3
pseudomonas 482.1
intrauterine (infective) 770.0
aspiration 770.1
Klebsiella pneumoniae 482.0
lipid, lipoid (exogenous) (interstitial) 507.1
endogenous 516.8
lobar (diplococcal) (disseminated) (double) (interstitial) (pneumococcal, any type) 481
with influenza 487.0
bacterial 482.9
specified type NEC 482.89
chronic (*see also* Fibrosis, lung) 515
Escherichia coli (E. coli) 482.82
Friedländer's bacillus 482.0
Hemophilus influenzae (H. influenzae) 482.2
hypostatic 514
influenzal 487.0
Klebsiella 482.0
ornithosis 073.0
Proteus 482.83
pseudomonas 482.1
psittacosis 073.0
specified organism NEC 483.8
bacterial NEC 482.89
staphylococcal 482.4
streptococcal—*see* Pneumonia, streptococcal
viral, virus (*see also* Pneumonia, viral) 480.9
lobular (confluent)—*see* Pneumonia, broncho-
Löffler's 518.3
massive—*see* Pneumonia, lobar
meconium 770.1
metastatic NEC 038.8 *[484.8]*
Mycoplasma (pneumoniae) 483.0
necrotic 513.0
nitrogen dioxide 506.9
orthostatic 514
parainfluenza virus 480.2
parenchymatous (*see also* Fibrosis, lung) 515
passive 514
patchy—*see* Pneumonia, broncho
Peptococcus 482.81
Peptostreptococcus 482.81
plasma cell 136.3
pleurolobar—*see* Pneumonia, lobar
pleuropneumonia-like organism (PPLO) 483.0
pneumococcal (broncho) (lobar) 481
Pneumocystis (carinii) 136.3
postinfectional NEC 136.9 *[484.8]*
postmeasles 055.1
postoperative 997.3
primary atypical 486
Proprionibacterium 482.81
Proteus 482.83
pseudomonas 482.1
psittacosis 073.0
radiation 508.0
respiratory syncytial virus 480.1
resulting from a procedure 997.3
rheumatic 390 *[517.1]*
Salmonella 003.22

Pneumonia—*continued*
segmented, segmental—*see* Pneumonia, broncho-
Serratia (marcescens) 482.83
specified
bacteria NEC 482.89
organism NEC 483.8
virus NEC 480.8
spirochetal 104.8 *[484.8]*
staphylococcal (broncho) (lobar) 482.4
static, stasis 514
streptococcal (broncho) (lobar) NEC 482.30
Group
A 482.31
B 482.32
specified NEC 482.39
pneumoniae 481
specified type NEC 482.39
Streptococcus pneumoniae 481
traumatic (complication) (early) (secondary) 958.8
tuberculous (any) (*see also* Tuberculosis) 011.6
tularemic 021.2
TWAR agent 078.88 *[484.8]*
varicella 052.1
Veillonella 482.81
viral, virus (broncho) (interstitial) (lobar) 480.9
with influenza, flu, or grippe 487.0
adenoviral 480.0
parainfluenza 480.2
respiratory syncytial 480.1
specified type NEC 480.8
white (congenital) 090.0
Pneumonic —*see* condition
Pneumonitis (acute) (primary) (*see also* Pneumonia) 486
allergic 495.9
specified type NEC 495.8
aspiration 507.0
due to fumes or gases 506.0
newborn 770.1
obstetric 668.0
chemical 506.0
due to fumes or gases 506.0
cholesterol 516.8
chronic (*see also* Fibrosis, lung) 515
congenital rubella 771.0
due to
fumes or vapors 506.0
inhalation
food (regurgitated), milk, vomitus 507.0
oils, essences 507.1
saliva 507.0
solids, liquids NEC 507.8
toxoplasmosis (acquired) 130.4
congenital (active) 771.2 *[484.8]*
eosinophilic 518.3
fetal aspiration 770.1
hypersensitivity 495.9
interstitial (chronic) (*see also* Fibrosis, lung) 515
lymphoid 516.8
lymphoid, interstitial 516.8
meconium 770.1
postanesthetic
correct substance properly administered 507.0
obstetric 668.0
overdose or wrong substance given 968.4
specified anesthetic—*see* Table of drugs and chemicals
postoperative 997.3
obstetric 668.0

Pneumonitis—*continued*
radiation 508.0
rubella, congenital 771.0
"ventilation" 495.7
wood-dust 495.8
Pneumonoconiosis —*see* Pneumoconiosis
Pneumoparotid 527.8
Pneumopathy NEC 518.89
alveolar 516.9
specified NEC 516.8
due to dust NEC 504
parietoalveolar 516.9
specified condition NEC 516.8
Pneumopericarditis (*see also* Pericarditis) 423.9
acute 420.90
Pneumopericardium —*see also* Pericarditis
congenital 770.2
fetus or newborn 770.2
traumatic (post) (*see also* Pneumothorax, traumatic) 860.0
with open wound into thorax 860.1
Pneumoperitoneum 568.89
fetus or newborn 770.2
Pneumophagia (psychogenic) 306.4
Pneumopleurisy, pneumopleuritis (*see also* Pneumonia) 486
Pneumopyopericardium 420.99
Pneumopyothorax (*see also* Pyopneumothorax) 510.9
with fistula 510.0
Pneumorrhagia 786.3
newborn 770.3
tuberculous (*see also* Tuberculosis, pulmonary) 011.9
Pneumosiderosis (occupational) 503
Pneumothorax (acute) (chronic) 512.8
congenital 770.2
due to operative injury of chest wall or lung 512.1
accidental puncture or laceration 512.1
fetus or newborn 770.2
iatrogenic 512.1
postoperative 512.1
spontaneous 512.8
fetus or newborn 770.2
tension 512.0
sucking 512.8
iatrogenic 512.1
postoperative 512.1
tense valvular, infectional 512.0
tension 512.0
iatrogenic 512.1
postoperative 512.1
spontaneous 512.0
traumatic 860.0
with
hemothorax 860.4
with open wound into thorax 860.5
open wound into thorax 860.1
tuberculous (*see also* Tuberculosis) 011.7
Pocket (s)
endocardial (*see also* Endocarditis) 424.90
periodontal 523.8
Podagra 274.9
Podencephalus 759.89
Poikilocytosis 790.0
Poikiloderma 709.09
Civatte's 709.09
congenital 757.33
vasculare atrophicans 696.2
Poikilodermatomyositis 710.3
Pointed ear 744.29
Poise imperfect 729.9
Poisoned —*see* Poisoning
Poisoning (acute)—*see also* Table of drugs and chemicals
Bacillus, B.
aertrycke (*see also* Infection, Salmonella) 003.9
botulinus 005.1
cholerae (suis) (*see also* Infection, Salmonella) 003.9
paratyphosus (*see also* Infection, Salmonella) 003.9
suipestifer (*see also* Infection, Salmonella) 003.9
bacterial toxins NEC 005.9
berries, noxious 988.2
blood (general)—*see* Septicemia
botulism 005.1
bread, moldy, mouldy—*see* Poisoning, food
damaged meat—*see* Poisoning, food
death-cap (Amanita phalloides) (Amanita verna) 988.1
decomposed food—*see* Poisoning, food
diseased food—*see* Poisoning, food
drug—*see* Table of drugs and chemicals
epidemic, fish, meat, or other food—*see* Poisoning, food
fava bean 282.2
fish (bacterial)—*see also* Poisoning, food
noxious 988.0
food (acute) (bacterial) (diseased) (infected) NEC 005.9
due to
Bacillus
aertrycke (*see also* Poisoning, food, due to Salmonella) 003.9
botulinus 005.1
cereus 005.89
choleraesuis (*see also* Poisoning, food, due to Salmonella) 003.9
paratyphosus (*see also* Poisoning, food, due to Salmonella) 003.9
suipestifer (*see also* Poisoning, food, due to Salmonella) 003.9
Clostridium 005.3
botulinum 005.1
perfringens 005.2
welchii 005.2
Salmonella (aertrycke) (callinarum) (choleraesuis) (enteritidis) (paratyphi) (suipestifer) 003.9
with
gastroenteritis 003.0
localized infection(s) (*see also* Infection, Salmonella) 003.20
septicemia 003.1
specified manifestation NEC 003.8
specified bacterium NEC 005.89
Staphylococcus 005.0
Streptococcus 005.8
Vibrio parahaemolyticus 005.4
Vibrio vulnificus 005.81
noxious or naturally toxic 988.0
berries 988.2
fish 988.0
mushroom 988.1
plants NEC 988.2
ice cream—*see* Poisoning, food
ichthyotoxism (bacterial) 005.9
kreotoxism, food 005.9
malarial—*see* Malaria
meat—*see* Poisoning, food

Poisoning—*continued*
mushroom (noxious) 988.1
mussel—*see also* Poisoning, food
noxious 988.0
noxious foodstuffs (*see also* Poisoning, food, noxious) 988.9
specified type NEC 988.8
plants, noxious 988.2
pork—*see also* Poisoning, food
specified NEC 988.8
Trichinosis 124
ptomaine—*see* Poisoning, food
putrefaction, food—*see* Poisoning, food
radiation 508.0
Salmonella (*see also* Infection, Salmonella) 003.9
sausage—*see also* Poisoning, food
Trichinosis 124
saxitoxin 988.0
shellfish—*see also* Poisoning, food
noxious 988.0
Staphylococcus, food 005.0
toxic, from disease NEC 799.8
truffles—*see* Poisoning, food
uremic—*see* Uremia
uric acid 274.9
Poison ivy, oak, sumac or other plant dermatitis 692.6
Poker spine 720.0
Policeman's disease 729.2
Polioencephalitis (acute) (bulbar) (*see also* Poliomyelitis, bulbar) 045.0
inferior 335.22
influenzal 487.8
superior hemorrhagic (acute) (Wernicke's) 265.1
Wernicke's (superior hemorrhagic) 265.1
Polioencephalomyelitis (acute) (anterior) (bulbar) (*see also* Polioencephalitis) 045.0
Polioencephalopathy, superior hemorrhagic 265.1
with
beriberi 265.0
pellagra 265.2
Poliomeningoencephalitis —*see* Meningoencephalitis
Poliomyelitis (acute) (anterior) (epidemic) 045.9

Note—Use the following fifth-digit subclassification with category 045:

0 poliovirus, unspecified type
1 poliovirus, type I
2 poliovirus, type II
3 poliovirus, type III

with
paralysis 045.1
bulbar 045.0
abortive 045.2
ascending 045.9
progressive 045.9
bulbar 045.0
cerebral 045.0
chronic 335.21
congenital 771.2
contact V01.2
deformities 138
exposure to V01.2
late effect 138
nonepidemic 045.9
nonparalytic 045.2
Poliomyelitis—*continued*
old with deformity 138
posterior, acute 053.19
residual 138
sequelae 138
spinal, acute 045.9
syphilitic (chronic) 094.89
vaccination, prophylactic (against) V04.0
Poliosis (eyebrow) (eyelashes) 704.3
circumscripta (congenital) 757.4
acquired 704.3
congenital 757.4
Pollakiuria 788.41
psychogenic 306.53
Pollinosis 477.0
Pollitzer's disease (hidradenitis suppurativa) 705.83
Polyadenitis (*see also* Adenitis) 289.3
malignant 020.0
Polyalgia 729.9
Polyangiitis (essential) 446.0
Polyarteritis (nodosa) (renal) 446.0
Polyarthralgia 719.49
psychogenic 306.0
Polyarthritis, polyarthropathy NEC 716.59
due to or associated with other specified conditions—*see* Arthritis, due to or associated with
endemic (*see also* Disease, Kaschin-Beck) 716.0
inflammatory 714.9
specified type NEC 714.89
juvenile (chronic) 714.30
acute 714.31
migratory—*see* Fever, rheumatic
rheumatic 714.0
fever (acute)—*see* Fever, rheumatic
Polycarential syndrome of infancy 260
Polychondritis (atrophic) (chronic) (relapsing) 733.99
Polycoria 743.46
Polycystic (congenital) (disease) 759.89
degeneration, kidney—*see* Polycystic, kidney
kidney (congenital) 753.12
adult type (APKD) 753.13
autosomal dominant 753.13
autosomal recessive 753.14
childhood type (CPKD) 753.14
infantile type 753.14
liver 751.62
lung 518.89
congenital 748.4
ovary, ovaries 256.4
spleen 759.0
Polycythemia (primary) (rubra) (vera) (M9950/1) 238.4
acquired 289.0
benign 289.0
familial 289.6
due to
donor twin 776.4
fall in plasma volume 289.0
high altitude 289.0
maternal-fetal transfusion 776.4
stress 289.0
emotional 289.0
erythropoietin 289.0
familial (benign) 289.6
Gaisböck's (hypertonica) 289.0
high altitude 289.0
hypertonica 289.0
hypoxemic 289.0

Polycythemia—*continued*
neonatorum 776.4
nephrogenous 289.0
relative 289.0
secondary 289.0
spurious 289.0
stress 289.0
Polycytosis cryptogenica 289.0
Polydactylism, polydactyly 755.00
fingers 755.01
toes 755.02
Polydipsia 783.5
Polydystrophic oligophrenia 277.5
Polyembryoma (M9072/3)—*see* Neoplasm, by site, malignant
Polygalactia 676.6
Polyglandular
deficiency 258.9
dyscrasia 258.9
dysfunction 258.9
syndrome 258.8
Polyhydramnios (*see also* Hydramnios) 657
Polymastia 757.6
Polymenorrhea 626.2
Polymicrogyria 742.2
Polymyalgia 725
arteritica 446.5
rheumatica 725
Polymyositis (acute) (chronic) (hemorrhagic) 710.4
with involvement of
lung 710.4 *[517.8]*
skin 710.3
ossificans (generalisata) (progressiva) 728.19
Wagner's (dermatomyositis) 710.3
Polyneuritis, polyneuritic (*see also* Polyneuropathy) 356.9
alcoholic 357.5
with psychosis 291.1
cranialis 352.6
diabetic 250.6 *[357.2]*
due to lack of vitamin NEC 269.2 *[357.4]*
endemic 265.0 *[357.4]*
erythredema 985.0
febrile 357.0
hereditary ataxic 356.3
idiopathic, acute 357.0
infective (acute) 357.0
nutritional 269.9 *[357.4]*
postinfectious 357.0
Polyneuropathy (peripheral) 356.9
alcoholic 357.5
amyloid 277.3 *[357.4]*
arsenical 357.7
diabetic 250.6 *[357.2]*
due to
antitetanus serum 357.6
arsenic 357.7
drug or medicinal substance 357.6
correct substance properly administered 357.6
overdose or wrong substance given or taken 977.9
specified drug—*see* Table of drugs and chemicals
lack of vitamin NEC 269.2 *[357.4]*
lead 357.7
organophosphate compounds 357.7
pellagra 265.2 *[357.4]*
porphyria 277.1 *[357.4]*
serum 357.6
Polyneuropathy—*continued*
toxic agent NEC 357.7
hereditary 356.0
idiopathic 356.9
progressive 356.4
in
amyloidosis 277.3 *[357.4]*
avitaminosis 269.2 *[357.4]*
specified NEC 269.1 *[357.4]*
beriberi 265.0 *[357.4]*
collagen vascular disease NEC 710.9 *[357.1]*
deficiency
B-complex NEC 266.2 *[357.4]*
vitamin B 266.9 *[357.4]*
vitamin B_6 266.1 *[357.4]*
diabetes 250.6 *[357.2]*
diphtheria (*see also* Diphtheria) 032.89 *[357.4]*
disseminated lupus erythematosus 710.0 *[357.1]*
herpes zoster 053.13
hypoglycemia 251.2 *[357.4]*
malignant neoplasm (M8000/3) NEC 199.1 *[357.3]*
mumps 072.72
pellagra 265.2 *[357.4]*
polyarteritis nodosa 446.0 *[357.1]*
porphyria 277.1 *[357.4]*
rheumatoid arthritis 714.0 *[357.1]*
sarcoidosis 135 *[357.4]*
uremia 585 *[357.4]*
lead 357.7
nutritional 269.9 *[357.4]*
specified NEC 269.8 *[357.4]*
postherpetic 053.13
progressive 356.4
sensory (hereditary) 356.2
Polyonychia 757.5
Polyopia 368.2
refractive 368.15
Polyorchism, polyorchidism (three testes) 752.8
Polyorrhymenitis (peritoneal) (*see also* Polyserositis) 568.82
pericardial 423.2
Polyostotic fibrous dysplasia 756.54
Polyotia 744.1
Polyp, polypus

Note—Polyps of organs or sites that do not appear in the list below should be coded to the residual category for diseases of the organ or site concerned.

accessory sinus 471.8
adenoid tissue 471.0
adenomatous (M8210/0)—*see also* Neoplasm, by site, benign
adenocarcinoma in (M8210/3)—*see* Neoplasm, by site, malignant
carcinoma in (M8210/3)—*see* Neoplasm, by site, malignant
multiple (M8221/0)—*see* Neoplasm, by site, benign
antrum 471.8
anus, anal (canal) 569.0
Bartholin's gland 624.6
bladder (M8120/1) 236.7
broad ligament 620.8

Polyp, polypus—*continued*
cervix (uteri) 622.7
adenomatous 219.0
in pregnancy or childbirth 654.6
affecting fetus or newborn 763.8
causing obstructed labor 660.2
mucous 622.7
nonneoplastic 622.7
choanal 471.0
cholesterol 575.6
clitoris 624.6
colon (M8210/0) (*see also* Polyp, adenomatous) 211.3
corpus uteri 621.0
dental 522.0
ear (middle) 385.30
endometrium 621.0
ethmoidal (sinus) 471.8
fallopian tube 620.8
female genital organs NEC 624.8
frontal (sinus) 471.8
gallbladder 575.6
gingiva 523.8
gum 523.8
labia 624.6
larynx (mucous) 478.4
malignant (M8000/3)—*see* Neoplasm, by site, malignant
maxillary (sinus) 471.8
middle ear 385.30
myometrium 621.0
nares
anterior 471.9
posterior 471.0
nasal (mucous) 471.9
cavity 471.0
septum 471.9
nasopharyngeal 471.0
neoplastic (M8210/0)—*see* Neoplasm, by site, benign
nose (mucous) 471.9
oviduct 620.8
paratubal 620.8
pharynx 478.29
congenital 750.29
placenta, placental 674.4
prostate 600
pudenda 624.6
pulp (dental) 522.0
rectum 569.0
septum (nasal) 471.9
sinus (accessory) (ethmoidal) (frontal) (maxillary) (sphenoidal) 471.8
sphenoidal (sinus) 471.8
stomach (M8210/0) 211.1
tube, fallopian 620.8
turbinate, mucous membrane 471.8
ureter 593.89
urethra 599.3
uterine
ligament 620.8
tube 620.8
uterus (body) (corpus) (mucous) 621.0
in pregnancy or childbirth 654.1
affecting fetus or newborn 763.8
causing obstructed labor 660.2
vagina 623.7
vocal cord (mucous) 478.4
vulva 624.6
Polyphagia 783.6
Polypoid —*see* condition
Polyposis —*see also* Polyp
coli (adenomatous) (M8220/0) 211.3
adenocarcinoma in (M8220/3) 153.9
carcinoma in (M8220/3) 153.9
familial (M8220/0) 211.3
intestinal (adenomatous) (M8220/0) 211.3
multiple (M8221/0)—*see* Neoplasm, by site, benign
Polyradiculitis (acute) 357.0
Polyradiculoneuropathy (acute) (segmentally demyelinating) 357.0
Polysarcia 278.00
Polyserositis (peritoneal) 568.82
due to pericarditis 423.2
paroxysmal (familial) 277.3
pericardial 423.2
periodic 277.3
pleural—*see* Pleurisy
recurrent 277.3
tuberculous (*see also* Tuberculosis, polyserositis) 018.9
Polysialia 527.7
Polysplenia syndrome 759.0
Polythelia 757.6
Polytrichia (*see also* Hypertrichosis) 704.1
Polyunguia (congenital) 757.5
acquired 703.8
Polyuria 788.42
Pompe's disease (glycogenosis II) 271.0
Pompholyx 705.81
Poncet's disease (tuberculous rheumatism) (*see also* Tuberculosis) 015.9
Pond fracture —*see* Fracture, skull, vault
Ponos 085.0
Pons, pontine —*see* condition
Poor
contractions, labor 661.2
affecting fetus or newborn 763.7
fetal growth NEC 764.9
affecting management of pregnancy 656.5
obstetrical history V23.4
sucking reflex (newborn) 796.1
vision NEC 369.9
Poradenitis, nostras 099.1
Porencephaly (congenital) (development) (true) 742.4
acquired 348.0
nondevelopmental 348.0
traumatic (post) 310.2
Porocephaliasis 134.1
Porokeratosis 757.39
Poroma, eccrine (M8402/0)—*see* Neoplasm, skin, benign
Porphyria (acute) (congenital) (constitutional) (erythropoietic) (familial) (hepatica) (idiopathic) (idiosyncratic) (intermittent) (latent) (mixed hepatic) (photosensitive) (South African genetic) (Swedish) 277.1
acquired 277.1
cutaneatarda
hereditaria 277.1
symptomatica 277.1
due to drugs
correct substance properly administered 277.1
overdose or wrong substance given or taken 977.9
specified drug—*see* Table of drugs and chemicals
secondary 277.1
toxic NEC 277.1
variegata 277.1

Porphyrinuria (acquired) (congenital) (secondary) 277.1
Porphyruria (acquired) (congenital) 277.1
Portal *—see* condition
Port wine nevus or mark 757.32
Posadas-Wernicke disease 114.9
Position
fetus, abnormal (*see also* Presentation, fetal) 652.9
teeth, faulty 524.3
Positive
culture (nonspecific) 795.3
AIDS virus V08
blood 790.7
HIV V08
human immunodeficiency virus V08
nose 795.3
skin lesion NEC 795.3
spinal fluid 792.0
sputum 795.3
stool 792.1
throat 795.3
urine 599.0
wound 795.3
HIV V08
human immunodeficiency virus (HIV) V08
PPD 795.5
serology
AIDS virus V08
inconclusive 795.71
HIV V08
inconclusive 795.71
human immunodeficiency virus V08
inconclusive 795.71
syphilis 097.1
with signs or symptoms—*see* Syphilis, by site and stage
false 795.6
skin test 795.7
tuberculin (without active tuberculosis) 795.5
VDRL 097.1
with signs or symptoms—*see* Syphilis, by site and stage
false 795.6
Wassermann reaction 097.1
false 795.6
Postcardiotomy syndrome 429.4
Postcaval ureter 753.4
Postcholecystectomy syndrome 576.0
Postclimacteric bleeding 627.1
Postcommissurotomy syndrome 429.4
Postconcussional syndrome 310.2
Postcontusional syndrome 310.2
Postcricoid region *—see* condition
Post-dates (pregnancy) 645
Postencephalitic *—see also* condition syndrome 310.8
Posterior *—see* condition
Posterolateral sclerosis (spinal cord)*—see* Degeneration, combined
Postexanthematous *—see* condition
Postfebrile *—see* condition
Postgastrectomy dumping syndrome 564.2
Posthemiplegic chorea 344.89
Posthemorrhagic anemia (chronic) 280.0
acute 285.1
newborn 776.5
Posthepatitis syndrome 780.7
Postherpetic neuralgia (intercostal) (syndrome) (zoster) 053.19
geniculate ganglion 053.11
ophthalmica 053.19
trigeminal 053.12
Posthitis 607.1
Postimmunization complication or reaction *—see* Complications, vaccination
Postinfectious *—see* condition
Postinfluenzal syndrome 780.7
Postlaminectomy syndrome 722.80
cervical, cervicothoracic 722.81
kyphosis 737.12
lumbar, lumbosacral 722.83
thoracic, thoracolumbar 722.82
Postleukotomy syndrome 310.0
Postlobectomy syndrome 310.0
Postmastectomy lymphedema (syndrome) 457.0
Postmaturity, postmature (fetus or newborn) 766.2
affecting management of pregnancy 645
syndrome 766.2
Postmeasles *—see also* condition
complication 055.8
specified NEC 055.79
Postmenopausal endometrium (atrophic) 627.8
suppurative (*see also* Endometritis) 615.9
Postnasal drip *—see* Sinusitis
Postnatal *—see* condition
Postoperative *—see also* condition
confusion state 293.9
psychosis 293.9
status NEC (*see also* Status (post)) V45.89
Postpancreatectomy hyperglycemia 251.3
Postpartum *—see also* condition
observation
immediately after delivery V24.0
routine follow-up V24.2
Postperfusion syndrome NEC 999.8
bone marrow 996.85
Postpoliomyelitic *—see* condition
Postsurgery status NEC (*see also* Status (post)) V45.89
Post-term (pregnancy) 645
infant (294 days or more gestation) 766.2
Posttraumatic *—see* condition
Posttraumatic brain syndrome, nonpsychotic 310.2
Post-typhoid abscess 002.0
Postures, hysterical 300.11
Postvaccinal reaction or complication *—see* Complications, vaccination
Postvagotomy syndrome 564.2
Postvalvulotomy syndrome 429.4
Postvasectomy sperm count V25.8
Potain's disease (pulmonary edema) 514
Potain's syndrome (gastrectasis with dyspepsia) 536.1
Pott's
curvature (spinal) (*see also* Tuberculosis) 015.0 *[737.43]*
disease or paraplegia (*see also* Tuberculosis) 015.0 *[730.88]*
fracture (closed) 824.4
open 824.5
gangrene 440.24
osteomyelitis (*see also* Tuberculosis) 015.0 *[730.88]*
spinal curvature (*see also* Tuberculosis) 015.0 *[737.43]*
tumor, puffy (*see also* Osteomyelitis) 730.2

Potter's
asthma 502
disease 753.0
facies 754.0
lung 502
syndrome (with renal agenesis) 753.0
Pouch
bronchus 748.3
Douglas'—*see* condition
esophagus, esophageal (congenital) 750.4
acquired 530.6
gastric 537.1
Hartmann's (abnormal sacculation of gallbladder neck) 575.8
pharynx, pharyngeal (congenital) 750.27
Poulet's disease 714.2
Poultrymen's itch 133.8
Poverty V60.2
Prader-Labhart-Willi-Fanconi syndrome (hypogenital dystrophy with diabetic tendency) 759.81
Prader-Willi syndrome (hypogenital dystrophy with diabetic tendency) 759.81
Preachers' voice 784.49
Pre-AIDS —*see* Human immunodeficiency virus (disease) (illness) (infection)
Preauricular appendage 744.1
Prebetalipoproteinemia (acquired) (essential) (familial) (hereditary) (primary) (secondary) 272.1
with chylomicronemia 272.3
Precipitate labor 661.3
affecting fetus or newborn 763.6
Preclimacteric bleeding 627.0
menorrhagia 627.0
Precocious
adrenarche 259.1
menarche 259.1
menstruation 626.8
pubarche 259.1
puberty NEC 259.1
sexual development NEC 259.1
thelarche 259.1
Precocity, sexual (constitutional) (cryptogenic) (female) (idiopathic) (male) NEC 259.1
with adrenal hyperplasia 255.2
Precordial pain 786.51
psychogenic 307.89
Predeciduous teeth 520.2
Prediabetes, prediabetic 790.2
complicating pregnancy, childbirth, or puerperium 648.8
fetus or newborn 775.8
Predislocation status of hip, at birth (*see also* Subluxation, congenital, hip) 754.32
Pre-eclampsia (mild) 642.4
with pre-existing hypertension 642.7
affecting fetus or newborn 760.0
severe 642.5
superimposed on pre-existing hypertensive disease 642.7
Preeruptive color change, teeth, tooth 520.8
Preexcitation 426.7
atrioventricular conduction 426.7
ventricular 426.7
Preglaucoma 365.00
Pregnancy (single) (uterine) (without sickness) V22.2

Note—Use the following fifth-digit subclassification with categories 640-648, 651-676:

0 unspecified as to episode of care
1 delivered, with or without mention of antepartum condition
2 delivered, with mention of postpartum complication
3 antepartum condition or complication
4 postpartum condition or complication

abdominal (ectopic) 633.0
affecting fetus or newborn 761.4
abnormal NEC 646.9
ampullar—*see* Pregnancy, tubal
broad ligament—*see* Pregnancy, cornual
cervical—*see* Pregnancy, cornual
combined (extrauterine and intrauterine)—*see* Pregnancy, cornual
complicated (by) 646.9
abnormal, abnormality NEC 646.9
cervix 654.6
cord (umbilical) 663.9
glucose tolerance (conditions classifiable to 790.2) 648.8
pelvic organs or tissues NEC 654.9
pelvis (bony) 653.0
perineum or vulva 654.8
placenta, placental (vessel) 656.7
position
cervix 654.4
placenta 641.1
without hemorrhage 641.0
uterus 654.4
size, fetus 653.5
uterus (congenital) 654.0
abscess or cellulitis
bladder 646.6
genitourinary tract (conditions classifiable to 590, 595, 597, 599.0, 614-616) 646.6
kidney 646.6
urinary tract NEC 646.6
air embolism 673.0
albuminuria 646.2
with hypertension—*see* Toxemia, of pregnancy
amnionitis 658.4
amniotic fluid embolism 673.1
anemia (conditions classifiable to 280-285) 648.2
atrophy, yellow (acute) (liver) (subacute) 646.7
bacilluria, asymptomatic 646.5
bacteriuria, asymptomatic 646.5
bicornis or bicornuate uterus 654.0
bone and joint disorders (conditions classifiable to 720-724 or conditions affecting lower limbs classifiable to 711-719, 725-738) 648.7
breech presentation 652.2
with successful version 652.1
cardiovascular disease (conditions classifiable to 390-398, 410-429) 648.6
congenital (conditions classifiable to 745-747) 648.5
cerebrovascular disorders conditions (classifiable to 430-434, 436-437) 674.0

Pregnancy—*continued*
kidney (conditions classifiable to 590.0-590.9) 646.6
urinary (tract) 646.6
asymptomatic 646.5
infective and parasitic diseases NEC 647.8
inflammation
bladder 646.6
genital organ (conditions classifiable to 614-616) 646.6
urinary tract NEC 646.6
injury 648.9
obstetrical NEC 665.9
insufficient weight gain 646.8
intrauterine fetal death (near term) NEC 656.4
early (before 22 completed weeks' gestation) 632
malaria (conditions classifiable to 084) 647.4
malformation, uterus (congenital) 654.0
malnutrition (conditions classifiable to 260-269) 648.9
malposition
fetus—*see* Pregnancy, complicated, malpresentation
uterus or cervix 654.4
malpresentation 652.9
with successful version 652.1
in multiple gestation 652.6
specified type NEC 652.8
marginal sinus hemorrhage or rupture 641.2
maternal obesity syndrome 646.1
menstruation 640.8
mental disorders (conditions classifiable to 290-303, 305-316, 317-319) 648.4
mentum presentation 652.4
missed
abortion 632
delivery (at or near term) 656.4
labor (at or near term) 656.4
necrosis
genital organ or tract (conditions classifiable to 614-616) 646.6
liver (conditions classifiable to 570) 646.7
renal, cortical 646.2
nephritis or nephrosis (conditions classifiable to 580-589) 646.2
with hypertension 642.1
nephropathy NEC 646.2
neuritis (peripheral) 646.4
nutritional deficiency (conditions classifiable to 260-269) 648.9
oblique lie or presentation 652.3
with successful version 652.1
obstetrical trauma NEC 665.9
oligohydramnios NEC 658.0
onset of contractions before 37 weeks 644.0
oversize fetus 653.5
papyraceous fetus 646.0
patent cervix 654.5
pelvic inflammatory disease (conditions classifiable to 614-616) 646.6
placenta, placental
abnormality 656.7
abruptio or ablatio 641.2
detachment 641.2
disease 656.7

Pregnancy—*continued*
infarct 656.7
low implantation 641.1
without hemorrhage 641.0
malformation 656.7
malposition 641.1
without hemorrhage 641.0
marginal sinus hemorrhage 641.2
previa 641.1
without hemorrhage 641.0
separation (premature) (undelivered) 641.2
placentitis 658.4
polyhydramnios 657
postmaturity 645
prediabetes 648.8
pre-eclampsia (mild) 642.4
severe 642.5
superimposed on pre-existing hypertensive disease 642.7
premature rupture of membranes 658.1
with delayed delivery 658.2
previous
infertility V23.0
nonobstetric condition V23.8
poor obstetrical history V23.4
premature delivery V23.4
trophoblastic disease (conditions classifiable to 630) V23.1
prolapse, uterus 654.4
proteinuria (gestational) 646.2
with hypertension—*see* Toxemia, of pregnancy
pruritus (neurogenic) 646.8
psychosis or psychoneurosis 648.4
ptyalism 646.8
pyelitis (conditions classifiable to 590.0-590.9) 646.6
renal disease or failure NEC 646.2
with secondary hypertension 642.1
hypertensive 642.2
retention, retained dead ovum 631
retroversion, uterus 654.3
Rh immunization, incompatibility, or sensitization 656.1
rubella (conditions classifiable to 056) 647.5
rupture
amnion (premature) 658.1
with delayed delivery 658.2
marginal sinus (hemorrhage) 641.2
membranes (premature) 658.1
with delayed delivery 658.2
uterus (before onset of labor) 665.0
salivation (excessive) 646.8
salpingo-oophoritis (conditions classifiable to 614.0-614.2) 646.6
septicemia (conditions classifiable to 038.0-038.9) 647.8
spasms, uterus (abnormal) 646.8
specified condition NEC 646.8
spurious labor pains 644.1
superfecundation 651.9
superfetation 651.9
syphilis (conditions classifiable to 090-097) 647.0
threatened
abortion 640.0
premature delivery 644.2
premature labor 644.0
thrombophlebitis (superficial) 671.2
deep 671.3

Pregnancy—*continued*
thrombosis 671.9
venous (superficial) 671.2
deep 671.3
thyroid dysfunction (conditions classifiable to 240-246) 648.1
thyroiditis 648.1
thyrotoxicosis 648.1
torsion of uterus 654.4
toxemia—*see* Toxemia, of pregnancy
transverse lie or presentation 652.3
with successful version 652.1
trauma 648.9
obstetrical 665.9
tuberculosis (conditions classifiable to 010-018) 647.3
tumor
cervix 654.6
ovary 654.4
pelvic organs or tissue NEC 654.4
uterus (body) 654.1
cervix 654.6
vagina 654.7
vulva 654.8
unstable lie 652.0
uremia—*see also* Pregnancy, complicated, renal disease
urethritis 646.6
vaginitis or vulvitis (conditions classifiable to 616.1) 646.6
varicose
placental vessels 656.7
veins (legs) 671.0
perineum 671.1
vulva 671.1
varicosity, labia or vulva 671.1
venereal disease NEC (conditions classifiable to 099) 647.2
viral disease NEC (conditions classifiable to 042, 050-055, 057-079) 647.6
vomiting (incoercible) (pernicious) (persistent) (uncontrollable) (vicious) 643.9
due to organic disease or other cause 643.8
early—*see* Hyperemesis, gravidarum
late (after 22 completed weeks gestation) 643.2
complications NEC 646.9
cornual 633.8
affecting fetus or newborn 761.4
death, maternal NEC 646.9
delivered—*see* Delivery
ectopic (ruptured) NEC 633.9
abdominal—*see* Pregnancy, abdominal
affecting fetus or newborn 761.4
combined (extrauterine and intrauterine)—*see* Pregnancy, cornual
ovarian—*see* Pregnancy, ovarian
specified type NEC 633.8
affecting fetus or newborn 761.4
tubal—*see* Pregnancy, tubal
examination, pregnancy not confirmed V72.4
extrauterine—*see* Pregnancy, ectopic
fallopian—*see* Pregnancy, tubal
false 300.11
labor (pains) 644.1
fatigue 646.8
illegitimate V61.6
incidental finding V22.2
in double uterus 654.0
interstitial—*see* Pregnancy, cornual
intraligamentous—*see* Pregnancy, cornual

Pregnancy—*continued*
intramural—*see* Pregnancy, cornual
intraperitoneal—*see* Pregnancy, abdominal
isthmian—*see* Pregnancy, tubal
management affected by
abnormal, abnormality
fetus (suspected) 655.9
specified NEC 655.8
placenta 656.7
advanced maternal age NEC 659.6
primigravida 659.5
antibodies (maternal)
anti-c 656.1
anti-d 656.1
anti-e 656.1
blood group (ABO) 656.2
Rh(esus) 656.1
elderly primigravida 659.5
fetal (suspected)
abnormality 655.9
acid-base balance 656.3
heart rate or rhythm 656.3
specified NEC 655.8
acidemia 656.3
anencephaly 655.0
bradycardia 656.3
central nervous system malformation 655.0
chromosomal abnormalities (conditions classifiable to 758.0-758.9) 655.1
damage from
drugs 655.5
obstetric, anesthetic, or sedative 655.5
environmental toxins 655.8
intrauterine contraceptive device 655.8
maternal
alcohol addiction 655.4
disease NEC 655.4
drug use 655.5
listeriosis 655.4
rubella 655.3
toxoplasmosis 655.4
viral infection 655.3
radiation 655.6
death (near term) 656.4
early (before 22 completed weeks gestation) 632
distress 656.3
excessive growth 656.6
growth retardation 656.5
hereditary disease 655.2
hydrocephalus 655.0
intrauterine death 656.4
poor growth 656.5
spina bifida (with myelomeningocele) 655.0
fetal-maternal hemorrhage 656.0
hereditary disease in family (possibly) affecting fetus 655.2
incompatibility, blood groups (ABO) 656.2
rh(esus) 656.1
insufficient prenatal care V23.7
intrauterine death 656.4
isoimmunization (ABO) 656.2
rh(esus) 656.1
large-for-dates fetus 656.6
light-for-dates fetus 656.5
meconium in liquor 656.3
mental disorder (conditions classifiable to 290-303, 305-316, 317-319) 648.4
multiparity (grand) 659.4
poor obstetric history V23.4

Primula dermatitis 692.6
Primus varus (bilateral) (metatarsus) 754.52
P.R.I.N.D. 436
Pringle's disease (tuberous sclerosis) 759.5
Prinzmetal's angina 413.1
Prinzmetal-Massumi syndrome (anterior chest wall) 786.52
Prizefighter ear 738.7
Problem (with) V49.9
academic V62.3
acculturation V62.4
adopted child V61.29
aged
in-law V61.3
parent V61.3
person NEC V61.8
alcoholism in family V61.41
anger reaction (*see also* Disturbance, conduct) 312.0
behavior, child 312.9
behavioral V40.9
specified NEC V40.3
betting V69.3
cardiorespiratory NEC V47.2
care of sick or handicapped person in family or household V61.49
career choice V62.2
child abuse, maltreatment or neglect V61.21
affecting the child 995.5
communication V40.1
conscience regarding medical care V62.6
delinquency (juvenile) 312.9
diet, inappropriate V69.1
digestive NEC V47.3
ear NEC V41.3
eating habits, inappropriate V69.1
economic V60.2
affecting care V60.9
specified type NEC V60.8
educational V62.3
enuresis, child 307.6
exercise, lack of V69.0
eye NEC V41.1
family V61.9
specified circumstance NEC V61.8
fear reaction, child 313.0
feeding (elderly) (infant) 783.3
newborn 779.3
nonorganic 307.50
fetal, affecting management of pregnancy 656.9
specified type NEC 656.8
financial V60.2
foster child V61.29
specified NEC V41.8
functional V41.9
specified type NEC V41.8
gambling V69.3
genital NEC V47.5
head V48.9
deficiency V48.0
disfigurement V48.6
mechanical V48.2
motor V48.2
movement of V48.2
sensory V48.4
specified condition NEC V48.8
hearing V41.2
high-risk sexual behavior V69.2

Problem—*continued*
influencing health status NEC V49.8
internal organ NEC V47.9
deficiency V47.0
mechanical or motor V47.1
interpersonal NEC V62.81
jealousy, child 313.3
learning V40.0
legal V62.5
life circumstance NEC V62.89
lifestyle V69.9
specified NEC V69.8
limb V49.9
deficiency V49.0
disfigurement V49.4
mechanical V49.1
motor V49.2
movement, involving
musculoskeletal system V49.1
nervous system V49.2
sensory V49.3
specified condition NEC V49.5
litigation V62.5
living alone V60.3
loneliness NEC V62.89
marital V61.1
involving
divorce V61.0
estrangement V61.0
psychosexual disorder 302.9
sexual function V41.7
mastication V41.6
medical care, within family V61.49
mental V40.9
specified NEC V40.2
mental hygiene, adult V40.9
multiparity V61.5
nail biting, child 307.9
neck V48.9
deficiency V48.1
disfigurement V48.7
mechanical V48.3
motor V48.3
movement V48.3
sensory V48.5
specified condition NEC V48.8
neurological NEC 781.9
none (feared complaint unfounded) V65.5
occupational V62.2
parent-child V61.20
partner V61.1
personal NEC V62.89
interpersonal conflict NEC V62.81
personality (*see also* Disorder, personality) 301.9
phase of life V62.89
placenta, affecting management of pregnancy 656.9
specified type NEC 656.8
poverty V60.2
presence of sick or handicapped person in family or household V61.49
psychiatric 300.9
psychosocial V62.9
specified type NEC V62.89
relational NEC V62.81
relationship, childhood 313.3
religious or spiritual belief
other than medical care V62.89
regarding medical care V62.6

Problem—*continued*
self-damaging behavior V69.8
sexual
behavior, high-risk V69.2
function NEC V41.7
sibling, relational V61.8
sight V41.0
sleep disorder, child 307.40
smell V41.5
speech V40.1
spite reaction, child (*see also* Disturbance, conduct) 312.0
spoiled child reaction (*see also* Disturbance, conduct) 312.1
swallowing V41.6
tantrum, child (*see also* Disturbance, conduct) 312.1
taste V41.5
thumb sucking, child 307.9
tic, child 307.21
trunk V48.9
deficiency V48.1
disfigurement V48.7
mechanical V48.3
motor V48.3
movement V48.3
sensory V48.5
specified condition NEC V48.8
unemployment V62.0
urinary NEC V47.4
voice production V41.4
Procedure (surgical) not done NEC V64.3
because of
contraindication V64.1
patient's decision V64.2
for reasons of conscience or religion V62.6
specified reason NEC V64.3
Procidentia
anus (sphincter) 569.1
rectum (sphincter) 569.1
stomach 537.89
uteri 618.1
Proctalgia 569.42
fugax 564.6
spasmodic 564.6
psychogenic 307.89
Proctitis 569.49
amebic 006.8
chlamydial 099.52
gonococcal 098.7
granulomatous 555.1
idiopathic 556.2
with ulcerative sigmoiditis 556.3
tuberculous (*see also* Tuberculosis) 014.8
ulcerative (chronic) (nonspecific) 556.2
with ulcerative sigmoiditis 556.3
Proctocele
female (without uterine prolapse) 618.0
with uterine prolapse 618.4
complete 618.3
incomplete 618.2
male 569.49
Proctocolitis, idiopathic 556.2
with ulcerative sigmoiditis 556.3
Proctoptosis 569.1
Proctosigmoiditis 569.89
ulcerative (chronic) 556.3
Proctospasm 564.6
psychogenic 306.4
Prodromal-AIDS —*see* Human immunodeficiency virus (disease) (illness) (infection)
Profichet's disease or syndrome 729.9
Progeria (adultorum) (syndrome) 259.8
Prognathism (mandibular) (maxillary) 524.00
Progonoma (melanotic) (M9363/0)—*see* Neoplasm, by site, benign
Progressive —*see* condition
Prolapse, prolapsed
anus, anal (canal) (sphincter) 569.1
arm or hand, complicating delivery 652.7
causing obstructed labor 660.0
affecting fetus or newborn 763.1
fetus or newborn 763.1
bladder (acquired) (mucosa) (sphincter)
congenital (female) (male) 753.8
female 618.0
male 596.8
breast implant (prosthetic) 996.54
cecostomy 569.69
cecum 569.89
cervix, cervical (stump) (hypertrophied) 618.1
anterior lip, obstructing labor 660.2
affecting fetus or newborn 763.1
congenital 752.49
postpartal (old) 618.1
ciliary body 871.1
colon (pedunculated) 569.89
colostomy 569.69
conjunctiva 372.73
cord—*see* Prolapse, umbilical cord
disc (intervertebral)—*see* Displacement, intervertebral disc
duodenum 537.89
eye implant (orbital) 996.59
lens (ocular) 996.53
fallopian tube 620.4
fetal extremity, complicating delivery 652.8
causing obstructed labor 660.0
fetus or newborn 763.1
funis—*see* Prolapse, umbilical cord
gastric (mucosa) 537.89
genital, female 618.9
specified NEC 618.8
globe 360 81
ileostomy bud 569.69
intervertebral disc—*see* Displacement, intervertebral disc
intestine (small) 569.89
iris 364.8
traumatic 871.1
kidney (*see also* Disease, renal) 593.0
congenital 753.3
laryngeal muscles or ventricle 478.79
leg, complicating delivery 652.8
causing obstructed labor 660.0
fetus or newborn 763.1
liver 573.8
meatus urinarius 599.5
mitral valve 424.0
ocular lens implant 996.53
organ or site, congenital NEC—*see* Malposition, congenital
ovary 620.4
pelvic (floor), female 618.8
perineum, female 618.8
pregnant uterus 654.4
rectum (mucosa) (sphincter) 569.1
due to Trichuris trichiuria 127.3
spleen 289.59
stomach 537.89

Prolapse, prolapsed—*continued*
umbilical cord
affecting fetus or newborn 762.4
complicating delivery 663.0
ureter 593.89
with obstruction 593.4
ureterovesical orifice 593.89
urethra (acquired) (infected) (mucosa) 599.5
congenital 753.8
uterovaginal 618.4
complete 618.3
incomplete 618.2
specified NEC 618.8
uterus (first degree) (second degree) (third degree) (complete) (without vaginal wall prolapse) 618.1
with mention of vaginal wall prolapse—*see* Prolapse, uterovaginal
congenital 752.3
in pregnancy or childbirth 654.4
affecting fetus or newborn 763.1
causing obstructed labor 660.2
affecting fetus or newborn 763.1
postpartal (old) 618.1
uveal 871.1
vagina (anterior) (posterior) (vault) (wall) (without uterine prolapse) 618.0
with uterine prolapse 618.4
complete 618.3
incomplete 618.2
posthysterectomy 618.5
vitreous (humor) 379.26
traumatic 871.1
womb—*see* Prolapse, uterus
Prolapsus, female 618.9
Proliferative —*see* condition
Prolinemia 270.8
Prolinuria 270.8
Prolonged, prolongation
bleeding time (*see also* Defect, coagulation) 790.92
"idiopathic" (in von Willebrand's disease) 286.4
coagulation time (*see also* Defect, coagulation) 790.92
gestation syndrome 766.2
labor 662.1
first stage 662.0
second stage 662.2
affecting fetus or newborn 763.8
PR interval 426.11
prothrombin time (*see also* Defect, coagulation) 790.92
rupture of membranes (24 hours or more prior to onset of labor) 658.2
uterine contractions in labor 661.4
affecting fetus or newborn 763.7
Prominauris 744.29
Prominence
auricle (ear) (congenital) 744.29
acquired 380.32
ischial spine or sacral promontory
with disproportion (fetopelvic) 653.3
affecting fetus or newborn 763.1
causing obstructed labor 660.1
affecting fetus or newborn 763.1
nose (congenital) 748.1
acquired 738.0
Pronation
ankle 736.79
foot 736.79
congenital 755.67
Prophylactic
administration of
antibiotics V07.39
antitoxin, any V07.2
antivenin V07.2
chemotherapeutic agent NEC V07.39
fluoride V07.31
diphtheria antitoxin V07.2
gamma globulin V07.2
immune sera (gamma globulin) V07.2
RhoGAM V07.2
tetanus antitoxin V07.2
chemotherapy NEC V07.39
fluoride V07.31
immunotherapy V07.2
measure V07.9
specified type NEC V07.8
sterilization V25.2
Proptosis (ocular) (*see also* Exophthalmos) 376.30
thyroid 242.0
Propulsion
eyeball 360.81
Prosecution, anxiety concerning V62.5
Prostate, prostatic —*see* condition
Prostatism 600
Prostatitis (congestive) (suppurative) 601.9
acute 601.0
cavitary 601.8
chlamydial 099.54
chronic 601.1
diverticular 601.8
due to Trichomonas (vaginalis) 131.03
fibrous 600
gonococcal (acute) 098.12
chronic or duration of 2 months or over 098.32
granulomatous 601.8
hypertrophic 600
specified type NEC 601.8
subacute 601.1
trichomonal 131.03
tuberculous (*see also* Tuberculosis) 016.5 *[601.4]*
Prostatocystitis 601.3
Prostatorrhea 602.8
Prostatoseminovesiculitis, trichomonal 131.03
Prostration 780.7
heat 992.5
anhydrotic 992.3
due to
salt (and water) depletion 992.4
water depletion 992.3
nervous 300.5
newborn 779.8
senile 797
Protanomaly 368.51
Protanopia (anomalous trichromat) (complete) (incomplete) 368.51
Protein
deficiency 260
malnutrition 260
sickness (prophylactic) (therapeutic) 999.5
Proteinemia 790.99
Proteinosis
alveolar, lung or pulmonary 516.0
lipid 272.8
lipoid (of Urbach) 272.8

- **Proteinuria** (*see also* Albuminuria) 791.0
  - Bence-Jones NEC 791.0
  - gestational 646.2
    - with hypertension—*see* Toxemia, of pregnancy
  - orthostatic 593.6
  - postural 593.6
- **Proteolysis, pathologic** 286.6
- **Protocoproporphyria** 277.1
- **Protoporphyria** (erythrohepatic) (erythropoietic) 277.1
- **Protrusio acetabuli** 718.65
- **Protrusion**
  - acetabulum (into pelvis) 718.65
  - device, implant, or graft—*see* Complications, mechanical
  - ear, congenital 744.29
  - intervertebral disc—*see* Displacement, intervertebral disc
  - nucleus pulposus—*see* Displacement, intervertebral disc
- **Proud flesh** 701.5
- **Prune belly** (syndrome) 756.7
- **Prurigo** (ferox) (gravis) (Hebra's) (hebrae) (mitis) (simplex) 698.2
  - agria 698.3
  - asthma syndrome 691.8
  - Besnier's (atopic dermatitis) (infantile eczema) 691.8
  - eczematodes allergicum 691.8
  - estivalis (Hutchinson's) 692.72
  - Hutchinson's 692.72
  - nodularis 698.3
  - psychogenic 306.3
- **Pruritus, pruritic** 698.9
  - ani 698.0
    - psychogenic 306.3
  - conditions NEC 698.9
    - psychogenic 306.3
  - due to Onchocerca volvulus 125.3
  - ear 698.9
  - essential 698.9
  - genital organ(s) 698.1
    - psychogenic 306.3
  - gravidarum 646.8
  - hiemalis 698.8
  - neurogenic (any site) 306.3
  - perianal 698.0
  - psychogenic (any site) 306.3
  - scrotum 698.1
    - psychogenic 306.3
  - senile, senilis 698.8
  - Trichomonas 131.9
  - vulva, vulvae 698.1
    - psychogenic 306.3
- **Psammocarcinoma** (M8140/3)—*see* Neoplasm, by site, malignant
- **Pseudarthrosis, pseudoarthrosis** (bone) 733.82
  - joint following fusion V45.4
- **Pseudoacanthosis**
  - nigricans 701.8
- **Pseudoaneurysm** —*see* Aneurysm
- **Pseudoangina** (pectoris)—*see* Angina
- **Pseudoangioma** 452
- **Pseudo-Argyll-Robertson pupil** 379.45
- **Pseudoarteriosus** 747.89
- **Pseudoarthrosis** —*see* Pseudarthrosis
- **Pseudoataxia** 799.8
- **Pseudobursa** 727.89
- **Pseudocholera** 025
- **Pseudochromidrosis** 705.89
- **Pseudocirrhosis, liver, pericardial** 423.2
- **Pseudocoarctation** 747.21
- **Pseudocowpox** 051.1
- **Pseudocoxalgia** 732.1
- **Pseudocroup** 478.75
- **Pseudocyesis** 300.11
- **Pseudocyst**
  - lung 518.89
  - pancreas 577.2
  - retina 361.19
- **Pseudodementia** 300.16
- **Pseudoelephantiasis neuroarthritica** 757.0
- **Pseudoemphysema** 518.89
- **Pseudoencephalitis**
  - superior (acute) hemorrhagic 265.1
- **Pseudoerosion cervix, congenital** 752.49
- **Pseudoexfoliation, lens capsule** 366.11
- **Pseudofracture** (idiopathic) (multiple) (spontaneous) (symmetrical) 268.2
- **Pseudoglanders** 025
- **Pseudoglioma** 360.44
- **Pseudogout** —*see* Chondrocalcinosis
- **Pseudohallucination** 780.1
- **Pseudohemianesthesia** 782.0
- **Pseudohemophilia** (Bernuth's) (hereditary) (type B) 286.4
  - type A 287.8
  - vascular 287.8
- **Pseudohermaphroditism** 752.7
  - with chromosomal anomaly—*see* Anomaly, chromosomal
  - adrenal 255.2
  - female (without adrenocortical disorder) 752.7
    - with adrenocortical disorder 255.2
    - adrenal 255.2
  - male (without gonadal disorder) 752.7
    - with
      - adrenocortical disorder 255.2
      - cleft scrotum 752.7
      - feminizing testis 257.8
      - gonadal disorder 257.9
    - adrenal 255.2
- **Pseudohole, macula** 362.54
- **Pseudo-Hurler's disease** (mucolipidosis III) 272.7
- **Pseudohydrocephalus** 348.2
- **Pseudohypertrophic muscular dystrophy** (Erb's) 359.1
- **Pseudohypertrophy, muscle** 359.1
- **Pseudohypoparathyroidism** 275.4
- **Pseudoinfluenza** 487.1
- **Pseudoinsomnia** 307.49
- **Pseudoleukemia** 288.8
  - infantile 285.8
- **Pseudomembranous** —*see* condition
- **Pseudomeningocele** (cerebral) (infective) (surgical) 349.2
  - spinal 349.2
- **Pseudomenstruation** 626.8
- **Pseudomucinous**
  - cyst (ovary) (M8470/0) 220
  - peritoneum 568.89
- **Pseudomyeloma** 273.1
- **Pseudomyxoma peritonei** (M8480/6) 197.6
- **Pseudoneuritis optic** (nerve) 377.24
  - papilla 377.24
    - congenital 743.57
- **Pseudoneuroma** —*see* Injury, nerve, by site
- **Pseudo-obstruction**
  - intestine 564.8
- **Pseudopapilledema** 377.24

Pseudoparalysis
arm or leg 781.4
atonic, congenital 358.8
Pseudopelade 704.09
Pseudophakia V43.1
Pseudopolycythemia 289.0
Pseudopolyposis, colon 556.4
Pseudoporencephaly 348.0
Pseudopseudohypoparathyroidism 275.4
Pseudopsychosis 300.16
Pseudopterygium 372.52
Pseudoptosis (eyelid) 374.34
Pseudorabies 078.89
Pseudoretinitis, pigmentosa 362.65
Pseudorickets 588.0
senile (Pozzi's) 731.0
Pseudorubella 057.8
Pseudoscarlatina 057.8
Pseudosclerema 778.1
Pseudosclerosis (brain)
Jakob's 046.1
of Westphal (-Strümpell) (hepatolenticular degeneration) 275.1
spastic 046.1
with dementia (*see also* Dementia, presenile) 290.10
Pseudotabes 799.8
diabetic 250.6 *[337.1]*
Pseudotetanus (*see also* Convulsions) 780.3
Pseudotetany 781.7
hysterical 300.11
Pseudothalassemia 285.0
Pseudotrichinosis 710.3
Pseudotruncus arteriosus 747.29
Pseudotuberculosis, pasteurella (infection) 027.2
Pseudotumor
cerebri 348.2
orbit (inflammatory) 376.11
Pseudo-Turner's syndrome 759.89
Pseudoxanthoma elasticum 757.39
Psilosis (sprue) (tropical) 579.1
Monilia 112.89
nontropical 579.0
not sprue 704.00
Psittacosis 073.9
Psoitis 728.89
Psora NEC 696.1
Psoriasis 696.1
any type, except arthropathic 696.1
arthritic, arthropathic 696.0
buccal 528.6
flexural 696.1
follicularis 696.1
guttate 696.1
inverse 696.1
mouth 528.6
nummularis 696.1
psychogenic 316 *[696.1]*
punctata 696.1
pustular 696.1
rupioides 696.1
vulgaris 696.1
Psorospermiasis 136.4
Psorospermosis 136.4
follicularis (vegetans) 757.39
Psychalgia 307.80
Psychasthenia 300.89
compulsive 300.3
mixed compulsive states 300.3
obsession 300.3
Psychiatric disorder or problem NEC 300.9
Psychogenic —*see also* condition
factors associated with physical conditions 316
Psychoneurosis, psychoneurotic (*see also* Neurosis) 300.9
anxiety (state) 300.00
climacteric 627.2
compensation 300.16
compulsion 300.3
conversion hysteria 300.11
depersonalization 300.6
depressive type 300.4
dissociative hysteria 300.15
hypochondriacal 300.7
hysteria 300.10
conversion type 300.11
dissociative type 300.15
mixed NEC 300.89
neurasthenic 300.5
obsessional 300.3
obsessive-compulsive 300.3
occupational 300.89
personality NEC 301.89
phobia 300.20
senile NEC 300.89
Psychopathic —*see also* condition
constitution, posttraumatic 310.2
with psychosis 293.9
personality 301.9
amoral trends 301.7
antisocial trends 301.7
asocial trends 301.7
mixed types 301.7
state 301.9
Psychopathy, sexual (*see also* Deviation, sexual) 302.9
Psychophysiologic, psychophysiological condition—*see* Reaction, psychophysiologic
Psychose passionelle 297.8
Psychosexual identity disorder 302.6
adult-life 302.85
childhood 302.6
Psychosis 298.9
acute hysterical 298.1
affecting management of pregnancy, childbirth, or puerperium 648.4
affective NEC 296.90

Note—Use the following fifth-digit subclassification with categories 296.0-296.6:

0 unspecified
1 mild
2 moderate
3 severe, without mention of psychotic behavior
4 severe, specified as with psychotic behavior
5 in partial or unspecified remission
6 in full remission

involutional 296.2
recurrent episode 296.3
single episode 296.2
manic-depressive 296.80
circular (alternating) 296.7
currently depressed 296.5
currently manic 296.4
depressed type 296.2
atypical 296.82
recurrent episode 296.3
single episode 296.2

Psychosis—*continued*
manic 296.0
atypical 296.81
recurrent episode 296.1
single episode 296.0
mixed type NEC 296.89
specified type NEC 296.89
senile 290.21
specified type NEC 296.99
alcoholic 291.9
with
anxiety 291.8
delirium tremens 291.0
delusions 291.5
dementia 291.2
hallucinosis 291.3
jealousy 291.5
mood disturbance 291.8
paranoia 291.5
persisting amnesia 291.1
sexual dysfunction 291.8
sleep disturbance 291.8
amnestic confabulatory 291.1
delirium tremens 291.0
hallucinosis 291.3
Korsakoff's, Korsakov's, Korsakow's 291.1
paranoid type 291.5
pathological intoxication 291.4
polyneuritic 291.1
specified type NEC 291.8
alternating (*see also* Psychosis, manic-depressive, circular) 296.7
anergastic (*see also* Psychosis, organic) 294.9
arteriosclerotic 290.40
with
acute confusional state 290.41
delirium 290.41
delusional features 290.42
depressive features 290.43
depressed type 290.43
paranoid type 290.42
simple type 290.40
uncomplicated 290.40
atypical 298.9
depressive 296.82
manic 296.81
borderline (schizophrenia) (*see also* Schizophrenia) 295.5
of childhood (*see also* Psychosis, childhood) 299.8
prepubertal 299.8
brief reactive 298.8
childhood, with origin specific to 299.9

Note—Use the following fifth-digit subclassification with category 299:

0 current or active state
1 residual state

atypical 299.8
specified type NEC 299.8
circular (*see also* Psychosis, manic-depressive, circular) 296.7
climacteric (*see also* Psychosis, involutional) 298.8
confusional 298.9
acute 293.0
reactive 298.2
subacute 293.1

Psychosis—*continued*
depressive (*see also* Psychosis, affective) 296.2
atypical 296.82
involutional 296.2
recurrent episode 296.3
single episode 296.2
psychogenic 298.0
reactive (emotional stress) (psychological trauma) 298.0
recurrent episode 296.3
with hypomania (bipolar II) 296.89
single episode 296.2
disintegrative (childhood) (*see also* Psychosis, childhood) 299.1
drug 292.9
with
affective syndrome 292.84
amnestic syndrome 292.83
anxiety 292.89
delirium 292.81
withdrawal 292.0
delusional syndrome 292.11
dementia 292.82
depressive state 292.84
hallucinosis 292.12
mood disturbance 292.84
organic personality syndrome NEC 292.89
sexual dysfunction 292.89
sleep disturbance 292.89
withdrawal syndrome (and delirium) 292.0
affective syndrome 292.84
delusional state 292.11
hallucinatory state 292.12
hallucinosis 292.12
paranoid state 292.11
specified type NEC 292.89
withdrawal syndrome (and delirium) 292.0
due to or associated with physical condition (*see also* Psychosis, organic) 294.9
epileptic NEC 294.8
excitation (psychogenic) (reactive) 298.1
exhaustive (*see also* Reaction, stress, acute) 308.9
hypomanic (*see also* Psychosis, affective) 296.0
recurrent episode 296.1
single episode 296.0
hysterical 298.8
acute 298.1
incipient 298.8
schizophrenic (*see also* Schizophrenia) 295.5
induced 297.3
infantile (*see also* Psychosis, childhood) 299.0
infective 293.9
acute 293.0
subacute 293.1
in pregnancy, childbirth, or puerperium 648.4
interactional (childhood) (*see also* Psychosis, childhood) 299.1
involutional 298.8
depressive (*see also* Psychosis, affective) 296.2
recurrent episode 296.3
single episode 296.2
melancholic 296.2
recurrent episode 296.3
single episode 296.2
paranoid state 297.2
paraphrenia 297.2

Psychosis—*continued*
Korsakoff's, Korakov's, Korsakow's (nonalcoholic) 294.0
alcoholic 291.1
mania (phase) (*see also* Psychosis, affective) 296.0
recurrent episode 296.1
single episode 296.0
manic (*see also* Psychosis, affective) 296.0
atypical 296.81
recurrent episode 296.1
single episode 296.0
manic-depressive 296.80
circular 296.7
currently
depressed 296.5
manic 296.4
mixed 296.6
depressive 296.2
recurrent episode 296.3
with hypomania (bipolar II) 296.89
single episode 296.2
hypomanic 296.0
recurrent episode 296.1
single episode 296.0
manic 296.0
atypical 296.81
recurrent episode 296.1
single episode 296.0
mixed NEC 296.89
perplexed 296.89
stuporous 296.89
menopausal (*see also* Psychosis, involutional) 298.8
mixed schizophrenic and affective (*see also* Schizophrenia) 295.7
multi-infarct (cerebrovascular) (*see also* Psychosis, arteriosclerotic) 290.40
organic NEC 294.9
due to or associated with
addiction
alcohol (*see also* Psychosis, alcoholic) 291.9
drug (*see also* Psychosis, drug) 292.9
alcohol intoxication, acute (*see also* Psychosis, alcoholic) 291.9
alcoholism (*see also* Psychosis, alcoholic) 291.9
arteriosclerosis (cerebral) (*see also* Psychosis, arteriosclerotic) 290.40
cerebrovascular disease
acute (psychosis) 293.0
arteriosclerotic (*see also* Psychosis, arteriosclerotic) 290.40
childbirth—*see* Psychosis, puerperal
conditions classified elsewhere 294.1
dependence
alcohol (*see also* Psychosis, alcoholic) 291.9
drug 292.9
disease
alcoholic liver (*see also* Psychosis, alcoholic) 291.9
brain
arteriosclerotic (*see also* Psychosis, arteriosclerotic) 290.40
cerebrovascular
acute (psychosis) 293.0
arteriosclerotic (*see also* Psychosis, arteriosclerotic) 290.40

Psychosis—*continued*
endocrine or metabolic 293.9
acute (psychosis) 293.0
subacute (psychosis) 293.1
Jakob-Creutzfeldt 290.10
liver, alcoholic (*see also* Psychosis, alcoholic) 291.9
disorder
cerebrovascular
acute (psychosis) 293.0
endocrine or metabolic 293.9
acute (psychosis) 293.0
subacute (psychosis) 293.1
epilepsy 294.1
transient (acute) 293.0
Huntington's chorea 294.1
infection
brain 293.9
acute (psychosis) 293.0
chronic 294.8
subacute (psychosis) 293.1
intracranial NEC 293.9
acute (psychosis) 293.0
chronic 294.8
subacute (psychosis) 293.1
intoxication
alcoholic (acute) (*see also* Psychosis, alcoholic) 291.9
pathological 291.4
drug (*see also* Psychosis, drug) 292.9
ischemia
cerebrovascular (generalized) (*see also* Psychosis, arteriosclerotic) 290.40
Jakob-Creutzfeldt disease or syndrome 290.10
multiple sclerosis 294.1
physical condition NEC 294.9
presenility 290.10
puerperium—*see* Psychosis, puerperal
sclerosis, multiple 294.1
senility 290.20
status epilepticus 294.1
trauma
brain (birth) (from electrical current) (surgical) 293.9
acute (psychosis) 293.0
chronic 294.8
subacute (psychosis) 293.1
unspecified physical condition 294.9
infective 293.9
acute (psychosis) 293.0
subacute 293.1
posttraumatic 293.9
acute 293.0
subacute 293.1
specified type NEC 294.8
transient 293.9
with
delusions 293.81
depression 293.83
hallucinations 293.82
depressive type 293.83
hallucinatory type 293.82
paranoid type 293.81
specified type NEC 293.89
paranoic 297.1

Puerperal
abscess
areola 675.1
Bartholin's gland 646.6
breast 675.1
cervix (uteri) 670
fallopian tube 670
genital organ 670
kidney 646.6
mammary 675.1
mesosalpinx 670
nabothian 646.6
nipple 675.0
ovary, ovarian 670
oviduct 670
parametric 670
para-uterine 670
pelvic 670
perimetric 670
periuterine 670
retro-uterine 670
subareolar 675.1
suprapelvic 670
tubal (ruptured) 670
tubo-ovarian 670
urinary tract NEC 646.6
uterine, uterus 670
vagina (wall) 646.6
vaginorectal 646.6
vulvovaginal gland 646.6
accident 674.9
adnexitis 670
afibrinogenemia, or other coagulation defect 666.3
albuminuria (acute) (subacute) 646.2
pre-eclamptic 642.4
anemia (conditions classifiable to 280-285) 648.2
anuria 669.3
apoplexy 674.0
asymptomatic bacteriuria 646.5
atrophy, breast 676.3
bacteremia 670
blood dyscrasia 666.3
caked breast 676.2
cardiomyopathy 674.8
cellulitis—*see* Puerperal, abscess
cerebrovascular disorder (conditions classifiable to 430-434, 436-437) 674.0
cervicitis (conditions classifiable to 616.0) 646.6
coagulopathy (any) 666.3
complications 674.9
specified type NEC 674.8
convulsions (eclamptic) (uremic) 642.6
with pre-existing hypertension 642.7
cracked nipple 676.1
cystitis 646.6
cystopyelitis 646.6
deciduitis (acute) 670
delirium NEC 293.9
diabetes (mellitus) (conditions classifiable to 250) 648.0
disease 674.9
breast NEC 676.3
cerebrovascular (acute) 674.0
nonobstetric NEC (*see also* Pregnancy, complicated, current disease or condition) 648.9
pelvis inflammatory 670
renal NEC 646.2
tubo-ovarian 670

Puerperal—*continued*
Valsuani's (progressive pernicious anemia) 648.2
disorder
lactation 676.9
specified type NEC 676.8
nonobstetric NEC (*see also* Pregnancy, complicated, current disease or condition) 648.9
disruption
cesarean wound 674.1
episiotomy wound 674.2
perineal laceration wound 674.2
drug dependence (conditions classifiable to 304) 648.3
eclampsia 642.6
with pre-existing hypertension 642.7
embolism (pulmonary) 673.2
air 673.0
amniotic fluid 673.1
blood-clot 673.2
brain or cerebral 674.0
cardiac 674.8
fat 673.8
intracranial sinus (venous) 671.5
pyemic 673.3
septic 673.3
spinal cord 671.5
endometritis (conditions classifiable to 615.0-615.9) 670
endophlebitis—*see* Puerperal, phlebitis
endotrachelitis 646.6
engorgement, breasts 676.2
erysipelas 670
failure
lactation 676.4
renal, acute 669.3
fever (meaning sepsis) 670
meaning pyrexia (of unknown origin) 672
fissure, nipple 676.1
fistula
breast 675.1
mammary gland 675.1
nipple 675.0
galactophoritis 675.2
galactorrhea 676.6
gangrene
gas 670
uterus 670
gonorrhea (conditions classifiable to 098) 647.1
hematoma, subdural 674.0
hematosalpinx, infectional 670
hemiplegia, cerebral 674.0
hemorrhage 666.1
brain 674.0
bulbar 674.0
cerebellar 674.0
cerebral 674.0
cortical 674.0
delayed (after 24 hours) (uterine) 666.2
extradural 674.0
internal capsule 674.0
intracranial 674.0
intrapontine 674.0
meningeal 674.0
pontine 674.0
subarachnoid 674.0
subcortical 674.0
subdural 674.0
uterine, delayed 666.2
ventricular 674.0

Puerperal—*continued*
pyo-oophoritis 670
pyosalpingitis 670
pyosalpinx 670
pyrexia (of unknown origin) 672
renal
disease NEC 646.2
failure, acute 669.3
retention
decidua (fragments) (with delayed hemorrhage) 666.2
without hemorrhage 667.1
placenta (fragments) (with delayed hemorrhage) 666.2
without hemorrhage 667.1
secundines (fragments) (with delayed hemorrhage) 666.2
without hemorrhage 667.1
retracted nipple 676.0
rubella (conditions classifiable to 056) 647.5
salpingitis 670
salpingo-oophoritis 670
salpingo-ovaritis 670
salpingoperitonitis 670
sapremia 670
secondary perineal tear 674.2
sepsis (pelvic) 670
septicemia 670
subinvolution (uterus) 674.8
sudden death (cause unknown) 674.9
suppuration—*see* Puerperal, abscess
syphilis (conditions classifiable to 090-097) 647.0
tetanus 670
thelitis 675.0
thrombocytopenia 666.3
thrombophlebitis (superficial) 671.2
deep 671.4
pelvic 671.4
specified site NEC 671.5
thrombosis (venous)—*see* Thrombosis, puerperal
thyroid dysfunction (conditions classifiable to 240-246) 648.1
toxemia (*see also* Toxemia, of pregnancy) 642.4
eclamptic 642.6
with pre-existing hypertension 642.7
pre-eclamptic (mild) 642.4
with
convulsions 642.6
pre-existing hypertension 642.7
severe 642.5
tuberculosis (conditions classifiable to 010-018) 647.3
uremia 669.3
vaginitis (conditions classifiable to 616.1) 646.6
varicose veins (legs) 671.0
vulva or perineum 671.1
vulvitis (conditions classifiable to 616.1) 646.6
vulvovaginitis (conditions classifiable to 616.1) 646.6
white leg 671.4
Pulled muscle —*see* Sprain, by site
Pulmolithiasis 518.89
Pulmonary —*see* condition
Pulmonitis (unknown etiology) 486
Pulpitis (acute) (anachoretic) (chronic) (hyperplastic) (putrescent) (suppurative) (ulcerative) 522.0
Pulpless tooth 522.9
Pulse
alternating 427.89
psychogenic 306.2
bigeminal 427.89
fast 785.0
feeble, rapid, due to shock following injury 958.4
rapid 785.0
slow 427.89
strong 785.9
trigeminal 427.89
water-hammer (*see also* Insufficiency, aortic) 424.1
weak 785.9
Pulseless disease 446.7
Pulsus
alternans or trigeminy 427.89
psychogenic 306.2
Punch drunk 310.2
Puncta lacrimalia occlusion 375.52
Punctiform hymen 752.49
Puncture (traumatic)—*see also* Wound, open, by site
accidental, complicating surgery 998.2
bladder, nontraumatic 596.6
by
device, implant, or graft—*see* Complications, mechanical
foreign body
internal organs—*see also* Injury, internal, by site
by ingested object—*see* Foreign body
left accidentally in operation wound 998.4
instrument (any) during a procedure, accidental 998.2
internal organs, abdomen, chest, or pelvis—*see* Injury, internal, by site
kidney, nontraumatic 593.89
Pupil —*see* condition
Pupillary membrane 364.74
persistent 743.46
Pupillotonia 379.46
pseudotabetic 379.46
Purpura 287.2
abdominal 287.0
allergic 287.0
anaphylactoid 287.0
annularis telangiectodes 709.1
arthritic 287.0
autoerythrocyte sensitization 287.2
autoimmune 287.0
bacterial 287.0
Bateman's (senile) 287.2
capillary fragility (hereditary) (idiopathic) 287.8
cryoglobulinemic 273.2
devil's pinches 287.2
fibrinolytic (*see also* Fibrinolysis) 286.6
fulminans, fulminous 286.6
gangrenous 287.0
hemorrhagic (*see also* Purpura, thrombocytopenic) 287.3
nodular 272.7
nonthrombocytopenic 287.0
thrombocytopenic 287.3
Henoch's (purpura nervosa) 287.0
Henoch-Schönlein (allergic) 287.0
hypergammaglobulinemic (benign primary) (Waldenström's) 273.0

Purpura—*continued*
idiopathic 287.3
nonthrombocytopenic 287.0
thrombocytopenic 287.3
infectious 287.0
malignant 287.0
neonatorum 772.6
nervosa 287.0
newborn NEC 772.6
nonthrombocytopenic 287.2
hemorrhagic 287.0
idiopathic 287.0
nonthrombopenic 287.2
peliosis rheumatica 287.0
pigmentaria, progressiva 709.09
posttransfusion 287.4
primary 287.0
primitive 287.0
red cell membrane sensitivity 287.2
rheumatica 287.0
Schönlein (-Henoch) (allergic) 287.0
scorbutic 267
senile 287.2
simplex 287.2
symptomatica 287.0
telangiectasia annularis 709.1
thrombocytopenic (congenital) (essential) (hereditary) (idiopathic) (primary) (*see also* Thrombocytopenia) 287.3
neonatal, transitory (*see also* Thrombocytopenia, neonatal transitory) 776.1
puerperal, postpartum 666.3
thrombotic 446.6
thrombohemolytic (*see also* Fibrinolysis) 286.6
thrombopenic (congenital) (essential) (*see also* Thrombocytopenia) 287.3
thrombotic 446.6
thrombocytic 446.6
thrombocytopenic 446.6
toxic 287.0
variolosa 050.0
vascular 287.0
visceral symptoms 287.0
Werlhof's (*see also* Purpura, thrombocytopenic) 287.3
Purpuric spots 782.7
Purulent —*see* condition
Pus
absorption, general—*see* Septicemia
in
stool 792.1
urine 599.0
tube (rupture) (*see also* Salpingo-oophoritis) 614.2
Pustular rash 782.1
Pustule 686.9
malignant 022.0
nonmalignant 686.9
Putnam's disease (subacute combined sclerosis with pernicious anemia) 281.0 *[336.2]*
Putnam-Dana syndrome (subacute combined sclerosis with pernicious anemia) 281.0 *[336.2]*
Putrefaction, intestinal 569.89
Putrescent pulp (dental) 522.1
Pyarthritis —*see* Pyarthrosis
Pyarthrosis (*see also* Arthritis, pyogenic) 711.0
tuberculous—*see* Tuberculosis, joint
Pycnoepilepsy, pycnolepsy (idiopathic) (*see also* Epilepsy) 345.0
Pyelectasia 593.89
Pyelectasis 593.89
Pyelitis (congenital) (uremic) 590.80
with
abortion—*see* Abortion, by type, with specified complication NEC
calculus or stones 592.9
contracted kidney 590.00
ectopic pregnancy (*see also* categories 633.0-633.9) 639.8
molar pregnancy (*see also* categories 630-632) 639.8
acute 590.10
with renal medullary necrosis 590.11
chronic 590.00
with
calculus 592.9
renal medullary necrosis 590.01
complicating pregnancy, childbirth, or puerperium 646.6
affecting fetus or newborn 760.1
cystica 590.3
following
abortion 639.8
ectopic or molar pregnancy 639.8
gonococcal 098.19
chronic or duration of 2 months or over 098.39
tuberculous (*see also* Tuberculosis) 016.0 *[590.81]*
Pyelocaliectasis 593.89
Pyelocystitis (*see also* Pyelitis) 590.80
Pyelohydronephrosis 591
Pyelonephritis (*see also* Pyelitis) 590.80
acute 590.10
with renal medullary necrosis 590.11
calculous 592.9
chronic 590.00
syphilitic (late) 095.4
tuberculous (*see also* Tuberculosis) 016.0 *[590.81]*
Pyelonephrosis (*see also* Pyelitis) 590.80
chronic 590.00
Pyelophlebitis 451.89
Pyelo-ureteritis cystica 590.3
Pyemia, pyemic (purulent) (*see also* Septicemia) 038.9
abscess—*see* Abscess
arthritis (*see also* Arthritis, pyogenic) 711.0
Bacillus coli 038.42
embolism—*see* Embolism, pyemic
fever 038.9
infection 038.9
joint (*see also* Arthritis, pyogenic) 711.0
liver 572.1
meningococcal 036.2
newborn 771.8
phlebitis—*see* Phlebitis
pneumococcal 038.2
portal 572.1
postvaccinal 999.3
specified organism NEC 038.8
staphylococcal 038.1
streptococcal 038.0
tuberculous—*see* Tuberculosis, miliary
Pygopagus 759.4
Pykno-epilepsy, pyknolepsy (idiopathic) (*see also* Epilepsy) 345.0
Pyle (-Cohn) disease (craniometaphyseal dysplasia) 756.89
Pylephlebitis (suppurative) 572.1
Pylethrombophlebitis 572.1
Pylethrombosis 572.1
Pyloritis (*see also* Gastritis) 535.5

Pylorospasm (reflex) 537.81
congenital or infantile 750.5
neurotic 306.4
newborn 750.5
psychogenic 306.4
Pylorus, pyloric —*see* condition
Pyoarthrosis —*see* Pyarthrosis
Pyocele
mastoid 383.00
sinus (accessory) (nasal) (*see also* Sinusitis) 473.9
turbinate (bone) 473.9
urethra (*see also* Urethritis) 597.0
Pyococcal dermatitis 686.0
Pyococcide, skin 686.0
Pyocolpos (*see also* Vaginitis) 616.10
Pyocyaneus dermatitis 686.0
Pyocystitis (*see also* Cystitis) 595.9
Pyoderma, pyodermia NEC 686.0
gangrenosum 686.0
vegetans 686.8
Pyodermatitis 686.0
vegetans 686.8
Pyogenic —*see* condition
Pyohemia —*see* Septicemia
Pyohydronephrosis (*see also* Pyelitis) 590.80
Pyometra 615.9
Pyometritis (*see also* Endometritis) 615.9
Pyometrium (*see also* Endometritis) 615.9
Pyomyositis 728.0
ossificans 728.19
tropical (bungpagga) 040.81
Pyonephritis (*see also* Pyelitis) 590.80
chronic 590.00
Pyonephrosis (congenital) (*see also* Pyelitis) 590.80
acute 590.10
Pyo-oophoritis (*see also* Salpingo-oophoritis) 614.2
Pyo-ovarium (*see also* Salpingo-oophoritis) 614.2
Pyopericarditis 420.99
Pyopericardium 420.99
Pyophlebitis —*see* Phlebitis
Pyopneumopericardium 420.99
Pyopneumothorax (infectional) 510.9
with fistula 510.0
subdiaphragmatic (*see also* Peritonitis) 567.2
subphrenic (*see also* Peritonitis) 567.2
tuberculous (*see also* Tuberculosis, pleura) 012.0
Pyorrhea (alveolar) (alveolaris) 523.4
degenerative 523.5
Pyosalpingitis (*see also* Salpingo-oophoritis) 614.2
Pyosalpinx (*see also* Salpingo-oophoritis) 614.2
Pyosepticemia —*see* Septicemia
Pyosis
Corlett's (impetigo) 684
Manson's (pemphigus contagiosus) 684
Pyothorax 510.9
with fistula 510.0
tuberculous (*see also* Tuberculosis, pleura) 012.0
Pyoureter 593.89
tuberculous (*see also* Tuberculosis) 016.2
Pyramidopallidonigral syndrome 332.0
Pyrexia (of unknown origin) (P.U.O.) 780.6
atmospheric 992.0
during labor 659.2
environmentally-induced
newborn 778.4
heat 992.0
newborn, environmentally-induced 778.4
puerperal 672
Pyroglobulinemia 273.8
Pyromania 312.33
Pyrosis 787.1
Pyrroloporphyria 277.1
Pyuria (bacterial) 599.0

Q

Q fever 083.0
with pneumonia 083.0 *[484.8]*
Quadricuspid aortic valve 746.89
Quadrilateral fever 083.0
Quadriparesis —*see* Quadriplegia
Quadriplegia 344.00
with fracture, vertebra (process)—*see* Fracture, vertebra, cervical, with spinal cord injury
brain (current episode) 437.8
cerebral (current episode) 437.8
C1-C4
complete 344.01
incomplete 344.02
C5-C7
complete 344.03
incomplete 344.04
congenital or infantile (cerebral) (spastic) (spinal) 343.2
cortical 437.8
embolic (current episode) (*see also* Embolism, brain) 434.1
infantile (cerebral) (spastic) (spinal) 343.2
newborn NEC 767.0
specified NEC 344.09
thrombotic (current episode) (*see also* Thrombosis, brain) 434.0
traumatic—*see* Injury, spinal, cervical
Quadruplet
affected by maternal complications of pregnancy 761.5
healthy liveborn—*see* Newborn, multiple
pregnancy (complicating delivery) NEC 651.8
with fetal loss and retention of one or more fetus(es) 651.5
Quarrelsomeness 301.3
Quartan
fever 084.2
malaria (fever) 084.2
Queensland fever 083.0
coastal 083.0
seven-day 100.89
Quervain's disease 727.04
thyroid (subacute granulomatous thyroiditis) 245.1
Queyrat's erythroplasia (M8080/2)
specified site—*see* Neoplasm, skin, in situ
unspecified site 233.5
Quincke's disease or edema —*see* Edema, angioneurotic
Quinquaud's disease (acne decalvans) 704.09
Quinsy (gangrenous) 475
Quintan fever 083.1
Quintuplet
affected by maternal complications of pregnancy 761.5
healthy liveborn—*see* Newborn, multiple
pregnancy (complicating delivery) NEC 651.2
with fetal loss and retention of one or more fetus(es) 651.6
Quotidian
fever 084.0
malaria (fever) 084.0

R

Rabbia 071
Rabbit fever (*see also* Tularemia) 021.9
Rabies 071
contact V01.5
exposure to V01.5
inoculation V04.5
reaction—*see* Complications, vaccination
vaccination, prophylactic (against) V04.5
Rachischisis (*see also* Spina bifida) 741.9
Rachitic —*see also* condition
deformities of spine 268.1
pelvis 268.1
with disproportion (fetopelvic) 653.2
affecting fetus or newborn 763.1
causing obstructed labor 660.1
affecting fetus or newborn 763.1
Rachitis, rachitism —*see also* Rickets
acute 268.0
fetalis 756.4
renalis 588.0
tarda 268.0
Racket nail 757.5
Radial nerve —*see* condition
Radiation effects or sickness —*see also* Effect, adverse, radiation
cataract 366.46
dermatitis 692.82
sunburn 692.71
Radiculitis (pressure) (vertebrogenic) 729.2
accessory nerve 723.4
anterior crural 724.4
arm 723.4
brachial 723.4
cervical NEC 723.4
due to displacement of intervertebral disc—*see* Neuritis, due to, displacement intervertebral disc
leg 724.4
lumbar NEC 724.4
lumbosacral 724.4
rheumatic 729.2
syphilitic 094.89
thoracic (with visceral pain) 724.4
Radiculomyelitis 357.0
toxic, due to
Clostridium tetani 037
Corynebacterium diphtheriae 032.89
Radiculopathy (*see also* Radiculitis) 729.2
Radioactive substances, adverse effect —*see* Effect, adverse, radioactive substance
Radiodermal burns (acute) (chronic) (occupational)—*see* Burn, by site
Radiodermatitis 692.82
Radionecrosis —*see* Effect, adverse, radiation
Radiotherapy session V58.0
Radium, adverse effect —*see* Effect, adverse, radioactive substance
Raeder-Harbitz syndrome (pulseless disease) 446.7
Rage (*see also* Disturbance, conduct) 312.0
meaning rabies 071
Rag sorters' disease 022.1
Raillietiniasis 123.8
Railroad neurosis 300.16
Railway spine 300.16
Raised —*see* Elevation
Raiva 071
Rake teeth, tooth 524.3

Rales 786.7
Ramifying renal pelvis 753.3
Ramsay Hunt syndrome (herpetic geniculate ganglionitis) 053.11
meaning dyssynergia cerebellaris myoclonica 334.2
Ranke's primary infiltration (*see also* Tuberculosis) 010.0
Ranula 527.6
congenital 750.26
Rape (*see also* nature and site of injury) 959.9
alleged, observation or examination V71.5
Rapid
feeble pulse, due to shock, following injury 958.4
heart (beat) 785.0
psychogenic 306.2
respiration 786.09
psychogenic 306.1
second stage (delivery) 661.3
affecting fetus or newborn 763.6
time-zone change syndrome 307.45
Rarefaction, bone 733.99
Rash 782.1
canker 034.1
diaper 691.0
drug (internal use) 693.0
contact 692.3
ECHO 9 virus 078.89
enema 692.89
food (*see also* Allergy, food) 693.1
heat 705.1
napkin 691.0
nettle 708.8
pustular 782.1
rose 782.1
epidemic 056.9
of infants 057.8
scarlet 034.1
serum (prophylactic) (therapeutic) 999.5
toxic 782.1
wandering tongue 529.1
Rasmussen's aneurysm (*see also* Tuberculosis) 011.2
Rat-bite fever 026.9
due to Streptobacillus moniliformis 026.1
spirochetal (morsus muris) 026.0
Rathke's pouch tumor (M9350/1) 237.0
Raymond (-Céstan) syndrome 433.8
Raynaud's
disease or syndrome (paroxysmal digital cyanosis) 443.0
gangrene (symmetric) 443.0 *[785.4]*
phenomenon (paroxysmal digital cyanosis) (secondary) 443.0
RDS 769
Reaction
acute situational maladjustment (*see also* Reaction, adjustment) 309.9
adaptation (*see also* Reaction, adjustment) 309.9
adjustment 309.9
with
anxious mood 309.24
with depressed mood 309.28
conduct disturbance 309.3
combined with disturbance of emotions 309.4
depressed mood 309.0
brief 309.0
with anxious mood 309.28
prolonged 309.1
Reaction—*continued*
elective mutism 309.83
mixed emotions and conduct 309.4
mutism, elective 309.83
physical symptoms 309.82
predominant disturbance (of)
conduct 309.3
emotions NEC 309.29
mixed 309.28
mixed, emotions and conduct 309.4
specified type NEC 309.89
specific academic or work inhibition 309.23
withdrawal 309.83
depressive 309.0
with conduct disturbance 309.4
brief 309.0
prolonged 309.1
specified type NEC 309.89
affective (*see also* Psychosis, affective) 296.90
specified type NEC 296.99
aggressive 301.3
unsocialized (*see also* Disturbance, conduct) 312.0
allergic (*see also* Allergy) 995.3
drug, medicinal substance, and biological—*see* Allergy, drug
food—*see* Allergy, food
serum 999.5
anaphylactic—*see* Shock, anaphylactic
anesthesia—*see* Anesthesia, complication
anger 312.0
antisocial 301.7
antitoxin (prophylactic) (therapeutic)—*see* Complications, vaccination
anxiety 300.00
asthenic 300.5
compulsive 300.3
conversion (anesthetic) (autonomic) (hyperkinetic) (mixed paralytic) (paresthetic) 300.11
deoxyribonuclease (DNA) (DNase) hypersensitivity NEC 287.2
depressive 300.4
acute 309.0
affective (*see also* Psychosis, affective) 296.2
recurrent episode 296.3
single episode 296.2
brief 309.0
manic (*see also* Psychosis, affective) 296.80
neurotic 300.4
psychoneurotic 300.4
psychotic 298.0
dissociative 300.15
drug NEC (*see also* Table of drugs and chemicals) 995.2
allergic—*see* Allergy, drug
correct substance properly administered 995.2
obstetric anesthetic or analgesic NEC 668.9
affecting fetus or newborn 763.5
specified drug—*see* Table of drugs and chemicals
overdose or poisoning 977.9
specified drug—*see* Table of drugs and chemicals
specific to newborn 779.4
transmitted via placenta or breast milk—*see* Absorption, drug, through placenta
withdrawal NEC 292.0
infant of dependent mother 779.5

Reaction—*continued*
wrong substance given or taken in error 977.9
specified drug—*see* Table of drugs and chemicals
dyssocial 301.7
erysipeloid 027.1
fear 300.20
child 313.0
fluid loss, cerebrospinal 349.0
food—*see also* Allergy, food
anaphylactic shock—*see* Anaphylactic shock, due to food
foreign
body NEC 728.82
in operative wound (inadvertently left) 998.4
due to surgical material intentionally left—*see* Complications, due to (presence of) any device, implant, or graft classified to 996.0-996.5 NEC
substance accidentally left during a procedure (chemical) (powder) (talc) 998.7
body or object (instrument) (sponge) (swab) 998.4
graft-versus-host (GVH) 996.85
grief (acute) (brief) 309.0
prolonged 309.1
gross stress (*see also* Reaction, stress, acute) 308.9
group delinquent (*see also* Disturbance, conduct) 312.2
Herxheimer's 995.0
hyperkinetic (*see also* Hyperkinesia) 314.9
hypochondriacal 300.7
hypoglycemic, due to insulin 251.0
therapeutic misadventure 962.3
hypomanic (*see also* Psychosis, affective) 296.0
recurrent episode 296.1
single episode 296.0
hysterical 300.10
conversion type 300.11
dissociative 300.15
id (bacterial cause) 692.89
immaturity NEC 301.89
aggressive 301.3
emotional instability 301.59
immunization—*see* Complications, vaccination
incompatibility
blood group (ABO) (infusion) (transfusion) 999.6
Rh (factor) (infusion) (transfusion) 999.7
inflammatory—*see* Infection
infusion—*see* Complications, infusion
inoculation (immune serum)—*see* Complications, vaccination
insulin 995.2
involutional
paranoid 297.2
psychotic (*see also* Psychosis, affective, depressive) 296.2
leukemoid (lymphocytic) (monocytic) (myelocytic) 288.8
LSD (*see also* Abuse, drugs, nondependent) 305.3
lumbar puncture 349.0
manic-depressive (*see also* Psychosis, affective) 296.80
depressed 296.2
recurrent episode 296.3
single episode 296.2
hypomanic 296.0
neurasthenic 300.5

Reaction—*continued*
neurogenic (*see also* Neurosis) 300.9
neurotic NEC 300.9
neurotic-depressive 300.4
nitritoid—*see* Crisis, nitritoid
obsessive (-compulsive) 300.3
organic 293.9
acute 293.0
subacute 293.1
overanxious, child or adolescent 313.0
paranoid (chronic) 297.9
acute 298.3
climacteric 297.2
involutional 297.2
menopausal 297.2
senile 290.20
simple 297.0
passive
aggressive 301.84
dependency 301.6
personality (*see also* Disorder, personality) 301.9
phobic 300.20
postradiation—*see* Effect, adverse, radiation
psychogenic NEC 300.9
psychoneurotic (*see also* Neurosis) 300.9
anxiety 300.00
compulsive 300.3
conversion 300.11
depersonalization 300.6
depressive 300.4
dissociative 300.15
hypochondriacal 300.7
hysterical 300.10
conversion type 300.11
dissociative type 300.15
neurasthenic 300.5
obsessive 300.3
obsessive-compulsive 300.3
phobic 300.20
tension state 300.9
psychophysiologic NEC (*see also* Disorder, psychosomatic) 306.9
cardiovascular 306.2
digestive 306.4
endocrine 306.6
gastrointestinal 306.4
genitourinary 306.50
heart 306.2
hemic 306.8
intestinal (large) (small) 306.4
laryngeal 306.1
lymphatic 306.8
musculoskeletal 306.0
pharyngeal 306.1
respiratory 306.1
skin 306.3
special sense organs 306.7
psychosomatic (*see also* Disorder, psychosomatic) 306.9
psychotic (*see also* Psychosis) 298.9
depressive 298.0
due to or associated with physical condition (*see also* Psychosis, organic) 294.9
involutional (*see also* Psychosis, affective) 296.2
recurrent episode 296.3
single episode 296.2
pupillary (myotonic) (tonic) 379.46
radiation—*see* Effect, adverse, radiation

Reaction—*continued*
runaway—*see also* Disturbance, conduct
socialized 312.2
undersocialized, unsocialized 312.1
scarlet fever toxin—*see* Complications, vaccination
schizophrenic (*see also* Schizophrenia) 295.9
latent 295.5
serological for syphilis—*see* Serology for syphilis
serum (prophylactic) (therapeutic) 999.5
immediate 999.4
situational (*see also* Reaction, adjustment) 309.9
acute, to stress 308.3
adjustment (*see also* Reaction, adjustment) 309.9
somatization (*see also* Disorder, psychosomatic) 306.9
spinal puncture 349.0
spite, child (*see also* Disturbance, conduct) 312.0
stress, acute 308.9
with predominant disturbance (of)
consciousness 308.1
emotions 308.0
mixed 308.4
psychomotor 308.2
specified type NEC 308.3
surgical procedure—*see* Complications, surgical procedure
tetanus antitoxin—*see* Complications, vaccination
toxin-antitoxin—*see* Complications, vaccination
transfusion (blood) (bone marrow) (lymphocytes) (allergic)—*see* Complications, transfusion
tuberculin skin test, nonspecific (without active tuberculosis) 795.5
positive (without active tuberculosis) 795.5
ultraviolet—*see* Effect, adverse, ultraviolet
undersocialized, unsocialized—*see also* Disturbance, conduct
aggressive (type) 312.0
unaggressive (type) 312.1
vaccination (any)—*see* Complications, vaccination
white graft (skin) 996.52
withdrawing, child or adolescent 313.22
x-ray—*see* Effect, adverse, x-rays
Reactive depression (*see also* Reaction, depressive) 300.4
neurotic 300.4
psychoneurotic 300.4
psychotic 298.0
Rebound tenderness 789.6
Recalcitrant patient V15.81
Recanalization, thrombus —*see* Thrombosis
Recession, receding
chamber angle (eye) 364.77
chin 524.06
gingival (generalized) (localized) (postinfective) (postoperative) 523.2
Recklinghausen's disease (M9540/1) 237.71
bones (osteitis fibrosa cystica) 252.0
Recklinghausen-Applebaum disease (hemochromatosis) 275.0
Reclus' disease (cystic) 610.1
Recrudescent typhus (fever) 081.1
Recruitment, auditory 388.44
Rectalgia 569.42
Rectitis 569.49
Rectocele
female (without uterine prolapse) 618.0
with uterine prolapse 618.4
complete 618.3
incomplete 618.2
in pregnancy or childbirth 654.4
causing obstructed labor 660.2
affecting fetus or newborn 763.1
male 569.49
vagina, vaginal (outlet) 618.0
Rectosigmoiditis 569.89
ulcerative (chronic) 556.3
Rectosigmoid junction —*see* condition
Rectourethral —*see* condition
Rectovaginal —*see* condition
Rectovesical —*see* condition
Rectum, rectal —*see* condition
Recurrent —*see* condition
Red bugs 133.8
Red cedar asthma 495.8
Redness
conjunctiva 379.93
eye 379.93
nose 478.1
Reduced ventilatory or vital capacity 794.2
Reduction
function
kidney (*see also* Disease, renal) 593.9
liver 573.8
ventilatory capacity 794.2
vital capacity 794.2
Redundant, redundancy
abdomen 701.9
anus 751.5
cardia 537.89
clitoris 624.2
colon (congenital) 751.5
foreskin (congenital) 605
intestine 751.5
labia 624.3
organ or site, congenital NEC—*see* Accessory
panniculus (abdominal) 278.1
prepuce (congenital) 605
pylorus 537.89
rectum 751.5
scrotum 608.89
sigmoid 751.5
skin (of face) 701.9
eyelids 374.30
stomach 537.89
uvula 528.9
vagina 623.8
Reduplication —*see* Duplication
Referral
adoption (agency) V68.89
nursing care V63.8
patient without examination or treatment V68.81
social services V63.8
Reflex —*see also* condition
blink, deficient 374.45
hyperactive gag 478.29
neurogenic bladder NEC 596.54
atonic 596.54
with cauda equina syndrome 344.61
vasoconstriction 443.9
vasovagal 780.2
Reflux
esophageal 530.81
esophagitis 530.11
gastroesophageal 530.81
mitral—*see* Insufficiency, mitral

Reflux—*continued*
ureteral —*see* Reflux, vesicoureteral
vesicoureteral 593.70
with
reflux nephropathy 593.73
bilateral 593.72
unilateral 593.71
Reformed gallbladder 576.0
Reforming, artificial openings (*see also* Attention to, artificial, opening) V55.9
Refractive error (*see also* Error, refractive) 367.9
Refsum's disease or syndrome (heredopathia atactica polyneuritiformis) 356.3
Refusal of
food 307.59
hysterical 300.11
treatment because of, due to
patient's decision NEC V64.2
reason of conscience or religion V62.6
Regaud
tumor (M8082/3)—*see* Neoplasm, nasopharynx, malignant
type carcinoma (M8082/3)—*see* Neoplasm, nasopharynx, malignant
Regional —*see* condition
Regulation feeding (elderly) (infant) 783.3
newborn 779.3
Regurgitated
food, choked on 933.1
stomach contents, choked on 933.1
Regurgitation
aortic (valve) (*see also* Insufficiency, aortic) 424.1
congenital 746.4
syphilitic 093.22
food—*see also* Vomiting
with reswallowing—*see* Rumination
newborn 779.3
gastric contents—*see* Vomiting
heart—*see* Endocarditis
mitral (valve)—*see also* Insufficiency, mitral
congenital 746.6
myocardial—*see* Endocarditis
pulmonary (heart) (valve) (*see also* Endocarditis, pulmonary) 424.3
stomach—*see* Vomiting
tricuspid—*see* Endocarditis, tricuspid
valve, valvular—*see* Endocarditis
vesicoureteral —*see* Reflux, vesicoureteral
Rehabilitation V57.9
multiple types V57.89
occupational V57.21
specified type NEC V57.89
speech V57.3
vocational V57.22
Reichmann's disease or syndrome (gastrosuccorrhea) 536.8
Reifenstein's syndrome (hereditary familial hypogonadism, male) 257.2
Reilly's syndrome or phenomenon (*see also* Neuropathy, peripheral, autonomic) 337.9
Reimann's periodic disease 277.3
Reinsertion, contraceptive device V25.42
Reiter's disease, syndrome, or urethritis 099.3
Rejection
food, hysterical 300.11
transplant 996.80
bone marrow 996.85
corneal 996.51

Rejection—*continued*
organ (immune or nonimmune cause) 996.80
bone marrow 996.85
heart 996.83
intestines 996.89
kidney 996.81
liver 996.82
lung 996.84
pancreas 996.86
specified NEC 996.89
skin 996.52
Relapsing fever 087.9
Carter's (Asiatic) 087.0
Dutton's (West African) 087.1
Koch's 087.9
louse-borne (epidemic) 087.0
Novy's (American) 087.1
Obermeyer's (European) 087.0
Spirillum 087.9
tick-borne (endemic) 087.1
Relaxation
anus (sphincter) 569.49
due to hysteria 300.11
arch (foot) 734
congenital 754.61
back ligaments 728.4
bladder (sphincter) 596.59
cardio-esophageal 530.89
cervix (*see also* Incompetency, cervix) 622.5
diaphragm 519.4
inguinal rings—*see* Hernia, inguinal
joint (capsule) (ligament) (paralytic) (*see also* Derangement, joint) 718.90
congenital 755.8
lumbosacral joint 724.6
pelvic floor 618.8
pelvis 618.8
perineum 618.8
posture 729.9
rectum (sphincter) 569.49
sacroiliac (joint) 724.6
scrotum 608.89
urethra (sphincter) 599.84
uterus (outlet) 618.8
vagina (outlet) 618.8
vesical 596.59
Remains
canal of Cloquet 743.51
capsule (opaque) 743.51
Remittent fever (malarial) 084.6
Remnant
canal of Cloquet 743.51
capsule (opaque) 743.51
cervix, cervical stump (acquired) (postoperative) 622.8
cystic duct, postcholecystectomy 576.0
fingernail 703.8
congenital 757.5
meniscus, knee 717.5
thyroglossal duct 759.2
tonsil 474.8
infected 474.0
urachus 753.7
Remote effect of cancer —*see* Condition
Removal (of)
catheter (urinary) (indwelling) V53.6
from artificial opening—*see* Attention to, artificial, opening
non-vascular V58.82
vascular V58.81

Removal (of)—*continued*
device—*see also* Fitting (of)
contraceptive V25.42
fixation
external V54.8
internal V54.0
traction V54.8
dressing V58.3
ileostomy V55.2
Kirschner wire V54.8
pin V54.0
plaster cast V54.8
plate (fracture) V54.0
rod V54.0
screw V54.0
splint, external V54.8
subdermal implantable contraceptive V25.43
suture V58.3
traction device, external V54.8
vascular catheter V58.81
Ren
arcuatus 753.3
mobile, mobilis (*see also* Disease, renal) 593.0
congenital 753.3
unguliformis 753.3
Renal —*see also* condition
glomerulohyalinosis-diabetic syndrome 250.4 *[581.81]*
Rendu-Osler-Weber disease or syndrome (familial hemorrhagic telangiectasia) 448.0
Reninoma (M8361/1) 236.91
Rénon-Delille syndrome 253.8
Repair
pelvic floor, previous, in pregnancy or childbirth 654.4
affecting fetus or newborn 763.8
scarred tissue V51
Replacement by artificial or mechanical device or prosthesis of (*see also* Fitting (of))
bladder V43.5
blood vessel V43.4
breast V43.82
eye globe V43.0
heart V43.2
valve V43.3
intestine V43.89
joint V43.60
ankle 43.66
elbow V43.62
finger V43.69
hip (partial) (total) V43.64
knee V43.65
shoulder V43.61
specified NEC V43.69
wrist V43.63
kidney V43.89
larynx V43.81
lens V43.1
limb(s) V43.7
liver V43.89
lung V43.89
organ NEC V43.89
pancreas V43.89
tissue NEC V43.89
Reprogramming
cardiac pacemaker V53.31
Request for expert evidence V68.2
Reserve, decreased or low
cardiac—*see* Disease, heart
kidney (*see also* Disease, renal) 593.9
Residual —*see also* condition
bladder 596.8
foreign body—*see* Retention, foreign body
state, schizophrenic (*see also* Schizophrenia) 295.6
urine 788.69
Resistance, resistant (to)

Note—Use the following subclassification for categories V09.5, V09.7, V09.8, V09.9.:

0 without mention of resistance to multiple drugs
1 with resistance to multiple drugs

V09.5 quinolones and fluoroquinolones
V09.7 antimycobacterial agents
V09.8 specified drugs NEC
V09.9 unspecified drugs

9 multiple sites

drugs by microorganisms V09.9
Amikacin V09.4
aminoglycosides V09.4
Amodiaquine V09.5
Amoxicillin V09.0
Ampicillin V09.0
antimycobacterial agents V09.7
Azithromycin V09.2
Azlocillin V09.0
Aztreonam V09.1
B-lactam antibiotics V09.1
Bacampicillin V09.0
Bacitracin V09.8
Benznidazole V09.8
Capreomycin V09.7
Carbenicillin V09.0
Cefaclor V09.1
Cefadroxil V09.1
Cefamandole V09.1
Cefatetan V09.1
Cefazolin V09.1
Cefixime V09.1
Cefonicid V09.1
Cefoperazone V09.1
Ceforanide V09.1
Cefotaxime V09.1
Cefoxitin V09.1
Ceftazidine V09.1
Ceftizoxime V09.1
Ceftriaxone V09.1
Cefuroxime V09.1
Cephalexin V09.1
Cephaloglycin V09.1
Cephaloridine V09.1
cephalosporins V09.1
Cephalothin V09.1
Cephapirin V09.1
Cephradine V09.1
Chloramphenicol V09.8
Chloraquine V09.5
Chlorguanide V09.8
Chlorproguanil V09.8
Chlortetracycline V09.3
Cinoxacin V09.5
Ciprofloxacin V09.5
Clarithromycin V09.2
Clindamycin V09.8
Clioquinol V09.5
Clofazimine V09.7
Cloxacillin V09.0

Resistance, resistant (to)—*continued*
Cyclacillin V09.0
Cycloserine V09.7
Dapsone [DZ] V09.7
Demeclocycline V09.3
Dicloxacillin V09.0
Doxycycline V09.3
Enoxacin V09.5
Erythromycin V09.2
Ethambutol [EMB] V09.7
Ethionamide [ETA] V09.7
fluoroquinolones NEC V09.5
Gentamicin V09.4
Halofantrine V09.8
ImipenemV09.1
Iodoquinol V09.5
Isoniazid [INH] V09.7
Kanamycin V09.4
macrolides V09.2
Mafenide V09.6
Mefloquine V09.8
Melassoprol V09.8
Methacillin V09.0
Methacycline V09.3
Methenamine V09.8
Metronidazole V09.8
Mezlocillin V09.0
Minocycline V09.3
Nafcillin V09.0
Nalidixic Acid V09.5
Natamycin V09.2
Neomycin V09.4
Netilmicin V09.4
Nimorazole V09.8
Nitrofurantoin V09.8
Nitrofurtimox V09.8
Norfloxacin V09.5
Nystatin V09.2
Ofloxacin V09.5
Oleandomycin V09.2
Oxacillin V09.0
Oxytetracycline V09.3
Para-amino salicylic acid [PAS] V09.7
Paromomycin V09.4
Penicillin (G)(V)(VK) V09.0
penicillins V09.0
Pentamidine V09.8
Piperacillin V09.0
Primaquine V09.5
Proguanil V09.8
Pyrazinamide [PZA] V09.7
Pyrimethamine/Sulfalene V09.8
Pyrimethamine/Sulfodoxine V09.8
Quinacrine V09.5
Quinidine V09.8
Quinine V09.8
quinolones V09.5
Rifabutin V09.7
Rifampin [RIF] V09.7
Rifamycin V09.7
Rolitetracycline V09.3
specified drugs NEC V09.8
Spectinomycin V09.8
Spiramycin V09.2
Streptomycin [SM] V09.4
Sulfacetamide V09.6
Sulfacytine V90.6
Sulfadiazine V09.6
Sulfadoxine V09.6
Sulfamethoxazole V09.6
Sulfapyridine V09.6

Resistance, resistant (to)—*continued*
Sulfasalizine V09.6
Sulfasoxazole V09.6
sulfonamides V09.6
Sulfoxone V09.7
Tetracycline V09.3
tetracyclines V09.3
Thiamphenicol V09.8
Ticarcillin V09.0
Tinidazole V09.8
Tobramycin V09.4
Triamphenicol V09.8
Trimethoprim V09.8
Vancomycin V09.8

Resorption
biliary 576.8
purulent or putrid (*see also* Cholecystitis) 576.8
dental (roots) 521.4
alveoli 525.8
septic—*see* Septicemia
teeth (external) (internal) (pathological) (roots) 521.4

Respiration
asymmetrical 786.09
bronchial 786.09
Cheyne-Stokes (periodic respiration) 786.09
decreased, due to shock following injury 958.4
disorder of 786.00
psychogenic 306.1
specified NEC 786.09
failure 518.81
newborn 770.8
insufficiency 786.09
acute 518.82
newborn NEC 770.8
Kussmaul (air hunger) 786.09
painful 786.52
periodic 786.09
poor 786.09
newborn NEC 770.8
sighing 786.7
psychogenic 306.1
wheezing 786.09

Respiratory —*see also* condition
distress 786.09
acute 518.82
fetus or newborn NEC 770.8
syndrome (newborn) 769
adult (following shock, surgery, or trauma) 518.5
specified NEC 518.82
failure (acute) (chronic) 518.81

Response
photoallergic 692.72
phototoxic 692.72

Rest, rests
mesonephric duct 752.8
fallopian tube 752.11
ovarian, in fallopian tubes 752.19
wolffian duct 752.8

Restless leg (syndrome) 333.99

Restlessness 799.2

Restoration of organ continuity from previous sterilization (tuboplasty) (vasoplasty) V26.0

Restriction of housing space V60.1

Restzustand, schizophrenic (*see also* Schizophrenia) 295.6

Retained —*see* Retention

Retardation
development, developmental, specific (*see also* Disorder, development, specific) 315.9
learning, specific 315.2
arithmetical 315.1
language (skills) 315.31
expressive 315.31
mixed receptive-expressive 315.31
mathematics 315.1
reading 315.00
phonological 315.39
written expression 315.2
motor 315.4
endochondral bone growth 733.91
growth (physical) 783.4
due to malnutrition 263.2
fetal (intrauterine) 764.9
affecting management of pregnancy 656.5
intrauterine growth 764.9
affecting management of pregnancy 656.5
mental 319
borderline V62.89
mild, IQ 50-70 317
moderate, IQ 35-49 318.0
profound, IQ under 20 318.2
severe, IQ 20-34 318.1
motor, specific 315.4
physical 783.4
child 783.4
due to malnutrition 263.2
fetus (intrauterine) 764.9
affecting management of pregnancy 656.5
psychomotor NEC 307.9
reading 315.00
Retching —*see* Vomiting
Retention, retained
bladder NEC (*see also* Retention, urine) 788.20
psychogenic 306.53
carbon dioxide 276.2
cyst—*see* Cyst
dead
fetus (after 22 completed weeks gestation) 656.4
early fetal death (before 22 completed weeks gestation) 632
ovum 631
decidua (following delivery) (fragments) (with hemorrhage) 666.2
without hemorrhage 667.1
deciduous tooth 520.6
dental root 525.3
fecal (*see also* Constipation) 564.0
fluid 276.6
foreign body—*see also* Foreign body, retained
bone 733.99
current trauma—*see* Foreign body, by site or type
middle ear 385.83
muscle 729.6
soft tissue NEC 729.6
gastric 536.8
membranes (following delivery) (with hemorrhage) 666.2
with abortion—*see* Abortion, by type
without hemorrhage 667.1
menses 626.8
milk (puerperal) 676.2
nitrogen, extrarenal 788.9

Retention, retained—*continued*
placenta (total) (with hemorrhage) 666.0
with abortion—*see* Abortion, by type
portions or fragments 666.2
without hemorrhage 667.1
without hemorrhage 667.0
products of conception
early pregnancy (fetal death before 22 completed weeks gestation) 632
following
abortion—*see* Abortion, by type
delivery 666.2
with hemorrhage 666.2
without hemorrhage 667.1
secundines (following delivery) (with hemorrhage) 666.2
with abortion—*see* Abortion, by type
complicating puerperium (delayed hemorrhage) 666.2
without hemorrhage 667.1
smegma, clitoris 624.8
urine NEC 788.20
bladder, incomplete emptying 788.21
psychogenic 306.53
specified NEC 788.29
water (in tissue) (*see also* Edema) 782.3
Reticulation, dust (occupational) 504
Reticulocytosis NEC 790.99
Reticuloendotheliosis
acute infantile (M9722/3) 202.5
leukemic (M9940/3) 202.4
malignant (M9720/3) 202.3
nonlipid (M9722/3) 202.5
Reticulohistiocytoma (giant cell) 277.8
Reticulohistiocytosis, multicentric 272.8
Reticulolymphosarcoma (diffuse) (M9613/3) 200.8
follicular (M9691/3) 202.0
nodular (M9691/3) 202.0
Reticulosarcoma (M9640/3) 200.0
odular (M9642/3) 200.0
pleomorphic cell type (M9641/3) 200.0
Reticulosis (skin)
acute of infancy (M9722/3) 202.5
histiocytic medullary (M9721/3) 202.3
lipomelanotic 695.89
malignant (M9720/3) 202.3
Sézary's (M9701/3) 202.2
Retina, retinal —*see* condition
Retinitis (*see also* Chorioretinitis) 363.20
albuminurica 585 *[363.10]*
arteriosclerotic 440.8 *[362.13]*
central angiospastic 362.41
Coat's 362.12
diabetic 250.5 *[362.01]*
disciformis 362.52
disseminated 363.10
metastatic 363.14
neurosyphilitic 094.83
pigment epitheliopathy 363.15
exudative 362.12
focal 363.00
in histoplasmosis 115.92
capsulatum 115.02
duboisii 115.12
juxtapapillary 363.05
macular 363.06
paramacular 363.06
peripheral 363.08
posterior pole NEC 363.07
gravidarum 646.8

Rhabdomyoma—*continued*
fetal (M8903/0)—*see* Neoplasm, connective tissue, benign
glycogenic (M8904/0)—*see* Neoplasm, connective tissue, benign
Rhabdomyosarcoma (M8900/3)—*see also* Neoplasm connective tissue, malignant
alveolar (M8920/3)—*see* Neoplasm, connective tissue, malignant
embryonal (M8910/3)—*see* Neoplasm, connective tissue malignant
mixed type (M8902/3)—*see* Neoplasm, connective tissue, malignant
pleomorphic (M8901/3)—*see* Neoplasm, connective tissue, malignant
Rhabdosarcoma (M8900/3)—*see* Rhabdomyosarcoma
Rhesus (factor) (Rh) incompatibility—*see* Rh, incompatibility
Rheumaticosis —*see* Rheumatism
Rheumatism, rheumatic (acute NEC) 729.0
adherent pericardium 393
arthritis
acute or subacute—*see* Fever, rheumatic
chronic 714.0
spine 720.0
articular (chronic) NEC (*see also* Arthritis) 716.9
acute or subacute—*see* Fever, rheumatic
back 724.9
blennorrhagic 098.59
carditis—*see* Disease, heart, rheumatic
cerebral—*see* Fever, rheumatic
chorea (acute)—*see* Chorea, rheumatic
chronic NEC 729.0
coronary arteritis 391.9
chronic 398.99
degeneration, myocardium (*see also* Degeneration, myocardium, with rheumatic fever) 398.0
desert 114.0
febrile—*see* Fever, rheumatic
fever—*see* Fever, rheumatic
gonococcal 098.59
gout 274.0
heart
disease (*see also* Disease, heart, rheumatic) 398.90
failure (chronic) (congestive) (inactive) 398.91
hemopericardium—*see* Rheumatic, pericarditis
hydropericardium—*see* Rheumatic, pericarditis
inflammatory (acute) (chronic) (subacute)—*see* Fever, rheumatic
intercostal 729.0
meaning Tietze's disease 733.6
joint (chronic) NEC (*see also* Arthritis) 716.9
acute—*see* Fever, rheumatic
mediastinopericarditis—*see* Rheumatic, pericarditis
muscular 729.0
myocardial degeneration (*see also* Degeneration, myocardium, with rheumatic fever) 398.0
myocarditis (chronic) (inactive) (with chorea) 398.0
active or acute 391.2
with chorea (acute) (rheumatic) (Sydenham's) 392.0
myositis 729.1
neck 724.9
neuralgic 729.0

Rheumatism, rheumatic—*continued*
neuritis (acute) (chronic) 729.2
neuromuscular 729.0
nodose—*see* Arthritis, nodosa
nonarticular 729.0
palindromic 719.30
ankle 719.37
elbow 719.32
foot 719.37
hand 719.34
hip 719.35
knee 719.36
multiple sites 719.39
pelvic region 719.35
shoulder (region) 719.31
specified site NEC 719.38
wrist 719.33
pancarditis, acute 391.8
with chorea (acute) (rheumatic) (Sydenham's) 392.0
chronic or inactive 398.99
pericarditis (active) (acute) (with effusion) (with pneumonia) 391.0
with chorea (acute) (rheumatic) (Sydenham's) 392.0
chronic or inactive 393
pericardium—*see* Rheumatic, pericarditis
pleuropericarditis—*see* Rheumatic, pericarditis
pneumonia 390 *[517.1]*
pneumonitis 390 *[517.1]*
pneumopericarditis—*see* Rheumatic, pericarditis
polyarthritis
acute or subacute—*see* Fever, rheumatic
chronic 714.0
polyarticular NEC (*see also* Arthritis) 716.9
psychogenic 306.0
radiculitis 729.2
sciatic 724.3
septic—*see* Fever, rheumatic
spine 724.9
subacute NEC 729.0
torticollis 723.5
tuberculous NEC (*see also* Tuberculosis) 015.9
typhoid fever 002.0
Rheumatoid —*see also* condition
lungs 714.81
Rhinitis (atrophic) (catarrhal) (chronic) (croupous) (fibrinous) (hyperplastic) (hypertrophic) (membranous) (purulent) (suppurative) (ulcerative) 472.0
with
hay fever (*see also* Fever, hay) 477.9
with asthma (bronchial) 493.0
sore throat—*see* Nasopharyngitis
acute 460
allergic (nonseasonal) (seasonal) (*see also* Fever, hay) 477.9
with asthma (*see also* Asthma) 493.0
granulomatous 472.0
infective 460
obstructive 472.0
pneumococcal 460
syphilitic 095.8
congenital 090.0
tuberculous (*see also* Tuberculosis) 012.8
vasomotor (*see also* Fever, hay) 477.9
Rhinoantritis (chronic) 473.0
acute 461.0
Rhinodacryolith 375.57
Rhinolalia (aperta) (clausa) (open) 784.49

Rhinolith 478.1
nasal sinus (*see also* Sinusitis) 473.9
Rhinomegaly 478.1
Rhinopharyngitis (acute) (subacute) (*see also* Nasopharyngitis) 460
chronic 472.2
destructive ulcerating 102.5
mutilans 102.5
Rhinophyma 695.3
Rhinorrhea 478.1
cerebrospinal (fluid) 349.81
paroxysmal (*see also* Fever, hay) 477.9
spasmodic (*see also* Fever, hay) 477.9
Rhinosalpingitis 381.50
acute 381.51
chronic 381.52
Rhinoscleroma 040.1
Rhinosporidiosis 117.0
Rhinovirus infection 079.3
Rhizomelique, pseudopolyarthritic 446.5
Rhoads and Bomford anemia (refractory) 284.9
Rhus
diversiloba dermatitis 692.6
radicans dermatitis 692.6
toxicodendron dermatitis 692.6
venenata dermatitis 692.6
verniciflua dermatitis 692.6
Rhythm
atrioventricular nodal 427.89
disorder 427.9
coronary sinus 427.89
ectopic 427.89
nodal 427.89
escape 427.89
heart, abnormal 427.9
idioventricular 426.89
accelerated 427.89
nodal 427.89
sleep, inversion 780.55
nonorganic origin 307.45
Rhytidosis facialis 701.8
Rib —*see also* condition
cervical 756.2
Riboflavin deficiency 266.0
Rice bodies (*see also* Loose, body, joint) 718.1
knee 717.6
Richter's hernia —*see* Hernia, Richter's
Ricinism 988.2
Rickets (active) (acute) (adolescent) (adult) (chest wall) (congenital) (current) (infantile) (intestinal) 268.0
celiac 579.0
fetal 756.4
hemorrhagic 267
hypophosphatemic with nephrotic-glycosuric dwarfism 270.0
kidney 588.0
late effect 268.1
renal 588.0
scurvy 267
vitamin D-resistant 275.3
Rickettsial disease 083.9
specified type NEC 083.8
Rickettsialpox 083.2
Rickettsiosis NEC 083.9
specified type NEC 083.8
tick-borne 082.9
specified type NEC 082.8
vesicular 083.2
Ricord's chancre 091.0
Riddoch's syndrome (visual disorientation) 368.16
Rider's
bone 733.99
chancre 091.0
Ridge, alveolus —*see also* condition
flabby 525.2
Ridged ear 744.29
Riedel's
disease (ligneous thyroiditis) 245.3
lobe, liver 751.69
struma (ligneous thyroiditis) 245.3
thyroiditis (ligneous) 245.3
Rieger's anomaly or syndrome (mesodermal dysgenesis, anterior ocular segment) 743.44
Riehl's melanosis 709.09
Rietti-Greppi-Micheli anemia or syndrome 282.4
Rieux's hernia —*see* Hernia, Rieux's
Rift Valley fever 066.3
Riga's disease (cachectic aphthae) 529.0
Riga-Fede disease (cachectic aphthae) 529.0
Riggs' disease (compound periodontitis) 523.4
Right middle lobe syndrome 518.0
Rigid, rigidity —*see also* condition
abdominal 789.4
articular, multiple congenital 754.89
back 724.8
cervix uteri
in pregnancy or childbirth 654.6
affecting fetus or newborn 763.8
causing obstructed labor 660.2
affecting fetus or newborn 763.1
hymen (acquired) (congenital) 623.3
nuchal 781.6
pelvic floor
in pregnancy or childbirth 654.4
affecting fetus or newborn 763.8
causing obstructed labor 660.2
affecting fetus or newborn 763.1
perineum or vulva
in pregnancy or childbirth 654.8
affecting fetus or newborn 763.8
causing obstructed labor 660.2
affecting fetus or newborn 763.1
spine 724.8
vagina
in pregnancy or childbirth 654.7
affecting fetus or newborn 763.8
causing obstructed labor 660.2
affecting fetus or newborn 763.1
Rigors 780.9
Riley-Day syndrome (familial dysautonomia) 742.8
Ring (s)
aorta 747.21
Bandl's, complicating delivery 661.4
affecting fetus or newborn 763.7
contraction, complicating delivery 661.4
affecting fetus or newborn 763.7
esophageal (congenital) 750.3
Fleischer (-Kayser) (cornea) 275.1 *[371.14]*
hymenal, tight (acquired) (congenital) 623.3
Kayser-Fleischer (cornea) 275.1 *[371.14]*
retraction, uterus, pathological 661.4
affecting fetus or newborn 763.7
Schatzki's (esophagus) (congenital) (lower) 750.3
acquired 530.3
Soemmering's 366.51
trachea, abnormal 748.3
vascular (congenital) 747.21
Vossius' 921.3
late effect 366.21

Ringed hair (congenital) 757.4
Ringing in the ear (*see also* Tinnitus) 388.30
Ringworm 110.9
beard 110.0
body 110.5
Burmese 110.9
corporeal 110.5
foot 110.4
groin 110.3
hand 110.2
honeycomb 110.0
nails 110.1
perianal (area) 110.3
scalp 110.0
specified site NEC 110.8
Tokelau 110.5
Rise, venous pressure 459.89
Risk
factor —*see* Problem
suicidal 300.9
Ritter's disease (dermatitis exfoliativa neonatorum) 695.81
Rivalry, sibling 313.3
Rivalta's disease (cervicofacial actinomycosis) 039.3
River blindness 125.3 *[360.13]*
Robert's pelvis 755.69
with disproportion (fetopelvic) 653.0
affecting fetus or newborn 763.1
causing obstructed labor 660.1
affecting fetus or newborn 763.1
Robin's syndrome 756.0
Robinson's (hidrotic) ectodermal dysplasia 757.31
Robles' disease (onchocerciasis) 125.3 *[360.13]*
Rochalimea —*see* Rickettsial disease
Rocky Mountain fever (spotted) 082.0
Rodent ulcer (M8090/3)—*see also* Neoplasm, skin, malignant
cornea 370.07
Roentgen ray, adverse effect —*see* Effect, adverse, x-ray
Roetheln 056.9
Roger's disease (congenital interventricular septal defect) 745.4
Rokitansky's
disease (*see also* Necrosis, liver) 570
tumor 620.2
Rokitansky-Aschoff sinuses (mucosal outpouching of gallbladder) (*see also* Disease, gallbladder) 575.8
Rokitansky-Kuster-Hauser syndrome (congenital absence vagina) 752.49
Rollet's chancre (syphilitic) 091.0
Rolling of head 781.0
Romano-Ward syndrome (prolonged Q-T interval) 794.31
Romanus lesion 720.1
Romberg's disease or syndrome 349.89
Roof, mouth —*see* condition
Rosacea 695.3
acne 695.3
keratitis 695.3 *[370.49]*
Rosary, rachitic 268.0
Rose
cold 477.0
fever 477.0
rash 782.1
epidemic 056.9
of infants 057.8
Rosen-Castleman-Liebow syndrome (pulmonary proteinosis) 516.0
Rosenbach's erysipelatoid or erysipeloid 027.1
Rosenthal's disease (factor XI deficiency) 286.2
Roseola 057.8
infantum, infantilis 057.8
Rossbach's disease (hyperchlorhydria) 536.8
psychogenic 306.4
Rössle-Urbach-Wiethe lipoproteinosis 272.8
Ross river fever 066.3
Rostan's asthma (cardiac) (*see also* Failure, ventricular, left) 428.1
Rot
Barcoo (*see also* Ulcer, skin) 707.9
knife-grinders' (*see also* Tuberculosis) 011.4
Rot-Bernhardt disease 355.1
Rotation
anomalous, incomplete or insufficient—*see* Malrotation
cecum (congenital) 751.4
colon (congenital) 751.4
manual, affecting fetus or newborn 763.8
spine, incomplete or insufficient 737.8
tooth, teeth 524.3
vertebra, incomplete or insufficient 737.8
Röteln 056.9
Roth's disease or meralgia 355.1
Roth-Bernhardt disease or syndrome 355.1
Rothmund (-Thomson) syndrome 757.33
Rotor's disease or syndrome (idiopathic hyperbilirubinemia) 277.4
Rotundum ulcus —*see* Ulcer, stomach
Round
back (with wedging of vertebrae) 737.10
late effect of rickets 268.1
hole, retina 361.31
with detachment 361.01
ulcer (stomach)—*see* Ulcer, stomach
worms (infestation) (large) NEC 127.0
Roussy-Lévy syndrome 334.3
Routine postpartum follow-up V24.2
Roy (-Jutras) syndrome (acropachyderma) 757.39
Rubella (German measles) 056.9
complicating pregnancy, childbirth, or puerperium 647.5
complication 056.8
neurological 056.00
encephalomyelitis 056.01
specified type NEC 056.09
specified type NEC 056.79
congenital 771.0
contact V01.4
exposure to V01.4
maternal
with suspected fetal damage affecting management of pregnancy 655.3
affecting fetus or newborn 760.2
manifest rubella in infant 771.0
specified complications NEC 056.79
vaccination, prophylactic (against) V04.3
Rubeola (measles) (*see also* Measles) 055.9
complicated 055.8
meaning rubella (*see also* Rubella) 056.9
scarlatinosis 057.8
Rubeosis iridis 364.42
diabetica 250.5 *[364.42]*
Rubinstein-Taybi's syndrome (brachydactylia, short stature and mental retardation) 759.89
Rud's syndrome (mental deficiency, epilepsy, and infantilism) 759.89

Rudimentary (congenital)—*see also* Agenesis
arm 755.22
bone 756.9
cervix uteri 752.49
eye (*see also* Microphthalmos) 743.10
fallopian tube 752.19
leg 755.32
lobule of ear 744.21
patella 755.64
respiratory organs in thoracopagus 759.4
tracheal bronchus 748.3
uterine horn 752.3
uterus 752.3
in male 752.7
solid or with cavity 752.3
vagina 752.49
Ruiter-Pompen (-Wyers) syndrome (angiokeratoma corporis diffusum) 272.7
Ruled out condition (*see also* Observation, suspected) V71.9
Rumination —*see also* Vomiting
neurotic 300.3
obsessional 300.3
psychogenic 307.53
Runaway reaction —*see also* Disturbance, conduct
socialized 312.2
undersocialized, unsocialized 312.1
Runeberg's disease (progressive pernicious anemia) 281.0
Runge's syndrome (postmaturity) 766.2
Rupia 091.3
congenital 090.0
tertiary 095.9
Rupture, ruptured 553.9
abdominal viscera NEC 799.8
obstetrical trauma 665.5
abscess (spontaneous)—*see* Abscess, by site
amnion—*see* Rupture, membranes
aneurysm—*see* Aneurysm
anus (sphincter)—*see* Laceration, anus
aorta, aortic 441.5
abdominal 441.3
arch 441.1
ascending 441.1
descending 441.5
abdominal 441.3
thoracic 441.1
syphilitic 093.0
thoracoabdominal 441.6
thorax, thoracic 441.1
transverse 441.1
traumatic (thoracic) 901.0
abdominal 902.0
valve or cusp (*see also* Endocarditis, aortic) 424.1
appendix (with peritonitis) 540.0
traumatic—*see* Injury, internal, gastrointestinal tract
with peritoneal abscess 540.1
arteriovenous fistula, brain (congenital) 430
artery 447.2
brain (*see also* Hemorrhage, brain) 431
coronary (*see also* Infarct, myocardium) 410.9
heart (*see also* Infarct, myocardium) 410.9
pulmonary 417.8
traumatic (complication) (*see also* Injury, blood vessel, by site) 904.9

Rupture, ruptured—*continued*
bile duct, except cystic (*see also* Disease, biliary) 576.3
cystic 575.4
traumatic—*see* Injury, internal, intra-abdominal
bladder (sphincter) 596.6
with
abortion—*see* Abortion, by type, with damage to pelvic organs
ectopic pregnancy (*see also* categories 633.0-633.9) 639.2
molar pregnancy (*see also* categories 630-632) 639.2
following
abortion 639.2
ectopic or molar pregnancy 639.2
nontraumatic 596.6
obstetrical trauma 665.5
spontaneous 596.6
traumatic—*see* Injury, internal, bladder
blood vessel (*see also* Hemorrhage) 459.0
brain (*see also* Hemorrhage, brain) 431
heart (*see also* Infarct, myocardium) 410.9
traumatic (complication) (*see also* Injury, blood vessel, by site) 904.9
bone—*see* Fracture, by site
bowel 569.89
traumatic—*see* Injury, internal, intestine
Bowman's membrane 371.31
brain
aneurysm (congenital) (*see also* Hemorrhage, subarachnoid) 430
late effect—*see* category 438
syphilitic 094.87
hemorrhagic (*see also* Hemorrhage, brain) 431
injury at birth 767.0
syphilitic 094.89
capillaries 448.9
cardiac (*see also* Infarct, myocardium) 410.9
cartilage (articular) (current)—*see also* Sprain, by site
knee—*see* Tear, meniscus
semilunar—*see* Tear, meniscus
cecum (with peritonitis) 540.0
traumatic 863.89
with open wound into cavity 863.99
with peritoneal abscess 540.1
cerebral aneurysm (congenital) (*see also* Hemorrhage, subarachnoid) 430
late effect—*see* category 438
cervix (uteri)
with
abortion—*see* Abortion, by type, with damage to pelvic organs
ectopic pregnancy (*see also* categories 633.0-633.9) 639.2
molar pregnancy (*see also* categories 630-632) 639.2
following
abortion 639.2
ectopic or molar pregnancy 639.2
obstetrical trauma 665.3
traumatic—*see* Injury, internal, cervix
chordae tendineae 429.5
choroid (direct) (indirect) (traumatic) 363.63
circle of Willis (*see also* Hemorrhage, subarachnoid) 430
late effect—*see* category 438
colon 569.89
traumatic—*see* Injury, internal, colon

Rupture, ruptured—*continued*
cornea (traumatic)—*see also* Rupture, eye
due to ulcer 370.00
coronary (artery) (thrombotic) (*see also* Infarct, myocardium) 410.9
corpus luteum (infected) (ovary) 620.1
cyst—*see* Cyst
cystic duct (*see also* Disease, gallbladder) 575.4
Descemet's membrane 371.33
traumatic—*see* Rupture, eye
diaphragm—*see also* Hernia, diaphragm
traumatic—*see* Injury, internal, diaphragm
diverticulum
bladder 596.3
intestine (large) (*see also* Diverticula) 562.10
small 562.00
duodenal stump 537.89
duodenum (ulcer)—*see* Ulcer, duodenum, with perforation
ear drum (*see also* Perforation, tympanum) 384.20
with otitis media—*see* Otitis media
traumatic—*see* Wound, open, ear
esophagus 530.4
traumatic 862.22
with open wound into cavity 862.32
cervical region—*see* Wound, open, esophagus
eye (without prolapse of intraocular tissue) 871.0
with
exposure of intraocular tissue 871.1
partial loss of intraocular tissue 871.2
prolapse of intraocular tissue 871.1
due to burn 940.5
fallopian tube 620.8
due to pregnancy—*see* Pregnancy, tubal
traumatic—*see* Injury, internal, fallopian tube
fontanel 767.3
free wall (ventricle) (*see also* Infarct, myocardium) 410.9
gallbladder or duct (*see also* Disease, gallbladder) 575.4
traumatic—*see* Injury, internal, gallbladder
gastric (*see also* Rupture, stomach) 537.89
vessel 459.0
globe (eye) (traumatic)—*see* Rupture, eye
graafian follicle (hematoma) 620.0
heart (auricle) (ventricle) (*see also* Infarct, myocardium) 410.9
infectional 422.90
traumatic—*see* Rupture, myocardium, traumatic
hymen 623.8
internal
organ, traumatic—*see also* Injury, internal, by site
heart—*see* Rupture, myocardium, traumatic
kidney—*see* Rupture, kidney
liver—*see* Rupture, liver
spleen—*see* Rupture, spleen, traumatic
semilunar cartilage—*see* Tear, meniscus
intervertebral disc—*see* Displacement, intervertebral disc
traumatic (current)—*see* Dislocation, vertebra
intestine 569.89
traumatic—*see* Injury, internal, intestine
intracranial, birth injury 767.0
iris 364.76
traumatic—*see* Rupture, eye
joint capsule—*see* Sprain, by site

Rupture, ruptured—*continued*
kidney (traumatic) 866.03
with open wound into cavity 866.13
due to birth injury 767.8
nontraumatic 593.89
lacrimal apparatus (traumatic) 870.2
lens (traumatic) 366.20
ligament—*see also* Sprain, by site
with open wound—*see* Wound, open, by site
old (*see also* Disorder, cartilage, articular) 718.0
liver (traumatic) 864.04
with open wound into cavity 864.14
due to birth injury 767.8
nontraumatic 573.8
lymphatic (node) (vessel) 457.8
marginal sinus (placental) (with hemorrhage) 641.2
affecting fetus or newborn 762.1
meaning hernia—*see* Hernia
membrana tympani (*see also* Perforation, tympanum) 384.20
with otitis media—*see* Otitis media
traumatic—*see* Wound, open, ear
membranes (spontaneous)
artificial
delayed delivery following 658.3
affecting fetus or newborn 761.1
fetus or newborn 761.1
delayed delivery following 658.2
affecting fetus or newborn 761.1
premature (less than 24 hours prior to onset of labor) 658.1
affecting fetus or newborn 761.1
delayed delivery following 658.2
affecting fetus or newborn 761.1
meningeal artery (*see also* Hemorrhage, subarachnoid) 430
late effect—*see* category 438
meniscus (knee)—*see also* Tear, meniscus
old (*see also* Derangement, meniscus) 717.5
site other than knee—*see* Disorder, cartilage, articular
site other than knee—*see* Sprain, by site
mesentery 568.89
traumatic—*see* Injury, internal, mesentery
mitral—*see* Insufficiency, mitral
muscle (traumatic) NEC—*see also* Sprain, by site
with open wound—*see* Wound, open, by site
nontraumatic 728.83
musculotendinous cuff (nontraumatic) (shoulder) 840.4
mycotic aneurysm, causing cerebral hemorrhage (*see also* Hemorrhage, subarachnoid) 430
late effect—*see* category 438
myocardium, myocardial (*see also* Infarct, myocardium) 410.9
traumatic 861.03
with open wound into thorax 861.13
nontraumatic (meaning hernia) (*see also* Hernia, by site) 553.9
obstructed (*see also* Hernia, by site, with obstruction) 552.9
gangrenous (*see also* Hernia, by site, with gangrene) 551.9
operation wound 998.3
ovary, ovarian 620.8
corpus luteum 620.1
follicle (graafian) 620.0

Rupture, ruptured—*continued*
oviduct 620.8
due to pregnancy—*see* Pregnancy, tubal
pancreas 577.8
traumatic—*see* Injury, internal, pancreas
papillary muscle (ventricular) 429.6
pelvic
floor, complicating delivery 664.1
organ NEC—*see* Injury, pelvic, organs
penis (traumatic)—*see* Wound, open, penis
perineum 624.8
during delivery (*see also* Laceration, perineum, complicating delivery) 664.4
pharynx (nontraumatic) (spontaneous) 478.29
postoperative 998.3
pregnant uterus (before onset of labor) 665.0
prostate (traumatic)—*see* Injury, internal, prostate
pulmonary
artery 417.8
valve (heart) (*see also* Endocarditis, pulmonary) 424.3
vein 417.8
vessel 417.8
pupil, sphincter 364.75
pus tube (*see also* Salpingo-oophoritis) 614.2
pyosalpinx (*see also* Salpingo-oophoritis) 614.2
rectum 569.49
traumatic—*see* Injury, internal, rectum
retina, retinal (traumatic) (without detachment) 361.30
with detachment (*see also* Detachment, retina, with retinal defect) 361.00
rotator cuff (capsule) (traumatic) 840.4
nontraumatic, complete 727.61
sclera 871.0
semilunar cartilage, knee (*see also* Tear, meniscus) 836.2
old (*see also* Derangement, meniscus) 717.5
septum (cardiac) 410.8
sigmoid 569.89
traumatic—*see* Injury, internal, colon, sigmoid
sinus of Valsalva 747.29
spinal cord—*see also* Injury, spinal, by site
due to injury at birth 767.4
fetus or newborn 767.4
syphilitic 094.89
traumatic—*see also* Injury, spinal, by site
with fracture—*see* Fracture, vertebra, by site, with spinal cord injury
spleen 289.59
congenital 767.8
due to injury at birth 767.8
malarial 084.9
nontraumatic 289.59
spontaneous 289.59
traumatic 865.04
with open wound into cavity 865.14
splenic vein 459.0
stomach 537.89
due to injury at birth 767.8
traumatic—*see* Injury, internal, stomach
ulcer—*see* Ulcer, stomach, with perforation
synovium 727.50
specified site NEC 727.59
tendon (traumatic)—*see also* Sprain, by site
with open wound—*see* Wound, open, by site
Achilles 845.09
nontraumatic 727.67
ankle 845.09
nontraumatic 727.68

Rupture, ruptured—*continued*
biceps (long bead) 840.8
nontraumatic 727.62
foot 845.10
interphalangeal (joint) 845.13
metatarsophalangeal (joint) 845.12
nontraumatic 727.68
specified site NEC 845.19
tarsometatarsal (joint) 845.11
hand 842.10
carpometacarpal (joint) 842.11
interphalangeal (joint) 842.13
metacarpophalangeal (joint) 842.12
nontraumatic 727.63
extensors 727.63
flexors 727.64
specified site NEC 842.19
nontraumatic 727.60
specified site NEC 727.69
patellar 844.8
nontraumatic 727.66
quadriceps 844.8
nontraumatic 727.65
rotator cuff (capsule) 840.4
nontraumatic, complete 727.61
wrist 842.00
carpal (joint) 842.01
nontraumatic 727.63
extensors 727.63
flexors 727.64
radiocarpal (joint) (ligament) 842.02
radioulnar (joint), distal 842.09
specified site NEC 842.09
testis (traumatic) 878.2
complicated 878.3
due to syphilis 095.8
thoracic duct 457.8
tonsil 474.8
traumatic
with open wound—*see* Wound, open, by site
aorta—*see* Rupture, aorta, traumatic
ear drum—*see* Wound, open, ear, drum
external site—*see* Wound, open, by site
eye 871.2
globe (eye)—*see* Wound, open, eyeball
internal organ (abdomen, chest, or pelvis)—*see also* Injury, internal, by site
heart—*see* Rupture, myocardium, traumatic
kidney—*see* Rupture, kidney
liver—*see* Rupture, liver
spleen—*see* Rupture, spleen, traumatic
ligament, muscle, or tendon—*see also* Sprain, by site
with open wound—*see* Wound, open, by site
meaning hernia—*see* Hernia
tricuspid (heart) (valve)—*see* Endocarditis, tricuspid
tube, tubal 620.8
abscess (*see also* Salpingo-oophoritis) 614.2
due to pregnancy—*see* Pregnancy, tubal
tympanum, tympanic (membrane) (*see also* Perforation, tympanum) 384.20
with otitis media—*see* Otitis media
traumatic—*see* Wound, open, ear, drum
umbilical cord 663.8
fetus or newborn 772.0
ureter (traumatic) (*see also* Injury, internal, ureter) 867.2
nontraumatic 593.89

Rupture, ruptured—*continued*
urethra 599.84
with
abortion—*see* Abortion, by type, with damage to pelvic organs
ectopic pregnancy (*see also* categories 633.0-633.9) 639.2
molar pregnancy (*see also* categories 630-632) 639.2
following
abortion 639.2
ectopic or molar pregnancy 639.2
obstetrical trauma 665.5
traumatic—*see* Injury, internal urethra
uterosacral ligament 620.8
uterus (traumatic)—*see also* Injury, internal uterus
affecting fetus or newborn 763.8
during labor 665.1
nonpuerperal, nontraumatic 621.8
nontraumatic 621.8
pregnant (during labor) 665.1
before labor 665.0
vaginal 878.6
complicated 878.7
complicating delivery—*see* Laceration, vagina, complicating delivery
valve, valvular (heart)—*see* Endocarditis
varicose vein—*see* Varicose, vein
varix—*see* Varix
vena cava 459.0
ventricle (free wall) (left) (*see also* Infarct, myocardium) 410.9
vesical (urinary) 596.6
traumatic—*see* Injury, internal, bladder
vessel (blood) 459.0
pulmonary 417.8
viscus 799.8
vulva 878.4
complicated 878.5
complicating delivery 664.0
Russell's dwarf (uterine dwarfism and craniofacial dysostosis) 759.89
Russell's dysentery 004.8
Russell (-Silver) syndrome (congenital hemihypertrophy and short stature) 759.89
Russian spring-summer type encephalitis 063.0
Rust's disease (tuberculous spondylitis) 015.0 *[720.81]*
Rustitskii's disease (multiple myeloma) (M9730/3) 203.0
Ruysch's disease (Hirschsprung's disease) 751.3
Rytand-Lipsitch syndrome (complete atrioventricular block) 426.0

S

Saber
shin 090.5
tibia 090.5
Sac, lacrimal —*see* condition
Saccharomyces infection (*see also* Candidiasis) 112.9
Saccharopinuria 270.7
Saccular —*see* condition
Sacculation
aorta (nonsyphilitic) (*see also* Aneurysm, aorta) 441.9
ruptured 441.5
syphilitic 093.0
bladder 596.3
colon 569.89
intralaryngeal (congenital) (ventricular) 748.3
larynx (congenital) (ventricular) 748.3
organ or site, congenital—*see* Distortion
pregnant uterus, complicating delivery 654.4
affecting fetus or newborn 763.1
causing obstructed labor 660.2
affecting fetus or newborn 763.1
rectosigmoid 569.89
sigmoid 569.89
ureter 593.89
urethra 599.2
vesical 596.3
Sachs (-Tay) disease (amaurotic familial idiocy) 330.1
Sacks-Libman disease 710.0 *[424.91]*
Sacralgia 724.6
Sacralization
fifth lumbar vertebra 756.15
incomplete (vertebra) 756.15
Sacrodynia 724.6
Sacroiliac joint —*see* condition
Sacroiliitis NEC 720.2
Sacrum —*see* condition
Saddle
back 737.8
embolus, aorta 444.0
nose 738.0
congenital 754.0
due to syphilis 090.5
Sadism (sexual) 302.84
Saemisch's ulcer 370.04
Saenger's syndrome 379.46
Sago spleen 277.3
Sailors' skin 692.74
Saint
Anthony's fire (*see also* Erysipelas) 035
Guy's dance—*see* Chorea
Louis-type encephalitis 062.3
triad (*see also* Hernia, diaphragm) 553.3
Vitus' dance—*see* Chorea
Salicylism
correct substance properly administered 535.4
overdose or wrong substance given or taken 965.1
Salivary duct or gland —*see also* condition
virus disease 078.5
Salivation (excessive) (*see also* Ptyalism) 527.7
Salmonella (aertrycke) (choleraesuis) (enteritidis) (gallinarum) (suipestifer) (typhimurium) (*see also* Infection, Salmonella) 003.9
arthritis 003.23
carrier (suspected) of V02.3
Salmonella—*continued*
meningitis 003.21
osteomyelitis 003.24
pneumonia 003.22
septicemia 003.1
typhosa 002.0
carrier (suspected) of V02.1
Salmonellosis 003.0
with pneumonia 003.22
Salpingitis (catarrhal) (fallopian tube) (nodular) (pseudofollicular) (purulent) (septic) (*see also* Salpingo-oophoritis) 614.2
ear 381.50
acute 381.51
chronic 381.52
Eustachian (tube) 381.50
acute 381.51
chronic 381.52
follicularis 614.1
gonococcal (chronic) 098.37
acute 098.17
interstitial, chronic 614.1
isthmica nodosa 614.1
old—*see* Salpingo-oophoritis, chronic
puerperal, postpartum, childbirth 670
specific (chronic) 098.37
acute 098.17
tuberculous (acute) (chronic) (*see also* Tuberculosis) 016.6
venereal (chronic) 098.37
acute 098.17
Salpingocele 620.4
Salpingo-oophoritis (catarrhal) (purulent) (ruptured) (septic) (suppurative) 614.2
acute 614.0
with
abortion—*see* Abortion, by type, with sepsis
ectopic pregnancy (*see also* categories 633.0-633.9) 639.0
molar pregnancy (*see also* categories 630-632) 639.0
following
abortion 639.0
ectopic or molar pregnancy 639.0
gonococcal 098.17
puerperal, postpartum, childbirth 670
tuberculous (*see also* Tuberculosis) 016.6
chronic 614.1
gonococcal 098.37
tuberculous (*see also* Tuberculosis) 016.6
complicating pregnancy 646.6
affecting fetus or newborn 760.8
gonococcal (chronic) 098.37
acute 098.17
old—*see* Salpingo-oophoritis, chronic
puerperal 670
specific—*see* Salpingo-oophoritis, gonococcal
subacute (*see also* Salpingo-oophoritis, acute) 614.0
tuberculous (acute) (chronic) (*see also* Tuberculosis) 016.6
venereal—*see* Salpingo-oophoritis, gonococcal
Salpingo-ovaritis (*see also* Salpingo-oophoritis) 614.2
Salpingoperitonitis (*see also* Salpingo-oophoritis) 614.2

Salt-losing
nephritis (*see also* Disease, renal) 593.9
syndrome (*see also* Disease, renal) 593.9
Salt-rheum (*see also* Eczema) 692.9
Salzmann's nodular dystrophy 371.46
Sampson's cyst or tumor 617.1
Sandblasters'
asthma 502
lung 502
Sander's disease (paranoia) 297.1
Sandfly fever 066.0
Sandhoff's disease 330.1
Sanfilippo's syndrome (mucopolysaccharidosis III) 277.5
Sanger-Brown's ataxia 334.2
San Joaquin Valley fever 114.0
São Paulo fever or typhus 082.0
Saponification, mesenteric 567.8
Sapremia —*see* Septicemia
Sarcocele (benign)
syphilitic 095.8
congenital 090.5
Sarcoepiplocele (*see also* Hernia) 553.9
Sarcoepiplomphalocele (*see also* Hernia, umbilicus) 553.1
Sarcoid (any site) 135
with lung involvement 135 *[517.8]*
Boeck's 135
Darier-Roussy 135
Spiegler-Fendt 686.8
Sarcoidosis 135
cardiac 135 *[425.8]*
lung 135 *[517.8]*
Sarcoma (M8800/3)—*see also* Neoplasm, connective tissue, malignant
alveolar soft part (M9581/3)—*see* Neoplasm, connective tissue, malignant
ameloblastic (M9330/3) 170.1
upper jaw (bone) 170.0
botryoid (M8910/3)—*see* Neoplasm, connective tissue, malignant
botryoides (M8910/3)—*see* Neoplasm, connective tissue, malignant
cerebellar (M9480/3) 191.6
circumscribed (arachnoidal) (M9471/3) 191.6
circumscribed (arachnoidal) cerebellar (M9471/3) 191.6
clear cell, of tendons and aponeuroses (M9044/3)—*see* Neoplasm, connective tissue, malignant
embryonal (M8991/3)—*see* Neoplasm, connective tissue, malignant
endometrial (stromal) (M8930/3) 182.0
isthmus 182.1
endothelial (M9130/3)—*see also* Neoplasm, connective tissue, malignant
bone (M9260/3)—*see* Neoplasm, bone, malignant
epithelioid cell (M8804/3)—*see* Neoplasm, connective tissue, malignant
Ewing's (M9260/3)—*see* Neoplasm, bone, malignant
germinoblastic (diffuse) (M9632/3) 202.8
follicular (M9697/3) 202.0
giant cell (M8802/3)—*see also* Neoplasm, connective tissue, malignant
bone (M9250/3)—*see* Neoplasm, bone, malignant
glomoid (M8710/3)—*see* Neoplasm, connective tissue, malignant

Sarcoma—*continued*
granulocytic (M9930/3) 205.3
hemangioendothelial (M9130/3)—*see* Neoplasm, connective tissue, malignant
hemorrhagic, multiple (M9140/3)—*see* Kaposi's, sarcoma
Hodgkin's (M9662/3) 201.2
immunoblastic (M9612/3) 200.8
Kaposi's (M9140/3)—*see* Kaposi's, sarcoma
Kupffer cell (M9124/3) 155.0
leptomeningeal (M9530/3)—*see* Neoplasm, meninges, malignant
lymphangioendothelial (M9170/3)—*see* Neoplasm, connective tissue, malignant
lymphoblastic (M9630/3) 200.1
lymphocytic (M9620/3) 200.1
mast cell (M9740/3) 202.6
melanotic (M8720/3)—*see* Melanoma
meningeal (M9530/3)—*see* Neoplasm, meninges, malignant
meningothelial (M9530/3)—*see* Neoplasm, meninges, malignant
mesenchymal (M8800/3)—*see also* Neoplasm, connective tissue, malignant
mixed (M8990/3)—*see* Neoplasm, connective tissue, malignant
mesothelial (M9050/3)—*see* Neoplasm, by site, malignant
monstrocellular (M9481/3)
specified site—*see* Neoplasm, by site, malignant
unspecified site 191.9
myeloid (M9930/3) 205.3
neurogenic (M9540/3)—*see* Neoplasm, connective tissue, malignant
odontogenic (M9270/3) 170.1
upper jaw (bone) 170.0
osteoblastic (M9180/3)—*see* Neoplasm, bone, malignant
osteogenic (M9180/3)—*see also* Neoplasm, bone, malignant
juxtacortical (M9190/3)—*see* Neoplasm, bone, malignant
periosteal (M9190/3)—*see* Neoplasm, bone, malignant
periosteal (M8812/3)—*see also* Neoplasm, bone, malignant
osteogenic (M9190/3)—*see* Neoplasm, bone, malignant
plasma cell (M9731/3) 203.8
pleomorphic cell (M8802/3)—*see* Neoplasm, connective tissue, malignant
reticuloendothelial (M9720/3) 202.3
reticulum cell (M9640/3) 200.0
nodular (M9642/3) 200.0
pleomorphic cell type (M9641/3) 200.0
round cell (M8803/3)—*see* Neoplasm, connective tissue, malignant
small cell (M8803/3)—*see* Neoplasm, connective tissue, malignant
spindle cell (M8801/3)—*see* Neoplasm, connective tissue, malignant
stromal (endometrial) (M8930/3) 182.0
isthmus 182.1
synovial (M9040/3)—*see also* Neoplasm, connective tissue, malignant
biphasic type (M9043/3)—*see* Neoplasm, connective tissue, malignant
epithelioid cell type (M9042/3)—*see* Neoplasm, connective tissue, malignant
spindle cell type (M9041/3)—*see* Neoplasm, connective tissue, malignant

Sarcomatosis
meningeal (M9539/3)—*see* Neoplasm, meninges, malignant
specified site NEC (M8800/3)—*see* Neoplasm, connective tissue, malignant
unspecified site (M8800/6) 171.9
Sarcosinemia 270.8
Sarcosporidiosis 136.5
Saturnine —*see* condition
Saturnism 984.9
specified type of lead—*see* Table of drugs and chemicals
Satyriasis 302.89
Sauriasis —*see* Ichthyosis
Sauriderma 757.39
Sauriosis —*see* Ichthyosis
Savill's disease (epidemic exfoliative dermatitis) 695.89
SBE (subacute bacterial endocarditis) 421.0
Scabies (any site) 133.0
Scabs 782.8
Scaglietti-Dagnini syndrome (acromegalic macrospondylitis) 253.0
Scald, scalded —*see also* Burn, by site
skin syndrome 695.1
Scalenus anticus (anterior) syndrome 353.0
Scales 782.8
Scalp —*see* condition
Scaphocephaly 756.0
Scaphoiditis, tarsal 732.5
Scapulalgia 733.90
Scapulohumeral myopathy 359.1
Scar, scarring (*see also* Cicatrix) 709.2
adherent 709.2
atrophic 709.2
cervix
in pregnancy or childbirth 654.6
affecting fetus or newborn 763.8
causing obstructed labor 660.2
affecting fetus or newborn 763.1
cheloid 701.4
chorioretinal 363.30
disseminated 363.35
macular 363.32
peripheral 363.34
posterior pole NEC 363.33
choroid (*see also* Scar, chorioretinal) 363.30
compression, pericardial 423.9
congenital 757.39
conjunctiva 372.64
cornea 371.00
xerophthalmic 264.6
due to previous cesarean delivery, complicating pregnancy or childbirth 654.2
affecting fetus or newborn 763.8
duodenal (bulb) (cap) 537.3
hypertrophic 701.4
keloid 701.4
labia 624.4
lung (base) 518.89
macula 363.32
disseminated 363.35
peripheral 363.34
muscle 728.89
myocardium, myocardial 412
painful 709.2
papillary muscle 429.81
posterior pole NEC 363.33
macular—*see* Scar, macula
postnecrotic (hepatic) (liver) 571.9

Scar, scarring—*continued*
psychic V15.4
retina (*see also* Scar, chorioretinal) 363.30
trachea 478.9
uterus 621.8
in pregnancy or childbirth NEC 654.9
affecting fetus or newborn 763.8
due to previous cesarean delivery 654.2
vulva 624.4
Scarabiasis 134.1
Scarlatina 034.1
anginosa 034.1
maligna 034.1
myocarditis, acute 034.1 *[422.0]*
old (*see also* Myocarditis) 429.0
otitis media 034.1 *[382.02]*
ulcerosa 034.1
Scarlatinella 057.8
Scarlet fever (albuminuria) (angina) (convulsions) (lesions of lid) (rash) 034.1
Schamberg's disease, dermatitis, or dermatosis (progressive pigmentary dermatosis) 709.09
Schatzki's ring (esophagus) (lower) (congenital) 750.3
acquired 530.3
Schaufenster krankheit 413.9
Schaumann's
benign lymphogranulomatosis 135
disease (sarcoidosis) 135
syndrome (sarcoidosis) 135
Scheie's syndrome (mucopolysaccharidosis IS) 277.5
Schenck's disease (sporotrichosis) 117.1
Scheuermann's disease or osteochondrosis 732.0
Scheuthauer-Marie-Sainton syndrome (cleidocranialis dysostosis) 755.59
Schilder (-Flatau) disease 341.1
Schilling-type monocytic leukemia (M9890/3) 206.9
Schimmelbusch's disease, cystic mastitis, or hyperplasia 610.1
Schirmer's syndrome (encephalocutaneous angiomatosis) 759.6
Schistocelia 756.7
Schistoglossia 750.13
Schistosoma infestation —*see* Infestation, Schistosoma
Schistosomiasis 120.9
Asiatic 120.2
bladder 120.0
chestermani 120.8
colon 120.1
cutaneous 120.3
due to
S. hematobium 120.0
S. japonicum 120.2
S. mansoni 120.1
S. mattheii 120.8
eastern 120.2
genitourinary tract 120.0
intestinal 120.1
lung 120.2
Manson's (intestinal) 120.1
Oriental 120.2
pulmonary 120.2
specified type NEC 120.8
vesical 120.0
Schizencephaly 742.4
Schizo-affective psychosis (*see also* Schizophrenia) 295.7
Schizodontia 520.2

Schizoid personality 301.20
introverted 301.21
schizotypal 301.22
Schizophrenia, schizophrenic (reaction) 295.9

Note—Use the following fifth-digit subclassification with category 295:

0 unspecified
1 subchronic
2 chronic
3 subchronic with acute exacerbation
4 chronic with acute exacerbation
5 in remission

acute (attack) NEC 295.8
episode 295.4
atypical form 295.8
borderline 295.5
catalepsy 295.2
catatonic (type) (acute) (excited) (withdrawn) 295.2
childhood (type) (*see also* Psychosis, childhood) 299.9
chronic NEC 295.6
coenesthesiopathic 295.8
cyclic (type) 295.7
disorganized (type) 295.1
flexibilitas cerea 295.2
hebephrenic (type) (acute) 295.1
incipient 295.5
latent 295.5
paranoid (type) (acute) 295.3
paraphrenic (acute) 295.3
prepsychotic 295.5
primary (acute) 295.0
prodromal 295.5
pseudoneurotic 295.5
pseudopsychopathic 295.5
reaction 295.9
residual (state) (type) 295.6
restzustand 295.6
schizo-affective (type) (depressed) (excited) 295.7
schizophreniform type 295.4
simple (type) (acute) 295.0
simplex (acute) 295.0
specified type NEC 295.8
syndrome of childhood NEC (*see also* Psychosis, childhood) 299.9
undifferentiated 295.9
acute 295.8
chronic 295.6
Schizothymia 301.20
introverted 301.21
schizotypal 301.22
Schlafkrankheit 086.5
Schlatter's tibia (osteochondrosis) 732.4
Schlatter-Osgood disease (osteochondrosis, tibial tubercle) 732.4
Schloffer's tumor (*see also* Peritonitis) 567.2
Schmidt's syndrome
sphallo-pharyngo-laryngeal hemiplegia 352.6
thyroid-adrenocortical insufficiency 258.1
vagoaccessory 352.6
Schmincke
carcinoma (M8082/3)—*see* Neoplasm, nasopharynx, malignant
tumor (M8082/3)—*see* Neoplasm, nasopharynx, malignant
Schmitz (-Stutzer) dysentery 004.0
Schmorl's disease or nodes 722.30
lumbar, lumbosacral 722.32
specified region NEC 722.39
thoracic, thoracolumbar 722.31
Schneider's syndrome 047.9
Schneiderian
carcinoma (M8121/3)
specified site—*see* Neoplasm, by site, malignant
unspecified site 160.0
papilloma (M8121/0)
specified site—*see* Neoplasm, by site, benign
unspecified site 212.0
Schoffer's tumor (*see also* Peritonitis) 567.2
Scholte's syndrome (malignant carcinoid) 259.2
Scholz's disease 330.0
Scholz (-Bielschowsky-Henneberg) syndrome 330.0
Schönlein (-Henoch) disease (primary) (purpura) (rheumatic) 287.0
School examination V70.3
Schottmüller's disease (*see also* Fever, paratyphoid) 002.9
Schroeder's syndrome (endocrine-hypertensive) 255.3
Schüller-Christian disease or syndrome (chronic histiocytosis X) 277.8
Schultz's disease or syndrome (agranulocytosis) 288.0
Schultze's acroparesthesia, simple 443.89
Schwalbe-Ziehen-Oppenheimer disease 333.6
Schwannoma (M9560/0)—*see also* Neoplasm, connective tissue, benign
malignant (M9560/3)—*see* Neoplasm, connective tissue, malignant
Schwartz (-Jampel) syndrome 756.89
Schwartz-Bartter syndrome (inappropriate secretion of antidiuretic hormone) 253.6
Schweninger-Buzzi disease (macular atrophy) 701.3
Sciatic —*see* condition
Sciatica (infectional) 724.3
due to
displacement of intervertebral disc 722.10
herniation, nucleus pulposus 722.10
Scimitar syndrome (anomalous venous drainage, right lung to inferior vena cava) 747.49
Sclera —*see* condition
Sclerectasia 379.11
Scleredema
adultorum 710.1
Buschke's 710.1
newborn 778.1
Sclerema
adiposum (newborn) 778.1
adultorum 710.1
edematosum (newborn) 778.1
neonatorum 778.1
newborn 778.1
Scleriasis —*see* Scleroderma
Scleritis 379.00
with corneal involvement 379.05
anterior (annular) (localized) 379.03
brawny 379.06
granulomatous 379.09
posterior 379.07
specified NEC 379.09
suppurative 379.09
syphilitic 095.0
tuberculous (nodular) (*see also* Tuberculosis) 017.3 *[379.09]*

Sclerochoroiditis (*see also* Scleritis) 379.00
Scleroconjunctivitis (*see also* Scleritis) 379.00
Sclerocystic ovary (syndrome) 256.4
Sclerodactylia 701.0
Scleroderma, sclerodermia (acrosclerotic) (diffuse) (generalized) (progressive) (pulmonary) 710.1
  circumscribed 701.0
  linear 701.0
  localized (linear) 701.0
  newborn 778.1
Sclerokeratitis 379.05
  meaning sclerosing keratitis 370.54
  tuberculous (*see also* Tuberculosis) 017.3 *[379.09]*
Scleroma, trachea 040.1
Scleromalacia
  multiple 731.0
  perforans 379.04
Scleromyxedema 701.8
Scleroperikeratitis 379.05
Sclerose en plaques 340
Sclerosis, sclerotic
  adrenal (gland) 255.8
  Alzheimer's 331.0
    with dementia—*see* Alzheimer's, demential
  amyotrophic (lateral) 335.20
  annularis fibrosi
    aortic 424.1
    mitral 424.0
  aorta, aortic 440.0
    valve (*see also* Endocarditis, aortic) 424.1
  artery, arterial, arteriolar, arteriovascular—*see* Arteriosclerosis
  ascending multiple 340
  Baló's (concentric) 341.1
  basilar—*see* Sclerosis, brain
  bone (localized) NEC 733.99
  brain (general) (lobular) 341.9
    Alzheimer's—*see* Alzheimer's dementia
    artery, arterial 437.0
    atrophic lobar 331.0
      with dementia 290.10
    diffuse 341.1
      familial (chronic) (infantile) 330.0
      infantile (chronic) (familial) 330.0
      Pelizaeus-Merzbacher type 330.0
    disseminated 340
    hereditary 334.2
    infantile, (degenerative) (diffuse) 330.0
    insular 340
    Krabbe's 330.0
    miliary 340
    multiple 340
    Pelizaeus-Merzbacher 330.0
    presenile (Alzheimer's) 331.0
      with dementia 290.10
    progressive familial 330.0
    senile 437.0
    tuberous 759.5
  bulbar, progressive 340
  bundle of His 426.50
    left 426.3
    right 426.4
  cardiac —*see* Arteriosclerosis, coronary
  cardiorenal (*see also* Hypertension, cardiorenal) 404.90
  cardiovascular (*see also* Disease, cardiovascular) 429.2
    renal (*see also* Hypertension, cardiorenal) 404.90

Sclerosis, sclerotic—*continued*
  centrolobar, familial 330.0
  cerebellar—*see* Sclerosis, brain
  cerebral—*see* Sclerosis, brain
  cerebrospinal 340
    disseminated 340
    multiple 340
  cerebrovascular 437.0
  choroid 363.40
    diffuse 363.56
  combined (spinal cord)—*see also* Degeneration, combined
    multiple 340
  concentric, Baló's 341.1
  cornea 370.54
  coronary (artery) —*see* Arteriosclerosis, coronary
  corpus cavernosum
    female 624.8
    male 607.89
  Dewitzky's
    aortic 424.1
    mitral 424.0
  diffuse NEC 341.1
  disease, heart —*see* Arteriosclerosis, coronary
  disseminated 340
  dorsal 340
  dorsolateral (spinal cord)—*see* Degeneration, combined
  endometrium 621.8
  extrapyramidal 333.90
  eye, nuclear (senile) 366.16
  Friedreich's (spinal cord) 334.0
  funicular (spermatic cord) 608.89
  gastritis 535.4
  general (vascular)—*see* Arteriosclerosis
  gland (lymphatic) 457.8
  hepatic 571.9
  hereditary
    cerebellar 334.2
    spinal 334.0
  idiopathic cortical (Garré's) (*see also* Osteomyelitis) 730.1
  ilium, piriform 733.5
  insular 340
    pancreas 251.8
  Islands of Langerhans 251.8
  kidney—*see* Sclerosis, renal
  larynx 478.79
  lateral 335.24
    amyotrophic 335.20
    descending 335.24
    primary 335.24
    spinal 335.24
  liver 571.9
  lobar, atrophic (of brain) 331.0
    with dementia 290.10
  lung (*see also* Fibrosis, lung) 515
  mastoid 383.1
  mitral—*see* Endocarditis, mitral
  Mönckeberg's (medial) (*see also* Arteriosclerosis, extremities) 440.20
  multiple (brain stem) (cerebral) (generalized) (spinal cord) 340
  myocardium, myocardial —*see* Arteriosclerosis, coronary
  nuclear (senile), eye 366.16
  ovary 620.8
  pancreas 577.8
  penis 607.89

Sclerosis, sclerotic—*continued*
peripheral arteries NEC (*see also* Arteriosclerosis, extremities) 440.20
plaques 340
pluriglandular 258.8
polyglandular 258.8
posterior (spinal cord) (syphilitic) 094.0
posterolateral (spinal cord)—*see* Degeneration, combined
prepuce 607.89
presenile (Alzheimer's) 331.0
with dementia 290.10
primary lateral 335.24
progressive systemic 710.1
pulmonary (*see also* Fibrosis, lung) 515
artery 416.0
valve (heart) (*see also* Endocarditis, pulmonary) 424.3
renal 587
with
cystine storage disease 270.0
hypertension (*see also* Hypertension, kidney) 403.90
hypertensive heart disease (conditions classifiable to 402) (*see also* Hypertension, cardiorenal) 404.90
arteriolar (hyaline) (*see also* Hypertension, kidney) 403.90
hyperplastic (*see also* Hypertension, kidney) 403.90
retina (senile) (vascular) 362.17
rheumatic
aortic valve 395.9
mitral valve 394.9
Schilder's 341.1
senile—*see* Arteriosclerosis
spinal (cord) (general) (progressive) (transverse) 336.8
ascending 357.0
combined—*see also* Degeneration, combined
multiple 340
syphilitic 094.89
disseminated 340
dorsolateral—*see* Degeneration, combined
hereditary (Friedreich's) (mixed form) 334.0
lateral (amyotrophic) 335.24
multiple 340
posterior (syphilitic) 094.0
stomach 537.89
subendocardial, congenital 425.3
systemic (progressive) 710.1
with lung involvement 710.1 *[517.2]*
tricuspid (heart) (valve)—*see* Endocarditis, tricuspid
tuberous (brain) 759.5
tympanic membrane (*see also* Tympanosclerosis) 385.00
valve, valvular (heart)—*see* Endocarditis
vascular—*see* Arteriosclerosis
vein 459.89
Sclerotenonitis 379.07
Sclerotitis (*see also* Scleritis) 379.00
syphilitic 095.0
tuberculous (*see also* Tuberculosis) 017.3 *[379.09]*
Scoliosis (acquired) (postural) 737.30
congenital 754.2
Scoliosis—*continued*
due to or associated with
Charcot-Marie-Tooth disease 356.1 *[737.43]*
mucopolysaccharidosis 277.5 *[737.43]*
neurofibromatosis 237.71 *[737.43]*
osteitis
deformans 731.0 *[737.43]*
fibrosa cystica 252.0 *[737.43]*
osteoporosis (*see also* Osteoporosis) 733.00 *[737.43]*
poliomyelitis 138 *[737.43]*
radiation 737.33
tuberculosis (*see also* Tuberculosis) 015.0 *[737.43]*
idiopathic 737.30
infantile
progressive 737.32
resolving 737.31
paralytic 737.39
rachitic 268.1
sciatic 724.3
specified NEC 737.39
thoracogenic 737.34
tuberculous (*see also* Tuberculosis) 015.0 *[737.43]*
Scoliotic pelvis 738.6
with disproportion (fetopelvic) 653.0
affecting fetus or newborn 763.1
causing obstructed labor 660.1
affecting fetus or newborn 763.1
Scorbutus, scorbutic 267
anemia 281.8
Scotoma (ring) 368.44
arcuate 368.43
Bjerrum 368.43
blind spot area 368.42
central 368.41
centrocecal 368.41
paracecal 368.42
paracentral 368.41
scintillating 368.12
Seidel 368.43
Scratch —*see* Injury, superficial, by site
Screening (for) V82.9
alcoholism V79.1
anemia, deficiency NEC V78.1
iron V78.0
anomaly, congenital V82.8
antenatal V28.9
alphafetoprotein levels, raised V28.1
based on amniocentesis V28.2
chromosomal anomalies V28.0
raised alpha-fetalprotein levels V28.1
fetal growth retardation using ultrasonics V28.4
isoimmunization V28.5
malformations using ultrasonics V28.3
raised alphafetoprotein levels V28.1
specified condition NEC V28.8
arterial hypertension V81.1
arthropod-borne viral disease NEC V73.5
asymptomatic bacteriuria V81.5
bacterial
conjunctivitis V74.4
disease V74.9
specified condition NEC V74.8
bacteriuria, asymptomatic V81.5
blood disorder NEC V78.9
specified type NEC V78.8
bronchitis, chronic V81.3

Screening (for)—*continued*
  brucellosis V74.8
  cancer—*see* Screening, malignant neoplasm
  cardiovascular disease NEC V81.2
  cataract V80.2
  Chagas' disease V75.3
  chemical poisoning V82.5
  cholera V74.0
  chromosomal
    anomalies
      by amniocentesis, antenatal V28.0
      postnatal V82.4
    athletes V70.3
  condition
    cardiovascular NEC V81.2
    eye NEC V80.2
    genitourinary NEC V81.6
    neurological V80.0
    respiratory NEC V81.4
    skin V82.0
    specified NEC V82.8
  congenital
    anomaly V82.8
      eye V80.2
    dislocation of hip V82.3
    eye condition or disease V80.2
  conjunctivitis, bacterial V74.4
  contamination NEC (*see also* Poisoning) V82.5
  coronary artery disease V81.0
  cystic fibrosis V77.6
  deficiency anemia NEC V78.1
    iron V78.0
  dengue fever V73.5
  depression V79.0
  developmental handicap V79.9
    in early childhood V79.3
    specified type NEC V79.8
  diabetes mellitus V77.1
  diphtheria V74.3
  disease or disorder V82.9
    bacterial V74.9
      specified NEC V74.8
    blood V78.9
      specified type NEC V78.8
    blood-forming organ V78.9
      specified type NEC V78.8
    cardiovascular NEC V81.2
      hypertensive V81.1
      ischemic V81.0
    Chagas' V75.3
    chlamydial V73.98
      specified NEC V73.88
    ear NEC V80.3
    endocrine NEC V77.9
    eye NEC V80.2
    genitourinary NEC V81.6
    heart NEC V81.2
      hypertensive V81.1
      ischemic V81.0
    immunity NEC V77.9
    infectious NEC V75.9
    mental V79.9
      specified type NEC V79.8
    metabolic NEC V77.9
      inborn NEC V77.7
    neurological V80.0
    nutritional NEC V77.9
    rheumatic NEC V82.2
    rickettsial V75.0
    sickle-cell V78.2
      trait V78.2

Screening (for)—*continued*
      specified type NEC V82.8
      thyroid V77.0
      vascular NEC V81.2
        ischemic V81.0
      venereal V74.5
      viral V73.99
        arthropod-borne NEC V73.5
        specified type NEC V73.89
  dislocation of hip, congenital V82.3
  drugs in athletes V70.3
  emphysema (chronic) V81.3
  encephalitis, viral (mosquito or tick borne) V73.5
  endocrine disorder NEC V77.9
  eye disorder NEC V80.2
    congenital V80.2
  fever
    dengue V73.5
    hemorrhagic V73.5
    yellow V73.4
  filariasis V75.6
  galactosemia V77.4
  genitourinary condition NEC V81.6
  glaucoma V80.1
  gonorrhea V74.5
  gout V77.5
  Hansen's disease V74.2
  heart disease NEC V81.2
    hypertensive V81.1
    ischemic V81.0
  heavy metal poisoning V82.5
  helminthiasis, intestinal V75.7
  hematopoietic malignancy V76.8
  hemoglobinopathies NEC V78.3
  hemorrhagic fever V73.5
  Hodgkin's disease V76.8
  hormones in athletes V70.3
  hypertension V81.1
  immunity disorder NEC V77.9
  inborn errors of metabolism NEC V77.7
  infection
    bacterial V74.9
      specified type NEC V74.8
    mycotic V75.4
    parasitic NEC V75.8
  infectious disease V75.9
    specified type NEC V75.8
  ingestion of radioactive substance V82.5
  intestinal helminthiasis V75.7
  iron deficiency anemia V78.0
  ischemic heart disease V81.0
  lead poisoning V82.5
  leishmaniasis V75.2
  leprosy V74.2
  leptospirosis V74.8
  leukemia V76.8
  lymphoma V76.8
  malaria V75.1
  malignant neoplasm (of) V76.9
    bladder V76.3
    blood V76.8
    breast V76.1
    cervix V76.2
    hematopoietic system V76.8
    lung V76.0
    lymph (glands) V76.8
    oral cavity V76.42
    rectum V76.41
    respiratory organs V76.0

Screening (for)—*continued*
skin V76.43
specified sites NEC V76.49
malnutrition V77.2
measles V73.2
mental
disorder V79.9
specified type NEC V79.8
retardation V79.2
metabolic errors, inborn V77.7
mucoviscidosis V77.6
multiphasic V82.6
mycosis V75.4
mycotic infection V75.4
nephropathy V81.5
neurological condition V80.0
nutritional disorder V77.9
obesity V77.8
parasitic infection NEC V75.8
phenylketonuria V77.3
plague V74.8
poisoning
chemical NEC V82.5
contaminated water supply V82.5
heavy metal V82.5
poliomyelitis V73.0
postnatal chromosomal anomalies V82.4
prenatal—*see* Screening, antenatal
pulmonary tuberculosis V74.1
radiation exposure V82.5
renal disease V81.5
respiratory condition NEC V81.4
rheumatic disorder NEC V82.2
rheumatoid arthritis V82.1
rickettsial disease V75.0
rubella V73.3
schistosomiasis V75.5
senile macular lesions of eye V80.2
sickle-cell anemia, disease, or trait V78.2
skin condition V82.0
sleeping sickness V75.3
smallpox V73.1
special V82.9
specified condition NEC V82.8
specified type NEC V82.8
spirochetal disease V74.9
specified type NEC V74.8
stimulants in athletes V70.3
syphilis V74.5
tetanus V74.8
thyroid disorder V77.0
trachoma V73.6
trypanosomiasis V75.3
tuberculosis, pulmonary V74.1
venereal disease V74.5
viral encephalitis
mosquito-borne V73.5
tick-borne V73.5
whooping cough V74.8
worms, intestinal V75.7
yaws V74.6
yellow fever V73.4
Scrofula (*see also* Tuberculosis) 017.2
Scrofulide (primary) (*see also* Tuberculosis) 017.0
Scrofuloderma, scrofulodermia (any site) (primary) (*see also* Tuberculosis) 017.0
Scrofulosis (universal) (*see also* Tuberculosis) 017.2
Scrofulosis lichen (primary) (*see also* Tuberculosis) 017.0
Scrofulous —*see* condition
Scrotal tongue 529.5
congenital 750.13
Scrotum —*see* condition
Scurvy (gum) (infantile) (rickets) (scorbutic) 267
Sea-blue histiocyte syndrome 272.7
Seabright-Bantam syndrome (pseudohypoparathyroidism) 275.4
Seasickness 994.6
Seatworm 127.4
Sebaceous
cyst (*see also* Cyst, sebaceous) 706.2
gland disease NEC 706.9
Sebocystomatosis 706.2
Seborrhea, seborrheic 706.3
adiposa 706.3
capitis 690.11
congestiva 695.4
corporis 706.3
dermatitis 690.10
infantile 690.12
diathesis in infants 695.89
eczema 690.18
infantile 690.12
keratosis 702.19
inflamed 702.11
nigricans 705.89
sicca 690.18
wart 702.19
inflamed 702.11
Seckel's syndrome 759.89
Seclusion pupil 364.74
Seclusiveness, child 313.22
Secondary —*see also* condition
neoplasm—*see* Neoplasm, by site, malignant, secondary
Secretan's disease or syndrome (posttraumatic edema) 782.3
Secretion
antidiuretic hormone, inappropriate (syndrome) 253.6
catecholamine, by pheochromocytoma 255.6
hormone
antidiuretic, inappropriate (syndrome) 253.6
by
carcinoid tumor 259.2
pheochromocytoma 255.6
ectopic NEC 259.3
urinary
excessive 788.42
suppression 788.5
Section
cesarean
affecting fetus or newborn 763.4
post mortem, affecting fetus or newborn 761.6
previous, in pregnancy or childbirth 654.2
affecting fetus or newborn 763.8
nerve, traumatic—*see* Injury, nerve, by site
Seeligmann's syndrome (ichthyosis congenita) 757.1
Segmentation, incomplete (congenital)—*see also* Fusion
bone NEC 756.9
lumbosacral (joint) 756.15
vertebra 756.15
lumbosacral 756.15
Seizure 780.3
akinetic (idiopathic) (*see also* Epilepsy) 345.0
psychomotor 345.4
apoplexy, apoplectic (*see also* Disease, cerebrovascular, acute) 436

Seizure—*continued*
atonic (*see also* Epilepsy) 345.0
autonomic 300.11
brain or cerebral (*see also* Disease, cerebrovascular, acute) 436
convulsive (*see also* Convulsions) 780.3
cortical (focal) (motor) (*see also* Epilepsy) 345.5
epilepsy, epileptic (cryptogenic) (*see also* Epilepsy) 345.9
epileptiform, epileptoid 780.3
focal (*see also* Epilepsy) 345.5
febrile 780.3
heart—*see* Disease, heart
hysterical 300.11
Jacksonian (focal) (*see also* Epilepsy) 345.5
motor type 345.5
sensory type 345.5
newborn 779.0
paralysis (*see also* Disease, cerebrovascular, acute) 436
recurrent 780.3
epileptic—*see* Epilepsy
repetitive 780.3
epileptic—*see* Epilepsy
salaam (*see also* Epilepsy) 345.6
uncinate (*see also* Epilepsy) 345.4
Self-mutilation 300.9
Semicoma 780.09
Semiconsciousness 780.09
Seminal
vesicle—*see* condition
vesiculitis (*see also* Vesiculitis) 608.0
Seminoma (M9061/3)
anaplastic type (M9062/3)
specified site—*see* Neoplasm, by site, malignant
unspecified site 186.9
specified site—*see* Neoplasm, by site, malignant
spermatocytic (M9063/3)
specified site—*see* Neoplasm, by site, malignant
unspecified site 186.9
unspecified site 186.9
Semliki Forest encephalitis 062.8
Senear-Usher disease or syndrome (pemphigus erythematosus) 694.4
Senecio jacobae dermatitis 692.6
Senectus 797
Senescence 797
Senile (*see also* condition) 797
cervix (atrophic) 622.8
degenerative atrophy, skin 701.3
endometrium (atrophic) 621.8
fallopian tube (atrophic) 620.3
heart (failure) 797
lung 492.8
ovary (atrophic) 620.3
syndrome 259.8
vagina, vaginitis (atrophic) 627.3
wart 702.0
Senility 797
with
acute confusional state 290.3
delirium 290.3
mental changes 290.9
psychosis NEC (*see also* Psychosis, senile) 290.20
premature (syndrome) 259.8
Sensation
burning (*see also* Disturbance, sensation) 782.0
tongue 529.6
choking 784.9
loss of (*see also* Disturbance, sensation) 782.0
prickling (*see also* Disturbance, sensation) 782.0
tingling (*see also* Disturbance, sensation) 782.0
Sense loss (touch) (*see also* Disturbance, sensation) 782.0
smell 781.1
taste 781.1
Sensibility disturbance NEC (cortical) (deep) (vibratory) (*see also* Disturbance, sensation) 782.0
Sensitive dentine 521.8
Sensitiver Beziehungswahn 297.8
Sensitivity, sensitization —*see also* Allergy
autoerythrocyte 287.2
carotid sinus 337.0
child (excessive) 313.21
cold, autoimmune 283.0
methemoglobin 289.7
suxamethonium 289.8
tuberculin, without clinical or radiological symptoms 795.5
Sensory
extinction 781.8
neglect 781.8
Separation
acromioclavicular—*see* Dislocation, shoulder
anxiety, abnormal 309.21
apophysis, traumatic—*see* Fracture, by site
choroid 363.70
hemorrhagic 363.72
serous 363.71
costochondral (simple) (traumatic)—*see* Dislocation, costochondral
epiphysis, epiphyseal
nontraumatic 732.9
upper femoral 732.2
traumatic—*see* Fracture, by site
fracture—*see* Fracture, by site
infundibulum cardiac from right ventricle by a partition 746.83
joint (current) (traumatic)—*see* Dislocation, by site
placenta (normally implanted)—*see* Placenta, separation
pubic bone, obstetrical trauma 665.6
retina, retinal (*see also* Detachment, retina) 361.9
layers 362.40
sensory (*see also* Retinoschisis) 361.10
pigment epithelium (exudative) 362.42
hemorrhagic 362.43
sternoclavicular (traumatic)—*see* Dislocation, sternoclavicular
symphysis pubis, obstetrical trauma 665.6
tracheal ring, incomplete (congenital) 748.3
Sepsis (generalized) (*see also* Septicemia) 038.9
with
abortion—*see* Abortion, by type, with sepsis
ectopic pregnancy (*see also* categories 633.0-633.9) 639.0
molar pregnancy (*see also* categories 630-632) 639.0
buccal 528.3
complicating labor 659.3
dental (pulpal origin) 522.4
female genital organ NEC 614.9

Sepsis—*continued*
fetus (intrauterine) 771.8
following
abortion 639.0
ectopic or molar pregnancy 639.0
infusion, perfusion, or transfusion 999.3
Friedländer's 038.49
intraocular 360.00
localized
in operation wound 998.5
skin (*see also* Abscess) 682.9
malleus 024
newborn (umbilical) (organism unspecified) NEC 771.8
of tracheostomy stoma 519.0
oral 528.3
puerperal, postpartum, childbirth (pelvic) 670
resulting from infusion, injection, transfusion, or vaccination 999.3
skin, localized (*see also* Abscess) 682.9
umbilical (newborn) (organism unspecified) 771.8
tetanus 771.3
urinary 599.0
Septate —*see also* Septum
Septic —*see also* condition
arm (with lymphangitis) 682.3
embolus—*see* Embolism
finger (with lymphangitis) 681.00
foot (with lymphangitis) 682.7
gallbladder (*see also* Cholecystitis) 575.8
hand (with lymphangitis) 682.4
joint (*see also* Arthritis, septic) 711.0
kidney (*see also* Infection, kidney) 590.9
leg (with lymphangitis) 682.6
mouth 528.3
nail 681.9
finger 681.02
toe 681.11
shock (endotoxic) 785.59
sore (*see also* Abscess) 682.9
throat 034.0
milk-borne 034.0
streptococcal 034.0
spleen (acute) 289.59
teeth (pulpal origin) 522.4
throat 034.0
thrombus—*see* Thrombosis
toe (with lymphangitis) 681.10
tonsils 474.0
umbilical cord (newborn) (organism unspecified) 771.8
uterus (*see also* Endometritis) 615.9
Septicemia, septicemic (generalized) (suppurative) 038.9
with
abortion—*see* Abortion, by type, with sepsis
ectopic pregnancy (*see also* categories 633.0-633.9) 639.0
molar pregnancy (*see also* categories 630-632) 639.0
Aerobacter aerogenes 038.49
anaerobic 038.3
anthrax 022.3
Bacillus coli 038.42
Bacteroides 038.3
Clostridium 038.3
complicating labor 659.3
cryptogenic 038.9
enteric gram-negative bacilli 038.40
Septicemia, septicemic—*continued*
Enterobacter aerogenes 038.49
Erysipelothrix (insidiosa) (rhusiopathiae) 027.1
Escherichia coli 038.42
following
abortion 639.0
ectopic or molar pregnancy 639.0
infusion, injection, transfusion, or vaccination 999.3
Friedländer's (bacillus) 038.49
gangrenous 038.9
gonococcal 098.89
gram-negative (organism) 038.40
anaerobic 038.3
Hemophilus influenzae 038.41
herpes (simplex) 054.5
herpetic 054.5
Listeria monocytogenes 027.0
meningeal—*see* Meningitis
meningococcal (chronic) (fulminating) 036.2
navel, newborn (organism unspecified) 771.8
newborn (umbilical) (organism unspecified) 771.8
plague 020.2
pneumococcal 038.2
postabortal 639.0
postoperative 998.5
Proteus vulgaris 038.49
Pseudomonas (aeruginosa) 038.43
puerperal, postpartum 670
Salmonella (aertrycke) (callinarum) (choleraesuis) (enteritidis) (suipestifer) 003.1
Serratia 038.44
Shigella (*see also* Dysentery, bacillary) 004.9
specified organism NEC 038.8
staphylococcal 038.1
streptococcal (anaerobic) 038.0
suipestifer 003.1
umbilicus, newborn (organism unspecified) 771.8
viral 079.99
Yersinia enterocolitica 038.49
Septum, septate (congenital)—*see also* Anomaly, specified type NEC
anal 751.2
aqueduct of Sylvius 742.3
with spina bifida (*see also* Spina bifida) 741.0
hymen 752.49
uterus (*see also* Double, uterus) 752.2
vagina 752.49
in pregnancy or childbirth 654.7
affecting fetus or newborn 763.8
causing obstructed labor 660.2
affecting fetus or newborn 763.1
Sequestration
lung (congenital) (extralobar) (intralobar) 748.5
orbit 376.10
pulmonary artery (congenital) 747.3
Sequestrum
bone (*see also* Osteomyelitis) 730.1
jaw 526.4
dental 525.8
jaw bone 526.4
sinus (accessory) (nasal) (*see also* Sinusitis) 473.9
maxillary 473.0
Sequoiosis asthma 495.8

Serology for syphilis
doubtful
with signs or symptoms—*see* Syphilis, by site and stage
follow-up of latent syphilis—*see* Syphilis, latent
false positive 795.6
negative, with signs or symptoms—*see* Syphilis, by site and stage
positive 097.1
with signs or symptoms—*see* Syphilis, by site and stage
false 795.6
follow-up of latent syphilis—*see* Syphilis, latent
only finding—*see* Syphilis, latent
reactivated 097.1
Seroma —*see* Hematoma
Seropurulent —*see* condition
Serositis, multiple 569.89
pericardial 423.2
peritoneal 568.82
pleural—*see* Pleurisy
Serotonin syndrome 333.99
Serous —*see* condition
Sertoli cell
adenoma (M8640/0)
specified site—*see* Neoplasm, by site, benign
unspecified site
female 220
male 222.0
carcinoma (M8640/3)
specified site—*see* Neoplasm, by site, malignant
unspecified site 186.9
syndrome (germinal aplasia) 606.0
tumor (M8640/0)
with lipid storage (M8641/0)
specified site—*see* Neoplasm, by site, benign
unspecified site
female 220
male 222.0
specified site—*see* Neoplasm, by site, benign
unspecified site
female 220
male 222.0
Sertoli-Leydig cell tumor (M8631/0)
specified site—*see* Neoplasm, by site, benign
unspecified site
female 220
male 222.0
Serum
allergy, allergic reaction 999.5
shock 999.4
arthritis 999.5 *[713.6]*
complication or reaction NEC 999.5
disease NEC 999.5
hepatitis—*see* Hepatitis, viral
carrier (suspected) of V02.6
intoxication 999.5
jaundice (homologous) *see* Hepatitis, viral
neuritis 999.5
poisoning NEC 999.5
rash NEC 999.5
reaction NEC 999.5
sickness NEC 999.5
Sesamoiditis 733.99
Seven-day fever 061
of
Japan 100.89
Queensland 100.89
Sever's disease or osteochondrosis (calcaneum) 732.5
Sex chromosome mosaics 758.8
Sextuplet
affected by maternal complications of pregnancy 761.5
healthy liveborn—*see* Newborn, multiple
pregnancy (complicating delivery) NEC 651.8
with fetal loss and retention of one or more fetus(es) 651.6
Sexual
anesthesia 302.72
deviation (*see also* Deviation, sexual) 302.9
disorder (*see also* Deviation, sexual) 302.9
frigidity (female) 302.72
function, disorder of (psychogenic) 302.70
specified type NEC 302.79
immaturity (female) (male) 259.0
impotence (psychogenic) 302.72
organic origin NEC 607.84
precocity (constitutional) (cryptogenic) (female) (idiopathic) (male) NEC 259.1
with adrenal hyperplasia 255.2
sadism 302.84
Sexuality, pathological (*see also* Deviation, sexual) 302.9
Sézary's disease, reticulosis, or syndrome (M9701/3) 202.2
Shadow, lung 793.1
Shaking
head (tremor) 781.0
palsy or paralysis (*see also* Parkinsonism) 332.0
Shallowness, acetabulum 736.39
Shaver's disease or syndrome (bauxite pneumoconiosis) 503
Sheath (tendon)—*see* condition
Shedding
nail 703.8
teeth, premature, primary (deciduous) 520.6
Sheehan's disease or syndrome (postpartum pituitary necrosis) 253.2
Shelf, rectal 569.49
Shell
shock (current) (*see also* Reaction, stress, acute) 308.9
lasting state 300.16
teeth 520.5
Shield kidney 753.3
Shift, mediastinal 793.2
Shifting
pacemaker 427.89
sleep-work schedule (affecting sleep) 307.45
Shiga's
bacillus 004.0
dysentery 004.0
Shigella (dysentery) (*see also* Dysentery, bacillary) 004.9
carrier (suspected) of V02.3
Shigellosis (*see also* Dysentery, bacillary) 004.9
Shingles (*see also* Herpes, zoster) 053.9
eye NEC 053.29
Shin splints 844.9
Shipyard eye or disease 077.1
Shirodkar suture, in pregnancy 654.5
Shock 785.50
with
abortion—*see* Abortion, by type, with shock
ectopic pregnancy (*see also* categories 633.0-633.9) 639.5
molar pregnancy (*see also* categories 630-632) 639.5

Shock—*continued*
allergic—*see* Shock, anaphylactic
anaclitic 309.21
anaphylactic 995.0
chemical—*see* Table of drugs and chemicals
correct medicinal substance properly administered 995.0
drug or medicinal substance
correct substance properly administered 995.0
overdose or wrong substance given or taken 977.9
specified drug—*see* Table of drugs and chemicals
food—*see* Anaphylactic shock, due to, food
following sting(s) 989.5
immunization 999.4
serum 999.4
anaphylactoid—*see* Shock, anaphylactic
anesthetic
correct substance properly administered 995.4
overdose or wrong substance given 968.4
specified anesthetic—*see* Table of drugs and chemicals
birth, fetus or newborn NEC 779.8
cardiogenic 785.51
chemical substance—*see* Table of drugs and chemicals
circulatory 785.59
complicating
abortion—*see* Abortion, by type, with shock
ectopic pregnancy (*see also* categories 633.0-633.9) 639.5
labor and delivery 669.1
molar pregnancy (*see also* categories 630-632) 639.5
culture 309.29
due to
drug 995.0
correct substance properly administered 995.0
overdose or wrong substance given or taken 977.9
specified drug—*see* Table of drugs and chemicals
food—*see* Anaphylactic shock, due to, food
during labor and delivery 669.1
electric 994.8
endotoxic 785.59
due to surgical procedure 998.0
following
abortion 639.5
ectopic or molar pregnancy 639.5
injury (immediate) (delayed) 958.4
labor and delivery 669.1
gram-negative 785.59
hematogenic 785.59
hemorrhagic
due to
disease 785.59
surgery (intraoperative) (postoperative) 998.0
trauma 958.4
hypovolemic NEC 785.59
surgical 998.0
traumatic 958.4
insulin 251.0
therapeutic misadventure 962.3
kidney 584.5
traumatic (following crushing) 958.5

Shock—*continued*
lightning 994.0
lung 518.5
nervous (*see also* Reaction, stress, acute) 308.9
obstetric 669.1
with
abortion—*see* Abortion, by type, with shock
ectopic pregnancy (*see also* categories 633.0-633.9) 639.5
molar pregnancy (*see also* categories 630-632) 639.5
following
abortion 639.5
ectopic or molar pregnancy 639.5
paralysis, paralytic (*see also* Disease, cerebrovascular, acute) 436
late effect—*see* category 438
pleural (surgical) 998.0
due to trauma 958.4
postoperative 998.0
with
abortion—*see* Abortion, by type, with shock
ectopic pregnancy (*see also* categories 633.0-633.9) 639.5
molar pregnancy (*see also* categories 630-632) 639.5
following
abortion 639.5
ectopic or molar pregnancy 639.5
psychic (*see also* Reaction, stress, acute) 308.9
past history (of) V15.4
psychogenic (*see also* Reaction, stress, acute) 308.9
septic 785.59
with
abortion—*see* Abortion, by type, with shock
ectopic pregnancy (*see also* categories 633.0-633.9) 639.5
molar pregnancy (*see also* categories 630-632) 639.5
due to
surgical procedure 998.0
transfusion NEC 999.8
bone marrow 996.85
following
abortion 639.5
ectopic or molar pregnancy 639.5
surgical procedure 998.0
transfusion NEC 999.8
bone marrow 996.85
spinal—*see also* Injury, spinal, by site
with spinal bone injury—*see* Fracture, vertebra, by site, with spinal cord injury
surgical 998.0
therapeutic misadventure NEC (*see also* Complications) 998.89
thyroxin 962.7
toxic 040.89
transfusion—*see* Complications, transfusion
traumatic (immediate) (delayed) 958.4
Shoemakers' chest 738.3
Short, shortening, shortness
Achilles tendon (acquired) 727.81
arm 736.89
congenital 755.20
back 737.9
bowel syndrome 579.3
breath 786.09
common bile duct, congenital 751.69
cord (umbilical) 663.4
affecting fetus or newborn 762.6

Short, shortening, shortness—*continued*
cystic duct, congenital 751.69
esophagus (congenital) 750.4
femur (acquired) 736.81
congenital 755.34
frenulum linguae 750.0
frenum, lingual 750.0
hamstrings 727.81
hip (acquired) 736.39
congenital 755.63
leg (acquired) 736.81
congenital 755.30
metatarsus (congenital) 754.79
acquired 736.79
organ or site, congenital NEC—*see* Distortion
palate (congenital) 750.26
P-R interval syndrome 426.81
radius (acquired) 736.09
congenital 755.26
round ligament 629.8
sleeper 307.49
stature, constitutional (hereditary) 783.4
tendon 727.81
Achilles (acquired) 727.81
congenital 754.79
congenital 756.89
thigh (acquired) 736.81
congenital 755.34
tibialis anticus 727.81
umbilical cord 663.4
affecting fetus or newborn 762.6
urethra 599.84
uvula (congenital) 750.26
vagina 623.8
Shortsightedness 367.1
Shoshin (acute fulminating beriberi) 265.0
Shoulder —*see* condition
Shovel-shaped incisors 520.2
Shower, thromboembolic —*see* Embolism
Shunt (status)
aortocoronary bypass V45.81
arterial-venous (dialysis) V45.1
arteriovenous, pulmonary (acquired) 417.0
congenital 747.3
traumatic (complication) 901.40
cerebral ventricle (communicating) in situ V45.2
coronary artery bypass V45.81
surgical, prosthetic, with complications—*see* Complications, shunt
vascular NEC V45.89
Shutdown
renal 586
with
abortion—*see* Abortion, by type, with renal failure
ectopic pregnancy (*see also* categories 633.0-633.9) 639.3
molar pregnancy (*see also* categories 630-632) 639.3
complicating
abortion 639.3
ectopic or molar pregnancy 639.3
following labor and delivery 669.3
Shwachman's syndrome 288.0
Shy-Drager syndrome (orthostatic hypotension with multisystem degeneration) 333.0
Sialadenitis (any gland) (chronic) (suppurative) 527.2
epidemic—*see* Mumps
Sialadenosis, periodic 527.2
Sialaporia 527.7
Sialectasia 527.8
Sialitis 527.2
Sialoadenitis (*see also* Sialadenitis) 527.2
Sialoangitis 527.2
Sialodochitis (fibrinosa) 527.2
Sialodocholithiasis 527.5
Sialolithiasis 527.5
Sialorrhea (*see also* Ptyalism) 527.7
periodic 527.2
Sialosis 527.8
rheumatic 710.2
Siamese twin 759.4
Sicard's syndrome 352.6
Sicca syndrome (keratoconjunctivitis) 710.2
Sick 799.9
cilia syndrome 759.89
or handicapped person in family V61.49
Sickle-cell
anemia (*see also* Disease, sickle-cell) 282.60
disease (*see also* Disease, sickle-cell) 282.60
hemoglobin
C disease 282.63
D disease 282.69
E disease 282.69
thalassemia 282.4
trait 282.5
Sicklemia (*see also* Disease, sickle-cell) 282.60
trait 282.5
Sickness
air (travel) 994.6
airplane 994.6
alpine 993.2
altitude 993.2
Andes 993.2
aviators' 993.2
balloon 993.2
car 994.6
compressed air 993.3
decompression 993.3
green 280.9
harvest 100.89
milk 988.8
morning 643.0
motion 994.6
mountain 993.2
acute 289.0
protein (*see also* Complications, vaccination) 999.5
radiation NEC 990
roundabout (motion) 994.6
sea 994.6
serum NEC 999.5
sleeping (African) 086.5
by Trypanosoma 086.5
gambiense 086.3
rhodesiense 086.4
Gambian 086.3
late effect 139.8
Rhodesian 086.4
sweating 078.2
swing (motion) 994.6
train (railway) (travel) 994.6
travel (any vehicle) 994.6
Sick sinus syndrome 427.81
Sideropenia (*see also* Anemia, iron deficiency) 280.9
Siderosis (lung) (occupational) 503
cornea 371.15
eye (bulbi) (vitreous) 360.23
lens 360.23
Siegal-Cattan-Mamou disease (periodic) 277.3

Siemens' syndrome
ectodermal dysplasia 757.31
keratosis follicularis spinulosa (decalvans) 757.39
Sighing respiration 786.7
Sigmoid
flexure—*see* condition
kidney 753.3
Sigmoiditis —*see* Enteritis
Silfverskiöld's syndrome 756.50
Silicosis, sillicotic (complicated) (occupational) (simple) 502
fibrosis, lung (confluent) (massive) (occupational) 502
non-nodular 503
pulmonum 502
Silicotuberculosis (*see also* Tuberculosis) 011.4
Silo fillers' disease 506.9
Silver's syndrome (congenital hemihypertrophy and short stature) 759.89
Silver wire arteries, retina 362.13
Silvestroni-Bianco syndrome (thalassemia minima) 282.4
Simian crease 757.2
Simmonds' cachexia or disease (pituitary cachexia) 253.2
Simons' disease or syndrome (progressive lipodystrophy) 272.6
Simple, simplex —*see* condition
Sinding-Larsen disease (juvenile osteopathia patellae) 732.4
Singapore hemorrhagic fever 065.4
Singers' node or nodule 478.5
Single
atrium 745.69
coronary artery 746.85
umbilical artery 747.5
ventricle 745.3
Singultus 786.8
epidemicus 078.89
Sinus —*see also* Fistula
abdominal 569.81
arrest 426.6
arrhythmia 427.89
bradycardia 427.89
chronic 427.81
branchial cleft (external) (internal) 744.41
coccygeal (infected) 685.1
with abscess 685.0
dental 522.7
dermal (congenital) 685.1
with abscess 685.0
draining—*see* Fistula
infected, skin NEC 686.9
marginal, ruptured or bleeding 641.2
affecting fetus or newborn 762.1
pause 426.6
pericranii 742.0
pilonidal (infected) (rectum) 685.1
with abscess 685.0
preauricular 744.46
rectovaginal 619.1
sacrococcygeal (dermoid) (infected) 685.1
with abscess 685.0
tachycardia 427.89
tarsi syndrome 355.5
testis 608.89
tract (postinfectional)—*see* Fistula
urachus 753.7
Sinuses, Rokitansky-Aschoff (*see also* Disease, gallbladder) 575.8
Sinusitis (accessory) (nasal) (hyperplastic) (nonpurulent) (purulent) (chronic) 473.9
with influenza, flu, or grippe 487.1
acute 461.9
ethmoidal 461.2
frontal 461.1
maxillary 461.0
specified type NEC 461.8
sphenoidal 461.3
allergic (*see also* Fever, hay) 477.9
antrum—*see* Sinusitis, maxillary
due to
fungus, any sinus 117.9
high altitude 993.1
ethmoidal 473.2
acute 461.2
frontal 473.1
acute 461.1
influenzal 478.1
maxillary 473.0
acute 461.0
specified site NEC 473.8
sphenoidal 473.3
acute 461.3
syphilitic, any sinus 095.8
tuberculous, any sinus (*see also* Tuberculosis) 012.8
Sinusitis-bronchiectasis-situs inversus (syndrome) (triad) 759.3
Sipple's syndrome (medullary thyroid carcinoma-pheochromocytoma) 193
Sirenomelia 759.89
Siriasis 992.0
Sirkari's disease 085.0
Siti 104.0
Sitophobia 300.29
Situation, psychiatric 300.9
Situational
disturbance (transient) (*see also* Reaction, adjustment) 309.9
acute 308.3
maladjustment, acute (*see also* Reaction, adjustment) 309.9
reaction (*see also* Reaction, adjustment) 309.9
acute 308.3
Situs inversus or transversus 759.3
abdominalis 759.3
thoracis 759.3
Sixth disease 057.8
Sjögren (-Gougerot) syndrome or disease (keratoconjunctivitis sicca) 710.2
with lung involvement 710.2 *[517.8]*
Sjögren-Larsson syndrome (ichthyosis congenita) 757.1
Skeletal —*see* condition
Skene's gland —*see* condition
Skenitis (*see also* Urethritis) 597.89
gonorrheal (acute) 098.0
chronic or duration of 2 months or over 098.2
Skerljevo 104.0
Skevas-Zerfus disease 989.5
Skin —*see also* condition
donor V59.1
hidebound 710.9
Slate-dressers' lung 502
Slate-miners' lung 502

Sleep
disorder 780.50
with apnea—*see* Apnea, sleep
child 307.40
nonorganic origin 307.40
specified type NEC 307.49
disturbance 780.50
with apnea—*see* Apnea, sleep
nonorganic origin 307.40
specified type NEC 307.49
drunkenness 307.47
paroxysmal 347
rhythm inversion 780.55
nonorganic origin 307.45
walking 307.46
hysterical 300.13
Sleeping sickness 086.5
late effect 139.8
Sleeplessness (*see also* Insomnia) 780.52
menopausal 627.2
nonorganic origin 307.41
Slipped, slipping
epiphysis (postinfectional) 732.9
traumatic (old) 732.9
current—*see* Fracture, by site
upper femoral (nontraumatic) 732.2
intervertebral disc—*see* Displacement, intervertebral disc
ligature, umbilical 772.3
patella 717.89
rib 733.99
sacroiliac joint 724.6
tendon 727.9
ulnar nerve, nontraumatic 354.2
vertebra NEC (*see also* Spondylolisthesis) 756.12
Slocumb's syndrome 255.3
Sloughing (multiple) (skin) 686.9
abscess—*see* Abscess, by site
appendix 543.9
bladder 596.8
fascia 728.9
graft—*see* Complications, graft
phagedena (*see also* Gangrene) 785.4
reattached extremity (*see also* Complications, reattached extremity) 996.90
rectum 569.49
scrotum 608.89
tendon 727.9
transplanted organ (*see also* Rejection, transplant, organ, by site) 996.80
ulcer (*see also* Ulcer, skin) 707.9
Slow
feeding newborn 779.3
fetal, growth NEC 764.9
affecting management of pregnancy 656.5
Slowing
heart 427.89
urinary stream 788.62
Sluder's neuralgia or syndrome 337.0
Slurred, slurring, speech 784.5
Small, smallness
cardiac reserve—*see* Disease, heart
for dates
fetus or newborn 764.0
with malnutrition 764.1
affecting management of pregnancy 656.5
infant, term 764.0
with malnutrition 764.1
affecting management of pregnancy 656.5
Small, smallness—*continued*
introitus, vagina 623.3
kidney, unknown cause 589.9
bilateral 589.1
unilateral 589.0
ovary 620.8
pelvis
with disproportion (fetopelvic) 653.1
affecting fetus or newborn 763.1
causing obstructed labor 660.1
affecting fetus or newborn 763.1
placenta—*see* Placenta, insufficiency
uterus 621.8
white kidney 582.9
Small-for-dates (*see also* Light-for-dates) 764.0
affecting management of pregnancy 656.5
Smallpox 050.9
contact V01.3
exposure to V01.3
hemorrhagic (pustular) 050.0
malignant 050.0
modified 050.2
vaccination
complications—*see* Complications, vaccination
prophylactic (against) V04.1
Smith's fracture (separation) (closed) 813.41
open 813.51
Smith-Lemli-Opitz syndrome (cerebrohepatorenal syndrome) 759.89
Smith-Strang disease (oasthouse urine) 270.2
Smokers'
bronchitis 491.0
cough 491.0
syndrome (*see also* Abuse, drugs, nondependent) 305.1
throat 472.1
tongue 528.6
Smothering spells 786.09
Snaggle teeth, tooth 524.3
Snapping
finger 727.05
hip 719.65
jaw 524.69
knee 717.9
thumb 727.05
Sneddon-Wilkinson disease or syndrome (subcorneal pustular dermatosis) 694.1
Sneezing 784.9
intractable 478.1
Sniffing
cocaine (*see also* Dependence) 304.2
ether (*see also* Dependence) 304.6
glue (airplane) (*see also* Dependence) 304.6
Snoring 786.09
Snow blindness 370.24
Snuffles (nonsyphilitic) 460
syphilitic (infant) 090.0
Social migrant V60.0
Sodoku 026.0
Soemmering's ring 366.51
Soft —*see also* condition
nails 703.8
Softening
bone 268.2
brain (necrotic) (progressive) 434.9
arteriosclerotic 437.0
congenital 742.4
embolic (*see also* Embolism, brain) 434.1
hemorrhagic (*see also* Hemorrhage, brain) 431

Softening—*continued*
occlusive 434.9
thrombotic (*see also* Thrombosis, brain) 434.0
cartilage 733.92
cerebellar—*see* Softening, brain
cerebral—*see* Softening, brain
cerebrospinal—*see* Softening, brain
myocardial, heart (*see also* Degeneration, myocardial) 429.1
nails 703.8
spinal cord 336.8
stomach 537.89
Solar fever 061
Soldier's
heart 306.2
patches 423.1
Solitary
cyst
bone 733.21
kidney 593.2
kidney (congenital) 753.0
tubercle, brain (*see also* Tuberculosis, brain) 013.2
ulcer, bladder 596.8
Somatization reaction, somatic reaction (*see also* Disorder, psychosomatic) 306.9
Somnambulism 307.46
hysterical 300.13
Somnolence 780.09
nonorganic origin 307.43
periodic 349.89
Sonne dysentery 004.3
Soor 112.0
Sore
Delhi 085.1
desert (*see also* Ulcer, skin) 707.9
eye 379.99
Lahore 085.1
mouth 528.9
canker 528.2
due to dentures 528.9
muscle 729.1
Naga (*see also* Ulcer, skin) 707.9
oriental 085.1
pressure 707.0
with gangrene 707.0 *[785.4]*
skin NEC 709.9
soft 099.0
throat 462
with influenza, flu, or grippe 487.1
acute 462
chronic 472.1
clergyman's 784.49
coxsackie (virus) 074.0
diphtheritic 032.0
epidemic 034.0
gangrenous 462
herpetic 054.79
influenzal 487.1
malignant 462
purulent 462
putrid 462
septic 034.0
streptococcal (ulcerative) 034.0
ulcerated 462
viral NEC 462
Coxsackie 074.0
tropical (*see also* Ulcer, skin) 707.9
veldt (*see also* Ulcer, skin) 707.9
Sotos' syndrome (cerebral gigantism) 253.0
Sounds
friction, pleural 786.7
succussion, chest 786.7
South African cardiomyopathy syndrome 425.2
South American
blastomycosis 116.1
trypanosomiasis—*see* Trypanosomiasis
Southeast Asian hemorrhagic fever 065.4
Spacing, teeth, abnormal 524.3
Spade-like hand (congenital) 754.89
Spading nail 703.8
congenital 757.5
Spanemia 285.9
Spanish collar 605
Sparganosis 123.5
Spasm, spastic, spasticity (*see also* condition) 781.0
accommodation 367.53
ampulla of Vater (*see also* Disease, gallbladder) 576.8
anus, ani (sphincter) (reflex) 564.6
psychogenic 306.4
artery NEC 443.9
basilar 435.0
carotid 435.8
cerebral 435.9
specified artery NEC 435.8
retinal (*see also* Occlusion, retinal, artery) 362.30
vertebral 435.1
vertebrobasilar 435.3
Bell's 351.0
bladder (sphincter, external or internal) 596.8
bowel 564.1
psychogenic 306.4
bronchus, bronchiole 519.1
cardia 530.0
cardiac—*see* Angina
carpopedal (*see also* Tetany) 781.7
cecum 564.1
psychogenic 306.4
cerebral (arteries) (vascular) 435.9
specified artery NEC 435.8
cerebrovascular 435.9
cervix, complicating delivery 661.4
affecting fetus or newborn 763.7
ciliary body (of accommodation) 367.53
colon 564.1
psychogenic 306.4
common duct (*see also* Disease, biliary) 576.8
compulsive 307.22
conjugate 378.82
convergence 378.84
coronary (artery)—*see* Angina
diaphragm (reflex) 786.8
psychogenic 306.1
duodenum, duodenal (bulb) 564.8
esophagus (diffuse) 530.5
psychogenic 306.4
facial 351.8
fallopian tube 620.8
gait 781.2
gastrointestinal (tract) 536.8
psychogenic 306.4
glottis 478.75
hysterical 300.11
psychogenic 306.1
specified as conversion reaction 300.11
reflex through recurrent laryngeal nerve 478.75

Spasm, spastic, spasticity—*continued*
habit 307.20
chronic 307.22
transient of childhood 307.21
heart—*see* Angina
hourglass—*see* Contraction, hourglass
hysterical 300.11
infantile (*see also* Epilepsy) 345.6
internal oblique, eye 378.51
intestinal 564.1
psychogenic 306.4
larynx, laryngeal 478.75
hysterical 300.11
psychogenic 306.1
specified as conversion reaction 300.11
levator palpebrae superioris 333.81
lightning (*see also* Epilepsy) 345.6
mobile 781.0
muscle 728.85
back 724.8
psychogenic 306.0
nerve, trigeminal 350.1
nervous 306.0
nodding 307.3
infantile (*see also* Epilepsy) 345.6
occupational 300.89
oculogyric 378.87
ophthalmic artery 362.30
orbicularis 781.0
perineal 625.8
peroneo-extensor (*see also* Flat, foot) 734
pharynx (reflex) 478.29
hysterical 300.11
psychogenic 306.1
specified as conversion reaction 300.11
pregnant uterus, complicating delivery 661.4
psychogenic 306.0
pylorus 537.81
adult hypertrophic 537.0
congenital or infantile 750.5
psychogenic 306.4
rectum (sphincter) 564.6
psychogenic 306.4
retinal artery NEC (*see also* Occlusion, retina, artery) 362.30
sacroiliac 724.6
salaam (infantile) (*see also* Epilepsy) 345.6
saltatory 781.0
sigmoid 564.1
psychogenic 306.4
sphincter of Oddi (*see also* Disease, gallbladder) 576.5
stomach 536.8
neurotic 306.4
throat 478.29
hysterical 300.11
psychogenic 306.1
specified as conversion reaction 300.11
tic 307.20
chronic 307.22
transient of childhood 307.21
tongue 529.8
torsion 333.6
trigeminal nerve 350.1
postherpetic 053.12
ureter 593.89
urethra (sphincter) 599.84

Spasm, spastic, spasticity—*continued*
uterus 625.8
complicating labor 661.4
affecting fetus or newborn 763.7
vagina 625.1
psychogenic 306.51
vascular NEC 443.9
vasomotor NEC 443.9
vein NEC 459.89
vesical (sphincter, external or internal) 596.8
viscera 789.0
Spasmodic —*see* condition
Spasmophilia (*see also* Tetany) 781.7
Spasmus nutans 307.3
Spastic —*see also* Spasm
child 343.9
Spasticity —*see also* Spasm
cerebral, child 343.9
Speakers' throat 784.49
Specific, specified —*see* condition
Speech
defect, disorder, disturbance, impediment NEC 784.5
psychogenic 307.9
therapy V57.3
Spells 780.3
breath-holding 786.9
Spencer's disease (epidemic vomiting) 078.82
Spens' syndrome (syncope with heart block) 426.9
Spermatic cord —*see* condition
Spermatocele 608.1
congenital 752.8
Spermatocystitis 608.4
Spermatocytoma (M9063/3)
specified site—*see* Neoplasm, by site, malignant
unspecified site 186.9
Spermatorrhea 608.89
Sperm counts V26.2
postvasectomy V25.8
Sphacelus (*see also* Gangrene) 785.4
Sphenoidal —*see* condition
Sphenoiditis (chronic) (*see also* Sinusitis, sphenoidal) 473.3
Sphenopalatine ganglion neuralgia 337.0
Sphericity, increased, lens 743.36
Spherocytosis (congenital) (familial) (hereditary) 282.0
hemoglobin disease 287.7
sickle-cell (disease) 282.60
Spherophakia 743.36
Sphincter —*see* condition
Sphincteritis, sphincter of Oddi (*see also* Cholecystitis) 576.8
Sphingolipidosis 272.7
Sphingolipodystrophy 272.7
Sphingomyelinosis 272.7
Spicule tooth 520.2
Spider
finger 755.59
nevus 448.1
vascular 448.1
Spiegler-Fendt sarcoid 686.8
Spielmeyer-Stock disease 330.1
Spielmeyer-Vogt disease 330.1

Spina bifida (aperta) 741.9

> Note—Use the following fifth-digit subclassification with category 741:
>
> *0 unspecified region*
> *1 cervical region*
> *2 dorsal [thoracic] region*
> *3 lumbar region*

with hydrocephalus 741.0
fetal (suspected), affecting management of pregnancy 655.0
occulta 756.17
Spindle, Krukenberg's 371.13
Spine, spinal —*see* condition
Spiradenoma (eccrine) (M8403/0)—*see* Neoplasm, skin, benign
Spirillosis NEC (*see also* Fever, relapsing) 087.9
Spirillum minus 026.0
Spirillum obermeieri infection 087.0
Spirochetal —*see* condition
Spirochetosis 104.9
arthritic, arthritica 104.9 *[711.8]*
bronchopulmonary 104.8
icterohemorrhagica 100.0
lung 104.8
Spitting blood (*see also* Hemoptysis) 786.3
Splanchnomegaly 569.89
Splanchnoptosis 569.89
Spleen, splenic —*see also* condition
agenesis 759.0
flexure syndrome 569.89
neutropenia syndrome 288.0
sequestration syndrome 282.60
Splenectasis (*see also* Splenomegaly) 789.2
Splenitis (interstitial) (malignant) (nonspecific) 289.59
malarial (*see also* Malaria) 084.6
tuberculous (*see also* Tuberculosis) 017.7
Splenocele 289.59
Splenomegalia —*see* Splenomegaly
Splenomegalic —*see* condition
Splenomegaly 789.2
Bengal 789.2
cirrhotic 289.51
congenital 759.0
congestive, chronic 289.51
cryptogenic 789.2
Egyptian 120.1
Gaucher's (cerebroside lipidosis) 272.7
idiopathic 789.2
malarial (*see also* Malaria) 084.6
neutropenic 288.0
Niemann-Pick (lipid histiocytosis) 272.7
siderotic 289.51
syphilitic 095.8
congenital 090.0
tropical (Bengal) (idiopathic) 789.2
Splenopathy 289.50
Splenopneumonia —*see* Pneumonia
Splenoptosis 289.59
Splinter —*see* Injury, superficial, by site
Split, splitting
heart sounds 427.89
lip, congenital (*see also* Cleft, lip) 749.10
nails 703.8
urinary stream 788.61
Spoiled child reaction (*see also* Disturbance, conduct) 312.1
Spondylarthritis (*see also* Spondylosis) 721.90
Spondylarthrosis (*see also* Spondylosis) 721.90
Spondylitis 720.9
ankylopoietica 720.0
ankylosing (chronic) 720.0
atrophic 720.9
ligamentous 720.9
chronic (traumatic) (*see also* Spondylosis) 721.90
deformans (chronic) (*see also* Spondylosis) 721.90
gonococcal 098.53
gouty 274.0
hypertrophic (*see also* Spondylosis) 721.90
infectious NEC 720.9
juvenile (adolescent) 720.0
Kümmell's 721.7
Marie-Strümpell (ankylosing) 720.0
muscularis 720.9
ossificans ligamentosa 721.6
osteoarthritica (*see also* Spondylosis) 721.90
posttraumatic 721.7
proliferative 720.0
rheumatoid 720.0
rhizomelica 720.0
sacroiliac NEC 720.2
senescent (*see also* Spondylosis) 721.90
senile (*see also* Spondylosis) 721.90
static (*see also* Spondylosis) 721.90
traumatic (chronic) (*see also* Spondylosis) 721.90
tuberculous (*see also* Tuberculosis) 015.0 *[720.81]*
typhosa 002.0 *[720.81]*
Spondyloarthrosis (*see also* Spondylosis) 721.90
Spondylolisthesis (congenital) (lumbosacral) 756.12
with disproportion (fetopelvic) 653.3
affecting fetus or newborn 763.1
causing obstructed labor 660.1
affecting fetus or newborn 763.1
acquired 738.4
degenerative 738.4
traumatic 756.12
acute (lumbar)—*see* Fracture, vertebra, lumbar
site other than lumbosacral—*see* Fracture, vertebra, by site
Spondylolysis (congenital) 756.11
acquired 738.4
cervical 756.19
lumbosacral region 756.11
with disproportion (fetopelvic) 653.3
affecting fetus or newborn 763.1
causing obstructed labor 660.1
affecting fetus or newborn 763.1
Spondylopathy
inflammatory 720.9
specified type NEC 720.89
traumatic 721.7
Spondylose rhizomelique 720.0
Spondylosis 721.90
with
disproportion 653.3
affecting fetus or newborn 763.1
causing obstructed labor 660.1
affecting fetus or newborn 763.1
myelopathy NEC 721.91
cervical, cervicodorsal 721.0
with myelopathy 721.1
inflammatory 720.9
lumbar, lumbosacral 721.3
with myelopathy 721.42

Spondylosis—*continued*
sacral 721.3
with myelopathy 721.42
thoracic 721.2
with myelopathy 721.41
traumatic 721.7
Sponge
divers' disease 989.5
inadvertently left in operation wound 998.4
kidney (medullary) 753.17
Spongioblastoma (M9422/3)
multiforme (M9440/3)
specified site—*see* Neoplasm, by site, malignant
unspecified site 191.9
polare (M9423/3)
specified site—*see* Neoplasm, by site, malignant
unspecified site 191.9
primitive polar (M9443/3)
specified site—*see* Neoplasm, by site, malignant
unspecified site 191.9
specified site—*see* Neoplasm, by site, malignant
unspecified site 191.9
Spongiocytoma (M9400/3)
specified site—*see* Neoplasm, by site, malignant
unspecified site 191.9
Spongioneuroblastoma (M9504/3)—*see* Neoplasm, by site, malignant
Spontaneous —*see also* condition
fracture—*see* Fracture, pathologic
Spoon nail 703.8
congenital 757.5
Sporadic —*see* condition
Sporotrichosis (bones) (cutaneous) (disseminated) (epidermal) (lymphatic) (lymphocutaneous) (mucous membranes) (pulmonary) (skeletal) (visceral) 117.1
Sporotrichum schenckii infection 117.1
Spots, spotting
atrophic (skin) 701.3
Bitôt's (in the young child) 264.1
café au lait 709.09
cayenne pepper 448.1
cotton wool (retina) 362.83
de Morgan's (senile angiomas) 448.1
Fúchs' black (myopic) 360.21
intermenstrual
irregular 626.6
regular 626.5
interpalpebral 372.53
Koplik's 055.9
liver 709.09
Mongolian (pigmented) 757.33
of pregnancy 641.9
purpuric 782.7
ruby 448.1
Spotted fever —*see* Fever, spotted
Sprain, strain (joint) (ligament) (muscle) (tendon) 848.9
abdominal wall (muscle) 848.8
Achilles tendon 845.09
acromioclavicular 840.0
ankle 845.00
and foot 845.00
anterior longitudinal, cervical 847.0
arm 840.9
upper 840.9
and shoulder 840.9

Sprain, strain—*continued*
astragalus 845.00
atlanto-axial 847.0
atlanto-occipital 847.0
atlas 847.0
axis 847.0
back (*see also* Sprain, spine) 847.9
breast bone 848.40
broad ligament—*see* Injury, internal, broad ligament
calcaneofibular 845.02
carpal 842.01
carpometacarpal 842.11
cartilage
costal, without mention of injury to sternum 848.3
involving sternum 848.42
ear 848.8
knee 844.9
with current tear (*see also* Tear, meniscus) 836.2
semilunar (knee) 844.8
with current tear (*see also* Tear, meniscus) 836.2
septal, nose 848.0
thyroid region 848.2
xiphoid 848.49
cervical, cervicodorsal, cervicothoracic 847.0
chondrocostal, without mention of injury to sternum 848.3
involving sternum 848.42
chondrosternal 848.42
chronic (joint)—*see* Derangement, joint
clavicle 840.9
coccyx 847.4
collar bone 840.9
collateral, knee (medial) (tibial) 844.1
lateral (fibular) 844.0
recurrent or old 717.89
lateral 717.81
medial 717.82
coracoacromial 840.8
coracoclavicular 840.1
coracohumeral 840.2
coracoid (process) 840.9
coronary, knee 844.8
costal cartilage, without mention of injury to sternum 848.3
involving sternum 848.42
cricoarytenoid articulation 848.2
cricothyroid articulation 848.2
cruciate
knee 844.2
old 717.89
anterior 717.83
posterior 717.84
deltoid
ankle 845.01
shoulder 840.8
dorsal (spine) 847.1
ear cartilage 848.8
elbow 841.9
and forearm 841.9
specified site NEC 841.8
femur (proximal end) 843.9
distal end 844.9
fibula (proximal end) 844.9
distal end 845.00
fibulocalcaneal 845.02
finger(s) 842.10

Sprain, strain—*continued*
foot 845.10
and ankle 845.00
forearm 841.9
and elbow 841.9
specified site NEC 841.8
glenoid (shoulder) 840.8
hand 842.10
hip 843.9
and thigh 843.9
humerus (proximal end) 840.9
distal end 841.9
iliofemoral 843.0
infraspinatus 840.3
innominate
acetabulum 843.9
pubic junction 848.5
sacral junction 846.1
internal
collateral, ankle 845.01
semilunar cartilage 844.8
with current tear (*see also* Tear, meniscus) 836.2
old 717.5
interphalangeal
finger 842.13
toe 845.13
ischiocapsular 843.1
jaw (cartilage) (meniscus) 848.1
old 524.69
knee 844.9
and leg 844.9
old 717.5
collateral
lateral 717.81
medial 717.82
cruciate
anterior 717.83
posterior 717.84
late effect—*see* Late, effects (of), sprain
lateral collateral, knee 844.0
old 717.81
leg 844.9
and knee 844.9
ligamentum teres femoris 843.8
low back 846.9
lumbar (spine) 847.2
lumbosacral 846.0
chronic or old 724.6
mandible 848.1
old 524.69
maxilla 848.1
medial collateral, knee 844.1
old 717.82
meniscus
jaw 848.1
old 524.69
knee 844.8
with current tear (*see also* Tear, meniscus) 836.2
old 717.5
mandible 848.1
old 524.69
specified site NEC 848.8
metacarpal 842.10
distal 842.12
proximal 842.11
metacarpophalangeal 842.12
metatarsal 845.10
metatarsophalangeal 845.12

Sprain, strain—*continued*
midcarpal 842.19
midtarsal 845.19
multiple sites, except fingers alone or toes alone 848.8
neck 847.0
nose (septal cartilage) 848.0
occiput from atlas 847.0
old—*see* Derangement, joint
orbicular, hip 843.8
patella(r) 844.8
old 717.89
pelvis 848.5
phalanx
finger 842.10
toe 845.10
radiocarpal 842.02
radiohumeral 841.2
radioulnar 841.9
distal 842.09
radius, radial (proximal end) 841.9
and ulna 841.9
distal 842.09
collateral 841.0
distal end 842.00
recurrent—*see* Sprain, by site
rib (cage), without mention of injury to sternum 848.3
involving sternum 848.42
rotator cuff (capsule) 840.4
round ligament—*see also* Injury, internal, round ligament
femur 843.8
sacral (spine) 847.3
sacrococcygeal 847.3
sacroiliac (region) 846.9
chronic or old 724.6
ligament 846.1
specified site NEC 846.8
sacrospinatus 846.2
sacrospinous 846.2
sacrotuberous 846.3
scaphoid bone, ankle 845.00
scapula(r) 840.9
semilunar cartilage (knee) 844.8
with current tear (*see also* Tear, meniscus) 836.2
old 717.5
septal cartilage (nose) 848.0
shoulder 840.9
and arm, upper 840.9
blade 840.9
specified site NEC 848.8
spine 847.9
cervical 847.0
coccyx 847.4
dorsal 847.1
lumbar 847.2
lumbosacral 846.0
chronic or old 724.6
sacral 847.3
sacroiliac (*see also* Sprain, sacroiliac) 846.9
chronic or old 724.6
thoracic 847.1
sternoclavicular 848.41
sternum 848.40
subglenoid 840.8
subscapularis 840.5
supraspinatus 840.6

Sprain, strain—*continued*
symphysis
jaw 848.1
old 524.69
mandibular 848.1
old 524.69
pubis 848.5
talofibular 845.09
tarsal 845.10
tarsometatarsal 845.11
temporomandibular 848.1
old 524.69
teres
ligamentum femoris 843.8
major or minor 840.8
thigh (proximal end) 843.9
and hip 843.9
distal end 844.9
thoracic (spine) 847.1
thorax 848.8
thumb 842.10
thyroid cartilage or region 848.2
tibia (proximal end) 844.9
distal end 845.00
tibiofibular
distal 845.03
superior 844.3
toe(s) 845.10
trachea 848.8
trapezoid 840.8
ulna, ulnar (proximal end) 841.9
collateral 841.1
distal end 842.00
ulnohumeral 841.3
vertebrae (*see also* Sprain, spine) 847.9
cervical, cervicodorsal, cervicothoracic 847.0
wrist (cuneiform) (scaphoid) (semilunar) 842.00
xiphoid cartilage 848.49
Sprengel's deformity (congenital) 755.52
Spring fever 309.23
Sprue 579.1
celiac 579.0
idiopathic 579.0
meaning thrush 112.0
nontropical 579.0
tropical 579.1
Spur —*see also* Exostosis
bone 726.91
calcaneal 726.73
calcaneal 726.73
iliac crest 726.5
nose (septum) 478.1
bone 726.91
septal 478.1
Spuria placenta —*see* Placenta, abnormal
Spurway's syndrome (brittle bones and blue sclera) 756.51
Sputum, abnormal (amount) (color) (excessive) (odor) (purulent) 786.4
bloody 786.3
Squamous —*see also* condition
cell metaplasia
bladder 596.8
cervix—*see* condition
epithelium in
cervical canal (congenital) 752.49
uterine mucosa (congenital) 752.3
metaplasia
bladder 596.8
cervix—*see* condition
Squashed nose 738.0
congenital 754.0
Squeeze, divers' 993.3
Squint (*see also* Strabismus) 378.9
accommodative (*see also* Esotropia) 378.00
concomitant (*see also* Heterotropia) 378.30
Stab —*see also* Wound, open, by site
internal organs—*see* Injury, internal, by site, with open wound
Staggering gait 781.2
hysterical 300.11
Staghorn calculus 592.0
Stähl's
ear 744.29
pigment line (cornea) 371.11
Stähli's pigment lines (cornea) 371.11
Stain
port wine 757.32
tooth, teeth (hard tissues) 521.7
due to
accretions 523.6
deposits (betel) (black) (green) (materia alba) (orange) (tobacco) 523.6
metals (copper) (silver) 521.7
nicotine 523.6
pulpal bleeding 521.7
tobacco 523.6
Stammering 307.0
Standstill
atrial 426.6
auricular 426.6
cardiac (*see also* Arrest, cardiac) 427.5
sinoatrial 426.6
sinus 426.6
ventricular (*see also* Arrest, cardiac) 427.5
Stannosis 503
Stanton's disease (melioidosis) 025
Staphylitis (acute) (catarrhal) (chronic) (gangrenous) (membranous) (suppurative) (ulcerative) 528.3
Staphylococcemia 038.1
Staphylococcus, staphylococcal —*see* condition
Staphyloderma (skin) 686.0
Staphyloma 379.11
anterior, localized 379.14
ciliary 379.11
cornea 371.73
equatorial 379.13
posterior 379.12
posticum 379.12
ring 379.15
sclera NEC 379.11
Starch eating 307.52
Stargardt's disease 362.75
Starvation (inanition) (due to lack of food) 994.2
edema 262
voluntary NEC 307.1
Stasis
bile (duct) (*see also* Disease, biliary) 576.8
bronchus (*see also* Bronchitis) 490
cardiac (*see also* Failure, heart, congestive) 428.0
cecum 564.8
colon 564.8
dermatitis (*see also* Varix, with stasis dermatitis) 454.1
duodenal 536.8
eczema (*see also* Varix, with stasis dermatitis) 454.1
foot 991.4
gastric 536.3
ileocecal coil 564.8

Status (post)—*continued*
defibrillator, automatic implantable cardiac V45.02
dialysis V45.1
donor V59.9
drug therapy or regimen V67.59
high-risk medication NEC V67.51
elbow prosthesis V43.62
enterostomy V44.4
epileptic, epilepticus (absence) (grand mal) (*see also* Epilepsy) 345.3
focal motor 345.7
partial 345.7
petit mal 345.2
psychomotor 345.7
temporal lobe 345.7
eye (adnexa) surgery V45.6
filtering bleb (eye) (postglaucoma) V45.6
with rupture or complication 997.99
postcataract extraction (complication) 997.99
finger joint prosthesis V43.69
gastrostomy V44.1
grand mal 345.3
heart valve prosthesis V43.3
hip prosthesis (joint) (partial) (total) V43.64
ileostomy V44.2
intestinal bypass V45.3
intrauterine contraceptive device V45.51
jejunostomy V44.4
knee joint prosthesis V43.65
lacunaris 437.8
lacunosis 437.8
lymphaticus 254.8
malignant neoplasm, ablated or excised—*see* History, malignant neoplasm
marmoratus 333.7
nephrostomy V44.6
neuropacemaker NEC V45.89
brain V45.89
carotid sinus V45.09
neurologic NEC V45.89
organ replacement
by artificial or mechanical device or prosthesis of
artery V43.4
bladder V43.5
blood vessel V43.4
breast V43.82
eye globe V43.0
heart V43.2
valve V43.3
intestine V43.89
joint V43.60
ankle V43.66
elbow V43.62
finger V43.69
hip (partial) (total) V43.64
knee V43.65
shoulder V43.61
specified NEC 43.69
wrist V43.63
kidney V43.89
larynx V43.81
lens V43.1
limb(s) V43.7
liver V43.89
lung V43.89
organ NEC V43.89
pancreas V43.89
tissue NEC V43.89
vein V43.4

Status (post)—*continued*
by organ transplant (heterologous) (homologous)—*see* Status, transplant
pacemaker
brain V45.89
cardiac V45.01
carotid sinus V45.09
neurologic NEC V45.89
specified site NEC V45.89
percutaneous transluminal coronary angioplasty V45.82
petit mal 345.2
postcommotio cerebri 310.2
postoperative NEC V45.89
postpartum NEC V24.2
care immediately following delivery V24.0
routine follow-up V24.2
postsurgical NEC V45.89
renal dialysis V45.1
reversed jejunal transposition (for bypass) V45.3
shoulder prosthesis V43.61
shunt
aortocoronary bypass V45.81
arteriovenous (for dialysis) V45.1
cerebrospinal fluid V45.2
vascular NEC V45.89
aortocoronary (bypass) V45.81
ventricular (communicating) (for drainage) V45.2
subdermal contraceptive device V45.52
thymicolymphaticus 254.8
thymicus 254.8
thymolymphaticus 254.8
tracheostomy V44.0
transplant
blood vessel V42.8
bone V42.4
marrow V42.8
cornea V42.5
heart V42.1
valve V42.2
intestine V42.8
kidney V42.0
liver V42.7
lung V42.6
organ V42.9
specified site NEC V42.8
pancreas V42.8
skin V42.3
tissue V42.9
specified type NEC V42.8
vessel, blood V42.8
ureterostomy V44.6
urethrostomy V44.6
vagina, artificial V44.7
vascular shunt NEC V45.89
aortocoronary (bypass) V45.81
wrist prosthesis V43.63
Stave fracture —*see* Fracture, metacarpus, metacarpal bone(s)
Steal
subclavian artery 435.2
vertebral artery 435.1
Stealing, solitary, child problem (*see also* Disturbance, conduct) 312.1
Steam burn —*see* Burn, by site
Steatocystoma multiplex 706.2
Steatoma (infected) 706.2
eyelid (cystic) 374.84
infected 373.13

Steatorrhea (chronic) 579.8
with lacteal obstruction 579.2
idiopathic 579.0
adult 579.0
infantile 579.0
pancreatic 579.4
primary 579.0
secondary 579.8
specified cause NEC 579.8
tropical 579.1
Steatosis 272.8
heart (*see also* Degeneration, myocardial) 429.1
kidney 593.89
liver 571.8
Stein's syndrome (polycystic ovary) 256.4
Stein-Leventhal syndrome (polycystic ovary) 256.4
Steinbrocker's syndrome (*see also* Neuropathy, peripheral, autonomic) 337.9
Steinert's disease 359.2
Stenocardia (*see also* Angina) 413.9
Stenocephaly 756.0
Stenosis (cicatricial)—*see also* Stricture
ampulla of Vater 576.2
with calculus, cholelithiasis, or stones—*see* Choledocholithiasis
anus, anal (canal) (sphincter) 569.2
congenital 751.2
aorta (ascending) 747.22
arch 747.10
arteriosclerotic 440.0
calcified 440.0
aortic (valve) 424.1
with
mitral (valve)
insufficiency or incompetence 396.2
stenosis or obstruction 396.0
atypical 396.0
congenital 746.3
rheumatic 395.0
with
insufficiency, incompetency or regurgitation 395.2
with mitral (valve) disease 396.8
mitral (valve)
disease (stenosis) 396.0
insufficiency or incompetence 396.2
stenosis or obstruction 396.0
specified cause, except rheumatic 424.1
syphilitic 093.22
aqueduct of Sylvius (congenital) 742.3
with spina bifida (*see also* Spina bifida) 741.0
acquired 331.4
artery NEC 447.1
basilar—*see* Narrowing, artery, basilar
carotid (common) (internal)—*see* Narrowing, artery, carotid
celiac 447.4
cerebral 437.0
due to
embolism (*see also* Embolism, brain) 434.1
thrombus (*see also* Thrombosis, brain) 434.0
precerebral—*see* Narrowing, artery, precerebral
pulmonary (congenital) 747.3
acquired 417.8
renal 440.1
vertebral—*see* Narrowing, artery, vertebral

Stenosis—*continued*
bile duct or biliary passage (*see also* Obstruction, biliary) 576.2
congenital 751.61
bladder neck (acquired) 596.0
congenital 753.6
brain 348.8
bronchus 519.1
syphilitic 095.8
cardia (stomach) 537.89
congenital 750.7
cardiovascular (*see also* Disease, cardiovascular) 429.2
carotid artery—*see* Narrowing, artery, carotid
cervix, cervical (canal) 622.4
congenital 752.49
in pregnancy or childbirth 654.6
affecting fetus or newborn 763.8
causing obstructed labor 660.2
affecting fetus or newborn 763.1
colon (*see also* Obstruction, intestine) 560.9
congenital 751.2
colostomy 569.69
common bile duct (*see also* Obstruction, biliary) 576.2
congenital 751.61
coronary (artery) —*see* Arteriosclerosis, coronary
cystic duct (*see also* Obstruction, gallbladder) 575.2
congenital 751.61
due to (presence of) any device, implant, or graft classifiable to 996.0-996.5—*see* Complications, due to (presence of) any device, implant, or graft classified to 996.0-996.5 NEC
duodenum 537.3
congenital 751.1
ejaculatory duct NEC 608.89
endocervical os—*see* Stenosis, cervix
enterostomy 569.69
esophagus 530.3
congenital 750.3
syphilitic 095.8
congenital 090.5
external ear canal 380.50
secondary to
inflammation 380.53
surgery 380.52
trauma 380.51
gallbladder (*see also* Obstruction, gallbladder) 575.2
glottis 478.74
heart valve (acquired)—*see also* Endocarditis
congenital NEC 746.89
aortic 746.3
mitral 746.5
pulmonary 746.02
tricuspid 746.1
hepatic duct (*see also* Obstruction, biliary) 576.2
hymen 623.3
hypertrophic subaortic (idiopathic) 425.1
infundibulum cardiac 746.83
intestine (*see also* Obstruction, intestine) 560.9
congenital (small) 751.1
large 751.2
lacrimal
canaliculi 375.53
duct 375.56
congenital 743.65

Stenosis—*continued*
punctum 375.52
congenital 743.65
sac 375.54
congenital 743.65
lacrimonasal duct 375.56
congenital 743.65
neonatal 375.55
larynx 478.74
congenital 748.3
syphilitic 095.8
congenital 090.5
mitral (valve) (chronic) (inactive) 394.0
with
aortic (valve)
disease (insufficiency) 396.1
insufficiency or incompetence 396.1
stenosis or obstruction 396.0
incompetency, insufficiency or regurgitation 394.2
with aortic valve disease 396.8
active or acute 391.1
with chorea (acute) (rheumatic) (Sydenham's) 392.0
congenital 746.5
specified cause, except rheumatic 424.0
syphilitic 093.21
myocardium, myocardial (*see also* Degeneration, myocardial) 429.1
hypertrophic subaortic (idiopathic) 425.1
nares (anterior) (posterior) 478.1
congenital 748.0
nasal duct 375.56
congenital 743.65
nasolacrimal duct 375.56
congenital 743.65
neonatal 375.55
organ or site, congenital NEC—*see* Atresia
papilla of Vater 576.2
with calculus, cholelithiasis, or stones—*see* Choledocholithiasis
pulmonary (artery) (congenital) 747.3
with ventricular septal defect, dextraposition of aorta and hypertrophy of right ventricle 745.2
acquired 417.8
infundibular 746.83
in tetralogy of Fallot 745.2
subvalvular 746.83
valve (*see also* Endocarditis, pulmonary) 424.3
congenital 746.02
vein 747.49
acquired 417.8
vessel NEC 417.8
pulmonic (congenital) 746.02
infundibular 746.83
subvalvular 746.83
pylorus (hypertrophic) 537.0
adult 537.0
congenital 750.5
infantile 750.5
rectum (sphincter) (*see also* Stricture, rectum) 569.2
renal artery 440.1
salivary duct (any) 527.8
sphincter of Oddi (*see also* Obstruction, biliary) 576.2
spinal 724.00
cervical 723.0
lumbar, lumbosacral 724.02

Stenosis—*continued*
nerve (root) NEC 724.9
specified region NEC 724.09
thoracic, thoracolumbar 724.01
stomach, hourglass 537.6
subaortic 746.81
hypertrophic (idiopathic) 425.1
supra (valvular)-aortic 747.22
trachea 519.1
congenital 748.3
syphilitic 095.8
tuberculous (*see also* Tuberculosis) 012.8
tracheostomy 519.0
tricuspid (valve) (*see also* Endocarditis, tricuspid) 397.0
congenital 746.1
nonrheumatic 424.2
tubal 628.2
ureter (*see also* Stricture, ureter) 593.3
congenital 753.2
urethra (*see also* Stricture, urethra) 598.9
vagina 623.2
congenital 752.49
in pregnancy or childbirth 654.7
affecting fetus or newborn 763.8
causing obstructed labor 660.2
affecting fetus or newborn 763.1
valve (cardiac) (heart) (*see also* Endocarditis) 424.90
congenital NEC 746.89
aortic 746.3
mitral 746.5
pulmonary 746.02
tricuspid 746.1
urethra 753.6
valvular (*see also* Endocarditis) 424.90
congenital NEC 746.89
urethra 753.6
vascular graft or shunt 996.1
atherosclerosis —*see* Arteriosclerosis, extremities
embolism 996.74
occlusion NEC 996.74
thrombus 996.74
vena cava (inferior) (superior) 459.2
congenital 747.49
ventricular shunt 996.2
vulva 624.8
Stercolith (*see also* Fecalith) 560.39
appendix 543.9
Stercoraceous, stercoral ulcer 569.82
anus or rectum 569.41
Stereopsis, defective
with fusion 368.33
without fusion 368.32
Stereotypies NEC 307.3
Sterility
female—*see* Infertility, female
male (*see also* Infertility, male) 606.9
Sterilization, admission for V25.2
Sternalgia (*see also* Angina) 413.9
Sternopagus 759.4
Sternum bifidum 756.3
Sternutation 784.9
Steroid
effects (adverse) (iatrogenic)
cushingoid
correct substance properly administered 255.0
overdose or wrong substance given or taken 962.0

Steroid—*continued*
diabetes
correct substance properly administered 251.8
overdose or wrong substance given or taken 962.0
due to
correct substance properly administered 255.8
overdose or wrong substance given or taken 962.0
fever
correct substance properly administered 780.6
overdose or wrong substance given or taken 962.0
withdrawal
correct substance properly administered 255.4
overdose or wrong substance given or taken 962.0
responder 365.03
Stevens-Johnson disease or syndrome (erythema multiforme exudativum) 695.1
Stewart-Morel syndrome (hyperostosis frontalis interna) 733.3
Sticker's disease (erythema infectiosum) 057.0
Sticky eye 372.03
Stieda's disease (calcification, knee joint) 726.62
Stiff
back 724.8
neck (*see also* Torticollis) 723.5
Stiff-man syndrome 333.91
Stiffness, joint NEC 719.50
ankle 719.57
back 724.8
elbow 719.52
finger 719.54
hip 719.55
knee 719.56
multiple sites 719.59
sacroiliac 724.6
shoulder 719.51
specified site NEC 719.58
spine 724.9
surgical fusion V45.4
wrist 719.53
Stigmata, congenital syphilis 090.5
Still's disease or syndrome 714.30
Still-Felty syndrome (rheumatoid arthritis with splenomegaly and leukopenia) 714.1
Stillbirth, stillborn NEC 779.9
Stiller's disease (asthenia) 780.7
Stilling-Türk-Duane syndrome (ocular retraction syndrome) 378.71
Stimulation, ovary 256.1
Sting (animal) (bee) (fish) (insect) (jellyfish) (Portuguese man-o-war) (wasp) (venomous) 989.5
anaphylactic shock or reaction 989.5
plant 692.6
Stippled epiphyses 756.59
Stitch
abscess 998.5
burst (in operation wound) 998.3
in back 724.5
Stojano's (subcostal) syndrome 098.86
Stokes' disease (exophthalmic goiter) 242.0
Stokes-Adams syndrome (syncope with heart block) 426.9
Stokvis' (-Talma) disease (enterogenous cyanosis) 289.7
Stomach —*see* condition
Stoma malfunction
colostomy 569.69
cystostomy 997.5
enterostomy 569.69
gastrostomy 997.4
ileostomy 569.69
nephrostomy 997.5
tracheostomy 519.0
ureterostomy 997.5
Stomatitis 528.0
angular 528.5
due to dietary or vitamin deficiency 266.0
aphthous 528.2
candidal 112.0
catarrhal 528.0
denture 528.9
diphtheritic (membranous) 032.0
due to
dietary deficiency 266.0
thrush 112.0
vitamin deficiency 266.0
epidemic 078.4
epizootic 078.4
follicular 528.0
gangrenous 528.1
herpetic 054.2
herpetiformis 528.2
malignant 528.0
membranous acute 528.0
monilial 112.0
mycotic 112.0
necrotic 528.1
ulcerative 101
necrotizing ulcerative 101
parasitic 112.0
septic 528.0
spirochetal 101
suppurative (acute) 528.0
ulcerative 528.0
necrotizing 101
ulceromembranous 101
vesicular 528.0
with exanthem 074.3
Vincent's 101
Stomatocytosis 282.8
Stomatomycosis 112.0
Stomatorrhagia 528.9
Stone (s)—*see also* Calculus
bladder 594.1
diverticulum 594.0
cystine 270.0
heart syndrome (*see also* Failure, ventricular, left) 428.1
kidney 592.0
prostate 602.0
pulp (dental) 522.2
renal 592.0
salivary duct or gland (any) 527.5
ureter 592.1
urethra (impacted) 594.2
urinary (duct) (impacted) (passage) 592.9
bladder 594.1
diverticulum 594.0
lower tract NEC 594.9
specified site 594.8
xanthine 277.2
Stonecutters' lung 502
tuberculous (*see also* Tuberculosis) 011.4

Stonemasons'
asthma, disease, or lung 502
tuberculous (*see also* Tuberculosis) 011.4
phthisis (*see also* Tuberculosis) 011.4
Stoppage
bowel (*see also* Obstruction, intestine) 560.9
heart (*see also* Arrest, cardiac) 427.5
intestine (*see also* Obstruction, intestine) 560.9
urine NEC (*see also* Retention, urine) 788.20
Storm, thyroid (apathetic) (*see also* Thyrotoxicosis) 242.9
Strabismus (alternating) (congenital) (nonparalytic) 378.9
concomitant (*see also* Heterotropia) 378.30
convergent (*see also* Esotropia) 378.00
divergent (*see also* Exotropia) 378.10
convergent (*see also* Esotropia) 378.00
divergent (*see also* Exotropia) 378.10
due to adhesions, scars—*see* Strabismus, mechanical
in neuromuscular disorder NEC 378.73
intermittent 378.20
vertical 378.31
latent 378.40
convergent (esophoria) 378.41
divergent (exophoria) 378.42
vertical 378.43
mechanical 378.60
due to
Brown's tendon sheath syndrome 378.61
specified musculofascial disorder NEC 378.62
paralytic 378.50
third or oculomotor nerve (partial) 378.51
total 378.52
fourth or trochlear nerve 378.53
sixth or abducens nerve 378.54
specified type NEC 378.73
vertical (hypertropia) 378.31
Strain —*see also* Sprain, by site
eye NEC 368.13
heart—*see* Disease, heart
meaning gonorrhea—*see* Gonorrhea
physical NEC V62.89
postural 729.9
psychological NEC V62.89
Strands
conjunctiva 372.62
vitreous humor 379.25
Strangulation, strangulated 994.7
appendix 543.9
asphyxiation or suffocation by 994.7
bladder neck 596.0
bowel—*see* Strangulation, intestine
colon—*see* Strangulation, intestine
cord (umbilical)—*see* Compression, umbilical cord
due to birth injury 767.8
food or foreign body (*see also* Asphyxia, food) 933.1
hemorrhoids 455.8
external 455.5
internal 455.2
hernia—*see also* Hernia, by site, with obstruction
gangrenous—*see* Hernia, by site, with gangrene
intestine (large) (small) 560.2
with hernia—*see also* Hernia, by site, with obstruction
Strangulation, strangulated—*continued*
gangrenous—*see* Hernia, by site, with gangrene
congenital (small) 751.1
large 751.2
mesentery 560.2
mucus (*see also* Asphyxia, mucus) 933.1
newborn 770.1
omentum 560.2
organ or site, congenital NEC—*see* Atresia
ovary 620.8
due to hernia 620.4
penis 607.89
foreign body 939.3
rupture (*see also* Hernia, by site, with obstruction) 552.9
gangrenous (*see also* Hernia, by site, with gangrene) 551.9
stomach, due to hernia (*see also* Hernia, by site, with obstruction) 552.9
with gangrene (*see also* Hernia, by site, with gangrene) 551.9
umbilical cord—*see* Compression, umbilical cord
vesicourethral orifice 596.0
Strangury 788.1
Strawberry
gallbladder (*see also* Disease, gallbladder) 575.6
mark 757.32
tongue (red) (white) 529.3
Straw itch 133.8
Streak, ovarian 752.0
Strephosymbolia 315.01
secondary to organic lesion 784.69
Streptobacillary fever 026.1
Streptobacillus moniliformis 026.1
Streptococcemia 038.0
Streptococcicosis —*see* Infection, streptococcal
Streptococcus, streptococcal —*see* condition
Streptoderma 686.0
Streptomycosis —*see* Actinomycosis
Streptothricosis —*see* Actinomycosis
Streptothrix —*see* Actinomycosis
Streptotrichosis —*see* Actinomycosis
Stress
fracture—*see* Fracture, pathologic
polycythemia 289.0
reaction (gross) (*see also* Reaction, stress, acute) 308.9
Stretching, nerve —*see* Injury, nerve, by site
Striae (albicantes) (atrophicae) (cutis distensae) (distensae) 701.3
Striations of nails 703.8
Stricture (*see also* Stenosis) 799.8
ampulla of Vater 576.2
with calculus, cholelithiasis, or stones—*see* Choledocholithiasis
anus (sphincter) 569.2
congenital 751.2
infantile 751.2
aorta (ascending) 747.22
arch 747.10
arteriosclerotic 440.0
calcified 440.0
aortic (valve) (*see also* Stenosis, aortic) 424.1
congenital 746.3
aqueduct of Sylvius (congenital) 742.3
with spina bifida (*see also* Spina bifida) 741.0
acquired 331.4

Stricture—*continued*
artery 447.1
basilar—*see* Narrowing, artery, basilar
carotid (common) (internal)—*see* Narrowing, artery, carotid
celiac 447.4
cerebral 437.0
congenital 747.81
due to
embolism (*see also* Embolism, brain) 434.1
thrombus (*see also* Thrombosis, brain) 434.0
congenital (peripheral) 747.60
cerebral 747.81
coronary 746.85
gastrointestinal 747.61
lower limb 747.64
renal 747.62
retinal 743.58
specified NEC 747.69
spinal 747.82
umbilical 747.5
upper limb 747.63
coronary —*see* Arteriosclerosis, coronary
congenital 746.85
precerebral—*see* Narrowing, artery, precerebral NEC
pulmonary (congenital) 747.3
acquired 417.8
renal 440.1
vertebral—*see* Narrowing, artery, vertebral
auditory canal (congenital) (external) 744.02
acquired (*see also* Stricture, ear canal, acquired) 380.50
bile duct or passage (any) (postoperative) (*see also* Obstruction, biliary) 576.2
congenital 751.61
bladder 596.8
congenital 753.6
neck 596.0
congenital 753.6
bowel (*see also* Obstruction, intestine) 560.9
brain 348.8
bronchus 519.1
syphilitic 095.8
cardia (stomach) 537.89
congenital 750.7
cardiac—*see also* Disease, heart
orifice (stomach) 537.89
cardiovascular (*see also* Disease, cardiovascular) 429.2
carotid artery—*see* Narrowing, artery, carotid
cecum (*see also* Obstruction, intestine) 560.9
cervix, cervical (canal) 622.4
congenital 752.49
in pregnancy or childbirth 654.6
affecting fetus or newborn 763.8
causing obstructed labor 660.2
affecting fetus or newborn 763.1
colon (*see also* Obstruction, intestine) 560.9
congenital 751.2
colostomy 569.69
common bile duct (*see also* Obstruction, biliary) 576.2
congenital 751.61
coronary (artery) —*see* Arteriosclerosis, coronary
congenital 746.85—
cystic duct (*see also* Obstruction, gallbladder) 575.2
congenital 751.61

Stricture—*continued*
cystostomy 997.5
digestive organs NEC, congenital 751.8
duodenum 537.3
congenital 751.1
ear canal (external) (congenital) 744.02
acquired 380.50
secondary to
inflammation 380.53
surgery 380.52
trauma 380.51
ejaculatory duct 608.85
enterostomy 569.69
esophagus (corrosive) (peptic) 530.3
congenital 750.3
syphilitic 095.8
congenital 090.5
Eustachian tube (*see also* Obstruction, Eustachian tube) 381.60
congenital 744.24
fallopian tube 628.2
gonococcal (chronic) 098.37
acute 098.17
tuberculous (*see also* Tuberculosis) 016.6
gallbladder (*see also* Obstruction, gallbladder) 575.2
congenital 751.69
glottis 478.74
heart—*see also* Disease, heart
congenital NEC 746.89
valve—*see also* Endocarditis
congenital NEC 746.89
aortic 746.3
mitral 746.5
pulmonary 746.02
tricuspid 746.1
hepatic duct (*see also* Obstruction, biliary) 576.2
hourglass, of stomach 537.6
hymen 623.3
hypopharynx 478.29
intestine (*see also* Obstruction, intestine) 560.9
congenital (small) 751.1
large 751.2
ischemic 557.1
lacrimal
canaliculi 375.53
congenital 743.65
punctum 375.52
congenital 743.65
sac 375.54
congenital 743.65
lacrimonasal duct 375.56
congenital 743.65
neonatal 375.55
larynx 478.79
congenital 748.3
syphilitic 095.8
congenital 090.5
lung 518.89
meatus
ear (congenital) 744.02
acquired (*see also* Stricture, ear canal, acquired) 380.50
osseous (congenital) (ear) 744.03
acquired (*see also* Stricture, ear canal, acquired) 380.50
urinarius (*see also* Stricture, urethra) 598.9
congenital 753.6
mitral (valve) (*see also* Stenosis, mitral) 394.0
congenital 746.5
specified cause, except rheumatic 424.0

Stricture—*continued*
myocardium, myocardial (*see also* Degeneration, myocardial) 429.1
hypertrophic subaortic (idiopathic) 425.1
nares (anterior) (posterior) 478.1
congenital 748.0
nasal duct 375.56
congenital 743.65
neonatal 375.55
nasolacrimal duct 375.56
congenital 743.65
neonatal 375.55
nasopharynx 478.29
syphilitic 095.8
nephrostomy 997.5
nose 478.1
congenital 748.0
nostril (anterior) (posterior) 478.1
congenital 748.0
organ or site, congenital NEC—*see* Atresia
osseous meatus (congenital) (ear) 744.03
acquired (*see also* Stricture, ear canal, acquired) 380.50
os uteri (*see also* Stricture, cervix) 622.4
oviduct—*see* Stricture, fallopian tube
pelviureteric junction 593.3
pharynx (dilation) 478.29
prostate 602.8
pulmonary, pulmonic
artery (congenital) 747.3
acquired 417.8
noncongenital 417.8
infundibulum (congenital) 746.83
valve (*see also* Endocarditis, pulmonary) 424.3
congenital 746.02
vein (congenital) 747.49
acquired 417.8
vessel NEC 417.8
punctum lacrimale 375.52
congenital 743.65
pylorus (hypertrophic) 537.0
adult 537.0
congenital 750.5
infantile 750.5
rectosigmoid 569.89
rectum (sphincter) 569.2
congenital 751.2
due to
chemical burn 947.3
irradiation 569.2
lymphogranuloma venereum 099.1
gonococcal 098.7
inflammatory 099.1
syphilitic 095.8
tuberculous (*see also* Tuberculosis) 014.8
renal artery 440.1
salivary duct or gland (any) 527.8
sigmoid (flexure) (*see also* Obstruction, intestine) 560.9
spermatic cord 608.85
stoma (following) (of)
colostomy 569.69
cystostomy 997.5
enterostomy 569.69
gastrostomy 997.4
ileostomy 569.69
nephrostomy 997.5
tracheostomy 519.0
ureterostomy 997.5
stomach 537.89
congenital 750.7

Stricture—*continued*
hourglass 537.6
subaortic 746.81
hypertrophic (acquired) (idiopathic) 425.1
subglottic 478.74
syphilitic NEC 095.8
tendon (sheath) 727.81
trachea 519.1
congenital 748.3
syphilitic 095.8
tuberculous (*see also* Tuberculosis) 012.8
tracheostomy 519.0
tricuspid (valve) (*see also* Endocarditis, tricuspid) 397.0
congenital 746.1
nonrheumatic 424.2
tunica vaginalis 608.85
ureter (postoperative) 593.3
congenital 753.2
tuberculous (*see also* Tuberculosis) 016.2
ureteropelvic junction 593.3
congenital 753.2
ureterovesical orifice 593.3
congenital 753.2
urethra (anterior) (meatal) (organic) (posterior) (spasmodic) 598.9
associated with schistosomiasis (*see also* Schistosomiasis) 120.9 *[598.01]*
congenital (valvular) 753.6
due to
infection 598.00
syphilis 095.8 *[598.01]*
trauma 598.1
gonococcal 098.2 *[598.01]*
gonorrheal 098.2 *[598.01]*
infective 598.00
late effect of injury 598.1
postcatheterization 598.2
postobstetric 598.1
postoperative 598.2
specified cause NEC 598.8
syphilitic 095.8 *[598.01]*
traumatic 598.1
valvular, congenital 753.6
urinary meatus (*see also* Stricture, urethra) 598.9
congenital 753.6
uterus, uterine 621.5
os (external) (internal)—*see* Stricture, cervix
vagina (outlet) 623.2
congenital 752.49
valve (cardiac) (heart) (*see also* Endocarditis) 424.90
congenital (cardiac) (heart) NEC 746.89
aortic 746.3
mitral 746.5
pulmonary 746.02
tricuspid 746.1
urethra 753.6
valvular (*see also* Endocarditis) 424.90
vascular graft or shunt 996.1
atherosclerosis —*see* Arteriosclerosis, extremities
embolism 996.74
occlusion NEC 996.74
thrombus 996.74
vas deferens 608.85
congenital 752.8
vein 459.2
vena cava (inferior) (superior) NEC 459.2
congenital 747.49

Stricture—*continued*
ventricular shunt 996.2
vesicourethral orifice 596.0
congenital 753.6
vulva (acquired) 624.8
Stridor 786.1
congenital (larynx) 748.3
Stridulous —*see* condition
Strippling of nails 703.8
Stroke (*see also* Disease, cerebrovascular, acute) 436
apoplectic (*see also* Disease, cerebrovascular, acute) 436
brain (*see also* Disease, cerebrovascular, acute) 436
epileptic—*see* Epilepsy
healed or old—*see also* category 438
without residuals V12.59
heart—*see* Disease, heart
heat 992.0
iatrogenic 997.02
in evolution 435.9
late effect—*see* category 438
lightning 994.0
paralytic (*see also* Disease, cerebrovascular, acute) 436
postoperative 997.02
progressive 435.9
Stromatosis, endometrial (M8931/1) 236.0
Strong pulse 785.9
Strongyloides stercoralis infestation 127.2
Strongyloidiasis 127.2
Strongyloidosis 127.2
Strongylus (gibsoni) infestation 127.7
Strophulus (newborn) 779.8
pruriginosus 698.2
Struck by lightning 994.0
Struma (*see also* Goiter) 240.9
fibrosa 245.3
Hashimoto (struma lymphomatosa) 245.2
lymphomatosa 245.2
nodosa (simplex) 241.9
endemic 241.9
multinodular 241.1
sporadic 241.9
toxic or with hyperthyroidism 242.3
multinodular 242.2
uninodular 242.1
toxicosa 242.3
multinodular 242.2
uninodular 242.1
uninodular 241.0
ovarii (M9090/0) 220
and carcinoid (M9091/1) 236.2
malignant (M9090/3) 183.0
Riedel's (ligneous thyroiditis) 245.3
scrofulous (*see also* Tuberculosis) 017.2
tuberculous (*see also* Tuberculosis) 017.2
abscess 017.2
adenitis 017.2
lymphangitis 017.2
ulcer 017.2
Strumipriva cachexia (*see also* Hypothyroidism) 244.9
Strümpell-Marie disease or spine (ankylosing spondylitis) 720.0
Strümpell-Westphal pseudosclerosis (hepatolenticular degeneration) 275.1
Stuart's disease (congenital factor X deficiency) (*see also* Defect, coagulation) 286.3
Stuart-Prower factor deficiency (congenital factor X deficiency) (*see also* Defect, coagulation) 286.3
Students' elbow 727.2
Stuffy nose 478.1
Stump —*see also* Amputation
cervix, cervical (healed) 622.8
Stupor 780.09
catatonic (*see also* Schizophrenia) 295.2
circular (*see also* Psychosis, manic-depressive, circular) 296.7
manic 296.89
manic-depressive (*see also* Psychosis, affective) 296.89
mental (anergic) (delusional) 298.9
psychogenic 298.8
reaction to exceptional stress (transient) 308.2
traumatic NEC—*see also* Injury, intracranial
with spinal (cord)
lesion—*see* Injury, spinal, by site
shock—*see* Injury, spinal, by site
Sturge (-Weber) (-Dimitri) disease or syndrome (encephalocutaneous angiomatosis) 759.6
Sturge-Kalischer-Weber syndrome (encephalocutaneous angiomatosis) 759.6
Stuttering 307.0
Sty, stye 373.11
external 373.11
internal 373.12
meibomian 373.12
Subacidity, gastric 536.8
psychogenic 306.4
Subacute —*see* condition
Subarachnoid —*see* condition
Subclavian steal syndrome 435.2
Subcortical —*see* condition
Subcostal syndrome 098.86
nerve compression 354.8
Subcutaneous, subcuticular —*see* condition
Subdelirium 293.1
Subdural —*see* condition
Subendocardium —*see* condition
Subependymoma (M9383/1) 237.5
Suberosis 495.3
Subglossitis —*see* Glossitis
Subhemophilia 286.0
Subinvolution (uterus) 621.1
breast (postlactational) (postpartum) 611.8
chronic 621.1
puerperal, postpartum 674.8
Sublingual —*see* condition
Sublinguitis 527.2
Subluxation —*see also* Dislocation, by site
congenital NEC—*see also* Malposition, congenital
hip (unilateral) 754.32
with dislocation of other hip 754.35
bilateral 754.33
joint
lower limb 755.69
shoulder 755.59
upper limb 755.59
lower limb (joint) 755.69
shoulder (joint) 755.59
upper limb (joint) 755.59
lens 379.32
anterior 379.33
posterior 379.34
rotary, cervical region of spine—*see* Fracture, vertebra, cervical
Submaxillary —*see* condition
Submersion (fatal) (nonfatal) 994.1

Submissiveness (undue), in child 313.0
Submucous —*see* condition
Subnormal, subnormality
accommodation (*see also* Disorder, accommodation) 367.9
mental (*see also* Retardation, mental) 319
mild 317
moderate 318.0
profound 318.2
severe 318.1
temperature (accidental) 991.6
not associated with low environmental temperature 780.9
Subphrenic —*see* condition
Subscapular nerve —*see* condition
Subseptus uterus 752.3
Subsiding appendicitis 542
Substernal thyroid (*see also* Goiter) 240.9
congenital 759.2
Substitution disorder 300.11
Subtentorial —*see* condition
Subtertian
fever 084.0
malaria (fever) 084.0
Subthyroidism (acquired) (*see also* Hypothyroidism) 244.9
congenital 243
Succenturiata placenta —*see* Placenta, abnormal
Succussion sounds, chest 786.7
Sucking thumb, child 307.9
Sudamen 705.1
Sudamina 705.1
Sudanese kala-azar 085.0
Sudden
death, cause unknown (less than 24 hours) 798.1
during childbirth 669.9
infant 798.0
puerperal, postpartum 674.9
hearing loss NEC 388.2
heart failure (*see also* Failure, heart) 428.9
infant death syndrome 798.0
Sudeck's atrophy, disease, or syndrome 733.7
SUDS (Sudden unexplained death) 798.2
Suffocation (*see also* Asphyxia) 799.0
by
bed clothes 994.7
bunny bag 994.7
cave-in 994.7
constriction 994.7
drowning 994.1
inhalation
food or foreign body (*see also* Asphyxia, food or foreign body) 933.1
oil or gasoline (*see also* Asphyxia, food or foreign body) 933.1
overlying 994.7
plastic bag 994.7
pressure 994.7
strangulation 994.7
during birth 768.1
mechanical 994.7
Sugar
blood
high 790.6
low 251.2
in urine 791.5
Suicide, suicidal (attempted)
by poisoning—*see* Table of drugs and chemicals
risk 300.9
tendencies 300.9
trauma NEC (*see also* nature and site of injury) 959.9
Suipestifer infection (*see also* Infection, Salmonella) 003.9
Sulfatidosis 330.0
Sulfhemoglobinemia, sulphemoglobinemia (acquired) (congenital) 289.7
Sumatran mite fever 081.2
Summer —*see* condition
Sunburn 692.71
dermatitis 692.71
Sunken
acetabulum 718.85
fontanels 756.0
Sunstroke 992.0
Superfecundation 651.9
with fetal loss and retention of one or more fetus(es) 651.6
Superfetation 651.9
with fetal loss and retention of one or more fetus(es) 651.6
Supernumerary (congenital)
aortic cusps 746.89
auditory ossicles 744.04
bone 756.9
breast 757.6
carpal bones 755.56
cusps, heart valve NEC 746.89
mitral 746.5
pulmonary 746.09
digit(s) 755.00
finger 755.01
toe 755.02
ear (lobule) 744.1
fallopian tube 752.19
finger 755.01
hymen 752.49
kidney 753.3
lacrimal glands 743.64
lacrimonasal duct 743.65
lobule (ear) 744.1
mitral cusps 746.5
muscle 756.82
nipples 757.6
organ or site NEC—*see* Accessory
ossicles, auditory 744.04
ovary 752.0
oviduct 752.19
pulmonic cusps 746.09
rib 756.3
cervical or first 756.2
syndrome 756.2
roots (of teeth) 520.2
spinal vertebra 756.19
spleen 759.0
tarsal bones 755.67
teeth 520.1
causing crowding 524.3
testis 752.8
thumb 755.01
toe 755.02
uterus 752.2
vagina 752.49
vertebra 756.19
Supervision (of)
contraceptive method previously prescribed V25.40
intrauterine device V25.42
oral contraceptive (pill) V25.41
specified type NEC V25.49
subdermal implantable contraceptive V25.43
dietary (for) V65.3
allergy (food) V65.3

Supervision—*continued*
colitis V65.3
diabetes mellitus V65.3
food allergy intolerance V65.3
gastritis V65.3
hypercholesterolemia V65.3
hypoglycemia V65.3
intolerance (food) V65.3
obesity V65.3
specified NEC V65.3
lactation V24.1
pregnancy—*see* Pregnancy, supervision of
Supplemental teeth 520.1
causing crowding 524.3
Suppression
binocular vision 368.31
lactation 676.5
menstruation 626.8
ovarian secretion 256.3
renal 586
urinary secretion 788.5
urine 788.5
Suppuration, suppurative —*see also* condition
accessory sinus (chronic) (*see also* Sinusitis) 473.9
adrenal gland 255.8
antrum (chronic) (*see also* Sinusitis, maxillary) 473.0
bladder (*see also* Cystitis) 595.89
bowel 569.89
brain 324.0
late effect 326
breast 611.0
puerperal, postpartum 675.1
dental periosteum 526.5
diffuse (skin) 686.0
ear (middle) (*see also* Otitis media) 382.4
external (*see also* Otitis, externa) 380.10
internal 386.33
ethmoidal (sinus) (chronic) (*see also* Sinusitis, ethmoidal) 473.2
fallopian tube (*see also* Salpingo-oophoritis) 614.2
frontal (sinus) (chronic) (*see also* Sinusitis, frontal) 473.1
gallbladder (*see also* Cholecystitis, acute) 575.0
gum 523.3
hernial sac—*see* Hernia, by site
intestine 569.89
joint (*see also* Arthritis, suppurative) 711.0
labyrinthine 386.33
lung 513.0
mammary gland 611.0
puerperal, postpartum 675.1
maxilla, maxillary 526.4
sinus (chronic) (*see also* Sinusitis, maxillary) 473.0
muscle 728.0
nasal sinus (chronic) (*see also* Sinusitis) 473.9
pancreas 577.0
parotid gland 527.2
pelvis, pelvic
female (*see also* Disease, pelvis, inflammatory) 614.4
acute 614.3
male (*see also* Peritonitis) 567.2
pericranial (*see also* Osteomyelitis) 730.2
salivary duct or gland (any) 527.2
sinus (nasal) (*see also* Sinusitis) 473.9
sphenoidal (sinus) (chronic) (*see also* Sinusitis, sphenoidal) 473.3
thymus (gland) 254.1
Suppuration, suppurative—*continued*
thyroid (gland) 245.0
tonsil 474.8
uterus (*see also* Endometritis) 615.9
vagina 616.10
wound—*see also* Wound, open, by site, complicated
dislocation—*see* Dislocation, by site, compound
fracture—*see* Fracture, by site, open
scratch or other superficial injury—*see* Injury, superficial, by site
Suprapubic drainage 596.8
Suprarenal (gland)—*see* condition
Suprascapular nerve —*see* condition
Suprasellar —*see* condition
Supraspinatus syndrome 726.10
Surfer knots 919.8
infected 919.9
Surgery
cosmetic NEC V50.1
following healed injury or operation V51
hair transplant V50.0
elective V50.9
breast augmentation reduction V50.1
circumcision, ritual or routine (in absence of medical indication) V50.2
cosmetic NEC V50.1
ear piercing V50.3
face-lift V50.1
following healed injury or operation V51
hair transplant V50.0
not done because of
contraindication V64.1
patient's decision V64.2
specified reason NEC V64.3
plastic
breast augmentation or reduction V50.1
cosmetic V50.1
face-lift V50.1
following healed injury or operation V51
repair of scarred tissue (following healed injury or operation) V51
specified type NEC V50.8
previous, in pregnancy or childbirth
cervix 654.6
affecting fetus or newborn 763.8
causing obstructed labor 660.2
affecting fetus or newborn 763.1
pelvic soft tissues NEC 654.9
affecting fetus or newborn 763.8
causing obstructed labor 660.2
affecting fetus or newborn 763.1
perineum or vulva 654.8
uterus NEC 654.9
affecting fetus or newborn 763.8
causing obstructed labor 660.2
affecting fetus or newborn 763.1
due to previous cesarean delivery 654.2
vagina 654.7
Surgical
abortion—*see* Abortion, legal
emphysema 998.81
kidney (*see also* Pyelitis) 590.80
operation NEC 799.9
procedures, complication or misadventure—*see* Complications, surgical procedure
shock 998.0
Suspected condition, ruled out (*see also* Observation, suspected) V71.9
specified condition NEC V71.8

Suspended uterus, in pregnancy or childbirth 654.4
affecting fetus or newborn 763.8
causing obstructed labor 660.2
affecting fetus or newborn 763.1
Sutton's disease 709.09
Sutton and Gull's disease (arteriolar nephrosclerosis) (*see also* Hypertension, kidney) 403.90
Suture
burst (in operation wound) 998.3
inadvertently left in operation wound 998.4
removal V58.3
Shirodkar, in pregnancy (with or without cervical incompetence) 654.5
Swab inadvertently left in operation wound 998.4
Swallowed, swallowing
difficulty (*see also* Dysphagia) 787.2
foreign body NEC (*see also* Foreign body) 938
Swamp fever 100.89
Swan neck hand (intrinsic) 736.09
Sweat (s), sweating
disease or sickness 078.2
excessive 780.8
fetid 705.89
fever 078.2
gland disease 705.9
specified type NEC 705.89
miliary 078.2
night 780.8
Sweeley-Klionsky disease (angiokeratoma corporis diffusum) 272.7
Sweet's syndrome (acute febrile neutrophilic dermatosis) 695.89
Swelling
abdominal (not referable to specific organ) 789.3
adrenal gland, cloudy 255.8
ankle 719.07
anus 787.99
arm 729.81
breast 611.72
Calabar 125.2
cervical gland 785.6
cheek 784.2
chest 786.6
ear 388.8
epigastric 789.3
extremity (lower) (upper) 729.81
eye 379.92
female genital organ 625.8
finger 729.81
foot 729.81
glands 785.6
gum 784.2
hand 729.81
head 784.2
inflammatory—*see* Inflammation
joint (*see also* Effusion, joint) 719.0
tuberculous—*see* Tuberculosis, joint
kidney, cloudy 593.89
leg 729.81
limb 729.81
liver 573.8
lung 786.6
lymph nodes 785.6
mediastinal 786.6
mouth 784.2
muscle (limb) 729.81
neck 784.2
Swelling—*continued*
nose or sinus 784.2
palate 784.2
pelvis 789.3
penis 607.83
perineum 625.8
rectum 787.99
scrotum 608.86
skin 782.2
splenic (*see also* Splenomegaly) 789.2
substernal 786.6
superficial, localized (skin) 782.2
testicle 608.86
throat 784.2
toe 729.81
tongue 784.2
tubular (*see also* Disease, renal) 593.9
umbilicus 789.3
uterus 625.8
vagina 625.8
vulva 625.8
wandering, due to Gnathostoma (spinigerum) 128.1
white—*see* Tuberculosis, arthritis
Swift's disease 985.0
Swimmers'
ear (acute) 380.12
itch 120.3
Swimming in the head 780.4
Swollen —*see also* Swelling
glands 785.6
Swyer-James syndrome (unilateral hyperlucent lung) 492.8
Swyer's syndrome (XY pure gonadal dysgenesis) 752.7
Sycosis 704.8
barbae (not parasitic) 704.8
contagiosa 110.0
lupoid 704.8
mycotic 110.0
parasitic 110.0
vulgaris 704.8
Sydenham's chorea —*see* Chorea, Sydenham's
Sylvatic yellow fever 060.0
Sylvest's disease (epidemic pleurodynia) 074.1
Symblepharon 372.63
congenital 743.62
Symonds' syndrome 348.2
Sympathetic —*see* condition
Sympatheticotonia (*see also* Neuropathy, peripheral, autonomic) 337.9
Sympathicoblastoma (M9500/3)
specified site—*see* Neoplasm, by site, malignant
unspecified site 194.0
Sympathicogonioma (M9500/3)—*see* Sympathicoblastoma
Sympathoblastoma (M9500/3)—*see* Sympathicoblastoma
Sympathogonioma (M9500/3)—*see* Sympathicoblastoma
Symphalangy (*see also* Syndactylism) 755.10
Symptoms, specified (general) NEC 780.9
abdomen NEC 789.9
bone NEC 733.90
breast NEC 611.79
cardiac NEC 785.9
cardiovascular NEC 785.9
chest NEC 786.9
development NEC 783.9
digestive system NEC 787.99

Symptoms, specified—*continued*
eye NEC 379.99
gastrointestinal tract NEC 787.99
genital organs NEC
female 625.9
male 608.9
head and neck NEC 784.9
heart NEC 785.9
joint NEC 719.60
ankle 719.67
elbow 719.62
foot 719.67
hand 719.64
hip 719.65
knee 719.66
multiple sites 719.69
pelvic region 719.65
shoulder (region) 719.61
specified site NEC 719.68
wrist 719.63
larynx NEC 784.9
limbs NEC 729.89
lymphatic system NEC 785.9
menopausal 627.2
metabolism NEC 783.9
mouth NEC 528.9
muscle NEC 728.9
musculoskeletal NEC 781.9
limbs NEC 729.89
nervous system NEC 781.9
neurotic NEC 300.9
nutrition, metabolism, and development NEC 783.9
pelvis NEC 789.9
female 625.9
peritoneum NEC 789.9
respiratory system NEC 786.9
skin and integument NEC 782.9
subcutaneous tissue NEC 782.9
throat NEC 784.9
tonsil NEC 784.9
urinary system NEC 788.9
vascular NEC 785.9
Sympus 759.89
Synarthrosis 719.80
ankle 719.87
elbow 719.82
foot 719.87
hand 719.84
hip 719.85
knee 719.86
multiple sites 719.89
pelvic region 719.85
shoulder (region) 719.81
specified site NEC 719.88
wrist 719.83
Syncephalus 759.4
Synchondrosis 756.9
abnormal (congenital) 756.9
ischiopubic (van Neck's) 732.1
Synchysis (senile) (vitreous humor) 379.21
scintillans 379.22
Syncope (near) (pre-) 780.2
anginosa 413.9
bradycardia 427.89
cardiac 780.2
carotid sinus 337.0
complicating delivery 669.2
due to lumbar puncture 349.0
fatal 798.1
Syncope—*continued*
heart 780.2
heat 992.1
laryngeal 786.2
tussive 786.2
vasoconstriction 780.2
vasodepressor 780.2
vasomotor 780.2
vasovagal 780.2
Syncytial infarct —*see* Placenta, abnormal
Syndactylism, syndactyly (multiple sites) 755.10
fingers (without fusion of bone) 755.11
with fusion of bone 755.12
toes (without fusion of bone) 755.13
with fusion of bone 755.14
Syndrome —*see also* Disease
abdominal
acute 789.0
migraine 346.2
muscle deficiency 756.7
Abercrombie's (amyloid degeneration) 277.3
abnormal innervation 374.43
abstinence
alcohol 291.8
drug 292.0
Abt-Letterer-Siwe (acute histiocytosis X) (M9722/3) 202.5
Achard-Thiers (adrenogenital) 255.2
acid pulmonary aspiration 997.3
obstetric (Mendelson's) 668.0
acquired immune deficiency 042
acquired immunodeficiency 042
acrocephalosyndactylism 755.55
acute abdominal 789.0
Adair-Dighton (brittle bones and blue sclera, deafness) 756.51
Adams-Stokes (-Morgagni) (syncope with heart block) 426.9
addisonian 255.4
Adie (-Holmes) (pupil) 379.46
adiposogenital 253.8
adrenal
hemorrhage 036.3
meningococcic 036.3
adrenocortical 255.3
adrenogenital (acquired) (congenital) 255.2
feminizing 255.2
iatrogenic 760.79
virilism (acquired) (congenital) 255.2
adult maltreatment (emotional) 995.81
affective organic NEC 293.89
drug-induced 292.84
afferent loop NEC 537.89
African macroglobulinemia 273.3
Ahumada-Del Castillo (nonpuerperal galactorrhea and amenorrhea) 253.1
air blast concussion—*see* Injury, internal, by site
Albright (-Martin) (pseudohypoparathyroidism) 275.4
Albright-McCune-Sternberg (osteitis fibrosa disseminata) 756.59
alcohol withdrawal 291.8
Alder's (leukocyte granulation anomaly) 288.2
Aldrich (-Wiskott) (eczema-thrombocytopenia) 279.12
Alibert-Bazin (mycosis, fungoides) (M9700/3) 202.1
Alice in Wonderland 293.89
Allen-Masters 620.6
Alligator baby (ichthyosis congenita) 757.1

Syndrome—*continued*
Alport's (hereditary hematuria-nephropathy-deafness) 759.89
Alvarez (transient cerebral ischemia) 435.9
alveolar capillary block 516.3
Alzheimer's 331.0
with dementia—*see* Alzheimer's, dementia
amnestic (confabulatory) 294.0
alcoholic 291.1
drug-induced 292.83
posttraumatic 294.0
amotivational 292.89
amyostatic 275.1
amyotrophic lateral sclerosis 335.20
angina (*see also* Angina) 413.9
ankyloglossia superior 750.0
anterior
chest wall 786.52
compartment (tibial) 958.8
spinal artery 433.8
compression 721.1
tibial (compartment) 958.8
antibody deficiency 279.00
agammaglobulinemic 279.00
congenital 279.04
hypogammaglobulinemic 279.00
antimongolism 758.3
Anton (-Babinski) (hemiasomatognosia) 307.9
anxiety (*see also* Anxiety) 300.00
aortic
arch 446.7
bifurcation (occlusion) 444.0
ring 747.21
Apert's (acrocephalosyndactyly) 755.55
Apert-Gallais (adrenogenital) 255.2
aphasia-apraxia-alexia 784.69
"approximate answers" 300.16
arcuate ligament (-celiac axis) 447.4
arcus aortae 446.7
arc-welders' 370.24
argentaffin, argintaffinoma 259.2
Argonz-Del Castillo (nonpuerperal galactorrhea and amenorrhea) 253.1
Argyll Robertson's (syphilitic) 094.89
nonsyphilitic 379.45
arm-shoulder (*see also* Neuropathy, peripheral, autonomic) 337.9
Arnold-Chiari (*see also* Spina bifida) 741.0
type I 348.4
type II 741.0
type III 742.0
type IV 742.2
Arrillaga-Ayerza (pulmonary artery sclerosis with pulmonary hypertension) 416.0
arteriomesenteric duodenum occlusion 537.89
arteriovenous steal 996.73
arteritis, young female (obliterative brachiocephalic) 446.7
aseptic meningitis—*see* Meningitis, aseptic
Asherman's 621.5
asphyctic (*see also* Anxiety) 300.00
aspiration, of newborn, massive or meconium 770.1
ataxia-telangiectasia 334.8
Audry's (acropachyderma) 757.39
auriculotemporal 350.8
autosomal—*see also* Abnormal, autosomes NEC
deletion 758.3
Avellis' 344.89
Axenfeld's 743.44

Syndrome—*continued*
Ayerza (-Arrillaga) (pulmonary artery sclerosis with pulmonary hypertension) 416.0
Baader's (erythema multiforme exudativum) 695.1
Baastrup's 721.5
Babinski (-Vaquez) (cardiovascular syphilis) 093.89
Babinski-Fröhlich (adiposogenital dystrophy) 253.8
Babinski-Nageotte 344.89
Bagratuni's (temporal arteritis) 446.5
Bakwin-Krida (craniometaphyseal dysplasia) 756.89
Balint's (psychic paralysis of visual disorientation) 368.16
Ballantyne (-Runge) (postmaturity) 766.2
ballooning posterior leaflet 424.0
Banti's—*see* Cirrhosis, liver
Bard-Pic's (carcinoma, head of pancreas) 157.0
Bardet-Biedl (obesity, polydactyly, and mental retardation) 759.89
Barlow's (mitral valve prolapse) 424.0
Barlow (-Möller) (infantile scurvy) 267
Baron Munchausen's 301.51
Barré-Guillain 357.0
Barré-Liéou (posterior cervical sympathetic) 723.2
Barrett's (chronic peptic ulcer of esophagus) 530.2
Bársony-Polgár (corkscrew esophagus) 530.5
Bársony-Teschendorf (corkscrew esophagus) 530.5
Bartter's (secondary hyperaldosteronism with juxtaglomerular hyperplasia) 255.1
Basedow's (exophthalmic goiter) 242.0
basilar artery 435.0
basofrontal 377.04
Bassen-Kornzweig (abetalipoproteinemia) 272.5
Batten-Steinert 359.2
battered
adult 995.81
baby or child 995.5
affecting parent or family V61.21
as reason for family seeking advice V61.21
history V61.21
specified person NEC 995.81
spouse 995.81
Baumgarten-Cruveilhier (cirrhosis of liver) 571.5
Bearn-Kunkel (-Slater) (lupoid hepatitis) 571.49
Beau's (*see also* Degeneration, myocardial) 429.1
Bechterew-Strümpell-Marie (ankylosing spondylitis) 720.0
Beck's (anterior spinal artery occlusion) 433.8
Beckwith (-Wiedemann) 759.89
Behçet's 136.1
Bekhterev-Strümpell-Marie (ankylosing spondylitis) 720.0
Benedikt's 344.89
Béquez César (-Steinbrinck-Chédiak-Higashi) (congenital gigantism of peroxidase granules) 288.2
Bernard-Horner (*see also* Neuropathy, peripheral, autonomic) 337.9
Bernard-Sergent (acute adrenocortical insufficiency) 255.4
Bernhardt-Roth 355.1
Bernheim's (*see also* Failure, heart, congestive) 428.0

Syndrome—*continued*
cervical (root) (spine) NEC 723.8
disc 722.71
posterior, sympathetic 723.2
rib 353.0
sympathetic paralysis 337.0
traumatic (acute) NEC 847.0
cervicobrachial (diffuse) 723.3
cervicocranial 723.2
cervicodorsal outlet 353.2
Céstan's 344.89
Céstan (-Raymond) 433.8
Céstan-Chenais 344.89
chancriform 114.1
Charcot's (intermittent claudication) 443.9
angina cruris 443.9
due to atherosclerosis 440.21
Charcot-Marie-Tooth 356.1
Charcot-Weiss-Baker 337.0
Cheadle (-Möller) (-Barlow) (infantile scurvy) 267
Chédiak-Higashi (-Steinbrinck) (congenital gigantism of peroxidase granules) 288.2
chest wall 786.52
Chiari's (hepatic vein thrombosis) 453.0
Chiari-Frommel 676.6
chiasmatic 368.41
Chilaiditi's (subphrenic displacement, colon) 751.4
child maltreatment (emotional) (nutritional) 995.5
affecting parent or family V61.21
history V61.21
chondroectodermal dysplasia 756.55
chorea-athetosis-agitans 275.1
Christian's (chronic histiocytosis X) 277.8
chromosome 4 short arm deletion 758.3
Clarke-Hadfield (pancreatic infantilism) 577.8
Claude's 352.6
Claude Bernard-Horner (*see also* Neuropathy, peripheral, autonomic) 337.9
Clérambault's
automatism 348.8
erotomania 297.8
Clifford's (postmaturity) 766.2
climacteric 627.2
Clouston's (hidrotic ectodermal dysplasia) 757.31
clumsiness 315.4
Cockayne's (microencephaly and dwarfism) 759.89
Cockayne-Weber (epidermolysis bullosa) 757.39
Cogan's (nonsyphilitic interstitial keratitis) 370.52
cold injury (newborn) 778.2
Collet (-Sicard) 352.6
combined immunity deficiency 279.2
compartment(al) (anterior) (deep) (posterior) (tibial) 958.8
compression 958.5
cauda equina 344.60
with neurogenic bladder 344.61
concussion 310.2
congenital
affecting more than one system 759.7
specified type NEC 759.89
facial diplegia 352.6
muscular hypertrophy-cerebral 759.89
congestion-fibrosis (pelvic) 625.5
conjunctivourethrosynovial 099.3
Conn (-Louis) (primary aldosteronism) 255.1

Syndrome—*continued*
Conradi (-Hünermann) (chondrodysplasia calcificans congenita) 756.59
conus medullaris 336.8
Cooke-Apert-Gallais (adrenogenital) 255.2
Cornelia de Lange's (Amsterdam dwarf, mental retardation, and brachycephaly) 759.8
coronary insufficiency or intermediate 411.1
cor pulmonale 416.9
corticosexual 255.2
Costen's (complex) 524.60
costochondral junction 733.6
costoclavicular 353.0
costovertebral 253.0
Cotard's (paranoia) 297.1
craniovertebral 723.2
Creutzfeldt-Jakob 046.1
with dementia 290.10
crib death 798.0
cricopharyngeal 787.2
cri-du-chat 758.3
Crigler-Najjar (congenital hyperbilirubinemia) 277.4
crocodile tears 351.8
Cronkhite-Canada 211.3
croup 464.4
CRST (cutaneous systemic sclerosis) 710.1
crush 958.5
crushed lung (*see also* Injury, internal, lung) 861.20
Cruveilhier-Baumgarten (cirrhosis of liver) 571.5
cubital tunnel 354.2
Cuiffini-Pancoast (M8010/3) (carcinoma, pulmonary apex) 162.3
Curschmann (-Batten) (-Steinert) 359.2
Cushing's (iatrogenic) (idiopathic) (pituitary basophilism) (pituitary-dependent) 255.0
overdose or wrong substance given or taken 962.0
Cyriax's (slipping rib) 733.99
cystic duct stump 576.0
Da Costa's (neurocirculatory asthenia) 306.2
Dameshek's (erythroblastic anemia) 282.4
Dana-Putnam (subacute combined sclerosis with pernicious anemia) 281.0 *[336.2]*
Danbolt (-Closs) (acrodermatitis enteropathica) 686.8
Dandy-Walker (atresia, foramen of Magendie) 742.3
with spina bifida (*see also* Spina bifida) 741.0
Danlos' 756.83
Davies-Colley (slipping rib) 733.99
dead fetus 641.3
defeminization 255.2
defibrination (*see also* Fibrinolysis) 286.6
Degos' 447.8
Deiters' nucleus 386.19
Déjérine-Roussy 348.8
Déjérine-Thomas 333.0
de Lange's (Amsterdam dwarf, mental retardation, and brachycephaly) (Cornelia) 759.89
Del Castillo's (germinal aplasia) 606.0
deletion chromosomes 758.3
delusional
induced by drug 292.11
dementia-aphonia, of childhood (*see also* Psychosis, childhood) 299.1
demyelinating NEC 341.9
denial visual hallucination 307.9

Syndrome—*continued*
depersonalization 300.6
Dercum's (adiposis dolorosa) 272.8
de Toni-Fanconi (-Debré) (cystinosis) 270.0
diabetes-dwarfism-obesity (juvenile) 258.1
diabetes mellitus-hypertension-nephrosis 250.4 *[581.81]*
diabetes mellitus in newborn infant 775.1
diabetes-nephrosis 250.4 *[581.81]*
diabetic amyotrophy 250.6 *[358.1]*
Diamond-Blackfan (congenital hypoplastic anemia) 284.0
Diamond-Gardener (autoerythrocyte sensitization) 287.2
DIC (diffuse or disseminated intravascular coagulopathy) (*see also* Fibrinolysis) 286.6
diencephalohypophyseal NEC 253.8
diffuse cervicobrachial 723.3
diffuse obstructive pulmonary 496
DiGeorge's (thymic hypoplasia) 279.11
Dighton's 756.51
Di Guglielmo's (erythremic myelosis) (M9841/3) 207.0
disc—*see* Displacement, intervertebral disc
discogenic—*see* Displacement, intervertebral disc
disequilibrium 276.9
disseminated platelet thrombosis 446.6
Ditthomska 307.81
Doan-Wiseman (primary splenic neutropenia) 288.0
Döhle body-panmyelopathic 288.2
Donohue's (leprechaunism) 259.8
dorsolateral medullary (*see also* Disease, cerebrovascular, acute) 436
double whammy 360.81
Down's (mongolism) 758.0
Dresbach's (elliptocytosis) 282.1
Dressler's (postmyocardial infarction) 411.0
hemoglobinuria 283.2
drug withdrawal, infant, of dependent mother 779.5
dry skin 701.1
eye 375.15
Duane's (retraction) 378.71
Duane-Stilling-Türk (ocular retraction syndrome) 378.71
Dubin-Johnson (constitutional hyperbilirubinemia) 277.4
Dubin-Sprinz (constitutional hyperbilirubinemia) 277.4
Duchenne's 335.22
due to abnormality
autosomal NEC (*see also* Abnormal, autosomes NEC) 758.5
13 758.1
18 758.2
21 or 22 758.0
D_1 758.1
E_3 758.2
G 758.0
chromosomal 758.9
sex 758.8
dumping 564.2
nonsurgical 536.8
Duplay's 726.2
Dupré's (meningism) 781.6
Dyke-Young (acquired macrocytic hemolytic anemia) 283.9
dyspraxia 315.4
dystocia, dystrophia 654.9

Syndrome—*continued*
Eales' 362.18
Eaton-Lambert (*see also* Neoplasm, by site, malignant) 199.1 *[358.1]*
Ebstein's (downward displacement, tricuspid valve into right ventricle) 746.2
ectopic ACTH secretion 255.0
eczema-thrombocytopenia 279.12
Eddowes' (brittle bones and blue sclera) 756.51
Edwards' 758.2
efferent loop 537.89
effort (aviators') (psychogenic) 306.2
Ehlers-Danlos 756.83
Eisenmenger's (ventricular septal defect) 745.4
Ekbom's (restless legs) 333.99
Ekman's (brittle bones and blue sclera) 756.51
electric feet 266.2
Ellison-Zollinger (gastric hypersecretion with pancreatic islet cell tumor) 251.5
Ellis-van Creveld (chondroectodermal dysplasia) 756.55
embryonic fixation 270.2
empty sella (turcica) 253.8
endocrine-hypertensive 255.3
Engel-von Recklinghausen (osteitis fibrosa cystica) 252.0
enteroarticular 099.3
entrapment—*see* Neuropathy, entrapment
eosinophilia myalgia 710.5
epidemic vomiting 078.82
Epstein's—*see* Nephrosis
Erb (-Oppenheim) -Goldflam 358.0
Erdheim's (acromegalic macrospondylitis) 253.0
Erlacher-Blount (tibia vara) 732.4
erythrocyte fragmentation 283.19
Evans' (thrombocytopenic purpura) 287.3
excess cortisol, iatrogenic 255.0
exhaustion 300.5
extrapyramidal 333.90
eyelid-malar-mandible 756.0
eye retraction 378.71
Faber's (achlorhydric anemia) 280.9
Fabry (-Anderson) (angiokeratoma corporis diffusum) 272.7
facet 724.8
Fallot's 745.2
falx (*see also* Hemorrhage, brain) 431
familial eczema-thrombocytopenia 279.12
Fanconi's (anemia) (congenital pancytopenia) 284.0
Fanconi (-de Toni) (-Debré) (cystinosis) 270.0
Farber (-Uzman) (disseminated lipogranulomatosis) 272.8
fatigue NEC 300.5
chronic 780.7
faulty bowel habit (idiopathic megacolon) 564.7
FDH (focal dermal hypoplasia) 757.39
fecal reservoir 560.39
Feil-Klippel (brevicollis) 756.16
Felty's (rheumatoid arthritis with splenomegaly and leukopenia) 714.1
fertile eunuch 257.2
fetal alcohol 760.71
late effect 760.71
fibrillation-flutter 427.32
fibrositis (periarticular) 729.0
Fiedler's (acute isolated myocarditis) 422.91
Fiessinger-Leroy (-Reiter) 099.3
Fiessinger-Rendu (erythema multiforme exudativum) 695.1
first arch 756.0

Syndrome—*continued*
Fisher's 357.0
Fitz's (acute hemorrhagic pancreatitis) 577.0
Fitz-Hugh and Curtis (gonococcal peritonitis) 098.86
Flajani (-Basedow) (exophthalmic goiter) 242.0
floppy
  infant 781.9
  valve (mitral) 424.0
flush 259.2
Foix-Alajouanine 336.1
Fong's (hereditary osteo-onychodysplasia) 756.89
foramen magnum 348.4
Forbes-Albright (nonpuerperal amenorrhea and lactation associated with pituitary tumor) 253.1
Foster-Kennedy 377.04
Foville's (peduncular) 344.89
Fragile X 759.83
Franceschetti's (mandibulofacial dysostosis) 756.0
Fraser's 759.89
Freeman-Sheldon 759.89
Frey's (auriculotemporal) 350.8
Friderichsen-Waterhouse 036.3
Friedrich-Erb-Arnold (acropachyderma) 757.39
Fröhlich's (adiposogenital dystrophy) 253.8
Froin's 336.8
Frommel-Chiari 676.6
frontal lobe 310.0
Fuller Albright's (osteitis fibrosa disseminata) 756.59
functional
  bowel 564.9
  prepubertal castrate 752.8
Gaisböck's (polycythemia hypertonica) 289.0
ganglion (basal, brain) 333.90
  geniculi 351.1
Ganser's, hysterical 300.16
Gardner-Diamond (autoerythrocyte sensitization) 287.2
gastroesophageal junction 530.0
gastroesophageal laceration-hemorrhage 530.7
gastrojejunal loop obstruction 537.89
Gayet-Wernicke's (superior hemorrhagic polioencephalitis) 265.1
Gee-Herter-Heubner (nontropical sprue) 579.0
Gélineau's 347
genito-anorectal 099.1
Gerhardt's (vocal cord paralysis) 478.30
Gerstmann's (finger agnosia) 784.69
Gilbert's 277.4
Gilford (-Hutchinson) (progeria) 259.8
Gilles de la Tourette's 307.23
Gillespie's (dysplasia oculodentodigitalis) 759.89
Glénard's (enteroptosis) 569.89
Glinski-Simmonds (pituitary cachexia) 253.2
glucuronyl transferase 277.4
glue ear 381.20
Goldberg (-Maxwell) (-Morris) (testicular feminization) 257.8
Goldenhar's (oculoauriculovertebral dysplasia) 756.0
Goldflam-Erb 358.0
Goltz-Gorlin (dermal hypoplasia) 757.39
Goodpasture's (pneumorenal) 446.21
Gopalan's (burning feet) 266.2
Gorlin-Chaudhry-Moss 759.89

Syndrome—*continued*
Gougerot (-Houwer) -Sjögren (keratoconjunctivitis sicca) 710.2
Gougerot-Blum (pigmented purpuric lichenoid dermatitis) 709.1
Gougerot-Carteaud (confluent reticulate papillomatosis) 701.8
Gouley's (constrictive pericarditis) 423.2
Gowers' (vasovagal attack) 780.2
Gowers-Paton-Kennedy 377.04
Gradenigo's 383.02
Gray or grey (chloramphenicol) (newborn) 779.4
Greig's (hypertelorism) 756.0
Gubler-Millard 344.89
Guérin-Stern (arthrogryposis multiplex congenita) 754.89
Guillain-Barré (-Strohl) 357.0
Gunn's (jaw-winking syndrome) 742.8
Günther's (congenital erythropoietic porphyria) 277.1
gustatory sweating 350.8
H_3O 759.81
Hadfield-Clarke (pancreatic infantilism) 577.8
Haglund-Läwen-Fründ 717.89
hairless women 257.8
Hallermann-Streiff 756.0
Hallervorden-Spatz 333.0
Hamman's (spontaneous mediastinal emphysema) 518.1
Hamman-Rich (diffuse interstitial pulmonary fibrosis) 516.3
Hand-Schüller-Christian (chronic histiocytosis X) 277.8
hand-foot 282.61
Hanot-Chauffard (-Troisier) (bronze diabetes) 275.0
Harada's 363.22
Hare's (M8010/3) (carcinoma, pulmonary apex) 162.3
Harkavy's 446.0
harlequin color change 779.8
Harris' (organic hyperinsulinism) 251.1
Hart's (pellagra-cerebellar ataxia-renal aminoaciduria) 270.0
Hayem-Faber (achlorhydric anemia) 280.9
Hayem-Widal (acquired hemolytic jaundice) 283.9
Heberden's (angina pectoris) 413.9
Hedinger's (malignant carcinoid) 259.2
Hegglin's 288.2
Heller's (infantile psychosis) (*see also* Psychosis, childhood) 299.1
H.E.L.L.P. 642.5
hemolytic-uremic (adult) (child) 283.11
Hench-Rosenberg (palindromic arthritis) (*see also* Rheumatism, palindromic) 719.3
Henoch-Schönlein (allergic purpura) 287.0
hepatic flexure 569.89
hepatorenal 572.4
  due to a procedure 997.4
  following delivery 674.8
hepatourologic 572.4
Herrick's (hemoglobin S disease) 282.61
Herter (-Gee) (nontropical sprue) 579.0
Heubner-Herter (nontropical sprue) 579.0
Heyd's (hepatorenal) 572.4
HHHO 759.81
Hilger's 337.0
Hoffa (-Kastert) (liposynovitis prepatellaris) 272.8
Hoffmann's 244.9 *[359.5]*

Syndrome—*continued*
Kalischer's (encephalocutaneous angiomatosis) 759.6
Kallmann's (hypogonadotropic hypogonadism with anosmia) 253.4
Kanner's (autism) (*see also* Psychosis, childhood) 299.0
Kartagener's (sinusitis, bronchiectasis, situs inversus) 759.3
Kasabach-Merritt (capillary hemangioma associated with thrombocytopenic purpura) 287.3
Kast's (dyschondroplasia with hemangiomas) 756.4
Kaznelson's (congenital hypoplastic anemia) 284.0
Kelly's (sideropenic dysphagia) 280.8
Kimmelstiel-Wilson (intercapillary glomerulosclerosis) 250.4 *[581.81]*
Klauder's (erythema multiforme exudativum) 695.1
Klein-Waardenburg (ptosis-epicanthus) 270.2
Kleine-Levin 349.89
Klinefelter's 758.7
Klippel-Feil (brevicollis) 756.16
Klippel-Trenaunay 759.89
Klumpke (-Déjérine) (injury to brachial plexus at birth) 767.6
Klüver-Bucy (-Terzian) 310.0
Köhler-Pellegrini-Stieda (calcification, knee joint) 726.62
König's 564.8
Korsakoff's (nonalcoholic) 294.0
alcoholic 291.1
Korsakoff (-Wernicke) (nonalcoholic) 294.0
alcoholic 291.1
Kostmann's (infantile genetic agranulocytosis) 288.0
Krabbe's
congenital muscle hypoplasia 756.89
cutaneocerebral angioma 759.6
Kunkel (lupoid hepatitis) 571.49
labyrinthine 386.50
laceration, broad ligament 620.6
Langdon Down (mongolism) 758.0
Larsen's (flattened facies and multiple congenital dislocations) 755.8
lateral
cutaneous nerve of thigh 355.1
medullary (*see also* Disease, cerebrovascular acute) 436
Launois' (pituitary gigantism) 253.0
Launois-Cléret (adiposogenital dystrophy) 253.8
Laurence-Moon (-Bardet) -Biedl (obesity, polydactyly, and mental retardation) 759.8
Lawford's (encephalocutaneous angiomatosis) 759.6
lazy
leukocyte 288.0
posture 728.3
Lederer-Brill (acquired infectious hemolytic anemia) 283.19
Legg-Calvé-Perthes (osteochondrosis capital femoral) 732.1
Lennox's (*see also* Epilepsy) 345.0
lenticular 275.1
Léopold-Lévi's (paroxysmal thyroid instability) 242.9
Lepore hemoglobin 282.4
Léri-Weill 756.59
Leriche's (aortic bifurcation occlusion) 444.0
Lermoyez's (*see also* Disease, Ménière's) 386.00
Lesch-Nyhan (hypoxanthine-guanine-phosphoribosyltransferase deficiency) 277.2
Lev's (acquired complete heart block) 426.0
Levi's (pituitary dwarfism) 253.3
Lévy-Roussy 334.3
Lichtheim's (subacute combined sclerosis with pernicious anemia) 281.0 *[336.2]*
Lightwood's (renal tubular acidosis) 588.8
Lignac (-de Toni) (-Fanconi) (-Debré) (cystinosis) 270.0
Likoff's (angina in menopausal women) 413.9
liver-kidney 572.4
Lloyd's 258.1
lobotomy 310.0
Löffler's (eosinophilic pneumonitis) 518.3
Löfgren's (sarcoidosis) 135
long arm 18 or 21 deletion 758.3
Looser (-Debray) -Milkman (osteomalacia with pseudofractures) 268.2
Lorain-Levi (pituitary dwarfism) 253.3
Louis-Bar (ataxia-telangiectasia) 334.8
low
atmospheric pressure 993.2
back 724.2
psychogenic 306.0
output (cardiac) (*see also* Failure, heart) 428.9
Lowe's (oculocerebrorenal dystrophy) 270.8
Lowe-Terrey-MacLachlan (oculocerebrorenal dystrophy) 270.8
lower radicular, newborn 767.4
Lown (-Ganong)-Levine (short P-R interval, normal QRS complex, and supraventricular tachycardia) 426.81
Lucey-Driscoll (jaundice due to delayed conjugation) 774.30
Luetscher's (dehydration) 276.5
lumbar vertebral 724.4
Lutembacher's (atrial septal defect with mitral stenosis) 745.5
Lyell's (toxic epidermal necrolysis) 695.1
due to drug
correct substance properly administered 695.1
overdose or wrong substance given or taken 977.9
specified drug—*see* Table of drugs and chemicals
MacLeod's 492.8
macrogenitosomia praecox 259.8
macroglobulinemia 273.3
Maffucci's (dyschondroplasia with hemangiomas) 756.4
Magenblase 306.4
magnesium-deficiency 781.7
malabsorption 579.9
postsurgical 579.3
spinal fluid 331.3
malignant carcinoid 259.2
Mallory-Weiss 530.7
mandibulofacial dysostosis 756.0
manic-depressive (*see also* Psychosis, affective) 296.80
Mankowsky's (familial dysplastic osteopathy) 731.2
maple syrup (urine) 270.3
Marable's (celiac artery compression) 447.4
Marchesani (-Weill) (brachymorphism and ectopia lentis) 759.89

Syndrome—*continued*
Marchiafava-Bignami 341.8
Marchiafava-Micheli (paroxysmal nocturnal hemoglobinuria) 283.2
Marcus Gunn's (jaw-winking syndrome) 742.8
Marfan's (arachnodactyly) 759.82
meaning congenital syphilis 090.49
with luxation of lens 090.49 *[379.32]*
Marie's (acromegaly) 253.0
primary or idiopathic (acropachyderma) 757.39
secondary (hypertrophic pulmonary osteoarthropathy) 731.2
Markus-Adie 379.46
Maroteaux-Lamy (mucopolysaccharidosis VI) 277.5
Martin's 715.27
Martin-Albright (pseudohypoparathyroidism) 275.4
Martorell-Fabré (pulseless disease) 446.7
massive aspiration of newborn 770.1
Masters-Allen 620.6
mastocytosis 757.33
maternal hypotension 669.2
maternal obesity 646.1
May (-Hegglin) 288.2
McArdle (-Schmid) (-Pearson) (glycogenosis V) 271.0
McCune-Albright (osteitis fibrosa disseminata) 756.59
McQuarrie's (idiopathic familial hypoglycemia) 251.2
meconium
aspiration 770.1
plug (newborn) NEC 777.1
median arcuate ligament 447.4
mediastinal fibrosis 519.3
Meekeren-Ehlers-Danlos 756.83
Meige (blepharospasm-oromandibular dystonia) 333.82
-Milroy (chronic hereditary edema) 757.0
Melkersson (-Rosenthal) 351.8
Mende's (ptosis-epicanthus) 270.2
Mendelson's (resulting from a procedure) 997.3
during labor 668.0
obstetric 668.0
Ménétrier's (hypertrophic gastritis) 535.2
Ménière's (*see also* Disease, Ménière's) 386.00
meningo-eruptive 047.1
Menkes' 759.89
glutamic acid 759.89
maple syrup (urine) disease 270.3
menopause 627.2
postartificial 627.4
menstruation 625.4
mesenteric
artery, superior 557.1
vascular insufficiency (with gangrene) 557.1
metastatic carcinoid 259.2
Meyenburg-Altherr-Uehlinger 733.99
Meyer-Schwickerath and Weyers (dysplasia oculodentodigitalis) 759.89
Micheli-Rietti (thalassemia minor) 282.4
Michotte's 721.5
micrognathia-glossoptosis 756.0
microphthalmos (congenital) 759.89
midbrain 348.8
middle
lobe (lung) (right) 518.0
radicular 353.0

Syndrome—*continued*
Miescher's
familial acanthosis nigricans 701.2
granulomatosis disciformis 709.3
Mieten's 759.89
migraine 346.0
Mikity-Wilson (pulmonary dysmaturity) 770.7
Mikulicz's (dryness of mouth, absent or decreased lacrimation) 527.1
milk alkali (milk drinkers') 999.9
Milkman (-Looser) (osteomalacia with pseudofractures) 268.2
Millard-Gubler 344.89
Miller Fisher's 357.0
Milles' (encephalocutaneous angiomatosis) 759.6
Minkowski-Chauffard (*see also* Spherocytosis) 282.0
Mirizzi's (hepatic duct stenosis) 576.2
with calculus, cholelithiasis, or stones—*see* Choledocholithiasis
mitral
click (-murmur) 785.2
valve prolapse 424.0
Möbius'
congenital oculofacial paralysis 352.6
ophthalmoplegic migraine 346.8
Mohr's (Types I and II) 759.89
monofixation 378.34
Moore's (*see also* Epilepsy) 345.5
Morel-Moore (hyperostosis frontalis interna) 733.3
Morel-Morgagni (hyperostosis frontalis interna) 733.3
Morgagni (-Stewart-Morel) (hyperostosis frontalis interna) 733.3
Morgagni-Adams-Stokes (syncope with heart block) 426.9
Morquio (-Brailsford) (-Ullrich) (mucopolysaccharidosis IV) 277.5
Morris (testicular feminization) 257.8
Morton's (foot) (metatarsalgia) (metatarsal neuralgia) (neuralgia) (neuroma) (toe) 355.6
Moschcowitz (-Singer-Symmers) (thrombotic thrombocytopenic purpura) 446.6
Mounier-Kuhn 494
Mucha-Haberman (acute parapsoriasis varioliformis) 696.2
mucocutaneous lymph node (acute) (febrile) (infantile) (MCLS) 446.1
multiple
deficiency 260
operations 301.51
Munchausen's 301.51
Münchmeyer's (exostosis luxurians) 728.11
Murchison-Sanderson—*see* Disease, Hodgkin's
myasthenic—*see* Myasthenia, syndrome
myelodysplastic 238.7
myeloproliferative (chronic) (M9960/1) 238.7
myofascial pain NEC 729.1
Naffziger's 353.0
Nager-de Reynier (dysostosis mandibularis) 756.0
nail-patella (hereditary osteo-onychodysplasia) 756.89
Nebécourt's 253.3
Neill-Dingwall (microencephaly and dwarfism) 759.89
nephrotic (*see also* Nephrosis) 581.9
diabetic 250.4 *[581.81]*
Netherton's (ichthyosiform erythroderma) 757.1

Syndrome—*continued*
Rett's 330.8
Reye's 331.81
Reye-Sheehan (postpartum pituitary necrosis) 253.2
Riddoch's (visual disorientation) 368.16
Ridley's (*see also* Failure, ventricular, left) 428.1
Rieger's (mesodermal dysgenesis, anterior ocular segment) 743.44
Rietti-Greppi-Micheli (thalassemia minor) 282.4
right ventricular obstruction—*see* Failure heart, congestive
Riley-Day (familial dysautonomia) 742.8
Robin's 756.0
Rokitansky-Kuster-Hauser (congenital absence, vagina) 752.49
Romano-Ward (prolonged Q-T interval) 794.31
Romberg's 349.89
Rosen-Castleman-Liebow (pulmonary proteinosis) 516.0
rotator cuff, shoulder 726.10
Roth's 355.1
Rothmund's (congenital poikiloderma) 757.33
Rotor's (idiopathic hyperbilirubinemia) 277.4
Roussy-Lévy 334.3
Roy (-Jutras) (acropachyderma) 757.39
rubella (congenital) 771.0
Rubinstein-Taybi's (brachydactylia, short stature, and mental retardation) 759.89
Rud's (mental deficiency, epilepsy, and infantilism) 759.89
Ruiter-Pompen (-Wyers) (angiokeratoma corporis diffusum) 272.7
Runge's (postmaturity) 766.2
Russell (-Silver) (congenital hemihypertrophy and short stature) 759.89
Rytand-Lipsitch (complete atrioventricular block) 426.0
sacralization-scoliosis-sciatica 756.15
sacroiliac 724.6
Saenger's 379.46
salt
depletion (*see also* Disease, renal) 593.9
due to heat NEC 992.8
causing heat exhaustion or prostration 992.4
low (*see also* Disease, renal) 593.9
salt-losing (*see also* Disease, renal) 593.9
Sanfilippo's (mucopolysaccharidosis III) 277.5
Scaglietti-Dagnini (acromegalic macrospondylitis) 253.0
scalded skin 695.1
scalenus anticus (anterior) 353.0
scapulocostal 354.8
scapuloperoneal 359.1
scapulovertebral 723.4
Schaumann's (sarcoidosis) 135
Scheie's (mucopolysaccharidosis IS) 277.5
Scheuthauer-Marie-Sainton (cleidocranialis dysostosis) 755.59
Schirmer's (encephalocutaneous angiomatosis) 759.6
schizophrenic, of childhood NEC (*see also* Psychosis, childhood) 299.9
Schmidt's
sphallo-pharyngo-laryngeal hemiplegia 352.6
thyroid-adrenocortical insufficiency 258.1
vagoaccessory 352.6
Schneider's 047.9
Scholte's (malignant carcinoid) 259.2
Scholz (-Bielschowsky-Henneberg) 330.0

Syndrome—*continued*
Schroeder's (endocrine-hypertensive) 255.3
Schüller-Christian (chronic histiocytosis X) 277.8
Schultz's (agranulocytosis) 288.0
Schwartz (-Jampel) 756.89
Schwartz-Bartter (inappropriate secretion of antidiuretic hormone) 253.6
Scimitar (anomalous venous drainage, right lung to inferior vena cave) 747.49
sclerocystic ovary 256.4
sea-blue histiocyte 272.7
Seabright-Bantam (pseudohypoparathyroidism) 275.4
Seckel's 759.89
Secretan's (posttraumatic edema) 782.3
secretoinhibitor (keratoconjunctivitis sicca) 710.2
Seeligmann's (ichthyosis congenita) 757.1
Senear-Usher (pemphigus erythematosus) 694.4
senilism 259.8
serotonin 333.99
serous meningitis 348.2
Sertoli cell (germinal aplasia) 606.0
sex chromosome mosaic 758.8
Sézary's (reticulosis) (M9701/3) 202.2
Shaver's (bauxite pneumoconiosis) 503
Sheehan's (postpartum pituitary necrosis) 253.2
shock (traumatic) 958.4
kidney 584.5
following crush injury 958.5
lung 518.5
neurogenic 308.9
psychic 308.9
short
bowel 579.3
P-R interval 426.81
shoulder-arm (*see also* Neuropathy, peripheral, autonomic) 337.9
shoulder-girdle 723.4
shoulder-hand (*see also* Neuropathy, peripheral, autonomic) 337.9
Shwachman's 288.0
Shy-Drager (orthostatic hypotension with multisystem degeneration) 333.0
Sicard's 352.6
sicca (keratoconjunctivitis) 710.2
sick
cell 276.1
cilia 759.89
sinus 427.81
sideropenic 280.8
Siemens'
ectodermal dysplasia 757.31
keratosis follicularis spinulosa (decalvans) 757.39
Silfverskiöld's (osteochondrodystrophy, extremities) 756.50
Silver's (congenital hemihypertrophy and short stature) 759.89
Silvestroni-Bianco (thalassemia minima) 282.4
Simons' (progressive lipodystrophy) 272.6
sinus tarsi 355.5
sinusitis-bronchiectasis-situs inversus 759.3
Sipple's (medullary thyroid carcinoma-pheochromocytoma) 193
Sjögren (-Gougerot) (keratoconjunctivitis sicca) 710.2
with lung involvement 710.2 *[517.8]*
Sjögren-Larsson (ichthyosis congenita) 757.1
Slocumb's 255.3
Sluder's 337.0

Syndrome—*continued*
Smith-Lemli-Opitz (cerebrohepatorenal syndrome) 759.89
smokers' 305.1
Sneddon-Wilkinson (subcorneal pustular dermatosis) 694.1
Sotos' (cerebral gigantism) 253.0
South African cardiomyopathy 425.2
spasmodic
upward movement, eyes(s) 378.82
winking 307.20
Spens' (syncope with heart block) 426.9
spherophakia-brachymorphia 759.89
spinal cord injury—*see also* Injury, spinal, by site
with fracture, vertebra—*see* Fracture, vertebra, by site, with spinal cord injury
cervical—*see* Injury, spinal, cervical
fluid malabsorption (acquired) 331.3
splenic
agenesis 759.0
flexure 569.89
neutropenia 288.0
sequestration 282.60
Spurway's (brittle bones and blue sclera) 756.51
staphylococcal scalded skin 695.1
Stein's (polycystic ovary) 256.4
Stein-Leventhal (polycystic ovary) 256.4
Steinbrocker's (*see also* Neuropathy, peripheral, autonomic) 337.9
Stevens-Johnson (erythema multiforme exudativum) 695.1
Stewart-Morel (hyperostosis frontalis interna) 733.3
stiff-man 333.91
Still's (juvenile rheumatoid arthritis) 714.30
Still-Felty (rheumatoid arthritis with splenomegaly and leukopenia) 714.1
Stilling-Türk-Duane (ocular retraction syndrome) 378.71
Stojano's (subcostal) 098.86
Stokes (-Adams) (syncope with heart block) 426.9
Stokvis-Talma (enterogenous cyanosis) 289.7
stone heart (*see also* Failure, ventricular, left) 428.1
straight-back 756.19
stroke (*see also* Disease, cerebrovascular, acute) 436
little 435.9
Sturge-Kalischer-Weber (encephalotrigeminal angiomatosis) 759.6
Sturge-Weber (-Dimitri) (encephalocutaneous angiomatosis) 759.6
subclavian-carotid obstruction (chronic) 446.7
subclavian steal 435.2
subcoracoid-pectoralis minor 447.8
subcostal 098.86
nerve compression 354.8
subperiosteal hematoma 267
subphrenic interposition 751.4
sudden infant death (SIDS) 798.0
Sudeck's 733.7
Sudeck-Leriche 733.7
superior
cerebellar artery (*see also* Disease, cerebrovascular, acute) 436
mesenteric artery 557.1
pulmonary sulcus (tumor) (M8010/3) 162.3
vena cava 459.2
suprarenal cortical 255.3

Syndrome—*continued*
supraspinatus 726.10
swallowed blood 777.3
sweat retention 705.1
Sweet's (acute febrile neutrophilic dermatosis) 695.89
Swyer-James (unilateral hyperlucent lung) 492.8
Swyer's (XY pure gonadal dysgenesis) 752.7
Symonds' 348.2
sympathetic
cervical paralysis 337.0
pelvic 625.5
syndactylic oxycephaly 755.55
syphilitic-cardiovascular 093.89
systemic fibrosclerosing 710.8
systolic click (-murmur) 785.2
Tabagism 305.1
tachycardia-bradycardia 427.81
Takayasu (-Onishi) (pulseless disease) 446.7
Tapia's 352.6
tarsal tunnel 355.5
Taussig-Bing (transposition, aorta and overriding pulmonary artery) 745.11
Taybi's (otopalatodigital) 759.89
Taylor's 625.5
teething 520.7
tegmental 344.89
telangiectasis-pigmentation-cataract 757.33
temporal 383.02
lobectomy behavior 310.0
temporomandibular joint-pain-dysfunction [TMJ] NEC 524.60
specified NEC 524.69
Terry's 362.21
testicular feminization 257.8
testis, nonvirilizing 257.8
tethered (spinal) cord 742.59
thalamic 348.8
Thibierge-Weissenbach (cutaneous systemic sclerosis) 710.1
Thiele 724.6
thoracic outlet (compression) 353.0
thoracogenous rheumatic (hypertrophic pulmonary osteoarthropathy) 731.2
Thorn's (*see also* Disease, renal) 593.9
Thorson-Biörck (malignant carcinoid) 259.2
thrombopenia-hemangioma 287.3
thyroid-adrenocortical insufficiency 258.1
Tietze's 733.6
time-zone (rapid) 307.45
Tobias' (carcinoma, pulmonary apex) (M8010/3) 162.3
toilet seat 926.0
Tolosa-Hunt 378.55
Toni-Fanconi (cystinosis) 270.0
Touraine's (hereditary osteo-onychodysplasia) 756.89
Touraine-Solente-Golé (acropachyderma) 757.39
toxic
oil 710.5
shock 040.89
transfusion
fetal-maternal 772.0
twin
donor (infant) 772.0
recipient (infant) 776.4
Treacher Collins' (incomplete mandibulofacial dysostosis) 756.0
trigeminal plate 259.8

Syphilis, syphilitic—*continued*
central nervous system (any site) (early) (late) (latent) (primary) (recurrent) (relapse) (secondary) (tertiary) 094.9
with
ataxia 094.0
paralysis, general 094.1
juvenile 090.40
paresis (general) 094.1
juvenile 090.40
tabes (dorsalis) 094.0
juvenile 090.40
taboparesis 094.1
juvenile 090.40
aneurysm (ruptured) 094.87
congenital 090.40
juvenile 090.40
remission in (sustained) 094.9
serology doubtful, negative, or positive 094.9
specified nature or site NEC 094.89
vascular 094.89
cerebral 094.89
meningovascular 094.2
nerves 094.89
sclerosis 094.89
thrombosis 094.89
cerebrospinal 094.89
tabetic 094.0
cerebrovascular 094.89
cervix 095.8
chancre (multiple) 091.0
extragenital 091.2
Rollet's 091.0
Charcot's joint 094.0 *[713.5]*
choked disc 094.89 *[377.00]*
chorioretinitis 091.51
congenital 090.0 *[363.13]*
late 094.83
choroiditis 091.51
congenital 090.0 *[363.13]*
late 094.83
prenatal 090.0 *[363.13]*
choroidoretinitis (secondary) 091.51
congenital 090.0 *[363.13]*
late 094.83
ciliary body (secondary) 091.52
late 095.8 *[364.11]*
colon (late) 095.8
combined sclerosis 094.89
complicating pregnancy, childbirth or puerperium 647.0
affecting fetus or newborn 760.2
condyloma (latum) 091.3
congenital 090.9
with
encephalitis 090.41
paresis (general) 090.40
tabes (dorsalis) 090.40
taboparesis 090.40
chorioretinitis, choroiditis 090.0 *[363.13]*
early or less than 2 years after birth NEC 090.2
with manifestations 090.0
latent (without manifestations) 090.1
negative spinal fluid test 090.1
serology, positive 090.1
symptomatic 090.0
interstitial keratitis 090.3
juvenile neurosyphilis 090.40

Syphilis, syphilitic—*continued*
late or 2 years or more after birth NEC 090.7
chorioretinitis, choroiditis 090.5 *[363.13]*
interstitial keratitis 090.3
juvenile neurosyphilis NEC 090.40
latent (without manifestations) 090.6
negative spinal fluid test 090.6
serology, positive 090.6
symptomatic or with manifestations NEC 090.5
interstitial keratitis 090.3
conjugal 097.9
tabes 094.0
conjunctiva 095.8 *[372.10]*
contact V01.6
cord, bladder 094.0
cornea, late 095.8 *[370.59]*
coronary (artery) 093.89
sclerosis 093.89
coryza 095.8
congenital 090.0
cranial nerve 094.89
cutaneous—*see* Syphilis, skin
dacryocystitis 095.8
degeneration, spinal cord 094.89
d'emblée 095.8
dementia 094.89
paralytica 094.1
juvenilis 090.40
destruction of bone 095.5
dilatation, aorta 093.0
due to blood transfusion 097.9
dura mater 094.89
ear 095.8
inner 095.8
nerve (eighth) 094.86
neurorecurrence 094.86
early NEC 091.0
cardiovascular 093.9
central nervous system 094.9
paresis 094.1
tabes 094.0
latent (without manifestations) (less than 2 years after infection) 092.9
negative spinal fluid test 092.9
serological relapse following treatment 092.0
serology positive 092.9
paresis 094.1
relapse (treated, untreated) 091.7
skin 091.3
symptomatic NEC 091.89
extragenital chancre 091.2
primary, except extragenital chancre 091.0
secondary (*see also* Syphilis, secondary) 091.3
relapse (treated, untreated) 091.7
tabes 094.0
ulcer 091.3
eighth nerve 094.86
endemic, nonvenereal 104.0
endocarditis 093.20
aortic 093.22
mitral 093.21
pulmonary 093.24
tricuspid 093.23
epididymis (late) 095.8
epiglottis 095.8
epiphysitis (congenital) 090.0
esophagus 095.8
Eustachian tube 095.8

Syphilis, syphilitic—*continued*
exposure to V01.6
eye 095.8 *[363.13]*
neuromuscular mechanism 094.85
eyelid 095.8 *[373.5]*
with gumma 095.8 *[373.5]*
ptosis 094.89
fallopian tube 095.8
fracture 095.5
gallbladder (late) 095.8
gastric 095.8
crisis 094.0
polyposis 095.8
general 097.9
paralysis 094.1
juvenile 090.40
genital (primary) 091.0
glaucoma 095.8
gumma (late) NEC 095.9
cardiovascular system 093.9
central nervous system 094.9
congenital 090.5
heart or artery 093.89
heart 093.89
block 093.89
decompensation 093.89
disease 093.89
failure 093.89
valve (*see also* Syphilis, endocarditis) 093.20
hemianesthesia 094.89
hemianopsia 095.8
hemiparesis 094.89
hemiplegia 094.89
hepatic artery 093.89
hepatitis 095.3
hepatomegaly 095.3
congenital 090.0
hereditaria tarda (*see also* Syphilis, congenital, late) 090.7
hereditary (*see also* Syphilis, congenital) 090.9
interstitial keratitis 090.3
Hutchinson's teeth 090.5
hyalitis 095.8
inactive—*see* Syphilis, latent
infantum NEC (*see also* Syphilis, congenital) 090.9
inherited—*see* Syphilis, congenital
internal ear 095.8
intestine (late) 095.8
iris, iritis (secondary) 091.52
late 095.8 *[364.11]*
joint (late) 095.8
keratitis (congenital) (early) (interstitial) (late) (parenchymatous) (punctata profunda) 090.3
kidney 095.4
lacrimal apparatus 095.8
laryngeal paralysis 095.8
larynx 095.8
late 097.0
cardiovascular 093.9
central nervous system 094.9
latent or 2 years or more after infection (without manifestations) 096
negative spinal fluid test 096
serology positive 096
paresis 094.1
specified site NEC 095.8
symptomatic or with symptoms 095.9
tabes 094.0

Syphilis, syphilitic—*continued*
latent 097.1
central nervous system 094.9
date of infection unspecified 097.1
early or less than 2 years after infection 092.9
late or 2 years or more after infection 096
serology
doubtful
follow-up of latent syphilis 097.1
central nervous system 094.9
date of infection unspecified 097.1
early or less than 2 years after infection 092.9
late or 2 years or more after infection 096
positive, only finding 097.1
date of infection unspecified 097.1
early or less than 2 years after infection 097.1
late or 2 years or more after infection 097.1
lens 095.8
leukoderma 091.3
late 095.8
lienis 095.8
lip 091.3
chancre 091.2
late 095.8
primary 091.2
Lissauer's paralysis 094.1
liver 095.3
secondary 091.62
locomotor ataxia 094.0
lung 095.1
lymphadenitis (secondary) 091.4
lymph gland (early) (secondary) 091.4
late 095.8
macular atrophy of skin 091.3
striated 095.8
maternal, affecting fetus or newborn 760.2
manifest syphilis in newborn—*see* Syphilis, congenital
mediastinum (late) 095.8
meninges (adhesive) (basilar) (brain) (spinal cord) 094.2
meningitis 094.2
acute 091.81
congenital 090.42
meningoencephalitis 094.2
meningovascular 094.2
congenital 090.49
mesarteritis 093.89
brain 094.89
spine 094.89
middle ear 095.8
mitral stenosis 093.21
monoplegia 094.89
mouth (secondary) 091.3
late 095.8
mucocutaneous 091.3
late 095.8
mucous
membrane 091.3
late 095.8
patches 091.3
congenital 090.0
mulberry molars 090.5
muscle 095.6
myocardium 093.82
myositis 095.6
nasal sinus 095.8
neonatorum NEC (*see also* Syphilis, congenital) 090.9

Syphilis, syphilitic—*continued*
spleen 095.8
splenomegaly 095.8
spondylitis 095.5
staphyloma 095.8
stigmata (congenital) 090.5
stomach 095.8
synovium (late) 095.7
tabes dorsalis (early) (late) 094.0
juvenile 090.40
tabetic type 094.0
juvenile 090.40
taboparesis 094.1
juvenile 090.40
tachycardia 093.89
tendon (late) 095.7
tertiary 097.0
with symptoms 095.8
cardiovascular 093.9
central nervous system 094.9
multiple NEC 095.8
specified site NEC 095.8
testis 095.8
thorax 095.8
throat 095.8
thymus (gland) 095.8
thyroid (late) 095.8
tongue 095.8
tonsil (lingual) 095.8
primary 091.2
secondary 091.3
trachea 095.8
tricuspid valve 093.23
tumor, brain 094.89
tunica vaginalis (late) 095.8
ulcer (any site) (early) (secondary) 091.3
late 095.9
perforating 095.9
foot 094.0
urethra (stricture) 095.8
urogenital 095.8
uterus 095.8
uveal tract (secondary) 091.50
late 095.8 *[363.13]*
uveitis (secondary) 091.50
late 095.8 *[363.13]*
uvula (late) 095.8
perforated 095.8
vagina 091.0
late 095.8
valvulitis NEC 093.20
vascular 093.89
brain or cerebral 094.89
vein 093.89
cerebral 094.89
ventriculi 095.8
vesicae urinariae 095.8
viscera (abdominal) 095.2
secondary 091.69
vitreous (hemorrhage) (opacities) 095.8
vulva 091.0
late 095.8
secondary 091.3
Syphiloma 095.9
cardiovascular system 093.9
central nervous system 094.9
circulatory system 093.9
congenital 090.5
Syphilophobia 300.29
Syringadenoma (M8400/0)—*see also* Neoplasm, skin, benign
papillary (M8406/0)—*see* Neoplasm, skin, benign
Syringobulbia 336.0
Syringocarcinoma (M8400/3)—*see* Neoplasm, skin, malignant
Syringocystadenoma (M8400/0)—*see also* Neoplasm, skin, benign
papillary (M8406/0)—*see* Neoplasm, skin, benign
Syringocystoma (M8407/0)—*see* Neoplasm, skin, benign
Syringoma (M8407/0)—*see also* Neoplasm, skin, benign
chondroid (M8940/0)—*see* Neoplasm, by site, benign
Syringomyelia 336.0
Syringomyelitis 323.9
late effect—*see* category 326
Syringomyelocele (*see also* Spina bifida) 741.9
Syringopontia 336.0
System, systemic —*see also* condition
disease, combined—*see* Degeneration, combined
fibrosclerosing syndrome 710.8
lupus erythematosus 710.0
inhibitor 286.5

T

Tab —*see* Tag
Tabacism 989.8
Tabacosis 989.8
Tabardillo 080
  flea-borne 081.0
  louse-borne 080
Tabes, tabetic
  with
    central nervous system syphilis 094.0
    Charcot's joint 094.0 *[713.5]*
    cord bladder 094.0
    crisis, viscera (any) 094.0
    paralysis, general 094.1
    paresis (general) 094.1
    perforating ulcer 094.0
  arthropathy 094.0 *[713.5]*
  bladder 094.0
  bone 094.0
  cerebrospinal 094.0
  congenital 090.40
  conjugal 094.0
  dorsalis 094.0
    neurosyphilis 094.0
  early 094.0
  juvenile 090.40
  latent 094.0
  mesenterica (*see also* Tuberculosis) 014.8
  paralysis insane, general 094.1
  peripheral (nonsyphilitic) 799.8
  spasmodic 094.0
    not dorsal or dorsalis 343.9
  syphilis (cerebrospinal) 094.0
Taboparalysis 094.1
Taboparesis (remission) 094.1
  with
    Charcot's joint 094.1 *[713.5]*
    cord bladder 094.1
    perforating ulcer 094.1
  juvenile 090.40
Tachyalimentation 579.3
Tachyarrhythmia, tachyrhythmia —*see also* Tachycardia
  paroxysmal with sinus bradycardia 427.81
Tachycardia 785.0
  atrial 427.89
  auricular 427.89
  nodal 427.89
    nonparoxysmal atrioventricular 426.89
  nonparoxysmal atrioventricular (nodal) 426.89
  paroxysmal 427.2
    with sinus bradycardia 427.81
    atrial (PAT) 427.0
      psychogenic 316 *[427.0]*
    atrioventricular (AV) 427.0
      psychogenic 316 *[427.0]*
    essential 427.2
    junctional 427.0
    nodal 427.0
    psychogenic 316 *[427.2]*
      atrial 316 *[427.0]*
      supraventricular 316 *[427.0]*
      ventricular 316 *[427.1]*
    supraventricular 427.0
      psychogenic 316 *[427.0]*
    ventricular 427.1
      psychogenic 316 *[427.1]*
  postoperative 997.1
Tachycardia—*continued*
  psychogenic 306.2
  sick sinus 427.81
  sinoauricular 427.89
  sinus 427.89
  supraventricular 427.89
  ventricular (paroxysmal) 427.1
    psychogenic 316 *[427.1]*
Tachypnea 786.09
  hysterical 300.11
  newborn (idiopathic) (transitory) 770.6
  psychogenic 306.1
  transitory, of newborn 770.6
Taenia (infection) (infestation) (*see also* Infestation, taenia) 123.3
  diminuta 123.6
  echinococcal infestation (*see also* Echinococcus) 122.9
  nana 123.6
  saginata infestation 123.2
  solium (intestinal form) 123.0
    larval form 123.1
Taeniasis (intestine) (*see also* Infestation, Taenia) 123.3
  saginata 123.2
  solium 123.0
Taenzer's disease 757.4
Tag (hypertrophied skin) (infected) 701.9
  adenoid 474.8
  anus 455.9
  endocardial (*see also* Endocarditis) 424.90
  hemorrhoidal 455.9
  hymen 623.8
  perineal 624.8
  preauricular 744.1
  rectum 455.9
  sentinel 455.9
  skin 701.9
    accessory 757.39
    anus 455.9
    congenital 757.39
    preauricular 744.1
    rectum 455.9
  tonsil 474.8
  urethra, urethral 599.84
  vulva 624.8
Tahyna fever 062.5
Takayasu (-Onishi) disease or syndrome (pulseless disease) 446.7
Talc granuloma 728.82
Talcosis 502
Talipes (congenital) 754.70
  acquired NEC 736.79
    planus 734
  asymmetric 754.79
    acquired 736.79
  calcaneovalgus 754.62
    acquired 736.76
  calcaneovarus 754.59
    acquired 736.76
  calcaneus 754.79
    acquired 736.76
  cavovarus 754.59
    acquired 736.75
  cavus 754.71
    acquired 736.73
  equinovalgus 754.69
    acquired 736.72

Talipes—*continued*
equinovarus 754.51
acquired 736.71
equinus 754.79
acquired, NEC 736.72
percavus 754.71
acquired 736.73
planovalgus 754.69
acquired 736.79
planus (acquired) (any degree) 734
congenital 754.61
due to rickets 268.1
valgus 754.60
acquired 736.79
varus 754.50
acquired 736.79
Talma's disease 728.85
Tamponade heart (Rose's) (*see also* Pericarditis) 423.9
Tanapox 078.89
Tangier disease (familial high-density lipoprotein deficiency) 272.5
Tank ear 380.12
Tantrum (childhood) (*see also* Disturbance, conduct) 312.1
Tapeworm (infection) (infestation) (*see also* Infestation, tapeworm) 123.9
Tapia's syndrome 352.6
Tarantism 297.8
Target-oval cell anemia 282.4
Tarlov's cyst 355.9
Tarral-Besnier disease (pityriasis rubra pilaris) 696.4
Tarsalgia 729.2
Tarsal tunnel syndrome 355.5
Tarsitis (eyelid) 373.00
syphilitic 095.8 *[373.00]*
tuberculous (*see also* Tuberculosis) 017.0 *[373.4]*
Tartar (teeth) 523.6
Tattoo (mark) 709.09
Taurodontism 520.2
Taussig-Bing defect, heart, or syndrome (transposition, aorta and overriding pulmonary artery) 745.11
Tay's choroiditis 363.41
Tay-Sachs
amaurotic familial idiocy 330.1
disease 330.1
Taybi's syndrome (otopalatodigital) 759.89
Taylor's
disease (diffuse idiopathic cutaneous atrophy) 701.8
syndrome 625.5
Tear, torn (traumatic)—*see also* Wound, open, by site
anus, anal (sphincter) 863.89
with open wound in cavity 863.99
complicating delivery 664.2
with mucosa 664.3
nontraumatic, nonpuerperal 565.0
articular cartilage, old (*see also* Disorder, cartilage, articular) 718.0
bladder
with
abortion—*see* Abortion, by type, with damage to pelvic organs
ectopic pregnancy (*see also* categories 633.0-633.9) 639.2
molar pregnancy (*see also* categories 630-632) 639.2

Tear, torn—*continued*
following
abortion 639.2
ectopic or molar pregnancy 639.2
obstetrical trauma 665.5
bowel
with
abortion—*see* Abortion, by type, with damage to pelvic organs
ectopic pregnancy (*see also* categories 633.0-633.9) 639.2
molar pregnancy (*see also* categories 630-632) 639.2
following
abortion 639.2
ectopic or molar pregnancy 639.2
obstetrical trauma 665.5
broad ligament
with
abortion—*see* Abortion, by type, with damage to pelvic organs
ectopic pregnancy (*see also* categories 633.0-633.9) 639.2
molar pregnancy (*see also* categories 630-632) 639.2
following
abortion 639.2
ectopic or molar pregnancy 639.2
obstetrical trauma 665.6
bucket handle (knee) (meniscus)—*see* Tear, meniscus
capsule
joint—*see* Sprain, by site
spleen—*see* Laceration, spleen, capsule
cartilage—*see also* Sprain, by site
articular, old (*see also* Disorder, cartilage, articular) 718.0
knee—*see* Tear, meniscus
semilunar (knee) (current injury)—*see* Tear, meniscus
cervix
with
abortion—*see* Abortion, by type, with damage to pelvic organs
ectopic pregnancy (*see also* categories 633.0-633.9) 639.2
molar pregnancy (*see also* categories 630-632) 639.2
following
abortion 639.2
ectopic or molar pregnancy 639.2
obstetrical trauma (current) 665.3
old 622.3
internal organ (abdomen, chest, or pelvis)—*see* Injury, internal, by site
ligament—*see also* Sprain, by site
with open wound—*see* Wound, open by site
meniscus (knee) (current injury) 836.2
bucket handle 836.0
old 717.0
lateral 836.1
anterior horn 836.1
old 717.42
bucket handle 836.1
old 717.41
old 717.40
posterior horn 836.1
old 717.43
specified site NEC 836.1
old 717.49

Tear, torn—*continued*
medial 836.0
anterior horn 836.0
old 717.1
bucket handle 836.0
old 717.0
old 717.3
posterior horn 836.0
old 717.2
old NEC 717.5
site other than knee—*see* Sprain, by site
muscle—*see also* Sprain, by site
with open wound—*see* Wound, open by site
pelvic
floor, complicating delivery 664.1
organ NEC
with
abortion—*see* Abortion, by type, with damage to pelvic organs
ectopic pregnancy (*see also* categories 633.0-633.9) 639.2
molar pregnancy (*see also* categories 630-632) 639.2
following
abortion 639.2
ectopic or molar pregnancy 639.2
obstetrical trauma 665.5
perineum—*see also* Laceration, perineum
obstetrical trauma 665.5
periurethral tissue
with
abortion—*see* Abortion, by type, with damage to pelvic organs
ectopic pregnancy (*see also* categories 633.0-633.9) 639.2
molar pregnancy (*see also* categories 630-632) 639.2
following
abortion 639.2
ectopic or molar pregnancy 639.2
obstetrical trauma 665.5
rectovaginal septum—*see* Laceration, rectovaginal septum
retina, retinal (recent) (with detachment) 361.00
without detachment 361.30
dialysis (juvenile) (with detachment) 361.04
giant (with detachment) 361.03
horseshoe (without detachment) 361.32
multiple (with detachment) 361.02
without detachment 361.33
old
delimited (partial) 361.06
partial 361.06
total or subtotal 361.07
partial (without detachment)
giant 361.03
multiple defects 361.02
old (delimited) 361.06
single defect 361.01
round hole (without detachment) 361.31
single defect (with detachment) 361.01
total or subtotal (recent) 361.05
old 361.07
rotator cuff 840.4
current injury 840.4
semilunar cartilage, knee (*see also* Tear, meniscus) 836.2
old 717.5
tendon—*see also* Sprain, by site
with open wound—*see* Wound, open by site
tentorial, at birth 767.0

Tear, torn—*continued*
umbilical cord
affecting fetus or newborn 772.0
complicating delivery 663.8
urethra
with
abortion—*see* Abortion, by type, with damage to pelvic organs
ectopic pregnancy (*see also* categories 633.0-633.9) 639.2
molar pregnancy (*see also* categories 630-632) 639.2
following
abortion 639.2
ectopic or molar pregnancy 639.2
obstetrical trauma 665.5
uterus—*see* Injury, internal, uterus
vagina—*see* Laceration, vagina
vessel, from catheter 998.2
vulva, complicating delivery 664.0
Tear stone 375.57
Teeth, tooth —*see also* condition
grinding 306.8
Teething 520.7
syndrome 520.7
Tegmental syndrome 344.89
Telangiectasia, telangiectasis (verrucous) 448.9
ataxic (cerebellar) 334.8
familial 448.0
hemorrhagic, hereditary (congenital) (senile) 448.0
hereditary hemorrhagic 448.0
retina 362.15
spider 448.1
Telecanthus (congenital) 743.63
Telescoped bowel or intestine (*see also* Intussusception) 560.0
Teletherapy, adverse effect NEC 990
Telogen effluvium 704.02
Temperature
body, high (of unknown origin) (*see also* Pyrexia) 780.6
cold, trauma from 991.9
newborn 778.2
specified effect NEC 991.8
high
body (of unknown origin) (*see also* Pyrexia) 780.6
trauma from—*see* Heat
Temper tantrum (childhood) (*see also* Disturbance, conduct) 312.1
Temple —*see* condition
Temporal —*see also* condition
lobe syndrome 310.0
Temporomandibular joint-pain-dysfunction syndrome 524.60
Temporosphenoidal —*see* condition
Tendency
bleeding (*see also* Defect, coagulation) 286.9
homosexual, ego-dystonic 302.0
paranoid 301.0
suicide 300.9
Tenderness
abdominal (generalized) (localized) 789.6
rebound 789.6
skin 782.0
Tendinitis, tendonitis (*see also* Tenosynovitis) 726.90
Achilles 726.71
adhesive 726.90
shoulder 726.0

Tendinitis, tendonitis—*continued*
calcific 727.82
shoulder 726.11
gluteal 726.5
patellar 726.64
peroneal 726.79
pes anserinus 726.61
psoas 726.5
tibialis (anterior) (posterior) 726.72
trochanteric 726.5
Tendon —*see* condition
Tendosynovitis —*see* Tenosynovitis
Tendovaginitis —*see* Tenosynovitis
Tenesmus 787.99
rectal 787.99
vesical 788.9
Tenia —*see* Taenia
Teniasis —*see* Taeniasis
Tennis elbow 726.32
Tenonitis —*see also* Tenosynovitis
eye (capsule) 376.04
Tenontosynovitis —*see* Tenosynovitis
Tenontothecitis —*see* Tenosynovitis
Tenophyte 727.9
Tenosynovitis 727.00
adhesive 726.90
shoulder 726.0
ankle 727.06
bicipital (calcifying) 726.12
buttock 727.09
due to crystals—*see* Arthritis, due to crystals
elbow 727.09
finger 727.05
foot 727.06
gonococcal 098.51
hand 727.05
hip 727.09
knee 727.09
radial styloid 727.04
shoulder 726.10
adhesive 726.0
spine 720.1
supraspinatus 726.10
toe 727.06
tuberculous—*see* Tuberculosis, tenosynovitis
wrist 727.05
Tenovaginitis —*see* Tenosynovitis
Tension
arterial, high (*see also* Hypertension) 401.9
without diagnosis of hypertension 796.2
headache 307.81
intraocular (elevated) 365.00
nervous 799.2
ocular (elevated) 365.00
pneumothorax 512.0
iatrogenic 512.1
postoperative 512.1
spontaneous 512.0
premenstrual 625.4
state 300.9
Tentorium —*see* condition
Teratencephalus 759.89
Teratism 759.7
Teratoblastoma (malignant) (M9080/3)—*see* Neoplasm, by site, malignant
Teratocarcinoma (M9081/3)—*see also* Neoplasm, by site, malignant
liver 155.0
Teratoma (solid) (M9080/1)—*see also* Neoplasm, by site, uncertain behavior
adult (cystic) (M9080/0)—*see* Neoplasm, by site, benign
and embryonal carcinoma, mixed (M9081/3)—*see* Neoplasm, by site, malignant
benign (M9080/0)—*see* Neoplasm, by site, benign
combined with choriocarcinoma (M9101/3)—*see* Neoplasm, by site, malignant
cystic (adult) (M9080/0)—*see* Neoplasm, by site, benign
differentiated type (M9080/0)—*see* Neoplasm, by site, benign
embryonal (M9080/3)—*see also* Neoplasm, by site, malignant
liver 155.0
fetal
sacral, causing fetopelvic disproportion 653.7
immature (M9080/3)—*see* Neoplasm, by site, malignant
liver (M9080/3) 155.0
adult, benign, cystic, differentiated type or mature (M9080/0) 211.5
malignant (M9080/3)—*see also* Neoplasm, by site, malignant
anaplastic type (M9082/3)—*see* Neoplasm, by site, malignant
intermediate type (M9083/3)—*see* Neoplasm, by site, malignant
liver (M9080/3) 155.0
trophoblastic (M9102/3)
specified site—*see* Neoplasm, by site, malignant
unspecified site 186.9
undifferentiated type (M9082/3)—*see* Neoplasm, by site, malignant
mature (M9080/0)—*see* Neoplasm, by site, benign
ovary (M9080/0) 220
embryonal, immature, or malignant (M9080/3) 183.0
suprasellar (M9080/3)—*see* Neoplasm, by site, malignant
testis (M9080/3) 186.9
adult, benign, cystic, differentiated type or mature (M9080/0) 222.0
undescended 186.0
Termination
anomalous—*see also* Malposition, congenital
portal vein 747.49
right pulmonary vein 747.42
pregnancy (legal) (therapeutic) (*see* Abortion, legal) 635.9
fetus NEC 779.6
illegal (*see also* Abortion, illegal) 636.9
Ternidens diminutus infestation 127.7
Terrors, night (child) 307.46
Terry's syndrome 362.21
Tertiary —*see* condition
Tessellated fundus, retina (tigroid) 362.89
Test(s)
AIDS virus V72.6
allergen V72.7
bacterial disease NEC (*see also* Screening, by name of disease) V74.9
basal metabolic rate V72.6
blood-alcohol V70.4

Test(s)—*continued*
blood-drug V70.4
developmental, infant or child V20.2
Dick V74.8
fertility V26.2
hearing V72.1
HIV V72.6
human immunodeficiency virus V72.6
Kveim V82.8
laboratory V72.6
for medicolegal reason V70.4
Mantoux (for tuberculosis) V74.1
mycotic organism V75.4
parasitic agent NEC V75.8
pregnancy
positive V22.1
first pregnancy V22.0
unconfirmed V72.4
preoperative V72.84
cardiovascular V72.81
respiratory V72.82
specified NEC V72.83
sarcoidosis V82.8
Schick V74.3
Schultz-Charlton V74.8
skin, diagnostic
allergy V72.7
bacterial agent NEC (*see also* Screening, by name of disease) V74.9
Dick V74.8
hypersensitivity V72.7
Kveim V82.8
Mantoux V74.1
mycotic organism V75.4
parasitic agent NEC V75.8
sarcoidosis V82.8
Schick V74.3
Schultz-Charlton V74.8
tuberculin V74.1
specified type NEC V72.85
tuberculin V74.1
vision V72.0
Wassermann
positive (*see also* Serology for syphilis, positive) 097.1
false 795.6
Testicle, testicular, testis —*see also* condition
feminization (syndrome) 257.8
Tetanus, tetanic (cephalic) (convulsions) 037
with
abortion—*see* Abortion, by type, with sepsis
ectopic pregnancy (*see also* categories 633.0-633.9) 639.0
molar pregnancy (*see* categories 630-632) 639.0
following
abortion 639.0
ectopic or molar pregnancy 639.0
inoculation V03.7
reaction (due to serum)—*see* Complications, vaccination
neonatorum 771.3
puerperal, postpartum, childbirth 670
Tetany, tetanic 781.7
alkalosis 276.3
associated with rickets 268.0
convulsions 781.7
hysterical 300.11
functional (hysterical) 300.11
hyperkinetic 781.7
hysterical 300.11

Tetany, tetanic—*continued*
hyperpnea 786.01
hysterical 300.11
psychogenic 306.1
hyperventilation 786.01
hysterical 300.11
psychogenic 306.1
hypocalcemic, neonatal 775.4
hysterical 300.11
neonatal 775.4
parathyroid (gland) 252.1
parathyroprival 252.1
postoperative 252.1
postthyroidectomy 252.1
pseudotetany 781.7
hysterical 300.11
psychogenic 306.1
specified as conversion reaction 300.11
Tetralogy of Fallot 745.2
Tetraplegia —*see* Quadriplegia
Thailand hemorrhagic fever 065.4
Thalassanemia 282.4
Thalassemia (alpha) (beta) (disease) (Hb-C) (Hb-D) (Hb-E) (Hb-H) (Hb-I) (Hb-S) (high fetal gene) (high fetal hemoglobin) (intermedia) (major) (minima) (minor) (mixed) (sickle-cell) (trait) (with other hemoglobinopathy) 282.4
Thalassemic variants 282.4
Thaysen-Gee disease (nontropical sprue) 579.0
Thecoma (M8600/0) 220
malignant (M8600/3) 183.0
Thelarche, precocious 259.1
Thelitis 611.0
puerperal, postpartum 675.0
Therapeutic —*see* condition
Therapy V57.9
blood transfusion, without reported diagnosis V58.2
breathing V57.0
chemotherapy V58.1
fluoride V07.31
prophylactic NEC V07.39
dialysis (intermittent) (treatment)
extracorporeal V56.0
peritoneal V56.8
renal V56.0
specified type NEC V56.8
exercise NEC V57.1
breathing V57.0
extracorporeal dialysis (renal) V56.0
fluoride prophylaxis V07.31
hemodialysis V56.0
occupational V57.21
orthoptic V57.4
orthotic V57.81
peritoneal dialysis V56.8
physical NEC V57.1
radiation V58.0
speech V57.3
vocational V57.22
Thermalgesia 782.0
Thermalgia 782.0
Thermanalgesia 782.0
Thermanesthesia 782.0
Thermic —*see* condition
Thermography (abnormal) 793.9
breast 793.8
Thermoplegia 992.0

Thesaurismosis
amyloid 277.3
bilirubin 277.4
calcium 275.4
cystine 270.0
glycogen (*see also* Disease, glycogen storage) 271.0
kerasin 272.7
lipoid 272.7
melanin 255.4
phosphatide 272.7
urate 274.9
Thiaminic deficiency 265.1
with beriberi 265.0
Thibierge-Weissenbach syndrome (cutaneous systemic sclerosis) 710.1
Thickening
bone 733.99
extremity 733.99
breast 611.79
hymen 623.3
larynx 478.79
nail 703.8
congenital 757.5
periosteal 733.99
pleura (*see also* Pleurisy) 511.0
skin 782.8
subepiglottic 478.79
tongue 529.8
valve, heart—*see* Endocarditis
Thiele syndrome 724.6
Thigh —*see* condition
Thinning vertebra (*see also* Osteoporosis) 733.00
Thirst, excessive 783.5
due to deprivation of water 994.3
Thomsen's disease 359.2
Thomson's disease (congenital poikiloderma) 757.33
Thoracic —*see also* condition
kidney 753.3
outlet syndrome 353.0
stomach—*see* Hernia, diaphragm
Thoracogastroschisis (congenital) 759.89
Thoracopagus 759.4
Thoracoschisis 756.3
Thorax —*see* condition
Thorn's syndrome (*see also* Disease, renal) 593.9
Thornwaldt's, Tornwaldt's
bursitis (pharyngeal) 478.29
cyst 478.26
disease (pharyngeal bursitis) 478.29
Thorson-Biörck syndrome (malignant carcinoid) 259.2
Threadworm (infection) (infestation) 127.4
Threatened
abortion or miscarriage 640.0
with subsequent abortion (*see also* Abortion, spontaneous) 634.9
affecting fetus 762.1
labor 644.1
affecting fetus or newborn 761.8
premature 644.0
miscarriage 640.0
affecting fetus 762.1
premature
delivery 644.2
affecting fetus or newborn 761.8
labor 644.0
before 22 completed weeks gestation 640.0
Three-day fever 066.0
Threshers' lung 495.0
Thrix annulata (congenital) 757.4
Throat —*see* condition
Thrombasthenia (Glanzmann's) (hemorrhagic) (hereditary) 287.1
Thromboangiitis 443.1
obliterans (general) 443.1
cerebral 437.1
vessels
brain 437.1
spinal cord 437.1
Thromboarteritis —*see* Arteritis
Thromboasthenia (Glanzmann's) (hemorrhagic) (hereditary) 287.1
Thrombocytasthenia (Glanzmann's) 287.1
Thrombocythemia (essential) (hemorrhagic) (primary) (M9962/1) 238.7
idiopathic (M9962/1) 238.7
Thrombocytopathy (dystrophic) (granulopenic) 287.1
Thrombocytopenia, thrombocytopenic 287.5
with giant hemangioma 287.3
amegakaryocytic, congenital 287.3
congenital 287.3
cyclic 287.3
dilutional 287.4
due to
drugs 287.4
extracorporeal circulation of blood 287.4
massive blood transfusion 287.4
platelet alloimmunization 287.4
essential 287.3
hereditary 287.3
Kasabach-Merritt 287.3
neonatal, transitory 776.1
due to
exchange transfusion 776.1
idiopathic maternal thrombocytopenia 776.1
isoimmunization 776.1
primary 287.3
puerperal, postpartum 666.3
purpura (*see also* Purpura, thrombocytopenic) 287.3
thrombotic 446.6
secondary 287.4
sex-linked 287.3
Thrombocytosis, essential 289.9
Thromboembolism —*see* Embolism
Thrombopathy (Bernard-Soulier) 287.1
constitutional 286.4
Willebrand-Jürgens (angiohemophilia) 286.4
Thrombopenia (*see also* Thrombocytopenia) 287.5
Thrombophlebitis 451.9
antecubital vein 451.82
antepartum (superficial) 671.2
affecting fetus or newborn 760.3
deep 671.3
arm 451.89
deep 451.83
superficial 451.82
breast, superficial 451.89
cavernous (venous) sinus—*see* Thrombophlebitis, intracranial venous sinus
cephalic vein 451.82
cerebral (sinus) (vein) 325
late effect—*see* category 326
nonpyogenic 437.6
in pregnancy or puerperium 671.5
late effect—*see* category 438

Thrombosis, thrombotic—*continued*
cardiac (*see also* Infarct, myocardium) 410.9
due to syphilis 093.89
healed or specified as old 412
valve—*see* Endocarditis
carotid (artery) (common) (internal) (*see also* Occlusion, artery, carotid) 433.1
with other precerebral artery 433.3
cavernous sinus (venous)—*see* Thrombosis, intracranial venous sinus
cerebellar artery (anterior inferior) (posterior inferior) (superior) 433.8
late effect—*see* category 438
cerebral (arteries) (*see also* Thrombosis, brain) 434.0
late effect—*see* category 438
coronary (artery) (*see also* Infarct, myocardium) 410.9
due to syphilis 093.89
healed or specified as old 412
without myocardial infarction 411.81
corpus cavernosum 607.82
cortical (*see also* Thrombosis, brain) 434.0
due to (presence of) any device, implant, or graft classifiable to 996.0-996.5—*see* Complications, due to (presence of) any device, implant, or graft classified to 996.0-996.5 NEC
effort 453.8
endocardial—*see* Infarct, myocardium
eye (*see also* Occlusion, retina) 362.30
femoral (vein) (deep) 453.8
with inflammation or phlebitis 451.11
artery 444.22
genital organ, male 608.83
heart (chamber) (*see also* Infarct, myocardium) 410.9
hepatic (vein) 453.0
artery 444.89
infectional or septic 572.1
iliac (vein) 453.8
with inflammation or phlebitis 451.81
artery (common) (external) (internal) 444.81
inflammation, vein—*see* Thrombophlebitis
internal carotid artery (*see also* Occlusion, artery, carotid) 433.1
with other precerebral artery 433.3
intestine (with gangrene) 557.0
intracranial (*see also* Thrombosis, brain) 434.0
venous sinus (any) 325
nonpyogenic origin 437.6
in pregnancy or puerperium 671.5
intramural (*see also* Infarct, myocardium) 410.9
without
cardiac condition 429.89
coronary artery disease 429.89
myocardial infarction 429.89
healed or specified as old 412
jugular (bulb) 453.8
kidney 593.81
artery 593.81
lateral sinus (venous)—*see* Thrombosis, intracranial venous sinus
leg 453.8
with inflammation or phlebitis—*see* Thrombophlebitis
deep (vessels) 453.8
superficial (vessels) 453.8
liver (venous) 453.0
artery 444.89
infectional or septic 572.1

Thrombosis, thrombotic—*continued*
portal vein 452
longitudinal sinus (venous)—*see* Thrombosis, intracranial venous sinus
lower extremity—*see* Thrombosis, leg
lung 415.19
iatrogenic 415.11
postoperative 415.11
marantic, dural sinus 437.6
meninges (brain) (*see also* Thrombosis, brain) 434.0
mesenteric (artery) (with gangrene) 557.0
vein (inferior) (superior) 452
mitral—*see* Insufficiency, mitral
mural (heart chamber) (*see also* Infarct, myocardium) 410.9
without
cardiac condition 429.89
coronary artery disease 429.89
myocardial infarction 429.89
due to syphilis 093.89
following myocardial infarction 429.79
healed or specified as old 412
omentum (with gangrene) 557.0
ophthalmic (artery) (*see also* Occlusion, retina) 362.30
pampiniform plexus (male) 608.83
female 620.8
parietal (*see also* Infarct, myocardium) 410.9
penis, penile 607.82
peripheral arteries 444.22
lower 444.22
upper 444.21
platelet 446.6
portal 452
due to syphilis 093.89
infectional or septic 572.1
precerebral artery—*see also* Occlusion, artery, precerebral NEC
pregnancy 671.9
deep (vein) 671.3
superficial (vein) 671.2
puerperal, postpartum, childbirth 671.9
brain (artery) 674.0
venous 671.5
cardiac 674.8
cerebral (artery) 674.0
venous 671.5
deep (vein) 671.4
intracranial sinus (nonpyogenic) (venous) 671.5
pelvic 671.4
pulmonary (artery) 673.2
specified site NEC 671.5
superficial 671.2
pulmonary (artery) (vein) 415.19
iatrogenic 415.11
postoperative 415.11
radial vein 451.83
renal (artery) 593.81
vein 453.3
resulting from presence of shunt or other internal prosthetic device—*see* Complications, due to (presence of) any device, implant, or graft classified to 996.0-996.5 NEC
retina, retinal (artery) 362.30
arterial branch 362.32
central 362.31
partial 362.33

Thrombosis, thrombotic—*continued*
vein
central 362.35
tributary (branch) 362.36
scrotum 608.83
seminal vesicle 608.83
sigmoid (venous) sinus (*see* Thrombosis, intracranial venous sinus) 325
silent NEC 453.9
sinus, intracranial (venous) (any) (*see also* Thrombosis, intracranial venous sinus) 325
softening, brain (*see also* Thrombosis, brain) 434.0
specified site NEC 453.8
spermatic cord 608.83
spinal cord 336.1
due to syphilis 094.89
in pregnancy or puerperium 671.5
pyogenic origin 324.1
late effect—*see* category 326
spleen, splenic 289.59
artery 444.89
testis 608.83
traumatic (complication) (early) (*see also* Injury, blood vessel, by site) 904.9
tricuspid—*see* Endocarditis, tricuspid
tunica vaginalis 608.83
umbilical cord (vessels) 663.6
affecting fetus or newborn 762.6
vas deferens 608.83
vena cava (inferior) (superior) 453.2
Thrombus —*see* Thrombosis
Thrush 112.0
newborn 771.7
Thumb —*see also* condition
gamekeeper's 842.12
sucking (child problem) 307.9
Thygeson's superficial punctate keratitis 370.21
Thymergasia (*see also* Psychosis, affective) 296.80
Thymitis 254.8
Thymoma (benign) (M8580/0) 212.6
malignant (M8580/3) 164.0
Thymus, thymic (gland)—*see* condition
Thyrocele (*see also* Goiter) 240.9
Thyroglossal —*see also* condition
cyst 759.2
duct, persistent 759.2
Thyroid (body) (gland)—*see also* condition
lingual 759.2
Thyroiditis 245.9
acute (pyogenic) (suppurative) 245.0
nonsuppurative 245.0
autoimmune 245.2
chronic (nonspecific) (sclerosing) 245.8
fibrous 245.3
lymphadenoid 245.2
lymphocytic 245.2
lymphoid 245.2
complicating pregnancy, childbirth, or puerperium 648.1
de Quervain's (subacute granulomatous) 245.1
fibrous (chronic) 245.3
giant (cell) (follicular) 245.1
granulomatous (de Quervain's) (subacute) 245.1
Hashimoto's (struma lymphomatosa) 245.2
iatrogenic 245.4
invasive (fibrous) 245.3
ligneous 245.3
lymphocytic (chronic) 245.2
Thyroiditis—*continued*
lymphoid 245.2
lymphomatous 245.2
pseudotuberculous 245.1
pyogenic 245.0
radiation 245.4
Riedel's (ligneous) 245.3
subacute 245.1
suppurative 245.0
tuberculous (*see also* Tuberculosis) 017.5
viral 245.1
woody 245.3
Thyrolingual duct, persistent 759.2
Thyromegaly 240.9
Thyrotoxic
crisis or storm (*see also* Thyrotoxicosis) 242.9
heart failure (*see also* Thyrotoxicosis) 242.9 *[425.7]*
Thyrotoxicosis 242.9

Note—Use the following fifth-digit subclassification with category 242:

0 without mention of thyrotoxic crisis or storm
1 with mention of thyrotoxic crisis or storm

with
goiter (diffuse) 242.0
adenomatous 242.3
multinodular 242.2
uninodular 242.1
nodular 242.3
multinodular 242.2
uninodular 242.1
infiltrative
dermopathy 242.0
ophthalmopathy 242.0
thyroid acropachy 242.0
complicating pregnancy, childbirth, or puerperium 648.1
due to
ectopic thyroid nodule 242.4
ingestion of (excessive) thyroid material 242.8
specified cause NEC 242.8
factitia 242.8
heart 242.9 *[425.7]*
neonatal (transient) 775.3
TIA (transient ischemic attack) 435.9
with transient neurologic deficit 435.9
late effect—*see* category 438
Tibia vara 732.4
Tic 307.20
breathing 307.20
child problem 307.21
compulsive 307.22
convulsive 307.20
degenerative (generalized) (localized) 333.3
facial 351.8
douloureux (*see also* Neuralgia, trigeminal) 350.1
atypical 350.2
habit 307.20
chronic (motor or vocal) 307.22
transient of childhood 307.21
lid 307.20
transient of childhood 307.21
motor-verbal 307.23
occupational 300.89
orbicularis 307.20
transient of childhood 307.21
organic origin 333.3
postchoreic—*see* Chorea

Tic —*continued*
psychogenic 307.20
compulsive 307.22
salaam 781.0
spasm 307.20
chronic (motor or vocal) 307.22
transient of childhood 307.21
Tick (-borne) fever NEC 066.1
American mountain 066.1
Colorado 066.1
hemorrhagic NEC 065.3
Crimean 065.0
Kyasanur Forest 065.2
Omsk 065.1
mountain 066.1
nonexanthematous 066.1
Tick-bite fever NEC 066.1
African 087.1
Colorado (virus) 066.1
Rocky Mountain 082.0
Tick paralysis 989.5
Tics and spasms, compulsive 307.22
Tietze's disease or syndrome 733.6
Tight, tightness
anus 564.8
chest 786.59
fascia (lata) 728.9
foreskin (congenital) 605
hymen 623.3
introitus (acquired) (congenital) 623.3
rectal sphincter 564.8
tendon 727.81
Achilles (heel) 727.81
urethral sphincter 598.9
Tilting vertebra 737.9
Timidity, child 313.21
Tinea (intersecta) (tarsi) 110.9
amiantacea 110.0
asbestina 110.0
barbae 110.0
beard 110.0
black dot 110.0
blanca 111.2
capitis 110.0
corporis 110.5
cruris 110.3
decalvans 704.09
flava 111.0
foot 110.4
furfuracea 111.0
imbricata (Tokelau) 110.5
lepothrix 039.0
manuum 110.2
microsporic (*see also* Dermatophytosis) 110.9
nigra 111.1
nodosa 111.2
pedis 110.4
scalp 110.0
specified site NEC 110.8
sycosis 110.0
tonsurans 110.0
trichophytic (*see also* Dermatophytosis) 110.9
unguium 110.1
versicolor 111.0
Tingling sensation (*see also* Disturbance, sensation) 782.0
Tin-miners' lung 503
Tinnitus (aurium) 388.30
audible 388.32
objective 388.32
subjective 388.31
Tipping pelvis 738.6
with disproportion (fetopelvic) 653.0
affecting fetus or newborn 763.1
causing obstructed labor 660.1
affecting fetus or newborn 763.1
Tiredness 780.7
Tissue —*see* condition
Tobacco
abuse (affecting health) NEC (*see also* Abuse, drugs, nondependent) 305.1
heart 989.8
Tobias' syndrome (carcinoma, pulmonary apex) (M8010/3) 162.3
Tocopherol deficiency 269.1
Todd's
cirrhosis—*see* Cirrhosis, biliary
paralysis (postepileptic transitory paralysis) 344.89
Toe —*see* condition
Toilet, artificial opening (*see also* Attention to, artificial, opening) V55.9
Tokelau ringworm 110.5
Tollwut 071
Tolosa-Hunt syndrome 378.55
Tommaselli's disease
correct substance properly administered 599.7
overdose or wrong substance given or taken 961.4
Tongue —*see also* condition
worms 134.1
Tongue tie 750.0
Toni-Fanconi syndrome (cystinosis) 270.0
Tonic pupil 379.46
Tonsil —*see* condition
Tonsillitis (acute) (catarrhal) (croupous) (follicular) (gangrenous) (infective) (lacunar) (lingual) (malignant) (membranous) (phlegmonous) (pneumococcal) (pseudomembranous) (purulent) (septic) (staphylococcal) (subacute) (suppurative) (toxic) (ulcerative) (vesicular) (viral) 463
with influenza, flu, or grippe 487.1
chronic 474.0
diphtheritic (membranous) 032.0
hypertrophic 474.0
influenzal 487.1
parenchymatous 475
streptococcal 034.0
tuberculous (*see also* Tuberculosis) 012.8
Vincent's 101
Tonsillopharyngitis 465.8
Tooth, teeth —*see* condition
Toothache 525.9
Topagnosis 782.0
Tophi (gouty) 274.0
ear 274.81
heart 274.82
specified site NEC 274.82
Torn —*see* Tear, torn
Tornwaldt's bursitis (disease) (pharyngeal bursitis) 478.29
cyst 478.26
Torpid liver 573.9
Torsion
accessory tube 620.5
adnexa (female) 620.5
aorta (congenital) 747.29
acquired 447.1
appendix epididymis 608.2

Torsion—*continued*
bile duct 576.8
with calculus, choledocholithiasis or stones—*see* Choledocholithiasis
congenital 751.69
bowel, colon, or intestine 560.2
cervix (*see also* Malposition, uterus) 621.6
duodenum 537.3
dystonia—*see* Dystonia, torsion
epididymis 608.2
appendix 608.2
fallopian tube 620.5
gallbladder (*see also* Disease, gallbladder) 575.8
congenital 751.69
gastric 537.89
hydatid of Morgagni (female) 620.5
kidney (pedicle) 593.89
Meckel's diverticulum (congenital) 751.0
mesentery 560.2
omentum 560.2
organ or site, congenital NEC—*see* Anomaly, specified type NEC
ovary (pedicle) 620.5
congenital 752.0
oviduct 620.5
penis 607.89
congenital 752.8
renal 593.89
spasm—*see* Dystonia, torsion
spermatic cord 608.2
spleen 289.59
testicle, testis 608.2
tibia 736.89
umbilical cord—*see* Compression, umbilical cord
uterus (*see also* Malposition, uterus) 621.6
Torticollis (intermittent) (spastic) 723.5
congenital 754.1
sternomastoid 754.1
due to birth injury 767.8
hysterical 300.11
psychogenic 306.0
specified as conversion reaction 300.11
rheumatic 723.5
rheumatoid 714.0
spasmodic 333.83
traumatic, current NEC 847.0
Tortuous
artery 447.1
fallopian tube 752.19
organ or site, congenital NEC—*see* Distortion
renal vessel, congenital 747.62
retina vessel (congenital) 743.58
acquired 362.17
ureter 593.4
urethra 599.84
vein—*see* Varicose, vein
Torula, torular (infection) 117.5
histolytica 117.5
lung 117.5
Torulosis 117.5
Torus
mandibularis 526.81
palatinus 526.81
Touch, vitreous 997.99
Touraine's syndrome (hereditary osteo-onychodysplasia) 756.89
Touraine-Solente-Golé syndrome (acropachyderma) 757.39
Tourette's disease (motor-verbal tic) 307.23
Tower skull 756.0
with exophthalmos 756.0
Toxemia 799.8
with
abortion—*see* Abortion, by type, with toxemia
bacterial—*see* Septicemia
biliary (*see also* Disease, biliary) 576.8
burn—*see* Burn, by site
congenital NEC 779.8
eclamptic 642.6
with pre-existing hypertension 642.7
erysipelatous (*see also* Erysipelas) 035
fatigue 799.8
fetus or newborn NEC 779.8
food (*see also* Poisoning, food) 005.9
gastric 537.89
gastrointestinal 558.2
intestinal 558.2
kidney (*see also* Disease, renal) 593.9
lung 518.89
malarial NEC (*see also* Malaria) 084.6
maternal (of pregnancy), affecting fetus or newborn 760.0
myocardial—*see* Myocarditis, toxic
of pregnancy (mild) (pre-eclamptic) 642.4
with
convulsions 642.6
pre-existing hypertension 642.7
affecting fetus or newborn 760.0
severe 642.5
pre-eclamptic—*see* Toxemia, of pregnancy
puerperal, postpartum—*see* Toxemia, of pregnancy
pulmonary 518.89
renal (*see also* Disease, renal) 593.9
septic (*see also* Septicemia) 038.9
small intestine 558.2
staphylococcal 038.1
due to food 005.0
stasis 799.8
stomach 537.89
uremic (*see also* Uremia) 586
urinary 586
Toxemica cerebropathia psychica (nonalcoholic) 294.0
alcoholic 291.1
Toxic (poisoning)—*see also* condition
from drug or poison—*see* Table of drugs and chemicals
oil syndrome 710.5
shock syndrome 040.89
thyroid (gland) (*see also* Thyrotoxicosis) 242.9
Toxicemia —*see* Toxemia
Toxicity
fava bean 282.2
from drug or poison—*see* Table of drugs and chemicals
Toxicosis (*see also* Toxemia) 799.8
capillary, hemorrhagic 287.0
Toxinfection 799.8
gastrointestinal 558.2
Toxocariasis 128.0
Toxoplasma infection, generalized 130.9
Toxoplasmosis (acquired) 130.9
with pneumonia 130.4
congenital, active 771.2
disseminated (multisystemic) 130.8
maternal
with suspected damage to fetus affecting management of pregnancy 655.4
affecting fetus or newborn 760.2
manifest toxoplasmosis in fetus or newborn 771.2
multiple sites 130.8

Toxoplasmosis—*continued*
multisystemic disseminated 130.8
specified site NEC 130.7
Trabeculation, bladder 596.8
Trachea —*see* condition
Tracheitis (acute) (catarrhal) (infantile) (membranous) (plastic) (pneumococcal) (septic) (suppurative) (viral) 464.10
with
bronchitis 490
acute or subacute 466.0
chronic 491.8
tuberculosis—*see* Tuberculosis, pulmonary
laryngitis (acute) 464.20
with obstruction 464.21
chronic 476.1
tuberculous (*see also* Tuberculosis, larynx) 012.3
obstruction 464.11
chronic 491.8
with
bronchitis (chronic) 491.8
laryngitis (chronic) 476.1
due to external agent—*see* Condition, respiratory, chronic, due to
diphtheritic (membranous) 032.3
due to external agent—*see* Inflammation, respiratory, upper, due to
edematous 464.11
influenzal 487.1
streptococcal 034.0
syphilitic 095.8
tuberculous (*see also* Tuberculosis) 012.8
Trachelitis (nonvenereal) (*see also* Cervicitis) 616.0
trichomonal 131.09
Tracheobronchial —*see* condition
Tracheobronchitis (*see also* Bronchitis) 490
acute or subacute 466.0
with bronchospasm or obstruction 466.0
chronic 491.8
influenzal 487.1
senile 491.8
Tracheobronchomegaly (congenital) 748.3
Tracheobronchopneumonitis —*see* Pneumonia, broncho
Tracheocele (external) (internal) 519.1
congenital 748.3
Tracheomalacia 519.1
congenital 748.3
Tracheopharyngitis (acute) 465.8
chronic 478.9
due to external agent—*see* Condition, respiratory, chronic, due to
due to external agent—*see* Inflammation, respiratory, upper, due to
Tracheostenosis 519.1
congenital 748.3
Tracheostomy
attention to V55.0
complication 519.0
hemorrhage 519.0
malfunctioning 519.0
obstruction 519.0
sepsis 519.0
status V44.0
stenosis 519.0
Trachoma, trachomatous 076.9
active (stage) 076.1
contraction of conjunctiva 076.1
dubium 076.0
Trachoma, trachomatous—*continued*
healed or late effect 139.1
initial (stage) 076.0
Türck's (chronic catarrhal laryngitis) 476.0
Trachyphonia 784.49
Training
orthoptic V57.4
orthotic V57.81
Train sickness 994.6
Trait
hemoglobin
abnormal NEC 282.7
with thalassemia 282.4
C (*see also* Disease, hemoglobin, C) 282.7
with elliptocytosis 282.7
S (Hb-S) 282.5
Lepore 282.4
with other abnormal hemoglobin NEC 282.4
paranoid 301.0
sickle-cell 282.5
with
elliptocytosis 282.5
spherocytosis 282.5
Traits, paranoid 301.0
Tramp V60.0
Trance 780.09
hysterical 300.13
Transaminasemia 790.4
Transfusion, blood
donor V59.01
stem cells V59.02
incompatible 999.6
reaction or complication—*see* Complications, transfusion
syndrome
fetomaternal 772.0
twin-to-twin
blood loss (donor twin) 772.0
recipient twin 776.4
without reported diagnosis V58.2
Transient —*see also* condition
alteration of awareness 780.02
blindness 368.12
deafness (ischemic) 388.02
global amnesia 437.7
person (homeless) NEC V60.0
Transitional, lumbosacral joint of vertebra 756.19
Translocation
autosomes NEC 758.5
13-15 758.1
16-18 758.2
21 or 22 758.0
balanced in normal individual 758.4
D_1 758.1
E_3 758.2
G 758.0
balanced autosomal in normal individual 758.4
chromosomes NEC 758.9
Down's syndrome 758.0
Translucency, iris 364.53
Transmission of chemical substances through the placenta
(affecting fetus or newborn) 760.70
alcohol 760.71
anti-infective agents 760.74
cocaine 760.75
"crack" 760.75
diethylstilbestrol [DES] 760.76
hallucinogenic agents 760.73
medicinal agents NEC 760.79

Treponema pallidum infection (*see also* Syphilis) 097.9
Treponematosis 102.9
due to
T. pallidum—*see* Syphilis
T. pertenue (yaws) (*see also* Yaws) 102.9
Triad
Kartagener's 759.3
Reiter's (complete) (incomplete) 099.3
Saint's (*see also* Hernia, diaphragm) 553.3
Trichiasis 704.2
cicatricial 704.2
eyelid 374.05
with entropion (*see also* Entropion) 374.00
Trichinella spiralis (infection) (infestation) 124
Trichinelliasis 124
Trichinellosis 124
Trichiniasis 124
Trichinosis 124
Trichobezoar 938
intestine 936
stomach 935.2
Trichocephaliasis 127.3
Trichocephalosis 127.3
Trichocephalus infestation 127.3
Trichoclasis 704.2
Trichoepithelioma (M8100/0)—*see also* Neoplasm, skin, benign
breast 217
genital organ NEC—*see* Neoplasm, by site, benign
malignant (M8100/3)—*see* Neoplasm, skin, malignant
Trichofolliculoma (M8101/0)—*see* Neoplasm, skin, benign
Tricholemmoma (M8102/0)—*see* Neoplasm, skin, benign
Trichomatosis 704.2
Trichomoniasis 131.9
bladder 131.09
cervix 131.09
intestinal 007.3
prostate 131.03
seminal vesicle 131.09
specified site NEC 131.8
urethra 131.02
urogenitalis 131.00
vagina 131.01
vulva 131.01
vulvovaginal 131.01
Trichomycosis 039.0
axillaris 039.0
nodosa 111.2
nodularis 111.2
rubra 039.0
Trichonocardiosis (axillaris) (palmellina) 039.0
Trichonodosis 704.2
Trichophytid, trichophyton infection (*see also* Dermatophytosis) 110.9
Trichophytide —*see* Dermatophytosis
Trichophytobezoar 938
intestine 936
stomach 935.2
Trichophytosis —*see* Dermatophytosis
Trichoptilosis 704.2
Trichorrhexis (nodosa) 704.2
Trichosporosis nodosa 111.2
Trichostasis spinulosa (congenital) 757.4
Trichostrongyliasis (small intestine) 127.6
Trichostrongylosis 127.6
Trichostrongylus (instabilis) infection 127.6
Trichotillomania 312.39
Trichromat, anomalous (congenital) 368.59
Trichromatopsia, anomalous (congenital) 368.59
Trichuriasis 127.3
Trichuris trichiuria (any site) (infection) (infestation) 127.3
Tricuspid (valve)—*see* condition
Trifid —*see also* Accessory
kidney (pelvis) 753.3
tongue 750.13
Trigeminal neuralgia (*see also* Neuralgia, trigeminal) 350.1
Trigeminoencephaloangiomatosis 759.6
Trigeminy 427.89
postoperative 997.1
Trigger finger (acquired) 727.03
congenital 756.89
Trigonitis (bladder) (chronic) (pseudomembranous) 595.3
tuberculous (*see also* Tuberculosis) 016.1
Trigonocephaly 756.0
Trihexosidosis 272.7
Trilobate placenta —*see* Placenta, abnormal
Trilocular heart 745.8
Tripartita placenta —*see* Placenta, abnormal
Triple —*see also* Accessory
kidneys 753.3
uteri 752.2
X female 758.8
Triplegia 344.89
congenital or infantile 343.8
Triplet
affected by maternal complications of pregnancy 761.5
healthy liveborn—*see* Newborn, multiple
pregnancy (complicating delivery) NEC 651.1
with fetal loss and retention of one or more fetus(es) 651.4
Triplex placenta —*see* Placenta, abnormal
Triplication —*see* Accessory
Trismus 781.0
neonatorum 771.3
newborn 771.3
Trisomy (syndrome) NEC 758.5
13 (partial) 758.1
16-18 758.2
18 (partial) 758.2
21 (partial) 758.0
22 758.0
autosomes NEC 758.5
D_1 758.1
E_3 758.2
G (group) 758.0
group D_1 758.1
group E 758.2
group G 758.0
Tritanomaly 368.53
Tritanopia 368.53
Troisier-Hanot-Chauffard syndrome (bronze diabetes) 275.0
Trombidiosis 133.8
Trophedema (hereditary) 757.0
congenital 757.0
Trophoblastic disease (*see also* Hydatidiform mole) 630
previous, affecting management of pregnancy V23.1
Tropholymphedema 757.0

Trophoneurosis NEC 356.9
arm NEC 354.9
disseminated 710.1
facial 349.89
leg NEC 355.8
lower extremity NEC 355.8
upper extremity NEC 354.9
Tropical —*see also* condition
maceration feet (syndrome) 991.4
wet foot (syndrome) 991.4
Trouble —*see also* Disease
bowel 569.9
heart—*see* Disease, heart
intestine 569.9
kidney (*see also* Disease, renal) 593.9
nervous 799.2
sinus (*see also* Sinusitis) 473.9
Trousseau's syndrome (thrombophlebitis migrans) 453.1
Truancy, childhood —*see also* Disturbance, conduct
socialized 312.2
undersocialized, unsocialized 312.1
Truncus
arteriosus (persistent) 745.0
common 745.0
communis 745.0
Trunk —*see* condition
Trychophytide —*see* Dermatophytosis
Trypanosoma infestation —*see* Trypanosomiasis
Trypanosomiasis 086.9
with meningoencephalitis 086.9 *[323.2]*
African 086.5
due to Trypanosoma 086.5
gambiense 086.3
rhodesiense 086.4
American 086.2
with
heart involvement 086.0
other organ involvement 086.1
without mention of organ involvement 086.2
Brazilian—*see* Trypanosomiasis, American
Chagas'—*see* Trypanosomiasis, American
due to Trypanosoma
cruzi—*see* Trypanosomiasis, American
gambiense 086.3
rhodesiense 086.4
gambiensis, Gambian 086.3
North American—*see* Trypanosomiasis, American
rhodesiensis, Rhodesian 086.4
South American—*see* Trypanosomiasis, American
T-shaped incisors 520.2
Tsutsugamushi fever 081.2
Tube, tubal, tubular —*see also* condition
ligation, admission for V25.2
Tubercle —*see also* Tuberculosis
brain, solitary 013.2
Darwin's 744.29
epithelioid noncaseating 135
Ghon, primary infection 010.0
Tuberculid, tuberculide (indurating) (lichenoid) (miliary) (papulonecrotic) (primary) (skin) (subcutaneous) (*see also* Tuberculosis) 017.0
Tuberculoma —*see also* Tuberculosis
brain (any part) 013.2
meninges (cerebral) (spinal) 013.1
spinal cord 013.4
Tuberculosis, tubercular, tuberculous (calcification) (calcified) (caseous) (chromogenic acid-fast bacilli) (congenital) (degeneration) (disease) (fibrocaseous) (fistula) (gangrene) (interstitial) (isolated circumscribed lesions) (necrosis) (parenchymatous) (ulcerative) 011.9

Note—Use the following fifth-digit subclassification with categories 010-018:

0 unspecified
1 bacteriological or histological examination not done
2 bacteriological or histological examination unknown (at present)
3 tubercle bacilli found (in sputum) by microscopy
4 tubercle bacilli not found (in sputum) by microscopy, but found by bacterial culture
5 tubercle bacilli not found by bacteriological examination, but tuberculosis confirmed histologically
6 tubercle bacilli not found by bacteriological or histological examination, but tuberculosis confirmed by other methods [inoculation of animals]

For tuberculous conditions specified as late effects or sequelae, see category 137.

abdomen 014.8
lymph gland 014.8
abscess 011.9
arm 017.9
bone (*see also* Osteomyelitis, due to, tuberculosis) 015.9 *[730.8]*
hip 015.1 *[730.85]*
knee 015.2 *[730.86]*
sacrum 015.0 *[730.88]*
specified site NEC 015.7 *[730.88]*
spinal 015.0 *[730.88]*
vertebra 015.0 *[730.88]*
brain 013.3
breast 017.9
Cowper's gland 016.5
dura (mater) 013.8
brain 013.3
spinal cord 013.5
epidural 013.8
brain 013.3
spinal cord 013.5
frontal sinus—*see* Tuberculosis, sinus
genital organs NEC 016.9
female 016.7
male 016.5
genitourinary NEC 016.9
gland (lymphatic)—*see* Tuberculosis, lymph gland
hip 015.1
iliopsoas 015.0 *[730.88]*
intestine 014.8
ischiorectal 014.8
joint 015.9
hip 015.1
knee 015.2
specified joint NEC 015.8
vertebral 015.0 *[730.88]*
kidney 016.0 *[590.81]*
knee 015.2
lumbar 015.0 *[730.88]*

Tuberculosis, tubercular, tuberculous—*cont.*
lung 011.2
primary, progressive 010.8
meninges (cerebral) (spinal) 013.0
pelvic 016.9
female 016.7
male 016.5
perianal 014.8
fistula 014.8
perinephritic 016.0 *[590.81]*
perineum 017.9
perirectal 014.8
psoas 015.0 *[730.88]*
rectum 014.8
retropharyngeal 012.8
sacrum 015.0 *[730.88]*
scrofulous 017.2
scrotum 016.5
skin 017.0
primary 017.0
spinal cord 013.5
spine or vertebra (column) 015.0 *[730.88]*
strumous 017.2
subdiaphragmatic 014.8
testis 016.5
thigh 017.9
urinary 016.3
kidney 016.0 *[590.81]*
uterus 016.7
accessory sinus—*see* Tuberculosis, sinus
Addison's disease 017.6
adenitis (*see also* Tuberculosis, lymph gland) 017.2
adenoids 012.8
adenopathy (*see also* Tuberculosis, lymph gland) 017.2
tracheobronchial 012.1
primary progressive 010.8
adherent pericardium 017.9 *[420.0]*
adnexa (uteri) 016.7
adrenal (capsule) (gland) 017.6
air passage NEC 012.8
alimentary canal 014.8
anemia 017.9
ankle (joint) 015.8
bone 015.5 *[730.87]*
anus 014.8
apex (*see also* Tuberculosis, pulmonary) 011.9
apical (*see also* Tuberculosis, pulmonary) 011.9
appendicitis 014.8
appendix 014.8
arachnoid 013.0
artery 017.9
arthritis (chronic) (synovial) 015.9 *[711.40]*
ankle 015.8 *[730.87]*
hip 015.1 *[711.45]*
knee 015.2 *[711.46]*
specified site NEC 015.8 *[711.48]*
spine or vertebra (column) 015.0 *[720.81]*
wrist 015.8 *[730.83]*
articular—*see* Tuberculosis, joint
ascites 014.0
asthma (*see also* Tuberculosis, pulmonary) 011.9
axilla, axillary 017.2
gland 017.2
bilateral (*see also* Tuberculosis, pulmonary) 011.9
bladder 016.1

Tuberculosis, tubercular, tuberculous—*cont.*
bone (*see also* Osteomyelitis, due to, tuberculosis) 015.9 *[730.8]*
hip 015.1 *[730.85]*
knee 015.2 *[730.86]*
limb NEC 015.5 *[730.88]*
sacrum 015.0 *[730.88]*
specified site NEC 015.7 *[730.88]*
spinal or vertebral column 015.0 *[730.88]*
bowel 014.8
miliary 018.9
brain 013.2
breast 017.9
broad ligament 016.7
bronchi, bronchial, bronchus 011.3
ectasia, ectasis 011.5
fistula 011.3
primary, progressive 010.8
gland 012.1
primary, progressive 010.8
isolated 012.2
lymph gland or node 012.1
primary, progressive 010.8
bronchiectasis 011.5
bronchitis 011.3
bronchopleural 012.0
bronchopneumonia, bronchopneumonic 011.6
bronchorrhagia 011.3
bronchotracheal 011.3
isolated 012.2
bronchus—*see* Tuberculosis, bronchi
bronze disease (Addison's) 017.6
buccal cavity 017.9
bulbourethral gland 016.5
bursa (*see also* Tuberculosis, joint) 015.9
cachexia NEC (*see also* Tuberculosis, pulmonary) 011.9
cardiomyopathy 017.9 *[425.8]*
caries (*see also* Tuberculosis, bone) 015.9 *[730.8]*
cartilage (*see also* Tuberculosis, bone) 015.9 *[730.8]*
intervertebral 015.0 *[730.88]*
catarrhal (*see also* Tuberculosis, pulmonary) 011.9
cecum 014.8
cellular tissue (primary) 017.0
cellulitis (primary) 017.0
central nervous system 013.9
specified site NEC 013.8
cerebellum (current) 013.2
cerebral (current) 013.2
meninges 013.0
cerebrospinal 013.6
meninges 013.0
cerebrum (current) 013.2
cervical 017.2
gland 017.2
lymph nodes 017.2
cervicitis (uteri) 016.7
cervix 016.7
chest (*see also* Tuberculosis, pulmonary) 011.9
childhood type or first infection 010.0
choroid 017.3 *[363.13]*
choroiditis 017.3 *[363.13]*
ciliary body 017.3 *[364.11]*
colitis 014.8
colliers' 011.4
colliquativa (primary) 017.0
colon 014.8
ulceration 014.8

Tuberculosis, tubercular, tuberculous—*cont.*
complex, primary 010.0
complicating pregnancy, childbirth, or puerperium 647.3
affecting fetus or newborn 760.2
congenital 771.2
conjunctiva 017.3 *[370.31]*
connective tissue 017.9
bone—*see* Tuberculosis, bone
contact V01.1
converter (tuberculin skin test) (without disease) 795.5
cornea (ulcer) 017.3 *[370.31]*
Cowper's gland 016.5
coxae 015.1 *[730.85]*
coxalgia 015.1 *[730.85]*
cul-de-sac of Douglas 014.8
curvature, spine 015.0 *[737.40]*
cutis (colliquativa) (primary) 017.0
cyst, ovary 016.6
cystitis 016.1
dacryocystitis 017.3 *[375.32]*
dactylitis 015.5
diarrhea 014.8
diffuse (*see also* Tuberculosis, miliary) 018.9
lung—*see* Tuberculosis, pulmonary
meninges 013.0
digestive tract 014.8
disseminated (*see also* Tuberculosis, miliary) 018.9
meninges 013.0
duodenum 014.8
dura (mater) 013.9
abscess 013.8
cerebral 013.3
spinal 013.5
dysentery 014.8
ear (inner) (middle) 017.4
bone 015.6
external (primary) 017.0
skin (primary) 017.0
elbow 015.8
emphysema—*see* Tuberculosis, pulmonary
empyema 012.0
encephalitis 013.6
endarteritis 017.9
endocarditis (any valve) 017.9 *[424.91]*
endocardium (any valve) 017.9 *[424.91]*
endocrine glands NEC 017.9
endometrium 016.7
enteric, enterica 014.8
enteritis 014.8
enterocolitis 014.8
epididymis 016.4
epididymitis 016.4
epidural abscess 013.8
brain 013.3
spinal cord 013.5
epiglottis 012.3
episcleritis 017.3 *[379.00]*
erythema (induratum) (nodosum) (primary) 017.1
esophagus 017.8
Eustachian tube 017.4
exposure to V01.1
exudative 012.0
primary, progressive 010.1
eye 017.3
glaucoma 017.3 *[365.62]*
eyelid (primary) 017.0
lupus 017.0 *[373.4]*

Tuberculosis, tubercular, tuberculous—*cont.*
fallopian tube 016.6
fascia 017.9
fauces 012.8
finger 017.9
first infection 010.0
fistula, perirectal 014.8
Florida 011.6
foot 017.9
funnel pelvis 137.3
gallbladder 017.9
galloping (*see also* Tuberculosis, pulmonary) 011.9
ganglionic 015.9
gastritis 017.9
gastrocolic fistula 014.8
gastroenteritis 014.8
gastrointestinal tract 014.8
general, generalized 018.9
acute 018.0
chronic 018.8
genital organs NEC 016.9
female 016.7
male 016.5
genitourinary NEC 016.9
genu 015.2
glandulae suprarenalis 017.6
glandular, general 017.2
glottis 012.3
grinders' 011.4
groin 017.2
gum 017.9
hand 017.9
heart 017.9 *[425.8]*
hematogenous—*see* Tuberculosis, miliary
hemoptysis (*see also* Tuberculosis, pulmonary) 011.9
hemorrhage NEC (*see also* Tuberculosis, pulmonary) 011.9
hemothorax 012.0
hepatitis 017.9
hilar lymph nodes 012.1
primary, progressive 010.8
hip (disease) (joint) 015.1
bone 015.1 *[730.85]*
hydrocephalus 013.8
hydropneumothorax 012.0
hydrothorax 012.0
hypoadrenalism 017.6
hypopharynx 012.8
ileocecal (hyperplastic) 014.8
ileocolitis 014.8
ileum 014.8
iliac spine (superior) 015.0 *[730.88]*
incipient NEC (*see also* Tuberculosis, pulmonary) 011.9
indurativa (primary) 017.1
infantile 010.0
infection NEC 011.9
without clinical manifestation 010.0
infraclavicular gland 017.2
inguinal gland 017.2
inguinalis 017.2
intestine (any part) 014.8
iris 017.3 *[364.11]*
iritis 017.3 *[364.11]*
ischiorectal 014.8
jaw 015.7 *[730.88]*
jejunum 014.8

Tuberculosis, tubercular, tuberculous—*cont.*
joint 015.9
hip 015.1
knee 015.2
specified site NEC 015.8
vertebral 015.0 *[730.88]*
keratitis 017.3 *[370.31]*
interstitial 017.3 *[370.59]*
keratoconjunctivitis 017.3 *[370.31]*
kidney 016.0
knee (joint) 015.2
kyphoscoliosis 015.0 *[737.43]*
kyphosis 015.0 *[737.41]*
lacrimal apparatus, gland 017.3
laryngitis 012.3
larynx 012.3
leptomeninges, leptomeningitis (cerebral) (spinal) 013.0
lichenoides (primary) 017.0
linguae 017.9
lip 017.9
liver 017.9
lordosis 015.0 *[737.42]*
lung—*see* Tuberculosis, pulmonary
luposa 017.0
eyelid 017.0 *[373.4]*
lymphadenitis—*see* Tuberculosis, lymph gland
lymphangitis—*see* Tuberculosis, lymph gland
lymphatic (gland) (vessel)—*see* Tuberculosis, lymph gland
lymph gland or node (peripheral) 017.2
abdomen 014.8
bronchial 012.1
primary, progressive 010.8
cervical 017.2
hilar 012.1
primary, progressive 010.8
intrathoracic 012.1
primary, progressive 010.8
mediastinal 012.1
primary, progressive 010.8
mesenteric 014.8
peripheral 017.2
retroperitoneal 014.8
tracheobronchial 012.1
primary, progressive 010.8
malignant NEC (*see also* Tuberculosis, pulmonary) 011.9
mammary gland 017.9
marasmus NEC (*see also* Tuberculosis, pulmonary) 011.9
mastoiditis 015.6
maternal, affecting fetus or newborn 760.2
mediastinal (lymph) gland or node 012.1
primary, progressive 010.8
mediastinitis 012.8
primary, progressive 010.8
mediastinopericarditis 017.9 *[420.0]*
mediastinum 012.8
primary, progressive 010.8
medulla 013.9
brain 013.2
spinal cord 013.4
melanosis, Addisonian 017.6
membrane, brain 013.0
meninges (cerebral) (spinal) 013.0
meningitis (basilar) (brain) (cerebral) (cerebrospinal) (spinal) 013.0
meningoencephalitis 013.0
mesentery, mesenteric 014.8
lymph gland or node 014.8

Tuberculosis, tubercular, tuberculous—*cont.*
miliary (any site) 018.9
acute 018.0
chronic 018.8
specified type NEC 018.8
millstone makers' 011.4
miners' 011.4
moulders' 011.4
mouth 017.9
multiple 018.9
acute 018.0
chronic 018.8
muscle 017.9
myelitis 013.6
myocarditis 017.9 *[422.0]*
myocardium 017.9 *[422.0]*
nasal (passage) (sinus) 012.8
nasopharynx 012.8
neck gland 017.2
nephritis 016.0 *[583.81]*
nerve 017.9
nose (septum) 012.8
ocular 017.3
old NEC 137.0
without residuals V12.01
omentum 014.8
oophoritis (acute) (chronic) 016.6
optic 017.3 *[377.39]*
nerve trunk 017.3 *[377.39]*
papilla, papillae 017.3 *[377.39]*
orbit 017.3
orchitis 016.5 *[608.81]*
organ, specified NEC 017.9
orificialis (primary) 017.0
osseous (*see also* Tuberculosis, bone) 015.9 *[730.8]*
osteitis (*see also* Tuberculosis, bone) 015.9 *[730.8]*
osteomyelitis (*see also* Tuberculosis, bone) 015.9 *[730.8]*
otitis (media) 017.4
ovaritis (acute) (chronic) 016.6
ovary (acute) (chronic) 016.6
oviducts (acute) (chronic) 016.6
pachymeningitis 013.0
palate (soft) 017.9
pancreas 017.9
papulonecrotic (primary) 017.0
parathyroid glands 017.9
paronychia (primary) 017.0
parotid gland or region 017.9
pelvic organ NEC 016.9
female 016.7
male 016.5
pelvis (bony) 015.7 *[730.85]*
penis 016.5
peribronchitis 011.3
pericarditis 017.9 *[420.0]*
pericardium 017.9 *[420.0]*
perichondritis, larynx 012.3
perineum 017.9
periostitis (*see also* Tuberculosis, bone) 015.9 *[730.8]*
periphlebitis 017.9
eye vessel 017.3 *[362.18]*
retina 017.3 *[362.18]*
perirectal fistula 014.8
peritoneal gland 014.8
peritoneum 014.0
peritonitis 014.0

Tuberculosis, tubercular, tuberculous—*cont.*
pernicious NEC (*see also* Tuberculosis, pulmonary) 011.9
pharyngitis 012.8
pharynx 012.8
phlyctenulosis (conjunctiva) 017.3 *[370.31]*
phthisis NEC (*see also* Tuberculosis, pulmonary) 011.9
pituitary gland 017.9
placenta 016.7
pleura, pleural, pleurisy, pleuritis (fibrinous) (obliterative) (purulent) (simple plastic) (with effusion) 012.0
primary, progressive 010.1
pneumonia, pneumonic 011.6
pneumothorax 011.7
polyserositis 018.9
acute 018.0
chronic 018.8
potters' 011.4
prepuce 016.5
primary 010.9
complex 010.0
complicated 010.8
with pleurisy or effusion 010.1
progressive 010.8
with pleurisy or effusion 010.1
skin 017.0
proctitis 014.8
prostate 016.5 *[601.4]*
prostatitis 016.5 *[601.4]*
pulmonaris (*see also* Tuberculosis, pulmonary) 011.9
pulmonary (artery) (incipient) (malignant) (multiple round foci) (pernicious) (reinfection stage) 011.9
cavitated or with cavitation 011.2
primary, progressive 010.8
childhood type or first infection 010.0
chromogenic acid-fast bacilli 795.3
fibrosis or fibrotic 011.4
infiltrative 011.0
primary, progressive 010.9
nodular 011.1
specified NEC 011.8
sputum positive only 795.3
status following surgical collapse of lung NEC 011.9
pyelitis 016.0 *[590.81]*
pyelonephritis 016.0 *[590.81]*
pyemia—*see* Tuberculosis, miliary
pyonephrosis 016.0
pyopneumothorax 012.0
pyothorax 012.0
rectum (with abscess) 014.8
fistula 014.8
reinfection stage (*see also* Tuberculosis, pulmonary) 011.9
renal 016.0
renis 016.0
reproductive organ 016.7
respiratory NEC (*see also* Tuberculosis, pulmonary) 011.9
specified site NEC 012.8
retina 017.3 *[363.13]*
retroperitoneal (lymph gland or node) 014.8
gland 014.8
retropharyngeal abscess 012.8
rheumatism 015.9
rhinitis 012.8
sacroiliac (joint) 015.8

Tuberculosis, tubercular, tuberculous—*cont.*
sacrum 015.0 *[730.88]*
salivary gland 017.9
salpingitis (acute) (chronic) 016.6
sandblasters' 011.4
sclera 017.3 *[379.09]*
scoliosis 015.0 *[737.43]*
scrofulous 017.2
scrotum 016.5
seminal tract or vesicle 016.5 *[608.81]*
senile NEC (*see also* Tuberculosis, pulmonary) 011.9
septic NEC (*see also* Tuberculosis, miliary) 018.9
shoulder 015.8
blade 015.7 *[730.8]*
sigmoid 014.8
sinus (accessory) (nasal) 012.8
bone 015.7 *[730.88]*
epididymis 016.4
skeletal NEC (*see also* Osteomyelitis, due to tuberculosis) 015.9 *[730.8]*
skin (any site) (primary) 017.0
small intestine 014.8
soft palate 017.9
spermatic cord 016.5
spinal
column 015.0 *[730.88]*
cord 013.4
disease 015.0 *[730.88]*
medulla 013.4
membrane 013.0
meninges 013.0
spine 015.0 *[730.88]*
spleen 017.7
splenitis 017.7
spondylitis 015.0 *[720.81]*
spontaneous pneumothorax—*see* Tuberculosis, pulmonary
sternoclavicular joint 015.8
stomach 017.9
stonemasons' 011.4
struma 017.2
subcutaneous tissue (cellular) (primary) 017.0
subcutis (primary) 017.0
subdeltoid bursa 017.9
submaxillary 017.9
region 017.9
supraclavicular gland 017.2
suprarenal (capsule) (gland) 017.6
swelling, joint (*see also* Tuberculosis, joint) 015.9
symphysis pubis 015.7 *[730.88]*
synovitis 015.9 *[727.01]*
hip 015.1 *[727.01]*
knee 015.2 *[727.01]*
specified site NEC 015.8 *[727.01]*
spine or vertebra 015.0 *[727.01]*
systemic—*see* Tuberculosis, miliary
tarsitis (eyelid) 017.0 *[373.4]*
ankle (bone) 015.5 *[730.87]*
tendon (sheath)—*see* Tuberculosis, tenosynovitis
tenosynovitis 015.9 *[727.01]*
hip 015.1 *[727.01]*
knee 015.2 *[727.01]*
specified site NEC 015.8 *[727.01]*
spine or vertebra 015.0 *[727.01]*
testis 016.5 *[608.81]*
throat 012.8
thymus gland 017.9

Tuberculosis, tubercular, tuberculous—*cont.*
thyroid gland 017.5
toe 017.9
tongue 017.9
tonsil (lingual) 012.8
tonsillitis 012.8
trachea, tracheal 012.8
gland 012.1
primary, progressive 010.8
isolated 012.2
tracheobronchial 011.3
glandular 012.1
primary, progressive 010.8
isolated 012.2
lymph gland or node 012.1
primary, progressive 010.8
tubal 016.6
tunica vaginalis 016.5
typhlitis 014.8
ulcer (primary) (skin) 017.0
bowel or intestine 014.8
specified site NEC—*see* Tuberculosis, by site
unspecified site—*see* Tuberculosis, pulmonary
ureter 016.2
urethra, urethral 016.3
urinary organ or tract 016.3
kidney 016.0
uterus 016.7
uveal tract 017.3 *[363.13]*
uvula 017.9
vaccination, prophylactic (against) V03.2
vagina 016.7
vas deferens 016.5
vein 017.9
verruca (primary) 017.0
verrucosa (cutis) (primary) 017.0
vertebra (column) 015.0 *[730.88]*
vesiculitis 016.5 *[608.81]*
viscera NEC 014.8
vulva 016.7 *[616.51]*
wrist (joint) 015.8
bone 015.5 *[730.83]*
Tuberculum
auriculae 744.29
occlusal 520.2
paramolare 520.2
Tuberous sclerosis (brain) 759.5
Tubo-ovarian —*see* condition
Tuboplasty, after previous sterilization V26.0
Tubotympanitis 381.10
Tularemia 021.9
with
conjunctivitis 021.3
pneumonia 021.2
bronchopneumonic 021.2
conjunctivitis 021.3
cryptogenic 021.1
disseminated 021.8
enteric 021.1
generalized 021.8
glandular 021.8
intestinal 021.1
oculoglandular 021.3
ophthalmic 021.3
pneumonia 021.2
pulmonary 021.2
specified NEC 021.8
typhoidal 021.1
ulceroglandular 021.0
vaccination, prophylactic (against) V03.4
Tularensis conjunctivitis 021.3
Tumefaction —*see also* Swelling
liver (*see also* Hypertrophy, liver) 789.1
Tumor (M8000/1)—*see also* Neoplasm, by site, unspecified nature
Abrikossov's (M9580/0)—*see also* Neoplasm, connective tissue, benign
malignant (M9580/3)—*see* Neoplasm, connective tissue, malignant
acinar cell (M8550/1)—*see* Neoplasm, by site, uncertain behavior
acinic cell (M8550/1)—*see* Neoplasm, by site, uncertain behavior
adenomatoid (M9054/0)—*see also* Neoplasm, by site, benign
odontogenic (M9300/0) 213.1
upper jaw (bone) 213.0
adnexal (skin) (M8390/0)—*see* Neoplasm, skin, benign
adrenal
cortical (benign) (M8370/0) 227.0
malignant (M8370/3) 194.0
rest (M8671/0)—*see* Neoplasm, by site, benign
alpha cell (M8152/0)
malignant (M8152/3)
pancreas 157.4
specified site NEC—*see* Neoplasm, by site, malignant
unspecified site 157.4
pancreas 211.7
specified site NEC—*see* Neoplasm, by site, benign
unspecified site 211.7
aneurysmal (*see also* Aneurysm) 442.9
aortic body (M8691/1) 237.3
malignant (M8691/3) 194.6
argentaffin (M8241/1)—*see* Neoplasm, by site, uncertain behavior
basal cell (M8090/1)—*see also* Neoplasm, skin, uncertain behavior
benign (M8000/0)—*see* Neoplasm, by site, benign
beta cell (M8151/0)
malignant (M8151/3)
pancreas 157.4
specified site—*see* Neoplasm, by site, malignant
unspecified site 157.4
pancreas 211.7
specified site NEC—*see* Neoplasm, by site, benign
unspecified site 211.7
blood—*see* Hematoma
brenner (M9000/0) 220
borderline malignancy (M9000/1) 236.2
malignant (M9000/3) 183.0
proliferating (M9000/1) 236.2
Brooke's (M8100/0)—*see* Neoplasm, skin, benign
brown fat (M8880/0)—*see* Lipoma, by site
Burkitt's (M9750/3) 200.2
calcifying epithelial odontogenic (M9340/0) 213.1
upper jaw (bone) 213.0
carcinoid (M8240/1)—*see* Carcinoid
carotid body (M8692/1) 237.3
malignant (M8692/3) 194.5
Castleman's (mediastinal lymph node hyperplasia) 785.6
cells (M8001/1)—*see also* Neoplasm, by site, unspecified nature

Tumor—*continued*
benign (M8001/0)—*see* Neoplasm, by site, benign
malignant (M8001/3)—*see* Neoplasm, by site, malignant
uncertain whether benign or malignant (M8001/1)—*see* Neoplasm, by site, uncertain nature
cervix
in pregnancy or childbirth 654.6
affecting fetus or newborn 763.8
causing obstructed labor 660.2
affecting fetus or newborn 763.1
chondromatous giant cell (M9230/0)—*see* Neoplasm, bone, benign
chromaffin (M8700/0)—*see also* Neoplasm, by site, benign
malignant (M8700/3)—*see* Neoplasm, by site, malignant
Cock's peculiar 706.2
Codman's (benign chondroblastoma) (M9230/0)—*see* Neoplasm, bone, benign
dentigerous, mixed (M9282/0) 213.1
upper jaw (bone) 213.0
dermoid (M9084/0)—*see* Neoplasm, by site, benign
with malignant transformation (M9084/3) 183.0
desmoid (extra-abdominal) (M8821/1)—*see also* Neoplasm, connective tissue, uncertain behavior
abdominal (M8822/1)—*see* Neoplasm, connective tissue, uncertain behavior
embryonal (mixed) (M9080/1)—*see also* Neoplasm, by site, uncertain behavior
liver (M9080/3) 155.0
endodermal sinus (M9071/3)
specified site—*see* Neoplasm, by site, malignant
unspecified site
female 183.0
male 186.9
epithelial
benign (M8010/0)—*see* Neoplasm, by site, benign
malignant (M8010/3)—*see* Neoplasm, by site, malignant
Ewing's (M9260/3)—*see* Neoplasm, bone, malignant
fatty—*see* Lipoma
fetal, causing disproportion 653.7
causing obstructed labor 660.1
fibroid (M8890/0)—*see* Leiomyoma
G cell (M8153/1)
malignant (M8153/3)
pancreas 157.4
specified site NEC—*see* Neoplasm, by site, malignant
unspecified site 157.4
specified site—*see* Neoplasm, by site, uncertain behavior
unspecified site 235.5
giant cell (type) (M8003/1)—*see also* Neoplasm, by site, unspecified nature
bone (M9250/1) 238.0
malignant (M9250/3)—*see* Neoplasm, bone, malignant
chondromatous (M9230/0)—*see* Neoplasm, bone, benign
malignant (M8003/3)—*see* Neoplasm, by site, malignant

Tumor—*continued*
peripheral (gingiva) 523.8
soft parts (M9251/1)—*see also* Neoplasm, connective tissue, uncertain behavior
malignant (M9251/3)—*see* Neoplasm, connective tissue, malignant
tendon sheath 727.02
glomus (M8711/0)—*see also* Hemangioma, by site
jugulare (M8690/1) 237.3
malignant (M8690/3) 194.6
gonadal stromal (M8590/1)—*see* Neoplasm, by site, uncertain behavior
granular cell (M9580/0)—*see also* Neoplasm, connective tissue, benign
malignant (M9580/3)—*see* Neoplasm, connective tissue, malignant
granulosa cell (M8620/1) 236.2
malignant (M8620/3) 183.0
granulosa cell-theca cell (M8621/1) 236.2
malignant (M8621/3) 183.0
Grawitz's (hypernephroma) (M8312/3) 189.0
hazard-crile (M8350/3) 193
hemorrhoidal—*see* Hemorrhoids
hilar cell (M8660/0) 220
hurthle cell (benign) (M8290/0) 226
malignant (M8290/3) 193
hydatid (*see also* Echinococcus) 122.9
hypernephroid (M8311/1)—*see also* Neoplasm, by site, uncertain behavior
interstitial cell (M8650/1)—*see also* Neoplasm, by site, uncertain behavior
benign (M8650/0)—*see* Neoplasm, by site, benign
malignant (M8650/3)—*see* Neoplasm, by site, malignant
islet cell (M8150/0)
malignant (M8150/3)
pancreas 157.4
specified site—*see* Neoplasm, by site, malignant
unspecified site 157.4
pancreas 211.7
specified site NEC—*see* Neoplasm, by site, benign
unspecified site 211.7
juxtaglomerular (M8361/1) 236.91
Krukenberg's (M8490/6) 198.6
Leydig cell (M8650/1)
benign (M8650/0)
specified site—*see* Neoplasm, by site, benign
unspecified site
female 220
male 220.0
malignant (M8650/3)
specified site—*see* Neoplasm, by site, malignant
unspecified site
female 183.0
male 186.9
specified site—*see* Neoplasm, by site, uncertain behavior
unspecified site
female 236.2
male 236.4
lipid cell, ovary (M8670/0) 220
lipoid cell, ovary (M8670/0) 220
lymphomatous, benign (M9590/0)—*see also* Neoplasm, by site, benign

Tumor—*continued*
Malherbe's (M8110/0)—*see* Neoplasm, skin, benign
malignant (M8000/3)—*see also* Neoplasm, by site, malignant
fusiform cell (type) (M8004/3)—*see* Neoplasm, by site, malignant
giant cell (type) (M8003/3)—*see* Neoplasm, by site, malignant
mixed NEC (M8940/3)—*see* Neoplasm, by site, malignant
small cell (type) (M8002/3)—*see* Neoplasm, by site, malignant
spindle cell (type) (M8004/3)—*see* Neoplasm, by site, malignant
mast cell (M9740/1) 238.5
malignant (M9740/3) 202.6
melanotic, neuroectodermal (M9363/0)—*see* Neoplasm, by site, benign
mesenchymal
malignant (M8800/3)—*see* Neoplasm, connective tissue, malignant
mixed (M8990/1)—*see* Neoplasm, connective tissue, uncertain behavior
mesodermal, mixed (M8951/3)—*see also* Neoplasm, by site, malignant
liver 155.0
mesonephric (M9110/1)—*see also* Neoplasm, by site, uncertain behavior
malignant (M9110/3)—*see* Neoplasm, by site, malignant
metastatic
from specified site (M8000/3)—*see* Neoplasm, by site, malignant
to specified site (M8000/6)—*see* Neoplasm, by site, malignant, secondary
mixed NEC (M8940/0)—*see also* Neoplasm, by site, benign
malignant (M8940/3)—*see* Neoplasm, by site, malignant
mucocarcinoid, malignant (M8243/3)—*see* Neoplasm, by site, malignant
mucoepidermoid (M8430/1)—*see* Neoplasm, by site, uncertain behavior
Mullerian, mixed (M8950/3)—*see* Neoplasm, by site, malignant
myoepithelial (M8982/0)—*see* Neoplasm, by site, benign
neurogenic olfactory (M9520/3) 160.0
nonencapsulated sclerosing (M8350/3) 193
odontogenic (M9270/1) 238.0
adenomatoid (M9300/0) 213.1
upper jaw (bone) 213.0
benign (M9270/0) 213.1
upper jaw (bone) 213.0
calcifying epithelial (M9340/0) 213.1
upper jaw (bone) 213.0
malignant (M9270/3) 170.1
upper jaw (bone) 170.0
squamous (M9312/0) 213.1
upper jaw (bone) 213.0
ovarian stromal (M8590/1) 236.2
ovary
in pregnancy or childbirth 654.4
affecting fetus or newborn 763.8
causing obstructed labor 660.2
affecting fetus or newborn 763.1
pacinian (M9507/0)—*see* Neoplasm, skin, benign
Pancoast's (M8010/3) 162.3
papillary—*see* Papilloma

Tumor—*continued*
pelvic, in pregnancy or childbirth 654.9
affecting fetus or newborn 763.8
causing obstructed labor 660.2
affecting fetus or newborn 763.1
phantom 300.11
plasma cell (M9731/1) 238.6
benign (M9731/0)—*see* Neoplasm, by site, benign
malignant (M9731/3) 203.8
polyvesicular vitelline (M9071/3)
specified site—*see* Neoplasm, by site, malignant
unspecified site
female 183.0
male 186.9
Pott's puffy (*see also* Osteomyelitis) 730.2
Rathke's pouch (M9350/1) 237.0
regaud's (M8082/3)—*see* Neoplasm, nasopharynx, malignant
rete cell (M8140/0) 222.0
retinal anlage (M9363/0)—*see* Neoplasm, by site, benign
Rokitansky's 620.2
salivary gland type, mixed (M8940/0)—*see also* Neoplasm, by site, benign
malignant (M8940/3)—*see* Neoplasm, by site, malignant
Sampson's 617.1
Schloffer's (*see also* Peritonitis) 567.2
Schmincke (M8082/3)—*see* Neoplasm, nasopharynx, malignant
sebaceous (*see also* Cyst, sebaceous) 706.2
secondary (M8000/6)—*see* Neoplasm, by site, secondary
Sertoli cell (M8640/0)
with lipid storage (M8641/0)
specified site—*see* Neoplasm, by site, benign
unspecified site
female 220
male 222.0
specified site—*see* Neoplasm, by site, benign
unspecified site
female 220
male 222.0
Sertoli-Leydig cell (M8631/0)
specified site—*see* Neoplasm, by site, benign
unspecified site
female 220
male 222.0
sex cord (-stromal) (M8590/1)—*see* Neoplasm, by site, uncertain behavior
skin appendage (M8390/0)—*see* Neoplasm, skin, benign
soft tissue
benign (M8800/0)—*see* Neoplasm, connective tissue, benign
malignant (M8800/3)—*see* Neoplasm, connective tissue, malignant
sternomastoid 754.1
superior sulcus (lung) (pulmonary) (syndrome) (M8010/3) 162.3
suprasulcus (M8010/3) 162.3
sweat gland (M8400/1)—*see also* Neoplasm, skin, uncertain behavior
benign (M8400/0)—*see* Neoplasm, skin, benign
malignant (M8400/3)—*see* Neoplasm, skin, malignant

Tumor—*continued*
syphilitic brain 094.89
congenital 090.49
testicular stromal (M8590/1) 236.4
theca cell (M8600/0) 220
theca cell-granulosa cell (M8621/1) 236.2
theca-lutein (M8610/0) 220
turban (M8200/0) 216.4
uterus
in pregnancy or childbirth 654.1
affecting fetus or newborn 763.8
causing obstructed labor 660.2
affecting fetus or newborn 763.1
vagina
in pregnancy or childbirth 654.7
affecting fetus or newborn 763.8
causing obstructed labor 660.2
affecting fetus or newborn 763.1
varicose (*see also* Varicose, vein) 454.9
von Recklinghausen's (M9540/1) 237.71
vulva
in pregnancy or childbirth 654.8
affecting fetus or newborn 763.8
causing obstructed labor 660.2
affecting fetus or newborn 763.1
Warthin's (salivary gland) (M8561/0) 210.2
white—*see also* Tuberculosis, arthritis
White-Darier 757.39
Wilms' (nephroblastoma) (M8960/3) 189.0
yolk sac (M9071/3)
specified site—*see* Neoplasm, by site, malignant
unspecified site
female 183.0
male 186.9
Tumorlet (M8040/1)—*see* Neoplasm, by site, uncertain behavior
Tungiasis 134.1
Tunica vasculosa lentis 743.39
Tunnel vision 368.45
Turban tumor (M8200/0) 216.4
Türck's trachoma (chronic catarrhal laryngitis) 476.0
Türk's syndrome (ocular retraction syndrome) 378.71
Turner's
hypoplasia (tooth) 520.4
syndrome 758.6
tooth 520.4
Turner-Kieser syndrome (hereditary osteo-onychodysplasia) 756.89
Turner-Varny syndrome 758.6
Turricephaly 756.0
Tussis convulsiva (*see also* Whooping cough) 033.9
Twin
affected by maternal complications of pregnancy 761.5
conjoined 759.4
healthy liveborn—*see* Newborn, twin
pregnancy (complicating delivery) NEC 651.0
with fetal loss and retention of one fetus 651.3
Twinning, teeth 520.2
Twist, twisted
bowel, colon, or intestine 560.2
hair (congenital) 757.4
mesentery 560.2
omentum 560.2
organ or site, congenital NEC—*see* Anomaly, specified type NEC
Twist, twisted—*continued*
ovarian pedicle 620.5
congenital 752.0
umbilical cord—*see* Compression, umbilical cord
Twitch 781.0
Tylosis 700
buccalis 528.6
gingiva 523.8
linguae 528.6
palmaris et plantaris 757.39
Tympanism 787.3
Tympanites (abdominal) (intestine) 787.3
Tympanitis —*see* Myringitis
Tympanosclerosis 385.00
involving
combined sites NEC 385.09
with tympanic membrane 385.03
tympanic membrane 385.01
with ossicles 385.02
and middle ear 385.03
Tympanum —*see* condition
Tympany
abdomen 787.3
chest 786.7
Typhlitis (*see also* Appendicitis) 541
Typhoenteritis 002.0
Typhogastric fever 002.0
Typhoid (abortive) (ambulant) (any site) (fever) (hemorrhagic) (infection) (intermittent) (malignant) (rheumatic) 002.0
with pneumonia 002.0 *[484.8]*
abdominal 002.0
carrier (suspected) of V02.1
cholecystitis (current) 002.0
clinical (Widal and blood test negative) 002.0
endocarditis 002.0 *[421.1]*
inoculation reaction—*see* Complications, vaccination
meningitis 002.0 *[320.7]*
mesenteric lymph nodes 002.0
myocarditis 002.0 *[422.0]*
osteomyelitis (*see also* Osteomyelitis, due to, typhoid) 002.0 *[730.8]*
perichondritis, larynx 002.0 *[478.71]*
pneumonia 002.0 *[484.8]*
spine 002.0 *[720.81]*
ulcer (perforating) 002.0
vaccination, prophylactic (against) V03.1
Widal negative 002.0
Typhomalaria (fever) (*see also* Malaria) 084.6
Typhomania 002.0
Typhoperitonitis 002.0
Typhus (fever) 081.9
abdominal, abdominalis 002.0
African tick 082.1
amarillic (*see also* Fever, Yellow) 060.9
brain 081.9
cerebral 081.9
classical 080
endemic (flea-borne) 081.0
epidemic (louse-borne) 080
exanthematic NEC 080
exanthematicus SAI 080
brillii SAI 081.1
Mexicanus SAI 081.0
pediculo vestimenti causa 080
typhus murinus 081.0
flea-borne 081.0
Indian tick 082.1

Typhus—*continued*
Kenya tick 082.1
louse-borne 080
Mexican 081.0
flea-borne 081.0
louse-borne 080
tabardillo 080
mite-borne 081.2
murine 081.0
North Asian tick-borne 082.2
petechial 081.9
Queensland tick 082.3
rat 081.0
recrudescent 081.1
recurrent (*see also* Fever, relapsing) 087.9
São Paulo 082.0
scrub (China) (India) (Malaya) (New Guinea) 081.2
shop (of Malaya) 081.0
Siberian tick 082.2
tick-borne NEC 082.9
tropical 081.2
vaccination, prophylactic (against) V05.8
Tyrosinosis (Medes) (Sakai) 270.2
Tyrosinuria 270.2
Tyrosyluria 270.2

U

Uehlinger's syndrome (acropachyderma) 757.39
Uhl's anomaly or disease (hypoplasia of myocardium, right ventricle) 746.84
Ulcer, ulcerated, ulcerating ulceration, ulcerative 707.9
with gangrene 707.9 *[785.4]*
abdomen (wall) (*see also* Ulcer, skin) 707.8
ala, nose 478.1
alveolar process 526.5
amebic (intestine) 006.9
skin 006.6
anastomotic—*see* Ulcer, gastrojejunal
anorectal 569.41
antral—*see* Ulcer, stomach
anus (sphincter) (solitary) 569.41
varicose—*see* Varicose, ulcer, anus
aphthous (oral) (recurrent) 528.2
genital organ(s)
female 616.8
male 608.89
mouth 528.2
arm (*see also* Ulcer, skin) 707.8
arteriosclerotic plaque—*see* Arteriosclerosis, by site
artery NEC 447.2
without rupture 447.8
atrophic NEC—*see* Ulcer, skin
Barrett's (chronic peptic ulcer of esophagus) 530.2
bile duct 576.8
bladder (solitary) (sphincter) 596.8
bilharzial (*see also* Schistosomiasis) 120.9 *[595.4]*
submucosal (*see also* Cystitis) 595.1
tuberculous (*see also* Tuberculosis) 016.1
bleeding NEC—*see* Ulcer, peptic, with hemorrhage
bone 730.9
bowel (*see also* Ulcer, intestine) 569.82
breast 611.0
bronchitis 491.8
bronchus 519.1
buccal (cavity) (traumatic) 528.9
burn (acute)—*see* Ulcer, duodenum
Buruli 031.1
buttock (*see also* Ulcer, skin) 707.8
decubitus (*see also* Ulcer, decubitus) 707.0
cancerous (M8000/3)—*see* Neoplasm, by site, malignant
cardia—*see* Ulcer, stomach
cardio-esophageal (peptic) 530.2
cecum (*see also* Ulcer, intestine) 569.82
cervix (uteri) (trophic) 622.0
with mention of cervicitis 616.0
chancroidal 099.0
chest (wall) (*see also* Ulcer, skin) 707.8
Chiclero 085.4
chin (pyogenic) (*see also* Ulcer, skin) 707.8
chronic (cause unknown)—*see also* Ulcer, skin
penis 607.89
Cochin-China 085.1
colitis —*see* Colitis, ulcerative
colon (*see also* Ulcer, intestine) 569.82
conjunctiva (acute) (postinfectional) 372.00

Ulcer, ulcerated, ulcerating—*continued*
cornea (infectional) 370.00
with perforation 370.06
annular 370.02
catarrhal 370.01
central 370.03
dendritic 054.42
marginal 370.01
mycotic 370.05
phlyctenular, tuberculous (*see also* Tuberculosis) 017.3 *[370.31]*
ring 370.02
rodent 370.07
serpent, serpiginous 370.04
superficial marginal 370.01
tuberculous (*see also* Tuberculosis) 017.3 *[370.31]*
corpus cavernosum (chronic) 607.89
crural—*see* Ulcer, lower extremity
Curling's—*see* Ulcer, duodenum
Cushing's—*see* Ulcer, peptic
cystitis (interstitial) 595.1
decubitus (any site) 707.0
with gangrene 707.0 *[785.4]*
dendritic 054.42
diabetes, diabetic (mellitus) 250.8 *[707.9]*
lower limb 250.8 *[707.1]*
specified site NEC 250.8 *[707.8]*
Dieulafoy's—*see* Ulcer, stomach
due to
infection NEC—*see* Ulcer, skin
radiation, radium—*see* Ulcer, by site
trophic disturbance (any region)—*see* Ulcer, skin
x-ray—*see* Ulcer, by site
duodenum, duodenal (eroded) (peptic) 532.9

Note—Use the following fifth-digit subclassification with categories 531-534:

0 without mention of obstruction
1 with obstruction

with
hemorrhage (chronic) 532.4
and perforation 532.6
perforation (chronic) 532.5
and hemorrhage 532.6
acute 532.3
with
hemorrhage 532.0
and perforation 532.2
perforation 532.1
and hemorrhage 532.2
bleeding (recurrent)—*see* Ulcer, duodenum, with hemorrhage
chronic 532.7
with
hemorrhage 532.4
and perforation 532.6
perforation 532.5
and hemorrhage 532.6
penetrating—*see* Ulcer, duodenum, with perforation
perforating—*see* Ulcer, duodenum, with perforation
dysenteric NEC 009.0
elusive 595.1

Ulcer, ulcerated, ulcerating—*continued*
endocarditis (any valve) (acute) (chronic) (subacute) 421.0
enteritis —*see* Colitis, ulcerative
enterocolitis 556.0
epiglottis 478.79
esophagus (peptic) 530.2
due to ingestion
aspirin 530.2
chemicals 530.2
medicinal agents 530.2
fungal 530.2
infectional 530.2
varicose (*see also* Varix, esophagus) 456.1
bleeding (*see also* Varix, esophagus, bleeding) 456.0
eye NEC 360.00
dendritic 054.42
eyelid (region) 373.01
face (*see also* Ulcer, skin) 707.8
fauces 478.29
Fenwick (-Hunner) (solitary) (*see also* Cystitis) 595.1
fistulous NEC—*see* Ulcer, skin
foot (indolent) (*see also* Ulcer, lower extremity) 707.1
perforating 707.1
leprous 030.1
syphilitic 094.0
trophic 707.1
varicose 454.0
inflamed or infected 454.2
frambesial, initial or primary 102.0
gallbladder or duct 575.8
gall duct 576.8
gangrenous (*see also* Gangrene) 785.4
gastric—*see* Ulcer, stomach
gastrocolic—*see* Ulcer, gastrojejunal
gastroduodenal—*see* Ulcer, peptic
gastroesophageal—*see* Ulcer, stomach
gastrohepatic—*see* Ulcer, stomach
gastrointestinal—*see* Ulcer, gastrojejunal
gastrojejunal (eroded) (peptic) 534.9

Note—Use the following fifth-digit subclassification with categories 531-534:

0 without mention of obstruction
1 with obstruction

with
hemorrhage (chronic) 534.4
and perforation 534.6
perforation 534.5
and hemorrhage 534.6
acute 534.3
with
hemorrhage 534.0
and perforation 534.2
perforation 534.1
and hemorrhage 534.2
bleeding (recurrent)—*see* Ulcer, gastrojejunal, with hemorrhage
chronic 534.7
with
hemorrhage 534.4
and perforation 534.6
perforation 534.5
and hemorrhage 534.6
penetrating—*see* Ulcer, gastrojejunal, with perforation

Ulcer, ulcerated, ulcerating—*continued*
perforating—*see* Ulcer, gastrojejunal, with perforation
gastrojejunocolic—*see* Ulcer, gastrojejunal
genital organ
female 629.8
male 608.89
gingiva 523.8
gingivitis 523.1
glottis 478.79
granuloma of pudenda 099.2
groin (*see also* Ulcer, skin) 707.8
gum 523.8
gumma, due to yaws 102.4
hand (*see also* Ulcer, skin) 707.8
hard palate 528.9
heel (*see also* Ulcer, lower extremity) 707.1
decubitus (*see also* Ulcer, decubitus) 707.0
hemorrhoids 455.8
external 455.5
internal 455.2
hip (*see also* Ulcer, skin) 707.8
decubitus (*see also* Ulcer, decubitus) 707.0
Hunner's 595.1
hypopharynx 478.29
hypopyon (chronic) (subacute) 370.04
hypostaticum—*see* Ulcer, varicose
ileocolitis 556.1
ileum (*see also* Ulcer, intestine) 569.82
intestine, intestinal 569.82
with perforation 569.83
amebic 006.9
duodenal—*see* Ulcer, duodenum
granulocytopenic (with hemorrhage) 288.0
marginal 569.82
perforating 569.83
small, primary 569.82
stercoraceous 569.82
stercoral 569.82
tuberculous (*see also* Tuberculosis) 014.8
typhoid (fever) 002.0
varicose 456.8
ischemic 707.9
lower extremity (*see also* Ulcer, lower extremity) 707.1
jejunum, jejunal—*see* Ulcer, gastrojejunal
keratitis (*see also* Ulcer, cornea) 370.00
knee—*see* Ulcer, lower extremity
labium (majus) (minus) 616.50
laryngitis (*see also* Laryngitis) 464.0
larynx (aphthous) (contact) 478.79
diphtheritic 032.3
leg—*see* Ulcer, lower extremity
lip 528.5
Lipschütz's 616.50
lower extremity (atrophic) (chronic) (neurogenic) (perforating) (pyogenic) (trophic) (tropical) 707.1
with gangrene 707.1 *[785.4]*
arteriosclerotic 440.24
arteriosclerotic 440.23
with gangrene 440.24
decubitus 707.0
with gangrene 707.0 *[785.4]*
varicose 454.0
inflamed or infected 454.2
luetic—*see* Ulcer, syphilitic
lung 518.89
tuberculous (*see also* Tuberculosis) 011.2
malignant (M8000/3)—*see* Neoplasm, by site, malignant

Ulcer, ulcerated, ulcerating—*continued*
marginal NEC—*see* Ulcer, gastrojejunal
meatus (urinarius) 597.89
Meckel's diverticulum 751.0
Meleney's (chronic undermining) 686.0
Mooren's (cornea) 370.07
mouth (traumatic) 528.9
mycobacterial (skin) 031.1
nasopharynx 478.29
navel cord (newborn) 771.4
neck (*see also* Ulcer, skin) 707.8
uterus 622.0
neurogenic NEC—*see* Ulcer, skin
nose, nasal (infectional) (passage) 478.1
septum 478.1
varicose 456.8
skin—*see* Ulcer, skin
spirochetal NEC 104.8
oral mucosa (traumatic) 528.9
palate (soft) 528.9
penetrating NEC—*see* Ulcer, peptic, with perforation
penis (chronic) 607.89
peptic (site unspecified) 533.9

> Note—Use the following fifth-digit subclassification with categories 531-534:
>
> *0 without mention of obstruction*
> *1 with obstruction*

with
hemorrhage 533.4
and perforation 533.6
perforation (chronic) 533.5
and hemorrhage 533.6
acute 533.3
with
hemorrhage 533.0
and perforation 533.2
perforation 533.1
and hemorrhage 533.2
bleeding (recurrent)—*see* Ulcer, peptic, with hemorrhage
chronic 533.7
with
hemorrhage 533.4
and perforation 533.6
perforation 533.5
and hemorrhage 533.6
penetrating—*see* Ulcer, peptic, with perforation
perforating NEC (*see also* Ulcer, peptic, with perforation) 533.5
skin 707.9
perineum (*see also* Ulcer, skin) 707.8
peritonsillar 474.8
phagedenic (tropical) NEC—*see* Ulcer, skin
pharynx 478.29
phlebitis—*see* Phlebitis
plaster (*see also* Ulcer, decubitus) 707.0
popliteal space—*see* Ulcer, lower extremity
postpyloric—*see* Ulcer, duodenum
prepuce 607.89
prepyloric—*see* Ulcer, stomach
pressure (*see also* Ulcer, decubitus) 707.0
primary of intestine 569.82
with perforation 569.83
proctitis 556.2
with ulcerative sigmoiditis 556.3
prostate 601.8
pseudopeptic—*see* Ulcer, peptic

Ulcer, ulcerated, ulcerating—*continued*
pyloric—*see* Ulcer, stomach
rectosigmoid 569.82
with perforation 569.83
rectum (sphincter) (solitary) 569.41
stercoraceous, stercoral 569.41
varicose—*see* Varicose, ulcer, anus
retina (*see also* Chorioretinitis) 363.20
rodent (M8090/3)—*see also* Neoplasm, skin, malignant
cornea 370.07
round—*see* Ulcer, stomach
sacrum (region) (*see also* Ulcer, skin) 707.8
Saemisch's 370.04
scalp (*see also* Ulcer, skin) 707.8
sclera 379.09
scrofulous (*see also* Tuberculosis) 017.2
scrotum 608.89
tuberculous (*see also* Tuberculosis) 016.5
varicose 456.4
seminal vesicle 608.89
sigmoid 569.82
with perforation 569.83
skin (atrophic) (chronic) (neurogenic) (perforating) (pyogenic) (trophic) 707.9
with gangrene 707.9 *[785.4]*
amebic 006.6
decubitus 707.0
with gangrene 707.0 *[785.4]*
in granulocytopenia 288.0
lower extremity (*see also* Ulcer, lower extremity) 707.1
with gangrene 707.1 *[785.4]*
arteriosclerotic 440.24
arteriosclerotic 440.23
with gangrene 440.24
mycobacterial 031.1
syphilitic (early) (secondary) 091.3
tuberculous (primary) (*see also* Tuberculosis) 017.0
varicose—*see* Ulcer, varicose
sloughing NEC—*see* Ulcer, skin
soft palate 528.9
solitary, anus or rectum (sphincter) 569.41
sore throat 462
streptococcal 034.0
spermatic cord 608.89
spine (tuberculous) 015.0 *[730.88]*
stasis (leg) (venous) 454.0
inflamed or infected 454.2
stercoral, stercoraceous 569.82
with perforation 569.83
anus or rectum 569.41
stoma, stomal—*see* Ulcer, gastrojejunal
stomach (eroded) (peptic) (round) 531.9

> Note—Use the following fifth-digit subclassification with categories 531-534:
>
> *0 without mention of obstruction*
> *1 with obstruction*

with
hemorrhage 531.4
and perforation 531.6
perforation (chronic) 531.5
and hemorrhage 531.6
acute 531.3
with
hemorrhage 531.0
and perforation 531.2

Ulcer, ulcerated, ulcerating—*continued*
perforation 531.1
and hemorrhage 531.2
bleeding (recurrent)—*see* Ulcer, stomach, with hemorrhage
chronic 531.7
with
hemorrhage 531.4
and perforation 531.6
perforation 531.5
and hemorrhage 531.6
penetrating—*see* Ulcer, stomach, with perforation
perforating—*see* Ulcer, stomach, with perforation
stomatitis 528.0
stress—*see* Ulcer, peptic
strumous (tuberculous) (*see also* Tuberculosis) 017.2
submental (*see also* Ulcer, skin) 707.8
submucosal, bladder 595.1
syphilitic (any site) (early) (secondary) 091.3
late 095.9
perforating 095.9
foot 094.0
testis 608.89
thigh—*see* Ulcer, lower extremity
throat 478.29
diphtheritic 032.0
toe—*see* Ulcer, lower extremity
tongue (traumatic) 529.0
tonsil 474.8
diphtheritic 032.0
trachea 519.1
trophic—*see* Ulcer, skin
tropical NEC (*see also* Ulcer, skin) 707.9
tuberculous—*see* Tuberculosis, ulcer
tunica vaginalis 608.89
turbinate 730.9
typhoid (fever) 002.0
perforating 002.0
umbilicus (newborn) 771.4
unspecified site NEC—*see* Ulcer, skin
urethra (meatus) (*see also* Urethritis) 597.89
uterus 621.8
cervix 622.0
with mention of cervicitis 616.0
neck 622.0
with mention of cervicitis 616.0
vagina 616.8
valve, heart 421.0
varicose (lower extremity, any part) 454.0
anus—*see* Varicose, ulcer, anus
broad ligament 456.5
esophagus (*see also* Varix, esophagus) 456.1
bleeding (*see also* Varix, esophagus, bleeding) 456.0
inflamed or infected 454.2
nasal septum 456.8
perineum 456.6
rectum—*see* Varicose, ulcer, anus
scrotum 456.4
specified site NEC 456.8
sublingual 456.3
vulva 456.6
vas deferens 608.89
vesical (*see also* Ulcer, bladder) 596.8
vulva (acute) (infectional) 616.50
Behçet's syndrome 136.1 *[616.51]*
herpetic 054.12
tuberculous 016.7 *[616.51]*

Ulcer, ulcerated, ulcerating—*continued*
vulvobuccal, recurring 616.50
x-ray—*see* Ulcer, by site
yaws 102.4
Ulcerosa scarlatina 034.1
Ulcus —*see also* Ulcer
cutis tuberculosum (*see also* Tuberculosis) 017.0
duodeni—*see* Ulcer, duodenum
durum 091.0
extragenital 091.2
gastrojejunale—*see* Ulcer, gastrojejunal
hypostaticum—*see* Ulcer, varicose
molle (cutis) (skin) 099.0
serpens cornea (pneumococcal) 370.04
ventriculi—*see* Ulcer, stomach
Ulegyria 742.4
Ulerythema
acneiforma 701.8
centrifugum 695.4
ophryogenes 757.4
Ullrich (-Bonnevie) (-Turner) syndrome 758.6
Ullrich-Feichtiger syndrome 759.89
Ulnar —*see* condition
Ulorrhagia 523.8
Ulorrhea 523.8
Umbilicus, umbilical —*see also* condition
cord necrosis, affecting fetus or newborn 762.6
Unavailability of medical facilities (at) V63.9
due to
investigation by social service agency V63.8
lack of services at home V63.1
remoteness from facility V63.0
waiting list V63.2
home V63.1
outpatient clinic V63.0
specified reason NEC V63.8
Uncinaria americana infestation 126.1
Uncinariasis (*see also* Ancylostomiasis) 126.9
Unconscious, unconsciousness 780.09
Underdevelopment —*see also* Undeveloped
sexual 259.0
Undernourishment 269.9
Undernutrition 269.9
Under observation —*see* Observation
Underweight 783.4
for gestational age—*see* Light-for-dates
Underwood's disease (sclerema neonatorum) 778.1
Undescended —*see also* Malposition, congenital
cecum 751.4
colon 751.4
testis 752.5
Undetermined diagnosis or cause 799.9
Undeveloped, undevelopment —*see also* Hypoplasia
brain (congenital) 742.1
cerebral (congenital) 742.1
fetus or newborn 764.9
heart 746.89
lung 748.5
testis 257.2
uterus 259.0
Undiagnosed (disease) 799.9
Undulant fever (*see also* Brucellosis) 023.9
Unemployment, anxiety concerning V62.0
Unequal leg (acquired) (length) 736.81
congenital 755.30
Unerupted teeth, tooth 520.6
Unextracted dental root 525.3
Unguis incarnatus 703.0
Unicornis uterus 752.3
Unicorporeus uterus 752.3

Uniformis uterus 752.3
Unilateral —*see also* condition
development, breast 611.8
organ or site, congenital NEC—*see* Agenesis
vagina 752.49
Unilateralis uterus 752.3
Unilocular heart 745.8
Uninhibited (neurogenic) bladder 596.54
with cauda equina syndrome 344.61
neurogenic—*see* Neurogenic, bladder 596.54
Union, abnormal —*see also* Fusion
divided tendon 727.89
larynx and trachea 748.3
Universal
joint, cervix 620.6
mesentery 751.4
Unknown
cause of death 799.9
diagnosis 799.9
Unna's disease (seborrheic dermatitis) 690.18
Unresponsiveness, adrenocorticotropin (ACTH) 255.4
Unsoundness of mind (*see also* Psychosis) 298.9
Unspecified cause of death 799.9
Unstable
back NEC 724.9
colon 569.89
joint—*see* Instability, joint
lie 652.0
affecting fetus or newborn (before labor) 761.7
causing obstructed labor 660.0
affecting fetus or newborn 763.1
lumbosacral joint (congenital) 756.19
acquired 724.6
sacroiliac 724.6
spine NEC 724.9
Untruthfulness, child problem (*see also* Disturbance, conduct) 312.0
Unverricht (-Lundborg) disease, syndrome, or epilepsy 333.2
Unverricht-Wagner syndrome (dermatomyositis) 710.3
Upper respiratory —*see* condition
Upset
gastric 536.8
psychogenic 306.4
gastrointestinal 536.8
psychogenic 306.4
virus (*see also* Enteritis, viral) 008.8
intestinal (large) (small) 564.9
psychogenic 306.4
menstruation 626.9
mental 300.9
stomach 536.8
psychogenic 306.4
Urachus —*see also* condition
patent 753.7
persistent 753.7
Uratic arthritis 274.0
Urbach's lipoid proteinosis 272.8
Urbach-Oppenheim disease or syndrome (necrobiosis lipoidica diabeticorum) 250.8 *[709.3]*
Urbach-Wiethe disease or syndrome (lipoid proteinosis) 272.8
Urban yellow fever 060.1
Urea, blood, high —*see* Uremia
Uremia, uremic (absorption) (amaurosis) (amblyopia) (aphasia) (apoplexy) (coma) (delirium) (dementia) (dropsy) (dyspnea) (fever) (intoxication) (mania) (paralysis) (poisoning) (toxemia) (vomiting) 586
with
abortion—*see* Abortion, by type, with renal failure
ectopic pregnancy (*see also* categories 633.0-633.9) 639.3
hypertension (*see also* Hypertension, kidney) 403.91
molar pregnancy (*see also* categories 630-632) 639.3
chronic 585
complicating
abortion 639.3
ectopic or molar pregnancy 639.3
hypertension (*see also* Hypertension, kidney) 403.91
labor and delivery 669.3
congenital 779.8
extrarenal 788.9
hypertensive (chronic) (*see also* Hypertension, kidney) 403.91
maternal NEC, affecting fetus or newborn 760.1
neuropathy 585 *[357.4]*
pericarditis 585 *[420.0]*
prerenal 788.9
pyelitic (*see also* Pyelitis) 590.80
Ureter, ureteral —*see* condition
Ureteralgia 788.0
Ureterectasis 593.89
Ureteritis 593.89
cystica 590.3
due to calculus 592.1
gonococcal (acute) 098.19
chronic or duration of 2 months or over 098.39
nonspecific 593.89
Ureterocele (acquired) 593.89
congenital 753.2
Ureterolith 592.1
Ureterolithiasis 592.1
Ureterostomy status V44.6
with complication 997.5
Urethra, urethral —*see* condition
Urethralgia 788.9
Urethritis (abacterial) (acute) (allergic) (anterior) (chronic) (nonvenereal) (posterior) (recurrent) (simple) (subacute) (ulcerative) (undifferentiated) 597.80
diplococcal (acute) 098.0
chronic or duration of 2 months or over 098.2
due to Trichomonas (vaginalis) 131.02
gonococcal (acute) 098.0
chronic or duration of 2 months or over 098.2
nongonococcal (sexually transmitted) 099.40
Chlamydia trachomatis 099.41
Reiter's 099.3
specified organism NEC 099.49
nonspecific (sexually transmitted) (*see also* Urethritis, nongonococcal) 099.40
not sexually transmitted 597.80
Reiter's 099.3
trichomonal or due to Trichomonas (vaginalis) 131.02
tuberculous (*see also* Tuberculosis) 016.3
venereal NEC (*see also* Urethritis, nongonococcal) 099.40

Uveitis—*continued*
due to
operation 360.11
toxoplasmosis (acquired) 130.2
congenital (active) 771.2
granulomatous 364.10
heterochromic 364.21
lens-induced 364.23
nongranulomatous 364.00
posterior 363.20
disseminated—*see* Chorioretinitis, disseminated
focal—*see* Chorioretinitis, focal
recurrent 364.02
sympathetic 360.11
syphilitic (secondary) 091.50
congenital 090.0 *[363.13]*
late 095.8 *[363.13]*
tuberculous (*see also* Tuberculosis) 017.3 *[364.11]*
Uveoencephalitis 363.22
Uveokeratitis (*see also* Iridocyclitis) 364.3
Uveoparotid fever 135
Uveoparotitis 135
Uvula —*see* condition
Uvulitis (acute) (catarrhal) (chronic) (gangrenous) (membranous) (suppurative) (ulcerative) 528.3

V

Varix (lower extremity) (ruptured) 454.9
with
inflammation or infection 454.1
with ulcer 454.2
stasis dermatitis 454.1
with ulcer 454.2
ulcer 454.0
with inflammation or infection 454.2
aneurysmal (*see also* Aneurysm) 442.9
anus—*see* Hemorrhoids
arteriovenous (congenital) (peripheral) NEC 747.60
gastrointestinal 747.61
lower limb 747.64
renal 747.62
specified NEC 747.69
spinal 747.82
upper limb 747.63
bladder 456.5
broad ligament 456.5
congenital (peripheral) NEC 747.60
esophagus (ulcerated) 456.1
bleeding 456.0
in
cirrhosis of liver 571.5 *[456.20]*
portal hypertension 572.3 *[456.20]*
congenital 747.69
in
cirrhosis of liver 571.5 *[456.21]*
with bleeding 571.5 *[456.20]*
portal hypertension 572.3 *[456.21]*
with bleeding 572.3 *[456.20]*
inflamed or infected 454.1
ulcerated 454.2
in pregnancy or puerperium 671.0
perineum 671.1
vulva 671.1
labia (majora) 456.6
orbit 456.8
congenital 747.69
ovary 456.5
papillary 448.1
pelvis 456.5
perineum 456.6
in pregnancy or puerperium 671.1
pharynx 456.8
placenta—*see* Placenta, abnormal
rectum—*see* Hemorrhoids
renal papilla 456.8
retina 362.17
scrotum (ulcerated) 456.4
sigmoid colon 456.8
specified site NEC 456.8
spinal (cord) (vessels) 456.8
spleen, splenic (vein) (with phlebolith) 456.8
sublingual 456.3
ulcerated 454.0
inflamed or infected 454.2
umbilical cord, affecting fetus or newborn 762.6
uterine ligament 456.5
vocal cord 456.8
vulva 456.6
in pregnancy, childbirth, or puerperium 671.1
Vasa previa 663.5
affecting fetus or newborn 762.6
hemorrhage from, affecting fetus or newborn 772.0
Vascular —*see also* condition
loop on papilla (optic) 743.51
sheathing, retina 362.13
spasm 443.9
spider 448.1
Vascularity, pulmonary, congenital 747.3
Vascularization
choroid 362.16
cornea 370.60
deep 370.63
localized 370.61
retina 362.16
subretinal 362.16
Vasculitis 447.6
allergic 287.0
cryoglobulinemic 273.2
disseminated 447.6
kidney 447.8
nodular 695.2
retinal 362.10
rheumatic—*see* Fever, rheumatic
Vas deferens —*see* condition
Vas deferentitis 608.4
Vasectomy, admission for V25.2
Vasitis 608.4
nodosa 608.4
scrotum 608.4
spermatic cord 608.4
testis 608.4
tuberculous (*see also* Tuberculosis) 016.5
tunica vaginalis 608.4
vas deferens 608.4
Vasodilation 443.9
Vasomotor —*see* condition
Vasoplasty, after previous sterilization V26.0
Vasoplegia, splanchnic (*see also* Neuropathy, peripheral, autonomic) 337.9
Vasospasm 443.9
cerebral (artery) 435.9
with transient neurologic deficit 435.9
nerve
arm NEC 354.9
autonomic 337.9
brachial plexus 353.0
cervical plexus 353.2
leg NEC 355.8
lower extremity NEC 355.8
peripheral NEC 355.9
spinal NEC 355.9
sympathetic 337.9
upper extremity NEC 354.9
peripheral NEC 443.9
retina (artery) (*see also* Occlusion, retinal, artery) 362.30
Vasospastic —*see* condition
Vasovagal attack (paroxysmal) 780.2
psychogenic 306.2
Vater's ampulla —*see* condition
VATER syndrome 759.89
Vegetation, vegetative
adenoid (nasal fossa) 474.2
consciousness (persistent) 780.03
endocarditis (acute) (any valve) (chronic) (subacute) 421.0
heart (mycotic) (valve) 421.0
state (persistent) 780.03
Veil
Jackson's 751.4
over face (causing asphyxia) 768.9
Vein, venous —*see* condition
Veldt sore (*see also* Ulcer, skin) 707.9
Velpeau's hernia —*see* Hernia, femoral

Venereal
balanitis NEC 099.8
bubo 099.1
disease 099.9
specified nature or type NEC 099.8
granuloma inguinale 099.2
lymphogranuloma (Durand-Nicolas-Favre), any site 099.1
salpingitis 098.37
urethritis (*see also* Urethritis, nongonococcal) 099.40
vaginitis NEC 099.8
warts 078.19
Vengefulness, in child (*see also* Disturbance, conduct) 312.0
Venofibrosis 459.89
Venom, venomous
bite or sting (animal or insect) 989.5
poisoning 989.5
Venous —*see* condition
Ventouse delivery NEC 669.5
affecting fetus or newborn 763.3
Ventral —*see* condition
Ventricle, ventricular —*see also* condition
escape 427.69
standstill (*see also* Arrest, cardiac) 427.5
Ventriculitis, cerebral (*see also* Meningitis) 322.9
Ventriculostomy status V45.2
Verbiest's syndrome (claudicatio intermittens spinalis) 435.1
Vernet's syndrome 352.6
Verneuil's disease (syphilitic bursitis) 095.7
Verruca (filiformis) 078.10
acuminata (any site) 078.11
necrogenica (primary) (*see also* Tuberculosis) 017.0
peruana 088.0
peruviana 088.0
plana (juvenilis) 078.19
plantaris 078.19
seborrheica 702.19
inflamed 702.11
senilis 702.0
tuberculosa (primary) (*see also* Tuberculosis) 017.0
venereal 078.19
viral NEC 078.10
Verrucosities (*see also* Verruca) 078.10
Verrucous endocarditis (acute) (any valve) (chronic) (subacute) 710.0 *[424.91]*
nonbacterial 710.0 *[424.91]*
Verruga
peruana 088.0
peruviana 088.0
Verse's disease (calcinosis intervertebralis) 275.4 *[722.90]*
Version
before labor, affecting fetus or newborn 761.7
cephalic (correcting previous malposition) 652.1
affecting fetus or newborn 763.1
cervix (*see also* Malposition, uterus) 621.6
uterus (postinfectional) (postpartal, old) (*see also* Malposition, uterus) 621.6
forward—*see* Anteversion, uterus
lateral—*see* Lateroversion, uterus
Vertebra, vertebral —*see* condition
Vertigo 780.4
auditory 386.19
aural 386.19
benign paroxysmal positional 386.11
Vertigo—*continued*
central origin 386.2
cerebral 386.2
Dix and Hallpike (epidemic) 386.12
endemic paralytic 078.81
epidemic 078.81
Dix and Hallpike 386.12
Gerlier's 078.81
Pedersen's 386.12
vestibular neuronitis 386.12
epileptic—*see* Epilepsy
Gerlier's (epidemic) 078.81
hysterical 300.11
labyrinthine 386.10
laryngeal 786.2
malignant positional 386.2
Ménière's (*see also* Disease, Ménière's) 386.00
menopausal 627.2
otogenic 386.19
paralytic 078.81
paroxysmal positional, benign 386.11
Pedersen's (epidemic) 386.12
peripheral 386.10
specified type NEC 386.19
positional
benign paroxysmal 386.11
malignant 386.2
Verumontanitis (chronic) (*see also* Urethritis) 597.89
Vesania (*see also* Psychosis) 298.9
Vesical —*see* condition
Vesicle
cutaneous 709.8
seminal—*see* condition
skin 709.8
Vesicocolic —*see* condition
Vesicoperineal —*see* condition
Vesicorectal —*see* condition
Vesicourethrorectal —*see* condition
Vesicovaginal —*see* condition
Vesicular —*see* condition
Vesiculitis (seminal) 608.0
amebic 006.8
gonorrheal (acute) 098.14
chronic or duration of 2 months or over 098.34
trichomonal 131.09
tuberculous (*see also* Tuberculosis) 016.5 *[608.81]*
Vestibulitis (ear) (*see also* Labyrinthitis) 386.30
nose (external) 478.1
vulvar 616.10
Vestibulopathy, acute peripheral (recurrent) 386.12
Vestige, vestigial —*see also* Persistence
branchial 744.41
structures in vitreous 743.51
Vibriosis NEC 027.9
Vidal's disease (lichen simplex chronicus) 698.3
Video display tube syndrome 723.8
Vienna type encephalitis 049.8
Villaret's syndrome 352.6
Villous —*see* condition
Vincent's
angina 101
bronchitis 101
disease 101
gingivitis 101
infection (any site) 101
laryngitis 101
stomatitis 101
tonsillitis 101

Vinson-Plummer syndrome (sideropenic dysphagia) 280.8
Viosterol deficiency (*see also* Deficiency, calciferol) 268.9
Virchow's disease 733.99
Viremia 790.8
Virilism (adrenal) (female) NEC 255.2
with
3-beta-hydroxysteroid dehydrogenase defect 255.2
11-hydroxylase defect 255.2
21-hydroxylase defect 255.2
adrenal
hyperplasia 255.2
insufficiency (congenital) 255.2
cortical hyperfunction 255.2
Virilization (female) (suprarenal) (*see also* Virilism) 255.2
isosexual 256.4
Virulent bubo 099.0
Virus, viral —*see also* condition
infection NEC (*see also* Infection, viral) 079.99
septicemia 079.99
Viscera, visceral —*see* condition
Visceroptosis 569.89
Visible peristalsis 787.4
Vision, visual
binocular, suppression 368.31
blurred, blurring 368.8
hysterical 300.11
defect, defective (*see also* Impaired, vision) 369.9
disorientation (syndrome) 368.16
disturbance NEC (*see also* Disturbance, vision) 368.9
hysterical 300.11
examination V72.0
field, limitation 368.40
fusion, with defective steropsis 368.33
hallucinations 368.16
halos 368.16
loss 369.9
both eyes (*see also* Blindness, both eyes) 369.3
complete (*see also* Blindness, both eyes) 369.00
one eye 369.8
sudden 368.16
low (both eyes) 369.20
one eye (other eye normal) (*see also* Impaired, vision) 369.70
blindness, other eye 369.10
perception, simultaneous without fusion 368.32
tunnel 368.45
Vitality, lack or want of 780.7
newborn 779.8
Vitamin deficiency NEC (*see also* Deficiency, vitamin) 269.2
Vitelline duct, persistent 751.0
Vitiligo 709.01
due to pinta (carate) 103.2
eyelid 374.53
vulva 624.8
Vitium cordis —*see* Disease, heart
Vitreous —*see also* condition
touch syndrome 997.99
Vocal cord —*see* condition
Vocational rehabilitation V57.22
Vogt's (Cecile) disease or syndrome 333.7
Vogt-Koyanagi syndrome 364.24
Vogt-Spielmeyer disease (amaurotic familial idiocy) 330.1
Voice
change (*see also* Dysphonia) 784.49
loss (*see also* Aphonia) 784.41
Volhard-Fahr disease (malignant nephrosclerosis) 403.00
Volhynian fever 083.1
Volkmann's ischemic contracture or paralysis (complicating trauma) 958.6
Voluntary starvation 307.1
Volvulus (bowel) (colon) (intestine) 560.2
with
hernia—*see also* Hernia, by site, with obstruction
gangrenous—*see* Hernia, by site, with gangrene
perforation 560.2
congenital 751.5
duodenum 537.3
fallopian tube 620.5
oviduct 620.5
stomach (due to absence of gastrocolic ligament) 537.89
Vomiting 787.03
with nausea 787.01
allergic 535.4
asphyxia 933.1
bilious (cause unknown) 787.0
following gastrointestinal surgery 564.3
blood (*see also* Hematemesis) 578.0
causing asphyxia, choking, or suffocation (*see also* Asphyxia, food) 933.1
cyclical 536.2
psychogenic 306.4
epidemic 078.82
fecal matter 569.89
following gastrointestinal surgery 564.3
functional 536.8
psychogenic 306.4
habit 536.2
hysterical 300.11
nervous 306.4
neurotic 306.4
newborn 779.3
of or complicating pregnancy 643.9
due to
organic disease 643.8
specific cause NEC 643.8
early—*see* Hyperemesis, gravidarum
late (after 22 completed weeks of gestation) 643.2
pernicious or persistent 536.2
complicating pregnancy—*see* Hyperemesis, gravidarum
psychogenic 306.4
physiological 787.0
psychic 306.4
psychogenic 307.54
stercoral 569.89
uncontrollable 536.2
psychogenic 306.4
uremic—*see* Uremia
winter 078.82
von Bechterew (-Strumpell) disease or syndrome (ankylosing spondylitis) 720.0
von Bezold's abscess 383.01
von Economo's disease (encephalitis lethargica) 049.8
von Eulenburg's disease (congenital paramyotonia) 359.2
von Gierke's disease (glycogenosis I) 271.0
von Gies' joint 095.8
von Graefe's disease or syndrome 378.72

von Hippel (-Lindau) disease or syndrome (retinocerebral angiomatosis) 759.6
von Jaksch's anemia or disease (pseudoleukemia infantum) 285.8
von Recklinghausen's
  disease or syndrome (nerves) (skin) (M9540/1) 237.71
    bones (osteitis fibrosa cystica) 252.0
  tumor (M9540/1) 237.71
von Recklinghausen-Applebaum disease (hemochromatosis) 275.0
von Schroetter's syndrome (intermittent venous claudication) 453.8
von Willebrand (-Jürgens) (-Minot) disease or syndrome (angiohemophilia) 286.4
von Zambusch's disease (lichen sclerosus et atrophicus) 701.0
Voorhoeve's disease or dyschondroplasia 756.4
Vossius' ring 921.3
  late effect 366.21
Voyeurism 302.82
Vrolik's disease (osteogenesis imperfecta) 756.51
Vulva —*see* condition
Vulvismus 625.1
Vulvitis (acute) (allergic) (aphthous) (chronic) (gangrenous) (hypertrophic) (intertriginous) 616.10
  with
    abortion—*see* Abortion, by type, with sepsis
    ectopic pregnancy (*see also* categories 633.0-633.9) 639.0
    molar pregnancy (*see also* categories 630-632) 639.0
  adhesive, congenital 752.49
  blennorrhagic (acute) 098.0
    chronic or duration of 2 months or over 098.2
  chlamydial 099.53
  complicating pregnancy or puerperium 646.6
  due to Ducrey's bacillus 099.0
  following
    abortion 639.0
    ectopic or molar pregnancy 639.0
  gonococcal (acute) 098.0
    chronic or duration of 2 months or over 098.2
  herpetic 054.11
  leukoplakic 624.0
  monilial 112.1
  puerperal, postpartum, childbirth 646.6
  syphilitic (early) 091.0
    late 095.8
  trichomonal 131.01
Vulvodynia 625.9
Vulvorectal —*see* condition
Vulvovaginitis (*see also* Vulvitis) 616.10
  amebic 006.8
  chlamydial 099.53
  gonococcal (acute) 098.0
    chronic or duration of 2 months or over 098.2
  herpetic 054.11
  monilial 112.1
  trichomonal (Trichomonas vaginalis) 131.01

W

Waardenburg's syndrome 756.89
meaning ptosis-epicanthus 270.2
Waardenburg-Klein syndrome (ptosis-epicanthus) 270.2
Wagner's disease (colloid milium) 709.3
Wagner (-Unverricht) syndrome (dermatomyositis) 710.3
Waiting list, person on V63.2
undergoing social agency investigation V63.8
Wakefulness disorder (*see also* Hypersomnia) 780.54
nonorganic origin 307.43
Waldenström's
disease (osteochondrosis, capital femoral) 732.1
hepatitis (lupoid hepatitis) 571.49
hypergammaglobulinemia 273.0
macroglobulinemia 273.3
purpura, hypergammaglobulinemic 273.0
syndrome (macroglobulinemia) 273.3
Waldenström-Kjellberg syndrome (sideropenic dysphagia) 280.8
Walking
difficulty 719.7
psychogenic 307.9
sleep 307.46
hysterical 300.13
Wall, abdominal —*see* condition
Wallenberg's syndrome (posterior inferior cerebellar artery) (*see also* Disease, cerebrovascular, acute) 436
Wallgren's
disease (obstruction of splenic vein with collateral circulation) 459.89
meningitis (*see also* Meningitis, aseptic) 047.9
Wandering
acetabulum 736.39
gallbladder 751.69
kidney, congenital 753.3
organ or site, congenital NEC—*see* Malposition, congenital
pacemaker (atrial) (heart) 427.89
spleen 289.59
Wardrop's disease (with lymphangitis) 681.9
finger 681.02
toe 681.11
War neurosis 300.16
Wart (common) (digitate) (filiform) (infectious) (juvenile) (plantar) (viral) 078.10
external genital organs (venereal) 078.19
fig 078.19
Hassall-Henle's (of cornea) 371.41
Henle's (of cornea) 371.41
juvenile 078.19
moist 078.10
Peruvian 088.0
plantar 078.19
prosector (*see also* Tuberculosis) 017.0
seborrheic 702.19
inflamed 702.11
senile 702.0
specified NEC 078.19
syphilitic 091.3
tuberculous (*see also* Tuberculosis) 017.0
venereal (female) (male) 078.19
Warthin's tumor (salivary gland) (M8561/0) 210.2
Washerwoman's itch 692.4
Wassilieff's disease (leptospiral jaundice) 100.0
Wasting
disease 799.4
due to malnutrition 261
extreme (due to malnutrition) 261
muscular NEC 728.2
palsy, paralysis 335.21
Water
clefts 366.12
deprivation of 994.3
in joint (*see also* Effusion, joint) 719.0
intoxication 276.6
itch 120.3
lack of 994.3
loading 276.6
on
brain—*see* Hydrocephalus
chest 511.8
poisoning 276.6
Waterbrash 787.1
Water-hammer pulse (*see also* Insufficiency, aortic) 424.1
Waterhouse (-Friderichsen) disease or syndrome 036.3
Water-losing nephritis 588.8
Wax in ear 380.4
Waxy
degeneration, any site 277.3
disease 277.3
kidney 277.3 *[583.81]*
liver (large) 277.3
spleen 277.3
Weak, weakness (generalized) 780.7
arches (acquired) 734
congenital 754.61
bladder sphincter 596.59
congenital 779.8
eye muscle—*see* Strabismus
foot (double)—*see* Weak, arches
heart, cardiac (*see also* Failure, heart) 428.9
congenital 746.9
mind 317
muscle 728.9
myocardium (*see also* Failure, heart) 428.9
newborn 779.8
pelvic fundus 618.8
pulse 785.9
senile 797
valvular—*see* Endocarditis
Wear, worn, tooth, teeth (approximal) (hard tissues) (interproximal) (occlusal) 521.1
Weather, weathered
effects of
cold NEC 991.9
specified effect NEC 991.8
hot (*see also* Heat) 992.9
skin 692.74
Web, webbed (congenital)—*see also* Anomaly, specified type NEC
canthus 743.63
digits (*see also* Syndactylism) 755.10
esophagus 750.3
fingers (*see also* Syndactylism, fingers) 755.11
larynx (glottic) (subglottic) 748.2
neck (pterygium colli) 744.5
Paterson-Kelly (sideropenic dysphagia) 280.8
popliteal syndrome 756.89
toes (*see also* Syndactylism, toes) 755.13

Weber's paralysis or syndrome 344.89
Weber-Christian disease or syndrome (nodular nonsuppurative panniculitis) 729.30
Weber-Cockayne syndrome (epidermolysis bullosa) 757.39
Weber-Dimitri syndrome 759.6
Weber-Gubler syndrome 344.89
Weber-Leyden syndrome 344.89
Weber-Osler syndrome (familial hemorrhagic telangiectasia) 448.0
Wedge-shaped or wedging vertebra (*see also* Osteoporosis) 733.00
Wegener's granulomatosis or syndrome 446.4
Wegner's disease (syphilitic osteochondritis) 090.0
Weight
  gain (abnormal) (excessive) 783.1
    during pregnancy 646.1
      insufficient 646.8
  less than 1000 grams at birth 765.0
  loss (cause unknown) 783.2
Weightlessness 994.9
Weil's disease (leptospiral jaundice) 100.00
Weill-Marchesani syndrome (brachymorphism and ectopia lentis) 759.89
Weingarten's syndrome (tropical eosinophilia) 518.3
Weir Mitchell's disease (erythromelalgia) 443.89
Weiss-Baker syndrome (carotid sinus syncope) 337.0
Weissenbach-Thibierge syndrome (cutaneous systemic sclerosis) 710.1
Wen (*see also* Cyst, sebaceous) 706.2
Wenckebach's phenomenon, heart block (second degree) 426.13
Werdnig-Hoffmann syndrome (muscular atrophy) 335.0
Werlhof's disease (*see also* Purpura, thrombocytopenic) 287.3
Werlhof-Wichmann syndrome (*see also* Purpura, thrombocytopenic) 287.3
Wermer's syndrome or disease (polyendocrine adenomatosis) 258.0
Werner's disease or syndrome (progeria adultorum) 259.8
Werner-His disease (trench fever) 083.1
Werner-Schultz disease (agranulocytosis) 288.0
Wernicke's encephalopathy, disease or syndrome (superior hemorrhagic polioencephalitis) 265.1
Wernicke-Korsakoff syndrome or psychosis (nonalcoholic) 294.0
  alcoholic 291.1
Wernicke-Posadas disease (*see also* Coccidioidomycosis) 114.9
Wesselsbron fever 066.3
West African fever 084.8
West Nile fever 066.3
Westphal-Strümpell syndrome (hepatolenticular degeneration) 275.1
Wet
  brain (alcoholic) (*see also* Alcoholism) 303.9
  feet, tropical (syndrome) (maceration) 991.4
  lung (syndrome)
    adult 518.5
    newborn 770.6
Wharton's duct —*see* condition
Wheal 709.8
Wheezing 786.09
Whiplash injury or syndrome 847.0
Whipple's disease or syndrome (intestinal lipodystrophy) 040.2
Whipworm 127.3
"Whistling face" syndrome (craniocarpotarsal dystrophy) 759.89
White —*see also* condition
  kidney
    large—*see* Nephrosis
    small 582.9
  leg, puerperal, postpartum, childbirth 671.4
    nonpuerperal 451.19
  mouth 112.0
  patches of mouth 528.6
  sponge nevus of oral mucosa 750.26
  spot lesions, teeth 521.0
White's disease (congenital) (keratosis follicularis) 757.39
Whitehead 706.2
Whitlow (with lymphangitis) 681.01
  herpetic 054.6
Whitmore's disease or fever (melioidosis) 025
Whooping cough 033.9
  with pneumonia 033.9 *[484.3]*
  due to
    Bordetella
      bronchoseptica 033.8
        with pneumonia 033.8 *[484.3]*
      parapertussis 033.1
        with pneumonia 033.1 *[484.3]*
      pertussis 033.0
        with pneumonia 033.0 *[484.3]*
    specified organism NEC 033.8
        with pneumonia 033.8 *[484.3]*
  vaccination, prophylactic (against) V03.6
Wichmann's asthma (laryngismus stridulus) 478.75
Widal (-Abrami) syndrome (acquired hemolytic jaundice) 283.9
Widening aorta (*see also* Aneurysm, aorta) 441.9
  ruptured 441.5
Wilkie's disease or syndrome 557.1
Wilkinson-Sneddon disease or syndrome (subcorneal pustular dermatosis) 694.1
Willan's lepra 696.1
Willan-Plumbe syndrome (psoriasis) 696.1
Willebrand (-Jürgens) syndrome or thrombopathy (angiohemophilia) 286.4
Willi-Prader syndrome (hypogenital dystrophy with diabetic tendency) 759.81
Willis' disease (diabetes mellitus) (*see also* Diabetes) 250.0
Wilms' tumor or neoplasm (nephroblastoma) (M8960/3) 189.0
Wilson's
  disease or syndrome (hepatolenticular degeneration) 275.1
  hepatolenticular degeneration 275.1
  lichen ruber 697.0
Wilson-Brocq disease (dermatitis exfoliativa) 695.89
Wilson-Mikity syndrome 770.7
Window —*see also* Imperfect, closure
  aorticopulmonary 745.0
Winged scapula 736.89
Winter —*see also* condition
  vomiting disease 078.82
Wise's disease 696.2
Wiskott-Aldrich syndrome (eczema-thrombocytopenia) 279.12

Withdrawal symptoms, syndrome
- alcohol 291.8
  - delirium (acute) 291.0
    - chronic 291.1
    - newborn 760.71
- drug or narcotic 292.0
- newborn, infant of dependent mother 779.5
- steroid NEC
  - correct substance properly administered 255.4
  - overdose or wrong substance given or taken 962.0

Withdrawing reaction, child or adolescent 313.22
Witts' anemia (achlorhydric anemia) 280.9
Witzelsucht 301.9
Woakes' syndrome (ethmoiditis) 471.1
Wohlfart-Kugelberg-Welander disease 335.11
Woillez's disease (acute idiopathic pulmonary congestion) 518.5
Wolff-Parkinson-White syndrome (anomalous atrioventricular excitation) 426.7
Wolhynian fever 083.1
Wolman's disease (primary familial xanthomatosis) 272.7
Wood asthma 495.8
Woolly, wooly hair (congenital) (nevus) 757.4
Wool-sorters' disease 022.1
Word
- blindness (congenital) (developmental) 315.01
  - secondary to organic lesion 784.61
- deafness (secondary to organic lesion) 784.69
  - developmental 315.31

Worm (s) (colic) (fever) (infection) (infestation) (*see also* Infestation) 128.9
- guinea 125.7
- in intestine NEC 127.9

Worm-eaten soles 102.3
Worn out (*see also* Exhaustion) 780.7
"Worried well" V65.5
Wound, open (by cutting or piercing instrument) (by firearms) (cut) (dissection) (incised) (laceration) (penetration) (perforating) (puncture) (with initial hemorrhage, not internal) 879.8

> Note—For fracture with open wound, see Fracture. For laceration, traumatic rupture, tear or penetrating wound of internal organs, such as heart, lung, liver, kidney, pelvic organs, etc., whether or not accompanied by open wound or fracture in the same region, see Injury, internal. For contused wound, see Contusion. For crush injury, see Crush. For abrasion, insect bite (nonvenomous), blister, or scratch, see Injury, superficial.
>
> Complicated includes wounds with:
> delayed healing
> delayed treatment
> foreign body
> primary infection
>
> For late effect of open wound, see Late, effect, wound, open, by site.

- abdomen, abdominal (external) (muscle) 879.2
  - complicated 879.3
  - wall (anterior) 879.2
    - complicated 879.3
    - lateral 879.4
      - complicated 879.5

Wound, open—*continued*
- alveolar (process) 873.62
  - complicated 873.72
- ankle 891.0
  - with tendon involvement 891.2
  - complicated 891.1
- anterior chamber, eye (*see also* Wound, open, intraocular) 871.9
- anus 879.6
  - complicated 879.7
- arm 884.0
  - with tendon involvement 884.2
  - complicated 884.1
  - forearm 881.00
    - with tendon involvement 881.20
    - complicated 881.10
  - multiple sites—*see* Wound, open, multiple, upper limb
  - upper 880.03
    - with tendon involvement 880.23
    - complicated 880.13
    - multiple sites (with axillary or shoulder regions) 880.09
      - with tendon involvement 880.29
      - complicated 880.19
- artery—*see* Injury, blood vessel, by site
- auditory
  - canal (external) (meatus) 872.02
    - complicated 872.12
  - ossicles (incus) (malleus) (stapes) 872.62
    - complicated 872.72
- auricle, ear 872.01
  - complicated 872.11
- axilla 880.02
  - with tendon involvement 880.22
  - complicated 880.12
    - with tendon involvement 880.29
  - involving other sites of upper arm 880.09
    - complicated 880.19
- back 876.0
  - complicated 876.1
- bladder—*see* Injury, internal, bladder
- blood vessel—*see* Injury, blood vessel, by site
- brain—*see* Injury, intracranial, with open intracranial wound
- breast 879.0
  - complicated 879.1
- brow 873.42
  - complicated 873.52
- buccal mucosa 873.61
  - complicated 873.71
- buttock 877.0
  - complicated 877.1
- calf 891.0
  - with tendon involvement 891.2
  - complicated 891.1
- canaliculus lacrimalis 870.8
  - with laceration of eyelid 870.2
- canthus, eye 870.8
  - laceration—*see* Laceration, eyelid
- cavernous sinus—*see* Injury, intracranial
- cerebellum—*see* Injury, intracranial
- cervical esophagus 874.4
  - complicated 874.5
- cervix—*see* Injury, internal, cervix
- cheek(s) (external) 873.41
  - complicated 873.51
  - internal 873.61
    - complicated 873.71
- chest (wall) (external) 875.0
  - complicated 875.1

Wound, open—*continued*
chin 873.44
complicated 873.54
choroid 363.63
ciliary body (eye) (*see also* Wound, open, intraocular) 871.9
clitoris 878.8
complicated 878.9
cochlea 872.64
complicated 872.74
complicated 879.9
conjunctiva—*see* Wound, open, intraocular
cornea (nonpenetrating) (*see also* Wound, open, intraocular) 871.9
costal region 875.0
complicated 875.1
Descemet's membrane (*see also* Wound, open, intraocular) 871.9
digit(s)
foot 893.0
with tendon involvement 893.2
complicated 893.1
hand 883.0
with tendon involvement 883.2
complicated 883.1
drumhead, ear 872.61
complicated 872.71
ear 872.8
canal 872.02
complicated 872.12
complicated 872.9
drum 872.61
complicated 872.71
external 872.00
complicated 872.10
multiple sites 872.69
complicated 872.79
ossicles (incus) (malleus) (stapes) 872.62
complicated 872.72
specified part NEC 872.69
complicated 872.79
elbow 881.01
with tendon involvement 881.21
complicated 881.11
epididymis 878.2
complicated 878.3
epigastric region 879.2
complicated 879.3
epiglottis 874.01
complicated 874.11
esophagus (cervical) 874.4
complicated 874.5
thoracic—*see* Injury, internal, esophagus
Eustachian tube 872.63
complicated 872.73
extremity
lower (multiple) NEC 894.0
with tendon involvement 894.2
complicated 894.1
upper (multiple) NEC 884.0
with tendon involvement 884.2
complicated 884.1
eye(s) (globe)—*see* Wound, open, intraocular
eyeball NEC 871.9
laceration (*see also* Laceration, eyeball) 871.4
penetrating (*see also* Penetrating wound, eyeball) 871.7
eyebrow 873.42
complicated 873.52
eyelid NEC 870.8
laceration—*see* Laceration, eyelid

Wound, open—*continued*
face 873.40
complicated 873.50
multiple sites 873.49
complicated 873.59
specified part NEC 873.49
complicated 873.59
fallopian tube—*see* Injury, internal, fallopian tube
finger(s) (nail) (subungual) 883.0
with tendon involvement 883.2
complicated 883.1
flank 879.4
complicated 879.5
foot (any part except toe(s) alone) 892.0
with tendon involvement 892.2
complicated 892.1
forearm 881.00
with tendon involvement 881.20
complicated 881.10
forehead 873.42
complicated 873.52
genital organs (external) NEC 878.8
complicated 878.9
internal—*see* Injury, internal, by site
globe (eye) (*see also* Wound, open, eyeball) 871.9
groin 879.4
complicated 879.5
gum(s) 873.62
complicated 873.72
hand (except finger(s) alone) 882.0
with tendon involvement 882.2
complicated 882.1
head NEC 873.8
with intracranial injury—*see* Injury, intracranial
due to or associated with skull fracture—*see* Fracture, skull
complicated 873.9
scalp—*see* Wound, open, scalp
heel 892.0
with tendon involvement 892.2
complicated 892.1
high-velocity (grease gun)—*see* Wound, open, complicated, by site
hip 890.0
with tendon involvement 890.2
complicated 890.1
hymen 878.6
complicated 878.7
hypochondrium 879.4
complicated 879.5
hypogastric region 879.2
complicated 879.3
iliac (region) 879.4
complicated 879.5
incidental to
dislocation—*see* Dislocation, open, by site
fracture—*see* Fracture, open, by site
intracranial injury—*see* Injury, intracranial, with open intracranial wound
nerve injury—*see* Injury, nerve, by site
inguinal region 879.4
complicated 879.5
instep 892.0
with tendon involvement 892.2
complicated 892.1
interscapular region 876.0
complicated 876.1

Wound, open—*continued*
intracranial—*see* Injury, intracranial, with open intracranial wound
intraocular 871.9
with
partial loss (of intraocular tissue) 871.2
prolapse or exposure (of intraocular tissue) 871.1
laceration (*see also* Laceration, eyeball) 871.4
penetrating 871.7
with foreign body (nonmagnetic) 871.6
magnetic 871.5
without prolapse (of intraocular tissue) 871.0
iris (*see also* Wound, open, eyeball) 871.9
jaw (fracture not involved) 873.44
with fracture—*see* Fracture, jaw
complicated 873.54
knee 891.0
with tendon involvement 891.2
complicated 891.1
labium (majus) (minus) 878.4
complicated 878.5
lacrimal apparatus, gland, or sac 870.8
with laceration of eyelid 870.2
larynx 874.01
with trachea 874.00
complicated 874.10
complicated 874.11
leg (multiple) 891.0
with tendon involvement 891.2
complicated 891.1
lower 891.0
with tendon involvement 891.2
complicated 891.1
thigh 890.0
with tendon involvement 890.2
complicated 890.1
upper 890.0
with tendon involvement 890.2
complicated 890.1
lens (eye) (alone) (*see also* Cataract, traumatic) 366.20
with involvement of other eye structures—*see* Wound, open, eyeball
limb
lower (multiple) NEC 894.0
with tendon involvement 894.2
complicated 894.1
upper (multiple) NEC 884.0
with tendon involvement 884.2
complicated 884.1
lip 873.43
complicated 873.53
loin 876.0
complicated 876.1
lumbar region 876.0
complicated 876.1
malar region 873.41
complicated 873.51
mastoid region 873.49
complicated 873.59
mediastinum—*see* Injury, internal, mediastinum
midthoracic region 875.0
complicated 875.1
mouth 873.60
complicated 873.70
floor 873.64
complicated 873.74
multiple sites 873.69
complicated 873.79

wound, open—*continued*
specified site NEC 873.69
complicated 873.79
multiple, unspecified site(s) 879.8

Note—Multiple open wounds of sites classifiable to the same four-digit category should be classified to that category unless they are in different limbs.

Multiple open wounds of sites classifiable to different four-digit categories, or to different limbs, should be coded separately.

complicated 879.9
lower limb(s) (one or both) (sites classifiable to more than one three-digit category in 890 to 893) 894.0
with tendon involvement 894.2
complicated 894.1
upper limb(s) (one or both) (sites classifiable to more than one three-digit category in 880 to 883) 884.0
with tendon involvement 884.2
complicated 884.1
muscle—*see* Sprain, by site
nail
finger(s) 883.0
complicated 883.1
thumb 883.0
complicated 883.1
toe(s) 893.0
complicated 893.1
nape (neck) 874.8
complicated 874.9
specified part NEC 874.8
complicated 874.9
nasal—*see also* Wound, open, nose
cavity 873.22
complicated 873.32
septum 873.21
complicated 873.31
sinuses 873.23
complicated 873.33
nasopharynx 873.22
complicated 873.32
neck 874.8
complicated 874.9
nape 874.8
complicated 874.9
specified part NEC 874.8
complicated 874.9
nerve—*see* Injury, nerve, by site
nose 873.20
complicated 873.30
multiple sites 873.29
complicated 873.39
septum 873.21
complicated 873.31
sinuses 873.23
complicated 873.33
occipital region—*see* Wound, open, scalp
ocular NEC 871.9
adnexa 870.9
specified region NEC 870.8
laceration (*see also* Laceration, ocular) 871.4
muscle (extraocular) 870.3
with foreign body 870.4
eyelid 870.1
intraocular—*see* Wound, open, eyeball
penetrating (*see also* Penetrating wound, ocular) 871.7

Wound, open—*continued*
vas deferens—*see* Injury, internal, vas deferens
vitreous (humor) 871.2
vulva 878.4
complicated 878.5
wrist 881.02
with tendon involvement 881.22
complicated 881.12
Wright's syndrome (hyperabduction) 447.8
pneumonia 390 *[517.1]*
Wringer injury —*see* Crush injury, by site
Wrinkling of skin 701.8
Wrist —*see also* condition
drop (acquired) 736.05
Wrong drug (given in error) NEC 977.9
specified drug or substance—*see* Table of drugs and chemicals
Wry neck —*see also* Torticollis
congenital 754.1
Wuchereria infestation 125.0
bancrofti 125.0
Brugia malayi 125.1
malayi 125.1
Wuchereriasis 125.0
Wuchereriosis 125.0
Wuchernde struma langhans (M8332/3) 193

X

Xanthelasma 272.2
eyelid 272.2 *[374.51]*
palpebrarum 272.2 *[374.51]*
Xanthelasmatosis (essential) 272.2
Xanthelasmoidea 757.33
Xanthine stones 277.2
Xanthinuria 277.2
Xanthofibroma (M8831/0)—*see* Neoplasm, connective tissue, benign
Xanthoma (s), xanthomatosis 272.2
with
hyperlipoproteinemia
type I 272.3
type III 272.2
type IV 272.1
type V 272.3
bone 272.7
craniohypophyseal 277.8
cutaneotendinous 272.7
diabeticorum 250.8 *[272.2]*
disseminatum 272.7
eruptive 272.2
eyelid 272.2 *[374.51]*
familial 272.7
hereditary 272.7
hypercholesterinemic 272.0
hypercholesterolemic 272.0
hyperlipemic 272.4
hyperlipidemic 272.4
infantile 272.7
joint 272.7
juvenile 272.7
multiple 272.7
multiplex 272.7
primary familial 272.7
tendon (sheath) 272.7
tuberosum 272.2
tuberous 272.2
tubo-eruptive 272.2
Xanthosis 709.09
surgical 998.81
Xenophobia 300.29
Xeroderma (congenital) 757.39
acquired 701.1
eyelid 373.33
eyelid 373.33
pigmentosum 757.33
vitamin A deficiency 264.8
Xerophthalmia 372.53
vitamin A deficiency 264.7
Xerosis
conjunctiva 372.53
with Bitôt's spot 372.53
vitamin A deficiency 264.1
vitamin A deficiency 264.0
cornea 371.40
with corneal ulceration 370.00
vitamin A deficiency 264.3
vitamin A deficiency 264.2
cutis 706.8
skin 706.8
Xerostomia 527.7
Xiphodynia 733.90
Xiphoidalgia 733.90
Xiphoiditis 733.99
Xiphopagus 759.4
XO syndrome 758.6
X-ray
effects, adverse, NEC 990
of chest
for suspected tuberculosis V71.2
routine V72.5
XXX syndrome 758.8
XXXXY syndrome 758.8
XXY syndrome 758.7
Xyloketosuria 271.8
Xylosuria 271.8
Xylulosuria 271.8
XYY syndrome 758.8

Y

Yawning 786.09
psychogenic 306.1
Yaws 102.9
bone or joint lesions 102.6
butter 102.1
chancre 102.0
cutaneous, less than five years after infection 102.2
early (cutaneous) (macular) (maculopapular) (micropapular) (papular) 102.2
frambeside 102.2
skin lesions NEC 102.2
eyelid 102.9 *[373.4]*
ganglion 102.6
gangosis, gangosa 102.5
gumma, gummata 102.4
bone 102.6
gummatous
frambeside 102.4
osteitis 102.6
periostitis 102.6
hydrarthrosis 102.6
hyperkeratosis (early) (late) (palmar) (plantar) 102.3
initial lesions 102.0
joint lesions 102.6
juxta-articular nodules 102.7
late nodular (ulcerated) 102.4
latent (without clinical manifestations) (with positive serology) 102.8
mother 102.0
mucosal 102.7
multiple papillomata 102.1
nodular, late (ulcerated) 102.4
osteitis 102.6
papilloma, papillomata (palmar) (plantar) 102.1
periostitis (hypertrophic) 102.6
ulcers 102.4
wet crab 102.1
Yeast infection (*see also* Candidiasis) 112.9
Yellow
atrophy (liver) 570
chronic 571.8
resulting from administration of blood, plasma, serum, or other biological substance (within 8 months of administration)—*see* Hepatitis, viral
fever—*see* Fever, yellow
jack (*see also* Fever, yellow) 060.9
jaundice (*see also* Jaundice) 782.4
Yersinia septica 027.8

Z

Zagari's disease (xerostomia) 527.7
Zahorsky's disease (exanthema subitum) 057.8
syndrome (herpangina) 074.0
Zenker's diverticulum (esophagus) 530.6
Ziehen-Oppenheim disease 333.6
Zieve's syndrome (jaundice, hyperlipemia, and hemolytic anemia) 571.1
Zika fever 066.3
Zollinger-Ellison syndrome (gastric hypersecretion with pancreatic islet cell tumor) 251.5
Zona (*see also* Herpes, zoster) 053.9
Zoophilia (erotica) 302.1
Zoophobia 300.29
Zoster (herpes) (*see also* Herpes, zoster) 053.9
Zuelzer (-Ogden) anemia or syndrome (nutritional megaloblastic anemia) 281.2
Zygodactyly (*see also* Syndactylism) 755.10
Zygomycosis 117.7
Zymotic —*see* condition

SECTION 2

ALPHABETIC INDEX TO POISONING AND EXTERNAL CAUSES OF ADVERSE EFFECTS OF DRUGS AND OTHER CHEMICAL SUBSTANCES

TABLE OF DRUGS AND CHEMICALS

This table contains a classification of drugs and other chemical substances to identify poisoning states and external causes of adverse effects.

Each of the listed substances in the table is assigned a code according to the poisoning classification (960–989). These codes are used when there is a statement of poisoning, overdose, wrong substance given or taken, or intoxication.

The table also contains a listing of external causes of adverse effects. An adverse effect is a pathologic manifestation due to ingestion or exposure to drugs or other chemical substances (e.g., dermatitis, hypersensitivity reaction, aspirin gastritis). The adverse effect is to be identified by the appropriate code found in Section 1, Index to Diseases and Injuries. An external cause code can then be used to identify the circumstances involved. The table headings pertaining to external causes are defined below:

Accidental poisoning (E850–E869)—accidental overdose of drug, wrong substance given or taken, drug taken inadvertently, accidents in the usage of drugs and biologicals in medical and surgical procedures, and to show external causes of poisonings classifiable to 980–989.

Therapeutic use (E930–E949)—a correct substance properly administered in therapeutic or prophylactic dosage as the external cause of adverse effects.

Suicide attempt (E950–E952)—instances in which self–inflicted injuries or poisonings are involved.

Assault (E961–E962)—injury or poisoning inflicted by another person with the intent to injure or kill.

Undetermined (E980–E982)—to be used when the intent of the poisoning or injury cannot be determined whether it was intentional or accidental.

The American Hospital Formulary Service list numbers are included in the table to help classify new drugs not identified in the table by name. The AHFS list numbers are keyed to the continually revised American Hospital Formulary Service (AHFS).* These listings are found in the table under the main term **Drug**.

Excluded from the table are radium and other radioactive substances. The classification of adverse effects and complications pertaining to these substances will be found in Section 1, Index to Diseases and Injuries, and Section 3, Index to External Causes of Injuries.

Although certain substances are indexed with one or more subentries, the majority are listed according to one use or state. It is recognized that many substances may be used in various ways, in medicine and in industry, and may cause adverse effects whatever the state of the agent (solid, liquid, or fumes arising from a liquid). In cases in which the reported data indicates a use or state not in the table, or which is clearly different from the one listed, an attempt should be made to classify the substance in the form which most nearly expresses the reported facts.

*American Hospital Formulary Service, 2 vol. (Washington, DC: American Society of Hospital Pharmacists, 1959-)

Substance	Poisoning	External Cause (E-Code)				
		Accident	Therapeutic Use	Suicide Attempt	Assault	Undetermined
1–propanol	980.3	E860.4	—	E950.9	E962.1	E980.9
2–propanol	980.2	E860.3	—	E950.9	E962.1	E980.9
2, 4–D (dichlorophenoxyacetic acid)	989.4	E863.5	—	E950.6	E962.1	E980.7
2, 4–toluene diisocyanate	983.0	E864.0	—	E950.7	E962.1	E980.6
2, 4, 5–T (trichlorophenoxyacetic acid)	989.2	E863.5	—	E950.6	E962.1	E980.7
14–hydroxydihydromorphinone	965.09	E850.2	E935.2	E950.0	E962.0	E980.0
ABOB	961.7	E857	E931.7	E950.4	E962.0	E980.4
Abrus (seed)	988.2	E865.3	—	E950.9	E962.1	E980.9
Absinthe	980.0	E860.1	—	E950.9	E962.1	E980.9
beverage	980.0	E860.0	—	E950.9	E962.1	E980.9
Acenocoumarin, acenocoumarol	964.2	E858.2	E934.2	E950.4	E962.0	E980.4
Acepromazine	969.1	E853.0	E939.1	E950.3	E962.0	E980.3
Acetal	982.8	E862.4	—	E950.9	E962.1	E980.9
Acetaldehyde (vapor)	987.8	E869.8	—	E952.8	E962.2	E982.8
liquid	989.8	E866.8	—	E950.9	E962.1	E980.9
Acetaminophen	965.4	E850.4	E935.4	E950.0	E962.0	E980.0
Acetaminosalol	965.1	E850.3	E935.3	E950.0	E962.0	E980.0
Acetanilid(e)	965.4	E850.4	E935.4	E950.0	E962.0	E980.0
Acetarsol, acetarsone	961.1	E857	E931.1	E950.4	E962.0	E980.4
Acetazolamide	974.2	E858.5	E944.2	E950.4	E962.0	E980.4
Acetic						
acid	983.1	E864.1	—	E950.7	E962.1	E980.6
with sodium acetate (ointment)	976.3	E858.7	E946.3	E950.4	E962.0	E980.4
irrigating solution	974.5	E858.5	E944.5	E950.4	E962.0	E980.4
lotion	976.2	E858.7	E946.2	E950.4	E962.0	E980.4
anhydride	983.1	E864.1	—	E950.7	E962.1	E980.6
ether (vapor)	982.8	E862.4	—	E950.9	E962.1	E980.9
Acetohexamide	962.3	E858.0	E932.3	E950.4	E962.0	E980.4
Acetomenaphthone	964.3	E858.2	E934.3	E950.4	E962.0	E980.4
Acetomorphine	965.01	E850.0	E935.0	E950.0	E962.0	E980.0
Acetone (oils) (vapor)	982.8	E862.4	—	E950.9	E962.1	E980.9
Acetophenazine (maleate)	969.1	E853.0	E939.1	E950.3	E962.0	E980.3
Acetophenetidin	965.4	E850.4	E935.4	E950.0	E962.0	E980.0
Acetophenone	982.0	E862.4	—	E950.9	E962.1	E980.9
Acetorphine	965.09	E850.2	E935.2	E950.0	E962.0	E980.0
Acetosulfone (sodium)	961.8	E857	E931.8	E950.4	E962.0	E980.4
Acetrizoate (sodium)	977.8	E858.8	E947.8	E950.4	E962.0	E980.4
Acetylcarbromal	967.3	E852.2	E937.3	E950.2	E962.0	E980.2
Acetylcholine (chloride)	971.0	E855.3	E941.0	E950.4	E962.0	E980.4
Acetylcysteine	975.5	E858.6	E945.5	E950.4	E962.0	E980.4
Acetyldigitoxin	972.1	E858.3	E942.1	E950.4	E962.0	E980.4
Acetyldihydrocodeine	965.09	E850.2	E935.2	E950.0	E962.0	E980.0
Acetyldihydrocodeinone	965.09	E850.2	E935.2	E950.0	E962.0	E980.0
Acetylene (gas) (industrial)	987.1	E868.1	—	E951.8	E962.2	E981.8
incomplete combustion of — *see* Carbon monoxide, fuel, utility						
tetrachloride (vapor)	982.3	E862.4	—	E950.9	E962.1	E980.9
Acetyliodosalicylic acid	965.1	E850.3	E935.3	E950.0	E962.0	E980.0
Acetylphenylhydrazine	965.8	E850.8	E935.8	E950.0	E962.0	E980.0
Acetylsalicylic acid	965.1	E850.3	E935.3	E950.0	E962.0	E980.0
Achromycin	960.4	E856	E930.4	E950.4	E962.0	E980.4
ophthalmic preparation	976.5	E858.7	E946.5	E950.4	E962.0	E980.4
topical NEC	976.0	E858.7	E946.0	E950.4	E962.0	E980.4
Acidifying agents	963.2	E858.1	E933.2	E950.4	E962.0	E980.4
Acids (corrosive) NEC	983.1	E864.1	—	E950.7	E962.1	E980.6
Aconite (wild)	988.2	E865.4	—	E950.9	E962.1	E980.9
Aconitine (liniment)	976.8	E858.7	E946.8	E950.4	E962.0	E980.4

Substance	Poisoning	External Cause (E-Code) Accident	Therapeutic Use	Suicide Attempt	Assault	Undetermined
Aconitum ferox	988.2	E865.4	—	E950.9	E962.1	E980.9
Acridine	983.0	E864.0	—	E950.7	E962.1	E980.6
vapor	987.8	E869.8	—	E952.8	E962.2	E982.8
Acriflavine	961.9	E857	E931.9	E950.4	E962.0	E980.4
Acrisorcin	976.0	E858.7	E946.0	E950.4	E962.0	E980.4
Acrolein (gas)	987.8	E869.8	—	E952.8	E962.2	E982.8
liquid	989.8	E866.8	—	E950.9	E962.1	E980.9
Actaea spicata	988.2	E865.4	—	E950.9	E962.1	E980.9
Acterol	961.5	E857	E931.5	E950.4	E962.0	E980.4
ACTH	962.4	E858.0	E932.4	E950.4	E962.0	E980.4
Acthar	962.4	E858.0	E932.4	E950.4	E962.0	E980.4
Actinomycin (C) (D)	960.7	E856	E930.7	E950.4	E962.0	E980.4
Adalin (acetyl)	967.3	E852.2	E937.3	E950.2	E962.0	E980.2
Adenosine (phosphate)	977.8	E858.8	E947.8	E950.4	E962.0	E980.4
Adhesives	989.8	E866.6	—	E950.9	E962.1	E980.9
ADH	962.5	E858.0	E932.5	E950.4	E962.0	E980.4
Adicillin	960.0	E856	E930.0	E950.4	E962.0	E980.4
Adiphenine	975.1	E855.6	E945.1	E950.4	E962.0	E980.4
Adjunct, pharmaceutical	977.4	E858.8	E947.4	E950.4	E962.0	E980.4
Adrenal (extract, cortex or medulla) (glucocorticoids) (hormones) (mineralocorticoids)	962.0	E858.0	E932.0	E950.4	E962.0	E980.4
ENT agent	976.6	E858.7	E946.6	E950.4	E962.0	E980.4
ophthalmic preparation	976.5	E858.7	E946.5	E950.4	E962.0	E980.4
topical NEC	976.0	E858.7	E946.0	E950.4	E962.0	E980.4
Adrenalin	971.2	E855.5	E941.2	E950.4	E962.0	E980.4
Adrenergic blocking agents	971.3	E855.6	E941.3	E950.4	E962.0	E980.4
Adrenergics	971.2	E855.5	E941.2	E950.4	E962.0	E980.4
Adrenochrome (derivatives)	972.8	E858.3	E942.8	E950.4	E962.0	E980.4
Adrenocorticotropic hormone	962.4	E858.0	E932.4	E950.4	E962.0	E980.4
Adrenocorticotropin	962.4	E858.0	E932.4	E950.4	E962.0	E980.4
Adriamycin	960.7	E856	E930.7	E950.4	E962.0	E980.4
Aerosol spray — *see* Sprays						
Aerosporin	960.8	E856	E930.8	E950.4	E962.0	E980.4
ENT agent	976.6	E858.7	E946.6	E950.4	E962.0	E980.4
ophthalmic preparation	976.5	E858.7	E946.5	E950.4	E962.0	E980.4
topical NEC	976.0	E858.7	E946.0	E950.4	E962.0	E980.4
Aethusa cynapium	988.2	E865.4	—	E950.9	E962.1	E980.9
Afghanistan black	969.6	E854.1	E939.6	E950.3	E962.0	E980.3
Aflatoxin	989.7	E865.9	—	E950.9	E962.1	E980.9
African boxwood	988.2	E865.4	—	E950.9	E962.1	E980.9
Agar (-agar)	973.3	E858.4	E943.3	E950.4	E962.0	E980.4
Agricultural agent NEC	989.8	E863.9	—	E950.6	E962.1	E980.7
Agrypnal	967.0	E851	E937.0	E950.1	E962.0	E980.1
Air contaminant(s), source or type not specified	987.9	E869.9	—	E952.9	E962.2	E982.9
specified type — *see* specific substance						
Akee	988.2	E865.4	—	E950.9	E962.1	E980.9
Akrinol	976.0	E858.7	E946.0	E950.4	E962.0	E980.4
Alantolactone	961.6	E857	E931.6	E950.4	E962.0	E980.4
Albamycin	960.8	E856	E930.8	E950.4	E962.0	E980.4
Albumin (normal human serum)	964.7	E858.2	E934.7	E950.4	E962.0	E980.4
Alcohol	980.9	E860.9	—	E950.9	E962.1	E980.9
absolute	980.0	E860.1	—	E950.9	E962.1	E980.9
beverage	980.0	E860.0	E947.8	E950.9	E962.1	E980.9
amyl	980.3	E860.4	—	E950.9	E962.1	E980.9
antifreeze	980.1	E860.2	—	E950.9	E962.1	E980.9

Substance	Poisoning	External Cause (E-Code)				
		Accident	Therapeutic Use	Suicide Attempt	Assault	Undetermined
butyl	980.3	E860.4	—	E950.9	E962.1	E980.9
dehydrated	980.0	E860.1	—	E950.9	E862.1	E980.9
beverage	980.0	E860.0	E947.8	E950.9	E962.1	E980.9
denatured	980.0	E860.1	—	E950.9	E962.1	E980.9
deterrents	977.3	E858.8	E947.3	E950.4	E962.0	E980.4
diagnostic (gastric function)	977.8	E858.8	E947.8	E950.4	E962.0	E980.4
ethyl	980.0	E860.1	—	E950.9	E962.1	E980.9
beverage	980.0	E860.0	E947.8	E950.9	E962.1	E980.9
grain	980.0	E860.1	—	E950.9	E962.1	E980.9
beverage	980.0	E860.0	E947.8	E950.9	E962.1	E980.9
industrial	980.9	E860.9	—	E950.9	E962.1	E980.9
isopropyl	980.2	E860.3	—	E950.9	E962.1	E980.9
methyl	980.1	E860.2	—	E950.9	E962.1	E980.9
preparation for consumption	980.0	E860.0	E947.8	E950.9	E962.1	E980.9
propyl	980.3	E860.4	—	E950.9	E962.1	E980.9
secondary	980.2	E860.3	—	E950.9	E962.1	E980.9
radiator	980.1	E860.2	—	E950.9	E962.1	E980.9
rubbing	980.2	E860.3	—	E950.9	E962.1	E980.9
specified type NEC	980.8	E860.8	—	E950.9	E962.1	E980.9
surgical	980.9	E860.9	—	E950.9	E962.1	E980.9
vapor (from any type of alcohol)	987.8	E869.8	—	E952.8	E962.2	E982.8
wood	980.1	E860.2	—	E950.9	E962.1	E980.9
Alcuronium chloride	975.2	E858.6	E945.2	E950.4	E962.0	E980.4
Aldactone	974.4	E858.5	E944.4	E950.4	E962.0	E980.4
Aldicarb	989.3	E863.2	—	E950.6	E962.1	E980.7
Aldomet	972.6	E858.3	E942.6	E950.4	E962.0	E980.4
Aldosterone	962.0	E858.0	E932.0	E950.4	E962.0	E980.4
Aldrin (dust)	989.2	E863.0	—	E950.6	E962.1	E980.7
Algeldrate	973.0	E858.4	E943.0	E950.4	E962.0	E980.4
Alidase	963.4	E858.1	E933.4	E950.4	E962.0	E980.4
Aliphatic thiocyanates	989.0	E866.8	—	E950.9	E962.1	E980.9
Alkaline antiseptic solution (aromatic)	976.6	E858.7	E946.6	E950.4	E962.0	E980.4
Alkalinizing agents (medicinal)	963.3	E858.1	E933.3	E950.4	E962.0	E980.4
Alkalis, caustic	983.2	E864.2	—	E950.7	E962.1	E980.6
Alkalizing agents (medicinal)	963.3	E858.1	E933.3	E950.4	E962.0	E980.4
Alka–seltzer	965.1	E850.3	E935.3	E950.0	E962.0	E980.0
Alkavervir	972.6	E858.3	E942.6	E950.4	E962.0	E980.4
Allegron	969.0	E854.0	E939.0	E950.3	E962.0	E980.3
Allobarbital, allobarbitone	967.0	E851	E937.0	E950.1	E962.0	E980.1
Allopurinol	974.7	E858.5	E944.7	E950.4	E962.0	E980.4
Allylestrenol	962.2	E858.0	E932.2	E950.4	E962.0	E980.4
Allylisopropylacetylurea	967.8	E852.8	E937.8	E950.2	E962.0	E980.2
Allylisopropylmalonylurea	967.0	E851	E937.0	E950.1	E962.0	E980.1
Allyltribromide	967.3	E852.2	E937.3	E950.2	E962.0	E980.2
Aloe, aloes, aloin	973.1	E858.4	E943.1	E950.4	E962.0	E980.4
Aloxidone	966.0	E855.0	E936.0	E950.4	E962.0	E980.4
Aloxiprin	965.1	E850.3	E935.3	E950.0	E962.0	E980.0
Alpha amylase	963.4	E858.1	E933.4	E950.4	E962.0	E980.4
Alphaprodine (hydrochloride)	965.09	E850.2	E935.2	E950.0	E962.0	E980.0
Alpha tocopherol	963.5	E858.1	E933.5	E950.4	E962.0	E980.4
Alseroxylon	972.6	E858.3	E942.6	E950.4	E962.0	E980.4
Alum (ammonium) (potassium)	983.2	E864.2	—	E950.7	E962.1	E980.6
medicinal (astringent) NEC	976.2	E858.7	E946.2	E950.4	E962.0	E980.4
Aluminium, aluminum (gel) (hydroxide)	973.0	E858.4	E943.0	E950.4	E962.0	E980.4
acetate solution	976.2	E858.7	E946.2	E950.4	E962.0	E980.4
aspirin	965.1	E850.3	E935.3	E950.0	E962.0	E980.0
carbonate	973.0	E858.4	E943.0	E950.4	E962.0	E980.4

Substance	Poisoning	External Cause (E-Code): Accident	Therapeutic Use	Suicide Attempt	Assault	Undetermined
glycinate	973.0	E858.4	E943.0	E950.4	E962.0	E980.4
nicotinate	972.2	E858.3	E942.2	E950.4	E962.0	E980.4
ointment (surgical) (topical)	976.3	E858.7	E946.3	E950.4	E962.0	E980.4
phosphate	973.0	E858.4	E943.0	E950.4	E962.0	E980.4
subacetate	976.2	E858.7	E946.2	E950.4	E962.0	E980.4
topical NEC	976.3	E858.7	E946.3	E950.4	E962.0	E980.4
Alurate	967.0	E851	E937.0	E950.1	E962.0	E980.1
Alverine (citrate)	975.1	E858.6	E945.1	E950.4	E962.0	E980.4
Alvodine	965.09	E850.2	E935.2	E950.0	E962.0	E980.0
Amanita phalloides	988.1	E865.5	—	E950.9	E962.1	E980.9
Amantadine (hydrochloride)	966.4	E855.0	E936.4	E950.4	E962.0	E980.4
Ambazone	961.9	E857	E931.9	E950.4	E962.0	E980.4
Ambenonium	971.0	E855.3	E941.0	E950.4	E962.0	E980.4
Ambutonium bromide	971.1	E855.4	E941.1	E950.4	E962.0	E980.4
Ametazole	977.8	E858.8	E947.8	E950.4	E962.0	E980.4
Amethocaine (infiltration) (topical)	968.5	E855.2	E938.5	E950.4	E962.0	E980.4
nerve block (peripheral) (plexus)	968.6	E855.2	E938.6	E950.4	E962.0	E980.4
spinal	968.7	E855.2	E938.7	E950.4	E962.0	E980.4
Amethopterin	963.1	E858.1	E933.1	E950.4	E962.0	E980.4
Amfepramone	977.0	E858.8	E947.0	E950.4	E962.0	E980.4
Amidon	965.02	E850.1	E935.1	E950.0	E962.0	E980.0
Amidopyrine	965.5	E850.5	E935.5	E950.0	E962.0	E980.0
Aminacrine	976.0	E858.7	E946.0	E950.4	E962.0	E980.4
Aminitrozole	961.5	E857	E931.5	E950.4	E962.0	E980.4
Aminoacetic acid	974.5	E858.5	E944.5	E950.4	E962.0	E980.4
Amino acids	974.5	E858.5	E944.5	E950.4	E962.0	E980.4
Aminocaproic acid	964.4	E858.2	E934.4	E950.4	E962.0	E980.4
Aminoethylisothiourium	963.8	E858.1	E933.8	E950.4	E962.0	E980.4
Aminoglutethimide	966.3	E855.0	E936.3	E950.4	E962.0	E980.4
Aminometradine	974.3	E858.5	E944.3	E950.4	E962.0	E980.4
Aminopentamide	971.1	E855.4	E941.1	E950.4	E962.0	E980.4
Aminophenazone	965.5	E850.5	E935.5	E950.0	E962.0	E980.0
Aminophenol	983.0	E864.0	—	E950.7	E962.1	E980.6
Aminophenylpyridone	969.5	E853.8	E939.5	E950.3	E962.0	E980.3
Aminophyllin	975.7	E858.6	E945.7	E950.4	E962.0	E980.4
Aminopterin	963.1	E858.1	E933.1	E950.4	E962.0	E980.4
Aminopyrine	965.5	E850.5	E935.5	E950.0	E962.0	E980.0
Aminosalicylic acid	961.8	E857	E931.8	E950.4	E962.0	E980.4
Amiphenazole	970.1	E854.3	E940.1	E950.4	E962.0	E980.4
Amiquinsin	972.6	E858.3	E942.6	E950.4	E962.0	E980.4
Amisometradine	974.3	E858.5	E944.3	E950.4	E962.0	E980.4
Amitriptyline	969.0	E854.0	E939.0	E950.3	E962.0	E980.3
Ammonia (fumes) (gas) (vapor)	987.8	E869.8	—	E952.8	E962.2	E982.8
liquid (household) NEC	983.2	E861.4	—	E950.7	E962.1	E980.6
spirit, aromatic	970.8	E854.3	E940.8	E950.4	E962.0	E980.4
Ammoniated mercury	976.0	E858.7	E946.0	E950.4	E962.0	E980.4
Ammonium						
carbonate	983.2	E864.2	—	E950.7	E962.1	E980.6
chloride (acidifying agent)	963.2	E858.1	E933.2	E950.4	E962.0	E980.4
expectorant	975.5	E858.6	E945.5	E950.4	E962.0	E980.4
compounds (household) NEC	983.2	E861.4	—	E950.7	E962.1	E980.6
fumes (any usage)	987.8	E869.8	—	E952.8	E962.2	E982.8
industrial	983.2	E864.2	—	E950.7	E962.1	E980.6
ichthyosulfonate	976.4	E858.7	E946.4	E950.4	E962.0	E980.4
mandelate	961.9	E857	E931.9	E950.4	E962.0	E980.4
Amobarbital	967.0	E851	E937.0	E950.1	E962.0	E980.1
Amodiaquin(e)	961.4	E857	E931.4	E950.4	E962.0	E980.4

Substance	Poisoning	Accident	Therapeutic Use	Suicide Attempt	Assault	Undetermined
		External Cause (E-Code)				
Amopyroquin(e)	961.4	E857	E931.4	E950.4	E962.0	E980.4
Amphenidone	969.5	E853.8	E939.5	E950.3	E962.0	E980.3
Amphetamine	969.7	E854.2	E939.7	E950.3	E962.0	E980.3
Amphomycin	960.8	E856	E930.8	E950.4	E962.0	E980.4
Amphotericin B	960.1	E856	E930.1	E950.4	E962.0	E980.4
topical	976.0	E858.7	E946.0	E950.4	E962.0	E980.4
Ampicillin	960.0	E856	E930.0	E950.4	E962.0	E980.4
Amprotropine	971.1	E855.4	E941.1	E950.4	E962.0	E980.4
Amygdalin	977.8	E858.8	E947.8	E950.4	E962.0	E980.4
Amyl						
acetate (vapor)	982.8	E862.4	—	E950.9	E962.1	E980.9
alcohol	980.3	E860.4	—	E950.9	E962.1	E980.9
nitrite (medicinal)	972.4	E858.3	E942.4	E950.4	E962.0	E980.4
Amylase (alpha)	963.4	E858.1	E933.4	E950.4	E962.0	E980.4
Amylene hydrate	980.8	E860.8	—	E950.9	E962.1	E980.9
Amylobarbitone	967.0	E851	E937.0	E950.1	E962.0	E980.1
Amylocaine	968.9	E855.2	E938.9	E950.4	E962.0	E980.4
infiltration (subcutaneous)	968.5	E855.2	E938.5	E950.4	E962.0	E980.4
nerve block (peripheral) (plexus)	968.6	E855.2	E938.6	E950.4	E962.0	E980.4
spinal	968.7	E855.2	E938.7	E950.4	E962.0	E980.4
topical (surface)	968.5	E855.2	E938.5	E950.4	E962.0	E980.4
Amytal (sodium)	967.0	E851	E937.0	E950.1	E962.0	E980.1
Analeptics	970.0	E854.3	E940.0	E950.4	E962.0	E980.4
Analgesics	965.9	E850.9	E935.9	E950.0	E962.0	E980.0
aromatic NEC	965.4	E850.4	E935.4	E950.0	E962.0	E980.0
non–narcotic NEC	965.7	E850.7	E935.7	E950.0	E962.0	E980.0
specified NEC	965.8	E850.8	E935.8	E950.0	E962.0	E980.0
Anamirta cocculus	988.2	E865.3	—	E950.9	E962.1	E980.9
Ancillin	960.0	E856	E930.0	E950.4	E962.0	E980.4
Androgens (anabolic congeners)	962.1	E858.0	E932.1	E950.4	E962.0	E980.4
Androstalone	962.1	E858.0	E932.1	E950.4	E962.0	E980.4
Androsterone	962.1	E858.0	E932.1	E950.4	E962.0	E980.4
Anemone pulsatilla	988.2	E865.4	—	E950.9	E962.1	E980.9
Anesthesia, anesthetic (general) NEC	968.4	E855.1	E938.4	E950.4	E962.0	E980.4
block (nerve) (plexus)	968.6	E855.2	E938.6	E950.4	E962.0	E980.4
gaseous NEC	968.2	E855.1	E938.2	E950.4	E962.0	E980.4
halogenated hydrocarbon derivatives NEC	968.2	E855.1	E938.2	E950.4	E962.0	E980.4
infiltration (intradermal) (subcutaneous) (submucosal)	968.5	E855.2	E938.5	E950.4	E962.0	E980.4
intravenous	968.3	E855.1	E938.3	E950.4	E962.0	E980.4
local NEC	968.9	E855.2	E938.9	E950.4	E962.0	E980.4
nerve blocking (peripheral) (plexus)	968.6	E855.2	E938.6	E950.4	E962.0	E980.4
rectal NEC	968.3	E855.1	E938.3	E950.4	E962.0	E980.4
spinal	968.7	E855.2	E938.7	E950.4	E962.0	E980.4
surface	968.5	E855.2	E938.5	E950.4	E962.0	E980.4
topical	968.5	E855.2	E938.5	E950.4	E962.0	E980.4
Aneurine	963.5	E858.1	E933.5	E950.4	E962.0	E980.4
Angio–Conray	977.8	E858.8	E947.8	E950.4	E962.0	E980.4
Angiotensin	971.2	E855.5	E941.2	E950.4	E962.0	E980.4
Anhydrohydroxyprogesterone	962.2	E858.0	E932.2	E950.4	E962.0	E980.4
Anhydron	974.3	E858.5	E944.3	E950.4	E962.0	E980.4
Anileridine	965.09	E850.2	E935.2	E950.0	E962.0	E980.0
Aniline (dye) (liquid)	983.0	E864.0	—	E950.7	E962.1	E980.6
analgesic	965.4	E850.4	E935.4	E950.0	E962.0	E980.0
derivatives, therapeutic NEC	965.4	E850.4	E935.4	E950.0	E962.0	E980.0
vapor	987.8	E869.8	—	E952.8	E962.2	E982.8

Substance	Poisoning	External Cause (E-Code) Accident	Therapeutic Use	Suicide Attempt	Assault	Undetermined
Anisindione	964.2	E858.2	E934.2	E950.4	E962.0	E980.4
Anisotropine	971.1	E855.4	E941.1	E950.4	E962.0	E980.4
Anorexic agents	977.0	E858.8	E947.0	E950.4	E962.0	E980.4
Ant (bite) (sting)	989.5	E905.5	—	E950.9	E962.1	E980.9
Antabuse	977.3	E858.8	E947.3	E950.4	E962.0	E980.4
Antacids	973.0	E858.4	E943.0	E950.4	E962.0	E980.4
Antazoline	963.0	E858.1	E933.0	E950.4	E962.0	E980.4
Anthelmintics	961.6	E857	E931.6	E950.4	E962.0	E980.4
Anthralin	976.4	E858.7	E946.4	E950.4	E962.0	E980.4
Anthramycin	960.7	E856	E930.7	E950.4	E962.0	E980.4
Antiadrenergics	971.3	E855.6	E941.3	E950.4	E962.0	E980.4
Antiallergic agents	963.0	E858.1	E933.0	E950.4	E962.0	E980.4
Antianemic agents NEC	964.1	E858.2	E934.1	E950.4	E962.0	E980.4
Antiaris toxicaria	988.2	E865.4	—	E950.9	E962.1	E980.9
Antiarteriosclerotic agents	972.2	E858.3	E942.2	E950.4	E962.0	E980.4
Antiasthmatics	975.7	E858.6	E945.7	E950.4	E962.0	E980.4
Antibiotics	960.9	E856	E930.9	E950.4	E962.0	E980.4
antifungal	960.1	E856	E930.1	E950.4	E962.0	E980.4
antimycobacterial	960.6	E856	E930.6	E950.4	E962.0	E980.4
antineoplastic	960.7	E856	E930.7	E950.4	E962.0	E980.4
cephalosporin (group)	960.5	E856	E930.5	E950.4	E962.0	E980.4
chloramphenicol (group)	960.2	E856	E930.2	E950.4	E962.0	E980.4
macrolides	960.3	E856	E930.3	E950.4	E962.0	E980.4
specified NEC	960.8	E856	E930.8	E950.4	E962.0	E980.4
tetracycline (group)	960.4	E856	E930.4	E950.4	E962.0	E980.4
Anticancer agents NEC	963.1	E858.1	E933.1	E950.4	E962.0	E980.4
antibiotics	960.7	E856	E930.7	E950.4	E962.0	E980.4
Anticholinergics	971.1	E855.4	E941.1	E950.4	E962.0	E980.4
Anticholinesterase (organophosphorus) (reversible)	971.0	E855.3	E941.0	E950.4	E962.0	E980.4
Anticoagulants	964.2	E858.2	E934.2	E950.4	E962.0	E980.4
antagonists	964.5	E858.2	E934.5	E950.4	E962.0	E980.4
Anti–common cold agents NEC	975.6	E858.6	E945.6	E950.4	E962.0	E980.4
Anticonvulsants NEC	966.3	E855.0	E936.3	E950.4	E962.0	E980.4
Antidepressants	969.0	E854.0	E939.0	E950.3	E962.0	E980.3
Antidiabetic agents	962.3	E858.0	E932.3	E950.4	E962.0	E980.4
Antidiarrheal agents	973.5	E858.4	E943.5	E950.4	E962.0	E980.4
Antidiuretic hormone	962.5	E858.0	E932.5	E950.4	E962.0	E980.4
Antidotes NEC	977.2	E858.8	E947.2	E950.4	E962.0	E980.4
Antiemetic agents	963.0	E858.1	E933.0	E950.4	E962.0	E980.4
Antiepilepsy agent NEC	966.3	E855.0	E936.3	E950.4	E962.0	E980.4
Antifertility pills	962.2	E858.0	E932.2	E950.4	E962.0	E980.4
Antiflatulents	973.8	E858.4	E943.8	E950.4	E962.0	E980.4
Antifreeze	989.8	E866.8	—	E950.9	E962.1	E980.9
alcohol	980.1	E860.2	—	E950.9	E962.1	E980.9
ethylene glycol	982.8	E862.4	—	E950.9	E962.1	E980.9
Antifungals (nonmedicinal) (sprays)	989.4	E863.6	—	E950.6	E962.1	E980.7
medicinal NEC	961.9	E857	E931.9	E950.4	E962.0	E980.4
antibiotic	960.1	E856	E930.1	E950.4	E962.0	E980.4
topical	976.0	E858.7	E946.0	E950.4	E962.0	E980.4
Antigastric secretion agents	973.0	E858.4	E943.0	E950.4	E962.0	E980.4
Antihelmintics	961.6	E857	E931.6	E950.4	E962.0	E980.4
Antihemophilic factor (human)	964.7	E858.2	E934.7	E950.4	E962.0	E980.4
Antihistamine	963.0	E858.1	E933.0	E950.4	E962.0	E980.4
Antihypertensive agents NEC	972.6	E858.3	E942.6	E950.4	E962.0	E980.4
Anti–infectives NEC	961.9	E857	E931.9	E950.4	E962.0	E980.4
antibiotics	960.9	E856	E930.9	E950.4	E962.0	E980.4

Substance	Poisoning	Accident	Therapeutic Use	Suicide Attempt	Assault	Undetermined
		External Cause (E-Code)				
specified NEC	960.8	E856	E930.8	E950.4	E962.0	E980.4
antihelmintic	961.6	E857	E931.6	E950.4	E962.0	E980.4
antimalarial	961.4	E857	E931.4	E950.4	E962.0	E980.4
antimycobacterial NEC	961.8	E857	E931.8	E950.4	E962.0	E980.4
antibiotics	960.6	E856	E930.6	E950.4	E962.0	E980.4
antiprotozoal NEC	961.5	E857	E931.5	E950.4	E962.0	E980.4
blood	961.4	E857	E931.4	E950.4	E962.0	E980.4
antiviral	961.7	E857	E931.7	E950.4	E962.0	E980.4
arsenical	961.1	E857	E931.1	E950.4	E962.0	E980.4
ENT agents	976.6	E858.7	E946.6	E950.4	E962.0	E980.4
heavy metals NEC	961.2	E857	E931.2	E950.4	E962.0	E980.4
local	976.0	E858.7	E946.0	E950.4	E962.0	E980.4
ophthalmic preparation	976.5	E858.7	E946.5	E950.4	E962.0	E980.4
topical NEC	976.0	E858.7	E946.0	E950.4	E962.0	E980.4
Anti–inflammatory agents (topical)	976.0	E858.7	E946.0	E950.4	E962.0	E980.4
Antiknock (tetraethyl lead)	984.1	E862.1	—	E950.9	E962.1	E980.9
Antilipemics	972.2	E858.3	E942.2	E950.4	E962.0	E980.4
Antimalarials	961.4	E857	E931.4	E950.4	E962.0	E980.4
Antimony (compounds) (vapor) NEC	985.4	E866.2	—	E950.9	E962.1	E980.9
anti–infectives	961.2	E857	E931.2	E950.4	E962.0	E980.4
pesticides (vapor)	985.4	E863.4	—	E950.6	E962.2	E980.7
potassium tartrate	961.2	E857	E931.2	E950.4	E962.0	E980.4
tartrated	961.2	E857	E931.2	E950.4	E962.0	E980.4
Antimuscarinic agents	971.1	E855.4	E941.1	E950.4	E962.0	E980.4
Antimycobacterials NEC	961.8	E857	E931.8	E950.4	E962.0	E980.4
antibiotics	960.6	E856	E930.6	E950.4	E962.0	E980.4
Antineoplastic agents	963.1	E858.1	E933.1	E950.4	E962.0	E980.4
antibiotics	960.7	E856	E930.7	E950.4	E962.0	E980.4
Anti–Parkinsonism agents	966.4	E855.0	E936.4	E950.4	E962.0	E980.4
Antiphlogistics	965.6	E850.6	E935.6	E950.0	E962.0	E980.0
Antiprotozoals NEC	961.5	E857	E931.5	E950.4	E962.0	E980.4
blood	961.4	E857	E931.4	E950.4	E962.0	E980.4
Antipruritics (local)	976.1	E858.7	E946.1	E950.4	E962.0	E980.4
Antipsychotic agents NEC	969.3	E853.8	E939.3	E950.3	E962.0	E980.3
Antipyretics	965.9	E850.9	E935.9	E950.0	E962.0	E980.0
specified NEC	965.8	E850.8	E935.8	E950.0	E962.0	E980.0
Antipyrine	965.5	E850.5	E935.5	E950.0	E962.0	E980.0
Antirabies serum (equine)	979.9	E858.8	E949.9	E950.4	E962.0	E980.4
Antirheumatics	965.6	E850.6	E935.6	E950.0	E962.0	E980.0
Antiseborrheics	976.4	E858.7	E946.4	E950.4	E962.0	E980.4
Antiseptics (external) (medicinal)	976.0	E858.7	E946.0	E950.4	E962.0	E980.4
Antistine	963.0	E858.1	E933.0	E950.4	E962.0	E980.4
Antithyroid agents	962.8	E858.0	E932.8	E950.4	E962.0	E980.4
Antitoxin, any	979.9	E858.8	E949.9	E950.4	E962.0	E980.4
Antituberculars	961.8	E857	E931.8	E950.4	E962.0	E980.4
antibiotics	960.6	E856	E930.6	E950.4	E962.0	E980.4
Antitussives	975.4	E858.6	E945.5	E950.4	E962.0	E980.4
Antivaricose agents (sclerosing)	972.7	E858.3	E942.7	E950.4	E962.0	E980.4
Antivenin (crotaline) (spider–bite)	979.9	E858.8	E949.9	E950.4	E962.0	E980.4
Antivert	963.0	E858.1	E933.0	E950.4	E962.0	E980.4
Antivirals NEC	961.7	E857	E931.7	E950.4	E962.0	E980.4
Ant poisons — *see* Pesticides						
Antrol	989.4	E863.4	—	E950.6	E962.1	E980.7
fungicide	989.4	E863.6	—	E950.6	E962.1	E980.7
Apomorphine hydrochloride (emetic)	973.6	E858.4	E943.6	E950.4	E962.0	E980.4
Appetite depressants, central	977.0	E858.8	E947.0	E950.4	E962.0	E980.4
Apresoline	972.6	E858.3	E942.6	E950.4	E962.0	E980.4

Substance	Poisoning	External Cause (E-Code)				
		Accident	Therapeutic Use	Suicide Attempt	Assault	Undetermined
Aprobarbital, aprobarbitone	967.0	E851	E937.0	E950.1	E962.0	E980.1
Apronalide	967.8	E852.8	E937.8	E950.2	E962.0	E980.2
Aqua fortis	983.1	E864.1	—	E950.7	E962.1	E980.6
Arachis oil (topical)	976.3	E858.7	E946.3	E950.4	E962.0	E980.4
cathartic	973.2	E858.4	E943.2	E950.4	E962.0	E980.4
Aralen	961.4	E857	E931.4	E950.4	E962.0	E980.4
Arginine salts	974.5	E858.5	E944.5	E950.4	E962.0	E980.4
Argyrol	976.0	E858.7	E946.0	E950.4	E962.0	E980.4
ENT agent	976.6	E858.7	E946.6	E950.4	E962.0	E980.4
ophthalmic preparation	976.5	E858.7	E946.5	E950.4	E962.0	E980.4
Aristocort	962.0	E858.0	E932.0	E950.4	E962.0	E980.4
ENT agent	976.6	E858.7	E946.6	E950.4	E962.0	E980.4
ophthalmic preparation	976.5	E858.7	E946.5	E950.4	E962.0	E980.4
topical NEC	976.0	E858.7	E946.0	E950.4	E962.0	E980.4
Aromatics, corrosive	983.0	E864.0	—	E950.7	E962.1	E980.6
disinfectants	983.0	E861.4	—	E950.7	E962.1	E980.6
Arsenate of lead (insecticide)	985.1	E863.4	—	E950.8	E962.1	E980.8
herbicide	985.1	E863.5	—	E950.8	E962.1	E980.8
Arsenic, arsenicals (compounds) (dust) (fumes) (vapor) NEC	985.1	E866.3	—	E950.8	E962.1	E980.8
anti–infectives	961.1	E857	E931.1	E950.4	E962.0	E980.4
pesticide (dust) (fumes)	985.1	E863.4	—	E950.8	E962.1	E980.8
Arsine (gas)	985.1	E866.3	—	E950.8	E962.1	E980.8
Arsphenamine (silver)	961.1	E857	E931.1	E950.4	E962.0	E980.4
Arsthinol	961.1	E857	E931.1	E950.4	E962.0	E980.4
Artane	971.1	E855.4	E941.1	E950.4	E962.0	E980.4
Arthropod (venomous) NEC	989.5	E905.5	—	E950.9	E962.1	E980.9
Ascaridole	961.6	E857	E931.6	E950.4	E962.0	E980.4
Ascorbic acid	963.5	E858.1	E933.5	E950.4	E962.0	E980.4
Asiaticoside	976.0	E858.7	E946.0	E950.4	E962.0	E980.4
Aspidium (oleoresin)	961.6	E857	E931.6	E950.4	E962.0	E980.4
Aspirin	965.1	E850.3	E935.3	E950.0	E962.0	E980.0
Astringents (local)	976.2	E858.7	E946.2	E950.4	E962.0	E980.4
Atabrine	961.3	E857	E931.3	E950.4	E962.0	E980.4
Ataractics	969.5	E853.8	E939.5	E950.3	E962.0	E980.3
Atonia drug, intestinal	973.3	E858.4	E943.3	E950.4	E962.0	E980.4
Atophan	974.7	E858.5	E944.7	E950.4	E962.0	E980.4
Atropine	971.1	E855.4	E941.1	E950.4	E962.0	E980.4
Attapulgite	973.5	E858.4	E943.5	E950.4	E962.0	E980.4
Attenuvax	979.4	E858.8	E949.4	E950.4	E962.0	E980.4
Aureomycin	960.4	E856	E930.4	E950.4	E962.0	E980.4
ophthalmic preparation	976.5	E858.7	E946.5	E950.4	E962.0	E980.4
topical NEC	976.0	E858.7	E946.0	E950.4	E962.0	E980.4
Aurothioglucose	965.6	E850.6	E935.6	E950.0	E962.0	E980.0
Aurothioglycanide	965.6	E850.6	E935.6	E950.0	E962.0	E980.0
Aurothiomalate	965.6	E850.6	E935.6	E950.0	E962.0	E980.0
Automobile fuel	981	E862.1	—	E950.9	E962.1	E980.9
Autonomic nervous system agents NEC	971.9	E855.9	E941.9	E950.4	E962.0	E980.4
Avlosulfon	961.8	E857	E931.8	E950.4	E962.0	E980.4
Avomine	967.8	E852.8	E937.8	E950.2	E962.0	E980.2
Azacyclonol	969.5	E853.8	E939.5	E950.3	E962.0	E980.3
Azapetine	971.3	E855.6	E941.3	E950.4	E962.0	E980.4
Azaribine	963.1	E858.1	E933.1	E950.4	E962.0	E980.4
Azaserine	960.7	E856	E930.7	E950.4	E962.0	E980.4
Azathioprine	963.1	E858.1	E933.1	E950.4	E962.0	E980.4
Azosulfamide	961.0	E857	E931.0	E950.4	E962.0	E980.4
Azulfidine	961.0	E857	E931.0	E950.4	E962.0	E980.4

Substance	Poisoning	External Cause (E-Code)				
		Accident	Therapeutic Use	Suicide Attempt	Assault	Undetermined
Azuresin	977.8	E858.8	E947.8	E950.4	E962.0	E980.4
Bacimycin	976.0	E858.7	E946.0	E950.4	E962.0	E980.4
ophthalmic preparation	976.5	E858.7	E946.5	E950.4	E962.0	E980.4
Bacitracin	960.8	E856	E930.8	E950.4	E962.0	E980.4
ENT agent	976.6	E858.7	E946.6	E950.4	E962.0	E980.4
ophthalmic preparation	976.5	E858.7	E946.5	E950.4	E962.0	E980.4
topical NEC	976.0	E858.7	E946.0	E950.4	E962.0	E980.4
Baking soda	963.3	E858.1	E933.3	E950.4	E962.0	E980.4
BAL	963.8	E858.1	E933.8	E950.4	E962.0	E980.4
Bamethan (sulfate)	972.5	E858.3	E942.5	E950.4	E962.0	E980.4
Bamipine	963.0	E858.1	E933.0	E950.4	E962.0	E980.4
Baneberry	988.2	E865.4	—	E950.9	E962.1	E980.9
Banewort	988.2	E865.4	—	E950.9	E962.1	E980.9
Barbenyl	967.0	E851	E937.0	E950.1	E962.0	E980.1
Barbital, barbitone	967.0	E851	E937.0	E950.1	E962.0	E980.1
Barbiturates, barbituric acid	967.0	E851	E937.0	E950.1	E962.0	E980.1
anesthetic (intravenous)	968.3	E855.1	E938.3	E950.4	E962.0	E980.4
Barium (carbonate) (chloride) (sulfate)	985.8	E866.4	—	E950.9	E962.1	E980.9
diagnostic agent	977.8	E858.8	E947.8	E950.4	E962.0	E980.4
pesticide	985.8	E863.4	—	E950.6	E962.1	E980.7
rodenticide	985.8	E863.7	—	E950.6	E962.1	E980.7
Barrier cream	976.3	E858.7	E946.3	E950.4	E962.0	E980.4
Battery acid or fluid	983.1	E864.1	—	E950.7	E962.1	E980.6
Bay rum	980.8	E860.8	—	E950.9	E962.1	E980.9
BCG vaccine	978.0	E858.8	E948.0	E950.4	E962.0	E980.4
Bearsfoot	988.2	E865.4	—	E950.9	E962.1	E980.9
Beclamide	966.3	E855.0	E936.3	E950.4	E962.0	E980.4
Bee (sting) (venom)	989.5	E905.3	—	E950.9	E962.1	E980.9
Belladonna (alkaloids)	971.1	E855.4	E941.1	E950.4	E962.0	E980.4
Bemegride	970.0	E854.3	E940.0	E950.4	E962.0	E980.4
Benactyzine	969.8	E855.8	E939.8	E950.3	E962.0	E980.3
Benadryl	963.0	E858.1	E933.0	E950.4	E962.0	E980.4
Bendrofluazide	974.3	E858.5	E944.3	E950.4	E962.0	E980.4
Bendroflumethiazide	974.3	E858.5	E944.3	E950.4	E962.0	E980.4
Benemid	974.7	E858.5	E944.7	E950.4	E962.0	E980.4
Benethamine penicillin G	960.0	E856	E930.0	E950.4	E962.0	E980.4
Benisone	976.0	E858.7	E946.0	E950.4	E962.0	E980.4
Benoquin	976.8	E858.7	E946.8	E950.4	E962.0	E980.4
Benoxinate	968.5	E855.2	E938.5	E950.4	E962.0	E980.4
Bentonite	976.3	E858.7	E946.3	E950.4	E962.0	E980.4
Benzalkonium (chloride)	976.0	E858.7	E946.0	E950.4	E962.0	E980.4
ophthalmic preparation	976.5	E858.7	E946.5	E950.4	E962.0	E980.4
Benzamidosalicylate (calcium)	961.8	E857	E931.8	E950.4	E962.0	E980.4
Benzathine penicillin	960.0	E856	E930.0	E950.4	E962.0	E980.4
Benzcarbimine	963.1	E858.1	E933.1	E950.4	E962.0	E980.4
Benzedrex	971.2	E855.5	E941.2	E950.4	E962.0	E980.4
Benzedrine (amphetamine)	969.7	E854.2	E939.7	E950.3	E962.0	E980.3
Benzene (acetyl) (dimethyl) (methyl) (solvent) (vapor)	982.0	E862.4	—	E950.9	E962.1	E980.9
hexachloride (gamma) (insecticide) (vapor)	989.2	E863.0	—	E950.6	E962.1	E980.7
Benzethonium	976.0	E858.7	E946.0	E950.4	E962.0	E980.4
Benzhexol (chloride)	966.4	E855.0	E936.4	E950.4	E962.0	E980.4
Benzilonium	971.1	E855.4	E941.1	E950.4	E962.0	E980.4
Benzin(e) — *see* Ligroin						
Benziodarone	972.4	E858.3	E942.4	E950.4	E962.0	E980.4
Benzocaine	968.5	E855.2	E938.5	E950.4	E962.0	E980.4

Substance	Poisoning	Accident	Therapeutic Use	Suicide Attempt	Assault	Undetermined
		External Cause (E-Code)				
Benzodiapin	969.4	E853.2	E939.4	E950.3	E962.0	E980.3
Benzodiazepines (tranquilizers) NEC	969.4	E853.2	E939.4	E950.3	E962.0	E980.3
Benzoic acid (with salicylic acid) (anti–infective)	976.0	E858.7	E946.0	E950.4	E962.0	E980.4
Benzoin	976.3	E858.7	E946.3	E950.4	E962.0	E980.4
Benzol (vapor)	982.0	E862.4	—	E950.9	E962.1	E980.9
Benzomorphan	965.09	E850.2	E935.2	E950.0	E962.0	E980.0
Benzonatate	975.4	E858.6	E945.4	E950.4	E962.0	E980.4
Benzothiadiazides	974.3	E858.5	E944.3	E950.4	E962.0	E980.4
Benzoylpas	961.8	E857	E931.8	E950.4	E962.0	E980.4
Benzperidol	969.5	E853.8	E939.5	E950.3	E962.0	E980.3
Benzphetamine	977.0	E858.8	E947.0	E950.4	E962.0	E980.4
Benzpyrinium	971.0	E855.3	E941.0	E950.4	E962.0	E980.4
Benzquinamide	963.0	E858.1	E933.0	E950.4	E962.0	E980.4
Benzthiazide	974.3	E858.5	E944.3	E950.4	E962.0	E980.4
Benztropine	971.1	E855.4	E941.1	E950.4	E962.0	E980.4
Benzyl						
acetate	982.8	E862.4	—	E950.9	E962.1	E980.9
benzoate (anti–infective)	976.0	E858.7	E946.0	E950.4	E962.0	E980.4
morphine	965.09	E850.2	E935.2	E950.0	E962.0	E980.0
penicillin	960.0	E856	E930.0	E950.4	E962.0	E980.4
Bephenium hydroxynapthoate	961.6	E857	E931.6	E950.4	E962.0	E980.4
Bergamot oil	989.8	E866.8	—	E950.9	E962.1	E980.9
Berries, poisonous	988.2	E865.3	—	E950.9	E962.1	E980.9
Beryllium (compounds) (fumes)	985.3	E866.4	—	E950.9	E962.1	E980.9
Beta–carotene	976.3	E858.7	E946.3	E950.4	E962.0	E980.4
Beta–Chlor	967.1	E852.0	E937.1	E950.2	E962.0	E980.2
Betamethasone	962.0	E858.0	E932.0	E950.4	E962.0	E980.4
topical	976.0	E858.7	E946.0	E950.4	E962.0	E980.4
Betazole	977.8	E858.8	E947.8	E950.4	E962.0	E980.4
Bethanechol	971.0	E855.3	E941.0	E950.4	E962.0	E980.4
Bethanidine	972.6	E858.3	E942.6	E950.4	E962.0	E980.4
Betula oil	976.3	E858.7	E946.3	E950.4	E962.0	E980.4
Bhang	969.6	E854.1	E939.6	E950.3	E962.0	E980.3
Bialamicol	961.5	E857	E931.5	E950.4	E962.0	E980.4
Bichloride of mercury — *see* Mercury, chloride						
Bichromates (calcium) (crystals) (potassium) (sodium)	983.9	E864.3	—	E950.7	E962.1	E980.6
fumes	987.8	E869.8	—	E952.8	E962.2	E982.8
Biguanide derivatives, oral	962.3	E858.0	E932.3	E950.4	E962.0	E980.4
Biligrafin	977.8	E858.8	E947.8	E950.4	E962.0	E980.4
Bilopaque	977.8	E858.8	E947.8	E950.4	E962.0	E980.4
Bioflavonoids	972.8	E858.3	E942.8	E950.4	E962.0	E980.4
Biological substance NEC	979.9	E858.8	E949.9	E950.4	E962.0	E980.4
Biperiden	966.4	E855.0	E936.4	E950.4	E962.0	E980.4
Bisacodyl	973.1	E858.4	E943.1	E950.4	E962.0	E980.4
Bishydroxycoumarin	964.2	E858.2	E934.2	E950.4	E962.0	E980.4
Bismarsen	961.1	E857	E931.1	E950.4	E962.0	E980.4
Bismuth (compounds) NEC	985.8	E866.4	—	E950.9	E962.1	E980.9
anti–infectives	961.2	E857	E931.2	E950.4	E962.0	E980.4
subcarbonate	973.5	E858.4	E943.5	E950.4	E962.0	E980.4
sulfarsphenamine	961.1	E857	E931.1	E950.4	E962.0	E980.4
Bithionol	961.6	E857	E931.6	E950.4	E962.0	E980.4
Bitter almond oil	989.0	E866.8	—	E950.9	E962.1	E980.9
Bittersweet	988.2	E865.4	—	E950.9	E962.1	E980.9
Black						

Substance	Poisoning	External Cause (E-Code) Accident	Therapeutic Use	Suicide Attempt	Assault	Undetermined
flag	989.4	E863.4	—	E950.6	E962.1	E980.7
henbane	988.2	E865.4	—	E950.9	E962.1	E980.9
leaf (40)	989.4	E863.4	—	E950.6	E962.1	E980.7
widow spider (bite)	989.5	E905.1	—	E950.9	E962.1	E980.9
antivenin	979.9	E858.8	E949.9	E950.4	E962.0	E980.4
Blast furnace gas (carbon monoxide from)	986	E868.8	—	E952.1	E962.2	E982.1
Bleach NEC	983.9	E864.3	—	E950.7	E962.1	E980.6
Bleaching solutions	983.9	E864.3	—	E950.7	E962.1	E980.6
Bleomycin (sulfate)	960.7	E856	E930.7	E950.4	E962.0	E980.4
Blockain	968.9	E855.2	E938.9	E950.4	E962.0	E980.4
infiltration (subcutaneous)	968.5	E855.2	E938.5	E950.4	E962.0	E980.4
nerve block (peripheral) (plexus)	968.6	E855.2	E938.6	E950.4	E962.0	E980.4
topical (surface)	968.5	E855.2	E938.5	E950.4	E962.0	E980.4
Blood (derivatives) (natural) (plasma) (whole)	964.7	E858.2	E934.7	E950.4	E962.0	E980.4
affecting agent	964.9	E858.2	E934.9	E950.4	E962.0	E980.4
specified NEC	964.8	E858.2	E934.8	E950.4	E962.0	E980.4
substitute (macromolecular)	964.8	E858.2	E934.8	E950.4	E962.0	E980.4
Blue velvet	965.09	E850.2	E935.2	E950.0	E962.0	E980.0
Bone meal	989.8	E866.5	—	E950.9	E962.1	E980.9
Bonine	963.0	E858.1	E933.0	E950.4	E962.0	E980.4
Boracic acid	976.0	E858.7	E946.0	E950.4	E962.0	E980.4
ENT agent	976.6	E858.7	E946.6	E950.4	E962.0	E980.4
ophthalmic preparation	976.5	E858.7	E946.5	E950.4	E962.0	E980.4
Borate (cleanser) (sodium)	989.6	E861.3	—	E950.9	E962.1	E980.9
Borax (cleanser)	989.6	E861.3	—	E950.9	E962.1	E980.9
Boric acid	976.0	E858.7	E946.0	E950.4	E962.0	E980.4
ENT agent	976.6	E858.7	E946.6	E950.4	E962.0	E980.4
ophthalmic preparation	976.5	E858.7	E946.5	E950.4	E962.0	E980.4
Boron hydride NEC	989.8	E866.8	—	E950.9	E962.1	E980.9
fumes or gas	987.8	E869.8	—	E952.8	E962.2	E982.8
Brake fluid vapor	987.8	E869.8	—	E952.8	E962.2	E982.8
Brass (compounds) (fumes)	985.8	E866.4	—	E950.9	E962.1	E980.9
Brasso	981	E861.3	—	E950.9	E962.1	E980.9
Bretylium (tosylate)	972.6	E858.3	E942.6	E950.4	E962.0	E980.4
Brevital (sodium)	968.3	E855.1	E938.3	E950.4	E962.0	E980.4
British antilewisite	963.8	E858.1	E933.8	E950.4	E962.0	E980.4
Bromal (hydrate)	967.3	E852.2	E937.3	E950.2	E962.0	E980.2
Bromelains	963.4	E858.1	E933.4	E950.4	E962.0	E980.4
Bromides NEC	967.3	E852.2	E937.3	E950.2	E962.0	E980.2
Bromine (vapor)	987.8	E869.8	—	E952.8	E962.2	E982.8
compounds (medicinal)	967.3	E852.2	E937.3	E950.2	E962.0	E980.2
Bromisovalum	967.3	E852.2	E937.3	E950.2	E962.0	E980.2
Bromobenzyl cyanide	987.5	E869.3	—	E952.8	E962.2	E982.8
Bromodiphenhydramine	963.0	E858.1	E933.0	E950.4	E962.0	E980.4
Bromoform	967.3	E852.2	E937.3	E950.2	E962.0	E980.2
Bromophenol blue reagent	977.8	E858.8	E947.8	E950.4	E962.0	E980.4
Bromosalicylhydroxamic acid	961.8	E857	E931.8	E950.4	E962.0	E980.4
Bromo–seltzer	965.4	E850.4	E935.4	E950.0	E962.0	E980.0
Brompheniramine	963.0	E858.1	E933.0	E950.4	E962.0	E980.4
Bromural	967.3	E852.2	E937.3	E950.2	E962.0	E980.2
Brown spider (bite) (venom)	989.5	E905.1	—	E950.9	E962.1	E980.9
Brucia	988.2	E865.3	—	E950.9	E962.1	E980.9
Brucine	989.1	E863.7	—	E950.6	E962.1	E980.7
Brunswick green — *see* Copper						
Bryonia (alba) (dioica)	988.2	E865.4	—	E950.9	E962.1	E980.9
Buclizine	969.5	E853.8	E939.5	E950.3	E962.0	E980.3

Substance	Poisoning	External Cause (E-Code) Accident	Therapeutic Use	Suicide Attempt	Assault	Undetermined
Bufferin	965.1	E850.3	E935.3	E950.0	E962.0	E980.0
Bufotenine	969.6	E854.1	E939.6	E950.3	E962.0	E980.3
Buphenine	971.2	E855.5	E941.2	E950.4	E962.0	E980.4
Bupivacaine	968.9	E855.2	E938.9	E950.4	E962.0	E980.4
infiltration (subcutaneous)	968.5	E855.2	E938.5	E950.4	E962.0	E980.4
nerve block (peripheral) (plexus)	968.6	E855.2	E938.6	E950.4	E962.0	E980.4
Busulfan	963.1	E858.1	E933.1	E950.4	E962.0	E980.4
Butabarbital (sodium)	967.0	E851	E937.0	E950.1	E962.0	E980.1
Butabarbitone	967.0	E851	E937.0	E950.1	E962.0	E980.1
Butabarpal	967.0	E851	E937.0	E950.1	E962.0	E980.1
Butacaine	968.5	E855.2	E938.5	E950.4	E962.0	E980.4
Butallylonal	967.0	E851	E937.0	E950.1	E962.0	E980.1
Butane (distributed in mobile container)	987.0	E868.0	—	E951.1	E962.2	E981.1
distributed through pipes	987.0	E867	—	E951.0	E962.2	E981.0
incomplete combustion of — *see* Carbon monoxide, butane						
Butanol	980.3	E860.4	—	E950.9	E962.1	E980.9
Butanone	982.8	E862.4	—	E950.9	E962.1	E980.9
Butaperazine	969.1	E853.0	E939.1	E950.3	E962.0	E980.3
Butazolidin	965.5	E850.5	E935.5	E950.0	E962.0	E980.0
Butethal	967.0	E851	E937.0	E950.1	E962.0	E980.1
Butethamate	971.1	E855.4	E941.1	E950.4	E962.0	E980.4
Buthalitone (sodium)	968.3	E855.1	E938.3	E950.4	E962.0	E980.4
Butisol (sodium)	967.0	E851	E937.0	E950.1	E962.0	E980.1
Butobarbital, butobarbitone	967.0	E851	E937.0	E950.1	E962.0	E980.1
Butriptyline	969.0	E854.0	E939.0	E950.3	E962.0	E980.3
Buttercups	988.2	E865.4	—	E950.9	E962.1	E980.9
Butter of antimony — *see* Antimony						
Butyl						
acetate (secondary)	982.8	E862.4	—	E950.9	E962.1	E980.9
alcohol	980.3	E860.4	—	E950.9	E962.1	E980.9
carbinol	980.8	E860.8	—	E950.9	E962.1	E980.9
carbitol	982.8	E862.4	—	E950.9	E962.1	E980.9
cellosolve	982.8	E862.4	—	E950.9	E962.1	E980.9
chloral (hydrate)	967.1	E852.0	E937.1	E950.2	E962.0	E980.2
formate	982.8	E862.4	—	E950.9	E962.1	E980.9
scopolammonium bromide	971.1	E855.4	E941.1	E950.4	E962.0	E980.4
Butyn	968.5	E855.2	E938.5	E950.4	E962.0	E980.4
Butyrophenone (–based tranquilizers)	969.2	E853.1	E939.2	E950.3	E962.0	E980.3
Cacodyl, cacodylic acid — *see* Arsenic						
Cactinomycin	960.7	E856	E930.7	E950.4	E962.0	E980.4
Cade oil	976.4	E858.7	E946.4	E950.4	E962.0	E980.4
Cadmium (chloride) (compounds) (dust) (fumes) (oxide)	985.5	E866.4	—	E950.9	E962.1	E980.9
sulfide (medicinal) NEC	976.4	E858.7	E946.4	E950.4	E962.0	E980.4
Caffeine	969.7	E854.2	E939.7	E950.3	E962.0	E980.3
Calabar bean	988.2	E865.4	—	E950.9	E962.1	E980.9
Caladium seguinium	988.2	E865.4	—	E950.9	E962.1	E980.9
Calamine (liniment) (lotion)	976.3	E858.7	E946.3	E950.4	E962.0	E980.4
Calciferol	963.5	E858.1	E933.5	E950.4	E962.0	E980.4
Calcium (salts) NEC	974.5	E858.5	E944.5	E950.4	E962.0	E980.4
acetylsalicylate	965.1	E850.3	E935.3	E950.0	E962.0	E980.0
benzamidosalicylate	961.8	E857	E931.8	E950.4	E962.0	E980.4
carbaspirin	965.1	E850.3	E935.3	E950.0	E962.0	E980.0
carbamide (citrated)	977.3	E858.8	E947.3	E950.4	E962.0	E980.4
carbonate (antacid)	973.0	E858.4	E943.0	E950.4	E962.0	E980.4
cyanide (citrated)	977.3	E858.8	E947.3	E950.4	E962.0	E980.4

Substance	Poisoning	External Cause (E-Code) Accident	Therapeutic Use	Suicide Attempt	Assault	Undetermined
dioctyl sulfosuccinate	973.2	E858.4	E943.2	E950.4	E962.0	E980.4
disodium edathamil	963.8	E858.1	E933.8	E950.4	E962.0	E980.4
disodium edetate	963.8	E858.1	E933.8	E950.4	E962.0	E980.4
EDTA	963.8	E858.1	E933.8	E950.4	E962.0	E980.4
hydrate, hydroxide	983.2	E864.2	—	E950.7	E962.1	E980.6
mandelate	961.9	E857	E931.9	E950.4	E962.0	E980.4
oxide	983.2	E864.2	—	E950.7	E962.1	E980.6
Calomel — *see* Mercury, chloride						
Caloric agents NEC	974.5	E858.5	E944.5	E950.4	E962.0	E980.4
Calusterone	963.1	E858.1	E933.1	E950.4	E962.0	E980.4
Camoquin	961.4	E857	E931.4	E950.4	E962.0	E980.4
Camphor (oil)	976.1	E858.7	E946.1	E950.4	E962.0	E980.4
Candeptin	976.0	E858.7	E946.0	E950.4	E962.0	E980.4
Candicidin	976.0	E858.7	E946.0	E950.4	E962.0	E980.4
Cannabinols	969.6	E854.1	E939.6	E950.3	E962.0	E980.3
Cannabis (derivatives) (indica) (sativa)	969.6	E854.1	E939.6	E950.3	E962.0	E980.3
Canned heat	980.1	E860.2	—	E950.9	E962.1	E980.9
Cantharides, cantharidin, cantharis	976.8	E858.7	E946.8	E950.4	E962.0	E980.4
Capillary agents	972.8	E858.3	E942.8	E950.4	E962.0	E980.4
Capreomycin	960.6	E856	E930.6	E950.4	E962.0	E980.4
Captodiame, captodiamine	969.5	E853.8	E939.5	E950.3	E962.0	E980.3
Caramiphen (hydrochloride)	971.1	E855.4	E941.1	E950.4	E962.0	E980.4
Carbachol	971.0	E855.3	E941.0	E950.4	E962.0	E980.4
Carbacrylamine resins	974.5	E858.5	E944.5	E950.4	E962.0	E980.4
Carbamate (sedative)	967.8	E852.8	E937.8	E950.2	E962.0	E980.2
herbicide	989.3	E863.5	—	E950.6	E962.1	E980.7
insecticide	989.3	E863.2	—	E950.6	E962.1	E980.7
Carbamazepine	966.3	E855.0	E936.3	E950.4	E962.0	E980.4
Carbamic esters	967.8	E852.8	E937.8	E950.2	E962.0	E980.2
Carbamide	974.4	E858.5	E944.4	E950.4	E962.0	E980.4
topical	976.8	E858.7	E946.8	E950.4	E962.0	E980.4
Carbamylcholine chloride	971.0	E855.3	E941.0	E950.4	E962.0	E980.4
Carbarsone	961.1	E857	E931.1	E950.4	E962.0	E980.4
Carbaryl	989.3	E863.2	—	E950.6	E962.1	E980.7
Carbaspirin	965.1	E850.3	E935.3	E950.0	E962.0	E980.0
Carbazochrome	972.8	E858.3	E942.8	E950.4	E962.0	E980.4
Carbenicillin	960.0	E856	E930.0	E950.4	E962.0	E980.4
Carbenoxolone	973.8	E858.4	E943.8	E950.4	E962.0	E980.4
Carbetapentane	975.4	E858.6	E945.4	E950.4	E962.0	E980.4
Carbimazole	962.8	E858.0	E932.8	E950.4	E962.0	E980.4
Carbinol	980.1	E860.2	—	E950.9	E962.1	E980.9
Carbinoxamine	963.0	E858.1	E933.0	E950.4	E962.0	E980.4
Carbitol	982.8	E862.4	—	E950.9	E962.1	E980.9
Carbocaine	968.9	E855.2	E938.9	E950.4	E962.0	E980.4
infiltration (subcutaneous)	968.5	E855.2	E938.5	E950.4	E962.0	E980.4
nerve block (peripheral) (plexus)	968.6	E855.2	E938.6	E950.4	E962.0	E980.4
topical (surface)	968.5	E855.2	E938.5	E950.4	E962.0	E980.4
Carbol-fuchsin solution	976.0	E858.7	E946.0	E950.4	E962.0	E980.4
Carbolic acid (*see also* Phenol)	983.0	E864.0	—	E950.7	E962.1	E980.6
Carbomycin	960.8	E856	E930.8	E950.4	E962.0	E980.4
Carbon						
bisulfide (liquid) (vapor)	982.2	E862.4	—	E950.9	E962.1	E980.9
dioxide (gas)	987.8	E869.8	—	E952.8	E962.2	E982.8
disulfide (liquid) (vapor)	982.2	E862.4	—	E950.9	E962.1	E980.9
monoxide (from incomplete combustion of) (in) NEC	986	E868.9	—	E952.1	E962.2	E982.1
blast furnace gas	986	E868.8	—	E952.1	E962.2	E982.1

Substance	Poisoning	Accident	Therapeutic Use	Suicide Attempt	Assault	Undetermined
		External Cause (E-Code)				
butane (distributed in mobile container)	986	E868.0	—	E951.1	E962.2	E981.1
distributed through pipes	986	E867	—	E951.0	E962.2	E981.0
charcoal fumes	986	E868.3	—	E952.1	E962.2	E982.1
coal						
gas (piped)	986	E867	—	E951.0	E962.2	E981.0
solid (in domestic stoves, fireplaces)	986	E868.3	—	E952.1	E962.2	E982.1
coke (in domestic stoves, fireplaces)	986	E868.3	—	E952.1	E962.2	E982.1
exhaust gas (motor) not in transit	986	E868.2	—	E952.0	E962.2	E982.0
combustion engine, any not in watercraft	986	E868.2	—	E952.0	E962.2	E982.0
farm tractor, not in transit	986	E868.2	—	E952.0	E962.2	E982.0
gas engine	986	E868.2	—	E952.0	E962.2	E982.0
motor pump	986	E868.2	—	E952.0	E962.2	E982.0
motor vehicle, not in transit	986	E868.2	—	E952.0	E962.2	E982.0
fuel (in domestic use)	986	E868.3	—	E952.1	E962.2	E982.1
gas (piped)	986	E867	—	E951.0	E962.2	E981.0
in mobile container	986	E868.0	—	E951.1	E962.2	E981.1
utility	986	E868.1	—	E951.8	E962.2	E981.1
in mobile container	986	E868.0	—	E951.1	E962.2	E981.1
piped (natural)	986	E867	—	E951.0	E962.2	E981.0
illuminating gas	986	E868.1	—	E951.8	E962.2	E981.8
industrial fuels or gases, any	986	E868.8	—	E952.1	E962.2	E982.1
kerosene (in domestic stoves, fireplaces)	986	E868.3	—	E952.1	E962.2	E982.1
kiln gas or vapor	986	E868.8	—	E952.1	E962.2	E982.1
motor exhaust gas, not in transit	986	E868.2	—	E952.0	E962.2	E982.0
piped gas (manufactured) (natural)	986	E867	—	E951.0	E962.2	E981.0
producer gas	986	E868.8	—	E952.1	E962.2	E982.1
propane (distributed in mobile container)	986	E868.0	—	E951.1	E962.2	E981.1
distributed through pipes	986	E867	—	E951.0	E962.2	E981.0
specified source NEC	986	E868.8	—	E952.1	E962.2	E982.1
stove gas	986	E868.1	—	E951.8	E962.2	E981.8
piped	986	E867	—	E951.0	E962.2	E981.0
utility gas	986	E868.1	—	E951.8	E962.2	E981.8
piped	986	E867	—	E951.0	E962.2	E981.0
water gas	986	E868.1	—	E951.8	E962.2	E981.8
wood (in domestic stoves, fireplaces)	986	E868.3	—	E952.1	E962.2	E982.1
tetrachloride (vapor) NEC	987.8	E869.8	—	E952.8	E962.2	E982.8
liquid (cleansing agent) NEC	982.1	E861.3	—	E950.9	E962.1	E980.9
solvent	982.1	E862.4	—	E950.9	E962.1	E980.9
Carbonic acid (gas)	987.8	E869.8	—	E952.8	E962.2	E982.8
anhydrase inhibitors	974.2	E858.5	E944.2	E950.4	E962.0	E980.4
Carbowax	976.3	E858.7	E946.3	E950.4	E962.0	E980.4
Carbrital	967.0	E851	E937.0	E950.1	E962.0	E980.1
Carbromal (derivatives)	967.3	E852.2	E937.3	E950.2	E962.0	E980.2
Cardiac						
depressants	972.0	E858.3	E942.0	E950.4	E962.0	E980.4
rhythm regulators	972.0	E858.3	E942.0	E950.4	E962.0	E980.4
Cardiografin	977.8	E858.8	E947.8	E950.4	E962.0	E980.4
Cardio-green	977.8	E858.8	E947.8	E950.4	E962.0	E980.4
Cardiotonic glycosides	972.1	E858.3	E942.1	E950.4	E962.0	E980.4
Cardiovascular agents NEC	972.9	E858.3	E942.9	E950.4	E962.0	E980.4
Cardrase	974.2	E858.5	E944.2	E950.4	E962.0	E980.4
Carfusin	976.0	E858.7	E946.0	E950.4	E962.0	E980.4

Substance	Poisoning	External Cause (E-Code)				
		Accident	Therapeutic Use	Suicide Attempt	Assault	Undetermined
Carisoprodol	968.0	E855.1	E938.0	E950.4	E962.0	E980.4
Carmustine	963.1	E858.1	E933.1	E950.4	E962.0	E980.4
Carotene	963.5	E858.1	E933.5	E950.4	E962.0	E980.4
Carphenazine (maleate)	969.1	E853.0	E939.1	E950.3	E962.0	E980.3
Carter's Little Pills	973.1	E858.4	E943.1	E950.4	E962.0	E980.4
Cascara (sagrada)	973.1	E858.4	E943.1	E950.4	E962.0	E980.4
Cassava	988.2	E865.4	—	E950.9	E962.1	E980.9
Castellani's paint	976.0	E858.7	E946.0	E950.4	E962.0	E980.4
Castor						
bean	988.2	E865.3	—	E950.9	E962.1	E980.9
oil	973.1	E858.4	E943.1	E950.4	E962.0	E980.4
Caterpillar (sting)	989.5	E905.5	—	E950.9	E962.1	E980.9
Catha (edulis)	970.8	E854.3	E940.8	E950.4	E962.0	E980.4
Cathartics NEC	973.3	E858.4	E943.3	E950.4	E962.0	E980.4
contact	973.1	E858.4	E943.1	E950.4	E962.0	E980.4
emollient	973.2	E858.4	E943.2	E950.4	E962.0	E980.4
intestinal irritants	973.1	E858.4	E943.1	E950.4	E962.0	E980.4
saline	973.3	E858.4	E943.3	E950.4	E962.0	E980.4
Cathomycin	960.8	E856	E930.8	E950.4	E962.0	E980.4
Caustic(s)	983.9	E864.4	—	E950.7	E962.1	E980.6
alkali	983.2	E864.2	—	E950.7	E962.1	E980.6
hydroxide	983.2	E864.2	—	E950.7	E962.1	E980.6
potash	983.2	E864.2	—	E950.7	E962.1	E980.6
soda	983.2	E864.2	—	E950.7	E962.1	E980.6
specified NEC	983.9	E864.3	—	E950.7	E962.1	E980.6
Ceepryn	976.0	E858.7	E946.0	E950.4	E962.0	E980.4
ENT agent	976.6	E858.7	E946.6	E950.4	E962.0	E980.4
lozenges	976.6	E858.7	E946.6	E950.4	E962.0	E980.4
Celestone	962.0	E858.0	E932.0	E950.4	E962.0	E980.4
topical	976.0	E858.7	E946.0	E950.4	E962.0	E980.4
Cellosolve	982.8	E862.4	—	E950.9	E962.1	E980.9
Cell stimulants and proliferants	976.8	E858.7	E946.8	E950.4	E962.0	E980.4
Cellulose derivatives, cathartic	973.3	E858.4	E943.3	E950.4	E962.0	E980.4
nitrates (topical)	976.3	E858.7	E946.3	E950.4	E962.0	E980.4
Centipede (bite)	989.5	E905.4	—	E950.9	E962.1	E980.9
Central nervous system						
depressants	968.4	E855.1	E938.4	E950.4	E962.0	E980.4
anesthetic (general) NEC	968.4	E855.1	E938.4	E950.4	E962.0	E980.4
gases NEC	968.2	E855.1	E938.2	E950.4	E962.0	E980.4
intravenous	968.3	E855.1	E938.3	E950.4	E962.0	E980.4
barbiturates	967.0	E851	E937.0	E950.1	E962.0	E980.1
bromides	967.3	E852.2	E937.3	E950.2	E962.0	E980.2
cannabis sativa	969.6	E854.1	E939.6	E950.3	E962.0	E980.3
chloral hydrate	967.1	E852.0	E937.1	E950.2	E962.0	E980.2
hallucinogenics	969.6	E854.1	E939.6	E950.3	E962.0	E980.3
hypnotics	967.9	E852.9	E937.9	E950.2	E962.0	E980.2
specified NEC	967.8	E852.8	E937.8	E950.2	E962.0	E980.2
muscle relaxants	968.0	E855.1	E938.0	E950.4	E962.0	E980.4
paraldehyde	967.2	E852.1	E937.2	E950.2	E962.0	E980.2
sedatives	967.9	E852.9	E937.9	E950.2	E962.0	E980.2
mixed NEC	967.6	E852.5	E937.6	E950.2	E962.0	E980.2
specified NEC	967.8	E852.8	E937.8	E950.2	E962.0	E980.2
muscle–tone depressants	968.0	E855.1	E938.0	E950.4	E962.0	E980.4
stimulants	970.9	E854.3	E940.9	E950.4	E962.0	E980.4
amphetamines	969.7	E854.2	E939.7	E950.3	E962.0	E980.3
analeptics	970.0	E854.3	E940.0	E950.4	E962.0	E980.4
antidepressants	969.0	E854.0	E939.0	E950.3	E962.0	E980.3

Substance	Poisoning	Accident	Therapeutic Use	Suicide Attempt	Assault	Undetermined
		External Cause (E-Code)				
opiate antagonists	970.1	E854.3	E940.0	E950.4	E962.0	E980.4
specified NEC	970.8	E854.3	E940.8	E950.4	E962.0	E980.4
Cephalexin	960.5	E856	E930.5	E950.4	E962.0	E980.4
Cephaloglycin	960.5	E856	E930.5	E950.4	E962.0	E980.4
Cephaloridine	960.5	E856	E930.5	E950.4	E962.0	E980.4
Cephalosporins NEC	960.5	E856	E930.5	E950.4	E962.0	E980.4
N (adicillin)	960.0	E856	E930.0	E950.4	E962.0	E980.4
Cephalothin (sodium)	960.5	E856	E930.5	E950.4	E962.0	E980.4
Cerbera (odallam)	988.2	E865.4	—	E950.9	E962.1	E980.9
Cerberin	972.1	E858.3	E942.1	E950.4	E962.0	E980.4
Cerebral stimulants	970.9	E854.3	E940.9	E950.4	E962.0	E980.4
psychotherapeutic	969.7	E854.2	E939.7	E950.3	E962.0	E980.3
specified NEC	970.8	E854.3	E940.8	E950.4	E962.0	E980.4
Cetalkonium (chloride)	976.0	E858.7	E946.0	E950.4	E962.0	E980.4
Cetoxime	963.0	E858.1	E933.0	E950.4	E962.0	E980.4
Cetrimide	976.2	E858.7	E946.2	E950.4	E962.0	E980.4
Cetylpyridinium	976.0	E858.7	E946.0	E950.4	E962.0	E980.4
ENT agent	976.6	E858.7	E946.6	E950.4	E962.0	E980.4
lozenges	976.6	E858.7	E946.6	E950.4	E962.0	E980.4
Cevadilla — *see* Sabadilla						
Cevitamic acid	963.5	E858.1	E933.5	E950.4	E962.0	E980.4
Chalk, precipitated	973.0	E858.4	E943.0	E950.4	E962.0	E980.4
Charcoal						
fumes (carbon monoxide)	986	E868.3	—	E952.1	E962.2	E982.1
industrial	986	E868.8	—	E952.1	E962.2	E982.1
medicinal (activated)	973.0	E858.4	E943.0	E950.4	E962.0	E980.4
Chelating agents NEC	977.2	E858.8	E947.2	E950.4	E962.0	E980.4
Chelidonium majus	988.2	E865.4	—	E950.9	E962.1	E980.9
Chemical substance	989.9	E866.9	—	E950.9	E962.1	E980.9
specified NEC	989.8	E866.8	—	E950.9	E962.1	E980.9
Chenopodium (oil)	961.6	E857	E931.6	E950.4	E962.0	E980.4
Cherry laurel	988.2	E865.4	—	E950.9	E962.1	E980.9
Chiniofon	961.3	E857	E931.3	E950.4	E962.0	E980.4
Chlophedianol	975.4	E858.6	E945.4	E950.4	E962.0	E980.4
Chloral (betaine) (formamide) (hydrate)	967.1	E852.0	E937.1	E950.2	E962.0	E980.2
Chloralamide	967.1	E852.0	E937.1	E950.2	E962.0	E980.2
Chlorambucil	963.1	E858.1	E933.1	E950.4	E962.0	E980.4
Chloramphenicol	960.2	E856	E930.2	E950.4	E962.0	E980.4
ENT agent	976.6	E858.7	E946.6	E950.4	E962.0	E980.4
ophthalmic preparation	976.5	E858.7	E946.5	E950.4	E962.0	E980.4
topical NEC	976.0	E858.7	E946.0	E950.4	E962.0	E980.4
Chlorate(s) (potassium) (sodium) NEC	983.9	E864.3	—	E950.7	E962.1	E980.6
herbicides	989.4	E863.5	—	E950.6	E962.1	E980.7
Chlorcyclizine	963.0	E858.1	E933.0	E950.4	E962.0	E980.4
Chlordan(e) (dust)	989.2	E863.0	—	E950.6	E962.1	E980.7
Chlordantoin	976.0	E858.7	E946.0	E950.4	E962.0	E980.4
Chlordiazepoxide	969.4	E853.2	E939.4	E950.3	E962.0	E980.3
Chloresium	976.8	E858.7	E946.8	E950.4	E962.0	E980.4
Chlorethiazol	967.1	E852.0	E937.1	E950.2	E962.0	E980.2
Chlorethyl — *see* Ethyl, chloride						
Chloretone	967.1	E852.0	E937.1	E950.2	E962.0	E980.2
Chlorex	982.3	E862.4	—	E950.9	E962.1	E980.9
Chlorhexadol	967.1	E852.0	E937.1	E950.2	E962.0	E980.2
Chlorhexidine (hydrochloride)	976.0	E858.7	E946.0	E950.4	E962.0	E980.4
Chlorhydroxyquinolin	976.0	E858.7	E946.0	E950.4	E962.0	E980.4
Chloride of lime (bleach)	983.9	E864.3	—	E950.7	E962.1	E980.6
Chlorinated						

Substance	Poisoning	External Cause (E-Code) Accident	Therapeutic Use	Suicide Attempt	Assault	Undetermined
camphene	989.2	E863.0	—	E950.6	E962.1	E980.7
diphenyl	989.8	E866.8	—	E950.9	E962.1	E980.9
hydrocarbons NEC	989.2	E863.0	—	E950.6	E962.1	E980.7
solvent	982.3	E862.4	—	E950.9	E962.1	E980.9
lime (bleach)	983.9	E864.3	—	E950.7	E962.1	E980.6
naphthalene — *see* Naphthalene						
pesticides NEC	989.2	E863.0	—	E950.6	E962.1	E980.7
soda — *see* Sodium, hypochlorite						
Chlorine (fumes) (gas)	987.6	E869.8	—	E952.8	E962.2	E982.8
bleach	983.9	E864.3	—	E950.7	E962.1	E980.6
compounds NEC	983.9	E864.3	—	E950.7	E962.1	E980.6
disinfectant	983.9	E861.4	—	E950.7	E962.1	E980.6
releasing agents NEC	983.9	E864.3	—	E950.7	E962.1	E980.6
Chlorisondamine	972.3	E858.3	E942.3	E950.4	E962.0	E980.4
Chlormadinone	962.2	E858.0	E932.2	E950.4	E962.0	E980.4
Chlormerodrin	974.0	E858.5	E944.0	E950.4	E962.0	E980.4
Chlormethiazole	967.1	E852.0	E937.1	E950.2	E962.0	E980.2
Chlormethylenecycline	960.4	E856	E930.4	E950.4	E962.0	E980.4
Chlormezanone	969.5	E853.8	E939.5	E950.3	E962.0	E980.3
Chloroacetophenone	987.5	E869.3	—	E952.8	E962.2	E982.8
Chloroaniline	983.0	E864.0	—	E950.7	E962.1	E980.6
Chlorobenzene, chlorobenzol	982.0	E862.4	—	E950.9	E962.1	E980.9
Chlorobutanol	967.1	E852.0	E937.1	E950.2	E962.0	E980.2
Chlorodinitrobenzene	983.0	E864.0	—	E950.7	E962.1	E980.6
dust or vapor	987.8	E869.8	—	E952.8	E962.2	E982.8
Chloroethane — *see* Ethyl, chloride						
Chloroform (fumes) (vapor)	987.8	E869.8	—	E952.8	E962.2	E982.8
anesthetic (gas)	968.2	E855.1	E938.2	E950.4	E962.0	E980.4
liquid NEC	968.4	E855.1	E938.4	E950.4	E962.0	E980.4
solvent	982.3	E862.4	—	E950.9	E962.1	E980.9
Chloroguanide	961.4	E857	E931.4	E950.4	E962.0	E980.4
Chloromycetin	960.2	E856	E930.2	E950.4	E962.0	E980.4
ENT agent	976.6	E858.7	E946.6	E950.4	E962.0	E980.4
ophthalmic preparation	976.5	E858.7	E946.5	E950.4	E962.0	E980.4
otic solution	976.6	E858.7	E946.6	E950.4	E962.0	E980.4
topical NEC	976.0	E858.7	E946.0	E950.4	E962.0	E980.4
Chloronitrobenzene	983.0	E864.0	—	E950.7	E962.1	E980.6
dust or vapor	987.8	E869.8	—	E952.8	E962.2	E982.8
Chlorophenol	983.0	E864.0	—	E950.7	E962.1	E980.6
Chlorophenothane	989.2	E863.0	—	E950.6	E962.1	E980.7
Chlorophyll (derivatives)	976.8	E858.7	E946.8	E950.4	E962.0	E980.4
Chloropicrin (fumes)	987.8	E869.8	—	E952.8	E962.2	E982.8
fumigant	989.4	E863.8	—	E950.6	E962.1	E980.7
fungicide	989.4	E863.6	—	E950.6	E962.1	E980.7
pesticide (fumes)	989.4	E863.4	—	E950.6	E962.1	E980.7
Chloroprocaine	968.9	E855.2	E938.9	E950.4	E962.0	E980.4
infiltration (subcutaneous)	968.5	E855.2	E938.5	E950.4	E962.0	E980.4
nerve block (peripheral) (plexus)	968.6	E855.2	E938.6	E950.4	E962.0	E980.4
Chloroptic	976.5	E858.7	E946.5	E950.4	E962.0	E980.4
Chloropurine	963.1	E858.1	E933.1	E950.4	E962.0	E980.4
Chloroquine (hydrochloride) (phosphate)	961.4	E857	E931.4	E950.4	E962.0	E980.4
Chlorothen	963.0	E858.1	E933.0	E950.4	E962.0	E980.4
Chlorothiazide	974.3	E858.5	E944.3	E950.4	E962.0	E980.4
Chlorotrianisene	962.2	E858.0	E932.2	E950.4	E962.0	E980.4
Chlorovinyldichloroarsine	985.1	E866.3	—	E950.8	E962.1	E980.8
Chloroxylenol	976.0	E858.7	E946.0	E950.4	E962.0	E980.4
Chlorphenesin (carbamate)	968.0	E855.1	E938.0	E950.4	E962.0	E980.4

Substance	Poisoning	Accident	Therapeutic Use	Suicide Attempt	Assault	Undetermined
		External Cause (E-Code)				
topical (antifungal)	976.0	E858.7	E946.0	E950.4	E962.0	E980.4
Chloropheniramine	963.0	E858.1	E933.0	E950.4	E962.0	E980.4
Chlorophenoxamine	966.4	E855.0	E936.4	E950.4	E962.0	E980.4
Chlorophentermine	977.0	E858.8	E947.0	E950.4	E962.0	E980.4
Chlorproguanil	961.4	E857	E931.4	E950.4	E962.0	E980.4
Chlorpromazine	969.1	E853.0	E939.1	E950.3	E962.0	E980.3
Chlorpropamide	962.3	E858.0	E932.3	E950.4	E962.0	E980.4
Chlorprothixene	969.3	E853.8	E939.3	E950.3	E962.0	E980.3
Chlorquinaldol	976.0	E858.7	E946.0	E950.4	E962.0	E980.4
Chlortetracycline	960.4	E856	E930.4	E950.4	E962.0	E980.4
Chlorthalidone	974.4	E858.5	E944.4	E950.4	E962.0	E980.4
Chlortrianisene	962.2	E858.0	E932.2	E950.4	E962.0	E980.4
Chlor–Trimeton	963.0	E858.1	E933.0	E950.4	E962.0	E980.4
Chlorzoxazone	968.0	E855.1	E938.0	E950.4	E962.0	E980.4
Choke damp	987.8	E869.8	—	E952.8	E962.2	E982.8
Cholebrine	977.8	E858.8	E947.8	E950.4	E962.0	E980.4
Cholera vaccine	978.2	E858.8	E948.2	E950.4	E962.0	E980.4
Cholesterol–lowering agents	972.2	E858.3	E942.2	E950.4	E962.0	E980.4
Cholestyramine (resin)	972.2	E858.3	E942.2	E950.4	E962.0	E980.4
Cholic acid	973.4	E858.4	E943.4	E950.4	E962.0	E980.4
Choline						
dihydrogen citrate	977.1	E858.8	E947.1	E950.4	E962.0	E980.4
salicylate	965.1	E850.3	E935.3	E950.0	E962.0	E980.0
theophyllinate	974.1	E858.5	E944.1	E950.4	E962.0	E980.4
Cholinergics	971.0	E855.3	E941.0	E950.4	E962.0	E980.4
Chografin	977.8	E858.8	E947.8	E950.4	E962.0	E980.4
Chorionic gonadotropin	962.4	E858.0	E932.4	E950.4	E962.0	E980.4
Chromates	983.9	E864.3	—	E950.7	E962.1	E980.6
dust or mist	987.8	E869.8	—	E952.8	E962.2	E982.8
lead	984.0	E866.0	—	E950.9	E962.1	E980.9
paint	984.0	E861.5	—	E950.9	E962.1	E980.9
Chromic acid	983.9	E864.3	—	E950.7	E962.1	E980.6
dust or mist	987.8	E869.8	—	E952.8	E962.2	E982.8
Chromium	985.6	E866.4	—	E950.9	E962.1	E980.9
compounds — *see* Chromates						
Chromonar	972.4	E858.3	E942.4	E950.4	E962.0	E980.4
Chromyl chloride	983.9	E864.3	—	E950.7	E962.1	E980.6
Chrysarobin (ointment)	976.4	E858.7	E946.4	E950.4	E962.0	E980.4
Chrysazin	973.1	E858.4	E943.1	E950.4	E962.0	E980.4
Chymar	963.4	E858.1	E933.4	E950.4	E962.0	E980.4
ophthalmic preparation	976.5	E858.7	E946.5	E950.4	E962.0	E980.4
Chymotrypsin	963.4	E858.1	E933.4	E950.4	E962.0	E980.4
ophthalmic preparation	976.5	E858.7	E946.5	E950.4	E962.0	E980.4
Cicuta maculata or virosa	988.2	E865.4	—	E950.9	E962.1	E980.9
Cigarette lighter fluid	981	E862.1	—	E950.9	E962.1	E980.9
Cinchocaine (spinal)	968.7	E855.2	E938.7	E950.4	E962.0	E980.4
topical (surface)	968.5	E855.2	E938.5	E950.4	E962.0	E980.4
Cinchona	961.4	E857	E931.4	E950.4	E962.0	E980.4
Cinchonine alkaloids	961.4	E857	E931.4	E950.4	E962.0	E980.4
Cinchophen	974.7	E858.5	E944.7	E950.4	E962.0	E980.4
Cinnarizine	963.0	E858.1	E933.0	E950.4	E962.0	E980.4
Citanest	968.9	E855.2	E938.9	E950.4	E962.0	E980.4
infiltration (subcutaneous)	968.5	E855.2	E938.5	E950.4	E962.0	E980.4
nerve block (peripheral) (plexus)	968.6	E855.2	E938.6	E950.4	E962.0	E980.4
Citric acid	989.8	E866.8	—	E950.9	E962.1	E980.9
Citrovorum factor	964.1	E858.2	E934.1	E950.4	E962.0	E980.4
Claviceps purpurea	988.2	E865.4	—	E950.9	E962.1	E980.9

Substance	Poisoning	Accident	Therapeutic Use	Suicide Attempt	Assault	Undetermined
		External Cause (E-Code)				
Cleaner, cleansing agent NEC	989.8	E861.3	—	E950.9	E962.1	E980.9
of paint or varnish	982.8	E862.9	—	E950.9	E962.1	E980.9
Clematis vitalba	988.2	E865.4	—	E950.9	E962.1	E980.9
Clemizole	963.0	E858.1	E933.0	E950.4	E962.0	E980.4
penicillin	960.0	E856	E930.0	E950.4	E962.0	E980.4
Clidinium	971.1	E855.4	E941.1	E950.4	E962.0	E980.4
Clindamycin	960.8	E856	E930.8	E950.4	E962.0	E980.4
Cliradon	965.09	E850.2	E935.2	E950.0	E962.0	E980.0
Clocortolone	962.0	E858.0	E932.0	E950.4	E962.0	E980.4
Clofedanol	975.4	E858.6	E945.4	E950.4	E962.0	E980.4
Clofibrate	972.2	E858.3	E942.2	E950.4	E962.0	E980.4
Clomethiazole	967.1	E852.0	E937.1	E950.2	E962.0	E980.2
Clomiphene	977.8	E858.8	E947.8	E950.4	E962.0	E980.4
Clonazepam	969.4	E853.2	E939.4	E950.3	E962.0	E980.3
Clonidine	972.6	E858.3	E942.6	E950.4	E962.0	E980.4
Clopamide	974.3	E858.5	E944.3	E950.4	E962.0	E980.4
Clorazepate	969.4	E853.2	E939.4	E950.3	E962.0	E980.3
Clorexolone	974.4	E858.5	E944.4	E950.4	E962.0	E980.4
Clorox (bleach)	983.9	E864.3	—	E950.7	E962.1	E980.6
Clortermine	977.0	E858.8	E947.0	E950.4	E962.0	E980.4
Clotrimazole	976.0	E858.7	E946.0	E950.4	E962.0	E980.4
Cloxacillin	960.0	E856	E930.0	E950.4	E962.0	E980.4
Coagulants NEC	964.5	E858.2	E934.5	E950.4	E962.0	E980.4
Coal (carbon monoxide from) — *see also* Carbon, monoxide, coal						
oil — *see* Kerosene						
tar NEC	983.0	E864.0	—	E950.7	E962.1	E980.6
fumes	987.8	E869.8	—	E952.8	E962.2	E982.8
medicinal (ointment)	976.4	E858.7	E946.4	E950.4	E962.0	E980.4
analgesics NEC	965.5	E850.5	E935.5	E950.0	E962.0	E980.0
naphtha (solvent)	981	E862.0	—	E950.9	E962.1	E980.9
Cobalt (fumes) (industrial)	985.8	E866.4	—	E950.9	E962.1	E980.9
Cobra (venom)	989.5	E905.0	—	E950.9	E962.1	E980.9
Coca (leaf)	970.8	E854.3	E940.8	E950.4	E962.0	E980.4
Cocaine (hydrochloride) (salt)	968.5	E855.2	E938.5	E950.4	E962.0	E980.4
Coccidioidin	977.8	E858.8	E947.8	E950.4	E962.0	E980.4
Cocculus indicus	988.2	E865.3	—	E950.9	E962.1	E980.9
Cochineal	989.8	E866.8	—	E950.9	E962.1	E980.9
medicinal products	977.4	E858.8	E947.4	E950.4	E962.0	E980.4
Codeine	965.09	E850.2	E935.2	E950.0	E962.0	E980.0
Coffee	989.8	E866.8	—	E950.9	E962.1	E980.9
Cogentin	971.1	E855.4	E941.1	E950.4	E962.0	E980.4
Coke fumes or gas (carbon monoxide)	986	E868.3	—	E952.1	E962.2	E982.1
industrial use	986	E868.8	—	E952.1	E962.2	E982.1
Colace	973.2	E858.4	E943.2	E950.4	E962.0	E980.4
Colchicine	974.7	E858.5	E944.7	E950.4	E962.0	E980.4
Colchicum	988.2	E865.3	—	E950.9	E962.1	E980.9
Cold cream	976.3	E858.7	E946.3	E950.4	E962.0	E980.4
Colestipol	972.2	E858.3	E942.2	E950.4	E962.0	E980.4
Colistimethate	960.8	E856	E930.8	E950.4	E962.0	E980.4
Colistin	960.8	E856	E930.8	E950.4	E962.0	E980.4
Collagenase	976.8	E858.7	E946.8	E950.4	E962.0	E980.4
Collodion (flexible)	976.3	E858.7	E946.3	E950.4	E962.0	E980.4
Colocynth	973.1	E858.4	E943.1	E950.4	E962.0	E980.4
Coloring matter — *see* Dye(s)						
Combustion gas — *see* Carbon, monoxide						
Compazine	969.1	E853.0	E939.1	E950.3	E962.0	E980.3

Substance	Poisoning	Accident	Therapeutic Use	Suicide Attempt	Assault	Undetermined
		External Cause (E-Code)				
Compound						
42 (warfarin)	989.4	E863.7	—	E950.6	E962.1	E980.7
269 (endrin)	989.2	E863.0	—	E950.6	E962.1	E980.7
497 (dieldrin)	989.2	E863.0	—	E950.6	E962.1	E980.7
1080 (sodium fluoroacetate)	989.4	E863.7	—	E950.6	E962.1	E980.7
3422 (parathion)	989.3	E863.1	—	E950.6	E962.1	E980.7
3911 (phorate)	989.3	E863.1	—	E950.6	E962.1	E980.7
3956 (toxaphene)	989.2	E863.0	—	E950.6	E962.1	E980.7
4049 (malathion)	989.3	E863.1	—	E950.6	E962.1	E980.7
4124 (dicapthon)	989.4	E863.4	—	E950.6	E962.1	E980.7
E (cortisone)	962.0	E858.0	E932.0	E950.4	E962.0	E980.4
F (hydrocortisone)	962.0	E858.0	E932.0	E950.4	E962.0	E980.4
Congo red	977.8	E858.8	E947.8	E950.4	E962.0	E980.4
Coniine, conine	965.7	E850.7	E935.7	E950.0	E962.0	E980.0
Conium (maculatum)	988.2	E865.4	—	E950.9	E962.1	E980.9
Conjugated estrogens (equine)	962.2	E858.0	E932.2	E950.4	E962.0	E980.4
Contac	975.6	E858.6	E945.6	E950.4	E962.0	E980.4
Contact lens solution	976.5	E858.7	E946.5	E950.4	E962.0	E980.4
Contraceptives (oral)	962.2	E858.0	E932.2	E950.4	E962.0	E980.4
vaginal	976.8	E858.7	E946.8	E950.4	E962.0	E980.4
Contrast media (roentgenographic)	977.8	E858.8	E947.8	E950.4	E962.0	E980.4
Convallaria majalis	988.2	E865.4	—	E950.9	E962.1	E980.9
Copper (dust) (fumes) (salts) NEC	985.8	E866.4	—	E950.9	E962.1	E980.9
arsenate, arsenite	985.1	E866.3	—	E950.8	E962.1	E980.8
insecticide	985.1	E863.4	—	E950.8	E962.1	E980.8
emetic	973.6	E858.4	E943.6	E950.4	E962.0	E980.4
fungicide	985.8	E863.6	—	E950.6	E962.1	E980.7
insecticide	985.8	E863.4	—	E950.6	E962.1	E980.7
oleate	976.0	E858.7	E946.0	E950.4	E962.0	E980.4
sulfate	983.9	E864.3	—	E950.7	E962.1	E980.6
fungicide	983.9	E863.6	—	E950.7	E962.1	E980.6
cupric	973.6	E858.4	E943.6	E950.4	E962.0	E980.4
cuprous	983.9	E864.3	—	E950.7	E962.1	E980.6
Copperhead snake (bite) (venom)	989.5	E905.0	—	E950.9	E962.1	E980.9
Coral (sting)	989.5	E905.6	—	E950.9	E962.1	E980.9
snake (bite) (venom)	989.5	E905.0	—	E950.9	E962.1	E980.9
Cordran	976.0	E858.7	E946.0	E950.4	E962.0	E980.4
Corn cures	976.4	E858.7	E946.4	E950.4	E962.0	E980.4
Cornhusker's lotion	976.3	E858.7	E946.3	E950.4	E962.0	E980.4
Corn starch	976.3	E858.7	E946.3	E950.4	E962.0	E980.4
Corrosive	983.9	E864.4	—	E950.7	E962.1	E980.6
acids NEC	983.1	E864.1	—	E950.7	E962.1	E980.6
aromatics	983.0	E864.0	—	E950.7	E962.1	E980.6
disinfectant	983.0	E861.4	—	E950.7	E962.1	E980.6
fumes NEC	987.9	E869.9	—	E952.9	E962.2	E982.9
specified NEC	983.9	E864.3	—	E950.7	E962.1	E980.6
sublimate — *see* Mercury, chloride						
Cortate	962.0	E858.0	E932.0	E950.4	E962.0	E980.4
Cort-Dome	962.0	E858.0	E932.0	E950.4	E962.0	E980.4
ENT agent	976.6	E858.7	E946.6	E950.4	E962.0	E980.4
ophthalmic preparation	976.5	E858.7	E946.5	E950.4	E962.0	E980.4
topical NEC	976.0	E858.7	E946.0	E950.4	E962.0	E980.4
Cortef	962.0	E858.0	E932.0	E950.4	E962.0	E980.4
ENT agent	976.6	E858.7	E946.6	E950.4	E962.0	E980.4
ophthalmic preparation	976.5	E858.7	E946.5	E950.4	E962.0	E980.4
topical NEC	976.0	E858.7	E946.0	E950.4	E962.0	E980.4
Corticosteroids (fluorinated)	962.0	E858.0	E932.0	E950.4	E962.0	E980.4

Substance	Poisoning	External Cause (E-Code) Accident	Therapeutic Use	Suicide Attempt	Assault	Undetermined
ENT agent	976.6	E858.7	E946.6	E950.4	E962.0	E980.4
ophthalmic preparation	976.5	E858.7	E946.5	E950.4	E962.0	E980.4
topical NEC	976.0	E858.7	E946.0	E950.4	E962.0	E980.4
Corticotropin	962.4	E858.0	E932.4	E950.4	E962.0	E980.4
Cortisol	962.0	E858.0	E932.0	E950.4	E962.0	E980.4
ENT agent	976.6	E858.7	E946.6	E950.4	E962.0	E980.4
ophthalmic preparation	976.5	E858.7	E946.5	E950.4	E962.0	E980.4
topical NEC	976.0	E858.7	E946.0	E950.4	E962.0	E980.4
Cortisone derivatives (acetate)	962.0	E858.0	E932.0	E950.4	E962.0	E980.4
ENT agent	976.6	E858.7	E946.6	E950.4	E962.0	E980.4
ophthalmic preparation	976.5	E858.7	E946.5	E950.4	E962.0	E980.4
topical NEC	976.0	E858.7	E946.0	E950.4	E962.0	E980.4
Cortogen	962.0	E858.0	E932.0	E950.4	E962.0	E980.4
ENT agent	976.6	E858.7	E946.6	E950.4	E962.0	E980.4
ophthalmic preparation	976.5	E858.7	E946.5	E950.4	E962.0	E980.4
Cortone	962.0	E858.0	E932.0	E950.4	E962.0	E980.4
ENT agent	976.6	E858.7	E946.6	E950.4	E962.0	E980.4
ophthalmic preparation	976.5	E858.7	E946.5	E950.4	E962.0	E980.4
Cortril	962.0	E858.0	E932.0	E950.4	E962.0	E980.4
ENT agent	976.6	E858.7	E946.6	E950.4	E962.0	E980.4
ophthalmic preparation	976.5	E858.7	E946.5	E950.4	E962.0	E980.4
topical NEC	976.0	E858.7	E946.0	E950.4	E962.0	E980.4
Cosmetics	989.8	E866.7	—	E950.9	E962.1	E980.9
Cosyntropin	977.8	E858.8	E947.8	E950.4	E962.0	E980.4
Cotarnine	964.5	E858.2	E934.5	E950.4	E962.0	E980.4
Cottonseed oil	976.3	E858.7	E946.3	E950.4	E962.0	E980.4
Cough mixtures (antitussives)	975.4	E858.6	E945.4	E950.4	E962.0	E980.4
containing opiates	965.09	E850.2	E935.2	E950.0	E962.0	E980.0
expectorants	975.5	E858.6	E945.5	E950.4	E962.0	E980.4
Coumadin	964.2	E858.2	E934.2	E950.4	E962.0	E980.4
rodenticide	989.4	E863.7	—	E950.6	E962.1	E980.7
Coumarin	964.2	E858.2	E934.2	E950.4	E962.0	E980.4
Coumetarol	964.2	E858.2	E934.2	E950.4	E962.0	E980.4
Cowbane	988.2	E865.4	—	E950.9	E962.1	E980.9
Cozyme	963.5	E858.1	E933.5	E950.4	E962.0	E980.4
Creolin	983.0	E864.0	—	E950.7	E962.1	E980.6
disinfectant	983.0	E861.4	—	E950.7	E962.1	E980.6
Creosol (compound)	983.0	E864.0	—	E950.7	E962.1	E980.6
Creosote (beechwood) (coal tar)	983.0	E864.0	—	E950.7	E962.1	E980.6
medicinal (expectorant)	975.5	E858.6	E945.5	E950.4	E962.0	E980.4
syrup	975.5	E858.6	E945.5	E950.4	E962.0	E980.4
Cresol	983.0	E864.0	—	E950.7	E962.1	E980.6
disinfectant	983.0	E861.4	—	E950.7	E962.1	E980.6
Cresylic acid	983.0	E864.0	—	E950.7	E962.1	E980.6
Cropropamide	965.7	E850.7	E935.7	E950.0	E962.0	E980.0
with crotethamide	970.0	E854.3	E940.0	E950.4	E962.0	E980.4
Crotamiton	976.0	E858.7	E946.0	E950.4	E962.0	E980.4
Crotethamide	965.7	E850.7	E935.7	E950.0	E962.0	E980.0
with cropropamide	970.0	E854.3	E940.0	E950.4	E962.0	E980.4
Croton (oil)	973.1	E858.4	E943.1	E950.4	E962.0	E980.4
chloral	967.1	E852.0	E937.1	E950.2	E962.0	E980.2
Crude oil	981	E862.1	—	E950.9	E962.1	E980.9
Cryogenine	965.8	E850.8	E935.8	E950.0	E962.0	E980.0
Cryolite (pesticide)	989.4	E863.4	—	E950.6	E962.1	E980.7
Cryptenamine	972.6	E858.3	E942.6	E950.4	E962.0	E980.4
Crystal violet	976.0	E858.7	E946.0	E950.4	E962.0	E980.4
Cuckoopint	988.2	E865.4	—	E950.9	E962.1	E980.9

Substance	Poisoning	Accident	Therapeutic Use	Suicide Attempt	Assault	Undetermined
		External Cause (E-Code)				
Cumetharol	964.2	E858.2	E934.2	E950.4	E962.0	E980.4
Cupric sulfate	973.6	E858.4	E943.6	E950.4	E962.0	E980.4
Cuprous sulfate	983.9	E864.3	—	E950.7	E962.1	E980.6
Curare, curarine	975.2	E858.6	E945.2	E950.4	E962.0	E980.4
Cyanic acid — *see* Cyanide(s)						
Cyanide(s) (compounds) (hydrogen) (potassium) (sodium) NEC	989.0	E866.8	—	E950.9	E962.1	E980.9
dust or gas (inhalation) NEC	987.7	E869.8	—	E952.8	E962.2	E982.8
fumigant	989.0	E863.8	—	E950.6	E962.1	E980.7
mercuric — *see* Mercury						
pesticide (dust) (fumes)	989.0	E863.4	—	E950.6	E962.1	E980.7
Cyanocobalamin	964.1	E858.2	E934.1	E950.4	E962.0	E980.4
Cyanogen (chloride) (gas) NEC	987.8	E869.8	—	E952.8	E962.2	E982.8
Cyclaine	968.5	E855.2	E938.5	E950.4	E962.0	E980.4
Cyclamen europaeum	988.2	E865.4	—	E950.9	E962.1	E980.9
Cyclandelate	972.5	E858.3	E942.5	E950.4	E962.0	E980.4
Cyclazocine	965.09	E850.2	E935.2	E950.0	E962.0	E980.0
Cyclizine	963.0	E858.1	E933.0	E950.4	E962.0	E980.4
Cyclobarbital, cyclobarbitone	967.0	E851	E937.0	E950.1	E962.0	E980.1
Cycloguanil	961.4	E857	E931.4	E950.4	E962.0	E980.4
Cyclohexane	982.0	E862.4	—	E950.9	E962.1	E980.9
Cyclohexanol	980.8	E860.8	—	E950.9	E962.1	E980.9
Cyclohexanone	982.8	E862.4	—	E950.9	E962.1	E980.9
Cyclomethycaine	968.5	E855.2	E938.5	E950.4	E962.0	E980.4
Cyclopentamine	971.2	E855.5	E941.2	E950.4	E962.0	E980.4
Cyclopenthiazide	974.3	E858.5	E944.3	E950.4	E962.0	E980.4
Cyclopentolate	971.1	E855.4	E941.1	E950.4	E962.0	E980.4
Cyclophosphamide	963.1	E858.1	E933.1	E950.4	E962.0	E980.4
Cyclopropane	968.2	E855.1	E938.2	E950.4	E962.0	E980.4
Cycloserine	960.6	E856	E930.6	E950.4	E962.0	E980.4
Cyclothiazide	974.3	E858.5	E944.3	E950.4	E962.0	E980.4
Cycrimine	966.4	E855.0	E936.4	E950.4	E962.0	E980.4
Cymarin	972.1	E858.3	E942.1	E950.4	E962.0	E980.4
Cyproheptadine	963.0	E858.1	E933.0	E950.4	E962.0	E980.4
Cyprolidol	969.0	E854.0	E939.0	E950.3	E962.0	E980.3
Cytarabine	963.1	E858.1	E933.1	E950.4	E962.0	E980.4
Cytisus						
laburnum	988.2	E865.4	—	E950.9	E962.1	E980.9
scoparius	988.2	E865.4	—	E950.9	E962.1	E980.9
Cytomel	962.7	E858.0	E932.7	E950.4	E962.0	E980.4
Cytosine (antineoplastic)	963.1	E858.1	E933.1	E950.4	E962.0	E980.4
Cytoxan	963.1	E858.1	E933.1	E950.4	E962.0	E980.4
Dacarbazine	963.1	E858.1	E933.1	E950.4	E962.0	E980.4
Dactinomycin	960.7	E856	E930.7	E950.4	E962.0	E980.4
DADPS	961.8	E857	E931.8	E950.4	E962.0	E980.4
Dakin's solution (external)	976.0	E858.7	E946.0	E950.4	E962.0	E980.4
Dalmane	969.4	E853.2	E939.4	E950.3	E962.0	E980.3
DAM	977.2	E858.8	E947.2	E950.4	E962.0	E980.4
Danilone	964.2	E858.2	E934.2	E950.4	E962.0	E980.4
Danthron	973.1	E858.4	E943.1	E950.4	E962.0	E980.4
Dantrolene	975.2	E858.6	E945.2	E950.4	E962.0	E980.4
Daphne (gnidium) (mezereum)	988.2	E865.4	—	E950.9	E962.1	E980.9
berry	988.2	E865.3	—	E950.9	E962.1	E980.9
Dapsone	961.8	E857	E931.8	E950.4	E962.0	E980.4
Daraprim	961.4	E857	E931.4	E950.4	E962.0	E980.4
Darnel	988.2	E865.3	—	E950.9	E962.1	E980.9
Darvon	965.8	E850.8	E935.8	E950.0	E962.0	E980.0

Substance	Poisoning	External Cause (E-Code)				
		Accident	Therapeutic Use	Suicide Attempt	Assault	Undetermined
Daunorubicin	960.7	E856	E930.7	E950.4	E962.0	E980.4
DBI	962.3	E858.0	E932.3	E950.4	E962.0	E980.4
D–Con (rodenticide)	989.4	E863.7	—	E950.6	E962.1	E980.7
DDS	961.8	E857	E931.8	E950.4	E962.0	E980.4
DDT	989.2	E863.0	—	E950.6	E962.1	E980.7
Deadly nightshade	988.2	E865.4	—	E950.9	E962.1	E980.9
berry	988.2	E865.3	—	E950.9	E962.1	E980.9
Deanol	969.7	E854.2	E939.7	E950.3	E962.0	E980.3
Debrisoquine	972.6	E858.3	E942.6	E950.4	E962.0	E980.4
Decaborane	989.8	E866.8	—	E950.9	E962.1	E980.9
fumes	987.8	E869.8	—	E952.8	E962.2	E982.8
Decadron	962.0	E858.0	E932.0	E950.4	E962.0	E980.4
ENT agent	976.6	E858.7	E946.6	E950.4	E962.0	E980.4
ophthalmic preparation	976.5	E858.7	E946.5	E950.4	E962.0	E980.4
topical NEC	976.0	E858.7	E946.0	E950.4	E962.0	E980.4
Decahydronaphthalene	982.0	E862.4	—	E950.9	E962.1	E980.9
Decalin	982.0	E862.4	—	E950.9	E962.1	E980.9
Decamethonium	975.2	E858.6	E945.2	E950.4	E962.0	E980.4
Decholin	973.4	E858.4	E943.4	E950.4	E962.0	E980.4
sodium (diagnostic)	977.8	E858.8	E947.8	E950.4	E962.0	E980.4
Declomycin	960.4	E856	E930.4	E950.4	E962.0	E980.4
Deferoxamine	963.8	E858.1	E933.8	E950.4	E962.0	E980.4
Dehydrocholic acid	973.4	E858.4	E943.4	E950.4	E962.0	E980.4
DeKalin	982.0	E862.4	—	E950.9	E962.1	E980.9
Delalutin	962.2	E858.0	E932.2	E950.4	E962.0	E980.4
Delphinium	988.2	E865.3	—	E950.9	E962.1	E980.9
Deltasone	962.0	E858.0	E932.0	E950.4	E962.0	E980.4
Deltra	962.0	E858.0	E932.0	E950.4	E962.0	E980.4
Delvinal	967.0	E851	E937.0	E950.1	E962.0	E980.1
Demecarium (bromide)	971.0	E855.3	E941.0	E950.4	E962.0	E980.4
Demeclocycline	960.4	E856	E930.4	E950.4	E962.0	E980.4
Demecolcine	963.1	E858.1	E933.1	E950.4	E962.0	E980.4
Demelanizing agents	976.8	E858.7	E946.8	E950.4	E962.0	E980.4
Demerol	965.09	E850.2	E935.2	E950.0	E962.0	E980.0
Demethylchlortetracycline	960.4	E856	E930.4	E950.4	E962.0	E980.4
Demethyltetracycline	960.4	E856	E930.4	E950.4	E962.0	E980.4
Demeton	989.3	E863.1	—	E950.6	E962.1	E980.7
Demulcents	976.3	E858.7	E946.3	E950.4	E962.0	E980.4
Demulen	962.2	E858.0	E932.2	E950.4	E962.0	E980.4
Denatured alcohol	980.0	E860.1	—	E950.9	E962.1	E980.9
Dendrid	976.5	E858.7	E946.5	E950.4	E962.0	E980.4
Dental agents, topical	976.7	E858.7	E946.7	E950.4	E962.0	E980.4
Deodorant spray (feminine hygiene)	976.8	E858.7	E946.8	E950.4	E962.0	E980.4
Deoxyribonuclease	963.4	E858.1	E933.4	E950.4	E962.0	E980.4
Depressants						
appetite, central	977.0	E858.8	E947.0	E950.4	E962.0	E980.4
cardiac	972.0	E858.3	E942.0	E950.4	E962.0	E980.4
central nervous system (anesthetic)	968.4	E855.1	E938.4	E950.4	E962.0	E980.4
psychotherapeutic	969.5	E853.9	E939.5	E950.3	E962.0	E980.3
Dequalinium	976.0	E858.7	E946.0	E950.4	E962.0	E980.4
Dermolate	976.2	E858.7	E946.2	E950.4	E962.0	E980.4
DES	962.2	E858.0	E932.2	E950.4	E962.0	E980.4
Desenex	976.0	E858.7	E946.0	E950.4	E962.0	E980.4
Deserpidine	972.6	E858.3	E942.6	E950.4	E962.0	E980.4
Desipramine	969.0	E854.0	E939.0	E950.3	E962.0	E980.3
Deslanoside	972.1	E858.3	E942.1	E950.4	E962.0	E980.4
Desocodeine	965.09	E850.2	E935.2	E950.0	E962.0	E980.0

Substance	Poisoning	External Cause (E-Code) Accident	Therapeutic Use	Suicide Attempt	Assault	Undetermined
Desomorphine	965.09	E850.2	E935.2	E950.0	E962.0	E980.0
Desonide	976.0	E858.7	E946.0	E950.4	E962.0	E980.4
Desoxycorticosterone derivatives	962.0	E858.0	E932.0	E950.4	E962.0	E980.4
Desoxyephedrine	969.7	E854.2	E939.7	E950.3	E962.0	E980.3
DET	969.6	E854.1	E939.6	E950.3	E962.0	E980.3
Detergents (ingested) (synthetic)	989.6	E861.0	—	E950.9	E962.1	E980.9
external medication	976.2	E858.7	E946.2	E950.4	E962.0	E980.4
Deterrent, alcohol	977.3	E858.8	E947.3	E950.4	E962.0	E980.4
Detrothyronine	962.7	E858.0	E932.7	E950.4	E962.0	E980.4
Dettol (external medication)	976.0	E858.7	E946.0	E950.4	E962.0	E980.4
Dexamethasone	962.0	E858.0	E932.0	E950.4	E962.0	E980.4
ENT agent	976.6	E858.7	E946.6	E950.4	E962.0	E980.4
ophthalmic preparation	976.5	E858.7	E946.5	E950.4	E962.0	E980.4
topical NEC	976.0	E858.7	E946.0	E950.4	E962.0	E980.4
Dexamphetamine	969.7	E854.2	E939.7	E950.3	E962.0	E980.3
Dexedrine	969.7	E854.2	E939.7	E950.3	E962.0	E980.3
Dexpanthenol	963.5	E858.1	E933.5	E950.4	E962.0	E980.4
Dextran	964.8	E858.2	E934.8	E950.4	E962.0	E980.4
Dextriferron	964.0	E858.2	E934.0	E950.4	E962.0	E980.4
Dextroamphetamine	969.7	E854.2	E939.7	E950.3	E962.0	E980.3
Dextro calcium pantothenate	963.5	E858.1	E933.5	E950.4	E962.0	E980.4
Dextromethorphan	975.4	E858.6	E945.4	E950.4	E962.0	E980.4
Dextromoramide	965.09	E850.2	E935.2	E950.0	E962.0	E980.0
Dextro pantothenyl alcohol	963.5	E858.1	E933.5	E950.4	E962.0	E980.4
topical	976.8	E858.7	E946.8	E950.4	E962.0	E980.4
Dextropropoxyphene (hydrochloride)	965.8	E850.8	E935.8	E950.0	E962.0	E980.0
Dextrorphan	965.09	E850.2	E935.2	E950.0	E962.0	E980.0
Dextrose NEC	974.5	E858.5	E944.5	E950.4	E962.0	E980.4
Dextrothyroxin	962.7	E858.0	E932.7	E950.4	E962.0	E980.4
DFP	971.0	E855.3	E941.0	E950.4	E962.0	E980.4
DHE-45	972.9	E858.3	E942.9	E950.4	E962.0	E980.4
Diabinese	962.3	E858.0	E932.3	E950.4	E962.0	E980.4
Diacetyl monoxime	977.2	E858.8	E947.2	E950.4	E962.0	E980.4
Diacetylmorphine	965.01	E850.0	E935.0	E950.0	E962.0	E980.0
Diagnostic agents	977.8	E858.8	E947.8	E950.4	E962.0	E980.4
Dial (soap)	976.2	E858.7	E946.2	E950.4	E962.0	E980.4
sedative	967.0	E851	E937.0	E950.1	E962.0	E980.1
Diallylbarbituric acid	967.0	E851	E937.0	E950.1	E962.0	E980.1
Diaminodiphenylsulfone	961.8	E857	E931.8	E950.4	E962.0	E980.4
Diamorphine	965.01	E850.0	E935.0	E950.0	E962.0	E980.0
Diamox	974.2	E858.5	E944.2	E950.4	E962.0	E980.4
Diamthazole	976.0	E858.7	E946.0	E950.4	E962.0	E980.4
Diaphenylsulfone	961.8	E857	E931.8	E950.4	E962.0	E980.4
Diasone (sodium)	961.8	E857	E931.8	E950.4	E962.0	E980.4
Diazepam	969.4	E853.2	E939.4	E950.3	E962.0	E980.3
Diazinon	989.3	E863.1	—	E950.6	E962.1	E980.7
Diazomethane (gas)	987.8	E869.8	—	E952.8	E962.2	E982.8
Diazoxide	972.5	E858.3	E942.5	E950.4	E962.0	E980.4
Dibenamine	971.3	E855.6	E941.3	E950.4	E962.0	E980.4
Dibenzheptropine	963.0	E858.1	E933.0	E950.4	E962.0	E980.4
Dibenzyline	971.3	E855.6	E941.3	E950.4	E962.0	E980.4
Diborane (gas)	987.8	E869.8	—	E952.8	E962.2	E982.8
Dibromomannitol	963.1	E858.1	E933.1	E950.4	E962.0	E980.4
Dibucaine (spinal)	968.7	E855.2	E938.7	E950.4	E962.0	E980.4
topical (surface)	968.5	E855.2	E938.5	E950.4	E962.0	E980.4
Dibunate sodium	975.4	E858.6	E945.4	E950.4	E962.0	E980.4
Dibutoline	971.1	E855.4	E941.1	E950.4	E962.0	E980.4

Substance	Poisoning	External Cause (E-Code) Accident	Therapeutic Use	Suicide Attempt	Assault	Undetermined
Dicapthon	989.4	E863.4	—	E950.6	E962.1	E980.7
Dichloralphenazone	967.1	E852.0	E937.1	E950.2	E962.0	E980.2
Dichlorodifluoromethane	987.4	E869.2	—	E952.8	E962.2	E982.8
Dichloroethane	982.3	E862.4	—	E950.9	E962.1	E980.9
Dichloroethylene	982.3	E862.4	—	E950.9	E962.1	E980.9
Dichloroethyl sulfide	987.8	E869.8	—	E952.8	E962.2	E982.8
Dichlorohydrin	982.3	E862.4	—	E950.9	E962.1	E980.9
Dichloromethane (solvent) (vapor)	982.3	E862.4	—	E950.9	E962.1	E980.9
Dichlorophen(e)	961.6	E857	E931.6	E950.4	E962.0	E980.4
Dichlorphenamide	974.2	E858.5	E944.2	E950.4	E962.0	E980.4
Dichlorvos	989.3	E863.1	—	E950.6	E962.1	E980.7
Dicoumarin, dicumarol	964.2	E858.2	E934.2	E950.4	E962.0	E980.4
Dicyanogen (gas)	987.8	E869.8	—	E952.8	E962.2	E982.8
Dicyclomine	971.1	E855.4	E941.1	E950.4	E962.0	E980.4
Dieldrin (vapor)	989.2	E863.0	—	E950.6	E962.1	E980.7
Dienestrol	962.2	E858.0	E932.2	E950.4	E962.0	E980.4
Dietetics	977.0	E858.8	E947.0	E950.4	E962.0	E980.4
Diethazine	966.4	E855.0	E936.4	E950.4	E962.0	E980.4
Diethyl						
barbituric acid	967.0	E851	E937.0	E950.1	E962.0	E980.1
carbamazine	961.6	E857	E931.6	E950.4	E962.0	E980.4
carbinol	980.8	E860.8	—	E950.9	E962.1	E980.9
carbonate	982.8	E862.4	—	E950.9	E962.1	E980.9
ether (vapor) — *see* Ether(s)						
propion	977.0	E858.8	E947.0	E950.4	E962.0	E980.4
stilbestrol	962.2	E858.0	E932.2	E950.4	E962.0	E980.4
Diethylene						
dioxide	982.8	E862.4	—	E950.9	E962.1	E980.9
glycol (monoacetate) (monoethyl ether)	982.8	E862.4	—	E950.9	E962.1	E980.9
Diethylsulfone–diethylmethane	967.8	E852.8	E937.8	E950.2	E962.0	E980.2
Difencloxazine	965.09	E850.2	E935.2	E950.0	E962.0	E980.0
Diffusin	963.4	E858.1	E933.4	E950.4	E962.0	E980.4
Diflos	971.0	E855.3	E941.0	E950.4	E962.0	E980.4
Digestants	973.4	E858.4	E943.4	E950.4	E962.0	E980.4
Digitalin(e)	972.1	E858.3	E942.1	E950.4	E962.0	E980.4
Digitalis glycosides	972.1	E858.3	E942.1	E950.4	E962.0	E980.4
Digitoxin	972.1	E858.3	E942.1	E950.4	E962.0	E980.4
Digoxin	972.1	E858.3	E942.1	E950.4	E962.0	E980.4
Dihydrocodeine	965.09	E850.2	E935.2	E950.0	E962.0	E980.0
Dihydrocodeinone	965.09	E850.2	E935.2	E950.0	E962.0	E980.0
Dihydroergocristine	972.9	E858.3	E942.9	E950.4	E962.0	E980.4
Dihydroergotamine	972.9	E858.3	E942.9	E950.4	E962.0	E980.4
Dihydroergotoxine	972.9	E858.3	E942.9	E950.4	E962.0	E980.4
Dihydrohydroxycodeinone	965.09	E850.2	E935.2	E950.0	E962.0	E980.0
Dihydrohydroxymorphinone	965.09	E850.2	E935.2	E950.0	E962.0	E980.0
Dihydroisocodeine	965.09	E850.2	E935.2	E950.0	E962.0	E980.0
Dihydromorphine	965.09	E850.2	E935.2	E950.0	E962.0	E980.0
Dihydromorphinone	965.09	E850.2	E935.2	E950.0	E962.0	E980.0
Dihydrostreptomycin	960.6	E856	E930.6	E950.4	E962.0	E980.4
Dihydrotachysterol	962.6	E858.0	E932.6	E950.4	E962.0	E980.4
Dihydroxyanthraquinone	973.1	E858.4	E943.1	E950.4	E962.0	E980.4
Dihydroxycodeinone	965.09	E850.2	E935.2	E950.0	E962.0	E980.0
Diiodohydroxyquin	961.3	E857	E931.3	E950.4	E962.0	E980.4
topical	976.0	E858.7	E946.0	E950.4	E962.0	E980.4
Diiodohydroxyquinoline	961.3	E857	E931.3	E950.4	E962.0	E980.4
Dilantin	966.1	E855.0	E936.1	E950.4	E962.0	E980.4
Dilaudid	965.09	E850.2	E935.2	E950.0	E962.0	E980.0

Substance		External Cause (E-Code)				
	Poisoning	Accident	Therapeutic Use	Suicide Attempt	Assault	Undetermined
Diloxanide	961.5	E857	E931.5	E950.4	E962.0	E980.4
Dimefline	970.0	E854.3	E940.0	E950.4	E962.0	E980.4
Dimenhydrinate	963.0	E858.1	E933.0	E950.4	E962.0	E980.4
Dimercaprol	963.8	E858.1	E933.8	E950.4	E962.0	E980.4
Dimercaptopropanol	963.8	E858.1	E933.8	E950.4	E962.0	E980.4
Dimetane	963.0	E858.1	E933.0	E950.4	E962.0	E980.4
Dimethicone	976.3	E858.7	E946.3	E950.4	E962.0	E980.4
Dimethindene	963.0	E858.1	E933.0	E950.4	E962.0	E980.4
Dimethisoquin	968.5	E855.2	E938.5	E950.4	E962.0	E980.4
Dimethisterone	962.2	E858.0	E932.2	E950.4	E962.0	E980.4
Dimethoxanate	975.4	E858.6	E945.4	E950.4	E962.0	E980.4
Dimethyl						
arsine, arsinic acid — *see* Arsenic						
carbinol	980.2	E860.3	—	E950.9	E962.1	E980.9
diguanide	962.3	E858.0	E932.3	E950.4	E962.0	E980.4
ketone	982.8	E862.4	—	E950.9	E962.1	E980.9
vapor	987.8	E869.8	—	E952.8	E962.2	E982.8
meperidine	965.09	E850.2	E935.2	E950.0	E962.0	E980.0
parathion	989.3	E863.1	—	E950.6	E962.1	E980.7
polysiloxane	973.8	E858.4	E943.8	E950.4	E962.0	E980.4
sulfate (fumes)	987.8	E869.8	—	E952.8	E962.2	E982.8
liquid	983.9	E864.3	—	E950.7	E962.1	E980.6
sulfoxide NEC	982.8	E862.4	—	E950.9	E962.1	E980.9
medicinal	976.4	E858.7	E946.4	E950.4	E962.0	E980.4
triptamine	969.6	E854.1	E939.6	E950.3	E962.0	E980.3
tubocurarine	975.2	E858.6	E945.2	E950.4	E962.0	E980.4
Dindevan	964.2	E858.2	E934.2	E950.4	E962.0	E980.4
Dinitro (–ortho–) cresol (herbicide) (spray)	989.4	E863.5	—	E950.6	E962.1	E980.7
insecticide	989.4	E863.4	—	E950.6	E962.1	E980.7
Dinitrobenzene	983.0	E864.0	—	E950.7	E962.1	E980.6
vapor	987.8	E869.8	—	E952.8	E962.2	E982.8
Dinitro–orthocresol (herbicide)	989.4	E863.5	—	E950.6	E962.1	E980.7
insecticide	989.4	E863.4	—	E950.6	E962.1	E980.7
Dinitrophenol (herbicide) (spray)	989.4	E863.5	—	E950.6	E962.1	E980.7
insecticide	989.4	E863.4	—	E950.6	E962.1	E980.7
Dinoprost	975.0	E858.6	E945.0	E950.4	E962.0	E980.4
Dioctyl sulfosuccinate (calcium) (sodium)	973.2	E858.4	E943.2	E950.4	E962.0	E980.4
Diodoquin	961.3	E857	E931.3	E950.4	E962.0	E980.4
Dione derivatives NEC	966.3	E855.0	E936.3	E950.4	E962.0	E980.4
Dionin	965.09	E850.2	E935.2	E950.0	E962.0	E980.0
Dioxane	982.8	E862.4	—	E950.9	E962.1	E980.9
Dioxyline	972.5	E858.3	E942.5	E950.4	E962.0	E980.4
Dipentene	982.8	E862.4	—	E950.9	E962.1	E980.9
Diphemanil	971.1	E855.4	E941.1	E950.4	E962.0	E980.4
Diphenadione	964.2	E858.2	E934.2	E950.4	E962.0	E980.4
Diphenhydramine	963.0	E858.1	E933.0	E950.4	E962.0	E980.4
Diphenidol	963.0	E858.1	E933.0	E950.4	E962.0	E980.4
Diphenoxylate	973.5	E858.4	E943.5	E950.4	E962.0	E980.4
Diphenylchloroarsine	985.1	E866.3	—	E950.8	E962.1	E980.8
Diphenylhydantoin (sodium)	966.1	E855.0	E936.1	E950.4	E962.0	E980.4
Diphenylpyraline	963.0	E858.1	E933.0	E950.4	E962.0	E980.4
Diphtheria						
antitoxin	979.9	E858.8	E949.9	E950.4	E962.0	E980.4
toxoid	978.5	E858.8	E948.5	E950.4	E962.0	E980.4
with tetanus toxoid	978.9	E858.8	E948.9	E950.4	E962.0	E980.4
with pertussis component	978.6	E858.8	E948.6	E950.4	E962.0	E980.4
vaccine	978.5	E858.8	E948.5	E950.4	E962.0	E980.4

Substance	Poisoning	External Cause (E-Code) Accident	Therapeutic Use	Suicide Attempt	Assault	Undetermined
Dipipanone	965.09	E850.2	E935.2	E950.0	E962.0	E980.0
Diplovax	979.5	E858.8	E949.5	E950.4	E962.0	E980.4
Diprophylline	975.1	E858.6	E945.1	E950.4	E962.0	E980.4
Dipyridamole	972.4	E858.3	E942.4	E950.4	E962.0	E980.4
Dipyrone	965.5	E850.5	E935.5	E950.0	E962.0	E980.0
Diquat	989.4	E863.5	—	E950.6	E962.1	E980.7
Disinfectant NEC	983.9	E861.4	—	E950.7	E962.1	E980.6
alkaline	983.2	E861.4	—	E950.7	E962.1	E980.6
aromatic	983.0	E861.4	—	E950.7	E962.1	E980.6
Disipal	966.4	E855.0	E936.4	E950.4	E962.0	E980.4
Disodium edetate	963.8	E858.1	E933.8	E950.4	E962.0	E980.4
Disulfamide	974.4	E858.5	E944.4	E950.4	E962.0	E980.4
Disulfanilamide	961.0	E857	E931.0	E950.4	E962.0	E980.4
Disulfiram	977.3	E858.8	E947.3	E950.4	E962.0	E980.4
Dithiazanine	961.6	E857	E931.6	E950.4	E962.0	E980.4
Dithioglycerol	963.8	E858.1	E933.8	E950.4	E962.0	E980.4
Dithranol	976.4	E858.7	E946.4	E950.4	E962.0	E980.4
Diucardin	974.3	E858.5	E944.3	E950.4	E962.0	E980.4
Diupres	974.3	E858.5	E944.3	E950.4	E962.0	E980.4
Diuretics NEC	974.4	E858.5	E944.4	E950.4	E962.0	E980.4
carbonic acid anhydrase inhibitors	974.2	E858.5	E944.2	E950.4	E962.0	E980.4
mercurial	974.0	E858.5	E944.0	E950.4	E962.0	E980.4
osmotic	974.4	E858.5	E944.4	E950.4	E962.0	E980.4
purine derivatives	974.1	E858.5	E944.1	E950.4	E962.0	E980.4
saluretic	974.3	E858.5	E944.3	E950.4	E962.0	E980.4
Diuril	974.3	E858.5	E944.3	E950.4	E962.0	E980.4
Divinyl ether	968.2	E855.1	E938.2	E950.4	E962.0	E980.4
D–lysergic acid diethylamide	969.6	E854.1	E939.6	E950.3	E962.0	E980.3
DMCT	960.4	E856	E930.4	E950.4	E962.0	E980.4
DMSO	982.8	E862.4	—	E950.9	E962.1	E980.9
DMT	969.6	E854.1	E939.6	E950.3	E962.0	E980.3
DNOC	989.4	E863.5	—	E950.6	E962.1	E980.7
DOCA	962.0	E858.0	E932.0	E950.4	E962.0	E980.4
Dolophine	965.02	E850.1	E935.1	E950.0	E962.0	E980.0
Doloxene	965.8	E850.8	E935.8	E950.0	E962.0	E980.0
DOM	969.6	E854.1	E939.6	E950.3	E962.0	E980.3
Domestic gas — *see* Gas, utility						
Domiphen (bromide) (lozenges)	976.6	E858.7	E946.6	E950.4	E962.0	E980.4
Dopa (levo)	966.4	E855.0	E936.4	E950.4	E962.0	E980.4
Dopamine	971.2	E855.5	E941.2	E950.4	E962.0	E980.4
Doriden	967.5	E852.4	E937.5	E950.2	E962.0	E980.2
Dormiral	967.0	E851	E937.0	E950.1	E962.0	E980.1
Dormison	967.8	E852.8	E937.8	E950.2	E962.0	E980.2
Dornase	963.4	E858.1	E933.4	E950.4	E962.0	E980.4
Dorsacaine	968.5	E855.2	E938.5	E950.4	E962.0	E980.4
Doxapram	970.0	E854.3	E940.0	E950.4	E962.0	E980.4
Doxepin	969.0	E854.0	E939.0	E950.3	E962.0	E980.3
Doxorubicin	960.7	E856	E930.7	E950.4	E962.0	E980.4
Doxycycline	960.4	E856	E930.4	E950.4	E962.0	E980.4
Doxylamine	963.0	E858.1	E933.0	E950.4	E962.0	E980.4
Dramamine	963.0	E858.1	E933.0	E950.4	E962.0	E980.4
Drano (drain cleaner)	983.2	E864.2	—	E950.7	E962.1	E980.6
Dromoran	965.09	E850.2	E935.2	E950.0	E962.0	E980.0
Dromostanolone	962.1	E858.0	E932.1	E950.4	E962.0	E980.4
Droperidol	969.2	E853.1	E939.2	E950.3	E962.0	E980.3
Drug	977.9	E858.9	E947.9	E950.5	E962.0	E980.5
specified NEC	977.8	E858.8	E947.8	E950.4	E962.0	E980.4

Substance	Poisoning	External Cause (E-Code)				
		Accident	Therapeutic Use	Suicide Attempt	Assault	Undetermined
AHFS List						
4:00 antihistamine drugs	963.0	E858.1	E933.0	E950.4	E962.0	E980.4
8:04 amebacides	961.5	E857	E931.5	E950.4	E962.0	E980.4
arsenical anti–infectives	961.1	E857	E931.1	E950.4	E962.0	E980.4
quinoline derivatives	961.3	E857	E931.3	E950.4	E962.0	E980.4
8:08 anthelmintics	961.6	E857	E931.6	E950.4	E962.0	E980.4
quinoline derivatives	961.3	E857	E931.3	E950.4	E962.0	E980.4
8:12.04 antifungal antibiotics	960.1	E856	E930.1	E950.4	E962.0	E980.4
8:12.06 cephalosporins	960.5	E856	E930.5	E950.4	E962.0	E980.4
8:12.08 chloramphenicol	960.2	E856	E930.2	E950.4	E962.0	E980.4
8:12.12 erythromycins	960.3	E856	E930.3	E950.4	E962.0	E980.4
8:12.16 penicillins	960.0	E856	E930.0	E950.4	E962.0	E980.4
8:12.20 streptomycins	960.6	E856	E930.6	E950.4	E962.0	E980.4
8:12.24 tetracyclines	960.4	E856	E930.4	E950.4	E962.0	E980.4
8:12.28 other antibiotics	960.8	E856	E930.8	E950.4	E962.0	E980.4
antimycobacterial	960.6	E856	E930.6	E950.4	E962.0	E980.4
macrolides	960.3	E856	E930.3	E950.4	E962.0	E980.4
8:16 antituberculars	961.8	E857	E931.8	E950.4	E962.0	E980.4
antibiotics	960.6	E856	E930.6	E950.4	E962.0	E980.4
8:18 antivirals	961.7	E857	E931.7	E950.4	E962.0	E980.4
8:20 plasmodicides (antimalarials)	961.4	E857	E931.4	E950.4	E962.0	E980.4
8:24 sulfonamides	961.0	E857	E931.0	E950.4	E962.0	E980.4
8:26 sulfones	961.8	E857	E931.8	E950.4	E962.0	E980.4
8:28 treponemicides	961.2	E857	E931.2	E950.4	E962.0	E980.4
8:32 trichomonacides	961.5	E857	E931.5	E950.4	E962.0	E980.4
quinoline derivatives	961.3	E857	E931.3	E950.4	E962.0	E980.4
nitrofuran derivatives	961.9	E857	E931.9	E950.4	E962.0	E980.4
8:36 urinary germicides	961.9	E857	E931.9	E950.4	E962.0	E980.4
quinoline derivatives	961.3	E857	E931.3	E950.4	E962.0	E980.4
8:40 other anti–infectives	961.9	E857	E931.9	E950.4	E962.0	E980.4
10:00 antineoplastic agents	963.1	E858.1	E933.1	E950.4	E962.0	E980.4
antibiotics	960.7	E856	E930.7	E950.4	E962.0	E980.4
progestogens	962.2	E858.0	E932.2	E950.4	E962.0	E980.4
12:04 parasympathomimetic (cholinergic) agents	971.0	E855.3	E941.0	E950.4	E962.0	E980.4
12:08 parasympatholytic (cholinergic –blocking) agents	971.1	E855.4	E941.1	E950.4	E962.0	E980.4
12:12 Sympathomimetic (adrenergic) agents	971.2	E855.5	E941.2	E950.4	E962.0	E980.4
12:16 sympatholytic (adrenergic– blocking) agents	971.3	E855.6	E941.3	E950.4	E962.0	E980.4
12:20 skeletal muscle relaxants						
central nervous system muscle-tone depressants	968.0	E855.1	E938.0	E950.4	E962.0	E980.4
myoneural blocking agents	975.2	E858.6	E945.2	E950.4	E962.0	E980.4
16:00 blood derivatives	964.7	E858.2	E934.7	E950.4	E962.0	E980.4
20:04 antianemia drugs	964.1	E858.2	E934.1	E950.4	E962.0	E980.4
20:04.04 iron preparations	964.0	E858.2	E934.0	E950.4	E962.0	E980.4
20:04.08 liver and stomach preparations	964.1	E858.2	E934.1	E950.4	E962.0	E980.4
20:12.04 anticoagulants	964.2	E858.2	E934.2	E950.4	E962.0	E980.4
20:12.08 antiheparin agents	964.5	E858.2	E934.5	E950.4	E962.0	E980.4
20:12.12 coagulants	964.5	E858.2	E934.5	E950.4	E962.0	E980.4
20:12.16 hemostatics NEC	964.5	E858.2	E934.5	E950.4	E962.0	E980.4
capillary active drugs	972.8	E858.3	E942.8	E950.4	E962.0	E980.4
24:04 cardiac drugs	972.9	E858.3	E942.9	E950.4	E962.0	E980.4
cardiotonic agents	972.1	E858.3	E942.1	E950.4	E962.0	E980.4
rhythm regulators	972.0	E858.3	E942.0	E950.4	E962.0	E980.4

Substance	Poisoning	Accident	Therapeutic Use	Suicide Attempt	Assault	Undetermined
		External Cause (E-Code)				
24:06 antilipemic agents	972.2	E858.3	E942.2	E950.4	E962.0	E980.4
thyroid derivatives	962.7	E858.0	E932.7	E950.4	E962.0	E980.4
24:08 hypotensive agents	972.6	E858.3	E942.6	E950.4	E962.0	E980.4
adrenergic blocking agents	971.3	E855.6	E941.3	E950.4	E962.0	E980.4
ganglion blocking agents	972.3	E858.3	E942.3	E950.4	E962.0	E980.4
vasodilators	972.5	E858.3	E942.5	E950.4	E962.0	E980.4
24:12 vasodilating agents NEC	972.5	E858.3	E942.5	E950.4	E962.0	E980.4
coronary	972.4	E858.3	E942.4	E950.4	E962.0	E980.4
nicotinic acid derivatives	972.2	E858.3	E942.2	E950.4	E962.0	E980.4
24:16 sclerosing agents	972.7	E858.3	E942.7	E950.4	E962.0	E980.4
28:04 general anesthetics	968.4	E855.1	E938.4	E950.4	E962.0	E980.4
gaseous anesthetics	968.2	E855.1	E938.2	E950.4	E962.0	E980.4
halothane	968.1	E855.1	E938.1	E950.4	E962.0	E980.4
intravenous anesthetics	968.3	E855.1	E938.3	E950.4	E962.0	E980.4
28:08 analgesics and antipyretics	965.9	E850.9	E935.9	E950.0	E962.0	E980.0
antirheumatics	965.6	E850.6	E935.6	E950.0	E962.0	E980.0
aromatic analgesics	965.4	E850.4	E935.4	E950.0	E962.0	E980.0
non–narcotic NEC	965.7	E850.7	E935.7	E950.0	E962.0	E980.0
opium alkaloids	965.00	E850.2	E935.2	E950.0	E962.0	E980.0
heroin	965.01	E850.0	E935.0	E950.0	E962.0	E980.0
methadone	965.02	E850.1	E935.1	E950.0	E962.0	E980.0
specified type NEC	965.09	E850.2	E935.2	E950.0	E962.0	E980.0
pyrazole derivatives	965.5	E850.5	E935.5	E950.0	E962.0	E980.0
salicylates	965.1	E850.3	E935.3	E950.0	E962.0	E980.0
specified NEC	965.8	E850.8	E935.8	E950.0	E962.0	E980.0
28:10 narcotic antagonists	970.1	E854.3	E940.1	E950.4	E962.0	E980.4
28:12 anticonvulsants	966.3	E855.0	E936.3	E950.4	E962.0	E980.4
barbiturates	967.0	E851	E937.0	E950.1	E962.0	E980.1
benzodiazepine–based tranquilizers	969.4	E853.4	E939.4	E950.3	E962.0	E980.3
bromides	967.3	E852.2	E937.3	E950.2	E962.0	E980.2
hydantoin derivatives	966.1	E855.0	E936.1	E950.4	E962.0	E980.4
oxazolidine (derivatives)	966.0	E855.0	E936.0	E950.4	E962.0	E980.4
succinimides	966.2	E855.0	E936.2	E950.4	E962.0	E980.4
28:16.04 antidepressants	969.0	E854.0	E939.0	E950.3	E962.0	E980.3
28:16.08 tranquilizers	969.5	E853.9	E939.5	E950.3	E962.0	E980.3
benzodiazepine–based	969.4	E853.2	E939.4	E950.3	E962.0	E980.3
butyrophenone–based	969.2	E853.1	E939.2	E950.3	E962.0	E980.3
major NEC	969.3	E853.8	E939.3	E950.3	E962.0	E980.3
phenothiazine–based	969.1	E853.0	E939.1	E950.3	E962.0	E980.3
28:16.12 other psychotherapeutic agents	969.8	E855.8	E939.8	E950.3	E962.0	E980.3
28:20 respiratory and cerebral stimulants	970.9	E854.3	E940.9	E950.4	E962.0	E980.4
analeptics	970.0	E854.3	E940.0	E950.4	E962.0	E980.4
anorexigenic agents	977.0	E858.8	E947.0	E950.4	E962.0	E980.4
psychostimulants	969.7	E854.2	E939.7	E950.3	E962.0	E980.3
specified NEC	970.8	E854.3	E940.8	E950.4	E962.0	E980.4
28:24 sedatives and hypnotics	967.9	E852.9	E937.9	E950.2	E962.0	E980.2
barbiturates	967.0	E851	E937.0	E950.1	E962.0	E980.1
benzodiazepine–based tranquilizers	969.4	E853.2	E939.4	E950.3	E962.0	E980.3
chloral hydrate (group)	967.1	E852.0	E937.1	E950.2	E962.0	E980.2
glutethamide group	967.5	E852.4	E937.5	E950.2	E962.0	E980.2
intravenous anesthetics	968.3	E855.1	E938.3	E950.4	E962.0	E980.4
methaqualone (compounds)	967.4	E852.3	E937.4	E950.2	E962.0	E980.2
paraldehyde	967.2	E852.1	E937.2	E950.2	E962.0	E980.2
phenothiazine–based tranquilizers	969.1	E853.0	E939.1	E950.3	E962.0	E980.3
specified NEC	967.8	E852.8	E937.8	E950.2	E962.0	E980.2
thiobarbiturates	968.3	E855.1	E938.3	E950.4	E962.0	E980.4

Substance	Poisoning	External Cause (E-Code)				
		Accident	Therapeutic Use	Suicide Attempt	Assault	Undetermined
tranquilizer NEC	969.5	E853.9	E939.5	E950.3	E962.0	E980.3
36:04 to 36:88 diagnostic agents	977.8	E858.8	E947.8	E950.4	E962.0	E980.4
40:00 electrolyte, caloric, and water balance agents NEC	974.5	E858.5	E944.5	E950.4	E962.0	E980.4
40:04 acidifying agents	963.2	E858.1	E933.2	E950.4	E962.0	E980.4
40:08 alkalinizing agents	963.3	E858.1	E933.3	E950.4	E962.0	E980.4
40:10 ammonia detoxicants	974.5	E858.5	E944.5	E950.4	E962.0	E980.4
40:12 replacement solutions	974.5	E858.5	E944.5	E950.4	E962.0	E980.4
plasma expanders	964.8	E858.2	E934.8	E950.4	E962.0	E980.4
40:16 sodium–removing resins	974.5	E858.5	E944.5	E950.4	E962.0	E980.4
40:18 potassium–removing resins	974.5	E858.5	E944.5	E950.4	E962.0	E980.4
40:20 caloric agents	974.5	E858.5	E944.5	E950.4	E962.0	E980.4
40:24 salt and sugar substitutes	974.5	E858.5	E944.5	E950.4	E962.0	E980.4
40:28 diuretics NEC	974.4	E858.5	E944.4	E950.4	E962.0	E980.4
carbonic acid anhydrase inhibitors	974.2	E858.5	E944.2	E950.4	E962.0	E980.4
mercurials	974.0	E858.5	E944.0	E950.4	E962.0	E980.4
purine derivatives	974.1	E858.5	E944.1	E950.4	E962.0	E980.4
saluretics	974.3	E858.5	E944.3	E950.4	E962.0	E980.4
thiazides	974.3	E858.5	E944.3	E950.4	E962.1	E980.4
40:36 irrigating solutions	974.5	E858.5	E944.5	E950.4	E962.0	E980.4
40:40 uricosuric agents	974.7	E858.5	E944.7	E950.4	E962.0	E980.4
44:00 enzymes	963.4	E858.1	E933.4	E950.4	E962.0	E980.4
fibrinolysis–affecting agents	964.4	E858.2	E934.4	E950.4	E962.0	E980.4
gastric agents	973.4	E858.4	E943.4	E950.4	E962.0	E980.4
48:00 expectorants and cough preparations						
antihistamine agents	963.0	E858.1	E933.0	E950.4	E962.0	E980.4
antitussives	975.4	E858.6	E945.4	E950.4	E962.0	E980.4
codeine derivatives	965.09	E850.2	E935.2	E950.0	E962.0	E980.0
expectorants	975.5	E858.6	E945.5	E950.4	E962.0	E980.4
narcotic agents NEC	965.09	E850.2	E935.2	E950.0	E962.0	E980.0
52:04 anti–infectives (EENT)						
ENT agent	976.6	E858.7	E946.6	E950.4	E962.0	E980.4
ophthalmic preparation	976.5	E858.7	E946.5	E950.4	E962.0	E980.4
52:04.04 antibiotics (EENT)						
ENT agent	976.6	E858.7	E946.6	E950.4	E962.0	E980.4
ophthalmic preparation	976.5	E858.7	E946.5	E950.4	E962.0	E980.4
52:04.06 antivirals (EENT)						
ENT agent	976.6	E858.7	E946.6	E950.4	E962.0	E980.4
ophthalmic preparation	976.5	E858.7	E946.5	E950.4	E962.0	E980.4
52:04.08 sulfonamides (EENT)						
ENT agent	976.6	E858.7	E946.6	E950.4	E962.0	E980.4
ophthalmic preparation	976.5	E858.7	E946.5	E950.4	E962.0	E980.4
52:04.12 miscellaneous anti–infectives (EENT)						
ENT agent	976.6	E858.7	E946.6	E950.4	E962.0	E980.4
ophthalmic preparation	976.5	E858.7	E946.5	E950.4	E962.0	E980.4
52:08 anti–inflammatory agents (EENT)						
ENT agent	976.6	E858.7	E946.6	E950.4	E962.0	E980.4
ophthalmic preparation	976.5	E858.7	E946.5	E950.4	E962.0	E980.4
52:10 carbonic anhydrase inhibitors	974.2	E858.5	E944.2	E950.4	E962.0	E980.4
52:12 contact lens solutions	976.5	E858.7	E946.5	E950.4	E962.0	E980.4
52:16 local anesthetics (EENT)	968.5	E855.2	E938.5	E950.4	E962.0	E980.4
52:20 miotics	971.0	E855.3	E941.0	E950.4	E962.0	E980.4
52:24 mydriatics						
adrenergics	971.2	E855.5	E941.2	E950.4	E962.0	E980.4
anticholinergics	971.1	E855.4	E941.1	E950.4	E962.0	E980.4
antimuscarinics	971.1	E855.4	E941.1	E950.4	E962.0	E980.4
parasympatholytics	971.1	E855.4	E941.1	E950.4	E962.0	E980.4

Substance		External Cause (E-Code)				
	Poisoning	Accident	Therapeutic Use	Suicide Attempt	Assault	Undetermined
spasmolytics	971.1	E855.4	E941.1	E950.4	E962.0	E980.4
sympathomimetics	971.2	E855.5	E941.2	E950.4	E962.0	E980.4
52:28 mouth washes and gargles	976.6	E858.7	E946.6	E950.4	E962.0	E980.4
52:32 vasoconstrictors (EENT)	971.2	E855.5	E941.2	E950.4	E962.0	E980.4
52:36 unclassified agents (EENT)						
ENT agent	976.6	E858.7	E946.6	E950.4	E962.0	E980.4
ophthalmic preparation	976.5	E858.7	E946.5	E950.4	E962.0	E980.4
56:04 antacids and adsorbents	973.0	E858.4	E943.0	E950.4	E962.0	E980.4
56:08 Antidiarrhea agents	973.5	E858.4	E943.5	E950.4	E962.0	E980.4
56:10 antiflatulents	973.8	E858.4	E943.8	E950.4	E962.0	E980.4
56:12 cathartics NEC	973.3	E858.4	E943.3	E950.4	E962.0	E980.4
emollients	973.2	E858.4	E943.2	E950.4	E962.0	E980.4
irritants	973.1	E858.4	E943.1	E950.4	E962.0	E980.4
56:16 digestants	973.4	E858.4	E943.4	E950.4	E962.0	E980.4
56:20 emetics and antiemetics						
antiemetics	963.0	E858.1	E933.0	E950.4	E962.0	E980.4
emetics	973.6	E858.4	E943.6	E950.4	E962.0	E980.4
56:24 lipotropic agents	977.1	E858.8	E947.1	E950.4	E962.0	E980.4
56:40 miscellaneous G.I. drugs	973.8	E858.4	E943.8	E950.4	E962.0	E980.4
60:00 gold compounds	965.6	E850.6	E935.6	E950.0	E962.0	E980.0
64:00 heavy metal antagonists	963.8	E858.1	E933.8	E950.4	E962.0	E980.4
68:04 adrenals	962.0	E858.0	E932.0	E950.4	E962.0	E980.4
68:08 androgens	962.1	E858.0	E932.1	E950.4	E962.0	E980.4
68:12 contraceptives, oral	962.2	E858.0	E932.2	E950.4	E962.0	E980.4
68:16 estrogens	962.2	E858.0	E932.2	E950.4	E962.0	E980.4
68:18 gonadotropins	962.4	E858.0	E932.4	E950.4	E962.0	E980.4
68:20 insulins and antidiabetic agents	962.3	E858.0	E932.3	E950.4	E962.0	E980.4
68:20.08 insulins	962.3	E858.0	E932.3	E950.4	E962.0	E980.4
68:24 parathyroid	962.6	E858.0	E932.6	E950.4	E962.0	E980.4
68:28 pituitary (posterior)	962.5	E858.0	E932.5	E950.4	E962.0	E980.4
anterior	962.4	E858.0	E932.4	E950.4	E962.0	E980.4
68:32 progestogens	962.2	E858.0	E932.2	E950.4	E962.0	E980.4
68:34 other corpus luteum hormones NEC	962.2	E858.0	E932.2	E950.4	E962.0	E980.4
68:36 thyroid and antithyroid						
antithyroid	962.8	E858.0	E932.8	E950.4	E962.0	E980.4
thyroid (derivatives)	962.7	E858.0	E932.7	E950.4	E962.0	E980.4
72:00 local anesthetics NEC	968.9	E855.2	E938.9	E950.4	E962.0	E980.4
topical (surface)	968.5	E855.2	E938.5	E950.4	E962.0	E980.4
infiltration (intradermal) (subcutaneous) (submucosal)	968.5	E855.2	E938.5	E950.4	E962.0	E980.4
nerve blocking (peripheral) (plexus) (regional)	968.6	E855.2	E938.6	E950.4	E962.0	E980.4
spinal	968.7	E855.2	E938.7	E950.4	E962.0	E980.4
76:00 oxytocics	975.0	E858.6	E945.0	E950.4	E962.0	E980.4
78:00 radioactive agents	990	—	—	—	—	—
80:04 serums NEC	979.9	E858.8	E949.9	E950.4	E962.0	E980.4
immune gamma globulin (human)	964.6	E858.2	E934.6	E950.4	E962.0	E980.4
80:08 toxoids NEC	978.8	E858.8	E948.8	E950.4	E962.0	E980.4
diphtheria	978.5	E858.8	E948.5	E950.4	E962.0	E980.4
and tetanus	978.9	E858.8	E948.9	E950.4	E962.0	E980.4
with pertussis component	978.6	E858.8	E948.6	E950.4	E962.0	E980.4
tetanus	978.4	E858.8	E948.4	E950.4	E962.0	E980.4
and diphtheria	978.9	E858.8	E948.9	E950.4	E962.0	E980.4
with pertussis component	978.6	E858.8	E948.6	E950.4	E962.0	E980.4
80:12 vaccines	979.9	E858.8	E949.9	E950.4	E962.0	E980.4
bacterial NEC	978.8	E858.8	E948.8	E950.4	E962.0	E980.4

Substance	Poisoning	Accident	Therapeutic Use	Suicide Attempt	Assault	Undetermined
		External Cause (E-Code)				
with						
other bacterial components	978.9	E858.8	E948.9	E950.4	E962.0	E980.4
pertussis component	978.6	E858.8	E948.6	E950.4	E962.0	E980.4
viral and rickettsial components	979.7	E858.8	E949.7	E950.4	E962.0	E980.4
rickettsial NEC	979.6	E858.8	E949.6	E950.4	E962.0	E980.4
with						
bacterial component	979.7	E858.8	E949.7	E950.4	E962.0	E980.4
pertussis component	978.6	E858.8	E948.6	E950.4	E962.0	E980.4
viral component	979.7	E858.8	E949.7	E950.4	E962.0	E980.4
viral NEC	979.6	E858.8	E949.6	E950.4	E962.0	E980.4
with						
bacterial component	979.7	E858.8	E949.7	E950.4	E962.0	E980.4
pertussis component	978.6	E858.8	E948.6	E950.4	E962.0	E980.4
rickettsial component	979.7	E858.8	E949.7	E950.4	E962.0	E980.4
84:04.04 antibiotics (skin and mucous membrane)	976.0	E858.7	E946.0	E950.4	E962.0	E980.4
84:04.08 fungicides (skin and mucous membrane)	976.0	E858.7	E946.0	E950.4	E962.0	E980.4
84:04.12 scabicides and pediculicides (skin and mucous membrane)	976.0	E858.7	E946.0	E950.4	E962.0	E980.4
84:04.16 miscellaneous local anti–infectives (skin and mucous membrane)	976.0	E858.7	E946.0	E950.4	E962.0	E980.4
84:06 anti–inflammatory agents (skin and mucous membrane)	976.0	E858.7	E946.0	E950.4	E962.0	E980.4
84:08 antipruritics and local anesthetics						
antipruritics	976.1	E858.7	E946.1	E950.4	E962.0	E980.4
local anesthetics	968.5	E855.2	E938.5	E950.4	E962.0	E980.4
84:12 astringents	976.2	E858.7	E946.2	E950.4	E962.0	E980.4
84:16 cell stimulants and proliferants	976.8	E858.7	E946.8	E950.4	E962.0	E980.4
84:20 detergents	976.2	E858.7	E946.2	E950.4	E962.0	E980.4
84:24 emollients, demulcents, and protectants	976.3	E858.7	E946.3	E950.4	E962.0	E980.4
84:28 keratolytic agents	976.4	E858.7	E946.4	E950.4	E962.0	E980.4
84:32 keratoplastic agents	976.4	E858.7	E946.4	E950.4	E962.0	E980.4
84:36 miscellaneous agents (skin and mucous membrane)	976.8	E858.7	E946.8	E950.4	E962.0	E980.4
86:00 spasmolytic agents	975.1	E858.6	E945.1	E950.4	E962.0	E980.4
antiasthmatics	975.7	E858.6	E945.7	E950.4	E962.0	E980.4
papaverine	972.5	E858.3	E942.5	E950.4	E962.0	E980.4
theophylline	974.1	E858.5	E944.1	E950.4	E962.0	E980.4
88:04 vitamin A	963.5	E858.1	E933.5	E950.4	E962.0	E980.4
88:08 vitamin B complex	963.5	E858.1	E933.5	E950.4	E962.0	E980.4
hematopoietic vitamin	964.1	E858.2	E934.1	E950.4	E962.0	E980.4
nicotinic acid derivatives	972.2	E858.3	E942.2	E950.4	E962.0	E980.4
88:12 vitamin C	963.5	E858.1	E933.5	E950.4	E962.0	E980.4
88:16 vitamin D	963.5	E858.1	E933.5	E950.4	E962.0	E980.4
88:20 vitamin E	963.5	E858.1	E933.5	E950.4	E962.0	E980.4
88:24 vitamin K activity	964.3	E858.2	E934.3	E950.4	E962.0	E980.4
88:28 multivitamin preparations	963.5	E858.1	E933.5	E950.4	E962.0	E980.4
92:00 unclassified therapeutic agents	977.8	E858.8	E947.8	E950.4	E962.0	E980.4
Duboisine	971.1	E855.4	E941.1	E950.4	E962.0	E980.4
Dulcolax	973.1	E858.4	E943.1	E950.4	E962.0	E980.4
Duponol (C) (EP)	976.2	E858.7	E946.2	E950.4	E962.0	E980.4
Durabolin	962.1	E858.0	E932.1	E950.4	E962.0	E980.4
Dyclone	968.5	E855.2	E938.5	E950.4	E962.0	E980.4

Substance	Poisoning	External Cause (E-Code) Accident	Therapeutic Use	Suicide Attempt	Assault	Undetermined
Dyclonine	968.5	E855.2	E938.5	E950.4	E962.0	E980.4
Dydrogesterone	962.2	E858.0	E932.2	E950.4	E962.0	E980.4
Dyes NEC	989.8	E866.8	—	E950.9	E962.1	E980.9
diagnostic agents	977.8	E858.8	E947.8	E950.4	E962.0	E980.4
pharmaceutical NEC	977.4	E858.8	E947.4	E950.4	E962.0	E980.4
Dyfols	971.0	E855.3	E941.0	E950.4	E962.0	E980.4
Dymelor	962.3	E858.0	E932.3	E950.4	E962.0	E980.4
Dynamite	989.8	E866.8	—	E950.9	E962.1	E980.9
fumes	987.8	E869.8	—	E952.8	E962.2	E982.8
Dyphylline	975.1	E858.6	E945.1	E950.4	E962.0	E980.4
Ear preparations	976.6	E858.7	E946.6	E950.4	E962.0	E980.4
Echothiopate, ecothiopate	971.0	E855.3	E941.0	E950.4	E962.0	E980.4
Ectylurea	967.8	E852.8	E937.8	E950.2	E962.0	E980.2
Edathamil disodium	963.8	E858.1	E933.8	E950.4	E962.0	E980.4
Edecrin	974.4	E858.5	E944.4	E950.4	E962.0	E980.4
Edetate, disodium (calcium)	963.8	E858.1	E933.8	E950.4	E962.0	E980.4
Edrophonium	971.0	E855.3	E941.0	E950.4	E962.0	E980.4
Elase	976.8	E858.7	E946.8	E950.4	E962.0	E980.4
Elaterium	973.1	E858.4	E943.1	E950.4	E962.0	E980.4
Elder	988.2	E865.4	—	E950.9	E962.1	E980.9
berry (unripe)	988.2	E865.3	—	E950.9	E962.1	E980.9
Electrolytes NEC	974.5	E858.5	E944.5	E950.4	E962.0	E980.4
Electrolytic agent NEC	974.5	E858.5	E944.5	E950.4	E962.0	E980.4
Embramine	963.0	E858.1	E933.0	E950.4	E962.0	E980.4
Emetics	973.6	E858.4	E943.6	E950.4	E962.0	E980.4
Emetine (hydrochloride)	961.5	E857	E931.5	E950.4	E962.0	E980.4
Emollients	976.3	E858.7	E946.3	E950.4	E962.0	E980.4
Emylcamate	969.5	E853.8	E939.5	E950.3	E962.0	E980.3
Encyprate	969.0	E854.0	E939.0	E950.3	E962.0	E980.3
Endocaine	968.5	E855.2	E938.5	E950.4	E962.0	E980.4
Endrin	989.2	E863.0	—	E950.6	E962.1	E980.7
Enflurane	968.2	E855.1	E938.2	E950.4	E962.0	E980.4
Enovid	962.2	E858.0	E932.2	E950.4	E962.0	E980.4
ENT preparations (anti–infectives)	976.6	E858.7	E946.6	E950.4	E962.0	E980.4
Enzodase	963.4	E858.1	E933.4	E950.4	E962.0	E980.4
Enzymes NEC	963.4	E858.1	E933.4	E950.4	E962.0	E980.4
Epanutin	966.1	E855.0	E936.1	E950.4	E962.0	E980.4
Ephedra (tincture)	971.2	E855.5	E941.2	E950.4	E962.0	E980.4
Ephedrine	971.2	E855.5	E941.2	E950.4	E962.0	E980.4
Epiestriol	962.2	E858.0	E932.2	E950.4	E962.0	E980.4
Epinephrine	971.2	E855.5	E941.2	E950.4	E962.0	E980.4
Epsom salt	973.3	E858.4	E943.3	E950.4	E962.0	E980.4
Equanil	969.5	E853.8	E939.5	E950.3	E962.0	E980.3
Equisetum (diuretic)	974.4	E858.5	E944.4	E950.4	E962.0	E980.4
Ergometrine	975.0	E858.6	E945.0	E950.4	E962.0	E980.4
Ergonovine	975.0	E858.6	E945.0	E950.4	E962.0	E980.4
Ergot NEC	988.2	E865.4	—	E950.9	E962.1	E980.9
medicinal (alkaloids)	975.0	E858.6	E945.0	E950.4	E962.0	E980.4
Ergotamine (tartrate) (for migraine) NEC	972.9	E858.3	E942.9	E950.4	E962.0	E980.4
Ergotrate	975.0	E858.6	E945.0	E950.4	E962.0	E980.4
Erythrityl tetranitrate	972.4	E858.3	E942.4	E950.4	E962.0	E980.4
Erythrol tetranitrate	972.4	E858.3	E942.4	E950.4	E962.0	E980.4
Erythromycin	960.3	E856	E930.3	E950.4	E962.0	E980.4
ophthalmic preparation	976.5	E858.7	E946.5	E950.4	E962.0	E980.4
topical NEC	976.0	E858.7	E946.0	E950.4	E962.0	E980.4
Eserine	971.0	E855.3	E941.0	E950.4	E962.0	E980.4
Eskabarb	967.0	E851	E937.0	E950.1	E962.0	E980.1

Substance	Poisoning	Accident	Therapeutic Use	Suicide Attempt	Assault	Undetermined
		External Cause (E-Code)				
Eskalith	969.8	E855.8	E939.8	E950.3	E962.0	E980.3
Estradiol (cypionate) (dipropionate) (valerate)	962.2	E858.0	E932.2	E950.4	E962.0	E980.4
Estriol	962.2	E858.0	E932.2	E950.4	E962.0	E980.4
Estrogens (with progestogens)	962.2	E858.0	E932.2	E950.4	E962.0	E980.4
Estrone	962.2	E858.0	E932.2	E950.4	E962.0	E980.4
Etafedrine	971.2	E855.5	E941.2	E950.4	E962.0	E980.4
Ethacrynate sodium	974.4	E858.5	E944.4	E950.4	E962.0	E980.4
Ethacrynic acid	974.4	E858.5	E944.4	E950.4	E962.0	E980.4
Ethambutol	961.8	E857	E931.8	E950.4	E962.0	E980.4
Ethamide	974.2	E858.5	E944.2	E950.4	E962.0	E980.4
Ethamivan	970.0	E854.3	E940.0	E950.4	E962.0	E980.4
Ethamsylate	964.5	E858.2	E934.5	E950.4	E962.0	E980.4
Ethanol	980.0	E860.1	—	E950.9	E962.1	E980.9
beverage	980.0	E860.0	—	E950.9	E962.1	E980.9
Ethchlorvynol	967.8	E852.8	E937.8	E950.2	E962.0	E980.2
Ethebenecid	974.7	E858.5	E944.7	E950.4	E962.0	E980.4
Ether(s) (diethyl) (ethyl) (vapor)	987.8	E869.8	—	E952.8	E962.2	E982.8
anesthetic	968.2	E855.1	E938.2	E950.4	E962.0	E980.4
petroleum — *see* Ligroin						
solvent	982.8	E862.4	—	E950.9	E962.1	E980.9
Ethidine chloride (vapor)	987.8	E869.8	—	E952.8	E962.2	E982.8
liquid (solvent)	982.3	E862.4	—	E950.9	E962.1	E980.9
Ethinamate	967.8	E852.8	E937.8	E950.2	E962.0	E980.2
Ethinylestradiol	962.2	E858.0	E932.2	E950.4	E962.0	E980.4
Ethionamide	961.8	E857	E931.8	E950.4	E962.0	E980.4
Ethisterone	962.2	E858.0	E932.2	E950.4	E962.0	E980.4
Ethobral	967.0	E851	E937.0	E950.1	E962.0	E980.1
Ethocaine (infiltration) (topical)	968.5	E855.2	E938.5	E950.4	E962.0	E980.4
nerve block (peripheral) (plexus)	968.6	E855.2	E938.6	E950.4	E962.0	E980.4
spinal	968.7	E855.2	E938.7	E950.4	E962.0	E980.4
Ethoheptazine (citrate)	965.7	E850.7	E935.7	E950.0	E962.0	E980.0
Ethopropazine	966.4	E855.0	E936.4	E950.4	E962.0	E980.4
Ethosuximide	966.2	E855.0	E936.2	E950.4	E962.0	E980.4
Ethotoin	966.1	E855.0	E936.1	E950.4	E962.0	E980.4
Ethoxazene	961.9	E857	E931.9	E950.4	E962.0	E980.4
Ethoxzolamide	974.2	E858.5	E944.2	E950.4	E962.0	E980.4
Ethyl						
acetate (vapor)	982.8	E862.4	—	E950.9	E962.1	E980.9
alcohol	980.0	E860.1	—	E950.9	E962.1	E980.9
beverage	980.0	E860.0	—	E950.9	E962.1	E980.9
aldehyde (vapor)	987.8	E869.8	—	E952.8	E962.2	E982.8
liquid	989.8	E866.8	—	E950.9	E962.1	E980.9
aminobenzoate	968.5	E855.2	E938.5	E950.4	E962.0	E980.4
biscoumacetate	964.2	E858.2	E934.2	E950.4	E962.0	E980.4
bromide (anesthetic)	968.2	E855.1	E938.2	E950.4	E962.0	E980.4
carbamate (antineoplastic)	963.1	E858.1	E933.1	E950.4	E962.0	E980.4
carbinol	980.3	E860.4	—	E950.9	E962.1	E980.9
chaulmoograte	961.8	E857	E931.8	E950.4	E962.0	E980.4
chloride (vapor)	987.8	E869.8	—	E952.8	E962.2	E982.8
anesthetic (local)	968.5	E855.2	E938.5	E950.4	E962.0	E980.4
inhaled	968.2	E855.1	E938.2	E950.4	E962.0	E980.4
solvent	982.3	E862.4	—	E950.9	E962.1	E980.9
estranol	962.1	E858.0	E932.1	E950.4	E962.0	E980.4
ether — *see* Ether(s)						
formate (solvent) NEC	982.8	E862.4	—	E950.9	E962.1	E980.9
iodoacetate	987.5	E869.3	—	E952.8	E962.2	E982.8

Substance	Poisoning	External Cause (E-Code) Accident	Therapeutic Use	Suicide Attempt	Assault	Undetermined
lactate (solvent) NEC	982.8	E862.4	—	E950.9	E962.1	E980.9
methylcarbinol	980.8	E860.8	—	E950.9	E962.1	E980.9
morphine	965.09	E850.2	E935.2	E950.0	E962.0	E980.0
Ethylene (gas)	987.1	E869.8	—	E952.8	E962.2	E982.8
anesthetic (general)	968.2	E855.1	E938.2	E950.4	E962.0	E980.4
chlorohydrin (vapor)	982.3	E862.4	—	E950.9	E962.1	E980.9
dichloride (vapor)	982.3	E862.4	—	E950.9	E962.1	E980.9
glycol(s) (any) (vapor)	982.8	E862.4	—	E950.9	E962.1	E980.9
Ethylidene						
chloride NEC	982.3	E862.4	—	E950.9	E962.1	E980.9
diethyl ether	982.8	E862.4	—	E950.9	E962.1	E980.9
Ethynodiol	962.2	E858.0	E932.2	E950.4	E962.0	E980.4
Etidocaine	968.9	E855.2	E938.9	E950.4	E962.0	E980.4
infiltration (subcutaneous)	968.5	E855.2	E938.5	E950.4	E962.0	E980.4
nerve (peripheral) (plexus)	968.6	E855.2	E938.6	E950.4	E962.0	E980.4
Etilfen	967.0	E851	E937.0	E950.1	E962.0	E980.1
Etomide	965.7	E850.7	E935.7	E950.0	E962.0	E980.0
Etorphine	965.09	E850.2	E935.2	E950.0	E962.0	E980.0
Etoval	967.0	E851	E937.0	E950.1	E962.0	E980.1
Etryptamine	969.0	E854.0	E939.0	E950.3	E962.0	E980.3
Eucaine	968.5	E855.2	E938.5	E950.4	E962.0	E980.4
Eucalyptus (oil) NEC	975.5	E858.6	E945.5	E950.4	E962.0	E980.4
Eucatropine	971.1	E855.4	E941.1	E950.4	E962.0	E980.4
Eucodal	965.09	E850.2	E935.2	E950.0	E962.0	E980.0
Euneryl	967.0	E851	E937.0	E950.1	E962.0	E980.1
Euphthalmine	971.1	E855.4	E941.1	E950.4	E962.0	E980.4
Eurax	976.0	E858.7	E946.0	E950.4	E962.0	E980.4
Euresol	976.4	E858.7	E946.4	E950.4	E962.0	E980.4
Euthroid	962.7	E858.0	E932.7	E950.4	E962.0	E980.4
Evans blue	977.8	E858.8	E947.8	E950.4	E962.0	E980.4
Evipal	967.0	E851	E937.0	E950.1	E962.0	E980.1
sodium	968.3	E855.1	E938.3	E950.4	E962.0	E980.4
Evipan	967.0	E851	E937.0	E950.1	E962.0	E980.1
sodium	968.3	E855.1	E938.3	E950.4	E962.0	E980.4
Exalgin	965.4	E850.4	E935.4	E950.0	E962.0	E980.0
Excipients, pharmaceutical	977.4	E858.8	E947.4	E950.4	E962.0	E980.4
Exhaust gas — *see* Carbon, monoxide						
Ex–Lax (phenolphthalein)	973.1	E858.4	E943.1	E950.4	E962.0	E980.4
Expectorants	975.5	E858.6	E945.5	E950.4	E962.0	E980.4
External medications (skin) (mucous membrane)	976.9	E858.7	E946.9	E950.4	E962.0	E980.4
dental agent	976.7	E858.7	E946.7	E950.4	E962.0	E980.4
ENT agent	976.6	E858.7	E946.6	E950.4	E962.0	E980.4
ophthalmic preparation	976.5	E858.7	E946.5	E950.4	E962.0	E980.4
specified NEC	976.8	E858.7	E946.8	E950.4	E962.0	E980.4
Eye agents (anti–infective)	976.5	E858.7	E946.5	E950.4	E962.0	E980.4
Factor IX complex (human)	964.5	E858.2	E934.5	E950.4	E962.0	E980.4
Fecal softeners	973.2	E858.4	E943.2	E950.4	E962.0	E980.4
Fenbutrazate	977.0	E858.8	E947.0	E950.4	E962.0	E980.4
Fencamfamin	970.8	E854.3	E940.8	E950.4	E962.0	E980.4
Fenfluramine	977.0	E858.8	E947.0	E950.4	E962.0	E980.4
Fenoprofen	965.6	E850.6	E935.6	E950.0	E962.0	E980.0
Fentanyl	965.09	E850.2	E935.2	E950.0	E962.0	E980.0
Fentazin	969.1	E853.0	E939.1	E950.3	E962.0	E980.3
Fenticlor, fentichlor	976.0	E858.7	E946.0	E950.4	E962.0	E980.4
Fer de lance (bite) (venom)	989.5	E905.0	—	E950.9	E962.1	E980.9
Ferric — *see* Iron						

Substance	Poisoning	Accident	Therapeutic Use	Suicide Attempt	Assault	Undetermined
		External Cause (E-Code)				
Ferrocholinate	964.0	E858.2	E934.0	E950.4	E962.0	E980.4
Ferrous fumerate, gluconate, lactate, salt NEC, sulfate (medicinal)	964.0	E858.2	E934.0	E950.4	E962.0	E980.4
Ferrum — *see* Iron						
Fertilizers NEC	989.8	E866.5	—	E950.9	E962.1	E980.4
with herbicide mixture	989.4	E863.5	—	E950.6	E962.1	E980.7
Fibrinogen (human)	964.7	E858.2	E934.7	E950.4	E962.0	E980.4
Fibrinolysin	964.4	E858.2	E934.4	E950.4	E962.0	E980.4
Fibrinolysis–affecting agents	964.4	E858.2	E934.4	E950.4	E962.0	E980.4
Filix mas	961.6	E857	E931.6	E950.4	E962.0	E980.4
Fiorinal	965.1	E850.3	E935.3	E950.0	E962.0	E980.0
Fire damp	987.1	E869.8	—	E952.8	E962.2	E982.8
Fish, nonbacterial or noxious	988.0	E865.2	—	E950.9	E962.1	E980.9
shell	988.0	E865.1	—	E950.9	E962.1	E980.9
Flagyl	961.5	E857	E931.5	E950.4	E962.0	E980.4
Flavoxate	975.1	E858.6	E945.1	E950.4	E962.0	E980.4
Flaxedil	975.2	E858.6	E945.2	E950.4	E962.0	E980.4
Flaxseed (medicinal)	976.3	E858.7	E946.3	E950.4	E962.0	E980.4
Florantyrone	973.4	E858.4	E943.4	E950.4	E962.0	E980.4
Floraquin	961.3	E857	E931.3	E950.4	E962.0	E980.4
Florinef	962.0	E858.0	E932.0	E950.4	E962.0	E980.4
ENT agent	976.6	E858.7	E946.6	E950.4	E962.0	E980.4
ophthalmic preparation	976.5	E858.7	E946.5	E950.4	E962.0	E980.4
topical NEC	976.0	E858.7	E946.0	E950.4	E962.0	E980.4
Flowers of sulfur	976.4	E858.7	E946.4	E950.4	E962.0	E980.4
Floxuridine	963.1	E858.1	E933.1	E950.4	E962.0	E980.4
Flucytosine	961.9	E857	E931.9	E950.4	E962.0	E980.4
Fludrocortisone	962.0	E858.0	E932.0	E950.4	E962.0	E980.4
ENT agent	976.6	E858.7	E946.6	E950.4	E962.0	E980.4
ophthalmic preparation	976.5	E858.7	E946.5	E950.4	E962.0	E980.4
topical NEC	976.0	E858.7	E946.0	E950.4	E962.0	E980.4
Flumethasone	976.0	E858.7	E946.0	E950.4	E962.0	E980.4
Flumethiazide	974.3	E858.5	E944.3	E950.4	E962.0	E980.4
Flumidin	961.7	E857	E931.7	E950.4	E962.0	E980.4
Fluocinolone	976.0	E858.7	E946.0	E950.4	E962.0	E980.4
Fluocortolone	962.0	E858.0	E932.0	E950.4	E962.0	E980.4
Fluohydrocortisone	962.0	E858.0	E932.0	E950.4	E962.0	E980.4
ENT agent	976.6	E858.7	E946.6	E950.4	E962.0	E980.4
ophthalmic preparation	976.5	E858.7	E946.5	E950.4	E962.0	E980.4
topical NEC	976.0	E858.7	E946.0	E950.4	E962.0	E980.4
Fluonid	976.0	E858.7	E946.0	E950.4	E962.0	E980.4
Fluopromazine	969.1	E853.0	E939.1	E950.3	E962.0	E980.3
Fluoracetate	989.4	E863.7	—	E950.6	E962.1	E980.7
Fluorescein (sodium)	977.8	E858.8	E947.8	E950.4	E962.0	E980.4
Fluoride(s) (pesticides) (sodium) NEC	989.4	E863.4	—	E950.6	E962.1	E980.7
hydrogen — *see* Hydrofluoric acid						
medicinal	976.7	E858.7	E946.7	E950.4	E962.0	E980.4
not pesticide NEC	983.9	E864.4	—	E950.7	E962.1	E980.6
stannous	976.7	E858.7	E946.7	E950.4	E962.0	E980.4
Fluorinated corticosteroids	962.0	E858.0	E932.0	E950.4	E962.0	E980.4
Fluorine (compounds) (gas)	987.8	E869.8	—	E952.8	E962.2	E982.8
salt — *see* Fluoride(s)						
Fluoristan	976.7	E858.7	E946.7	E950.4	E962.0	E980.4
Fluoroacetate	989.4	E863.7	—	E950.6	E962.1	E980.7
Fluorodeoxyuridine	963.1	E858.1	E933.1	E950.4	E962.0	E980.4
Fluorometholone (topical) NEC	976.0	E858.7	E946.0	E950.4	E962.0	E980.4
ophthalmic preparation	976.5	E858.7	E946.5	E950.4	E962.0	E980.4

Substance		External Cause (E-Code)				
	Poisoning	Accident	Therapeutic Use	Suicide Attempt	Assault	Undetermined
Fluorouracil	963.1	E858.1	E933.1	E950.4	E962.0	E980.4
Fluothane	968.1	E855.1	E938.1	E950.4	E962.0	E980.4
Fluoxymesterone	962.1	E858.0	E932.1	E950.4	E962.0	E980.4
Fluphenazine	969.1	E853.0	E939.1	E950.3	E962.0	E980.3
Fluprednisolone	962.0	E858.0	E932.0	E950.4	E962.0	E980.4
Flurandrenolide	976.0	E858.7	E946.0	E950.4	E962.0	E980.4
Flurazepam (hydrochloride)	969.4	E853.2	E939.4	E950.3	E962.0	E980.3
Flurobate	976.0	E858.7	E946.0	E950.4	E962.0	E980.4
Flurothyl	969.8	E855.8	E939.8	E950.3	E962.0	E980.3
Fluroxene	968.2	E855.1	E938.2	E950.4	E962.0	E980.4
Folacin	964.1	E858.2	E934.1	E950.4	E962.0	E980.4
Folic acid	964.1	E858.2	E934.1	E950.4	E962.0	E980.4
Follicle stimulating hormone	962.4	E858.0	E932.4	E950.4	E962.0	E980.4
Food, foodstuffs, nonbacterial or noxious	988.9	E865.9	—	E950.9	E962.1	E980.9
berries, seeds	988.2	E865.3	—	E950.9	E962.1	E980.9
fish	988.0	E865.2	—	E950.9	E962.1	E980.9
mushrooms	988.1	E865.5	—	E950.9	E962.1	E980.9
plants	988.2	E865.9	—	E950.9	E962.1	E980.9
specified type NEC	988.2	E865.4	—	E950.9	E962.1	E980.9
shellfish	988.0	E865.1	—	E950.9	E962.1	E980.9
specified NEC	988.8	E865.8	—	E950.9	E962.1	E980.9
Fool's parsley	988.2	E865.4	—	E950.9	E962.1	E980.9
Formaldehyde (solution)	989.8	E861.4	—	E950.9	E962.1	E980.9
fungicide	989.4	E863.6	—	E950.6	E962.1	E980.7
gas or vapor	987.8	E869.8	—	E952.8	E962.2	E982.8
Formalin	989.8	E861.4	—	E950.9	E962.1	E980.9
fungicide	989.4	E863.6	—	E950.6	E962.1	E980.7
vapor	987.8	E869.8	—	E952.8	E962.2	E982.8
Formic acid	983.1	E864.1	—	E950.7	E962.1	E980.6
vapor	987.8	E869.8	—	E952.8	E962.2	E982.8
Fowler's solution	985.1	E866.3	—	E950.8	E962.1	E980.8
Foxglove	988.2	E865.4	—	E950.9	E962.1	E980.9
Fox green	977.8	E858.8	E947.8	E950.4	E962.0	E980.4
Framycetin	960.8	E856	E930.8	E950.4	E962.0	E980.4
Frangula (extract)	973.1	E858.4	E943.1	E950.4	E962.0	E980.4
Frei antigen	977.8	E858.8	E947.8	E950.4	E962.0	E980.4
Freons	987.4	E869.2	—	E952.8	E962.2	E982.8
Fructose	974.5	E858.5	E944.5	E950.4	E962.0	E980.4
Frusemide	974.4	E858.5	E944.4	E950.4	E962.0	E980.4
FSH	962.4	E858.0	E932.4	E950.4	E962.0	E980.4
Fuel						
automobile	981	E862.1	—	E950.9	E962.1	E980.9
exhaust gas, not in transit	986	E868.2	—	E952.0	E962.2	E982.0
vapor NEC	987.1	E869.8	—	E952.8	E962.2	E982.8
gas (domestic use) — *see also* Carbon, monoxide, fuel						
utility	987.1	E868.1	—	E951.8	E962.2	E981.8
incomplete combustion of — *see* Carbon, monoxide, fuel, utility						
in mobile container	987.0	E868.0	—	E951.1	E962.2	E981.1
piped (natural)	987.1	E867	—	E951.0	E962.2	E981.0
industrial, incomplete combustion	986	E868.3	—	E952.1	E962.2	E982.1
Fugillin	960.8	E856	E930.8	E950.4	E962.0	E980.4
Fulminate of mercury	985.0	E866.1	—	E950.9	E962.1	E980.9
Fulvicin	960.1	E856	E930.1	E950.4	E962.0	E980.4
Fumadil	960.8	E856	E930.8	E950.4	E962.0	E980.4
Fumagillin	960.8	E856	E930.8	E950.4	E962.0	E980.4

Substance	Poisoning	External Cause (E-Code)				
		Accident	Therapeutic Use	Suicide Attempt	Assault	Undetermined
Fumes (from)	987.9	E869.9	—	E952.9	E962.2	E982.9
carbon monoxide — *see* Carbon, monoxide						
charcoal (domestic use)	986	E868.3	—	E952.1	E962.2	E982.1
chloroform — *see* Chloroform						
coke (in domestic stoves, fireplaces)	986	E868.3	—	E952.1	E962.2	E982.1
corrosive NEC	987.8	E869.8	—	E952.8	E962.2	E982.8
ether — *see* Ether(s)						
freons	987.4	E869.2	—	E952.8	E962.2	E982.8
hydrocarbons	987.1	E869.8	—	E952.8	E962.2	E982.8
petroleum (liquefied)	987.0	E868.0	—	E951.1	E962.2	E981.1
distributed through pipes (pure or mixed with air)	987.0	E867	—	E951.0	E962.2	E981.0
lead — *see* Lead						
metals — *see* specified metal						
nitrogen dioxide	987.2	E869.0	—	E952.8	E962.2	E982.8
pesticides — *see* Pesticides						
petroleum (liquefied)	987.0	E868.0	—	E951.1	E962.2	E981.1
distributed through pipes (pure or mixed with air)	987.0	E867	—	E951.0	E962.2	E981.0
polyester	987.8	E869.8	—	E952.8	E962.2	E982.8
specified source, other (see also substance specified)	987.8	E869.8	—	E952.8	E962.2	E982.8
sulfur dioxide	987.3	E869.1	—	E952.8	E962.2	E982.8
Fumigants	989.4	E863.8	—	E950.6	E962.1	E980.7
Fungi, noxious, used as food	988.1	E865.5	—	E950.9	E962.1	E980.9
Fungicides (*see also* Antifungals)	989.4	E863.6	—	E950.6	E962.1	E980.7
Fungizone	960.1	E856	E930.1	E950.4	E962.0	E980.4
topical	976.0	E858.7	E946.0	E950.4	E962.0	E980.4
Furacin	976.0	E858.7	E946.0	E950.4	E962.0	E980.4
Furadantin	961.9	E857	E931.9	E950.4	E962.0	E980.4
Furazolidone	961.9	E857	E931.9	E950.4	E962.0	E980.4
Furnace (coal burning) (domestic), gas from	986	E868.3	—	E952.1	E962.2	E982.1
industrial	986	E868.8	—	E952.1	E962.2	E982.1
Furniture polish	989.8	E861.2	—	E950.9	E962.1	E980.9
Furosemide	974.4	E858.5	E944.4	E950.4	E962.0	E980.4
Furoxone	961.9	E857	E931.9	E950.4	E962.0	E980.4
Fusel oil (amyl) (butyl) (propyl)	980.3	E860.4	—	E950.9	E962.1	E980.9
Fusidic acid	960.8	E856	E930.8	E950.4	E962.0	E980.4
Gallamine	975.2	E858.6	E945.2	E950.4	E962.0	E980.4
Gallotannic acid	976.2	E858.7	E946.2	E950.4	E962.0	E980.4
Gamboge	973.1	E858.4	E943.1	E950.4	E962.0	E980.4
Gamimune	964.6	E858.2	E934.6	E950.4	E962.0	E980.4
Gamma–benzene hexachloride (vapor)	989.2	E863.0	—	E950.6	E962.1	E980.7
Gamma globulin	964.6	E858.2	E934.6	E950.4	E962.0	E980.4
Gamulin	964.6	E858.2	E934.6	E950.4	E962.0	E980.4
Ganglionic blocking agents	972.3	E858.3	E942.3	E950.4	E962.0	E980.4
Ganja	969.6	E854.1	E939.6	E950.3	E962.0	E980.3
Garamycin	960.8	E856	E930.8	E950.4	E962.0	E980.4
ophthalmic preparation	976.5	E858.7	E946.5	E950.4	E962.0	E980.4
topical NEC	976.0	E858.7	E946.0	E950.4	E962.0	E980.4
Gardenal	967.0	E851	E937.0	E950.1	E962.0	E980.1
Gardepanyl	967.0	E851	E937.0	E950.1	E962.0	E980.1
Gas	987.9	E869.9	—	E952.9	E962.2	E982.9
acetylene	987.1	E868.1	—	E951.8	E962.2	E981.8
incomplete combustion of — *see* Carbon, monoxide, fuel, utility						

Substance	Poisoning	External Cause (E-Code)				
		Accident	Therapeutic Use	Suicide Attempt	Assault	Undetermined
air contaminants, source or type not specified	987.9	E869.9	—	E952.9	E962.2	E982.9
anesthetic (general) NEC	968.2	E855.1	E938.2	E950.4	E962.0	E980.4
blast furnace	986	E868.8	—	E952.1	E962.2	E982.1
butane — *see* Butane						
carbon monoxide — *see* Carbon, monoxide						
chlorine	987.6	E869.8	—	E952.8	E962.2	E982.8
coal — *see* Carbon, monoxide, coal						
cyanide	987.7	E869.8	—	E952.8	E962.2	E982.8
dicyanogen	987.8	E869.8	—	E952.8	E962.2	E982.8
domestic — *see* Gas, utility						
exhaust — *see* Carbon, monoxide, exhaust gas						
from wood– or coal–burning stove or fireplace	986	E868.3	—	E952.1	E962.2	E982.1
fuel (domestic use) — *see also* Carbon, monoxide, fuel						
industrial use	986	E868.8	—	E952.1	E962.2	E982.1
utility	987.1	E868.1	—	E951.8	E962.2	E981.8
incomplete combustion of — *see* Carbon, monoxide, fuel, utility						
in mobile container	987.0	E868.0	—	E951.1	E962.2	E981.1
piped (natural)	987.1	E867	—	E951.0	E962.2	E981.0
garage	986	E868.2	—	E952.0	E962.2	E982.0
hydrocarbon NEC	987.1	E869.8	—	E952.8	E962.2	E982.8
incomplete combustion of — *see* Carbon, monoxide, fuel, utility						
liquefied (mobile container)	987.0	E868.0	—	E951.1	E962.2	E981.1
piped	987.0	E867	—	E951.0	E962.2	E981.0
hydrocyanic acid	987.7	E869.8	—	E952.8	E962.2	E982.8
illuminating — *see* Gas, utility						
incomplete combustion, any — *see* Carbon, monoxide						
kiln	986	E868.8	—	E952.1	E962.2	E982.1
lacrimogenic	987.5	E869.3	—	E952.8	E962.2	E982.8
marsh	987.1	E869.8	—	E952.8	E962.2	E982.8
motor exhaust, not in transit	986	E868.8	—	E952.1	E962.2	E982.1
mustard — *see* Mustard, gas						
natural	987.1	E867	—	E951.0	E962.2	E981.0
nerve (war)	987.9	E869.9	—	E952.9	E962.2	E982.9
oils	981	E862.1	—	E950.9	E962.1	E980.9
petroleum (liquefied) (distributed in mobile containers)	987.0	E868.0	—	E951.1	E962.2	E981.1
piped (pure or mixed with air)	987.0	E867	—	E951.1	E962.2	E981.1
piped (manufactured) (natural) NEC	987.1	E867	—	E951.0	E962.2	E981.0
producer	986	E868.8	—	E952.1	E962.2	E982.1
propane — *see* Propane						
refrigerant (freon)	987.4	E869.2	—	E952.8	E962.2	E982.8
not freon	987.9	E869.9	—	E952.9	E962.2	E982.9
sewer	987.8	E869.8	—	E952.8	E962.2	E982.8
specified source NEC (*see also* substance specified)	987.8	E869.8	—	E952.8	E962.2	E982.8
stove — *see* Gas, utility						
tear	987.5	E869.3	—	E952.8	E962.2	E982.8
utility (for cooking, heating, or lighting) (piped) NEC	987.1	E868.1	—	E951.8	E962.2	E981.8
incomplete combustion of — *see* Carbon, monoxide, fuel, utility						

Substance	Poisoning	External Cause (E-Code)				
		Accident	Therapeutic Use	Suicide Attempt	Assault	Undetermined
in mobile container	987.0	E868.0	—	E951.1	E962.2	E981.1
piped (natural)	987.1	E867	—	E951.0	E962.2	E981.0
water	987.1	E868.1	—	E951.8	E962.2	E981.8
incomplete combustion of — *see* Carbon, monoxide, fuel, utility						
Gaseous substance — *see* Gas						
Gasoline, gasolene	981	E862.1	—	E950.9	E962.1	E980.9
vapor	987.1	E869.8	—	E952.8	E962.2	E982.8
Gastric enzymes	973.4	E858.4	E943.4	E950.4	E962.0	E980.4
Gastrografin	977.8	E858.8	E947.8	E950.4	E962.0	E980.4
Gastrointestinal agents	973.9	E858.4	E943.9	E950.4	E962.0	E980.4
specified NEC	973.8	E858.4	E943.8	E950.4	E962.0	E980.4
Gaultheria procumbens	988.2	E865.4	—	E950.9	E962.1	E980.9
Gelatin (intravenous)	964.8	E858.2	E934.8	E950.4	E962.0	E980.4
absorbable (sponge)	964.5	E858.2	E934.5	E950.4	E962.0	E980.4
Gelfilm	976.8	E858.7	E946.8	E950.4	E962.0	E980.4
Gelfoam	964.5	E858.2	E934.5	E950.4	E962.0	E980.4
Gelsemine	970.8	E854.3	E940.8	E950.4	E962.0	E980.4
Gelsemium (sempervirens)	988.2	E865.4	—	E950.9	E962.1	E980.9
Gemonil	967.0	E851	E937.0	E950.1	E962.0	E980.1
Gentamicin	960.8	E856	E930.8	E950.4	E962.0	E980.4
ophthalmic preparation	976.5	E858.7	E946.5	E950.4	E962.0	E980.4
topical NEC	976.0	E858.7	E946.0	E950.4	E962.0	E980.4
Gentian violet	976.0	E858.7	E946.0	E950.4	E962.0	E980.4
Gexane	976.0	E858.7	E946.0	E950.4	E962.0	E980.4
Gila monster (venom)	989.5	E905.0	—	E950.9	E962.1	E980.9
Ginger, Jamaica	989.8	E866.8	—	E950.9	E962.1	E980.9
Gitalin	972.1	E858.3	E942.1	E950.4	E962.0	E980.4
Gitoxin	972.1	E858.3	E942.1	E950.4	E962.0	E980.4
Glandular extract (medicinal) NEC	977.9	E858.9	E947.9	E950.5	E962.0	E980.5
Glaucarubin	961.5	E857	E931.5	E950.4	E962.0	E980.4
Globin zinc insulin	962.3	E858.0	E932.3	E950.4	E962.0	E980.4
Glucagon	962.3	E858.0	E932.3	E950.4	E962.0	E980.4
Glucochloral	967.1	E852.0	E937.1	E950.2	E962.0	E980.2
Glucocorticoids	962.0	E858.0	E932.0	E950.4	E962.0	E980.4
Glucose	974.5	E858.5	E944.5	E950.4	E962.0	E980.4
oxidase reagent	977.8	E858.8	E947.8	E950.4	E962.0	E980.4
Glucosulfone sodium	961.8	E857	E931.8	E950.4	E962.0	E980.4
Glue(s)	989.8	E866.6	—	E950.9	E962.1	E980.9
Glutamic acid (hydrochloride)	973.4	E858.4	E943.4	E950.4	E962.0	E980.4
Glutathione	963.8	E858.1	E933.8	E950.4	E962.0	E980.4
Glutethimide (group)	967.5	E852.4	E937.5	E950.2	E962.0	E980.2
Glycerin (lotion)	976.3	E858.7	E946.3	E950.4	E962.0	E980.4
Glycerol (topical)	976.3	E858.7	E946.3	E950.4	E962.0	E980.4
Glyceryl						
guaiacolate	975.5	E858.6	E945.5	E950.4	E962.0	E980.4
triacetate (topical)	976.0	E858.7	E946.0	E950.4	E962.0	E980.4
trinitrate	972.4	E858.3	E942.4	E950.4	E962.0	E980.4
Glycine	974.5	E858.5	E944.5	E950.4	E962.0	E980.4
Glycobiarsol	961.1	E857	E931.1	E950.4	E962.0	E980.4
Glycols (ether)	982.8	E862.4	—	E950.9	E962.1	E980.9
Glycopyrrolate	971.1	E855.4	E941.1	E950.4	E962.0	E980.4
Glymidine	962.3	E858.0	E932.3	E950.4	E962.0	E980.4
Gold (compounds) (salts)	965.6	E850.6	E935.6	E950.0	E962.0	E980.0
Golden sulfide of antimony	985.4	E866.2	—	E950.9	E962.1	E980.9
Goldylocks	988.2	E865.4	—	E950.9	E962.1	E980.9
Gonadal tissue extract	962.9	E858.0	E932.9	E950.4	E962.0	E980.4

Substance	Poisoning	External Cause (E-Code) Accident	Therapeutic Use	Suicide Attempt	Assault	Undetermined
female	962.2	E858.0	E932.2	E950.4	E962.0	E980.4
male	962.1	E858.0	E932.1	E950.4	E962.0	E980.4
Gonadotropin	962.4	E858.0	E932.4	E950.4	E962.0	E980.4
Grain alcohol	980.0	E860.1	—	E950.9	E962.1	E980.9
beverage	980.0	E860.0	—	E950.9	E962.1	E980.9
Gramicidin	960.8	E856	E930.8	E950.4	E962.0	E980.4
Gratiola officinalis	988.2	E865.4	—	E950.9	E962.1	E980.9
Grease	989.8	E866.8	—	E950.9	E962.1	E980.9
Green hellebore	988.2	E865.4	—	E950.9	E962.1	E980.9
Green soap	976.2	E858.7	E946.2	E950.4	E962.0	E980.4
Grifulvin	960.1	E856	E930.1	E950.4	E962.0	E980.4
Griseofulvin	960.1	E856	E930.1	E950.4	E962.0	E980.4
Growth hormone	962.4	E858.0	E932.4	E950.4	E962.0	E980.4
Guaiacol	975.5	E858.6	E945.5	E950.4	E962.0	E980.4
Guaiac reagent	977.8	E858.8	E947.8	E950.4	E962.0	E980.4
Guaifenesin	975.5	E858.6	E945.5	E950.4	E962.0	E980.4
Guaiphenesin	975.5	E858.6	E945.5	E950.4	E962.0	E980.4
Guanatol	961.4	E857	E931.4	E950.4	E962.0	E980.4
Guanethidine	972.6	E858.3	E942.6	E950.4	E962.0	E980.4
Guano	989.8	E866.5	—	E950.9	E962.1	E980.9
Guanochlor	972.6	E858.3	E942.6	E950.4	E962.0	E980.4
Guanoctine	972.6	E858.3	E942.6	E950.4	E962.0	E980.4
Guanoxan	972.6	E858.3	E942.6	E950.4	E962.0	E980.4
Hair treatment agent NEC	976.4	E858.7	E946.4	E950.4	E962.0	E980.4
Halcinonide	976.0	E858.7	E946.0	E950.4	E962.0	E980.4
Halethazole	976.0	E858.7	E946.0	E950.4	E962.0	E980.4
Hallucinogens	969.6	E854.1	E939.6	E950.3	E962.0	E980.3
Haloperidol	969.2	E853.1	E939.2	E950.3	E962.0	E980.3
Haloprogin	976.0	E858.7	E946.0	E950.4	E962.0	E980.4
Halotex	976.0	E858.7	E946.0	E950.4	E962.0	E980.4
Halothane	968.1	E855.1	E938.1	E950.4	E962.0	E980.4
Halquinols	976.0	E858.7	E946.0	E950.4	E962.0	E980.4
Harmonyl	972.6	E858.3	E942.6	E950.4	E962.0	E980.4
Hartmann's solution	974.5	E858.5	E944.5	E950.4	E962.0	E980.4
Hashish	969.6	E854.1	E939.6	E950.3	E962.0	E980.3
Hawaiian wood rose seeds	969.6	E854.1	E939.6	E950.3	E962.0	E980.3
Headache cures, drugs, powders NEC	977.9	E858.9	E947.9	E950.5	E962.0	E980.9
Heavenly Blue (morning glory)	969.6	E854.1	E939.6	E950.3	E962.0	E980.3
Heavy metal						
antagonists	963.8	E858.1	E933.8	E950.4	E962.0	E980.4
anti–infectives	961.2	E857	E931.2	E950.4	E962.0	E980.4
Hedaquinium	976.0	E858.7	E946.0	E950.4	E962.0	E980.4
Hedge hyssop	988.2	E865.4	—	E950.9	E962.1	E980.9
Heet	976.8	E858.7	E946.8	E950.4	E962.0	E980.4
Helenin	961.6	E857	E931.6	E950.4	E962.0	E980.4
Hellebore (black) (green) (white)	988.2	E865.4	—	E950.9	E962.1	E980.9
Hemlock	988.2	E865.4	—	E950.9	E962.1	E980.9
Hemostatics	964.5	E858.2	E934.5	E950.4	E962.0	E980.4
capillary active drugs	972.8	E858.3	E942.8	E950.4	E962.0	E980.4
Henbane	988.2	E865.4	—	E950.9	E962.1	E980.9
Heparin (sodium)	964.2	E858.2	E934.2	E950.4	E962.0	E980.4
Heptabarbital, heptabarbitone	967.0	E851	E937.0	E950.1	E962.0	E980.1
Heptachlor	989.2	E863.0	—	E950.6	E962.1	E980.7
Heptalgin	965.09	E850.2	E935.2	E950.0	E962.0	E980.0
Herbicides	989.4	E863.5	—	E950.6	E962.1	E980.7
Heroin	965.01	E850.0	E935.0	E950.0	E962.0	E980.0
Herplex	976.5	E858.7	E946.5	E950.4	E962.0	E980.4

Substance	Poisoning	Accident	Therapeutic Use	Suicide Attempt	Assault	Undetermined
		External Cause (E-Code)				
HES	964.8	E858.2	E934.8	E950.4	E962.0	E980.4
Hetastarch	964.8	E858.2	E934.8	E950.4	E962.0	E980.4
Hexachlorocyclohexane	989.2	E863.0	—	E950.6	E962.1	E980.7
Hexachlorophene	976.2	E858.7	E946.2	E950.4	E962.0	E980.4
Hexadimethrine (bromide)	964.5	E858.2	E934.5	E950.4	E962.0	E980.4
Hexafluorenium	975.2	E858.6	E945.2	E950.4	E962.0	E980.4
Hexa–germ	976.2	E858.7	E946.2	E950.4	E962.0	E980.4
Hexahydrophenol	980.8	E860.8	—	E950.9	E962.1	E980.9
Hexalin	980.8	E860.8	—	E950.9	E962.1	E980.9
Hexamethonium	972.3	E858.3	E942.3	E950.4	E962.0	E980.4
Hexamethyleneamine	961.9	E857	E931.9	E950.4	E962.0	E980.4
Hexamine	961.9	E857	E931.9	E950.4	E962.0	E980.4
Hexanone	982.8	E862.4	—	E950.9	E962.1	E980.9
Hexapropymate	967.8	E852.8	E937.8	E950.2	E962.0	E980.2
Hexestrol	962.2	E858.0	E932.2	E950.4	E962.0	E980.4
Hexethal (sodium)	967.0	E851	E937.0	E950.1	E962.0	E980.1
Hexetidine	976.0	E858.7	E946.0	E950.4	E962.0	E980.4
Hexobarbital, hexobarbitone	967.0	E851	E937.0	E950.1	E962.0	E980.1
sodium (anesthetic)	968.3	E855.1	E938.3	E950.4	E962.0	E980.4
soluble	968.3	E855.1	E938.3	E950.4	E962.0	E980.4
Hexocyclium	971.1	E855.4	E941.1	E950.4	E962.0	E980.4
Hexoestrol	962.2	E858.0	E932.2	E950.4	E962.0	E980.4
Hexone	982.8	E862.4	—	E950.9	E962.1	E980.9
Hexylcaine	968.5	E855.2	E938.5	E950.4	E962.0	E980.4
Hexylresorcinol	961.6	E857	E931.6	E950.4	E962.0	E980.4
Hinkle's pills	973.1	E858.4	E943.1	E950.4	E962.0	E980.4
Histalog	977.8	E858.8	E947.8	E950.4	E962.0	E980.4
Histamine (phosphate)	972.5	E858.3	E942.5	E950.4	E962.0	E980.4
Histoplasmin	977.8	E858.8	E947.8	E950.4	E962.0	E980.4
Holly berries	988.2	E865.3	—	E950.9	E962.1	E980.9
Homatropine	971.1	E855.4	E941.1	E950.4	E962.0	E980.4
Homo–tet	964.6	E858.2	E934.6	E950.4	E962.0	E980.4
Hormones (synthetic substitute) NEC	962.9	E858.0	E932.9	E950.4	E962.0	E980.4
adrenal cortical steroids	962.0	E858.0	E932.0	E950.4	E962.0	E980.4
antidiabetic agents	962.3	E858.0	E932.3	E950.4	E962.0	E980.4
follicle stimulating	962.4	E858.0	E932.4	E950.4	E962.0	E980.4
gonadotropic	962.4	E858.0	E932.4	E950.4	E962.0	E980.4
growth	962.4	E858.0	E932.4	E950.4	E962.0	E980.4
ovarian (substitutes)	962.2	E858.0	E932.2	E950.4	E962.0	E980.4
parathyroid (derivatives)	962.6	E858.0	E932.6	E950.4	E962.0	E980.4
pituitary (posterior)	962.5	E858.0	E932.5	E950.4	E962.0	E980.4
anterior	962.4	E858.0	E932.4	E950.4	E962.0	E980.4
thyroid (derivative)	962.7	E858.0	E932.7	E950.4	E962.0	E980.4
Hornet (sting)	989.5	E905.3	—	E950.9	E962.1	E980.9
Horticulture agent NEC	989.4	E863.9	—	E950.6	E962.1	E980.7
Hyaluronidase	963.4	E858.1	E933.4	E950.4	E962.0	E980.4
Hyazyme	963.4	E858.1	E933.4	E950.4	E962.0	E980.4
Hycodan	965.09	E850.2	E935.2	E950.0	E962.0	E980.0
Hydantoin derivatives	966.1	E855.0	E936.1	E950.4	E962.0	E980.4
Hydeltra	962.0	E858.0	E932.0	E950.4	E962.0	E980.4
Hydergine	971.3	E855.6	E941.3	E950.4	E962.0	E980.4
Hydrabamine penicillin	960.0	E856	E930.0	E950.4	E962.0	E980.4
Hydralazine, hydrallazine	972.6	E858.3	E942.6	E950.4	E962.0	E980.4
Hydrargaphen	976.0	E858.7	E946.0	E950.4	E962.0	E980.4
Hydrazine	983.9	E864.3	—	E950.7	E962.1	E980.6
Hydriodic acid	975.5	E858.6	E945.5	E950.4	E962.0	E980.4
Hydrocarbon gas	987.1	E869.8	—	E952.8	E962.2	E982.8

Substance	Poisoning	External Cause (E-Code)				
		Accident	Therapeutic Use	Suicide Attempt	Assault	Undetermined
incomplete combustion of — *see* Carbon, monoxide, fuel, utility						
liquefied (mobile container)	987.0	E868.0	—	E951.1	E962.2	E981.1
piped (natural)	987.0	E867	—	E951.0	E962.2	E981.0
Hydrochloric acid (liquid)	983.1	E864.1	—	E950.7	E962.1	E980.6
medicinal	973.4	E858.4	E943.4	E950.4	E962.0	E980.4
vapor	987.8	E869.8	—	E952.8	E962.2	E982.8
Hydrochlorothiazide	974.3	E858.5	E944.3	E950.4	E962.0	E980.4
Hydrocodone	965.09	E850.2	E935.2	E950.0	E962.0	E980.0
Hydrocortisone	962.0	E858.0	E932.0	E950.4	E962.0	E980.4
ENT agent	976.6	E858.7	E946.6	E950.4	E962.0	E980.4
ophthalmic preparation	976.5	E858.7	E946.5	E950.4	E962.0	E980.4
topical NEC	976.0	E858.7	E946.0	E950.4	E962.0	E980.4
Hydrocortone	962.0	E858.0	E932.0	E950.4	E962.0	E980.4
ENT agent	976.6	E858.7	E946.6	E950.4	E962.0	E980.4
ophthalmic preparation	976.5	E858.7	E946.5	E950.4	E962.0	E980.4
topical NEC	976.0	E858.7	E946.0	E950.4	E962.0	E980.4
Hydrocyanic acid — *see* Cyanide(s)						
Hydroflumethiazide	974.3	E858.5	E944.3	E950.4	E962.0	E980.4
Hydrofluoric acid (liquid)	983.1	E864.1	—	E950.7	E962.1	E980.6
vapor	987.8	E869.8	—	E952.8	E962.2	E982.8
Hydrogen	987.8	E869.8	—	E952.8	E962.2	E982.8
arsenide	985.1	E866.3	—	E950.8	E962.1	E980.8
arseniureted	985.1	E866.3	—	E950.8	E962.1	E980.8
cyanide (salts)	989.0	E866.8	—	E950.9	E962.1	E980.9
gas	987.7	E869.8	—	E952.8	E962.2	E982.8
fluoride (liquid)	983.1	E864.1	—	E950.7	E962.1	E980.6
vapor	987.8	E869.8	—	E952.8	E962.2	E982.8
peroxide (solution)	976.6	E858.7	E946.6	E950.4	E962.0	E980.4
phosphureted	987.8	E869.8	—	E952.8	E962.2	E982.8
sulfide (gas)	987.8	E869.8	—	E952.8	E962.2	E982.8
arseniureted	985.1	E866.3	—	E950.8	E962.1	E980.8
sulfureted	987.8	E869.8	—	E952.8	E962.2	E982.8
Hydromorphinol	965.09	E850.2	E935.2	E950.0	E962.0	E980.0
Hydromorphinone	965.09	E850.2	E935.2	E950.0	E962.0	E980.0
Hydromorphone	965.09	E850.2	E935.2	E950.0	E962.0	E980.0
Hydromox	974.3	E858.5	E944.3	E950.4	E962.0	E980.4
Hydrophilic lotion	976.3	E858.7	E946.3	E950.4	E962.0	E980.4
Hydroquinone	983.0	E864.0	—	E950.7	E962.1	E980.6
vapor	987.8	E869.8	—	E952.8	E962.2	E982.8
Hydrosulfuric acid (gas)	987.8	E869.8	—	E952.8	E962.2	E982.8
Hydrous wool fat (lotion)	976.3	E858.7	E946.3	E950.4	E962.0	E980.4
Hydroxide, caustic	983.2	E864.2	—	E950.7	E962.1	E980.6
Hydroxocobalamin	964.1	E858.2	E934.1	E950.4	E962.0	E980.4
Hydroxyamphetamine	971.2	E855.5	E941.2	E950.4	E962.0	E980.4
Hydroxychloroquine	961.4	E857	E931.4	E950.4	E962.0	E980.4
Hydroxydihydrocodeinone	965.09	E850.2	E935.2	E950.0	E962.0	E980.0
Hydroxyethyl starch	964.8	E858.2	E934.8	E950.4	E962.0	E980.4
Hydroxyphenamate	969.5	E853.8	E939.5	E950.3	E962.0	E980.3
Hydroxyphenylbutazone	965.5	E850.5	E935.5	E950.0	E962.0	E980.0
Hydroxyprogesterone	962.2	E858.0	E932.2	E950.4	E962.0	E980.4
Hydroxyquinoline derivatives	961.3	E857	E931.3	E950.4	E962.0	E980.4
Hydroxystilbamidine	961.5	E857	E931.5	E950.4	E962.0	E980.4
Hydroxyurea	963.1	E858.1	E933.1	E950.4	E962.0	E980.4
Hydroxyzine	969.5	E853.8	E939.5	E950.3	E962.0	E980.3
Hyoscine (hydrobromide)	971.1	E855.4	E941.1	E950.4	E962.0	E980.4
Hyoscyamine	971.1	E855.4	E941.1	E950.4	E962.0	E980.4

Substance	Poisoning	Accident	Therapeutic Use	Suicide Attempt	Assault	Undetermined
		External Cause (E-Code)				
Hyoscyamus (albus) (niger)	988.2	E865.4	—	E950.9	E962.1	E980.9
Hypaque	977.8	E858.8	E947.8	E950.4	E962.0	E980.4
Hypertussis	964.6	E858.2	E934.6	E950.4	E962.0	E980.4
Hypnotics NEC	967.9	E852.9	E937.9	E950.2	E962.0	E980.2
Hypochlorites — *see* Sodium, hypochlorite						
Hypotensive agents NEC	972.6	E858.3	E942.6	E950.4	E962.0	E980.4
Ibufenac	965.6	E850.6	E935.6	E950.0	E962.0	E980.0
Ibuprofen	965.6	E850.6	E935.6	E950.0	E962.0	E980.0
ICG	977.8	E858.8	E947.8	E950.4	E962.0	E980.4
Ichthammol	976.4	E858.7	E946.4	E950.4	E962.0	E980.4
Ichthyol	976.4	E858.7	E946.4	E950.4	E962.0	E980.4
Idoxuridine	976.5	E858.7	E946.5	E950.4	E962.0	E980.4
IDU	976.5	E858.7	E946.5	E950.4	E962.0	E980.4
Iletin	962.3	E858.0	E932.3	E950.4	E962.0	E980.4
Ilex	988.2	E865.4	—	E950.9	E962.1	E980.9
Illuminating gas — *see* Gas, utility						
Ilopan	963.5	E858.1	E933.5	E950.4	E962.0	E980.4
Ilotycin	960.3	E856	E930.3	E950.4	E962.0	E980.4
ophthalmic preparation	976.5	E858.7	E946.5	E950.4	E962.0	E980.4
topical NEC	976.0	E858.7	E946.0	E950.4	E962.0	E980.4
Imipramine	969.0	E854.0	E939.0	E950.3	E962.0	E980.3
Immu–G	964.6	E858.2	E934.6	E950.4	E962.0	E980.4
Immuglobin	964.6	E858.2	E934.6	E950.4	E962.0	E980.4
Immune serum globulin	964.6	E858.2	E934.6	E950.4	E962.0	E980.4
Immunosuppressive agents	963.1	E858.1	E933.1	E950.4	E962.0	E980.4
Immu–tetanus	964.6	E858.2	E934.6	E950.4	E962.0	E980.4
Indandione (derivatives)	964.2	E858.2	E934.2	E950.4	E962.0	E980.4
Inderal	972.0	E858.3	E942.0	E950.4	E962.0	E980.4
Indian						
hemp	969.6	E854.1	E939.6	E950.3	E962.0	E980.3
tobacco	988.2	E865.4	—	E950.9	E962.1	E980.9
Indigo carmine	977.8	E858.8	E947.8	E950.4	E962.0	E980.4
Indocin	965.6	E850.6	E935.6	E950.0	E962.0	E980.0
Indocyanine green	977.8	E858.8	E947.8	E950.4	E962.0	E980.4
Indomethacin	965.6	E850.6	E935.6	E950.0	E962.0	E980.0
Industrial						
alcohol	980.9	E860.9	—	E950.9	E962.1	E980.9
fumes	987.8	E869.8	—	E952.8	E962.2	E982.8
solvents (fumes) (vapors)	982.8	E862.9	—	E950.9	E962.1	E980.9
Influenza vaccine	979.6	E858.8	E949.6	E950.4	E962.0	E982.8
Ingested substances NEC	989.9	E866.9	—	E950.9	E962.1	E980.9
INH (isoniazid)	961.8	E857	E931.8	E950.4	E962.0	E980.4
Inhalation, gas (noxious) — *see* Gas						
Ink	989.8	E866.8	—	E950.9	E962.1	E980.9
Innovar	967.6	E852.5	E937.6	E950.2	E962.0	E980.2
Inositol niacinate	972.2	E858.3	E942.2	E950.4	E962.0	E980.4
Inproquone	963.1	E858.1	E933.1	E950.4	E962.0	E980.4
Insect (sting), venomous	989.5	E905.5	—	E950.9	E962.1	E980.9
Insecticides (*see also* Pesticides)	989.4	E863.4	—	E950.6	E962.1	E980.7
chlorinated	989.2	E863.0	—	E950.6	E962.1	E980.7
mixtures	989.4	E863.3	—	E950.6	E962.1	E980.7
organochlorine (compounds)	989.2	E863.0	—	E950.6	E962.1	E980.7
organophosphorus (compounds)	989.3	E863.1	—	E950.6	E962.1	E980.7
Insular tissue extract	962.3	E858.0	E932.3	E950.4	E962.0	E980.4
Insulin (amorphous) (globin) (isophane) (Lente) (NPH) (protamine) (Semilente) (Ultralente) (zinc)	962.3	E858.0	E932.3	E950.4	E962.0	E980.4

Substance	Poisoning	Accident	Therapeutic Use	Suicide Attempt	Assault	Undetermined
		External Cause (E-Code)				
Intranarcon	968.3	E855.1	E938.3	E950.4	E962.0	E980.4
Inulin	977.8	E858.8	E947.8	E950.4	E962.0	E980.4
Invert sugar	974.5	E858.5	E944.5	E950.4	E962.0	E980.4
Iodide NEC (*see also* Iodine)	976.0	E858.7	E946.0	E950.4	E962.0	E980.4
mercury (ointment)	976.0	E858.7	E946.0	E950.4	E962.0	E980.4
methylate	976.0	E858.7	E946.0	E950.4	E962.0	E980.4
potassium (expectorant) NEC	975.5	E858.6	E945.5	E950.4	E962.0	E980.4
Iodinated glycerol	975.5	E858.6	E945.5	E950.4	E962.0	E980.4
Iodine (antiseptic, external) (tincture) NEC	976.0	E858.7	E946.0	E950.4	E962.0	E980.4
diagnostic	977.8	E858.8	E947.8	E950.4	E962.0	E980.4
for thyroid conditions (antithyroid)	962.8	E858.0	E932.8	E950.4	E962.0	E980.4
vapor	987.8	E869.8	—	E952.8	E962.2	E982.8
Iodized oil	977.8	E858.8	E947.8	E950.4	E962.0	E980.4
Iodobismitol	961.2	E857	E931.2	E950.4	E962.0	E980.4
Iodochlorhydroxyquin	961.3	E857	E931.3	E950.4	E962.0	E980.4
topical	976.0	E858.7	E946.0	E950.4	E962.0	E980.4
Iodoform	976.0	E858.7	E946.0	E950.4	E962.0	E980.4
Iodopanoic acid	977.8	E858.8	E947.8	E950.4	E962.0	E980.4
Iodophthalein	977.8	E858.8	E947.8	E950.4	E962.0	E980.4
Ion exchange resins	974.5	E858.5	E944.5	E950.4	E962.0	E980.4
Iopanoic acid	977.8	E858.8	E947.8	E950.4	E962.0	E980.4
Iophendylate	977.8	E858.8	E947.8	E950.4	E962.0	E980.4
Iothiouracil	962.8	E858.0	E932.8	E950.4	E962.0	E980.4
Ipecac	973.6	E858.4	E943.6	E950.4	E962.0	E980.4
Ipecacuanha	973.6	E858.4	E943.6	E950.4	E962.0	E980.4
Ipodate	977.8	E858.8	E947.8	E950.4	E962.0	E980.4
Ipral	967.0	E851	E937.0	E950.1	E962.0	E980.1
Iproniazid	969.0	E854.0	E939.0	E950.3	E962.0	E980.3
Iron (compounds) (medicinal) (preparations)	964.0	E858.2	E934.0	E950.4	E962.0	E980.4
dextran	964.0	E858.2	E934.0	E950.4	E962.0	E980.4
nonmedicinal (dust) (fumes) NEC	985.8	E866.4	—	E950.9	E962.1	E980.9
Irritant drug	977.9	E858.9	E947.9	E950.5	E962.0	E980.5
Ismelin	972.6	E858.3	E942.6	E950.4	E962.0	E980.4
Isoamyl nitrite	972.4	E858.3	E942.4	E950.4	E962.0	E980.4
Isobutyl acetate	982.8	E862.4	—	E950.9	E962.1	E980.9
Isocarboxazid	969.0	E854.0	E939.0	E950.3	E962.0	E980.3
Isoephedrine	971.2	E855.5	E941.2	E950.4	E962.0	E980.4
Isoetharine	971.2	E855.5	E941.2	E950.4	E962.0	E980.4
Isofluorophate	971.0	E855.3	E941.0	E950.4	E962.0	E980.4
Isoniazid (INH)	961.8	E857	E931.8	E950.4	E962.0	E980.4
Isopentaquine	961.4	E857	E931.4	E950.4	E962.0	E980.4
Isophane insulin	962.3	E858.0	E932.3	E950.4	E962.0	E980.4
Isopregnenone	962.2	E858.0	E932.2	E950.4	E962.0	E980.4
Isoprenaline	971.2	E855.5	E941.2	E950.4	E962.0	E980.4
Isopropamide	971.1	E855.4	E941.1	E950.4	E962.0	E980.4
Isopropanol	980.2	E860.3	—	E950.9	E962.1	E980.9
topical (germicide)	976.0	E858.7	E946.0	E950.4	E962.0	E980.4
Isopropyl						
acetate	982.8	E862.4	—	E950.9	E962.1	E980.9
alcohol	980.2	E860.3	—	E950.9	E962.1	E980.9
topical (germicide)	976.0	E858.7	E946.0	E950.4	E962.0	E980.4
ether	982.8	E862.4	—	E950.9	E962.1	E980.9
Isoproterenol	971.2	E855.5	E941.2	E950.4	E962.0	E980.4
Isosorbide dinitrate	972.4	E858.3	E942.4	E950.4	E962.0	E980.4
Isothipendyl	963.0	E858.1	E933.0	E950.4	E962.0	E980.4

Substance	Poisoning	Accident	Therapeutic Use	Suicide Attempt	Assault	Undetermined
		External Cause (E-Code)				
Isoxazolyl penicillin	960.0	E856	E930.0	E950.4	E962.0	E980.4
Isoxsuprine hydrochloride	972.5	E858.3	E942.5	E950.4	E962.0	E980.4
I–thyroxine sodium	962.7	E858.0	E932.7	E950.4	E962.0	E980.4
Jaborandi (pilocarpus) (extract)	971.0	E855.3	E941.0	E950.4	E962.0	E980.4
Jalap	973.1	E858.4	E943.1	E950.4	E962.0	E980.4
Jamaica						
dogwood (bark)	965.7	E850.7	E935.7	E950.0	E962.0	E980.0
ginger	989.8	E866.8	—	E950.9	E962.1	E980.9
Jatropha	988.2	E865.4	—	E950.9	E962.1	E980.9
curcas	988.2	E865.3	—	E950.9	E962.1	E980.9
Jectofer	964.0	E858.2	E934.0	E950.4	E962.0	E980.4
Jellyfish (sting)	989.5	E905.6	—	E950.9	E962.1	E980.9
Jequirity (bean)	988.2	E865.3	—	E950.9	E962.1	E980.9
Jimson weed	988.2	E865.4	—	E950.9	E962.1	E980.9
seeds	988.2	E865.3	—	E950.9	E962.1	E980.9
Juniper tar (oil) (ointment)	976.4	E858.7	E946.4	E950.4	E962.0	E980.4
Kallikrein	972.5	E858.3	E942.5	E950.4	E962.0	E980.4
Kanamycin	960.6	E856	E930.6	E950.4	E962.0	E980.4
Kantrex	960.6	E856	E930.6	E950.4	E962.0	E980.4
Kaolin	973.5	E858.4	E943.5	E950.4	E962.0	E980.4
Karaya (gum)	973.3	E858.4	E943.3	E950.4	E962.0	E980.4
Kemithal	968.3	E855.1	E938.3	E950.4	E962.0	E980.4
Kenacort	962.0	E858.0	E932.0	E950.4	E962.0	E980.4
Keratolytics	976.4	E858.7	E946.4	E950.4	E962.0	E980.4
Keratoplastics	976.4	E858.7	E946.4	E950.4	E962.0	E980.4
Kerosene, kerosine (fuel) (solvent) NEC	981	E862.1	—	E950.9	E962.1	E980.9
insecticide	981	E863.4	—	E950.6	E962.1	E980.7
vapor	987.1	E869.8	—	E952.8	E962.2	E982.8
Ketamine	968.3	E855.1	E938.3	E950.4	E962.0	E980.4
Ketobemidone	965.09	E850.2	E935.2	E950.0	E962.0	E980.0
Ketols	982.8	E862.4	—	E950.9	E962.1	E980.9
Ketone oils	982.8	E862.4	—	E950.9	E962.1	E980.9
Kiln gas or vapor (carbon monoxide)	986	E868.8	—	E952.1	E962.2	E982.1
Konsyl	973.3	E858.4	E943.3	E950.4	E962.0	E980.4
Kosam seed	988.2	E865.3	—	E950.9	E962.1	E980.9
Krait (venom)	989.5	E905.0	—	E950.9	E962.1	E980.9
Kwell (insecticide)	989.2	E863.0	—	E950.6	E962.1	E980.7
anti–infective (topical)	976.0	E858.7	E946.0	E950.4	E962.0	E980.4
Laburnum (flowers) (seeds)	988.2	E865.3	—	E950.9	E962.1	E980.9
leaves	988.2	E865.4	—	E950.9	E962.1	E980.9
Lacquers	989.8	E861.6	—	E950.9	E962.1	E980.9
Lacrimogenic gas	987.5	E869.3	—	E952.8	E962.2	E982.8
Lactic acid	983.1	E864.1	—	E950.7	E962.1	E980.6
Lactobacillus acidophilus	973.5	E858.4	E943.5	E950.4	E962.0	E980.4
Lactoflavin	963.5	E858.1	E933.5	E950.4	E962.0	E980.4
Lactuca (virosa) (extract)	967.8	E852.8	E937.8	E950.2	E962.0	E980.2
Lactucarium	967.8	E852.8	E937.8	E950.2	E962.0	E980.2
Laevulose	974.5	E858.5	E944.5	E950.4	E962.0	E980.4
Lanatoside(C)	972.1	E858.3	E942.1	E950.4	E962.0	E980.4
Lanolin (lotion)	976.3	E858.7	E946.3	E950.4	E962.0	E980.4
Largactil	969.1	E853.0	E939.1	E950.3	E962.0	E980.3
Larkspur	988.2	E865.3	—	E950.9	E962.1	E980.9
Laroxyl	969.0	E854.0	E939.0	E950.3	E962.0	E980.3
Lasix	974.4	E858.5	E944.4	E950.4	E962.0	E980.4
Lathyrus (seed)	988.2	E865.3	—	E950.9	E962.1	E980.9
Laudanum	965.09	E850.2	E935.2	E950.0	E962.0	E980.0
Laudexium	975.2	E858.6	E945.2	E950.4	E962.0	E980.4

Substance	Poisoning	Accident	Therapeutic Use	Suicide Attempt	Assault	Undetermined
		External Cause (E-Code)				
Laurel, black or cherry	988.2	E865.4	—	E950.9	E962.1	E980.9
Laurolinium	976.0	E858.7	E946.0	E950.4	E962.0	E980.4
Lauryl sulfoacetate	976.2	E858.7	E946.2	E950.4	E962.0	E980.4
Laxatives NEC	973.3	E858.4	E943.3	E950.4	E962.0	E980.4
emollient	973.2	E858.4	E943.2	E950.4	E962.0	E980.4
L–dopa	966.4	E855.0	E936.4	E950.4	E962.0	E980.4
Lead (dust) (fumes) (vapor) NEC	984.9	E866.0	—	E950.9	E962.1	E980.9
acetate (dust)	984.1	E866.0	—	E950.9	E962.1	E980.9
anti–infectives	961.2	E857	E931.2	E950.4	E962.0	E980.4
antiknock compound (tetraethyl)	984.1	E862.1	—	E950.9	E962.1	E980.9
arsenate, arsenite (dust) (insecticide) (vapor)	985.1	E863.4	—	E950.8	E962.1	E980.8
herbicide	985.1	E863.5	—	E950.8	E962.1	E980.8
carbonate	984.0	E866.0	—	E950.9	E962.1	E980.9
paint	984.0	E861.5	—	E950.9	E962.1	E980.9
chromate	984.0	E866.0	—	E950.9	E962.1	E980.9
paint	984.0	E861.5	—	E950.9	E962.1	E980.9
dioxide	984.0	E866.0	—	E950.9	E962.1	E980.9
inorganic (compound)	984.0	E866.0	—	E950.9	E962.1	E980.9
paint	984.0	E861.5	—	E950.9	E962.1	E980.9
iodine	984.0	E866.0	—	E950.9	E962.1	E980.9
pigment (paint)	984.0	E861.5	—	E950.9	E962.1	E980.9
monoxide (dust)	984.0	E866.0	—	E950.9	E962.1	E980.9
paint	984.0	E861.5	—	E950.9	E962.1	E980.9
organic	984.1	E866.0	—	E950.9	E962.1	E980.9
oxide	984.0	E866.0	—	E950.9	E962.1	E980.9
paint	984.0	E861.5	—	E950.9	E962.1	E980.9
paint	984.0	E861.5	—	E950.9	E962.1	E980.9
salts	984.0	E866.0	—	E950.9	E962.1	E980.9
specified compound NEC	984.8	E866.0	—	E950.9	E962.1	E980.9
tetra–ethyl	984.1	E862.1	—	E950.9	E962.1	E980.9
Lebanese red	969.6	E854.1	E939.6	E950.3	E962.0	E980.3
Lente Iletin (insulin)	962.3	E858.0	E932.3	E950.4	E962.0	E980.4
Leptazol	970.0	E854.3	E940.0	E950.4	E962.0	E980.4
Leritine	965.09	E850.2	E935.2	E950.0	E962.0	E980.0
Letter	962.7	E858.0	E932.7	E950.4	E962.0	E980.4
Lettuce opium	967.8	E852.8	E937.8	E950.2	E962.0	E980.2
Leucovorin (factor)	964.1	E858.2	E934.1	E950.4	E962.0	E980.4
Leukeran	963.1	E858.1	E933.1	E950.4	E962.0	E980.4
Levallorphan	970.1	E854.3	E940.1	E950.4	E962.0	E980.4
Levanil	967.8	E852.8	E937.8	E950.2	E962.0	E980.2
Levarterenol	971.2	E855.5	E941.2	E950.4	E962.0	E980.4
Levodopa	966.4	E855.0	E936.4	E950.4	E962.0	E980.4
Levo–dromoran	965.09	E850.2	E935.2	E950.0	E962.0	E980.0
Levoid	962.7	E858.0	E932.7	E950.4	E962.0	E980.4
Levo–iso–methadone	965.02	E850.1	E935.1	E950.0	E962.0	E980.0
Levomepromazine	967.8	E852.8	E937.8	E950.2	E962.0	E980.2
Levoprome	967.8	E852.8	E937.8	E950.2	E962.0	E980.2
Levopropoxyphene	975.4	E858.6	E945.4	E950.4	E962.0	E980.4
Levorphan, levophanol	965.09	E850.2	E935.2	E950.0	E962.0	E980.0
Levothyroxine (sodium)	962.7	E858.0	E932.7	E950.4	E962.0	E980.4
Levsin	971.1	E855.4	E941.1	E950.4	E962.0	E980.4
Levulose	974.5	E858.5	E944.5	E950.4	E962.0	E980.4
Lewisite (gas)	985.1	E866.3	—	E950.8	E962.1	E980.8
Librium	969.4	E853.2	E939.4	E950.3	E962.0	E980.3
Lidex	976.0	E858.7	E946.0	E950.4	E962.0	E980.4
Lidocaine (infiltration) (topical)	968.5	E855.2	E938.5	E950.4	E962.0	E980.4

Substance	Poisoning	Accident	Therapeutic Use	Suicide Attempt	Assault	Undetermined
		External Cause (E-Code)				
nerve block (peripheral) (plexus)	968.6	E855.2	E938.6	E950.4	E962.0	E980.4
spinal	968.7	E855.2	E938.7	E950.4	E962.0	E980.4
Lighter fluid	981	E862.1	—	E950.9	E962.1	E980.9
Lignocaine (infiltration) (topical)	968.5	E855.2	E938.5	E950.4	E962.0	E980.4
nerve block (peripheral) (plexus)	968.6	E855.2	E938.6	E950.4	E962.0	E980.4
spinal	968.7	E855.2	E938.7	E950.4	E962.0	E980.4
Ligroin(e) (solvent)	981	E862.0	—	E950.9	E962.1	E980.9
vapor	987.1	E869.8	—	E952.8	E962.2	E982.8
Ligustrum vulgare	988.2	E865.3	—	E950.9	E962.1	E980.9
Lily of the valley	988.2	E865.4	—	E950.9	E962.1	E980.9
Lime (chloride)	983.2	E864.2	—	E950.7	E962.1	E980.6
solution, sulferated	976.4	E858.7	E946.4	E950.4	E962.0	E980.4
Limonene	982.8	E862.4	—	E950.9	E962.1	E980.9
Lincomycin	960.8	E856	E930.8	E950.4	E962.0	E980.4
Lindane (insecticide) (vapor)	989.2	E863.0	—	E950.6	E962.1	E980.7
anti–infective (topical)	976.0	E858.7	E946.0	E950.4	E962.0	E980.4
Liniments NEC	976.9	E858.7	E946.9	E950.4	E962.0	E980.4
Linoleic acid	972.2	E858.3	E942.2	E950.4	E962.0	E980.4
Liothyronine	962.7	E858.0	E932.7	E950.4	E962.0	E980.4
Liotrix	962.7	E858.0	E932.7	E950.4	E962.0	E980.4
Lipancreatin	973.4	E858.4	E943.4	E950.4	E962.0	E980.4
Lipo–Lutin	962.2	E858.0	E932.2	E950.4	E962.0	E980.4
Lipotropic agents	977.1	E858.8	E947.1	E950.4	E962.0	E980.4
Liquefied petroleum gases	987.0	E868.0	—	E951.1	E962.2	E981.1
piped (pure or mixed with air)	987.0	E867	—	E951.0	E962.2	E981.0
Liquid						
petrolatum	973.2	E858.4	E943.2	E950.4	E962.0	E980.4
substance	989.9	E866.9	—	E950.9	E962.1	E980.9
specified NEC	989.8	E866.8	—	E950.9	E962.1	E980.9
Lirugen	979.4	E858.8	E949.4	E950.4	E962.0	E980.4
Lithane	969.8	E855.8	E939.8	E950.3	E962.0	E980.3
Lithium	985.8	E866.4	—	E950.9	E962.1	E980.9
carbonate	969.8	E855.8	E939.8	E950.3	E962.0	E980.3
Lithonate	969.8	E855.8	E939.8	E950.3	E962.0	E980.3
Liver (extract) (injection) (preparations)	964.1	E858.2	E934.1	E950.4	E962.0	E980.4
Lizard (bite) (venom)	989.5	E905.0	—	E950.9	E962.1	E980.9
LMD	964.8	E858.2	E934.8	E950.4	E962.0	E980.4
Lobelia	988.2	E865.4	—	E950.9	E962.1	E980.9
Lobeline	970.0	E854.3	E940.0	E950.4	E962.0	E980.4
Locorten	976.0	E858.7	E946.0	E950.4	E962.0	E980.4
Lolium temulentum	988.2	E865.3	—	E950.9	E962.1	E980.9
Lomotil	973.5	E858.4	E943.5	E950.4	E962.0	E980.4
Lomustine	963.1	E858.1	E933.1	E950.4	E962.0	E980.4
Lophophora williamsii	969.6	E854.1	E939.6	E950.3	E962.0	E980.3
Lorazepam	969.4	E853.2	E939.4	E950.3	E962.0	E980.3
Lotions NEC	976.9	E858.7	E946.9	E950.4	E962.0	E980.4
Lotusate	967.0	E851	E937.0	E950.1	E962.0	E980.1
Lowila	976.2	E858.7	E946.2	E950.4	E962.0	E980.4
Loxapine	969.3	E853.8	E939.3	E950.3	E962.0	E980.3
Lozenges (throat)	976.6	E858.7	E946.6	E950.4	E962.0	E980.4
LSD (25)	969.6	E854.1	E939.6	E950.3	E962.0	E980.3
Lubricating oil NEC	981	E862.2	—	E950.9	E962.1	E980.9
Lucanthone	961.6	E857	E931.6	E950.4	E962.0	E980.4
Luminal	967.0	E851	E937.0	E950.1	E962.0	E980.1
Lung irritant (gas) NEC	987.9	E869.9	—	E952.9	E962.2	E982.9
Lutocylol	962.2	E858.0	E932.2	E950.4	E962.0	E980.4
Lutromone	962.2	E858.0	E932.2	E950.4	E962.0	E980.4

Substance	Poisoning	Accident	Therapeutic Use	Suicide Attempt	Assault	Undetermined
		External Cause (E-Code)				
Lututrin	975.0	E858.6	E945.0	E950.4	E962.0	E980.4
Lye (concentrated)	983.2	E864.2	—	E950.7	E962.1	E980.6
Lygranum (skin test)	977.8	E858.8	E947.8	E950.4	E962.0	E980.4
Lymecycline	960.4	E856	E930.4	E950.4	E962.0	E980.4
Lymphogranuloma venereum antigen	977.8	E858.8	E947.8	E950.4	E962.0	E980.4
Lynestrenol	962.2	E858.0	E932.2	E950.4	E962.0	E980.4
Lyovac Sodium Edecrin	974.4	E858.5	E944.4	E950.4	E962.0	E980.4
Lypressin	962.5	E858.0	E932.5	E950.4	E962.0	E980.4
Lysergic acid (amide) (diethylamide)	969.6	E854.1	E939.6	E950.3	E962.0	E980.3
Lysergide	969.6	E854.1	E939.6	E950.3	E962.0	E980.3
Lysine vasopressin	962.5	E858.0	E932.5	E950.4	E962.0	E980.4
Lysol	983.0	E864.0	—	E950.7	E962.1	E980.6
Lytta (vitatta)	976.8	E858.7	E946.8	E950.4	E962.0	E980.4
Mace	987.5	E869.3	—	E952.8	E962.2	E982.8
Macrolides (antibiotics)	960.3	E856	E930.3	E950.4	E962.0	E980.4
Mafenide	976.0	E858.7	E946.0	E950.4	E962.0	E980.4
Magaldrate	973.0	E858.4	E943.0	E950.4	E962.0	E980.4
Magic mushroom	969.6	E854.1	E939.6	E950.3	E962.0	E980.3
Magnamycin	960.8	E856	E930.8	E950.4	E962.0	E980.4
Magnesia magma	973.0	E858.4	E943.0	E950.4	E962.0	E980.4
Magnesium (compounds) (fumes) NEC	985.8	E866.4	—	E950.9	E962.1	E980.9
antacid	973.0	E858.4	E943.0	E950.4	E962.0	E980.4
carbonate	973.0	E858.4	E943.0	E950.4	E962.0	E980.4
cathartic	973.3	E858.4	E943.3	E950.4	E962.0	E980.4
citrate	973.3	E858.4	E943.3	E950.4	E962.0	E980.4
hydroxide	973.0	E858.4	E943.0	E950.4	E962.0	E980.4
oxide	973.0	E858.4	E943.0	E950.4	E962.0	E980.4
sulfate (oral)	973.3	E858.4	E943.3	E950.4	E962.0	E980.4
intravenous	966.3	E855.0	E936.3	E950.4	E962.0	E980.4
trisilicate	973.0	E858.4	E943.0	E950.4	E962.0	E980.4
Malathion (insecticide)	989.3	E863.1	—	E950.6	E962.1	E980.7
Male fern (oleoresin)	961.6	E857	E931.6	E950.4	E962.0	E980.4
Mandelic acid	961.9	E857	E931.9	E950.4	E962.0	E980.4
Manganese compounds (fumes) NEC	985.2	E866.4	—	E950.9	E962.1	E980.9
Mannitol (diuretic) (medicinal) NEC	974.4	E858.5	E944.4	E950.4	E962.0	E980.4
hexanitrate	972.4	E858.3	E942.4	E950.4	E962.0	E980.4
mustard	963.1	E858.1	E933.1	E950.4	E962.0	E980.4
Mannomustine	963.1	E858.1	E933.1	E950.4	E962.0	E980.4
MAO inhibitors	969.0	E854.0	E939.0	E950.3	E962.0	E980.3
Mapharsen	961.1	E857	E931.1	E950.4	E962.0	E980.4
Marcaine	968.9	E855.2	E938.9	E950.4	E962.0	E980.4
infiltration (subcutaneous)	968.5	E855.2	E938.5	E950.4	E962.0	E980.4
nerve block (peripheral) (plexus)	968.6	E855.2	E938.6	E950.4	E962.0	E980.4
Marezine	963.0	E858.1	E933.0	E950.4	E962.0	E980.4
Marihuana, marijuana (derivatives)	969.6	E854.1	E939.6	E950.3	E962.0	E980.3
Marine animals or plants (sting)	989.5	E905.6	—	E950.9	E962.1	E980.9
Marplan	969.0	E854.0	E939.0	E950.3	E962.0	E980.3
Marsh gas	987.1	E869.8	—	E952.8	E962.2	E982.8
Marsilid	969.0	E854.0	E939.0	E950.3	E962.0	E980.3
Matulane	963.1	E858.1	E933.1	E950.4	E962.0	E980.4
Mazindol	977.0	E858.8	E947.0	E950.4	E962.0	E980.4
Meadow saffron	988.2	E865.3	—	E950.9	E962.1	E980.9
Measles vaccine	979.4	E858.8	E949.4	E950.4	E962.0	E980.4
Meat, noxious or nonbacterial	988.8	E865.0	—	E950.9	E962.1	E980.9
Mebanazine	969.0	E854.0	E939.0	E950.3	E962.0	E980.3
Mebaral	967.0	E851	E937.0	E950.1	E962.0	E980.1
Mebendazole	961.6	E857	E931.6	E950.4	E962.0	E980.4

Substance	Poisoning	External Cause (E-Code) Accident	Therapeutic Use	Suicide Attempt	Assault	Undetermined
Mebeverine	975.1	E858.6	E945.1	E950.4	E962.0	E980.4
Mebhydroline	963.0	E858.1	E933.0	E950.4	E962.0	E980.4
Mebrophenhydramine	963.0	E858.1	E933.0	E950.4	E962.0	E980.4
Mebutamate	969.5	E853.8	E939.5	E950.3	E962.0	E980.3
Mecamylamine (chloride)	972.3	E858.3	E942.3	E950.4	E962.0	E980.4
Mechlorethamine hydrochloride	963.1	E858.1	E933.1	E950.4	E962.0	E980.4
Meclizene (hydrochloride)	963.0	E858.1	E933.0	E950.4	E962.0	E980.4
Meclofenoxate	970.0	E854.3	E940.0	E950.4	E962.0	E980.4
Meclozine (hydrochloride)	963.0	E858.1	E933.0	E950.4	E962.0	E980.4
Medazepam	969.4	E853.2	E939.4	E950.3	E962.0	E980.3
Medicine, medicinal substance	977.9	E858.9	E947.9	E950.5	E962.0	E980.5
specified NEC	977.8	E858.8	E947.8	E950.4	E962.0	E980.4
Medinal	967.0	E851	E937.0	E950.1	E962.0	E980.1
Medomin	967.0	E851	E937.0	E950.1	E962.0	E980.1
Medroxyprogesterone	962.2	E858.0	E932.2	E950.4	E962.0	E980.4
Medrysone	976.5	E858.7	E946.5	E950.4	E962.0	E980.4
Mefenamic acid	965.7	E850.7	E935.7	E950.0	E962.0	E980.0
Megahallucinogen	969.6	E854.1	E939.6	E950.3	E962.0	E980.3
Megestrol	962.2	E858.0	E932.2	E950.4	E962.0	E980.4
Meglumine	977.8	E858.8	E947.8	E950.4	E962.0	E980.4
Meladinin	976.3	E858.7	E946.3	E950.4	E962.0	E980.4
Melanizing agents	976.3	E858.7	E946.3	E950.4	E962.0	E980.4
Melarsoprol	961.1	E857	E931.1	E950.4	E962.0	E980.4
Melia azedarach	988.2	E865.3	—	E950.9	E962.1	E980.9
Mellaril	969.1	E853.0	E939.1	E950.3	E962.0	E980.3
Meloxine	976.3	E858.7	E946.3	E950.4	E962.0	E980.4
Melphalan	963.1	E858.1	E933.1	E950.4	E962.0	E980.4
Menadiol sodium diphosphate	964.3	E858.2	E934.3	E950.4	E962.0	E980.4
Menadione (sodium bisulfate)	964.3	E858.2	E934.3	E950.4	E962.0	E980.4
Menaphthone	964.3	E858.2	E934.3	E950.4	E962.0	E980.4
Meningococcal vaccine	978.8	E858.8	E948.8	E950.4	E962.0	E980.4
Menningovax–C	978.8	E858.8	E948.8	E950.4	E962.0	E980.4
Menotropins	962.4	E858.0	E932.4	E950.4	E962.0	E980.4
Menthol NEC	976.1	E858.7	E946.1	E950.4	E962.0	E980.4
Mepacrine	961.3	E857	E931.3	E950.4	E962.0	E980.4
Meparfynol	967.8	E852.8	E937.8	E950.2	E962.0	E980.2
Mepazine	969.1	E853.0	E939.1	E950.3	E962.0	E980.3
Mepenzolate	971.1	E855.4	E941.1	E950.4	E962.0	E980.4
Meperidine	965.09	E850.2	E935.2	E950.0	E962.0	E980.0
Mephenamin(e)	966.4	E855.0	E936.4	E950.4	E962.0	E980.4
Mephenesin (carbamate)	968.0	E855.1	E938.0	E950.4	E962.0	E980.4
Mephenoxalone	969.5	E853.8	E939.5	E950.3	E962.0	E980.3
Mephentermine	971.2	E855.5	E941.2	E950.4	E962.0	E980.4
Mephenytoin	966.1	E855.0	E936.1	E950.4	E962.0	E980.4
Mephobarbital	967.0	E851	E937.0	E950.1	E962.0	E980.1
Mepiperphenidol	971.1	E855.4	E941.1	E950.4	E962.0	E980.4
Mepivacaine	968.9	E855.2	E938.9	E950.4	E962.0	E980.4
infiltration (subcutaneous)	968.5	E855.2	E938.5	E950.4	E962.0	E980.4
nerve block (peripheral) (plexus)	968.6	E855.2	E938.6	E950.4	E962.0	E980.4
topical (surface)	968.5	E855.2	E938.5	E950.4	E962.0	E980.4
Meprednisone	962.0	E858.0	E932.0	E950.4	E962.0	E980.4
Meprobam	969.5	E853.8	E939.5	E950.3	E962.0	E980.3
Meprobamate	969.5	E853.8	E939.5	E950.3	E962.0	E980.3
Mepyramine (maleate)	963.0	E858.1	E933.0	E950.4	E962.0	E980.4
Meralluride	974.0	E858.5	E944.0	E950.4	E962.0	E980.4
Merbaphen	974.0	E858.5	E944.0	E950.4	E962.0	E980.4
Merbromin	976.0	E858.7	E946.0	E950.4	E962.0	E980.4

Substance	Poisoning	External Cause (E-Code) Accident	Therapeutic Use	Suicide Attempt	Assault	Undetermined
Mercaptomerin	974.0	E858.5	E944.0	E950.4	E962.0	E980.4
Mercaptopurine	963.1	E858.1	E933.1	E950.4	E962.0	E980.4
Mercumatilin	974.0	E858.5	E944.0	E950.4	E962.0	E980.4
Mercuramide	974.0	E858.5	E944.0	E950.4	E962.0	E980.4
Mercuranin	976.0	E858.7	E946.0	E950.4	E962.0	E980.4
Mercurochrome	976.0	E858.7	E946.0	E950.4	E962.0	E980.4
Mercury, mercuric, mercurous (compounds) (cyanide) (fumes) (nonmedicinal) (vapor) NEC	985.0	E866.1	—	E950.9	E962.1	E980.9
ammoniated	976.0	E858.7	E946.0	E950.4	E962.0	E980.4
anti-infective	961.2	E857	E931.2	E950.4	E962.0	E980.4
topical	976.0	E858.7	E946.0	E950.4	E962.0	E980.4
chloride (antiseptic) NEC	976.0	E858.7	E946.0	E950.4	E962.0	E980.4
fungicide	985.0	E863.6	—	E950.6	E962.1	E980.7
diuretic compounds	974.0	E858.5	E944.0	E950.4	E962.0	E980.4
fungicide	985.0	E863.6	—	E950.6	E962.1	E980.7
organic (fungicide)	985.0	E863.6	—	E950.6	E962.1	E980.7
Merethoxylline	974.0	E858.5	E944.0	E950.4	E962.0	E980.4
Mersalyl	974.0	E858.5	E944.0	E950.4	E962.0	E980.4
Merthiolate (topical)	976.0	E858.7	E946.0	E950.4	E962.0	E980.4
ophthalmic preparation	976.5	E858.7	E946.5	E950.4	E962.0	E980.4
Meruvax	979.4	E858.8	E949.4	E950.4	E962.0	E980.4
Mescal buttons	969.6	E854.1	E939.6	E950.3	E962.0	E980.3
Mescaline (salts)	969.6	E854.1	E939.6	E950.3	E962.0	E980.3
Mesoridazine besylate	969.1	E853.0	E939.1	E950.3	E962.0	E980.3
Mestanolone	962.1	E858.0	E932.1	E950.4	E962.0	E980.4
Mestranol	962.2	E858.0	E932.2	E950.4	E962.0	E980.4
Metacresylacetate	976.0	E858.7	E946.0	E950.4	E962.0	E980.4
Metaldehyde (snail killer) NEC	989.4	E863.4	—	E950.6	E962.1	E980.7
Metals (heavy) (nonmedicinal) NEC	985.9	E866.4	—	E950.9	E962.1	E980.9
dust, fumes, or vapor NEC	985.9	E866.4	—	E950.9	E962.1	E980.9
light NEC	985.9	E866.4	—	E950.9	E962.1	E980.9
dust, fumes, or vapor NEC	985.9	E866.4	—	E950.9	E962.1	E980.9
pesticides (dust) (vapor)	985.9	E863.4	—	E950.6	E962.1	E980.7
Metamucil	973.3	E858.4	E943.3	E950.4	E962.0	E980.4
Metaphen	976.0	E858.7	E946.0	E950.4	E962.0	E980.4
Metaproterenol	975.1	E858.6	E945.1	E950.4	E962.0	E980.4
Metaraminol	972.8	E858.3	E942.8	E950.4	E962.0	E980.4
Metaxalone	968.0	E855.1	E938.0	E950.4	E962.0	E980.4
Metformin	962.3	E858.0	E932.3	E950.4	E962.0	E980.4
Methacycline	960.4	E856	E930.4	E950.4	E962.0	E980.4
Methadone	965.02	E850.1	E935.1	E950.0	E962.0	E980.0
Methallenestril	962.2	E858.0	E932.2	E950.4	E962.0	E980.4
Methamphetamine	969.7	E854.2	E939.7	E950.3	E962.0	E980.3
Methandienone	962.1	E858.0	E932.1	E950.4	E962.0	E980.4
Methandriol	962.1	E858.0	E932.1	E950.4	E962.0	E980.4
Methandrostenolone	962.1	E858.0	E932.1	E950.4	E962.0	E980.4
Methane gas	987.1	E869.8	—	E952.8	E962.2	E982.8
Methanol	980.1	E860.2	—	E950.9	E962.1	E980.9
vapor	987.8	E869.8	—	E952.8	E962.2	E982.8
Methantheline	971.1	E855.4	E941.1	E950.4	E962.0	E980.4
Methaphenilene	963.0	E858.1	E933.0	E950.4	E962.0	E980.4
Methapyrilene	963.0	E858.1	E933.0	E950.4	E962.0	E980.4
Methaqualone (compounds)	967.4	E852.3	E937.4	E950.2	E962.0	E980.2
Metharbital, metharbitone	967.0	E851	E937.0	E950.1	E962.0	E980.1
Methazolamide	974.2	E858.5	E944.2	E950.4	E962.0	E980.4
Methdilazine	963.0	E858.1	E933.0	E950.4	E962.0	E980.4

Substance	Poisoning	Accident	Therapeutic Use	Suicide Attempt	Assault	Undetermined
		External Cause (E-Code)				
Methedrine	969.7	E854.2	E939.7	E950.3	E962.0	E980.3
Methenamine (mandelate)	961.9	E857	E931.9	E950.4	E962.0	E980.4
Methenolone	962.1	E858.0	E932.1	E950.4	E962.0	E980.4
Methergine	975.0	E858.6	E945.0	E950.4	E962.0	E980.4
Methiacil	962.8	E858.0	E932.8	E950.4	E962.0	E980.4
Methicillin (sodium)	960.0	E856	E930.0	E950.4	E962.0	E980.4
Methimazole	962.8	E858.0	E932.8	E950.4	E962.0	E980.4
Methionine	977.1	E858.8	E947.1	E950.4	E962.0	E980.4
Methisazone	961.7	E857	E931.7	E950.4	E962.0	E980.4
Methitural	967.0	E851	E937.0	E950.1	E962.0	E980.1
Methixene	971.1	E855.4	E941.1	E950.4	E962.0	E980.4
Methobarbital, methobarbitone	967.0	E851	E937.0	E950.1	E962.0	E980.1
Methocarbamol	968.0	E855.1	E938.0	E950.4	E962.0	E980.4
Methohexital, methohexitone (sodium)	968.3	E855.1	E938.3	E950.4	E962.0	E980.4
Methoin	966.1	E855.0	E936.1	E950.4	E962.0	E980.4
Methopholine	965.7	E850.7	E935.7	E950.0	E962.0	E980.0
Methorate	975.4	E858.6	E945.4	E950.4	E962.0	E980.4
Methoserpidine	972.6	E858.3	E942.6	E950.4	E962.0	E980.4
Methotrexate	963.1	E858.1	E933.1	E950.4	E962.0	E980.4
Methotrimeprazine	967.8	E852.8	E937.8	E950.2	E962.0	E980.2
Methoxa–Dome	976.3	E858.7	E946.3	E950.4	E962.0	E980.4
Methoxamine	971.2	E855.5	E941.2	E950.4	E962.0	E980.4
Methoxsalen	976.3	E858.7	E946.3	E950.4	E962.0	E980.4
Methoxybenzyl penicillin	960.0	E856	E930.0	E950.4	E962.0	E980.4
Methoxychlor	989.2	E863.0	—	E950.6	E962.1	E980.7
Methoxyflurane	968.2	E855.1	E938.2	E950.4	E962.0	E980.4
Methoxyphenamine	971.2	E855.5	E941.2	E950.4	E962.0	E980.4
Methoxypromazine	969.1	E853.0	E939.1	E950.3	E962.0	E980.3
Methoxypsoralen	976.3	E858.7	E946.3	E950.4	E962.0	E980.4
Methscopolamine (bromide)	971.1	E855.4	E941.1	E950.4	E962.0	E980.4
Methsuximide	966.2	E855.0	E936.2	E950.4	E962.0	E980.4
Methyclothiazide	974.3	E858.5	E944.3	E950.4	E962.0	E980.4
Methyl						
acetate	982.8	E862.4	—	E950.9	E962.1	E980.9
acetone	982.8	E862.4	—	E950.9	E962.1	E980.9
alcohol	980.1	E860.2	—	E950.9	E962.1	E980.9
amphetamine	969.7	E854.2	E939.7	E950.3	E962.0	E980.3
androstanolone	962.1	E858.0	E932.1	E950.4	E962.0	E980.4
atropine	971.1	E855.4	E941.1	E950.4	E962.0	E980.4
benzene	982.0	E862.4	—	E950.9	E962.1	E980.9
bromide (gas)	987.8	E869.8	—	E952.8	E962.2	E982.8
fumigant	987.8	E863.8	—	E950.6	E962.2	E980.7
butanol	980.8	E860.8	—	E950.9	E962.1	E980.9
carbinol	980.1	E860.2	—	E950.9	E962.1	E980.9
cellosolve	982.8	E862.4	—	E950.9	E962.1	E980.9
cellulose	973.3	E858.4	E943.3	E950.4	E962.0	E980.4
chloride (gas)	987.8	E869.8	—	E952.8	E962.2	E982.8
cyclohexane	982.8	E862.4	—	E950.9	E962.1	E980.9
cyclohexanone	982.8	E862.4	—	E950.9	E962.1	E980.9
dihydromorphinone	965.09	E850.2	E935.2	E950.0	E962.0	E980.0
ergometrine	975.0	E858.6	E945.0	E950.4	E962.0	E980.4
ergonovine	975.0	E858.6	E945.0	E950.4	E962.0	E980.4
ethyl ketone	982.8	E862.4	—	E950.9	E962.1	E980.9
hydrazine	983.9	E864.3	—	E950.7	E962.1	E980.6
isobutyl ketone	982.8	E862.4	—	E950.9	E962.1	E980.9
morphine NEC	965.09	E850.2	E935.2	E950.0	E962.0	E980.0
parafynol	967.8	E852.8	E937.8	E950.2	E962.0	E980.2

Substance	Poisoning	Accident	Therapeutic Use	Suicide Attempt	Assault	Undetermined
		External Cause (E-Code)				
parathion	989.3	E863.1	—	E950.6	E962.1	E980.7
pentynol NEC	967.8	E852.8	E937.8	E950.2	E962.0	E980.2
peridol	969.2	E853.1	E939.2	E950.3	E962.0	E980.3
phenidate	969.7	E854.2	E939.7	E950.3	E962.0	E980.3
prednisolone	962.0	E858.0	E932.0	E950.4	E962.0	E980.4
ENT agent	976.6	E858.7	E946.6	E950.4	E962.0	E980.4
ophthalmic preparation	976.5	E858.7	E946.5	E950.4	E962.0	E980.4
topical NEC	976.0	E858.7	E946.0	E950.4	E962.0	E980.4
propylcarbinol	980.8	E860.8	—	E950.9	E962.1	E980.9
rosaniline NEC	976.0	E858.7	E946.0	E950.4	E962.0	E980.4
salicylate NEC	976.3	E858.7	E946.3	E950.4	E962.0	E980.4
sulfate (fumes)	987.8	E869.8	—	E952.8	E962.2	E982.8
liquid	983.9	E864.3	—	E950.7	E962.1	E980.6
sulfonal	967.8	E852.8	E937.8	E950.2	E962.0	E980.2
testosterone	962.1	E858.0	E932.1	E950.4	E962.0	E980.4
thiouracil	962.8	E858.0	E932.8	E950.4	E962.0	E980.4
Methylated spirit	980.0	E860.1	—	E950.9	E962.1	E980.9
Methyldopa	972.6	E858.3	E942.6	E950.4	E962.0	E980.4
Methylene						
blue	961.9	E857	E931.9	E950.4	E962.0	E980.4
chloride or dichloride (solvent) NEC	982.3	E862.4	—	E950.9	E962.1	E980.9
Methylhexabital	967.0	E851	E937.0	E950.1	E962.0	E980.1
Methylparaben (ophthalmic)	976.5	E858.7	E946.5	E950.4	E962.0	E980.4
Methyprylon	967.5	E852.4	E937.5	E950.2	E962.0	E980.2
Methysergide	971.3	E855.6	E941.3	E950.4	E962.0	E980.4
Metoclopramide	963.0	E858.1	E933.0	E950.4	E962.0	E980.4
Metofoline	965.7	E850.7	E935.7	E950.0	E962.0	E980.0
Metopon	965.09	E850.2	E935.2	E950.0	E962.0	E980.0
Metronidazole	961.5	E857	E931.5	E950.4	E962.0	E980.4
Metycaine	968.9	E855.2	E938.9	E950.4	E962.0	E980.4
infiltration (subcutaneous)	968.5	E855.2	E938.5	E950.4	E962.0	E980.4
nerve block (peripheral) (plexus)	968.6	E855.2	E938.6	E950.4	E962.0	E980.4
topical (surface)	968.5	E855.2	E938.5	E950.4	E962.0	E980.4
Metyrapone	977.8	E858.8	E947.8	E950.4	E962.0	E980.4
Mevinphos	989.3	E863.1	—	E950.6	E962.1	E980.7
Mezereon (berries)	988.2	E865.3	—	E950.9	E962.1	E980.9
Micatin	976.0	E858.7	E946.0	E950.4	E962.0	E980.4
Miconazole	976.0	E858.7	E946.0	E950.4	E962.0	E980.4
Midol	965.1	E850.3	E935.3	E950.0	E962.0	E980.0
Milk of magnesia	973.0	E858.4	E943.0	E950.4	E962.0	E980.4
Millipede (tropical) (venomous)	989.5	E905.4	—	E950.9	E962.1	E980.9
Miltown	969.5	E853.8	E939.5	E950.3	E962.0	E980.3
Mineral						
oil (medicinal)	973.2	E858.4	E943.2	E950.4	E962.0	E980.4
nonmedicinal	981	E862.1	—	E950.9	E962.1	E980.9
topical	976.3	E858.7	E946.3	E950.4	E962.0	E980.4
salts NEC	974.6	E858.5	E944.6	E950.4	E962.0	E980.4
spirits	981	E862.0	—	E950.9	E962.1	E980.9
Minocycline	960.4	E856	E930.4	E950.4	E962.0	E980.4
Mithramycin (antineoplastic)	960.7	E856	E930.7	E950.4	E962.0	E980.4
Mitobronitol	963.1	E858.1	E933.1	E950.4	E962.0	E980.4
Mitomycin (antineoplastic)	960.7	E856	E930.7	E950.4	E962.0	E980.4
Mitotane	963.1	E858.1	E933.1	E950.4	E962.0	E980.4
Moderil	972.6	E858.3	E942.6	E950.4	E962.0	E980.4
Molindone	969.3	E853.8	E939.3	E950.3	E962.0	E980.3
Monistat	976.0	E858.7	E946.0	E950.4	E962.0	E980.4
Monkshood	988.2	E865.4	—	E950.9	E962.1	E980.9

Substance	Poisoning	Accident	Therapeutic Use	Suicide Attempt	Assault	Undetermined
		External Cause (E-Code)				
Monoamine oxidase inhibitors	969.0	E854.0	E939.0	E950.3	E962.0	E980.3
Monochlorobenzene	982.0	E862.4	—	E950.9	E962.1	E980.9
Monosodium glutamate	989.8	E866.8	—	E950.9	E962.1	E980.9
Monoxide, carbon — *see* Carbon, monoxide						
Moperone	969.2	E853.1	E939.2	E950.3	E962.0	E980.3
Morning glory seeds	969.6	E854.1	E939.6	E950.3	E962.0	E980.3
Moroxydine (hydrochloride)	961.7	E857	E931.7	E950.4	E962.0	E980.4
Morphazinamide	961.8	E857	E931.8	E950.4	E962.0	E980.4
Morphinans	965.09	E850.2	E935.2	E950.0	E962.0	E980.0
Morphine NEC	965.09	E850.2	E935.2	E950.0	E962.0	E980.0
antagonists	970.1	E854.3	E940.1	E950.4	E962.0	E980.4
Morpholinylethylmorphine	965.09	E850.2	E935.2	E950.0	E962.0	E980.0
Morrhuate sodium	972.7	E858.3	E942.7	E950.4	E962.0	E980.4
Moth balls *(see also* Pesticides)	989.4	E863.4	—	E950.6	E962.1	E980.7
naphthalene	983.0	E863.4	—	E950.7	E962.1	E980.6
Motor exhaust gas — *see* Carbon, monoxide, exhaust gas						
Mouth wash	976.6	E858.7	E946.6	E950.4	E962.0	E980.4
Mucolytic agent	975.5	E858.6	E945.5	E950.4	E962.0	E980.4
Mucomyst	975.5	E858.6	E945.5	E950.4	E962.0	E980.4
Mucous membrane agents (external)	976.9	E858.7	E946.9	E950.4	E962.0	E980.4
specified NEC	976.8	E858.7	E946.8	E950.4	E962.0	E980.4
Mumps						
immune globulin (human)	964.6	E858.2	E934.6	E950.4	E962.0	E980.4
skin test antigen	977.8	E858.8	E947.8	E950.4	E962.0	E980.4
vaccine	979.6	E858.8	E949.6	E950.4	E962.0	E980.4
Mumpsvax	979.6	E858.8	E949.6	E950.4	E962.0	E980.4
Muriatic acid — *see* Hydrochloric acid						
Muscarine	971.0	E855.3	E941.0	E950.4	E962.0	E980.4
Muscle affecting agents NEC	975.3	E858.6	E945.3	E950.4	E962.0	E980.4
oxytocic	975.0	E858.6	E945.0	E950.4	E962.0	E980.4
relaxants	975.3	E858.6	E945.3	E950.4	E962.0	E980.4
central nervous system	968.0	E855.1	E938.0	E950.4	E962.0	E980.4
skeletal	975.2	E858.6	E945.2	E950.4	E962.0	E980.4
smooth	975.1	E858.6	E945.1	E950.4	E962.0	E980.4
Mushrooms, noxious	988.1	E865.5	—	E950.9	E962.1	E980.9
Mussel, noxious	988.0	E865.1	—	E950.9	E962.1	E980.9
Mustard (emetic)	973.6	E858.4	E943.6	E950.4	E962.0	E980.4
gas	987.8	E869.8	—	E952.8	E962.2	E982.8
nitrogen	963.1	E858.1	E933.1	E950.4	E962.0	E980.4
Mustine	963.1	E858.1	E933.1	E950.4	E962.0	E980.4
M-vac	979.4	E858.8	E949.4	E950.4	E962.0	E980.4
Mycifradin	960.8	E856	E930.8	E950.4	E962.0	E980.4
topical	976.0	E858.7	E946.0	E950.4	E962.0	E980.4
Mycitracin	960.8	E856	E930.8	E950.4	E962.0	E980.4
ophthalmic preparation	976.5	E858.7	E946.5	E950.4	E962.0	E980.4
Mycostatin	960.1	E856	E930.1	E950.4	E962.0	E980.4
topical	976.0	E858.7	E946.0	E950.4	E962.0	E980.4
Mydriacyl	971.1	E855.4	E941.1	E950.4	E962.0	E980.4
Myelobromal	963.1	E858.1	E933.1	E950.4	E962.0	E980.4
Myleran	963.1	E858.1	E933.1	E950.4	E962.0	E980.4
Myochrysin(e)	965.6	E850.6	E935.6	E950.0	E962.0	E980.0
Myoneural blocking agents	975.2	E858.6	E945.2	E950.4	E962.0	E980.4
Myristica fragrans	988.2	E865.3	—	E950.9	E962.1	E980.9
Myristicin	988.2	E865.3	—	E950.9	E962.1	E980.9
Mysoline	966.3	E855.0	E936.3	E950.4	E962.0	E980.4
Nafcillin (sodium)	960.0	E856	E930.0	E950.4	E962.0	E980.4

Substance	Poisoning	External Cause (E-Code)				
		Accident	Therapeutic Use	Suicide Attempt	Assault	Undetermined
Nalidixic acid	961.9	E857	E931.9	E950.4	E962.0	E980.4
Nalorphine	970.1	E854.3	E940.1	E950.4	E962.0	E980.4
Naloxone	970.1	E854.3	E940.1	E950.4	E962.0	E980.4
Nandrolone (decanoate) (phenproprioate)	962.1	E858.0	E932.1	E950.4	E962.0	E980.4
Naphazoline	971.2	E855.5	E941.2	E950.4	E962.0	E980.4
Naphtha (painter's) (petroleum)	981	E862.0	—	E950.9	E962.1	E980.9
solvent	981	E862.0	—	E950.9	E962.1	E980.9
vapor	987.1	E869.8	—	E952.8	E962.2	E982.8
Naphthalene (chlorinated)	983.0	E864.0	—	E950.7	E962.1	E980.6
insecticide or moth repellent	983.0	E863.4	—	E950.7	E962.1	E980.6
vapor	987.8	E869.8	—	E952.8	E962.2	E982.8
Naphthol	983.0	E864.0	—	E950.7	E962.1	E980.6
Naphthylamine	983.0	E864.0	—	E950.7	E962.1	E980.6
Naproxen	965.6	E850.6	E935.6	E950.0	E962.0	E980.0
Narcotic (drug)	967.9	E852.9	E937.9	E950.2	E962.0	E980.2
analgesic NEC	965.8	E850.8	E935.8	E950.0	E962.0	E980.0
antagonist	970.1	E854.3	E940.1	E950.4	E962.0	E980.4
specified NEC	967.8	E852.8	E937.8	E950.2	E962.0	E980.2
Narcotine	975.4	E858.6	E945.4	E950.4	E962.0	E980.4
Nardil	969.0	E854.0	E939.0	E950.3	E962.0	E980.3
Natrium cyanide — *see* Cyanide(s)						
Natural						
blood (product)	964.7	E858.2	E934.7	E950.4	E962.0	E980.4
gas (piped)	987.1	E867	—	E951.0	E962.2	E981.0
incomplete combustion	986	E867	—	E951.0	E962.2	E981.0
Nealbarbital, nealbarbitone	967.0	E851	E937.0	E950.1	E962.0	E980.1
Nectadon	975.4	E858.6	E945.4	E950.4	E962.0	E980.4
Nematocyst (sting)	989.5	E905.6	—	E950.9	E962.1	E980.9
Nembutal	967.0	E851	E937.0	E950.1	E962.0	E980.1
Neoarsphenamine	961.1	E857	E931.1	E950.4	E962.0	E980.4
Neocinchophen	974.7	E858.5	E944.7	E950.4	E962.0	E980.4
Neomycin	960.8	E856	E930.8	E950.4	E962.0	E980.4
ENT agent	976.6	E858.7	E946.6	E950.4	E962.0	E980.4
ophthalmic preparation	976.5	E858.7	E946.5	E950.4	E962.0	E980.4
topical NEC	976.0	E858.7	E946.0	E950.4	E962.0	E980.4
Neonal	967.0	E851	E937.0	E950.1	E962.0	E980.1
Neoprontosil	961.0	E857	E931.0	E950.4	E962.0	E980.4
Neosalvarsan	961.1	E857	E931.1	E950.4	E962.0	E980.4
Neosilversalvarsan	961.1	E857	E931.1	E950.4	E962.0	E980.4
Neosporin	960.8	E856	E930.8	E950.4	E962.0	E980.4
ENT agent	976.6	E858.7	E946.6	E950.4	E962.0	E980.4
ophthalmic preparation	976.5	E858.7	E946.5	E950.4	E962.0	E980.4
topical NEC	976.0	E858.7	E946.0	E950.4	E962.0	E980.4
Neostigmine	971.0	E855.3	E941.0	E950.4	E962.0	E980.4
Neraval	967.0	E851	E937.0	E950.1	E962.0	E980.1
Neravan	967.0	E851	E937.0	E950.1	E962.0	E980.1
Nerium oleander	988.2	E865.4	—	E950.9	E962.1	E980.9
Nerve gases (war)	987.9	E869.9	—	E952.9	E962.2	E982.9
Nesacaine	968.9	E855.2	E938.9	E950.4	E962.0	E980.4
infiltration (subcutaneous)	968.5	E855.2	E938.5	E950.4	E962.0	E980.4
nerve block (peripheral) (plexus)	968.6	E855.2	E938.6	E950.4	E962.0	E980.4
Neurobarb	967.0	E851	E937.0	E950.1	E962.0	E980.1
Neuroleptics NEC	969.3	E853.8	E939.3	E950.3	E962.0	E980.3
Neutral spirits	980.0	E860.1	—	E950.9	E962.1	E980.9
beverage	980.0	E860.0	—	E950.9	E962.1	E980.9
Niacin, niacinamide	972.2	E858.3	E942.2	E950.4	E962.0	E980.4
Nialamide	969.0	E854.0	E939.0	E950.3	E962.0	E980.3

Substance	Poisoning	External Cause (E-Code) Accident	Therapeutic Use	Suicide Attempt	Assault	Undetermined
Nickle (carbonyl) (compounds) (fumes) (tetracarbonyl) (vapor)	985.8	E866.4	—	E950.9	E962.1	E980.9
Niclosamide	961.6	E857	E931.6	E950.4	E962.0	E980.4
Nicomorphine	965.09	E850.2	E935.2	E950.0	E962.0	E980.0
Nicotinamide	972.2	E858.3	E942.2	E950.4	E962.0	E980.4
Nicotine (insecticide) (spray) (sulfate) NEC	989.4	E863.4	—	E950.6	E962.1	E980.7
not insecticide	989.8	E866.8	—	E950.9	E962.1	E980.9
Nicotinic acid (derivatives)	972.2	E858.3	E942.2	E950.4	E962.0	E980.4
Nicotinyl alcohol	972.2	E858.3	E942.2	E950.4	E962.0	E980.4
Nicoumalone	964.2	E858.2	E934.2	E950.4	E962.0	E980.4
Nifenazone	965.5	E850.5	E935.5	E950.0	E962.0	E980.0
Nifuraldezone	961.9	E857	E931.9	E950.4	E962.0	E980.4
Nightshade (deadly)	988.2	E865.4	—	E950.9	E962.1	E980.9
Nikethamide	970.0	E854.3	E940.0	E950.4	E962.0	E980.4
Nilstat	960.1	E856	E930.1	E950.4	E962.0	E980.4
topical	976.0	E858.7	E946.0	E950.4	E962.0	E980.4
Niridazole	961.6	E857	E931.6	E950.4	E962.0	E980.4
Nisentil	965.09	E850.2	E935.2	E950.0	E962.0	E980.0
Nitrates	972.4	E858.3	E942.4	E950.4	E962.0	E980.4
Nitrazepam	969.4	E853.2	E939.4	E950.3	E962.0	E980.3
Nitric						
acid (liquid)	983.1	E864.1	—	E950.7	E962.1	E980.6
vapor	987.8	E869.8	—	E952.8	E962.2	E982.8
oxide (gas)	987.2	E869.0	—	E952.8	E962.2	E982.8
Nitrite, amyl (medicinal) (vapor)	972.4	E858.3	E942.4	E950.4	E962.0	E980.4
Nitroaniline	983.0	E864.0	—	E950.7	E962.1	E980.6
vapor	987.8	E869.8	—	E952.8	E962.2	E982.8
Nitrobenzene, nitrobenzol	983.0	E864.0	—	E950.7	E962.1	E980.6
vapor	987.8	E869.8	—	E952.8	E962.2	E982.8
Nitrocellulose	976.3	E858.7	E946.3	E950.4	E962.0	E980.4
Nitrofuran derivatives	961.9	E857	E931.9	E950.4	E962.0	E980.4
Nitrofurantoin	961.9	E857	E931.9	E950.4	E962.0	E980.4
Nitrofurazone	976.0	E858.7	E946.0	E950.4	E962.0	E980.4
Nitrogen (dioxide) (gas) (oxide)	987.2	E869.0	—	E952.8	E962.2	E982.8
mustard (antineoplastic)	963.1	E858.1	E933.1	E950.4	E962.0	E980.4
Nitroglycerin, nitroglycerol (medicinal)	972.4	E858.3	E942.4	E950.4	E962.0	E980.4
nonmedicinal	989.8	E866.8	—	E950.9	E962.1	E980.9
fumes	987.8	E869.8	—	E952.8	E962.2	E982.8
Nitrohydrochloric acid	983.1	E864.1	—	E950.7	E962.1	E980.6
Nitromersol	976.0	E858.7	E946.0	E950.4	E962.0	E980.4
Nitronaphthalene	983.0	E864.0	—	E950.7	E962.2	E980.6
Nitrophenol	983.0	E864.0	—	E950.7	E962.2	E980.6
Nitrothiazol	961.6	E857	E931.6	E950.4	E962.0	E980.4
Nitrotoluene, nitrotoluol	983.0	E864.0	—	E950.7	E962.1	E980.6
vapor	987.8	E869.8	—	E952.8	E962.2	E982.8
Nitrous	968.2	E855.1	E938.2	E950.4	E962.0	E980.4
acid (liquid)	983.1	E864.1	—	E950.7	E962.1	E980.6
fumes	987.2	E869.0	—	E952.8	E962.2	E982.8
oxide (anesthetic) NEC	968.2	E855.1	E938.2	E950.4	E962.0	E980.4
Nitrozone	976.0	E858.7	E946.0	E950.4	E962.0	E980.4
Noctec	967.1	E852.0	E937.1	E950.2	E962.0	E980.2
Noludar	967.5	E852.4	E937.5	E950.2	E962.0	E980.2
Noptil	967.0	E851	E937.0	E950.1	E962.0	E980.1
Noradrenalin	971.2	E855.5	E941.2	E950.4	E962.0	E980.4
Noramidopyrine	965.5	E850.5	E935.5	E950.0	E962.0	E980.0
Norepinephrine	971.2	E855.5	E941.2	E950.4	E962.0	E980.4
Norethandrolone	962.1	E858.0	E932.1	E950.4	E962.0	E980.4

Substance	Poisoning	External Cause (E-Code) Accident	Therapeutic Use	Suicide Attempt	Assault	Undetermined
Norethindrone	962.2	E858.0	E932.2	E950.4	E962.0	E980.4
Norethisterone	962.2	E858.0	E932.2	E950.4	E962.0	E980.4
Norethynodrel	962.2	E858.0	E932.2	E950.4	E962.0	E980.4
Norlestrin	962.2	E858.0	E932.2	E950.4	E962.0	E980.4
Norlutin	962.2	E858.0	E932.2	E950.4	E962.0	E980.4
Normorphine	965.09	E850.2	E935.2	E950.0	E962.0	E980.0
Nortriptyline	969.0	E854.0	E939.0	E950.3	E962.0	E980.3
Noscapine	975.4	E858.6	E945.4	E950.4	E962.0	E980.4
Nose preparations	976.6	E858.7	E946.6	E950.4	E962.0	E980.4
Novobiocin	960.8	E856	E930.8	E950.4	E962.0	E980.4
Novocain (infiltration) (topical)	968.5	E855.2	E938.5	E950.4	E962.0	E980.4
nerve block (peripheral) (plexus)	968.6	E855.2	E938.6	E950.4	E962.0	E980.4
spinal	968.7	E855.2	E938.7	E950.4	E962.0	E980.4
Noxythiolin	961.9	E857	E931.9	E950.4	E962.0	E980.4
NPH Iletin (insulin)	962.3	E858.0	E932.3	E950.4	E962.0	E980.4
Numorphan	965.09	E850.2	E935.2	E950.0	E962.0	E980.0
Nunol	967.0	E851	E937.0	E950.1	E962.0	E980.1
Nupercaine (spinal anesthetic)	968.7	E855.2	E938.7	E950.4	E962.0	E980.4
topical (surface)	968.5	E855.2	E938.5	E950.4	E962.0	E980.4
Nutmeg oil (liniment)	976.3	E858.7	E946.3	E950.4	E962.0	E980.4
Nux vomica	989.1	E863.7	—	E950.6	E962.1	E980.7
Nydrazid	961.8	E857	E931.8	E950.4	E962.0	E980.4
Nylidrin	971.2	E855.5	E941.2	E950.4	E962.0	E980.4
Nystatin	960.1	E856	E930.1	E950.4	E962.0	E980.4
topical	976.0	E858.7	E946.0	E950.4	E962.0	E980.4
Nytol	963.0	E858.1	E933.0	E950.4	E962.0	E980.4
Oblivion	967.8	E852.8	E937.8	E950.2	E962.0	E980.2
Octyl nitrite	972.4	E858.3	E942.4	E950.4	E962.0	E980.4
Oestradiol (cypionate) (dipropionate) (valerate)	962.2	E858.0	E932.2	E950.4	E962.0	E980.4
Oestriol	962.2	E858.0	E932.2	E950.4	E962.0	E980.4
Oestrone	962.2	E858.0	E932.2	E950.4	E962.0	E980.4
Oil (of) NEC	989.8	E866.8	—	E950.9	E962.1	E980.9
bitter almond	989.0	E866.8	—	E950.9	E962.1	E980.9
camphor	976.1	E858.7	E946.1	E950.4	E962.0	E980.4
colors	989.8	E861.6	—	E950.9	E962.1	E980.9
fumes	987.8	E869.8	—	E952.8	E962.2	E982.8
lubricating	981	E862.2	—	E950.9	E962.1	E980.9
specified source, other — *see* substance specified						
vitriol (liquid)	983.1	E864.1	—	E950.7	E962.1	E980.6
fumes	987.8	E869.8	—	E952.8	E962.2	E982.8
wintergreen (bitter) NEC	976.3	E858.7	E946.3	E950.4	E962.0	E980.4
Ointments NEC	976.9	E858.7	E946.9	E950.4	E962.0	E980.4
Oleander	988.2	E865.4	—	E950.9	E962.1	E980.9
Oleandomycin	960.3	E856	E930.3	E950.4	E962.0	E980.4
Oleovitamin A	963.5	E858.1	E933.5	E950.4	E962.0	E980.4
Oleum ricini	973.1	E858.4	E943.1	E950.4	E962.0	E980.4
Olive oil (medicinal) NEC	973.2	E858.4	E943.2	E950.4	E962.0	E980.4
OMPA	989.3	E863.1	—	E950.6	E962.1	E980.7
Oncovin	963.1	E858.1	E933.1	E950.4	E962.0	E980.4
Ophthaine	968.5	E855.2	E938.5	E950.4	E962.0	E980.4
Ophthetic	968.5	E855.2	E938.5	E950.4	E962.0	E980.4
Opiates, opioids, opium NEC	965.00	E850.2	E935.2	E950.0	E962.0	E980.0
antagonists	970.1	E854.3	E940.1	E950.4	E962.0	E980.4
Oracon	962.2	E858.0	E932.2	E950.4	E962.0	E980.4
Oragrafin	977.8	E858.8	E947.8	E950.4	E962.0	E980.4

Substance	Poisoning	Accident	Therapeutic Use	Suicide Attempt	Assault	Undetermined
		External Cause (E-Code)				
Oral contraceptives	962.2	E858.0	E932.2	E950.4	E962.0	E980.4
Orciprenaline	975.1	E858.6	E945.1	E950.4	E962.0	E980.4
Organidin	975.5	E858.6	E945.5	E950.4	E962.0	E980.4
Organophosphates	989.3	E863.1	—	E950.6	E962.1	E980.7
Orimune	979.5	E858.8	E949.5	E950.4	E962.0	E980.4
Orinase	962.3	E858.0	E932.3	E950.4	E962.0	E980.4
Orphenadrine	966.4	E855.0	E936.4	E950.4	E962.0	E980.4
Ortal (sodium)	967.0	E851	E937.0	E950.1	E962.0	E980.1
Orthoboric acid	976.0	E858.7	E946.0	E950.4	E962.0	E980.4
ENT agent	976.6	E858.7	E946.6	E950.4	E962.0	E980.4
ophthalmic preparation	976.5	E858.7	E946.5	E950.4	E962.0	E980.4
Orthocaine	968.5	E855.2	E938.5	E950.4	E962.0	E980.4
Ortho–Novum	962.2	E858.0	E932.2	E950.4	E962.0	E980.4
Orthotolidine (reagent)	977.8	E858.8	E947.8	E950.4	E962.0	E980.4
Osmic acid (liquid)	983.1	E864.1	—	E950.7	E962.1	E980.6
fumes	987.8	E869.8	—	E952.8	E962.2	E982.8
Osmotic diuretics	974.4	E858.5	E944.4	E950.4	E962.0	E980.4
Ouabain	972.1	E858.3	E942.1	E950.4	E962.0	E980.4
Ovarian hormones (synthetic substitutes)	962.2	E858.0	E932.2	E950.4	E962.0	E980.4
Ovral	962.2	E858.0	E932.2	E950.4	E962.0	E980.4
Ovulation suppressants	962.2	E858.0	E932.2	E950.4	E962.0	E980.4
Ovulen	962.2	E858.0	E932.2	E950.4	E962.0	E980.4
Oxacillin (sodium)	960.0	E856	E930.0	E950.4	E962.0	E980.4
Oxalic acid	983.1	E864.1	—	E950.7	E962.1	E980.6
Oxanamide	969.5	E853.8	E939.5	E950.3	E962.0	E980.3
Oxandrolone	962.1	E858.0	E932.1	E950.4	E962.0	E980.4
Oxazepam	969.4	E853.2	E939.4	E950.3	E962.0	E980.3
Oxazolidine derivatives	966.0	E855.0	E936.0	E950.4	E962.0	E980.4
Ox bile extract	973.4	E858.4	E943.4	E950.4	E962.0	E980.4
Oxedrine	971.2	E855.5	E941.2	E950.4	E962.0	E980.4
Oxeladin	975.4	E858.6	E945.4	E950.4	E962.0	E980.4
Oxethazaine NEC	968.5	E855.2	E938.5	E950.4	E962.0	E980.4
Oxidizing agents NEC	983.9	E864.3	—	E950.7	E962.1	E980.6
Oxolinic acid	961.3	E857	E931.3	E950.4	E962.0	E980.4
Oxophenarsine	961.1	E857	E931.1	E950.4	E962.0	E980.4
Oxsoralen	976.3	E858.7	E946.3	E950.4	E962.0	E980.4
Oxtriphylline	975.7	E858.6	E945.7	E950.4	E962.0	E980.4
Oxybuprocaine	968.5	E855.2	E938.5	E950.4	E962.0	E980.4
Oxybutynin	975.1	E858.6	E945.1	E950.4	E962.0	E980.4
Oxycodone	965.09	E850.2	E935.2	E950.0	E962.0	E980.0
Oxygen	987.8	E869.8	—	E952.8	E962.2	E982.8
Oxylone	976.0	E858.7	E946.0	E950.4	E962.0	E980.4
ophthalmic preparation	976.5	E858.7	E946.5	E950.4	E962.0	E980.4
Oxymesterone	962.1	E858.0	E932.1	E950.4	E962.0	E980.4
Oxymetazoline	971.2	E855.5	E941.2	E950.4	E962.0	E980.4
Oxymetholone	962.1	E858.0	E932.1	E950.4	E962.0	E980.4
Oxymorphone	965.09	E850.2	E935.2	E950.0	E962.0	E980.0
Oxypertine	969.0	E854.0	E939.0	E950.3	E962.0	E980.3
Oxyphenbutazone	965.5	E850.5	E935.5	E950.0	E962.0	E980.0
Oxyphencyclimine	971.1	E855.4	E941.1	E950.4	E962.0	E980.4
Oxyphenisatin	973.1	E858.4	E943.1	E950.4	E962.0	E980.4
Oxyphenonium	971.1	E855.4	E941.1	E950.4	E962.0	E980.4
Oxyquinoline	961.3	E857	E931.3	E950.4	E962.0	E980.4
Oxytetracycline	960.4	E856	E930.4	E950.4	E962.0	E980.4
Oxytocics	975.0	E858.6	E945.0	E950.4	E962.0	E980.4
Oxytocin	975.0	E858.6	E945.0	E950.4	E962.0	E980.4
Ozone	987.8	E869.8	—	E952.8	E962.2	E982.8

Substance	Poisoning	Accident	Therapeutic Use	Suicide Attempt	Assault	Undetermined
		External Cause (E-Code)				
PABA	976.3	E858.7	E946.3	E950.4	E962.0	E980.4
Packed red cells	964.7	E858.2	E934.7	E950.4	E962.0	E980.4
Paint NEC	989.8	E861.6	—	E950.9	E962.1	E980.9
cleaner	982.8	E862.9	—	E950.9	E962.1	E980.9
fumes NEC	987.8	E869.8	—	E952.8	E962.1	E982.8
lead (fumes)	984.0	E861.5	—	E950.9	E962.1	E980.9
solvent NEC	982.8	E862.9	—	E950.9	E962.1	E980.9
stripper	982.8	E862.9	—	E950.9	E962.1	E980.9
Palfium	965.09	E850.2	E935.2	E950.0	E962.0	E980.0
Paludrine	961.4	E857	E931.4	E950.4	E962.0	E980.4
PAM	977.2	E855.8	E947.2	E950.4	E962.0	E980.4
Pamaquine (naphthoate)	961.4	E857	E931.4	E950.4	E962.0	E980.4
Pamprin	965.1	E850.3	E935.3	E950.0	E962.0	E980.0
Panadol	965.4	E850.4	E935.4	E950.0	E962.0	E980.0
Pancreatic dornase (mucolytic)	963.4	E858.1	E933.4	E950.4	E962.0	E980.4
Pancreatin	973.4	E858.4	E943.4	E950.4	E962.0	E980.4
Pancrelipase	973.4	E858.4	E943.4	E950.4	E962.0	E980.4
Pangamic acid	963.5	E858.1	E933.5	E950.4	E962.0	E980.4
Panthenol	963.5	E858.1	E933.5	E950.4	E962.0	E980.4
topical	976.8	E858.7	E946.8	E950.4	E962.0	E980.4
Pantopaque	977.8	E858.8	E947.8	E950.4	E962.0	E980.4
Pantopon	965.00	E850.2	E935.2	E950.0	E962.0	E980.0
Pantothenic acid	963.5	E858.1	E933.5	E950.4	E962.0	E980.4
Panwarfin	964.2	E858.2	E934.2	E950.4	E962.0	E980.4
Papain	973.4	E858.4	E943.4	E950.4	E962.0	E980.4
Papaverine	972.5	E858.3	E942.5	E950.4	E962.0	E980.4
Para–aminobenzoic acid	976.3	E858.7	E946.3	E950.4	E962.0	E980.4
Para–aminophenol derivatives	965.4	E850.4	E935.4	E950.0	E962.0	E980.0
Para–aminosalicylic acid (derivatives)	961.8	E857	E931.8	E950.4	E962.0	E980.4
Paracetaldehyde (medicinal)	967.2	E852.1	E937.2	E950.2	E962.0	E980.2
Paracetamol	965.4	E850.4	E935.4	E950.0	E962.0	E980.0
Paracodin	965.09	E850.2	E935.2	E950.0	E962.0	E980.0
Paradione	966.0	E855.0	E936.0	E950.4	E962.0	E980.4
Paraffin(s) (wax)	981	E862.3	—	E950.9	E962.1	E980.9
liquid (medicinal)	973.2	E858.4	E943.2	E950.4	E962.0	E980.4
nonmedicinal (oil)	981	E962.1	—	E950.9	E962.1	E980.9
Paraldehyde (medicinal)	967.2	E852.1	E937.2	E950.2	E962.0	E980.2
Paramethadione	966.0	E855.0	E936.0	E950.4	E962.0	E980.4
Paramethasone	962.0	E858.0	E932.0	E950.4	E962.0	E980.4
Paraquat	989.4	E863.5	—	E950.6	E962.1	E980.7
Parasympatholytics	971.1	E855.4	E941.1	E950.4	E962.0	E980.4
Parasympathomimetics	971.0	E855.3	E941.0	E950.4	E962.0	E980.4
Parathion	989.3	E863.1	—	E950.6	E962.1	E980.7
Parathormone	962.6	E858.0	E932.6	E950.4	E962.0	E980.4
Parathyroid (derivatives)	962.6	E858.0	E932.6	E950.4	E962.0	E980.4
Paratyphoid vaccine	978.1	E858.8	E948.1	E950.4	E962.0	E980.4
Paredrine	971.2	E855.5	E941.2	E950.4	E962.0	E980.4
Paregoric	965.00	E850.2	E935.2	E950.0	E962.0	E980.0
Pargyline	972.3	E858.3	E942.3	E950.4	E962.0	E980.4
Paris green	985.1	E866.3	—	E950.8	E962.1	E980.8
insecticide	985.1	E863.4	—	E950.8	E962.1	E980.8
Parnate	969.0	E854.0	E939.0	E950.3	E962.0	E980.3
Paromomycin	960.8	E856	E930.8	E950.4	E962.0	E980.4
Paroxypropione	963.1	E858.1	E933.1	E950.4	E962.0	E980.4
Parzone	965.09	E850.2	E935.2	E950.0	E962.0	E980.0
PAS	961.8	E857	E931.8	E950.4	E962.0	E980.4
PCP (pentachlorophenol)	989.4	E863.6	—	E950.6	E962.1	E980.7

Substance	Poisoning	Accident	Therapeutic Use	Suicide Attempt	Assault	Undetermined
		External Cause (E-Code)				
herbicide	989.4	E863.5	—	E950.6	E962.1	E980.7
insecticide	989.4	E863.4	—	E950.6	E962.1	E980.7
phencyclidine	968.3	E855.1	E938.3	E950.4	E962.0	E980.4
Peach kernel oil (emulsion)	973.2	E858.4	E943.2	E950.4	E962.0	E980.4
Peanut oil (emulsion) NEC	973.2	E858.4	E943.2	E950.4	E962.0	E980.4
topical	976.3	E858.7	E946.3	E950.4	E962.0	E980.4
Pearly Gates (morning glory seeds)	969.6	E854.1	E939.6	E950.3	E962.0	E980.3
Pecazine	969.1	E853.0	E939.1	E950.3	E962.0	E980.3
Pecilocin	960.1	E856	E930.1	E950.4	E962.0	E980.4
Pectin (with kaolin) NEC	973.5	E858.4	E943.5	E950.4	E962.0	E980.4
Pelletierine tannate	961.6	E857	E931.6	E950.4	E962.0	E980.4
Pemoline	969.7	E854.2	E939.7	E950.3	E962.0	E980.3
Pempidine	972.3	E858.3	E942.3	E950.4	E962.0	E980.4
Penamecillin	960.0	E856	E930.0	E950.4	E962.0	E980.4
Penethamate hydriodide	960.0	E856	E930.0	E950.4	E962.0	E980.4
Penicillamine	963.8	E858.1	E933.8	E950.4	E962.0	E980.4
Penicillin (any type)	960.0	E856	E930.0	E950.4	E962.0	E980.4
Penicillinase	963.4	E858.1	E933.4	E950.4	E962.0	E980.4
Pentachlorophenol (fungicide)	989.4	E863.6	—	E950.6	E962.1	E980.7
herbicide	989.4	E863.5	—	E950.6	E962.1	E980.7
insecticide	989.4	E863.4	—	E950.6	E962.1	E980.7
Pentaerythritol	972.4	E858.3	E942.4	E950.4	E962.0	E980.4
chloral	967.1	E852.0	E937.1	E950.2	E962.0	E980.2
tetranitrate NEC	972.4	E858.3	E942.4	E950.4	E962.0	E980.4
Pentagastrin	977.8	E858.8	E947.8	E950.4	E962.0	E980.4
Pentalin	982.3	E862.4	—	E950.9	E962.1	E980.9
Pentamethonium (bromide)	972.3	E858.3	E942.3	E950.4	E962.0	E980.4
Pentamidine	961.5	E857	E931.5	E950.4	E962.0	E980.4
Pentanol	980.8	E860.8	—	E950.9	E962.1	E980.9
Pentaquine	961.4	E857	E931.4	E950.4	E962.0	E980.4
Pentazocine	965.8	E850.8	E935.8	E950.0	E962.0	E980.0
Penthienate	971.1	E855.4	E941.1	E950.4	E962.0	E980.4
Pentobarbital, pentobarbitone (sodium)	967.0	E851	E937.0	E950.1	E962.0	E980.1
Pentolinium (tartrate)	972.3	E858.3	E942.3	E950.4	E962.0	E980.4
Pentothal	968.3	E855.1	E938.3	E950.4	E962.0	E980.4
Pentylenetetrazol	970.0	E854.3	E940.0	E950.4	E962.0	E980.4
Pentylsalicylamide	961.8	E857	E931.8	E950.4	E962.0	E980.4
Pepsin	973.4	E858.4	E943.4	E950.4	E962.0	E980.4
Peptavlon	977.8	E858.8	E947.8	E950.4	E962.0	E980.4
Percaine (spinal)	968.7	E855.2	E938.7	E950.4	E962.0	E980.4
topical (surface)	968.5	E855.2	E938.5	E950.4	E962.0	E980.4
Perchloroethylene (vapor)	982.3	E862.4	—	E950.9	E962.1	E980.9
medicinal	961.6	E857	E931.6	E950.4	E962.0	E980.4
Percodan	965.09	E850.2	E935.2	E950.0	E962.0	E980.0
Percogesic	965.09	E850.2	E935.2	E950.0	E962.0	E980.0
Percorten	962.0	E858.0	E932.0	E950.4	E962.0	E980.4
Pergonal	962.4	E858.0	E932.4	E950.4	E962.0	E980.4
Perhexiline	972.4	E858.3	E942.4	E950.4	E962.0	E980.4
Periactin	963.0	E858.1	E933.0	E950.4	E962.0	E980.4
Periclor	967.1	E852.0	E937.1	E950.2	E962.0	E980.2
Pericyazine	969.1	E853.0	E939.1	E950.3	E962.0	E980.3
Peritrate	972.4	E858.3	E942.4	E950.4	E962.0	E980.4
Permanganates NEC	983.9	E864.3	—	E950.7	E962.1	E980.6
potassium (topical)	976.0	E858.7	E946.0	E950.4	E962.0	E980.4
Pernocton	967.0	E851	E937.0	E950.1	E962.0	E980.1
Pernoston	967.0	E851	E937.0	E950.1	E962.0	E980.1
Peronin(e)	965.09	E850.2	E935.2	E950.0	E962.0	E980.0

Substance	Poisoning	External Cause (E-Code) Accident	Therapeutic Use	Suicide Attempt	Assault	Undetermined
Perphenazine	969.1	E853.0	E939.1	E950.3	E962.0	E980.3
Pertofrane	969.0	E854	E939.0	E950.3	E962.0	E980.3
Pertussis						
immune serum (human)	964.6	E858.2	E934.6	E950.4	E962.0	E980.4
vaccine (with diphtheria toxoid) (with tetanus toxoid)	978.6	E858.8	E948.6	E950.4	E962.0	E980.4
Peruvian balsam	976.8	E858.7	E946.8	E950.4	E962.0	E980.4
Pesticides (dust) (fumes) (vapor)	989.4	E863.4	—	E950.6	E962.1	E980.7
arsenic	985.1	E863.4	—	E950.8	E962.1	E980.8
chlorinated	989.2	E863.0	—	E950.6	E962.1	E980.7
cyanide	989.0	E863.4	—	E950.6	E962.1	E980.7
kerosene	981	E863.4	—	E950.6	E962.1	E980.7
mixture (of compounds)	989.4	E863.3	—	E950.6	E962.1	E980.7
naphthalene	983.0	E863.4	—	E950.7	E962.1	E980.6
organochlorine (compounds)	989.2	E863.0	—	E950.6	E962.1	E980.7
petroleum (distillate) (products) NEC	981	E863.4	—	E950.6	E962.1	E980.7
specified ingredient NEC	989.4	E863.4	—	E950.6	E962.1	E980.7
strychnine	989.1	E863.4	—	E950.6	E962.1	E980.7
thallium	985.8	E863.7	—	E950.6	E962.1	E980.7
Pethidine (hydrochloride)	965.09	E850.2	E935.2	E950.0	E962.0	E980.0
Petrichloral	967.1	E852.0	E937.1	E950.2	E962.0	E980.2
Petrol	981	E862.1	—	E950.9	E962.1	E980.9
vapor	987.1	E869.8	—	E952.8	E962.2	E982.8
Petrolatum (jelly) (ointment)	976.3	E858.7	E946.3	E950.4	E962.0	E980.4
hydrophilic	976.3	E858.7	E946.3	E950.4	E962.0	E980.4
liquid	973.2	E858.4	E943.2	E950.4	E962.0	E980.4
topical	976.3	E858.7	E946.3	E950.4	E962.0	E980.4
nonmedicinal	981	E862.1	—	E950.9	E962.1	E980.9
Petroleum (cleaners) (fuels) (products) NEC	981	E862.1	—	E950.9	E962.1	E980.9
benzin(e) — *see* Ligroin						
ether — *see* Ligroin						
jelly — *see* Petrolatum						
naphtha — *see* Ligroin						
pesticide	981	E863.4	—	E950.6	E962.1	E980.7
solids	981	E862.3	—	E950.9	E962.1	E980.9
solvents	981	E862.0	—	E950.9	E962.1	E980.9
vapor	987.1	E869.8	—	E952.8	E962.2	E982.8
Peyote	969.6	E854.1	E939.6	E950.3	E962.0	E980.3
Phanodorm, phanodorn	967.0	E851	E937.0	E950.1	E962.0	E980.1
Phanquinone, phanquone	961.5	E857	E931.5	E950.4	E962.0	E980.4
Pharmaceutical excipient or adjunct	977.4	E858.8	E947.4	E950.4	E962.0	E980.4
Phenacemide	966.3	E855.0	E936.3	E950.4	E962.0	E980.4
Phenacetin	965.4	E850.4	E935.4	E950.0	E962.0	E980.0
Phenadoxone	965.09	E850.2	E935.2	E950.0	E962.0	E980.0
Phenaglycodol	969.5	E853.8	E939.5	E950.3	E962.0	E980.3
Phenantoin	966.1	E855.0	E936.1	E950.4	E962.0	E980.4
Phenaphthazine reagent	977.8	E858.8	E947.8	E950.4	E962.0	E980.4
Phenazocine	965.09	E850.2	E935.2	E950.0	E962.0	E980.0
Phenazone	965.5	E850.5	E935.5	E950.0	E962.0	E980.0
Phenazopyridine	976.1	E858.7	E946.1	E950.4	E962.0	E980.4
Phenbenicillin	960.0	E856	E930.0	E950.4	E962.0	E980.4
Phenbutrazate	977.0	E858.8	E947.0	E950.4	E962.0	E980.4
Phencyclidine	968.3	E855.1	E938.3	E950.4	E962.0	E980.4
Phendimetrazine	977.0	E858.8	E947.0	E950.4	E962.0	E980.4
Phenelzine	969.0	E854.0	E939.0	E950.3	E962.0	E980.3

Substance	Poisoning	External Cause (E-Code) Accident	Therapeutic Use	Suicide Attempt	Assault	Undetermined
Phenergan	967.8	E852.8	E937.8	E950.2	E962.0	E980.2
Phenethicillin (potassium)	960.0	E856	E930.0	E950.4	E962.0	E980.4
Phenetsal	965.1	E850.3	E935.3	E950.0	E962.0	E980.0
Pheneturide	966.3	E855.0	E936.3	E950.4	E962.0	E980.4
Phenformin	962.3	E858.0	E932.3	E950.4	E962.0	E980.4
Phenglutarimide	971.1	E855.4	E941.1	E950.4	E962.0	E980.4
Phenicarbazide	965.8	E850.8	E935.8	E950.0	E962.0	E980.0
Phenindamine (tartrate)	963.0	E858.1	E933.0	E950.4	E962.0	E980.4
Phenindione	964.2	E858.2	E934.2	E950.4	E962.0	E980.4
Pheniprazine	969.0	E854.0	E939.0	E950.3	E962.0	E980.3
Pheniramine (maleate)	963.0	E858.1	E933.0	E950.4	E962.0	E980.4
Phenmetrazine	977.0	E858.8	E947.0	E950.4	E962.0	E980.4
Phenobal	967.0	E851	E937.0	E950.1	E962.0	E980.1
Phenobarbital	967.0	E851	E937.0	E950.1	E962.0	E980.1
Phenobarbitone	967.0	E851	E937.0	E950.1	E962.0	E980.1
Phenoctide	976.0	E858.7	E946.0	E950.4	E962.0	E980.4
Phenol (derivatives) NEC	983.0	E864.0	—	E950.7	E962.1	E980.6
disinfectant	983.0	E864.0	—	E950.7	E962.1	E980.6
pesticide	989.4	E863.4	—	E950.6	E962.1	E980.7
red	977.8	E858.8	E947.8	E950.4	E962.0	E980.4
Phenolphthalein	973.1	E858.4	E943.1	E950.4	E962.0	E980.4
Phenolsulfonphthalein	977.8	E858.8	E947.8	E950.4	E962.0	E980.4
Phenomorphan	965.09	E850.2	E935.2	E950.0	E962.0	E980.0
Phenonyl	967.0	E851	E937.0	E950.1	E962.0	E980.1
Phenoperidine	965.09	E850.2	E935.2	E950.0	E962.0	E980.0
Phenoquin	974.7	E858.5	E944.7	E950.4	E962.0	E980.4
Phenothiazines (tranquilizers) NEC	969.1	E853.0	E939.1	E950.3	E962.0	E980.3
insecticide	989.3	E863.4	—	E950.6	E962.1	E980.7
Phenoxybenzamine	971.3	E855.6	E941.3	E950.4	E962.0	E980.4
Phenoxymethyl penicillin	960.0	E856	E930.0	E950.4	E962.0	E980.4
Phenprocoumon	964.2	E858.2	E934.2	E950.4	E962.0	E980.4
Phensuximide	966.2	E855.0	E936.2	E950.4	E962.0	E980.4
Phentermine	977.0	E858.8	E947.0	E950.4	E962.0	E980.4
Phentolamine	971.3	E855.6	E941.3	E950.4	E962.0	E980.4
Phenyl						
butazone	965.5	E850.5	E935.5	E950.0	E962.0	E980.0
enediamine	983.0	E864.0	—	E950.7	E962.1	E980.6
hydrazine	983.0	E864.0	—	E950.7	E962.1	E980.6
antineoplastic	963.1	E858.1	E933.1	E950.4	E962.0	E980.4
mercuric compounds — *see* Mercury						
salicylate	976.3	E858.7	E946.3	E950.4	E962.0	E980.4
Phenylephrin	971.2	E855.5	E941.2	E950.4	E962.0	E980.4
Phenylethybiguanide	962.3	E858.0	E932.3	E950.4	E962.0	E980.4
Phenylpropanolamine	971.2	E855.5	E941.2	E950.4	E962.0	E980.4
Phenylsulfthion	989.3	E863.1	—	E950.6	E962.1	E980.7
Phenyramidol, phenyramidon	965.7	E850.7	E935.7	E950.0	E962.0	E980.0
Phenytoin	966.1	E855.0	E936.1	E950.4	E962.0	E980.4
pHisoHex	976.2	E858.7	E946.2	E950.4	E962.0	E980.4
Pholcodine	965.09	E850.2	E935.2	E950.0	E962.0	E980.0
Phorate	989.3	E863.1	—	E950.6	E962.1	E980.7
Phosdrin	989.3	E863.1	—	E950.6	E962.1	E980.7
Phosgene (gas)	987.8	E869.8	—	E952.8	E962.2	E982.8
Phosphate (tricresyl)	989.8	E866.8	—	E950.9	E962.1	E980.9
organic	989.3	E863.1	—	E950.6	E962.1	E980.7
solvent	982.8	E862.4	—	E950.9	E926.1	E980.9
Phosphine	987.8	E869.8	—	E952.8	E962.2	E982.8
fumigant	987.8	E863.8	—	E950.6	E962.2	E980.7

Substance	Poisoning	External Cause (E-Code) Accident	Therapeutic Use	Suicide Attempt	Assault	Undetermined
Phospholine	971.0	E855.3	E941.0	E950.4	E962.0	E980.4
Phosphoric acid	983.1	E864.1	—	E950.7	E962.1	E980.6
Phosphorus (compounds) NEC	983.9	E864.3	—	E950.7	E962.1	E980.6
rodenticide	983.9	E863.7	—	E950.7	E962.1	E980.6
Phthalimidogluarimide	967.8	E852.8	E937.8	E950.2	E962.0	E980.2
Phthalylsulfathiazole	961.0	E857	E931.0	E950.4	E962.0	E980.4
Phylloquinone	964.3	E858.2	E934.3	E950.4	E962.0	E980.4
Physeptone	965.02	E850.1	E935.1	E950.0	E962.0	E980.0
Physostigma venenosum	988.2	E865.4	—	E950.9	E962.1	E980.9
Physostigmine	971.0	E855.3	E941.0	E950.4	E962.0	E980.4
Phytolacca decandra	988.2	E865.4	—	E950.9	E962.1	E980.9
Phytomenadione	964.3	E858.2	E934.3	E950.4	E962.0	E980.4
Phytonadione	964.3	E858.2	E934.3	E950.4	E962.0	E980.4
Picric (acid)	983.0	E864.0	—	E950.7	E962.1	E980.6
Picrotoxin	970.0	E854.3	E940.0	E950.4	E962.0	E980.4
Pilocarpine	971.0	E855.3	E941.0	E950.4	E962.0	E980.4
Pilocarpus (jaborandi) extract	971.0	E855.3	E941.0	E950.4	E962.0	E980.4
Pimaricin	960.1	E856	E930.1	E950.4	E962.0	E980.4
Piminodine	965.09	E850.2	E935.2	E950.0	E962.0	E980.0
Pine oil, pinesol (disinfectant)	983.9	E861.4	—	E950.7	E962.1	E980.6
Pinkroot	961.6	E857	E931.6	E950.4	E962.0	E980.4
Pipadone	965.09	E850.2	E935.2	E950.0	E962.0	E980.0
Pipamazine	963.0	E858.1	E933.0	E950.4	E962.0	E980.4
Pipazethate	975.4	E858.6	E945.4	E950.4	E962.0	E980.4
Pipenzolate	971.1	E855.4	E941.1	E950.4	E962.0	E980.4
Piperacetazine	969.1	E853.0	E939.1	E950.3	E962.0	E980.3
Piperazine NEC	961.6	E857	E931.6	E950.4	E962.0	E980.4
estrone sulfate	962.2	E858.0	E932.2	E950.4	E962.0	E980.4
Piper cubeba	988.2	E865.4	—	E950.9	E962.1	E980.9
Piperidione	975.4	E858.6	E945.4	E950.4	E962.0	E980.4
Piperidolate	971.1	E855.4	E941.1	E950.4	E962.0	E980.4
Piperocaine	968.9	E855.2	E938.9	E950.4	E962.0	E980.4
infiltration (subcutaneous)	968.5	E855.2	E938.5	E950.4	E962.0	E980.4
nerve block (peripheral) (plexus)	968.6	E855.2	E938.6	E950.4	E962.0	E980.4
topical (surface)	968.5	E855.2	E938.5	E950.4	E962.0	E980.4
Pipobroman	963.1	E858.1	E933.1	E950.4	E962.0	E980.4
Pipradrol	970.8	E854.3	E940.8	E950.4	E962.0	E980.4
Piscidia (bark) (erythrina)	965.7	E850.7	E935.7	E950.0	E962.0	E980.0
Pitch	983.0	E864.0	—	E950.7	E962.1	E980.6
Pitkin's solution	968.7	E855.2	E938.7	E950.4	E962.0	E980.4
Pitocin	975.0	E858.6	E945.0	E950.4	E962.0	E980.4
Pitressin (tannate)	962.5	E858.0	E932.5	E950.4	E962.0	E980.4
Pituitary extracts (posterior)	962.5	E858.0	E932.5	E950.4	E962.0	E980.4
anterior	962.4	E858.0	E932.4	E950.4	E962.0	E980.4
Pituitrin	962.5	E858.0	E932.5	E950.4	E962.0	E980.4
Placental extract	962.9	E858.0	E932.9	E950.4	E962.0	E980.4
Placidyl	967.8	E852.8	E937.8	E950.2	E962.0	E980.2
Plague vaccine	978.3	E858.8	E948.3	E950.4	E962.0	E980.4
Plant foods or fertilizers NEC	989.8	E866.5	—	E950.9	E962.1	E980.9
mixed with herbicides	989.4	E863.5	—	E950.6	E962.1	E980.7
Plants, noxious, used as food	988.2	E865.9	—	E950.9	E962.1	E980.9
berries and seeds	988.2	E865.3	—	E950.9	E962.1	E980.9
specified type NEC	988.2	E865.4	—	E950.9	E962.1	E980.9
Plasma (blood)	964.7	E858.2	E934.7	E950.4	E962.0	E980.4
expanders	964.8	E858.2	E934.8	E950.4	E962.0	E980.4
Plasmanate	964.7	E858.2	E934.7	E950.4	E962.0	E980.4
Plegicil	969.1	E853.0	E939.1	E950.3	E962.0	E980.3

Substance	Poisoning	Accident	Therapeutic Use	Suicide Attempt	Assault	Undetermined
		External Cause (E-Code)				
Podophyllin	976.4	E858.7	E946.4	E950.4	E962.0	E980.4
Podophyllum resin	976.4	E858.7	E946.4	E950.4	E962.0	E980.4
Poison NEC	989.9	E866.9	—	E950.9	E962.1	E980.9
Poisonous berries	988.2	E865.3	—	E950.9	E962.1	E980.9
Pokeweed (any part)	988.2	E865.4	—	E950.9	E962.1	E980.9
Poldine	971.1	E855.4	E941.1	E950.4	E962.0	E980.4
Poliomyelitis vaccine	979.5	E858.8	E949.5	E950.4	E962.0	E980.4
Poliovirus vaccine	979.5	E858.8	E949.5	E950.4	E962.0	E980.4
Polish (car) (floor) (furniture) (metal) (silver)	989.8	E861.2	—	E950.9	E962.1	E980.9
abrasive	989.8	E861.3	—	E950.9	E962.1	E980.9
porcelain	989.8	E861.3	—	E950.9	E962.1	E980.9
Poloxalkol	973.2	E858.4	E943.2	E950.4	E962.0	E980.4
Polyaminostyrene resins	974.5	E858.5	E944.5	E950.4	E962.0	E980.4
Polycycline	960.4	E856	E930.4	E950.4	E962.0	E980.4
Polyester resin hardener	982.8	E862.4	—	E950.9	E962.1	E980.9
fumes	987.8	E869.8	—	E952.8	E962.2	E982.8
Polyestradiol (phosphate)	962.2	E858.0	E932.2	E950.4	E962.0	E980.4
Polyethanolamine alkyl sulfate	976.2	E858.7	E946.2	E950.4	E962.0	E980.4
Polyethylene glycol	976.3	E858.7	E946.3	E950.4	E962.0	E980.4
Polyferose	964.0	E858.2	E934.0	E950.4	E962.0	E980.4
Polymyxin B	960.8	E856	E930.8	E950.4	E962.0	E980.4
ENT agent	976.6	E858.7	E946.6	E950.4	E962.0	E980.4
ophthalmic preparation	976.5	E858.7	E946.5	E950.4	E962.0	E980.4
topical NEC	976.0	E858.7	E946.0	E950.4	E962.0	E980.4
Polynoxylin(e)	976.0	E858.7	E946.0	E950.4	E962.0	E980.4
Polyoxymethyleneurea	976.0	E858.7	E946.0	E950.4	E962.0	E980.4
Polytetrafluoroethylene (inhaled)	987.8	E869.8	—	E952.8	E962.2	E982.8
Polythiazide	974.3	E858.5	E944.3	E950.4	E962.0	E980.4
Polyvinylpyrrolidone	964.8	E858.2	E934.8	E950.4	E962.0	E980.4
Pontocaine (hydrochloride) (infiltration) (topical)	968.5	E855.2	E938.5	E950.4	E962.0	E980.4
nerve block (peripheral) (plexus)	968.6	E855.2	E938.6	E950.4	E962.0	E980.4
spinal	968.7	E855.2	E938.7	E950.4	E962.0	E980.4
Pot	969.6	E854.1	E939.6	E950.3	E962.0	E980.3
Potash (caustic)	983.2	E864.2	—	E950.7	E962.1	E980.6
Potassic saline injection (lactated)	974.5	E858.5	E944.5	E950.4	E962.0	E980.4
Potassium (salts) NEC	974.5	E858.5	E944.5	E950.4	E962.0	E980.4
aminosalicylate	961.8	E857	E931.8	E950.4	E962.0	E980.4
arsenite (solution)	985.1	E866.3	—	E950.8	E962.1	E980.8
bichromate	983.9	E864.3	—	E950.7	E962.1	E980.6
bisulfate	983.9	E864.3	—	E950.7	E962.1	E980.6
bromide (medicinal) NEC	967.3	E852.2	E937.3	E950.2	E962.0	E980.2
carbonate	983.2	E864.2	—	E950.7	E962.1	E980.6
chlorate NEC	983.9	E864.3	—	E950.7	E962.1	E980.6
cyanide — *see* Cyanide						
hydroxide	983.2	E864.2	—	E950.7	E962.1	E980.6
iodide (expectorant) NEC	975.5	E858.6	E945.5	E950.4	E962.0	E980.4
nitrate	989.8	E866.8	—	E950.9	E962.1	E980.9
oxalate	983.9	E864.3	—	E950.7	E962.1	E980.6
perchlorate NEC	977.8	E858.8	E947.8	E950.4	E962.0	E980.4
antithyroid	962.8	E858.0	E932.8	E950.4	E962.0	E980.4
permanganate	976.0	E858.7	E946.0	E950.4	E962.0	E980.4
nonmedicinal	983.9	E864.3	—	E950.7	E962.1	E980.6
Povidone–iodine (anti–infective) NEC	976.0	E858.7	E946.0	E950.4	E962.0	E980.4
Practolol	972.0	E858.3	E942.0	E950.4	E962.0	E980.4
Pralidoxime (chloride)	977.2	E858.8	E947.2	E950.4	E962.0	E980.4

Substance	Poisoning	Accident	Therapeutic Use	Suicide Attempt	Assault	Undetermined
		External Cause (E-Code)				
Pramoxine	968.5	E855.2	E938.5	E950.4	E962.0	E980.4
Prazosin	972.6	E858.3	E942.6	E950.4	E962.0	E980.4
Prednisolone	962.0	E858.0	E932.0	E950.4	E962.0	E980.4
ENT agent	976.6	E858.7	E946.6	E950.4	E962.0	E980.4
ophthalmic preparation	976.5	E858.7	E946.5	E950.4	E962.0	E980.4
topical NEC	976.0	E858.7	E946.0	E950.4	E962.0	E980.4
Prednisone	962.0	E858.0	E932.0	E950.4	E962.0	E980.4
Pregnanediol	962.2	E858.0	E932.2	E950.4	E962.0	E980.4
Pregneninolone	962.2	E858.0	E932.2	E950.4	E962.0	E980.4
Preludin	977.0	E858.8	E947.0	E950.4	E962.0	E980.4
Premarin	962.2	E858.0	E932.2	E950.4	E962.0	E980.4
Prenylamine	972.4	E858.3	E942.4	E950.4	E962.0	E980.4
Preparation H	976.8	E858.7	E946.8	E950.4	E962.0	E980.4
Preservatives	989.8	E866.8	—	E950.9	E962.1	E980.9
Pride of China	988.2	E865.3	—	E950.9	E962.1	E980.9
Prilocaine	968.9	E855.2	E938.9	E950.4	E962.0	E980.4
infiltration (subcutaneous)	968.5	E855.2	E938.5	E950.4	E962.0	E980.4
nerve block (peripheral) (plexus)	968.6	E855.2	E938.6	E950.4	E962.0	E980.4
Primaquine	961.4	E857	E931.4	E950.4	E962.0	E980.4
Primidone	966.3	E855.0	E936.3	E950.4	E962.0	E980.4
Primula (veris)	988.2	E865.4	—	E950.9	E962.1	E980.9
Prinadol	965.09	E850.2	E935.2	E950.0	E962.0	E980.0
Priscol, Priscoline	971.3	E855.6	E941.3	E950.4	E962.0	E980.4
Privet	988.2	E865.4	—	E950.9	E962.1	E980.9
Privine	971.2	E855.5	E941.2	E950.4	E962.0	E980.4
Pro–Banthine	971.1	E855.4	E941.1	E950.4	E962.0	E980.4
Probarbital	967.0	E851	E937.0	E950.1	E962.0	E980.1
Probenecid	974.7	E858.5	E944.7	E950.4	E962.0	E980.4
Procainamide (hydrochloride)	972.0	E858.3	E942.0	E950.4	E962.0	E980.4
Procaine (hydrochloride) (infiltration) (topical)	968.5	E855.2	E938.5	E950.4	E962.0	E980.4
nerve block (peripheral) (plexus)	968.6	E855.2	E938.6	E950.4	E962.0	E980.4
penicillin G	960.0	E856	E930.0	E950.4	E962.0	E980.4
spinal	968.7	E855.2	E938.7	E950.4	E962.0	E980.4
Procalmidol	969.5	E853.8	E939.5	E950.3	E962.0	E980.3
Procarbazine	963.1	E858.1	E933.1	E950.4	E962.0	E980.4
Prochlorperazine	969.1	E853.0	E939.1	E950.3	E962.0	E980.3
Procyclidine	966.4	E855.0	E936.4	E950.4	E962.0	E980.4
Producer gas	986	E868.8	—	E952.1	E962.2	E982.1
Profenamine	966.4	E855.0	E936.4	E950.4	E962.0	E980.4
Profenil	975.1	E858.6	E945.1	E950.4	E962.0	E980.4
Progesterones	962.2	E858.0	E932.2	E950.4	E962.0	E980.4
Progestin	962.2	E858.0	E932.2	E950.4	E962.0	E980.4
Progestogens (with estrogens)	962.2	E858.0	E932.2	E950.4	E962.0	E980.4
Progestone	962.2	E858.0	E932.2	E950.4	E962.0	E980.4
Proguanil	961.4	E857	E931.4	E950.4	E962.0	E980.4
Prolactin	962.4	E858.0	E932.4	E950.4	E962.0	E980.4
Proloid	962.7	E858.0	E932.7	E950.4	E962.0	E980.4
Proluton	962.2	E858.0	E932.2	E950.4	E962.0	E980.4
Promacetin	961.8	E857	E931.8	E950.4	E962.0	E980.4
Promazine	969.1	E853.0	E939.1	E950.3	E962.0	E980.3
Promedol	965.09	E850.2	E935.2	E950.0	E962.0	E980.0
Promethazine	967.8	E852.8	E937.8	E950.2	E962.0	E980.2
Promin	961.8	E857	E931.8	E950.4	E962.0	E980.4
Pronestyl (hydrochloride)	972.0	E858.3	E942.0	E950.4	E962.0	E980.4
Pronetalol, pronethalol	972.0	E858.3	E942.0	E950.4	E962.0	E980.4
Prontosil	961.0	E857	E931.0	E950.4	E962.0	E980.4

Substance	Poisoning	Accident	Therapeutic Use	Suicide Attempt	Assault	Undetermined
		External Cause (E-Code)				
Propamidine isethionate	961.5	E857	E931.5	E950.4	E962.0	E980.4
Propanal (medicinal)	967.8	E852.8	E937.8	E950.2	E962.0	E980.2
Propane (gas) (distributed in mobile container)	987.0	E868.0	—	E951.1	E962.2	E981.1
distributed through pipes	987.0	E867	—	E951.0	E962.2	E981.0
incomplete combustion of – *see* Carbon monoxide, Propane						
Propanidid	968.3	E855.1	E938.3	E950.4	E962.0	E980.4
Propanol	980.3	E860.4	—	E950.9	E962.1	E980.9
Propantheline	971.1	E855.4	E941.1	E950.4	E962.0	E980.4
Proparacaine	968.5	E855.2	E938.5	E950.4	E962.0	E980.4
Propatyl nitrate	972.4	E858.3	E942.4	E950.4	E962.0	E980.4
Propicillin	960.0	E856	E930.0	E950.4	E962.0	E980.4
Propiolactone (vapor)	987.8	E869.8	—	E952.8	E962.2	E982.8
Propiomazine	967.8	E852.8	E937.8	E950.2	E962.0	E980.2
Propionaldehyde (medicinal)	967.8	E852.8	E937.8	E950.2	E962.0	E980.2
Propionate compound	976.0	E858.7	E946.0	E950.4	E962.0	E980.4
Propion gel	976.0	E858.7	E946.0	E950.4	E962.0	E980.4
Propitocaine	968.9	E855.2	E938.9	E950.4	E962.0	E980.4
infiltration (subcutaneous)	968.5	E855.2	E938.5	E950.4	E962.0	E980.4
nerve block (peripheral) (plexus)	968.6	E855.2	E938.6	E950.4	E962.0	E980.4
Propoxur	989.3	E863.2	—	E950.6	E962.1	E980.7
Propoxycaine	968.9	E855.2	E938.9	E950.4	E962.0	E980.4
infiltration (subcutaneous)	968.5	E855.2	E938.5	E950.4	E962.0	E980.4
nerve block (peripheral) (plexus)	968.6	E855.2	E938.6	E950.4	E962.0	E980.4
topical (surface)	968.5	E855.2	E938.5	E950.4	E962.0	E980.4
Propoxyphene (hydrochloride)	965.8	E850.8	E935.8	E950.0	E962.0	E980.0
Propranolol	972.0	E858.3	E942.0	E950.4	E962.0	E980.4
Propyl						
alcohol	980.3	E860.4	—	E950.9	E962.1	E980.9
carbinol	980.3	E860.4	—	E950.9	E962.1	E980.9
hexadrine	971.2	E855.5	E941.2	E950.4	E962.0	E980.4
iodone	977.8	E858.8	E947.8	E950.4	E962.0	E980.4
thiouracil	962.8	E858.0	E932.8	E950.4	E962.0	E980.4
Propylene	987.1	E869.8	—	E952.8	E962.2	E982.8
Propylparaben (ophthalmic)	976.5	E858.7	E946.5	E950.4	E962.0	E980.4
Proscillaridin	972.1	E858.3	E942.1	E950.4	E962.0	E980.4
Prostaglandins	975.0	E858.6	E945.0	E950.4	E962.0	E980.4
Prostigmin	971.0	E855.3	E941.0	E950.4	E962.0	E980.4
Protamine (sulfate)	964.5	E858.2	E934.5	E950.4	E962.0	E980.4
zinc insulin	962.3	E858.0	E932.3	E950.4	E962.0	E980.4
Protectants (topical)	976.3	E858.7	E946.3	E950.4	E962.0	E980.4
Protein hydrolysate	974.5	E858.5	E944.5	E950.4	E962.0	E980.4
Prothionamide	961.8	E857	E931.8	E950.4	E962.0	E980.4
Prothipendyl	969.5	E853.8	E939.5	E950.3	E962.0	E980.3
Protokylol	971.2	E855.5	E941.2	E950.4	E962.0	E980.4
Protopam	977.2	E858.8	E947.2	E950.4	E962.0	E980.4
Protoveratrine(s) (A) (B)	972.6	E858.3	E942.6	E950.4	E962.0	E980.4
Protriptyline	969.0	E854.0	E939.0	E950.3	E962.0	E980.3
Provera	962.2	E858.0	E932.2	E950.4	E962.0	E980.4
Provitamin A	963.5	E858.1	E933.5	E950.4	E962.0	E980.4
Proxymetacaine	968.5	E855.2	E938.5	E950.4	E962.0	E980.4
Proxyphylline	975.1	E858.6	E945.1	E950.4	E962.0	E980.4
Prunus						
laurocerasus	988.2	E865.4	—	E950.9	E962.1	E980.9
virginiana	988.2	E865.4	—	E950.9	E962.1	E980.9
Prussic acid	989.0	E866.8	—	E950.9	E962.1	E980.9

Substance	Poisoning	Accident	Therapeutic Use	Suicide Attempt	Assault	Undetermined
		External Cause (E-Code)				
vapor	987.7	E869.8	—	E952.8	E962.2	E982.8
Pseudoephedrine	971.2	E855.5	E941.2	E950.4	E962.0	E980.4
Psilocin	969.6	E854.1	E939.6	E950.3	E962.0	E980.3
Psilocybin	969.6	E854.1	E939.6	E950.3	E962.0	E980.3
PSP	977.8	E858.8	E947.8	E950.4	E962.0	E980.4
Psychedelic agents	969.6	E854.1	E939.6	E950.3	E962.0	E980.3
Psychodysleptics	969.6	E854.1	E939.6	E950.3	E962.0	E980.3
Psychostimulants	969.7	E854.2	E939.7	E950.3	E962.0	E980.3
Psychotherapeutic agents	969.9	E855.9	E939.9	E950.3	E962.0	E980.3
antidepressants	969.0	E854.0	E939.0	E950.3	E962.0	E980.3
specified NEC	969.8	E855.8	E939.8	E950.3	E962.0	E980.3
tranquilizers NEC	969.5	E853.9	E939.5	E950.3	E962.0	E980.3
Psychotomimetic agents	969.6	E854.1	E939.6	E950.3	E962.0	E980.3
Psychotropic agents	969.9	E855.9	E939.9	E950.3	E962.0	E980.3
specified NEC	969.8	E855.8	E939.8	E950.3	E962.0	E980.3
Psyllium	973.3	E858.4	E943.3	E950.4	E962.0	E980.4
Pteroylglutamic acid	964.1	E858.2	E934.1	E950.4	E962.0	E980.4
Pteroyltriglutamate	963.1	E858.1	E933.1	E950.4	E962.0	E980.4
PTFE	987.8	E869.8	—	E952.8	E962.2	E982.8
Pulsatilla	988.2	E865.4	—	E950.9	E962.1	E980.9
Purex (bleach)	983.9	E864.3	—	E950.7	E962.1	E980.6
Purine diuretics	974.1	E858.5	E944.1	E950.4	E962.0	E980.4
Purinethol	963.1	E858.1	E933.1	E950.4	E962.0	E980.4
PVP	964.8	E858.2	E934.8	E950.4	E962.0	E980.4
Pyrabital	965.7	E850.7	E935.7	E950.0	E962.0	E980.0
Pyramidon	965.5	E850.5	E935.5	E950.0	E962.0	E980.0
Pyrantel (pamoate)	961.6	E857	E931.6	E950.4	E962.0	E980.4
Pyrathiazine	963.0	E858.1	E933.0	E950.4	E962.0	E980.4
Pyrazinamide	961.8	E857	E931.8	E950.4	E962.0	E980.4
Pyrazinoic acid (amide)	961.8	E857	E931.8	E950.4	E962.0	E980.4
Pyrazole (derivatives)	965.5	E850.5	E935.5	E950.0	E962.0	E980.0
Pyrazolone (analgesics)	965.5	E850.5	E935.5	E950.0	E962.0	E980.0
Pyrethrins, pyrethrum	989.4	E863.4	—	E950.6	E962.1	E980.7
Pyribenzamine	963.0	E858.1	E933.0	E950.4	E962.0	E980.4
Pyridine (liquid) (vapor)	982.0	E862.4	—	E950.9	E962.1	E980.9
aldoxime chloride	977.2	E858.8	E947.2	E950.4	E962.0	E980.4
Pyridium	976.1	E858.7	E946.1	E950.4	E962.0	E980.4
Pyridostigmine	971.0	E855.3	E941.0	E950.4	E962.0	E980.4
Pyridoxine	963.5	E858.1	E933.5	E950.4	E962.0	E980.4
Pyrilamine	963.0	E858.1	E933.0	E950.4	E962.0	E980.4
Pyrimethamine	961.4	E857	E931.4	E950.4	E962.0	E980.4
Pyrogallic acid	983.0	E864.0	—	E950.7	E962.1	E980.6
Pyroxylin	976.3	E858.7	E946.3	E950.4	E962.0	E980.4
Pyrrobutamine	963.0	E858.1	E933.0	E950.4	E962.0	E980.4
Pyrrocaine	968.5	E855.2	E938.5	E950.4	E962.0	E980.4
Pyrvinium (pamoate)	961.6	E857	E931.6	E950.4	E962.0	E980.4
PZI	962.3	E858.0	E932.3	E950.4	E962.0	E980.4
Quaalude	967.4	E852.3	E937.4	E950.2	E962.0	E980.2
Quaternary ammonium derivatives	971.1	E855.4	E941.1	E950.4	E962.0	E980.4
Quicklime	983.2	E864.2	—	E950.7	E962.1	E980.6
Quinacrine	961.3	E857	E931.3	E950.4	E962.0	E980.4
Quinaglute	972.0	E858.3	E942.0	E950.4	E962.0	E980.4
Quinalbarbitone	967.0	E851	E937.0	E950.1	E962.0	E980.1
Quinestradiol	962.2	E858.0	E932.2	E950.4	E962.0	E980.4
Quinethazone	974.3	E858.5	E944.3	E950.4	E962.0	E980.4
Quinidine (gluconate) (polygalacturonate) (salts) (sulfate)	972.0	E858.3	E942.0	E950.4	E962.0	E980.4

Substance	Poisoning	External Cause (E-Code) Accident	Therapeutic Use	Suicide Attempt	Assault	Undetermined
Quinine	961.4	E857	E931.4	E950.4	E962.0	E980.4
Quiniobine	961.3	E857	E931.3	E950.4	E962.0	E980.4
Quinolines	961.3	E857	E931.3	E950.4	E962.0	E980.4
Quotane	968.5	E855.2	E938.5	E950.4	E962.0	E980.4
Rabies						
immune globulin (human)	964.6	E858.2	E934.6	E950.4	E962.0	E980.4
vaccine	979.1	E858.8	E949.1	E950.4	E962.0	E980.4
Racemoramide	965.09	E850.2	E935.2	E950.0	E962.0	E980.0
Racemorphan	965.09	E850.2	E935.2	E950.0	E962.0	E980.0
Radiator alcohol	980.1	E860.2	—	E950.9	E962.1	E980.9
Radio–opaque (drugs) (materials)	977.8	E858.8	E947.8	E950.4	E962.0	E980.4
Ranunculus	988.2	E865.4	—	E950.9	E962.1	E980.9
Rat poison	989.4	E863.7	—	E950.6	E962.1	E980.7
Rattlesnake (venom)	989.5	E905.0	—	E950.9	E962.1	E980.9
Raudixin	972.6	E858.3	E942.6	E950.4	E962.0	E980.4
Rautensin	972.6	E858.3	E942.6	E950.4	E962.0	E980.4
Rautina	972.6	E858.3	E942.6	E950.4	E962.0	E980.4
Rautotal	972.6	E858.3	E942.6	E950.4	E962.0	E980.4
Rauwiloid	972.6	E858.3	E942.6	E950.4	E962.0	E980.4
Rauwoldin	972.6	E858.3	E942.6	E950.4	E962.0	E980.4
Rauwolfia (alkaloids)	972.6	E858.3	E942.6	E950.4	E962.0	E980.4
Realgar	985.1	E866.3	—	E950.8	E962.1	E980.8
Red cells, packed	964.7	E858.2	E934.7	E950.4	E962.0	E980.4
Reducing agents, industrial NEC	983.9	E864.3	—	E950.7	E962.1	E980.6
Refrigerant gas (freon)	987.4	E869.2	—	E952.8	E962.2	E982.8
not freon	987.9	E869.9	—	E952.9	E962.2	E982.9
Regroton	974.4	E858.5	E944.4	E950.4	E962.0	E980.4
Rela	968.0	E855.1	E938.0	E950.4	E962.0	E980.4
Relaxants, skeletal muscle (autonomic)	975.2	E858.6	E945.2	E950.4	E962.0	E980.4
central nervous system	968.0	E855.1	E938.0	E950.4	E962.0	E980.4
Renese	974.3	E858.5	E944.3	E950.4	E962.0	E980.4
Renografin	977.8	E858.8	E947.8	E950.4	E962.0	E980.4
Replacement solutions	974.5	E858.5	E944.5	E950.4	E962.0	E980.4
Rescinnamine	972.6	E858.3	E942.6	E950.4	E962.0	E980.4
Reserpine	972.6	E858.3	E942.6	E950.4	E962.0	E980.4
Resorcin, resorcinol	976.4	E858.7	E946.4	E950.4	E962.0	E980.4
Respaire	975.5	E858.6	E945.5	E950.4	E962.0	E980.4
Respiratory agents NEC	975.8	E858.6	E945.8	E950.4	E962.0	E980.4
Retinoic acid	976.8	E858.7	E946.8	E950.4	E962.0	E980.4
Retinol	963.5	E858.1	E933.5	E950.4	E962.0	E980.4
Rho (D) immune globulin (human)	964.6	E858.2	E934.6	E950.4	E962.0	E980.4
Rhodine	965.1	E850.3	E935.3	E950.0	E962.0	E980.0
RhoGAM	964.6	E858.2	E934.6	E950.4	E962.0	E980.4
Riboflavin	963.5	E858.1	E933.5	E950.4	E962.0	E980.4
Ricin	989.8	E866.8	—	E950.9	E962.1	E980.9
Ricinus communis	988.2	E865.3	—	E950.9	E962.1	E980.9
Rickettsial vaccine NEC	979.6	E858.8	E949.6	E950.4	E962.0	E980.4
with viral and bacterial vaccine	979.7	E858.8	E949.7	E950.4	E962.0	E980.4
Rifampin	960.6	E856	E930.6	E950.4	E962.0	E980.4
Rimifon	961.8	E857	E931.8	E950.4	E962.0	E980.4
Ringer's injection (lactated)	974.5	E858.5	E944.5	E950.4	E962.0	E980.4
Ristocetin	960.8	E856	E930.8	E950.4	E962.0	E980.4
Ritalin	969.7	E854.2	E939.7	E950.3	E962.0	E980.3
Roach killers — *see* Pesticides						
Rocky Mountain spotted fever vaccine	979.6	E858.8	E949.6	E950.4	E962.0	E980.4
Rodenticides	989.4	E863.7	—	E950.6	E962.1	E980.7
Rolaids	973.0	E858.4	E943.0	E950.4	E962.0	E980.4

Substance	Poisoning	External Cause (E-Code): Accident	Therapeutic Use	Suicide Attempt	Assault	Undetermined
Rolitetracycline	960.4	E856	E930.4	E950.4	E962.0	E980.4
Romilar	975.4	E858.6	E945.4	E950.4	E962.0	E980.4
Rose water ointment	976.3	E858.7	E946.3	E950.4	E962.0	E980.4
Rotenone	989.4	E863.7	—	E950.6	E962.1	E980.7
Rotoxamine	963.0	E858.1	E933.0	E950.4	E962.0	E980.4
Rough–on–rats	989.4	E863.7	—	E950.6	E962.1	E980.7
Rubbing alcohol	980.2	E860.3	—	E950.9	E962.1	E980.9
Rubella virus vaccine	979.4	E858.8	E949.4	E950.4	E962.0	E980.4
Rubelogen	979.4	E858.8	E949.4	E950.4	E962.0	E980.4
Rubeovax	979.4	E858.8	E949.4	E950.4	E962.0	E980.4
Rubidomycin	960.7	E856	E930.7	E950.4	E962.0	E980.4
Rue	988.2	E965.4	—	E950.9	E962.1	E980.9
Ruta	988.2	E865.4	—	E950.9	E962.1	E980.9
Sabadilla (medicinal)	976.0	E858.7	E946.0	E950.4	E962.0	E980.4
pesticide	989.4	E863.4	—	E950.6	E962.1	E980.7
Sabin oral vaccine	979.5	E858.8	E949.5	E950.4	E962.0	E980.4
Saccharated iron oxide	964.0	E858.2	E934.0	E950.4	E962.0	E980.4
Saccharin	974.5	E858.5	E944.5	E950.4	E962.0	E980.4
Safflower oil	972.2	E858.3	E942.2	E950.4	E962.0	E980.4
Salicylamide	965.1	E850.3	E935.3	E950.0	E962.0	E980.0
Salicylate(s)	965.1	E850.3	E935.3	E950.0	E962.0	E980.0
methyl	976.3	E858.7	E946.3	E950.4	E962.0	E980.4
theobromine calcium	974.1	E858.5	E944.1	E950.4	E962.0	E980.4
Salicylazosulfapyridine	961.0	E857	E931.0	E950.4	E962.0	E980.4
Salicylhydroxamic acid	976.0	E858.7	E946.0	E950.4	E962.0	E980.4
Salicylic acid (keratolytic) NEC	976.4	E858.7	E946.4	E950.4	E962.0	E980.4
congeners	965.1	E850.3	E935.3	E950.0	E962.0	E980.0
salts	965.1	E850.3	E935.3	E950.0	E962.0	E980.0
Saliniazid	961.8	E857	E931.8	E950.4	E962.0	E980.4
Salol	976.3	E858.7	E946.3	E950.4	E962.0	E980.4
Salt (substitute) NEC	974.5	E858.5	E944.5	E950.4	E962.0	E980.4
Saluretics	974.3	E858.5	E944.3	E950.4	E962.0	E980.4
Saluron	974.3	E858.5	E944.3	E950.4	E962.0	E980.4
Salvarsan 606 (neosilver) (silver)	961.1	E857	E931.1	E950.4	E962.0	E980.4
Sambucus canadensis	988.2	E865.4	—	E950.9	E962.1	E980.9
berry	988.2	E865.3	—	E950.9	E962.1	E980.9
Sandril	972.6	E858.3	E942.6	E950.4	E962.0	E980.4
Sanguinaria canadensis	988.2	E865.4	—	E950.9	E962.1	E980.9
Saniflush (cleaner)	983.9	E861.3	—	E950.7	E962.1	E980.6
Santonin	961.6	E857	E931.6	E950.4	E962.0	E980.4
Santyl	976.8	E858.7	E946.8	E950.4	E962.0	E980.4
Sarkomycin	960.7	E856	E930.7	E950.4	E962.0	E980.4
Saroten	969.0	E854.0	E939.0	E950.3	E962.0	E980.3
Saturnine – *see* Lead						
Savin (oil)	976.4	E858.7	E946.4	E950.4	E962.0	E980.4
Scammony	973.1	E858.4	E943.1	E950.4	E962.0	E980.4
Scarlet red	976.8	E858.7	E946.8	E950.4	E962.0	E980.4
Scheele's green	985.1	E866.3	—	E950.8	E962.1	E980.8
insecticide	985.1	E863.4	—	E950.8	E962.1	E980.8
Schradan	989.3	E863.1	—	E950.6	E962.1	E980.7
Schweinfurt (h) green	985.1	E866.3	—	E950.8	E962.1	E980.8
insecticide	985.1	E863.4	—	E950.8	E962.1	E980.8
Scilla — *see* Squill						
Sclerosing agents	972.7	E858.3	E942.7	E950.4	E962.0	E980.4
Scopolamine	971.1	E855.4	E941.1	E950.4	E962.0	E980.4
Scouring powder	989.8	E861.3	—	E950.9	E962.1	E980.9
Sea						

Substance	Poisoning	Accident	Therapeutic Use	Suicide Attempt	Assault	Undetermined
		External Cause (E-Code)				
anemone (sting)	989.5	E905.6	—	E950.9	E962.1	E980.9
cucumber (sting)	989.5	E905.6	—	E950.9	E962.1	E980.9
snake (bite) (venom)	989.5	E905.0	—	E950.9	E962.1	E980.9
urchin spine (puncture)	989.5	E905.6	—	E950.9	E962.1	E980.9
Secbutabarbital	967.0	E851	E937.0	E950.1	E962.0	E980.1
Secbutabaritone	967.0	E851	E937.0	E950.1	E962.0	E980.1
Secobarbital	967.0	E851	E937.0	E950.1	E962.0	E980.1
Seconal	967.0	E851	E937.0	E950.1	E962.0	E980.1
Secretin	977.8	E858.8	E947.8	E950.4	E962.0	E980.4
Sedatives, nonbarbiturate	967.9	E852.9	E937.9	E950.2	E962.0	E980.2
specified NEC	967.8	E852.8	E937.8	E950.2	E962.0	E980.2
Sedormid	967.8	E852.8	E937.8	E950.2	E962.0	E980.2
Seed (plant)	988.2	E865.3	—	E950.9	E962.1	E980.9
disinfectant or dressing	989.8	E866.5	—	E950.9	E962.1	E980.9
Selenium (fumes) NEC	985.8	E866.4	—	E950.9	E962.1	E980.9
disulfide or sulfide	976.4	E858.7	E946.4	E950.4	E962.0	E980.4
Selsun	976.4	E858.7	E946.4	E950.4	E962.0	E980.4
Senna	973.1	E858.4	E943.1	E950.4	E962.0	E980.4
Septisol	976.2	E858.7	E946.2	E950.4	E962.0	E980.4
Serax	969.4	E853.2	E939.4	E950.3	E962.0	E980.3
Serenesil	967.8	E852.8	E937.8	E950.2	E962.0	E980.2
Serenium (hydrochloride)	961.9	E857	E931.9	E950.4	E962.0	E980.4
Sernyl	968.3	E855.1	E938.3	E950.4	E962.0	E980.4
Serotonin	977.8	E858.8	E947.8	E950.4	E962.0	E980.4
Serpasil	972.6	E858.3	E942.6	E950.4	E962.0	E980.4
Sewer gas	987.8	E869.8	—	E952.8	E962.2	E982.8
Shampoo	989.6	E861.0	—	E950.9	E962.1	E980.9
Shellfish, nonbacterial or noxious	988.0	E865.1	—	E950.9	E962.1	E980.9
Silicones NEC	989.8	E866.8	E947.8	E950.9	E962.1	E980.9
Silvadene	976.0	E858.7	E946.0	E950.4	E962.0	E980.4
Silver (compound) (medicinal) NEC	976.0	E858.7	E946.0	E950.4	E962.0	E980.4
anti–infectives	976.0	E858.7	E946.0	E950.4	E962.0	E980.4
arsphenamine	961.1	E857	E931.1	E950.4	E962.0	E980.4
nitrate	976.0	E858.7	E946.0	E950.4	E962.0	E980.4
ophthalmic preparation	976.5	E858.7	E946.5	E950.4	E962.0	E980.4
toughened (keratolytic)	976.4	E858.7	E946.4	E950.4	E962.0	E980.4
nonmedicinal (dust)	985.8	E866.4	—	E950.9	E962.1	E980.9
protein (mild) (strong)	976.0	E858.7	E946.0	E950.4	E962.0	E980.4
salvarsan	961.1	E857	E931.1	E950.4	E962.0	E980.4
Simethicone	973.8	E858.4	E943.8	E950.4	E962.0	E980.4
Sinequan	969.0	E854.0	E939.0	E950.3	E962.0	E980.3
Singoserp	972.6	E858.3	E942.6	E950.4	E962.0	E980.4
Sintrom	964.2	E858.2	E934.2	E950.4	E962.0	E980.4
Sitosterols	972.2	E858.3	E942.2	E950.4	E962.0	E980.4
Skeletal muscle relaxants	975.2	E858.6	E945.2	E950.4	E962.0	E980.4
Skin						
agents (external)	976.9	E858.7	E946.9	E950.4	E962.0	E980.4
specified NEC	976.8	E858.7	E946.8	E950.4	E962.0	E980.4
test antigen	977.8	E858.8	E947.8	E950.4	E962.0	E980.4
Sleep–eze	963.0	E858.1	E933.0	E950.4	E962.0	E980.4
Sleeping draught (drug) (pill) (tablet)	967.9	E852.9	E937.9	E950.2	E962.0	E980.2
Smallpox vaccine	979.0	E858.8	E949.0	E950.4	E962.0	E980.4
Smelter fumes NEC	985.9	E866.4	—	E950.9	E962.1	E980.9
Smog	987.3	E869.1	—	E952.8	E962.2	E982.8
Smoke NEC	987.9	E869.9	—	E952.9	E962.2	E982.9
Smooth muscle relaxant	975.1	E858.6	E945.1	E950.4	E962.0	E980.4
Snail killer	989.4	E863.4	—	E950.6	E962.1	E980.7

Substance	Poisoning	Accident	Therapeutic Use	Suicide Attempt	Assault	Undetermined
		External Cause (E-Code)				
Snake (bite) (venom)	989.5	E905.0	—	E950.9	E962.1	E980.9
Snuff	989.8	E866.8	—	E950.9	E962.1	E980.9
Soap (powder) (product)	989.6	E861.1	—	E950.9	E962.1	E980.9
medicinal, soft	976.2	E858.7	E946.2	E950.4	E962.0	E980.4
Soda (caustic)	983.2	E864.2	—	E950.7	E962.1	E980.6
bicarb	963.3	E858.1	E933.3	E950.4	E962.0	E980.4
chlorinated — *see* Sodium, hypochlorite						
Sodium						
acetosulfone	961.8	E857	E931.8	E950.4	E962.0	E980.4
acetrizoate	977.8	E858.8	E947.8	E950.4	E962.0	E980.4
amytal	967.0	E851	E937.0	E950.1	E962.0	E980.1
arsenate — *see* Arsenic						
bicarbonate	963.3	E858.1	E933.3	E950.4	E962.0	E980.4
bichromate	983.9	E864.3	—	E950.7	E962.1	E980.6
biphosphate	963.2	E858.1	E933.2	E950.4	E962.0	E980.4
bisulfate	983.9	E864.3	—	E950.7	E962.1	E980.6
borate (cleanser)	989.6	E861.3	—	E950.9	E962.1	E980.9
bromide NEC	967.3	E852.2	E937.3	E950.2	E962.0	E980.2
cacodylate (nonmedicinal) NEC	978.8	E858.8	E948.8	E950.4	E962.0	E980.4
anti–infective	961.1	E857	E931.1	E950.4	E962.0	E980.4
herbicide	989.4	E863.5	—	E950.6	E962.1	E980.7
calcium edetate	963.8	E858.1	E933.8	E950.4	E962.0	E980.4
carbonate NEC	983.2	E864.2	—	E950.7	E962.1	E980.6
chlorate NEC	983.9	E864.3	—	E950.7	E962.1	E980.6
herbicide	983.9	E863.5	—	E950.7	E962.1	E980.6
chloride NEC	974.5	E858.5	E944.5	E950.4	E962.0	E980.4
chromate	983.9	E864.3	—	E950.7	E962.1	E980.6
citrate	963.3	E858.1	E933.3	E950.4	E962.0	E980.4
cyanide — *see* Cyanide(s)						
cyclamate	974.5	E858.5	E944.5	E950.4	E962.0	E980.4
diatrizoate	977.8	E858.8	E947.8	E950.4	E962.0	E980.4
dibunate	975.4	E858.6	E945.4	E950.4	E962.0	E980.4
dioctyl sulfosuccinate	973.2	E858.4	E943.2	E950.4	E962.0	E980.4
edetate	963.8	E858.1	E933.8	E950.4	E962.0	E980.4
ethacrynate	974.4	E858.5	E944.4	E950.4	E962.0	E980.4
fluoracetate (dust) (rodenticide)	989.4	E863.7	—	E950.6	E962.1	E980.7
fluoride — *see* Fluoride(s)						
free salt	974.5	E858.5	E944.5	E950.4	E962.0	E980.4
glucosulfone	961.8	E857	E931.8	E950.4	E962.0	E980.4
hydroxide	983.2	E864.2	—	E950.7	E962.1	E980.6
hypochlorite (bleach) NEC	983.9	E864.3	—	E950.7	E962.1	E980.6
disinfectant	983.9	E861.4	—	E950.7	E962.1	E980.6
medicinal (anti–infective) (external)	976.0	E858.7	E946.0	E950.4	E962.0	E980.4
vapor	987.8	E869.8	—	E952.8	E962.2	E982.8
hyposulfite	976.0	E858.7	E946.0	E950.4	E962.0	E980.4
indigotindisulfonate	977.8	E858.8	E947.8	E950.4	E962.0	E980.4
iodide	977.8	E858.8	E947.8	E950.4	E962.0	E980.4
iothalamate	977.8	E858.8	E947.8	E950.4	E962.0	E980.4
iron edetate	964.0	E858.2	E934.0	E950.4	E962.0	E980.4
lactate	963.3	E858.1	E933.3	E950.4	E962.0	E980.4
lauryl sulfate	976.2	E858.7	E946.2	E950.4	E962.0	E980.4
L–triiodothyronine	962.7	E858.0	E932.7	E950.4	E962.0	E980.4
metrizoate	977.8	E858.8	E947.8	E950.4	E962.0	E980.4
monofluoracetate (dust) (rodenticide)	989.4	E863.7	—	E950.6	E962.1	E980.7
morrhuate	972.7	E858.3	E942.7	E950.4	E962.0	E980.4
nafcillin	960.0	E856	E930.0	E950.4	E962.0	E980.4
nitrate (oxidizing agent)	983.9	E864.3	—	E950.7	E962.1	E980.6

Substance	Poisoning	External Cause (E-Code) Accident	Therapeutic Use	Suicide Attempt	Assault	Undetermined
nitrite (medicinal)	972.4	E858.3	E942.4	E950.4	E962.0	E980.4
nitroferricyanide	972.6	E858.3	E942.6	E950.4	E962.0	E980.4
nitroprusside	972.6	E858.3	E942.6	E950.4	E962.0	E980.4
para–aminohippurate	977.8	E858.8	E947.8	E950.4	E962.0	E980.4
perborate (nonmedicinal) NEC	989.8	E866.8	—	E950.9	E962.1	E980.9
medicinal	976.6	E858.7	E946.6	E950.4	E962.0	E980.4
soap	989.6	E861.1	—	E950.9	E962.1	E980.9
percarbonate — *see* Sodium, perborate						
phosphate	973.3	E858.4	E943.3	E950.4	E962.0	E980.4
polystyrene sulfonate	974.5	E858.5	E944.5	E950.4	E962.0	E980.4
propionate	976.0	E858.7	E946.0	E950.4	E962.0	E980.4
psylliate	972.7	E858.3	E942.7	E950.4	E962.0	E980.4
removing resins	974.5	E858.5	E944.5	E950.4	E962.0	E980.4
salicylate	965.1	E850.3	E935.3	E950.0	E962.0	E980.0
sulfate	973.3	E858.4	E943.3	E950.4	E962.0	E980.4
sulfoxone	961.8	E857	E931.8	E950.4	E962.0	E980.4
tetradecyl sulfate	972.7	E858.3	E942.7	E950.4	E962.0	E980.4
thiopental	968.3	E855.1	E938.3	E950.4	E962.0	E980.4
thiosalicylate	965.1	E850.3	E935.3	E950.0	E962.0	E980.0
thiosulfate	976.0	E858.7	E946.0	E950.4	E962.0	E980.4
tolbutamide	977.8	E858.8	E947.8	E950.4	E962.0	E980.4
tyropanoate	977.8	E858.8	E947.8	E950.4	E962.0	E980.4
Solanine	977.8	E858.8	E947.8	E950.4	E962.0	E980.4
Solanum dulcamara	988.2	E865.4	—	E950.9	E962.1	E980.9
Solapsone	961.8	E857	E931.8	E950.4	E962.0	E980.4
Solasulfone	961.8	E857	E931.8	E950.4	E962.0	E980.4
Soldering fluid	983.1	E864.1	—	E950.7	E962.1	E980.6
Solid substance	989.9	E866.9	—	E950.9	E962.1	E980.9
specified NEC	989.9	E866.8	—	E950.9	E962.1	E980.9
Solvents, industrial	982.8	E862.9	—	E950.9	E962.1	E980.9
naphtha	981	E862.0	—	E950.9	E962.1	E980.9
petroleum	981	E862.0	—	E950.9	E962.1	E980.9
specified NEC	982.8	E862.4	—	E950.9	E962.1	E980.9
Soma	968.0	E855.1	E938.0	E950.4	E962.0	E980.4
Somatotropin	962.4	E858.0	E932.4	E950.4	E962.0	E980.4
Sominex	963.0	E858.1	E933.0	E950.4	E962.0	E980.4
Somnos	967.1	E852.0	E937.1	E950.2	E962.0	E980.2
Somonal	967.0	E851	E937.0	E950.1	E962.0	E980.1
Soneryl	967.0	E851	E937.0	E950.1	E962.0	E980.1
Soothing syrup	977.9	E858.9	E947.9	E950.5	E962.0	E980.5
Sopor	967.4	E852.3	E937.4	E950.2	E962.0	E980.2
Soporific drug	967.9	E852.9	E937.9	E950.2	E962.0	E980.2
specified type NEC	967.8	E852.8	E937.8	E950.2	E962.0	E980.2
Sorbitol NEC	977.4	E858.8	E947.4	E950.4	E962.0	E980.4
Sotradecol	972.7	E858.3	E942.7	E950.4	E962.0	E980.4
Spacoline	975.1	E858.6	E945.1	E950.4	E962.0	E980.4
Spanish fly	976.8	E858.7	E946.8	E950.4	E962.0	E980.4
Sparine	969.1	E853.0	E939.1	E950.3	E962.0	E980.3
Sparteine	975.0	E858.6	E945.0	E950.4	E962.0	E980.4
Spasmolytics	975.1	E858.6	E945.1	E950.4	E962.0	E980.4
anticholinergics	971.1	E855.4	E941.1	E950.4	E962.0	E980.4
Spectinomycin	960.8	E856	E930.8	E950.4	E962.0	E980.4
Speed	969.7	E854.2	E939.7	E950.3	E962.0	E980.3
Spermicides	976.8	E858.7	E946.8	E950.4	E962.0	E980.4
Spider (bite) (venom)	989.5	E905.1	—	E950.9	E962.1	E980.9
antivenin	979.9	E858.8	E949.9	E950.4	E962.0	E980.4
Spigelia (root)	961.6	E857	E931.6	E950.4	E962.0	E980.4

Substance	Poisoning	Accident	Therapeutic Use	Suicide Attempt	Assault	Undetermined
		External Cause (E-Code)				
Spiperone	969.2	E853.1	E939.2	E950.3	E962.0	E980.3
Spiramycin	960.3	E856	E930.3	E950.4	E962.0	E980.4
Spirilene	969.5	E853.8	E939.5	E950.3	E962.0	E980.3
Spirit(s) (neutral) NEC	980.0	E860.1	—	E950.9	E962.1	E980.9
beverage	980.0	E860.0	—	E950.9	E962.1	E980.9
industrial	980.9	E860.9	—	E950.9	E962.1	E980.9
mineral	981	E862.0	—	E950.9	E962.1	E980.9
of salt — *see* Hydrochloric acid						
surgical	980.9	E860.9	—	E950.9	E962.1	E980.9
Spironolactone	974.4	E858.5	E944.4	E950.4	E962.0	E980.4
Sponge, absorbable (gelatin)	964.5	E858.2	E934.5	E950.4	E962.0	E980.4
Sporostacin	976.0	E858.7	E946.0	E950.4	E962.0	E980.4
Sprays (aerosol)	989.8	E866.8	—	E950.9	E962.1	E980.9
cosmetic	989.8	E866.7	—	E950.9	E962.1	E980.9
medicinal NEC	977.9	E858.9	E947.9	E950.5	E962.0	E980.5
pesticides — *see* Pesticides						
specified content — *see* substance specified						
Spurge flax	988.2	E865.4	—	E950.9	E962.1	E980.9
Spurges	988.2	E865.4	—	E950.9	E962.1	E980.9
Squill (expectorant) NEC	975.5	E858.6	E945.5	E950.4	E962.0	E980.4
rat poison	989.4	E863.7	—	E950.6	E962.1	E980.7
Squirting cucumber (cathartic)	973.1	E858.4	E943.1	E950.4	E962.0	E980.4
Stains	989.8	E866.8	—	E950.9	E962.1	E980.9
Stannous — *see also* Tin						
fluoride	976.7	E858.7	E946.7	E950.4	E962.0	E980.4
Stanolone	962.1	E858.0	E932.1	E950.4	E962.0	E980.4
Stanozolol	962.1	E853.0	E932.1	E950.4	E962.0	E980.4
Staphisagria or stavesacre (pediculicide)	976.0	E858.7	E946.0	E950.4	E962.0	E980.4
Stelazine	969.1	E853.0	E939.1	E950.3	E962.0	E980.3
Stemetil	969.1	E853.0	E939.1	E950.3	E962.0	E980.3
Sterculia (cathartic) (gum)	973.3	E858.4	E943.3	E950.4	E962.0	E980.4
Sternutator gas	987.8	E869.8	—	E952.8	E962.2	E982.8
Steroids NEC	962.0	E858.0	E932.0	E950.4	E962.0	E980.4
ENT agent	976.6	E858.7	E946.6	E950.4	E962.0	E980.4
ophthalmic preparation	976.5	E858.7	E946.5	E950.4	E962.0	E980.4
topical NEC	976.0	E858.7	E946.0	E950.4	E962.0	E980.4
Stibine	985.8	E866.4	—	E950.9	E962.1	E980.9
Stibophen	961.2	E857	E931.2	E950.4	E962.0	E980.4
Stilbamide, stilbamidine	961.5	E857	E931.5	E950.4	E962.0	E980.4
Stilbestrol	962.2	E858.0	E932.2	E950.4	E962.0	E980.4
Stimulants (central nervous system)	970.9	E854.3	E940.9	E950.4	E962.0	E980.4
analeptics	970.0	E854.3	E940.0	E950.4	E962.0	E980.4
opiate antagonist	970.1	E854.3	E940.1	E950.4	E962.0	E980.4
psychotherapeutic NEC	969.0	E854.0	E939.0	E950.3	E962.0	E980.3
specified NEC	970.8	E854.3	E940.8	E950.4	E962.0	E980.4
Storage batteries (acid) (cells)	983.1	E864.1	—	E950.7	E962.1	E980.6
Stovaine	968.9	E855.2	E938.9	E950.4	E962.0	E980.4
infiltration (subcutaneous)	968.5	E855.2	E938.5	E950.4	E962.0	E980.4
nerve block (peripheral) (plexus)	968.6	E855.2	E938.6	E950.5	E962.0	E980.4
spinal	968.7	E855.2	E938.7	E950.4	E962.0	E980.4
topical (surface)	968.5	E855.2	E938.5	E950.4	E962.0	E980.4
Stovarsal	961.1	E857	E931.1	E950.4	E962.0	E980.4
Stove gas — *see* Gas, utility						
Stoxil	976.5	E858.7	E946.5	E950.4	E962.0	E980.4
STP	969.6	E854.1	E939.6	E950.3	E962.0	E980.3
Stramonium (medicinal) NEC	971.1	E855.4	E941.1	E950.4	E962.0	E980.4

Substance	Poisoning	External Cause (E-Code)				
		Accident	Therapeutic Use	Suicide Attempt	Assault	Undetermined
natural state	988.2	E865.4	—	E950.9	E962.1	E980.9
Streptodornase	964.4	E858.2	E934.4	E950.4	E962.0	E980.4
Streptoduocin	960.6	E856	E930.6	E950.4	E962.0	E980.4
Streptokinase	964.4	E858.2	E934.4	E950.4	E962.0	E980.4
Streptomycin	960.6	E856	E930.6	E950.4	E962.0	E980.4
Streptozocin	960.7	E856	E930.7	E950.4	E962.0	E980.4
Stripper (paint) (solvent)	982.8	E862.9	—	E950.9	E962.1	E980.9
Strobane	989.2	E863.0	—	E950.6	E962.1	E980.7
Strophanthin	972.1	E858.3	E942.1	E950.4	E962.0	E980.4
Strophanthus hispidus or kombe	988.2	E865.4	—	E950.9	E962.1	E980.9
Strychnine (rodenticide) (salts)	989.1	E863.7	—	E950.6	E962.1	E980.7
medicinal NEC	970.8	E854.3	E940.8	E950.4	E962.0	E980.4
Strychnos (ignatii) — *see* Strychnine						
Styramate	968.0	E855.1	E938.0	E950.4	E962.0	E980.4
Styrene	983.0	E864.0	—	E950.7	E962.1	E980.6
Succinimide (anticonvulsant)	966.2	E855.0	E936.2	E950.4	E962.0	E980.4
mercuric — *see* Mercury						
Succinylcholine	975.2	E858.6	E945.2	E950.4	E962.0	E980.4
Succinylsulfathiazole	961.0	E857	E931.0	E950.4	E962.0	E980.4
Sucrose	974.5	E858.5	E944.5	E950.4	E962.0	E980.4
Sulfacetamide	961.0	E857	E931.0	E950.4	E962.0	E980.4
ophthalmic preparation	976.5	E858.7	E946.5	E950.4	E962.0	E980.4
Sulfachlorpyridazine	961.0	E857	E931.0	E950.4	E962.0	E980.4
Sulfacytine	961.0	E857	E931.0	E950.4	E962.0	E980.4
Sulfadiazine	961.0	E857	E931.0	E950.4	E962.0	E980.4
silver (topical)	976.0	E858.7	E946.0	E950.4	E962.0	E980.4
Sulfadimethoxine	961.0	E857	E931.0	E950.4	E962.0	E980.4
Sulfadimidine	961.0	E857	E931.0	E950.4	E962.0	E980.4
Sulfaethidole	961.0	E857	E931.0	E950.4	E962.0	E980.4
Sulfafurazole	961.0	E857	E931.0	E950.4	E962.0	E980.4
Sulfaguanidine	961.0	E857	E931.0	E950.4	E962.0	E980.4
Sulfamerazine	961.0	E857	E931.0	E950.4	E962.0	E980.4
Sulfameter	961.0	E857	E931.0	E950.4	E962.0	E980.4
Sulfamethizole	961.0	E857	E931.0	E950.4	E962.0	E980.4
Sulfamethoxazole	961.0	E857	E931.0	E950.4	E962.0	E980.4
Sulfamethoxydiazine	961.0	E857	E931.0	E950.4	E962.0	E980.4
Sulfamethoxypyridazine	961.0	E857	E931.0	E950.4	E962.0	E980.4
Sulfamethylthiazole	961.0	E857	E931.0	E950.4	E962.0	E980.4
Sulfamylon	976.0	E858.7	E946.0	E950.4	E962.0	E980.4
Sulfan blue (diagnostic dye)	977.8	E858.8	E947.8	E950.4	E962.0	E980.4
Sulfanilamide	961.0	E857	E931.0	E950.4	E962.0	E980.4
Sulfanilylguanidine	961.0	E857	E931.0	E950.4	E962.0	E980.4
Sulfaphenazole	961.0	E857	E931.0	E950.4	E962.0	E980.4
Sulfaphenylthiazole	961.0	E857	E931.0	E950.4	E962.0	E980.4
Sulfaproxyline	961.0	E857	E931.0	E950.4	E962.0	E980.4
Sulfapyridine	961.0	E857	E931.0	E950.4	E962.0	E980.4
Sulfapyrimidine	961.0	E857	E931.0	E950.4	E962.0	E980.4
Sulfarsphenamine	961.1	E857	E931.1	E950.4	E962.0	E980.4
Sulfasalazine	961.0	E857	E931.0	E950.4	E962.0	E980.4
Sulfasomizole	961.0	E857	E931.0	E950.4	E962.0	E980.4
Sulfasuxidine	961.0	E857	E931.0	E950.4	E962.0	E980.4
Sulfinpyrazone	974.7	E858.5	E944.7	E950.4	E962.0	E980.4
Sulfisoxazole	961.0	E857	E931.0	E950.4	E962.0	E980.4
ophthalmic preparation	976.5	E858.7	E946.5	E950.4	E962.0	E980.4
Sulfomyxin	960.8	E856	E930.8	E950.4	E962.0	E980.4
Sulfonal	967.8	E852.8	E937.8	E950.2	E962.0	E980.2
Sulfonamides (mixtures)	961.0	E857	E931.0	E950.4	E962.0	E980.4

Substance	Poisoning	External Cause (E-Code)				
		Accident	Therapeutic Use	Suicide Attempt	Assault	Undetermined
Sulfones	961.8	E857	E931.8	E950.4	E962.0	E980.4
Sulfonethylmethane	967.8	E852.8	E937.8	E950.2	E962.0	E980.2
Sulfonmethane	967.8	E852.8	E937.8	E950.2	E962.0	E980.2
Sulfonphthal, sulfonphthol	977.8	E858.8	E947.8	E950.4	E962.0	E980.4
Sulfonylurea derivatives, oral	962.3	E858.0	E932.3	E950.4	E962.0	E980.4
Sulfoxone	961.8	E857	E931.8	E950.4	E962.0	E980.4
Sulfur, sulfureted, sulfuric, sulfurous, sulfuryl (compounds) NEC	989.8	E866.8	—	E950.9	E962.1	E980.9
acid	983.1	E864.1	—	E950.7	E962.1	E980.6
dioxide	987.3	E869.1	—	E952.8	E962.2	E982.8
ether — *see* Ether(s)						
hydrogen	987.8	E869.8	—	E952.8	E962.2	E982.8
medicinal (keratolytic) (ointment) NEC	976.4	E858.7	E946.4	E950.4	E962.0	E980.4
pesticide (vapor)	989.4	E863.4	—	E950.6	E962.1	E980.7
vapor NEC	987.8	E869.8	—	E952.8	E962.2	E982.8
Sulkowitch's reagent	977.8	E858.8	E947.8	E950.4	E962.0	E980.4
Sulph — *see also* Sulf–						
Sulphadione	961.8	E857	E931.8	E950.4	E962.0	E980.4
Sulthiame, sultiame	966.3	E855.0	E936.3	E950.4	E962.0	E980.4
Superinone	975.5	E858.6	E945.5	E950.4	E962.0	E980.4
Suramin	961.5	E857	E931.5	E950.4	E962.0	E980.4
Surfacaine	968.5	E855.2	E938.5	E950.4	E962.0	E980.4
Surital	968.3	E855.1	E938.3	E950.4	E962.0	E980.4
Sutilains	976.8	E858.7	E946.8	E950.4	E962.0	E980.4
Suxamethoniam (bromide) (chloride) (iodide)	975.2	E858.6	E945.2	E950.4	E962.0	E980.4
Suxethonium (bromide)	975.2	E858.6	E945.2	E950.4	E962.0	E980.4
Sweet oil (birch)	976.3	E858.7	E946.3	E950.4	E962.0	E980.4
Sym–dichloroethyl ether	982.3	E862.4	—	E950.9	E962.1	E980.9
Sympatholytics	971.3	E855.6	E941.3	E950.4	E962.0	E980.4
Sympathomimetics	971.2	E855.5	E941.2	E950.4	E962.0	E980.4
Synalar	976.0	E858.7	E946.0	E950.4	E962.0	E980.4
Synthroid	962.7	E858.0	E932.7	E950.4	E962.0	E980.4
Syntocinon	975.0	E858.6	E945.0	E950.4	E962.0	E950.4
Syrosingopine	972.6	E858.3	E942.6	E950.4	E962.0	E980.4
Systemic agents (primarily)	963.9	E858.1	E933.9	E950.4	E962.0	E980.4
specified NEC	963.8	E858.1	E933.8	E950.4	E962.0	E980.4
Tablets (see also specified substance)	977.9	E858.9	E947.9	E950.5	E962.0	E980.5
Tace	962.2	E858.0	E932.2	E950.4	E962.0	E980.4
Tacrine	971.0	E855.3	E941.0	E950.4	E962.0	E980.4
Talbutal	967.0	E851	E937.0	E950.1	E962.0	E980.1
Talc	976.3	E858.7	E946.3	E950.4	E962.0	E980.4
Talcum	976.3	E858.7	E946.3	E950.4	E962.0	E980.4
Tandearil, tanderil	965.5	E850.5	E935.5	E950.0	E962.0	E980.0
Tannic acid	983.1	E864.1	—	E950.7	E962.1	E980.6
medicinal (astringent)	976.2	E858.7	E946.2	E950.4	E962.0	E980.4
Tannin — *see* Tannic acid						
Tansy	988.2	E865.4	—	E950.9	E962.1	E980.9
TAO	960.3	E856	E930.3	E950.4	E962.0	E980.4
Tapazole	962.8	E858.0	E932.8	E950.4	E962.0	E980.4
Tar NEC	983.0	E864.0	—	E950.7	E962.1	E980.6
camphor — *see* Naphthalene						
fumes	987.8	E869.8	—	E952.8	E962.2	E982.8
Taractan	969.3	E853.8	E939.3	E950.3	E962.0	E980.3
Tarantula (venomous)	989.5	E905.1	—	E950.9	E962.1	E980.9
Tartar emetic (anti–infective)	961.2	E857	E931.2	E950.4	E962.0	E980.4
Tartaric acid	983.1	E864.1	—	E950.7	E962.1	E980.6

Substance	Poisoning	Accident	Therapeutic Use	Suicide Attempt	Assault	Undetermined
		External Cause (E-Code)				
Tartrated antimony (anti–infective)	961.2	E857	E931.2	E950.4	E962.0	E980.4
TCA — *see* Trichloroacetic acid						
TDI	983.0	E864.0	—	E950.7	E962.1	E980.6
vapor	987.8	E869.8	—	E952.8	E962.2	E982.8
Tear gas	987.5	E869.3	—	E952.8	E962.2	E982.8
Teclothiazide	974.3	E858.5	E944.3	E950.4	E962.0	E980.4
Tegretol	966.3	E855.0	E936.3	E950.4	E962.0	E980.4
Telepaque	977.8	E858.8	E947.8	E950.4	E962.0	E980.4
Tellurium	985.8	E866.4	—	E950.9	E962.1	E980.9
fumes	985.8	E866.4	—	E950.9	E962.1	E980.9
TEM	963.1	E858.1	E933.1	E950.4	E962.0	E980.4
TEPA	963.1	E858.1	E933.1	E950.4	E962.0	E980.4
TEPP	989.3	E863.1	—	E950.6	E962.1	E980.7
Terbutaline	971.2	E855.5	E941.2	E950.4	E962.0	E980.4
Teroxalene	961.6	E857	E931.6	E950.4	E962.0	E980.4
Terpin hydrate	975.5	E858.6	E945.5	E950.4	E962.0	E980.4
Terramycin	960.4	E856	E930.4	E950.4	E962.0	E980.4
Tessalon	975.4	E858.6	E945.4	E950.4	E962.0	E980.4
Testosterone	962.1	E858.0	E932.1	E950.4	E962.0	E980.4
Tetanus (vaccine)	978.4	E858.8	E948.4	E950.4	E962.0	E980.4
antitoxin	979.9	E858.8	E949.9	E950.4	E962.0	E980.4
immune globulin (human)	964.6	E858.2	E934.6	E950.4	E962.0	E980.4
toxoid	978.4	E858.8	E948.4	E950.4	E962.0	E980.4
with diphtheria toxoid	978.9	E858.8	E948.9	E950.4	E962.0	E980.4
with pertussis	978.6	E858.8	E948.6	E950.4	E962.0	E980.4
Tetrabenazine	969.5	E853.8	E939.5	E950.3	E962.0	E980.3
Tetracaine (infiltration) (topical)	968.5	E855.2	E938.5	E950.4	E962.0	E980.4
nerve block (peripheral) (plexus)	968.6	E855.2	E938.6	E950.4	E962.0	E980.4
spinal	968.7	E855.2	E938.7	E950.4	E962.0	E980.4
Tetrachlorethylene—*see* Tetrachloroethylene						
Tetrachlormethiazide	974.3	E858.5	E944.3	E950.4	E962.0	E980.4
Tetrachloroethane (liquid) (vapor).	982.3	E862.4	—	E950.9	E962.1	E980.9
paint or varnish	982.3	E861.6	—	E950.9	E962.1	E980.9
Tetrachloroethylene (liquid) (vapor)	982.3	E862.4	—	E950.9	E962.1	E980.9
medicinal	961.6	E857	E931.6	E950.4	E962.0	E980.4
Tetrachloromethane — *see* Carbon, tetrachloride						
Tetracycline	960.4	E856	E930.4	E950.4	E962.0	E980.4
ophthalmic preparation	976.5	E858.7	E946.5	E950.4	E962.0	E980.4
topical NEC	976.0	E858.7	E946.0	E950.4	E962.0	E980.4
Tetraethylammonium chloride	972.3	E858.3	E942.3	E950.4	E962.0	E980.4
Tetraethyl lead (antiknock compound)	984.1	E862.1	—	E950.9	E962.1	E980.9
Tetraethyl pyrophosphate	989.3	E863.1	—	E950.6	E962.1	E980.7
Tetraethylthiuram disulfide	977.3	E858.8	E947.3	E950.4	E962.0	E980.4
Tetrahydroaminoacridine	971.0	E855.3	E941.0	E950.4	E962.0	E980.4
Tetrahydrocannabinol	969.6	E854.1	E939.6	E950.3	E962.0	E980.3
Tetrahydronaphthalene	982.0	E862.4	—	E950.9	E962.1	E980.9
Tetrahydrozoline	971.2	E855.5	E941.2	E950.4	E962.0	E980.4
Tetralin	982.0	E862.4	—	E950.9	E962.1	E980.9
Tetramethylthiuram (disulfide) NEC	989.4	E863.6	—	E950.6	E962.1	E980.7
medicinal	976.2	E858.7	E946.2	E950.4	E962.0	E980.4
Tetronal	967.8	E852.8	E937.8	E950.2	E962.0	E980.2
Tetryl	983.0	E864.0	—	E950.7	E962.1	E980.6
Thalidomide	967.8	E852.8	E937.8	E950.2	E962.0	E980.2
Thallium (compounds) (dust) NEC	985.8	E866.4	—	E950.9	E962.1	E980.9
pesticide (rodenticide)	985.8	E863.7	—	E950.6	E962.1	E980.7
THC	969.6	E854.1	E939.6	E950.3	E962.0	E980.3

Substance	Poisoning	External Cause (E-Code) Accident	Therapeutic Use	Suicide Attempt	Assault	Undetermined
Thebacon	965.09	E850.2	E935.2	E950.0	E962.0	E980.0
Thebaine	965.09	E850.2	E935.2	E950.0	E962.0	E980.0
Theobromine (calcium salicylate)	974.1	E858.5	E944.1	E950.4	E962.0	E980.4
Theophylline (diuretic)	974.1	E858.5	E944.1	E950.4	E962.0	E980.4
ethylenediamine	975.7	E858.6	E945.7	E950.4	E962.0	E980.4
Thiabendazole	961.6	E857	E931.6	E950.4	E962.0	E980.4
Thialbarbital, thialbarbitone	968.3	E855.1	E938.3	E950.4	E962.0	E980.4
Thiamine	963.5	E858.1	E933.5	E950.4	E962.0	E980.4
Thiamylal (sodium)	968.3	E855.1	E938.3	E950.4	E962.0	E980.4
Thiazesim	969.0	E854.0	E939.0	E950.3	E962.0	E980.3
Thiazides (diuretics)	974.3	E858.5	E944.3	E950.4	E962.0	E980.4
Thiethylperazine	963.0	E858.1	E933.0	E950.4	E962.0	E980.4
Thimerosal (topical)	976.0	E858.7	E946.0	E950.4	E962.0	E980.4
ophthalmic preparation	976.5	E858.7	E946.5	E950.4	E962.0	E980.4
Thioacetazone	961.8	E857	E931.8	E950.4	E962.0	E980.4
Thiobarbiturates	968.3	E855.1	E938.3	E950.4	E962.0	E980.4
Thiobismol	961.2	E857	E931.2	E950.4	E962.0	E980.4
Thiocarbamide	962.8	E858.0	E932.8	E950.4	E962.0	E980.4
Thiocarbarsone	961.1	E857	E931.1	E950.4	E962.0	E980.4
Thiocarlide	961.8	E857	E931.8	E950.4	E962.0	E980.4
Thioguanine	963.1	E858.1	E933.1	E950.4	E962.0	E980.4
Thiomercaptomerin	974.0	E858.5	E944.0	E950.4	E962.0	E980.4
Thiomerin	974.0	E858.5	E944.0	E950.4	E962.0	E980.4
Thiopental, thiopentone (sodium)	968.3	E855.1	E938.3	E950.4	E962.0	E980.4
Thiopropazate	969.1	E853.0	E939.1	E950.3	E962.0	E980.3
Thioproperazine	969.1	E853.0	E939.1	E950.3	E962.0	E980.3
Thioridazine	969.1	E853.0	E939.1	E950.3	E962.0	E980.3
Thio–TEPA, thiotepa	963.1	E858.1	E933.1	E950.4	E962.0	E980.4
Thiothixene	969.3	E853.8	E939.3	E950.3	E962.0	E980.3
Thiouracil	962.8	E858.0	E932.8	E950.4	E962.0	E980.4
Thiourea	962.8	E858.0	E932.8	E950.4	E962.0	E980.4
Thiphenamil	971.1	E855.4	E941.1	E950.4	E962.0	E980.4
Thiram NEC	989.4	E863.6	—	E950.6	E962.1	E980.7
medicinal	976.2	E858.7	E946.2	E950.4	E962.0	E980.4
Thonzylamine	963.0	E858.1	E933.0	E950.4	E962.0	E980.4
Thorazine	969.1	E853.0	E939.1	E950.3	E962.0	E980.3
Thornapple	988.2	E865.4	—	E950.9	E962.1	E980.9
Throat preparation (lozenges) NEC	976.6	E858.7	E946.6	E950.4	E962.0	E980.4
Thrombin	964.5	E858.2	E934.5	E950.4	E962.0	E980.4
Thrombolysin	964.4	E858.2	E934.4	E950.4	E962.0	E980.4
Thymol	983.0	E864.0	—	E950.7	E962.1	E980.6
Thymus extract	962.9	E858.0	E932.9	E950.4	E962.0	E980.4
Thyroglobulin	962.7	E858.0	E932.7	E950.4	E962.0	E980.4
Thyroid (derivatives) (extract)	962.7	E858.0	E932.7	E950.4	E962.0	E980.4
Thyrolar	962.7	E858.0	E932.7	E950.4	E962.0	E980.4
Thyrothrophin, thyrotropin	977.8	E858.8	E947.8	E950.4	E962.0	E980.4
Thyroxin(e)	962.7	E858.0	E932.7	E950.4	E962.0	E980.4
Tigan	963.0	E858.1	E933.0	E950.4	E962.0	E980.4
Tigloidine	968.0	E855.1	E938.0	E950.4	E962.0	E980.4
Tin (chloride) (dust) (oxide) NEC	985.8	E866.4	—	E950.9	E962.1	E980.9
anti–infectives	961.2	E857	E931.2	E950.4	E962.0	E980.4
Tinactin	976.0	E858.7	E946.0	E950.4	E962.0	E980.4
Tincture, iodine — *see* Iodine						
Tindal	969.1	E853.0	E939.1	E950.3	E962.0	E980.3
Titanium (compounds) (vapor)	985.8	E866.4	—	E950.9	E962.1	E980.9
ointment	976.3	E858.7	E946.3	E950.4	E962.0	E980.4
Titroid	962.7	E858.0	E932.7	E950.4	E962.0	E980.4

Substance	Poisoning	Accident	Therapeutic Use	Suicide Attempt	Assault	Undetermined
		External Cause (E-Code)				
TMTD — *see* Tetramethylthiuram disulfide						
TNT	989.8	E866.8	—	E950.9	E962.1	E980.9
fumes	987.8	E869.8	—	E952.8	E962.2	E982.8
Toadstool	988.1	E865.5	—	E950.9	E962.1	E980.9
Tobacco NEC	989.8	E866.8	—	E950.9	E962.1	E980.9
Indian	988.2	E865.4	—	E950.9	E962.1	E980.9
smoke, second-hand	987.8	E869.4	—	—	—	—
Tocopherol	963.5	E858.1	E933.5	E950.4	E962.0	E980.4
Tocosamine	975.0	E858.6	E945.0	E950.4	E962.0	E980.4
Tofranil	969.0	E854.0	E939.0	E950.3	E962.0	E980.3
Toilet deodorizer	989.8	E866.8	—	E950.9	E962.1	E980.9
Tolazamide	962.3	E858.0	E932.3	E950.4	E962.0	E980.4
Tolazoline	971.3	E855.6	E941.3	E950.4	E962.0	E980.4
Tolbutamide	962.3	E858.0	E932.3	E950.4	E962.0	E980.4
sodium	977.8	E858.8	E947.8	E950.4	E962.0	E980.4
Tolmetin	965.6	E856.0	E935.6	E950.0	E962.0	E980.0
Tolnaftate	976.0	E858.7	E946.0	E950.4	E962.0	E980.4
Tolpropamine	976.1	E858.7	E946.1	E950.4	E962.0	E980.4
Tolserol	968.0	E855.1	E938.0	E950.4	E962.0	E980.4
Toluene (liquid) (vapor)	982.0	E862.4	—	E950.9	E962.1	E980.9
diisocyanate	983.0	E864.0	—	E950.7	E962.1	E980.6
Toluidine	983.0	E864.0	—	E950.7	E962.1	E980.6
vapor	987.8	E869.8	—	E952.8	E962.2	E982.8
Toluol (liquid) (vapor)	982.0	E862.4	—	E950.9	E962.1	E980.9
Tolylene-2,4-diisocyanate	983.0	E864.0	—	E950.7	E962.1	E980.6
Tonics, cardiac	972.1	E858.3	E942.1	E950.4	E962.0	E980.4
Toxaphene (dust) (spray)	989.2	E863.0	—	E950.6	E962.1	E980.7
Toxoids NEC	978.8	E858.8	E948.8	E950.4	E962.0	E980.4
Tractor fuel NEC	981	E862.1	—	E950.9	E962.1	E980.9
Tragacanth	973.3	E858.4	E943.3	E950.4	E962.0	E980.4
Tramazoline	971.2	E855.5	E941.2	E950.4	E962.0	E980.4
Tranquilizers	969.5	E853.9	E939.5	E950.3	E962.0	E980.3
benzodiazepine-based	969.4	E853.2	E939.4	E950.3	E962.0	E980.3
butyrophenone-based	969.2	E853.1	E939.2	E950.3	E962.0	E980.3
major NEC	969.3	E853.8	E939.3	E950.3	E962.0	E980.3
phenothiazine-based	969.1	E853.0	E939.1	E950.3	E962.0	E980.3
specified NEC	969.5	E853.8	E939.5	E950.3	E962.0	E980.3
Trantoin	961.9	E857	E931.9	E950.4	E962.0	E980.4
Tranxene	969.4	E853.2	E939.4	E950.3	E962.0	E980.3
Tranylcypromine (sulfate)	969.0	E854.0	E939.0	E950.3	E962.0	E980.3
Trasentine	975.1	E858.6	E945.1	E950.4	E962.0	E980.4
Travert	974.5	E858.5	E944.5	E950.4	E962.0	E980.4
Trecator	961.8	E857	E931.8	E950.4	E962.0	E980.4
Tretinoin	976.8	E858.7	E946.8	E950.4	E962.0	E980.4
Triacetin	976.0	E858.7	E946.0	E950.4	E962.0	E980.4
Triacetyloleandomycin	960.3	E856	E930.3	E950.4	E962.0	E980.4
Triamcinolone	962.0	E858.0	E932.0	E950.4	E962.0	E980.4
ENT agent	976.6	E858.7	E946.6	E950.4	E962.0	E980.4
ophthalmic preparation	976.5	E858.7	E946.5	E950.4	E962.0	E980.4
topical NEC	976.0	E858.7	E946.0	E950.4	E962.0	E980.4
Triamterene	974.4	E858.5	E944.4	E950.4	E962.0	E980.4
Triaziquone	963.1	E858.1	E933.1	E950.4	E962.0	E980.4
Tribromacetaldehyde	967.3	E852.2	E937.3	E950.2	E962.0	E980.2
Tribromoethanol	968.2	E855.1	E938.2	E950.4	E962.0	E980.4
Tribromomethane	967.3	E852.2	E937.3	E950.2	E962.0	E980.2
Trichlorethane	982.3	E862.4	—	E950.9	E962.1	E980.9
Trichlormethiazide	974.3	E858.5	E944.3	E950.4	E962.0	E980.4

Substance	Poisoning	External Cause (E-Code) Accident	Therapeutic Use	Suicide Attempt	Assault	Undetermined
Trichloroacetic acid	983.1	E864.1	—	E950.7	E962.1	E980.6
medicinal (keratolytic)	976.4	E858.7	E946.4	E950.4	E962.0	E980.4
Trichloroethanol	967.1	E852.0	E937.1	E950.2	E962.0	E980.2
Trichloroethylene (liquid) (vapor)	982.3	E862.4	—	E950.9	E962.1	E980.9
anesthetic (gas)	968.2	E855.1	E938.2	E950.4	E962.0	E980.4
Trichloroethyl phosphate	967.1	E852.0	E937.1	E950.2	E962.0	E980.2
Trichlorofluoromethane NEC	987.4	E869.2	—	E952.8	E962.2	E982.8
Trichlorotriethylamine	963.1	E858.1	E933.1	E950.4	E962.0	E980.4
Trichomonacides NEC	961.5	E857	E931.5	E950.4	E962.0	E980.4
Trichomycin	960.1	E856	E930.1	E950.4	E962.0	E980.4
Triclofos	967.1	E852.0	E937.1	E950.2	E962.0	E980.2
Tricresyl phosphate	989.8	E866.8	—	E950.9	E962.1	E980.9
solvent	982.8	E862.4	—	E950.9	E962.1	E980.9
Tricyclamol	966.4	E855.0	E936.4	E950.4	E962.0	E980.4
Tridesilon	976.0	E858.7	E946.0	E950.4	E962.0	E980.4
Tridihexethyl	971.1	E855.4	E941.1	E950.4	E962.0	E980.4
Tridione	966.0	E855.0	E936.0	E950.4	E962.0	E980.4
Triethanolamine NEC	983.2	E864.2	—	E950.7	E962.1	E980.6
detergent	983.2	E861.0	—	E950.7	E962.1	E980.6
trinitrate	972.4	E858.3	E942.4	E950.4	E962.0	E980.4
Triethanomelamine	963.1	E858.1	E933.1	E950.4	E962.0	E980.4
Triethylene melamine	963.1	E858.1	E933.1	E950.4	E962.0	E980.4
Triethylenephosphoramide	963.1	E858.1	E933.1	E950.4	E962.0	E980.4
Triethylenethiophosphoramide	963.1	E858.1	E933.1	E950.4	E962.0	E980.4
Trifluoperazine	969.1	E853.0	E939.1	E950.3	E962.0	E980.3
Trifluperidol	969.2	E853.1	E939.2	E950.3	E962.0	E980.3
Triflupromazine	969.1	E853.0	E939.1	E950.3	E962.0	E980.3
Trihexyphenidyl	971.1	E855.4	E941.1	E950.4	E962.0	E980.4
Triiodothyronine	962.7	E858.0	E932.7	E950.4	E962.0	E980.4
Trilene	968.2	E855.1	E938.2	E950.4	E962.0	E980.4
Trimeprazine	963.0	E858.1	E933.0	E950.4	E962.0	E980.4
Trimetazidine	972.4	E858.3	E942.4	E950.4	E962.0	E980.4
Trimethadione	966.0	E855.0	E936.0	E950.4	E962.0	E980.4
Trimethaphan	972.3	E858.3	E942.3	E950.4	E962.0	E980.4
Trimethidinium	972.3	E858.3	E942.3	E950.4	E962.0	E980.4
Trimethobenzamide	963.0	E858.1	E933.0	E950.4	E962.0	E980.4
Trimethylcarbinol	980.8	E860.8	—	E950.9	E962.1	E980.9
Trimethylpsoralen	976.3	E858.7	E946.3	E950.4	E962.0	E980.4
Trimeton	963.0	E858.1	E933.0	E950.4	E962.0	E980.4
Trimipramine	969.0	E854.0	E939.0	E950.3	E962.0	E980.3
Trimustine	963.1	E858.1	E933.1	E950.4	E962.0	E980.4
Trinitrin	972.4	E858.3	E942.4	E950.4	E962.0	E980.4
Trinitrophenol	983.0	E864.0	—	E950.7	E962.1	E980.6
Trinitrotoluene	989.8	E866.8	—	E950.9	E962.1	E980.9
fumes	987.8	E869.8	—	E952.8	E962.2	E982.8
Trional	967.8	E852.8	E937.8	E950.2	E962.0	E980.2
Trioxide of arsenic — *see* Arsenic						
Trioxsalen	976.3	E858.7	E946.3	E950.4	E962.0	E980.4
Tripelennamine	963.0	E858.1	E933.0	E950.4	E962.0	E980.4
Triperidol	969.2	E853.1	E939.2	E950.3	E962.0	E980.3
Triprolidine	963.0	E858.1	E933.0	E950.4	E962.0	E980.4
Trisoralen	976.3	E858.7	E946.3	E950.4	E962.0	E980.4
Troleandomycin	960.3	E856	E930.3	E950.4	E962.0	E980.4
Trolnitrate (phosphate)	972.4	E858.3	E942.4	E950.4	E962.0	E980.4
Trometamol	963.3	E858.1	E933.3	E950.4	E962.0	E980.4
Tromethamine	963.3	E858.1	E933.3	E950.4	E962.0	E980.4
Tronothane	968.5	E855.2	E938.5	E950.4	E962.0	E980.4

Substance	Poisoning	Accident	Therapeutic Use	Suicide Attempt	Assault	Undetermined
		External Cause (E-Code)				
Tropicamide	971.1	E855.4	E941.1	E950.4	E962.0	E980.4
Troxidone	966.0	E855.0	E936.0	E950.4	E962.0	E980.4
Tryparsamide	961.1	E857	E931.1	E950.4	E962.0	E980.4
Trypsin	963.4	E858.1	E933.4	E950.4	E962.0	E980.4
Tryptizol	969.0	E854.0	E939.0	E950.3	E962.0	E980.3
Tuaminoheptane	971.2	E855.5	E941.2	E950.4	E962.0	E980.4
Tuberculin (old)	977.8	E858.8	E947.8	E950.4	E962.0	E980.4
Tubocurare	975.2	E858.6	E945.2	E950.4	E962.0	E980.4
Tubocurarine	975.2	E858.6	E945.2	E950.4	E962.0	E980.4
Turkish green	969.6	E854.1	E939.6	E950.3	E962.0	E980.3
Turpentine (spirits of) (liquid) (vapor)	982.8	E862.4	—	E950.9	E962.1	E980.9
Tybamate	969.5	E853.8	E939.5	E950.3	E962.0	E980.3
Tyloxapol	975.5	E858.6	E945.5	E950.4	E962.0	E980.4
Tymazoline	971.2	E855.5	E941.2	E950.4	E962.0	E980.4
Typhoid vaccine	978.1	E858.8	E948.1	E950.4	E962.0	E980.4
Typhus vaccine	979.2	E858.8	E949.2	E950.4	E962.0	E980.4
Tyrothricin	976.0	E858.7	E946.0	E950.4	E962.0	E980.4
ENT agent	976.6	E858.7	E946.6	E950.4	E962.0	E980.4
ophthalmic preparation	976.5	E858.7	E946.5	E950.4	E962.0	E980.4
Undecenoic acid	976.0	E858.7	E946.0	E950.4	E962.0	E980.4
Undecylenic acid	976.0	E858.7	E946.0	E950.4	E962.0	E980.4
Unna's boot	976.3	E858.7	E946.3	E950.4	E962.0	E980.4
Uracil mustard	963.1	E858.1	E933.1	E950.4	E962.0	E980.4
Uramustine	963.1	E858.1	E933.1	E950.4	E962.0	E980.4
Urari	975.2	E858.6	E945.2	E950.4	E962.0	E980.4
Urea	974.4	E858.5	E944.4	E950.4	E962.0	E980.4
topical	976.8	E858.7	E946.8	E950.4	E962.0	E980.4
Urethan(e) (antineoplastic)	963.1	E858.1	E933.1	E950.4	E962.0	E980.4
Urginea (maritima) (scilla) — *see* Squill						
Uric acid metabolism agents NEC	974.7	E858.5	E944.7	E950.4	E962.0	E980.4
Urokinase	964.4	E858.2	E934.4	E950.4	E962.0	E980.4
Urokon	977.8	E858.8	E947.8	E950.4	E962.0	E980.4
Urotropin	961.9	E857	E931.9	E950.4	E962.0	E980.4
Urtica	988.2	E865.4	—	E950.9	E962.1	E980.9
Utility gas — *see* Gas, utility						
Vaccine NEC	979.9	E858.8	E949.9	E950.4	E962.0	E980.4
bacterial NEC	978.8	E858.8	E948.8	E950.4	E962.0	E980.4
with						
other bacterial component	978.9	E858.8	E948.9	E950.4	E962.0	E980.4
pertussis component	978.6	E858.8	E948.6	E950.4	E962.0	E980.4
viral–rickettsial component	979.7	E858.8	E949.7	E950.4	E962.0	E980.4
mixed NEC	978.9	E858.8	E948.9	E950.4	E962.0	E980.4
BCG	978.0	E858.8	E948.0	E950.4	E962.0	E980.4
cholera	978.2	E858.8	E948.2	E950.4	E962.0	E980.4
diphtheria	978.5	E858.8	E948.5	E950.4	E962.0	E980.4
influenza	979.6	E858.8	E949.6	E950.4	E962.0	E980.4
measles	979.4	E858.8	E949.4	E950.4	E962.0	E980.4
meningococcal	978.8	E858.8	E948.8	E950.4	E962.0	E980.4
mumps	979.6	E858.8	E949.6	E950.4	E962.0	E980.4
paratyphoid	978.1	E858.8	E948.1	E950.4	E962.0	E980.4
pertussis (with diphtheria toxoid) (with tetanus toxoid)	978.6	E858.8	E948.6	E950.4	E962.0	E980.4
plague	978.3	E858.8	E948.3	E950.4	E962.0	E980.4
poliomyelitis	979.5	E858.8	E949.5	E950.4	E962.0	E980.4
poliovirus	979.5	E858.8	E949.5	E950.4	E962.0	E980.4
rabies	979.1	E858.8	E949.1	E950.4	E962.0	E980.4

Substance	Poisoning	External Cause (E-Code)				
		Accident	Therapeutic Use	Suicide Attempt	Assault	Undetermined
rickettsial NEC	979.6	E858.8	E949.6	E950.4	E962.0	E980.4
with						
bacterial component	979.7	E858.8	E949.7	E950.4	E962.0	E980.4
pertussis component	978.6	E858.8	E948.6	E950.4	E962.0	E980.4
viral component	979.7	E858.8	E949.7	E950.4	E962.0	E980.4
Rocky mountain spotted fever	979.6	E858.8	E949.6	E950.4	E962.0	E980.4
rubella virus	979.4	E858.8	E949.4	E950.4	E962.0	E980.4
sabin oral	979.5	E858.8	E949.5	E950.4	E962.0	E980.4
smallpox	979.0	E858.8	E949.0	E950.4	E962.0	E980.4
tetanus	978.4	E858.8	E948.4	E950.4	E962.0	E980.4
typhoid	978.1	E858.8	E948.1	E950.4	E962.0	E980.4
typhus	979.2	E858.8	E949.2	E950.4	E962.0	E980.4
viral NEC	979.6	E858.8	E949.6	E950.4	E962.0	E980.4
with						
bacterial component	979.7	E858.8	E949.7	E950.4	E962.0	E980.4
pertussis component	978.6	E858.8	E948.6	E950.4	E962.0	E980.4
rickettsial component	979.7	E858.8	E949.7	E950.4	E962.0	E980.4
yellow fever	979.3	E858.8	E949.3	E950.4	E962.0	E980.4
Vaccinia immune globulin (human)	964.6	E858.2	E934.6	E950.4	E962.0	E980.4
Vaginal contraceptives	976.8	E858.7	E946.8	E950.4	E962.0	E980.4
Valethamate	971.1	E855.4	E941.1	E950.4	E962.0	E980.4
Valisone	976.0	E858.7	E946.0	E950.4	E962.0	E980.4
Valium	969.4	E853.2	E939.4	E950.3	E962.0	E980.3
Valmid	967.8	E852.8	E937.8	E950.2	E962.0	E980.2
Vanadium	985.8	E866.4	—	E950.9	E962.1	E980.9
Vancomycin	960.8	E856	E930.8	E950.4	E962.0	E980.4
Vapor (*see also* Gas)	987.9	E869.9	—	E952.9	E962.2	E982.9
kiln (carbon monoxide)	986	E868.8	—	E952.1	E962.2	E982.1
lead — *see* Lead						
specified source NEC (*see also* specific substance)	987.8	E869.8	—	E952.8	E962.2	E982.8
Varidase	964.4	E858.2	E934.4	E950.4	E962.0	E980.4
Varnish	989.8	E861.6	—	E950.9	E962.1	E980.9
cleaner	982.8	E862.9	—	E950.9	E962.1	E980.9
Vaseline	976.3	E858.7	E946.3	E950.4	E962.0	E980.4
Vasodilan	972.5	E858.3	E942.5	E950.4	E962.0	E980.4
Vasodilators NEC	972.5	E858.3	E942.5	E950.4	E962.0	E980.0
coronary	972.4	E858.3	E942.4	E950.4	E962.0	E980.4
Vasopressin	962.5	E858.0	E932.5	E950.4	E962.0	E980.4
Vasopressor drugs	962.5	E858.0	E932.5	E950.4	E962.0	E980.4
Venom, venomous (bite) (sting)	989.5	E905.9	—	E950.9	E962.1	E980.9
arthropod NEC	989.5	E905.5	—	E950.9	E962.1	E980.9
bee	989.5	E905.3	—	E950.9	E962.1	E980.9
centipede	989.5	E905.4	—	E950.9	E962.1	E980.9
hornet	989.5	E905.3	—	E950.9	E962.1	E980.9
lizard	989.5	E905.0	—	E950.9	E962.1	E980.9
marine animals or plants	989.5	E905.6	—	E950.9	E962.1	E980.9
millipede (topical)	989.5	E905.4	—	E950.9	E962.1	E980.9
plant NEC	989.5	E905.7	—	E950.9	E962.1	E980.9
marine	989.5	E905.6	—	E950.9	E962.1	E980.9
scorpion	989.5	E905.2	—	E950.9	E962.1	E980.9
snake	989.5	E905.0	—	E950.9	E962.1	E980.9
specified NEC	989.5	E905.8	—	E950.9	E962.1	E980.9
spider	989.5	E905.1	—	E950.9	E962.1	E980.9
wasp	989.5	E905.3	—	E950.9	E962.1	E980.9
Veramon	967.0	E851	E937.0	E950.1	E962.0	E980.1

Substance	Poisoning	Accident	Therapeutic Use	Suicide Attempt	Assault	Undetermined
		External Cause (E-Code)				
Veratrum						
album	988.2	E865.4	—	E950.9	E962.1	E980.9
alkaloids	972.6	E858.3	E942.6	E950.4	E962.0	E980.4
viride	988.2	E865.4	—	E950.9	E962.1	E980.9
Verdigris (*see also* Copper)	985.8	E866.4	—	E950.9	E962.1	E980.9
Veronal	967.0	E851	E937.0	E950.1	E962.0	E980.1
Veroxil	961.6	E857	E931.6	E950.4	E962.0	E980.4
Versidyne	965.7	E850.7	E935.7	E950.0	E962.0	E980.0
Vienna						
green	985.1	E866.3	—	E950.8	E962.1	E980.8
insecticide	985.1	E863.4	—	E950.6	E962.1	E980.7
red	989.8	E866.8	—	E950.9	E962.1	E980.9
pharmaceutical dye	977.4	E858.8	E947.4	E950.4	E962.0	E980.4
Vinbarbital, vinbarbitone	967.0	E851	E937.0	E950.1	E962.0	E980.1
Vinblastine	963.1	E858.1	E933.1	E950.4	E962.0	E980.4
Vincristine	963.1	E858.1	E933.1	E950.4	E962.0	E980.4
Vinesthene, vinethene	968.2	E855.1	E938.2	E950.4	E962.0	E980.4
Vinyl						
bital	967.0	E851	E937.0	E950.1	E962.0	E980.1
ether	968.2	E855.1	E938.2	E950.4	E962.0	E980.4
Vioform	961.3	E857	E931.3	E950.4	E962.0	E980.4
topical	976.0	E858.7	E946.0	E950.4	E962.0	E980.4
Viomycin	960.6	E856	E930.6	E950.4	E962.0	E980.4
Viosterol	963.5	E858.1	E933.5	E950.4	E962.0	E980.4
Viper (venom)	989.5	E905.0	—	E950.9	E962.1	E980.9
Viprynium (embonate)	961.6	E857	E931.6	E950.4	E962.0	E980.4
Virugon	961.7	E857	E931.7	E950.4	E962.0	E980.4
Visine	976.5	E858.7	E946.5	E950.4	E962.0	E980.4
Vitamins NEC	963.5	E858.1	E933.5	E950.4	E962.0	E980.4
B_{12}	964.1	E858.2	E934.1	E950.4	E962.0	E980.4
hematopoietic	964.1	E858.2	E934.1	E950.4	E962.0	E980.4
K	964.3	E858.2	E934.3	E950.4	E962.0	E980.4
Vleminckx's solution	976.4	E858.7	E946.4	E950.4	E962.0	E980.4
Warfarin (potassium) (sodium)	964.2	E858.2	E934.2	E950.4	E962.0	E980.4
rodenticide	989.4	E863.7	—	E950.6	E962.1	E980.7
Wasp (sting)	989.5	E905.3	—	E950.9	E962.1	E980.9
Water						
balance agents NEC	974.5	E858.5	E944.5	E950.4	E962.0	E980.4
gas	987.1	E868.1	—	E951.8	E962.2	E981.8
incomplete combustion of — *see* Carbon, monoxide, fuel, utility						
hemlock	988.2	E865.4	—	E950.9	E962.1	E980.9
moccasin (venom)	989.5	E905.0	—	E950.9	E962.1	E980.9
Wax (paraffin) (petroleum)	981	E862.3	—	E950.9	E962.1	E980.9
automobile	989.8	E861.2	—	E950.9	E962.1	E980.9
floor	981	E862.0	—	E950.9	E962.1	E980.9
Weed killers NEC	989.4	E863.5	—	E950.6	E962.1	E980.7
Welldorm	967.1	E852.0	E937.1	E950.2	E962.0	E980.2
White						
arsenic — *see* Arsenic						
hellebore	988.2	E865.4	—	E950.9	E962.1	E980.9
lotion (keratolytic)	976.4	E858.7	E946.4	E950.4	E962.0	E980.4
spirit	981	E862.0	—	E950.9	E962.1	E980.9
Whitewashes	989.8	E861.6	—	E950.9	E962.1	E980.9
Whole blood	964.7	E858.2	E934.7	E950.4	E962.0	E980.4
Wild						
black cherry	988.2	E865.4	—	E950.9	E962.1	E980.9

Substance	Poisoning	Accident	Therapeutic Use	Suicide Attempt	Assault	Undetermined
		External Cause (E-Code)				
poisonous plants NEC	988.2	E865.4	—	E950.9	E962.1	E980.9
Window cleaning fluid	989.8	E861.3	—	E950.9	E962.1	E980.9
Wintergreen (oil)	976.3	E858.7	E946.3	E950.4	E962.0	E980.4
Witch hazel	976.2	E858.7	E946.2	E950.4	E962.0	E980.4
Wood						
alcohol	980.1	E860.2	—	E950.9	E962.1	E980.9
spirit	980.1	E860.2	—	E950.9	E962.1	E980.9
Woorali	975.2	E858.6	E945.2	E950.4	E962.0	E980.4
Wormseed, American	961.6	E857	E931.6	E950.4	E962.0	E980.4
Xanthine diuretics	974.1	E858.5	E944.1	E950.4	E962.0	E980.4
Xanthocillin	960.0	E856	E930.0	E950.4	E962.0	E980.4
Xanthotoxin	976.3	E858.7	E946.3	E950.4	E962.0	E980.4
Xylene (liquid) (vapor)	982.0	E862.4	—	E950.9	E962.1	E980.9
Xylocaine (infiltration) (topical)	968.5	E855.2	E938.5	E950.4	E962.0	E980.4
nerve block (peripheral) (plexus)	968.6	E855.2	E938.6	E950.4	E962.0	E980.4
spinal	968.7	E855.2	E938.7	E950.4	E962.0	E980.4
Xylol (liquid) (vapor)	982.0	E862.4	—	E950.9	E962.1	E980.9
Xylometazoline	971.2	E855.5	E941.2	E950.4	E962.0	E980.4
Yellow						
fever vaccine	979.3	E858.8	E949.3	E950.4	E962.0	E980.4
jasmine	988.2	E865.4	—	E950.9	E962.1	E980.9
Yew	988.2	E865.4	—	E950.9	E962.1	E980.9
Zactane	965.7	E850.7	E935.7	E950.0	E962.0	E980.0
Zaroxolyn	974.3	E858.5	E944.3	E950.4	E962.0	E980.4
Zephiran (topical)	976.0	E858.7	E946.0	E950.4	E962.0	E980.4
ophthalmic preparation	976.5	E858.7	E946.5	E950.4	E962.0	E980.4
Zerone	980.1	E860.2	—	E950.9	E962.1	E980.9
Zinc (compounds) (fumes) (salts) (vapor) NEC	985.8	E866.4	—	E950.9	E962.1	E980.9
anti–infectives	976.0	E858.7	E946.0	E950.4	E962.0	E980.4
antivaricose	972.7	E858.3	E942.7	E950.4	E962.0	E980.4
bacitracin	976.0	E858.7	E946.0	E950.4	E962.0	E980.4
chloride	976.2	E858.7	E946.2	E950.4	E962.0	E980.4
gelatin	976.3	E858.7	E946.3	E950.4	E962.0	E980.4
oxide	976.3	E858.7	E946.3	E950.4	E962.0	E980.4
peroxide	976.0	E858.7	E946.0	E950.4	E962.0	E980.4
pesticides	985.8	E863.4	—	E950.6	E962.1	E980.7
phosphide (rodenticide)	985.8	E863.7	—	E950.6	E962.1	E980.7
stearate	976.3	E858.7	E946.3	E950.4	E962.0	E980.4
sulfate (antivaricose)	972.7	E858.3	E942.7	E950.4	E962.0	E980.4
ENT agent	976.6	E858.7	E946.6	E950.4	E962.0	E980.4
ophthalmic solution	976.5	E858.7	E946.5	E950.4	E962.0	E980.4
topical NEC	976.0	E858.7	E946.0	E950.4	E962.0	E980.4
undecylenate	976.0	E858.7	E946.0	E950.4	E962.0	E980.4
Zoxazolamine	968.0	E855.1	E938.0	E950.4	E962.0	E980.4
Zygadenus (venenosus)	988.2	E865.4	—	E950.9	E962.1	E980.9

SECTION 3

ALPHABETIC INDEX TO EXTERNAL CAUSES OF INJURY AND POISONING (E CODE)

This section contains the index to the codes which classify environmental events, circumstances, and other conditions as the cause of injury and other adverse effects. Where a code from the section Supplementary Classification of External Causes of Injury and Poisoning (E800-E998) is applicable, it is intended that the E code shall be used in addition to a code form the main body of the classification, Chapters 1-17.

The alphabetic index to the E codes is organized by main terms which describe the *accident, circumstance, event,* or specific *agent* which caused the injury or other adverse effect.

Note—Transport accidents (E800-E848) include accidents involving:
aircraft and space craft (E840-E845)
watercraft (E830-E838)
motor vehicle (E810-E825)
railway (E800-E807)
other road vehicles (E826-E829)

For definitions and examples related to transport accidents—see Volume 1, pages 477-491.

The fourth-digit subdivisions for use with categories E800-E848 to identify the injured person are found on pages 1343-1348.

For identifying the place in which an accident or poisoning occurred (circumstances classifiable to categories E850-E869 and E880-E928)— see the listing in this section under "Accident, occurring."

See the Table of Drugs and Chemicals (Section 2 of this volume) for identifying the specific agent involved in drug overdose or a wrong substance given or taken in error, and for intoxication or poisoning by a drug or other chemical substance.

The specific adverse effect, reaction, or localized toxic effect to a correct drug or substance properly administered in therapeutic or prophylactic dosage should be classified according to the nature of the adverse effect (e.g.: allergy, dermatitis, tachycardia) listed in Section 1 of this volume.

A

Accident—*continued*
spinning E919.8
weaving E919.8
natural factor NEC E928.9
overhead plane E919.4
plane E920.4
overhead E919.4
powered
hand tool NEC E920.1
saw E919.4
hand E920.1
printing machine E919.8
pulley (block) E919.2
agricultural operations E919.0
mining operations E919.1
transmission E919.6
radial saw E919.4
radiation—*see* Radiation
reaper E919.0
road scraper E919.7
when in transport under its own power—*see* categories E810—E825
roller coaster E919.8
sander E919.4
saw E920.4
band E919.4
bench E919.4
chain E920.1
circular E919.4
hand E920.4
powered E920.1
powered, except hand E919.4
radial E919.4
sawing machine, metal E919.3
shaft
hoist E919.1
lift E919.1
transmission E919.6
shears E920.4
hand E920.4
powered E920.1
mechanical E919.3
shovel E920.4
steam E919.7
spinning machine E919.8
steam—*see also* Burning, steam
engine E919.5
shovel E919.7
thresher E919.0
thunderbolt NEC E907
tractor E919.0
when in transport under its own power—*see* categories E810-E825
transmission belt, cable, chain, gear, pinion, pulley, shaft E919.6
turbine (gas) (water driven) E919.5
under-cutter E919.1
weaving machine E919.8
winch E919.2
agricultural operations E919.0
mining operations E919.1
diving E883.0
with insufficient air supply E913.2
glider (hang) (*see also* Collision, aircraft, unpowered) E842
hovercraft
on
land—*see* Accident, motor vehicle
water—*see* Accident, watercraft
ice yacht (*see also* Accident, vehicle NEC) E848

Accident—*continued*
in
medical, surgical procedure
as, or due to misadventure—*see* Misadventure
causing an abnormal reaction or later complication without mention of misadventure—*see* Reaction, abnormal
kite carrying a person (*see also* Collision, aircraft, unpowered) E842
land yacht (*see also* Accident, vehicle NEC) E848
late effect of—*see* Late effect
launching pad E845
machine, machinery (*see also* Accident, caused by, due to, by specific type of machine) E919.9
agricultural including animal-powered E919.0
earth-drilling E919.1
earth moving or scraping E919.7
excavating E919.7
involving transport under own power on highway or transport vehicle—*see* categories E810-E825, E840-E845
lifting (appliances) E919.2
metalworking E919.3
mining E919.1
prime movers, except electric motors E919.5
electric motors—*see* Accident, machine, by specific type of machine
recreational E919.8
specified type NEC E919.8
transmission E919.6
watercraft (deck) (engine room) (galley) (laundry) (loading) E836
woodworking or forming E919.4
motor vehicle (on public highway) (traffic) E819
due to cataclysm—*see* categories E908, E909
involving
collision (*see also* Collision, motor vehicle) E812
nontraffic, not on public highway—*see* categories E820-E825
not involving collision—*see* categories E816-E819
nonmotor vehicle NEC E829
nonroad—*see* Accident, vehicle NEC
road, except pedal cycle, animal-drawn vehicle, or animal being ridden E829
nonroad vehicle NEC—*see* Accident, vehicle NEC
not elsewhere classifiable involving
cable car (not on rails) E847
on rails E829
coal car in mine E846
hand truck—*see* Accident, vehicle NEC
logging car E846
sled(ge), meaning snow or ice vehicle E848
tram, mine or quarry E846
truck
mine or quarry E846
self-propelled, industrial E846
station baggage E846
tub, mine or quarry E846

Accident—*continued*
vehicle NEC E848
snow and ice E848
used only on industrial premises E846
wheelbarrow E848
occurring (at) (in)
apartment E849.0
baseball field, diamond E849.4
construction site, any E849.3
dock E849.8
yard E849.3
dormitory E849.7
factory (building) (premises) E849.3
farm E849.1
buildings E849.1
house E849.0
football field E849.4
forest E849.8
garage (place of work) E849.3
private (home) E849.0
gravel pit E849.2
gymnasium E849.4
highway E849.5
home (private) (residential) E849.0
institutional E849.7
hospital E849.7
hotel E849.6
house (private) (residential) E849.0
movie E849.6
public E849.6
institution, residential E849.7
jail E849.7
mine E849.2
motel E849.6
movie house E849.6
office (building) E849.6
orphanage E849.7
park (public) E849.4
mobile home E849.8
trailer E849.8
parking lot or place E849.8
place
industrial NEC E849.3
parking E849.8
public E849.8
specified place NEC E849.5
recreational NEC E849.4
sport NEC E849.4
playground (park) (school) E849.4
prison E849.6
public building NEC E849.6
quarry E849.2
railway
line NEC E849.8
yard E849.3
residence
home (private) E849.0
resort (beach) (lake) (mountain) (seashore) (vacation) E849.4
restaurant E849.6
sand pit E849.2
school (building) (private) (public) (state) E849.6
reform E849.7
riding E849.4
seashore E849.8
resort E849.4
shop (place of work) E849.3
commercial E849.6
skating rink E849.4
sports palace E849.4

Accident—*continued*
stadium E849.4
store E849.6
street E849.5
swimming pool (public) E849.4
private home or garden E849.0
tennis court E849.4
theatre, theater E849.6
trailer court E849.8
tunnel E849.8
under construction E849.2
warehouse E849.3
yard
dock E849.3
industrial E849.3
private (home) E849.0
railway E849.3
off-road type motor vehicle (not on public highway) NEC E821
on public highway—*see* categories E810-E819
pedal cycle E826
railway E807
due to cataclysm—*see* categories E908, E909
involving
burning by engine, locomotive, train (*see also* Explosion, railway engine) E803
collision (*see also* Collision, railway) E800
derailment (*see also* Derailment, railway) E802
explosion (*see also* Explosion, railway engine) E803
fall (*see also* Fall, from, railway rolling stock) E804
fire (*see also* Explosion, railway engine) E803
hitting by, being struck by
object falling in, on, from, rolling stock, train, vehicle E806
rolling stock, train, vehicle E805
overturning, railway rolling stock, train, vehicle (*see also* Derailment, railway) E802
running off rails, railway (*see also* Derailment, railway) E802
specified circumstances NEC E806
train or vehicle hit by
avalanche E909
falling object (earth, rock, tree) E806
due to cataclysm—*see* categories E908, E909
landslide E909
ski(ing) E885
jump E884.9
lift or tow (with chair or gondola) E847
snow vehicle, motor driven (not on public highway) E820
on public highway—*see* categories E810-E819
spacecraft E845
specified cause NEC E928.8
street car E829
traffic NEC E819
vehicle NEC (with pedestrian) E848
battery powered
airport passenger vehicle E846
truck (baggage) (mail) E846

Accident—*continued*
powered commercial or industrial (with other vehicle or object within commercial or industrial premises) E846
watercraft E838
with
drowning or submersion resulting from
accident other than to watercraft E832
accident to watercraft E830
injury, except drowning or submersion, resulting from
accident other than to watercraft—*see* categories E833-E838
accident to watercraft E831
due to, caused by cataclysm—*see* categories E908, E909
machinery E836
Acid throwing E961
Acosta syndrome E902.0
Aeroneurosis E902.1
Aero-otitis media —*see* Effects of, air pressure
Aerosinusitis —*see* Effects of, air pressure
After-effect, late —*see* Late effect
Air
blast in war operations E933
embolism (traumatic) NEC E928.9
in
infusion or transfusion E874.1
perfusion E874.2
sickness E903
Alpine sickness E902.0
Altitude sickness —*see* Effects of, air pressure
Anaphylactic shock, anaphylaxis (*see also* Table of drugs and chemicals) E947.9
due to bite or sting (venomous)—*see* Bite, venomous
Andes disease E902.0
Apoplexy
heat—*see* Heat
Arachnidism E905.1
Arson E968.0
Asphyxia, asphyxiation
by
chemical in war operations E997.2
explosion—*see* Explosion
food (bone) (regurgitated food) (seed) E911
foreign object, except food E912
fumes in war operations E997.2
gas—*see also* Table of drugs and chemicals
in war operations E997.2
legal
execution E978
intervention (tear) E972
tear E972
mechanical means (*see also* Suffocation) E913.9
from
conflagration—*see* Conflagration
fire—*see also* Fire
in war operations E990.9
ignition—*see* Ignition
Aspiration
foreign body—*see* Foreign body, aspiration
mucus, not of newborn (with asphyxia, obstruction respiratory passage, suffocation) E912
phlegm (with asphyxia, obstruction respiratory passage, suffocation) E912

Aspiration—*continued*
vomitus (with asphyxia, obstruction respiratory passage, suffocation) (*see also* Foreign body, aspiration, food) E911
Assassination (attempt) (*see also* Assault) E968.9
Assault (homicidal) (by) (in) E968.9
acid E961
swallowed E962.1
bite (of human being) E968.8
bomb ((placed in) car or house) E965.8
antipersonnel E965.5
letter E965.7
petrol E965.7
brawl (hand) (fists) (foot) E960.0
burning, burns (by fire) E968.0
acid E961
swallowed E962.1
caustic, corrosive substance E961
swallowed E962.1
chemical from swallowing caustic, corrosive substance NEC E962.1
hot liquid E968.3
scalding E968.3
vitriol E961
swallowed E962.1
caustic, corrosive substance E961
swallowed E962.1
cut, any part of body E966
dagger E966
drowning E964
explosive(s) E965.9
bomb (*see also* Assault, bomb) E965.8
dynamite E965.8
fight (hand) (fists) (foot) E960.0
with weapon E968.9
blunt or thrown E968.2
cutting or piercing E966
firearm—*see* Shooting, homicide
fire E968.0
firearm(s)—*see* Shooting, homicide
garrotting E963
gunshot (wound)—*see* Shooting, homicide
hanging E963
injury NEC E968.9
to child due to criminal abortion E968.8
knife E966
late effect of E969
ligature E963
poisoning E962.9
drugs or medicinals E962.0
gas(es) or vapors, except drugs and medicinals E962.2
solid or liquid substances, except drugs and medicinals E962.1
puncture, any part of body E966
pushing
before moving object, train, vehicle E968.8
from high place E968.1
rape E960.1
scalding E968.3
shooting—*see* Shooting, homicide
stab, any part of body E966
strangulation E963
submersion E964
suffocation E963
transport vehicle E968.5
violence NEC E968.9
vitriol E961
swallowed E962.1

Assault—*continued*
weapon E968.9
blunt or thrown E968.2
cutting or piercing E966
firearm—*see* Shooting, homicide
wound E968.9
cutting E966
gunshot—*see* Shooting, homicide
knife E966
piercing E966
puncture E966
stab E966
Attack by animal NEC E906.9
Avalanche E909.2
falling on or hitting
motor vehicle (in motion) (on public highway) E909
railway train E909
Aviators' disease E902.1

B

Barotitis, barodontalgia, barosinusitis, barotrauma (otitic) (sinus)—*see* Effects of, air pressure
Battered
baby or child (syndrome)—*see* Abuse, child
person other than baby or child—*see* Assault
Bayonet wound (*see also* Cut, by bayonet) E920.3
in
legal intervention E974
war operations E995
Bean in nose E912
Bed set on fire NEC E898.0
Beheading (by guillotine)
homicide E966
legal execution E978
Bending, injury in E927
Bends E902.0
Bite
animal (nonvenomous) NEC E906.5
venomous NEC E905.9
arthropod (nonvenomous) NEC E906.4
venomous—*see* Sting
black widow spider E905.1
cat E906.3
centipede E905.4
cobra E905.0
copperhead snake E905.0
coral snake E905.0
dog E906.0
fer de lance E905.0
gila monster E905.0
human being E968.8
insect (nonvenomous) E906.4
venomous—*see* Sting
krait E905.0
late effect of—*see* Late effect
lizard E906.2
venomous E905.0
mamba E905.0
marine animal
nonvenomous E906.3
snake E906.2
venomous E905.6
snake E905.0
millipede E906.4
venomous E905.4
moray eel E906.3

Bite —*continued*
rat E906.1
rattlesnake E905.0
rodent, except rat E906.3
serpent—*see* Bite, snake
shark E906.3
snake (venomous) E905.0
nonvenomous E906.2
sea E905.0
spider E905.1
nonvenomous E906.4
tarantula (venomous) E905.1
venomous NEC E905.9
by specific animal—*see* category E905
viper E905.0
water moccasin E905.0
Blast (air) in war operations E993
from nuclear explosion E996
underwater E992
Blizzard E908.3
Blow E928.9
by law-enforcing agent, police (on duty) E975
with blunt object (baton) (nightstick) (stave) (truncheon) E973
Blowing up (*see also* Explosion) E923.9
Brawl (hand) (fists) (foot) E960.0
Breakage (accidental)
cable of cable car not on rails E847
ladder (causing fall) E881.0
part (any) of
animal-drawn vehicle E827
ladder (causing fall) E881.0
motor vehicle
in motion (on public highway) E818
not on public highway E825
nonmotor road vehicle, except animal-drawn vehicle or pedal cycle E829
off-road type motor vehicle (not on public highway) NEC E821
on public highway E818
pedal cycle E826
scaffolding (causing fall) E881.1
snow vehicle, motor-driven (not on public highway) E820
on public highway E818
vehicle NEC—*see* Accident, vehicle
Broken
glass, injury by E920.8
power line (causing electric shock) E925.1
Bumping against, into (accidentally)
object (moving) (projected) (stationary) E917.9
with fall E888
caused by crowd (with fall) E917.1
in
running water E917.2
sports E917.0
person(s) E917.9
with fall E886.9
in sports E886.0
as, or caused by, a crowd (with fall) E917.1
in sports E917.0
with fall E886.0
Burning, burns (accidental) (by) (from) (on) E899
acid (any kind) E924.1
swallowed—*see* Table of drugs and chemicals
bedclothes (*see also* Fire, specified NEC) E898.0

Burning, burns—*continued*
blowlamp (*see also* Fire, specified NEC) E898.1
blowtorch (*see also* Fire, specified NEC) E898.1
boat, ship, watercraft—*see* categories E830, E831, E837
bonfire (controlled) E897
uncontrolled E892
candle (*see also* Fire, specified NEC) E898.1
caustic liquid, substance E924.1
swallowed—*see* Table of drugs and chemicals
chemical E924.1
from swallowing caustic, corrosive substance—*see* Table of drugs and chemicals
in war operations E997.2
cigar(s) or cigarette(s) (*see also* Fire, specified NEC) E898.1
clothes, clothing, nightdress—*see* Ignition, clothes
with conflagration—*see* Conflagration
conflagration—*see* Conflagration
corrosive liquid, substance E924.1
swallowed—*see* Table of drugs and chemicals
electric current (*see also* Electric shock) E925.9
fire, flames (*see also* Fire) E899
flare, Verey pistol E922.8
heat
from appliance (electrical) E924.8
in local application or packing during medical or surgical procedure E873.5
homicide (attempt) (*see also* Assault, burning) E968.0
hot
liquid E924.0
caustic or corrosive E924.1
object (not producing fire or flames) E924.8
substance E924.9
caustic or corrosive E924.1
liquid (metal) NEC E924.0
specified type NEC E924.8
tap water E924.2
ignition—*see also* Ignition
clothes, clothing, nightdress—*see also* Ignition, clothes
with conflagration—*see* Conflagration
highly inflammable material (benzine) (fat) (gasoline) (kerosine) (paraffin) (petrol) E894
inflicted by other person
stated as
homicidal, intentional (*see also* Assault, burning) E968.0
undetermined whether accidental or intentional (*see also* Burn, stated as undetermined whether accidental or intentional) E988.1
internal, from swallowed caustic, corrosive liquid, substance—*see* Table of drugs and chemicals
in war operations (from fire-producing device or conventional weapon) E990.9
from nuclear explosion E996
petrol bomb E990.0
lamp (*see also* Fire, specified NEC) E898.1
late effect of NEC E929.4

Burning, burns—*continued*
lighter (cigar) (cigarette) (*see also* Fire, specified NEC) E898.1
lightning E907
liquid (boiling) (hot) (molten) E924.0
caustic, corrosive (external) E924.1
swallowed—*see* Table of drugs and chemicals
local application of externally applied substance in medical or surgical care E873.5
machinery—*see* Accident, machine
matches (*see also* Fire, specified NEC) E898.1
medicament, externally applied E873.5
metal, molten E924.0
object (hot) E924.8
producing fire or flames—*see* Fire
pipe (smoking) (*see also* Fire, specified NEC) E898.1
radiation—*see* Radiation
railway engine, locomotive, train (*see also* Explosion, railway engine) E803
self-inflicted (unspecified whether accidental or intentional) E988.1
caustic or corrosive substance NEC E988.7
stated as intentional, purposeful E958.1
caustic or corrosive substance NEC E958.7
stated as undetermined whether accidental or intentional E988.1
caustic or corrosive substance NEC E988.7
steam E924.0
pipe E924.8
substance (hot) E924.9
boiling or molten E924.0
caustic, corrosive (external) E924.1
swallowed—*see* Table of drugs and chemicals
suicidal (attempt) NEC E958.1
caustic substance E958.7
late effect of E959
therapeutic misadventure
overdose of radiation E873.2
torch, welding (*see also* Fire, specified NEC) E898.1
trash fire (*see also* Burning, bonfire) E897
vapor E924.0
vitriol E924.1
x-rays E926.3
in medical, surgical procedure—*see* Misadventure, failure, in dosage, radiation
Butted by animal E906.8

C

Cachexia, lead or saturnine E866.0
from pesticide NEC (*see also* Table of drugs and chemicals) E863.4
Caisson disease E902.2
Capital punishment (any means) E978
Car sickness E903
Casualty (not due to war) NEC E928.9
war (*see also* War operations) E995
Cat
bite E906.3
scratch E906.8
Cataclysmic (any injury)
earth surface movement or eruption E909.9
storm or flood resulting from storm E908.9
Catching fire —*see* Ignition
Caught
between
objects (moving) (stationary and moving) E918
and machinery—*see* Accident, machine
by cable car, not on rails E847
in
machinery (moving parts of)—*see* Accident, machine
object E918
Cave-in (causing asphyxia, suffocation (by pressure)) (*see also* Suffocation, due to, cave-in) E913.3
with injury other than asphyxia or suffocation E916
with asphyxia or suffocation (*see also* Suffocation, due to, cave-in) E913.3
struck or crushed by E916
with asphyxia or suffocation (*see also* Suffocation, due to, cave-in) E913.3
Change(s) in air pressure—*see also* Effects of, air pressure
sudden, in aircraft (ascent) (descent) (causing aeroneurosis or aviators' disease) E902.1
Chilblains E901.0
due to manmade conditions E901.1
Choking (on) (any object except food or vomitus) E912
apple E911
bone E911
food, any type (regurgitated) E911
mucus or phlegm E912
seed E911
Civil insurrection —*see* War operations
Cloudburst (any injury) E908
Cold, exposure to (accidental) (excessive) (extreme) (place) E901.9
causing chilblains or immersion foot E901.0
due to
manmade conditions E901.1
specified cause NEC E901.8
weather (conditions) E901.0
late effect of NEC E929.5
self-inflicted (undetermined whether accidental or intentional) E988.3
suicidal E958.3
suicide E958.3
Colic, lead, painters', or saturnine —*see* category E866
Collapse
building E916
burning E891.8
private E890.8
dam E909.3
due to heat—*see* Heat
machinery—*see* Accident, machine
man-made structure E909.3
postoperative NEC E878.9
structure, burning NEC E891.8
Collision (accidental)

Note—In the case of collisions between different types of vehicles, persons and objects, priority in classification is in the following order:

Aircraft
Watercraft
Motor vehicle
Railway vehicle
Pedal Cycle
Animal-drawn vehicle
Animal being ridden
Streetcar or other nonmotor road vehicle
Other vehicle
Pedestrian or person using pedestrian conveyance
Object (except where falling from or set in motion by vehicle etc. listed above)

In the listing below, the combinations are listed only under the vehicle etc. having priority. For definitions, see Volume 1, page 477.

aircraft (with object or vehicle) (fixed) (movable) (moving) E841
with
person (while landing, taking off) (without accident to aircraft) E844
powered (in transit) (with unpowered aircraft) E841
while landing, taking off E840
unpowered E842
while landing, taking off E840
animal being ridden (in sport or transport) E828
and
animal (being ridden) (herded) (unattended) E828
nonmotor road vehicle, except pedal cycle or animal-drawn vehicle E828
object (fallen) (fixed) (movable) (moving) not falling from or set in motion by vehicle of higher priority E828
pedestrian (conveyance or vehicle) E828
animal-drawn vehicle E827
and
animal (being ridden) (herded) (unattended) E827
nonmotor road vehicle, except pedal cycle E827
object (fallen) (fixed) (movable) (moving) not falling from or set in motion by vehicle of higher priority E827
pedestrian (conveyance or vehicle) E827
streetcar E827
motor vehicle (on public highway) (traffic accident) E812
after leaving, running off, public highway (without antecedent collision) (without re-entry) E816

Collision—*continued*
with antecedent collision on public highway—*see* categories E810-E815
with re-entrance collision with another motor vehicle E811
and
abutment (bridge) (overpass) E815
animal (herded) (unattended) E815
carrying person, property E813
animal-drawn vehicle E813
another motor vehicle (abandoned) (disabled) (parked) (stalled) (stopped) E812
with, involving re-entrance (on same roadway) (across median strip) E811
any object, person, or vehicle off the public highway resulting from a noncollision motor vehicle nontraffic accident E816
avalanche, fallen or not moving E815
falling E909
boundary fence E815
culvert E815
fallen
stone E815
tree E815
guard post or guard rail E815
inter-highway divider E815
landslide, fallen or not moving E815
moving E909
machinery (road) E815
nonmotor road vehicle NEC E813
object (any object, person, or vehicle off the public highway resulting from a noncollision motor vehicle nontraffic accident) E815
off, normally not on, public highway resulting from a noncollision motor vehicle traffic accident E816
pedal cycle E813
pedestrian (conveyance) E814
person (using pedestrian conveyance) E814
post or pole (lamp) (light) (signal) (telephone) (utility) E815
railway rolling stock, train, vehicle E810
safety island E815
street car E813
traffic signal, sign, or marker (temporary) E815
tree E815
tricycle E813
wall of cut made for road E815
due to cataclysm—*see* categories E908, E909
not on public highway, nontraffic accident E822
and
animal (carrying person, property) (herded) (unattended) E822
animal-drawn vehicle E822
another motor vehicle (moving), except off-road motor vehicle E822
stationary E823
avalanche, fallen, not moving E823
moving E909
landslide, fallen, not moving E823
moving E909
nonmotor vehicle (moving) E822
stationary E823

Collision—*continued*
object (fallen) (normally) (fixed) (movable but not in motion) (stationary) E823
moving, except when falling from, set in motion by, aircraft or cataclysm E822
pedal cycle (moving) E822
stationary E823
pedestrian (conveyance) E822
person (using pedestrian conveyance) E822
railway rolling stock, train, vehicle (moving) E822
stationary E823
road vehicle (any) (moving) E822
stationary E823
tricycle (moving) E822
stationary E823
off-road type motor vehicle (not on public highway) E821
and
animal (being ridden) (-drawn vehicle) E821
another off-road motor vehicle, except snow vehicle E821
other motor vehicle, not on public highway E821
other object or vehicle NEC, fixed or movable, not set in motion by aircraft, motor vehicle on highway, or snow vehicle, motor-driven E821
pedal cycle E821
pedestrian (conveyance) E821
railway train E821
on public highway—*see* Collision, motor vehicle
pedal cycle E826
and
animal (carrying person, property) (herded) (unherded) E826
animal-drawn vehicle E826
another pedal cycle E826
nonmotor road vehicle E826
object (fallen) (fixed) (movable) (moving) not falling from or set in motion by aircraft, motor vehicle, or railway train NEC E826
pedestrian (conveyance) E826
person (using pedestrian conveyance) E826
street car E826
pedestrian(s) (conveyance) E917.9
with fall E886.9
in sports E886.0
and
crowd, human stampede (with fall) E917.1
machinery—*see* Accident, machine
object (fallen) (moving) (projected) (stationary) not falling from or set in motion by any vehicle classifiable to E800-E848 E917.9
with fall E888
caused by a crowd E917.1
in
running water E917.2
with drowning or submersion—*see* Submersion
sports E917.0
vehicle, nonmotor, nonroad E848
in
running water E917.2

Collision—*continued*
with drowning or submersion—*see* Submersion
sports E917.0
with fall E886.0
person(s) (using pedestrian conveyance) (*see also* Collision, pedestrian) E917.9
railway (rolling stock) (train) (vehicle) (with (subsequent) derailment, explosion, fall or fire) E800
with antecedent derailment E802
and
animal (carrying person) (herded) (unattended) E801
another railway train or vehicle E800
buffers E801
fallen tree on railway E801
farm machinery, nonmotor (in transport) (stationary) E801
gates E801
nonmotor vehicle E801
object (fallen) (fixed) (movable) (moving) not falling from, set in motion by, aircraft or motor vehicle NEC E801
pedal cycle E801
pedestrian (conveyance) E805
person (using pedestrian conveyance) E805
platform E801
rock on railway E801
street car E801
snow vehicle, motor-driven (not on public highway) E820
and
animal (being ridden) (-drawn vehicle) E820
another off-road motor vehicle E820
other motor vehicle, not on public highway E820
other object or vehicle NEC, fixed or movable, not set in motion by aircraft or motor vehicle on highway E820
pedal cycle E820
pedestrian (conveyance) E820
railway train E820
on public highway—*see* Collision, motor vehicle
street car(s) E829
and
animal, herded, not being ridden, unattended E829
nonmotor road vehicle NEC E829
object (fallen) (fixed) (movable) (moving) not falling from or set in motion by aircraft, animal-drawn vehicle, animal being ridden, motor vehicle, pedal cycle, or railway train E829
pedestrian (conveyance) E829
person (using pedestrian conveyance) E829
vehicle
animal-drawn—*see* Collision, animal-drawn vehicle
motor—*see* Collision, motor vehicle
nonmotor
nonroad E848
and
another nonmotor, nonroad vehicle E848

Collision—*continued*
object (fallen) (fixed) (movable) (moving) not falling from or set in motion by aircraft, animal-drawn vehicle, animal being ridden, motor vehicle, nonmotor road vehicle, pedal cycle, railway train, or streetcar E848
road, except animal being ridden, animal-drawn vehicle, or pedal cycle E829
and
animal, herded, not being ridden, unattended E829
another nonmotor road vehicle, except animal being ridden, animal-drawn vehicle, or pedal cycle E829
object (fallen) (fixed) (movable) (moving) not falling from or set in motion by, aircraft, animal-drawn vehicle, animal being ridden, motor vehicle, pedal cycle, or railway train E829
pedestrian (conveyance) E829
person (using pedestrian conveyance) E829
vehicle, nonmotor, nonroad E829
watercraft E838
and
person swimming or water skiing E838
causing
drowning, submersion E830
injury except drowning, submersion E831
Combustion, spontaneous —*see* Ignition
Complication of medical or surgical procedure or treatment
as an abnormal reaction—*see* Reaction, abnormal
delayed, without mention of misadventure—*see* Reaction, abnormal
due to misadventure—*see* Misadventure
Compression
divers' squeeze E902.2
trachea by
food E911
foreign body, except food E912
Conflagration
building or structure, except private dwelling (barn) (church) (convalescent or residential home) (factory) (farm outbuilding) (hospital) (hotel) (institution) (educational) (dormitory) (residential) (school) (shop) (store) (theatre) E891.9
with or causing (injury due to)
accident or injury NEC E891.9
specified circumstance NEC E891.8
burns, burning E891.3
carbon monoxide E891.2
fumes E891.2
polyvinylchloride (PVC) or similar material E891.1
smoke E891.2
causing explosion E891.0
not in building or structure E892
private dwelling (apartment) (boarding house) (camping place) (caravan) (farmhouse) (home (private)) (house) (lodging house) (private garage) (rooming house) (tenement) E890.9

Conflagration—*continued*
with or causing (injury due to)
accident or injury NEC E890.9
specified circumstance NEC E890.8
burns, burning E890.3
carbon monoxide E890.2
fumes E890.2
polyvinylchloride (PVC) or similar material E890.1
smoke E890.2
causing explosion E890.0
Contact with
dry ice E901.1
liquid air, hydrogen, nitrogen E901.1
Cramp(s)
Heat—*see* Heat
swimmers (*see also* category E910) E910.2
not in recreation or sport E910.3
Cranking (car) (truck) (bus) (engine), injury by E917.9
Crash
aircraft (in transit) (powered) E841
at landing, take-off E840
in war operations E994
on runway NEC E840
stated as
homicidal E968.8
suicidal E968.8
undetermined whether accidental or intentional E988.6
unpowered E842
glider E842
motor vehicle—*see also* Accident, motor vehicle
homicidal E968.8
suicidal E958.5
undetermined whether accidental or intentional E988.5
Crushed (accidentally) E928.9
between
boat(s), ship(s), watercraft (and dock or pier) (without accident to watercraft) E838
after accident to, or collision, watercraft E831
objects (moving) (stationary and moving) E918
by
avalanche NEC E909.2
boat, ship, watercraft after accident to, collision, watercraft E831
cave-in E916
with asphyxiation or suffocation (*see also* Suffocation, due to, cave-in) E913.3
crowd, human stampede E917.1
falling
aircraft (*see also* Accident, aircraft) E841
in war operations E994
earth, material E916
with asphyxiation or suffocation (*see also* Suffocation, due to, cave-in) E913.3
object E916
on ship, watercraft E838
while loading, unloading watercraft E838
landslide NEC E909.2
lifeboat after abandoning ship E831
machinery—*see* Accident, machine
railway rolling stock, train, vehicle (part of) E805
Crushed—*continued*
street car E829
vehicle NEC—*see* Accident, vehicle NEC
in
machinery—*see* Accident, machine
object E918
transport accident—*see* categories E800-E848
late effect of NEC E929.9
Cut, cutting (any part of body) (accidental) E920.9
by
arrow E920.8
axe E920.4
bayonet (*see also* Bayonet wound) E920.3
blender E920.2
broken glass E920.8
can opener E920.4
powered E920.2
chisel E920.4
circular saw E919.4
cutting or piercing instrument—*see also* category E920
late effect of E929.8
dagger E920.3
dart E920.8
drill—*see* Accident, caused by drill
edge of stiff paper E920.8
electric
beater E920.2
fan E920.2
knife E920.2
mixer E920.2
fork E920.4
garden fork E920.4
hand saw or tool (not powered) E920.4
powered E920.1
hedge clipper E920.4
powered E920.1
hoe E920.4
ice pick E920.4
knife E920.3
electric E920.2
lathe turnings E920.8
lawn mower E920.4
powered E920.0
riding E919.8
machine—*see* Accident, machine
meat
grinder E919.8
slicer E919.8
nails E920.8
needle E920.4
hypodermic E920.5
object, edged, pointed, sharp—*see* category E920
paper cutter E920.4
piercing instrument—*see also* category E920
late effect of E929.8
pitchfork E920.4
powered
can opener E920.2
garden cultivator E920.1
riding E919.8
hand saw E920.1
hand tool NEC E920.1
hedge clipper E920.1
household appliance or implement E920.2
lawn mower (hand) E920.0
riding E919.8

Cut, cutting—*continued*
rivet gun E920.1
staple gun E920.1
rake E920.4
saw
circular E919.4
hand E920.4
scissors E920.4
screwdriver E920.4
sewing machine (electric) (powered) E920.2
not powered E920.4
shears E920.4
shovel E920.4
spade E920.4
splinters E920.8
sword E920.3
tin can lid E920.8
wood slivers E920.8
homicide (attempt) E966
inflicted by other person
stated as
intentional, homicidal E966
undetermined whether accidental or intentional E986
late effect of NEC E929.8
legal
execution E978
intervention E974
self-inflicted (unspecified whether accidental or intentional) E986
stated as intentional, purposeful E956
stated as undetermined whether accidental or intentional E986
suicidal (attempt) E956
war operations E995
Cyclone (any injury) E908

D

Death due to injury occurring one year or more previous —*see* Late effect
Decapitation (accidental circumstances) NEC E928.9
homicidal E966
legal execution (by guillotine) E978
Deprivation —*see also* Privation
homicidal intent E968.4
Derailment (accidental)
railway (rolling stock) (train) (vehicle) (with subsequent collision) E802
with
collision (antecedent) (*see also* Collision, railway) E800
explosion (subsequent) (without antecedent collision) E802
antecedent collision E803
fall (without collision (antecedent)) E802
fire (without collision (antecedent)) E802
street car E829
Descent
parachute (voluntary) (without accident to aircraft) E844
due to accident to aircraft—*see* categories E840-E842
Desertion
child, with intent to injure or kill E968.4
helpless person, infant, newborn E904.0
with intent to injure or kill E968.4
Destitution —*see* Privation
Disability, late effect or sequela of injury —*see* Late effect
Disease
Andes E902.0
aviators' E902.1
caisson E902.2
range E902.0
Divers' disease, palsy, paralysis, squeeze E902.0
Dog bite E906.0
Dragged by
cable car (not on rails) E847
on rails E829
motor vehicle (on highway) E814
not on highway, nontraffic accident E825
street car E829
Drinking poison (accidental) —*see* Table of drugs and chemicals
Drowning —*see* Submersion
Dust in eye E914

E

Earth falling (on) (with asphyxia or suffocation (by pressure)) (*see also* Suffocation, due to, cave-in) E913.3
as, or due to, a cataclysm (involving any transport vehicle)—*see* categories E908, E909
not due to cataclysmic action E913.3
motor vehicle (in motion) (on public highway) E818
not on public highway E825
nonmotor road vehicle NEC E829
pedal cycle E826
railway rolling stock, train, vehicle E806
street car E829
struck or crushed by E916
with asphyxiation or suffocation E913.3
with injury other than asphyxia, suffocation E916
Earthquake (any injury) E909.0
Effect(s) (adverse) of
air pressure E902.9
at high altitude E902.9
in aircraft E902.1
residence or prolonged visit (causing conditions classifiable to E902.0) E902.0
due to
diving E902.2
specified cause NEC E902.8
in aircraft E902.1
cold, excessive (exposure to) (*see also* Cold, exposure to) E901.9
heat (excessive) (*see also* Heat) E900.9
hot
place—*see* Heat
weather E900.0
insulation—*see* Heat
late—*see* Late effect of
motion E903
nuclear explosion or weapon in war operations (blast) (fireball) (heat) (radiation) (direct) (secondary) E996
radiation—*see* Radiation
travel E903

Electric shock, electrocution (accidental) (from exposed wire, faulty appliance, high voltage cable, live rail, open socket) (by) (in) E925.9
appliance or wiring
domestic E925.0
factory E925.2
farm (building) E925.8
house E925.0
home E925.0
industrial (conductor) (control apparatus) (transformer) E925.2
outdoors E925.8
public building E925.8
residential institution E925.8
school E925.8
specified place NEC E925.8
caused by other person
stated as
intentional, homicidal E968.8
undetermined whether accidental or intentional E988.4
electric power generating plant, distribution station E925.1
homicidal (attempt) E968.8
legal execution E978
lightning E907
machinery E925.9
domestic E925.0
factory E925.2
farm E925.8
home E925.0
misadventure in medical or surgical procedure
in electroshock therapy E873.4
self-inflicted (undetermined whether accidental or intentional) E988.4
stated as intentional E958.4
stated as undetermined whether accidental or intentional E988.4
suicidal (attempt) E958.4
transmission line E925.1
Electrocution —*see* Electric shock
Embolism
air (traumatic) NEC—*see* Air, embolism
Encephalitis
lead or saturnine E866.0
from pesticide NEC E863.4
Entanglement
in
bedclothes, causing suffocation E913.0
wheel of pedal cycle E826
Entry of foreign body, material, any —*see* Foreign body
Execution, legal (any method) E978
Exhaustion
cold—*see* Cold, exposure to
due to excessive exertion E927
heat—*see* Heat
Explosion (accidental) (in) (of) (on) E923.9
acetylene E923.2
aerosol can E921.8
aircraft (in transit) (powered) E841
at landing, take-off E840
in war operations E994
unpowered E842
air tank (compressed) (in machinery) E921.1
anesthetic gas in operating theatre E923.2
automobile tire NEC E921.8
causing transport accident—*see* categories E810-E825

Explosion—*continued*
blasting (cap) (materials) E923.1
boiler (machinery), not on transport vehicle E921.0
steamship—*see* Explosion, watercraft
bomb E923.8
in war operations E993
after cessation of hostilities E998
atom, hydrogen or nuclear E996
injury by fragments from E991.9
antipersonnel bomb E991.3
butane E923.2
caused by
other person
stated as
intentional, homicidal—*see* Assault, explosive
undetermined whether accidental or homicidal E985.5
coal gas E923.2
detonator E923.1
dynamite E923.1
explosive (material) NEC E923.9
gas(es) E923.2
missile E923.8
in war operations E993
injury by fragments from E991.9
antipersonnel bomb E991.3
used in blasting operations E923.1
fire-damp E923.2
fireworks E923.0
gas E923.2
cylinder (in machinery) E921.1
pressure tank (in machinery) E921.1
gasoline (fumes) (tank) not in moving motor vehicle E923.2
grain store (military) (munitions) E923.8
grenade E923.8
in war operations E993
injury by fragments from E991.9
homicide (attempt)—*see* Assault, explosive
hot water heater, tank (in machinery) E921.0
in mine (of explosive gases) NEC E923.2
late effect of NEC E929.8
machinery—*see also* Accident, machine
pressure vessel—*see* Explosion, pressure vessel
methane E923.2
missile E923.8
in war operations E993
injury by fragments from E991.9
motor vehicle (part of)
in motion (on public highway) E818
not on public highway E825
munitions (dump) (factory) E923.8
in war operations E993
of mine E923.8
in war operations
after cessation of hostilities E998
at sea or in harbor E992
land E993
after cessation of hostilities E998
injury by fragments from E991.9
marine E992
own weapons in war operations E993
injury by fragments from E991.9
antipersonnel bomb E991.3

Explosion—*continued*
pressure
cooker E921.8
gas tank (in machinery) E921.1
vessel (in machinery) E921.9
on transport vehicle—*see* categories E800-E848
specified type NEC E921.8
propane E923.2
railway engine, locomotive, train (boiler) (with subsequent collision, derailment, fall) E803
with
collision (antecedent) (*see also* Collision, railway) E800
derailment (antecedent) E802
fire (without antecedent collision or derailment) E803
secondary fire resulting from—*see* Fire
self-inflicted (unspecified whether accidental or intentional) E985.5
stated as intentional, purposeful E955.5
shell (artillery) E923.8
in war operations E993
injury by fragments from E991.9
stated as undetermined whether caused accidentally or purposely inflicted E985.5
steam or water lines (in machinery) E921.0
suicide (attempted) E955.5
torpedo E923.8
in war operations E992
transport accident—*see* categories E800-E848
war operations—*see* War operations, explosion
watercraft (boiler) E837
causing drowning, submersion (after jumping from watercraft) E830
Exposure (weather) (conditions) (rain) (wind) E904.3
with homicidal intent E968.4
excessive E904.3
cold (*see also* Cold, exposure to) E901.9
self-inflicted—*see* Cold, exposure to, self-inflicted
heat (*see also* Heat) E900.9
helpless person, infant, newborn due to abandonment or neglect E904.0
noise E928.1
prolonged in deep-freeze unit or refrigerator E901.1
radiation—*see* Radiation
resulting from transport accident—*see* categories E800-E848
smoke from, due to
fire —*see* Fire
tobacco, second-hand E869.4
vibration E928.2

F

Fall, falling (accidental) E888
building E916
burning E891.8
private E890.8
down
escalator E880.0
ladder E881.0
in boat, ship, watercraft E833
staircase E880.9
stairs, steps—*see* Fall, from, stairs
earth (with asphyxia or suffocation (by pressure)) (*see also* Earth, falling) E913.3
from, off
aircraft (at landing, take-off) (in-transit) (while alighting, boarding) E843
resulting from accident to aircraft—*see* categories E840-E842
animal (in sport or transport) E828
animal-drawn vehicle E827
balcony E882
bed E884.4
bicycle E826
boat, ship, watercraft (into water) E832
after accident to, collision, fire on E830
and subsequently struck by (part of) boat E831
and subsequently struck by (part of) boat E838
burning, crushed, sinking E830
and subsequently struck by (part of) boat E831
bridge E882
building E882
burning E891.8
private E890.8
bunk in boat, ship, watercraft E834
due to accident to watercraft E831
cable car (not on rails) E847
on rails E829
car—*see* Fall from motor vehicle
chair E884.2
cliff E884.1
commode E884.6
curb (sidewalk) E880.1
elevation aboard ship E834
due to accident to ship E831
embankment E884.9
escalator E880.0
flagpole E882
furniture NEC E884.5
gangplank (into water) (*see also* Fall, from, boat) E832
to deck, dock E834
hammock on ship E834
due to accident to watercraft E831
haystack E884.9
high place NEC E884.9
stated as undetermined whether accidental or intentional—*see* Jumping, from, high place
horse (in sport or transport) E828
ladder E881.0
in boat, ship, watercraft E833
due to accident to watercraft E831
machinery—*see also* accident, machine
not in operation E884.9
motor vehicle (in motion) (on public highway) E818
not on public highway E825

Fall, falling—*continued*
stationary, except while alighting, boarding, entering, leaving E884.9
while alighting, boarding, entering, leaving E824
stationary, except while alighting, boarding, entering, leaving E884.9
while alighting, boarding, entering, leaving, except off-road type motor vehicle E817
off-road type—*see* Fall, from, off-road type motor vehicle
nonmotor road vehicle (while alighting, boarding) NEC E829
stationary, except while alighting, boarding, entering, leaving E884.9
off road type motor vehicle (not on public highway) NEC E821
on public highway E818
while alighting, boarding, entering, leaving E817
snow vehicle—*see* Fall from snow vehicle, motor-driven
one
deck to another on ship E834
due to accident to ship E831
level to another NEC E884.9
boat, ship, or watercraft E834
due to accident to watercraft E831
pedal cycle E826
playground equipment E884.0
railway rolling stock, train, vehicle (while alighting, boarding) E804
with
collision (*see also* Collision, railway) E800
derailment (*see also* Derailment, railway) E802
explosion (*see also* Explosion, railway engine) E803
rigging (aboard ship) E834
due to accident to watercraft E831
scaffolding E881.1
sidewalk (curb) E880.1
snow vehicle, motor-driven (not on public highway) E820
on public highway E818
while alighting, boarding, entering, leaving E817
stairs, steps E880.9
boat, ship, watercraft E833
due to accident to watercraft E831
motor bus, motor vehicle—*see* Fall, from, motor vehicle, while alighting, boarding
street car E829
stationary vehicle NEC E884.9
stepladder E881.0
street car (while boarding, alighting) E829
stationary, except while boarding or alighting E884.9
structure NEC E882
burning E891.8
table E884.9
toilet E884.6
tower E882
tree E884.9
turret E882
vehicle NEC—*see also* Accident, vehicle NEC
stationary E884.9
viaduct E882

Fall, falling—*continued*
wall E882
wheelchair E884.3
window E882
in, on
aircraft (at landing, take-off) (in-transit) E843
resulting from accident to aircraft—*see* categories E840-E842
boat, ship, watercraft E835
due to accident to watercraft E831
one level to another NEC E834
on ladder, stairs E833
cutting or piercing instrument or machine—*see* Cut
deck (of boat, ship, watercraft) E835
due to accident to watercraft E831
escalator E880.0
gangplank E835
glass, broken E920.8
knife—*see* Cut, knife
ladder E881.0
in boat, ship, watercraft E833
due to accident to watercraft E831
object, edged, pointed or sharp—*see* Cut
pitchfork E920.4
railway rolling stock, train, vehicle (while alighting, boarding) E804
with
collision (*see also* Collision, railway) E800
derailment (*see also* Derailment, railway) E802
explosion (*see also* Explosion, railway engine) E803
scaffolding E881.1
scissors E920.4
staircase, stairs, steps (*see also* Fall, from, stairs) E880.9
street car E829
water transport (*see also* Fall, in, boat) E835
into
cavity E883.9
dock E883.9
from boat, ship, watercraft (*see also* Fall, from, boat) E832
hold (of ship) E834
due to accident to watercraft E831
hole E883.9
manhole E883.2
moving part of machinery—*see* Accident, machine
opening in surface NEC E883.9
pit E883.9
quarry E883.9
shaft E883.9
storm drain E883.2
tank E883.9
water (with drowning or submersion) E910.9
well E883.1
late effect of NEC E929.3
object (*see also* Hit by, object, falling) E916
over
animal E885
cliff E884.1
embankment E884.9
small object E885
overboard (*see also* Fall, from, boat) E832
rock E916

Fireball effects from nuclear explosion in war operations E996
Fireworks (explosion) E923.0
Flash burns from explosion (*see also* Explosion) E923.9
Flood (any injury) (resulting from storm) E908.2
caused by collapse of dam or manmade structure E909.3
Forced landing (aircraft) E840
Foreign body, object or material (entrance into (accidental))
air passage (causing injury) E915
with asphyxia, obstruction, suffocation E912
food or vomitus E911
nose (with asphyxia, obstruction, suffocation) E912
causing injury without asphyxia, obstruction, suffocation E915
alimentary canal (causing injury) (with obstruction) E915
with asphyxia, obstruction respiratory passage, suffocation E912
food E911
mouth E915
with asphyxia, obstruction, suffocation E912
food E911
pharynx E915
with asphyxia, obstruction, suffocation E912
food E911
aspiration (with asphyxia, obstruction respiratory passage, suffocation) E912
causing injury without asphyxia, obstruction respiratory passage, suffocation E915
food (regurgitated) (vomited) E911
causing injury without asphyxia, obstruction respiratory passage, suffocation E915
mucus (not of newborn) E912
phlegm E912
bladder (causing injury or obstruction) E915
bronchus, bronchi—*see* Foreign body, air passages
conjunctival sac E914
digestive system—*see* Foreign body, alimentary canal
ear (causing injury or obstruction) E915
esophagus (causing injury or obstruction) (*see also* Foreign body, alimentary canal) E915
eye (any part) E914
eyelid E914
hairball (stomach) (with obstruction) E915
ingestion—*see* Foreign body, alimentary canal
inhalation—*see* Foreign body, aspiration
intestine (causing injury or obstruction) E915
iris E914
lacrimal apparatus E914
larynx—*see* Foreign body, air passage
late effect of NEC E929.8
lung—*see* Foreign body, air passage
mouth—*see* Foreign body, alimentary canal, mouth
nasal passage—*see* Foreign body, air passage, nose
nose—*see* Foreign body, air passage, nose
ocular muscle E914
operation wound (left in)—*see* Misadventure, foreign object
Foreign body, object or material—*continued*
orbit E914
pharynx—*see* Foreign body, alimentary canal, pharynx
rectum (causing injury or obstruction) E915
stomach (hairball) (causing injury or obstruction) E915
tear ducts or glands E914
trachea—*see* Foreign body, air passage
urethra (causing injury or obstruction) E915
vagina (causing injury or obstruction) E915
Found dead, injured
from exposure (to)—*see* Exposure
on
public highway E819
railway right of way E807
Fracture (circumstances unknown or unspecified) E887
due to specified external means—*see* manner of accident
late effect of NEC E929.3
occurring in water transport NEC E835
Freezing —*see* Cold, exposure to
Frostbite E901.0
due to manmade conditions E901.1
Frozen —*see* Cold, exposure to

G

Garrotting, homicidal (attempted) E963
Gored E906.8
Gunshot wound (*see also* Shooting) E922.9

H

Hailstones, injury by E904.3
Hairball (stomach) (with obstruction) E915
Hanged himself (*see also* Hanging, self-inflicted) E983.0
Hang gliding E842
Hanging (accidental) E913.8
caused by other person
in accidental circumstances E913.8
stated as
intentional, homicidal E963
undetermined whether accidental or intentional E983.0
homicide (attempt) E963
in bed or cradle E913.0
legal execution E978
self-inflicted (unspecified whether accidental or intentional) E983.0
in accidental circumstances E913.8
stated as intentional, purposeful E953.0
stated as undetermined whether accidental or intentional E983.0
suicidal (attempt) E953.0
Heat (apoplexy) (collapse) (cramps) (effects of) (excessive) (exhaustion) (fever) (prostration) (stroke) E900.9
due to
manmade conditions (listed in E900.1, except boat, ship, watercraft) E900.1
weather (conditions) E900.0
from
electric heating apparatus causing burning E924.8
nuclear explosion in war operations E996

I

Ictus
caloris—*see* Heat
solaris E900.0
Ignition (accidental)
anesthetic gas in operating theatre E923.2
bedclothes
with
conflagration—*see* Conflagration
ignition (of)
clothing—*see* Ignition, clothes
highly inflammable material (benzine) (fat) (gasoline) (kerosene) (paraffin) (petrol) E894
benzine E894
clothes, clothing (from controlled fire) (in building) E893.9
with conflagration—*see* Conflagration
from
bonfire E893.2
highly inflammable material E894
sources or material as listed in E893.8
trash fire E893.2
uncontrolled fire—*see* Conflagration
in
private dwelling E893.0
specified building or structure, except private dwelling E893.1
not in building or structure E893.2
explosive material—*see* Explosion
fat E894
gasoline E894
kerosene E894
material
explosive—*see* Explosion
highly inflammable E894
with conflagration—*see* Conflagration
with explosion E923.2
nightdress—*see* Ignition, clothes
paraffin E894
petrol E894
Immersion —*see* Submersion
Implantation of quills of porcupine E906.8
Inanition (from) E904.9
hunger—*see* Lack of, food
resulting from homicidal intent E968.4
thirst—*see* Lack of, water
Inattention after, at birth E904.0
homicidal, infanticidal intent E968.4
Infanticide (*see also* Assault)
Ingestion
foreign body (causing injury) (with obstruction)—*see* Foreign body, alimentary canal
poisonous substance NEC—*see* Table of drugs and chemicals
Inhalation
excessively cold substance, manmade E901.1
foreign body—*see* Foreign body, aspiration
liquid air, hydrogen, nitrogen E901.1
mucus, not of newborn (with asphyxia, obstruction respiratory passage, suffocation) E912
phlegm (with asphyxia, obstruction respiratory passage, suffocation) E912
poisonous gas—*see* Table of drugs and chemicals
Inhalation—*continued*
smoke from, due to
fire —*see* Fire
tobacco, second-hand E869.4
vomitus (with asphyxia, obstruction respiratory passage, suffocation) E911
Injury, injured (accidental(ly)) NEC E928.9
by, caused by, from
air rifle (B-B gun) E917.9
animal (not being ridden) NEC E906.9
being ridden (in sport or transport) E828
assault (*see also* Assault) E968.9
avalanche E909.2
bayonet (*see also* Bayonet wound) E920.3
being thrown against some part of, or object in
motor vehicle (in motion) (on public highway) E818
not on public highway E825
nonmotor road vehicle NEC E829
off-road motor vehicle NEC E821
railway train E806
snow vehicle, motor-driven E820
street car E829
bending E927
broken glass E920.8
bullet—*see* Shooting
cave-in (*see also* Suffocation, due to, cave-in) E913.3
earth surface movement or eruption E909
storm E908
without asphyxiation or suffocation E916
cloudburst E908
cutting or piercing instrument (*see also* Cut) E920.9
cyclone E908
earthquake E909.0
electric current (*see also* Electric shock) E925.9
explosion (*see also* Explosion) E923.9
fire—*see* Fire
flare, Very pistol E922.8
flood E908.2
foreign body—*see* Foreign body
hailstones E904.3
hurricane E908.0
landslide E909.2
law-enforcing agent, police, in course of legal intervention—*see* Legal intervention
lightning E907
live rail or live wire—*see* Electric shock
machinery—*see also* Accident, machine
aircraft, without accident to aircraft E844
boat, ship, watercraft (deck) (engine room) (galley) (laundry) (loading) E836
missile
explosive E923.8
firearm—*see* Shooting
in war operations—*see* War operations, missile
moving part of motor vehicle (in motion) (on public highway) E818
not on public highway, nontraffic accident E825
while alighting, boarding, entering, leaving—*see* Fall, from, motor vehicle, while alighting, boarding
nail E920.8
needle (sewing) E920.4
hypodermic E920.5

Injury, injured—*continued*
noise E928.1
object
fallen on
motor vehicle (in motion) (on public highway) E818
not on public highway E825
falling—*see* Hit by, object, falling
radiation—*see* Radiation
railway rolling stock, train, vehicle (part of) E805
door or window E806
rotating propeller, aircraft E844
rough landing of off-road type motor vehicle (after leaving ground or rough terrain) E821
snow vehicle E820
saber (*see also* Wound, saber) E920.3
shot—*see* Shooting
sound waves E928.1
splinter or sliver, wood E920.8
straining E927
street car (door) E829
suicide (attempt) E958.9
sword E920.3
third rail—*see* Electric shock
thunderbolt E907
tidal wave E909.4
caused by storm E908
tornado E908.1
torrential rain E908.2
twisting E927
vehicle NEC—*see* Accident, vehicle NEC
vibration E928.2
volcanic eruption E909.1
weapon burst, in war operations E993
weightlessness (in spacecraft, real or simulated) E928.0
wood splinter or sliver E920.8
due to
civil insurrection—*see* War operations
occurring after cessation of hostilities E998
war operations—*see* War operations
occurring after cessation of hostilities E998
homicidal (*see also* Assault) E968.9
in, on
civil insurrection—*see* War operations
fight E960.0
parachute descent (voluntary) (without accident to aircraft) E844
with accident to aircraft—*see* categories E840-E842
public highway E819
railway right of way E807
war operations—*see* War operations
inflicted (by)
in course of arrest (attempted), suppression of disturbance, maintenance of order, by law-enforcing agents—*see* Legal intervention
law-enforcing agent (on duty)—*see* Legal intervention
other person
stated as
accidental E928.9
homicidal, intentional—*see* Assault
undetermined whether accidental or intentional—*see* Injury, stated as undetermined

Injury, injured—*continued*
police (on duty)—*see* Legal intervention
late effect of E929.9
purposely (inflicted) by other person(s)—*see* Assault
self-inflicted (unspecified whether accidental or intentional) E988.9
stated as
accidental E928.9
intentionally, purposely E958.9
specified cause NEC E928.8
stated as
undetermined whether accidentally or purposely inflicted (by) E988.9
cut (any part of body) E986
cutting or piercing instrument (classifiable to E920) E986
drowning E984
explosive(s) (missile) E985.5
falling from high place E987.9
manmade structure, except residential E987.1
natural site E987.2
residential premises E987.0
hanging E983.0
knife E986
late effect of E989
puncture (any part of body) E986
shooting—*see* Shooting, stated as undetermined whether accidental or intentional
specified means NEC E988.8
stab (any part of body) E986
strangulation—*see* Suffocation, stated as undetermined whether accidental or intentional
submersion E984
suffocation—*see* Suffocation, stated as undetermined whether accidental or intentional
to child due to criminal abortion E968.8
Insufficient nourishment —*see also* Lack of, food
homicidal intent E968.4
Insulation, effects —*see* Heat
Interruption of respiration by
food lodged in esophagus E911
foreign body, except food, in esophagus E912
Intervention, legal —*see* Legal intervention
Intoxication, drug or poison —*see* Table of drugs and chemicals
Irradiation —*see* Radiation

J

Jammed (accidentally)
between objects (moving) (stationary and moving) E918
in object E918
Jumped or fell from high place, so stated —*see* Jumping, from, high place, stated as in undetermined circumstances
Jumping
before train, vehicle or other moving object (unspecified whether accidental or intentional) E988.0
stated as
intentional, purposeful E958.0
suicidal (attempt) E958.0

Jumping—*continued*
from
aircraft
by parachute (voluntarily) (without accident to aircraft) E844
due to accident to aircraft—*see* categories E840-E842
boat, ship, watercraft (into water)
after accident to, fire on, watercraft E830
and subsequently struck by (part of) boat E831
burning, crushed, sinking E830
and subsequently struck by (part of) boat E831
voluntarily, without accident (to boat) with injury other than drowning or submersion E883.0
building
burning E891.8
private E890.8
cable car (not on rails) E847
on rails E829
high place
in accidental circumstances or in sport—*see* categories E880-E884
stated as
with intent to injure self E957.9
man-made structures NEC E957.1
natural sites E957.2
residential premises E957.0
in undetermined circumstances E987.9
man-made structures NEC E987.1
natural sites E987.2
residential premises E987.0
suicidal (attempt) E957.9
man-made structures NEC E957.1
natural sites E957.1
residential premises E957.0
motor vehicle (in motion) (on public highway)—*see* Fall, from, motor vehicle
nonmotor road vehicle NEC E829
street car E829
structure, burning NEC E891.8
into water
with injury other than drowning or submersion E883.0
drowning or submersion—*see* Submersion
from, off, watercraft—*see* Jumping, from, boat
Justifiable homicide —*see* Assault

K

Kicked by
animal E906.8
person(s) (accidentally) E917.9
with intent to injure or kill E960.0
as, or caused by a crowd (with fall) E917.1
in fight E960.0
in sports (with fall) E917.0
Kicking against
object (moving) (projected) (stationary) E917.9
in sports E917.0
person—*see* Striking against, person
Killed, killing (accidentally) NEC (*see also* Injury) E928.9
in
action—*see* War operations
brawl, fight (hand) (fists) (foot) E960.0
by weapon—*see also* Assault
cutting, piercing E966
firearm—*see* Shooting, homicide
self
stated as
accident E928.9
suicide—*see* Suicide
unspecified whether accidental or suicidal E988.9
Knocked down (accidentally) (by) NEC E928.9
animal (not being ridden) E906.8
being ridden (in sport or transport) E828
blast from explosion (*see also* Explosion) E923.9
crowd, human stampede E917.1
late effect of—*see* Late effect
person (accidentally) E917.9
in brawl, fight E960.0
in sports E917.0
transport vehicle—*see* vehicle involved under Hit by
while boxing E917.0

L

Laceration NEC E928.9
Lack of
air (refrigerator or closed place), suffocation by E913.2
care (helpless person) (infant) (newborn) E904.0
homicidal intent E968.4
food except as result of transport accident E904.1
helpless person, infant, newborn due to abandonment or neglect E904.0
water except as result of transport accident E904.2
helpless person, infant, newborn due to abandonment or neglect E904.0
Landslide E909.2
falling on, hitting
motor vehicle (any) (in motion) (on or off public highway) E909
railway rolling stock, train, vehicle E909
Late effect of
accident NEC (accident classifiable to E928.9) E929.9
specified NEC (accident classifiable to E910-E928.8) E929.8
assault E969
fall, accidental (accident classifiable to E880-E888) E929.3
fire, accident caused by (accident classifiable to E890-E899) E929.4
homicide, attempt (any means) E969
injury undetermined whether accidentally or purposely inflicted (injury classifiable to E980-E988) E989
legal intervention (injury classifiable to E970-E976) E977
medical or surgical procedure, test or therapy
as, or resulting in, or from

Late effect of—*continued*
abnormal or delayed reaction or complication—*see* Reaction, abnormal
misadventure—*see* Misadventure
motor vehicle accident (accident classifiable to E810-E825) E929.0
natural or environmental factor, accident due to (accident classifiable to E900-E909) E929.5
poisoning, accidental (accident classifiable to E850-E858, E860-E869) E929.2
suicide, attempt (any means) E959
transport accident NEC (accident classifiable to E800-E807, E826-E838, E840-E848) E929.1
war operations, injury due to (injury classifiable to E990-E998) E999
Launching pad accident E845
Legal
execution, any method E978
intervention (by) (injury from) E976
baton E973
bayonet E974
blow E975
blunt object (baton) (nightstick) (stave) (truncheon) E973
cutting or piercing instrument E974
dynamite E971
execution, any method E973
explosive(s) (shell) E971
firearms(s) E970
gas (asphyxiation) (poisoning) (tear) E972
grenade E971
late effect of E977
machine gun E970
manhandling E975
mortar bomb E971
nightstick E973
revolver E970
rifle E970
specified means NEC E975
stabbing E974
stave E973
truncheon E973
Lifting, injury in E927
Lightning (shock) (stroke) (struck by) E907
Liquid (noncorrosive) in eye E914
corrosive E924.1
Loss of control
motor vehicle (on public highway) (without antecedent collision) E816
with
antecedent collision on public highway—*see* Collision, motor vehicle
involving any object, person or vehicle not on public highway E816
on public highway—*see* Collision, motor vehicle
not on public highway, nontraffic accident E825
with antecedent collision—*see* Collision, motor vehicle, not on public highway
off-road type motor vehicle (not on public highway) E821
on public highway—*see* Loss of control, motor vehicle
snow vehicle, motor-driven (not on public highway) E820
on public highway—*see* Loss of control, motor vehicle
Lost at sea E832
with accident to watercraft E830
in war operations E995
Low
pressure, effects—*see* Effects of, air pressure
temperature, effects—*see* Cold, exposure to
Lying before train, vehicle or other moving object (unspecified whether accidental or intentional) E988.0
stated as intentional, purposeful, suicidal (attempt) E958.0
Lynching (*see also* Assault) E968.9

M

Malfunction, atomic power plant in water transport E838
Mangled (accidentally) NEC E928.9
Manhandling (in brawl, fight) E960.0
legal intervention E975
Manslaughter (nonaccidental)—*see* Assault
Marble in nose E912
Mauled by animal E906.8
Medical procedure, complication of
delayed or as an abnormal reaction without mention of misadventure—*see* Reaction, abnormal
due to or as a result of misadventure—*see* Misadventure
Minamata disease E865.2
Misadventure(s) to patient(s) during surgical or medical care E876.9
contaminated blood, fluid, drug or biological substance (presence of agents and toxins as listed in E875) E875.9
administered (by) NEC E875.9
infusion E875.0
injection E875.1
specified means NEC E875.2
transfusion E875.0
vaccination E875.1
cut, cutting, puncture, perforation or hemorrhage (accidental) (inadvertent) (inappropriate) (during) E870.9
aspiration of fluid or tissue (by puncture or catheterization, except heart) E870.5
biopsy E870.8
needle (aspirating) E870.5
blood sampling E870.5
catheterization E870.5
heart E870.6
dialysis (kidney) E870.2
endoscopic examination E870.4
enema E870.7
infusion E870.1
injection E870.3
lumbar puncture E870.5
needle biopsy E870.5
paracentesis, abdominal E870.5
perfusion E870.2
specified procedure NEC E870.8
surgical operation E870.0
thoracentesis E870.5
transfusion E870.1
vaccination E870.3
excessive amount of blood or other fluid during transfusion or infusion E873.0

Misadventures—*continued*
failure
in dosage E873.9
electroshock therapy E873.4
inappropriate temperature (too hot or too cold) in local application and packing E873.5
infusion
excessive amount of fluid E873.0
incorrect dilution of fluid E873.1
insulin-shock therapy E873.4
nonadministration of necessary drug or medicinal E873.6
overdose—*see also* Overdose
radiation, in therapy E873.2
radiation
inadvertent exposure of patient (receiving radiation for test or therapy) E873.3
not receiving radiation for test or therapy—*see* Radiation
overdose E873.2
specified procedure NEC 873.8
transfusion
excessive amount of blood E873.0
mechanical, of instrument or apparatus (during procedure) E874.9
aspiration of fluid or tissue (by puncture or catheterization, except of heart) E874.4
biopsy E874.8
needle (aspirating) E874.4
blood sampling E874.4
catheterization E874.4
heart E874.5
dialysis (kidney) E874.2
endoscopic examination E874.3
enema E874.8
infusion E874.1
injection E874.8
lumbar puncture E874.4
needle biopsy E874.4
paracentesis, abdominal E874.4
perfusion E874.2
specified procedure NEC E874.8
surgical operation E874.0
thoracentesis E874.4
transfusion E874.1
vaccination E874.8
sterile precautions (during procedure) E872.9
aspiration of fluid or tissue (by puncture or catheterization, except heart) E872.5
biopsy E872.8
needle (aspirating) E872.5
blood sampling E872.5
catheterization E872.5
heart E872.6
dialysis (kidney) E872.2
endoscopic examination E872.4
enema E872.8
infusion E872.1
injection E872.3
lumbar puncture E872.5
needle biopsy E872.5
paracentesis, abdominal E872.5
perfusion E872.2
removal of catheter or packing E872.8
specified procedure NEC E872.8
surgical operation E872.0

Misadventures—*continued*
thoracentesis E872.5
transfusion E872.1
vaccination E872.3
suture or ligature during surgical procedure E876.2
to introduce or to remove tube or instrument E876.4
foreign object left in body—*see* Misadventure, foreign object
foreign object left in body (during procedure) E871.9
aspiration of fluid or tissue (by puncture or catheterization, except heart) E871.5
biopsy E871.8
needle (aspirating) E871.5
blood sampling E871.5
catheterization E871.5
heart E871.6
dialysis (kidney) E871.2
endoscopic examination E871.4
enema E871.8
infusion E871.1
injection E871.3
lumbar puncture E871.5
needle biopsy E871.5
paracentesis, abdominal E871.5
perfusion E871.2
removal of catheter or packing E871.7
specified procedure NEC E871.8
surgical operation E871.0
thoracentesis E871.5
transfusion E871.1
vaccination E871.3
hemorrhage—*see* Misadventure, cut
inadvertent exposure of patient to radiation (being received for test or therapy) E873.3
inappropriate
operation performed E876.5
temperature (too hot or too cold) in local application or packing E873.5
infusion—*see also* Misadventure, by specific type, infusion
excessive amount of fluid E873.0
incorrect dilution of fluid E873.1
wrong fluid E876.1
mismatched blood in transfusion E876.0
nonadministration of necessary drug or medicinal E873.6
overdose—*see also* Overdose
radiation, in therapy E873.2
perforation—*see* Misadventure, cut
performance of inappropriate operation E876.5
puncture—*see* Misadventure, cut
specified type NEC E876.8
failure
suture or ligature during surgical operation E876.2
to introduce or to remove tube or instrument E876.4
foreign object left in body E871.9
infusion of wrong fluid E876.1
performance of inappropriate operation E876.5
transfusion of mismatched blood E876.0
wrong
fluid in infusion E876.1
placement of endotracheal tube during anesthetic procedure E876.3

Misadventures—*continued*
transfusion—*see also* Misadventure, by specific type, transfusion
excessive amount of blood E873.0
mismatched blood E876.0
wrong
drug given in error—*see* Table of drugs and chemicals
fluid in infusion E876.1
placement of endotracheal tube during anesthetic procedure E876.3
Motion (effects) E903
sickness E903
Mountain sickness E902.0
Mucus aspiration or inhalation, not of newborn (with asphyxia, obstruction respiratory passage, suffocation) E912
Mudslide of cataclysmic nature E909.2
Murder (attempt) (*see also* Assault) E968.9

N

Nail, injury by E920.8
Needlestick E920.4
Neglect —*see also* Privation
criminal E968.4
homicidal intent E968.4
Noise (causing injury) (pollution) E928.1

O

Object
falling
from, in, on, hitting
aircraft E844
due to accident to aircraft—*see* categories E840-E842
machinery—*see also* Accident, machine
not in operation E916
motor vehicle (in motion) (on public highway) E818
not on public highway E825
stationary E916
nonmotor road vehicle NEC E829
pedal cycle E826
person E916
railway rolling stock, train, vehicle E806
street car E829
watercraft E838
due to accident to watercraft E831
set in motion by
accidental explosion of pressure vessel—*see* category E921
firearm—*see* category E922
machine(ry)—*see* Accident, machine
transport vehicle—*see* categories E800-E848
thrown from, in, on, towards
aircraft E844
cable car (not on rails) E847
on rails E829
motor vehicle (in motion) (on public highway) E818
not on public highway E825
nonmotor road vehicle NEC E829
pedal cycle E826
street car E829
vehicle NEC—*see* Accident, vehicle NEC
Obstruction
air passages, larynx, respiratory passages
by
external means NEC—*see* Suffocation
food, any type (regurgitated) (vomited) E911
material or object, except food E912
mucus E912
phlegm E912
vomitus E911
digestive tract, except mouth or pharynx
by
food, any type E915
foreign body (any) E915
esophagus
food E911
foreign body, except food E912
without asphyxia or obstruction of respiratory passage E915
mouth or pharynx
by
food, any type E911
material or object, except food E912
respiration—*see* Obstruction, air passages
Oil in eye E914
Overdose
anesthetic (drug)—*see* Table of drugs and chemicals
drug—*see* Table of drugs and chemicals
Overexertion (lifting) (pulling) (pushing) E927
Overexposure (accidental) (to)
cold (*see also* Cold, exposure to) E901.9
due to manmade conditions E901.1
heat (*see also* Heat) E900.9
radiation—*see* Radiation
radioactivity—*see* Radiation
sun, except sunburn E900.0
weather—*see* Exposure
wind—*see* Exposure
Overheated (*see also* Heat) E900.9
Overlaid E913.0
Overturning (accidental)
animal-drawn vehicle E827
boat, ship, watercraft
causing
drowning, submersion E830
injury except drowning, submersion E831
machinery—*see* Accident, machine
motor vehicle (*see also* Loss of control, motor vehicle) E816
with antecedent collision on public highway—*see* Collision, motor vehicle
not on public highway, nontraffic accident E825
with antecedent collision—*see* Collision, motor vehicle, not on public highway
nonmotor road vehicle NEC E829
off-road type motor vehicle—*see* Loss of control, off-road type motor vehicle
pedal cycle E826
railway rolling stock, train, vehicle (*see also* Derailment, railway) E802
street car E829
vehicle NEC—*see* Accident, vehicle NEC

P

Palsy, divers' E902.2
Parachuting (voluntary) (without accident to aircraft) E844
  due to accident to aircraft—*see* categories E840-E842
Paralysis
  divers' E902.2
  lead or saturnine E866.0
    from pesticide NEC E863.4
Pecked by bird E906.8
Phlegm aspiration or inhalation (with asphyxia, obstruction respiratory passage, suffocation) E912
Piercing (*see also* Cut) E920.9
Pinched
  between objects (moving) (stationary and moving) E918
  in object E918
Pinned under
  machine(ry)—*see* Accident, machine
Place of occurrence of accident —*see* Accident (to), occurring (at) (in)
Plumbism E866.0
  from insecticide NEC E863.4
Poisoning (accidental) (by)—*see also* Table of drugs and chemicals
  carbon monoxide
    generated by
      aircraft in transit E844
      motor vehicle
        in motion (on public highway) E818
          not on public highway E825
      watercraft (in transit) (not in transit) E838
  caused by injection of poisons or toxins into or through skin by plant thorns, spines, or other mechanism E905.7
    marine or sea plants E905.6
  fumes or smoke due to
    conflagration—*see* Conflagration
    explosion or fire—*see* Fire
    ignition—*see* Ignition
  gas
    in legal intervention E972
    legal execution, by E978
    on watercraft E838
    used as anesthetic—*see* Table of drugs and chemicals
  in war operations E997.2
  late effect of—*see* Late effect
  legal
    execution E978
    intervention
      by gas E972
Pressure, external, causing asphyxia, suffocation (*see also* Suffocation) E913.9
Privation E904.9
  food (*see also* Lack of, food) E904.1
  helpless person, infant, newborn due to abandonment or neglect E904.0
  late effect of NEC E929.5
  resulting from transport accident—*see* categories E800-E848
  water (*see also* Lack of, water) E904.2
Projected objects, striking against or struck by —*see* Striking against, object
Prolonged stay in
  high altitude (causing conditions as listed in E902.0) E902.0
  weightless environment E928.0
Prostration
  heat—*see* Heat
Pulling, injury in E927
Puncture, puncturing (*see also* Cut) E920.9
  by
    plant thorns or spines E920.8
      toxic reaction E905.7
        marine or sea plants E905.6
    sea-urchin spine E905.6
Pushing (injury in) (overexertion) E927
  by other person(s) (accidental) E917.9
    as, or caused by, a crowd, human stampede (with fall) E917.1
    before moving vehicle or object
      stated as
        intentional, homicidal E968.8
        undetermined whether accidental or intentional E988.8
    from
      high place
        in accidental circumstances—*see* categories E880-E884
        stated as
          intentional, homicidal E968.1
          undetermined whether accidental or intentional E987.9
            man-made structure, except residential E987.1
            natural site E987.2
            residential E987.0
      motor vehicle (*see also* Fall, from, motor vehicle) E818
        stated as
          intentional, homicidal E968.8
          undetermined whether accidental or intentional E988.8
    in sports E917.0
      with fall E886.0
    with fall E886.9
      in sports E886.0

R

Radiation (exposure to) E926.9
  abnormal reaction to medical test or therapy E879.2
  arc lamps E926.2
  atomic power plant (malfunction) NEC E926.9
    in water transport E838
  electromagnetic, ionizing E926.3
  gamma rays E926.3
  in
    war operations (from or following nuclear explosion) (direct) (secondary) E996
      laser(s) E997.0
    water transport E838
  inadvertent exposure of patient (receiving test or therapy) E873.3
  infrared (heaters and lamps) E926.1
    excessive heat E900.1
  ionized, ionizing (particles, artificially accelerated) E926.8
    electromagnetic E926.3
  isotopes, radioactive—*see* Radiation, radioactive isotopes

S

Shooting, shot—*continued*
  self-inflicted (unspecified whether accidental or intentional) E985.4
    hand gun (pistol) (revolver) E985.0
    military firearm, except hand gun E985.3
      hand gun (pistol) (revolver) E985.0
    rifle (hunting) E985.2
      military E985.3
    shotgun (automatic) E985.1
    specified firearm NEC E985.4
    stated as
      accidental E922.9
        hand gun (pistol) (revolver) E922.0
        military firearm, except hand gun E922.3
          hand gun (pistol) (revolver) E922.0
        rifle (hunting) E922.2
          military E922.3
        shotgun (automatic) E922.1
        specified firearm NEC E922.8
        Verey pistol E922.8
      intentional, purposeful E955.4
        hand gun (pistol) (revolver) E955.0
        military firearm, except hand gun E955.3
          hand gun (pistol) (revolver) E955.0
        rifle (hunting) E955.2
          military E955.3
        shotgun (automatic) E955.1
        specified firearm NEC E955.4
        Verey pistol E955.4
  shotgun (automatic) E922.1
  specified firearm NEC E922.8
  stated as undetermined whether accidental or intentional E985.4
    hand gun (pistol) (revolver) E985.0
    military firearm, except hand gun E985.3
      hand gun (pistol) (revolver) E985.0
    rifle (hunting) E985.2
      military E985.3
    shotgun (automatic) E985.1
    specified firearm NEC E985.4
    Verey pistol E985.4
  suicidal (attempt) E955.4
    hand gun (pistol) (revolver) E955.0
    military firearm, except hand gun E955.3
      hand gun (pistol) (revolver) E955.0
    rifle (hunting) E955.2
      military E955.3
    shotgun (automatic) E955.1
    specified firearm NEC E955.4
    Verey pistol E955.4
  Verey pistol E922.8
Shoving (accidentally) by other person (*see also* Pushing by other person) E917.9
Sickness
  air E903
  alpine E902.0
  car E903
  motion E903
  mountain E902.0
  sea E903
  travel E903
Sinking (accidental)
  boat, ship, watercraft (causing drowning, submersion) E830
    causing injury except drowning, submersion E831
Siriasis E900.0
Skydiving E844
Slashed wrists (*see also* Cut, self-inflicted) E986
Slipping (accidental)
  on
    deck (of boat, ship, watercraft) (icy) (oily) (wet) E835
    ice E885
    ladder of ship E833
      due to accident to watercraft E831
    mud E885
    oil E885
    snow E885
    stairs of ship E833
      due to accident to watercraft E831
    surface
      slippery E885
      wet E885
Sliver, wood, injury by E920.8
Smothering, smothered (*see also* Suffocation) E913.9
Solid substance in eye (any part) or adnexa E914
Sound waves (causing injury) E928.1
Splinter, injury by E920.8
Stab, stabbing E966
  accidental—*see* Cut
Starvation E904.1
  helpless person, infant, newborn—*see* Lack of food
  homicidal intent E968.4
  late effect of NEC E929.5
  resulting from accident connected with transport—*see* categories E800-E848
Stepped on
  by
    animal (not being ridden) E906.8
      being ridden (in sport or transport) E828
    crowd E917.1
    person E917.9
      in sports E917.0
  in sports E917.0
Stepping on
  object (moving) (projected) (stationary) E917.9
    with fall E888
    in sports E917.0
  person E917.9
    by crowd E917.1
    in sports E917.0
Sting E905.9
  ant E905.5
  bee E905.3
  caterpillar E905.5
  coral E905.6
  hornet E905.3
  insect NEC E905.5
  jelly fish E905.6
  marine animal or plant E905.6
  nematocysts E905.6
  scorpion E905.2
  sea anemone E905.6
  sea cucumber E905.6
  wasp E905.3
  yellow jacket E905.3
Storm (causing flood) E908.9
  dust E908.4
Straining, injury in E927
Strangling —*see* Suffocation
Strangulation —*see* Suffocation
Strenuous movements (in recreational or other activities) E927

Suffocation—*continued*
due to, by
avalanche E909.2
bedclothes E913.0
bib E913.0
blanket E913.0
cave-in E913.3
caused by cataclysmic earth surface movement or eruption E909.9
conflagration—*see* Conflagration
explosion—*see* Explosion
falling earth, other substance E913.3
fire—*see* Fire
food, any type (ingestion) (inhalation) (regurgitated) (vomited) E911
foreign body, except food (ingestion) (inhalation) E912
ignition—*see* Ignition
landslide E909.2
machine(ry)—*see* Accident, machine
material, object except food entering by nose or mouth, ingested, inhaled E912
mucus (aspiration) (inhalation), not of newborn E912
phlegm (aspiration) (inhalation) E912
pillow E913.0
plastic bag—*see* Suffocation, in, plastic bag
sheet (plastic) E913.0
specified means NEC E913.8
vomitus (aspiration) (inhalation) E911
homicidal (attempt) E963
in
airtight enclosed place E913.2
baby carriage E913.0
bed E913.0
closed place E913.2
cot, cradle E913.0
perambulator E913.0
plastic bag (in accidental circumstances) E913.1
homicidal, purposely inflicted by other person E963
self-inflicted (unspecified whether accidental or intentional) E983.1
in accidental circumstances E913.1
intentional, suicidal E953.1
stated as undetermined whether accidentally or purposely inflicted E983.1
suicidal, purposely self-inflicted E953.1
refrigerator E913.2
self-inflicted—*see also* Suffocation, stated as undetermined whether accidental or intentional E953.9
in accidental circumstances—*see* category E913
stated as intentional, purposeful—*see* Suicide, suffocation
stated as undetermined whether accidental or intentional E983.9
by, in
hanging E983.0
plastic bag E983.1
specified means NEC E983.8
suicidal—*see* Suicide, suffocation

Suicide, suicidal (attempted) (by) E958.9
burning, burns E958.1
caustic substance E958.7
poisoning E950.7
swallowed E950.7
cold, extreme E958.3
cut (any part of body) E956
cutting or piercing instrument (classifiable to E920) E956
drowning E954
electrocution E958.4
explosive(s) (classifiable to E923) E955.5
fire E958.1
firearm (classifiable to E922)—*see* Shooting, suicidal
hanging E953.0
jumping
before moving object, train, vehicle E958.0
from high place—*see* Jumping, from, high place, stated as, suicidal
knife E956
late effect of E959
motor vehicle, crashing of E958.5
poisoning—*see* Table of drugs and chemicals
puncture (any part of body) E956
scald E958.2
shooting—*see* Shooting, suicidal
specified means NEC E958.8
stab (any part of body) E956
strangulation—*see* Suicide, suffocation
submersion E954
suffocation E953.9
by, in
hanging E953.0
plastic bag E953.1
specified means NEC E953.8
wound NEC E958.9
Sunburn E926.2
Sunstroke E900.0
Supersonic waves (causing injury) E928.1
Surgical procedure, complication of
delayed or as an abnormal reaction without mention of misadventure—*see* Reaction, abnormal
due to or as a result of misadventure—*see* Misadventure
Swallowed, swallowing
foreign body—*see* Foreign body, alimentary canal
poison—*see* Table of drugs and chemicals
substance
caustic—*see* Table of drugs and chemicals
corrosive—*see* Table of drugs and chemicals
poisonous—*see* Table of drugs and chemicals
Swimmers cramp (*see also* category E910) E910.2
not in recreation or sport E910.3
Syndrome, battered
baby or child—*see* Abuse, child
wife—*see* Assault

T

Tackle in sport E886.0
Thermic fever E900.9
Thermoplegia E900.9
Thirst —*see also* Lack of water
  resulting from accident connected with transport—*see* categories E800-E848
Thrown (accidentally)
  against object in or part of vehicle
    by motion of vehicle
      aircraft E844
      boat, ship, watercraft E838
      motor vehicle (on public highway) E818
        not on public highway E825
        off-road type (not on public highway) E821
          on public highway E818
          snow vehicle E820
            on public highway E818
    nonmotor road vehicle NEC E829
    railway rolling stock, train, vehicle E806
    street car E829
  from
    animal (being ridden) (in sport or transport) E828
    high place, homicide (attempt) E968.1
    machinery—*see* Accident, machine
    vehicle NEC—*see* Accident, vehicle NEC
  off—*see* Thrown, from
  overboard (by motion of boat, ship, watercraft) E832
    by accident to boat, ship, watercraft E830
Thunderbolt NEC E907
Tidal wave (any injury) E909.4
  caused by storm E908
Took
  overdose of drug—*see* Table of drugs and chemicals
  poison—*see* Table of drugs and chemicals
Tornado (any injury) E908.1
Torrential rain (any injury) E908
Traffic accident NEC E819
Trampled by animal E906.8
  being ridden (in sport or transport) E828
Trapped (accidentally)
  between
    objects (moving) (stationary and moving) E918
  by
    door of
      elevator E918
      motor vehicle (on public highway) (while alighting, boarding)—*see* Fall, from, motor vehicle, while alighting
      railway train (underground) E806
      street car E829
      subway train E806
  in object E918
Travel (effects) E903
  sickness E903
Tree
  falling on or hitting E916
    motor vehicle (in motion) (on public highway) E818
      not on public highway E825
    nonmotor road vehicle NEC E829
    pedal cycle E826
    person E916
    railway rolling stock, train, vehicle E806
    street car E829
Trench foot E901.0
Tripping over animal, carpet, curb, rug, or small object (with fall) E885
  without fall—*see* Striking against, object
Tsunami E909.4
Twisting, injury in E927

V

Violence, nonaccidental (*see also* Assault) E968.9
Volcanic eruption (any injury) E909.1
Vomitus in air passages (with asphyxia, obstruction or suffocation) E911

W

War operations (during hostilities) (injury) (by) (in) E995
  after cessation of hostilities, injury due to E998
  air blast E993
  aircraft burned, destroyed, exploded, shot down E994
  asphyxia from
    chemical E997.2
    fire, conflagration (caused by fire-producing device or conventional weapon) E990.9
      from nuclear explosion E996
      petrol bomb E990.0
    fumes E997.2
    gas E997.2
  battle wound NEC E995
  bayonet E995
  biological warfare agents E997.1
  blast (air) (effects) E993
    from nuclear explosion E996
    underwater E992
  bomb (mortar) (explosion) E993
    after cessation of hostilities E998
    fragments, injury by E991.9
      antipersonnel E991.3
  bullet(s) (from carbine, machine gun, pistol, rifle, shotgun) E991.2
    rubber E991.0
  burn from
    chemical E997.2
    fire, conflagration (caused by fire-producing device or conventional weapon) E990.9
      from nuclear explosion E996
      petrol bomb E990.0
    gas E997.2
  burning aircraft E994
  chemical E997.2
  chlorine E997.2
  conventional warfare, specified form NEC E995
  crushing by falling aircraft E994
  depth charge E992
  destruction of aircraft E994
  disability as sequela one year or more after injury E999
  drowning E995
  effect (direct) (secondary) nuclear weapon E996
  explosion (artillery shell) (breech block) (cannon shell) E993
    after cessation of hostilities of bomb, mine placed in war E998

War operations—*continued*
aircraft E994
bomb (mortar) E993
atom E996
hydrogen E996
injury by fragments from E991.9
antipersonnel E991.3
nuclear E996
depth charge E992
injury by fragments from E991.9
antipersonnel E991.3
marine weapon E992
mine
at sea or in harbor E992
land E993
injury by fragments from E991.9
marine E992
munitions (accidental) (being used in war) (dump) (factory) E993
nuclear (weapon) E996
own weapons (accidental) E993
injury by fragments from E991.9
antipersonnel E991.3
sea-based artillery shell E992
torpedo E992
exposure to ionizing radiation from nuclear explosion E996
falling aircraft E994
fire or fire-producing device E990.9
petrol bomb E990.0
fireball effects from nuclear explosion E996
fragments from
antipersonnel bomb E991.3
artillery shell, bomb NEC, grenade, guided missile, land mine, rocket, shell, shrapnel E991.9
fumes E997.2
gas E997.2
grenade (explosion) E993
fragments, injury by E991.9
guided missile (explosion) E993
fragments, injury by E991.9
nuclear E996
heat from nuclear explosion E996
injury due to, but occurring after cessation of hostilities E998
lacrimator (gas) (chemical) E997.2
land mine (explosion) E993
after cessation of hostilities E998
fragments, injury by E991.9
laser(s) E997.0
late effect of E999
lewisite E997.2
lung irritant (chemical) (fumes) (gas) E997.2
marine mine E992
mine
after cessation of hostilities E998
at sea E992
in harbor E992
land (explosion) E993
fragments, injury by E991.9
marine E992
missile (guided) (explosion) E993
fragments, injury by E991.9
marine E992
nuclear E996
mortar bomb (explosion) E993
fragments, injury by E991.9
mustard gas E997.2
nerve gas E997.2
phosgene E997.2

War operations—*continued*
poisoning (chemical) (fumes) (gas) E997.2
radiation, ionizing from nuclear explosion E996
rocket (explosion) E993
fragments, injury by E991.9
saber, sabre E995
screening smoke E997.8
shell (aircraft) (artillery) (cannon) (land based) (explosion) E993
fragments, injury by E991.9
sea-based E992
shooting E991.2
after cessation of hostilities E998
bullet(s) E991.2
rubber E991.0
pellet(s) (rifle) E991.1
shrapnel E991.9
submersion E995
torpedo E992
unconventional warfare, except by nuclear weapon E997.9
biological (warfare) E997.1
gas, fumes, chemicals E997.2
laser(s) E997.0
specified type NEC E997.8
underwater blast E992
vesicant (chemical) (fumes) (gas) E997.2
weapon burst E993
Washed
away by flood—*see* Flood
away by tidal wave—*see* Tidal wave
off road by storm (transport vehicle) E908
overboard E832
Weather exposure —*see also* Exposure
cold E901.0
hot E900.0
Weightlessness (causing injury) (effects of) (in spacecraft, real or simulated) E928.0
Wound (accidental) NEC (*see also* Injury) E928.9
battle (*see also* War operation) E995
bayonet E920.3
in
legal intervention E974
war operations E995
gunshot—*see* Shooting
incised—*see* Cut
saber, sabre E920.3
in war operations E995 categories (633.0-633.9) 639.3

RAILWAY ACCIDENTS (E800–E807)

The following fourth–digit subdivisions are for use with categories E800–E807 to identify the injured person.

.0 Railway employee

Any person who by virtue of his employment in connection with a railway, whether by the railway company or not, is at increased risk of involvement in a railway accident, such as:

catering staff on train
driver
guard
porter
postal staff on train
railway fireman
shunter
sleeping car attendant

.1 Passenger on railway

Any authorized person traveling on a train, except a railway employee

Excludes: intending passenger waiting at station (.8)
unauthorized rider on railway vehicle (.8)

.2 Pedestrian

See definition (r), Vol. 1, page 479

.3 Pedal cyclist

See definition (p), Vol. 1, page 479

.8 Other specified person

Intending passenger waiting at station

Unauthorized rider on railway vehicle

.9 Unspecified person

MOTOR VEHICLE TRAFFIC AND NONTRAFFIC ACCIDENTS (E810–825)

The following fourth–digit subdivisions are for use with categories E810–E819 and E820–E825 to identify the injured person:

.0 Driver of motor vehicle other than motorcycle

See definition (l), Vol. 1, page 479

.1 Passenger in motor vehicle other than motorcycle

See definition (l), Vol. 1, page 479

.2 Motorcyclist

See definition (l), Vol. 1, page 479

.3 Passenger on motorcycle

See definition (l), Vol. 1, page 479

.4 Occupant of streetcar

.5 Rider of animal; occupant of animal–drawn vehicle

.6 Pedal cyclist

See definition (p), Vol. 1, page 479

.7 Pedestrian

See definition (r), Vol. 1, page 479

.8 Other specified person

Occupant of vehicle other than above

Person in railway train involved in accident

Unauthorized rider of motor vehicle

.9 Unspecified person

OTHER ROAD VEHICLE ACCIDENTS (E826–E829)

(animal–drawn vehicle, streetcar, pedal cycle, and other nonmotor road vehicle accidents)

The following fourth–digit subdivisions are for use with categories E826–E829 to identify the injured person:

.0 Pedestrian

See definition (r), Vol. 1, page 479

.1 Pedal cyclist (does not apply to codes E827, E828, E829)

See definition (p), Vol. 1, page 479

.2 Rider of animal (does not apply to code E829)

.3 Occupant of animal–drawn vehicle (does not apply to codes E828, E829)

.4 Occupant of streetcar

.8 Other specified person

.9 Unspecified person

WATER TRANSPORT ACCIDENTS (E830–E838)

The following fourth–digit subdivisions are for use with categories E830–E838 to identify the injured person:

.0 Occupant of small boat, unpowered

.1 Occupant of small boat, powered

See definition (t), Vol. 1, page 479

Excludes: water skier (.4)

.2 Occupant of other watercraft — crew

Persons:

engaged in operation of watercraft

providing passenger services [cabin attendants, ship's physician, catering personnel]

working on ship during voyage in other capacity [musician in band, operators of shops and beauty parlors]

.3 Occupant of other watercraft — other than crew

Passenger

Occupant of lifeboat, other than crew, after abandoning ship

.4 Water skier

.5 Swimmer

.6 Dockers, stevedores

Longshoreman employed on the dock in loading and unloading ships

.8 Other specified person

Immigration and custom officials on board ship

Person:

accompanying passenger or member of crew

visiting boat

Pilot (guiding ship into port)

.9 Unspecified person

AIR AND SPACE TRANSPORT ACCIDENTS (E840–E845)

The following fourth–digit subdivisions are for use with categories E840–E845 to identify the injured person:

.0 Occupant of spacecraft

.1 Occupant of military aircraft, any

Crew Passenger (civilian) (military) Troops	in military aircraft [air force] [army] [national guard] [navy]

Excludes: occupants of aircraft operated under jurisdiction of police departments (.5)
parachutist (.7).

.2 Crew of commercial aircraft (powered) in surface to surface transport

.3 Other occupant of commercial aircraft (powered) in surface to surface transport

Flight personnel:

not part of crew
on familiarization flight

Passenger on aircraft (powered) NOS

.4 Occupant of commercial aircraft (powered) in surface to air transport

Occupant [crew] [passenger] of aircraft (powered) engaged in activities, such as:

aerial spraying (crops) (fire retardants)
air drops of emergency supplies
air drops of parachutists, except from military craft
crop dusting
lowering of construction material [bridge or telephone pole]
sky writing

.5 Occupant of other powered aircraft

Occupant [crew] [passenger] of aircraft (powered) engaged in activities, such as:

aerobatic flying
aircraft racing
rescue operation
storm surveillance
traffic surveillance

Occupant of private plane NOS

.6 Occupant of unpowered aircraft, except parachutist

Occupant of aircraft classifiable to E842

.7 Parachutist (military) (other)

Person making voluntary descent

Excludes: person making descent after accident to aircraft (.1–.6)

.8 Ground crew, airline employee

Persons employed at airfields (civil) (military) or launching pads, not occupants of aircraft

.9 Other person

SUMMARY OF ADDITIONS, DELETIONS, AND REVISIONS TO VOLUME 1

NOTE **All "code also" notes were changed to "code first" notes throughout text**

005.81 **Food poisoning due to Vibrio vulnificus**
New code

005.89 **Other bacterial food poisoning**
New code

009.3 **Diarrhea of presumed infectious origin**
Exclusion revised

038 **Septicemia**
Exclusion revised

041.84 **Other anaerobes**
Exclusion added

041.86 **Helicobacter pylori (H. pylori)**
New code

079.5 **Retrovirus**
Exclusion revised

079.81 **Hantavirus**
New code

278.00 **Obesity unspecified**
New code

278.01 **Morbid obesity**
New code

249.1 **Dementia in conditions classified elsewhere**
"Use additional" deleted; "Code first" added

317 **Mild mental retardation**
Description deleted

318.0 **Moderate mental retardation**
Description deleted

318.2 **Profound mental retardation**
Description deleted

349.2 **Disorders of meninges, not elsewhere classified**
Description added

349.81 **Cerebrospinal fluid rhinorrhea**
Description deleted

362.53 **Cystoid macular degeneration**
Description added

363.13 **Disseminated choroiditis and chorioretinitis, generalized**
"Use additional" deleted; "Code first" added

366.31 **Glaucomatous flecks (subcapsular)**
"Use additional" deleted; "Code first" added

366.32 **Cataract in inflammatory disorders**
"Use additional" deleted; "Code first" added

366.33 **Cataract with neovascularization**
"Use additional" deleted; "Code first" added

366.34 **Cataract in degenerative disorders**
"Use additional" deleted; "Code first" added

415.11 **Iatrogenic pulmonary embolism and infarction**
New code

415.19 **Other**
New code

425 **Cardiomyopathy**
Exclusion deleted

435.3 **Vertebrobasilar artery syndrome**
New code

440.24 **Atherosclerosis of the extremities with gangrene**
Description revised, exclusion added

441.0 **Dissection of aorta**
Code revised

458.2 **Iatrogenic hypotension**
New code

558.9 **Other and unspecified noninfectious gastroenteritis and colitis**
Description deleted

560.81 **Intestinal or peritoneal adhesions with obstruction (postoperative) (postinfection)**
Code revised

564.4 **Other postoperative functional disorders**
Exclusion revised

564.5 **Functional diarrhea**
Exclusion revised

567.8 **Other specified peritonitis**
Exclusion deleted

568.0 **Peritoneal adhesions (postoperative) (postinfection)**
Code revised

569.6 **Colostomy and enterostomy complications**
Code revised

569.60 **Unspecified complication**
New code

569.61 **Infection of colostomy or enterostomy**
New code

569.69 **Other complication**
New code

590-599 **OTHER DISEASES OF URINARY SYSTEM**
Exclusion deleted

599.0 **Urinary tract infection, site not specified**
Description deleted

614.6 **Pelvic peritoneal adhesions, female (postoperative) (postinfection)**
Code revised

630-633 **ECTOPIC AND MOLAR PREGNANCY**
"Use additional code" added

646 **Other complications of pregnancy, NEC**
"Use additional code" added

646.7 **Liver disorders in pregnancy**
Exclusion added

647 **Infectious and parasitic conditions in the mother classifiable elsewhere, but complicating pregnancy, childbirth or the puerperium**
"Use additional code" added

648 **Other current conditions in the mother classifiable elsewhere, but complicating pregnancy, childbirth or the puerperium**
"Use additional code" added

648.6 **Other cardiovascular diseases**
Description revised

650 **Normal delivery**
Code revised

668 **Complications of the administration of anesthetic or other sedation in labor and delivery**
"Use additional code" added

686.8 **Other specified local infections of skin and subcutaneous tissue**
Exclusion revised

690 **Erythematosquamous dermatosis**
Description deleted

690.1 **Seborrheic dermatitis**
New subcategory

690.10 **Seborrheic dermatitis, unspecified**
New code

690.11 **Seborrhea capitis**
New code

690.12 **Seborrheic infantile dermatitis**
New code

690.18 **Other seborrheic dermatitis**
New code

690.8 **Other erythematosquamous dermatosis**
New code

696.5 **Other and unspecified pityriasis**
Exclusion revised

704.8 **Other specified diseases of hair and hair follicles**
Description deleted

719.1 **Hemarthrosis**
Exclusion deleted

728.8 **Other disorders of muscle, ligament, and fascia**
Code revised

728.86 **Necrotizing fasciitis**
New code

729.4 **Fasciitis, unspecified**
Exclusion added

733.6 **Tietze's disease**
Description added

760-779 **CERTAIN CONDITIONS ORIGINATING IN THE PERINATAL PERIOD**
"Use additional code" added

771 **Infections specific to the perinatal period**
Exclusion revised

780.6 **Fever**
Code revised, description added

787 **Symptoms involving digestive system**
Exclusion deleted

787.91 **Diarrhea**
New code

787.99 **Other**
New code

789.0 **Abdominal pain**
Description deleted

800-999 **INJURY AND POISONING**
"Use additional code" added

989.81 **Asbestos**
New code

989.82 **Latex**
New code

989.83 **Silicone**
New code

989.84 **Tobacco**
New code

989.89 **Other**
New code

995.6 **Anaphylactic shock due to adverse food reaction**
Description added

997.0 **Nervous system complications**
Code revised

997.99 **Nervous system complication, unspecified**
New code

997.01 **Central nervous system complication**
New code

997.02 **Iatrogenic cerebrovascular infarction or hemorrhage**
New code

997.09 **Other nervous system complications**
New code

997.3 **Respiratory complications**
Exclusion added

997.4 **Digestive system complications**
Code revised

997.91 **Hypertension**
New code

997.99 **Other**
New code

998.5 **Postoperative infection**
"Use additional code" added

999.2 **Other vascular complications**
Exclusion revised

V01-V06 **PERSONS WITH POTENTIAL HEALTH HAZARDS RELATED TO COMMUNICABLE DISEASES**
Inclusive code numbers revised

V07-V09 **PERSONS WITH NEED FOR ISOLATION, OTHER POTENTIAL HEALTH HAZARDS AND PROPHYLACTIC MEASURES**
New subject heading

V12.50 **Unspecified circulatory disease**
New code

V12.51 **Venous thrombosis and embolism**
New code

V12.52 **Thrombophlebitis**
New code

V12.59 **Other**
New code

V15.84 **Exposure to asbestos**
New code

V15.85 **Exposure to potentially hazardous body fluids**
New code

V15.86 **Exposure to lead**
New code

V43.8 **Other organ or tissue**
Description deleted

V43.81 **Larynx**
New code

V43.82 **Breast**
New code

V43.89 **Other**
New code

V45.83 **Breast implant removal status**
New code

V52 **Fitting and adjustment of prosthetic device and implant**
Code revised

V52.4 **Breast prosthesis and implant**
Code revised

V53.5 **Other intestinal appliance**
Code revised

V53.6 **Urinary device**
Description and exclusions added

V53.7 **Orthopedic devices**
Exclusion added

V54 **Other orthopedic aftercare**
Exclusion added

V56 **Encounter for dialysis and dialysis catheter care**
Code revised

V56.1 **Fitting and adjustment of dialysis (extracorporeal) (peritoneal) catheter**
New code

V58.5 **Orthodontics**
Exclusion added

V58.6 **Long-term (current) drug use**
New category

V58.61 **Long-term (current) use of anticoagulants**
New code

V58.69 **Long-term (current) use of other medications**
New code

V58.8 **Other specified procedures and aftercare**
Code revised

V58.81 **Fitting and adjustment of vascular catheter**
Code revised

V58.82 **Fitting and adjustment of non-vascular catheter NEC**
New code

V59 **Donors**
Exclusion added

V59.01 **Whole blood donor**
New code

V59.02 **Stem cell donor**
New code

V59.09 **Other donor**
New code

V59.6 **Liver donor**
New code

V67.51 **Following completed treatment with high-risk medications, not elsewhere classified**
Code revised

E854.8 **Other psychotropic agents**
New code

E865 **Accidental poisoning from poisonous foodstuffs and poisonous plants**
Code revised

E880.1 **Fall on or from sidewalk curb**
New code

E884.2 **Fall from chair**
Code revised

E884.3 **Fall from wheelchair**
New code

E884.4 **Fall from bed**
New code

E884.5 **Fall from other furniture**
New code

E884.6 **Fall from commode**
New code

E906.5 **Bite by unspecified animal**
New code

E908 **Cataclysmic storms, and floods resulting from storms**
Description deleted, exclusion revised

E908.0 **Hurricane**
New code

E908.1 **Tornado**
New code

E908.2 **Floods**
New code

E908.3 **Blizzard**
New code

E908.4 **Dust storm**
New code

E908.8 **Other cataclysmic storms**
New code

E908.9 **Unspecified cataclysmic storms, and floods resulting from storms**
New code

E909 **Cataclysmic earth surface movements and eruptions**
Description deleted

E909.0 **Earthquakes**
New code

E909.1 **Volcanic eruptions**
New code

E909.2 **Avalanche, landslide or mudslide**
New code

E909.3 **Collapse of dam or man-made structure**
New code

E909.4 **Tidalwave caused by earthquake**
New code

E909.8 **Other cataclysmic earth surface movements and eruptions**
New code

E909.9 **Unspecified cataclysmic earth surface movements and eruptions**
New code

E920.4 **Other hand tools and implements**
Description revised

E920.5 Hypodermic needle
New code

E924.0 Hot liquids and vapors, including steam
Exclusion added

E924.2 Hot (boiling) tap water
New code

E929 LATE EFFECTS OF ACCIDENTAL INJURY
Note revised

E959 Late effects of self-inflicted injury
Note revised

E968.5 Transport vehicle
New code

E969 Late effects of injury purposely inflicted by other person
Note revised

E977 Late effects of injuries due to legal intervention
Note revised

E989 Late effects of injury undetermined whether accidentally or purposely inflicted
Note revised

E999 Late effect of injury due to war operations
Note revised